Handbuch der experimentellen Pharmakologie
Handbook of Experimental Pharmacology

Heffter-Heubner New Series

XXXVIII/2

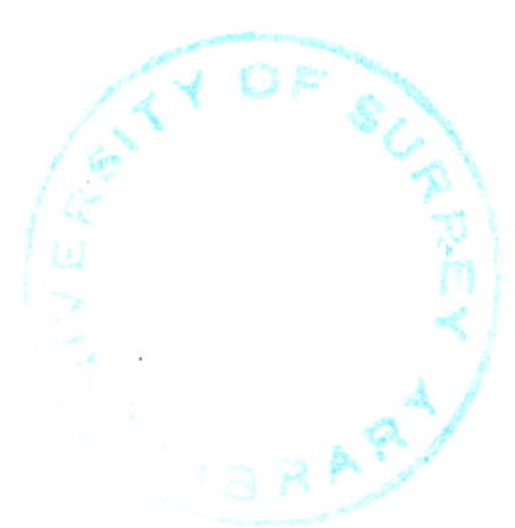

UNIVERSITY OF SURREY
LIBRARY

Antineoplastic and Immunosuppressive Agents
Part II

Contributors

H. T. Abelson · R. H. Adamson · K. C. Agarwal · K. C. Agrawal · L. L. Bennett
J. R. Bertino · B. K. Bhuyan · T. A. Connors · W. A. Creasey · T. L. Dao
L. S. Dietrich · A. DiMarco · G. B. Elion · B. W. Fox · S. Frederiksen
E. J. Freireich · G. R. Gale · G. F. Gause · I. H. Goldberg · B. Goz
A. P. Grollman · M. M. Hart · C. Heidelberger · R. Hilf · G. H. Hitchings
D. H. W. Ho · S. B. Horwitz · C. J. Kensler · H. Kersten · H. Klenow · I. H. Krakoff
W. B. Kremer · P. F. Kruse · J. Laszlo · G. A. LePage · T. L. Loo
D. B. Ludlum . E. Mihich · R. J. Milholland · C. A. Nichol · H. F. Oettgen
B. W. O'Malley · R. E. Parks · A. R. P. Paterson · M. K. Patterson · S. Penman
D. H. Petering · H. G. Petering · P. Pietsch · C. C. Price · W. H. Prusoff
D. J. Reed · F. Rosen · A. C. Sartorelli · J. Škoda · C. G. Smith
C. A. Strott · J. A. Straw · D. M. Tidd · D. W. Visser · G. P. Wheeler
J. L. Wittliff · D. W. Yesair

Editors

Alan C. Sartorelli and David G. Johns

With 128 Figures

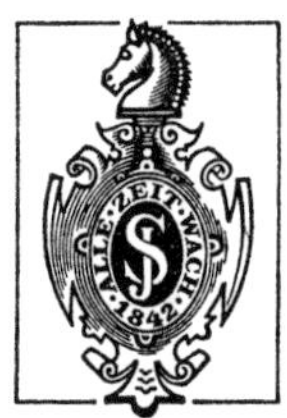

Springer-Verlag Berlin · Heidelberg · New York 1975

ALAN C. SARTORELLI, Professor, Department of Pharmacology, Yale University School of Medicine, New Haven, Connecticut 06510/USA

DAVID G. JOHNS, M. D., Laboratory of Chemical Pharmacology, National Cancer Institute, National Institutes of Health, Bethesda, Maryland 20014/USA

This book was co-edited by DAVID G. JOHNS in his private capacity. No official support or endorsement by the Department of Health, Education and Welfare is intended or should be inferred.

ISBN 3-540-06633-0 Springer-Verlag Berlin · Heidelberg · New York
ISBN 0-387-06633-0 Springer-Verlag New York · Heidelberg · Berlin

Type setting, printing and binding: Brühlsche Universitätsdruckerei Gießen

Preface

Over the past two decades a number of attempts have been made, with varying degrees of success, to collect in a single treatise available information on the basic and applied pharmacology and biochemical mechanism of action of antineoplastic and immunosuppressive agents. The logarithmic growth of knowledge in this field has made it progressively more difficult to do justice to all aspects of this topic, and it is possible that the present handbook, more than four years in preparation, may be the last attempt to survey in a single volume the entire field of drugs employed in cancer chemotherapy and immunosuppression. Even in the present instance, it has proved necessary for practical reasons to publish the material in two parts, although the plan of the work constitutes, at least in the editors' view, a single integrated treatment of this research area.

A number of factors have contributed to the continuous expansion of research in the areas of cancer chemotherapy and immunosuppression. Active compounds have been emerging at ever-increasing rates from experimental tumor screening systems maintained by a variety of private and governmental laboratories throughout the world. At the molecular level, knowledge of the modes of action of established agents has continued to expand, and has permitted rational drug design to play a significantly greater role in a process which, in its early years, depended almost completely upon empirical and fortuitous observations. In addition, the rapid expansion in our knowledge of cancer etiology has begun to afford opportunities for the development of new types of agents with the capacity to inhibit the neoplastic process. Recent advances in our knowledge of viral carcinogenesis, and the consequent expansion of the field of cancer chemotherapy to agents which affect the processes of viral replication and virus-induced transformation of mammalian cells, are factors which are already having a profound influence on drug design and development. Modification and enhancement by pharmacological means of immune defenses to neoplastic growth is another area which is only beginning to be exploited by the chemotherapist. Many major advances still remain to be made to take full advantage of potential synergistic interactions between chemotherapy and surgery and/or radiation therapy: these three major modalities have devloped almost independently despite the continuing efforts of several outstanding groups of investigators to bridge the gap between them at both the experimental and applied levels.

In addition to the rapid growth of these research areas, a second feature which strikes the editor who attempts to survey cancer chemotherapy and immunotherapy is the frequency with which, as in so many other areas of science, fundamental advances have been made unexpectedly, seemingly almost fortuitously. While such random progress may be expected to be a characteristic of the early development of any new research field, it appears to have played an unusually large role in cancer research, and the recent history of cancer chemotherapy shows that major findings have continued to emerge unpredictably, despite retrospective attempts of scientific historians to detect a previously discernable rationale in such developments. The unusually prominent role of chance in the development of antineoplastic and immunosuppressive agents may be a reflection of the slow and difficult progress in our knowledge of cancer etiology: when the location of a target is still shrouded in darkness, it is probably inevitable that direct hits will continue to be a consequence of accident rather than design. It is to be hoped that the current efforts of public and private research funding agencies to superimpose order and modern management techniques on the apparently random development of this and other biomedical sciences will not have the paradoxical effect of slowing the progress they are designed to enhance.

The volume is divided into two parts. The first, has two major sections on general considerations in the areas of antineoplastic and immunosuppressive agents, with chapters included on (a) test systems for both classes of drugs, (b) the clinical utility of both classes of drugs in suppressing the growth of cancer and the immune responses, (c) design of new agents in several major chemical and biochemical classes, (d) the role of cell cycle kinetics in the utility of these therapeutic agents, (e) pharmacologic factors of importance in their optimal utility, (f) selective toxicity, (g) tests predictive of cytotoxic potency, (h) mechanisms of resistance, (i) combination chemotherapy, and (j) among the related modalities, radiation therapy and immunotherapy.

The second part of the volume describes the agents of importance in the treatment of these disease states. It includes major sections on alkylating agents, hormones, antimetabolites and a variety of other cytotoxic compounds, including inhibitors of protein and RNA synthesis, antibiotics and alkaloids, a variety of important synthetic agents and cytotoxic metal-containing compounds.

The Editors wish to express their deepest gratitude to their collaborators who have not only contributed important chapters, but have cooperated fully in the final preparation of this volume. They are also most appreciative of the invaluable editorial assistance provided by Dr. Barbara Renkin and the important secretarial help they have received from Miss Lenora Antinozzi and Miss Lynn A. Bon Tempo. Special thanks go to Dr. William A. Creasey who has compiled the subject index for this volume. It is our deepest hope that research workers in cancer, immunosuppression and other scientific disciplines will find this volume of use in both their intellectual and laboratory endeavors and that it may aid in the accomplishment of further advances in science for the benefit of man.

New Haven and Bethesda
Winter, 1974/75

Alan C. Sartorelli
David G. Johns

Part II Table of Contents

Section C: Alkylating Agents

Chapter 30

Chemistry of Alkylation. CHARLES C. PRICE

Introduction 1

Reaction Mechanism 1

References 5

Chapter 31

Molecular Biology of Alkylation: An Overview. DAVID B. LUDLUM. With 5 Figures

Introduction 6

Alkylation of DNA 6

Effects of Alkylating Agents on Bacteriophage 9

Cellular Modification of Damaged DNA 11

Functional Capacity of Alkylated Template 14

References 15

Chapter 32

Mechanism of Action of 2-Chloroethylamine Derivatives, Sulfur Mustards, Epoxides, and Aziridines. T. A. CONNORS. With 2 Figures

Introduction 18

The Mechanism of Alkylation 19

Mechanism of Action at the Cellular Level 20

A. Long Term Effects of the Alkylating Agents 22

B. Antineoplastic Effects 22

C. Effects on Hemopoietic Tissue 23

D. Effects on Spermatogenesis 23

E. Effects on the Immune Response 24

Mechanism of Action at the Macromolecular Level 24

A. Reactions with Enzymes and Coenzymes 25

B. Reaction with Nucleic Acids 25

Distribution and Metabolism of Alkylating Agents 28

Conclusions 29

References 30

Chapter 33

Mechanism of Action of Methanesulfonates. BRIAN W. FOX. With 1 Figure

Introduction 35

Whole Tissue Studies 35

A. Antitumor Activity 35

B. Spermatogenesis 37

C. Hemopoietic Effects 37
D. Immunosuppressive Properties 38
E. Miscellaneous Effects 38
Metabolism and Distribution Studies 39
Cellular Studies 40
Studies at the Molecular Level 41
Mutagenic Action 41
Conclusions 42
References 42

Chapter 34

Mechanism of Action of Mitomycins. HELGA KERSTEN. With 7 Figures

Introduction 47
Molecular Mechanism of Action 48
A. Interaction with DNA *in Vitro* 48
B. Interaction with DNA in Intact Cells (DNA Damage and Repair) 52
C. DNA Synthesis and Degradation 53
D. RNA Metabolism 54
E. Synthesis of Enzymes 56
Biological Effects of Mitomycins Related to Molecular Mechanism of Action 56
A. Mutagenicity 56
B. Chromosome Breakage 56
C. Viruses, Phage, and Episomal DNA 57
D. Mitosis 59
E. Immunological Aspects 59
References 60

Chapter 35

Mechanism of Action of Nitrosoureas. GLYNN P. WHEELER

Introduction 65
Chemistry 65
Pharmacological Considerations 69
Reactions with Biological Materials 69
A. Alkylation 69
B. Carbamoylation 72
Biochemical Effects 73
A. Synthesis of Macromolecules 73
B. Enzyme Levels and Inactivation of Enzymes 75
Biological Effects 76
A. Effects upon Cell Cycle and Cytotoxicity during the Cycle 76
B. Genetic Effects 78
Conclusions 79
References 79

Section D: Hormones

Chapter 36

Mechanism of Action of Glucocorticoids. FRED ROSEN and RICHARD J. MILHOLLAND

Introduction 85

Biochemical Effects of Glucocorticoids on Lymphoid Tissues 86
A. DNA Metabolism 86
B. RNA and Protein Metabolism 88
C. Carbohydrate Metabolism 91
D. Changes in Enzyme Activity 94
Glucocorticoid Receptors 94
A. Studies in Animals 96
B. Whole Cell Studies *in Vitro* 96
C. Broken-Cell System 98
Possible Mechanism of Action and Basis for Resistance to Glucocorticoids 98
References 100

Chapter 37

Mechanisms of Action of Estrogens. RUSSELL HILF and JAMES L. WITTLIFF. With 5 Figures

Introduction 104
Chemical Structure and Steroidogenesis 104
Actions on Target Organs 108
A. Accessory Sex Organs 108
B. Pituitary and Hypothalamus 108
C. Lipogenesis and Cholesterol 109
D. Antiestrogens 109
E. Breast and Breast Cancer 111
F. Additional Effects of Estrogens 113
Biochemical Basis of Action 113
A. Specific Estrogen Binding Proteins 113
B. Macromolecular Synthesis 118
C. Carbohydrate Metabolism 122
References 125

Chapter 38

Mechanism of Action of Androgens. RUSSELL HILF. With 1 Figure

Introduction 139
Biosynthesis of Androgens 139
Relative Potency of Androgens 142
Actions on Target Organs 142
A. Testis and Male Accessory Sex Organs 142
B. Ovaries and Female Accessory Sex Organs 143
C. Pituitary 143
D. Breast and Breast Cancer 144
E. Metabolic Actions 145
F. Antiandrogens 145
Mechanisms of Action 146
A. Effects of Androgens on Synthesis of Macromolecules 147
B. Androgen Receptor Macromolecules 149
C. Energy Metabolism and Enzyme Changes 151
References 153

Chapter 39

Mechanism of Action of Progesterone. Bert W. O'Malley and Charles A. Strott. With 1 Figure

Biologic Responses to Progesterone 158
The Uptake and Metabolism of Progesterone 159
Binding of Progesterone to Target Cells 162
Sequence of Events in the Action of Progesterone 163
References 167

Chapter 40

Pharmacology and Clinical Utility of Hormones in Hormone Related Neoplasms. Thomas L. Dao

Introduction 170
Hormone-Induced Tissue Growth and Neoplasia 171
Antineoplastic Property of Steroid Hormones as Related to Their Biological Activities. 172
A. Estrogens and Antiandrogenic Effect 172
B. Androgen and its Antiestrogenic Effect 173
C. Antineoplastic Effect of Estrogen and Hypothalamic-Pituitary Regulation of Prolactin 174
D. Effect of Progestogens on Endometrium, Mammary Gland, and Kidney, and Their Antitumor Activity 174
E. Corticosteroids and Their Antitumor Activity 175
F. Direct Effect of Steroid Hormones on Tumor Growth 176
Metabolism of Steroids in Cancer 177
A. Metabolism of Estrogens 177
B. Metabolism of Androgens 179
Clinical Use of Hormonal Steroids in the Treatment of Cancer 179
A. Cancer of the Prostate 179
I. Diethylstilbestrol (α,α'-diethyl-4,4'-stilbenediol) 179
II. Chlorotrianisene (tri-p-anisylchloroethylene, TACE) 180
III. Corticosteroid Therapy 180
B. Cancer of the Breast 180
I. Androgen Therapy 181
1. Testosterone 181
2. Dihydrotestosterone (Stanolone, Androstanolone, Androstan-17β-ol-3-one) 181
3. 17α-Methyltestosterone 182
4. Fluoxymestrone (9α-fluoro-11β-hydroxy-17α-methyltestosterone, Halotestin) 182
5. 19-Nor-Testosterone 182
6. Δ^1-Testololactone (Teslac) 182
7. Other Synthetic Androgens 183
II. Estrogen Therapy 183
III. Adrenocorticoid Therapy 184
IV. Progesterone 185
C. Endometrial Carcinoma 186
D. Carcinoma of the Kidney 186
E. Lymphomas and Leukemia 187
Conclusions 187
References 188

Section E: Antimetabolites

Chapter 41

Fluorinated Pyrimidines and Their Nucleosides. CHARLES HEIDELBERGER. With 10 Figures

Introduction . . . 193
Rationale . . . 193
Syntheses . . . 195
Physical, Chemical, and Conformational Properties . . . 197
Tumor-Inhibitory Properties . . . 198
Other Biological Effects . . . 199
A. Inhibition of the Growth of Cultured Cells . . . 199
B. Antiviral Activity . . . 199
C. Mutagenic Activity . . . 200
D. Teratogenic Activity . . . 200
E. Effects on Chromosomes . . . 200
F. Effects on Bacterial Cell Walls . . . 201
G. Antifungal Effects . . . 201
H. Immunosuppression . . . 201
Biochemical Summary . . . 201
A. Metabolic Degradation of the Pyrimidine Ring . . . 202
B. Anabolic Reactions along the Ribonucleotide Pathway . . . 202
C. Anabolic Reactions along the Deoxyribonucleotide Pathway . . . 203
D. Nucleoside Catabolic Reactions . . . 203
Inhibition of DNA Synthesis . . . 203
A. Cellular . . . 203
B. Enzymatic Mechanism . . . 204
Incorporation into DNA . . . 204
Effects on RNA Synthesis . . . 205
A. Mammalian . . . 205
B. Microorganisms . . . 206
C. Effects on Ribosome Biosynthesis . . . 206
Incorporation into RNA . . . 207
A. Total Cellular . . . 207
B. Viral RNA . . . 208
C. Transfer RNA . . . 209
D. Ribosomal RNA . . . 210
E. Messenger RNA . . . 210
Consequences of Incorporation into RNA . . . 211
A. Mutagenesis to RNA Viruses . . . 211
B. Effects on Protein Synthesis . . . 211
C. Effects on Enzyme Induction . . . 212
D. Coding Properties . . . 213
E. Translational Errors . . . 214
Pathways of Activation and Resistance . . . 215
A. Role of Catabolism . . . 215
B. Activation . . . 216
C. Resistance . . . 217
Effects on the Cell Cycle . . . 217

Preclinical Pharmacology 219
Clinical Use 219
Clinical Pharmacology 221
References 223

Chapter 42

Arabinosylcytosine. William A. Creasey. With 1 Figure

Introduction 232
Synthesis and Structure-Activity Relationships of the Arabinosides 232
Assay Methods for Arabinosylcytosine 234
Biological Actions 235
A. Antitumor Effects in Experimental Systems 235
B. Other Biological Effects 236
Metabolic Fate of Arabinosylcytosine 237
Biochemical Studies with Arabinosylcytosine 239
A. Uptake and Phosphorylation of Ara-C 239
B. Inhibition of DNA Biosynthesis 241
C. Ribonucleoside Diphosphate Reductase 242
D. DNA Polymerase 243
E. Incorporation of Ara-C into Nucleic Acids 244
F. Miscellaneous Biochemical Effects 245
G. Resistance to Arabinosylcytosine 246
Conclusions 248
References 249

Chapter 43

Clinical Pharmacology of Arabinosylcytosine. D. H. W. Ho and Emil J Freireich. With 1 Figure

Introduction 257
Effect of Route of Administration 257
A. Intravenous Administration — Single Dose 257
I. Volume of Distribution 257
II. Half-Life 258
III. Metabolism 259
1. Plasma 259
2. Leukemic Cells 259
IV. Excretion 259
B. Oral Administration 259
I. Absorption 259
II. Effect of 1-(β-D-ribofuranosyl)-4-hydroxy-3,4,5,6-tetrahydropyrimidine-2-(1H)one (Tetrahydrouridine, THU) 259
C. Intrathecal Administration 260
D. Intramuscular and Subcutaneous Administration 260
Toxicity 260
A. Myelosuppression 260
B. Megaloblastosis and Unbalanced Growth 261
C. Chromosomal Aberrations and Teratogenesis 261
D. Other Toxic Effects 261
Effect of Schedule, Dose, and Strategy of Treatment 261
A. Effect of Duration of Continuous Infusion on Clinical Toxicity 261

B. Effect of Dose and Schedule on Pharmacological Findings 262
I. Dose 262
II. Schedule 262
C. Clinical Results for Acute Leukemia and the Relationship of Schedule to Effectiveness 263

Combination Chemotherapy 263
A. Ara-C and Cyclophosphamide 263
B. Ara-C and 1,3-*bis*(2-Chloroethyl)-1-Nitrosourea (BCNU) 264
C. Ara-C and 6-Thioguanine (TG) 264
D. Ara-C and Methyl Mitomycin (Porfiromycin) 264

Resistance to Ara-C as Related to Kinase: Deaminase Ratios and to Intracellular Ribonucleotide Concentrations 264

Perspectives 266
A. Tetrahydrouridine (THU) 266
B. 1-β-D-Arabinofuranosylcytosine 5′-Adamantoate (AdO-Ara-C) 266
C. Other Ara-C Analogs 266
I. 2,2′-O-Cyclocytidine (Cyclocytidine) 266
II. Arabinosylcytosine 3-N-Oxide (Ara-C-3-N-Oxide) 267
D. Sparing Action by Uridine 267

References 267

Chapter 44

Halogenated Pyrimidine Deoxyribonucleosides. WILLIAM H. PRUSOFF and BARRY GOZ. With 4 Figures

Introduction 272

Chemistry 272
A. Synthesis 272
I. Synthesis of Nucleosides Halogenated in the Pyrimidine Moiety 272
II. Synthesis of Radioactive Halogenated Nucleosides and Nucleotides 273
III. Synthesis of Nucleosides Halogenated in the Sugar Moiety 273
IV. Synthesis of Nucleotides Halogenated in the Pyrimidine Moiety 274
V. Synthesis of Halogenated Nucleic Acid 274
B. Stability of Nucleosides 275
C. Steric Effects 277
D. Ionization Effects 277
E. Molecular Conformation 278

Metabolism 279
A. Anabolism 279
B. Catabolism 282
C. Enzyme Inhibition 285
D. Augmentation of Utilization of Halogenated Deoxyribonucleosides 288
I. Inhibition of Thymidylate Synthetase 288
II. Inhibition of Nucleoside Phosphorylase 289
III. Inhibition of Pyrimidine Degradation 290
IV. Complex Formation 291
V. Alteration of Structure 291
VI. Improved Regimens 291

Physical Effects of Incorporation of Halogenated Uracil Derivatives into DNA 292
A. Increased Lability to Stress 292
B. Increased Density 292
C. Increased Temperature (Tm) for DNA Denaturation 292
D. Decreased pH for DNA Denaturation 294
E. Increased Sensitivity to Heat Degradation 294

Biological Consequences of Incorporation of Halogenated Uracil Derivatives into DNA 295
A. Mutagenic Effects 295
B. Inhibition of Cellular Division. . . . 297
I. Cell Culture 297
II. Animals 300
C. Inhibition of Viral Replication 302
D. Effect on Oncogenic Viruses 307
E. Effects on Transformation, Conjugation, and Transduction 308
F. Inhibition of Antibody Production. . . . 309
G. Effects on Embryonic Development and Differentiation 310
H. Toxicity 313
Marker Function 314
Radiosensitization. . . . 318
Clinical Use. . . . 322
Mode of Inhibition 325
Conclusions. . . . 326
References 327

Chapter 45

Azapyrimidine Nucleosides. J. Škoda. With 3 Figures

Introduction 348
Review of Existing Azapyrimidine Nucleosides 348
A. 6-Azapyrimidine Nucleosides 348
B. 5-Azapyrimidine Nucleosides 350
C. 6-Azauridine 351
I. Molecular Mechanism of Inhibitory Effects 351
II. Biological Effects 354
1. Virostatic Activity 354
2. Antineoplastic Effects. . . . 355
3. Immunosuppressive Activity. . . . 356
4. Cholesterol and Lipid Changes Induced by 6-Azauridine. . . . 356
5. Embryotoxic Effects 356
III. Pharmacological Studies 358
IV. Clinical Application 360
1. Virostatic Effects. . . . 360
2. Antineoplastic and Antihyperplastic Effects 360
3. Effect on Psoriasis 361
D. 5-Azacytidine. . . . 361
I. Molecular Mechanism of Inhibitory Action 361
II. Biological Effects in Animal Systems 362
III. Clinical Studies 363
References 364

Chapter 46

Showdomycin, 5-Hydroxyuridine, and 5-Aminouridine. D. W. Visser. With 1 Figure

Introduction 373
Chemistry of Showdomycin. . . . 373
Metabolism of Showdomycin 373
Inhibitory Effects of Showdomycin 374
Chemistry and Metabolism of 5-Hydroxyuridine. . . . 376
Inhibitory Effects of 5-Hydroxyuridine. . . . 377

Chemistry, Metabolism, and Inhibitory Effects of 5-Aminouridine 379
References 381

Chapter 47

6-Thiopurines. A. R. P. Paterson and David M. Tidd. With 1 Figure

Introduction 384
Metabolism of 6-Mercaptopurine and 6-Methylthioinosine 385
A. Anabolism 385
I. 6-Thioinosinate 385
II. 6-Methylthioinosinate 385
III. 6-Thioxanthylate 386
IV. Other Anabolites of 6-Mercaptopurine 386
V. 6-Thioinosine 387
B. Catabolism 387
Metabolism of 6-Thioguanine 387
A. Anabolism 387
I. 6-Thioguanosine Phosphates 387
II. Deoxythioguanosine Phosphates 388
III. Other Anabolites of 6-Thioguanine 388
IV. 6-Thioguanosine and β-2′-Deoxythioguanosine 388
B. Catabolism 389
Metabolic Effects of 6-Mercaptopurine and 6-Methylthioinosine 389
A. The Free Base, 6-Mercaptopurine 389
B. Nucleotide Anabolites 390
I. Inhibition of Purine Ribonucleotide Synthesis *de novo* 390
II. Inhibition of Purine Ribonucleotide Interconversions 392
III. Incorporation into DNA 392
IV. Resistance to 6-Mercaptopurine 393
V. Conclusions 393
Metabolic Effects of 6-Thioguanine 393
A. The Free Base, 6-Thioguanine 394
B. Nucleotide Anabolites 394
I. Inhibition of Purine Ribonucleotide Synthesis *de novo* 394
II. Inhibition of Purine Ribonucleotide Interconversions 395
III. Incorporation into DNA 395
IV. Delayed Cytotoxicity 396
V. Conclusions 396
Combination Chemotherapy 397
References 397

Chapter 48

Azathioprine. Gertrude B. Elion and George H. Hitchings

Introduction (Basic Aspects) 404
Biochemical Effects 404
Biological Effects 405
A. Classes of Lymphocytes and Their Interactions 405
B. Effects on Cells *in Vitro* 405
C. Effects on the Immune Response 407
I. Antibody Formation 407
II. Cell-Borne Immunity 407
D. Antitumor Effects 408
I. In Rodents 408
II. In Man 408
E. Comparison of 6-Mercaptopurine and Azathioprine 409

Clinical Pharmacology . . . 409
A. Toxicity . . . 409
B. Tissue Distribution . . . 411
C. Metabolism of Azathioprine . . . 411
I. Introduction . . . 411
II. Urinary Metabolites . . . 411
1. ^{35}S-Azathioprine . . . 411
2. ^{14}C-Azathioprine . . . 412
III. Blood Levels . . . 413
1. ^{35}S-Azathioprine . . . 413
2. ^{14}C-Azathioprine . . . 413
3. Rosette Inhibitory Activity (RIA) . . . 413
IV. Effect of Disease Conditions . . . 414
1. Renal Insufficiency . . . 414
2. Gout . . . 414
3. Lesch-Nyhan Syndrome . . . 414
4. Liver Disease . . . 414
D. Teratology . . . 415
I. Chromosome Studies . . . 415
II. Teratogenesis in Laboratory Animals . . . 415
III. Clinical Experience . . . 415
E. Effects on Immunological Status . . . 416
I. Tests for Immunological Reactivity . . . 416
II. Infections . . . 416
III. Carcinogenesis . . . 417
Conclusions . . . 418
References . . . 419

Chapter 49

Purine Arabinosides, Xylosides, and Lyxosides. G. A. LePage. With 1 Figure

Introduction . . . 426
9-β-D-Arabinofuranosyladenine (Ara-A) . . . 427
9-β-D-Arabinofuranosylguanine (Ara-G) . . . 428
9-β-D-Arabinofuranosylhypoxanthine (Ara-H) . . . 429
9-β-D-Arabinofuranosyl-6-Mercaptopurine (Ara-6-MP) . . . 429
9-β-D-Arabinofuranosyl-6-Thioguanine (Ara-TG) . . . 430
9-β-D-Xylofuranosyladenine (Xyl-A) . . . 430
9-β-D-Xylofuranosyl-6-Mercaptopurine (Xyl-6-MP) . . . 430
9-β-D-Xylofuranosyl-6-Thioguanine (Xyl-TG) . . . 431
9-β-D-Lyxofuranosyladenine (Lys-A) . . . 431
9-β-D-Lyxofuranosyl-6-Mercaptopurine (Lyx-6-MP) . . . 431
References . . . 431

Chapter 50

Antibiotics Resembling Adenosine: Tubercidin, Toyocamycin, Sangivamycin, Formycin, Psicofuranine, and Decoyinine. Charles A. Nichol. With 3 Figures

Introduction . . . 434
Pyrrolopyrimidine Nucleosides: Tubercidin, Toyocamycin, and Sangivamycin . . . 435
A. Common Pathway of Biosynthesis . . . 435
B. Tubercidin: An Anabolic Analog of Adenosine . . . 436
C. Biochemical Basis for the Cytotoxicity of Tubercidin . . . 437

I. Feedback Inhibition of Purine Nucleotide Biosynthesis by Tubercidin Monophosphate . . . 437
II. Impairment of Some Vital Function of ATP . . . 437
III. Formation of an Analog of Cyclic AMP . . . 438
IV. Impairment of Some Reaction Depending on NAD Cofactors . . . 438
V. Formation of Fraudulent Macromolecules that can Impede Protein or Nucleic Acid Synthesis . . . 438
VI. Different Action of Tubercidin in Cells of Different Origin . . . 439
D. Comparison of Toyocamycin and Sangivamycin with Tubercidin . . . 439
E. Potential for Chemotherapy . . . 440

Formycin . . . 441
A. Enzymatic Studies . . . 442
B. Biopolymers Containing Formycin . . . 443
C. Potential for Chemotherapy . . . 444

Inosine Analogs: Formycin B and 7-Deazainosine . . . 444
A. Formycin B . . . 444
B. 7-Deazainosine . . . 445

Psicofuranine, Decoyinine, and Mycophenolic Acid . . . 445
A. Rediscovered Antibiotics . . . 446
B. Biochemical Sites of Action . . . 447
I. Psicofuranine . . . 448
II. Decoyinine . . . 449
III. Mycophenolic Acid (MPA) . . . 449
C. Potential for Chemotherapy . . . 451

Concluding Comments . . . 451

References . . . 452

Chapter 51

8-Azaguanine. R. E. Parks, Jr., and K. C. Agarwal

Introduction . . . 458

Early Investigations . . . 458

Pharmacological Behavior . . . 459

Effect of 8-Azaguanine and Its Derivatives on Enzymes . . . 459
A. Degradative Enzymes . . . 459
B. Anabolic Enzymes . . . 460
C. Metabolic Enzymes . . . 461
D. RNA Polymerase, DNA Polymerase, and Ribonuclease (RNAase) . . . 462

Effects of 8-Azaguanine on Protein Synthesis . . . 463

Incorporation of 8-Azaguanine into Nucleic Acids . . . 463

References . . . 464

Chapter 52

Folate Antagonists. Joseph R. Bertino. With 2 Figures

Basic Considerations . . . 468
A. Structure and Mechanism of Action of Folate Antagonists . . . 468
B. Mechanism of Cell Death . . . 469

Pharmacology of Folate Antagonists . . . 471
A. Absorption . . . 471
B. Transport . . . 471
C. Distribution of Folate Antagonists . . . 472
D. Metabolism . . . 472

E. Excretion . . . 473
F. Mechanisms of Drug Resistance . . . 473

Clinical Application . . . 474
A. General Considerations . . . 474
B. Toxic Effects . . . 474
C. Treatment of Neoplastic Disease: General Principles . . . 475
D. Treatment of Specific Tumors . . . 476
I. Choriocarcinoma . . . 476
II. Acute Leukemia . . . 476
III. Head and Neck Cancer . . . 477
IV. Breast Cancer . . . 477
V. Lung Cancer . . . 477
VI. Lymphoma . . . 478
VII. Brain Tumors . . . 478
VIII. Primary or Metastatic Liver Tumors . . . 478
IX. Mycosis Fungoides . . . 478
X. Miscellaneous Solid Tumors . . . 478
XI. Nonneoplastic Diseases . . . 479

References . . . 479

Chapter 53

Glutamine Antagonists. L. L. Bennett, Jr.

Introduction . . . 484

Metabolic Effects of Glutamine Analogs . . . 485
A. Azaserine and DON . . . 485
I. Isolation and General Biological Activity . . . 485
II. Inhibition of Purine Biosynthesis . . . 486
III. Inhibition of Pyrimidine Biosynthesis . . . 489
IV. Inhibition of Synthesis of NAD . . . 491
V. Inhibition of Synthesis of Glucosamine . . . 491
VI. Inhibition of Synthesis of Asparagine . . . 491
VII. Inhibition of Synthesis of Anthranilic Acid and *p*-Aminobenzoic Acid . . . 492
VIII. Synthesis of Histidine . . . 492
IX. Effects on Glutaminase and Glutamine Synthetase . . . 492
X. Other Actions . . . 493
XI. Mechanism of Growth Inhibition by Azaserine and DON . . . 494
B. Conjugates of DON . . . 496
C. Amide Derivatives of Glutamine: γ-Glutamylhydrazide and γ-*N*-Benzylglutamine 496
D. *O*-Carbamyl-L-Serine and *O*-Carbazyl-L-Serine . . . 497
E. *S*-Carbamyl-L-Cysteine . . . 497
F. Albizziin . . . 498

Agents Affecting Synthesis and Degradation of Glutamine . . . 498
A. Inhibitors of Glutamine Synthetase . . . 498
B. Glutaminase . . . 499

Glutamine Analogs as Antitumor Agents . . . 499

Glutamine Analogs as Immunosuppressive Agents . . . 502

References . . . 502

Chapter 54

Cytotoxic Amino Acid Analogs. Paul F. Kruse, Jr.

Introduction . . . 512

Amino Acid Analogs and Anticancer Properties . . . 513
A. Aspartic Acid and Asparagine . . . 513

B. Basic Amino Acids 515
I. Arginine 515
II. Histidine 517
III. Lysine 518
C. Aromatic Amino Acids 519
I. Phenylalanine 519
II. Tyrosine 520
III. Tryptophan 521
D. Sulfur-Containing Amino Acids 521
I. Methionine 521
II. Cysteine and Cystine 522
E. Leucine, Isoleucine, Valine, and Other Amino Acids 523
I. Leucine, Isoleucine, and Valine 523
II. Other Amino Acids 524
Amino Acid Analogs and Immunosuppression 525
Future Considerations 528
References 529

Chapter 55

Cytotoxic Analogs of Pyridine Nucleotide Coenzymes. L. S. Dietrich. With 2 Figures
Introduction 539
Analogs of NAD 540
References 542

Chapter 56

Triazenoimidazole Derivatives. Ti Li Loo. With 3 Figures
Introduction 544
Chemistry 544
5-(3,3-Dimethyl-1-Triazene) Imidazole-4-Carboxamide (DIC, NSC-45388) 545
5-[3,3-*bis*(2-Chloroethyl)-1-Triazeno]Imidazole-4-Carboxamide (BIC, NSC-82196) . . . 548
Structure-Activity Relationships 549
References 550

Section F: Additional Cytotoxic Agents

Chapter 57

Cytotoxic Inhibitors of Protein Synthesis. Arthur P. Grollman. With 10 Figures
Introduction 554
Classification of Inhibitors 554
Effects on Protein Synthesis and Polyribosome Structure 555
Inhibitors 556
A. Harringtonine 556
I. General 556
II. Mechanism of Action 556
III. Other Cephalotaxus Alkaloids 557
B. Pactamycin 557
I. General 557
II. Mechanism of Action 557
C. Emetine 558
I. General 558
II. Mechanism of Action 559
III. Structure-Activity Relationships 560

IV. Effects on Synthesis of RNA . . . 560
V. Mechanism of Cytotoxicity . . . 560
D. Cycloheximide . . . 561
I. General . . . 561
II. Mechanism of Action . . . 561
III. Structure-Activity Relationships . . . 562
IV. Topological Similarity to the Ipecac Alkaloids . . . 562
V. Effects on Synthesis of RNA . . . 563
E. Tylocrebrine . . . 564
I. General . . . 564
II. Mechanism of Action . . . 564
F. Anisomycin . . . 564
I. General . . . 564
II. Mechanism of Action . . . 565
III. Structure-Activity Relationships . . . 565
G. Sparsomycin . . . 565
I. General . . . 565
II. Mechanism of Action . . . 566
H. Paederin . . . 566
I. General . . . 566
II. Mechanism of Action . . . 566
References . . . 567

Chapter 58

Selective Interruption of RNA Metabolism by Chemotherapeutic Agents. HERBERT T. ABELSON and SHELDON PENMAN. With 2 Figures

Introduction . . . 571
Nucleolus . . . 572
Nuclear Heterogeneous RNA (HnRNA) and Messenger RNA (mRNA) . . . 574
4S and 5S RNA . . . 576
Mitochondrial RNA . . . 577
Some Examples of the Use of Selective Inhibitors . . . 578
References . . . 579

Chapter 59

Actinomycin D. IRVING H. GOLDBERG. With 2 Figures

Introduction . . . 582
Site of Action in Mammalian Cells . . . 583
Structural Features Required for Biological Activity . . . 584
Models of Actinomycin Binding Site on DNA . . . 586
Clinical Uses of Actinomycin D . . . 589
Carcinogenicity of Actinomycin D . . . 589
References . . . 589

Chapter 60

Daunomycin (Daunorubicin) and Adriamycin. A. DIMARCO. With 17 Figures

Introduction . . . 593
Chemistry . . . 593
Activity on Normal and Neoplastic Cells *in Vitro* . . . 594
Activity on Experimental Tumors . . . 597

Biochemical Effects and Mechanisms of Action 597
Resistance to Daunomycin 606
Antiviral Activity 606
Pharmacological and Toxicological Studies 608
References 611

Chapter 61

Chromomycin, Olivomycin, and Mithramycin. G. F. GAUSE. With 2 Figures
Chemistry and Mechanism of Action 615
Antitumor Activity 617
Pharmacology 619
Clinical Investigations 621
References 621

Chapter 62

Nogalamycin. B. K. BHUYAN and C. G. SMITH. With 1 Figure
Introduction 623
Chemistry of Nogalamycin 623
In Vitro Studies 623
A. Antibacterial Activity 623
B. Cytotoxicity to Mammalian Cells 624
C. Characteristics of Nogalamycin — DNA Interaction 624
D. Effects of Nogalamycin on RNA Synthesis 628
E. Other Activities Inhibited by Nogalamycin 629
F. Phase Specificity of Nogalamycin 629
G. Comparative Biological Activity of Nogalamycin and Its Derivatives 629
In Vivo Studies 630
A. Enzyme Synthesis in Regenerating Liver 630
B. Whole Animal Toxicity 631
C. Antitumor Activity 631
References 631

Chapter 63

Streptonigrin. WILLIAM B. KREMER and JOHN LASZLO. With 4 Figures
Introduction 633
Biological Properties 634
Biochemical Effects 634
Clinical Studies 638
Derivatives of Streptonigrin 639
References 640

Chapter 64

Anthramycin. SUSAN B. HORWITZ. With 2 Figures
Introduction 642
Cytotoxic, Antimicrobial, and Chemosterilant Properties 642

Effects on Macromolecular Synthesis in Cultured Cells 644
Interaction of Anthramycin with DNA 644
Structure-Activity Relationships 646
Conclusions 647
References 647

Chapter 65

Camptothecin. SUSAN B. HORWITZ. With 5 Figures

Introduction 649
Pharmacokinetics 650
Antitumor Properties 650
Effects on Cultured Cells 651
Effects on Mammalian Viruses 654
Structure-Activity Relationships 654
Mechanism of Action 654
Conclusions 655
References 655

Chapter 66

3′-Deoxyadenosine and Other Polynucleotide Chain Terminators. SUNE FREDERIKSEN and HANS KLENOW

Introduction 657
Enzymatic Studies 658
A. Deamination 658
B. Phosphorylation 658
Effects of Phosphorylated Derivatives 659
Effects on Whole Cells 660
A. Growth 660
I. 3′-Deoxyadenosine and 3′-Amino-3′-Deoxyadenosine 660
II. 3′-Deoxyinosine and 3′-Deoxyadenosine N^1-Oxide 661
III. Other 3′-Deoxyribonucleosides 661
IV. 3′-Amino Substituted Compounds 661
V. 3′-Halogen Substituted Compounds 661
VI. 2′,3′-Dideoxyribonucleosides 662
B. Mitosis and Chromosomes 662
C. Uptake and Metabolism 662
RNA Synthesis 663
A. Ehrlich Ascites Cells 663
B. HeLa Cells 664
C. H.Ep. Cells 664
References 664

Chapter 67

Vinca Alkaloids and Colchicine. WILLIAM A. CREASEY. With 2 Figures

Introduction 670
Basic Considerations 671
A. Chemical Nature and Structure-Activity Relationships 671

I. Vinca Alkaloids . . . 671
II. Colchicine Derivatives . . . 672
III. Podophyllotoxin and Griseofulvin . . . 673
B. Biological Activity . . . 673
I. Mitotic Arrest . . . 673
II. Antitumor Effects . . . 675
III. Anti-Inflammatory Action . . . 675
VI. Other Biological Effects . . . 675
C. Microtubule Interaction . . . 676
D. Biochemical Effects . . . 679
I. Nucleic Acid Biosynthesis . . . 679
II. Protein Biosynthesis . . . 681
III. Lipid Metabolism . . . 682
IV. Miscellaneous Biochemical Effects . . . 682
E. Metabolism and Distribution . . . 683
Clinical Considerations . . . 684
A. Drugs, Dosage, and Administration . . . 685
B. Toxicity . . . 686
The Place of the Vinca Alkaloids in the Chemotherapy of Cancer . . . 687
References . . . 687

Chapter 68

L-Asparaginase: Basic Aspects. M. K. PATTERSON, JR.

Introduction . . . 695
Assay of Enzyme Activity . . . 696
Distribution and Antitumor Activity . . . 697
Isolation and Purification . . . 698
Properties and Structure . . . 699
A. D-Asparagine . . . 700
B. Glutamine . . . 701
C. 5-Diazo-4-Oxo-L-Norvaline (DONV) . . . 701
D. L-β-Cyanoalanine . . . 701
E. β-Aspartylhydroxamate . . . 701
F. β-Methyl-L-Aspartate . . . 701
G. Macromolecules . . . 701
Pharmacological Effects . . . 703
Immunological Studies . . . 705
Biochemical Studies . . . 708
Toxicological Effects . . . 710
Asparagine Synthetase . . . 711
References . . . 713

Chapter 69

L-Asparaginase: Current Status of Clinical Evaluation. HERBERT F. OETTGEN

Introduction . . . 723
Properties of the Enzyme Preparation . . . 723
Distribution and Elimination . . . 724
Dose and Route of Administration . . . 725
Effects of Asparaginase Therapy on Plasma Amino Acid Levels . . . 725
Therapeutic Effects . . . 725

A. Spectrum of Response . . . 725
B. Relation of Incidence and Duration of Remissions to Dose and Schedule of Administration of Asparaginase . . . 730
C. Central Nervous System Leukemia . . . 732
D. Combination Therapy . . . 732
E. Resistance . . . 733
Toxic Effects . . . 734
Conclusions . . . 739
Appendix . . . 740
References . . . 742

Chapter 70

Procarbazine. DONALD J. REED. With 2 Figures

Introduction . . . 747
Tumor Inhibition . . . 747
Chemical Properties . . . 747
Pharmacology . . . 751
Metabolism . . . 753
Mode of Action of Procarbazine . . . 756
Clinical Aspects . . . 759
References . . . 760

Chapter 71

***Bis*-Guanylhydrazones.** E. MIHICH. With 2 Figures

Introduction . . . 766
Methylglyoxal-*bis*-(Guanylhydrazone) and Aliphatic Derivatives . . . 766
A. Effects on Experimental Tumors . . . 767
I. Tumor Sensitivity . . . 767
II. Structure-Activity Relationships . . . 768
III. Combination Treatments . . . 768
B. Effects on Microorganisms . . . 769
I. Bacteria and Protozoa . . . 769
II. Viruses . . . 769
C. Pharmacological Studies . . . 769
I. Toxicological Effects . . . 769
II. Disposition and Cellular Uptake . . . 770
III. Therapeutic Effects in Man . . . 772
D. Mechanism of Action . . . 773
I. Relationships to Spermidine . . . 776
II. Relationships to Nucleic Acids . . . 776
III. Relationships to Mitochondrial Functions . . . 776
4,4′-Diacetyl-Diphenyl-Urea-*bis*(Guanylhydrazone) (DDUG) and Other Aromatic *bis*-(Guanylhydrazones) . . . 777
A. Effects on Experimental Tumors . . . 777
I. Spectrum of Tumor Sensitivity . . . 777
II. Structure-Activity Relationships . . . 778
III. Combination Treatments . . . 779
B. Pharmacological Studies . . . 780
I. Toxicological Effects . . . 780
II. Disposition and Cellular Uptake . . . 780
C. Mechanism of Action . . . 781
Conclusions . . . 782
References . . . 783

Chapter 72

Clinical and Pharmacologic Effects of Hydroxyurea. IRWIN H. KRAKOFF

Introduction . . . 789
Fate and Distribution . . . 789
Teratogenic Effects . . . 790
Mechanism of Action . . . 790
Cell Cycle Specificity . . . 791
Conclusions . . . 791
References . . . 791

Chapter 73

α-(N)-Heterocyclic Carboxaldehyde Thiosemicarbazones. KRISHNA C. AGRAWAL and ALAN C. SARTORELLI. With 2 Figures

Introduction . . . 793
Antineoplastic Activity . . . 793
A. Correlation of Ring Substitution with Tumor-Inhibitory Potency . . . 795
B. Correlative Studies of Chelating Potential with Antitumor Activity . . . 798
C. Combination Chemotherapy . . . 799
D. Clinical Studies . . . 799
Antiviral Activity . . . 800
Distribution and Metabolism . . . 800
Biochemical Mechanism of Action . . . 802
Conclusions . . . 804
References . . . 804

Chapter 74

1-(*o*-Chlorophenyl)-1-(*p*-Chlorophenyl)-2,2-Dichloroethane (*o,p'*-DDD), an Adrenocorticolytic Agent. JAMES A. STRAW and MICHAEL M. HART. With 1 Figure

Introduction . . . 808
Pharmacology . . . 809
A. Absorption . . . 809
B. Distribution . . . 809
C. Metabolism . . . 810
D. Excretion . . . 810
Effects on Adrenocortical Tissue . . . 810
A. Histologic and Ultrastructural Changes . . . 810
B. Effects on Steroid Production . . . 811
C. Mechanism of Action of *o,p'*-DDD . . . 812
Extra-Adrenal Effects . . . 813
A. Effects on Steroid Metabolism . . . 813
B. Effects on Drug Metabolism . . . 813
C. Effects on Thyroxine Binding Globulin . . . 814
Clinical Studies . . . 814
A. Patient Population . . . 815
B. Drug Treatment . . . 815
C. Clinical Results . . . 815
D. Side Effects and Toxicity . . . 817
References . . . 817

Chapter 75

The Phthalanilides. DAVID W. YESAIR and CHARLES J. KENSLER. With 2 Figures

Introduction 820
Tumor-Inhibitory Activity and Toxicity 820
Metabolism 822
Biochemical Mechanism of Action 823
Conclusions 826
References 826

Chapter 76

Platinum Compounds. GLEN R. GALE. With 1 Figure

Introduction 829
Tumor-Inhibitory Activity 830
Toxicity of Platinum Compounds 831
Distribution of Tumor-Inhibitory Platinum Compounds 832
Biochemical Mechanism of Action 833
Addendum 836
References 839

Chapter 77

Metal Chelates of 3-Ethoxy-2-Oxobutyraldehyde *bis* (Thiosemicarbazone), H_2KTS. DAVID H. PETERING and HAROLD G. PETERING. With 1 Figure

Introduction 841
Antineoplastic Activity of H_2KTS 842
Metal Chelation and Antitumor Activity of H_2KTS (Activity of Cu(II) KTS and ZnKTS) 843
Studies on the Mechanisms of Action of Cu(II)KTS 845
References 847

Chapter 78

Phleomycin and Bleomycin. PAUL PIETSCH. With 7 Figures

Introduction 850
General Properties 851
A. Composition 851
B. Physical Properties 852
C. Spectral Features 852
D. Permeability 855
E. Range of Biological Activity 855
Actions 856
A. Selective Inhibition of DNA Synthesis 856
B. Receptivity of Target Sites 858
C. Selective Inhibition of Cell Division 859
D. Inhibition of Replicative RNA 859
E. Arrest of Transcription 860
F. Toxicity 860
G. Effects on Genes 862
Reactions with DNA and Considerations of Mechanisms 862
A. Reactions 862

B. Polyphleomycin Model . . . 866
C. Cleaving of DNA . . . 868
Bleomycin in Cancer Chemotherapy . . . 869
References . . . 871

Chapter 79

Pharmacology of Newer Antineoplastic Agents. RICHARD H. ADAMSON. With 9 Figures
Introduction . . . 877
Guanazole . . . 877
Gallium . . . 879
Hycanthone . . . 879
Ellipticine and 9-Methoxyellipticine . . . 881
Alanosine . . . 882
Rifamycin SV and Derivatives . . . 882
Tilorone Hydrochloride . . . 884
ICRF 159 . . . 885
Isophosphamide . . . 886
Cyclocytidine . . . 886
References . . . 887

Addendum to

Cytotoxic Analogs of Pyridine Nucleotide Coenzymes. L. S. DIETRICH . . . 891

Author Index . . . 893

Subject Index . . . 1035

Part II Contributors

HERBERT T. ABELSON, Department of Biology, Massachusetts Institute of Technology, Cambridge, MA 02139/USA

RICHARD H. ADAMSON, Section of Pharmacology and Experimental Therapeutics, National Cancer Institute, National Institutes of Health, Bethesda, MD 20014/USA

K. C. AGARWAL, Division of Biological and Medical Sciences, Brown University, Providence, RI 02912/USA

KRISHNA C. AGRAWAL, Department of Pharmacology, Yale University, School of Medicine, 333 Cedar Street, New Haven, CT 06510/USA

L. L. BENNETT, JR., Biochemistry Research, Southern Research Institute, 2000 Ninth Avenue South, Birmingham, AL 35205/USA

JOSEPH R. BERTINO, Department of Pharmacology, Yale University, School of Medicine, 333 Cedar Street, New Haven, CT 06510/USA

B. K. BHUYAN, The Upjohn Company, Kalamazoo, MI 49001/USA

T. A. CONNORS, Chester Beatty Research Institute, Fulham Road, London SW3/ Great Britain

WILLIAM A. CREASEY, Department of Internal Medicine and Pharmacology, Yale University School of Medicine, 333 Cedar Street, New Haven, CT 06510/USA

THOMAS L. DAO, Department of Breast Surgery and Endocrine Research Laboratory, Roswell Park Memorial Institute, 666 Elm Street, Buffalo, NY 14203/USA

L. S. DIETRICH†, Department of Biochemistry, University of Miami, School of Medicine, Biscayne Avenue, Miami, FL 33152/USA

A. DIMARCO, Instituto Nazionale, Per Lo Studio e La Aura Dei Tumori, Via Venezia 1, 20133-Milano/Italy

GERTRUDE B. ELION, The Wellcome Research Laboratories, Burroughs Wellcome Company, 3030 Cornwallis Road, Research Triangle Park, NC 27709/USA

BRIAN W. FOX, Cristie Hospital and Holt Radium Institute, Paterson Laboratories, Manchester 20 Lancaster/Great Britain

SUNE FREDERIKSEN, Universitetes Biokemiske Inst. B, Juliane Maries vej 30, DK-2100 Copenhagen/Denmark

EMIL J FREIREICH, Department of Developmental Therapeutics, The University of Texas, M. D. Anderson Hospital and Tumor Institute, Houston, TX 77025/USA

CLEN R. GALE, Department of Pharmacology, Medical University of South Carolina, 80 Barre Street, Charleston, SC 29401/USA

G. F. GAUSE, Academy of Medical Sciences of USSR, Institute of New Antibiotics, Bolshaia Pirogovskaia, 11, Moscow/USSR

IRVING H. GOLDBERG, Department of Pharmacology, Harvard Medical School, Boston, MA 02115/USA

BARRY GOZ, Department of Pharmacology, University of North Carolina, School of Medicine, Chapel Hill, NC 27514/USA

ARTHUR P. GROLLMAN, Department of Pharmacology, Albert Einstein College of Medicine and Yeshiva University, 1300 Morris Park Avenue, Bronx, NY 10461/USA

MICHAEL M. HART, Laboratory of Chemical Pharmacology, National Cancer Institute, National Institutes of Health, Bethesda, MD 20014/USA

CHARLES HEIDELBERGER, McArdle Laboratory for Cancer Research, University of Wisconsin, 450 N. Randell Avenue, Madison, WI 53706/USA

RUSSELL HILF, The University of Rochester, School of Medicine and Dentistry and Strong Memorial Hospital, 260 Crittenden Boulevard, Rochester, NY 14642/USA

GEORGE H. HITCHINGS, The Wellcome Research Laboratories, Burroughs Wellcome Company, Research Triangle Park, NC 27709/USA

DAH HSI W. HO, Department of Developmental Therapeutics, The University of Texas, M.D. Anderson Hospital and Tumor Institute, Houston, TX 77025/USA

SUSAN B. HORWITZ, Department of Pharmacology, Albert Einstein College of Medicine, New York, NY 10461/USA

CHARLES J. KENSLER, Life Sciences Division, Arthur D. Little, Inc., Cambridge, MA 02140/USA

HELGA KERSTEN, Physiologisch-Chemisches Institut der Universität Erlangen-Nürnberg, Wasserturmstraße 5, 8520 Erlangen/Federal Republic of Germany

HANS KLENOW, Universitetes Biokemiske Institute B, Juiane Maries vej 30, DK-2100, Copenhagen, Denmark

IRWIN H. KRAKOFF, Sloan-Kettering Institute for Cancer Research, 444 East 68 Street, New York, NY 10021/USA

W. B. KREMER, Veterans Administration Hospital and Duke University, Medical Center, Fulton Street and Erwin Road, Durham, NC 27706/USA

PAUL F. KRUSE, JR.†, Biomedical Division, The Samuel Roberts Noble Foundation Inc., P.O. Box 878, Ardmore, OK 73401/USA

JOHN LASZLO, Veterans Administration Hospital and Duke University Medical Center, Fulton Street and Erwin Road, Durham, NC 27706/USA

G. A. LEPAGE, University of Alberta, Cancer Research Unit, McEachern Laboratory, Edmonton 7 Alberta/Canada

TI LI LOO, Department of Developmental Therapeutics, The University of Texas, M.D. Anderson Hospital and Tumor Institute, Houston, TX 77025/USA

DAVID B. LUDLUM, Department of Cell Biology and Pharmacology, University of Maryland, School of Medicine, 660 West Redwood Street, Baltimore, MD 21201/USA

ENRICO MIHICH, Cancer Drug Center, Roswell Park Memorial Institute, 666 Elm Street, Buffalo, NY 14203/USA

R. J. MILHOLLAND, Cancer Drug Center, Roswell Park Memorial Institute, 666 Elm Street, Buffalo, NY 14203/USA

CHARLES A. NICHOL, Wellcome Research Laboratories, 3030 Cornwallis Road, Research Triangle Park, NC 27709/USA

HERBERT F. OETTGEN, Institut für Immunbiologie, 7800 Freiburg (Brsg.) Federal Republic of Germany

BERT W. O'MALLEY, Department of Cell Biology, Baylor College of Medicine, Houston, TX 77025/USA

ROBERT E. PARKS, JR., Division of Biological and Medical Sciences, Brown University, Providence, RI 02912/USA

A. R. P. PATERSON, University of Alberta, Cancer Research Unit., Edmonton 7, Alberta/Canada

M. K. PATTERSON, JR., Biomedical Division, The Samuel Roberts Noble Foundation Inc., Ardmore, OK 73401/USA

SHELDON PENMAN, Department of Biology, Massachusetts Institute of Technology, Cambridge, MA 02139/USA

DAVID H. PETERING, Department of Chemistry, University of Wisconsin-Milwaukee, Milwaukee, WI/USA

HAROLD G. PETERING, Department of Environmental Health and Biological Chemistry, University of Cincinnati, Cincinnati, OH/USA

PAUL PIETSCH, Division of Optometry, Indiana University, 800 East Atwater, Bloomington, IN 47401/USA

CHARLES C. PRICE, Department of Chemistry, University of Pennsylvania, Philadelphia, PA 19104/USA

WILLIAM H. PRUSOFF, Department of Pharmacology, Yale University School of Medicine, 333 Cedar Street, New Haven, CT 06510/USA

DONALD J. REED, Department of Biochemistry and Biophysics, Oregon State University, Corvallis, OR 97331/USA

FRED ROSEN, Cancer Drug Center, Roswell Park Memorial Institute, 666 Elm Street, Buffalo, NY 14203/USA

ALAN C. SARTORELLI, Department of Pharmacology, Yale University, School of Medicine, 333 Cedar Street, New Haven, CT 06510/USA

JAN ŠKODA, Department of Molecular Biology, Institute of Organic Chemistry and Biochemistry, Czechoslovak Academy of Sciences, Flemingovo nam. 2, Prague 6, Dejvice/Czechoslovakia

Charles G. Smith, E. R. Squibb & Sons, Inc., Princeton, N. J. 08540/USA

James A. Straw, Department of Pharmacology, The George Washington University School of Medicine, 1331 H Street NW, Washington, DC 20005/USA

Charles A. Strott, National Institute for Child Health and Human Development, National Institutes of Health, Bethesda, MD 20014/USA

David M. Tidd, Churchill Hospital Research Institute, Headington, Oxford, OX3 7LJ/Great Britain

Donald W. Visser, Department of Biochemistry, University of Southern California, School of Medicine, Los Angeles, CA 90033/USA

Glynn P. Wheeler, Cancer Biochemistry Division, Southern Research Institute, 2000 Ninth Avenue South, Birmingham, AL 35205/USA

James L. Wittliff, School of Medicine and Dentistry and Strong Memorial Hospital, The University of Rochester, 260 Crittenden Boulevard, Rochester, NY 14642/USA

David W. Yesair, Life Sciences Division, Arthur D. Little Inc., Cambridge, MA 02140/USA

Part I Table of Contents

Section A: General Considerations: Antineoplastic Agents

Chapter 1 Agents of Choice in Neoplastic Disease. C. GORDON ZUBROD
Chapter 2 Evaluation of Antineoplastic Activity: Requirements of Test Systems. ABRAHAM GOLDIN, STEPHEN CARTER, and NATHAN MANTEL
Chapter 3 Rational Design of Alkylating Agents. W. C. J. ROSS
Chapter 4 Rational Design of Folic Acid Antagonists. J. A. R. MEAD. With 2 Figures
Chapter 5 Rational Design of Purine Nucleoside Analogs. JOHN A. MONTGOMERY
Chapter 6 Rational Design of Pyrimidine Nucleoside Analogs. LEROY B. TOWNSEND and C. C. CHENG
Chapter 7 Basic Concepts of Cell Population Kinetics. L. F. LAMERTON. With 5 Figures
Chapter 8 Clinical Applications of Cell Cycle Kinetics. BAYARD CLARKSON. With 3 Figures
Chapter 9 Metabolic Events in the Regulation of Cell Reproduction. ELTON STUBBLEFIELD and SANDRA MURPHREE. With 1 Figure
Chapter 10 Site of Action of Cytotoxic Agents in the Cell Life Cycle. H. MADOC-JONES and F. MAURO. With 3 Figures
Chapter 11 Pharmacokinetic Models for Antineoplastic Agents. DANIEL S. ZAHARKO and ROBERT L. DEDRICK. With 4 Figures
Chapter 12 Absorption, Distribution, and Excretion of Antineoplastic and Immunosuppressive Agents. VINCENT T. OLIVERIO. With 3 Figures
Chapter 13 Transport of Antineoplastic Agents. M. T. HAKALA
Chapter 14 Metabolism of Cancer Chemotherapeutic Agents via Pathways Utilized by Endogenous Substrates. DAVID G. JOHNS. With 7 Figures
Chapter 15 Metabolism of Cancer Chemotherapeutic Agents via Pathways Utilized by Xenobiotics. A. M. GUARINO and C. L. LITTERST. With 3 Figures
Chapter 16 Theoretical Considerations in the Chemotherapy of Brain Tumors. ALAN L. COWLES and JOSEPH D. FENSTERMACHER
Chapter 17 The Constancy of the Product of Concentration and Time. L. B. MELLETT. With 5 Figures
Chapter 18 Biochemical Aspects of Selective Toxicity. J. FRANK HENDERSON
Chapter 19 Mechanisms of Resistance. R. W. BROCKMAN. With 7 Figures
Chapter 20 Combination Chemotherapy: Basic Considerations. ABRAHAM GOLDIN, JOHN M. VENDITTI, and NATHAN MANTEL. With 6 Figures
Chapter 21 Combination Chemotherapy: Clinical Considerations. EMIL FREI, III and JEFFREY A. GOTTLIEB
Chapter 22 Tests Predictive of Cytotoxic Activity. THOMAS C. HALL
Chapter 23 Metabolic Changes Induced by Ionizing Radiations. PAUL TODD. With 2 Figures
Chapter 24 Radiation Research: Survival Kinetics. L. J. TOLMACH and L. E. HOPWOOD. With 7 Figures
Chapter 25 Clinical and Laboratory Investigation of Combination Radiation and Chemical Therapy. R. L. SCOTTE DOGGETT and MALCOLM A. BAGSHAW. With 1 Figure
Chapter 26 Tumor Immunotherapy. A. FEFER

Section B: General Considerations: Immunosuppressive Agents

Chapter 27 Evaluation of Immunosuppressive Agents. MALCOLM S. MITCHELL. With 2 Figures
Chapter 28 Immunosuppressive Agents. EVAN M. HERSH
Chapter 29 Clinical Utility of Immunosuppressive Agents. JULES E. HARRIS and RAMESH C. BAGAI

Author Index

Subject Index

Chapter 30

Chemistry of Alkylation

CHARLES C. PRICE

Introduction

The alkylation reaction may be defined as the conversion

$$H-X+R-Y \longrightarrow R-X+H^{+}+Y^{-}, \tag{1}$$

where R represents an alkyl or substituted alkyl group. In the biological context, the substrate X is usually a nucleic acid or protein molecule, which is alkylated on nitrogen, sulfur, or oxygen. This chapter will consider the chemical mechanisms by which such conversions may be accomplished and the effect of the detailed structure of R, X, and Y on the course of the conversion (for earlier reviews, see PRICE, 1958, 1967, 1969). Normally, the solvent medium can seriously affect the course of alkylation reactions, but in the biological context we are concerned solely with aqueous media and therefore changes due to solvent are negligible.

Reaction Mechanism

The reaction (1) depends on the nucleophilicity of the atom in X undergoing alkylation. This ability of X to donate electrons is greatly enhanced under conditions where H − X is ionized:

$$H-X \rightleftharpoons H^{+}+X:^{-} \tag{2}$$

$$X:^{-}+R-Y \longrightarrow X-R+:Y^{-}. \tag{3}$$

There are two extreme courses for the nucleophilic substitution step (3). At one extreme (S_N2), the process proceeds essentially as represented in (3), with X^- attacking the alkylating agent and expelling Y^-. This limiting case follows second order kinetics, the rate being directly dependent on the concentrations of both reagents.

At the other extreme, the process proceeds stepwise, involving a slow solvent assisted ionization of the alkylating agent followed by rapid reaction of the resulting carbenium ion (also frequently called a "carbonium" ion).

$$R-Y \xrightarrow[\text{(slow)}]{\text{solv}} R^{+}{}_{\text{solv}}+Y^{-}{}_{\text{solv}} \tag{4}$$

$$R^{+}{}_{\text{solv}}+X\text{—}H \xrightarrow[\text{(fast)}]{} R\text{—}X+H^{+} \tag{5}$$

If indeed the initial ionization (4) is fast (compared to subsequent reactions of R^+) then the rate of this process is independent of the concentration of the substrate, H−X. The process follows first-order kinetics and is referred to as S_N1.

Even for the case of simple alkyl groups, it is clear that there is no sharp dividing line between S_N2 and S_N1 reactions. Many refinements are now recognized, involving the role of solvent in promoting separation of R and Y, first to "tight" ion pairs, then to "solvent-separated" ion pairs and finally to free ions.

A second important refinement is the role of "neighboring groups" in the process of displacing Y from R. Classical examples of this factor are the nitrogen and sulfur mustards, where a β-nitrogen or sulfur participates in the process of displacing Y.

$$RSCH_2CH_2Cl \xrightarrow{\text{solv}} R\overset{+}{S}\begin{matrix} / CH_2 \\ | \\ \backslash CH_2 \end{matrix} + Cl^-_{\text{solv}} \quad (6)$$

$$Et_2NCH_2CH_2Cl \xrightarrow{\text{solv}} Et_2\overset{+}{N}\begin{matrix} / CH_2 \\ | \\ \backslash CH_2 \end{matrix} + Cl^-_{\text{solv}} \quad (7)$$

The role of a polar solvent in stabilizing the ions formed in such cyclization reactions is most important and in nonpolar solvents such as ether (and presumably also in body lipids) this activating cyclization reaction does not occur.

The strained three membered rings produced in reactions (6) and (7) are chemically reactive alkylating agents and may attack the nucleophilic centers, H–X or X^-.

$$Et_2\overset{+}{N}\begin{matrix} / CH_2 \\ | \\ \backslash CH_2 \end{matrix} + X^- \xrightarrow{k_x} Et_2NCH_2CH_2X \quad (8)$$

$$k_w \downarrow H_2O$$

$$Et_2NCH_2CH_2OH + H^+ \quad (9)$$

There are two important considerations about the proceeding of these reactions via neighboring group participation. One is that the cyclization process most closely resembles the S_N2 process, except that the nucleophile X is now part of the R group. The second is that the overall kinetics of reactions proceeding through cyclic intermediates will depend on the relative rates of cyclization (6) and (7) and subsequent reaction with a nucleophile X, or H–X (8) and (9).

At one extreme are the sulfur mustards (6), where the cyclization is slow, compared to the ring opening nucleophilic attack of even such a weak nucleophile as water. In this instance, the cyclic intermediate ethylene sulfonium ion will be rapidly destroyed, its steady state concentration will be very low, and the overall kinetics will be first-order with respect to the alkylating agent and independent of the nucleophile. This resemblance to the limiting S_N1 case is, however, formal only, as no reactive carbenium ion intermediate is involved.

The other extreme is the case of β-chloroethyl diethyl amine, a nitrogen mustard (7). With this particular nitrogen mustard, the cyclization reaction (7) is very rapid, being complete in approximately one minute at 0° and pH 10. (The latter condition is necessary to remove the proton from the basic amine group).

$$(Et_2\overset{H}{N}CH_2CH_2Cl)^+ + OH^- \rightleftharpoons Et_2NCH_2CH_2Cl + H_2O \quad (10)$$

Furthermore, the ring-opening reactions (8) and (9) are relatively slow. For example, the reaction with water takes place to the extent of only a few percent in one week at room temperature. In this case, the cyclic aziridinium salt accumulates and its presence can be detected and quantitatively measured, e.g. by *nmr* spectra (SOWA, 1969).

One interesting question which has not been unequivocally answered for the mustard-type alkylating agents is the possible unimolecular ring opening of the cyclic intermediates in (6) and (7) to carbenium ions, as indicated in (11).

$$R_2\overset{+}{N}\begin{matrix} / CH_2 \\ | \\ \backslash CR'_2 \end{matrix} \overset{\text{solv}}{\rightleftharpoons} R_2NCH_2\overset{+}{C}R'_2 \quad (11)$$

Leonard and his colleagues (see CRUST and LEONARD, 1969) have extensively studied reactions of complex aziridinium ions and proposed that such a mechanism is possible, especially when the carbenium ion would be the more stable tertiary structure and the attacking reagent Y is a weak nucleophile. However, extensive stereochemical studies of an analogous and presumably even easier possible ring opening of this kind, as is involved in cationic polymerization of epoxides, has shown that the nucleophilic attack on the cyclic oxonium ion by as weak a nucleophile as an epoxide always proceeds with inversion of configuration at the carbon atom undergoing nucleophilic attack. Since a carbenium ion would lose configuration stability, this evidence indicates that such an intermediate cannot be invoked in this case.

$$\sim\!\sim\!\sim \overset{+}{O}\!\!<\!\!\begin{array}{l}CH(CH_3)\\ |\\ CH(CH_3)\end{array} + O\!\!<\!\!\begin{array}{l}CH(CH_3)\\ |\\ CH(CH_3)\end{array} \xrightarrow{S_N2} \sim\!\sim\!\sim OCH(CH_3)-CH(CH_3)\overset{+}{O}\!\!<\!\!\begin{array}{l}CH(CH_3)\\ |\\ CH(CH_3)\end{array} \qquad (12)$$

It thus appears unclear whether an unequivocal case of ring opening as represented by (11) has yet been established for a nucleophilic substitution reaction. In any event, for the important step in biological alkylations, which is the actual attack on the nucleophilic group in nucleic acid or protein, all available evidence indicates the reaction is of the S_N2 type involving either the original molecule (α-haloacetate, sulfonate esters) or a cyclic ion derived from it (nitrogen and sulfur mustards). For this reason, it is instructive to recognize the factors in R, Y, and X that facilitate such S_N2 reactions.

In the case of one simple S_N2 displacement, i.e.

$$I^- + RCl \longrightarrow IR + Cl^-, \qquad (13)$$

changes in relative reactivity with changes in the structure of R are summarized in Table 1.

Table 1. *Variation of reactivity for the reaction* $I^- + RCl \longrightarrow IR + Cl^-$

R	$k_R/k_{n\text{-}Bu}$	R	$k_R/k_{n\text{-}Bu}$
CH_3	120[a]		
C_2H_5	1.94		
$CH_3CH_2CH_2CH_2$	(1.00)		
$CH_3(CH_2)_{10}CH_2$	1.00		
$CH_3(CH_2)_{28}CH_2$	0.88		
$(CH_3)_2CH$	0.015	$CH_2{=}CH{-}CH_2$	80
$(CH_3)_2CHCH_2$	0.15[a]	$C_6H_5CH_2$	195
$(CH_3)_3C$	0.018	CH_3OCH_2	918
$(CH_3)_3CCH_2$	0.000026[a]	EtO_2CCH_2	2800
		CH_3COCH_2	35700
Cyclohexyl	<0.0001	$C_6H_5COCH_2$	105100

[a] For the reaction $Cl^- + RBr \rightarrow RCl + Br^-$ in acetone. (From: PRICE 1958, p. 664)

The great importance of the nucleophilic center is seen in Table 2, summarizing data on the relative reactivities of a number of nucleophiles in reactions with methyl bromide.

$$X^- + CH_3Br \longrightarrow XCH_3 + Br^- \qquad (14)$$

It is convenient to represent such relative reactivities in comparison to the reactivity of water as a nucleophile. This is especially significant biologically since the reaction medium is usually water. The relative rates in Table 2 are expressed in terms of the equation

$$\log(k_x/k_w) = sn\,, \tag{15}$$

where s is defined as 1.00 for methyl bromide and n is the relative nucleophilicity of the reagent X (defined as 0.00 for water). Note that n is logarithmic, so that when $n = 6$, this means the nucleophile X is 10^6 times more reactive than water.

Table 2. *Nucleophilic constants, n, according to* (15)

Nucleophile	n	Nucleophile	n
ClO_3^-, ClO_4^-, BrO_3^-, IO_3^-	<0	Br^-	3.89
H_2O	0.00	N_3^-	4.00
p-$CH_3C_6H_4SO_3^-$	<1.0	$(NH_2)_2CS$	4.1
NO_3^-	1.03	HO^-	4.20
$Picrate^-$	1.9	$C_6H_5NH_2$	4.49
F^-	2.0	SCN^-	4.77
$SO_4^=$	2.5	I^-	5.04
$CH_3CO_2^-$	2.72	CN^-	5.1
Cl^-	3.04	SH^-	5.1
C_5H_5N	3.6	$SO_3^=$	5.1
HCO_3^-	3.8	$S_2O_3^=$	6.36
$HPO_4^=$	3.8	$HPSO_3^-$	6.6

(From: Thornton, 1964, p. 163)

Table 3. *Leaving-group constants, L, according to* (16)

Y	L	pK_a of HY
$OClO_3$	3.34	$>H_2SO_4$
OSO_2OCH_3	1.57	$>HOSO_2C_6H_4CH_3$—p
$OSO_2C_6H_4CH_3$—p	0.63	$>HBr$
Br	0.00	-7.74
I	-0.04	-10.74
OH_2^+	-0.17	-1.74
Cl	-1.61	-7.1, -4.74
ONO_2	-1.90	-1.34
$OSOOCH_3$	-2.05	1.77
$S(CH_3)_2^+$	-3.01	—
$N(CH_3)_3^+$	-3.54	9.91
F	-3.60	3.14
SSO_2O^-	-3.72	1.21
OSO_2O^-	-4.58	1.70
$OCOCH_3$	-4.68	4.72
OCH_3	<-6.45	14.4

(From Thornton, 1964, p. 165)

A third important factor influencing S_N2 displacement is the nature of the leaving group, Y. An equation similar to (15) has been proposed for the purpose of correlating data of this kind.

$$\log(k_y/k_{Br}) = \gamma L \tag{16}$$

In (16), γ is characteristic of the nucleophile and is designated as 1.00 for CH_3O^- and the "standard" leaving group is defined as Br, for which $L = 0.00$.

$$CH_3O^- + CH_3Y \longrightarrow CH_3OCH_3 + Y^- \quad (17)$$

Note that there is a general parallel between the nucleophilicity factor (L) for Y^- and the acidity (pK_a) of H–Y (except where Y is positively charged).

Two other types of biological alkylating agents deserve brief mention. One group consists of olefinic compounds with a double bond activated toward nucleophilic addition by a strong electron withdrawing group such as NO_2, CN, CO_2Et, COPh, or SO_2R. For example, divinyl sulfone has biological properties very similar to sulfur mustard, presumably because it can alkylate the same kinds of nucleophilic groups that sulfur mustard does.

$$2\,X^- + (CH_2{=}CH)_2SO_2 + 2\,H^+ \longrightarrow (XCH_2CH_2)_2SO_2 \quad (18)$$

Since in this reaction, the nucleophile is attacking an electron deficient carbon atom, relative reactivities of nucleophiles presumably parallel those for S_N2 reactions.

$$CH_2{=}CH{-}\underset{\substack{|\\Ph}}{C}{=}O \longleftrightarrow \overset{\delta+}{CH_2}{-}CH{=}\underset{\substack{|\\Ph}}{C}{-}\overset{\delta-}{O} \quad (19)$$

$$CH_3{-}X \longleftrightarrow \overset{\delta+}{CH_3}\overset{\delta-}{X} \quad (20)$$

A second quite different type of alkylation process is that involving diazoalkanes. Diazomethane, for example, shows a very different selectivity for DNA bases, preferring the very weakly nucleophilic thymine, rather than guanine or adenine preferred by S_N2 type reagents (see Price et al., 1968). In this case, the reaction appears to proceed through a carbenium ion intermediate, which reacts with the closest available nucleophilic center, the X^- of the H–X which generated the carbenium ion.

$$\begin{matrix} CH_2N_2 \\ + \\ H{-}X \end{matrix} \longrightarrow \begin{bmatrix} CH_3N_2^+ \\ \\ X^- \end{bmatrix} \xrightarrow{-N_2} \begin{bmatrix} CH_3^+ \\ \\ X^- \end{bmatrix} \longrightarrow CH_3X \quad (21)$$

References

Crist, D. R., Leonard, N. J.: Small charged heterocycles. Angew. Chem. 8, 962—974 (1969).

Price, C. C.: Fundamental mechanisms of alkylation. Ann. N. Y. Acad. Sci. **68**, 663—668 (1958).

Price, C. C., Gaucher, G. M., Koneru, P., Shibakawa, R., Sowa, J. R., Yamaguchi, M.: Relative reactivities for monofunctional nitrogen mustard alkylation of nucleic acid components. Biochim. biophys. Acta (Amst.) **166**, 327—359 (1968).

Price, C. C., Gaucher, G. M., Koneru, P., Shibakawa, R., Sowa, J. R., Yamaguchi, M.: Mechanism of action of alkylating agents. Ann. N. Y. Acad. Sci. **163**, 593—600 (1969).

Price, C. C., Yamaguchi, M., Sowa, J. R., Rao, K. P., Gaucher, G. M., Shibakawa, R.: Mechanism of action of alkylating agents. In: Brodsky, I., Kahn, S. B. (Eds.): Cancer chemotherapy. New York: Grune and Stratton 1967.

Sowa, J. R., Price, C. C.: Nitrogen mustard reactions by nuclear magnetic resonance spectroscopy. J. org. Chem. **34**, 474—476 (1969).

Thornton, E. R.: Solvolysis mechanisms. New York: Ronald Press 1964.

Chapter 31

Molecular Biology of Alkylation: An Overview

DAVID B. LUDLUM

With 5 Figures

Introduction

To explain the actions of an alkylating agent at a molecular level, changes in chemical structure produced by the agent must be related to specific biological effects. It is obvious that this easily stated objective is extremely difficult to achieve in practice. Not only do the alkylating agents react with virtually every cell component, but they produce a large number of important biological effects. Clearly, a working hypothesis must be adopted and the one discussed here is widely accepted – namely, that the alkylating agents produce their cytotoxic, mutagenic, and carcinogenic effects by reacting with cellular DNA. Some data do not fit into this scheme easily, and other hypotheses are probably still tenable. Indeed, different agents could act by different mechanisms, or different biological effects could be produced in different ways. Nevertheless, the suggestion that DNA is the primary target of alkylation has two important points in its favor: it correlates observations on a wide range of biological systems, and many of its fundamental features can be investigated experimentally. Recently, in a technique which serves to emphasize DNA alkylation, CASPERSSON et al. (1968) have used fluorescent alkylating agents to visualize chromosomal material.

In this chapter, data relevant to the hypothesis that DNA is the primary target of alkylation will be reviewed, placing special emphasis on the experimental techniques involved. Alternate hypotheses, as well as a further discussion of this one, may be found in recent review articles and collected works on alkylating agents (DRAKE, 1970; KARNOFSKY, 1958; KIHLMAN, 1966; LAWLEY, 1966; LOVELESS, 1966; OCHOA and HIRSCHBERG, 1967; ROSS, 1962; VAN DUUREN, 1969; WARWICK, 1963; WHEELER, 1962, 1963).

Alkylation of DNA

Several steps may be interposed between the exposure of a cell to an alkylating agent and the biological expression of damage to its DNA. There is already considerable evidence for all of the steps shown in Fig. 1.

This scheme consists basically of two parts: the formation of a definitive lesion in DNA and the subsequent malfunction of the damaged template. Much of the recent experimental work in this field has been concerned either with establishing an overall correlation between alkylation of DNA and particular biological effects, or with elucidating individual steps in the process shown in Fig. 1.

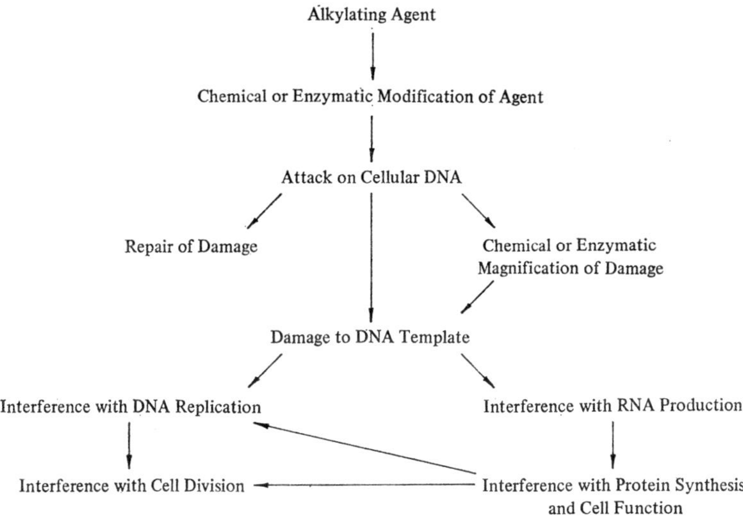

Fig. 1. Steps involved in the production and expression of damage to DNA

The organic chemistry of alkylation has been described in Chapter 30. The major types of damage to DNA, which may be of importance in modifying its biological function, are classified in Fig. 2.

1. Single substitution reactions
   a) Base substitution
   b) Phosphate esterification
2. Difunctional substitution reactions
   a) Interstrand crosslinks
   b) Intrastrand crosslinks
3. Depurination reactions
4. Single strand breaks
5. Double strand breaks

Fig. 2. Classification of damage to DNA

Attack on DNA by a monofunctional alkylating agent results in a single substitution reaction. Extensive studies by Brookes and Lawley (1961), Lawley and Brookes (1963), Lawley (1966), and other investigators have identified the base positions shown in Fig. 3 as primary sites of attack.

Substitution at the 7 position of guanine usually accounts for about 90% of the total alkylation. Smaller amounts of the other derivatives are formed, but these may be even more significant biologically. Thus, Loveless (1969) has recently drawn attention to alkylation at the *O*-6 position of guanine, Lawley et al. (1972) to alkylation at the *N*-3 position of guanine, and other workers (Ludlum and Wilhelm, 1968; Singer and Fraenkel-Conrat, 1969b) have stressed the possible importance of cytosine substitution. It is also becoming clear from recent studies that different alkylating agents may produce somewhat different distributions of minor alkylation products (Singer and Fraenkel-Conrat, 1969a; Lawley and Thatcher, 1970).

There is less agreement about esterification of phosphate groups because experimental difficulties are encountered in isolating the expected derivatives from DNA hydrolysates. However, recent studies on model compounds have shown that phosphate esterification probably does occur (LUDLUM, 1967; RHAESE and FREESE, 1969). Nevertheless, the biological effect of this attack is somewhat hard to assess; it could lead to chain scission, but would presumably lack the specificity of base substitution.

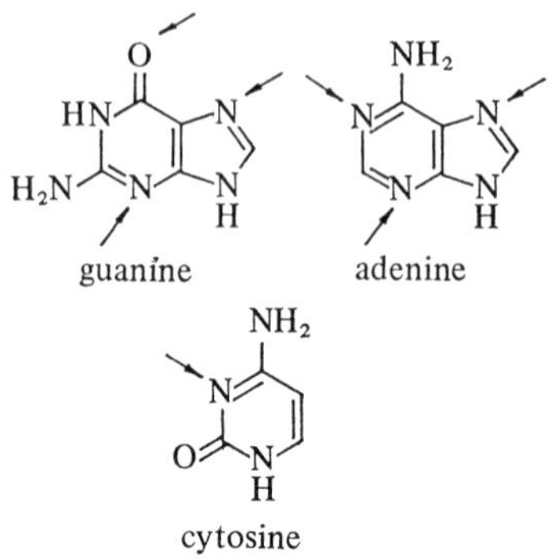

guanine adenine

cytosine

Fig. 3. Sites of base alkylation in DNA

Although the main chemical features of alkylation have been elucidated, specific details of the process may be very important. LAWLEY and BROOKES (1963) have shown that the secondary structure of DNA influences the site of alkylation; studies with polynucleotides (LUDLUM, 1965) have shown that this influence is very marked indeed. Changes in secondary structure during replication may well explain the special sensitivity of replicating cells to alkylation (LUDLUM, 1965; CERDÁ-OLMEDA et al., 1968), and more work should be done in this area.

The most effective alkylating agents from the standpoint of cytotoxicity have two reactive groups. Such compounds can result in single substitutions if one group on the alkylating agent is rendered inactive by hydrolysis. In addition, however, bifunctional compounds can form interstrand crosslinks in a double-stranded DNA helix, or intrastrand crosslinks within a single strand of DNA. Presumably, such crosslinks arise from an attack on neighboring guanines, since derivatives consisting of two guanines linked together by the residue of an alkylating agent have been isolated from DNA hydrolysates (LAWLEY and BROOKES, 1963).

Physical evidence for the existence of interstrand crosslinks is obtained by reversible denaturation experiments (GEIDUSCHEK, 1961; KOHN et al., 1966). When DNA is heated to a temperature sufficient to separate the two strands, and then cooled to room temperature, it will renature if the two strands are held in register by crosslinks. Such renaturation is detected by the melting behavior of the DNA, or by its buoyant density in a cesium chloride gradient.

Bases which either contain a single substitution or are involved in a crosslink may remain in DNA and lead to the mispairing phenomena discussed below. Alternatively, since the glycosidic bond is weakened by this substitution, the alkylated base may be released. This process of depurination leaves a gap in the sequence of DNA bases which, again, may lead to mispairing phenomena.

Finally, depurination weakens the sugar-phosphate backbone and may lead to chain scission. Enzymatic attack at the site of alkylation can also cause breaks in DNA as discussed below. If only one strand is involved in the helix, such breaks will be single-stranded. Double strand breaks will be produced occasionally if two single strand breaks occur independently opposite each other, or if both ends of an interstrand crosslink are converted to single strand breaks. Double strand breaks are significant in that they can probably not be repaired by enzymatic action, whereas single strand breaks can be.

These, then, are the major types of damage to DNA. At the molecular level, such damage is ultimately expressed as interference with the base-pairing process. Base-pairing may be prevented altogether, or it may occur incorrectly between bases which are not normally pairs in the Watson-Crick sense. In the first case, the template may be rendered totally inactive, or synthesis of the new strand may be terminated at the site of an alkylation or strand break. In any case, a non-functioning or misfunctioning product may result.

With respect to cancer chemotherapy, we are interested primarily in the mechanisms by which these agents produce cellular toxicity. However, the central position of base-pairing in expressing damage to DNA is a unifying feature in comparing data on the cytotoxic, mutagenic, and carcinogenic effects of these agents. Data on mutagenic effects, in particular, provide direct information on the cellular response to altered DNA. In a few cases (Yanofsky et al., 1966), the amino acid sequence of a protein produced by an alkylated DNA has been determined. In such cases, one can say that the biological effect of alkylation is completely determined at a molecular level.

The following sections will include a discussion of the effects of alkylating agents on bacteriophage, a discussion of enzymatic modification of the original DNA lesion in bacterial cells, a summary of similar data obtained on mammalian cells, and, finally, experiments which yield information on the mispairing of alkylated bases.

Correlations between DNA alkylation and lethality can be firmly established in bacteriophage systems where DNA can be isolated intact for analytical studies, and survival can be assayed on the bacterial host. Accordingly, some of the most precise data on cytotoxicity have been obtained in such systems.

Effects of Alkylating Agents on Bacteriophage

The lethal action of an alkylating agent is commonly expressed in the form of a dose-response curve like the hypothetical one in Fig. 4. These curves are constructed to show the dependence of log survival on alkylating agent concentration. A linear relationship indicates a one-hit process – i.e., a noncooperative lethal action by individual alkylations. A shoulder, such as the one shown, can result from a multiple hit process; more frequently, however, it indicates repair by enzymes in the host bacteria.

Data of the type shown in Fig. 4 are obtained when alkylated phage are assayed for viability immediately after treatment. Loveless and Stock (1959) showed that a further decrease in viability occurred when the phage were stored for a period of time before assay. Later, Ronen (1968) demonstrated that the delayed inactivation of phage T_4 by ethyl methanesulfonate was a kinetically distinct reaction from immediate inactivation, suggesting that the two were different chemical processes. Immediate inactivation is usually attributed to base alkylation or some other initial chemical reaction, whereas delayed inactivation seems to be related to depurination, at least for monofunctional agents.

YAMAMOTO et al. (1966) compared the cytotoxicity of mono and difunctional nitrogen mustards on bacteriophage which contained either single or double-stranded DNA or single-stranded RNA. The greater biological activity of bifunctional compounds was clearly demonstrated in these studies. This was true in all

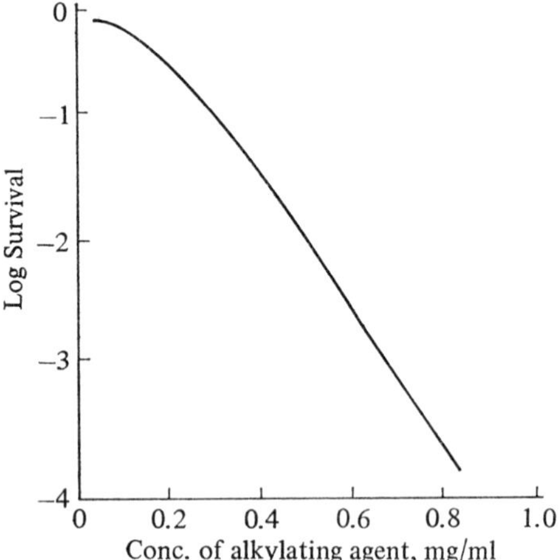

Fig. 4. Dependence of bacteriophage survival on alkylating agent concentration for a hypothetical compound

cases, emphasizing the possible importance of intrastrand as well as interstrand crosslinks in causing lethality. LOVELESS (1966) also indicated that bifunctional agents have an increased lethality towards bacteriophage which contain either single or double-stranded DNA.

Recently, detailed studies have been performed on the T_7 phage, which contains a smaller, more easily studied DNA molecule. LAWLEY et al. (1969) compared the actions of sulfur mustard [di-(2-chloroethyl)sulfide] and half sulfur mustard (2-chloroethyl-2-hydroxyethyl sulfide) on this bacteriophage. As expected, the bifunctional compound was much more effective than half sulfur mustard in causing immediate inactivation. At the mean lethal dose of sulfur mustard, there were about 1.3 moles of di-(guanin-7-yl-ethyl) sulfide and 7 moles of monoalkylation products per mole of DNA polymer, whereas 280 moles of monoalkylation products were formed at the mean lethal dose of half sulfur mustard. Formation of a crosslink was clearly much more damaging than a single substitution reaction. Physical data indicated that approximately one quarter of these were interstrand crosslinks, and the remainder were intrastrand in nature.

Delayed inactivation was relatively unimportant following reaction with sulfur mustard, but accounted for extensive inactivation after treatment with half mustard. Delayed inactivation in the latter case was associated with depurination of the alkylated residues.

VERLY and BRAKIER (1969) and BRAKIER and VERLY (1970) have studied the action of ethyl methanesulfonate, nitrogen mustard, myleran, and diepoxybutane on the same T_7 bacteriophage. Their results on the monofunctional compound, ethyl methanesulfonate, are qualitatively very similar to those of LAWLEY et al. (1969) on half sulfur mustard. Crosslinks were again associated with lethality for the difunctional nitrogen mustard, but the dependence was rather complex. When the phage were incubated for varying periods of time before assay, lethality first increased and subsequently decreased. During the later part of this period, the number of crosslinks also decreased; presumably, one end of the diguaninyl bridge was released by depurination.

There was no evidence for interstrand crosslinks when the T_7 phage was treated with myleran, another bifunctional agent. In fact, the behavior of this compound was in many ways similar to that of ethyl methanesulfonate. Although the possibility of intrastrand crosslinks was not ruled out, some other factor might explain the difference between the action of these two compounds on higher organisms. The final compound studied, diepoxybutane, formed a few crosslinks, but evidently produced some lethality by a monofunctional mechanism.

There are many other excellent studies which correlate damage to DNA with lethality to microorganisms. Unfortunately, there is insufficient space to mention all of these in this section; reference may be made to LOVELESS' book (1966) for a complete coverage of earlier work in this area.

The identity of biologically important lesions in DNA can be partially elucidated from studies of point mutations. Genetic data on reversion frequencies, or analyses of amino acid substitutions in the gene product, will often identify the base pair which is affected by a particular alkylating agent. Some uncertainty remains about the details of the mispairing process involved in these changes, however, since the change in chemical structure produced at the significant point within the DNA molecule cannot be identified with certainty.

TESSMAN et al. (1964) studied mutations which were produced in S_{13}, a single-stranded DNA phage, by ethyl methanesulfonate. Their data indicated that all four bases could be altered by this alkylating agent, but that $G \rightarrow A$ and $C \rightarrow T$ changes occurred most frequently. The earlier data of BAUTZ and FREESE (1960) and of KRIEG (1963) on T_4, and the more recent studies by OSBORN et al. (1967) with bacteria, suggest that $GC \rightarrow AT$ transitions are caused by alkylating agents. Studies by YANOFSKY et al. (1966) on amino acid replacements in the A protein of tryptophane synthetase did not, however, result in a totally unambiguous assignment of base changes produced by alkylating agents. In summary, then, data obtained from mutants suggest that a GC pair is changed to an AT pair most frequently, but that other changes can also occur.

Cellular Modification of Damaged DNA

The inactivation of the T_7 phage mentioned above occurred by one-hit kinetics, and there was no evidence for repair of initial damage to the DNA by host enzymes. However, there is an extensive and rapidly growing literature on cellular mechanisms, which, in bacteria, repair damage either to host cell DNA or to DNA of phage grown in the appropriate bacteria. Similar, but not as extensively studied, mechanisms are found in mammalian cells. Reviews by STRAUSS (1968) and HOWARD-FLANDERS (1968) cover the basic material in this area, but it remains a field of extremely active investigation.

Several classes of *E. coli* mutants have been selected on the basis of sensitivity to ultraviolet light. Frequently, these mutants are also deficient in their ability to repair alkylation damage. The following types are recognized. (1) HCR mutants. These bacteria, in addition to having a diminished ability to repair UV-induced lesions in their own DNA, have lost the ability to repair damage to phage DNA by a process known as host cell reactivation. (2) UVR mutants. These are UV sensitive mutants which are still able to repair UV-induced damage to phage DNA

(3) REC mutants. These UV-sensitive mutants are characterized by deficiencies in their ability to undergo genetic recombination.

Relationships among these different phenotypes, and the different mechanisms of repair which are implied by their existence, are extremely complex. The best established model is the excision-repair process for UV damage proposed independently by Setlow and Carrier (1964) and by Boyce and Howard-Flanders (1964). This model is particularly important because some repair of alkylation damage probably follows a similar pathway. This process, sketched in Fig. 5, consists of the following steps:

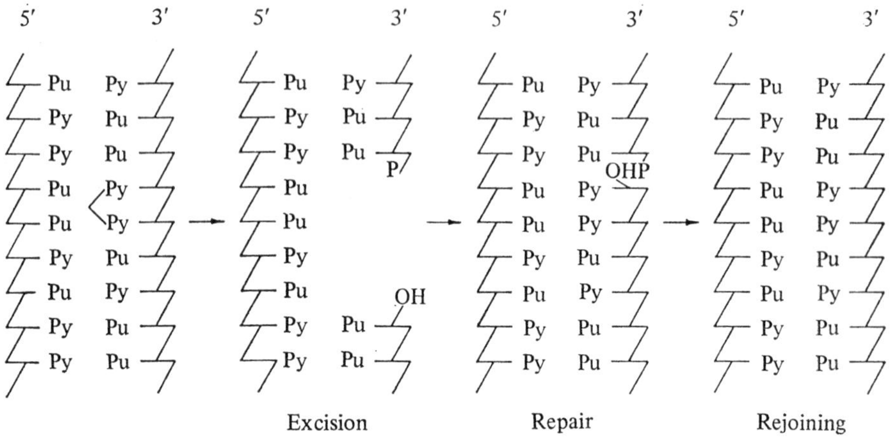

Fig. 5. Excision-repair process for UV-induced damage to DNA. *Pu* represents a purine base, and *Py*, a pyrimidine base. Sugar-phosphate bonds are drawn in the conventional manner. $\widehat{PyPy}$ represents a pyrimidine dimer located in a section of DNA

1. *Excision.* Repair is initiated when an endonuclease recognizes an abnormal region in the DNA and excises it. In the case of UV damage, this abnormal region is a pyrimidine dimer produced by the radiation; in the case of alkylation, it is presumably an alkylated base or a crosslink. Recognition of an abnormality may be based on local disturbances in the secondary structure of DNA rather than on changes in the primary structure. Following the initial excision, several neighboring deoxyribonucleoside 5′-phosphates are released.

2. *Repair Synthesis.* The correct nucleotides are replaced by an enzymatic process which presumably uses deoxyribonucleoside 5′-triphosphates as substrates and the other strand of DNA as template.

3. *Rejoining.* The final nucleotide bond is completed by a ligase enzyme which leaves the repaired strand intact.

Repair synthesis may be demonstrated by the simultaneous use of a density and radioactive pulse label in a method which distinguishes it from semiconservative synthesis. Thus, ^{3}H-labeled bromodeoxyuridine may be substituted for thymidine during a brief period of DNA synthesis. Since UV damage occurs along both strands of DNA, excision and repair of these regions will distribute small amounts of ^{3}H-labeled bromodeoxyuridine throughout the entire double-stranded DNA helix. Therefore, both strands of repaired DNA will band together in an alkaline cesium chloride gradient at a density which is not detectably greater than that occupied by normal single-stranded DNA. This is in sharp contrast to the situation after semiconservative (replicative) synthesis where all of the bromodeoxyuridine is concentrated in one strand of DNA, causing that strand to band at a much higher density. Since there may not have been time to replicate the entire strand of DNA, the resolution of this method may be increased by shearing the double-stranded DNA before banding it.

Damage caused by both monofunctional and bifunctional alkylating agents can evidently be repaired by a process similar to the one described above. Loss of sulfur mustard alkylation products from the DNA of *E. coli* was demonstrated by PAPIRMEISTER and DAVIDSON (1964); as these products were eliminated, the bacteria gradually regained their ability to synthesize DNA and divide. Repair synthesis was demonstrated after treatment with a monofunctional agent (methyl methanesulfonate) by REITER and STRAUSS (1965) and after treatment with a bifunctional agent by HANAWALT and HAYNES (1965). LAWLEY and BROOKES (1965) and KOHN et al. (1965) obtained evidence that crosslinks were eliminated in *E. coli B/r*, but not in *E. coli* B_{s-1}.

Thus, under certain conditions, the cell is evidently able to repair alkylation damage. Under other conditions, however, the original damage may be magnified by cellular enzymes. STRAUSS et al. (1969) have recently summarized their studies on the enzymatic degradation of methylated DNA. They have described an endonuclease which apparently attacks some, but not all, methylated sites. Recent work by PAPIRMEISTER et al. (1970) suggests that the DNA of T_1 bacteriophage is sensitized to attack by adenine alkylation rather than the more prevalent guanine alkylation. There is a real possibility, therefore, that alkylations which are not particularly damaging in themselves may lead to significant enzymatic degradation. If the excised portions are not replaced by a repair mechanism, the original damage would be greatly magnified by this process.

The ability of a cell either to repair or to magnify the original chemical lesion may help to explain the development of cell lines resistant to alkylating agents. Tumor cells frequently become resistant to treatment, and this is a common clinical problem with these compounds. Clearly, resistance could develop from the loss of enzymes which magnify the original lesion, or from the development of an enhanced repair capability. Again, this is an active area for current research.

The importance of DNA alkylation and the repair of such damage were both first demonstrated in bacterial cells and their viruses. Many investigators have now demonstrated that mammalian cells show similar behavior. Unfortunately, it is not possible to cover all of this work here, but a few representative studies will be mentioned.

ROBERTS et al. (1968) have investigated the toxic effects of sulfur mustard and half mustard on HeLa cells. DNA synthesis was selectively affected by low concentrations of these compounds, and the bifunctional agents were much more toxic than the monofunctional one. Since mammalian cells synthesize DNA during a portion of their cell cycle only, cell growth was synchronized for a detailed investigation of this effect. Different stages of cell growth were found to have different sensitivities to alkylation damage; treatment of cells in the late G_1 (postmitotic) or early S (DNA synthetic) phases, particularly, resulted in a delay in cell division. Some recovery occurred by later cycles, and this was attributed to repair of alkylated DNA, a process which was accompanied by release of low molecular weight derivatives of the alkylating agent.

More recently, BALL and ROBERTS (1970) have reported a quantitative investigation of repair in sensitive and resistant Yoshida cells. Both lines were able to excise alkylated moieties from DNA and to carry out repair synthesis, and it was not possible to explain the differences in sensitivity on the basis of overall differences in repair. However, other steps in the repair process may be involved, or a particular, minor lesion may exert an overriding influence on survival.

Repair or modification of initial damage to DNA has also been studied in HeLa and Chinese hamster cells by ROBERTS et al. (1971a, b), in L cells by REID and WALKER (1969), and in Ehrlich ascites cells by CHUN et al. (1969). The latter authors and WALKER (1971) have also pointed out that many of the crosslinks in mammalian cell DNA may be intrastrand in nature. For this reason, release of diguaninyl compounds cannot be equated with the elimination of interstrand crosslinks.

Functional Capacity of Alkylated Template

Thus, DNA is alkylated and, to some extent, repaired in many different types of cells. Referring back to Fig. 1, however, it is clear that we must still determine how this affects cellular function. At a molecular level, we must show how damage to DNA is expressed during replication and transcription. Presumably, a fragmented template will lead to an inactive or malfunctioning product, but it is less clear how a slightly modified template – e.g., one containing a single substituted base – will be interpreted.

This problem can be studied with simple polynucleotide templates in the model systems shown in Table 1. Each of these systems uses the information contained in the template at the left to direct the synthesis of the polymer at the right. A polynucleotide containing a particular substituted base can be incubated with the required enzyme or cell extract, and its performance compared with that of a similar polynucleotide which does not contain the odd base. Thus, the mispairing associated with a particular base substitution can be observed directly.

Table 1. *Model systems for testing base-pairing relationships*

System	Enzyme
DNA → DNA	DNA polymerase
DNA → RNA	RNA polymerase
RNA → RNA	RNA polymerase
RNA → protein	cell extract

The author and his colleagues have introduced this approach in studies of simple methylating and ethylating agents. Concentrating first on the substituted base found most frequently after treatment with a methylating agent, WILHELM and LUDLUM (1966) investigated polypeptide synthesis directed by 7-methylguanine-containing polyribonucleotides. These experiments were designed to detect amino acid incorporation which would occur if 7-methylguanine resembled adenine in its base-pairing properties. No such misincorporation was observed, but the overall ability of the 7-methylguanine-containing templates to promote polypeptide synthesis was diminished.

More extensive studies of the mispairing process have been performed with the enzyme, RNA polymerase. This enzyme can use either a DNA or RNA strand to direct the synthesis of a daughter strand. Experiments with synthetic RNA templates have progressed further than experiments with synthetic DNA templates because the former are somewhat easier to synthesize. However, the base-pairing properties of the synthetic polydeoxyribonucleotides have, in general, resembled those of the ribose series. Accordingly, one would expect abnormal base-pairing behavior in one series of polymers to occur in the other series as well.

Experiments with polyribonucleotide templates show, first of all, that 7-methylguanine retains the base-pairing properties of guanine (LUDLUM, 1970a). On the other hand, 3-methyl and 3-ethylcytosine, compounds which are produced in much smaller amounts when cellular DNA is alkylated, cause marked misincorporation of uridylic and adenylic acid into daughter polynucleotides (LUDLUM and WILHELM, 1968; LUDLUM, 1970b; SINGER and FRAENKEL-CONRAT, 1970). This finding has now been verified in experiments with polydeoxyribonucleotide templates (LUDLUM, 1971). Although no molecular explanation for this misincorporation has yet been devised, studies by SINGER and FRAENKEL-CONRAT (1969) emphasize the possible biological importance of cytosine substitution in explaining mutational events in TMV RNA. Thus, the biological significance of relatively minor substitution products may sometimes exceed that of guanine alkylation. Additional studies are in progress to delineate the effects of other base alterations, including crosslinking reactions.

To summarize our present state of knowledge, therefore, there is a considerable body of evidence which relates alkylation of DNA to important biological effects. The most significant lesions in DNA have not been identified with certainty, but the production of intra and interstrand crosslinks seems to be especially important in explaining the cytotoxicity of bifunctional agents. Finally, the original lesions produced in the DNA are probably modified or repaired with some frequency, but the exact mechanism by which the remaining lesions produce cellular dysfunction is not yet completely elucidated.

References

BALL, C. R., ROBERTS, J. J.: DNA repair after mustard gas alkylation by sensitive and resistant Yoshida sarcoma cells *in vitro*. Chem. Biol. Interact. **2**, 321—329 (1970).

BAUTZ, E., FREESE, E.: On the mutagenic effect of alkylating agents. Proc. nat. Acad. Sci. (Wash.) **46**, 1585—1594 (1960).

BOYCE, R. P., HOWARD-FLANDERS, P.: Release of ultraviolet light-induced thymine dimers from DNA in *E. coli* K-12. Proc. nat. Acad. Sci. (Wash.) **51**, 293—300 (1964).

BRAKIER, L., VERLY, W. G.: The lethal action of ethyl methanesulfonate, nitrogen mustard, and myleran on the T_7 coliphage. Biochim. biophys. Acta **213**, 296—311 (1970).

BROOKES, P., LAWLEY, P. D.: The reaction of mono- and difunctional alkylating agents with nucleic acids. Biochem. J. **80**, 495—503 (1961).

CASPERSSON, T., FARBER, S., FOLEY, G. E., KUDYNOWSKI, J., MODEST, E. J., SIMONSSON, E., WAGH, U., ZECH, L.: Chemical differentiation along metaphase chromosomes. Exp. cell Res. **49**, 219—222 (1968).

CERDÁ-OLMEDA, E., HANAWALT, P. C., GUEROLA, N.: Mutagenesis of the replication point by nitrosoguanidine: map and patterns of replication of the *Escherichia coli* chromosome. J. molec. Biol. **33**, 705—719 (1968).

CHUN, E. H. L., GONZALES, L., LEWIS, F. S., JONES, J., RUTMAN, R. J.: Differences in the *in vivo* alkylation and cross-linking of nitrogen-mustard-sensitive and -resistant lines of Lettré-Ehrlich ascites tumours. Cancer Res. **29**, 1184—1194 (1969).

DRAKE, J. W.: The molecular basis of mutation. San Francisco: Holden-Day 1970.

GEIDUSCHEK, P.: "Reversible" DNA. Proc. nat. Acad. Sci. (Wash.) **47**, 950—955 (1961).

HANAWALT, P., HAYNES, R.: Repair replication of DNA in bacteria: irrelevance of chemical nature of base defect. Biochem. biophys. Res. Commun. **19**, 462—467 (1965).

HOWARD-FLANDERS, P.: DNA repair. Ann. Rev. Biochem. **37**, 175—200 (1968).

KARNOFSKY, D. A. (Ed.): Comparative clinical and biological effects of alkylating agents. Ann. N. Y. Acad. Sci. **68**, 657—1266 (1958).

KIHLMAN, B. A.: Actions of chemicals on dividing cells. Englewood Cliffs, N. J.: Prentice-Hall 1966.

KOHN, K. W., SPEARS, C. L., DOTY, P.: Inter-strand crosslinking of DNA by nitrogen mustard. J. molec. Biol. **19**, 266—288 (1966).

KOHN, K.W., STEIGBIGEL, N., SPEARS, C.: Cross linking and repair of DNA in sensitive and resistant strains of *E. coli* treated with nitrogen mustard. Proc. Nat. Acad. Sci. (Wash.) **53**, 1154—1161 (1965).
KRIEG, D.R.: Ethyl methanesulfonate-induced reversion of bacteriophage T_4r II mutants. Genetics **48**, 561—580 (1963).
LAWLEY, P.D.: Effects of some chemical mutagens and carcinogens on nucleic acids. Progr. nucleic Acid. Res. **5**, 89—131 (1966).
LAWLEY, P.D., BROOKES, P.: Further studies on the alkylation of nucleic acids and their constituent nucleotides. Biochem. J. **89**, 127—144 (1963).
LAWLEY, P.D., BROOKES, P.: Molecular mechanism of the cytotoxic action of difunctional alkylating agents and of resistance to this action. Nature (Lond.) **206**, 480—483 (1965).
LAWLEY, P.D., LETHBRIDGE, J.H., EDWARDS, P.A., SHOOTER, K.V.: Inactivation of bacteriophage T_7 by mono- and difunctional sulphur mustards in relation to cross-linking and depurination of bacteriophage DNA. J. molec. Biol. **39**, 181—198 (1969).
LAWLEY, P.D., ORR, D.J., SHAH, S.A.: Reaction of alkylating mutagens and carcinogens with nucleic acids: N-3 of guanine as a site of alkylation by N-methyl-N-nitrosourea and dimethyl sulfate. Chem. biol. Interact. **4**, 431—434 (1971/72).
LAWLEY, P.D., THATCHER, C.J.: Methylation of deoxyribonucleic acid in cultured mammalian cells by *N*-methyl-*N'*-nitro-*N*-nitrosoguanidine. Biochem. J. **116**, 693—707 (1970).
LOVELESS, A.: Genetic and allied effects of alkylating agents. University Park and London: Pennsylvania State University Press 1966.
LOVELESS, A.: Possible relevance of *O*-6 alkylation of deoxyguanosine to the mutagenicity and carcinogenicity of nitrosamines and nitrosamides. Nature (Lond.) **223**, 206—207 (1969).
LOVELESS, A., STOCK, J.C.: The influence of radiomimetic substances on deoxyribonucleic acid synthesis and function studied in *Escherichia coli* phage systems. I. The nature of the inactivation of T_2 phage *in vitro* by certain alkylating agents. Proc. roy. Soc. B **150**, 423—445 (1959).
LUDLUM, D.B.: Alkylation of polynucleotide complexes. Biochim. biophys. Acta **95**, 674—676 (1965).
LUDLUM, D.B.: Reaction of nitrogen mustard with synthetic polynucleotides. Biochim. biophys. Acta **142**, 282—284 (1967).
LUDLUM, D.B.: The properties of 7-methylguanine-containing templates for ribonucleic acid polymerase. J. biol. Chem. **245**, 477—482 (1970a).
LUDLUM, D.B.: Alkylated polycytidylic acid templates for RNA polymerase. Biochim. biophys. Acta **213**, 142—148 (1970b).
LUDLUM, D.B.: Methylated polydeoxyribocytidylic acid templates for RNA polymerase. Biochim. biophys. Acta **247**, 412—418 (1971).
LUDLUM, D.B., WILHELM, R.C.: Ribonucleic acid polymerase reactions with methylated polycytidylic acid templates. J. biol. Chem. **243**, 2750—2753 (1968).
OCHOA, M., JR., HIRSCHBERG, E.: Alkylating agents. In: SCHNITZER, R.J., HAWKING, F. (Eds.): Experimental chemotherapy, Vol. 5, pp. 1—132. New York and London: Academic Press 1967.
OSBORN, M., PERSON, S., PHILLIPS, S., FUNK, F.: A determination of mutagen specificity in bacteria using nonsense mutants of bacteriophage T_4. J. molec. Biol. **26**, 437—447 (1967).
PAPIRMEISTER, B., DAVIDSON, C.L.: Elimination of sulfur-mustard-induced products from DNA of *Escherichia coli*. Biochem. biophys. Res. Commun. **17**, 608—617 (1964).
PAPIRMEISTER, B., DORSEY, J.K., DAVIDSON, C.L., GROSS, C.L.: Sensitization of DNA to endonuclease by adenine alkylation and its biological significance. Fed. Proc. **29**, 726 (1970).
REID, B.D., WALKER, I.G.: The response of mammalian cells to alkylating agents. II. On the mechanism of the removal of sulphur-mustard-induced cross-links. Biochim. biophys. Acta **179**, 179—188 (1969).
REITER, H., STRAUSS, B.: Repair of damage induced by a monofunctional alkylating agent in a transformable, ultraviolet-sensitive strain of *Bacillus subtilis*. J. molec. Biol. **14**, 179—194 (1965).
RHAESE, H.J., FREESE, E.: Chemical analysis of DNA alterations. IV. Reactions of oligodeoxynucleotides with monofunctional alkylating agents leading to backbone breakage. Biochim. biophys. Acta **190**, 418—433 (1969).
ROBERTS, J.J., BRENT, T.P., CRATHORN, A.R.: The mechanism of the cytotoxic action of alkylating agents on mammalian cells. In: CAMPBELL, P.N. (Ed.): The interaction of drugs and subcellular components in animal cells, pp. 5—27. London: Churchill 1968.
ROBERTS, J.J., PASCOE, J.M., PLANT, J.E., STURROCK, J.E., CRATHORN, A.R.: Quantitative aspects of the repair of alkylated DNA in cultured mammalian cells. I. The effect on HeLa and Chinese hamster cell survival of alkylation of cellular macromolecules. Chem. biol. Interact. **3**, 29—47 (1971a).

ROBERTS, J. J., PASCOE, J. M., SMITH, B. A., CRATHORN, A. R.: Quantitative aspects of the repair of alkylated DNA in cultured mammalian cells. II. Non-semiconservative DNA synthesis (repair synthesis) in HeLa and Chinese hamster cells following treatment with alkylating agents. Chem. biol. Interact. **3**, 49—68 (1971b).
RONEN, A.: Inactivation of phage T_4 by ethylmethane sulfonate. Biochem. biophys. Res. Commun. **33**, 190—196 (1968).
ROSS, W. C. J.: Biological alkylating agents. London: Butterworth 1962.
SETLOW, R. B., CARRIER, W. L.: The disappearance of thymine dimers from DNA: an error-correcting mechanism. Proc. nat. Acad. Sci. (Wash.) **51**, 226—231 (1964).
SINGER, B., FRAENKEL-CONRAT, H.: Chemical modifications of viral ribonucleic acid. VII. The action of methylating agents and nitrosoguanidine on polynucleotides including tobacco mosiac virus ribonucleic acid. Biochemistry **8**, 3260—3266 (1969a).
SINGER, B., FRAENKEL-CONRAT, H.: Chemical modification of viral ribonucleic acid. VIII. The chemical and biochemical effects of methylating agents and nitrosoguanidine on tobacco mosiac virus. Biochemistry **8**, 3266—3269 (1969b).
SINGER, B., FRAENKEL-CONRAT, H.: Messenger and template activities of chemically modified polynucleotides. Biochemistry **9**, 3694—3701 (1970).
STRAUSS, B. S.: DNA repair mechanisms and their relation to mutation and recombination. Curr. Top. Microbiol. and Immunol. **44**, 1—85 (1968).
STRAUSS, B., COYLE, M., ROBBINS, M.: Consequences of alkylation for the behavior of DNA. Ann. N. Y. Acad. Sci. **163**, 765—787 (1969).
TESSMAN, I., PODDAR, R. K., KUMAR, S.: Identification of the altered bases in mutated single-stranded DNA. J. molec. Biol. **9**, 352—363 (1964).
VAN DUUREN, B. L. (Ed.): Biological effects of alkylating agents. Ann. N. Y. Acad. Sci. **163**, 589—1029 (1969).
VERLY, W. G., BRAKIER, L.: The lethal action of monofunctional and bifunctional alkylating agents on T_7 coliphage. Biochim. biophys. Acta **174**, 674—685 (1969).
WALKER, I. G.: Intrastrand bifunctional alkylation of DNA in mammalian cells treated with mustard gas. Can. J. Biochem. **49**, 332—336 (1971).
WARWICK, G. P.: The mechanism of action of alkylating agents. Cancer Res. **23**, 1315—1333 (1963).
WHEELER, G. P.: Studies related to the mechanism of action of cytotoxic alkylating agents. A review. Cancer Res. **22**, 651—688 (1962).
WHEELER, G. P.: Studies related to mechanisms of resistance to biological alkylating agents. Cancer Res. **23**, 1334—1349 (1963).
WILHELM, R. C., LUDLUM, D. B.: Coding properties of 7-methylguanine. Science **153**, 1403—1405 (1966).
YAMAMOTO, N., NAITO, T., SHIMKIN, M. B.: Mechanism of inactivation of DNA and RNA bacteriophages by alkylating agents *in vitro*. Cancer Res. **26**, 2301—2306 (1966).
YANOFSKY, C., ITO, J., HORN, V.: Amino acid replacement and the genetic code. Sympos. quant. Biol. **31**, 151—162 (1966).

Chapter 32

Mechanism of Action of 2-Chloroethylamine Derivatives, Sulfur Mustards, Epoxides, and Aziridines

T. A. Connors

With 2 Figures

Introduction

The first recorded observations on the biological effects of alkylating agents appeared in the literature at the turn of the century (Meyer, 1887), one of the earliest observations being made, appropriately enough, by Paul Ehrlich, the founder of modern chemotherapy (see the collected papers of Paul Ehrlich, 1956). Although it was initially their vesicant properties that excited most attention and led to their intensive investigation and limited use as chemical warfare agents, it was appreciated very early that these chemicals could have effects on different tissues at sites distant from the area of application (Lynch et al., 1918; Krumbhaar and Krumbhaar, 1919; Warthin and Weller, 1919; Pappenheimer and Vance, 1920; Flury and Wieland, 1921). Almost forty years ago it was known that sulfur mustard had antitumor effects in experimental animals, and it was used clinically in the treatment of a solid tumor by direct injection into the tumor (Berenblum, 1935; Adair and Bagg, 1931). However, the extreme toxicity of these early alkylating agents, and their use in chemical warfare, never suggested that they might prove generally useful in the treatment of cancer. The advent of the second World War necessitated a detailed study of the properties of sulfur mustard and the synthesis and testing of many related derivatives. The experience gained in the handling of the agents during this period, and the synthesis of less vesicant analogs was followed by the demonstration that many alkylating agents had relatively selective effects on lymphoid tissue and other rapidly dividing cells. These findings led to the suggestion, obvious in retrospect but imaginative at the time, that they might be useful in the treatment of tumors of the lymphoid system. Preliminary experiments in tumor-bearing animals, followed by cautious clinical trials, revealed that methyl-di-2-chloroethylamine had useful properties in the treatment of Hodgkin's disease and certain lymphosarcomas. These results were published in 1946 to 1948 in a series of papers, and the first one in the series (Gilman and Philips, 1946) marks the beginning of fundamental and applied studies on the biological properties of the alkylating agents and their mechanism of action. Since 1946, studies on these agents have increased exponentially, and the results of screening many thousands of derivatives for their antitumor action have been published (e.g. Bratzel et al., 1963; Schmidt et al., 1965; Cancer Research Supplements, 1953–1967).

By 1957, the clinical and experimental antitumor effects of a wide variety of alkylating agents had been investigated in detail, and it was recognized that they had properties in common with x-rays, and that, under certain conditions, they could be carcinogenic, mutagenic and teratogenic (Ann. N. Y. Acad. Sci. Symposium, 1958). A follow-up symposium ten years later (Ann. N. Y. Acad. Sci., 1969), while still concerned with the evaluation of new alkylating derivatives for their antitumor activity, also devoted much of its time to the study of alkylating agents in many other areas of research.

The past fifteen years have seen the first successes in the clinical treatment of cancer using alkylating agents, whether alone or in combination with other agents (LIVINGSTON and CARTER, 1970; AARON, 1970). Their present day status in clinical chemotherapy has been the subject of many reviews (LARIONOV, 1965; BOESEN and DAVIS, 1969; COLE, 1970; SELLEI et al., 1970; ELKERBOUT et al., 1971). It is maintained by some that all alkylating agents are so similar in their mechanism of action that there is no point in their further study or in the synthesis of new types in attempts to obtain better antitumor agents. Others maintain that an ever increasing knowledge of the mechanism of action of these agents, combined with a greater knowledge of the biochemistry of cancer cells, will ultimately lead to the design of alkylating agents with selective toxicity for all forms of cancer.

The Mechanism of Alkylation

Fundamental to a study of the mechanism of action of the alkylating agents is a knowledge of the chemistry of alkylation. This has been the subject of a number of reviews (GOLUMBIC et al., 1946; ROSS, 1953, 1962; PRICE, 1958; WARWICK, 1963; PRICE et al., 1969), and is dealt with in more detail elsewhere in this volume. In the majority of cases the mechanism of alkylation is quite clear, and proceeds through a second order nucleophilic substitution (S_N2) as in the case of epoxides:

$$\underset{\diagdown O \diagup}{R \cdot CH \cdot CH_2} + A^- \xrightarrow{H_2O} R \cdot CH(OH)CH_2A + OH^- ,$$

or in the case of ethyleneimines (aziridines) or ethyleneimides:

$$R \cdot N\left\langle \begin{matrix} CH_2 \\ | \\ CH_2 \end{matrix} \right. + A^- \xrightarrow{H_2O} R \cdot NH \cdot CH_2 \cdot CH_2 \cdot A + OH^- .$$

Protonation of the nitrogen leads to increased reactivity, and both ethyleneimines and epoxides are more reactive under acid conditions. Since both classes act by a bimolecular mechanism their rate of reaction with nucleophilic centers will be dependent on the concentration of such centers.

The basic aliphatic nitrogen mustards act by a similar mechanism following formation of a cyclic immonium ion:

$$R_2N \cdot CH_2CH_2Cl \rightleftharpoons R_2 \cdot \overset{+}{N}\left\langle \begin{matrix} CH_2 \\ | \\ CH_2 \end{matrix} \right. + Cl^- \xrightarrow{A^-} R_2N \cdot CH_2CH_2A .$$

The unimolecular conversion to the immonium ion is relatively fast, and alkylation of the nucleophilic center (A^-) by the immonium ion then proceeds by a bimolecular reaction dependent on the concentration of reacting centers. In contrast to the ethyleneimines and epoxides, the alkylating properties of nitrogen mustards are depressed in acid solution.

It is only in the case of the less basic aromatic nitrogen mustards and the sulfur mustards that there has been any question concerning their mechanism of alkylation. With these compounds, the lower basicity of the nitrogen or sulfur atom does not allow the formation of a stable cyclic immonium ion analogous to the aliphatic nitrogen mustards. These compounds follow first order kinetics in their alkylation reactions, the rate of alkylation being independent of the concentration of nucleophilic centers. This finding, and the observation that chloride and hydrogen ions were always simultaneously liberated in equivalent quantities upon hydrolysis, led ROSS (1962, 1963) to propose that these alkylating agents react through a carbonium ion formed by unimolecular loss of a chloride ion (Pathway 1, Fig. 1), rather than by formation of a cyclic intermediate analogous to the aliphatic nitrogen mustards (Pathway 2, Fig. 1).

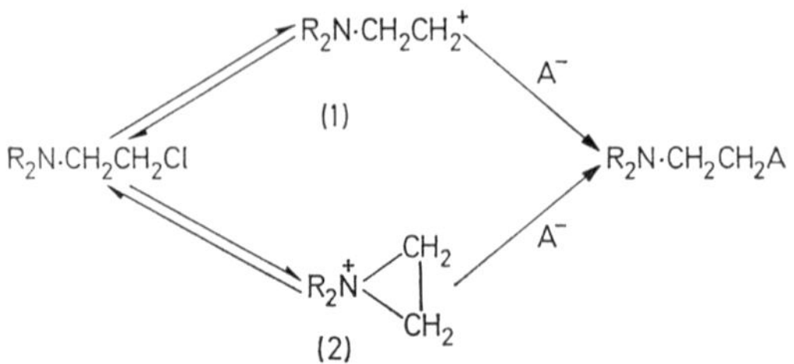

Fig. 1. Mechanisms of Alkylation

This assumption of a different mechanism of alkylation for the less basic nitrogen mustards has been questioned by some authors (TRIGGLE, 1964; PRICE et al., 1969; BARDOS et al., 1969). Evidence has also been obtained that at least one aromatic nitrogen mustard may, under the appropriate conditions, form a relatively stable reactive intermediate, and may also release chloride at a significantly faster rate than alkylating activity disappears (WILLIAMSON and WITTEN, 1967).

Probably all authors now agree that the aromatic nitrogen mustards act similarly to other alkylating agents, but that their mechanism of alkylation superficially resembles an S_N1 nucleophilic substitution. For these agents, cyclization is very slow compared to ring opening (by hydrolysis or by alkylation of a nucleophilic center). There will therefore be no accumulation of a cyclic intermediate and the rate determining step will be first-order ionization of the halogen atom.

The important difference for the biologist is that the majority of alkylating agents act by a bimolecular mechanism and their rate of alkylation depends on the concentration of nucleophilic centers. The aromatic nitrogen mustards, however, have a rate of alkylation independent of substrate concentration. A knowledge of these mechanistic differences can explain observed differences in biological effects between aliphatic and aromatic nitrogen mustards (CONNORS et al., 1964b).

Mechanism of Action at the Cellular Level

While individual alkylating agents may have effects on tissues such as liver, kidney, and mature lymphocytes which normally have a low mitotic index, the evidence is overwhelming that they are most cytotoxic to rapidly proliferating tissues which have a large proportion of cells in cycle. It has often been demonstrated that cells which vary markedly in their *in vivo* response to alkylating agents are of the same order of sensitivity when adapted to growing in culture and in log phase growth. The alkylating agents may react extensively with nondividing cells but cytotoxicity is only seen if these cells are stimulated to divide (PITTILLO et al.,

1970; SKIPPER, 1971). Alkylation in itself may be considered to be a relatively non-cytotoxic event. However, if cells are forced into division before repair of alkylations can take place, cytotoxicity results.

The effects of alkylating agents on the cell nucleus have been well known for a number of years (AUERBACH et al., 1947; KOLLER, 1947) and literature reports on the nucleotoxic effects of the alkylating agents are extensive (see reviews of WHEELER, 1962; OCHOA and HIRSCHBERG, 1967). Following administration of alkylating agents, many nuclear degenerative changes are observed *in vivo* or *in vitro*. These changes include chromosomal aberrations, enlargement of nuclei, and nucleoli with vacuolation, *pyknosis*, and *karyolysis*. An interesting phenomenon sometimes seen with low levels of alkylating agents is the development of giant cells with enlarged nuclei often containing several times the normal amount of nucleic acids and protein (COHEN and STUDZINSKI, 1967; CASPERSSON, 1963). Cellular gigantism has also been observed in man after chronic administration of alkylating agents (KOSS, 1969). It has been proposed that cell death, following minimal lethal doses of alkylating agent, is the result of unbalanced growth, the various stages of RNA and protein synthesis being out of phase with DNA synthesis. Similar unbalanced growth is seen in cells treated with a variety of toxic agents (RUECKERT and MUELLER, 1960; KIM and EIDINOFF, 1965) and is very similar to the "thymineless" death observed in bacteria (COHEN and BARNER, 1955).

Although many of the cellular effects of the alkylating agents involve the nucleus, one can also observe considerable damage, in the cytoplasm of dividing cells, to mitochondria, cellular membranes, and endoplasmic reticulum. It is hardly surprising that at the cellular level there is considerable damage to many structures. Once the initial lesion has occurred, malfunction of all subcellular components is to be expected in the dying cell. The importance of studies of this kind does not lie in describing the events that take place in the lethally alkylated cell but rather in identifying the site of the initial lesion.

The effects of these agents are not, of course, confined to mammalian tissues, and their cytotoxicity has been described in a wide variety of organisms including bacteria, yeasts, slime molds, higher plants, and invertebrates (WHEELER, 1962; OCHOA and HIRSCHBERG, 1967). In every case the most sensitive cells are those that are in cycle. Root tips, seedlings, or growing shoots of plants are most sensitive, for example, while bacteria in exponential growth are more affected than the same organisms growing slowly in a minimal medium (PAPIRMEISTER and DAVIDSON, 1965).

Using spleen colony techniques it has been shown that nitrogen mustards (and probably epoxides and ethyleneimines) are proliferation dependent but not phase specific[1] (BRUCE et al., 1966; VAN PUTTEN and LELIEVELD, 1971). Hydroxyurea and cytosine arabinoside, for example, are only toxic to cells in the DNA synthetic phase of the cell cycle and are therefore phase specific, but alkylating agents can act on cells at any stage in the cycle. Quantitative differences have been shown to exist, with a mustard derivative, depending on the phase of the cycle a cell is in when the alkylating agent is applied. Synchronously growing HeLa cells are more sensitive if alkylated in late G_1 or S than in G_2, mitosis, or early G_1. Effects observed were primarily a reduction in the rate of DNA synthesis and a delay before the next S period (ROBERTS et al., 1968). This particular sensitivity of the S phase to alkylation is also shown in other experiments where cells alkylated in G_2 by

1 BRUCE, using lymphoma cells and bone marrow cells, singles out nitrogen mustard (HN2) as the exception to the general rule that alkylating agents are proliferation dependent. However, VAN PUTTEN and LELIEVELD, using both slowly and rapidly growing bone marrow cells, show that HN2 is proliferation dependent.

nitrogen mustard show no major toxicity until the commencement of the succeeding S phase (LEVIS et al., 1965). The high sensitivity of cells in S to alkylating agents has been attributed to the particular sensitivity of DNA to these agents during this phase of the cell cycle (LUDLUM, 1965). In an unpaired state, it is known that polynucleotides are more susceptible to alkylation than when in the helical form. When DNA is replicating during the S phase it is at least partially in an unpaired state and likely to be more susceptible to alkylation than when in the form of the double helix.

A. Long Term Effects of the Alkylating Agents

The long term effects of the alkylating agents are dealt with in detail elsewhere; they are carcinogenesis, mutagenesis, and teratogenesis and are most probably a consequence of the nonlethal alkylation of genetic material (FAHMY and FAHMY, 1959; LOVELESS, 1966; VOGEL and ROHRBORN, 1970; BROOKES and LAWLEY, 1964; DIPAOLO, 1969). The finding that these agents can have such serious long term effects must make one cautious when they are administered to man. While they are justifiably used as a last resort in the treatment of advanced cancer, or specifically in the treatment of cancers which are known to respond, they should never be administered before a conclusive diagnosis of cancer is established, especially where young people are concerned. Furthermore, their use in the treatment of nonlethal conditions such as psoriasis, should never be undertaken lightly, while their projected use as insect chemosterilants and epilating agents should involve long term research on their pollutant aspects before even being considered for use on a large scale.

B. Antineoplastic Effects

The success of nitrogen mustard in the treatment of certain human cancers was initially responsible for the present day prominence of the alkylating agents in many fields of both fundamental and applied research. New types are continually being tested in experimental models in the search for more selective antitumor agents and reference has already been made to some of the vast amount of literature on the effects of alkylating agents in animals and man. The rapidly growing transplanted tumors such as the L1210 leukemia, the Walker 256 carcinosarcoma and the Yoshida sarcoma have been most often selected as the primary screening models for alkylating agents because they are known to be sensitive to this type of compound and thus are unlikely to give any false negative results. Besides these models, many alkylating agents have been tested in a variety of other systems including spontaneous and induced tumors, cells in culture and simple cell-free systems (CONNORS and ROE, 1964). It is quite clear that no experimental technique is very reliable or predictive as a model for human cancer. As a consequence, the translation of findings from animals to man is one area where many potentially useful alkylating agents are presumably lost because of the failure to employ them against the most appropriate human tumor.

Because of the predominant action of the alkylating agents on cells in cycle and the use in the laboratory of animal tumors, which have the majority of their cells rapidly cycling, it has been suggested that more reliable results may be obtained by using tumors with longer generation times. Such tumors would kinetically be a much better model of human cancer and they might select alkylating agents with a specific effect on slowly growing or even nondividing cells. Agents with these properties might be active in man against the solid carcinomas, presently untreatable, which probably contain many nondividing cells or cells with relatively long generation times.

The assumption is often made that all rapidly dividing cells are sensitive to alkylating agents (SKIPPER, 1969). Nevertheless, it is well known that some rapidly dividing animal tumors are quite insensitive, while others, that are initially sensitive may rapidly acquire resistance with no change in their cell kinetics (BALL et al., 1967). The proliferation rate of a cell is obviously not the only determinant of sensitivity to alkylating agents. Certain biochemical properties of cells can markedly affect the amount of drug which reaches the target site and can lead to large differences in sensitivity between similarly growing cells.

C. Effects on Hemopoietic Tissue

The half-life of bone marrow granulocytes is no longer than a few hours in man (MAUER et al., 1960) and it is not surprising that the rapidly dividing tissues necessary in maintaining a normal blood level of granulocytes are extremely sensitive to the alkylating agents. Various side effects are encountered with the use of individual alkylating agents, ranging from neurotoxicity and alopecia to cystitis and gastrointestinal disturbances. However, all alkylating agents have in common a myelosuppressive action, and this is usually the major limiting toxicity in man. Their effects on peripheral blood have been reviewed by ELSON (1963). Nitrogen mustards, epoxides, and ethyleneimines have qualitatively similar effects causing a rapid depression in the numbers of lymphocytes and granulocytes in peripheral blood. In rats the minimum values occur about four days after administration and are frequently followed by a massive neutrophilia. Effects on platelets are usually less pronounced while the depression of hemoglobin is rarely important. Important quantitative differences are seen between various agents in the degree of inhibition of lymphocytes and neutrophils. Aminochlorambucil at one end of the scale, has a much greater effect on lymphocytes than neutrophils (inhibition ratio 1.93), while at the other end of the scale, merophan has an inhibition ratio of 0.59 (ELSON, 1963). Quantitative differences such as these are often an important indication of the potential clinical usefulness of an agent and whether it is likely to be more useful in the treatment of myeloid leukemia where selective suppression of neutrophils is required or lymphoblastic leukemia where suppression of lymphocytes is important.

More detailed kinetic studies of the action of these agents on the bone marrow have been carried out by methods such as the spleen colony forming technique (TILL and McCULLOCH, 1961). Injection of the bone marrow of rats into suitably irradiated recipients leads to the formation of germinal centers in the spleen arising from viable stem cells in the injected bone marrow. A comparison of the colony forming ability of bone marrow, from control animals and animals treated with alkylating agents, and histological study of the colonies, gives considerable information on the effects of these agents on the various bone marrow cells. Kinetic studies of this kind have revealed that the situation is a complicated one and that some of the alkylating agents may have indirect effects on bone marrow cells (DUNNE, 1971).

D. Effects on Spermatogenesis

Alkylating agents, particularly ethyleneimines and sulfonoxyalkanes, can have pronounced and specific effects on various stages of spermatogenesis. A detailed knowledge of the spermatogenic process in rats and the time required for cells to pass through the various stages of differentiation (CLERMONT and HARVEY, 1967) has enabled the development of a test system which can measure the effects of chemicals on defined stages of spermatogenesis (JACKSON, 1969). By using a serial mating technique and measuring the occurrence of periods of infertility, cells that were in a particular stage of development at the time of administration of the agent and that are selectively killed may be identified. TEM (triethylene melamine) has been shown to have highly selective effects on the development of spermatogonia through spermatocytes and spermatids into spermatozoa. From the time of occurrence of infertility, after administration of a small single dose of this agent, it has been concluded that it interferes with the maturation of spermatocytes. A five day course of injections of TEM has additional effects on mature sperm in the epididymis (JACKSON, 1959). The effects of aliphatic nitrogen mustards were less well defined, apparently causing complete cessation of spermatogenesis in contrast to two aromatic nitrogen mustards (melphalan and chlorambucil) which, even at high dose levels, had little effect on male fertility. These properties have led to a study of the possible application of the alkylating agents in pest control as insect chemosterilants (BORKOVEC, 1967) and the suggestion has even been made that agents of this sort may be used as male contraceptives.

E. Effects on the Immune Response

Alkylating agents, particularly the bifunctional derivatives, cause marked changes in lymphoid tissues such as bone marrow, spleen, thymus, lymph nodes, and PEYER's patches. It is not unexpected, therefore, that they have profound effects on the immune response, and many alkylating agents depress the formation of antibodies induced by various antigenic stimuli. Some compounds, such as TEM and thioTEPA (N,N',N''-triethylenethiophosphoramide) only prevent the normal development of antibodies at near lethal doses, but others, such as cyclophosphamide, cause a significant reduction of the immune response at doses well below the lethal range (BERENBAUM and BROWN, 1964). This effect is known to be markedly dependent on timing, alkylating agents (with some exceptions in the sulfonoxyalkane series) having maximum effects if given one to two days after administration of the antigen. This probably coincides with the period of rapid multiplication of immunologically competent cells in response to the antigenic stimulus (BERENBAUM, 1962, 1971; BUSKIRK et al., 1965; HITCHINGS and ELION, 1963). The immunosuppressive effects of cyclophosphamide and nitrogen mustard (HN2) have also been demonstrated by measurement of the levels of 7S and 15S immunoglobulins following administration of an antigen (VAN DEN BROEK, 1971). The immunosuppressive properties of the alkylating agents have led to their use, particularly cyclophosphamide, in the prolongation of tissue homografts and in the treatment of autoimmune diseases. It is not likely that this property is a desirable one when alkylating agents are used in cancer chemotherapy, but because of the importance of timing in determining suppression of antibody formation, it is not obvious whether this property diminishes their antitumor effectiveness. It has certainly been shown, in experimental systems, that a nonspecific immunostimulant can potentiate the antitumor action of cyclophosphamide, but once again there is an important factor of timing involved (CURRIE and BAGSHAWE, 1970).

Mechanism of Action at the Macromolecular Level

It is frequently pointed out in studies on the mechanism of action of the alkylating agents that these chemicals are very reactive electrophilic reagents. They will bind readily, covalently, and irreversibly to a large number of nucleophilic centers, especially acids, thiols, and amino groups. It is to be expected that under appropriate conditions, considerable binding will take place with any of a large variety of cellular constituents that contain nucleophilic centers, such as small molecular weight materials, amino acids, lipids, structural proteins, enzymes, coenzymes, and nucleic acids. It is possible that alkylation of any one of a number of sites can cause cytotoxicity, but it is more probable in view of the similar and predictable properties of a wide chemical range of alkylating agents that toxicity at minimum lethal doses is a result of reaction at one highly sensitive site.

A. Reactions with Enzymes and Coenzymes

Early studies on *in vitro* systems using cell homogenates or purified extracts showed that a large variety of enzymes could be inhibited by alkylating agents. In view of the present day knowledge of the chemistry of alkylating agents, these results are hardly surprising and contribute little to a knowledge of their mechanism of action at physiological dose levels. Much of this early work has been well documented in reviews (Ross, 1962; Wheeler, 1962; Warwick, 1963; Ochoa and Hirschberg, 1967). More quantitative studies showed that many alkylating agents could cause death at extremely low intracellular concentrations. It follows that the target sites must react readily with the alkylating agents and also be few in number. Most normal cellular enzyme concentrations are such that even if they were inactivated by stoichiometric reaction with alkylating agents, there would still be an excess of noninactivated enzyme molecules. Some enzyme activity is undoubtedly depressed after administration of alkylating agents, but this may be secondary to alkylation of other sites and not necessarily a direct reaction.

The literature of the last five years only rarely considers that inhibition of protein synthesis is a primary mechanism of action of the alkylating agents. However, interest in the coenzyme NAD as a principal target site for alkylating agents is still evident (Fussganger et al., 1967). Respiration and glycolysis are two important pathways which have certainly been shown to be sensitive to a variety of alkylating agents in a wide variety of circumstances (Wheeler, 1962; Ochoa and Hirschberg, 1967). Tumor cells, with their emphasis on anaerobic glycolysis, have NAD levels which are readily depressed by alkylating agents, causing interference with glycolysis at the stage of the conversion of 3-phosphoglyceraldehyde to 1,3-diphosphoglyceric acid. In some experiments NAD levels in tumor cells were reduced by concentrations of alkylating agents which had little effect on other sensitive sites (Wheeler, 1962; Dold et al., 1962). However, in direct contrast, other workers have claimed that using almost identical methods, inhibition of DNA synthesis can be demonstrated at dose levels of alkylating agents which have no effect on NAD or glycolysis (Liss and Palme, 1964). While effects on enzymes can often be demonstrated, following administration of the alkylating agents, it seems that enzyme inhibition is not the major cause of toxicity. Certain enzymatic pathways, such as respiration and glycolysis, are apparently very sensitive to alkylating agents, and the coenzyme NAD appears to be particularly susceptible. However, inhibition of glycolysis and depression of NAD levels is by no means a general occurrence in cells treated with alkylating agents. It is therefore unlikely that the cytotoxic effects of the alkylating agents are due primarily to effects on glycolysis and NAD levels, although they may be important contributory factors.

B. Reaction with Nucleic Acids

Nucleic acid synthesis, particularly DNA synthesis, can be shown to be readily inhibited in many cell types after exposure to small amounts of alkylating agents (Lutwak-Mann, 1951; Pardee, 1954; Katchman et al., 1959; Levis et al., 1963; Smith and Busch, 1964; Lawley and Brookes, 1965; Roberts et al., 1968).

Inhibition of DNA synthesis, at dose levels that have no detectable effect on the synthesis or function of other macromolecules, has been demonstrated for a wide variety of cells *in vivo* and *in vitro*. Figures 2a and 2b show that whereas many anticancer agents, e.g. 6-mercaptopurine, may affect both protein and nucleic acids at physiological dose levels, DNA is particularly sensitive to alkylating agents.

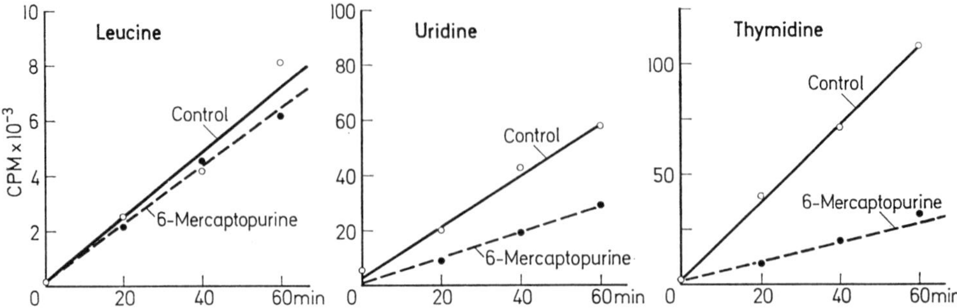

Fig. 2a. The effect of the antimetabolite, 6-mercaptopurine, on protein and nucleic acid synthesis of Walker carcinosarcoma ascites tumor cells *in vitro*. Incorporation of radioactive labeled precursors into both DNA and RNA are inhibited at minimum lethal dose levels of the agent

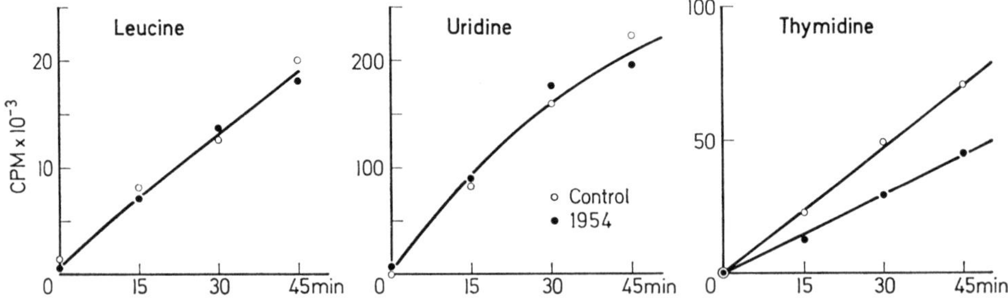

Fig. 2b. The effect of the alkylating agent, CB 1954, on protein and nucleic acid synthesis of Walker carcinosarcoma ascites tumor cells *in vitro*. Incorporation of labeled thymidine into DNA is selectively inhibited at toxic dose levels of the agent that have no effect on the incorporation of radioactive leucine or uridine into protein and RNA, respectively. (From: MANDEL, MERAI, and CONNORS, unpublished results)

Much attention has therefore been focussed on DNA as the primary target site, and attempts have been made to identify the areas of DNA most sensitive to alkylation (LAWLEY and WALLICK, 1957; REINER and ZAMENHOF, 1957; WACKER and EBERT, 1959; BROOKES and LAWLEY, 1960; WALKER and WATSON, 1961). Studies on DNA *in vitro* showed that, while there are a large number of sites of varying nucleophilicity, the most commonly alkylated site is the N_7 atom of guanine (LAWLEY and WALLICK, 1957; WALKER and WATSON, 1961) with lesser alkylation of other bases. Guanine in DNA is markedly more reactive to alkylating agents than any of the monomeric guanine nucleosides or nucleotides due to the arrangement of the purine ring system in the double helical structure (PRICE et al., 1969). From model experiments, it appears that the order of reactivity of the bases in DNA to alkylating agents is guanine $>$ adenine $>$ cytosine $>$ thymine and uracil. These findings are in good agreement with the amounts of alkylated bases isolated from cells treated with alkylating agents *in vivo* and demonstrates that model systems can give information on events likely to occur *in vivo*. One limitation to these experiments is the result of the procedures used, which involve acid hydrolysis to isolate the free bases and nucleosides. Techniques such as these would remove less stable, but perhaps no less important, DNA alkylations and it has, in fact, been shown that O_6 alkylation of guanine, which is acid labile, does occur and may play an important role in the mutagenicity of the alkylating agents (LOVELESS, 1969). Similarly, although there is no direct evidence for alkylation of phosphate groups, the possibility has not been entirely excluded that alkylation of the bases takes place in some cases by initial phosphate esterification followed by transalkylation. Milder hydrolytic methods are required to investigate the products of DNA and alkylating agents.

DNA as a primary target site of the alkylating agents offers a satisfactory explanation for a number of their properties. The sensitivity of cells in cycle and the effects on DNA synthesis are readily explained and can also be related to the mutagenic and carcinogenic properties of the alkylating agents which almost certainly involve some form of interaction with genetic material. Very low levels of alkylating agents can be cytotoxic, but because of the large molecular weight of DNA the alkylation of this material, expressed on a molar basis, is some ten to fifty times higher than the alkylation of protein (ROBERTS et al., 1968; VENITT, 1971). Reaction with DNA also offers an explanation of one essential feature of tumor inhibitory alkylating agents. In order to have optimum antitumor effects, they must be at least bifunctional, having a minimum of two alkylating centers in each molecule. It is well known that bifunctional alkylating agents can crosslink DNA, either by linking one strand in adjacent areas, or by joining together opposite strands of the helix (BROOKES and LAWLEY, 1961; LAWLEY and BROOKES, 1967). By assuming that crosslinking is a much more toxic lesion for tumor cells than simple monoalkylation, one can explain the pronounced antitumor action of these compounds.

Following the demonstration that alkylating agents interacted with DNA *in vitro*, a number of papers were published showing that damage to DNA or alkylation of DNA could not be detected in cells exposed to low, but lethal, concentrations of alkylating agents (TRAMS et al., 1961; LORKIEWICZ and SZYBALSKI, 1961; BREWER and ARONOW, 1963; WHEELER and STEPHENS, 1965; MILNER et al., 1965). However, the fact that DNA alkylation cannot be demonstrated in this situation, does not allow the conclusion to be drawn that reaction with DNA *in vivo* is not an important cytotoxic event. Present day techniques are certainly not sensitive enough to demonstrate low levels of crosslinking which, in the finely balanced cell, may be sufficient to cause profound disturbances in metabolism. The actual amount of alkylating agent covalently bound to DNA represents only a small quantity of the total bound material and in experiments using radioactively labeled material, if the specific activity is low, it may be quite insufficient to detect the low levels of crosslinking which are known to be cytotoxic (MILNER et al., 1965).

Nevertheless, in whole animal experiments, no good correlation has ever been seen between the binding of an agent to cellular DNA and the sensitivity of that cell to alkylation. Many tumors of widely differing sensitivity have been shown to have their DNA alkylated to the same extent. While the repair of DNA alkylation is obviously a complicating factor, it would seem essential to demonstrate a correlation between binding to one site of DNA and sensitivity, before it can be accepted unequivocally that DNA crosslinking is the major toxic event that occurs in cells exposed to alkylating agents.

Distribution and Metabolism of Alkylating Agents

The distribution, metabolism, and excretion of almost every alkylating agent of interest has been studied in small mammals and also quite frequently in man (MANDEL, 1959; OLIVERIO and ZUBROD, 1965; OCHOA and HIRSCHBERG, 1967). Most commonly used techniques have employed radioactively labeled material or have used colorimetric reactions specific for alkylating function. Neither method is entirely specific for the administered agent and either may measure various metabolites. However, these methods combined with attempts to isolate and identify the active and inactive metabolites have given a broad general picture of the fate of many alkylating agents *in vivo*. Many alkylating agents disappear rapidly from the plasma after injection and very few have biological half-lives of more than a few hours. Usually the major route of excretion is the kidney with lesser amounts found in the feces and occasionally in the expired air. A general finding is that the alkylating agents show little selective localization, the concentration in sensitive organs, such as the tumor and bone marrow, being no higher than the levels in resistant organs, such as the liver and kidney. Similarly, there is a fairly uniform distribution among cellular particles and macromolecules, indicating a general alkylation of many sites. It is not unexpected that these chemically reactive agents should bind to many cellular sites. Expressed in terms of amount bound per mg of dry weight, there is little difference seen in the level of most alkylating agents bound to DNA, RNA, or protein. Differences only become apparent when binding is expressed in terms of drug bound per mole of macromolecule and is a reflection of the higher molecular weight of DNA.

One interesting and consistent difference in the distribution of alkylating agents comes from studies on sensitive and resistant tumors. It has been shown for many tumors that lines resistant to alkylating agents take up less drug than the sensitive tumor (HIRONO et al., 1962; YAMADA et al., 1963; CHUN et al., 1969; WOLPERT and RUDDON, 1969; POYNTER, 1970; INABA and SAKURAI, 1971; HILL et al., 1971; FOX, 1971). The difference in drug concentration between the two lines is usually about two fold and, while this cannot account directly for the degree of resistance, which in some cases may be a hundred fold or more, it appears to be a general finding associated with resistance to alkylating agents. Little is known about the mechanism(s) by which resistance develops to alkylating agents (BALL, 1969), and this phenomenon requires further study.

The physical and chemical properties of individual alkylating agents can sometimes endow them with unique biological properties. A series of alkylating sulfonamides, for example, while having typical properties of alkylating agents, also has properties strongly suggesting that they interfere with folate metabolism (HAWKINS et al., 1963). There is also evidence that chlorambucil is an atypical agent exerting its toxicity at the cell surface rather than by an alkylation of intracellular components (LINFORD et al., 1963; KUMMER and OCHS, 1970). The degree of binding of an agent to serum protein also may affect considerably its biological properties (LINFORD, 1963), and agents that have the property of passing the blood brain barrier are likely to be of considerable importance in the search for drugs for the treatment of advanced cancer with involvement of the nervous system.

Some alkylating agents may be excreted largely in unchanged form. The low toxicity of mannitol myleran is due to its excretion as 90% unchanged drug. In the presence of agents causing anuria, which results in retention of mannitol myleran in the body, there is a ten fold increase in toxicity (CONNORS et al., 1964a). However, considerable metabolism of alkylating agents usually occurs, although this may vary markedly for any one agent, from species to species (OCHOA and

HIRSCHBERG, 1967). Large numbers of metabolites are frequently identified, some of which may be more active than the administered agent and others of which may be inactive detoxication products.

Sometimes alkylating agents are purposely synthesized to be chemically unreactive and therefore of low toxicity, but of such a structure that they could be converted *in vivo* by a known metabolic pathway to a highly reactive and cytotoxic metabolite (ROSS, 1962). In the optimal situation, the activating enzymes would be located predominantly in the cells of the cancer. Attempts to design latent compounds have included azo-derivatives to be reduced to active amines (ROSS and WARWICK, 1955), carbamates designed to release active phenolic mustards (BARDOS et al., 1969), and acetylamino derivatives to be activated by deacetylation (HEBBORN and DANIELLI, 1958). By far the most outstanding compound to result from attempts to design latently active agents has been cyclophosphamide, Endoxan (ARNOLD and BOURSEAUX, 1958). It is now well known that, although it was made to be activated by tumors high in phosphatase and phosphoramidase activities (GOMORI, 1948), the initial activation takes place in the liver (ARNOLD et al., 1958; FOLEY et al., 1961; BROCK and HOHORST, 1967). Since cyclophosphamide is one of the most effective and safest alkylating agents in clinical use, there have naturally been attempts to elucidate its metabolism to the active agent. However, despite its relatively simple structure, and intensive efforts by groups of research workers all over the world, the nature of the active metabolite of cyclophosphamide still eludes identification. A number of metabolites have been isolated from the urine and serum of animals and from *in vitro* systems. Their identification has shown that cyclophosphamide is metabolized by many pathways, giving rise to ring oxidation, ring opened products, and small fragments of the original molecule. However, there is no unequivocal evidence that any of these is the active metabolite of cyclophosphamide *in vivo* (HILL et al., 1970; HOHORST et al., 1971; STRUCK et al., 1971).

Conclusions

Results obtained in the clinic with the first alkylating agents marked the emergence of chemotherapy as an alternative to surgery and irradiation. However, even today little is known in detail of the mechanisms by which these chemicals cause cell death. Early suggestions that they released hydrochloric acid intracellularly, or that they inhibited choline metabolism, were soon discounted. Other theories that these agents have a direct effect on cell membranes, cause lysosome fragility, activate prophage, or act as antimetabolites may be important for certain alkylating agents in certain situations, but no general explanation is available for the basic mechanism of action of alkylating agents. A general theory must take into account the essential bifunctional nature of these agents, their high efficiency, and the sensitivity of cells in cycle. Since tumor lines with acquired resistance to one alkylating agent are in most instances cross-resistant to all other alkylating agents it is probable that all alkylating agents act in essentially the same way.

The likely target site remains DNA where low levels of alkylation could be expected to cause considerable toxicity. The bifunctionality is explained by a crosslinking reaction which is more toxic than a monofunctional alkylation. Whether crosslinking is more toxic when it is between two nucleophilic centers in one strand (intrastrand crosslinking) or in adjacent strand (interstrand crosslinking) is still not certain, although both reactions occur *in vivo*. A further type of crosslinking that has been demonstrated, involves nucleophilic centers on DNA and protein (KLATT et al., 1969; PUSCHENDORF et al., 1971). There seems to be no doubt that, in some cases, this type of crosslinking takes place at low dose levels, but its role in causing cytotoxicity is obscure. It is likely that alkylation of DNA is not, in itself, a lethal event. Resting cells only alkylated to a small extent may repair their DNA before irreversible damage has taken place. However, if the cell is in cycle it is likely that there will be irreversible damage, hence the differential sensitivity of resting and dividing cells to alkylating agents.

Although all alkylating agents act in the same way there is a large variation in their selectivity as antitumor agents. While some may kill the host at dose levels which have little antitumor effect, others may cause tumor inhibition at dose levels only 1/300th of the LD_{50}. Selectivity of action of an agent is not determined by its alkylating ability, but on the amount that reaches its target site in the tumor cell compared with the quantity that reaches the target site of the most sensitive of the host cells. For the alkylating agents, where it is assumed that DNA is the target site, the drug must be taken up by the cell and pass through the cytoplasm to the nucleus before any lethal alkylation takes place. Differences in cell permeability, in degree of activation or deactivation of the agent before it reaches DNA, the presence or absence of repair mechanisms, and the cell cycle time, combine to determine the actual sensitivity of each cell.

For this reason, new alkylating agents continue to be studied for their antitumor action. Their mechanism of action, particularly those that show high selectivity as antineoplastic agents, continue to be investigated. As more is learned about the ways in which alkylating agents can be highly selective for cancer cells, more effective agents can be introduced into the clinic.

References

AARON, H.: The choice of therapy in the treatment of cancer. Med. Let. **12**, 13—20 (1970).

ADAIR, F. E., BAGG, H. J.: Experimental and clinical studies on the treatment of cancer by dichloroethylsulfide. Ann. Surg. **93**, 190—199 (1931).

Ann. N.Y. Acad. Sci. Comparative clinical and biological effects of alkylating agents. **68**, 657—1266 (1958).

Ann. N. Y. Acad. Sci. Biological effects of alkylating agents. **163**, 589—1029 (1969).

ARNOLD, H., BOURSEAUX, F.: Synthese und Abbau cytostatisch wirksamer cyclischer *N*-Phosphamidester des *Bis*(β-chlorathyl)-amins. Angew. Chem. **70**, 539—544 (1958).

ARNOLD, H., BOURSEAUX, F., BROCK, N.: Chemotherapeutic action of a cyclic nitrogen mustard phosphamide ester in tumours of the rat. Nature (Lond.) **181**, 931 (1958).

AUERBACH, C., ROBSON, J. M., CARR, J. G.: The chemical production of mutation. Science **105**, 243—247 (1947).

BALL, C. R.: Intracellular factors influencing the response of tumours to chemotherapeutic agents. In: MATHÉ, G. (Ed.): Scientific basis of cancer chemotherapy. Recent results in cancer research, Vol. 21, pp. 26—40. London: Heinemann, and Berlin: Springer 1969.

BALL, C. R., CONNORS, T. A., COOPER, E. H., TOPPING, N. E.: Comparison of nitrogen mustard sensitive and resistant Yoshida sarcomas. II. Effect of treatment on cell kinetics. Neoplasma **14**, 253—263 (1967).

BARDOS, T. J., CHMIELEWICZ, Z. F., HEBBORN, P.: Structure activity relationships of alkylating agents in cancer chemotherapy. Ann. N. Y. Acad. Sci. **163**, 1006—1025 (1969).

BERENBAUM, M. C.: A screen for agents inhibiting the immune response and the growth of tumours. Nature (Lond.) **196**, 384—385 (1962).

BERENBAUM, M. C.: Suppression of specific immunity by non-specific agents. In: SAMTER (Ed.): Immunological diseases, pp. 118—135. Boston: Little, Brown & Company 1971.

BERENBAUM, M. C., BROWN, I. N.: Dose response relationships for agents inhibiting the immune response. Immunology **7**, 65—71 (1964).

BERENBLUM, I.: Experimental inhibition of tumour induction by mustard gas and other compounds. J. Path. Bact. **40**, 549—558 (1935).

BOESEN, E., DAVIS, W.: Cytotoxic drugs in the treatment of cancer. London: Arnold 1969.

BORKOVEC, A. B.: Insect chemosterilants. New York: Wiley 1967.

BRATZEL, R. P., ROSS, R. B., GOODRIDGE, T. H., HUNTRESS, W. T., FLATHER, M. T., JOHNSON, D. E.: A survey of alkylating agents. Cancer Chemother. Rep. **26**, 1—509 (1963).

BREWER, H. B., ARONOW, L.: Effects of nitrogen mustard on the physico-chemical properties of mouse fibroblast deoxyribonucleic acid. Cancer Res. **23**, 285—290 (1963).
BROCK, N., HOHORST, H. J.: Metabolism of cyclophosphamide. Cancer **20**, 900—904 (1967).
BROOKES, P., LAWLEY, P. D.: The reaction of mustard gas with nucleic acids *in vivo* and *in vitro*. Biochem. J. **77**, 478—484 (1960).
BROOKES, P., LAWLEY, P. D.: The reaction of mono and di-functional alkylating agents with nucleic acids. Biochem. J. **80**, 496—503 (1961).
BROOKES, P., LAWLEY, P. D.: Alkylating agents. Brit. med. Bull. **20**, 91—95 (1964).
BRUCE, W. R., MEEKER, B. E., VALERIOTE, F. A.: Comparison of the sensitivity of normal haematopoietic and transplanted lymphoma colony-forming cells to chemotherapeutic agents administered *in vivo*. J. nat. Cancer. Inst. **37**, 233—245 (1966).
BUSKIRK, H. H., CRIM, J. A., PETERING, H. G., MERRIT, K., JOHNSON, A. G.: Effect of uracil mustard on the primary antibody response in rats and mice. J. nat. Cancer Inst. **34**, 747—758 (1965).
Cancer Research Supplements I—LIV, 1953—1967.
CASPERSSON, T., FARBER, S., FOLEY, G. E., KILLANDER, D.: Cytochemical observations on the nucleolus-ribosome system. Effects of actinomycin D and nitrogen mustard. Exp. cell Res. **32**, 529—552 (1963).
CHUN, E. H. L., GONZALES, L., LEWIS, F. S., JONES, J., RUTMAN, R. J.: Differences in the *in vivo* alkylation and cross-linking of nitrogen mustard-sensitive and -resistant lines of Lettré-Ehrlich ascites tumours. Cancer Res. **29**, 1184—1194 (1969).
CLERMONT, Y., HARVEY, S. C.: Effects of hormones on spermatogenesis in the rat. In: Endocrinology of the testis. CIBA foundation colloquia on endocrinology, Vol. 16, pp. 173—189. London: J. A. Churchill 1967.
COHEN, S. S., BARNER, H. D.: The death of bacteria as a function of unbalanced growth. Pediatrics **16**, 704—708 (1955).
COHEN, L. S., STUDZINSKI, G. P.: Correlation between cell enlargement and nucleic acid and protein content of HeLa cells in unbalanced growth produced by inhibitors of DNA synthesis. J. cell. Physiol. **69**, 331—339 (1967).
COLE, W. H.: Chemotherapy of cancer. Philadelphia: Lea and Febiger 1970.
CONNORS, T. A., ELSON, L. A., LEESE, C. L.: The effect of glucose pretreatment on the anti-tumour action of mannitol myleran. Biochem. Pharmacol. **13**, 963—968 (1964a).
CONNORS, T. A., JENEY, A., JONES, M.: Reduction of the toxicity of "radiomimetic" alkylating agents in rats by thiol pretreatment. Biochem. Pharmacol. **13**, 1545—1550 (1964b).
CONNORS, T. A., ROE, F. J. C.: Anti-tumour agents. In: LAURENCE, D. R., BACHARACH, A. L. (Eds.): Evaluation of drug activities: pharmacometrics, Vol. 2, pp. 827—874. London and New York: Academic Press 1964.
CURRIE, G. A., BAGSHAWE, K. D.: Active immunotherapy with *coryne bacterium parvum* and chemotherapy in murine fibrosarcomas. Brit. med. J. **1**, 541—544 (1970).
DIPAOLO, J. A.: Teratogenic agents: mammalian test systems and chemicals. Ann. N. Y. Acad. Sci. **163**, 801—812 (1969).
DOLD, U., MIELSCH, M., HOLZER, H.: DPN-Gehalt, Nucleinsäuregehalt und Zellstruktur von Ascites-Tumorzellen nach Einwirkung alkylierender Cytostatica. Z. Krebsforsch. **65**, 139—146 (1962).
DUNNE, C. R.: personal communication.
EHRLICH, P.: In: HIMMELWEIT, F. (Ed.): The collected papers of PAUL EHRLICH, I, pp. 596—618. Oxford: Pergamon Press 1956.
ELKERBOUT, F., THOMAS, P., ZWAVELING, A.: Cancer chemotherapy. Leiden: Leiden University Press 1971.
ELSON, L. A.: Radiation and radiomimetic chemicals: comparative physiological effects. London: Butterworths 1963.
FAHMY, O. G., FAHMY, M.: The genetic effects of the biological alkylating agents with reference to the pesticides. Ann. N. Y. Acad. Sci. **160**, 228—243 (1969).
FLURY, F., WIELAND, H.: The pharmacologic action of *bis*(β-chloroethyl)sulfide. Z. exp. Med. **13**, 367—483 (1921).
FOLEY, G. E., FRIEDMAN, O. M., DROLET, B. P.: Studies on the mechanism of action of cytoxan. Evidence of activation *in vivo* and *in vitro*. Cancer Res. **21**, 57—63 (1961).
FOX, B. W.: Uptake studies of ^{14}C-methylene dimethane sulphonate in bilaterally transplanted sensitive and resistant Yoshida sarcomas. Chem. biol. Interact. **3**, 149—156 (1971).
FUSSGANGER, R., DOLD, U., HOLZER, H.: The influence of trenimon on the content of nicotinic acid and nicotinamide in Ehrlich ascites cells. Z. Krebsforsch. **69**, 275—282 (1967).
GILMAN, A., PHILIPS, F. S.: The biological actions and therapeutic applications of the β-chloroethylamines and sulfides. Science **103**, 409—415 (1946).
GOLUMBIC, C., FRUTON, J. S., BERGMANN, M.: Chemical reactions of the nitrogen mustard gases, I—VIII. J. Org. Chem. **11**, 518—591 (1946).

Gomori, G.: Histochemical demonstration of sites of phosphamidase activity. Proc. Soc. exp. biol. Med. **69**, 407—409 (1948).
Hawkins, R., Owen, L.N., Danielli, J.F.: The toxicity and anti-tumour action of some alkylating sulphonamides. J. theor. Biol. **5**, 236—248 (1963).
Hebborn, P., Danielli, J.F.: The increased tumour inhibitory effect of enzyme-activated nitrogen mustards. Biochem. Pharmacol. **1**, 19—24 (1958).
Hill, B.T., Jarman, M., Harrap, K.R.: The selectivity of action of alkylating agents and drug resistance. J. med. Chem. **14**, 614—618 (1971).
Hill, D.L., Kirk, M.C., Struck, R.F.: Isolation and identification of 4-ketocyclophosphamide, a possible active form of the anti-tumour agent cyclophosphamide. J. Amer. chem. Soc. **92**, 3207—3208 (1970).
Hirono, I., Kachi, H., Ohashi, A.: Mechanism of natural and acquired resistance to methyl-bis-(2-chloroethyl)amine-N-oxide in ascites tumors. II. Permeability of tumour cells to alkylating agents. Gann **53**, 73—80 (1962).
Hitchings, G.H., Elion, G.B.: Chemical suppression of the immune response. Pharmacol. Rev. **15**, 365—405 (1963).
Hohorst, H.J., Ziemann, A., Brock, N.: 4-Ketocyclophosphamide, a metabolite of cyclophosphamide. Arzneimittel-Forsch. **21**, 1254—1257 (1971).
Inaba, M., Sakurai, Y.: Mechanism of resistance of Yoshida sarcoma to nitrogen mustard. Int. J. Cancer **7**, 430—435 (1971).
Jackson, H.: Antifertility substances. Pharmacol. Rev. **11**, 135—172 (1959).
Jackson, H.: Chemical interference with spermatogenesis and fertility. In: McLaren, A. (Ed.): Advances in reproductive physiology, Vol. 4, pp. 65—97. London: Logospress 1969.
Jae Ho Kim, Eidinoff, M.L.: Action of 1-β-D-arabinofuranosylcytosine on the nucleic metabolism and viability of HeLa cells. Cancer Res. **25**, 698—702 (1965).
Katchman, B.J., Fetty, W.O., Busch, K.A.: Effect of cell division inhibition on the phosphorus metabolism of growing cultures of *Saccharomyces cerevisiae*. J. Bact. **77**, 331—338 (1959).
Klatt, O., Stehlin, J.S., McBride, C., Griffin, A.C.: The effect of nitrogen mustard treatment on the deoxyribonucleic acid of sensitive and resistant Ehrlich tumour cells. Cancer Res. **29**, 286—290 (1969).
Koller, P.C.: Experimental modification of nucleic acid systems in the cell. I. Nucleic acid. Symp. Soc. Exp. Biol. No. 1, 270—290 (1947).
Koss, G.L.: Some effects of alkylating agents on epithelia in man and in an experimental system in the rat. Ann. N.Y. Acad. Sci. **163**, 931—935 (1969).
Krumbhaar, E.B., Krumbhaar, H.D.: The blood and bone marrow in yellow cross gas (mustard gas) poisoning. Changes produced in the bone marrow in fatal cases. J. med. Res. **40**, 497—507 (1919).
Kummer, D., Ochs, H.D.: Differentiation of reaction mechanisms of alkylating cytostatics on Ehrlich ascites carcinoma and lymphatic leukemic cells. Z. Krebsforsch. **73**, 315—328 (1970).
Larionov, L.F.: Cancer chemotherapy. London: Pergamon Press 1965.
Lawley, P.D., Brookes, P.: Molecular mechanism of the cytotoxic action of difunctional alkylating agents and of resistance to this action. Nature (Lond.) **206**, 480—483 (1965).
Lawley, P.D., Brookes, P.: Interstrand cross-linking of DNA by difunctional alkylating agents. J. molec. Biol. **25**, 143—160 (1967).
Lawley, P.D., Wallick, C.A.: The action of alkylating agents on deoxyribonucleic acid and guanylic acid. Chem. and Ind. 633 (1957).
Levis, A.G., Danieli, G.A., Piccinni, E.: Nucleic acid synthesis and the mitotic cycle in mammalian cells treated with nitrogen mustard in culture. Nature (Lond.) **207**, 608—610 (1965).
Levis, A.G., Spanio, L., DeNadai, A.: Radiomimetic effects of a nitrogen mustard on survival, growth, protein and nucleic acid synthesis of mammalian cells *in vitro*. Exp. cell Res. **31**, 19—30 (1963).
Linford, J.H.: The role of adsorption in controlling the rate of reaction of chlorambucil with protein. Can. J. biochem. Physiol. **41**, 931—939 (1963).
Linford, J.H., Froese, A., Israels, L.G.: Interaction of chlorambucil with cell surfaces. Nature (Lond.) **197**, 1068—1070 (1963).
Liss, E., Palme, G.: Der Einfluß von alkylierenden Cytostatica auf den Nucleinsäurestoffwechsel von Ehrlich-Ascites-Tumorzellen. Z. Krebsforsch. **66**, 196—206 (1964).
Livingston, R.B., Carter, S.K.: Single agents in cancer chemotherapy. London and New York: Plenum 1970.
Lorkiewicz, Z., Szybalski, W.: Mechanism of chemical mutagenesis. IV. Reaction between triethylene melamine and nucleic acid components. J. Bact. **82**, 195—201 (1961).
Loveless, A.: Genetic and allied effects of alkylating agents. London: Butterworths 1966.

LOVELESS, A.: Possible relevance of O-6 alkylation of deoxyguanosine to the mutagenicity and carcinogenicity of nitrosamines and nitrosamides. Nature (Lond.) **223**, 206—207 (1969).
LUDLUM, D. B.: Alkylation of polynucleotide complexes. Biochim. biophys. Acta **95**, 674—676 (1965).
LUTWAK-MANN, C.: Some aspects of phosphorous metabolism in bone marrow. Biochem. J. **49**, 300—310 (1951).
LYNCH, V., SMITH, M. W., MARSHALL, E. K.: Dichloroethyl sulfide. Mustard Gas I. The systemic effects and mechanism of action. J. Pharmacol. exp. Therap. **12**, 265—290 (1918).
MANDEL, H. G.: The physiological disposition of some anticancer agents. Pharmacol. Rev. **11**, 743—837 (1959).
MAUER, A. M., ATHENS, J. W., ASHENBRUCKER, H., CARTWRIGHT, G. E., WINTROBE, M. M.: Leukokinetic studies II. J. clin. Invest. **39**, 1481—1486 (1960).
MEYER, V.: Versuche über die Haltbarkeit von Sublimatlosungen. Berichte der Deutschen Chemischen Gesellschaft **1**, 1725—1739 (1887).
MILNER, A. N., KLATT, D., YOUNG, S. E., STEHUN, J. S., JR.: The biochemical mechanism of action of L-phenylalanine mustard. I. Distribution of L-phenylalanine mustard-H^3 in tumor bearing rats. Cancer Res. **25**, 259—264 (1965).
OCHOA, M., JR., HIRSCHBERG, E.: Alkylating Agents in Experimental Chemotherapy, pp. 1—32. SCHNITZER, R. J., HAWKING, F. (Ed.): London and New York: Academic Press 1967.
OLIVERIO, V. T., ZUBROD, C. G.: Clinical pharmacology of the effective anti-tumour drugs. Ann. Rev. Pharmacol. **5**, 335—356 (1965).
PAPIRMEISTER, B., DAVISON, C. L.: Unbalanced growth and latent killing of *E. coli* following exposure to sulfur mustard. Biochim. biophys. Acta **103**, 70—92 (1965).
PAPPENHEIMER, A. M., VANCE, M. J.: Effects of intravenous injection of dichloroethyl sulfide in rabbits with special reference to its leucotoxic action. J. exp. Med. **31**, 71—94 (1920).
PARDEE, A. B.: Nucleic acid precursors and protein synthesis. Proc. nat. Acad. Sci. (Wash.) **40**, 263—270 (1954).
PITTILLO, R. F., SCHABEL, F. M., JR., SKIPPER, H. E.: The "sensitivity" of resting and dividing cells. Cancer Chemother. Rep. **54**, 137—142 (1970).
POYNTER, R. W.: Studies on the mechanism of resistance to alkylating agents of three ascites tumours in the rat. Biochem. Pharmacol. **19**, 1387—1397 (1970).
PRICE, C. C.: Fundamental mechanisms of alkylation. Ann. N. Y. Acad. Sci. **68**, 663—668 (1958).
PRICE, C. C., GAUCHER, G. M., KONERU, P., SHIBAKAWA, R., SOWA, J. R., YAMAGUCHI, M.: Mechanism of action of alkylating agents. Ann. N. Y. Acad. Sci. **163**, 593—600 (1969).
PUSCHENDORF, B., WOLF, H., GRUNICKE, H.: Effect of the alkylating agent trisethyleneiminobenzoquinone (trenimon) on the template activity of chromatin and DNA in RNA and DNA polymerase systems. Biochem. Pharmacol. **20**, 3039—3050 (1971).
REINER, B., ZAMENHOF, S.: Studies on the chemically reactive groups of deoxyribonucleic acids. J. biol. Chem. **228**, 475—486 (1957).
ROBERTS, J. J., BRENT, T. P., CRATHORN, A. R.: The mechanism of the cytotoxic action of alkylating agents on mammalian cells. In: CAMPBELL, P. N. (Ed.): Interaction of drugs and sub-cellular components in animal cells, pp. 5—27. London: J. & A. Churchill 1968.
ROSS, W. C. J.: The chemistry of cytotoxic alkylating agents. Advanc. Cancer Res. **1**, 397—449 (1953).
ROSS, W. C. J.: Biological alkylating agents. London: Butterworths 1962.
ROSS, W. C. J., WARWICK, G. P.: Reduction of cytotoxic azo compounds by hydrazine and by the xanthine oxidase-xanthine system. Nature (Lond.) **176**, 298—299 (1955).
RUECKERT, R. R., MUELLER, G. C.: Studies on unbalanced growth in tissue culture. Cancer Res. **20**, 1584—1591 (1960).
SCHMIDT, L. H., FRADKIN, R., SULLIVAN, R., FLOWERS, A.: Comparative pharmacology of alkylating agents. Cancer Chemother. Rep. suppl. 2, pts. I, II, III (1965).
SELLEI, C., ECKHARDT, S., NEMETH, L.: Chemotherapy of Neoplastic Diseases. Budapest: Akademiai Kiado 1970.
SKIPPER, H. E.: Improvement of the model systems. Cancer Res. **29**, 2329—2333 (1969).
SKIPPER, H. E.: The cell cycle and the chemotherapy of cancer. In: BASERGA, R. (Ed.): The cell cycle and cancer, pp. 355—387. New York: Marcel Dekker 1971.
SMITH, S. J., BUSCH, H.: Effects of uracil mustard on *in vivo* incorporation of precursors into nucleic acids of the Walker tumour. Texas Rep. Biol. and Med. **22**, 731—740 (1964).
STRUCK, R. F., KIRK, M. C., MELLET, L. B., DAREER, S., HILL, D. L.: Urinary metabolites of the anti-tumour agent cyclophosphamide. Molec. Pharmacol. **7**, 519—529 (1971).
TILL, J. E., MCCULLOCH, E. A.: A direct measurement of the radiation sensitivity of normal mouse bone marrow cells. Radiat. Res. **14**, 213—222 (1961).
TRAMS, E. G., NADKARNI, M. V., SMITH, R. K.: On the mechanism of action of the alkylating agents. II. Effects of nitrogen mustard, myleran and x-irradiation on nucleic acid biosynthesis. Cancer Res. **21**, 567—570 (1961).

TRIGGLE, D. J.: The reaction mechanisms, selectivity and specificity of action of 2-halogeno-ethylamines: an analysis. J. theor. Biol. **7**, 241—275 (1964).

VAN DEN BROEK, A. A.: Immune suppression and histophysiology of the immune response. Ph. D. dissertation, Rijksuniversiteit te Groningen, Drukkerij van Denderen, Groningen, 1971.

VAN PUTTEN, L. M., LELIEVELD, P.: Factors determining cell killing by chemotherapeutic agents *in vivo*. II. Melphalan, chlorambucil and nitrogen mustard. Europ. J. Cancer **7**, 11—16 (1971).

VENNITT, S.: The differential response of resistant and sensitive strains of *Escherichia coli* to the cytotoxic effects of 5-aziridino-2,4-dinitrobenzamide (CB 1954). Chem. biol. Interact. **3**, 177—191 (1971).

VOGEL, F., ROHRBORN, G. (Eds.): Chemical mutagenesis in mammals and man. Berlin-Heidelberg-New York: Springer 1970.

WACKER, A., EBERT, M.: Über die Methylierung des Adenosins mit Dimethylsulfat. Z. Naturforsch. **14** B, 709—712 (1959).

WALKER, I. G., WATSON, W. J.: The reaction of mustard gas with the purine portion of deoxyribonucleic acid. Can. J. Biochem. **39**, 365—376 (1961).

WARTHIN, A. S., WELLER, C. V.: The medical aspects of mustard gas poisoning. St. Louis: C. V. Mosby & Co. 1919.

WARWICK, G. P.: The mechanism of action of alkylating agents. Cancer Res. **23**, 1315—1333 (1963).

WHEELER, G. P.: Studies related to the mechanism of action of cytotoxic alkylating agents: a review. Cancer Res. **22**, 651—688 (1962).

WHEELER, G. P., STEPHENS, Z. H.: Studies with mustards. VII. Effects of alkylating agents *in vitro* and *in vivo* upon the thermal properties of deoxyribonucleic acids from sensitive and resistant plasmacytomas. Cancer Res. **25**, 410—416 (1965).

WILLIAMSON, C. E., WITTEN, B.: Reaction mechanism of some aromatic nitrogen mustards. Cancer Res. **27**, 33—38 (1967).

WOLPERT, M. K., RUDDON, R. W.: A study on the mechanism of resistance to nitrogen mustard (HN_2) in Ehrlich ascites tumour cells. Comparison of uptake of HN_2-^{14}C into sensitive and resistant cells. Cancer Res. **29**, 873—879 (1969).

YAMADA, T., IWANAMI, Y., BABA, T.: The transport of ^{14}C-labelled nitrogen mustard N-oxide through cellular membranes treated with Tween 80 *in vitro*. Gann **54**, 171—176 (1963).

Chapter 33

Mechanism of Action of Methanesulfonates

Brian W. Fox

With 1 Figure

Introduction

The methane sulfonate esters of dihydric and polyhydric alcohols are biological alkylating agents since their alkyl-oxygen bonds undergo fission and react within the intracellular milieu. The structure of the alkyl group of these esters may vary around the carbon atom adjacent to the oxygen atom where fission is likely to occur. This means that the alkyl group will tend to favor entry into the confines of a sterically favorable nucleophilic site, unlike the ethylene immonium series whose chemically variable grouping will always be separated from the nucleophilic site by a three atom chain and hence exert less of an influence on it. The local structural characteristics of the nucleophile itself would thus assist in conferring a degree of selectivity on the action of the alkane sulfonates.

The importance of these factors in conferring variability in the nature of the biological action produced is not only shown in the antitumor action of these polysulfonate esters, but also in normal steady state systems, e.g. spermatogenesis, hemopoiesis, lymphopoiesis, etc., especially with the lower homologs of the series. The most important of the alkane sulfonate esters from the point of view of the experimental oncologist and immunologist are the di- and polyfunctional derivatives; these agents show marked antitumor activity, but have not been exploited clinically. A considerable literature exists concerning the mutagenic and other molecular aspects of the interaction of the monofunctional esters (for review, see Ochoa and Hirschberg, 1967). These esters, however, will not be considered in this chapter.

Whole Tissue Studies

A. Antitumor Activity

The straight chain diesters (Fig. 1a) exhibit a variety of responses in biological systems, including marked preferences for different experimental tumor systems. The simplest member of the series, methylene dimethanesulfonate (MDMS, Fig. 1a, $n = 1$), has shown antitumor activity against the Yoshida sarcoma, in both solid and ascitic forms, in Wistar rats (Fox and Jackson, 1965; Fox, 1969), but is less effective against the Walker carcinoma. Ethylene dimethanesulfonate (EDS, Fig. 1a, $n = 2$), on the other hand, shows a greater effectiveness against the Walker carcinoma (Edwards et al., 1969, 1970a). The tetramethylene diester (Fig. 1a, $n = 4$, busulfan, myleran) shows a similar difference in sensitivity in these latter tumors. This compound has found considerable clinical use in the treatment of chronic myeloid leukemia (Kurrle, 1955; Galton, 1956; Galton et al., 1958).

Dimethyl busulfan (Fig. 1b) has also been examined and appears to be comparable to busulfan in its action against chronic myeloid leukemia (GALTON et al., 1958; BIERMAN et al., 1958). Nonamethylene sulfonate (Fig. 1a, $n = 9$, Nonane) is also an active antitumor agent and has been employed in the clinical treatment of malignant disease (MILLER, 1961). Although preliminary histological work (STERNBERG et al., 1958) and limited experimental work have been done in hamsters (SUGIURA et al., 1971), little is known about the action of this agent.

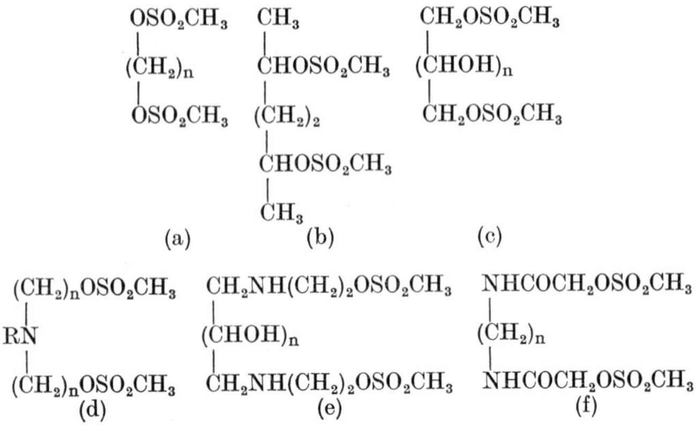

(a) OSO_2CH_3 — $(CH_2)_n$ — OSO_2CH_3

(b) CH_3 — $CHOSO_2CH_3$ — $(CH_2)_2$ — $CHOSO_2CH_3$ — CH_3

(c) $CH_2OSO_2CH_3$ — $(CHOH)_n$ — $CH_2OSO_2CH_3$

(d) $RN[(CH_2)_nOSO_2CH_3]_2$

(e) $CH_2NH(CH_2)_2OSO_2CH_3$ — $(CHOH)_n$ — $CH_2NH(CH_2)_2OSO_2CH_3$

(f) $NHCOCH_2OSO_2CH_3$ — $(CH_2)_n$ — $NHCOCH_2OSO_2CH_3$

Fig. 1

Among several carbohydrate dimethanesulfonates, D-mannitol-1,6-dimethanesulfonate (Fig. 1c, $n = 4$, mannitol myleran, mannogranol) has been used successfully in clinical practice (ECKHARDT et al., 1967) despite its relative inactivity in animal tumors. Its tumor-inhibiting action has been investigated (HADDOW et al., 1958) in pulmonary tumors in strain A mice (SHIMKIN et al., 1966), as well as in a variety of rat and mouse tumors (SUGIURA and STOCK, 1967).

1,2,5,6-Tetramethanesulfonyl-D-mannitol (Zitostop, R52), was prepared by VARGHA and BALO (1971), and has also been shown to be a potentially important clinical tool (see the symposium report by KENDRAY, 1968). The agent has also been tried with some success in canine tumors (LAPIS, 1968) and with polycythemia vera (NAGY et al., 1971). Further clinical trials have also been initiated (SZENTKLARAY and SELLEI, 1971).

A number of other diesters have been synthesized and subjected to preclinical testing (EL-MERZABANI and SAKURAI, 1965a, b, 1967; GOLDIN and WOOD, 1969). These included compounds based on nitrogen mustard [Fig. 1d, R=H, CH_3, $n = 3$; R=$ON(C_6H_4)$, $n = 2$] which showed some activity in both Yoshida sarcoma and L1210 leukemia. The diester, R74 (Fig. 1e, $n = 2$) has been studied both from the point of view of its toxicological and tumor-inhibitory effects (KELLNER and NEMETH, 1967—1968). This compound showed significant activity against L1210 leukemia cells implanted into BDF_1 male mice when given as eight doses of 3.75 mg/kg every 3 h (SANDBERG and GOLDIN, 1969).

The serious disadvantage in the use of the tumor systems, especially in the solid subcutaneous form in drug testing with this series, is the difficulty experienced in relating chemical structure to biological activity. This is primarily due to the very wide variation in cell types of unknown interrelationships that occur in the tumor tissue. In order to achieve a clearer understanding of any selectivity of drug action on different cell types, more detailed studies have been conducted in other normal, steady-state systems such as spermatogenesis and hemopoiesis.

B. Spermatogenesis

A quantitative assessment of the activity of different diesters is possible in the spermatogenic epithelium of the rodent, where the sequence and timing of the events are known with considerable accuracy in both the rat (LEBLOND and CLERMONT, 1952) and the mouse (OAKBERG, 1956). Busulfan induces sterility in the male rat (JACKSON et al., 1959, 1961), and it can be shown that its action is directed towards the first of the mitotic divisions of the spermatogonial stages (PARTINGTON et al., 1964). This division stage would appear to be associated with the conversion of a cell from the stem cell compartment into one of the steady state systems of spermatogenesis. This stage has been investigated in the rat, mouse, and golden hamster using busulfan as a tool (DEROOIJ and KRAMER, 1968). Many of the properties of this diester suggest that its primary action may be exerted on a general humoral system responsible for the triggering of stem cells into the steady state differentiated cell systems which they serve.

The antispermatogenic activities of MDMS and EDS do not mimic that of busulfan, which suggests that the fundamental biochemical lesions involved in their actions are different. MDMS exerts an action on an early stage of spermatogonial division as well as an action on the spermatozoa in the distal regions of the epididymis (FOX and JACKSON, 1965). The evidence suggests, however, that the action on the early spermatogonial cells may differ in detail from that observed after busulfan treatment since a single dose fails to exert an action long enough for it to be observed by routine fertility tests. Multiple doses are necessary to produce a period of sterility which can be observed by the usual routine mating procedures (FOX and JACKSON, 1964, 1965). EDS, however, appears to inhibit spermatogenesis in the same way as does hypophysectomy (COOPER and JACKSON, 1970), being associated with involution of the prostate and epididymis, with spermatoceles occurring in the latter. Trimethylene dimethanesulfonate (PDMS, Fig. 1a, $n = 3$), on the other hand, resembles busulfan in this system, except that, to induce a similar effect, the dose of the former was several times greater than the latter. This agent resembles x-irradiation in its action on the spermatozoa of the mosquito, *Culex pipiens* (JOST and AMIRKHANIAN, 1971). The *N*,*N*-*bis*(methane sulfonyloxyacetal)-1,10-diamino decane (Fig. 1f, $n = 10$) has also been shown to possess properties similar to busulfan on rodent spermatogonesis, inhibiting an early stage of spermatogonial division (SKINNER and JOHANSSON, 1970).

C. Hemopoietic Effects

STERNBERG et al. (1958) examined a number of tissues from busulfan treated rats and recorded histological changes. In the light of more recent kinetic knowledge of the systems examined, the changes observed suggest that the development of a very early cell type is being inhibited, often resulting in an effect on the differentiated cell population at a time significantly later than that observed after such agents as nitrogen and sulfur mustard. This is particularly true for the histological changes in the small and large intestine, stomach and kidney. The bone marrow showed very marked delayed effects and this system has been extensively investigated by ELSON (1958), especially with regard to busulfan treatment. It was primarily the protracted action of this agent on the hemopoietic system that led to its successful use against chronic myeloid leukemia (HADDOW and TIMMIS, 1953; GALTON et al., 1958). ELSON (1958, 1963) investigated the hemopoietic action of the diesters (Fig. 1a, $n = 2-8$) mainly by studying changes in the peripheral blood elements. It is still not clear whether in these circumstances it is permissable to extrapolate information obtained on peripheral cell counts to effects on progenitor cells in the bone marrow, due to the transient nature of the former population and other humoral and hormonal factors that could influence both the timing and degree of change observed in the peripheral cell counts. However, comparative information has been obtained and has provided useful insight into the mode of action of these agents on the hemopoietic system.

The main action of busulfan is directed towards the early stages of the development of the granulocyte and other myeloid elements with very little effect on the lymphopoietic system. Elson et al. (1958) suggested that an intermitotic delay is imposed by the drug on all cells, but that this delay was proportionately longer for those cells that divide infrequently. More recent findings (Dunn and Elson, 1970a, b) have suggested that since the number of colony forming units in the femur decreases to low levels for a prolonged period, the cell type affected was originally in the resting, or G_0 phase, at the time at which damage by the drug occurred. This result is in contrast to those obtained with agents like vinblastine and aminochlorambucil which do not significantly affect the G_0 phase. A similar behavior of stem cells was observed after busulfan treatment of dogs (Israels et al., 1962) and an interference with the development of the cells at an early stage was again suggested. EDS does not affect bone marrow cellularity even though studies of spermatogenesis suggested that an effect on a humoral system had occurred (Jackson and Craig, 1969). MDMS, on the other hand, produced a marked and rapid diminution in peripheral blood elements following administration (Fox and Jackson, 1965; James, 1966). The depression in leucocytes brought about by some of these agents appears to be reduced by concomitant administration of erythropoietin (Medici et al., 1965), bone marrow cells (Weston et al., 1957; Talbot and Elson, 1958) or yeast ribonucleic acid (Maisin et al., 1962). Dimethyl busulfan (Fig. 1b) has also been studied in some detail with regard to its action on the peripheral blood elements. It has the advantage of being more soluble in water than busulfan and also has a shorter half-life of hydrolysis. The hemopoietic effects were also studied by Elson (1958) and were found to be qualitatively similar to those of busulfan but required a lower dose (4 mg/kg) in rats to exert a comparable effect. The time of maximum depression of both granulocytes and platelets was some four to six days earlier than with busulfan, suggesting that a later stage in the development of these series of cell types may be inhibited by this drug.

D. Immunosuppressive Properties

The immunosuppressive activity of the representatives of the diester series (Fig. 1a, $n = 3,4,5,6,8$) has been investigated by Berenbaum et al. (1967). The degree of immunosuppression depended upon the interval between administration of the drug and administration of antigen, as well as on the value of n. Among the disulfonates investigated, the maximum interval for optimum immunosuppression was observed with busulfan, i.e. 5 days. These authors noted that the size of the interval in the mouse was directly related to the lipid-water partition coefficient for each drug. Cysteine potentiated the immunosuppressive activity of busulfan (Addison and Berenbaum, 1971) unlike the protection it afforded against nitrogen mustard and cyclophosphamide.

E. Miscellaneous Effects

The teratogenic activity of busulfan is well known in clinical practice (Diamond et al., 1960; Williams, 1966) and it has been studied in rats (Hemsworth and

JACKSON, 1962). In the latter species, the drug activity is directed towards the gonocytes and not the supporting cells, both of which divide at comparable rates. The period of maximum sensitivity towards the alkylating agents appears to be around day 15 of the gestation period in the rat. The production of sterile offspring following treatment of pregnant rats, 5 to 7 days before parturition, was first described by BOLLAG (1954). Both male (HEMSWORTH and JACKSON, 1963a) and female (HEMSWORTH and JACKSON, 1963b) fetuses demonstrate similar sensitivity to busulfan in the later stages of gestation. HEMSWORTH (1968) examined the teratogenic effects of the first four members of the straight chain dimethanesulfonate series (Fig. 1a, $n = 1$ to 4). MDMS produced a very high incidence of limb defects compared with the ethylene and propylene diesters, when administered on the 13th day of pregnancy in the rat. Busulfan also inhibited osteogenesis in the mouse embryo (PINTO-MACHADO, 1969).

A number of toxic side effects mainly concerning epithelia (KOSS, 1969) have been observed during the clinical use of busulfan. An often reported effect of protracted treatment during maintenance therapy is that of a syndrome resembling adrenal cortical deficiency (KYLE et al., 1961; NELSON and ANDREWS, 1964; WARD et al., 1965; HARROLD, 1966). It was noted that a selective pituitary insufficiency was sometimes observed following its use (VIVACQUA et al., 1967). These observations suggest that any action on hormonally mediated triggering mechanisms could be effected via the pituitary. Ovarian dysgenesis has also been observed in both the rat and man (HELLER and JONES, 1964). Other side effects in clinical practice include a pulmonary fibrosis known as "Busulfan Lung" (LEAKE et al., 1963; HEARD and COOKE, 1968; FEINGOLD and KOSS, 1969; LITTLER and OGILVIE, 1970) as well as pigmentation phenomena (SPRUNT and RIZZA, 1966).

In rats, prolonged therapy with busulfan induced polyploidy in the lens epithelium (GRIMES and SALLMANN, 1966), cataract formation (LIGHT, 1967), and a shortening of life span (DUNJIC, 1964). Prenatal administration to rats produces a hypoplastic thymus in the postnatal animal (PINTO-MACHADO, 1970).

Metabolism and Distribution Studies

The fate of S^{35} labeled busulfan has been studied in the rat (PENG, 1957; TRAMS et al., 1957; FOX et al., 1960), in the mouse and rabbit (FOX et al., 1960), and in man (NADKARNI et al., 1959). The main product in each case was methane sulfonic acid-^{35}S in the urine, but varying levels of unchanged busulfan-^{35}S and other unidentified components have been described. Using this isotope, only the degree and rate of destruction of the molecule can be assessed; the fate of the alkylating portion requires the labeling of the butylene chain. Attempts to study the distribution of the ^{14}C-labeled molecule in the rat (TRAMS et al., 1957) and in man (NADKARNI et al., 1959), resulted only in a complex mixture of at least 12 urinary products. These remained unidentified until ROBERTS and WARWICK (1959a, b, 1961) showed that the main urinary product in the mouse was 3-hydroxytetrahydrothiophene-1,1-dioxide, which they considered to be produced by interaction of the dimethanesulfonate with a sulfhydryl group, which was cleaved after the diester interacted with a single sulfhydryl group, a so-called "sulfur stripping" process. This process was independently confirmed by investigating the direct chemical interaction of busulfan with l-cysteine ethyl ester (PARHAM and WILBUR, 1959, 1961); these investigators also suggested that a cyclic sulfonium intermediate could be involved in the pharmacological action of this agent. This product is almost certainly due to its detoxication via glutathione. The interaction of this agent with nucleic acids will be discussed later.

The synthesis of tritiated busulfan was first described by Koch et al. (1959a, b). It was used to investigate the uptake of the drug into the mouse testis (Moutschen and Ezell, 1960), using liquid scintillation counting of solubilized testis homogenate, and these authors concluded that the uptake reached a maximum approximately twenty minutes after intraperitoneal administration. The elimination of radioactivity over fifteen days followed the degeneration of the testis due to the damaging level of the drug used. Chevremont (1961) referred to autoradiographic evidence that the agent was taken up by the chromosomes of cultured cells; its selective uptake into *Vicia faba* root tip nuclei has been described by Moutschen et al. (1960). An investigation of the distribution of the tritium labeled drug has also been undertaken in humans (Vodopick et al., 1969). These latter authors noted that the drug was cleared from the plasma in a biphasic fashion, rapidly at first ($t_{\frac{1}{2}} = 1$ day) then more slowly ($t_{\frac{1}{2}} = 5$ days). Repeated doses, however, caused an accumulation of radioactivity in the circulating plasma. The urinary clearance was less than 50% of the administered dose.

Both ^{14}C and ^{35}S labeled methylene dimethanesulfonate have been studied in rats and mice (Edwards et al., 1970b). In both species, *N*-formyl cysteine-^{14}C and *N,N'*-diformyl cystine-^{14}C were identified as urinary products. The ready incorporation of the methylene group into the one carbon pool, however, makes it difficult to distinguish *in vivo* the products that are different from those that would be produced from ^{14}C-formaldehyde. The uptake of a higher specific activity ^{14}C-MDMS was studied in rats bearing bilaterally transplanted Yoshida tumors, one very sensitive and the other resistant to the drug (Fox, 1971). The uptake into the sensitive tumor was somewhat greater than in the resistant one, but only for a short time after administration, suggesting that the *initial* alkylation may be greater in the sensitive tumor. In cell culture experiments with the same tumors, no such difference was observed, even though the cell lines retained their relative sensitivities to the drug. The distribution of ^{14}C-ethylene dimethanesulfonate has also been studied (Edwards et al., 1969; Edwards and Jackson, 1970a) in the rat and mouse and was found to be excreted unchanged in the urine together with ^{14}C-*S*-(2-hydroxyethyl) cysteine-*N*-acetate and ^{14}C-*S*-(2-hydroxyethyl) cysteine-*N*-acetate-*S*-oxide. The metabolism of ^{14}C-EDS was found to be similar to that of ^{14}C ethylene dibromide, but the latter was more completely converted into the two metabolites. Both compounds undergo a "sulfur stripping" process with sulfhydryl groups *in vitro* and exhibit some differences in their distribution among the various tissues. Most of these results suggest that a major detoxication route of these agents may be interaction with glutathione sulfhydryl, a frequent detoxication pathway for alkane sulfonates. The importance of this interaction as a primary biological site of action *in vivo* is yet to be assessed, and it is possible that important physiological regulatory systems could be affected (Niskanen, 1967).

Cellular Studies

Not many investigations into the action of busulfan have been carried out in cell culture systems because of the low solubility of the agent in the media used. Dimethyl busulfan, however, has been studied in a radioresistant, a radiosensitive diploid, and a tetraploid line of leukemia L5178Y (Goldenberg and Alexander, 1965). Whereas the radioresistant and radiosensitive lines showed a parallel response to dimethyl busulfan, the tetraploid line showed an increased sensitivity. Cell division occurred for some time after treatment. An attempt to locate repair of sublethal damage using split dose recovery data failed (Goldenberg, 1968). It was found, however, that bromodeoxyuridine, which is known to sensitize mammalian cell lines to x-irradiation, also sensitized a P815Y cell line to dimethyl busulfan (SCHINDLER et al., 1966). The mechanism of this sensitization is not understood.

The development of resistance to alkane sulfonates in tumor cell lines by selection in culture appears to be very difficult to achieve. However, resistance *in vivo* is more easily produced, and transfer of these cells to culture conditions has not significantly altered their resistance to the drugs *in vitro*. Cross sensitivity experiments towards other agents are thus possible, and some indication of the nature of the biological action may be deduced. Yoshida sarcoma cells in culture showing resistance to methylene dimethanesulfonate also show resistance to ultraviolet light and nitrogen mustard, but not to x-irradiation and methyl methanesulfonate (FOX and FOX, 1971). Similar differences between the four last mentioned agents have been reported for bacteria (BRIDGES and MUNSON, 1966) and yeast (BRENDEL et al., 1970).

Studies at the Molecular Level

The similarity in pattern of sensitivity between the mammalian cell systems and the bacterial systems suggests that similar genetic differences may be involved. It is considered that in the latter, different loci are involved with repair of UV-like and x-ray-like damage. The x-ray-like damage is considered to be primarily single strand breaks, whereas the UV-like damage is due primarily to intrastrand crosslinking (FOX and FOX, 1971). Whether these same lesions occur *in vivo* is of course not proven, but the striking similarity of the bacterial and mammalian results suggests that interaction with DNA is an important lesion not far removed from the primary lesion.

Using ^{14}C-busulfan, BROOKES and LAWLEY (1961) demonstrated that both 7-(4′-hydroxybutyl) guanine and 1′,4′-di(guanin-7-yl)butane could be isolated from a direct reaction at 37° with DNA in phosphate (0.03M) or acetate (0.05M) buffer at neutral pH. This product could be due to either inter or intrastrand crosslinking of the alkylating agent with the guanine moieties of the DNA. By studying the denaturation resistance following alkylation, KOHN et al. (1966) showed that busulfan did not produce such resistance, suggesting that no interstrand crosslinking occurred. It would thus appear from this data that intrastrand crosslinking only was occurring. Work in T_7 coliphage (BRAKIER and VERLY, 1970) essentially confirmed this conclusion and studies were extended to include dimethyl busulfan.

Mutagenic Action

In common with the other biologically active alkylating agents, the alkane sulfonates are active mutagenic agents. The genetic and allied effects have been reviewed by LOVELESS (1966) in a general work on the alkylating agents. The alkane sulfonates have long been recognized as powerful mutagens, especially the simple methyl and ethyl methanesulfonates. The mutagenic action of busulfan in *Drosophila melanogaster* was studied by FAHMY and FAHMY (1956) and RÖHRBORN (1959a, b). GEBHART (1969) studied chromosome aberrations in mouse lymphocyte cultures, following busulfan and cysteine treatment. The mutagenic action of this same alkane sulfonate in mice had previously been studied by MOUTSCHEN (1961). Busulfan induced a low frequency of chromosome aberrations and mutations in barley *(Hordeum sativum)* (MOUTSCHEN and MOUTSCHEN-DAHMEN, 1958; NATARAJAN and RAMANNA, 1966; RAMANNA and NATARAJAN, 1966) and in *Vicia faba* (RIEGER and MICHAELIS, 1960; MICHAELIS and RIEGER, 1960). L-Threitol-1,4-dimethanesulfonate, first synthezised by FEIT (1964) was also shown to be an important plant mutagen and more useful by virtue of its increased solubility. Its mutagenic action on *Vicia faba* (MOUTSCHEN and REEKMANS, 1964; MOUTSCHEN, 1965; MOUTSCHEN et al., 1966, 1967) and on barley (MATAGNE, 1969) has been investigated and the L-isomer shown to be 10 to 20 times more effective than the D and *meso* forms. Its possible conversion to diepoxybutane *in vivo* has been considered to be the primary cause of its mutagenic action (DAVIS and ROSS, 1963) even though the latter is less effective as a mutagen (MOUTSCHEN-DAHMEN et al., 1963). The stereochemical aspects of the sugar molecule derivatives particularly lend themselves to structure-activity investigations. Further "fixation" of the reactive alkane sulfonate ester groups has also been achieved by synthesis of the isomers of cyclohexane dimethanesulfonates (JACKSON, 1970).

Conclusions

The dimethanesulfonates offer a potentially wide spectrum of biologically active agents, whose action is considered to be due to the diverse manner in which the chemical structures, introduced by alkylation onto a nucleophilic site, possess greater scope for steric variability than those derived from nitrogen mustard or aziridine linkages. This is born out not only in the antitumor properties of these agents, but also in their action on the normal steady state systems such as spermatogenesis and hematopoiesis. There is a high probability that the biologically important primary target is closely related to DNA, if not DNA itself, but the importance of other nucleophilic interactions has yet to be appreciated. None have been shown to crosslink DNA by interstrand crosslinking mechanisms, but intrastrand crosslinks do occur and are probably biologically important, especially in bacteriophage. Resistance to these agents in certain rodent tumors has occurred, but no definite conclusions as to the mechanism of this resistance have been reached. Detoxication, especially with the lower members of the series, appears to be accompanied by the "sulfur stripping" process, i.e. the removal of a sulfhydryl group of proteins and peptides by the two prong attack of these esters. It remains to be seen whether this process is an important one in the physiological regulation of cellular dynamics and thus a potentially important site for the action of these agents.

References

ADDISON, I. E., BERENBAUM, M. C.: The effect of cysteine on the immunosuppressive activity of busulphan, cyclophosphamide, and nitrogen mustard. Brit. J. Cancer **25**, 172—181 (1971).

BERENBAUM, M. C., TIMMIS, G. M., BROWN, I. N.: The relation between physico-chemical properties and immunodepressive effects of an homologous series of sulphonic acid esters. Immunology **13**, 517—522 (1967).

BIERMAN, H. R., KELLY, K. H., MAEKAWA, T., TIMMIS, G. M.: The influence of 1,4-dimethylsulfonoxy-1,4-dimethyl-butane (CB 2348, Dimethylmyleran) in neoplastic disease. Ann. N.Y. Acad. Sci. **68**, 1211—1222 (1958).

BOLLAG, W.: Cytostatica in der Schwangerschaft. Schweiz. med. Wschr. **84**, 393—395 (1954).

BRAKIER, L., VERLY, W. G.: The lethal action of ethyl methanesulfonate, nitrogen mustard and myleran on the T_7 coliphage. Biochim. biophys. Acta (Amst.) **213**, 296—311 (1970).

BRENDEL, M., KHAN, N. A., HAYNES, R. H.: Common steps in the repair of alkylation and radiation damage in yeast. Molec. gen. Genetics **106**, 289—295 (1970).

BRIDGES, B. A., MUNSON, R. J.: Excision-repair of DNA in an auxotropic strain of *Escherichia coli*. Biochem. biophys. Res. Commun. **22**, 268—273 (1966).

BROOKES, P., LAWLEY, P. D.: The reaction of mono- and di-functional alkylating agents with nucleic acids. Biochem. J. **80**, 496—503 (1961).

CHEVREMONT, M.: Le mécanisme de l'action antimitotique. Pathol-Biologie **9**, 973—1004 (1961).

COOPER, E. R. A., JACKSON, H.: Comparative effects of methylene, ethylene and propylene dimethanesulfonates on the male rat reproductive system. J. Reprod. Fert. **23**, 103—108 (1970).

DAVIS, W., ROSS, W. C. J.: The formation of epoxides from cytotoxic polyol methane sulfonates under physiological conditions. Biochem. Pharmacol. **12**, 915—917 (1963).

DEROOIJ, D. G., KRAMER, M. F.: Spermatogonial stem cell renewal in the rat, mouse and golden hamster. A study with the alkylating agent myleran. Z. Zellforsch. mikrosk. Anat. **92**, 400—405 (1968).

DIAMOND, I., ANDERSON, M. M., MCCREADIE, S. R.: Transplacental transmission of busulfan (myleran) in a mother with leukemia: production of fetal malformation and cytomegaly. Pediatrics, Springfield **25**, 85—90 (1960).

DUNJIC, A.: Shortening of the span of life of rats by "myleran." Nature (Lond.) **203**, 887—888 (1964).

DUNN, C. D. R., ELSON, L. A.: The effect of a homologous series of dimethane sulfonoxyalkanes on hemopoietic colony forming units in the rat. Chem. biol. Interact. **2**, 273—280 (1970a).

DUNN, C. D. R., ELSON, L. A.: The comparative effect of busulfan ("myleran") and aminochlorambucil on hemopoietic colony forming units in the rat. Cell. Tissue Kinet. **3**, 131—141 (1970b).

ECKHARDT, S., SELLEI, C., HINDY, I.: Mannogranol treatment of neoplastic diseases. Jap. Cancer Assoc., Gann Monograph 2, Tokyo: Maruzen Co. 1967.

EDWARDS, K., CRAIG, A. W., JACKSON, H., JONES, A. R.: Studies with alkylating esters. I. The fate of ethylene dimethane sulfonate. Biochem. Pharmacol. **18**, 1693—1700 (1969).

EDWARDS, K., JACKSON, H.: Studies with alkylating esters. II. A chemical interpretation through metabolic studies of the antifertility effects of ethylene dimethane sulfonate and ethylene dibromide. Biochem. Pharmacol. **19**, 1783—1789 (1970a).

EDWARDS, K., JACKSON, H., JONES, A. R.: Studies with alkylating esters. III. The metabolism and fate of methylene dimethane sulfonate. Biochem. Pharmacol. **19**, 1791—1795 (1970b).

EL-MERZABANI, M. M., SAKURAI, Y.: Inhibition of tumor growth by new sulfonic acid esters of amino glycols. Gann **56**, 575—587 (1965a).

EL-MERZABANI, M. M., SAKURAI, Y.: A new alkylating antitumor agent effective on experimental tumors resistant to nitrogen mustard. Gann **56**, 589—598 (1965b).

EL-MERZABANI, M. M., SAKURAI, Y.: Anticancer activities of methane sulfonic esters of amino glycols against leukemia L1210. Gann **58**, 199—201 (1967).

ELSON, L. A.: The effects of myleran (1 : 4-dimethanesulfonoxybutane) and homologous compounds on the blood. Biochem. Pharmac. **1**, 39—47 (1958).

ELSON, L. A.: Radiation and Radiomimetic Chemicals, 1st. ed. London: Butterworths 1963.

ELSON, L. A., GALTON, D. A. G., TILL, M.: The action of chlorambucil (CB1348) and busulfan (myleran) on the hemopoietic organs of the rat. Brit. J. Hematol. **4**, 355—374 (1958).

FAHMY, O. G., FAHMY, M. J.: Mutagenicity of 2-chloroethyl methanesulfonate in Drosophila melanogaster. Nature (Lond.) **177**, 996—997 (1956).

FEINGOLD, M. L., KOSS, L. G.: Effects of long term administration of busulfan. Report of a case with generalized nuclear abnormalities, carcinoma of vulva and pulmonary fibrosis. Arch. intern. Med. **124**, 66—71 (1969).

FEIT, P. W.: 1,4-Bismethanesulfonates of the stereoisomeric butanetetraols and related compounds. J. med. Chem. **7**, 14—17 (1964).

FOX, B. W.: The sensitivity of a Yoshida sarcoma to methylene dimethane sulfonate. Int. J. Cancer **4**, 54—60 (1969).

FOX, B. W.: Uptake studies of [^{14}C] methylene dimethane sulphonate in bilaterally transplanted sensitive and resistant Yoshida sarcoma. Chem. biol. Interact. **3**, 149—156 (1971).

FOX, B. W., CRAIG, A. W., JACKSON, H.: The comparative metabolism of myleran-^{35}S in the rat, mouse and rabbit. Biochem. Pharmacol. **5**, 27—29 (1960).

FOX, B. W., JACKSON, H.: Antifertility agents. In: Evaluation of drug activities: Pharmacometrics, 1st ed. London—New York: Academic Press 1964.

FOX, B. W., JACKSON, H.: *In vivo* effects of methylene dimethane sulfonate on proliferating cell systems. Brit. J. Pharmacol. Chemother. **24**, 24—28 (1965).

FOX, M., FOX, B. W.: The establishment of cloned cell lines from Yoshida sarcomas having differential sensitivities to methylene dimethane sulfonate *in vivo* and their cross-sensitivity to x-rays, UV and other alkylating agents. Chem. biol. Interact. **4**, 363—376 (1971/72).

GALTON, D. A. G.: The use of myleran and similar agents in chronic leukemias. Advanc. Cancer Res. **4**, 73—112 (1956).

GALTON, D. A. G., TILL, M., WILTSHAW, E.: Busulfan (1,4-dimethane sulfonyl oxybutane, myleran): summary of clinical results. Ann. N.Y. Acad. Sci. **68**, 967—973 (1958).

GEBHART, E.: Zur Beeinflussung der Wirkung von Myleran auf menschliche Chromosomen durch L-Cystein. Mutation Res. **7**, 254—257 (1969).

GOLDENBERG, G. J.: Repair of sub-lethal damage of L5178Y lymphoblasts *in vitro* treated with dimethyl myleran and nitrogen mustard. Biochem. Pharmacol. **17**, 820—824 (1968).

GOLDENBERG, G. J., ALEXANDER, P.: The effects of nitrogen mustard and dimethyl myleran on murine leukemia cell lines of different radiosensitivity *in vivo*. Cancer Res. **25**, 1401—1409 (1965).
GOLDIN, A., WOOD, H. B., JR.: Preclinical investigation of alkylating agents in cancer chemotherapy. Ann. N.Y. Acad. Sci. **163**, 954—1005 (1969).
GRIMES, P., VON SALLMANN, L.: Interference with cell proliferation and induction of polyploidy in rat lens epithelium during prolonged myleran treatment. Exp. cell. Res. **42**, 265—273 (1966).
HADDOW, A., TIMMIS, G. M.: Myleran in chronic myeloid leukemia; chemical constitution and biological action. Lancet I, 207—208 (1953).
HADDOW, A., TIMMIS, G. M., BROWN, S. S.: Tumor inhibiting action of 1,6-dimethanesulfonyl D-mannitol. Nature (Lond.) **182**, 1164—1165 (1958).
HAGY, G., BALAZS, C., PETRANYI, G.: Therapeutic use of zitostop in polycythemia vera. Therapia Hungarica **1**, 16—18 (1971).
HARROLD, B. P.: Syndrome resembling ADDISON's disease following prolonged treatment with busulfan. Brit. med. J. **5485**, 463—464 (1966).
HEARD, B. E., COOKE, R. A.: Busulfan Lung. Thorax **23**, 187—193 (1968).
HELLER, R. H., JONES, H. W.: Production of ovarian dysgenesis in the rat and human by busulfan. Amer. J. Obstet. Gynecol. **89**, 414—420 (1964).
HEMSWORTH, B. N.: Embryopathies in the rat due to alkane sulfonates. J. Reprod. Fert. **17**, 325—334 (1968).
HEMSWORTH, B. N., JACKSON, H.: Effect of busulfan on the fetal gonad. Nature (Lond.) **195**, 816—817 (1962).
HEMSWORTH, B. N., JACKSON, H.: Effect of busulfan on the developing gonad of the male rat. J. Reprod. Fertil. **5**, 187—194 (1963a).
HEMSWORTH, B. N., JACKSON, H.: Effect of busulfan on the developing ovary in the rat. J. Reprod. Fertil. **6**, 229—233 (1963b).
ISRAELS, L. G., SINCLAIR, C., GRAF, J., ZIPURSKY, A.: Comparative effects of nitrogen mustard (HN_2), chlorambucil (CB1348) and busulfan (myleran) on the peripheral blood and the ferrokinetic patterns in dogs. Can. J. Biochem. Physiol. **40**, 667—677 (1962).
JACKSON, H.: Nonsteroidal antifertility agents in the male. In: DICZFALUSY, E., BORELL, U. (Eds.): Control of human fertility. Nobel Symposium No. 19, pp. 119—130. Stockholm, New York—London—Sydney: Almqvist and Wiksell, John Wiley and Sons 1970.
JACKSON, H., CRAIG, A. W.: Effects of alkylating chemicals on reproductive cells. Ann. N.Y. Acad. Sci. **160**, 215—227 (1969).
JACKSON, H., FOX, B. W., CRAIG, A. W.: The effect of alkylating agents on male rat fertility. Brit. J. Pharmacol. Chemother. **14**, 149—157 (1959).
JACKSON, H., FOX, B. W., CRAIG, A. W.: Antifertility substances and their assessment in the male rodent. J. Reprod. Fertil. **2**, 447—465 (1961).
JAMES, R. M. V.: Hematological studies with methylene dimethane sulfonate (dimethanesulfonoxy methane). Brit. J. Haematol. **12**, 546—554 (1966).
JOST, E., AMIRKHANIAN, J. D.: Comparative studies of the effect of x-rays and 1,3-propanediol-dimethane sulfonate on the mosquito Culex pipiens L. Mutation Res. **13**, 49—57 (1971).
KELLNER, B., NÉMETH, L.: R-74 toxicologiai es daganatgatlo hatasanak vizsgalata (investigation of the toxicological and tumor inhibitory action of R-74). Budapest: Rep. Res. Inst., Pharm. Inst. 1967—1968, cited in Chemotherapy of neoplastic diseases.
KENDREY, G.: Tetramesylmannitol symposium. Budapest: Nat. Oncol. Inst. 1968.
KOCH, G.: Preparation de myleran tritié. Bull. soc. Chim. Belges **68**, 59 (1959a).
KOCH, G., VERLY, W. G., BACQ, Z. M.: Synthese de myleran tritié. Arch. int. Physiol. **67**, 117—121 (1959b).
KOHN, K. W., SPEARS, C. L., DOTY, P.: Inter-strand cross linking of DNA by nitrogen mustard. J. molec. Biol. **19**, 266—288 (1966).
KOSS, L. G.: Effects of alkylating agents on epithelia in man and in an experimental system in the rat. Ann. N.Y. Acad. Sci. **163**, 931—935 (1969).
KURRLE, G. R.: "Myleran"; a review of its action and a report on its use in chronic myeloid leukemia. Med. J. Aust. **42**, 636—641 (1955).
KYLE, R. A., SCHWARTZ, R. S., DAMESHEK, W.: A syndrome resembling adrenal cortical insufficiency associated with long term busulfan (myleran) therapy. Blood **18**, 497—510 (1961).
LAPIS, K.: Report addressed to the Research Institute of the Pharmaceutical Industry, 1968; cited in SZENTKLARAY and SELLEI, 1971.
LEAKE, E., SMITH, W. G., WOODLIFF, H. J.: Diffuse interstitial pulmonary fibrosis after busulfan therapy. Lancet II, 432—434 (1963).
LEBLOND, C. P., CLERMONT, Y.: Definition of the stages of the cycle of the seminiferous epithelium in the rat. Ann. N.Y. Acad. Sci. **55**, 548—573 (1952).

Light, A. E.: Additional observations on the effects of busulfan on cataract formation, duration of anesthesia, and reproduction in rats. Toxic. appl. Pharmacol. **10**, 459—466 (1967).
Littler, W. A., Ogilvie, C.: Lung function in patients receiving busulfan. Brit. med. J. **4**, 530—532 (1970).
Loveless, A.: Genetic and allied effects of alkylating agents. London: Butterworths 1966.
Maisin, J. A., Dunjic, A., Dumont, P.: Restorative action of yeast ribonucleic acid and its mixed nucleotides on bone marrow death induced in rats by myleran. J. Radiat. Biol. **5**, 291—300 (1962).
Matagne, R.: Induction of chromosomal aberrations and mutations with isomeric forms of L-threitol-1,4-*bis* methane sulfonate in plant materials. Mutation Res. **7**, 241—247 (1969).
Medici, P. T., Hurst, J. M., Pillero, S. J.: Protective effects of erythropoietin against myleran induced hematodepression. Acta haemat. (Basel) **33**, 167—177 (1965).
Michaelis, A., Rieger, R.: Einige experimentelle Ergebnisse zur Wirkung von Myleran auf die Chromosomen von Vicia faba L. Der Züchter **30**, 150—163 (1960).
Miller, E.: The effects of nonane on malignant disease. Cancer Chemother. Rep. **14**, 11—21 (1961).
Moutschen, J.: Differential sensitivity of mouse spermatogenesis to alkylating agents. Genetics **46**, 291—299 (1961).
Moutschen, J.: Analyse des effects due l-threitol-1,4-bismethanesulfonate sur les chromosomes de Vicia faba L. Cellule **65**, 161—189 (1965).
Moutschen, J., Matagne, R., Gilot, J.: Chromosome breakage with two isomers of R-threitol 1,4-bismethanesulfonate in plants. Nature (Lond.) **210**, 262—763 (1966).
Moutschen, J., Matagne, R., Gilot, J.: Sur les differences de sensibilité des chromosomes aux isomeres d'un agent d'alkylation de threitol-1,4-bis(methane sulfonate). Bull. Soc. roy. botan. Belg. **100**, 11—21 (1967).
Moutschen, J., Moutschen-Dahmen, M.: L'action due myleran sur les chromosomes chez Hordeum salivum et chez Vicia faba. Hereditas **44**, 18—36 (1958).
Moutschen, J., Moutschen-Dahmen, M., Verly, W. G., Koch, G.: Autoradiograms with tritiated myleran. Exp. cell. Res. **20**, 585—588 (1960).
Moutschen, J., Reekmans, M.: Effects of L-threitol-1,4-*bis* methane sulfonate on chromosomes. Caryologica **17**, 495—508 (1964).
Moutschen-Dahman, J., Moutschen-Dahmen, M., Loppes, R.; Differential mutagenic activity of L(+) and D(—) diepoxybutane. Nature (Lond.) **199**, 406—407 (1963).
Nadkarni, V. M., Trams, E. G., Smith, P. K.: Preliminary studies on the distribution and fate of TEM, TEPA and myleran in the human. Cancer Res. **19**, 713—718 (1959).
Natarajan, A. T., Ramanna, M. S.: Modification of relative mutagenic efficiency in barley of mesyloxyesters by different treatments. Nature (Lond.) **211**, 1099—1100 (1966).
Nelson, B. M., Andrews, G. A.: Breast cancer and cytological dysplasia in many organs after busulfan (myleran). Amer. J. clin. Path. **42**, 37—44 (1964).
Niskanen, E.: Bone marrow cell proliferation after busulfan treatment and its relation to humoral control mechanisms. Acta path. microbiol. Scand. **70**, 1—93 (1967).
Oakberg, E. F.: Duration of spermatogenesis in the mouse and timing of stages of the cycle of the seminiferous epithelium. Amer. J. Anat. **99**, 507—516 (1956).
Ochoa, M., Jr., Hirschberg, E.: Alkylating Agents. In: Schnitzer, R. J., Hawking, F. (Eds.): Experimental chemotherapy, Vol. 5, pp. 1—132. New York-London: Academic Press 1967.
Parham, W. E., Wilbur, J. M., Jr.: The reaction of myleran with L-cysteine ethyl ester. J. Amer. chem. Soc. **81**, 6071—6072 (1959).
Parham, W. E., Wilbur, J. M., Jr.: The mechanisms of action of bisalkylating agents in cancer chemotherapy II. The reaction of myleran with mercaptans. J. org. Chem. **26**, 1569—1572 (1961).
Partington, M., Fox, B. W., Jackson, H.: Comparative action of some methane sulfonic esters on the cell population of the rat testis. Exp. cell. Res. **33**, 78—88 (1964).
Peng, C. T.: Distribution and metabolic fate of ^{35}S labelled myleran (busulfan) in normal and tumor bearing rats. J. Pharmac. exp. Therap. **120**, 229—238 (1957).
Pinto-Machado, J.: Inhibition of osteogenesis induced in the mouse embryo by busulfan. Demonstration by alizarin. C.r. Seanc. Soc. Biol. **163**, 1712—1715 (1969).
Pinto-Machado, J.: Influence of prenatal administration of busulfan on the postnatal development of mice. Production of a syndrome including hypoplasia of the thymus. Teratology **3**, 363—369 (1970).
Ramanna, M. S., Natarajan, A. T.: Chromosome breakage induced by alkyl alkane sulfonates under different physical treatment conditions. Chromosoma **18**, 44—59 (1966).
Rieger, R., Michaelis, A.: Chromatidenaberratonen nach Einwirkung von Athylmethanesulfonate (Methansulfonsäureäthylester) auf Primärwurzeln von *Vicia faba*. Kulturpflanze **8**, 230—243 (1960).

Roberts, J. J., Warwick, G. P.: Metabolism of myleran (1 : 4-dimethane sulfonyl-oxybutane). Nature (Lond.) **183**, 1509—1510 (1959a).
Roberts, J. J., Warwick, G. P.: Metabolic and chemical studies of "myleran": formation of 3-hydroxytetrahydrothiophene-1,1-dioxide *in vivo*, and reactions with thiols *in vitro*. Nature (Lond.) **184**, 1288—1289 (1959b).
Roberts, J. J., Warwick, G. P.: The mode of action of alkylating agents. III. The formation of 3-hydroxytetrahydrothiophen-1:1-dioxide from 1:4-dimethane sulfonoxybutane (myleran), *S*,β-L-alanyl tetrahydrothiophenium mesylate, tetrahydrothiophene, and tetrahydrothiophene-1:1-dioxide in the rat, rabbit, and mouse. Biochem. Pharmacol. **6**, 217—227 (1961).
Röhrborn, G.: Untersuchungen zur Frage der genetischen Wirksamkeit von Myleran an Drosophila melanogaster. Z. Vererblehre **90**, 116—131 (1959a).
Röhrborn, G.: Mutagenitätsuntersuchungen mit 1,4-dimethylsulfonoxy-1,4-dimethylbutan an Drosophila melanogaster. Z. Vererblehre **90**, 457—462 (1959b).
Sandberg, J., Goldin, A.: Antileukemic action of a new sugar derivative dimethane sulfonate (NSC-122402) and related compounds in mice. Cancer Chemother. Rep. **53**, 367—376 (1969).
Schindler, R. L., Ramseier, L., Grieder, A.: Increased sensitivity of mammalian cell cultures to radiomimetic alkylating agents following incorporation of 5-bromodeoxyuridine into cellular DNA. Biochem. Pharmacol. **15**, 2013—2023 (1966).
Shimkin, M. B., Weisburger, J. H., Weisburger, E. K., Gubareff, N., Suntzeff, V.: Bioassay of 29 alkylating chemicals by the pulmonary-tumor response in strain A mice. J. nat. Cancer Inst. **36**, 915—935 (1966).
Skinner, W. A., Johansson, J. G.: Effect of organic compounds on reproductive processes. VIII. Methane sulfonyloxyacetyl derivatives of diamines. J. med. Chem. **13**, 319—320 (1970).
Sprunt, J. G., Rizza, C. R.: Pigmentation and busulfan therapy. Brit. med. J. **5489**, 736—737 (1966).
Sternberg, S. S., Philips, F. S., Scholler, J.: Pharmacological and pathological effects of alkylating agents. Ann. N.Y. Acad. Sci. **68**, 811—825 (1958).
Sugiura, K., Schmid, F. A., Brown, G. F., Gonzalez, R.: Chemotherapy of hamster tumors. Cancer Chemother. Rep. **2**, 141—175 (1971).
Sugiura, K., Stock, C. C.: Studies in a tumor spectrum V. The effects of esters of sulfonic acids on the growth of a variety of mouse and rat tumours. Cancer **10**, 596—605 (1967).
Szentklaray, J., Sellei, C.: Clinical study of tetramesylmannitol in neoplastic disease. Therapia Hungarica **1**, 12—15 (1971).
Talbot, T. R., Elson, L. A.: Protection of August rats against lethal doses of dimethyl homologue of myleran by isologous bone marrow. Nature (Lond.) **181**, 684—686 (1958).
Trams, E. G., Salvador, R. A., Maemgwyn-Davies, G., DeQuattro, V.: Studies on the uptake, distribution and metabolic fate of 1,4-dimethane sulfonoxybutane (myleran) in the rat. Proc. Am. Ass. Cancer Res. **2**, 256 (1957).
Vargha, L., Balo, J.: Chemistry and bioassay of zitostop. Therapia Hungarica **1**, 10—11 (1971).
Vivacqua, R. J., Haurani, I., Ersley, A. J.: "Selective" pituitary insufficiency secondary to busulfan. Ann. intern. Med. **67**, 380—387 (1967).
Vodopick, H., Hamilton, A. E., Jackson, H. L., Peng, C. T., Sheets, R. F.: Metabolic fate of tritiated busulfan in man. J. Lab. clin. Med. **73**, 266—282 (1969).
Ward, H. N., Konikov, N., Reinhard, E. H.: Cytologic dysplasias occurring after busulfan (myleran) therapy. A syndrome resembling adreno-cortical insufficiency and atrophic bronchitis. Ann. intern. Med. **63**, 654—660 (1965).
Weston, J. K., Maxwell, R. E., Lee, M., Funzle, J., Fisher, R. A.: Curative effect of rat bone marrow transfusions in aplastic (severe hypoplastic) anemia in rats induced by myleran, a radiomimetic chemical. Fed. Proc. **16**, 377 (1957).
Williams, D. W.: Busulfan in early pregnancy. Obstet. Gynecol. **27**, 738—740 (1966).

Chapter 34

Mechanism of Action of Mitomycins

H. KERSTEN

With 7 Figures

Introduction

The mitomycins were discovered by HATA et al. (1956) in *Streptomyces caespitosus* and isolated by WAKAKI et al. (1958) as deep violet crystals. Porfiromycin produced by *Streptomyces ardus* (DEBOER et al., 1961) also belongs to the group of mitomycin antibiotics. The two unidentified antibiotics, G 253 B and G 253 C, from *Streptomyces reticuli* var. *shimofasuensis* described by HATA et al. (1966) resemble the mitomycins in molecular weight, absorption spectra, and elemental analysis.

The chemical structures of the mitomycins, shown in Fig. 1, were elucidated by WEBB et al. (1962). All mitomycins including porfiromycin have in common structure I, differing only in minor substituents.

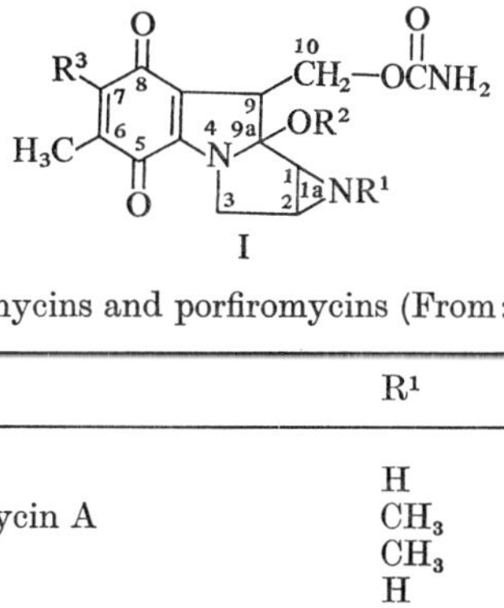

Fig. 1. Structure of mitomycins and porfiromycins (From: WEBB, J.S., et al., 1962)

	R^1	R^2	R^3
Mitomycin A	H	CH_3	H_3CO
N-Methyl-mitomycin A	CH_3	CH_3	H_3CO
Mitomycin B	CH_3	H	H_3CO
Mitomycin C	H	CH_3	H_2N
Porfiromycin (*N*-methyl-mitomycin C)	CH_3	CH_3	H_2N
7-Hydroxy-porfiromycin	CH_3	CH_3	HO

The mitomycins represent the first naturally occurring compounds containing an aziridine ring, a pyrrolo(1,2-a)indole ring system, an amino (or methoxybenzoquinone) and pyrrolizidine residue. All members of the mitomycins have three typical carcinostatic groups, i.e. aziridine, quinone, and urethane. In contrast to the usual synthetic ethyleneimine rings, the aziridine ring is stable and inactive in the native form of the mitomycin molecule (SCHWARTZ et al., 1963).

Conversion to the active state occurs by a reductive process (Schwartz et al., 1963; Patrick et al., 1964; Szybalski and Arneson, 1965). The alkylating properties of the mitomycins are strictly dependent on the aziridine ring system.

Depending on the concentration, the mitomycins exhibit a variety of inhibitory effects. At very low, noninhibitory concentrations, they suppress the ability of recipient *Diplococcus pneumoniae* cells to integrate transforming DNA. Slightly higher, but noncidal concentrations inhibit cell division of several bacterial species, and also cell division of mammalian cells. Still higher mitomycin concentrations result in bacteriostasis and in rapid cidal effects. The mitomycins have been shown to be active against some viruses, to exhibit mutagenicity, to induce lysogenic phages, and to cause the production of colicins. Mitomycins interfere with DNA and RNA metabolism in bacteria as well as in higher organisms. Furthermore, several observations indicate that the mitomycins affect the activity or the synthesis of some enzymes. (For summary see the review by Szybalski and Iyer, 1967.)

Mitomycin C suppresses transformation of normal plant cells by the crown-gall organism *Agrobacterium tumefaciens* without macroscopically observable phytotoxic effects when applied on *Kalachoe daigremontiana in vivo* (Gribnau and Veldstra, 1969). Among several groups of carcinostatic substances, the mitomycins constitute a most powerful group (see the review by Carter, 1968; Moore, 1968).

Molecular Mechanism of Action

As has already been discussed, the mitomycins contain three main functional groups. The antibiotics might therefore interact differently with certain cell components. Possibly the nutritional environment of the cells determines which functional group of the molecule becomes active. Thus, some selectivity for one or another inhibitory effect should be considered. As a consequence, the mechanism of action may not be unique and could depend on (1) the cell type, (2) the physiological state of the cells, and (3) their environment. The following sections are an attempt to discuss how far the proposed mechanism of action can explain the biological effects, rather than a complete review covering the whole literature on mitomycins, which was summarized excellently up to 1966 by Szybalski and Iyer (1966).

The discussion on the mechanism of action of mitomycins presented here will include some derivatives of the mitomycins not containing the aziridine ring system, but with the quinone and urethane side chain unchanged. These compounds are still biologically active (Roth et al., 1966).

A. Interaction with DNA *in Vitro*

In vitro the mitomycins react with purified DNA in the presence of reducing agents or NADPH and a quinone reductase. DNA treated in this way, on heat denaturation and rapid chilling, renatures spontaneously, retaining its native-like hypochromicity, transforming activity, and buoyant density in cesium chloride or cesium sulfate gradients. Iyer and Szybalski (1963, 1964) concluded from their results, that activated forms of mitomycins alkylate DNA, thereby forming crosslinks between the two strands of the DNA molecule.

Among several bacterial DNAs tested, the greatest susceptibility to mitomycin crosslinking was observed with *Sarcina lutea* DNA (70% G + C) and the least susceptibility with DNA from *Cytophaga johnsonii* (32% G + C). These results indicate that either guanine or cytosine or both might preferentially react with the mitomycins, since the degree of crosslinking increases with increasing G + C content. Alternatively one can argue that only the structural features of DNA with high G + C content favor the binding of mitomycins, and crosslinking of the two strands of DNA.

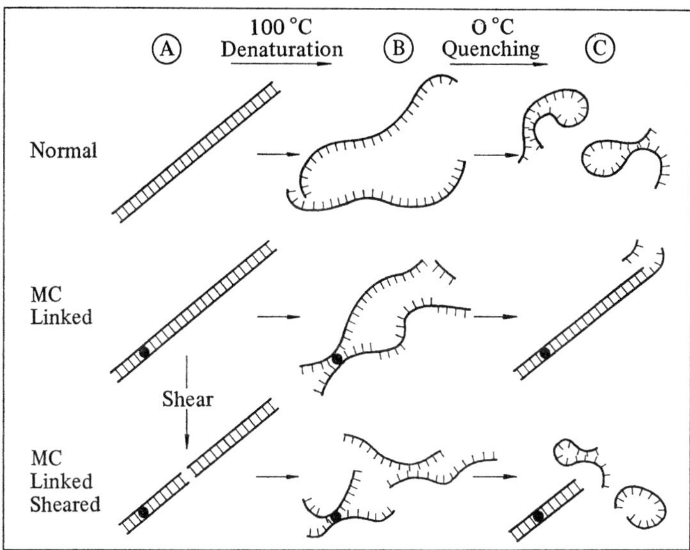

Fig. 2. Schematic presentation of molecular events following denaturation (A to B) and rapid cooling (B to C) of DNA. *Top row:* normal DNA extracted from control cells. *Middle row:* crosslinked DNA extracted from mitomycin C(MC)-inactivated cells. The possibility of hydrolytic cleavage of the phosphate ester bonds and its consequences are illustrated for denaturated (B) and spontaneously renatured, quenched form (C). *Bottom row:* crosslinked DNA extracted from mitomycin inactivated cells and subsequently exposed to shearing forces with resulting double-strand break. Upon heating and rapid cooling only the crosslink bearing fragment renatures spontaneously. (From IYER and SZYBALSKI, 1963)

SZYBALSKI and IYER (1964a, b) exposed purified *Bacillus subtilis* DNA in the presence of a reducing agent to radioactively labeled *N*-methyl-mitomycin and calculated the average number of crosslinks per molecule. At a concentration of 20 μg of *N*-methyl-mitomycin per 200 μg of DNA, the amount of radioactivity in DNA, purified by alcohol precipitation and by cesium chloride gradient fractionation, corresponded to one mitomycin molecule per 2.5 nucleotide pairs, i.e. per molecular weight of 1.5×10^6 daltons. From these results it could be calculated that only one out of five to ten antibiotic molecules participated in the crosslinks and the others reacted with one strand only. The mitomycins were visualized as interacting with DNA like the bifunctional alkylating agents studied by LAWLEY and BROOKES (1963, 1967).

WEISSBACH and LISIO (1965) reported on the alkylation of nucleic acids by mitomycin C and porfiromycin and showed that up to one antibiotic molecule was bound per 500 nucleotide residues using DNA from *E. coli*. Ribonucleic acids and ribosomes are also alkylated, but to a lesser degree than DNA. Bovine plasma albumin, starch, and glycogen can also be alkylated by mitomycins under comparable conditions, but not to the same extent as nucleic acids. The site of alkylation of nucleic acids by mitomycins was studied by LIPSETT and WEISSBACH (1965).

Experiments with synthetic polyribonucleotides showed that alkylation with ^{3}H-mitomycin or ^{14}C-porfiromycin proceeds at least four times as easily on guanine as on the other common bases. Alkylation of tRNA with porfiromycin and subsequent hydrolysis was demonstrated to yield both monoguaninyl and diguaninyl porfiromycin. It was suggested that the diguaninyl product probably arose from interstrand crosslinking. However, analogous experiments with DNA were not reported by these authors.

Interstrand crosslinking of DNA by bifunctional alkylating agents has been extensively studied. LAWLEY and BROOKES (1967) found that only double-stranded but not single-stranded DNA, when reacted *in vitro* with bifunctional alkylating agents such as nitrogen mustard, results upon hydrolysis in di-(7-guaninyl) derivatives. It was concluded that the product formed must originate from interstrand cross-links. In addition to cross-linking, the bifunctional alkylating agents alkylate N_7 of guanine in the same way as do monofunctional alkylating agents. Small amounts of 1-alkyladenine and 3-alkyladenine have also been observed. Since mitomycin shows preference in binding for G + C base pairs, it was suggested that diguaninyl-mitomycin participates in interstrand crosslinking. By using space-filling models of DNA and of mitomycin, it is extremely difficult to fit the mitomycin molecule as a cross-link between the complementary strands of DNA, without assuming a large distortion of the double-helix. The best fit with the models was obtained by postulating links between two O_6 groups of the nearest guanines on the opposite strands (SZYBALSKI and IYER, 1967).

A novel assay of 7-alkylation of guanine residues in DNA has been described by TOMASZ (1970). This assay is based upon the finding that methylation of the N_7 position of guanine derivatives renders the C_8 hydrogen extremely labile. This lability is manifested by a rapid deuterium or tritium exchange of the C_8 hydrogen with the solvent, under physiological conditions. The method has been used to analyze the interaction of DNA with three drugs, the bifunctional nitrogen mustard, methyl-(*bis*-β-chlorethyl)amine, the synthetic mutagen, triethylenemelamine, and the antibiotic, mitomycin C. Nitrogen mustard showed a stoichiometric correspondence between the amount of guanine alkylated and the amount of tritium released into the medium. Triethylenemelamine caused substantial release of tritium. There was, however, no detectable tritium release with mitomycin C under the optimal conditions for covalent binding of the drug to DNA *in vitro*. These findings indicate that, contrary to earlier suggestions, mitomycin differs in its interaction with DNA from the bifunctional alkylating agents. Since the experiments of LIPSETT and WEISSBACH (1965) were carried out with synthetic polyribonucleotides or soluble RNA, there was, up to the present time, no precise information on the site of alkylation of DNA by mitomycins. The question of the nature of the crosslink induced by mitomycin on DNA remains to be solved.

KODOMA (1967) reported low, but considerable direct, interactions of mitomycins and DNA, which did not involve a reductive step. The methods used to show this interaction were flow dichroism, difference spectra, and viscosity measurements. From the results of flow dichroism, the authors concluded that mitomycin is oriented parallel to the planes of the DNA bases. Furthermore, an increase in viscosity was found upon interaction of mitomycin with DNA. The authors suggested some form of intercalation of mitomycin between the base-pairs of DNA. More conclusive evidence is necessary to prove this proposed mechanism of mitomycin-DNA interaction.

The active alkylating species of reduced mitomycin is not known with certainty. The proposed mechanism of activation is shown in Fig. 2 (for details see SZYBALSKI and IYER, 1967). The reduction of the quinone moiety of mitomycin is followed by spontaneous elimination of the tertiary methoxy group and formation of an aromatic indole system with two active centers. The reactive sites are probably the opened aziridine ring and the CH_2 group of the methyl urethane side chain. The substituent in position 7 of the quinone ring might also be involved in the interaction with DNA.

An electronic mechanism of crosslinkage formation was discussed extensively by MURAKAMI (1966). The mitomycins are completely inert in their native form; reduction results in the extension of a π-electron system in their molecular structures. The sensitivity of the aziridine ring during the activation reaction is

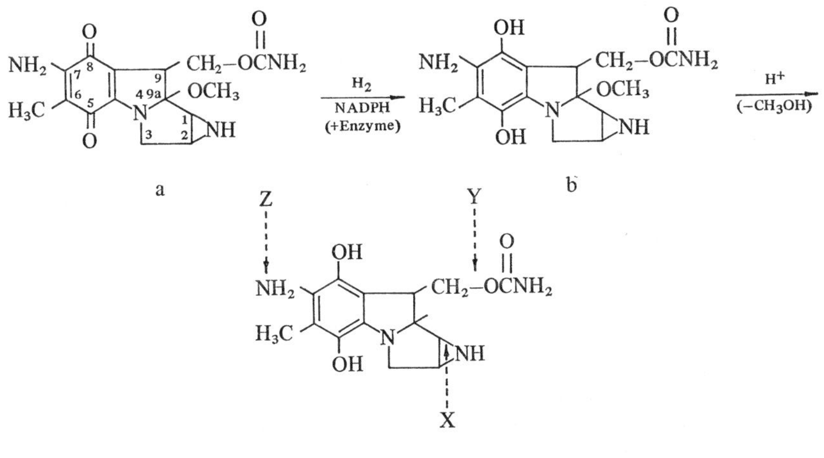

Fig. 3. Structure of mitomycin (a), the primary product after chemical or enzymatic reduction (b), postulated structure after secondary rearrangement (c), X and Y and Z are the possible reaction sites of the difunctional alkylating product (From SZYBALSKI and IYER, 1967)

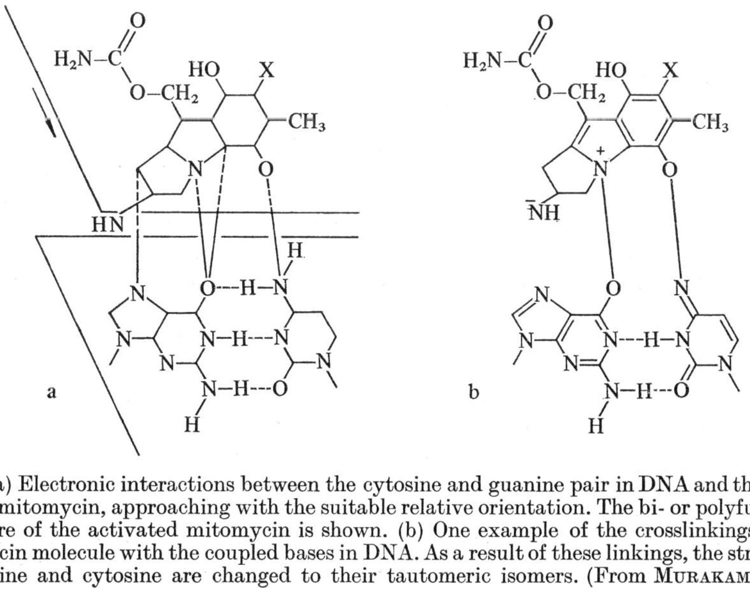

Fig. 4. (a) Electronic interactions between the cytosine and guanine pair in DNA and the active form of mitomycin, approaching with the suitable relative orientation. The bi- or polyfunctional feature of the activated mitomycin is shown. (b) One example of the crosslinkings of the mitomycin molecule with the coupled bases in DNA. As a result of these linkings, the structures of guanine and cytosine are changed to their tautomeric isomers. (From MURAKAMI, 1966)

considered to be caused by an electronic effect on that ring. This theory explains the high reactivity of the proposed ionized radical system of the activated molecule, corresponding to the intermediary semiquinoid form. This form of the mitomycin molecule exhibits, as the author states, "beautiful harmony, with the known electronic features of the coupled bases in DNA and hence interacts with them as a bi- or even polyfunctional agent." The ability of the mitomycin molecule to form the crosslinkage on the double strands of DNA is interpreted on the basis of a radical mechanism including the electronic transformations mentioned above.

This proposed scheme of crosslinkage formation results in a structural change of the purine and pyrimidine bases in DNA, corresponding to their tautomeric isomerism. The greater tendency towards such isomerization in cytosine and guanine, as compared to thymine and adenine, is thought to provide the basis for explaining the experimentally observed preferential contribution of cytosine and guanine to the crosslinking reactions. This proposed mechanism of formation of crosslinks does not involve covalent binding of mitomycin to the N_7 of guanine. Thus, this model can help to explain the more recent findings of TOMASZ (1970) that mitomycins do not alkylate – like other bifunctional alkylating agents – the N_7 position of the guanine residues in DNA.

B. Interaction with DNA in Intact Cells (DNA Damage and Repair)

The renaturation following rapid cooling of heat-denatured DNA extracted from mitomycin treated microorganisms was demonstrated by IYER and SZYBALSKI (1964), indicating that mitomycins cause crosslinks *in vivo*, as well as *in vitro*. Exposure of *B. subtilis* cells to *N*-methylmitomycin-^{14}C resulted in a binding of the antibiotic to intracellular DNA. Changes in the physicochemical properties of DNA, isolated from mitomycin treated cells, were reported by WHITE and WHITE (1965). IYER and SZYBALSKI (1964) studied the transforming activity of DNA, isolated from mitomycin treated *B. subtilis*. Even when the crosslinking was quite extensive, as much as 20% of the original transforming activity was still retained by the molecules. Furthermore, the biological activity of the linked DNA, unlike the activity of normal DNA, was not critically and abruptly destroyed over a narrow temperature range. This remarkable heat stability of DNA isolated from mitomycin treated cells indicates that residual transforming activity is primarily associated with the crosslinked DNA molecules. Prolonged exposure to mitomycin can result in a loss of all detectable transforming activity of the DNA (TERAWAKI and GREENBERG, 1966). The transforming activity of DNA from streptococci was also found to be depressed upon prolonged treatment of the cells with mitomycin C (TERESHIN, 1969).

It is now well established, that damage caused in DNA by x-irradiation, UV-irradiation, mono- or bifunctional alkylating agents, and mitomycin can be repaired. For a summary of available literature see SETLOW (1968), HOWARD-FLANDERS (1968), HANAWALT (1968), STRAUSS (1968), and RAUTH (1966). X-irradiation results in chemical changes of the pyrimidines. UV-irradiation leads to formation of covalently linked pyrimidine dimers, mainly thymine dimers (BEUKERS and BERENDS, 1960; WACKER, 1963). Damage by mono and bifunctional alkylating agents is mainly directed towards the N_7 of guanine, however, other bases or even the phosphate groups might be alkylated (FREESE, 1969).

The different types of damage can be repaired. One type of DNA repair involves the following steps: (1) the recognition of the damage by special recognition enzymes; (2) incision at the damaged locations by an endonuclease;

(3) the repair process itself which involves the action of three additional enzymes, an exonuclease to remove the damaged bases and contiguous nucleotides (excision), the DNA polymerase to replace the excised bases, and a ligase to join the newly synthesized strand with the old one.

If a single mechanism of repair were to operate for all types of lesions, then UV resistant mutants should also be resistant to monofunctional or difunctional alkylating agents or mitomycins. Several mutants that are sensitive to UV, mitomycin (Mahler, 1966), or alkylating agents have been isolated. Okubo and Romig (1966) presented experimental evidence suggesting that in one mutational step *B. subtilis* can acquire sensitivity to mitomycin and UV, and that this mutation impairs at least one reaction involved in the process of recombination. On the other hand, organisms exist that are unable to repair UV damages, but can repair lesions induced by alkylating agents or mitomycins (Boyce and Howard-Flanders, 1964; Kohn et al., 1965; Setlow and Carrier, 1966).

C. DNA Synthesis and Degradation

The selective inhibitory effect of mitomycin C on the synthesis of DNA was discovered first in *E. coli* by Shiba et al. (1958, 1959). Also, in higher organisms, including plant cells and tumor cells, mitomycins preferentially inhibit the synthesis of DNA (Reich and Franklin, 1961; Albach and Shaffer, 1967; Reimer and Yoshida, 1968). The effect of mitomycin on DNA synthesis in virus host systems will be discussed extensively in a following section.

Mitomycin C has become an important tool for inhibiting the synthesis of DNA and studying the processes that depend on DNA synthesis. The inhibitory effect of mitomycin on DNA synthesis appears to be a consequence of the crosslinking effect of mitomycin which prevents the separation of the two strands of DNA during the replication process (Szybalski and Iyer, 1964a). Another potent inhibitor of DNA synthesis is streptonigrin (Fig. 5), which resembles mitomycin C with respect to the aminobenzoquinone ring.

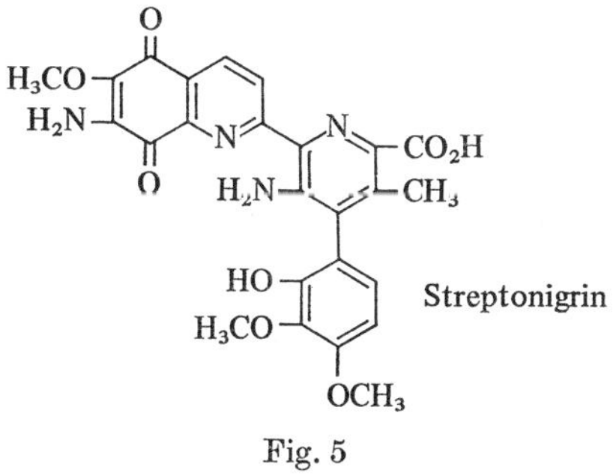

Streptonigrin

Fig. 5

Streptonigrin does not form crosslinks, therefore, it is not yet clear whether crosslinkage or a streptonigrin analogous interaction of mitomycin with DNA, or both types of interaction are responsible for the inhibitory effect of mitomycins on the synthesis of DNA within intact cells.

In certain types of cells it is difficult to measure the inhibition of DNA synthesis, because mitomycins also induce DNA breakdown, so that concurrent depolymerization and synthesis can take place. A depolymerization of DNA in mitomycin treated microorganisms or mammalian cells has been observed (KERSTEN, 1962, a, b; SHATKIN et al., 1962; MATSUMOTO et al., 1966). The depolymerization of DNA in mitomycin exposed microorganisms depends on the concentration of magnesium ions in the culture medium (KERSTEN et al., 1963) and leads to the formation of mononucleotides and free bases (REICH et al., 1961; SHIIO et al., 1962). Little, if any, mitomycin induced DNA breakdown was noticed in other mammalian or bacterial cultures (MAGEE and MILLER, 1962; IYER and SZYBALSKI, 1963; BOYCE and HOWARD-FLANDERS, 1964; ALBACH and SHAFFER, 1969). The depolymerization of DNA in mitomycin exposed cells is most probably dependent on the capacity of these cells to repair DNA, i.e. the activity and amount of repair enzymes. *E. coli uvr*-mutants, hypersensitive to mitomycins, do not show significant breakdown of DNA at bacteriocidal concentrations of the antibiotic, whereas in mitomycin-resistant *uvr*$^{+}$ mutants, DNA becomes partially degraded. The excision-repair accompanied degradation of DNA is enhanced by chlor amphenicol, indicating that only DNA degradation (excision) can occur in the absence of protein synthesis, but not the subsequent steps of the repair process, i.e. "DNA synthesis" (PAPIRMEISTER and DAVISON, 1964). This could explain the findings of KERSTEN and KERSTEN (1963) and CONSTANTOPOULOS and TCHEN (1964), that the mitomycin induced breakdown of DNA in the resistant line of *E. coli* B is markedly enhanced by chloramphenicol.

Different nucleases are involved in the initial stages of repair. In bacterial extracts nucleases have been found with specificity for alkylation or mitomycin induced damages (STRAUSS and RUBBINS, 1968). An increase in the activity of DNA degrading enzymes in mitomycin treated microorganisms was observed by NAKATA et al. (1962), KERSTEN and KERSTEN (1963), KERSTEN et al. (1964) and LEOPOLD et al. (1965). Elevation of deoxyribonuclease activities also occurs in mammalian cells (NIITANI et al., 1964). STUDZINSKI and COHEN (1966) and STUDZINSKI et al. (1966) have found mitomycin induced increases in the activities of acid DNAase and alkaline DNAase in HeLa cells. Enzyme systems capable of repairing DNA have been shown to be operative in HeLa cells, as well as in microorganisms (RASMUSSEN and PAINTER, 1966). It seems plausible that the increased activities of DNAases in mitomycin treated HeLa cells are related to repair processes.

D. RNA Metabolism

The mitomycins not only interfere with DNA and DNA metabolism, but also affect RNA metabolism. SMITH-KIELLAND (1966a, b) has reported on the effect of mitomycins on RNA synthesis in a wild strain of *E. coli* under conditions which completely arrested the synthesis of DNA. An increased rate of total RNA synthesis was found during the first thirty minutes after the addition of the inhibitor, the result of increased synthesis of soluble RNA. No concomitant increase in ribosomal RNA synthesis occurred. Upon exposure of the cell cultures to the drug for longer periods, the rate of soluble RNA synthesis also decreased. Furthermore, total RNA became degraded. Messenger RNAs, labeled with 2-^{14}C-uracil after pulses of 15 or 30 seconds, were less efficient in forming hybrids with denatured DNA, compared with control messenger RNA. The mechanism by which mitomycin causes an increased rate of RNA synthesis is unexplained.

On prolonged treatment of *E. coli* with mitomycin C, ribosomes, ribosomal RNA, and tRNA become degraded (KERSTEN and KERSTEN, 1963; KERSTEN et al., 1964; LEOPOLD et al., 1965). Besides a degradation of ribosomes, SUZUKI and KILGORE (1964) observed a reduced rate of ribosomal RNA synthesis upon mitomycin treatment of *E. coli*. Simultaneous synthesis and degradation, i.e. a rapid turnover of RNA, occurs in the presence of mitomycin, as described by KATO et al. (1969), under conditions where DNA remained unaffected during the treatment. These authors present evidence to suggest that RNAase I does not participate in this degradation of ribosomes. In a mutant strain of *Alcaligenes faecalis*, not containing RNAase I, RNA and ribosomes were also degraded (NATORI et al., 1967). Thus, it does not seem probable that RNAase I participates in the degradation of RNA, though increased overall RNAase activity in cell extracts from mitomycin treated *E. coli* has been found (KERSTEN and KERSTEN, 1969).

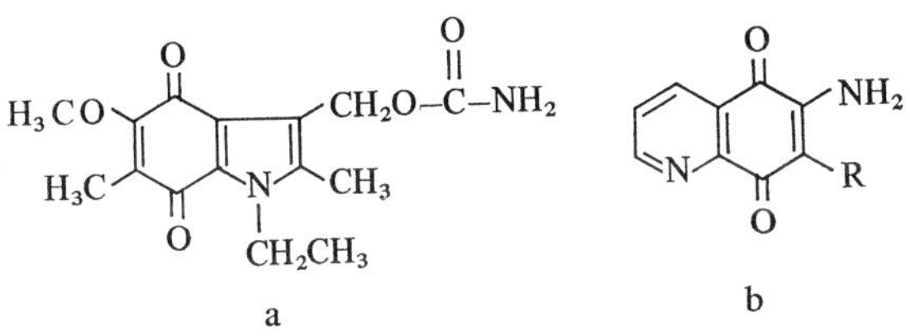

Fig. 6. (a) Mitomycin derivative not containing the aziridine ring, (b) Synthetic quinone (Bayer)

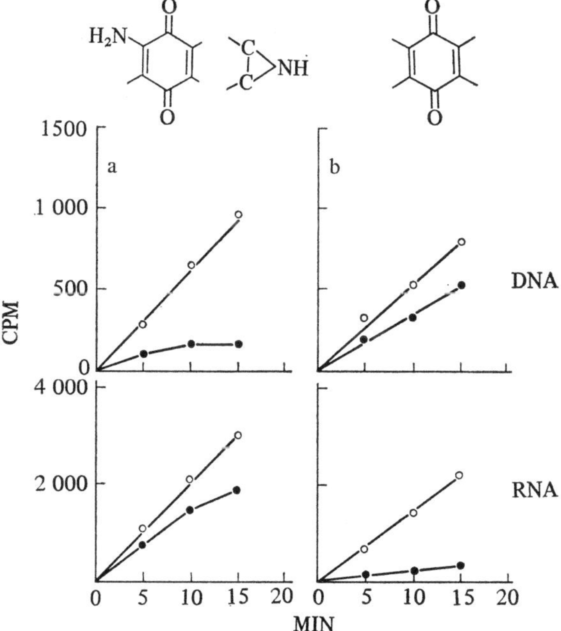

Fig. 7. Inhibition of DNA and RNA synthesis in *B. subtilis* by a mitomycin derivative containing the aziridine ring (a) and a synthetic quinone (b). ○—○, Control; •—•, Treated

The inhibitory effect of mitomycins on the synthesis of RNA has been postulated by KERSTEN and KERSTEN (1969) to involve the quinone ring, since mitomycin derivatives not containing the alkylating aziridine group, and synthetic quinones (see Fig. 6), have been found to inhibit immediately and reversibly the synthesis of RNA in microorganisms (Fig. 7).

The inhibitory effect of quinones on the synthesis of RNA can be reversed totally by a mixture of amino acids (cysteine omitted). OGILVIE et al. (1972) observed that quinones interfere with the control of RNA synthesis by amino acids. This control has been shown to operate in both prokaryotes (for summary see Cold Spring Harbour Symposium on Quantitative Biology **35**, 1970) and eukaryotes (WANNEMACHER et al., 1971).

E. Synthesis of Enzymes

Mitomycins inhibit the synthesis of induced enzymes (CHEER and TCHEN, 1962, 1963; CUMMINGS, 1965; COLES and GROSS, 1965; KIT et al., 1963; SHIBA et al., 1958; TAKAGI, 1963). This inhibitory effect of mitomycins on the induced synthesis of penicillinase, for example, occurs at concentrations of drug, and at a time following inhibition of the synthesis of DNA, when RNA synthesis is arrested. According to BASU et al. (1965), it seems likely that the inhibition of induced β-galactosidase synthesis by mitomycin C is a case of enhanced catabolite repression, which has often been observed to be associated with nonspecific nuclear damage to cells (MCFALL, 1961). Since catabolite repression of β-galactosidase synthesis appears to take place through inhibition of the transcription of the lac-gene, the effect of mitomycin on the rate of β-galactosidase messenger RNA synthesis is followed by a decrease in enzyme synthesis. Mitomycin causes appreciable reduction of the transcription of the lac-gene in the presence of glycerol, but stimulates the transcription nearly twofold in its absence.

Mitomycin activates thymidine kinase in two day old human embryonic lung cells in culture. Additional treatment with an inhibitor of protein synthesis such as puromycin, in combination with mitomycin, prevents the elevation of thymidine kinase activity. This indicates that mitomycin in some way induces the synthesis of this enzyme (ROSS and SOLYMOSI, 1967).

LERMAN and BENYUMOVICH (1965) studied the effect of mitomycin C on overall protein synthesis in human neoplastic cell lines. These authors found a rapid inhibition of protein synthesis following addition of mitomycin which was comparable to that obtained with puromycin. No other reports exist, however, which indicate that mitomycin preferentially acts on protein synthesis.

Biological Effects of Mitomycins Related to Molecular Mechanism of Action

This section is concerned with the question as to whether it is possible to explain the biological effects exhibited by mitomycin antibiotics on the basis of their actions on DNA, RNA, or protein metabolism.

A. Mutagenicity

The mitomycins are mutagenic for bacteria (SZYBALSKI, 1958; IIJIMA and HAGAWARA, 1960; TSUKAMURA and TSUKAMURA, 1962). The mutagenic effect of the mitomycins can easily be explained by a direct interaction with cellular DNA. The precise nature of the damage to DNA responsible for the mutagenic effect remains to be determined.

B. Chromosome Breakage

Mitomycins frequently produce cytologically detectable "translocation-like" cross configurations in dividing leucocytes (COHEN and SHAW, 1964). Similar results were obtained by NOWELL (1964) following treatment of leucocyte cultures with mitomycin. From the cytological data, SHAW and COHEN (1965) suggested that a process analogous to somatic crossing-over, as well as reciprocal translocations between nonhomologous autosomes, can be induced by mitomycin. A cytogenic effect of mitomycin C on chromosomes in cultured human cells was described by SINKUS (1969). Mitomycins cause mitotic inhibition and chromosome damage, involving chromosomes 1, 9, and 16 in the paracentromeric region of the long arms. GERMAN and LAROCK (1969) also have described the effects of the mitomycins on chromosomes and stated that these antibiotics are potential recombinogens in mammalian cell genetics. Mitomycins also produce localized chromosome breaks in plants in the heterochromatin segments of *Vicia* root cells (ARORA et al., 1969).

The stimulation of chromosomal exchanges and crossing-over and the increased rate of genetic recombination observed in mitomycin treated organisms favor the hypothesis that the biological effects of mitomycins on chromosomes involve DNA specific enzymes and are probably not caused by random alkylation of bases or crosslinks in the DNA molecule. Fragmentation of chromosomes is most probably the result of enzymatic DNA breakdown.

C. Viruses, Phage, and Episomal DNA

Mitomycins induce lysogenic phage (KORN and WEISSBACH, 1962; LEIN et al., 1962; LEVINE, 1961; OTSUJI, 1961, 1962). *E. coli* K_{12} (λ) lyse upon treatment with mitomycin within 90 minutes with optimal production of phage particles.

Various phage inducing agents, like UV light, cause damage to DNA. The development of phage stops when the damaged DNA is repaired by the excision repair mechanism. TAKENO (1968) reported that mitomycin induced phage formation and lysis of cells can be suppressed when *E. coli* K_{12} (λ) cells are exposed to light. The mechanism of this photosuppression of mitomycin induced λ phage development is the result of DNA repair by the photo-activated enzyme.

B. subtilis 168 and related strains have been reported to carry defective phage referred to as PBSX by SEAMAN et al. (1964), phage μ by IONESCO et al. (1964), and "phage-like particles" by STICKLER et al. (1965). For the purposes of this chapter the term "phage-like particles" will be used. No bacterial strain has been found to support the growth of these particles, although the particles kill certain sensitive *B. subtilis* strains. Thus, these particles seem to share properties of both bacteriocines and temperate phages. The "phage-like particles" can be induced in the absence of DNA synthesis, suggesting that the majority of DNA in the phage particles originates from the bacterial chromosomes (SEAMAN et al., 1964). OKAMOTO et al. (1968a, b) studied in more detail the "phage-like particles" obtained by mitomycin treatment of *B. subtilis*. The "particles" have been purified by sucrose gradient and cesium chloride density gradient centrifugations. They adsorb only to cells of sensitive strains, resulting in a killing pattern resembling a single-hit process. There is no detectable injection of DNA of the particles into the bacteria. The DNA within the phage heads has a high degree of size homogeneity with a sedimentation coefficient S^0_{20w} of 22. DNA-DNA hybridization and transformation experiments indicate that most, if not all, of the DNA in the "phage-like particles" is of bacterial origin.

These results clearly show that, after induction with mitomycin, bacterial DNA is degraded, converted into fragments of homogeneous size, and wrapped into coat proteins. As much as 50% of the prelabeled bacterial DNA can be incorporated into the "phage-like particles" (OKAMOTO, 1968b).

The fact that chloramphenicol inhibits the appearance of $22S$ DNA indicates that, for the specific breakdown of DNA, the synthesis of some protein is necessary. Evidence has been presented that synthesis of this specific protein starts between 30 and 40 minutes after the addition of mitomycin. The formation of the "phage-like particles" can be explained by the induction of a specific DNA degrading enzyme by mitomycin. The enzyme responsible for the conversion of host DNA to $22S$ DNA remains to be identified and characterized.

As early as 1957 FREDERICO (1957) recognized the similarities between colicinogenic factors and lysogenic phage, and suggested that the process of colicin induction involved a vegetative multiplication of colicinogenic factors. DE WITT and HELSINKI (1965) presented experimental evidence which showed that the colicinogenic factor E_1 (col E_1) from *E. coli* is a satellite DNA which increases in amount under conditions of induction by mitomycin C. Furthermore, a rough proportionality exists between the magnitude of the increase in col E_1 and colicin production. The striking analogy between the induction of replication of col E_1 and the induced multiplication of bacteriophage favors the view that the increased production of colicin E_1 is at least partly due to an increase in copies of the genetic determinants of col E_1.

Colicinogenic factors are autonomous DNAs. The replication of this DNA conceivably can start immediately upon inhibition of host cell DNA synthesis by mitomycin C. These results can be explained best by assuming a different sensitivity of viral or episomal DNA, as compared with host DNA, to mitomycin and mitomycin-induced DNA degrading enzymes.

Differential sensitivity to mitomycin of episomal DNA versus host DNA has been found; mitomycin inhibits the synthesis of both nuclear DNA and episomal DNA in an *E. coli* strain containing the sex factor F^+. The host cell DNA becomes degraded, whereas F^+ DNA is resistant to degradation (DRISKELL-ZAMENHOF and ADELBERG, 1963). Several virus/host systems have been described in which the sensitivity of host DNA and virus DNA differ (for summary see the review by SZYBALSKI and IYER, 1967). Thus, the inducing effect of mitomycin on the release of lysogenic phage, the production of "phage-like particles", and the formation of colicins is most probably related to the specific inhibitory effect of mitomycin on the synthesis of host DNA and the induction of specific host DNA degrading enzymes. In support of this view are the findings of LINDQVIST and SINSHEIMER (1966) who observed selective inhibition of host DNA synthesis in mitomycin treated repair-deficient hcr^- *E. coli* mutants without inhibition by this agent of the synthesis of viral DNA ($\Phi \times 174$).

Some RNA viruses containing single-stranded RNA can be produced in the presence of mitomycin (REICH and FRANKLIN, 1961; COOPER and ZINDER, 1962; KNOLLE and KAUDEWITZ, 1964). ROTT et al. (1965) showed that mitomycin inhibits the growth of the double-stranded RNA of fowl plague myxovirus and VIGIER and GOLDE (1964a, b) found the RNA Rous sarcoma virus to be sensitive to mitomycin.

The inhibitory action of mitomycins on RNA viruses either depends on a direct effect of the mitomycins on viral RNA synthesis or may be due to rapid degradation as a consequence of the induction of ribonuclease. If the virus RNA is replicated by the intermediate formation of an RNA-like DNA by an RNA-dependent DNA polymerase (TEMIN and MIZUTANI 1970), mitomycin could theoretically effect viral RNA synthesis by interacting with the intermediate DNA.

D. Mitosis

That certain chemicals have different toxicities with respect to various stages of the cell division cycle, has been observed in several types of mammalian cells in culture, for vinblastine by BRUCHOVSKY et al. (1965), for hydroxyurea by SINCLAIR (1965), and for 5-bromodeoxyuridine by KIM et al. (1967). During the division cycle, HeLa cells were found to be most susceptible to mitomycin during the G_1 phase, whereas their sensitivity to actinomycin D was most pronounced in the S phase. Though a good correlation exists between crosslinking and the lethal action of mitomycin C in bacteria, very little crosslinking was found in DNA isolated from mammalian cell lines (DJORDJEVIC and KIM, 1968).

PARKIN and CHIGA (1966) investigated the effect of mitomycin on hepatic regeneration. It was found that under certain experimental conditions, mitomycin allowed DNA synthesis to take place in rat liver after partial hepatectomy, but blocked mitosis completely. The inhibition of mitosis by mitomycin C is thus not mediated by an inhibitory effect on DNA synthesis.

The precise mechanisms involved in the process of mitosis are not yet known. Therefore, the mechanism by which several antibiotics interfere with mitosis cannot be explained. It has been postulated that the cell membrane is the key structural component involved in the initiation of cell division. Some authors speculate that mitomycin may alkylate membranes or other cytoplasmic components involved in mitosis (SZYBALSKI, 1964; DJORDJEVIC and KIM, 1968; GRULA et al., 1968). An interesting observation in this regard was described by STEIN and ROTHSTEIN (1968) who reported that mitomycin blocks mitosis in cultured frog lens tissue, even when the drug was added to the system after peak DNA synthesis. The authors suggested that the mitotic inhibition produced by the antibiotic may be due to an effect on the synthesis of RNA.

E. Immunological Aspects

Many agents clinically useful in the treatment of cancer possess immunosuppressive activity. The action of mitomycin on DNA synthesis and thus cellular proliferation would account for its bone marrow depressive activity and would additionally suggest immunosuppressive activity. It has been shown conclusively by SAKUCHI and DE WITT (1967) that mitomycin inhibits antibody production when given in minute doses at the time of antigenic stimulation, but not when given at the height of the immune response. These observations confirm the absence of any direct mitomycin action on the production of protein. LEMMEL and GOOD (1969) studied the tolerance of cell mediated immunoresponse after *in vitro* treatment of competent cells with mitomycin C. Their findings indicate that *in vitro* treatment of lymphoid cells with mitomycin C prevents graft-versus-host reactivity, as tested by injection into appropriate recipients. The treated cells seemed to survive *in vivo*, however, and to maintain cellular reactivity towards partial antigens as detected by appropriate transfer studies. The findings indicate that mitomycin can induce a temporary blockage of certain cellular activities in treated cell populations which permits recovery of at least some of the injected cells and the development by these cells of a specific tolerance toward the recipient antigens. In accordance with the immunosuppressive action of mitomycin is the observation (VINCENT et al., 1967) that mitomycin causes a decrease in total globulin without significant changes in serum albumin or in total protein.

References

Albach, H. R., Shaffer, J. G.: Effect of mitomycin C metabolism on thymidine-methyl-H^3 utilization by Entamoeba histolytica in CLG medium. J. Protozool. **14**, 60a (1967).

Arora, O. P., Shah, V. C., Rao, S. R. V.: Studies on micronuclei induced by mitomycin C in the root cells of Vicia faba. Exp. cell Res. **56**, 443—448 (1969).

Basu, S. K., Chakrabarty, A. M., Roy, S. C.: Enhancement of catabolite repression by mitomycin C in the induced-synthesis of β-galactosidase. Biochim. biophys. Acta. (Amst.) **108**, 713—716 (1965).

Beukers, R., Berends, A.: Isolation and identification of the irradiation product of thymine. Biochim. biophys. Acta (Amst.) **41**, 550—551 (1960).

Boyce, R. P., Howard-Flanders, P.: Genetic control of DNA breakdown and repair in *E. coli* K-12 treated with mitomycin C or ultraviolet light. Z. Vererbungslehre **95**, 345—350 (1964).

Bruchovsky, N., Owen, A. A., Becher, A. J., Till, J. E.: Effects of vinblastine on the proliferative capacity of L cells and their progress through the division cycle. Cancer Res. **25**, 1232—1237 (1965).

Carter, S. K.: Mitomycin C. Cancer Chemother. Rep. **1**, 99 (1968).

Cheer, S., Tchen, T. T.: Effect of mitomycin C on the synthesis of induced β-galactosidase in *E. coli*. Biochem. biophys. Res. Com. **9**, 271—274 (1962).

Cheer, S., Tchen, T. T.: Effect of mitomycin C on induced enzyme synthesis in *E. coli*. Bacteriol. Proc. **6**, 38 (1963).

Cohen, M. M., Shaw, M. W.: Effects of mitomycin C on human chromosomes. J. cell Biol. **23**, 386—395 (1964).

Coles, N. W., Gross, R.: The effect of mitomycin C on the induced synthesis of penicillinase in Staphylococcus aureus. Biochem. biophys. Res. Com. **20**, 366—371 (1965).

Constantopoulos, G., Tchen, T. T.: Enhancement of mitomycin C induced breakdown of DNA by inhibitors of protein synthesis. Biochem. biophys. Acta (Amst.) **80**, 456—462 (1964).

Cooper, S., Zinder, N. D.: The growth of an RNA bacteriophage: the role of DNA synthesis. Virology 18, 405—411 (1962).

Cummings, D. J.: Macromolecular synthesis during synchronous growth of *E. coli B/r*. Biochim. biophys. Acta (Amst.) **85**, 341—350 (1965).

DeBoer, D., Dietz, A., Lummis, N. E., Savage, G. M.: Porfiromycin, a new antibiotic. I. Discovery and biological activities. Antimicrob. Agents Annual 1960, pp. 17—22. New York: Plenum Press 1961.

DeWitt, W., Helsinki, D. R.: Characterization of colicinogenic factor E_1 from a non-induced and a mitomycin C-induced Proteus strain. J. molec. Biol. **13**, 692—703 (1965).

Djordjevic, B., Kim, J. H.: Different lethal effects of mitomycin C and actinomycin D during the division cycle of HeLa cells. J. cell Biol. **38**, 477 (1968).

Driskell-Zamenhof, P. J., Adelberg, E. A.: Studies on the chemical nature and size of sex factors of *E. coli* K_{12}. J. molec. Biol. **6**, 483—497 (1963).

Federicq, P.: Colicins. Ann. Rev. Microbiol. **11**, 7—22 (1957).

Freese, E.: Hereditary DNA alterations. Angew. Chemie Int. Ed. 8, 12—20 (1969).

German, J., LaRock, J.: Chromosomal effects of mitomycin, a potential recombinogen in mammalian cell genetics. Texas Rep. biol. Med. **27**, 409—418 (1969).

Gribnau, A. G. M., Veldstra, H.: The influence of mitomycin C on the induction of crown-gall-tumors. FEBS Let. **3**, 115—117 (1969).

Grula, E. A., Smith, G. L., Grula, M.: Cell division in Erwinia: inhibition of nuclear body division in filaments grown in penicillin or mitomycin C. Science **161**, 164 (1968).

Hanawalt, P. C.: Cellular recovery from photochemical damage. In: Giese, A. C. (Ed.): Photophysiology, Vol. 4, p. 203. New York: Academic Press 1968.

Hata, T., Nomura, S., Umesawa, I.: Antitumor activity of antibiotic G-253. Antimicr. Agents and Chemother. *S* **543** (1966).

Hata, T., Sano, Y., Sugawara, R., Matsuma, A., Kanamori, K., Shima, T., Hoshi, T.: Mitomycin, a new antibiotic from streptomyces. J. Antibiot. (Tokyo) **9**, 141 (1956).

Higuchi, M., Goto, K., Fujimoto, M., Namiki, O., Kiguchi, G.: Effect of inhibitors of nucleic acid and protein synthesis on the induced synthesis of bacteriochlorophyll and δ-aminolevulinic acid synthetase by *Rhodopseudomonas spheroides*. Biochim. biophys. Acta (Amst.) **95**, 94—110 (1965).

Howard-Flanders, P.: DNA repair. Ann. Rev. Biochem. **37**, 175—200 (1968).

Iijima, T., Hagawara, A.: Mutagenic action of mitomycin C on *E. coli*. Nature (Lond.) **185**, 395—396 (1960).

IONESCO, M., RYTER, A., SCHAEFFER, P.: Sur une bactériophage hérbérge par la souche marburg de *bacillus subtilis*. Ann. Inst. Pasteur **107**, 764—776 (1964).

IYER, V. N., SZYBALSKI, W.: A molecular mechanism of mitomycin action: linking of complementary DNA strands. Proc. nat. Acad. Sci. (Wash.) **50**, 355—362 (1963).

IYER, V. N., SZYBALSKI, W.: Mitomycins and porfiromycins: chemical mechanism of activation and cross-linking of DNA. Science **145**, 55—58 (1964).

KATO, N., OKABAYASHI, K., MIZUNO, H.: The degradation of ribosomal RNA in *E. coli* by mitomycin C and AF-5, preferential inhibitors of DNA synthesis. J. Biochem. **67**, 175—184 (1970).

KERSTEN, H.: Action of mitomycin C on nucleic acid metabolism in tumor and bacterial cells. Biochim. biophys. Acta (Amst.) **55**, 558—560 (1962a).

KERSTEN, H.: Zur Wirkungsweise von Mitomycin C. I. Einfluß von Mitomycin C auf den Desoxyribonucleinsäure-Abbau in ruhenden Bakterien. Hoppe-Seyler's Z. physiol. Chemie **329**, 31—39 (1962b).

KERSTEN, H., KERSTEN, W.: Zur Wirkungsweise von Mitomycin C. II. Einfluß von Mitomycin, Chloramphenicol and Mg^{2+} auf den RNA- und DNA-Stoffwechsel in Bakterien. Hoppe-Seyler's Z. physiol. Chemie **334**, 141—153 (1963).

KERSTEN, H., KERSTEN, W.: Inhibitors acting on DNA and their use to study DNA replication and repair. In: BÜCHER, T., SIES, H. (Eds.): Inhibitor tools in cell research, p. 11. Berlin-Heidelberg-New York: Springer 1969.

KERSTEN, H., KERSTEN, W., LEOPOLD, G., SCHNIEDERS, B.: Effect of mitomycin C on DNAase and RNA in *E. coli*. Biochim. biophys. Acta (Amst.) **80**, 521—523 (1964).

KIM, J. H., GELBARD, A. S., PEREZ, A. G., EIDINOFF, M. L.: Effect of 5-bromo-deoxyuridine on nucleic acid and protein synthesis and viability in HeLa cells. Biochim. biophys. Acta (Amst.) **134**, 388—394 (1967).

KIT, S., PIEKARSKI, J. L., DUBBS, D. R.: Effects of 5-fluorouracil, actinomycin D and mitomycin C on the induction of thymidine kinase by vaccinia-infected L-cells. J. molec. Biol. **7**, 497—510 (1963).

KNOLLE, P., KAUDEWITZ, F.: Degree of host control on RNA production of an RNA phage. Abstracts, VI Internat. Congr. Biochem. **3**, 234 (1964).

KODOMA, M.: The interaction of mitomycin C with deoxyribonucleic acid in vitro. J. Biochem. (Tokyo) **61**, 162—167 (1967).

KOHN, K. W., STEIGBIGEL, N. H., SPEARS, C. L.: Crosslinking and repair of DNA in sensitive and resistant strains of *E. coli* treated with nitrogen mustard. Proc. nat. Acad. Sci. (Wash.) **53**, 1154—1161 (1965).

KORN, D., WEISSBACH, A.: Thymineless induction in *E. coli* $K_{12}\lambda$. Biochim. biophys. Acta (Amst.) **61**, 775—790 (1962).

LAWLEY, P. D., BROOKES, P.: Further studies on the alkylation of nucleic acids and the constituent nucleotides. Biochem. J. **89**, 127—138 (1963).

LAWLEY, P. D., BROOKES, P.: Interstrand cross-linking of DNA by difunctional alkylating agents. J. molec. Biol. **25**, 143—160 (1967).

LEIN, J., HEINEMANN, B., GOUREVITCH, A.: Induction of lysogenic bacteria as a method of detecting potential antitumor agents. Nature (Lond.) **196**, 783—784 (1962).

LEMMEL, E. M., GOOD, R. A.: Tolerance of cell mediated immune responses after in vitro treatment of competent cells with mitomycin C. Nature (Lond.) **221**, 1164—1165 (1969).

LEOPOLD, G., SCHNIEDERS, B., KERSTEN, H., KERSTEN, W.: The effect of mitomycin C on ribosomes and soluble ribonucleic acid in *Escherichia coli*. Biochemische Zeitschrift **343**, 423—432 (1965).

LERMAN, M. I., BENYUMOVICH, M. S.: Effect of mitomycin C on protein synthesis in human neoplastic cell lines. Nature (Lond.) **206**, 1231—1232 (1965).

LEVINE, M.: Effect of mitomycin C on interactions between temperate phages and bacteria. Virology **13**, 493—499 (1961).

LINDQVIST, B., SINSHEIMER, R. L.: The use of mitomycin C as a selective inhibitor of host DNA synthesis in ΦX 174-infected HCr^- cells. Fed. Proc. **25**, 651 (1966).

LIPSETT, M. N., WEISSBACH, A.: The site of alkylation of nucleic acids by mitomycin. Biochemistry **4**, 206—211 (1965).

MAGEE, W. E., MILLER, O. V.: Dissociation of the synthesis of host and viral deoxyribonucleic acid. Biochim. biophys. Acta (Amst.) **55**, 818—826 (1962).

MAHLER, I.: Effect of mitomycin C on five excision-repair mutants of *B. subtilis*. Biochem. biophys. Res. Com. **25**, 73—79 (1966).

MATSUNOTO, I., KOZAKA, M., TAKAGI, Y.: Analysis of the acid-soluble deoxyribosidic compounds accumulated in mitomycin C treated bacteria. J. Biochemistry (Tokyo) **60**, 653—659 (1966).

MCFALL, E.: Effects of ^{32}P decay on enzyme synthesis. J. molec. Biol. 3, 219—224 (1961).
MOORE, G. E.: Effects of mitomycin C in 346 patients with advanced cancer. Cancer Chemother. Rep. 52, 672—684 (1968).
MURAKAMI, H.: Electron aspects of the mode of action of the mitomycin molecule. J. Theor. Biol. 10, 236—250 (1966).
NAKATA, Y., NAKATA, K., SAKAMOTO, Y.: On the action mechanism of mitomycin C. Biochem. biophys. Res. Comm. 6, 339—343 (1962).
NATORI, S., HORIGUCHI, T., MIZUNO, D.: Absence of ribonuclease in *Alcaligenes faecalis* and a possible mechanism of RNA degradation in this bacterium. Biochem. biophys. Acta (Amst.) 134, 337—346 (1967).
NIITANI, H., SUZUKI, A., SHIMOYAMA, M., KIMURA, K.: Effect of mitomycin C injection on lysosomal enzymic activities of Yoshida ascites sarcoma. Gann 55, 447—449 (1964).
NOWELL, P. C.: Mitotic inhibition and chromosome damage by mitomycin in human leucocyte cultures. Exp. cell Res. 33, 445—449 (1964).
OGILVIE, A., KERSTEN, W., KERSTEN, H.: Involvement of the ⟨rel gene⟩ in the transient depression of stable RNA synthesis by quinones. Arch. int. Physiol. Biochim. 80, 611—612 (1972).
OKAMOTO, K., MUDD, J. A., MANGAN, J., HUANG, W. M., SUBBAIAH, T. V., MARMUR, J.: Properties of the defective phage of *B. subtilis*. J. molec. Biol. 34, 413—428 (1968a).
OKAMOTO, K., MUDD, J. A., MARMUR, J.: Conversion of *B. subtilis* DNA to phage DNA following mitomycin C induction. J. molec. Biol. 34, 429—437 (1968b).
OKUBO, S., ROMIG, W. R.: Impaired transformability of *B. subtilis* mutant sensitive to mitomycin C and ultraviolet radiation. J. molec. Biol. 15, 440—454 (1966).
OTSUJI, N.: The effect of glucose on the induction of lambda phage formation by mitomycin C. Biken's J. 4, 235—241 (1961).
OTSUJI, N.: DNA synthesis and lambda phage development in a lysogenic strain of *E. coli* K_{12}. Biken's J. 5, 9—19 (1962).
PAPIRMEISTER, B., DAVISON, C.: Unbalanced growth and latent killing of *E. coli* following exposure to sulfur mustard. Biochim. biophys. Acta (Amst.) 103, 70—92 (1965).
PARKIN, I. L., CHIGA, M.: Dissociation of DNA synthesis and mitosis by mitomycin C in regenerating rat liver. Fed. Proc. 25, 480 (1966).
PATRICK, J. B., WILLIAMS, R. P., MEYER, W. E., FULMOR, W., COSULICH, D. B., BROSCHARD, R. W., WEBB, J. S.: Aziridinomitosenes: a new class of antibiotics related to the mitomycins. J. Amer. chem. Soc. 86, 1889—1890 (1964).
RASMUSSEN, R. E., PAINTER, R. B.: Radiation stimulated DNA synthesis in cultured mammalian cells. J. cell. Biol. 29, 11—19 (1966).
RAUTH, A. M.: Evidence for the dark reactivation of mitomycin C anti-infection damage in mouse cells. Ned. Tijdschr. Geneesh. 110, 101 (1966).
REICH, E., FRANKLIN, R. M.: Effect of mitomycin C on the growth of some animal viruses. Proc. nat. Acad. Sci. (Wash.) 47, 1212—1217 (1961).
ROSS, V. C., SOLYMOSI, J.: Induction of thymidine kinase in L-132 cells: dependence of protein synthesis and time of mitomycin action. Fed. Proc. 26, 291 (1967).
ROTH, R. H., REMERS, W. A., WEISS, M. J.: The mitomycin antibiotics. Synthetic studies. XIII. Indoloquinone analogs with variation at C-5. J. org. Chem. 31, 1012—1015 (1966).
ROTT, R., SABER, S., SCHOLTISSEK, C.: Effect on myxovirus of mitomycin C, actinomycin D and pretreatment of the host cell with ultraviolet light. Nature (Lond.) 205, 1187—1190 (1965).
RUNNER, M. N., YOSHIDA, S.: Differential depression of DNA synthesis in the isolated embryo. Teratology 1, 221 (1968).
SAKUCHI, G., DEWITT, C. W.: Immunosuppressive activity of mitomycin C. Transplantation 5, 248—255 (1967).
SCHWARTZ, H. S., SODERGREN, J. E., PHILIPS, F. S.: Mitomycin C: chemical and biological studies on alkylation. Science 142, 1181—1183 (1963).
SEAMAN, E., TARMY, E., MARMUR, J.: Inducible phages of *B. subtilis*. Biochemistry 3, 607—613 (1964).
SETLOW, R. B.: The photochemistry, photobiology and repair of polynucleotides. Progr. Nucleic acid Res. 8, 257—295 (1968).
SETLOW, R. B., CARRIER, W.: Pyrimidine dimers in ultraviolet-irradiated DNAs. J. molec. Biol. 17, 237—254 (1966).
SHATKIN, A. H., REICH, E., FRANKLIN, R. M., TATUM, E. L.: Effect of mitomycin C on mammalian cells in culture. Biochim. biophys. Acta (Amst.) 55, 277—289 (1962).
SHAW, M. W., COHEN, M. M.: Chromosome exchanges in human leucocytes induced by mitomycin C. Genetics 51, 181—190 (1965).

SHIBA, S., TERAWAKI, A., TAGUCHI, T., KAWAMATA, J.: Studies on the effect of mitomycin C on nucleic acid metabolism in *E. coli* strain B. Biken's J. **1**, 179—193 (1958).

SHIIO, T., WEINBAUM, G., TAKAHASHI, H., MARUO, B.: Chromatographic analysis of nucleotidic compounds in *Bacillus subtilis*. J. gen. appl. Microbiol. 8, 178 (1962).

SINCLAIR, W. K.: Hydroxyurea: differential lethal effects on cultured mammalian cells during the cell cycle. Science **150**, 1729—1731 (1965).

SINKUS, A. G.: Effects of mitomycin C on chromosomes in the human cell culture. Tsitologiya **11**, 933 (1969).

SMITH-KIELLAND, I.: The effect of mitomycin C on deoxyribonucleic acid and messenger ribonucleic acid in *E. coli*. Biochim. biophys. Acta (Amst.) **114**, 254—263 (1966a).

SMITH-KIELLAND, I.: The effect of mitomycin C on ribonucleic acid synthesis in growing cultures of *E. coli*. Biochim. biophys. Acta (Amst.) **119**, 486—491 (1966b).

STEIN, G. S., ROTHSTEIN, H.: Mitomycin C may inhibit mitosis by reducing "G_2" RNA synthesis. Curr. Mod. Biology **2**, 254—263 (1968).

STICKLER, D. J., TUCHER, R. G., KAY, D.: Bacteriophage-like particles released from *Bacillus subtilis* after induction with hydrogen peroxide. Virology **26**, 142—145 (1965).

STRAUSS, B. S.: DNA repair mechanisms and their relation to mutation and recombination. Curr. Top. Microbiol. Immunol. **44**, 1—85 (1968).

STRAUSS, B. S., RUBBINS, M.: DNA methylated in vitro by a monofunctional alkylating agent as a substrate for a specific nuclease from *Micrococcus lysodeikticus*. Biochim. biophys. Acta (Amst.) **161**, 68—75 (1968).

STUDZINSKI, G. P., COHEN, L. S.: Mitomycin C induced increases in the activities of the deoxyribonucleases of HeLa cells. Biochem. biophys. Res. Commun. **23**, 506—512 (1966).

STUDZINSKI, G. P., COHEN, L. S., ROSEMAN, J., SCHWEITZER, L.: Elevation of deoxyribonuclease activities in HeLa cells treated with selective inhibitors of DNA synthesis. Biochem. biophys. Res. Comm. **25**, 313—319 (1966).

SUZUKI, H., KILGORE, W. W.: Mitomycin C: effect on ribosomes of *E. coli*. Science **146**, 1585—1587 (1964).

SZYBALSKI, W.: Special microbiological systems. II. Observation on chemical mutagenesis in microorganisms. Ann. N. Y. Acad. Sci. **76**, 475—489 (1958).

SZYBALSKI, W.: Chemical reactivity of chromosomal DNA as related to mutagenicity: studies with human cell lines. Cold Spring Harbor Symposia quant. Biol. **29**, 151—159 (1964).

SZYBALSKI, W., ARNESON, V. G.: Reductive activation and inactivation of mitomycin as studied with human and bacterial cell cultures. Molec. Pharmacol. **1**, 202—204 (1965).

SZYBALSKI, W., IYER, V. N.: Cross-linking of DNA by enzymatically or chemically activated mitomycins and porfiromycins, bifunctionally "alkylating" antibiotics. Fed. Proc. **23**, 946—951 (1964a).

SZYBALSKI, W., IYER, V. N.: Binding of C^{14}-labeled mitomycin or porfiromycin to nucleic acids. Microbial Genetics Bull. **21**, 16 (1964b).

SZYBALSKI, W., IYER, V. N.: The mitomycins and porfiromycins. In: Antibiotics, vol. I. (D. GOTTLIEB and P. D. SHAW, Eds.) Berlin-Heidelberg-New York: Springer 1967.

TAKAGI, Y.: Action of mitomycin C. Japan. J. med. Sci. Biol. **16**, 246—249 (1963).

TAKENO, T., NAGATA, T., MIZUNOYA, T.: Photosuppression of mitomycin-induced lambda-phage development. Nature (Lond.) **218**, 295—296 (1968).

TEMIN, H. A., MIZUTANI, S.: RNA-dependent DNA-polymerase in virions of Rous sarcoma virus. Nature (Lond.) **226**, 1211—1213 (1970).

TERAWAKI, A., GREENBERG, J.: Post-treatment breakage of mitomycin C induced cross-links in deoxyribonucleic acid of *E. coli*, Biochim. biophys. Acta (Amst.) **119**, 540—546 (1966).

TERESHIN, I. M.: On mechanism of action of mitomycin C on genetic transformation in hemolytic streptococci. Antibiotiki **9**, 796 (1969).

TOMASZ, M.: Novel assay of 7-alkylation of guanine residues in DNA application to nitrogen mustard, triethylenemelanine and mitomycin C. Biochim. biophys. Acta (Amst.) **213**, 288—295 (1970).

TSUKAMURA, M., TSUKAMURA, S.: Mutagenic effect of mitomycin C on Mycobacterium and its combined effect with ultraviolet irradiation. Japan. J. Microbiol. **6**, 53—58 (1962).

VIGIER, P., GOLDE, A.: Action de l'actinomycine D et de la mitomycine C sur le dévelopment du virus de Rous. Compt. Rend. Acad. Sci. **258**, 389—392 (1964a).

VIGIER, P., GOLDE, A.: Effects of actinomycin D and mitomycin C on development of Rous sarcoma virus. Virology **23**, 511—519 (1964b).

VINCENT, P. C., REEVE, T. S., BRITTLE, N., NICHOLIS, A., RICHARDS, M.: The effect of cytotoxic drugs on serum albumin in the rat. Aust. J. exp. biol. med. Sci. **45**, 427—435 (1967).

WACKER, A.: Molecular mechanisms of radiation effects. Progr. nucleic acid Res. molec. Biol. **1**, 369—399 (1963).

WAKAKI, S., MARUMO, H., TOMIOKA, K., SHIMIZU, G., KATO, E., KAMADA, H., KUDO, S., FUJIMOTO, Y.: Isolation of new fractions of antitumor mitomycins. Antibiot. and Chemother. 8, 228 (1958).

WANNEMACHER, R. W., WANNEMACHER, C. F., YATVIN, M. B.: Amino acid regulation of synthesis of ribonucleic acid and protein in the liver of rats. Biochem. J. **124**, 385—392 (1971).

WEBB, J. S., COSULICH, D. B., MOWAT, J. H., PATRICK, J. B., BROSCHARD, R. W., MEYER, W. E., WILLIAMS, R. P., WOLF, C. F., FULMOR, W., PIDACKS, C., LANCASTER, J. E.: The structures of mitomycin A, B and C, and porfiromycin. Part I. J. Amer. chem. Soc. **84**, 3185—3187 (1962).

WEISSBACH, A., LISIO, A.: Alkylation of nucleic acids by mitomycin C and porfiromycin. Biochemistry **4**, 196—200 (1965).

WHITE, H. L., WHITE, J. R.: The binding of porfiromycin to the deoxyribonucleic acid. J. Elisha Mitchell Sci. Soc. **81**, 37 (1965).

Chapter 35

Mechanism of Action of Nitrosoureas

GLYNN P. WHEELER

Introduction

The material that is presented in this chapter is limited to that which relates directly or indirectly to the mechanism of action of the nitrosoureas. For a review of the results of experimental and clinical therapeutic trials with these agents, the reader is referred to other sections of this volume and to the review by CARTER et al. (1972).

Many substituted *N*-nitrosoureas have been synthesized and tested for activity against L1210 leukemia implanted both intraperitoneally and intracerebrally (JOHNSTON et al., 1963, 1966, 1971; SCHABEL et al., 1963; JOHNSTON and OPLIGER, 1967). In general, the most active compounds in these two experimental systems were 1-(2-haloethyl)-1-nitrosoureas substituted in the 3 position by a 2-haloethyl, an alicyclic, or a heteroalicyclic group, the halogen atoms being either chlorine or fluorine (JOHNSTON et al., 1971), but 1-methyl-1-nitrosoureas were somewhat active (JOHNSTON et al., 1963). Therefore, this chapter concerns only synthetic nitrosoureas having a 2-haloethyl or a methyl group on *N*-1 and the antibiotic streptozotocin (VAVRA et al., 1959), which has structure I (HERR et al., 1967).

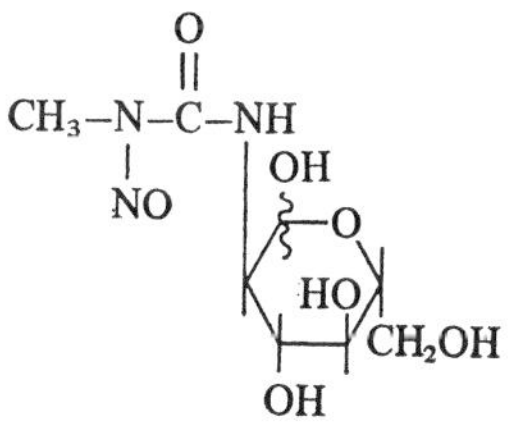

O
||
CH_3–N–C–NH
NO
OH
O
HO
CH_2OH
OH

(I)

Chemistry

N-Alkyl-*N*-nitrosoureas are unstable in aqueous media under physiological conditions of temperature and hydrogen ion concentration. The half-life of streptozotocin is about one hour at pH 7 and 37° (GARRETT, 1960), that of 1-methyl-1-nitrosourea is 32 min at pH 6.8 and 35° (GARRETT et al., 1965), and those of several 1-(2-haloethyl)-3-substituted-1-nitrosoureas are within the range of 20 to 200 min at 37° (LOO et al., 1966; MONTGOMERY et al., 1967; JOHNSTON, unpublished). The decomposition is catalyzed by the monohydrogen phosphate ion (GARRETT, 1965; MONTGOMERY et al., 1967), and in phosphate buffer the range for the half lives mentioned above is 20 to 68 min. Although thiols accelerate the rate of decomposition of the structurally and chemically similar 1-methyl-3-nitro-1-

nitrosoguanidine, MNNG (Lawley and Thatcher, 1970), cysteine does not accelerate the decomposition of 1-methyl-1-nitrosourea or three 1-(2-haloethyl)-3-alkyl-1-nitrosoureas (Wheeler and Bowdon, 1972).

McKay and Wright (1947) observed that, when an aqueous solution of MNNG and an alkyl or aryl amine was allowed to stand at or below room temperature, the major reaction product was a 1-alkyl (or aryl)-3-nitroguanidine and that MNNG served as a useful reagent for preparing such substituted nitroguanidines. Henry (1950) studied the reaction of MNNG with aniline and identified the products as 1-phenyl-3-nitroguanidine and *N*-methylaniline. Since this methylation occurred under conditions in which diazomethane does not methylate aniline, he suggested that methyl diazohydroxide might be an intermediate that could serve as a methylating agent. He also obtained an 87% yield of phenylurea and a 26% yield of *N*-methylaniline after allowing a mixture of 1-methyl-1-nitrosourea and excess aniline in 50% aqueous ethanol to stand at 10° for 60 h, and he assumed that the reactions occurring with 1-methyl-1-nitrosourea were analogous to those that occurred with MNNG. Garrett et al. (1965) suggested a scheme whereby 1,3-disubstituted-1-nitrosoureas might decompose to yield an isocyanate and a precursor of a diazoalkane. Montgomery et al. (1967) presented evidence

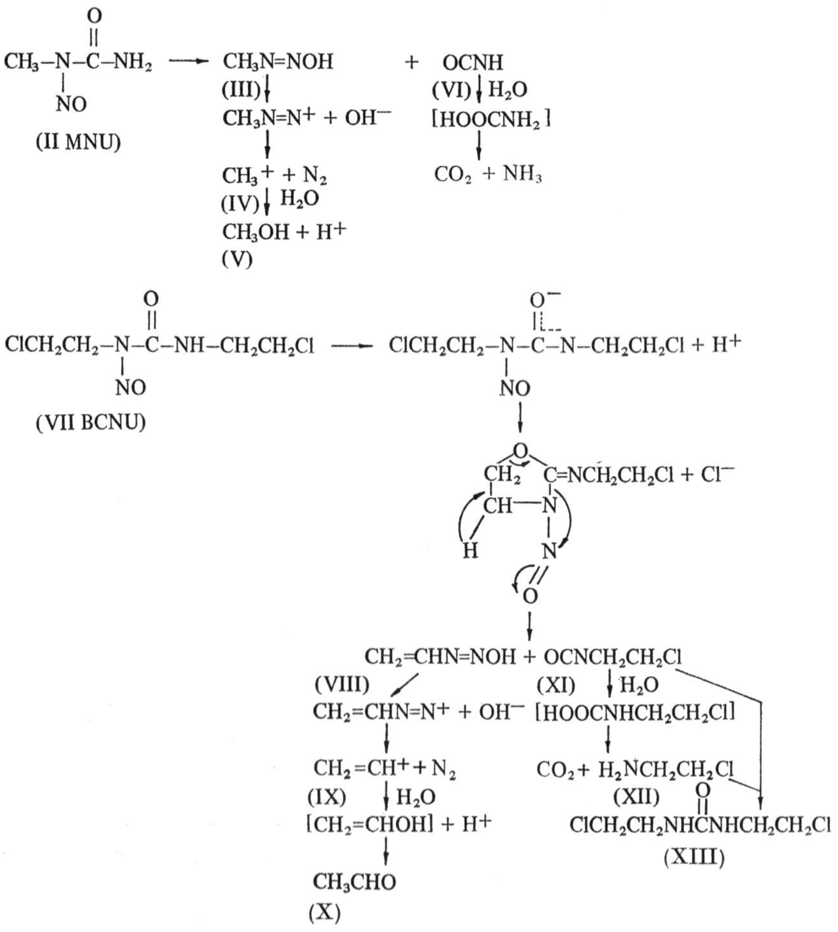

$CH_3{-}N(NO){-}C(=O){-}NH_2$ (II MNU) $\longrightarrow$ $CH_3N{=}NOH$ (III) + $OCNH$ (VI)

(III) $\downarrow$ $CH_3N{=}N^+ + OH^-$ $\downarrow$ $CH_3^+ + N_2$ (IV) $\downarrow H_2O$ $CH_3OH + H^+$ (V)

(VI) $\downarrow H_2O$ $[HOOCNH_2]$ $\downarrow$ $CO_2 + NH_3$

$ClCH_2CH_2{-}N(NO){-}C(=O){-}NH{-}CH_2CH_2Cl$ (VII BCNU) $\longrightarrow$ $ClCH_2CH_2{-}N(NO){-}C(O^-){=}N{-}CH_2CH_2Cl + H^+$

$\downarrow$

cyclic intermediate: CH_2–O–$C{=}NCH_2CH_2Cl$, $CH{-}N$, H, N=O $+ Cl^-$

$\downarrow$

$CH_2{=}CHN{=}NOH$ (VIII) + $OCNCH_2CH_2Cl$ (XI)

(VIII) $\downarrow$ $CH_2{=}CHN{=}N^+ + OH^-$ $\downarrow$ $CH_2{=}CH^+ + N_2$ (IX) $\downarrow H_2O$ $[CH_2{=}CHOH] + H^+$ $\downarrow$ CH_3CHO (X)

(XI) $\downarrow H_2O$ $[HOOCNHCH_2CH_2Cl]$ $\downarrow$ $CO_2 + H_2NCH_2CH_2Cl$ (XII)

(XI) + (XII) $\longrightarrow$ $ClCH_2CH_2NHC(=O)NHCH_2CH_2Cl$ (XIII) that supports the view that 1-alkyl-1-nitrosoureas decompose at physiological conditions to yield alkyl diazohydroxides, which are progenitors of carbonium ions, and isocyanic acid or alkyl isocyanates (if there is an alkyl group on N-3 of the nitrosourea), which can undergo further reactions. The specific substituents on *N*-1 and *N*-3 of the nitrosourea determine the mechanism of the decomposition in water and the chemical reactivities of the generated entities, and therefore these substituents may significantly influence the biological effects of the nitrosoureas. The following schemes (MONTGOMERY et al., 1967) show some of the differences for the decomposition and subsequent reactions in aqueous media for 1-methyl-1-nitrosourea (MNU; II), 1,3-*bis*(2-chloroethyl)-1-nitrosourea (BCNU; VII), 1-(2-chloroethyl)-3-cyclohexyl-1-nitrosourea (CCNU; XIV), and 1,3-*bis*(2-fluoroethyl)-1-nitrosourea (BFNU; XXI).

Each of these nitrosoureas decomposes to yield an alkyl diazohydroxide (III, VIII, XV, XXII) and isocyanic acid (VI) or an alkyl isocyanate (XI, XVIII, XXV), but the mode of generation of these compounds from MNU and BFNU differs from that of BCNU and CCNU. (The first three steps in the decomposition of CCNU are similar to those for BCNU.) The decomposition of MNU and BFNU occurs by the normal mechanism for substituted nitrosoureas, while BCNU and CCNU decompose by an abnormal mechanism. Neither of these mechanisms is a requisite for anticancer activity. It would be expected that the chemical reactivities of the methyl (IV), vinyl (IX and XVI), and 2-fluoroethyl (XXIII) carbonium ions would be different, and their reactions with water yield, respectively, methanol, acetaldehyde, and 2-fluoroethanol, which would be expected to produce different physiological effects. The isocyanic acid (VI) and the three isocyanates

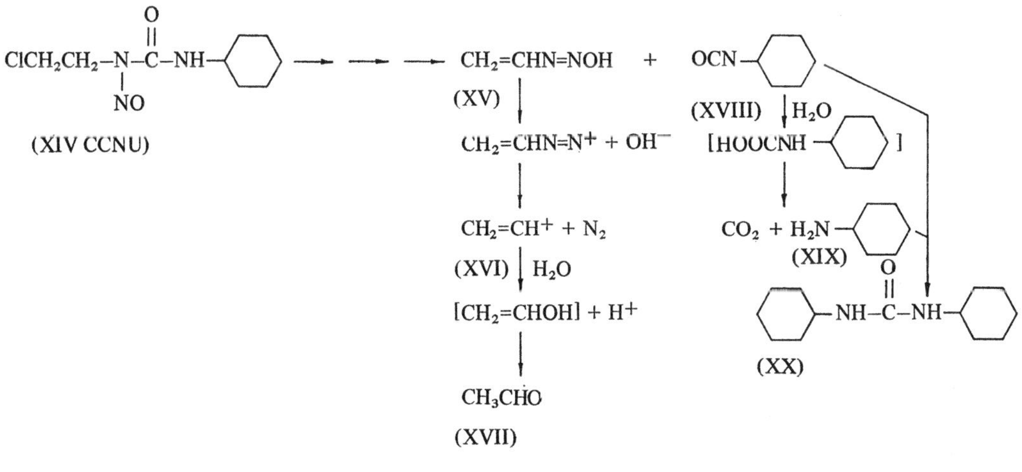

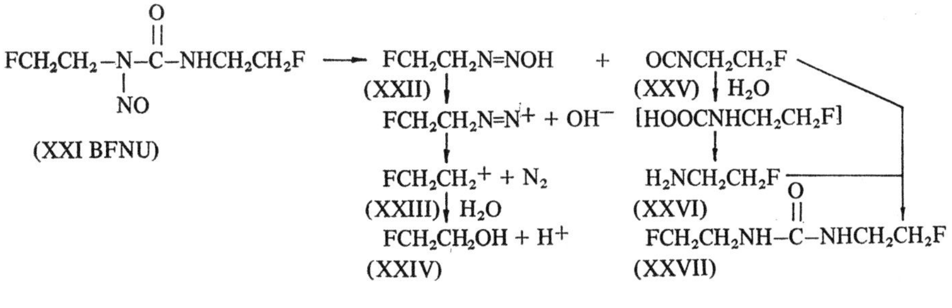

$ClCH_2CH_2{-}N(NO){-}C(=O){-}NH{-}C_6H_{11}$ (XIV CCNU) → → → $CH_2{=}CHN{=}NOH$ (XV) + $OCN{-}C_6H_{11}$ (XVIII)

(XV) → $CH_2{=}CHN{=}N^+ + OH^-$ → $CH_2{=}CH^+ + N_2$ (XVI) $\xrightarrow{H_2O}$ $[CH_2{=}CHOH] + H^+$ → CH_3CHO (XVII)

(XVIII) $\xrightarrow{H_2O}$ $[HOOCNH{-}C_6H_{11}]$ → $CO_2 + H_2N{-}C_6H_{11}$ (XIX); (XIX) + (XVIII) → $C_6H_{11}{-}NH{-}C(=O){-}NH{-}C_6H_{11}$ (XX)

$FCH_2CH_2{-}N(NO){-}C(=O){-}NHCH_2CH_2F$ (XXI BFNU) → $FCH_2CH_2N{=}NOH$ (XXII) + $OCNCH_2CH_2F$ (XXV)

(XXII) → $FCH_2CH_2N{=}N^+ + OH^-$ → $FCH_2CH_2^+ + N_2$ (XXIII) $\xrightarrow{H_2O}$ $FCH_2CH_2OH + H^+$ (XXIV)

(XXV) $\xrightarrow{H_2O}$ $[HOOCNHCH_2CH_2F]$ → $H_2NCH_2CH_2F$ (XXVI); (XXVI) + (XXV) → $FCH_2CH_2NH{-}C(=O){-}NHCH_2CH_2F$ (XXVII)

(XI, XVIII, and XXV) probably react with water at different rates to form the corresponding carbamic acids, which decompose to yield, respectively, ammonia, 2-chloroethylamine (XII), cyclohexylamine (XIX), or 2-fluoroethylamine (XXVI). If the initial concentrations of the nitrosoureas are high, these amines react with the respective newly generated isocyanates to yield the corresponding symmetrical ureas (XIII, XX, XXVII). At lower initial concentrations (probably analogous to therapeutic use in animals) the yield of the symmetrical ureas would probably be quite low.

The carbonium ions that are generated from the 1-alkyl-1-nitrosoureas can react with a number of chemical groups that occur in biological material to effect alkylation of those groups. It is for this reason that these agents are commonly considered to be alkylating agents. The 4-(*p*-nitrobenzyl) pyridine test has been used to compare the alkylating activities of MNU, BCNU, CCNU, and BFNU (Wheeler and Chumley, 1967). The reactivity of BCNU was much greater than those of MNU, CCNU, and BFNU, and the reactivities of these latter three compounds were about equal. (Although the published data show CCNU and BFNU to be more reactive than MNU, more recently obtained data show these compounds to be about equally reactive.) The greater reactivity of BCNU is due to the 2-chloroethylamine (XII) that is generated from it, as is evidenced by the fact that 2-chloroethyl isocyanate (XI) and 2-chloroethylamine (XII) yielded about as much color as BCNU in the tests. The 2-chloroethylamine might be considered to be a monofunctional nitrogen mustard that can function as an alkylating agent, perhaps with the intermediate formation of ethylenimine (Chan and Leh, 1966). The 2-fluoroethylamine (XXVI) might also be considered to be a monofunctional nitrogen mustard, but it is converted to ethylenimine much less readily than is 2-chloroethylamine (Levins and Papanastassiou, 1965), and its alkylating activity is much less than that of 2-chloroethylamine (Wheeler and Chumley, 1967). Since cyclohexylamine (XIX), which derives from CCNU, has no alkylating activity, the alkylating activity observed for CCNU must be due to the vinyl carbonium ion (XVI) derived from it. It is assumed that other 1-(2-chloroethyl)-3-alicyclic (or heteroalicyclic)-1-nitrosoureas decompose similarly to CCNU and that any observed alkylating activity observed for them would also be due to the generated vinyl carbonium ion. Since a number of 1-(2-chloroethyl)-3-alicyclic (or heteroalicyclic)-1-nitrosoureas are known to be active antileukemic agents against L 1210 leukemia (Schabel et al., 1963; Johnston et al., 1963, 1966, 1971; Johnston and Opliger, 1967), the supplemental alkylating activity that is specifically characteristic of BCNU is not essential for antineoplastic activity.

If the nitrosoureas decompose in the presence of biological materials, the isocyanic acid (VI) or isocyanates (e.g. XI, XVIII, XXV) might react with amino, sulfhydryl, or hydroxyl groups of the biological material to alter the functional abilities of such materials. Such reactions might occur extensively (see below), and it has been suggested that such reactions might account for the physiological effects of these agents to a significant extent (Wheeler, 1962; Montgomery et al., 1967; Bray et al., 1971; Cheng et al., 1972). Some preliminary evidence that 1-(2-chloroethyl)-1-nitrosoureas having various alicyclic substituents on N-3 yield significantly different isocyanate reactivities has been obtained (Wheeler and Bowdon, unpublished results).

It is evident from the facts presented above that the chemical properties of various 1-(2-haloethyl)-3-(substituted)-1-nitrosoureas might be quite different and that it is necessary to consider the properties of the individual compound in trying to define the reason for its biological effects.

Pharmacological Considerations

As would be expected from consideration of the chemical reactivities of the nitrosoureas, the biological half-lives of these agents are short. SCHEIN (1969a) observed that 5 min after the administration of MNU to mice at a dosage of 100 mg/kg, 85% of the dose could be accounted for in serum with a half-life of 25 min, and that 3.6% was in the liver with a half-life of 12 min. SWANN (1968) could not detect MNU in the blood of the rat 15 min after an intravenous dose of 100 mg/kg. The half-life of BCNU in the mouse (DE VITA et al., 1967), the plasma of the dog (LOO et al., 1966), and the cerebrospinal fluid of the dog (LOO et al., 1966; DE VITA et al., 1967), the monkey and human (DE VITA et al., 1967) was 15 min or less. However, SCHABEL (1970) reported that effective antineoplastic activity against intraperitoneally implanted leukemia L 1210 was evident 60 min following the intraperitoneal or oral administration of an LD_{10} dose of BCNU. OLIVERIO et al. (1970) observed that the degradation of CCNU in the plasma of the mouse and in the plasma and cerebrospinal fluid of the dog occurred in two exponential phases, the first indicating a half-life of 5 min and the second a half-life of more than 60 min.

Following the administration of ^{14}C-labeled BCNU or CCNU to mice, dogs, monkeys, and humans, most of the radioactivity was excreted in the urine as decomposition products or reaction products, while 6 to 20% was expired as carbon dioxide (LOO et al., 1966, DE VITA et al., 1967; OLIVERIO et al., 1970). Radioactivity from 1-[^{14}C]methyl-1-nitrosourea (KLEIHUES and PATZSCHKE, 1971), 1,3-*bis*(2-chloro[^{14}C]ethyl)-1-nitrosourea (WHEELER et al., 1964; DE VITA et al., 1967), 1,3-*bis*(2-chloroethyl)-1-nitroso[^{14}C]urea (WHEELER et al., 1964), 1-(2-chloro[^{14}C]ethyl)-3-cyclohexyl-1-nitrosourea, 1-(2-chloroethyl)-3-[^{14}C]cyclohexyl-1-nitrosourea, and 1-(2-chloroethyl)-3-cyclohexyl-1-nitroso[^{14}C]urea (OLIVERIO et al., 1970) was widely distributed among tissues, including brain and nerve tissue, of experimental animals within a few minutes following administration of the radioactive compound. Radioactivity was present in subcutaneous plasmacytomas of hamsters (WHEELER et al., 1964) and in subcutaneous and intracerebral gliomas of mice (LEVIN et al., 1970), and the quantities of radioactivity present were similar in the intracerebral tumors and the nontumorous portions of the brain. In most instances the ^{14}C-containing compounds present in the various tissues were not characterized or identified, but the observed activity of nitrosoureas against intracerebrally implanted neoplasms in animals (SCHABEL et al., 1963; ROSSO, 1967; SCHABEL, 1970; SHAPIRO et al., 1970) and brain tumors and other brain involved neoplasms in man (IRIARTE et al., 1966; WALKER and HURWITZ, 1970; WILSON et al., 1970; WALKER et al., 1971) indicates that the intact nitrosourea or an active material derived from it reached these neoplasms. Perhaps the ease with which these compounds can cross the "blood-brain barrier" results from their being uncharged and lipid-soluble (SCHABEL et al., 1963). The apparent ease of crossing this barrier and affecting neoplasms of the tissues of the nervous system places the nitrosoureas in a favored position relative to a number of other recognized anticancer agents.

Reactions with Biological Materials

A. Alkylation

The substituents on *N*-1 of the 1-alkyl-1-nitrosoureas are converted to carbonium ions, as shown in the above schemes, which can react with nucleophilic centers in molecules of biological interest to yield alkylated materials. Most of the experimental evidence for alkylation of molecules by the carbonium ions derived from nitrosoureas has been limited to reactions of MNU and 1-ethyl-1-nitrosourea (ENU), and little such evidence has been obtained with the more chemotherapeutically active compounds, such as BCNU and CCNU. This situation arises from the fact that the modes of action of MNU and ENU have been avidly investigated by workers who are primarily interested in mutagenesis and carcinogenesis, for which MNU and ENU are active agents. These investigations have also been concerned with the reactions of other compounds, including 1-methyl-3-nitro-1-nitrosoguanidine, dialkylnitrosamines, nitrosourethanes, and 1-aryl-3,3-dialkyltriazenes, which can give rise to alkyl diazohydroxides either by direct breakdown or by breakdown following enzymatic alteration (Druckrey et al., 1969; Preussman et al., 1969a; Magee, 1969; Lawley and Thatcher, 1970; Lingens et al., 1971). These alkyl diazohydroxides are identical or analogous to those derived from the nitrosoureas, and therefore it is of interest to consider here also the alkylations that have been observed in experiments with these agents. It is necessary, however, to be aware that the physiological effects of the various agents might be different because of their chemical and pharmacological properties and the necessity that some of them be enzymatically activated.

Incubation of DNA with MNU at approximate neutrality at 37° or below, and subsequent hydrolysis of the treated DNA yielded chiefly 7-methylguanine (Loveless and Hampton, 1969; Serebryanyi et al., 1969a; Wunderlich et al., 1970) with smaller quantities of 3-methyladenine and possibly 3(1)-methylcytosine (Loveless and Hampton, 1969); only 7-ethylguanine was detected when ENU was used instead of MNU (Loveless and Hampton, 1969). When deoxyguanosine was similarly incubated with MNU and with ENU and care was taken in hydrolyzing the treated deoxyguanosine, significant quantities of deoxy-(O-6)-methylguanosine and deoxy-(O-6)-ethylguanosine were detected (Loveless, 1969). After treatment of cultured cells with 1-[^{3}H]methyl-1-nitrosourea, there was as much, or more, ^{3}H associated with the RNA as with the DNA, and a smaller quantity associated with the protein; 7-methylguanine was isolated from the nucleic acids (Roberts et al., 1971a). 7-Methylguanine was also found in the DNA and RNA following the incubation of liver mitochondria with MNU and in the DNA following incubation of liver nuclei with MNU (Wunderlich et al., 1970). Following the administration of MNU to rats, the DNA and/or RNA of the liver, kidney, heart, lung, small intestine, large intestine, stomach, brain, and Walker carcinosarcoma contained 7-methylguanine (Swann and Magee, 1968; Krüger et al., 1968, 1970; Wunderlich et al., 1970). Although *in vivo* formation of 7-methylguanine of RNA occurred in brain, liver, and kidney of rats after the administration of MNU, no analogous alkylation was detected after the administration of ENU (Krüger et al., 1968). Wunderlich et al. (1970) observed that *in vivo* the alkylation of the mitochondrial DNA of liver occurred more extensively than the alkylation of the nuclear DNA.

Cheng et al. (1972) used 1-(2-chloro[^{14}C]ethyl)-3-cyclohexyl-1-nitrosourea to treat intact animals, suspended leukemia L 1210 cells, and dissolved nucleic acids and proteins, and observed that the ^{14}C became bound to the nucleic acids and proteins under all of these conditions.

Several investigators have studied alkylation of nucleic acids and related compounds by MNNG. Lingens et al. (1968) incubated mixtures of MNNG with free bases, ribonucleosides, ribonucleotides, and synthetic polyribonucleotides at pH 5.5 and room temperature or 37°; in each mixture the concentration of the MNNG was ten times that of the other compound. 1-Methyladenine and 3-methyladenine were obtained after incubation of MNNG with adenine, adenosine, AMP, and polyadenylic acid, and *N*-6-methyladenine also was obtained after incubation with adenine and polyadenylic acid. After incubation of MNNG with guanosine, GMP, and polyuridylguanylic acid the product was 7-methylguanine, with cytosine the products were 1-methylcytosine and 3-methylcytosine, and with polycytidylic acid the product was 1-methylcytosine. SINGER and FRAENKEL-CONRAT (1969a, b) obtained 1-methyladenine, 3-methyladenine, and 7-methyladenine after incubation of MNNG with polyadenylic acid, and these derivatives of adenine in addition to 7-methylguanine and 3-methylcytidylic acid after incubation with tobacco mosaic virus-RNA or intact tobacco mosaic virus; 7-methylguanine was the major product. *In vitro* reactions of MNNG with DNA also yielded 7-methylguanine as a major product with smaller quantities of 3-methyladenine and 1-methyladenine (McCALLA, 1968; LAWLEY, 1968; CRADDOCK, 1969). When DNA or intact L-cells were treated with MNNG and care was taken in hydrolysis of the DNA, about 70% of the alkylation was accounted for as 7-methylguanine, 7% as 3-methyladenine, and 6% as *O*-6-methylguanine (LAWLEY and THATCHER, 1970). Studies with 1-trideuteromethyl-3-nitro-1-nitrosoguanidine showed that the reaction of MNNG with high molecular weight DNA and with the DNA of intact *Escherichia coli* yielded 7-methylguanine and that the methyl group was transferred intact, thus, diazomethane could not be an intermediate in the process (LINGENS et al., 1971).

Following the *in vivo* administration of dimethylnitrosamine, 7-methylguanine was isolated from the RNA and DNA of the liver, kidney, pancreas, lung, and spleen of rats (MAGEE and FARBER, 1962; LEE et al., 1964; SWANN and MAGEE, 1968) and from the RNA of liver of mice, hamsters, and guinea pigs (LEE et al., 1964). Data obtained in a subsequent study showed that although approximately 80 to 90% of the methylation that occurred in rat liver could be accounted for as 7-methylguanine, there were also present small quantities of 1-methyladenine, 3-methyladenine, and 1-methylcytosine (LAWLEY et al., 1968). With the use of deuterated dimethylnitrosamine LIJINSKY et al. (1968) showed that the methyl group was transferred intact, and therefore diazomethane was not an intermediate in the alkylation process. KRÜGER et al. (1970) detected no 7-methylguanine in the RNA of the Walker tumor in the rat following the administration of dimethylnitrosamine, but did detect it following the administration of MNU.

SCHOENTAL (1967) administered *N*-[^{14}C]methyl-*N*-nitrosourethane intragastrically to rats and then detected 7-methylguanine in the hydrolysate of the total nucleic acids of the liver. Incubation of DNA with *N*-methyl-*N*-nitrosourethane and subsequent hydrolysis yielded 7-methylguanine and 3-methyladenine (SCHOENTAL, 1967; LAWLEY, 1968).

PREUSSMANN et al. (1969b) showed that 1-phenyl-3,3-dimethyltriazene and 1-phenyl-3,3-diethyltriazene are converted to the corresponding 1-phenyl-3-methyltriazene and 1-phenyl-3-ethyltriazene by enzymatic oxidation and subsequent hydrolysis, and suggested that these compounds decompose to yield methyl and ethyl diazohydroxides, respectively, which in turn decompose to generate methyl and ethyl carbonium ions. PREUSSMANN and HODENBERG (1970) isolated 7-methylguanine and 7-ethylguanine following incubation of guanosine, DNA, or RNA with 1-phenyl-3-methyltriazene or 1-phenyl-3-ethyltriazene. SKIBBA et al. (1970) administered 4(5)-(3,3-di[^{14}C]methyl-1-triazeno)imidazole-5(4)-carboxamide to a rat and subsequently isolated 7-methylguanine from the RNA and DNA of the liver.

Although the evidence indicates that the bases of RNA and DNA are the major targets of alkylation with the agents considered above, some alkylation of sulfhydryl groups and histidine may also occur. No report of alkylation of these groups by substituted 1-nitrosoureas under physiological conditions has been found, but there have been studies of such alkylation with three of the compounds considered above. Reaction of MNNG with cysteine at neutrality and room temperature yielded a small quantity of *S*-methylcysteine (SCHULZ and McCALLA, 1969), and ^{14}C from 1-[^{14}C]methyl-3-nitro-1-nitrosoguanidine became fixed to albumin when these two materials were allowed to react at room temperature and pH 7 (McCALLA and REUVERS, 1968). Methylation of protein also occurred when cultured mammalian cells were treated with 1-[^{14}C]methyl-3-nitro-1-nitrosoguanidine (LAWLEY and THATCHER, 1970). After incubation of rat liver slices and rat kidney slices with [^{14}C]dimethylnitrosamine, MAGEE and HULTIN (1962) isolated 1-methylhistidine and 3-methylhistidine from the protein. CRADDOCK (1965) administered [^{14}C]dimethylnitrosamine to rats and subsequently isolated *S*-[^{14}C]methylcysteine from the acid-soluble fraction and the protein of the liver and 1-[^{14}C]methylhistidine and 3-[^{14}C]methylhistidine from the protein of the liver. The extent of methylation of histidine exceeded that of cysteine. SCHOENTAL and RIVE (1965) isolated *S*-methylcysteine and *S*-methylglutathione after treating cysteine and glutathione, respectively, with *N*-methyl-*N*-nitrosourethane. In all of the experiments with these three alkylating agents the extents of alkylation of the cysteine and histidine moieties have been quite small compared to the extent of alkylation of nucleic acids that occurs under similar conditions.

B. Carbamoylation

The isocyanic acid (VI) derived from 1-alkyl-1-nitrosoureas conceivably could react with a number of functional groups present in biological materials. Cyanate, which is a progenitor of isocyanic acid, reacts with cysteine and cysteine moieties of proteins to yield *S*-carbamoyl derivatives, which are unstable and decompose reversibly at pH values above 6 and have a half-life of 1 to 2 h at pH 6.8 and 30° (STARK, 1964). Cyanate also reacts reversibly with imidazole to form *N*-carbamoylimidazole (STARK, 1965a) and with carboxyl groups to form mixed anhydrides (STARK, 1965b). Cyanate does not react to any significant extent with the hydroxyl groups of serine, threonine, dipeptides of serine, ethanol, or glycolic acid at pH 7 (STARK, 1965c). However, reaction of cyanate with amino groups of amino acids and peptides to form carbamoyl derivatives does occur (STARK, 1965b). At pH 7 or below, reaction with the α-amino group of peptides occurs more extensively than reaction with the ε-amino group of lysine moieties. STARK (1965b) concluded: "Of all adducts of cyanate with the functional groups of proteins, a carbamylamino group, stable to alkali at room temperature, is the only one that does not decompose readily".

OLIVERIO et al. (1970) observed that following the administration of 1-(2-chloroethyl)-3-[^{14}C]cyclohexyl-1-nitrosourea to dogs there was extensive fixation of ^{14}C to the plasma proteins, but similar fixation did not occur following the administration of 1-(2-[^{14}C]chloroethyl)-3-cyclohexyl-1-nitrosourea. CHENG et al. (1972) studied the fixation of ^{14}C from [^{14}C]CCNU labeled in either the 2-chloroethyl group or the cyclohexyl group in intact mice, in suspensions of leukemia L 1210 cells, and in incubation mixtures containing nucleic acids and proteins. In all of these systems there was extensive labeling of the proteins, but not of the nucleic acids when the CCNU was labeled in the cyclohexyl group. When the ^{14}C was in the 2-chloroethyl group of CCNU, there was labeling of both the proteins and the nucleic acids, but the total amount of labeling was much less than when the cyclohexyl group contained ^{14}C. In the *in vitro* experiments with several macromolecules, fixation of ^{14}C from cyclohexyl-labeled CCNU was greatest with polylysine and albumin, and that of ^{14}C from 2-chloroethyl-labeled CCNU was greatest with polyguanylic acid, polycytidylic acid, and tRNA.

BOWDON and WHEELER (1971) have studied the fixation and reactions of BCNU labeled with ^{14}C in the two 2-chloroethyl groups or the carbonyl group. After incubation of leukemia L 1210 cells with either labeled compound there was fixation of ^{14}C to the crude protein fraction of the cells. After incubation of the labeled BCNU with DNA, with nucleohistone, or with histone, the largest amount of ^{14}C was associated with the histone. Incubation of carbonyl-labeled BCNU with lysine yielded a product that behaved chromatographically and electrophoretically similar to N^6-(2-chloroethylcarbamoyl)lysine that was obtained by the reaction of 2-chloroethyl isocyanate with lysine. A similar product was a major component obtained following the enzymatic degradation of histone that had been incubated with carbonyl-labeled BCNU. What appears to be the same material has been isolated from the protein of leukemia cells that had been incubated with carbonyl-labeled BCNU.

This carbamoylation of lysine moieties of proteins upon treatment with BCNU is analogous to that discussed above for MNU and is analogous to the formation of nitrohomoarginine from the lysine moieties when albumin (MCCALLA and REUVERS, 1968) and histone (NAGAO et al., 1969) are incubated with MNNG.

The observations of BROWN and WOLD (1971) concerning the specificity of *in vitro* deactivation of enzymes by alkylisocyanates is pertinent to the possible biochemical effects of nitrosoureas. These investigators observed that octyl isocyanate reacted with chymotrypsin to inactivate the enzyme, but it did not react with or deactivate elastase, although both enzymes contain serine and it is believed that the deactivations result from carbamoylation of the hydroxyl group of serine. On the other hand, butyl isocyanate inactivated both chymotrypsin and elastase but showed a greater potency toward elastase. These specificities are believed to be due to differences in the sizes of the "binding pocket" into which the alkyl chain of the alkyl isocyanate might fit. Thus, the size and properties of the group bearing an isocyanate might have a great influence upon the extent and effects of carbamoylation of proteins. It is also of interest that in the experiments of BROWN and WOLD the isocyanates reacted with the hydroxyl groups rather than with the amino groups of the lysine moieties that are present in these enzymes.

SEREBRYANYI et al. (1969b) incubated 1-methyl-1-nitroso[^{14}C]urea with rat spleen DNA and observed fixation of the ^{14}C to the DNA. They concluded that carbamoylation of the phosphate moieties had occurred and suggested that carbamoylation of the bases might have also taken place, but they did not obtain direct evidence for the latter reaction.

Biochemical Effects

A. Synthesis of Macromolecules

MNU inhibited the biosynthesis of DNA more than the synthesis of RNA and of protein in *Escherichia coli* (ROSENKRANZ et al., 1968), and it interfered with the biosynthesis of DNA in several organs of the rat following intraperitoneal administration (KLEIHUES, 1969). Streptozotocin and streptozotocin tetraacetate inhibited the formation of DNA more than the synthesis of RNA and of protein in cultured leukemia L 1210 cells (BHUYAN, 1970). However, ROSENKRANZ and CARR (1970) concluded from studies with *Escherichia coli* that the modes of action of MNU and streptozotocin are different, because MNU inhibited the synthesis of

DNA, RNA, and protein, and streptozotocin primarily inhibited the synthesis of DNA.

In experiments in which GORBACHEVA and KUKUSHKINA (1970) administered 1-propyl-1-nitrosourea to mice bearing Ehrlich ascites carcinoma or a hepatoma, and 22 and 30 min later injected ^{14}C-formate, there was stimulation of the synthesis of RNA and inhibition of the synthesis of DNA in the tumors after low dosages, and inhibition of the synthesis of both RNA and DNA after larger doses. In the livers and spleens of these animals there was stimulation of the synthesis of both RNA and DNA after low dosages and inhibition after larger doses. In *in vitro* experiments with leukemia L 1210 cells and Ehrlich ascites carcinoma cells, the pattern of stimulation and inhibition of synthesis of RNA and DNA was similar to that obtained with the Ehrlich ascites carcinoma *in vivo*; there was also inhibition of the synthesis of arginine-rich histones and stimulation of the synthesis of lysine-rich histones at both the low and high concentrations of the agent.

Treatment of *Saccharomyces cerevisiae* with BCNU reduced the concentrations of protein, DNA, insoluble RNA, and soluble RNA in the cells, and the reduction in the level of DNA was somewhat greater than for the other macromolecules (GALE, 1965).

Administration of BCNU to mice bearing subcutaneously implanted solid leukemia L 1210 tumors inhibited the incorporation of ^{14}C from formate-^{14}C and adenine-8-^{14}C into both the RNA and DNA of the tumors; the inhibition was greater for DNA than for RNA and the inhibition of the incorporation of ^{14}C from formate-^{14}C was greater than that from adenine-8-^{14}C (WHEELER and BOWDON, 1965). With elevated doses of BCNU there was inhibition of the *de novo* synthesis of purine ribonucleotides, but not of the conversion of adenine-8-^{14}C to purine nucleotides; there was also a small inhibition of the incorporation of DL-leucine-4,5-^{3}H into protein. Similar effects upon the *in vivo* metabolism and fixation of ^{14}C from formate-^{14}C and adenine-8-^{14}C were observed for hamster plasmacytomas. Maximum inhibition of the synthesis of RNA and DNA in L 1210 solid tumor (WHEELER and BOWDON, 1965) and of DNA in murine bone marrow, spleen, lymph node, and sarcoma 180 (MIZUNO and HUMPHREY, 1969) occurred 16 to 24 h after a single dose of BCNU. The bone marrow, spleen, and lymph node recovered from this inhibition more rapidly than did sarcoma 180. In the L 1210 solid tumors stimulation of the synthesis of RNA, DNA, and protein occurred during the first few hours after administration of the BCNU and preceded the inhibition mentioned above. Low concentrations of BCNU stimulated the *in vitro* incorporation of ^{14}C from formate-^{14}C and adenine-8-^{14}C into the RNA and DNA of L 1210 ascites cells, and higher concentrations inhibited such incorporation; both the stimulations and the inhibitions were greater for formate-^{14}C than for adenine-8-^{14}C (WHEELER and BOWDON, 1965). In *in vitro* experiments with Ehrlich ascites cells, BCNU at concentrations comparable to those obtainable *in vivo* caused stimulation of the synthesis of RNA, inhibition of the synthesis of DNA, and little effect upon the synthesis of protein; at higher concentrations there was inhibition of all three types of synthesis (GALE, 1965b). GROTH et al. (1971) observed that BCNU stimulated the *in vitro* incorporation of ^{14}C from formate-^{14}C and serine-3-^{14}C into adenine and guanine, but not thymine, of nucleic acids of human leukemic cells and L 1210 ascites cells, but there was inhibition of the incorporation of ^{14}C from histidine-2-^{14}C into the purines. They suggested that these effects may be due to interference with the formation or utilization of N^5-formiminotetrahydrofolic acid by BCNU.

Incubation of crude cell-free preparations from L 1210 ascites cells with BCNU or CCNU caused decreases in the DNA nucleotidyltransferase activity of the preparation, but 1-(2-chloroethyl)-1-nitrosourea and 1-methyl-1-nitrosourea had much less effect (WHEELER and BOWDON, 1968). 2-Chloroethyl isocyanate caused as much decrease as BCNU or CCNU, and it was suggested that the apparent deactivation of the enzyme by BCNU and CCNU was due chiefly to the reactions of the isocyanates generated from them. Incubation of commercial DNA with BCNU did not significantly alter its activity as a primer for the DNA nucleotidyltransferase system. Incubation of intact L 1210 cells with 2.5×10^{-3}M BCNU caused a decrease in the synthesis of DNA by the cells and also a decrease in the DNA nucleotidyltransferase activity of the crude enzyme preparation prepared from these cells, but did not alter the primer activity of the DNA isolated from these cells. At a concentration of 1×10^{-3}M, BCNU inhibited the synthesis of DNA by the intact cells, but did not reduce the DNA nucleotidyltransferase activity of the crude preparation from these same cells. Treatment of tumor-bearing mice with BCNU inhibited the *in vivo* synthesis of DNA by solid or ascitic L 1210 leukemia without altering the DNA nucleotidyltransferase activity of the cell-free preparation or the primer activity of the DNA derived from these same tissues. It was concluded that, although under certain conditions BCNU can cause decreases in the DNA nucleotidyltransferase activity, deactivation of this enzyme is probably not the cause of the decreased rate of synthesis of DNA *in vivo*. Such a conclusion is consistent with the possibility that the DNA nucleotidyltransferase that is measured in this assay is a repair enzyme rather than an enzyme for normal replication of DNA. The possible role of the isocyanate reactions in inhibiting repair of damaged DNA is yet to be investigated.

Exposure of cultured L 1210 cells to BCNU caused a preferential inhibition of the synthesis of nucleolar RNA, an increase in the average size of the nucleoplasmic RNA molecules synthesized, and an interference with the processing of the nucleolar RNA (KANN et al., 1971).

B. Enzyme Levels and Inactivation of Enzymes

Some information relating to levels of enzymes involved in the synthesis of nucleic acids and precursors of nucleic acids and to deactivation of some of these enzymes has been given above.

BHUYAN (1970) reported that treatment of extracts of cultured L 1210 cells with streptozotocin and streptozotocin tetraacetate deactivated thymidine kinase, deoxycytidine kinase, thymidylate synthetase, and DNA polymerase only moderately at concentrations that were high relative to concentrations that were toxic to the cells. The levels of activity of thymidine kinase, thymidylate synthetase, and DNA polymerase were only slightly lower, or no lower, in L 1210 cells treated with streptozotocin or streptozotocin tetraacetate than in untreated cells.

Streptozotocin caused decreases in the concentrations of oxidized and reduced nicotinamide adenine dinucleotide in mouse liver, and prior administration of nicotinamide prevented such decrease (SCHEIN and LOFTUS, 1968). These investigators suggested that streptozotocin inhibits the synthesis of pyridine nucleotides. 1-Methyl-1-nitrosourea decreased the nicotinamide adenine dinucleotide (NAD) content of mouse liver and L 1210 ascites cells and caused an early increase in liver nicotinamide adenine dinucleotide glycohydrolase (NADase) but no significant change in NAD pyrophosphorylase (SCHEIN, 1969a). Nicotinamide prevented the decrease in NAD, but did not alter the toxicity or the anticancer activity of MNU. There was a decrease in the concentration of NAD in the brain at a time following the administration of MNU at which there was no change in the level of NADase; streptozotocin was not detected in the brain, and it caused no depression of NAD (SCHEIN, 1969b). Low concentrations of BCNU caused an increase in the content of NAD in Ehrlich ascites tumor cells during incubation *in vitro*, but higher concentrations caused decreases (GALE, 1965b).

GREEN (1966) reported that BCNU increased the NADase activity of Ehrlich ascites carcinoma, sarcoma 180 (solid and ascitic), Taper liver tumor (solid and ascitic), Walker carcinosarcoma 256, Murphy-Sturm lymphosarcoma and THF thyroid tumor, but did not increase the NADase activity of the liver, kidney, spleen, lung, intestine, and brain of the host animals. Other investigators (TSUKAGOSHI et al., 1968) studied the effects of BCNU upon the NADase activity of several tissues of normal and leukemic (L 1210) mice. There was a transient increase of activity in the spleen followed by a decrease reaching a nadir at 8 to 11 days after treatment. Delayed decreases also occurred in the brain, lung, liver, and kidney. Exposure of homogenates of brain, spleen, and liver to relatively high concentrations of BCNU did not cause decreases in NADase activity. This fact plus the delayed *in vivo* decrease indicates that the decreases must not be due to direct deactivation of the enzyme.

The mechanisms responsible for producing the above mentioned increases and decreases in NAD and NADase and the significance of these alterations in relation to the anticancer effects of nitrosoureas are not presently known. It is of interest that BCNU inhibited anaerobic glycolysis in *Saccharomyces cerevisiae*; when the concentration of BCNU was 100 μg/ml, growth was inhibited 47%, carbon dioxide release was reduced 49%, and NAD synthesis was inhibited 36%, while protein synthesis was inhibited 63% (GALE, 1965a). Also, streptozotocin administration to rats caused a large reduction in *in vitro* oxidation of glucose by the islets of Langerhans (WYSE and DULIN, 1971).

Biological Effects

A. Effects upon Cell Cycle and Cytotoxicity during the Cycle

Experiments with normal and lymphoma colony-forming cells led to the conclusion that BCNU is more toxic to actively proliferating cells than to nonproliferating (G_0) cells, but that cells in all phases of the cycle are about equally sensitive (BRUCE and VALERIOTE, 1968). A lack of phase-specificity was also indicated by the first order kill kinetics of BCNU for cultured L 1210 cells (WILKOFF et al., 1967) and exponential dose-response curves for MNU, BCNU, and streptozotocin with cultured DON cells (BHUYAN, 1970; BHUYAN et al., 1970; ROBERTS et al., 1971a), for BCNU with cultured H. Ep. No. 2 cells (WHEELER et al., 1970), and for cultured Chinese hamster ovary cells (BARRANCO and HUMPHREY, 1971). In contrast to the conclusion of BRUCE and VALERIOTE (1968), THATCHER and WALKER (1969) observed that stationary phase cultures of embryonic hamster cells were as sensitive to BCNU as actively proliferating cells, but they suggested that the nonproliferative state of these cells might differ from such a state with the lymphoma cells *in vivo*. Cells of a heterogeneous population of L 1210 cells suspended in ascitic fluid at 35° (and thus considered to be "resting") were sensitive to BCNU according to the first order kill kinetics, whereas they were insensitive to several agents that are considered to be phase-specific (SCHABEL et al., 1965). On the other hand, there is evidence that cells are not equally sensitive to BCNU in all phases of the cycle. Cultured Chinese ovary cells are most sensitive to BCNU in mid-S-phase (BARRANCO and HUMPHREY, 1971), and cultured DON cells were most sensitive to BCNU and CCNU at the G_1/S boundary (BHUYAN et al., 1971).

A variety of cell lines and techniques have been used to determine the effects of nitrosoureas upon the progression of cells through the cycle. Streptozotocin prevented the progression of cultured L 1210 cells to mitosis and subsequent proliferation at concentrations that were considerably less than that required to inhibit the synthesis of DNA; the block in progression appeared to be in G_2 (BHUYAN, 1970). Results obtained by applying the double-labeling technique to L 1210 cells *in vivo* indicated that BCNU (SHIRAKAWA and FREI, 1970; YOUNG and DEVITA, 1970; BRAY et al., 1971) and CCNU (BRAY et al., 1971) caused an increase in the S-phase of cells that were lethally affected; BCNU had much less effect upon the S-phase of BCNU-resistant L 1210. Cyclohexyl isocyanate affected the S-phase of sensitive cells in a manner similar to that of CCNU, but cyclohexylamine, 1,3-dicyclohexylurea, and cyclophosphamide did not (BRAY et al., 1971). A lengthening of S-phase also resulted when a primary culture of mouse embryo cells was treated with MNU (FREI, 1970). The labeling index of the L 1210 cells was not altered by BCNU, CCNU, cyclophosphamide, cyclohexyl isocyanate, cyclohexylamine, or 1,3-dicyclohexylurea (BRAY et al., 1971).

A modified colcemid-block method was used to determine the effect of BCNU and some chemically related compounds upon progression of nonsynchronized H.Ep.No. 2 cells through the cycle (WHEELER et al., 1970). The progression to metaphase of cells in the last half of G_2, when exposed to BCNU at a concentration of 25 μg/ml, was not inhibited, but the progression to metaphase of cells initially in the first part of G_2, in S, and in G_1, was delayed or prevented. The labeling of cells initially in S at the time of exposure to BCNU was partially inhibited, and the progression into S of cells initially in the first half of G_1 was inhibited or delayed. At equimolar concentrations, CCNU had much less effect than BCNU, and BFNU and MNU were almost without effect on cell progression. Also, 2-chloroethyl isocyanate and 2-chloroethylamine were as active as, or more active than BCNU, while cyclohexylisocyanate was inactive. These results indicate that a large portion of the effects of BCNU upon the progression of cells through the cycle is probably due to the 2-chloroethylamine that is generated from it, but the N-(2-chloroethyl)-N-nitrosamino portion of the molecule also contributed to the effect. [BCNU was considerably more active than 1-methyl-3-(2-chloroethyl)-1-nitrosourea.] The relative cytotoxicities of these various compounds corresponded to their relative potencies upon the progression of cells through the cycle.

BARRANCO and HUMPHREY (1971) treated synchronized hamster ovary cells in various phases of the cycle with BCNU at a concentration of 100 μg/ml and determined the effects upon subsequent progression through the cycle. Cells in G_2 did not progress to mitosis, and mitotic cells did not proceed to divide. The progress of cells from S into G_2 and from G_1 into S was also delayed. The cells eventually overcame all of these delays in progression even though the treatment was lethal to 95% of the cells.

Treatment of synchronized HeLa cells with MNU during G_1, S, or G_2 did not delay progression through the cycle, nor inhibit the synthesis of DNA during the concurrent cycle, but cells treated during G_1 or S did exhibit a dose dependent depression of the synthesis of DNA during the next cycle; cells treated during G_2 divided two times before a depression in the rate of synthesis of DNA occurred (PLANT and ROBERTS, 1970a). On the other hand, treatment of Chinese hamster cells with MNU during G_1 caused a delay in progression into S without significantly altering the rate or extent of synthesis of DNA during S, this was accompanied by a corresponding delay in reaching mitosis (PLANT and ROBERTS, 1971b). Treatment of hamster cells during S caused an immediate decrease in the rate of synthesis of DNA, thus causing an elongation of the S-phase during which the normal quantity of DNA was synthesized. For the hamster cells treated during G_1 or S there was a depression in the rate of synthesis of DNA during the next cycle. The sensitivities of the two cell lines to either MNU or MNNG differed greatly. MNU and MNNG were about 50 and 100 times, respectively, more toxic to HeLa cells than to hamster cells, and at equitoxic levels the extents of alkylation of DNA in hamster cells were 20 and 50 times, respectively, as great as the extent of alkylation of DNA in HeLa cells (ROBERTS et al., 1971a). There appear to be differences in the abilities of the two kinds of cells to repair the damage caused by alkylation, but the repair probably involves some process in addition to the classical "repair synthesis" (ROBERTS et al., 1971b). HeLa cells were about 8 times as sensitive to methyl methane sulfonate as hamster cells, but the two kinds of cells were about equally sensitive to mustard gas and half mustard gas (ROBERTS et al., 1971a). The experiments of ROBERTS and coworkers show that levels of alkylation of DNA, RNA, and protein corresponding to toxic concentrations of the agents, and the resulting effects upon progression through the cell cycle, differ for various alkylating agents and cell lines. More information concerning these phenomena will be required before they can be satisfactorily explained.

There is evidence that cultured carcinoma 755 cells (SIMPSON-HERREN et al., 1966) and leukemia L 1210 cells *in vivo* (YOUNG and DEVITA, 1970), that survive exposure to BCNU, have normal generation times.

B. Genetic Effects

Streptozotocin is mutagenic to *Arabidopsis thalina* (GICHNER et al., 1968). 1-Methyl, 1-ethyl, 1-butyl, 1-isobutyl, and 1-allyl-1-nitrosourea are also mutagenic to this species (GICHNER and VELEMINSKY, 1967), and 1-methyl-1-nitrosourea is a more active mutagen than 1-methyl-3-methyl-1-nitrosourea, which in turn is more active than 1-methyl-3,3-dimethyl-1-nitrosourea (GICHNER et al., 1969). Exposure to MNU results in mutagenesis in *Saccharomyces cerevisiae* (MARQUARDT et al., 1963), *Drosophila melanogaster* (PASTERNAK, 1964), and Chinese hamster ovary cells (KAO and PUCK, 1971). Both MNU and 1-ethyl-1-nitrosourea are mutagenic to coliphage T_2, which is interesting in view of the fact that ethyl methanesulfonate is mutagenic in this system but methyl methanesulfonate is not (LOVELESS, 1959; LOVELESS and HAMPTON, 1969). In this system with these four agents there is a correlation between the extent of formation of O^6-methylguanine and mutagenicity (LOVELESS, 1969).

Both MNU and 1-ethyl-1-nitrosourea are teratogenic (KREYBIG, 1965; JOBST, 1967; GIVELBER and DIPAOLO, 1969; DIPAOLO, 1969).

Streptozotocin (BERMAN et al., 1971) and a number of alkyl nitrosoureas (DURCKREY et al., 1967) are potent carcinogens, and it is of particular interest that the latter give a high incidence of tumors in the brain, spinal cord, and peripheral nervous system. Tumors of the nervous system occurred following intravenous (JANISH and SCHREIBER, 1967), intraperitoneal (THOMAS and SIERRA, 1968), and oral (THOMAS and SIERRA, 1967) administration of MNU. Topical application of MNU yielded skin tumors (GRAFFI et al., 1967). Treatment of cultured cells with MNU produced "converted" cells that formed multilayer colonies and caused nodules when implanted into the cheeks of hamsters (SANDERS and BURFORD, 1967). Transplacental carcinogenesis was also caused by treatment of pregnant mice with MNU (RICE, 1969).

Since it is generally thought that mutagenesis, teratogenesis, and carcinogenesis are results of alterations of the genetic apparatus, these phenomena reinforce the likelihood that reaction of breakdown products of nitrosoureas with nucleic acids occurs.

Cross-resistance of a drug-resistant strain of a biological species to other agents implies that the agents might have some biochemical mechanisms of action in common, or that the agents are deactivated or reversed by a common mechanism. A strain of *Escherichia coli* selected for resistance to MNNG was resistant to MNU, and a strain selected for resistance to MNU was resistant to MNNG (KILGORE et al., 1960). A strain of *E. coli* resistant to BCNU was also resistant to MNU, MNNG, mitomycin C, porfiromycin, nitrogen mustard, myleran, azaserine, 6-diazo-5-oxo-L-norleucine, a terephthalanilide, and ionizing and ultraviolet radiation, but not to 6-mercaptopurine or methotrexate; strains selected for resistance to mitomycin C, porfiromycin, nitrogen mustard, or azaserine were cross-resistant to BCNU (PITTILLO et al., 1964). A cyclophosphamide-resistant line of a hamster plasmacytoma was also resistant to MNU and BCNU (SCHABEL et al., 1963). Whereas a variant of leukemia L 1210 resistant to 5-[3,3-*bis*(2-chloroethyl)-1-triazeno]imidazole-4-carboxamide was also resistant to seven nitrosoureas, including streptozotocin, MNU, BCNU, and CCNU, a variant resistant to 5-(3,3-dimethyl-1-triazeno)imidazole-4-carboxamide retained sensitivity to MNU, BCNU, and CCNU (KLINE et al., 1971). The former variant was also sensitive to cyclophosphamide, phosphoramide mustard, L-phenylalanine mustard, *o*-DL-phenylalanine mustard, thio-TEPA, and to a lesser extent to nitrogen mustard, and the latter variant retained sensitivity to cyclophosphamide and phosphoramide mustard. The reasons for the cross-resistance or lack of cross-resistance observed with these various agents and biological systems are not known at present, but the observations arouse interest and provoke additional experimentation.

Conclusions

The biological and biochemical effects of the nitrosoureas are undoubtedly dependent upon the limited chemical stability of these compounds and the high chemical reactivities of the products of their decomposition. The evidence indicates that the carbonium ions that derive from the alkyl group on the nitrosated nitrogen react primarily with the bases of nucleic acids and that the derived isocyanates (or isocyanic acid) react mainly with proteins or low molecular weight molecules. If there is a 2-chloroethyl group on *N*-3 of the nitrosourea, formation of 2-chloroethylamine can occur, and it in turn can act as an alkylating agent. It appears that alkylation reactions might account to a large extent for the mutagenic, teratogenic, carcinogenic, and cytotoxic effects of these agents, but it is considered quite likely that carbamoylation reactions also might contribute significantly to their cytotoxicity. Since the rates of decomposition of the nitrosoureas, the reactivities of the carbonium ions and alkyl isocyanates, and the lipid solubility are influenced by the nature of the specific substituents on the two nitrogen atoms, the various nitrosoureas can differ considerably in their usefulness as therapeutic agents. Therefore, one must be cautious in making generalizations about the biochemical and biological effects of the nitrosoureas.

References

BARRANCO, S. C., HUMPHREY, R. M.: The effects of 1,3-*bis*(2-chloroethyl)-1-nitrosourea on survival and cell progression in Chinese hamster cells. Cancer Res. **31**, 191—195 (1971).

BERMAN, L. D., HAYES, J., SIBAY, T.: The oncogenicity of the drug streptozotocin in the Chinese hamster. Proc. Amer. Ass. Cancer Res. **12**, 86 (1971).

BHUYAN, B. K.: The action of streptozotocin on mammalian cells. Cancer Res. **30**, 2017—2023 (1970).

BHUYAN, B. K., SCHEIDT, L. G., FRASER, T. J.: Cell cycle specificity of several antitumor agents. Proc. Amer. Ass. Cancer Res. **11**, 8 (1970).

BHUYAN, B. K., SCHEIDT, L. G., FRASER, T. J.: Cell-cycle phase specificity of antitumor agents. Proc. Amer. Ass. Cancer Res. **12**, 88 (1971).

BOWDON, B. J., WHEELER, G. P.: Reaction of 1,3-*bis*(2-chloroethyl)-1-nitrosourea (BCNU) with protein. Proc. Amer. Ass. Cancer Res. **12**, 67 (1971).

BRAY, D. A., DEVITA, V. T., ADAMSON, R. H., OLIVERIO, V. T.: Effects of 1-(2-chloroethyl)-3-cyclohexyl-1-nitrosourea (CCNU; NSC-79037) and its degradation products on progression of L1210 cells through the cell cycle. Cancer Chemother. Rep. **55**, 215—220 (1971).

BROWN, W. E., WOLD, F.: Alkyl isocyanates as active site-specific inhibitors of chymotrypsin and elastase. Science **174**, 608—610 (1971).

BRUCE, W. R., VALERIOTE, F. A.: Normal and malignant stem cells and chemotherapy. In: The Proliferation and Spread of Neoplastic Cells, pp. 409—420. The University of Texas M. D. Anderson Hospital and Tumor Institute at Houston. Baltimore: The Williams and Wilkins Company, 1968.

CARTER, S. K., SCHABEL, F. M., JR., BRODER, L., JOHNSTON, T. P.: BCNU and other nitrosoureas: a review. Advanc. Cancer Res., **16**, 273—332 (1972).

CHAN, S. C., LEH, F.: The release of halide ions from some primary haloalkylamines. Austral. J. Chem. **19**, 2271—2279 (1966).

CHENG, C. J., FUJIMURA, S., GRUNBERGER, D., WEINSTEIN, I. B.: Interaction of 1-(2-chloroethyl)-3-cyclohexyl-1-nitrosourea (NSC 79037) with nucleic acids and proteins *in vivo* and *in vitro*. Cancer Res. **32**, 22—27 (1972).

CRADDOCK, V. M.: Reaction of the carcinogen dimethylnitrosamine with proteins and with thiol compounds in the intact animal. Biochem. J. **94**, 323—330 (1965).

CRADDOCK, V. M.: Study of the methylation and lack of deamination of deoxyribonucleic acid by *N*-methyl-*N'*-nitro-*N*-nitrosoguanidine. Biochem. J. **111**, 615—620 (1969).

DEVITA, V. T., DENHAM, C., DAVIDSON, J. D., OLIVERIO, V. T.: The physiological disposition of the carcinostatic 1,3-*bis*(2-chloroethyl)-1-nitrosourea (BCNU) in man and animals. Clin. Pharmacol. Ther. **8**, 566—577 (1967).

DIPAOLO, J. A.: Teratogenic agents: mammalian test systems and chemicals. Ann. N. Y. Acad. Sci. **163**, 801—812 (1969).

DRUCKREY, H., PREUSSMANN, R., IVANKOVIC, S.: *N*-Nitroso compounds in organotropic and transplacental carcinogenesis. Ann. N.Y. Acad. Sci. **163**, 676—695 (1969).

DRUCKREY, H., PREUSSMANN, R., IVANKOVIC, S., SCHMÄHL, D., AFKHAM, J., BLUM, G., MENNEL, H. D., MÜLLER, M., PETROPOULAS, P., SCHNEIDER, H.: Organotrope carcinogene Wirkungen bei 64 verschiedenen *N*-Nitroso-Verbindungen an BD-Ratten. Z. Krebsforsch. **69**, 103—201 (1967).

FREI, J. V.: Approach to transformation of mouse embryo cells by methylnitrosourea (MNUA). Proc. Amer. Ass. Cancer Res. **11**, 27 (1970).

GALE, G. R.: Effect of 1,3-*bis*(2-chloroethyl)-1-nitrosourea on *Saccharomyces cerevisiae*. Proc. Soc. exp. Biol. (N.Y.) **119**, 1004—1010 (1965a).

GALE, G. R.: Effect of 1,3-*bis*-(2-chloroethyl)-1-nitrosourea on Ehrlich ascites tumor cells. Biochem. Pharmacol. **14**, 1707—1712 (1965b).

GARRETT, E. R.: Prediction of stability in pharmaceutical preparations. VII. The solution degradation of the antibiotic streptozotocin. J. Amer. Pharm. Ass., sci. Ed. **49**, 767—777 (1960).

GARRETT, E. R., GOTO, S., STUBBINS, J. F.: Kinetics of solvolysis of various *N*-alkyl-*N*-nitrosoureas in neutral and alkaline solutions. J. pharm. Sci. **54**, 119—123 (1965).

GICHNER, T., VELEMÍNSKÝ, J.: The mutagenic activity of 1-alkyl-1-nitrosoureas and 1-alkyl-3-nitro-1-nitrosoguanidines. Mutation Res. **4**, 207—212 (1967).

GICHNER, T., VELEMÍNSKÝ, J., KŘEPINSKÝ, J.: Strong mutagenic activity of streptozotocin—an antibiotic with an alkylnitroso group. Molec. gen. Genet. **102**, 184—186 (1968).

GICHNER, T., VELEMÍNSKÝ, J., POKORNÝ, V.: Comparison of the mutagenic activity of N-methylnitrosourea, *N,N'*-dimethylnitrosourea and *N,N',N'*-trimethylnitrosourea. Arzneimittel-Forsch. **19**, 1053—1055 (1969).

GIVELBER, H. M., DIPAOLO, J. A.: Teratogenic effects of *N*-ethyl-*N*-nitrosourea in the Syrian hamster. Cancer Res. **29**, 1151—1155 (1969).

GORBACHEVA, L. B., KUKUSHKINA, G. V.: Some aspects of the mechanism of action of 1-propyl-1-nitrosourea. Biochem. Pharmacol. **19**, 1561—1568 (1970).

GRAFFI, A., HOFFMAN, F., SCHÜTT, M.: *N*-Methyl-*N*-nitrosourea as a strong topical carcinogen when painted on skin of rodents. Nature (Lond.) **214**, 611 (1967).

GREEN, S.: The effect of 1,3-*bis*(2-chloroethyl)-1-nitrosourea on nicotinamide adenine dinucleotide glycohydrolase of mouse and rat neoplastic and normal tissues. Cancer Res. **26**, 2481—2484 (1966).

GROTH, D. P., D'ANGELO, J. M., VOGLER, W. R., MINGIOLI, E. S., BETZ, B.: Selective metabolic effects of 1,3-*bis*(2-chloroethyl)-1-nitrosourea upon *de novo* purine biosynthesis. Cancer Res. **31**, 332—336 (1971).

HENRY, R. A.: The reaction of amines with *N*-methyl-*N*-nitroso-*N'*-nitroguanidine. J. Amer. chem. Soc. **72**, 3287—3289 (1950).

HERR, R. R., JAHNKE, H. K., ARGOUDELIS, A. D.: The structure of streptozotocin. J. Amer. chem. Soc. **89**, 4808—4809 (1967).

IRIARTE, P. V., HANANIAN, J., CORTNER, J. A.: Central nervous system leukemia and solid tumors of childhood — Treatment with 1,3-*bis*(2-chloroethyl)-1-nitrosourea (BCNU). Cancer (Philad.) **19**, 1187—1194 (1966).

JÄNISH, W., SCHREIBER, D.: Experimentelle Hirngeschwülste bei Kaninchen nach Injektion von Methylnitrosoharnstoff. Naturwissenschaften **54**, 171—172 (1967).

JOBST, K.: Teratogenous changes and tumors in rats following treatment with methylnitrosourea (MNU). Neoplasma (Bratisl.) **14**, 435—436 (1967).

JOHNSTON, T. P., MCCALEB, G. S., MONTGOMERY, J. A.: The synthesis of antineoplastic agents. XXXII. *N*-Nitrosoureas. I. J. med. Chem. **6**, 669—681 (1963).

JOHNSTON, T. P., MCCALEB, G. S., OPLIGER, P. S., LASTER, W. R., MONTGOMERY, J. A.: Synthesis of potential anticancer agents. 38. N-Nitrosoureas. 4. Further synthesis and evaluation of haloethyl derivatives. J. med. Chem. **14**, 600—614 (1971).

JOHNSTON, T. P., MCCALEB, G. S., OPLIGER, P. S., MONTGOMERY, J. A.: The synthesis of potential anticancer agents. XXXVI. *N*-Nitrosoureas. II. Haloalkyl derivatives. J. med. Chem. **9**, 892—911 (1966).

JOHNSTON, T. P., OPLIGER, P. S.: The synthesis of potential anticancer agents. XXXVII. N-Nitrosoureas. III. 1,5-*Bis*(2-chloroethyl)-1-nitrosobiuret and related derivatives of biurets, biureas, and carboxamides. J. med. Chem. **10**, 675—681 (1967).

KANN, H. E., JR., SNYDER, A. L., KOHN, K. W.: Effects of chemotherapeutic agents on RNA synthesis in L1210 cells. Proc. Amer. Ass. Cancer Res. **12**, 59 (1971).

KAO, F-T., PUCK, T. T.: Genetics of somatic mammalian cells XII: mutagenesis by carcinogenic nitroso compounds. J. cell. Physiol. **78**, 139—144 (1971).

KILGORE, W. W., MORRIS, J. E., GREENBERG, J.: Effect of diazoalkane-yielding compounds on strains of *Escherichia coli* resistant to 1-methyl-3-nitro-1-nitrosoguanidine. Proc. Soc. exp. Biol. (N.Y.) **105**, 469—473 (1960).

KLEIHUES, P.: Blockierung der DNS-Synthese durch *N*-Methyl-*N*-Nitrosoharnstoff *in vivo*. Arzneimittel-Forsch. **19**, 1041—1043 (1969).

KLEIHUES, P., PATZSCHKE, K.: Verteilung von *N*-[^{14}C]Methyl-*N*-nitrosoharnstoff in der Ratte nach systemischer Applikation. Z. Krebsforsch. **75**, 193—200 (1971).

KLINE, I., WOODMAN, R. J., GANG, M., VENDITTI, J. M.: Effectiveness of antileukemic agents in mice inoculated with leukemia L1210 variants resistant to 5-(3,3-dimethyl-1-triazeno)-imidazole-4-carboxamide (NSC-45388) or 5-[3,3-bis(2-chloroethyl)-1-triazeno]imidazole-4-carboxamide (NSC-82196). Cancer Chemother. Rept., Pt. 1, **55**, 9—28 (1971).

KREYBIG, T. VON: Die Wirkung einer carcinogenen Methyl-nitroso-Harnstoffdosis auf die Embryonalentwicklung der Ratte. Z. Krebsforsch. **67**, 46—50 (1965).

KRÜGER, F. W., BALLWEG, H., MAIER-BORST, W.: Untersuchungen über die alkylierende Wirkung von ^{14}C-Methylnitrosoharnstoff und 1-^{14}C-Äthylnitrosoharnstoff. Experientia (Basel) **24**, 592—593 (1968).

KRÜGER, F. W., OSSWALD, H., WALKER, G., SCHELTEN, E.: Untersuchungen zur Organotropie der alkylierenden Wirkung von Dimethylnitrosamin (DMNA) und Nitrosomethylharnstoff (NMH) *in vivo*. Z. Krebsforsch. **74**, 434—447 (1970).

LAWLEY, P. D.: Methylation of DNA by *N*-methyl-*N*-nitrosourethane and *N*-methyl-*N*-nitroso-*N'*-nitroguanidine. Nature (Lond.) **218**, 580—581 (1968).

LAWLEY, P. D., BROOKES, P., MAGEE, P. N., CRADDOCK, V. M., SWANN, P. F.: Methylated bases in liver nucleic acids from rats treated with dimethylnitrosamine. Biochim. biophys. Acta (Amst.) **157**, 646—648 (1948).

LAWLEY, P. D., THATCHER, C. J.: Methylation of deoxyribonucleic acid in cultured mammalian cells by *N*-methyl-*N'*-nitro-*N*-nitrosoguanidine. The influence of cellular thiol concentrations on the extent of methylation and the 6-oxygen atom of guanine as a site of methylation. Biochem. J. **116**, 693—707 (1970).

LEE, K. Y., LIJINSKY, W., MAGEE, P. N.: Methylation of ribonucleic acids of liver and other organs in different species treated with C^{14}- and H^{3}-dimethylnitrosamines *in vivo*. J. nat. Cancer Inst. **32**, 65—76 (1964).

LEVIN, V. A., SHAPIRO, W. R., CLANCY, T. P., OLIVERIO, V. T.: The uptake, distribution, and antitumor activity of 1-(2-chloroethyl)-3-cyclohexyl-1-nitrosourea in the murine glioma. Cancer Res. **30**, 2451—2455 (1970).

LEVINS, P. L., PAPANASTASSIOU, Z. B.: A nuclear magnetic resonance study of the 2-haloethylamines. J. Amer. chem. Soc. **87**, 826—831 (1965).

Lijinsky, W., Loo, J., Ross, A. E.: Mechanism of alkylation of nucleic acids by nitrosodimethylamine. Nature (Lond.) **218**, 1174—1175 (1968).

Lingens, F., Haerlin, R., Süssmuth, R.: Mechanism of mutagenesis by *N*-methyl-*N'*-nitro-*N*-nitrosoguanidine (MNNG). Methylation of nucleic acids by *N*-trideuteromethyl-*N'*-nitro-*N*-nitrosoguanidine (D_3-MNNG) in the presence of cysteine and in cells of *Escherichia coli*. FEBS Let. **13**, 241—242 (1971).

Lingens, F., Rau, J., Süssmuth, R.: Zum Wirkungsmechanismus von 1-Nitroso-3-nitro-1-methyl-guanidin bei der Mutationsauslösung. II. Produkte der Reaktion von 1-Nitroso-3-nitro-1-methyl-guanidin mit Nucleobasen, Nucleosiden, Nucleosidphosphaten und Homopolyribonucleinsäuren. Z. Naturforsch. **23** b, 1565—1570 (1968).

Loo, T. L., Dion, R. L., Dixon, R. L., Rall, D. P.: The antitumor agent, 1,3-*bis*(2-chloroethyl)-1-nitrosourea. J. pharm. Sci. **55**, 492—497 (1966).

Loveless, A.: Possible relevance of *O*-6-alkylation of deoxyguanosine to the mutagenicity and carcinogenicity of nitrosamines and nitrosamides. Nature (Lond.) **223**, 206—207 (1969).

Loveless, A., Hampton, C. L.: Inactivation and mutation of coliphage T_2 by *N*-methyl- and *N*-ethyl-*N*-nitrosourea. Mutation Res. **7**, 1—12 (1969).

Magee, P. N.: *In vivo* reactions of nitroso compounds. Ann. N.Y. Acad. Sci. **163**, 717—729 (1969).

Magee, P. N., Farber, E.: Toxic liver injury and carcinogenesis — Methylation of rat-liver nucleic acids by dimethylnitrosamine *in vivo*. Biochem. J. **83**, 114—124 (1962).

Magee, P. N., Hultin, T.: Toxic liver injury and carcinogenesis — Methylation of proteins of rat-liver slices by dimethylnitrosamine *in vitro*. Biochem. J. **83**, 106—114 (1962).

Marquardt, H., Zimmermann, F. K., Schwaier, R.: Nitrosamide als mutagene Agentien. Naturwissenschaften **50**, 625 (1963).

McCalla, D. R.: Reaction of *N*-methyl-*N'*-nitro-*N*-nitrosoguanidine and *N*-methyl-*N*-nitroso-*p*-toluenesulfonamide with DNA *in vitro*. Biochim. biophys. Acta (Amst.) **155**, 114—120 (1968).

McCalla, D. R., Reuvers, A.: Reaction of *N*-methyl-*N'*-nitro-*N*-nitrosoguanidine with protein: formation of nitroguanido derivatives. Canad. J. Biochem. **46**, 1411—1415 (1968).

McKay, A. F., Wright, G. F.: Preparation and properties of *N*-methyl-*N*-nitroso-*N'*-nitroguanidine. J. Amer. chem. Soc. **69**, 3028—3030 (1947).

Mizuno, N. S., Humphrey, E. W.: Effect of combined therapy with cytosine arabinoside (NSC-63878) and 1,3-*bis*(2-chloroethyl)-1-nitrosourea (NSC-409962) on sarcoma 180 and L 1210 *in vivo*. Cancer Chemother. Rep. **53**, 215—221 (1969).

Montgomery, J. A., James, R., McCaleb, G. S., Johnston, T. P.: The modes of decomposition of 1,3-*bis*(2-chloroethyl)-1-nitrosourea and related compounds. J. med. Chem. **10**, 668—674 (1967).

Nagao, M., Yokoshima, T., Hosoi, H., Sugimura, T.: Interaction of *N*-methyl-*N'*-nitro-*N*-nitrosoguanidine with ascites hepatoma cells *in vitro*. Biochim. biophys. Acta (Amst.) **192**, 191—199 (1969).

Oliverio, V. T., Vietzke, W. M., Williams, M. K., Adamson, R. H.: The absorption, distribution, excretion, and biotransformation of the carcinostatic 1-(2-chloroethyl)-3-cyclohexyl-1-nitrosourea in animals. Cancer Res. **30**, 1330—1337 (1970).

Pasternak, L.: Untersuchungen über die mutagene Wirkung verschiedener Nitrosamin- und Nitrosamid-Verbindungen. Arzneimittel-Forsch. **14**, 802—804 (1964).

Pittillo, R. F., Narkates, A. N., Burns, J.: Microbiological evaluation of 1,3-*bis*(2-chloroethyl)-1 nitrosourea. Cancer Res. **24**, 1222—1228 (1964).

Plant, J. E., Roberts, J. J.: A novel mechanism for the inhibition of DNA synthesis following methylation: the effect of *N*-methyl-*N*-nitrosourea on HeLa cells. Chem. biol. Interact. **3**, 337—342 (1971a).

Plant, J. E., Roberts, J. J.: Extension of the pre-DNA synthetic phase of the cell cycle as a consequence of DNA alkylation in Chinese hamster cells: a possible mechanism of DNA repair. Chem. biol. Interact. **3**, 343—351 (1971b).

Preussmann, R., Druckrey, H., Ivankovic, S., Hodenberg, A. v.: Chemical structure and carcinogenicity of aliphatic hydrazo, azo, and azoxy compounds and of triazenes, potential *in vivo* alkylating agents. Ann. N. Y. Acad. Sci. **163**, 697—714 (1969a).

Preussmann, R., Hodenberg, A. v.: Mechanism of carcinogenesis with 1-aryl-3,3-dialkyltriazenes. II. *In vitro* alkylation of guanosine, RNA and DNA with aryl-monoalkyltriazenes to form 7-alkylguanine. Biochem. Pharmacol. **19**, 1505—1508 (1970).

Preussmann, R., Hodenberg, A. v., Hengy, H.: Mechanism of carcinogenesis with 1-aryl-3,3-dialkyltriazenes. Enzymatic dealkylation by rat liver microsomal fraction *in vitro*. Biochem. Pharmacol. **18**, 1—13 (1969b).

Rice, J. M.: Transplacental carcinogenesis in mice by 1-ethyl-1-nitrosourea. Ann. N. Y. Acad. Sci. **163**, 813—826 (1969).

ROBERTS, J. J., PASCOE, J. M., PLANT, J. E., STURROCK, J. E., CRATHORN, A. R.: Quantitative aspects of the repair of alkylated DNA in cultured mammalian cells. I. The effect on HeLa and Chinese hamster cell survival of alkylation of cellular macromolecules. Chem. biol. Interact. **3**, 29—47 (1971a).

ROBERTS, J. J., PASCOE, J. M., SMITH, B. A., CRATHORN, A. R.: Quantitative aspects of the repair of alkylated DNA in cultured mammalian cells. II. Non-semiconservative DNA synthesis ("repair synthesis") in HeLa and Chinese hamster cells following treatment with alkylating agents. Chem. biol. Interact. **3**, 49—68 (1971b).

ROSENKRANZ, H. S., BITOON, M., SCHMIDT, R. M.: Biological and metabolic effects of nitrosomethylurea and nitrosomethylurethan. J. nat. Cancer Inst. **41**, 1099—1109 (1968).

ROSENKRANZ, H. S., CARR, H. S.: Differences in the action of nitrosomethylurea and streptozotocin. Cancer Res. **30**, 112—117 (1970).

ROSSO, R., DONNELLI, M. G., INNOCENTI, I. R. D., GARATTINI, S.: Chemotherapy of tumors transplanted intracerebrally. Europ. J. Cancer **3**, 125—137 (1967).

SANDERS, F. K., BURFORD, B. O.: Morphological conversion of cells *in vitro* by *N*-nitrosomethylurea. Nature (Lond.) **213**, 1171—1173 (1967).

SCHABEL, F. M., Jr.: BCNU, 1,3-*bis*(2-chloroethyl)-1-nitrosourea. Development, antitumor activity, and mechanism of action. In: CARTER, S. K. (Ed.): Proceedings of the chemotherapy conference on the chemotherapy of solid tumors: an appraisal of 5-fluorouracil and BCNU, pp. 159—180. Bethesda, Maryland: Cancer Therapy Evaluation Branch, National Cancer Institute, 1970.

SCHABEL, F. M., Jr., JOHNSTON, T. P., MCCALEB, G. S., MONTGOMERY, J. A., LASTER, W. R., SKIPPER, H. E.: Experimental evaluation of potential anticancer agents. VIII. Effects of certain nitrosoureas on intracerebral L 1210 leukemia. Cancer Res. **23**, 725—733 (1963).

SCHABEL, F. M., Jr., SKIPPER, H. E., TRADER, M. W., WILCOX, W. S.: Experimental evaluation of potential anticancer agents. XIX. Sensitivity of nondividing leukemic cell populations to certain classes of drugs *in vivo*. Cancer Chemother. Rept. **48**, 17—30 (1965).

SCHEIN, P. S.: 1-Methyl-1-nitrosourea and dialkylnitrosamine depression of nicotinamide adenine dinucleotide. Cancer Res. **29**, 1226—1232 (1969a).

SCHEIN, P. S.: 1-Methyl-1-nitrosourea depression of brain nicotinamide adenine dinucleotide in the production of neurologic toxicity. Proc. Soc. exp. Biol. (N. Y.) **131**, 517—520 (1969b).

SCHEIN, P. S., LOFTUS, S.: Streptozotocin: depression of mouse liver pyridine nucleotides. Cancer Res. **28**, 1501—1506 (1968).

SCHOENTAL, R.: Methylation of nucleic acids by *N*[^{14}C]-methyl-*N*-nitrosourethane *in vitro* and *in vivo*. Biochem. J. **102**, 5c—7c (1967).

SCHOENTAL, R., RIVE, D. J.: Interaction of *N*-alkyl-*N*-nitrosourethanes with thiols. Biochem. J. **97**, 466—474 (1965).

SCHULZ, U., MCCALLA, D. R.: Reactions of cysteine with *N*-methyl-*N*-nitroso-*p*-toluenesulfonamide and *N*-methyl-*N'*-nitro-*N*-nitrosoguanidine. Canad. J. Chem. **47**, 2021—2027 (1969).

SEREBRYANYI, A. M., SMOTRYAEVA, M. A., KRUGLYAKOVA, K. E.: Methylation of DNA by *N*-nitroso-*N*-methylurea. Izv. Akad. Nauk SSSR, Ser. Biol. 607—608 (1969a).

SEREBRYANYI, A. M., SMOTRYAEVA, M. A., KRUGLYAKOVA, K. E., KOSTYANOVSKII, R. G.: Carbamoylation of DNA by *N*-nitroso-*N*-methylurea. Dokl. Akad. Nauk SSSR. **185**, 847—849 (1969b).

SHAPIRO, W. R., AUSMAN, J. I., RALL, D. P.: Studies on the chemotherapy of experimental brain tumors: evaluation of 1,3-*bis*(2-chloroethyl)-1-nitrosourea, cyclophosphamide, mithramycin, and methotrexate. Cancer Res. **30**, 2401—2413 (1970).

SHIRAKAWA, S., FREI, E. III, : Comparative effects of the antitumor agents 5-(dimethyltriazeno)-imidazole-4-carboxamide and 1,3-*bis*(2-chloroethyl)-1-nitrosourea on cell cycle of L 1210 leukemia cells *in vivo*. Cancer Res. **30**, 2173—2179 (1970).

SIMPSON-HERREN, L., SKIPPER, H. E., BLOW, J. G.: Kinetics of cell growth and death following treatment with 1,3-*bis*(2-chloroethyl)-1-nitrosourea. Proc. Amer. Ass. Cancer Res. **7**, 65 (1966).

SINGER, B., FRAENKEL-CONRAT, H.: Chemical modification of viral ribonucleic acid. VII. The action of methylating agents and nitrosoguanidine on polynucleotides including tobacco mosaic virus ribonucleic acid. Biochemistry 8, 3260—3266 (1969a).

SINGER, B., FRAENKEL-CONRAT, H.: Chemical modification of viral ribonucleic acid. VIII. The chemical and biological effects of methylating agents and nitrosoguanidine on tobacco mosaic virus. Biochemistry 8, 3266—3269 (1969b).

SKIBBA, J. L., JOHNSON, R. O., BRYAN, G. T.: Carcinogenicity and possible mode of action of 4(5)-(3,3-dimethyl-1-triazeno)imidazole-5(4)-carboxamide (NSC-45388, DIC). Proc. Amer. Ass. Cancer Res. **11**, 73 (1970).

STARK, G. R.: On the reversible reaction of cyanate with sulfhydryl groups and the determination of NH_2-terminal cysteine and cystine in proteins. J. biol. Chem. **239**, 1411—1414 (1964).

STARK, G. R.: Reactions of cyanate with functional groups of proteins. II. Formation, decomposition, and properties of *N*-carbamylimidazole. Biochemistry **4**, 588—595 (1965a).
STARK, G. R.: Reactions of cyanate with functional groups of proteins. III. Reactions with amino and carboxyl groups. Biochemistry **4**, 1030—1036 (1965b).
STARK, G. R.: Reactions of cyanate with functional groups of proteins. IV. Inertness of aliphatic hydroxyl groups. Formation of carbamyl- and acylhydantoins. Biochemistry **4**, 2363—2367 (1965c).
SWANN, P. F.: The rate of breakdown of methyl methanesulphonate, dimethyl sulphate and *N*-methyl-*N*-nitrosourea in the rat. Biochem. J. **110**, 49—52 (1968).
SWANN, P. F., MAGEE, P. N.: Nitrosamine-induced carcinogenesis. The alkylation of nucleic acids of the rat by *N*-methyl-*N*-nitrosourea, dimethylnitrosamine, dimethyl sulphate and methyl methanesulphonate. Biochem. J. **110**, 39—47 (1968).
THATCHER, C. J., WALKER, I. G.: Sensitivity of confluent and cycling embryonic hamster cells to sulfur mustard, 1,3-*bis*(2-chloroethyl)-1-nitrosourea, and actinomycin D. J. nat. Cancer Inst. **42**, 363—368 (1969).
THOMAS, C., SIERRA, J. L.: Hirntumoren bei Ratten nach oraler Gabe von *N*-Nitroso-*N*-methyl-Harnstoff. Naturwissenschaften **54**, 228 (1967).
THOMAS, C., SIERRA, J. L.: Neurogene Tumoren bei Ratten nach intraperitonealer Applikation von *N*-Nitroso-*N*-methyl-Harnstoff. Naturwissenschaften **55**, 183 (1968).
TSUKAGOSHI, S., KAO, M. H., GOLDIN, A.: Effect of 1,3-*bis*(2-chloroethyl)-1-nitrosourea (NSC-409962) and cyclophosphamide (NSC-26271) on nicotinamide adenine dinucleotide glycohydrolase in normal and leukemic mouse tissues. Cancer Chemother. Rept. **52**, 569—578 (1968).
VAVRA, J. J., DEBOER, C., DIETZ, A., HANKA, L. J., SOKOLSKI, W. T.: Streptozotocin, a new antibacterial antibiotic. Antibiot. Ann. 230—235 (1959—1960).
WALKER, M. D., HURWITZ, B. S.: BCNU (1,3-*bis*(2-chloroethyl)-1-nitrosourea; NSC-409962) in the treatment of malignant brain tumor — A preliminary report. Cancer Chemother. Rept. **54**, 263—271 (1970).
WALKER, M. D., ROSENBLUM, M. L., SMITH, K. A., REYNOLDS, A. F., Jr.: The treatment of brain tumor with 1-(2-chloroethyl)-3-cyclohexyl-1-nitrosourea (CCNU). Proc. Amer. Ass. Cancer Res. **12**, 51 (1971).
WHEELER, G. P.: Studies related to the mechanisms of action of cytotoxic alkylating agents. A review. Cancer Res. **22**, 651—688 (1962).
WHEELER, G. P., BOWDON, B. J.: Some effects of 1,3-*bis*(2-chloroethyl)-1-nitrosourea upon the synthesis of protein and nucleic acids *in vivo* and *in vitro*. Cancer Res. **25**, 1770—1778 (1965).
WHEELER, G. P., BOWDON, B. J.: Effects of 1,3-*bis*(2-chloroethyl)-1-nitrosourea and related compounds upon the synthesis of DNA by cell-free systems. Cancer Res. **28**, 52—59 (1968).
WHEELER, G. P., BOWDON, B. J.: Comparison of the effects of cysteine upon the decomposition of nitrosoureas and of 1-methyl-3-nitro-1-nitrosoguanidine. Biochem. Pharmacol. **21**, 265—267 (1972).
WHEELER, G. P., BOWDON, B. J., ADAMSON, D. J., VAIL, M. H.: Effects of 1,3-*bis*(2-chloroethyl)-1-nitrosourea and some chemically related compounds upon the progression of cultured H. Ep. No. 2 cells through the cell cycle. Cancer Res. **30**, 1817—1827 (1970).
WHEELER, G. P., BOWDON, B. J., HERREN, T. C.: Distribution of C^{14} from C^{14}-labeled 1,3-*bis*-(2-chloroethyl)-1-nitrosourea (NSC-409962) in tissues of mice and hamsters after intraperitoneal administration of the agent. Cancer Chemotherapy Repts. **42**, 9—12 (1964).
WHEELER, G. P., CHUMLEY, S.: Alkylating activity of 1,3-*bis*(2-chloroethyl)-1-nitrosourea and related compounds. J. med. Chem. **10**, 259—261 (1967).
WILKOFF, L. J., DIXON, G. J., DULMADGE, E. A., SCHABEL, F. M., Jr.: Effect of 1,3-*bis*(2-chloroethyl)-1-nitrosourea (NSC-409962) and nitrogen mustard (NSC-762) on kinetic behavior of cultured L 1210 cells. Cancer Chemotherapy Repts. **51**, 7—18 (1967).
WILSON, C. B., BOLDREY, E. B., ENOT, K. J.: 1,3-*Bis*(2-chloroethyl)-1-nitrosourea (NSC-409962) in the treatment of brain tumors. Cancer Chemotherapy Repts. **54**, 273—281 (1970).
WUNDERLICH, V., SCHÜTT, M., BÖTTGER, M., GRAFFI, A.: Preferential alkylation of mitochondrial deoxyribonucleic acid by *N*-methyl-*N*-nitrosourea. Biocem. J. **118**, 99—109 (1970).
WYSE, B. M., DULIN, W. E.: The effects of streptozotocin on glucose oxidation by isolated islets of Langerhans. Proc. Soc. exp. Biol. (N.Y.) **136**, 70—72 (1971).
YOUNG, R. C., DEVITA, V. T.: The effect of chemotherapy on the growth characteristics and cellular kinetics of leukemia L 1210. Cancer Res. **30**, 1789—1794 (1970).

Chapter 36

Mechanism of Action of Glucocorticoids

FRED ROSEN and RICHARD J. MILHOLLAND

Introduction

Although recent advances in our knowledge of hormone action have been impressive, there is at present no clear understanding of how any hormone acts at the molecular level. This is one of the major unsolved problems in biology today. It seems evident that one or more hormones are involved in the growth and metabolism of most normal tissues. The fact that certain tumors are hormone dependent or responsive also indicates that hormones may play an important role in the etiology and treatment of cancer. There is little doubt that knowledge concerning hormone action is likely to yield new insight and provide different approaches to the treatment of various diseases, including cancer.

Many reports during the past decade have revealed that steroid hormones affect their target tissues by altering the rate of synthesis of nucleic acids and proteins. The action of glucocorticoids on these processes is tissue specific. In liver, treatment with adrenal corticoids stimulates the incorporation of specific radioactive precursors into RNA and protein, whereas in normal and malignant lymphoid cells glucocorticoid administration depresses the incorporation of labeled precursors into nucleic acids and protein. The ultimate objective of studies concerned with the metabolic effects of hormones on target tissues is to describe the initial biochemical event which mediates the subsequent or secondary effects elicited by the hormone, e.g., alterations in the biosynthesis of macromolecules.

A direct approach to the study of hormone action is to demonstrate the presence and function of "receptor" macromolecules in target tissues, which bind the hormone tightly and specifically. So far, the effort expended in this area has clearly revealed the presence of protein receptors for estrogens (JENSEN and JACOBSON, 1962), androgens (BRUCHOVSKY and WILSON, 1968), progesterone (SHERMAN et al., 1970), aldosterone (HERMAN et al., 1968), and glucocorticoids (WIRA and MUNCK, 1970), each in tissues highly responsive to the hormone. For some of these steroids, the initial hormone-receptor complex which is formed in the cytoplasm undergoes a modification in structure prior to entering the nucleus. Recent studies have indicated that the estrogen-receptor complex is capable of stimulating RNA synthesis in isolated uterine nuclei (E.V. JENSEN, personal communication), and that the progesterone-receptor complex binds to an acidic protein fraction in chick oviduct nuclei (SPELSBERG et al., 1971). The role established for the "receptor" in the intracellular transport of steroid hormones, and the activity of the estrogen-receptor complex in stimulating RNA transcription suggests that this approach to the study of hormone action is likely to be very productive.

Within the past five years remarkable advances have been made concerning the basis for the selective action of steroid hormones in target tissues, and in describing the biochemical effects elicited by these hormones. Much of this work has been carried out in normal tissues and has been descriptive rather than interpretative. In the area of cancer, a number of questions must be considered. What determines acquired or inherent resistance of malignant cells to steroid therapy? Why is the growth of certain tumors dependent on and others independent of steroids? What is the subcellular locus of action of steroid hormones? These are a few questions which serve to highlight some of the unsolved problems in this field of research.

Early studies by DOUGHERTY and WHITE (1945) demonstrated that the regression and dissolution of lymphoid tissues observed after glucocorticoid administration were accompanied by an inhibition of mitosis, and the occurrence of pycnosis and karyorrhexis of lymphocyte nuclei. It is the purpose of this chapter to direct attention to the biochemical basis for the selective action of adrenal corticoids on normal and malignant lymphoid tissues. No attempt will be made to review findings in liver, with the realization that much exciting work in this important area cannot be cited. This presentation deals mainly with rat thymus and the cortisol sensitive and resistant lines of mouse lymphosarcoma P1798. These lymphoid tissues have been studied extensively in recent years, and provide examples of differences between normal and neoplastic tissue, as well as of the problems which remain in this area of research. The references were selected with the intent of citing illustrative examples of the concepts discussed rather than to provide complete documentation.

Biochemical Effects of Glucocorticoids on Lymphoid Tissues

WHITE et al. (1948) demonstrated that the loss of cellular protein from lymphoid organs was not a catabolic effect of adrenal steroids, but rather an antianabolic action. This conclusion was soon confirmed in studies which showed that treatment with glucocorticoids significantly reduced the incorporation of ^{32}P and ^{15}N-glycine into nucleic acids and protein of various types of lymphoid tissues (HULL and WHITE, 1952; KIT et al., 1954; CLARK and STOERK, 1956). More recently, glucocorticoid-responsive lymphoid tissues obtained from animals previously treated with adrenal steroids or exposed to these steroids *in vitro* have been found to undergo an impairment of glucose uptake (MORITA and MUNCK, 1964), inhibition of incorporation of specific radioactive precursors into nucleic acids (MAKMAN et al., 1967) and protein (YOUNG, 1969), and alterations in the activity of several enzymes (ROSEN, 1963). Some of these effects occur rapidly, within 30 min, while others require several days of treatment before they are evident. It is not yet clear which of these effects is causally related to lymphoid tissue atrophy.

The development of techniques to study the effects of glucocorticoids *in vitro* has stimulated investigations of their action in lymphoid tissues. The *in vitro* systems provide a degree of reproducibility and sensitivity which cannot be achieved in studies in the whole animal. MORITA and MUNCK (1964) and MAKMAN et al. (1966) were the first to demonstrate that physiological concentrations of corticosteroids *in vitro* were able to produce biochemical changes in rat thymocytes; similar findings were reported by GABOUREL and ARONOW (1962) in cultured mouse lymphoma cells and in cell suspensions of the cortisol sensitive and resistant lines of lymphosarcoma P1798 (J. ROSEN et al., 1970a).

A. DNA Metabolism

Administration of glucocorticoids to animals or their addition *in vitro* markedly inhibits the incorporation of radioactive thymidine into DNA in both normal

(MORITA and MUNCK, 1964) and malignant lymphoid tissues (J. ROSEN et al., 1970a, b). A similar effect of glucocorticoids has been observed in mouse lymphoma ML 388 (GABOUREL and ARONOW, 1962), mouse fibroblasts grown in culture (PRATT and ARONOW, 1960), and spleen (STEVENS and DOUGHERTY, 1967). Treatment of mice bearing established implants of lymphosarcoma P1798 with cortisol led to a marked reduction of ^{3}H-thymidine incorporation into tumor DNA only in the glucocorticoid-sensitive tumor (J. ROSEN et al., 1970c). Thus cortisol-mediated inhibition of DNA biosynthesis could be correlated with the inhibition of growth and subsequent dissolution of the responsive P1798 tumor. The effect of cortisol on thymidine incorporation in rat thymocytes (MUNCK and WIRA, 1971) and the P1798 tumor (J. ROSEN et al., 1970a) is preceded in time by the impairment of glucose uptake into these cells.

Attempts have been made to explain the selective action and mechanism by which adrenal corticoids affect DNA metabolism in the P1798 tumor (J. ROSEN et al., 1970c). When the purine and pyrimidine precursors of DNA were compared, it was found that cortisol significantly reduced the incorporation of radioactive thymidine and deoxycytidine into DNA. However, only minimal effects on the incorporation of purine precursors into DNA were observed. The low incorporation of deoxyadenosine and deoxyguanosine into tumor DNA suggested that the pool size of these precursors was large or that they were metabolized or diverted into other pathways in addition to that of DNA synthesis. Of interest was the finding that in the tumor, thymidine was a better precursor than deoxycytidine, whereas in rat thymus the opposite was observed.

In other studies on lymphosarcoma P1798, it was possible to rule out inhibition of DNA polymerase activity, alterations in pool size of thymidine, and a decrease in the cellular uptake of ^{3}H-thymidine as factors involved in the depression of DNA metabolism produced by glucocorticoids (J. ROSEN et al., 1970c). Although cortisol, when given to tumor-bearing mice, failed to alter DNA polymerase activity measured in an *in vitro* system with added template, it is conceivable that the hormone could influence the polymerization of deoxynucleoside triphosphates by reacting with the chromatin template. When ^{3}H-thymidine with high specific activity was used as a precursor, cortisol treatment inhibited its transport into rat thymus (MAKMAN et al., 1968), but not into the P1798 tumor (J. ROSEN et al., 1970c); however, the uptake of thymidine with low specific activity into the tumor was impaired by cortisol. Thus, transport might be rate limiting only when blood levels of the nucleoside precursors are high. Under normal conditions, when blood levels of the nucleoside precursor are low, uptake may have little significance since most of the precursor is being synthesized *de novo*. The rate-limiting step in ^{3}H-thymidine incorporation into DNA may be its phosphorylation by specific nucleoside and nucleotide kinases. However, PRATT and ARONOW (1960) have reported no difference in the conversion of thymidine to thymidine triphosphate (TTP) in control and steroid treated mouse fibroblasts. It seems that further studies are necessary in thymus and malignant lymphoid tumors to resolve this problem.

In rats pretreated with cortisol, slices of thymus gland released several times more DNA into the incubation medium than did slices from untreated animals (HAYNES and SUTHERLAND III, 1968). Also, slices of thymus obtained from rats 2 h after cortisol treatment incorporated ^{3}H-thymidine into DNA at only about 50% of the rate of control tissue when 0.01 mM labeled thymidine was added to the incubation medium. However, when ^{3}H-thymidine was present at a concentration of 1 mM in the medium there was no depression in its incorporation into thymus DNA after cortisol was given. MAKMAN et al. (1968) observed that cortisol, added to a suspension of rat thymocytes, impaired the uptake of radioactive thymidine into the TCA-soluble fraction. *In vitro*, cortisol inhibited the uptake of ^{3}H-thymidine into the DNA of P 1798 cells by about 50%, and exerted a smaller (16%) but significant effect on the transport of this pyrimidine.

The effect of steroids on DNA metabolism in lymphoid tissues (J. Rosen et al., 1970c) and fibroblasts (Pratt and Aronow, 1960) has been shown to be specific for compounds with glucocorticoid activity. Treatments of mice bearing the P1798 tumor with large doses of cortisol, testosterone, desoxycorticosterone acetate (DOCA), and estrogen were compared for their effects on DNA metabolism. None of these steroids affected the cellular uptake of ^{3}H-thymidine, and only cortisol significantly depressed the incorporation of this precursor into DNA. Treatment with DOCA stimulated the incorporation of ^{3}H-thymidine into DNA; this may be due to its known feedback inhibition of ACTH release and a consequent suppression of corticosterone secretion from the adrenals (Harding et al., 1961). Estradiol also caused a slight increase in ^{3}H-thymidine uptake into DNA, whereas testosterone was inactive in this regard.

B. RNA and Protein Metabolism

There is a large body of experimental evidence which indicates that hormones are involved in the control of RNA and protein metabolism in responsive tissues. In some instances it appears that hormones act directly on DNA to affect its use as a template for the transcription of RNA, in others the evidence suggests that hormones can influence RNA polymerase activity or the translation of RNA into protein. In target tissues which undergo growth (Gorski et al., 1965) or enzyme induction (Lang and Sekeris, 1964) following hormone administration there is a concomitant stimulation of RNA polymerase activity and an increase in the incorporation of specific precursors into RNA. In contrast, a depression in polymerase activity and RNA biosynthesis is observed in lymphoid tissues which undergo dissolution following exposure to glucocorticoids (Fox and Gabourel, 1967). Actinomycin D, which inhibits DNA mediated RNA synthesis, has been found to prevent many of the characteristic physiological responses elicited by hormones. Although numerous studies with this antibiotic neglected biochemical actions other than its effect on RNA synthesis, it seems evident nevertheless that new RNA synthesis is required for certain responses to hormones.

At present it is not possible to account for differences in the control of RNA and protein synthesis by steroid and peptide hormones, by various hormones in the same class, or even by a single hormone acting on different tissues. Thus, in rat liver, cortisol causes a net increase in the synthesis of rapidly labeled RNA (Kenney et al., 1965) and in the activity of certain adaptive enzymes (Kenney and Kull, 1963), whereas in lymphoid cells there is a catabolic effect on RNA and protein synthesis (J. Rosen et al., 1972). These selective effects argue against a general action of glucocorticoids, for example, on a single enzyme such as RNA polymerase.

Kidson (1965) reported that cortisol (10^{-5} M) exerted an inhibitory effect on RNA synthesis within 5 min after its addition to a suspension of rabbit mesenteric lymph nodes. More complete studies in the same system later revealed that the action of cortisol on RNA synthesis occurred rapidly, and that after a lag period of several minutes, there was a "burst" of protein synthesis, maximal after 15 to 20 min, followed by a decrease in protein synthesis (Kidson, 1967). Subsequent studies by Makman et al. (1966, 1968), employing a suspension of rat thymocytes exposed to physiological concentrations of cortisol (10^{-8} to 10^{-6}M), indicated that this steroid inhibited the incorporation of radioactive precursors into DNA, RNA, and protein, 1 to 3 h after exposure. MAKMAN and coworkers (1966, 1967, 1968) also demonstrated an inhibitory effect of corticosteroids on amino acid transport and on the intracellular accumulation of labeled nucleotides. These results indicate that in rat thymocytes one locus of cortisol action is on the cell membrane, although the question of whether this is a direct or indirect effect needs to be resolved. Moreover, these results suggest that impairment of the cellular uptake of the precursors of nucleic acids and protein can, in part, account for the inhibitory effect of corticosteroids on the biosynthesis of these macromolecules in rat thymocytes.

NAKAGAWA and WHITE (1968) have reported that cortisol administration *in vivo* decreased labeled uridine triphosphate (UTP) incorporation into RNA of isolated thymus nuclei as early as 30 min after treatment. Thus, cortisol appears to have an effect on RNA synthesis, as well as on the cellular uptake of uridine (MAKMAN et al., 1967). A diminished activity of aggregate RNA polymerase (i.e., enzyme plus chromatin template) following cortisol treatment was demonstrated by FOX and GABOUREL (1967). However, the earliest significant inhibition was observed 6 h after administration of 50 mg/kg of cortisol to adrenalectomized rats. In subsequent studies, FOX and GABOUREL (1971) reported that cortisol was influencing the amount or activity of the RNA polymerase enzyme, rather than the chromatin template activity. These results were obtained 12 h after treatment. It is possible that their technique could not detect subtle changes in chromatin template activity. For example, ALLFREY et al. (1966) have demonstrated an inhibitory effect of cortisol *in vitro* on calf thymus histone acetylation, and AMBROSE (1970) has reported an increased binding of actinomycin D to DNA following the exposure of chromatin to cortisol *in vitro*. The physiological significance of both of these studies is uncertain, due to the large concentrations of steroid needed to produce these effects, but they do suggest a possible influence of cortisol on chromatin template activity.

Studies from several laboratories concerning the inhibition of protein synthesis in lymphoid tissue produced by hydrocortisone have indicated an inhibitory effect of this hormone on the microsomal incorporation of labeled amino acids into protein. Thus, decreased capacity to incorporate amino acids into protein has been demonstrated in microsomes of rat thymus 3 h after treatment (PENA et al., 1964), in microsomes of ML-388 lymphoma cells 12 h after treatment (GABOUREL and COMSTOCK, 1964), and in the microsomes of the corticoid sensitive lympho sarcoma P1798 18 h after treatment (HOLLANDER et al., 1967). In the experiments of PENA et al. (1964) the steroid effect was manifested in both the high speed supernatant and the ribosomal fraction, while in those of GABOUREL and COMSTOCK (1964) the biochemical lesion was only found in the ribosomal fraction. Furthermore, GABOUREL and FOX (1965) reported that cortisol treatment led to a decrease in polysome aggregation 6 to 12 h after hormone administration. This phenomenon was not observed by PENA et al. (1964) 3 h after treatment. The reasons for these discrepancies are unclear, but they could reflect the different times following treatment at which these measurements were performed. Studies by UETE (1968) have shown that administration of glucocorticoids to rats inhibited the incorporation of amino acids into proteins of all subcellular fractions of thymus cells, including the nuclei, mitochondria, and microsomes. This effect became apparent within 2 h and could be duplicated in isolated nuclei after exposure to glucocorticoids at concentrations of 10^{-4} to 10^{-6}M. It was concluded that an inhibition of nuclear protein synthesis may play an important role in adrenal corticoid action.

Although synthetic messenger RNA could not overcome the inhibitory effect of adrenal corticoids on microsomal protein synthesis, it has been suggested that RNA synthesis was affected prior to any change in protein synthesis. Thus, KIDSON (1967) has proposed that the first effect of cortisol would be a reduction in the rate of synthesis of rapidly labeled RNA. FEIGELSON and FEIGELSON (1966) have reported a decreased rate of purine nucleotide biosynthesis in thymus and spleen within 2 h after cortisone administration, and a decrease in glycine incorporation into RNA after 2 to 4 h. STEVENS et al. (1969) have demonstrated a decreased incorporation of uridine into both 18S and 28S ribosomal RNA of the corticoid-sensitive lymphosarcoma P1798, at 6 and 18 h after treatment. More recently, STEVENS et al. (1970) have reported a decrease in the *in vivo* labeling of nuclear RNA 6 h after treatment with 9α-fluoroprednisolone, but this effect was not seen when the RNA was labeled *in vitro*. These changes appeared to precede those previously mentioned on microsomal protein synthesis. It has also been reported that the decrease in protein synthesis in rat thymus was accompanied by a decrease in total cytoplasmic particulate RNA (GABOUREL and FOX, 1965). In addition, the data of PRATT et al. (1967) indicated that the cortisol effect on uridine incorporation into RNA in thymocytes was not secondary to dilution of precursor specific activity by an increased intracellular precursor pool. The inhibition of uridine incorporation into RNA was constant at both high and low levels of precursor specific activity. In contrast, the inhibition of deoxycytidine incorporation into DNA was not seen when the labeled precursor was diluted with large amounts of the unlabeled compound. Thus, an effect of cortisol on the pool size of DNA precursors, but not on RNA precursors, was suggested. The effect of cortisol on uridine incorporation into RNA, therefore, represents a true inhibition of RNA synthesis, possibly leading to an inhibition of ribosome assembly from a 45S precursor (STEVENS et al., 1969), and subsequent ribosomal aggregation. In support of this hypothesis, DREWS (1969) reported that glucocorticoids, besides causing a general inhibition of RNA synthesis in thymus, exerted a more specific preferential reduction in the formation of ribosomal RNA. In this study, it was not possible to demonstrate the appearance of new RNA species by DNA-RNA hybridization experiments, or explain the inhibitory effects of cortisol by a dilution of the precursor pool or by an acceleration of RNA breakdown.

Recently, the effect of cortisol *in vitro* on the incorporation of specific precursors into RNA and protein in both the cortisol-sensitive and -resistant lines of lymphosarcoma P1798 has been determined (J. ROSEN et al., 1972). Marked inhibition of ^{3}H-uridine incorporation into RNA (52%) and of ^{14}C-leucine into protein (44%) occurred in the sensitive cells incubated for 3 h in RPMI 1640 (MOORE et al., 1967) culture medium containing cortisol (10^{-6}M). Minimal changes were seen in the incorporation of leucine into protein in cells obtained from the resistant tumor, although a significant effect on uridine uptake (16%) was evident. The effect of cortisol on uridine and leucine incorporation into RNA and protein was shown to be dose dependent and specific for steroids with glucocorticoid activity. In contrast to the failure of cortisol to influence the uptake of ^{3}H-thymidine (J. ROSEN et al., 1970a) or ^{14}C-leucine into the TCA-soluble fraction of P1798 cells, an inhibitory effect of this hormone on ^{3}H-uridine transport into these cells was observed and this effect could be correlated with the inhibition of incorporation of uridine into RNA (J. ROSEN et al., 1972).

Studies on the cellular transport of precursors of macromolecules are extremely difficult to interpret. An investigation of the kinetics of uptake of uridine and leucine into P1798 cells has shown that the entry of these precursors is very rapid. Maximum TCA-soluble radioactivity was found within 5 to 10 min after exposure to labeled precursors. Significant uptake was even observed at 4°. Uptake after a 30 min pulse, therefore, may represent both the cellular influx and efflux of radioactivity. This problem is further complicated because these precursors are metabolized, as well as incorporated into RNA and protein (J. ROSEN et al., 1972).

C. Carbohydrate Metabolism

In as much as maintenance of the structure and function of lymphoid tissues is probably dependent upon energy producing reactions, a number of early investigations were concerned with the effects of steroids on carbohydrate metabolism in normal and malignant tissues. The effects of steroids on anaerobic (BACILA and BARRON, 1954) and aerobic (MILLER, 1954) glycolysis of lymphoid tissue, as well as on the respiration of other tissues (GORDAN et al., 1951) have been described. Hydrocortisone and deoxycorticosterone were compared at unphysiologically high concentrations ($>10^{-5}$M) for their action on several aspects of carbohydrate metabolism in lymphoid cells obtained from rat lymph nodes and thymus, and the Murphy-Sturm lymphosarcoma (JEDEIKIN and WHITE, 1958). In cells derived from each of these sources, both of these steroids, when added *in vitro*, significantly inhibited glucose oxidation, oxygen consumption, and endogenous respiration. Although the administration of deoxycorticosterone does not alter thymus growth or histology, this steroid as well as hydrocortisone, when injected into rats, markedly suppressed the oxidation of ^{14}C-glucose by a suspension of thymocytes, prepared from the steroid treated animals. This finding, and the appreciable influence on carbohydrate metabolism produced by other steroids without glucocorticoid activity, which were examined in this study, suggest that the effects noted were the consequence of the unusually large concentrations of steroids used, and thus are of minimal physiological significance.

The current status and the physiological significance of glucocorticoid-induced changes in glucose utilization in various tissues have recently been discussed in an excellent review by MUNCK (1971). Two observations made in the early 1960's indicated the profound changes in glucose metabolism that could be obtained by cortisol administration: (1) cortisol injected into fasted, adrenalectomized rats produced a sharp increase in blood glucose that was seen in 80 to 100 min (MUNCK and KORITZ, 1962), and (2) cortisol treatment caused a decreased incorporation of radioactivity from glucose into rat thymus gland (BARTLETT et al., 1962). Since then, there have been many reports indicating that physiological amounts of glucocorticoids can exert a significant inhibitory effect on glucose utilization in normal and malignant cells. A similar action of glucocorticoids has been reported for adipose tissue (MUNCK, 1962), mouse ear preparations (MATSUI and PLAGER, 1969), cultured chick duodenum (HIJMANS and MCCARTY, 1969), and mouse fibroblasts grown in culture (GRAY et al., 1970).

Impairment of glucose uptake occurs within 15 to 20 min in rat thymocytes (MUNCK, 1968) and somewhat later (30 to 60 min) in P1798 cells exposed to cortisol (J. ROSEN et al., 1970a). This lag effect is not seen in cultured Novikoff rat hepatoma cells in which prednisolone acts immediately and as a competitive inhibitor of glucose uptake (PLAGEMANN and RENNER, 1972). At present it appears that the earliest biochemical change elicited by glucocorticoids in lymphoid cells is on glucose transport; this precedes the action of this steroid on the incorporation of radioactivity from specific precursors into macromolecules. Studies in several laboratories have demonstrated a requirement for glucose in the incubation medium for maximal incorporation of labeled precursors into protein and nucleic acids (MAKMAN et al., 1967). YOUNG (1969) noted that added glucose was required for continued maximal levels of incorporation of amino acids into protein in rat thymocytes, and that this requirement was only partially satisfied by other readily metabolized carbohydrate substrates such as lactate and pyruvate. In this study, the effect of the hormone was associated with a decreased ability of glucose and other carbohydrates to generate ATP, the effects on ATP in some cases preceding those on incorporation of amino acids into protein. With glucose as a substrate, these effects could be attributed to a prior inhibition of glucose uptake by cortisol. The precise relationship of the small depression in total ATP concentration (10 to 20%) to the inhibition of incorporation of precursors into macromolecules remains uncertain.

Differences exist between thymocytes and cortisol-sensitive P1798 cells with respect to cellular uptake and incorporation of radioactive precursors into nucleic acids, and the extent to which these effects are modified by cortisol and glucose. Incubation of thymocytes in a medium without glucose produced a marked, and essentially similar, depression in the incorporation of ^{3}H-uridine into both the trichloracetic acid-soluble and -insoluble fractions; cortisol added to this system had no significant effect on the cellular transport or incorporation of uridine into RNA (MAKMAN et al., 1968). However, omission of glucose markedly decreased both uridine-^{3}H uptake and incorporation into the TCA-soluble and -insoluble fractions in untreated cell suspensions of the P1798 tumor (J. ROSEN et al., 1972). Thus, glucose is required for the transport and possibly the phosphorylation of uridine in P1798 cells. In a medium lacking glucose, the incorporation of radioactive thymidine into DNA of P1798 cells was inhibited by more than 80%, whereas the uptake of this precursor into the TCA-soluble fraction was reduced by 26%, in comparison to the values obtained when the cells were incubated in a complete medium (J. ROSEN et al., 1970a). When thymocytes were incubated in a complete medium containing cortisol, inhibition of uptake of radioactivity from uridine and thymidine into both the TCA-soluble and -insoluble fractions was approximately equal (MAKMAN et al., 1968).

Table 1 summarizes the role of glucose on the incorporation of precursors into DNA, RNA, and protein of cortisol-sensitive P1798 cells. Cell suspensions were incubated in RPMI 1640 medium containing 2 mg% glucose, or lacking glucose, for 3 h at 37° in an atmosphere of 95% O_2 −5% CO_2 in a metabolic shaking incubator. Omission of glucose from the medium resulted in a 94% reduction of thymidine incorporation into DNA, an 87% reduction of uridine incorporation into RNA, and an 85% reduction of leucine incorporation into protein. The data also show that the maximal inhibitory effect of cortisol on precursor incorporation

Table 1. *Effect of cortisol and glucose on the incorporation of precursors into nucleic acids and protein in the corticosteroid-sensitive lymphosarcoma P 1798*

Precursor[a]	Medium	Control	10^{-6}M Cortisol	Inhibition
		(cpm/10^8 cells)	(cpm/10^8 cells)	
Thymidine-^{3}H, 1 μc	Complete	18,320[b] ± 1,130	9,570 ± 850	48 (p <0.01)
	+Glucose	1,010 ± 60 (−94%)	850 ± 65	16[c]
Uridine-^{3}H, 1 μc	Complete	8,160 ± 450	4,630 ± 160	43 (p <0.01)
	+Glucose	1,030 ± 80 (−87%)	810 ± 60	21 (p <0.05)
Leucine-^{14}C, 0.5 μc	Complete	38,870 ± 340	23,960 ± 420	38 (p <0.01)
	+Glucose	5,800 ± 120 (−85%)	4,420 ± 100	24 (p <0.01)

[a] Added 30 min prior to end of 3 h incubation.
[b] Each value represents the mean of 3 to 5 individual determinations.
[c] Not significant p >0.05.

occurred in glucose enriched medium. It can be concluded that a source of energy is required to maintain optimum rates of nucleic acid and protein biosynthesis, and to obtain a significant catabolic effect of glucocorticoids on the synthesis of these macromolecules in P1798 cells.

It has been proposed that adrenal corticoids act either directly or indirectly on glucose uptake or phosphorylation in various target tissues. Young (1969) has reported that cortisol in thymocytes causes a small but reproducible drop in intracellular ATP levels. Thus, an effect of glucocorticoids on intracellular glucose phosphorylation as suggested by Munck (1968) might be due to the reduced availability of ATP for the conversion of glucose to glucose-6-phosphate, rather than to a direct effect of the hormone on hexokinase activity. J. Rosen et al. (1970b) have reported that there is no change in lymphosarcoma P1798 hexokinase activity at times when there is a significant impairment of ^{14}C-deoxyglucose uptake, after both *in vivo* or *in vitro* exposure of these cells to dexamethasone. In the same study, it was observed that the ATP concentration decreased by 10 to 20% in P1798 cells within 3 h after exposure to the hormone, but that at 1 h no significant changes in ATP levels could be detected. Since the inhibitory effect of glucocorticoids on glucose uptake is seen within 1 h it is not clear whether the reduction in ATP content is the cause of, or results from, reduced glucose uptake.

There is evidence from studies in yeast that a membrane phosphorylating system, which utilizes a polyphosphate donor, is associated with an active transport system for glucose (van Steveninck, 1958). Such a mechanism is different from the earlier view of a passive transport of glucose followed by intracellular phosphorylation by the hexokinase enzyme. A phosphotransferase system has also been described for bacteria (Kundig et al., 1966; Simoni et al., 1967), and appears to be involved in transmembrane sugar transport. Thus, an effect of glucocorticoids on membrane phosphorylation cannot be ruled out.

Transport changes could also depend indirectly on the synthesis of specific RNA species which direct the synthesis of one or more proteins affecting the cell membrane. These proteins may be specific carrier proteins, or enzymes directly involved in energy production. This hypothesis has been advanced to explain the stimulatory action of testosterone on glucose and amino acid uptake into rat sex accessory tissues (Mills and Spaziani, 1968). Smith and Gorski (1968) have shown that estradiol stimulates glucose uptake into rat uterus and that cycloheximide abolished this effect, implying the requirement for prior protein synthesis. Also, Kono (1969) has reported that the insulin mediated glucose transport system in isolated fat cells is dependent on a rapidly renewable peptide located on the cell surface. Further support for the validity of this concept in lymphoid cells comes from recent reports by Makman et al. (1971) and Hallahan et al. (1971) indicating that the action of cortisol on the uptake of hexoses, including 2-deoxyglucose, in rat thymocytes is mediated through the induction of a specific protein inhibitor or inhibitors. In contrast, data obtained in P1798 cells suggest that inhibition of protein synthesis may be involved in the mechanism by which cortisol influences the transport of glucose into these cells (J. Rosen et al., 1972). In the absence of cortisol, Makman et al. (1971) did not observe an inhibitory effect of cycloheximide and actinomycin D on the uptake of 2-deoxyglucose into rat thymocytes, but this was clearly the case with P1798 cells. In the presence of cortisol, these antibiotics either prevented or reversed the inhibitory action of the steroid on the transport of several compounds into thymocytes (Makman et al., 1971), but did not significantly alter the effect of cortisol on 2-deoxyglucose uptake by P1798 cells (J. Rosen et al., 1972). It remains to be determined if differences in methodology (e.g., in studies on the P1798 tumor a complete tissue culture medium was used, whereas the rat thymocytes were incubated in a balanced salt solution containing glucose) can account for these striking differences between normal and malignant lymphoid cells in their response to certain antibiotics.

D. Changes in Enzyme Activity

Certain enzymes in liver which are inducible by adrenal corticoids also increase in activity in thymus and lymphosarcoma P1798 following cortisol administration. For example, this was the case with alanine-α-ketoglutarate transaminase. Aspartate-α-ketoglutarate transaminase, however, was unresponsive to cortisol treatment in these tissues. Changes in alanine transaminase which occur in various physiological and pathological conditions, as well as after glucocorticoid administration, may indicate that this enzyme is involved in the regulation of growth of target tissues (ROSEN, 1963). The increase in alanine transaminase activity observed in these tissues, however, occurred only after four daily treatments with the steroid and therefore its significance with respect to cortisol mediated lymphocytolysis is unclear.

Numerous investigators have attempted to explain the reduced incorporation of precursors into nucleic acids and protein following glucocorticoid administration by an increase in lysosomal hydrolases. A relationship between tumor regression and acid ribonuclease activity in lymphosarcoma P1798 following glucocorticoid treatment has been demonstrated (MCLEOD et al., 1963; AMBELLAN and HOLLANDER, 1966). Ribonuclease activity was enhanced significantly 18 h following a 25 mg/kg dose of 9α-fluoroprednisolone in the corticoid-sensitive tumor, but was only minimally affected in the resistant tumor. Other therapeutic agents, including vinblastine, 5-fluorouracil, and methotrexate, were also shown to cause an increase in ribonuclease activity in the appropriate subline of the tumor that underwent regression. WIERNIK (1970) has recently disputed the conclusion that increased ribonuclease activity is necessary for tumor regression. He observed no increase in ribonuclease activity during vinblastine-induced or starvation-induced regression. NAKAGAWA et al. (1968) were unable to detect changes in either acid or alkaline ribonuclease activity in rat thymus three hours after treatment with cortisol. However, in this study, the activity of β-glucuronidase, deoxyribonuclease II, and acid phosphatase was elevated at 3 h in the 700 × g supernatant fraction, and after 20 h a marked elevation of all of these enzymes was seen in both the supernatant and 700 × g pellet. CSEH et al. (1958) have also demonstrated a doubling in deoxyribonuclease II in thymus and lymph nodes of rats 24 h following a large i.p. dose of cortisol. RAINA and ROSEN (1969) have observed a two-fold elevation in deoxyribonuclease II in the cortisol-sensitive lymphosarcoma P1798, and no significant change in the resistant tumor, 16 h after cortisol treatment. NAKAGAWA and coworkers (1968) have suggested that the changes in hydrolase activity induced by corticosteroids are due to an increased release from the lysosomal fraction, and an apparent selective retention of these enzymes when extensive tissue protein loss is taking place. They have also indicated that the increase in deoxyribonuclease activity occurred in the cytoplasm and not in the nucleus, and have suggested that alterations in hydrolase levels in response to cortisol injection were a consequence of an influx of significant numbers of cell types other than lymphocytes in response to the initiation of lymphokaryorrhexis.

Glucocorticoid Receptors

The foregoing discussion clearly reveals that adrenal corticoids can exert multiple biochemical effects on lymphoid tissues. The earliest biochemical alteration yet noticed appears to be an inhibition of glucose transport, followed by inhibition of incorporation of radioactivity from specific precursors into DNA, RNA, and protein. This sequence of effects places impairment of glucose transport in a key position with regard to the later effects on nucleic acid and protein metabolism, but does not reveal the primary action of the hormone which initiates these events.

It is becoming increasingly evident that the primary action of hormones is mediated by interaction with specific receptor molecules in cells of target tissues. A major advance in this area of hormone research was made by GLASCOCK and HOEKSTRA in 1959 and JENSEN and JACOBSON in 1960 when they prepared tritium labeled estrogens of extremely high specific activity. Both groups reported that when physiological doses of ^{3}H-17β-estradiol were administered to immature rats, target tissues such as uterus and vagina showed greater uptake and more prolonged retention of the hormone than nontarget tissues such as blood and liver, which showed an initial uptake, followed by a rapid loss of the labeled steroid. The association of estradiol with its target tissues showed specificity since the bound radioactivity could be reduced by estrone and estradiol but not by non-estrogenic steroids such as progesterone, cortisol, and testosterone. Furthermore, the binding of estrogen in uterus was blocked by certain antiuterotrophic compounds such as nafoxidine (Upjohn 11,100) and ethamoxytriphetol (Mer-25), and this effect probably explains the inhibition of uterine growth when these substances are administered with estradiol (JENSEN et al., 1967).

Although much of our basic information on steroid receptor molecules was obtained with the estradiol-uterine tissue model system, the generality of these observations is apparent from recent reports on other steroid hormones. The macromolecular component which binds estradiol as well as other steroid hormones appears to be protein in nature, since incubation of the receptor-hormone complex with proteolytic enzymes, but not with DNase or RNase, leads to the release of free hormone (KIRKPATRICK et al., 1971). Differential centrifugation has been used to demonstrate the presence of steroid hormone-receptor complexes in both the cytoplasmic and nuclear fractions, whereas protein hormones bind to receptors located at the cell surface (KONO and BARHAM, 1971). The initial binding of the steroid occurs in the cytosol, but within minutes the steroid-receptor complex can be detected in the nucleus (MUNCK and WIRA, 1971). In target tissues obtained from rats, the cytoplasmic steroid hormone-receptor complexes sediment in a 5 to 20% sucrose density gradient at 6.5 to 8S and 3.5 to 4S under conditions of low salt, and at 3.5 to 4S when 0.15 to 0.3 M salt is used for extraction (GIANNOPOULOS and GORSKI, 1971). Steroid-receptor complexes in the nucleus sediment at 3.5 to 5S, following extraction with a medium containing a high concentration of salt. A temperature dependent "two-step" mechanism for the transfer of hormone bound in the cytosol to the nucleus was first demonstrated for estradiol by JENSEN et al. (1968), and appears to be operative for other steroid hormones as well. The results of these studies are compatible with the suggestion (JENSEN et al., 1972) that the hormone-receptor (3.5 to 5S) isolated from the nucleus is derived from the 3.5 to 4S subunit of the 6.5 to 8S receptor in the cytoplasm. Evidence for such a mechanism has also come from *in vitro* experiments in which the cytoplasmic steroid-macromolecular complex is transferred to the nuclei of the same tissue when these fractions are incubated together at 37°.

Several possibilities have been proposed to explain the functional role of the "receptor" molecule in mediating the action of steroid hormones. The "receptor" may function as a repressor in the nucleus, and its attachment to the steroid is required for its transport from the cytoplasm to the nucleus. Conversely, the "receptor" may function as a messenger for the transfer of the steroid into the nucleus, where after dissociation from the "receptor" the hormone acts directly on chromatin. The most likely explanation is that the hormone-receptor complex is functionally active in the nucleus. The recent investigations by E. V. Jensen (personal communication) which indicate that the estradiol-receptor complex of the cytosol can stimulate RNA synthesis in uterine nuclei strongly supports this mode of action. The fact that the progesterone-receptor complex of chick cytosol binds specifically to chick oviduct nuclei also suggests that the complex rather than either of its components is the biologically active molecule (Spelsberg et al., 1971).

The demonstration and characterization of steroid hormone receptors has been investigated *in vivo*, in whole cell studies *in vitro*, and in cell-free studies *in vitro*. At each of these levels of investigation certain criteria must be met to insure that the steroid is interacting specifically and, if possible, with the macromolecular component that may be involved in its physiological action. For example, the tissues of an animal contain a variety of potential steroid binding components. Macromolecules which can specifically bind steroid hormones, but which are unrelated to the physiological response, include proteins involved in the transport of the steroid to the cell such as the corticosteroid-binding globulin (transcortin) of serum (Westphal and de Venuto, 1966) or enzymes involved in the metabolism of steroid. Cellular components which may bind nonspecifically include lipid or membrane components in which the steroid is dissolved, or serum albumin which binds most steroid hormones (Westphal, 1971). In addition, animal studies are complicated by differences in distribution of steroids due to variations in vascularity of tissues which might limit steroid uptake.

A. Studies in Animals

It has been difficult so far to demonstrate selective uptake and retention of radioactive glucocorticoids in target tissues in whole animal experiments. Bottoms and Goetsch (1967) studied the distribution of ^{3}H-corticosterone in the brain, thymus, heart, and liver of rats 30 min after the steroid was injected intravenously. A comparison of the tissue/blood ratio of radioactivity of thymus with tissues (brain and heart) not recognized as being responsive to this hormone indicated that the thymus had the lowest ratio. Similar studies were performed by Bellamy et al. (1962); 30 min after the injection of ^{3}H-cortisol into rats, the highest levels of radioactivity were present in liver and kidney, whereas the submaxillary and parotid glands, skeletal muscle, and brain contained significantly less. Munck (1968) has reported that the magnitude of total steroid uptake by thymocytes shows no correlation with glucocorticoid activity. Based on these findings, he has recently concluded that the inability to show differences between target and nontarget tissues *in vivo* is due to the high degree of nonspecific binding of glucocorticoids to these tissues and/or to the fact that most tissues are somewhat responsive to the adrenal corticoids (Munck, 1968).

B. Whole Cell Studies in Vitro

Glucocorticoid binding has been studied in HeLa cells, which show induction of alkaline phosphatase following exposure to corticosteroids (Melnykovych and Bishop, 1971). At 1° the major portion of the specifically bound steroid was localized in the cytosol, whereas at 37° the radioactivity was found mainly in the nucleus. Wira and Munck (1970) recently reported that most of the specific binding of glucocorticoids in thymocytes occurs in the nuclear fraction when the cells are incubated at 37°. Schaumberg (1970), using different methods, also has shown that at 37° nearly all of the corticosterone binding component in rat thymocytes is located in the nucleus, while at 4° a substantial amount of the steroid-receptor complex is retained in the cytoplasm. Even after incubation for 16 h at 4°, there was no additional increase in nuclear binding. The results of these studies are essentially similar to those described above for estradiol, with regard to the intracellular localization and temperature-dependent movement of the steroid-receptor complex into the nucleus.

HACKNEY et al. (1970) have reported that glucocorticoid-resistant mouse fibroblasts grown in culture, bind less ^{3}H-triamcinolone acetonide in a specific manner than the sensitive line of these cells. Specificity of binding was determined by displacement of bound radioactive triamcinolone acetonide by cortisol, but not by its inactive isomer 11α-cortisol. The binding component became saturated between 10^{-8} and 5×10^{-8}M triamcinolone acetonide, a concentration range which also gave maximum inhibition of growth of these fibroblasts. BAXTER et al. (1971) have presented evidence for the existence of glucocorticoid receptors in lymphoid derived cells grown in tissue culture. To maintain the viability of these cells in culture, the binding studies were done in a medium containing serum proteins including transcortin which is known to bind glucocorticoids specifically. The presence of serum proteins in tissue culture media makes it difficult to evaluate the specificity of binding achieved in these experiments. The possibility also exists that at 37° some of the steroids used in this work might undergo metabolism to yield metabolites with altered affinity constants for the binding components.

With the use of ^{3}H-triamcinolone acetonide of high specific activity, it was possible to determine the sedimentation coefficients of glucocorticoid-binding macromolecules in rat thymocytes (KAISER et al., 1972). Cells incubated at 0° or 37°, and extracted with a high salt buffer, yielded a glucocorticoid-receptor complex with a coefficient of $\sim$4S, whereas cells incubated at 0° and extracted with low salt buffer yielded two components with sedimentation coefficients of $\sim$3.5S and 6.5S. When the cells were incubated at 37° and extracted with the low salt medium, no glucocorticoid-receptor complex could be demonstrated. However, when the $27{,}000 \times g$ pellet of this low salt preparation was treated with high salt, a 3.5S complex was found. Thus, like other steroid hormones, the distribution and sedimentation coefficients of the glucocorticoid-receptor complexes in rat thymocytes are dependent on the ionic strength of the medium and the incubation temperature.

Employing essentially the methodology described by HACKNEY et al. (1970), studies in the cortisol-sensitive and -resistant lines of the P1798 tumor revealed the specificity, distribution, and certain of the characteristics of the macromolecular component which formed a complex with ^{3}H-triamcinolone acetonide (KIRKPATRICK et al., 1971). Cell suspensions used in these studies were isolated from solid tumors, and were washed and incubated in RPMI 1640 culture medium that did not contain serum protein, thus avoiding the problem of specific binding that can occur with transcortin. Of the total ^{3}H-triamcinolone acetonide bound specifically in the sensitive tumor, more than 70% was present in the high speed ($105000 \times g$) supernatant fraction, and the remainder in the sediment of this fraction which contained 98% of the cellular DNA. In adrenalectomized mice there was a significantly greater amount of total triamcinolone bound to the soluble macromolecular fraction. The binding of cortisol, indicated by the displacement of ^{3}H-triamcinolone acetonide, appeared to be related to the concentration of this steroid required to inhibit deoxyglucose uptake and thymidine incorporation into tumor DNA. When the cells were incubated at 4°, about 75% of the bound ^{3}H-triamcinolone acetonide was recovered in the cytoplasmic fraction, whereas at 37° about 70% of the radioactivity was found in the nuclear fraction. The distribution of the receptor-^{3}H-triamcinolone acetonide complex was essentially the same in the resistant and sensitive neoplasms, but in the resistant tumor only 30 to 55% of the total labeled steroid was bound.

C. Broken-Cell System

The advantages of a cell-free system for studying steroid receptors are as follows: (1) the data would not be dependent on the metabolic state of the cells, (2) it would obviate the influence of steroid transport through the cell membrane on intracellular binding, (3) if carried out at low temperatures, it would rule out the metabolism of the steroid as a basis for differences in binding, and (4) it could be used for measuring the binding of glucocorticoids to various human lymphoid tumors which are difficult to prepare as cell suspensions and to maintain in a viable state. The instability of glucocorticoid-binding macromolecules in cell-free systems derived from lymphoid tissues has been observed in several laboratories. Schaumberg (1970) noted in rat thymus that the velocity of dissociation of the corticosterone-macromolecular complex was greater in cell-free preparations than in whole cells. Wira and Munck (1970) were unable to show a significant amount of binding of cortisol to the "receptor" isolated from rat thymus. Recently, Hackney and Pratt (1971) were unable to accomplish rebinding of triamcinolone acetonide to the specific binding component partially purified from mouse fibroblasts.

Studies on lymphosarcoma P1798 by Hollander and Chiu (1966) indicated that cortisol bound in a cell-free system was not displaceable by the potent glucocorticoid, 9α-fluoroprednisolone. When attempts were made to develop a cell-free system for studying glucocorticoid binding in the P1798 tumor (Kirkpatrick et al., 1972), it was noted that the $105000 \times g$ supernatant fraction bound less than 5% of the amount bound when whole cells were incubated with the steroid at 37°. However, when triamcinolone acetonide was present in the medium at the time of cell breakage at 4°, or added immediately after the cells were broken, it protected the binding component from spontaneous degradation. It is unlikely that stabilization with the steroid is due to protection of the binding component from enzymatic digestion since the incubation is carried out at 4°. For this reason, it appears that in the absence of steroid there is a conformational change in the glucocorticoid binding component, leading to a loss in this binding capacity. The specificity of this system with regard to displacement of the bound triamcinolone acetonide by cortisol and 11α-cortisol was comparable to that seen in whole cells. Thus, adrenalectomy caused a significant increase in specific binding, and the resistant tumor bound only 64% as much triamcinolone acetonide as the sensitive neoplasm, in the cell-free system. Of considerable interest was the finding that in the broken cell preparations of target and nontarget organs, tissue specific binding could be detected. Thus, thymus of either mouse or rat bound about 3 times more ^{3}H-triamcinolone acetonide than the corresponding fraction from either testis or cerebral cortex.

Possible Mechanism of Action and Basis for Resistance to Glucocorticoids

Although an impressive amount of new information on the biochemical effects and on the distribution and physical characteristics of the glucocorticoid "receptor" in lymphoid tissues including tumors has been accumulated in recent years, it is still not possible to relate these findings to the mode of action of this class of steroids. The data which are available at present, both for thymus and P1798 cells, are consistent with the following sequence of events: (1) binding of the steroid to its specific "receptor" and movement of this complex into the nucleus, (2) an effect of the steroid-receptor complex on chromatin, possibly to alter the synthesis or activity of a substance involved in glucose uptake, and (3) as a consequence of impaired glucose metabolism, the inhibition of nucleic acid and protein biosynthesis leading to cell lysis. The site of action of glucocorticoids and other steroid hormones appears to be in the nucleus, and at the level of transcription. The specificity of the interaction of the progesterone-receptor complex with the acidic proteins but not with the histones bound to chick oviduct chromatin, represents a significant advance in our understanding of hormone action at the molecular level (SPELSBERG et al., 1971). Further progress in this area awaits the development of very sensitive methods for detecting minor changes in chromatin template activity.

A better understanding of the role of the hormone-receptor complex may come from additional studies on the mechanism by which inactive analogs of steroid hormones act as steroid antagonists. The present evidence suggests that these compounds compete with the biologically active hormone for a site on the receptor molecule. Subsequent to this interaction, the fate of such a complex is unknown. For example, does it penetrate the nucleus but lack the required structural conformation for biological activity? Apart from the potential of such agents in hormone mechanism studies, their therapeutic possibilities in preventing the adverse effects of increased hormone secretion or in impairing the growth of hormone-dependent tumors should not be overlooked. In addition, any treatment which blocks the formation of the hormone-receptor complex or which might stimulate biosynthesis of the "receptor" deserves study.

The availability of cell lines in culture (HACKNEY et al., 1970; BAXTER et al., 1971) and of lymphosarcoma P1798, which are both sensitive and resistant to glucocorticoids, provide experimental systems in which the biochemical changes, seen following exposure to the hormone, can be related to the inhibition of cell growth. Use of resistant cells serves as a control for the nonspecific and nonphysiological responses to glucocorticoid treatment.

Previous studies in our laboratory (CHANG et al., 1964) and by HOLLANDER and CHIU (1966) have shown that the glucocorticoid sensitivity and resistance of the two lines of lymphosarcoma P1798 could not be explained by differences in uptake, subcellular distribution, or metabolism of cortisol. The metabolic sensitivities of the responsive and resistant P1798 tumors to the same concentration of cortisol have been shown to differ by a factor larger than the difference between the relative number of binding sites in these tumors (KIRKPATRICK et al., 1972). In view of this relationship, it cannot be concluded that steroid resistance is due solely to the lack of specific binding sites. However, such a mechanism has recently been proposed to explain the dependency on estradiol for the sustained growth of the DMBA induced mammary rat tumor, and the lack of this hormonal requirement by the R3230AC mammary tumor (MCGUIRE et al., 1971). Other mechanisms which could explain resistance to a hormone include (1) an altered physical conformation of the receptor, either before or after binding by the hormone, (2) failure of the receptor-hormone complex to penetrate the nucleus and (3) failure of the steroid receptor complex to interact with a specific component (e.g. acidic protein) in chromatin. The recently acquired information on hormone action has led to questions which appear to be relevant to the problem of hormone dependency and resistance in endocrine tumors, as well as to the solution of other contemporary problems in endocrinology.

References

Allfrey, V. G., Pogo, B. G. T., Pogo, A. O., Kleinsmith, L. J., Mirsky, A. E.: The metabolic behaviour of chromatin. In: Histones: their role in the transfer of genetic information. Boston: Little, Brown and Co. 1966.

Ambellan, E., Hollander, V. P.: The role of ribonuclease in regression of lymphosarcoma P1798. Cancer Res. **26**, 903—909 (1966).

Ambrose, C. T.: Optical rotary dispersion (ORD) measurements of actinomycin D (AD) binding to chromatin and DNA in the presence of cortisol and other steroids. Fed. Proc. **29**, 470 (1970).

Bacila, M., Barron, E. S. G.: The effect of adrenal cortical hormones on the anaerobic glycolysis and hexokinase activity. Endocrinology **54**, 591—603 (1954).

Bartlett, D., Morita, Y., Munck, A.: Rapid inhibition by cortisol of incorporation of glucose *in vivo* into the thymus of the rat. Nature (Lond.) **196**, 897—898 (1962).

Baxter, J. D., Harris, A. W., Tomkins, G. M., Cohn, M.: Glucocorticoid receptors in lymphoma cells in culture: relationship to glucocorticoid killing activity. Science **171**, 189—191 (1971).

Bellamy, D., Phillips, J. G., Jones, I. C., Leonard, R. A.: The uptake of cortisol by rat tissues. Biochem. J. **85**, 537—545 (1962).

Bottoms, G., Goetsch, D. D.: Subcellular distribution of the (^{3}H) corticosterone fraction in brain, thymus, heart, and liver of the rat. Proc. Soc. exp. Biol. (N. Y.) **124**, 662—665 (1967).

Bruchovsky, N., Wilson, J. D.: The conversion of testosterone to 5α-androstan-17β-ol-3-one by rat prostate *in vivo* and *in vitro*. J. biol. Chem. **243**, 2012—2021 (1968).

Chang, E., Mittelman, A., Rosen, F.: The metabolism *in vitro* of 4-^{14}C cortisone by lymphosarcoma P1798. Biochim. biophys. Acta (Amst.) **90**, 600—605 (1964).

Clark, I., Stoerk, H. C.: The uptake of P^{32} by nucleic acids of lymphoid tissue undergoing atrophy. J. biol. Chem. **222**, 285—292 (1956).

Cseh, G., Marosvari, I., Harmath, A.: Effect of corticosteroids on deoxyribonuclease in lymphoid organs. Acta Physiol. (Budapest) **14**, 115—126 (1958).

Dougherty, T. F., White, A.: Functional alterations in lymphoid tissue induced by adrenal corticoid secretion. Amer. J. Anat. **77**, 81—116 (1945).

Drews, J.: The effect of prednisolone injected *in vivo* on RNA synthesis in rat thymus cells. European J. Biochem. **7**, 200—208 (1969).

Feigelson, M., Feigelson, P.: Relationships between hepatic enzyme induction, glutamate formation, and purine nucleotide biosynthesis in glucocorticoid action. J. biol. Chem. **241**, 5819—5826 (1966).

Fox, K. E., Gabourel, J. D.: Effect of cortisol on the RNA polymerase systems of rat thymus. Molec. Pharmacol. **3**, 479—486 (1967).

Gabourel, J. D., Aronow, L.: Growth inhibitory effects of hydrocortisone on mouse lymphoma ML-388 *in vitro*. J. pharmacol. exp. Ther. **136**, 213—221 (1962).

Gabourel, J. D., Comstock, J. P.: Effect of hydrocortisone on amino acid incorporation by microsomes isolated from mouse lymphoma ML-388 cells and rat thymus. Biochem. Pharmacol. **13**, 1369—1376 (1964).

Gabourel, J. D., Fox, K. E.: Effect of hydrocortisone on the size of rat thymus polysomes. Biochem. biophys. Res. Comm. **18**, 81—86 (1965).

Gabourel, J. D., Fox, K. E.: On the site of cortisol inhibition of thymus ribonucleic acid synthesis. Biochem. Pharmacol. **20**, 885—895 (1971).

Giannopoulos, G., Gorski, J.: Estrogen-binding protein of the rat uterus. Different molecular forms associated with nuclear uptake of estradiol. J. biol. Chem. **246**, 2530—2536 (1971).

Glascock, R. F., Hoekstra, W. G.: Selective accumulation of tritium-labelled hexoestrol by the reproductive organs of immature female goats and sheep. Biochem. J. **72**, 673—682 (1959).

Gordan, G. S., Bentinck, R. C., Eisenberg, E.: The influence of steroids on cerebral metabolism. Ann. N. Y. Acad. Sci. **54**, 575—607 (1951).

Gorski, J., Noteboom, W. D., Nicolette, J. A.: Estrogen control of the synthesis of RNA and protein in the uterus. J. cell. comp. Physiol. **66**, 91—110 (1965).

Gray, J. G., Aronow, L., Pratt, W. B.: Effect of glucocorticoids on hexose uptake in mouse fibroblasts. Proc. Amer. Assoc. Cancer Res. **11**, 32 (1970).

Hackney, J. F., Gross, S. R., Aronow, L., Pratt, W. B.: Specific glucocorticoid-binding macromolecules from mouse fibroblasts growing *in vitro*. A possible steroid receptor for growth inhibition. Molec. Pharmacol. **6**, 500—512 (1970).

Hackney, J. F., Pratt, W. B.: Characterization and partial purification of the specific glucocorticoid-binding component from mouse fibroblasts. Biochemistry **10**, 3002—3008 (1971).

Hallahan, C., Young, D. A., Munck, A.: Evidence for a protein synthetic step in the early action of cortisol on glucose uptake in rat thymus tissue. Fed. Proc. **30**, 308 (1971).

HARDING, H. R., ROSEN, F., NICHOL, C. A.: Inhibition of hepatic alanine transaminase activity in response to treatment with 11-deoxycorticosterone. Proc. Soc. exp. Biol. (N.Y.) **108**, 96—99 (1961).
HAYNES, R. C., Jr., SUTHERLAND III, E. W.: Altered metabolism of DNA in rat thymus, an early response to cortisol. Endocrinology **80**, 297—301 (1967).
HERMAN, T. S., FIMOGNARI, G. M., EDELMAN, I. S.: Studies in renal aldosterone-binding proteins. J. biol. Chem. **243**, 3849—3856 (1968).
HIJMANS, J. C., MCCARTY, K. S.: Effect of hydrocortisone on chick duodenum cultured in chemically defined medium. Proc. Soc. exp. Biol. (N.Y.) **131**, 1407—1412 (1969).
HOFERT, J. F., WHITE, A.: Effect of a single injection of cortisol on the incorporation of ^{3}H-thymidine and ^{3}H-deoxycytidine into lymphatic tissue DNA of adrenalectomized rats. Endocrinology **82**, 767—776 (1968).
HOLLANDER, N., CHIU, Y. W.: *In vitro* binding of cortisol-1,2-^{3}H by a substance in the supernatant fraction of P1798 mouse lymphosarcoma. Biochem. biophys. Res. Commun. **25**, 291—297 (1966).
HOLLANDER, V. P., GORDON, C., HOLLANDER, N.: Effects of corticoid injection and of adrenalectomy on *in vitro* amino acid incorporation into microsomes of P1798 lymphosarcoma. Nature (Lond.) **213**, 1036—1037 (1967).
HULL, W., WHITE, A.: Effects of adrenocorticotrophic hormone on the phosphorous metabolism of lymphoid tissue. Endocrinology **51**, 210—216 (1952).
JEDEIKIN, L. A., WHITE, A.: *In vitro* and *in vivo* effects of steroids on glucose oxidation and respiration by normal and malignant lymphoid tissue. Endocrinology **63**, 226—236 (1958).
JENSEN, E. V., BLOCK, G. E., SMITH, S., KYSER, K., DE SOMBRE, E. R.: Estrogen receptors and hormone dependency. In: Estrogen target tissues and neoplasia. Chicago: University of Chicago Press 1972.
JENSEN, E. V., DE SOMBRE, E. R., JUNGBLUT, P. W.: Interaction of estrogens with receptor sites *in vivo* and *in vitro*. In: Proceedings of the second international congress on hormonal steroids, Milan 1966. Amsterdam: Excerpta Medica Foundation 1967.
JENSEN, E. V., JACOBSON, H. I.: Fate of steroid estrogens in target tissues. In: Biological activity of steroids in relation to cancer. New York: Academic Press 1960.
JENSEN, E. V., JACOBSON, H. I.: Basic guides to the mechanism of estrogen action. Rec. Progr. Hormone Res. **18**, 387—414 (1962).
KAISER, N., KIRKPATRICK, A. F., MILHOLLAND, R. J., ROSEN, F.: Sedimentation coefficients of glucocorticoid-binding macromolecules in rat thymocytes. Fed. Proc. (1972).
KENNEY, T., KULL, F. J.: Hydrocortisone-stimulated synthesis of nuclear RNA in enzyme induction. Proc. nat. Acad. Sci. (Wash.) **50**, 493—499 (1963).
KENNEY, F. T., WICKS, W. D., GREENMAN, D. L.: Hydrocortisone stimulation of RNA synthesis in induction of hepatic enzymes. J. cell. comp. Physiol. **66**, 125—136 (1965).
KIDSON, C.: Kinetics of cortisol action on RNA synthesis. Biochem. biophys. Res. Comm. **21**, 283—289 (1965).
KIDSON, C.: Cortisol in the regulation of RNA and protein synthesis. Nature (Lond.) **213**, 779—782 (1967).
KIRKPATRICK, A. F., MILHOLLAND, R. J., ROSEN, F.: Stereospecific glucocorticoid binding to subcellular fractions of the sensitive and resistant lymphosarcoma P 1798. Nature (Lond.) **232**, 216—218 (1971).
KIRKPATRICK, A. F., KAISER, N., MILHOLLAND, R. J., ROSEN, F.: Glucocorticoid-binding macromolecules in normal tissues and tumors. Stabilization of the specific binding component. J. biol. Chem. **247**, 70—74 (1972).
KIT, S., BACILA, M., BARRON, E. S. G.: The incorporation of ^{32}P into the nucleic acids of lymphatic cells *in vitro*. Effect of adrenal cortical hormones (Compound F). Biochim. biophys. Acta (Amst.) **13**, 516—524 (1954).
KONO, T.: Destruction and restoration of the insulin effector system of isolated fat cells. J. biol. Chem. **244**, 5777—5784 (1969).
KONO, T., BARHAM, F. W.: Insulin-like effects of trypsin on fat cells. Localization of the metabolic steps and the cellular site affected by the enzyme. J. biol. Chem. **246**, 6204—6209 (1971).
KUNDIG, W., KUNDIG, F. D., ANDERSON, B., ROSEMAN, S.: Restoration of active transport of glycosides in *Escherichia coli* by a component of a phosphotransferase system. J. biol. Chem. **241**, 3243—3246 (1966).
LANG, N., SEKERIS, C. E.: Stimulation of RNA-polymerase activity in rat liver by cortisol. Life Sci. **3**, 391—393 (1964).
LUNDIN, P. M.: Anterior pituitary gland and lymphoid tissue growth. Acta Endocrinol. Suppl. **40**, 1—80 (1958).
MACLEOD, R. M., KING, C. E., HOLLANDER, V. P.: Effect of corticosteroids on ribonuclease and nucleic acid content in lymphosarcoma P1798. Cancer Res. **23**, 1045—1050 (1963).

Makman, M. H., Dvorkin, B., White, A.: Alterations in protein and nucleic acid metabolism of thymocytes produced by adrenal steroids *in vitro*. J. biol. Chem. **241**, 1646—1648 (1966).
Makman, M. H., Dvorkin, B., White, A.: Influence of cortisol on the utilization of precursors of nucleic acids and protein by lymphoid cells *in vitro*. J. biol. Chem. **243**, 1485—1497 (1968).
Makman, M. H., Dvorkin, B., White, A.: Evidence for induction by cortisol *in vitro* of a protein inhibitor of transport and phosphorylation processes in rat thymocytes. Proc. nat. Acad. Sci. (Wash.) **68**, 1269—1273 (1971).
Makman, M. H., Nakagawa, S., White, A.: Studies of the mode of action of adrenal steroids on lymphocytes. Rec. Progr. Hormone Res. **23**, 195—227 (1967).
Matsui, N., Plager, J. E.: "Anti-insulin" action of cortisol. I. Influence of cortisol on the metabolism of specifically labeled glucose, pyruvate and glucose-6-phosphate. Endocrinology **84**, 1439—1449 (1969).
McGuire, W. L., Julian, J. A., Chamness, G. C.: A dissociation between ovarian dependent growth and estrogen sensitivity in mammary carcinoma. Endocrinology **89**, 969—973 (1971).
Melnykovych, G., Bishop, C. F.: Specific binding of cortisol in subcellular fractions of HeLa cells: temperature dependence and effects of inhibitors. Endocrinology **88**, 450—455 (1971).
Miller, Z.: A study of the lymphocytolytic action of an adrenal cortical extract *in vitro*. Endocrinology **54**, 431—436 (1954).
Mills, T. M., Spaziani, E.: The influence of testosterone on penetration of α-aminoisobutyric acid and 2-deoxyglucose in male rat accessory tissues. Biochim. biophys. Acta (Amst.) **150**, 435—445 (1968).
Moore, G. E., Gerner, R. E., Franklin, H. A.: Culture of normal human leukocytes. J. Amer. med. Ass. **199**, 519—524 (1967).
Morita, Y., Munck, A.: Effect of glucocorticoids *in vivo* and *in vitro* on net glucose uptake and amino acid incorporation by rat-thymus cells. Biochim. biophys. Acta (Amst.) **93**, 150—157 (1964).
Munck, A.: Studies on the mode of action of glucocorticoid in rats. II. The effects *in vivo* and *in vitro* on net glucose uptake by isolated adipose tissue. Biochim. biophys. Acta (Amst.) **57**, 318—326 (1962).
Munck, A.: Steroid concentration and tissue integrity as factors determining the physiological significance of effects of adrenal steroids *in vitro*. Endocrinology **77**, 356—360 (1965).
Munck, A.: Metabolic site and time course of cortisol action on glucose uptake, lactic acid output, and glucose-6-phosphate levels of rat thymus cells *in vitro*. J. biol. Chem. **243**, 1039—1042 (1968).
Munck, A.: Glucocorticoid inhibition of glucose uptake by peripheral tissues: old and new evidence, molecular mechanisms, and physiological significance. Perspect. Biol. Med. **14**, 265—289 (1970).
Munck, A., Koritz, S. B.: Studies on the mode of action of glucocorticoids in rats. I. Early effects of cortisol on blood glucose and on glucose entry into muscle, liver, and adipose tissue. Biochim. biophys. Acta (Amst.) **57**, 310—317 (1962).
Munck, A., Wira, C.: Glucocorticoid receptor in rat thymus cells. In: Advances in the biosciences. Vol. 7. New York: Pergamon Press 1971.
Nakagawa, S., Dvorkin, B., White, A.: Response of some hydrolases in thymus and lymphosarcoma of rats to injection of adrenal steroid hormones. Yale J. biol. Med. **41**, 120—132 (1968).
Nakagawa, S., White, A.: Acute decrease in RNA polymerase activity of rat thymus in response to cortisol injection. Proc. nat. Acad Sci. (Wash.) **55**, 900—904 (1968).
Pena, A., Dvorkin, B., White, A.: Acute effect of a single *in vivo* injection of cortisol on *in vitro* amino acid incorporating activity of rat liver and thymic preparations. Biochem. biophys. Res. Comm. **16**, 449—454 (1964).
Plagemann, P. G. W., Renner, E. D.: Glucocorticoids: competitive inhibition of glucose transport. Biochem. biophys. Res. Comm. **46**, 816—823 (1972).
Pratt, W. B., Aronow, L.: The effect of glucocorticoids on protein and nucleic acid synthesis in mouse fibroblasts growing *in vitro*. J. biol. Chem. **241**, 5244—5250 (1960).
Pratt, W. B., Edelman, S., Aronow, L.: The effect of cortisol, administered *in vivo*, on the *in vitro* incorporation of DNA and RNA precursors by rat thymus cells. Molec. Pharmacol. **3**, 219—224 (1967).
Raina, P. N., Rosen, F.: Selective effect of cortisol on deoxyribonuclease II activity of lymphosarcoma P1798. Arch. Int. Pharmacodyn. **182**, 14—23 (1969).
Rosen, F.: Enzymes in tissues responsive to corticosteroids. Cancer Res. **23**, 1447—1458 (1963).
Rosen, J., Fina, J. J., Milholland, R. J., Rosen, F.: Inhibition of glucose uptake in lymphosarcoma P1798 by cortisol and its relationship to the biosynthesis of deoxyribonucleic acid. J. biol. Chem. **245**, 2074—2080 (1970a).

ROSEN, J.M., FINA, J., MILHOLLAND, R.J., ROSEN, F.: Inhibitory effect of cortisol *in vitro* on 2-deoxyglucose uptake and RNA and protein metabolism in lymphosarcoma P 1798. Cancer Res. **32**, 350—355 (1972).
ROSEN, J.M., MILHOLLAND, R.J., ROSEN, F.: A comparison of the effect of glucocorticoids on glucose uptake and hexokinase activity in lymphosarcoma P1798. Biochim. biophys. Acta (Amst.) **219**, 447—454 (1970b).
ROSEN, J.M., ROSEN, F., MILHOLLAND, R.J., NICHOL, C.A.: Effect of cortisol on DNA metabolism in the sensitive and resistant lines of mouse lymphoma P1798. Cancer Res. **30**, 1129—1136 (1970c).
SCHAUMBERG, B.P.: Studies of the glucocorticoid-binding protein from thymocytes I. Localization in the cell and some properties of the protein. Biochim. biophys. Acta (Amst.) **214**, 520—532 (1970).
SHERMAN, M.R., CORVOL, P.L., O'MALLEY, B.W.: Progesterone-binding components of chick oviduct I. Preliminary characterization of cytoplasmic components. J. biol. Chem. **245**, 6085—6096 (1970).
SIMONI, R.D., LEVINTHAL, M., KUNDIG, F.D., KUNDIG, W., ANDERSON, B., HARTMAN, P.E., ROSEMAN, S.: Genetic evidence for the role of a bacterial phosphotransferase system in sugar transport. Proc. nat. Acad. Sci. (Wash.) **58**, 1963—1970 (1967).
SMITH, D.E., GORSKI, J.: Estrogen control of uterine glucose metabolism. An analysis based on transport and phosphorylation of 2-deoxyglucose. J. biol. Chem. **243**, 4169—4174 (1968).
SPELSBERG, T.C., STEGGLES, A.W., O'MALLEY, B.W.: Progesterone-binding components of chick oviduct. III. Chromatin acceptor sites. J. biol. Chem. **246**, 4188—4197 (1971).
STEVENS, J., MASHBURN, L.T., HOLLANDER, V.P.: Effect of 9α-fluoroprednisolone and L-asparaginase on uridine incorporation into ribosomal RNA of P1798 lymphosarcoma. Biochim. biophys. Acta (Amst.) **186**, 332—339 (1969).
STEVENS, J., MASHBURN, L.T., HOLLANDER, V.P.: Inhibition of uridine incorporation into P1798 lymphosarcoma nuclear RNA by L-asparaginase and 9α-fluoroprednisolone. Proc. Amer. Ass. Cancer Res. **11**, 75 (1970).
STEVENS, W., COLESSIDES, C., DOUGHERTY, T.F.: Effects of cortisol on the incorporation of thymidine-2-^{14}C into nucleic acids of lymphatic tissue from adrenalectomized CBA mice. Endocrinology **76**, 1100—1108 (1965).
STEVENS, W., COLESSIDES, C., DOUGHERTY, T.F.: A time study on the effect of cortisol on the incorporation of thymidine-2-^{14}C into nucleic acids of mouse lymphatic tissue. Endocrinology **78**, 600—604 (1966).
STEVENS, W., DOUGHERTY, T.F.: Effect of continued treatment with cortisol on thymidine incorporation into mouse lymphatic tissue nucleic acid. Proc. Soc. exp. Biol. (N.Y.) **124**, 542—545 (1967).
UETE, T.: Mode of action of adrenal cortical hormones. I. Effect of corticosteroids on amino acid incorporation into proteins of thymus and liver subcellular components in cell-free systems. J. Biochem. **63**, 176—185 (1968).
VAN STEVENINCK, J.: Transport and transport-associated phosphorylation of 2-deoxy-*O*-glucose in yeast. Biochim. biophys. Acta (Amst.) **163**, 386—394 (1968).
WESTPHAL, U.: Steroid-protein interactions. New York: Springer-Verlag 1971.
WESTPHAL, U., DEVENUTO, F.: Steroid-protein interactions. XI. Electrophoretic characterization of corticosteroid-binding proteins in serum of rat, man and other species. Biochim. biophys. Acta (Amst.) **115**, 187—196 (1966).
WHITE, A., HOBERMAN, H.D., SZEGO, C.M.: Influence of adrenalectomy and fasting on the incorporation of isotopic nitrogen into the tissues of mice. J. biol. Chem. **174**, 1049—1050 (1948).
WIERNIK, P.H.: Effect of starvation of intact and adrenalectomized mice bearing lymphosarcoma P1798 on tumor regression and ribonuclease activity. Cancer Res. **30**, 280—282 (1970).
WIERNIK, P.H., MACLEOD, R.M.: Vinblastine effect on nucleic acids and ribonuclease of lymphoid tissue. Proc. Soc. exp. Biol. (N.Y.) **119**, 118—120 (1965a).
WIERNIK, P.H., MACLEOD, R.M.: The effect of a single large dose of 9α-fluoroprednisolone on nucleodepolymerase activity and nucleic acid content of the rat thymus. Acta Endocrinol. **49**, 138—144 (1965b).
WIRA, C., MUNCK, A.: Specific glucocorticoid receptors in thymus cells. Localization in the nucleus and extraction of the cortisol-receptor complex. J. biol. Chem. **245**, 3436—3438 (1970).
YOUNG, D.A.: Glucocorticoid action of rat thymus cells. Interrelationships between carbohydrate, protein, and adenine nucleotide metabolism and cortisol effects on these functions *in vitro*. J. biol. Chem. **244**, 2210—2217 (1969).

Chapter 37

Mechanisms of Action of Estrogens

RUSSELL HILF and JAMES L. WITTLIFF

With 5 Figures

Introduction

Among the sex hormones, no greater variety of chemical structure exists than among those possessing estrogenic activity. The naturally occurring steroid estrogens, the synthetic diphenolic stilbene derivatives, numerous triphenolic compounds, and the estrogens derived from plants are all capable of inducing cornification of the vaginal epithelium and of increasing the weight of the uterus. It, therefore, seems somewhat surprising that the first clear-cut demonstration of a highly specific receptor molecule for estrogens was reported in the uterus. It should be pointed out that the biochemical studies on the mechanism of action of estrogens have been the pace-setters for most of the investigations of hormones at the cellular and molecular levels (JENSEN et al., 1971b). The authors of the present chapter have attempted to summarize the current status of knowledge in the area of estrogen action; in so doing, we are aware of our inability to pay due credit to all of the investigators who have contributed to the rapidly growing literature in this field. The readers interested in gaining more detailed information are referred to the classical volumes comprising *Marshall's Physiology of Reproduction*, edited by PARKES (1966) and the following treatises: *The Ovary*, edited by ZUCKERMAN (1962), *Sex and Internal Secretions*, edited by YOUNG (1961), and *Reproductive Biology*, edited by BALIN and GLASSER (1972).

Chemical Structure and Steroidogenesis

The naturally occurring estrogens, estrone, estriol, and estradiol, are steroids containing 18 carbons. With the development of a reliable, sensitive bioassay by ALLEN and DOISY (1924), two laboratories simultaneously isolated crystalline estrone in 1929 (DOISY et al., 1929; BUTENANDT, 1929). Shortly thereafter, MARRION (1930) and BUTENANDT (1930) isolated from human pregnancy urine the hydrated estrogen, estriol. It was not until 1935 that Doisy and coworkers isolated estradiol from the ovary (MACCORQUODALE et al., 1935); estradiol is the most potent of the naturally occurring steroidal estrogens. One of the major controversies in the literature, leading to some confusion, related to the configuration at the carbon-17 position. It is now clear that the hydroxyl group in estradiol is in the β configuration, as the 17α epimer of estradiol is considerably less potent (less than 1/1000 the potency of estradiol-17β). Similarly, weak potency is found in estriol, which possesses a 16α hydroxyl group on the D-ring. The structures of the naturally occurring steroids are shown in Fig. 1.

The first demonstration of estrogenic activity in a synthetic compound not possessing the phenanthrene nucleus was reported in 1933 (Cook et al., 1933). The intensive work by Dodds and his coworkers led to the synthesis of many diphenolic and triphenolic compounds, culminating in the elucidation and synthesis of diethylstilbestrol in 1938 (Dodds and Lawson, 1936, 1937; Dodds et al., 1938a). Extensive synthetic modification of this stilbene has failed to produce an increase in estrogenic activity above that seen in stilbestrol (Fig. 1). Dodds et al. (1938b) synthesized two other derivatives, hexestrol and dienestrol, which have been utilized clinically because of their high estrogenic potency.

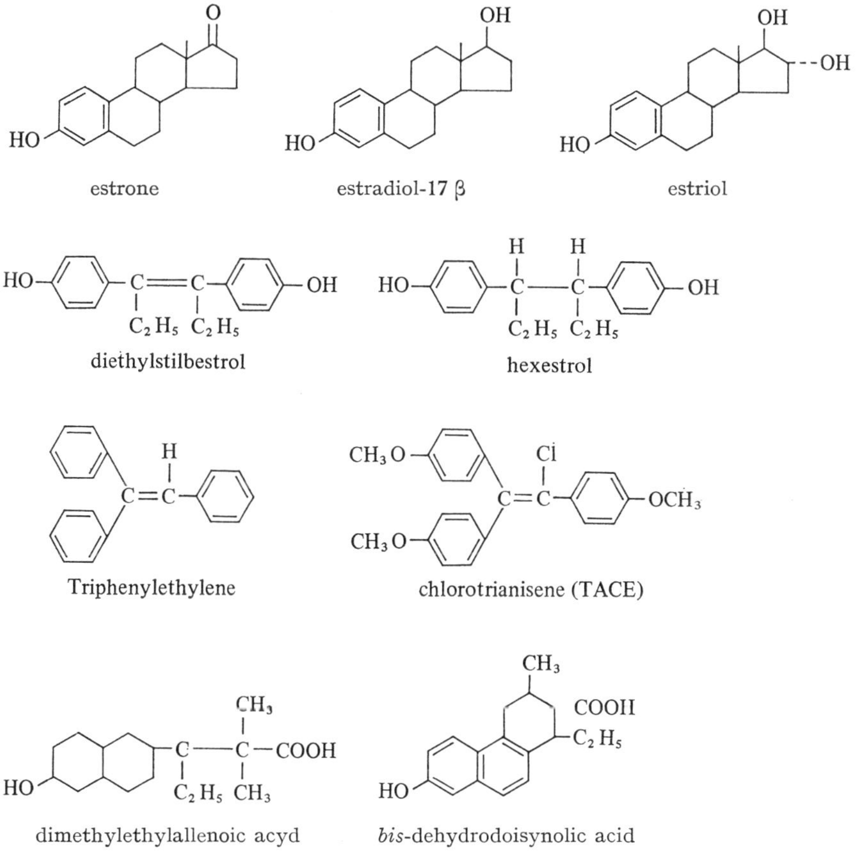

estrone estradiol-17 β estriol

diethylstilbestrol hexestrol

Triphenylethylene chlorotrianisene (TACE)

dimethylethylallenoic acyd *bis*-dehydrodoisynolic acid

Fig. 1. Structure of various estrogens

In 1937, Robson and Schonberg demonstrated estrogenic activity with triphenylethylene. As with the stilbenes, synthetic derivatives were made resulting in the appearance of many derivatives of triphenylethylene possessing estrogenic activities. One such modification was a halogenated derivative, chlorotrianisene or TACE (Thompson and Werner, 1951; Shelton, 1953). With this lead, additional modifications of chlorotrianisene have produced such compounds as chlomiphene (Holtkamp et al., 1960) and triparinol (Blohm et al., 1959).

Other non-steroidal estrogens have been synthesized, such as allenoic acid, dimethylallenoic acid, doisynolic acid, and bis dehydrodoisynolic acid, some of which are shown in Fig. 1 (HEER et al., 1945; MIESCHER, 1944). These compounds bear some structural resemblance to the phenanthrene nucleus.

There are numerous naturally occurring compounds that do not possess the phenanthrene ring but are estrogenic. For example, compounds such as genistein, daidzein, and coumestrol are chemicals with conjugated ring systems which are estrogenic. These compounds have been isolated from clover, alfalfa, peas, and beans. Although most of these plant estrogens are rather weak in potency, there is reason to believe that more potent naturally occurring estrogens exist.

Studies *in vitro* have shown that estrone and estradiol-17β are produced from ^{14}C-labeled acetate in the ovaries of the human (HAMMERSTEIN et al., 1964; O'DONNELL and CRAIG, 1959; RABINOWITZ, 1956; RYAN and SMITH, 1961a; SWEAT et al., 1960; WOTIZ et al., 1955), of the dog (RABINOWITZ and DOWBEN, 1955), of the cat (RABINOWITZ, 1956), and of the pig (WERTHESSEN et al., 1953), as well as in the testes of the human, dog, cat, and stallion (RABINOWITZ, 1956; NYMAN et al., 1959). Administration of labeled acetate to the pregnant mare leads to recovery of labeled estrone, equilin, and equilenin (HEARD et al., 1956). Pregnenolone or progesterone may act as a precursor for estrone and estradiol-17β in the ovaries of many species (AXELROD and GOLDZIEHER, 1962a; RYAN, 1966; RYAN and SMITH, 1961). Tissues such as the placenta, ovaries, testes, and adrenal cortex are capable of converting androstenedione and testosterone to estrogens (BAGGETT et al., 1956, 1959; GRIFFITHS et al., 1964; MARSH et al., 1962; HUANG and PEARLMAN, 1962; WOTIZ et al., 1956).

A summary of biosynthetic pathways for production of estrogens is presented in Fig. 2. The biosynthesis of estrogens in the ovary occurs in the cells lining the follicles and these cells, therefore, possess the enzymes necessary for 17-hydroxylation, *C*-21 side chain cleavage, and aromatization of ring A. In contrast, the

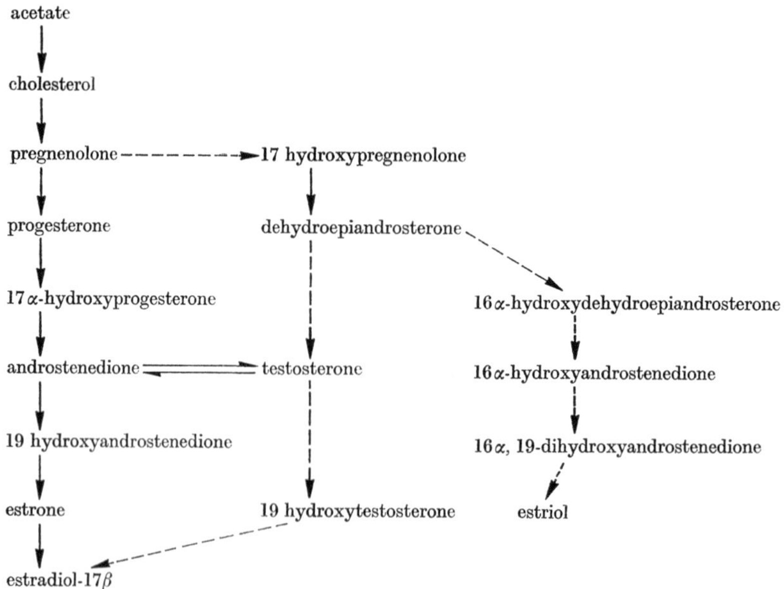

Fig. 2. Biosynthesis of estrogens

cells of the corpus luteum primarily produce progesterone and, in the mare (SHORT, 1962), are not capable of producing estrogens. SHORT (1962) proposed a "two cell type" theory, which postulated that the theca interna cells are responsible for estrogen production and the luteinized granulosa cells are primarily involved in the synthesis of progesterone. However, MARSH et al. (1962) have reported the conversion of testosterone to estrogen by a granulosa cell tumor that had no theca cells.

Pathways not involving progesterone may be of some slight significance (RYAN and SMITH, 1961b). SHORT (1961) found dehydroepiandrosterone in equine follicular fluid, suggesting an alternate pathway in the conversion of pregnenolone to androstenedione. Additionally, GRIFFITHS et al. (1964) observed that a granulosatheca cell tumor could not utilize progesterone as a precursor for estrogens although androstenedione did serve as a precursor to some estrogen.

The final aromatization of the A ring has been investigated using tritium and ^{14}C-labeled derivatives of androstenedione and testosterone (AXELROD and GOLDZIEHER, 1962b). Following hydroxylation at C-19, there appears to be a simultaneous elimination of the C-19 group together with a hydrogen from C-1, forming a 3-keto, 1,4-diene, which then undergoes spontaneous aromatization to give the 3-hydroxy, 1,3,5 (10)-triene. By using tritium label at the 1α position, these investigators could determine if the α or β hydrogen was removed by following the reduction in radioactivity. Since the tritium label was indeed reduced, it would appear that there occurs a preferential removal of the α hydrogen (axial) at C-1. Acetylation of the product, which also had originally contained a tritium label at the 2α position, did not further reduce the radioactivity, suggesting that the 2β (axial) hydrogen forms the hydroxyl group at C-3.

In a series of extensive and careful studies, DICZFALUSY and his colleagues (BOLTE et al., 1964a, b, c) have demonstrated that steroids such as dehydroepiandrosterone, androstenedione, and testosterone undergo extensive conversion to estrogens during pregnancy. The placenta was shown to produce estrone and estradiol-17β, but not estriol; the latter is formed by the fetal-placental unit. It would seem that estrone and estradiol-17β proceed to the fetus, where 16α-hydroxylation occurs and the 16α-hydroxylated steroid then returns to the placenta for the final conversion to estriol.

The interconversion of estrone, estriol, and estradiol-17β has been studied by experiments utilizing liver and kidney slices *in vitro* (RYAN and ENGEL, 1953a; VELLE and ERICKSON, 1960). The enzymes involved in the interconversion of the estrogens have also been demonstrated to be present in the ovary, placenta, intestine, mammary gland, and red cells (RYAN and ENGEL, 1953b). For the conversion of estrone to estradiol-17β, NADP is a required cofactor for the 17β-dehydrogenase (MIGEON et al., 1962). The outline presented (Fig. 3) shows the various conversions among the estrogens. It is still not certain that estriol is the

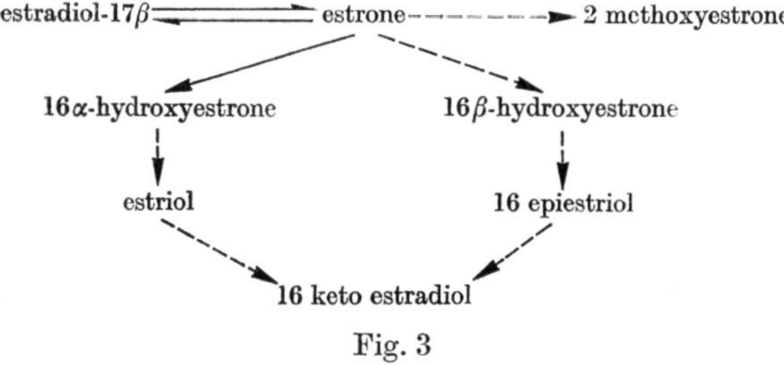

Fig. 3

last stage for inactivation of estrogens, as not all of the labeled estradiol-17β administered can be accounted for in the urine (BEER and GALLAGHER, 1955; JELLINCK, 1959).

Actions on Target Organs

A. Accessory Sex Organs

Removal of the ovary from an animal, before puberty, arrests the development of the uterus, vagina, and mammary glands, and the cyclic changes constituting the estrus cycle do not appear (LONG and EVANS, 1922; ALLEN, 1922). In the adult female rat, oophorectomy caused uterine atrophy, which was pronounced at 14 days following removal of the ovaries (LANGSTON and ROBINSON, 1935). The maximum atrophy of the uterus was observed at 49 days after oophorectomy, and the atrophy was greatest in the endometrium and least in the myometrium. The regression of the myometrium results in a decreased spontaneous contractility of the uterus (ROBSON, 1933).

The biological activity of estrogenic substances, which consists of hyperemia, cellular growth, cellular division, and edema in specific target organs, can be readily demonstrated in ovariectomized or hypophysectomized rats. Administration of estrogens to these hypogonadal animals produced histologic and physiologic changes in the vulva, vagina, uterus, and fallopian tubes that are comparable to those changes observed during the normal estrus period. Mice, rats, hamsters, guinea pigs, rabbits, cats, dogs, monkeys, and humans have all been studied to ascertain the effects of endogenous and exogenous estrogens.

Swelling of the vulva occurs at estrus and it has been thought that such a change might facilitate coitus. In the rat and the mouse, opening of the vagina occurs with first estrus; administration of estrogens to induce vaginal opening has been used as a bioassay (ALLEN and DOISY, 1924). One of the most sensitive parameters of estrogen action is the effect on stratification and subsequent cornification of the epithelium of the vagina. Indeed, one can define an estrogen as a substance capable of this action on the vagina (EMMENS, 1957). ALLEN et al. (1924) employed this as a routine assay for estrogens and this test enabled investigators to make the advances in isolation and identification of naturally occurring estrogens. Vaginal cornification in response to estrogens occurs in humans, monkeys, dogs, hamsters, mice, and rats.

The uterotrophic activity of estrogens is also a commonly utilized measure of estrogenic potency. In a very careful study, ASTWOOD (1938) reported that hyperemia of the rat uterus occurred within 4 h after administration of 0.1 μg of estradiol, accounting for a total weight increase within 6 h. A peak uterotrophic response was found to occur at 30 h after the single injection of estradiol. Histologically, estradiol stimulated the division of endometrial cells followed by secretion into the lumen. There was noted an increase in the growth of the myometrium and in uterine motility.

Estrogens also control the nature of the mucus secretion from the cervix. Under estrogen stimulation, the cervical mucus is thin, clear, and flows more readily, whereas progesterone causes a thickening of the mucus.

B. Pituitary and Hypothalamus

Although the secretion and release of pituitary gonadotropins are directly controlled by the hypothalamus, estrogens markedly influence the levels of these pituitary hormones. Low doses of estrogen have been demonstrated to increase plasma levels of luteinizing hormone (LH), and larger doses will cause the opposite effect (CALLENTINE et al., 1966a; McCANN and RAMIREZ, 1964). This dichotomy of action is important as estrogens can stimulate LH to, in turn, stimulate organ steroidogenesis and, thereby, further elevate the levels of circulating steroids. These elevations in estrogenic hormones can then block the release of LH. It is also known that estrogens can increase the sensitivity of the ovary to respond to gonadotropins (BRADBURY, 1961), as well as cause follicular development in the immature hypophysectomized rat. It thus appears that estrogens and gonadotropins play an integrated role in both maturation and ovulation processes of the ovary.

The role of estrogens in control of FSH (follicle-stimulating hormone) is less clear. Although high doses of estrogen can block secretion of FSH from the pituitary, small doses apparently do not inhibit FSH secretion (PARLOW, 1964). Apparently, release of FSH is stimulated by cessation of progesterone secretion by the corpus luteum and/or low levels of estrogen, since urinary levels of FSH are high during menses and decline towards the middle of the cycle (VORYS et al., 1965).

It should be noted that estrogens can act synergistically with progesterone to affect pituitary function. For example, small doses of estrogen and progesterone administered simultaneously can effectively lower luteinizing hormone (LH) to levels which would require larger doses of estrogen alone (McCANN and RAMIREZ, 1964).

C. Lipogenesis and Cholesterol

Relatively large doses of estrogen will produce a significant decrease in the cholesterol concentration in serum and adrenal glands of the rat (LEVIN, 1945; BOYD and McGUIRE, 1956). STEINBERG et al. (1967) have shown that the hypocholesterolemic response in serum was related to the dose of estradiol administered subcutaneously. However, this effect was shown to be dependent on the presence of the pituitary gland (STEINBERG, 1969). Estrogen administration has been shown to decrease cholesterol biosynthesis in rat liver (FILLIOS et al., 1958; BOYD, 1962; MUKHERJEE et al., 1967). Although the exact site of the hormonal effect is not known, it has been suggested that it occurs between acetate and mevalonate, or at the point of decarboxylation of mevalonate. In a recent study, MUKHERJEE and BHOSE (1968) presented evidence that estrogen inhibited cholesterol biosynthesis by depressing the enzymes responsible for formation of hydroxymethyl glutamyl-CoA and mevalonic acid.

D. Antiestrogens

In recent years, considerable interest has arisen from investigation of compounds possessing antiestrogenic activity. To be accurate, one should be quite specific in stating the exact hormonal activity that is antagonized by the compound designated as an antiestrogen. A general definition, as stated by LERNER (1964), defines an antagonist as a compound capable of inhibiting hormonal activity at one or more sites regardless of the route of administration or the dose employed.

Inhibition of estrogen induced responses in estrogen target organs is a property of many naturally occurring substances. It has been well established that weak estrogens antagonize strong estrogens (HISAW et al., 1954; VELARDO and STURGIS, 1955), and certain progestogens, androgens, and glucocorticoids are capable of antagonizing estrogen-induced uterotrophic responses (ROBSON, 1938; SZEGO and

ROBERTS, 1948; HUGGINS and JENSEN, 1955; EDGREN and CALHOUN, 1957; VELARDO et al., 1955). A deficient nutritional state or use of a folic acid antagonist has been shown to prevent the full estrogenic response in experimental animals (HERTZ and SEBRELL, 1944; DAVIS et al., 1956; LERNER and TURKHEIMER, 1965; HILF et al., 1963).

The most desirable antiestrogenic agent is one which possesses little or no inherent hormonal or metabolic activity, but is capable of antagonizing specifically the effects of estrogens at the target organ site. Since weakly active estrogens can antagonize stronger estrogens, such as estradiol, it seemed logical that examination of compounds structurally related to estrogens would be a sound and fruitful approach to the discovery of antiestrogens. One of the first such compounds was reported by LERNER et al. (1958). This compound, ethamoxytriphetol or MER-25, is structurally related to chlorotrianisene, a nonsteroidal estrogen. In an incisive study, LERNER et al. (1958) demonstrated that MER-25 was capable of antagonizing estrogen-induced responses in the uterus, vagina, and pituitary of rats, mice, monkeys, chicks, and rabbits. Furthermore, MER-25 was not by itself estrogenic, androgenic, antiandrogenic, progestational, antiprogestational, or gonadotrophin-like, although MER-25 did possess slight uterotrophic and antigonadotrophic activities. These results led Lerner to conclude that MER-25 was probably a competitive antagonist at the target site, a result later confirmed by JENSEN et al. (1969a) utilizing the binding of labeled estradiol to estrogen receptors in the uterus as a discrete assay system.

Emmens and his coworkers have extensively studied analogs of diethylstilbestrol as potential antiestrogenic compounds (EMMENS et al., 1962; MARTIN et al., 1961). Dimethylstilbestrol proved to be an active antiestrogen in preventing vaginal cornification induced by estrogens, when dimethylstilbestrol was administered intravaginally at the same time as the estrogen. However, dimethylstilbestrol was estrogenic as reflected by the vaginal response when the compound was administered subcutaneously (MARTIN, 1969). Since it has been shown that dimethylstilbestrol can compete with estradiol for binding to uterine receptors, MARTIN (1969) has suggested that certain competitors of estrogen can act as estrogens themselves if sufficient levels are attained *in vivo*; these conclusions would account for the inability of finding to date, an estrogen antagonist totally devoid of some inherent estrogenic activity.

In searching for additional antiestrogens, particularly agents demonstrating this action when administered orally, DUNCAN et al. (1962, 1963) reported that certain diphenyldehydronaphthalene derivatives inhibited pregnancy when given prior to ovum implantation. These compounds, U11100A and U11555A, demonstrated antiuterotrophic activities when administered concomitantly with estradiol-17β; when administered alone, U11100A and U11555A produced a slight uterotrophic response, suggestive of the results seen with MER-25. CALLENTINE et al. (1966b) reported on a compound, CN-55945-27, somewhat related to the above agents, which also possessed antiestrogenic activity as assayed by inhibition of estrogen induced uterotrophic response. All of these compounds possess a similar spectrum of biological activity: weak uterotrophic activity, antiuterotrophic activity against exogenous estradiol administration, inhibition or stimulation of pituitary gonadotrophins depending on dose employed, inhibition of pregnancy probably by preventing implantation, and inhibition of estradiol binding to estrogen receptor molecules in the uterus. This latter property has made these compounds invaluable tools for the investigation of mechanisms of action of estrogens, which will be discussed later (see Fig. 4).

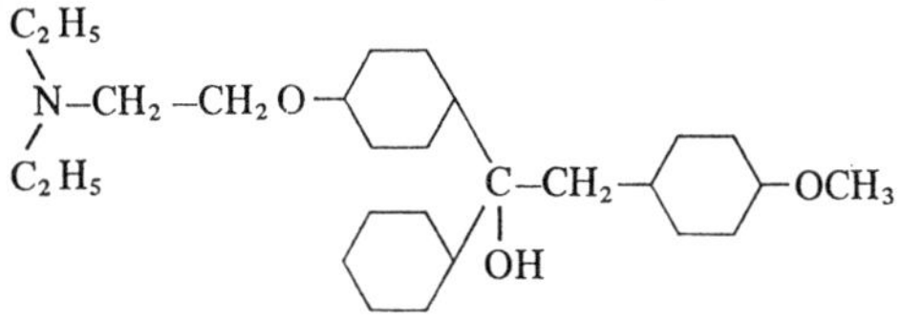

ethamoxytriphetol (MER-25)

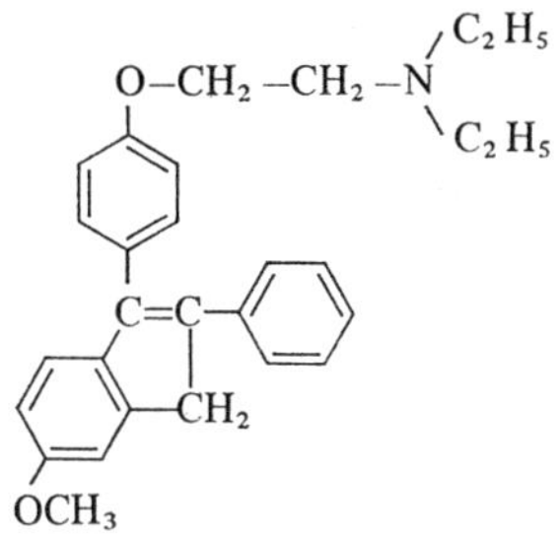

U 11555 A

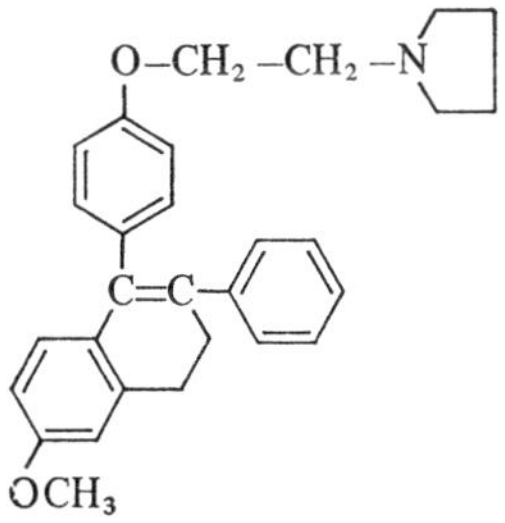

U 11100 A

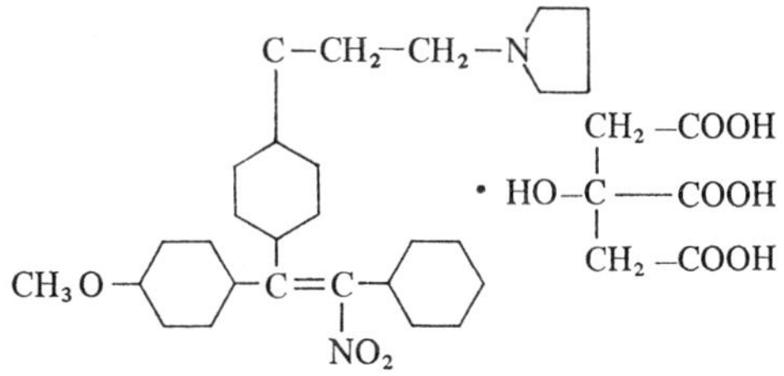

CN - 55,945-27 (citrate salt)

Fig. 4. Structures of various anti-estrogens

E. Breast and Breast Cancer

Estrogens cause duct proliferation in the breast of the ovariectomized rat. In order to achieve full lobulo-alveolar growth, progesterone is required along with estrogen in the rat. FOLLEY (1956) has divided mammals into three categories in terms of hormonally induced responses in the mammary gland. The first group, comprising the mouse, rat, rabbit, and human, responds to estrogen by demonstrating duct development with little alveolar growth. The second group, including the monkey, guinea pig, cow, and goat, shows both duct development and considerable lobulo-alveolar development in response to the administration of estrogens. In the third group, which is comprised of the dog, estrogen produces only slight growth of the mammary gland duct system. There is no doubt that the pituitary hormones play an essential role, since maximal stimulation of the breasts is achieved by the steroids in the presence of the pituitary (LYONS et al., 1958). Optimal growth of the breasts of ovariectomized, adrenalectomized, hypophysectomized rats can be achieved by the administration of estrogen, progesterone, growth hormone, and prolactin along with maintenance doses of thyroid and adrenal hormones.

The role of estrogen in breast cancer has been the subject of a great number of studies. From a therapeutic view, removal of estrogens by oophorectomy and/or adrenalectomy results in a significant temporary remission of breast cancer in women, the figure approximating 40%. This hormone-dependency of breast cancer has been known since the late 1800's (SCHINZINGER, 1889; BEATSON, 1896), and removal of the ovaries of premenopausal women with disseminated breast cancer seems to be a justifiable primary maneuver. Adrenalectomy has been shown to alter the course of breast cancer; some investigators have reported approximately 40% of the patients demonstrated objective remission after adrenalectomy (Dao, 1967). It is of interest that some patients who have failed to respond to oophorectomy will demonstrate a response to adrenalectomy, suggesting that hormone dependence of breast cancer may not be simply related to estrogens.

Administration of estrogen to postmenopausal women with disseminated breast cancer results in objective remission of the disease in about 3 of 10 patients (Kennedy, 1965). Here, one is again faced with what appears to be a paradox in the role of estrogens in breast cancer. However, the effects of removal of physiologic levels of estrogens versus the effects of pharmacologic doses of estrogenic hormones may reflect a difference in action at the extremes of the hormonal spectrum. One might invoke the pituitary inhibitory actions of superphysiologic doses of estrogen, particularly inhibition of prolactin, along with a direct action of estrogens at the tumor cell level.

These latter proposals have some validity on the basis of experimental mammary tumor studies in rats. Induction of mammary carcinoma by carcinogens, such as methylcholanthrene or 7,12-dimethylbenz(a)anthracene (DMBA), occurs in the intact rat, is reduced in the ovariectomized rat, and does not occur in the hypophysectomized rat (Shay et al., 1952; Huggins et al., 1959; Dao and Sunderland, 1959). Although pregnancy accelerated the growth of carcinogen-induced mammary tumors, the well-differentiated mammary gland resulting from pregnancy or administration of gestational hormones was considerably less susceptible to cancer induction by these carcinogens (Dao et al., 1960; Huggins et al., 1959). Recent studies by Pearson and coworkers (Sterental et al., 1963; Pearson et al., 1969; Butler and Pearson, 1971) have clearly shown that the DMBA-induced carcinoma was dependent on prolactin for continued growth; good correlations were observed between alterations of prolactin secretion, as influenced by drugs, and the growth rate of the neoplasias. If all human breast cancer was similar to the DMBA-induced rat model, hypophysectomy should result in 100 % regression of the disease. Since this is not the case, one must conclude that the DMBA-induced tumor is representative of just one class of human breast cancer.

Hilf (1971) has attempted to categorize rodent mammary tumors by examining numerous biochemical characteristics of hormone-dependent, hormone-responsive, and hormone-independent carcinomas. One of these tumors, the transplantable R3230AC neoplasm, responded to estrogen therapy, as well as to administration of androgens (Hilf, 1967). The response to estrogen was most intriguing; pharmacologic doses of estrogenic hormones resulted in the induction of secretion in the neoplasms, and the secretions contained casein and lactose, two unique components of milk. It would appear that modifying the hormonal milieu to create a highly differentiated cellular state resulted in a slowing of the growth of the tumor. Another interesting finding in these studies was the observation that the ratio of activities of glucose-6-phosphate dehydrogenase to α-glycerol-phosphate dehydrogenase appeared to correlate with hormonal status of a variety of rodent tumors (Hilf, 1971). For example, the ratio was lowest in the quiescent normal breast, and reached very high values in hormone-independent tumors, with hormone-dependent and hormone-responsive tumors being intermediate. Since human infiltrating ductal carcinomas were shown to possess the entire spectrum of enzyme ratios (Hilf et al., 1970), it is intriguing to speculate that specific metabolic characteristics are possessed by mammary carcinomas related to their hormonal state, making possible a predictive identification of each neoplasm. Studies of the presence of specific estrogen binding proteins in breast carcinomas, and correlation with the clinical course of the disease, provide another approach to identifying hormone-dependent neoplasia; these will be discussed later.

F. Additional Effects of Estrogens

In rats, administration of estrogens results in retardation of body growth (BORGART et al., 1944). In contrast, increased growth occurs in lambs and heifers after administration of estrogens (ANDREWS et al., 1949; DINUSSON et al., 1950), resulting in less fat but more protein in the carcass. Estrogenization of poultry, however, produces more fat in the carcass. These effects of estrogens have led to the use of hormonal agents to increase edible meat yields in the above animals.

Estrogens play a role in calcium metabolism. Skeletal maturation, as reflected by bone calcification, occurs more rapidly in the female rat and mouse and in women. Some concern has been expressed over the use of oophorectomy in women with disseminated breast cancer, since one commonly observes a hypercalcemia in this disease and removal of endogenous estrogens may enhance the decreased calcification of the skeletal bones.

Finally, estrogens are used in the treatment of disseminated prostatic cancer. It is not known if remission of this disease is a result of a direct antiandrogenic action of estrogen at the prostatic level, or of the ability of estrogens to inhibit pituitary gonadotrophins, or of a combination of both actions.

Biochemical Basis of Action

A. Specific Estrogen Binding Proteins

Although the effects of small doses of estrogenic hormones on the growth and function of certain target organs and tissues have been known for sometime, the exact mechanism by which these steroids exert their effects awaits elucidation.

Earlier attempts to demonstrate the fate of physiological doses of estradiol-17β or its derivatives met with little success, since most of these studies utilized microgram quantities of ^{14}C-labeled hormone possessing low specific radioactivity (TWOMBLY and SCHOENEWALDT, 1951; BUDY, 1955). In 1958, DODDS et al. (1958) administered microgram doses of ^{3}H-labeled hexoestrol to rats and rabbits and followed the excretion patterns of radioactivity; no attempt was made to trace the compound's fate in the tissues of the animals. However, after injection of physiological doses of ^{3}H-hexoestrol to young sheep and goats, GLASCOCK and HOEKSTRA (1959) demonstrated that radioactive estrogen was selectively distributed either in the physiological target organs, e.g. uterus, vagina, mammary glands, and pituitary gland, or in those organs which excrete or reabsorb the hormone, e.g. kidney, liver, and intestine. Simultaneously, JENSEN (1958) and JENSEN and JACOBSON (1960) showed that 6,7-^{3}H-estradiol-17β of high specific radioactivity (prepared by the catalytic reduction of 6-dehydroestradiol with carrier-free tritium gas) was taken up and retained by organs of the rat, which respond to estrogen treatment *in vivo*. Furthermore, retention of the labeled hormone by the target tissue occurred against a large concentration gradient with the blood. Extraction of isotopically labeled steroid retained by the uterus revealed that estradiol-17β had not undergone metabolic transformation (JENSEN and JACOBSON, 1960, 1962). Using ^{14}C-labeled estradiol-17β, NOALL and ALLEN (1961) were first to report that uteri from rabbits accumulated the radioactive hormone when incubated *in vitro*. The observation that the uterus and vagina have the ability to concentrate and retain radioactive estrogens after administration *in vivo* or incubation *in vitro* was confirmed and extended by many investigators (STONE et al., 1963; STONE, 1963, 1964; DAVIS et al., 1963; MARTIN and BAGGETT, 1964; STONE and MARTIN, 1964; MARTIN, 1964; STONE and BAGGETT, 1965a,b; TERENIUS 1965, 1966, 1969; ROY et al., 1964; TALWAR et al., 1964; KING et al.,

1965; NOTEBOOM and GORSKI, 1965; EISENFELD and AXELROD, 1965, 1966; KING and GORDON, 1966; MICHAEL, 1962, 1965; FLESHER, 1965). Data from these laboratories and JENSEN'S (JENSEN and JACOBSON, 1960, 1962; JENSEN, 1963, 1965a, b; JENSEN et al., 1966) had established that estrogen responsive tissues contain components that specifically bind estradiol-17β, 17-methylestradiol, 17-ethynylestradiol, and hexoestrol with a very high affinity. Antiuterotrophic agents, such as U11100A (nafoxidine) (JENSEN et al., 1966), MER-25 (ethamoxytriphetol) (STONE, 1964; JENSEN et al., 1966) and clomiphene (ROY et al., 1964) administered *in vivo* block the association of estrogens with target tissues. The inhibition was dose-responsive and was seen only in those tissues that have an affinity for estrogen, e.g., uterus, vagina, and anterior pituitary, providing further evidence for the presence of specific receptor sites (JENSEN et al., 1966, 1967a, b). Since administration of actinomycin D or puromycin did not inhibit the uptake of the hormone, Jensen concluded that these substances exerted their effects at some later stage in the sequence of events following hormone administration (JENSEN et al., 1966). Thus, the uptake and retention of estradiol-17β by the uterus is an early step in the uterotrophic response, preceding any alterations in the rates of biosynthetic reactions known to be inhibited by actinomycin D or puromycin, i.e. ribonucleic acid and protein synthesis.

In addition to the aforementioned studies, numerous workers have provided autoradiographic data concerning the cellular distribution of the hormones (DE PAEPE, 1960; MOBBS, 1968; ULLBERG and BENGTSSON, 1963; KING et al., 1965; INMAN et al., 1965; ATTRAMADAL, 1964; MICHAEL, 1965; JENSEN et al., 1967a, b, 1969; STUMPF, 1968, 1969, 1970). Most of these studies indicated that the nucleus was the major site of ^{3}H-estradiol-17β localization in uteri, although a substantial portion (15 to 40 %) was also found in the cytoplasm. The ratio of the distribution of labeled estradiol-17β in nuclei versus cytoplasm agreed well with results obtained by cellular fractionation techniques (TALWAR et al., 1968; BAULIEU et al., 1967; KING et al., 1965; KING and GORDON, 1966; NOTEBOOM and GORSKI, 1965; JENSEN et al., 1967a, 1969a; STUMPF, 1968; TOFT and GORSKI, 1966; TOFT et al., 1967).

Evidence that estradiol-17β was associated with a macromolecular component was first shown by TALWAR et al. (1964) using Sephadex G-75 and G-100 chromatography. However, the important findings of TOFT and GORSKI (1966) and TOFT et al. (1967) that labeled estradiol receptor complex of the cytoplasm could be separated by ultracentrifugation in sucrose gradients, set the stage for intensive investigation of hormone receptor molecules. The receptor was thought to be a protein since the hormone-receptor complex was sensitive to treatment with proteolytic enzymes, but was stable to treatment with ribonuclease or deoxyribonuclease. The labeled steroid was bound to a protein or proteins displaying a discrete peak with a sedimentation coefficient of approximately 9.5 Svedbergs. Later studies (JENSEN et al., 1968, 1969a, b; ERDOS, 1968; ERDOS et al., 1968; ROCHEFORT and BAULIEU, 1968) indicated that the cytoplasmic binding-protein has a sedimentation coefficient closer to 8 S. The hormone-receptor complex was unstable in the presence of detergents, such as sodium dodecyl sulfate or taurocholate (TOFT et al., 1967), or sulfhydryl-reacting agents, such as *p*-chloromercuribenzoate or *N*-ethylmaleimide (TOFT et al., 1967; JENSEN et al., 1967a, b).

Presently, there are several methods available for measurement of the estrogen binding capacity by a tissue using a cell-free preparation. These procedures include: Sephadex gel-filtration (KING and GORDON, 1966; ERDOS et al., 1968; PUCA and BRESCIANI, 1968, 1969; SOLOFF and SZEGO, 1969; VONDERHAAR et al., 1970); equilibrium dialysis (ERDOS et al., 1968; BAULIEU and RAYNAUD, 1970);

protamine precipitation (STEGGLES and KING, 1970); adsorption to glass pellets (CLARK and GORSKI, 1969; NOTIDES, 1970), to dextran-coated charcoal (BAULIEU et al., 1971; MÉŠTER et al., 1970) or to hydroxyapatite (ERDOS et al., 1970); and sucrose gradient analysis (TOFT and GORSKI, 1966; TOFT et al., 1967; JENSEN et al. 1967a, 1969a; BROOKS and WITTLIFF, 1973). In most cases, determination of the binding constants and the number of binding sites in a tissue preparation were calculated using either a Lineweaver-Burk plot (LINEWEAVER and BURK, 1934), a Scatchard plot (SCATCHARD, 1949), or the proportional graph of BAULIEU and RAYNAUD (1970). Affinity constants in the range of 10^9 to 10^{11} M^{-1} have been reported for the 8 S cytosol receptor of a number of species (see WILLIAMS-ASHMAN and REDDI, 1971).

In 1967, JENSEN and coworkers made several important contributions towards an understanding of the relationship between hormone receptor interaction and the uterotrophic response. First, it appeared that the uptake and retention of labeled estradiol-17β by uterine cells were interrelated processes. This was substantiated by the finding that another receptor sedimenting at approximately 5 S could be isolated from the nucleus (DESOMBRE et al., 1967). SHYAMALA and GORSKI (1967) found that deoxyribonuclease treatment of purified uterine nuclei prior to extraction with 0.3 M KCl also provided evidence of a nuclear receptor having a sedimentation coefficient of 5 S. Subsequent experiments indicated that this nuclear receptor was bound to chromatin. Secondly, JENSEN et al. (1967a) made the initial effort to isolate the receptor by passing extracts of calf uteri over an estradiol-azobenzylcellulose column. A protein, which retained receptor activity, was isolated and injected into rabbits to produce antibodies. Subsequent examination of the antiserum revealed the presence of precipitating antibodies (JENSEN et al., 1967a). Later studies (GORSKI et al., 1968; ERDOS, 1968; KOREMAN and RAO, 1968; JENSEN et al., 1969a, b) have shown that the 8 S cytoplasmic estrogen-receptor complex will dissociate in the presence of 0.3 to 0.4 M KCl into subunits having sedimentation coefficients of approximately 4 S. These subunits retain the ability to bind estradiol-17β. Stabilization of the uterine 4 S subunit with calcium ions under conditions of high ionic strength has enabled a 5000-fold purification of the 4 S subunit by using salt precipitation, gel filtration, and ion-exchange chromatography (DESOMBRE et al., 1969a, b, 1971). Using procedures *in vitro*, Gorski and his coworkers (GORSKI et al., 1968; SHYAMALA and GORSKI, 1969) have shown that there was a temperature dependent translocation of labeled hormone from the 8 S cytoplasmic receptor to the 5 S nuclear receptor. Recently, JENSEN et al. (1968, 1969a) have proposed a two step sequential mechanism for the uptake and retention of estradiol-17β. JENSEN has postulated that estradiol-17β first interacts without chemical alteration with a 4 S binding unit of the 8 S cytoplasmic protein. This interaction is followed by a transformation (which is temperature dependent) to the 5 S form, and then by migration of the estradiol-receptor complex into the nucleus. It is not known whether these events are sequential or simultaneous. It is this nuclear form of the receptor that interacts with some nuclear acceptor site and produces the stimulation of biosynthetic processes leading to growth and differentiation. A similar model has been proposed (GORSKI et al., 1968) (see Fig. 5).

There is some question as to the exact levels of specific estrogen receptors in target organs, since the circulating levels of estrogen change during the cycle and are never really zero, even under special conditions, such as in the immature or ovariectomized animals. Therefore, most binding assays using labeled steroids exclude those receptor sites already occupied by endogenous estradiol. Recently, MCGUIRE and LISK (1968) have shown that, in intact female rats, target tissues such as the uterus, pituitary, and hypothalamus, preferentially accumulate labeled estradiol-17β in a manner inversely proportional to the expected circulating level of the steroid. Furthermore, they suggested that the estrogen receptor degenerates in the absence of estrogenic steroids and that the measured hormone retention by the cell may be the result of new receptor activity. Earlier, a comparison of the uptake and retention of ^{3}H-estradiol-17β by target tissues of the immature,

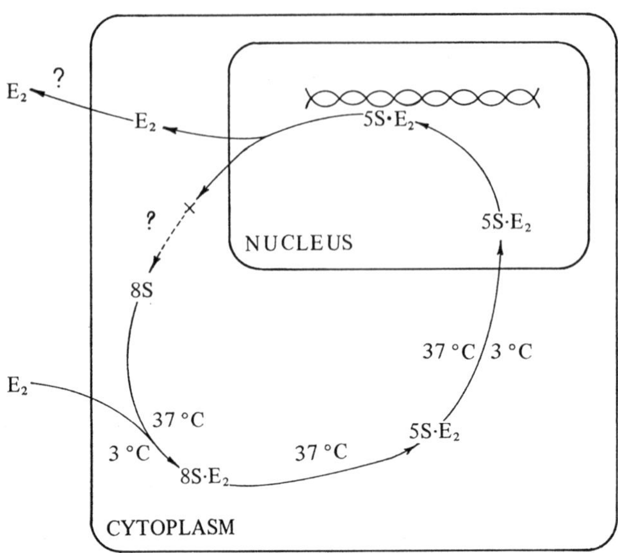

Fig. 5. Proposed model for interaction of estrogen with a target cell. E_2 = estradiol-17β; S = Svedberg

mature intact, and mature ovariectomized female rat led EISENFELD and AXELROD (1966) to the conclusion that, while the distribution of the steroid was similar, there was a lower concentration but higher content in the uterus of intact, mature females. In confirmation of the findings of JENSEN and JACOBSON (1962), administration of estradiol-17β to ovariectomized rats increased the estrogen-binding capacity of the uterus. FEHERTY et al. (1970) argue that the concentration of receptors in the uterus does not reflect alterations in the levels of cytoplasmic protein but rather the concentration is influenced by the hormonal state of the animal. Changes in the concentration of receptor activity were observed during the estrus cycle, pseudopregnancy, pregnancy, and after ovariectomy. Low receptor activity in the uteri of ovariectomized females could be restored by treatment with estradiol-17β. FEHERTY et al. (1970) have suggested that there is little contribution to binding by endogenous steroid in view of the high concentration of available receptor sites.

Studies on the ontogeny of the estrogen receptor in the rodent uterus by CLARK and GORSKI (1970) have shown that there are increases in the concentration of estrogen-binding sites between 1 and 10 days following birth. After that time, the number of binding sites/cell decreased slightly and remained constant up to 22 days of life. They suggest that the estrogen binding protein is an autonomous property of the uterine cell. LEE and JACOBSON (1971) studied the levels of estrogen receptors in rats 21 to 45 days of age. Their results indicated that the concentration of available receptors in the uterus is under direct or indirect hormonal control as evidenced by cyclic fluctuation in the amount of receptor during the estrus cycle. SARFF and GORSKI (1971) have proposed that there are three events determining the concentration of cytoplasmic estrogen receptor, following the administration of physiological amounts of hormone. These are (1) depletion, (2) macromolecular synthesis, and (3) replenishment. These investigators also found that uterine estrogen receptor had a half-life of 5 to 6 days, which is considerably longer than that of most uterine proteins (20 to 22 h) (GORSKI and NOTIDES, 1969).

As pointed out previously, evidence has been presented which indicates that specific estrogen binding proteins are found in the uterus (TOFT and GORSKI, 1966; JENSEN et al., 1967a), vagina (JENSEN et al., 1960, 1962; STONE and BAGGETT, 1965b; TERENIUS, 1968), corpora lutea (SCOTT and RENNIE, 1971; LEE et al., 1971), pituitary gland (EISENFELD and AXELROD, 1965, 1966; KATO and VILLEE, 1967; KAHWANAGO et al., 1970; NOTIDES, 1970), hypothalamus (EISENFELD, 1967, 1970; KATO and VILLEE, 1967; KAHWANAGO et al., 1970), and mammary gland (SANDER, 1968a, b; PUCA and BRESCIANI, 1969; WITTLIFF et al., 1972b). Specific estrogen binding proteins have now been reported in uterine preparations from the rat (GORSKI et al., 1968); mouse (TERENIUS, 1968); rabbit (KORENMAN, 1968); calf (DESOMBRE et al., 1969b), seal, black bear, mink, and armadillo, (O'FARRELL and DANIEL, 1971), and man (EVANS and HAHNEL, 1971).

The role of estrogens in breast cancer is being pursued actively, and with the elucidation provided by the biochemical approach to hormone action, new insight has been gained toward the goal of better therapy. Although there are many studies (SANDER, 1968a, b, c; DESHPANDE et al., 1967; PUCA and BRESCIANI, 1969; SANDER and ATTRAMADAL, 1968a) indicating that mammary cells bind tritiated estradiol-17β, isolation of the receptor-hormone complex was only recently reported (WITTLIFF et al., 1972b). Investigation of normal breast tissue from pre- and post-menopausal women (WITTLIFF et al., 1972c) indicated that estrogen-binding proteins were apparently not present; however, the high concentration of adipose cells may have prohibited accurate measurements.

Several studies of the uptake and retention of labeled estrogens by mammary carcinomas have been conducted. A number of investigators (SANDER and ATTRAMADAL, 1968b; KING et al., 1965; MOBBS, 1966, 1968; JUNGBLUT et al., 1967; JENSEN et al., 1967a; TERENIUS, 1968; KYSER, 1970) have shown that the rat mammary carcinomas induced by 7,12-dimethylbenz(a)anthracene (HUGGINS et al., 1961, 1964) contain specific receptors for estrogen. It is certainly of interest that, in a tumor which regresses after ovariectomy, the estrogen receptor is present and that the interaction of estradiol-17β with receptor proceeds by a two-step mechanism similar to that described for the uterus (KYSER, 1970). Recently (MCGUIRE et al., 1971; WITTLIFF et al., 1972b), a specific receptor for estrogens has been described in the estrogen-responsive transplantable R3230AC mammary carcinoma of the rat (HILF et al., 1967a).

Studies are being conducted to establish the relationship between the uptake of labeled estrogen by human mammary carcinomas and metastatic lesions and the patient's response to endocrine ablative surgery or steroid therapy (LEMON, 1970; SANDER, 1968; BRAUNSBERG et al., 1967; DESHPANDE et al., 1968; KORENMAN and DUKES, 1970; PEARLMAN et al., 1969; JOHANSSON et al., 1970; JENSEN et al., 1971a, WITTLIFF et al., 1971, 1972c). These studies are based on the important observation by FOLCA et al. (1961) that, following injection of tritiated-hexoestrol into patients with breast cancer, the estrogen was taken up to a greater extent by the neoplasms from four patients who later experienced remission, than by tumors from six patients who did not respond to ablative surgery. Presently, several studies (see Table 1) indicate that approximately one half of the primary tumors from patients with infiltrating ductal carcinoma of the breast contain specific receptors for estrogens. Since one can anticipate that 30 to 40 % of the patient population presents with breast cancer that will regress after removal of endogenous estrogens (oophorectomy or adrenalectomy), information on the hormonal characteristics of a tumor, i.e. dependent, responsive, or independent, would be invaluable for predicting the response of the neoplasm in the patient. Preliminary data have been obtained by JENSEN et al. (1971 a) to indicate that remission of breast cancer after adrenalectomy occurred more often in patients having breast tumors possessing estrogen receptors than in those patients whose carcinomas did not have measurable estrogen binding proteins.

Table 1. Incidence of estrogen-binding in human breast carcinoma

Investigator	No. of Tumors examined	No. of Tumors exhibiting estrogen-binding
KORENMAN and DUKES (1970)	15	7
JOHANSSON et al. (1970)	31	14
JENSEN et al. (1971 a)	84	46
WITTLIFF et al. (1971, 1972 c)	51	28
Total	181	95

B. Macromolecular Synthesis

Since the pioneering studies of MUELLER and his colleagues (MUELLER et al., 1958; AIZAWA and MUELLER, 1961) describing alterations in the incorporation of radioactive precursors into phospholipid, nucleic acid, and protein, a great volume of information has accumulated concerning the sequence of events following the administration of estradiol-17β. Although the exact mechanism by which this steroid hormone exerts its rapid and diverse effects is not known, a better understanding of the temporal relationships has emerged within the past few years. As discussed earlier, the specific binding proteins for the estrogens appear to be essential for a response at the macromolecular level in a target cell. Inhibition of binding prevents the subsequent alterations in the syntheses of deoxyribonucleic acid (DNA) and ribonucleic acid (RNA), and in protein biosynthesis, which are required for growth and differentiation. The events following localization of the steroid in the nucleus will be addressed in the following section. However, the reader is referred to several excellent reviews containing many of the details which are unavoidably deleted in this chapter (HECHTER and HALKERSTON, 1964; WILLIAMS-ASHMAN and LIAO, 1964; MUELLER, 1965, 1971; HAMILTON, 1968, 1971; WILLIAMS-ASHMAN and REDDI, 1971).

As early as 1953, TELFER reported on the elevation of RNA in the uterus of the rat following estradiol-17β administration. However, MUELLER et al. (1958) and AIZAWA and MUELLER (1961) provided the first evidence that the steroid hormone initiated a series of time related changes in the uterus. The earliest alteration was an increase in phospholipid synthesis followed by an increase in RNA synthesis 6 h after administration of the hormone. Eighteen hours after treatment with estradiol-17β, the rate of protein synthesis was elevated; the level of DNA, however, was unaltered during the first 24 h. The increased incorporation of labeled amino acids into proteins of the estrogen stimulated uteri was correlated with an increase in the activities of several aminoacyl-transfer RNA synthetases (McCorquodale and Mueller, 1958). Data from several laboratories (Mueller et al., 1961; Hamilton, 1963; Gorski and Axman, 1964; Hilf et al., 1967; Nicolette and Gorski, 1964) indicate that the estrogen-induced response in protein synthesis was prevented by the administration of either puromycin or cycloheximide. Furthermore, administration of actinomycin D, an inhibitor of transcription, almost completely abolished the effect of estrogen on phospholipid and protein synthesis (Ui and Mueller, 1963; Hamilton, 1964; Nicolette and Mueller, 1966; De Angelo and Gorski, 1970). Thus, it appears that the initiation of growth and differentiation of the uterus by estradiol-17β is correlated with alterations in genetic expression, which are manifest in accelerated synthesis and transport of nuclear RNA species. Subsequent elevations in cellular activity apparently result from the increased availability of messenger RNA, transfer RNA, and ribosomes.

Following the uptake and retention of estradiol-17β by a target cell, numerous investigators (Talwar and Segal, 1963; Hamilton et al., 1965, 1968a; Trachewsky and Segal, 1968; O'Malley, 1969; Raynaud-Jammet and Baulieu, 1969; Gorski et al., 1969; DeAngelo and Gorski, 1970; Church and McCarthy, 1970; Hamilton, 1971) have concluded that the primary site of action of the steroid hormone is at the level of transcription. This is not to imply that the exact mechanism of hormonal induction is known or that the steroid interacts directly with the genome. In fact, it is the answer to this question which is presently the subject of many active investigations.

It has been shown that the activity of the DNA-dependent RNA polymerase in isolated uterine nuclei from estrogen treated immature or ovariectomized rats was increased when assayed under conditions of low ionic strength (Noteboom and Gorski, 1963; Gorski, 1964; Hamilton et al., 1965). However, protein synthesis appeared to be a prerequisite for the estrogen effect on uterine RNA polymerase, since the elevation in polymerase activity was shown to require a temperature dependent process and could be prevented by cycloheximide and puromycin (Noteboom and Gorski, 1963; Nicolette and Mueller, 1966; Gorski et al., 1965; Gorski and Morgan, 1967; Nicolette et al., 1968).

Hamilton and coworkers (Means and Hamilton, 1966a, b; Hamilton et al., 1968a, b) have investigated the effects of estrogen on the synthesis of nuclear RNA in the uterus and found that the incorporation of ^{3}H-uridine into nuclear RNA was stimulated by 40% within 2 min after a single injection of estradiol-17β to ovariectomized rats. Twenty minutes after hormone treatment, the incorporation of labeled precursor was elevated five fold. Further studies by Hamilton et al. (1965, 1968a, b) indicated that there were at least two DNA-dependent polymerases in isolated uterine nuclei. The product of one reaction, which was Mg^{++} activated, was ribosomal in nature, i.e., $A+U/G+C = 0.8$; the product of the second, Mn^{++} activated polymerase, was more DNA like ($A+U/G+C = 1.0$). The activity of the Mn^{++} activated polymerase was not elevated until 12 h after estrogen administration. However, the Mg^{++} activated reaction was significantly stimulated within 1 h, confirming the earlier report of Gorski (1964).

The increase in the rate of RNA synthesis has been attributed to increased amounts of genetic template undergoing transcription. Several laboratories (Barker and Warren, 1966b; Teng and Hamilton, 1968; Church and McCarthy, 1970) have shown that the template capacity of uterine chromatin isolated after estrogen treatment was significantly elevated over the control value. However, Barry and Gorski (1971) have recently presented convincing evidence that estrogen does not cause a change in the number of growing chains, but does elevate the rate of chain elongation. Their data imply that the activity, and not the concentration, of polymerase molecules has changed in response to estrogen. Additionally, little of the estrogen effect was due to transcription of additional template, although DEANGELO and GORSKI (1970) reported earlier that there was a small change in the population of templates.

It is known that the labeling of cytoplasmic RNA species is preceded by an increase in the incorporation of radioactive precursors into nuclear RNA in estrogen stimulated uteri, indicating that RNA is transported from the nucleus to the cytoplasm. However, the central question of whether estradiol-17β increases the rate of transport across the nuclear membrane deserves mention. HAMILTON (1971) has suggested that the labeling of all cytoplasmic species of RNA was accelerated by estradiol-17β, indicating a general effect on the rate of transport from the nucleus. Recently, LUCK and HAMILTON (1972) have provided evidence that estrogen stimulated not only the rate of synthesis of ribosomal RNA in the uterus, but also the rate of processing of precursor RNA of higher molecular weight. Earlier, BILLING et al. (1969) had reported that an elevation in the synthesis of ribosomal precursor was the first change observed in the immature rat uterus in response to administration of estradiol-17β. These data extend the observation made by MOORE and HAMILTON (1964) that estradiol-17β stimulated both the rate of synthesis and the cytoplasmic concentration of ribosomes in the uterus. Simultaneously, GREENMAN and KENNEY (1964) reported that both the number and the capacity of uterine ribosomes to stimulate amino acid incorporation into protein *in vitro* were dependent upon estrogen. Thus, it appears that the synthesis of specific nuclear RNA species, particularly the precursor of ribosomal RNA, is an early and essential response to the administration of estradiol-17β. Enhancement of protein synthesis is correlated with the appearance of new ribosomes in the cytoplasm.

In addition to the early action of estradiol-17β on the synthesis of stable species of RNA, several workers (NOTIDES and GORSKI, 1966; MAYOL and THAYER, 1970; DEANGELO and GORSKI, 1970) have reported evidence for the induction of specific acidic proteins in the uterus of the immature rat. However, treatment with actinomycin D abolished the hormonal induction, indicating a requirement for RNA synthesis. TENG and HAMILTON (1970) recently reported that estrogen induced the synthesis of a specific nuclear acidic protein in the uterus. Although the identity of these proteins is unknown presently, it is of interest that all are acidic in nature.

It has been observed by many investigators that elevations in the levels of certain serum components, such as lipid, calcium, phosphorus, and protein, occur during periods of vitellogenesis (yolk protein formation) in various species of oviparous vertebrates (HESS et al., 1928; LASKOWSKI, 1935, 1936; ZWARENSTEIN and SHAPIRO, 1933; DESSAUER et al., 1956; DESSAUER and FOX, 1959; CLARK, 1967; ROEPKE and HUGHES, 1935; VANSTONE et al., 1955; MCINDOE, 1959; URIST and SCHJEIDE, 1961). More conclusive studies have shown that these striking changes in the serum can be produced in nonvitellogenic females or, more interestingly, in males by the administration of estradiol-17β or an analog (MCDONALD and RIDDLE, 1945; CLEGG et al., 1951; SCHJEIDE and URIST, 1956; VANSTONE et al., 1957; SCHJEIDE et al., 1963; GREENGARD et al., 1964, 1965; CLARK, 1967; HAHN, 1967; GRUBER, 1967; WALLACE and JARED, 1968a, b; WALLACE and DUMONT, 1968; FOLLETT and REDSHAW, 1968; FOLLETT et al., 1968; REDSHAW et al., 1969; BEUVING and GRUBER, 1971a, b; WITTLIFF and KENNEY, 1972; ZELSON and WITTLIFF, 1973). Several investigators (SCHJEIDE et al., 1963; HAHN,

1967; NICHOLLS et al., 1968) have also shown that there are changes in the cytology of the liver associated with the vitellogenic state.

Although COMMON and MOK (1959) and MOK et al. (1961) provided the first evidence for the probable identity of egg and serum phosphoproteins, the report from HEALD and McLACHLAN (1963) revealed a striking chemical similarity between egg phosvitin (a yolk protein) and the phosphoprotein obtained from the blood of untreated laying hens. These studies and others (SCHJEIDE and URIST, 1960; McCULLY and COMMON, 1961; HEALD and McLACHLAN, 1964) suggested that the serum phosphoprotein of the chicken exists as a calcium-lipophosphoprotein complex, which contains phosvitin. In the amphibia, WALLACE and JARED (1968a, 1969), WALLACE and DUMONT (1968), and WALLACE (1970) have shown that the phosphoprotein, which appears in the serum of vitellogenic females or estrogen treated males, has a molecular weight of 460000 and a lipid and protein-phosphorus content of 12 and 14 %, respectively. WALLACE (1970) proposed that this phosphoprotein complex, which he termed vitellogenin, is composed of a covalently bound complex of one lipovitellin dimer (lipovitellin is a protein component of yolk) and two phosvitin molecules; this complex is the immediate precursor of these yolk proteins. Supporting data for this proposal have been provided by FOLLETT et al. (1968), MUNDAY et al. (1968), and WITTLIFF and KENNEY (1972). Synthesis of the yolk proteins is apparently limited to the liver (HEALD and McLACHLAN, 1964; GREENGARD et al., 1965; RUDACK and WALLACE, 1968; WITTLIFF and KENNEY, 1972), although its subsequent secretion into the serum is rapid (ZELSON and WITTLIFF, 1973).

Because of the unique nature of the response to estrogens by oviparous vertebrates, many investigators have chosen this system to study the mechanism of hormonal induction of the synthesis of ribonucleic acid and protein (CARLSEN et al., 1964; GREENGARD et al., 1964, 1965; COOLSMA and GRUBER, 1968; HAHN et al., 1969a, b; MÄENPÄÄ and BERNFELD, 1969, 1970; BECK et al., 1970; WITTLIFF and KENNEY, 1972; WITTLIFF et al., 1972a).

Estrogens are also known to cause certain morphological changes in the chick oviduct (HERTZ et al., 1947). Administration of the hormone stimulates the growth of the oviduct and the synthesis of ovalbumin (O'MALLEY, 1967; DINGMAN et al., 1969). Later studies by HAHN et al. (1968), using DNA-RNA hybridization techniques, and by DINGMAN et al. (1969), using polyacrylamide gel procedures, revealed that new RNA species were synthesized by the oviduct after treatment with estrogen. PALMITER et al. (1970) found that there was a secondary elevation in the synthesis of certain oviduct proteins induced by estradiol-17β, resulting from the reassembly of polysomes from preexisting ribosomes.

In the chicken, estrogen presumably increased the formation of transfer-RNA specific for serine (CARLSEN et al., 1964; MÄENPÄÄ and BERNFELD, 1969) and phosphoserine (MÄENPÄÄ and BERNFELD, 1970), which are related to the induction of phosvitin synthesis by the liver. DINGMAN et al. (1969) have also reported an increase in nuclear transfer-RNA isolated from the oviducts of chicks treated with diethylstilbesterol. Earlier O'MALLEY et al. (1968) had shown that amino acid acceptor activity was elevated simultaneously with an accumulation of 4 S RNA in the oviducts of immature chicks treated with estrogen. In a brief report, HACKER (1969) suggested that long term treatment of chicks with diethylstilbesterol resulted in elevated tRNA methylase activity. Using the amphibian, WITTLIFF et al. (1972a) have shown that there was no alteration in the charging capacity or in the distribution of isoaccepting species of seryl-tRNA at a time when hepatic yolk protein synthesis was elevated.

C. Carbohydrate Metabolism

In the preceding sections, we have dealt with the immediate metabolic events that occur in the uterus in response to an estrogenic stimulus. Following the very rapid interaction between hormone and receptor, the target tissue initiates a sequence of gene directe devents, which result in the classical uterotrophic response. Since both endogenous and synthetic estrogens are effective in stimulating growth and secretion in the uterus, it is logical that energy will be required for such synthetic processes. Numerous studies have been conducted to investigate this aspect of hormone action and particular attention will be given to changes in carbohydrate metabolism resulting from the administration of estrogens. While it is not likely that many of these changes would be involved in the very early action of the hormone on its target tissue, it is certainly important to ascertain the role of those pathways associated with carbohydrate metabolism that are influenced by treatment with hormones. It is certainly pertinent that data have been reported suggesting that abnormalities in carbohydrate metabolism of the endometrium of women occur in patients demonstrating fertility problems or habitual abortion (HUGHES and RUBULIS, 1966).

Much use has been made of inhibitors of protein and RNA synthesis to ascertain the basis for the estrogen induced alterations in enzyme activity. Substances such as actinomycin D, which inhibits DNA-directed RNA synthesis, and cycloheximide, which inhibits protein synthesis, have been employed extensively in experiments designed to demonstrate inhibition of hormone induced responses when the inhibitor was administered concomitant with or immediately preceding treatment with the hormone. Caution must be exercised, however, in reaching definitive conclusions from these experiments, as generalized toxicity attendant on the use of these inhibitors may account for or mask the desired specificity of the inhibition. It has been shown by LERNER et al. (1965) that although actinomycin D was capable of inhibiting the estrogen induced uterotrophic response in immature rats, generalized toxicity as reflected by reduced body weight gain was observed in animals at most of the doses of actinomycin D employed. More credence may be given to results of experiments in which dose-related inhibitions are observed. Additionally, conclusions from studies *in vitro*, in which inhibitors have been used at considerable doses, i.e. level of drug relative to the amount of tissue, also present certain problems in translating data from experiments *in vitro* to the studies *in vivo*. Certainly, the use of specific antiestrogens, such as those discussed in an earlier section, may give more meaningful interpretations, as the basis of inhibition would be primarily competition for estrogen receptor sites.

The central role of glucose-6-phosphate in carbohydrate metabolism has prompted numerous studies of enzymes utilizing this phosphorylated sugar as a substrate. SZEGO and ROBERTS (1953) demonstrated that glucose uptake in uteri was elevated as early as 4 h after injection of estrogen. Glycogen formation (WALAAS, 1952) and increased glucose-6-phosphate dehydrogenase (G6PD) activity (SCOTT and LISI, 1960) were shown to be increased at 12 h after administration of estradiol. Since G6PD catalyzes metabolic reactions that lead to the production of ribose, which can be utilized for RNA synthesis, as well as the production of NADPH, a cofactor essential for lipogenesis and certain steroid transformations, it seemed logical to study in detail the response of G6PD in the uterus after the administration of uterotrophic steroids. It was found that a dose related elevation in the activity of G6PD, as well as in the activities of NADP-malate dehydrogenase and to a lesser extent in NADP-isocitrate dehydrogenase, occurred after the injection of estradiol to immature rats (LERNER, 1964; LERNER et al., 1966a, b). Concomitant administration of the antiestrogen, MER-25, prevented the estradiol induced increase in the activities of G6PD and NADP-malate dehydrogenase, although MER-25 alone had no significant effect on the activities of these enzymes. HILF et al. (1965b, 1967b) had shown that actinomycin D or cycloheximide could prevent the estrogen induced increases in the activities of G6PD and NADP-malate dehydrogenase, suggesting that these dose related inhibitions of the hormone-induced responses were probably a result of protein synthesis *de novo*. Using human endometrium samples, WILSON (1959) demonstrated estrogen induced increases in G6PD activity *in vitro*, and actinomycin D blocked the hormone induced effects. Another target tissue that showed a response to estrogen administration with an increase in G6PD activity in the rat was the breast (HILF et al., 1967a); during early pregnancy there was observed an elevation in G6PD, which may be due to the elevation in endogenous estrogen during the first trimester (BALDWIN and MILLIGAN, 1966; RICHARDS and HILF, 1971b). In contrast, KITAY (1965, 1966) has shown that estradiol decreased the activity of G6PD in the rat adrenal gland, although the hormone produced an increase in corticosterone production.

Glucose-6-phosphate dehydrogenase activity in the uterus varied at different stages of the rat estrus cycle, with a significant increase occurring during estrus (NOACK and SCHMIDT, 1968). No changes were found in the activities of isocitrate dehydrogenase and malate dehydrogenase by these investigators. Several investigators have examined the time course of the estrogen induced changes in enzyme activities of the uterus after injection of a single dose of estradiol. SCHMIDT et al. (1966, 1967) demonstrated that uterine G6PD activity was elevated at 12 h after treatment with estradiol benzoate and continued to rise up to 96 h, whereas no significant change in the activities of isocitrate dehydrogenase, aldolase, and leucine aminopeptidase occurred until 24 to 48 h after administration of the hormone. ECKSTEIN and VILLEE (1966) found that G6PD activity in the uterus was elevated at 24 h after administration of estradiol-17β, whereas none of the enzymes of the citric acid cycle was affected by hormone treatment up to 96 h after injection of estrogen. In uteri from immature rats, LERNER et al. (1966a) and HARRIS et al. (1968) demonstrated a significant estrogen induced increase in G6PD activity at 4 h after treatment with estradiol-17β; glucose phosphate isomerase activity was unchanged at this time. The results on glucose phosphate isomerase are in contrast to the report of SINGHAL et al. (1967) that this isomerase was elevated at 4 h after treatment with estrogen. However, it should be noted that SINGHAL et al. (1967) employed a dose of estrogen that was 40 times higher than the amount of estrogen used in the studies of LERNER et al. (1967a) and HARRIS et al. (1968).

Estrogen can produce elevations in G6PD activity in mammary tumors. HILF et al. (1965a, 1966, 1968) have demonstrated an estrogen induced increase in G6PD activity in the R3230AC and 13762 mammary adenocarcinomas, as well as in the primary breast cancers induced by 7,12-dimethylbenz(a)anthracene or by 3-methylcholanthrene (HILF et al., 1969). In contrast, a mammary tumor unresponsive to hormonal therapy, the HMC carcinoma, did not display any alteration in enzyme activities after the administration of pharmacologic doses of estrogen (HILF, 1970). Further studies of these neoplasms have demonstrated that the estrogen induced elevation of G6PD activity in the R3230AC tumor was prevented by concomitant administration of actinomycin D or of cycloheximide (HILF et al., 1965b, 1967b) suggesting that the response of the enzyme in the tumor, as well as in the uterus, was due to enzyme synthesis *de novo*. In contrast, removal of the ovaries of animals bearing the 7,12-dimethylbenz(a)-

anthracene induced hormone dependent tumors resulted in a decrease in G6PD activity (HILF et al., 1971a), the decrease occurring prior to a regression of the neoplasm (HILF et al., 1971b). More recent studies of RICHARDS and HILF (1971a, 1972) have indicated that two isoenzymes of G6PD exist in the quiescent mammary gland, the R3230AC tumor and the 7,12-dimethylbenz(a)anthracene induced carcinoma. Administration of estrogen produced a striking increase in only one isoenzyme species in the normal breast and in the R3230AC tumor; ovariectomy caused a dramatic decrease in only one isoenzyme in the carcinogen-induced carcinoma. In the uterus, there appeared to be at least three isoenzyme species of G6PD; only the fastest migrating isoenzyme demonstrated a dose related increase in activity after estrogen was administered (HILF et al., 1972). HORI and MATSUI (1967) found that liver contained 7 isoenzymes of G6PD, only one of which increased after treatment of the animals with estrogen. It would appear that estrogen can produce a rapid elevation in the activity of G6PD in both normal and neoplastic target tissues and that the hormonal effect may be primarily limited to certain discrete isoenzyme species.

BARKER and his coworkers (BARKER and WARREN, 1966a; BARKER, 1967) have suggested that the estrogen induced increase in G6PD may be due, at least in part, to a regulatory role of NADP. Intrauterine application of NADP produced an increase in G6PD activity, as early as 2 h after introduction of the cofactor, whereas administration of estradiol-17β via the same route did not increase G6PD activity until 6 h after application of the hormone. It is of interest that the NADP-induced enzyme elevation was not inhibited by actinomycin D, but was inhibited by cycloheximide, compared with the ability of both inhibitors to prevent the estrogen-induced changes in enzyme activity. These investigators (O'DORISIO and BARKER, 1970) propose that the increased level of NADP, seen first at 4 h after estradiol-17β was administered, may interact with a nascent form of G6PD enzyme, resulting in a configurational change that would be required for enzyme activity (KIRKMAN, 1962; NIELSON and WARREN, 1965). These most interesting results will require further studies to delineate this proposed sequence of events.

NICOLETTE and GORSKI (1964) found an increased incorporation of uniformly labeled glucose into uterine CO_2, protein, RNA, and lipid as early as 1 to 2 h after administration of 5 μg of estradiol-17β to immature rats; the increased activities were blocked by actinomycin D and cycloheximide. This rapid metabolism of glucose to CO_2 suggested early changes in glucose metabolism resulting from administration of the hormone. SMITH and GORSKI (1967) reported that hexokinase and G6PD activities demonstrated similar responses in the uterus, increasing in activity by 8 h after administration of 5 μg of estradiol-17β to immature rats. They concluded that these changes in enzyme activity were too late to be a causal event in the early effects of estrogen on glucose metabolism. SINGHAL et al. (1967) and VALADARES et al. (1968a) reported that estradiol-17β increased the uterine activities of phosphofructokinase and hexokinase relative to the dose of hormone used. Using a very large dose of estradiol-17β (0.1 mg/kg), VALADARES et al. (1968b) reported a significant increase in the activities of these enzymes as early as 4h after administration of the hormone with a peak activity occurring at 16 h. Concomitant administration of actinomycin D, puromycin, cycloheximide, or ethionine prevented the hormone induced elevations in enzyme activity. Recently, DEASUA et al. (1968) reported an estrogen induced increase in pyruvate kinase activity in uteri, a response that was prevented by inhibitors of protein and RNA synthesis. Hexokinase activity, in this study, showed similar but less marked responses to administration of estradiol-17β. It should be noted that DEASUA et al. (1968) found that pyruvate kinase activity was elevated during the estrus phase of the cycle. In the chicken oviduct, CAMPBELL et al. (1971) showed that estrogen produced a significant increase in the activities of phosphofructokinase and aldolase, and to a lesser extent, in the activity of fructose-1,6-diphosphatase. However, the doses of estrogen employed were quite large (9.6 mg per chick over a 12 day period). Nevertheless, the growth resulting in the uterus and oviduct after hormonal stimulation suggests a major role for glycolysis and further work will be required to ascertain the role of these enzymes in more physiological circumstances.

Glycogen content in the human endometrium varies at different stages of the menstrual cycle. RUBULIS et al. (1965) showed that glycogen synthetase activity was highest midway through the cycle, a time coinciding with maximal estrogen excretion, and glycogen synthetase activity was markedly elevated in samples from patients receiving diethylstilbestrol treatment. Similar data were obtained for rat uterus by these investigators (RUBULIS et al., 1965), which contrasts with the earlier report of BO and SMITH (1963) that glycogen synthetase activity was not demonstrable in uteri of rats after treatment with estrogen. A most interesting observation was made by BITMAN et al. (1966) and CECIL and BITMAN (1966), showing that cycloheximide stimulated glycogen synthesis in the rat uterus. However, the antibiotic was capable of preventing the early estrogen induced increase in glycogen synthesis. These findings were confirmed by VALADARES et al. (1968b) and were also shown to occur with administration of ethionine and actinomycin D. Since BITMAN et al. (1966) showed that cycloheximide caused a marked glycogenolysis in the liver and a resulting elevation in blood and uterine glucose levels, they concluded that the additional availability of the glucose substrate stimulated glycogen synthesis. These data again indicate the need for caution when interpreting data from experiments employing general inhibitors of the synthesis of macromolecules.

References

AIZAWA, Y., MUELLER, G.C.: The effect *in vivo* and *in vitro* of estrogens on lipid synthesis in the rat uterus. J. biol. Chem. **236**, 381—386 (1961).

ALLEN, E.: The estrus cycle in the mouse. Amer. J. Anat. **30**, 297—371 (1922).

ALLEN, E., DOISY, E.A.: The induction of a sexually mature condition in immature females by injection of the ovarian follicular hormone. Amer. J. Physiol. **69**, 577—588 (1924).

ALLEN, E., FRANCIS, B.F., ROBERTSON, L.L., COLGATE, C.E., JOHNSTON, C.G., DOISY, E.A., KOUNTZ, W.B., GIBSON, H.V.: The hormone of the ovarian follicle; its localization and action in test animals and additional points bearing upon the internal secretion of the ovary. Amer. J. Anat. **34**, 133—181 (1924).

ANDREWS, F.N., BEESON, W.M., HARPER, C.: The effect of stilbestrol and testosterone on the growth and fattening of lambs. J. Animal Sci. **8**, 579 (1949).

ASTWOOD, E.B.: A six-hour assay for the quantitative determination of estrogen. Endocrinology **23**, 25—31 (1938).

ATTRAMADAL, A.: The uptake and intracellular localization of oestradiol-17β-6,7-H^3 in the anterior pituitary and hypothalamus of the rat. Acta. pathol. Microbiol. Scand. **61**, 151—152 (1964).

AXELROD, L.R., GOLDZIEHER, J.W.: The polycystic ovary. III. Steroid biosynthesis in normal and polycystic ovarian tissue. J. clin. Endocrinol. **22**, 431—440 (1962a).

AXELROD, L.R., GOLDZIEHER, J.W.: Mechanism of biochemical aromatization of steroids. J. clin. Endocrinol. **22**, 537—542 (1962b).

BAGGETT, B., ENGEL, L.L., BOLDERAS, L., LANONAN, G.: Conversion of C^{14}-testosterone to C^{14}-estrogenic steroids by endocrine tissues. Endocrinology **64**, 600—608 (1959).

BALDWIN, R.L., MILLIGAN, L.P.: Enzymatic changes associated with the initiation and maintenance of lactation in the rat. J. biol. Chem. **241**, 59—70 (1966).

BALIN, H., GLASSER, S.: Reproductive biology. Amsterdam: Excerpta Medica 1972.

BARKER, K.L.: Cofactor induced synthesis of D-glucose-6-phosphate: NADP oxidoreductase in the uterus. Endocrinology **81**, 791—797 (1967).

Barker, K. L., Warren, J. C.: Estrogen control of carbohydrate metabolism in the rat uterus: pathways of glucose metabolism. Endocrinology **78**, 1205—1212 (1966a).
Barker, K. L., Warren, J. C.: Template capacity of uterine chromatin: control by estradiol. Proc. nat. Acad. Sci. (Wash.) **56**, 1298—1302 (1966b).
Barry, J., Gorski, J.: Uterine ribonucleic acid polymerase. Effect of estrogen on nucleotide incorporation into 3′ chain termini. Biochemistry **10**, 2384—2390 (1971).
Baulieu, E. E., Alberga, A., Jung, I.: Recepteurs hormonaux. Liaison de divers oestrogénes á des proteines utérines. Une méthode de dosage de l' oestradiol. C. R. Acad. Sci. Paris, T. **265**, 501—504 (1967).
Baulieu, E. E., Alberga, A., Jung, I., LeBeau, M. C., Mercier-Bodard, C., Milgrom, E., Raynaud, J. P., Raynaud-Jammet, C., Rochefort, H., Truong, H., Robel, P.: Metabolism and protein-binding of sex steroids in target organs: an approach to the mechanism of hormone action. Rec. Progr. Hormone Res. **27**, 351—419 (1971).
Baulieu, E. E., Raynaud, J. P.: A "proportion graph" method for measuring binding systems. Europ. J. Biochem. **13**, 293—304 (1970).
Beatson, G. T.: On the treatment of inoperable cases of carcinoma of the mamma. Suggestion for a new method of treatment with illustrative cases. Lancet **2**, 104—107 (1896).
Beck, G., Hentzen, D., Ebel, J.-P.: Essais de mise en évidence d'une regulation hormonale au niveau des RNA de transfert. I. Étude comparative des RNA de transfert de foie de poules immature et de poules en ponte. Biochim. biophys. Acta (Amst.) **213**, 55—67 (1970).
Beer, C. T., Gallagher, T. F.: Excretion of estrogen metabolites by humans I. The fate of small doses of estrone and estradiol-17β. J. biol. Chem. **214**, 335—349 (1955).
Beuving, G., Gruber, M.: Isolation of phosvitin from plasma of estrogenized roosters. Biochim. biophys. Acta (Amst.) **232**, 524—528 (1971a).
Beuving, G., Gruber, M.: Induction of phosvitin synthesis in roosters by estradiol injection. Biochim. biophys. Acta (Amst.) **232**, 529—536 (1971b).
Billing, R. J., Barbiroli, B., Smellie, R. M. S.: Changes in the patterns of synthesis of ribonucleic acid species in immature rat uterus in response to oestradiol-17β. Biochem. J. **112**, 563—569 (1969).
Bitman, J., Trezise, L. A., Cecil, H. C.: Effect of cycloheximide (actidione) on the glycogen content of the rat uterus. Arch. Biochem. Biophys. **114**, 414—420 (1966).
Blohm, T. R., Kariya, T., Laughlin, M. W.: Effects of MER-29, a cholesterol-synthesis inhibitor, on mammalian tissue lipids. Arch. Biochem. Biophys. **85**, 250—263 (1959).
Bo, W., Smith, M. S.: Comparison of UDPG-glycogen synthetase activity of the tongue and uterus. Proc. Soc. exp. Biol. (N.Y.) **113**, 812—814 (1963).
Bogart, R., Lesley, J. F., Mayer, D. T.: Influence of reproductive hormones upon growth in ovariectomized and normal female rats. Endocrinology **35**, 173—181 (1944).
Bolte, E., Mancuso, S., Eriksson, G., Wiqvist, N., Diczfalusy, E.: Studies on the aromatization of neutral steroids in pregnant women. I. Aromatization of C-19 steroids by placentas perfused in situ. Acta Endocrinol. **45**, 535—559 (1964a).
Bolte, E., Mancuso, S., Eriksson, G., Wiqvist, N., Diczfalusy, E.: Studies on the aromatization of neutral steroids in pregnant women. 2. Aromatization of dehydroepiandrosterone and of its sulphate administered simultaneously in a uterine artery. Acta Endocrinol. **45**, 560—575 (1964b).
Bolte, E., Mancuso, S., Eriksson, G., Wiqvist, N., Diczfalusy, E.: Studies on the aromatization of neutral steroids in pregnant women. 3. Over-all aromatization of dehydroepiandrosterone sulphate circulating in the foetal and maternal compartments. Acta Endocrinol. **45**, 576—599 (1964c).
Boyd, G. S.: Effect of linoleate and estrogen on cholesterol metabolism. Fed. Proc. **21**, 86—92 (1962).
Boyd, G. S., McGuire, W. B.: The effect of hexoestrol on cholesterol metabolism in the rat. Biochem. J. **62**, 19P (1956).
Bradbury, J. T.: Direct action of estrogen on the ovary of the immature rat. Endocrinology **68**, 115—120 (1961).
Braunsberg, H., Irvine, W. T., James, V. H. T.: A comparison of steroid hormone concentrations in human tissues including breast cancer. Brit. J. Cancer **21**, 714—726 (1967).
Brooks, W. F., Jr., Wittliff, J. L.: Quantitation of radio-ligand binding data using a desk-top calculator in the program mode. Anal. Biochem. **54**, 464—476 (1973).
Budy, A. M.: Metabolism, excretion, and retention of C^{14} labeled estrone in immature mice. Arch. int. Pharmacodyn. **103**, 435—452 (1955).
Butenandt, A.: Progynon, a crystalline female sexual hormone. Naturwissensch. **17**, 879 (1929).
Butenandt, A.: Über physikalische und chemische Eigenschaften des krystallisierten Follikelhormons. Untersuchungen über das weibliche Sexualhormon. Z. Physiol. **191**, 140—156 (1930).

BUTLER, T.P., PEARSON, O.H.: Regression of prolactin-dependent rat mammary carcinoma in response to antihormone treatment. Cancer Res. **31**, 817—820 (1971).

CALLENTINE, M.R., HUMPHREY, R.R., LEE, S.L., WINDSOR, B.L., SCHOTTIN, N.H., O'BRIEN, O.P.: Action of an estrogen antagonist on reproductive mechanisms in the rat. Endocrinology **79**, 153—167 (1966b).

CALLENTINE, M.R., HUMPHREY, R.R., NESSET, B.L.: LH release by 17β estradiol in the rat. Endocrinology **79**, 455—456 (1966a).

CAMPBELL, L.D., YU, J.Y.-L., STOTHERS, S.C., MARQUARDT, R.R.: Sex hormone control mechanisms. II. Influence of estrogen and progesterone on the activities of key enzymes involved in the carbohydrate metabolism of chicken oviducts. Can. J. Biochem. **49**, 201—206 (1971).

CARLSEN, E.N., TRELLE, G.J., SCHJEIDE, O.A.: Transfer ribonucleic acids. Nature (Lond.) **202**, 984—986 (1964).

CECIL, H.C., BITMAN, J.: Inhibition of estrogen-induced glycogen synthesis in the rat uterus by cycloheximide. Arch. Biochem. Biophys. **119**, 105—109 (1967).

CHURCH, R.H., MCCARTHY, B.J.: Unstable nuclear RNA synthesis following estrogen stimulation. Biochim. biophys. Acta. (Amst.) **199**, 103—114 (1970).

CLARK, J.H., GORSKI, J.: Estrogen receptors: An evaluation of cytoplasmic nuclear interactions in a cell-free system and a method for assay. Biochim. biophys. Acta (Amst.) **192**, 508—515 (1969).

CLARK, J.H., GORSKI, J.: Ontogeny of the estrogen receptor during early uterine development. Science **169**, 76—78 (1970).

CLARK, N.B.: Influence of estrogens upon serum calcium, phosphate and protein concentrations of fresh-water turtles. Comp. biochem. Physiol. **20**, 823—834 (1967).

CLEGG, R.E., SANFORD, R.E., HEIN, P.E., ANDREWS, R.E., HUGHES, A.C., MUELLER, C.D.: Electrophoretic comparison of the serum proteins of normal and diethylstilbestrol-treated cockerels. Science **114**, 437—438 (1951).

COMMON, R.H., MOK, C.C.: Phosvitin in the serum of the hen. Nature (Lond.) **183**, 1811—1812 (1959).

COOK, J.W., DODDS, E.C., HEWETT, C.L.: Synthetic oestrus-exciting compound. Nature (Lond.) **131**, 56—57 (1933).

COOLSMA, J.W., GRUBER, M., GRUBER, T.: RNA synthesis in rooster liver. Biochim. biophys. Acta (Amst.) **169**, 306—315 (1968).

DAO, T.L.: Some current thoughts on adrenalectomy. In: SEGALOFF, A., MEYER, K.K., DEBAKEY, S., Eds.: Current concepts of breast cancer, pp. 189—199. Baltimore: Williams & Wilkins 1967.

DAO, T.L., BOCK, F.G., GREINER, M.: Mammary carcinogenesis by 3-methylcholanthrene. II. Inhibitory effect of pregnancy and lactation on tumor induction. J. nat. Cancer Inst. **25**, 991—1003 (1960).

DAO, T.L., SUNDERLAND, H.: Mammary carcinogenesis by 3-methylcholanthrene. I. Hormonal aspects in tumor induction and growth. J. nat. Cancer Inst. **23**, 567—585 (1959).

DAVIS, J.S., MEYER, R.K., MCSHAN, W.H.: The effects of aminopterin and estrogen on the phosphate metabolism of rat uterus. Endocrinology **59**, 505—515 (1956).

DAVIS, M.E., WIENER, M., JACOBSON, H.I., JENSEN, E.V.: Estradiol metabolism in pregnant and non-pregnant women. Amer. J. Obstet. Gynecol. **87**, 979—990 (1963).

DEANGELO, A.B., GORSKI, J.: Role of RNA synthesis in the estrogen induction of a specific uterine protein. Proc. nat. Acad. Sci. (Wash.) **66**, 693—700 (1970).

DEASUA, L.J., ROZENGURT, E., CARMINATTI, H.: Estradiol induction of pyruvate kinase in the rat uterus. Biochim. biophys. Acta (Amst.) **170**, 254—262 (1968).

DEPAEPE, J.C.: An autoradiographic study of the distribution in mice of oestrogens labeled with carbon-14 and tritium. Nature (Lond.) **185**, 264—265 (1960).

DESHPANDE, N., JENSEN, V., BULBROOK, R.D., BERNE, T., ELLIS, F.: Accumulation of tritiated oestradiol by human breast tissue. Steroids **10**, 219—232 (1967).

DESOMBRE, E.R., CHABAUD, J.P., PUCA, G.A., JENSEN, E.V.: Purification and properties of an estrogen-binding protein from calf uterus. J. steroid Biochem. **2**, 95—103 (1971).

DESOMBRE, E.R., HURST, D., KAWASHIMA, T., JUNGBLUT, P.W., JENSEN, E.V.: Sulfhydryl groups and estradiol-receptor interaction. Fed. Proc. **26**, 536 (1967).

DESOMBRE, E.R., PUCA, G.A., JENSEN, E.V.: Purification of an oestrophilic protein from calf uterus. Biochem. J. **115**, 47 (1969a).

DESOMBRE, E.R., PUCA, G.A., JENSEN, E.V.: Purification of an estrophilic protein from calf uterus. Proc. nat. Acad. Sci. (Wash.) **64**, 148—154 (1969b).

DESSAUER, H.C., FOX, W.: Changes in ovarian follicle composition with plasma levels of snakes during estrus. Amer. J. Physiol. **197**, 360—366 (1959).

Dessauer, H.C., Fox, W., Gilbert, N.L.: Plasma calcium, magnesium and protein of viviparous colubrid snakes during estrous cycle. Proc. Soc. exp. Biol. (N.Y.) **92**, 299—301 (1956).
Dingman, C.W., Aronow, A., Bunting, S.L., Peacock, A.C., O'Malley, B.W.: Changes in chick oviduct ribonucleic acid following hormonal stimulation. Biochemistry **8**, 489—495 (1969).
Dinusson, W.E., Andrews, F.N., Beeson, W.M.: The effects of stilbestrol, testosterone, thyroid alteration and spaying on the growth and fattening of beef heifers. J. animal Sci. **9**, 321 (1950).
Dodds, E.C., Folley, S.J., Glascock, R.F., Lawson, W.: The excretion of microgram doses of hexoestrol by rabbits and rats. Biochem. J. **68**, 161—167 (1958).
Dodds, E.C., Goldberg, L., Lawson, W., Robinson, R.: Oestrogenic activity of certain synthetic compounds. Nature (Lond.) **141**, 247—248 (1938a).
Dodds, E.C., Goldberg, L., Lawson, W., Robinson, R.: Oestrogenic activity of alkylated stilboestrols. Nature (Lond.) **142**, 34 (1938b).
Dodds, E.C., Lawson, W.: Synthetic oestrogenic agents without the phenanthrene nucleus. Nature (Lond.) **137**, 996 (1936).
Dodds, E.C., Lawson, W.: A simple aromatic oestrogenic agent with an activity of the same order as that of oestrone. Nature (Lond.) **139**, 627—628 (1937).
Doisy, E.A., Veler, C.D., Thayer, S.A.: Folliculin from urine of pregnant women. Amer. J. Physiol. **90**, 329—330 (1929).
Duncan, G.W., Lyster, S.C., Clark, J.J., Lednicer, D.: Antifertility activities of two diphenyldehydronaphthalene derivatives. Proc. Soc. exp. Biol. (N.Y.) **112**, 439—442 (1963).
Duncan, G.W., Stucki, J.C., Lyster, S.C., Lednicer, D.: An orally effective mammalian antifertility agent. Proc. Soc. exp. Biol. (N.Y.) **109**, 163—166 (1962).
Eckstein, B., Villee, C.A.: Effect of estradiol on enzymes of carbohydrate metabolism in rat uterus. Endocrinology **78**, 409—411 (1966).
Edgren, R.A., Calhoun, D.W.: Estrogen antagonisms: Inhibition of estrone-induced uterine growth by testosterone propionate, progesterone and 17-ethyl-19-nortestosterone. Proc. Soc. exp. Biol. (N.Y.) **94**, 537—539 (1957).
Eisenfeld, A.J.: Computer analysis of the distribution of ^{3}H estradiol. Biochim. biophys. Acta (Amst.) **136**, 498—507 (1967).
Eisenfeld, A.J.: ^{3}H-estradiol: *In Vitro* binding to macromolecules from the rat hypothalamus, anterior pituitary and uterus. Endocrinology **86**, 1313—1318 (1970).
Eisenfeld, A.J., Axelrod, J.: Selectivity of estrogen distribution in tissues. J. Pharmacol. exp. Ther. **150**, 469—475 (1965).
Eisenfeld, A.J., Axelrod, J.: Effect of steroid hormones, ovariectomy, estrogen pretreatment, sex and immaturity on the distribution of ^{3}H-estradiol. Endocrinology **79**, 38—42 (1966).
Emmens, C.W.: Some properties of methylethylstilboestrol. J. Endocrinology **16**, 148—155 (1957).
Emmens, C.W., Cox, R.I., Martin, L.: Antiestrogens. Rec. Progr. Hormone Res. **18**, 415—466 (1962).
Erdos, T.: Properties of a uterine oestradiol receptor. Biochem. biophys. Res. Commun. **32**, 338—343 (1968).
Erdos, T., Best-Belpomme, M., Bessada, R.: A rapid assay for binding estradiol to uterine receptor(s). Anal. Biochem. **37**, 244—252 (1970).
Erdos, T., Gospodarowicz, D., Bessada, R., Fries, J.: Propriétés d'un récepteur utérin de L'oestradiol. Compt. Rend. Acad. Sci. Paris: **266**, 2164—2167 (1968).
Evans, L.H., Hähnel, R.: Oestrogen receptors in human uterine tissue. J. Endocrinol. **50**, 209—229 (1971).
Feherty, P., Robertson, D.M., Waynforth, H.B., Kellie, A.E.: Changes in the concentration of high-affinity oestradiol receptors in rat uterine supernatant preparations during the oestrous cycle, pseudopregnancy, pregnancy, maturation and after ovariectomy. Biochem. J. **120**, 837—844 (1970).
Fillios, L.C., Kaplan, R., Martin, R.S., Stare, F.: Some aspects of the gonadal regulation of cholesterol metabolism. Amer. J. Physiol. **193**, 47—51 (1958).
Flesher, J.W.: Preferential uptake of 6,7-H^{3} estradiol by the endometrium of the rat uterus. Steroids **5**, 737—742 (1965).
Folca, P.J., Glascock, R.F., Irvine, W.T.: Studies with tritium-labeled hexoestrol in advanced breast cancer. Lancet **2**, 796—798 (1961).
Folley, S.J.: The physiology and biochemistry of lactation. Edinburgh: Oliver and Boyd (1956).
Follett, B.K., Nicholls, T.J., Redshaw, M.R.: The vitellogenic response in the south african clawed toad (*Xenopus laevis* Daudin). J. cell. Physiol. **72**, 91—102 (1968).

FOLLETT, B. K., REDSHAW, M. R.: The effects of oestrogen and gonadotrophins on lipid and protein metabolism in *Xenopus laevis* Daudin. J. Endocrinol. **40**, 439—456 (1968).

GLASCOCK, R. F., HOEKSTRA, W. G.: Selective accumulation of tritium-labeled hexoestrol by the reproductive organs of immature female goats and sheep. Biochem. J. **72**, 673—682 (1959).

GORSKI, J.: Early estrogen effects on the activity of uterine ribonucleic acid polymerase. J. biol. Chem. **239**, 889—892 (1964).

GORSKI, J., AXMAN, M. C.: Cycloheximide (actidione) inhibition of protein synthesis and the uterine response to estrogen. Arch. biochem. Biophys. **105**, 517—520 (1964).

GORSKI, J., MORGAN, M. S.: Estrogen effects on uterine metabolism: reversal by inhibitors of protein synthesis. Biochim. biophys. Acta. (Amst.) **149**, 282—287 (1967).

GORSKI, J., NOTEBOOM, W. D., NICOLETTE, J. A.: Estrogen control of the synthesis of RNA and protein in the uterus. J. cell comp. Physiol. **66**, 91—110 (1965).

GORSKI, J., NOTIDES, A. C.: Estrogen control of uterine growth: synthesis of specific uterine proteins. In: BASERGA, R. (Ed.): Biochemistry of cell division, pp. 57—76. Springfield, Charles C. Thomas 1969.

GORSKI, J., SHYAMALA, G., TOFT, D. O.: Interrelationships of nuclear and cytoplasmic estrogen receptors. Curr. Top. Develop. Biol. **4**, 149—167 (1969).

GORSKI, J., TOFT, D., SHYAMALA, G., SMITH, D., NOTIDES, A.: Hormone receptors: studies on the interaction of estrogen with the uterus. Rec. Progr. Hormone Res. **24**, 45—80 (1968).

GREENGARD, O., GORDON, M., SMITH, M. A., ACS, G.: Studies on the mechanism of diethylstilbestrol-induced formation of phosphoprotein in male chickens. J. biol. Chem. **239**, 2079—2082 (1964).

GREENGARD, O., SENTENAC, A., ACS, G.: Induced formation of phosphoprotein in tissues of cockerels *in vivo* and *in vitro*. J. biol. Chem. **240**, 1687—1691 (1965).

GREENMAN, D. L., KENNEY, F. T.: Effects of alterations in hormonal status on ribosomes of rat uterus. Arch. biochem. Biophys. **107**, 1—6 (1964).

GRIFFITHS, K., GRANT, J. K., SYMINGTON, T.: Steroid biosynthesis *in vitro* by granulosa-theca cell tumour tissue. J. Endocrinol. **30**, 247—254 (1964).

GRUBER, M.: Regulation of protein synthesis in chicken liver: the action of estradiol. In: KONISBERGER, V. V., BOSCH, L. (Eds.): Regulation of nucleic acid and protein biosynthesis, pp. 383—387. Amsterdam: Elsevier Publishing Co. 1967.

HACKER, B.: Estrogen-induced transfer RNA methylase activity in chick oviduct. Biochim. biophys. Acta (Amst.) **186**, 214—216 (1969).

HAHN, W. E.: Estradiol-induced vitellogenesis and concomitant fat mobilization in the lizard *Uta stansburiana*. Comp. Biochem. Physiol. **23**, 83—93 (1967).

HAHN, W. E., CHURCH, R. B., GORBMAN, A., WILMOT, L.: Estrone- and progesterone-induced synthesis of new RNA species in the chick oviduct. Gen. Comp. Endocr. **10**, 438—442 (1968).

HAHN, W. E., CHURCH, R. B., GORBMAN, A.: Synthesis of new RNA species prior to estradiol-induced vitellogenesis. Endocrinology **84**, 738—745 (1969a).

HAHN, W. E., SCHJEIDE, O. A., GORBMAN, A.: Organ-specific estrogen-induced RNA synthesis resolved by DNA-RNA hybridization in the domestic fowl. Proc. nat. Acad. Sci. (Wash.) **62**, 112—119 (1969b).

HAMILTON, T. H.: Isotopic studies on estrogen-induced alterations of ribonucleic acid and protein synthesis. Proc. nat. Acad. Sci (Wash.) **49**, 373—379 (1963).

HAMILTON, T. H.: Sequences of RNA and protein synthesis during early estrogen action. Proc. nat. Acad. Sci. (Wash.) **51**, 83—89 (1964).

HAMILTON, T. H.: Control by estrogen of genetic transcription and translation. Science **161**, 649—661 (1968).

HAMILTON, T. H.: Steroid hormones, ribonucleic acid synthesis and transport and the regulation of cytoplasmic translation. In: SMELLIE, R. M. S. (Ed.): The biochemistry of steroid hormone action, pp. 49—84. New York: Academic Press 1971.

HAMILTON, T. H., TENG, C. S., MEANS, A. R.: Early estrogen action: nuclear synthesis and accumulation of protein correlated with enhancement of two-DNA dependent RNA polymerase activities. Proc. nat. Acad. Sci. (Wash.) **59**, 1265—1272 (1968 a).

HAMILTON, T. H., WIDNELL, C. C., TATA, J. R.: Sequential stimulations by oestrogen of nuclear RNA synthesis and DNA-dependent RNA polymerase activities in rat uterus. Biochim. biophys. Acta. **108**, 168—172 (1965).

HAMILTON, T. H., WIDNELL, C. C., TATA, J. R.: Synthesis of ribonucleic acid during early estrogen action. J. biol. Chem. **243**, 408—417 (1968b).

HAMMERSTEIN, J., RICE, B. F., SAVARD, K.: Steroid formation in the human ovary. I. Identification of steroids formed *in vitro* from acetate-1-^{14}C in the corpus luteum. J. clin. Endocrinol. **24**, 597—605 (1964).

HARRIS, D. N., LERNER, L. J., HILF, R.: The effect of progesterone and ethamoxytriphetol on estradiol- induced changes in the immature rat uterus. Trans. N.Y. Acad. Sci. **30**, 774—782 (1968).
HEALD, P. J., MCLACHLAN, P. M.: Isolation of phosvitin from the plasma of the laying hen. Biochem. J. **87**, 571—576 (1963).
HEALD, P. J., MCLACHLAN, P. M.: The isolation of phosvitin from the plasma of the oestrogen-treated immature pullet. Biochem. J. **92**, 51—55 (1964).
HEARD, R. D., BLIGH, E. G., CANN, M. C., JELLINCK, P. H., O'DONNELL, V. J., RAO, B. G., WEBB, J. L.: Steroid biogenesis. Rec. Progr. Hormone Res. **12**, 45—77 (1956).
HECHTER, O., HALKERSTON, I. D. K.: On the action of mammalian hormones. In: PINCUS, G., THIMANN, K. V., ASTWOOD, E. B. (Eds.): The hormones, Vol. V, pp. 697—825. New York: Academic Press 1964.
HEER, J., BILLETER, J. R., MIESCHER, K.: Bisdehydro-Marrianol und Bisdehydro-doisynolsäuren. Über oestrogene carbon-säuren III. Helv. chim. Acta. **28**, 991—1003 (1945).
HERTZ, R., LARSEN, C. D., TULLNER, W.: Inhibition of estrogen-induced tissue growth with progesterone. J. nat. Cancer Inst. **8**, 123—126 (1947).
HERTZ, R., SEBRELL, W. H.: Impairment of response to stilbestrol in the oviduct of chicks deficient in L. casei factor ("Folic acid"). Science **100**, 293—294 (1944).
HESS, A. F., BILLS, C. E., WEINSTOCK, M., RINKIN, H.: Differences in calcium level of the blood between the male and female cod. Proc. Soc. exp. Biol. (N.Y.) **25**, 349—350 (1928).
HILF, R.: Investigation of experimental mammary tumors. In: BIANCHI, C. P., HILF, R. (Eds.): Protein metabolism and biological function, pp. 251—261. New Brunswick: Rutgers University Press 1970.
HILF, R.: Will the best model of breast cancer please come forward? Nat. Cancer Inst. Monograph No. 34, pp. 43—54, 1971.
HILF, R., BATTAGLINI, J. W., DELMEZ, J. A., COHEN, N., RECTOR, W. D.: Some biochemical changes preceding regression of 7,12-dimethylbenz(a)anthracene-induced mammary tumors following oophorectomy. Cancer Res. **31**, 1195—1200 (1971b).
HILF, R., BELL, C., MICHEL, I.: Biochemical and morphological responses of normal and neoplastic mammary tissue to hormonal treatment. Rec. Progr. Hormone Res. **23**, 229—295 (1967a).
HILF, R., GOLDENBERG, H., BELL, C.: Effect of actidione (cycloheximide) on estrogen-induced biochemical changes in R3230AC mammary tumors, uteri and mammary glands. Cancer Res. **27**, 1485—1493 (1967b).
HILF, R., GOLDENBERG, H., MICHEL, I., CARRINGTON, M. J., BELL, C., GRUENSTEIN, M., MERANZE, D. R., SHIMKIN, M. B.: Biochemical characteristics of mammary glands and mammary tumors of rats induced by 3-methylcholanthrene and 7,12-dimethylbenz(a)anthracene. Cancer Res. **29**, 977—988 (1969).
HILF, R., GOLDENBERG, H., MICHEL, I., GRUENSTEIN, M., MERANZE, D. R., SHIMKIN, M. B.: Biochemical events associated with regression of 7,12-dimethylbenz(a)anthracene-induced mammary carcinomas after ovariectomy. Cancer Res. **31**, 52—58 (1971a).
HILF, R., LERNER, L. J., LANG, E., BORMAN, A.: The effect of progressive sarcoma 180 growth upon the uterotrophic response to estrogen in mice. Cancer Res. **23**, 304—309 (1963).
HILF, R., MCDONALD, E., SARTINI, J., RECTOR, W. D., RICHARDS, A. H.: Response of uterine glucose-6-phosphate dehydrogenase isoenzymes to estrogen. Endocrinology **91**, 280—286 (1972).
HILF, R., MICHEL, I., BELL, C.: Dose responses of R3230AC mammary tumor and mammary tissue to estrogen: enzymes, nucleic acids and lipids. Cancer Res. **26**, 865—870 (1966).
HILF, R., MICHEL, I., BELL, C., FREEMAN, J. J., BORMAN, A.: Biochemical and morphological properties of a new lactating mammary tumor line in the rat. Cancer Res. **25**, 286—299 (1965a).
HILF, R., MICHEL, I., SILVERSTEIN, G., BELL, C.: Effect of actinomycin D on estrogen-induced changes in enzymes and nucleic acids of R3230AC mammary tumors, uteri and mammary glands. Cancer Res. **25**, 1854—1859 (1965b).
HILF, R., SEGALOFF, A., LERNER, L. J.: Influence of hormonal treatment of Fischer rats on the biochemistry of a transplantable dimethylbenz(a)anthracene-induced mammary carcinoma and its sublines. Cancer Res. **28**, 1550—1558 (1968).
HISAW, F. L., VELARDO, J. T., GOOLSBY, C. M.: Interaction of estrogens on uterine growth. J. clin. Endocrinol. **14**, 1134—1143 (1954).
HOLTKAMP, D. E., GRESLIN, J. G., ROOT, C. A., LERNER, L. J.: Gonadotrophin inhibiting and anti-fecundity effects of chloromiphene. Proc. Soc. exp. Biol. (N.Y.) **105**, 197—201 (1960).
HORI, S. H., MATSUI, S.: Effects of hormones on hepatic glucose-6-phosphate dehydrogenase of rat. J. Histochem. Cytochem. **15**, 530—534 (1967).
HUANG, W. Y., PEARLMAN, W. H.: The corpus luteum and steroid hormone formation. I. Studies on luteinized rat ovarian tissue *in vitro*. J. biol. Chem. **237**, 1060—1065 (1962).

HUGGINS, C., BRIZIARELLI, G., SUTTON, H., JR.: Rapid induction of mammary carcinoma in the rat and the influence of hormones on the tumors. J. exp. Med. **109**, 25—42 (1959).

HUGGINS, C., GRAND, L. C., BRILLANTES, F. P.: Mammary cancer induced by feeding of polynuclear hydrocarbons, and its suppression. Nature (Lond.) **189**, 204—207 (1961).

HUGGINS, C., GRAND, L., FUKUNISHI, R.: Aromatic influences on the yields of mammary cancers following administration of 7,12-dimethylbenz(a)anthracene. Proc. nat. Acad. Sci. (Wash.) **51**, 737—742 (1964).

HUGGINS, C., JENSEN, E. V.: The depression of growth of the uterus, adrenals and ovaries by fluorinated steroids in the pregnane series. J. exp. Med. **102**, 347—359 (1955).

HUGHES, E. C., RUBULIS, A.: Carbohydrate defects in the endometrium. Proceedings of the 5th world congress on fertility and sterility, 453—460 (1966).

INMAN, D. R., BANFIELD, R. E. W., KING, R. J. B.: Autoradiographic localization of oestrogen in rat tissues. J. Endocrinol. **32**, 17—22 (1965).

JENSEN, E. V.: Studies of growth phenomena using tritium-labeled steroids. Proceedings of the 4th international congress of biochemistry, Vienna, Vol. 15, p. 119. London: Pergamon Press 1958.

JENSEN, E. V.: Comments on Dr. Pearlman's paper; comparison of androgens and estrogens as to their fate in target tissues. Nat. Cancer Inst. Monograph **12**, 317—322 (1963).

JENSEN, E. V.: Metabolic fate of sex hormones in target tissues with regard to tissue specificity. Proc. 2nd intern. congr. endocrinol. p. 420. London (1964). Excerpta Med. Found. Congr. Ser. No. 83 Amsterdam: (1965a).

JENSEN, E. V.: Mechanism of estrogen action in relation to carcinogenesis. Proc. Can. Cancer Res. Conf. **6**, 143—165 (1965b).

JENSEN, E. V., BLOCK, G. E., SMITH, S., KYSER, K., DESOMBRE, E. R.: Estrogen receptors and breast cancer response to adrenalectomy. Nat. Cancer Inst. Monograph **34**, 55—79 (1971a).

JENSEN, E. V., DESOMBRE, E. R., HURST, D. J., KAWASHIMA, T., JUNGBLUT, P. W.: Estrogen-receptor interactions in target tissues. Arch. anat. micr. Morph. exp. **56**, 547—569 (1967b).

JENSEN, E. V., DESOMBRE, E. R., JUNGBLUT, P. W.: Estrogen receptors in hormone-responsive tissues and tumors. In: WISSLER, R. W., DAO, T. L., WOOD, S. (Eds.): Endogenous factors influencing host-tumor balance, pp. 15—30. Chicago: University of Chicago Press, 1967a.

JENSEN, E, V., JACOBSON, H. I.: Fate of steroid estrogens in target tissues. In: PINCUS, G., VOLLMER, E. P. (Eds.): Biological activities of steroids in relation to cancer, pp. 161—178. New York: Academic Press 1960.

JENSEN, E. V., JACOBSON, H. I.: Basic guides to the mechanism of estrogen action. Rec. Progr. Hormone Res. **18**, 387—414 (1962).

JENSEN, E. V., JACOBSON, H. I., FLESHER, J. W., SAHA, N. N., GUPTA, G. N., SMITH, S., COLUCCI, V., SHIPLACOFF, D., NEUMANN, H. G., DESOMBRE, E. R., JUNGBLUT, P. W.: Estrogen receptors in target tissues. In: NAKAO, T., PINCUS, G., TAIT, J. (Eds.): Steroid dynamics, pp. 133—157. New York: Academic Press 1966.

JENSEN, E. V., NUMATA, M., BRECHER, P. I., DESOMBRE, E. R.: Hormone-receptor interaction as a guide to biochemical mechanism. In: SMELLIE, R. M. S. (Ed.): The biochemistry of steroid hormone action, 133—159. New York: Academic Press 1971b.

JENSEN, E. V., NUMATA, M., SMITH, S., SUZUKI, T., BRECHER, P. I., DESOMBRE, E. R.: Estrogen-receptor interaction in target tissues. Develop. Biol. **3**, 151—171 (1969a).

JENSEN, E. V., SUZUKI, T., KAWASHIMA, T., STUMPF, W. E., JUNGBLUT, P. W., DESOMBRE, E. R.: A two-step mechanism for the interaction of estradiol with rat uterus. Proc. nat. Acad. Sci. **59**, 632—638 (1968).

JENSEN, E. V., SUZUKI, T., NUMATA, M., SMITH, S., DESOMBRE, E. R.: Estrogen-binding substances of target tissues. Steroids **13**, 417—427 (1969b).

JELLINCK, P. H.: The metabolism of (16-^{14}C) oestrone *in vitro*. Biochem. J. **71**, 665—670 (1959).

JOHANSSON, H., TERENIUS, L., THOREN, L.: The binding of estradiol-17β to human breast cancers and other tissues *in vitro*. Cancer Res. **30**, 692—698 (1970).

JUNGBLUT, P. W., DESOMBRE, E. R., JENSEN, E. V.: Estrogen receptors in induced rat mammary tumor. In: GUMMEL, H., KRAATZ, H., BACIGALUPO, G. (Eds.): Hormone in Genese und Therapie des Mammacarcinoms, pp. 109—122. Berlin: Adademie-Verlag 1967.

KAHWANAGO, I., HEINRICKS, W. L., HERRMANN, W. L.: Estradiol receptors in hypothalamus and anterior pituitary gland: inhibition of estradiol binding by SH-group blocking agents and clomiphene citrate. Endocrinology **86**, 1319—1326 (1970).

KATO, J., VILLEE, C. A.: Preferential uptake of estradiol by the anterior hypothalamus of the rat. Endocrinology **80**, 567—575 (1967).

KENNEDY, B. J.: Hormone therapy for advanced breast cancer. Cancer **18**, 1551—1557 (1965).

KING, R. J. B., GORDON, J.: The localization of (6,7-^{3}H) oestradiol-17β in rat uterus. J. Endocrinol. **34**, 431—437 (1966).

KING, R. J. B., GORDON, J., MARTIN, L.: The association of (6,7-$^{3}H_2$) oestradiol with nuclear chromatin. Biochem. J. **97**, 28P (1965).

KIRKMAN, H.N.: Glucose-6-phosphate dehydrogenase from human erythrocytes. I. Further purification and characterization. J. biol. Chem. **237**, 2364—2370 (1962).
KITAY, J.I.: Effects of oophorectomy and various doses of estradiol-17β on corticosterone production by rat adrenal slices. Proc. Soc. Exp. biol. Med. **120**, 193—196 (1965).
KITAY, J.I.: Effects of oestradiol in adrenal corticoidogenesis: an additional step in steroid biosynthesis. Nature (Lond.) **209**, 808—809 (1966).
KORENMAN, S.G.: Radio-ligand binding assay of specific estrogens using a soluble uterine macromolecule. J. clin. Endocrinol. **28**, 127—130 (1968).
KORENMAN, S.G., DUKES, B.A.: Specific estrogen binding by the cytoplasm of human breast carcinoma. J. clin. Endocrinol. **30**, 639—645 (1970).
KORENMAN, S.G., RAO, C.R.: Reversible disaggregation of the cytosol estrogen binding protein of uterine cytosol. Proc. nat. Acad. Sci. (Wash.) **61**, 1028—1033 (1968).
KYSER, K.A.: The tissue, subcellular and molecular binding of estradiol to dimethylbenzanthracene-induced rat mammary tumor. Ph. D. Dissertation, Dept. of Physiology, University of Chicago. March, 1970.
LANGSTON, W.C., ROBINSON, B.L.: Castration atrophy. A chronological study of uterine changes following bilateral ovariectomy in the albino rat. Endocrinol. **19**, 51—62 (1935).
LASKOWSKI, M.: Über die Phosphorverbindungen im Blutplasma der Legehenne. Biochem. Z. **275**, 293—300 (1935).
LASKOWSKI, M.: Über das Vorkommen des Serumvitellins im Blute der Wirbeltiere. Biochem. Z. **284**, 318—321 (1936).
LEE, C., JACOBSON, H.I.: Uterine estrogen receptor in rats during pubescence and the estrous cycle. Endocrinology 88, 596—601 (1971).
LEE, C., KEYES, P.L., JACOBSON, H.I.: Estrogen receptor in the rabbit corpus luteum. Science **173**, 1032—1033 (1971).
LEMON, H.M.: Abnormal estrogen metabolism and tissue estrogen receptor proteins in breast cancer. Cancer **25**, 423—435 (1970).
LERNER, L.J.: Hormone antagonists: inhibitors of specific activities of estrogen and androgen. Rec. Progr. Hormone Res. **20**, 435—490 (1964).
LERNER, L.J., HARRIS, D.N., HILF, R., BIANCHI, A., RASKIN, B.K.: Responses of the rat uterus and oviduct to sex steroids as influenced by time and antagonists. Proc. 2nd int. Congr. hormon. Steroids, 628—636 (1966a).
LERNER, L.J., HILF, R., TÜRKHEIMER, A.R., MICHEL, I.: Effect of small doses of actinomycin D on oestrogen-induced uterine changes in the immature rat. J. Endocrinol. **33**, 531—532 (1965).
LERNER, L.J., HILF, R., TÜRKHEIMER, A.R., MICHEL, I., ENGEL, S.L.: Effects of hormone antagonists on morphological and biochemical changes induced by hormonal steroids in the immature rat uterus. Endocrinology **78**, 111—124 (1966b).
LERNER, L.J., HOLTHAUS, F.J., JR., THOMPSON, C.R.: A non-steroidal estrogen antagonist 1-(*p*-2-diethylaminoethoxyphenyl)-1-phenyl-2-*p*-methyoxyphenyl ethanol. Endocrinology **63**, 295—318 (1958).
LERNER, L.J., TÜRKHEIMER, A.R.: Effect of the lack of dietary protein on the uterine response to estrogen in the mouse. Endocrinology **76**, 539—542 (1965).
LEVIN, L.: The effects of several varieties of stress on the cholesterol content of the adrenal glands and of the serum of rats. Endocrinology **37**, 34—43 (1945).
LINEWEAVER, H., BURK, D.: The determination of enzyme dissociation constants. J. Amer. chem. Soc. **56**, 658—666 (1934).
LONG, J.A., EVANS, H.M.: The estrus cycle in the rat and its associated phenomena. Mem. Univ. Calif. **6**, 1—148 (1922).
LUCK, D.N., HAMILTON, T.H.: Early estrogen action: stimulation of the metabolism of high molecular weight and ribosomal RNA's. Proc. nat. Acad. Sci. (Wash.) 157—161 (1972).
LYONS, W.R., LI, C.H., JOHNSON, R.E.: The hormonal control of mammary growth and development. Rec. Progr. Hormone Res. **14**, 219—254 (1958).
MACCORQUODALE, D.W., THAYER, S.A., DOISY, E.A.: The crystalline ovarian follicular hormone. Proc. Soc. exp. Biol. (N.Y.) **32**, 1182 (1935).
MÄENPÄÄ, P.H., BERNFELD, M.R.: Quantitative variation in serine transfer ribonucleic acid during estrogen-induced phosphoprotein synthesis in rooster liver. Biochemistry 8, 4926—4934 (1969).
MÄENPÄÄ, P.H., BERNFELD, M.R.: A specific rooster liver tRNA containing phosphoserine. Fed. Proc. **29**, 468 (1970).
MARRIAN, G.F.: II. The chemistry of oestrin. III. An improved method of preparation and the isolation of active crystalline material. Biochem. J. **24**, 435—445 (1930).
MARSH, J.M., SAVARD, K., BAGGETT, B., VAN WYCK, J.J., TALBOT, L.M.: Estrogen synthesis in a feminizing ovarian granulosa cell tumor. J. clin. Endocrinol. **22**, 1196—1200 (1962).

MARTIN, L.: The uptake of locally applied (6:7-^{3}H) oestradiol-17β by the vagina of the ovariectomized mouse. J. Endocrinol. **30**, 337—346 (1964).

MARTIN, L.: Dimethylstilbestrol and 16-oxoestradiol: anti-estrogens or estrogens? Steroids **13**, 1—10 (1969).

MARTIN, L., BAGGETT, B.: The uptake of locally applied (6:7-^{3}H) oestrone by the vagina of the ovariectomized mouse. J. Endocrinol. **30**, 41—51 (1964).

MARTIN, L., COX, R.I., ENIMENS, C.W.: The rate of uptake of locally applied oestrone by the vaginal epithelium of the mouse. J. Endocrinol. **22**, 129—132 (1961).

MAYOL, R.F., THAYER, S.A.: Synthesis of estrogen-specific proteins in the uterus of the immature rat. Biochemistry **9**, 2484—2489 (1970).

MCCANN, S.M., RAMIREZ, V.D.: Neuroendocrine regulation of hypophyseal luteinizing hormone secretion. Rec. Progr. Hormone Res. **20**, 131—181 (1964).

MCCORQUODALE, D.J., MUELLER, G.C.: Effect of estradiol on the level of amino acid activating enzymes in the rat uterus. J. biol. Chem. **232**, 31—42 (1958).

MCCULLY, K.A., COMMON, R.H.: Zone electrophoresis of protein-bound phosphorous of fowl's serum. Can. J. Biochem. Physiol. **39**, 1451—1466 (1961).

MCDONALD, M.R., RIDDLE, O.: The effect of reproduction and estrogen administration on the partition of calcium, phosphorus, and nitrogen in pigeon plasma. J. biol. Chem. **159**, 445—464 (1945).

MCGUIRE, J.L., LISK, R.D.: Estrogen receptors in the intact rat. Proc. nat. Acad. Sci. (Wash.) **61**, 497—503 (1968).

MCGUIRE, W.L., JULIAN, J.A., CHAMNESS, G.C.: A dissociation between ovarian dependent growth and estrogen sensitivity in mammary carcinoma. Endocrinology **89**, 969—973 (1971).

MCINDOE, W.M.: A lipophosphoprotein complex in hen plasma associated with yolk production. Biochem. J. **72**, 153—159 (1959).

MEANS, A.R., HAMILTON, T.H.: Evidence for depression of nuclear protein synthesis and concomitant stimulation of nuclear RNA synthesis during early estrogen action. Proc. nat. Acad. Sci. (Wash.) **56**, 686—693 (1966a).

MEANS, A.R., HAMILTON, T.H.: Early estrogen action: concomitant stimulations within two minutes of nuclear RNA synthesis and uptake of RNA precursor by the uterus. Proc. nat. Acad. Sci. (Wash.) **56**, 1594—1598 (1966b).

MÉŠTER, J., ROBERTSON, D.M., FEHERTY, P., KELLIE, A.E.: Determination of high-affinity oestrogen receptor sites in uterine supernatant preparations. Biochem. J. **120**, 831—836 (1970).

MICHAEL, R.P.: Oestrogen sensitive systems in mammalian brains. Proc. 22nd. Intern. Physiol. Congr. Leyden **1** (part 2), 650—652 (1962).

MICHAEL, R.P.: Oestrogens in the central nervous system. Brit. med. Bull. **21**, 87—90 (1965).

MIESCHER, K.: Konstitution und synthese hochwirksamer abkommeinge Oestrogener Hormone. Helv. chim. Acta **27**, 1727—1735 (1944).

MIGEON, C.J., LESCURE, O.L., ZINKHAM, W.H., SIDBURY, J.B.: *In vitro* interconversion of 16-C^{14} estrone and 16-C^{14} estradiol-17β by erythrocytes from normal subjects and from subjects with a deficiency of red cell glucose-6-phosphate dehydrogenase activity. J. clin. Invest. **41**, 2025—2035 (1962).

MOBBS, B.G.: The uptake of tritiated oestradiol by dimethylbenz anthracene-induced mammary tumours of the rat. J. Endocrinol. **36**, 409—414 (1966).

MOBBS, B.G.: The uptake of simultaneously administered (^{3}H) oestradiol and (^{14}C) progesterone by dimethylbenzanthracene-induced rat mammary tumours. J. Endocrinol. **41**, 339—344 (1968).

MOK, C.-C., MARTIN, W.G., COMMON, R.H.: A comparison of phosvitins prepared from hen's serum and from hen's egg yolk. Can. J. biochem. Physiol. **39**, 109—117 (1961).

MOORE, R.J., HAMILTON, T.H.: Estrogen-induced formation of uterine ribosomes. Proc. nat. Acad. Sci. (Wash.) **52**, 439—446 (1964).

MUELLER, G.C.: The role of RNA and protein synthesis in estrogen action. In: KARLSON, P. (Ed.): Mechanisms of hormone action, pp. 228—245. New York: Academic Press 1965.

MUELLER, G.C.: Estrogen action: a study of the influence of steroid hormones on genetic expression. In: SMELLIE, R.M.S. (Ed.): The biochemistry of steroid hormone action, pp. 1—29. New York: Academic Press 1971.

MUELLER, G.C., HERRANEN, A.M., JERNELL, K.F.: Studies on the mechanism of action of estrogens. In: PINCUS, G. (Ed.): Recent prog. hormone res., pp. 95—139. New York: Academic Press 1958.

MUELLER, G.C., GORSKI, J., AIZAWA, Y.: The role of protein synthesis in early estrogen action. Proc. nat. Acad. Sci. (Wash.) **47**, 164—169 (1961).

MUKHERJEE, S., BHOSE, A.: Studies on estrogen regulation of cholesterol biosynthesis in rat liver microsomes. Biochim. biophys. Acta (Amst.) **164**, 357—368 (1968).

Mukherjee, S., Gupta, S., Bhose, A.: Effects of gonadal hormones on cholesterol metabolism in the rat. J. Atheroscler. Res. 7, 435—452 (1967).
Munday, K. A., Ansari, A. Q., Oldroyd, D., Akhtar, M.: Oestrogen-induced calcium-binding protein in *Xenopus laevis*. Biochim. biophys. Acta (Amst.) **166**, 748—751 (1968).
Nicholls, T. J., Follett, B. K., Evennett, P. J.: The effects of oestrogens and other steroid hormones on the ultrastructure of the liver of *Xenopus laevis* Daudin. Z. Zellforsch. **90**, 19—27 (1968).
Nicolette, J. A., Gorski, J.: Effect of estradiol on glucose-U-C^{14} metabolism in the rat uterus. Arch. Biochem. Biophys. **107**, 279—283 (1964).
Nicolette, J. A., Lemahiew, M. A., Mueller, G. C.: A role of estrogens in the regulation of RNA polymerase in surviving rat uteri. Biochim. biophys. Acta (Amst.) **166**, 403—409 (1968).
Nicolette, J. A., Mueller, G. C.: Effect of actinomycin D on the estrogen response in uteri of adrenalectomized rats. Endocrinology **79**, 1162—1165 (1966).
Nielson, M. N., Warren, J. C.: Steroid effects on glucose-6-phosphate dehydrogenase from bovine corpora lutea. Biochim. biophys. Acta (Amst.) **97**, 532—541 (1965).
Noack, V. I., Schmidt, H.: Cyclische Bewegungen biochemischer Parameter im Uterus der Ratte. Endokrinologie **53**, 291—321 (1968).
Noall, M. W., Allen, W. M.: Early stimulation by estradiol of amino acid penetration in rabbit uterus. J. biol. Chem. **236**, 2987—2990 (1961).
Noteboom, W. D., Gorski, J.: An early effect of estrogen on protein synthesis. Proc. nat. Acad. Sci. (Wash.) **50**, 250—255 (1963).
Noteboom, W. D., Gorski, J.: Stereospecific binding of estrogens in the rat uterus. Arch. Biochem. Biophys. **111**, 559—568 (1965).
Notides, A. C.: Binding affinity and specificity of the estrogen receptor of the rat uterus and anterior pituitary. Endocrinology **87**, 987—992 (1970).
Notides, A., Gorski, J.: Estrogen-induced synthesis of a specific uterine protein. Proc. nat. Acad. Sci. (Wash.) **56**, 230—235 (1966).
Nyman, M. A., Geiger, J., Goldzieher, J. W.: Biosynthesis of estrogen by the perfused stallion testis. J. biol. Chem. **234**, 16—18 (1959).
O'Donnell, V. J., McCaig, J. G.: Biosynthesis of steroids by human ovaries. Biochem. J. **71**, 9P (1959).
O'Dorisio, M. S., Barker, K. L.: Effects of estradiol on the levels of pyridine nucleotide coenzymes in the rat uterus. Endocrinology **86**, 1118—1126 (1970).
O'Farrell, P. H., Daniel, J. C., Jr.: Estrogen binding in the uteri of mammals with delayed implantation. Endocrinology **88**, 1104—1106 (1971).
O'Malley, B. W.: *In vitro* hormonal induction of a specific protein (Avidin) in chick oviduct. Biochemistry **6**, 2546—2551 (1967).
O'Malley, B. W.: Hormonal regulation of nucleic acid and protein synthesis. Trans. N.Y. Acad. Sci. **31**, 478—503 (1969).
O'Malley, B. W., Aronow, A., Peacock, A., Dingman, E. W.: Estrogen dependent increase in transfer RNA during differentiation of the chick oviduct. Science **162**, 567—568 (1968).
Palmiter, R., Christensen, A. K., Schimke, R. T.: Organization of polysomes from pre-existing ribosomes in chick oviduct by a secondary administration of either estradiol or progesterone. J. biol. Chem. **245**, 833—845 (1970).
Parkes, A. S.: Marshall's physiology of reproduction. Boston: Little, Brown and Co. 1966.
Parlow, A.: Differential action of small doses of estradiol on gonadotrophins in the rat. Endocrinology **75**, 1—8 (1964).
Pearlman, W. H., DeHertogh, R., Laumas, K. R., Pearlman, M. R. J.: Metabolism and tissue uptake of estrogen in women with advanced carcinoma of the breast. J. clin. Endocrinol. **29**, 707—720 (1969).
Pearson, O. H., Llerana, O., Llerana, L., Molina, A., Butler, T.: Prolactin-dependent rat mammary cancer: a model for man? Trans. Assoc. Amer. Physicians **82**, 225—238 (1969).
Puca, G. A., Bresciani, F.: Receptor molecule for oestrogens from rat uterus. Nature (Lond.) **218**, 967—969 (1968).
Puca, G. A., Bresciani, F.: Interactions of 6,7-^{3}H-17β-estradiol with mammary gland and other organs of the C3H mouse *in vivo*. Endocrinol. **85**, 1—10 (1969).
Rabinowitz, J. C.: The biosynthesis of radioactive 17β-estradiol. II. Synthesis by testicular and ovarian homogenates. Arch. Biochem. Biophys. **64**, 285—290 (1956).
Rabinowitz, J. C., Dowben, R. M.: The biosynthesis of radioactive estradiol. I. Synthesis by surviving tissue slices and cell-free homogenates of dog ovary. Biochim. biophys. Acta (Amst.) **16**, 96—98 (1955).
Raynaud-Jammet, M., Baulieu, E.-E.: Action de l'oestradiol *in vitro:* augmentation de la biosynthèse d'acide ribonucléique dans les noyaux utérins. C. R. Acad. Sci. Paris **268**, 3211—3214 (1969).

REDSHAW, M. R., FOLLET, B. K., NICHOLLS, T. J.: Comparative effects of the estrogens and other steroid hormones on serum lipids and proteins in *Xenopus laevis* Daudin. J. Endocrinol. **43**, 47—53 (1969).

RICHARDS, A. H., HILF, R.: Glucose-6-phosphate and lactate dehydrogenase isoenzymes in rodent mammary carcinomas and the effect of oophorectomy. Biochim. biophys. Acta (Amst.) **232**, 753—756 (1971a).

RICHARDS, A. H., HILF, R.: Glucose-6-phosphate (G6PD) and lactate (LDH) isoenzymes in several states of differentiation of the rat mammary gland. Fed. Proc. **30**, 1172 (1971b).

RICHARDS, A. H., HILF, R.: Effect of estrogen administration on glucose-6-phosphate dehydrogenase and lactate dehydrogenase isoenzymes in rodent mammary tumors and normal mammary glands. Cancer Res. **32**, 611—616 (1972).

ROBSON, J. M.: Effect of oestrin on the reactivity and spontaneous activity of the rabbit's uterus. J. Physiol. **79**, 139—151 (1933).

ROBSON, J. M.: Quantitative data on the inhibition of oestrus by testosterone, progesterone and certain other compounds. J. Physiol. **92**, 371—382 (1938).

ROBSON, J. M., SCHONBERG, A.: Oestrus reactions, including mating, produced by triphenyl ethylene. Nature (Lond.) **140**, 106 (1937).

ROCHEFORT, H., BAULIEU, E. E.: Récepteurs hormonaux: relations entre les "récepteurs" utérins de l'oestradiol. Compt. Rend. Acad. Sci. (Paris) **267**, 662—665 (1968).

ROEPKE, R. R., HUGHES, J. S.: Phosphorous partition in the blood serum of laying hens. J. biol. Chem. **108**, 79—83 (1935).

ROY, S., MAHESH, V. B., GREENBLATT, R. B.: Inhibition of uptake of radioactive estradiol by the uterus and pituitary gland of immature rats. Acta Endocrinol. **47**, 669—675 (1964).

RUBULIS, A., JACOBS, R. D., HUGHES, E. C.: Glycogen synthetase in mammalian uterus. Biochim. biophys. Acta (Amst.) **99**, 584—586 (1965).

RUDACK, D., WALLACE, R. A.: On the site of phosvitin synthesis in *Xenopus laevis*. Biochim. biophys. Acta (Amst.) **155**, 299—301 (1968).

RYAN, K. J.: The conversion of prenenolone-7-^{3}H and progesterone-4-^{14}C to oestradiol by a corpus luteum of pregnancy. Acta Endocrinol. **44**, 81—89 (1963).

RYAN, K. J., ENGEL, L. L.: The interconversion of estrone and estradiol-17β by rat liver slices. Endocrinology **52**, 277—286 (1953a).

RYAN, K. J., ENGEL, L. L.: The interconversion of estrone and estradiol by human tissue slices. Endocrinology **52**, 287—291 (1953b).

RYAN, K. J., SMITH, O. W.: Biogenesis of estrogens by the human ovary. I. Conversion of acetate-1-C^{14} to estrone and estradiol. J. biol. Chem. **236**, 705—709 (1961a).

RYAN, K. J., SMITH, O. W.: Biogenesis of estrogens by the human ovary. II. Conversion of progesterone-4-C^{14} to esterone and estradiol. J. biol. Chem. **236**, 710—714 (1961b).

SANDER, S.: The uptake of 17β-oestradiol in breast tissue of female rats. Acta Endocrinol. **58**, 49—56 (1968a).

SANDER, S.: The uptake of 17β-oestradiol in breast tissue of rats following hypophysectomy. Acta Endocrinol. **59**, 235—238 (1968b).

SANDER, S.: The *in vitro* uptake of oestradiol in biopsies from 25 breast cancer patients. Acta path. Microbiol. scand. **74**, 301—302 (1968c).

SANDER, S., ATTRAMADAL, A.: An autoradiographic study of oestradiol incorporation into the breast tissue of female rats. Acta Endocrinol. **58**, 235—242 (1968a)

SANDER, S., ATTRAMADAL, A.: The *in vivo* uptake of oestradiol-17β by hormone responsive and unresponsive breast tumours of the rat. Acta. path. Microbiol. scand. **74**, 169—178 (1968b).

SARFF, M., GORSKI, J.: Control of estrogen binding protein concentration under basal conditions and after estrogen administration. Biochemistry **10**, 2557—2563 (1971).

SCATCHARD, G.: The attractions of proteins for small molecules and ions. Ann. N. Y. Acad. Sci. **51**, 660—672 (1949).

SCHINZINGER, A.: Über carcinoma mammae. Bericht über die Verhandlungen der Deutschen Gesellschaft für Chirurgie, 18. Kongreß als Beilage zum Centralblatt f. Chir. **29**, 55 (1889).

SCHJEIDE, O. A., URIST, M. R.: Proteins and calcium in serums of estrogen-treated roosters. Science **124**, 1242—1244 (1956).

SCHJEIDE, O. A., URIST, M. R.: Proteins induced in plasma by oestrogens. Nature (Lond.) **188**, 291—294 (1960).

SCHJEIDE, O. A., WILKENS, M., MCCANDLESS, R. G., MUNN, R., PETERSON, M., CARLSEN, E.: Liver synthesis, plasma transport and structural alterations accompanying passage of yolk proteins. Amer. Zool. **3**, 167—184 (1963).

SCHMIDT, H., NOACK, I., WALTHER, H., VOIGT, K. D.: Einfluß von Cyclus und exogener Hormonzufuhr auf Stoffwechselvorgänge des Rattenuterus. Acta Endocrinol. **56**, 231—243 (1967).

Schmidt, H., Walther, H., Voigt, K. D.: Der Einfluß von Ostradiol auf den Gehalt des Rattenuterus an Nucleinsäuren, Protein und Enzymaktivitäten. Enzymol. biol. Clin. **7**, 239—248 (1966).
Scott, D. B. M., Lisi, A. G.: Changes in enzymes of the uterus of the ovariectomized rat after treatment with oestradiol. Biochem. J. **77**, 52—63 (1960).
Scott, R. S., Rennie, P. I. C.: An estrogen receptor in the corpora lutea of the pseudo-pregnant rabbit. Endocrinology **89**, 297—301 (1971).
Shay, H., Harris, C., Gruenstein, M.: Influence of sex hormones on the incidence and form of tumors produced in male or female rats by gastric instillation of methylcholanthrene. J. nat. Cancer Inst. **13**, 307—332 (1952).
Shelton, R. S., Vancampen, M. G., Jr., Meisner, D. F., Parmerter, S. M., Andrews, E. R., Allen, R. E., Wyckoff, K. K.: Synthetic estrogens. Halotriphenyl ethylene derivatives. J. Amer. chem. Soc. **75**, 5491—5493 (1953).
Short, R. V.: Δ^5-3β-Hydroxy steroids in the follicular fluid of the mare. J. Endocrinol. **23**, 277—283 (1961).
Short, R. V.: Steroids in the follicular fluid and the corpus luteum of the mare. A "two cell type" theory of ovarian steroid synthesis. J. Endocrinol. **24**, 59—63 (1962).
Shyamala, G., Gorski, J.: Interrelationship of estrogen receptors in the nucleus and cytosol. J. cell Biol. **35**, 125A (1967).
Shyamala, G., Gorski, J.: Estrogen receptors in the rat uterus. Studies on the interaction of cytosol and nuclear binding sites. J. biol. Chem. **244**, 1097—1103 (1969).
Singhal, R. L., Valadares, J. R. E.: The effect of estrogen administration on phosphofructokinase activity in the rat uterus. Life Sci. **5**, 1299—1307 (1966).
Singhal, R. L., Valadares, J. R. E., Ling, G. M.: Estrogen induced increase in phosphohexose isomerase activity in the rat uterus. Metabolism **16**, 271—277 (1967).
Smith, D. E., Gorski, J.: The effect of estrogen on the activity of glucose phosphorylating enzymes in the rat uterus. Life Sci. **6**, 1263—1268 (1967).
Soloff, M. S., Szego, C. M.: Purification of estradiol receptor from rat uterus and blockade of its estrogen-binding function by specific antibody. Biochem. biophys. Res. Commun. **34**, 141—147 (1969).
Steggles, A. W., King, R. J. B.: The use of protamine to study (6,7-^{3}H) oestradiol-17β binding in rat uterus. Biochem. J. **118**, 695—701 (1970).
Steinberg, M.: Hypophyseal mediation of estrogen-induced hypocholesterolemia. Advanc. exp. med. Biol. **4**, 521—529 (1969).
Steinberg, M., Tolksdorf, S., Gordon, A. S.: Relation of the adrenal and pituitary to the hypocholesterolemic effect of estrogen in rats. Endocrinology **81**, 340—344 (1967).
Sterental, A., Dominguez, J. M., Weissman, C., Pearson, O. H.: Pituitary role in the estrogen dependency of experimental mammary cancer. Cancer Res. **23**, 481—484 (1963).
Stone, G. M.: The uptake of tritiated oestrogens by various organs of the ovariectomized mouse following subcutaneous administration. J. Endocrinol. **27**, 281—288 (1963).
Stone, G. M.: The radioactive compounds in various tissues of the ovariectomized mouse following the systemic administration of tritiated oestradiol and oestrone. Acta Endocrinol. **47**, 433—443 (1964).
Stone, G. M., Baggett, B.: The *in vitro* uptake of tritiated estradiol and estrone by the uterus and vagina of the ovariectomized mouse. Steroids **5**, 809—826 (1965a).
Stone, G. M., Baggett, B.: The uptake of some tritiated estrogenic and non-estrogenic steroids by the mouse uterus and vagina *in vivo* and *in vitro*. Steroids **6**, 277—299 (1965b).
Stone, G. M., Baggett, B., Donnelly, R. B.: The uptake of tritiated oestrogens by various organs of the ovariectomized mouse following intravenous administration. J. Endocrinol. **27**, 271—280 (1963).
Stone, G. M., Martin, L.: The uptake of tritiated oestradiol and oestrone by the uterus of the ovariectomized mouse following local application. Steroids **3**, 699—706 (1964).
Stumpf, W. E.: Cellular and subcellular ^{3}H-estradiol localization in the pituitary by autoradiography. Z. Zellforsch. Mikrosk. Anat. **92**, 23—33 (1968).
Stumpf, W. E.: Nuclear concentration of ^{3}H-estradiol in target tissues. Dry-mount autoradiography of vagina, ovary, testis, mammary tumor, liver and adrenal. Endocrinology **85**, 31—37 (1969).
Stumpf, W. E.: Localization of hormones by autoradiography and other histochemical techniques. J. Histochem. Cytochem. **18**, 21—29 (1970).
Sweat, M. L., Berliner, D. L., Bryson, M. J., Nabors, C., Haskell, J., Holmstrom, E. G.: The synthesis and metabolism of progesterone in the human and bovine ovary. Biochim. biophys. Acta (Amst.) **40**, 289—296 (1960).
Szego, C. M., Roberts, S.: Pituitary-adrenal cortical antagonism to estrogenic stimulation of the uterus of the ovariectomized rat. Am. J. Physiol. **152**, 131—140 (1948).

SZEGO, C., ROBERTS, S.: Steroid action and interaction in uterine metabolism. Rec. Progr. Hormone Res. 8, 419—469 (1953).
TALWAR, G. P., SEGAL, S. J.: Prevention of hormone action by local application of actinomycin D. Proc. nat. Acad. Sci. (Wash.) **50**, 226—230 (1963).
TALWAR, G. P., SEGAL, S. J., EVANS, A., DAVIDSON, O. W.: The binding of estradiol in the uterus: a mechanism for derepression of RNA synthesis. Proc. nat. Acad. Sci. (Wash.) **52**, 1059—1066 (1964).
TALWAR, G. P., SOPORI, M. L., BISWAS, D. K., SEGAL, S. J.: Nature and characteristics of the binding of oestradiol-17β to a uterine macromolecular fraction. Biochem. J. **107**, 765—774 (1968).
TELFER, M. A.: Influences of estradiol on nucleic acids, respiratory enzymes and the distribution of nitrogen in the rat uterus. Arch. Biochem. Biophys. **44**, 111—119 (1953).
TENG, C. S., HAMILTON, T. H.: The role of chromatin in estrogen action in the uterus. I. The control of template capacity and chemical composition and the binding of H^3-estradiol-17β. Proc. nat. Acad. Sci. (Wash.) **60**, 1410—1417 (1968).
TENG, C. S., HAMILTON, T. H.: Regulation by estrogen of organ specific synthesis of a nuclear acidic protein. Biochem. biophys. Res. Commun. **40**, 1231—1238 (1970).
TERENIUS, L.: Uptake of radioactive oestradiol in some organs of immature mice. Acta Endocrinol. **50**, 584—596 (1965).
TERENIUS, L.: Specific uptake of oestrogens by the mouse uterus *in vitro*. Acta Endocrinol. **53**, 611—618 (1966).
TERENIUS, L.: Selective retention of estrogen isomers in estrogen dependent breast tumors of rats demonstrated by *in vitro* methods. Cancer Res. **28**, 328—337 (1968).
TERENIUS, L.: The effect of steroidal hormones on the binding of 17β-estradiol by the mouse uterus and vagina. Steroids **13**, 311—325 (1969).
THOMPSON, C. R., WERNER, H. W.: Studies on estrogen tri-*p*-anisylchloroethylene. Proc. Soc. exp. Biol. (N.Y.) **77**, 494—497 (1951).
TOFT, D., GORSKI, J.: A receptor molecule for estrogens: Isolation from the rat uterus and preliminary characterization. Proc. nat. Acad. Sci. (Wash.) **55**, 1574—1581 (1966).
TOFT, D., SHYAMALA, G., GORSKI, J.: A receptor molecule for estrogens: Studies using a cell-free system. Proc. nat. Acad. Sci. (Wash.) **57**, 1740—1743 (1967).
TRACHEWSKY, D., SEGAL, S. J.: Differential synthesis of ribonucleic acid in uterine nuclei: evidence for selective gene transcription induced by estrogens. Europ. J. Biochem. **4**, 279—285 (1968).
TWOMBLY, G. H., SCHOENEWALDT, E. F.: Tissue localization and excretion routes of radioactive diethylstilbestrol. Cancer **4**, 296—302 (1951).
UI, H., MUELLER, G. C.: The role of RNA synthesis in early estrogen action. Proc. nat. Acad. Sci. (Wash.) **50**, 256—260 (1963).
ULLBERG, S., BENGTSSON, G.: Autoradiographic distribution studies with natural estrogens. Acta Endocrinol. **43**, 75—86 (1963).
URIST, M. R., SCHJEIDE, A. O.: The partition of calcium and protein in the blood of oviparous vertebrates during estrus. J. gen. Physiol. **44**, 743—756 (1961).
VALADARES, J. R. E., SINGHAL, R. L., PARULEKAR, M. R.: 17β-estradiol: Inducer of uterine hexokinase. Science **159**, 990—991 (1968a).
VALADARES, J. R. E., SINGHAL, R. L., PARULEKAR, M. R.: Influence of actinomycin, cycloheximide, ethionine and 5-fluorouracil on glycogen synthesis in the rat uterus. Arch. Biochem. Biophys. **123**, 417—419 (1968b).
VANSTONE, W. E., DALE, D. G., OLIVER, W. F., COMMON, R. H.: Sites of formation of plasma, phosphoprotein and phospholipid in the estrogenized cockerel. Can. J. biochem. Physiol. **35**, 659—665 (1957).
VANSTONE, W. E., MAW, W. A., COMMON, R. H.: Levels and partition of the fowl's serum proteins in relation to age and egg production. Can. J. biochem. Physiol. **33**, 891—903 (1955).
VELARDO, J. T., HISAW, F. L., BEVER, A. F.: Inhibition of estradiol-17β-induced uterine growth in rats by desoxycorticosterone acetate, testosterone and cortisone acetate. Anat. Rec. **117**, 552 (1955).
VELARDO, J. T., STURGIS, S. H.: Interaction of 16 epi-estriol and estradiol-17β on uterine growth. Proc. Soc. exp. Biol. (N.Y.) **90**, 609—610 (1955).
VELLE, W., ERICHSEN, S.: Studies on oestrogens in cattle. Conversions of oestrogens by bovine kidney cells *in vitro*. Acta. Endocrinol. **33**, 277—286 (1960).
VONDERHAAR, B. K., KIM, U. H., MUELLER, G. C.: The subunit character of soluble estrogen receptors from rat uteri and their modification *in vitro*. Biochim. Biophys. Acta **215**, 125—133 (1970).
VORYS, N., ULLERY, J. C., STEVENS, V.: Effects of sex steroids on gonadotrophins. Amer. J. Obstet. Gynecol. **93**, 641—658 (1965).

Walaas, O.: Effect of oestrogens on the glycogen content of the rat uterus. Acta Endocrinol. **10**, 175—192 (1952).
Wallace, R. A.: Studies on amphibian yolk. IX. *Xenopus* vitellogenin. Biochim. biophys. Acta (Amst.) **215**, 176—183 (1970).
Wallace, R. A., Dumont, J. N.: The induced synthesis and transport of yolk proteins and their accumulation by the oocyte in *Xenopus laevis*. J. cell. Physiol. **72**, 73—89 (1968).
Wallace, R. A., Jared, D. W.: Studies on amphibian yolk. VII. Serum phosphoprotein synthesis by vitellogenic females and estrogen-treated males of *Xenopus laevis*. Can. J. Biochem. **46**, 953—959 (1968a).
Wallace, R. A., Jared, D. W.: Estrogen induced lipophosphoprotein in serum of male *Xenopus laevis*. Science **160**, 91—92 (1968b).
Wallace, R. A., Jared, D. W.: Studies on amphibian yolk. VIII. The estrogen-induced hepatic synthesis of a serum lipophosphoprotein and its selective uptake by the ovary and transformation into yolk platelet proteins in *Xenopus laevis*. Develop. Biol. **19**, 498—526 (1969).
Werthessen, N. T., Schwenk, E., Baker, C.: Biosynthesis of estrone and β-estradiol in the perfused ovary. Science **117**, 380—381 (1953).
Williams-Ashman, H. G., Liao, S.: Sex hormones and hydrogen transport by isolated enzyme systems. In: Kritchevsky, D., Litwack, G. (Eds.): Actions of hormones on molecular processes, pp. 482—508. New York: John Wiley and Sons 1964.
Williams-Ashman, H. G., Reddi, A. H.: Actions of vertebrate sex hormones. Ann. Rev. Physiol. **33**, 31—83 (1971).
Wilson, E. W.: The effect of oestradiol-17β on enzymes concerned with metabolism of carbohydrate in human endometrium *in vitro*. J. Endocrinol. **44**, 63—68 (1969).
Wittliff, J. L., Gardner, D. G., Battema, W., Gilbert, P. J.: Specific estrogen-receptors in the neoplastic and lactating mammary gland of the rat. Biochem. biophys. Res. Commun. **48**, 119—125 (1972b).
Wittliff, J. L., Hilf, R., Brooks, W. F., Jr.: Specific binding of estradiol-17β by normal and neoplastic breast tissues from humans. Proc. Amer. Assoc. Cancer Res. **12**, 47 (1971).
Wittliff, J. L., Hilf, R., Brooks, W. F., Jr., Savlov, E. D., Hall, T. C., Orlando, R. A.: Specific estrogen-binding capacity of the cytoplasmic receptor in normal and neoplastic breast tissues of humans. Cancer Res. **32**, 1983—1992 (1972c).
Wittliff, J. L., Kenney, F. T.: Regulation of yolk protein synthesis in amphibian liver. I. Induction of lipovitellin synthesis by estrogen. Biochim. biophys. Acta (Amst.) **269**, 485—492 (1972).
Wittliff, J. L., Lee, K. L., Kenney, F. T.: Regulation of yolk protein synthesis in amphibian liver. II. Elevation of ribonucleic acid synthesis by estrogen. Biochim. biophys. Acta (Amst.) **269**, 493—504 (1972a).
Wotiz, H. H., Davis, J. W., Lemon, H. M.: Steroid biosynthesis by surviving testicular tumor tissue. J. biol. Chem. **216**, 677—687 (1955).
Wotiz, H. H., Davis, J. W., Lemon, H. M., Gut, M.: Studies in steroid metabolism. V. The conversion of testosterone-4-C^{14} to estrogen by human ovarian tissue. J. biol. Chem. **222**, 487—495 (1956).
Young, W. C.: Sex and internal secretions. Baltimore: Williams and Wilkins 1961.
Zelson, P. R., Wittliff, J. L.: Secretion of lipovitellin into serum following induction of synthesis in the liver by estradiol-17β. Endocrinology **93**, 256—258 (1973).
Zuckerman, S.: The ovary. New York: Academic Press 1962.
Zwarenstein, H., Shapiro, H. A.: Metabolic changes associated with endocrine activity and the reproductive cycle in *Xenopus laevis*. III. Changes in the calcium content of serum associated with capacity and the normal reproductive cycle. J. exp. Biol. **10**, 372—378 (1933).

Chapter 38

Mechanism of Action of Androgens

RUSSELL HILF

With 1 Figure

Introduction

Almost 85 years elapsed between the proposal of the existence of testicular secretions affecting male secondary sex characteristics and the isolation and synthesis of testosterone in 1935. The availability of synthetic androgens was quickly followed by a profusion of now classical morphologic and physiologic studies of the effects of administration of these compounds to a large array of experimental animals. Thus, a solid foundation was laid for the biochemist to begin his explorations into the mechanisms whereby androgens produce their dramatic effects on the accessory sex organs. The information presented here can survey only briefly the many aspects of our knowledge of androgens and the author is keenly aware of the many investigators whose scientific contributions could not be acknowledged in the space allotted. The reader wishing to obtain more detailed information is referred to the very thorough treatise of DORFMAN and SHIPLEY (1956), and to the more recent books by YOUNG (1961), EIK-NES (1970), and ROSEMBERG and PAULSEN (1970).

Biosynthesis of Androgens

It is now well established that the production of testosterone arises from cholesterol via several enzymatic conversions. Cholesterol is hydroxylated to 20α-hydroxycholesterol (CONSTANTOPOULOS and TCHEN, 1961; SHIMIZU et al., 1961b), thence to 20α, 22ξ-dihydroxycholesterol (SHIMIZU et al., 1961a). This latter compound is converted to pregnenolone, with the side chain released as isocaproic aldehyde (SATOH et al., 1966; CONSTANTOPOULOS et al., 1966). Although recent data suggest that the above sequence may not necessarily be correct (BURSTEIN and GUT, 1969), all of these steps can take place in the mitochondria of the testis, as well as in the adrenal and ovary (HALKERSTON et al., 1961; TOREN et al., 1964; SULIMOVICI and BOYD, 1969).

The enzymes involved in the conversion of cholesterol to pregnenolone occur in the mitochondria, require NADPH as a cofactor and oxygen for the hydroxylation (HALKERSTON et al., 1961). While some investigators have reservations about the necessity of the second hydroxylation of cholesterol prior to side chain cleavage, there is little doubt that hydroxylation does precede side chain cleavage of cholesterol for the production of pregnenolone. Some concern has been expressed regarding the specificity of the enzymes causing hydroxylation of cholesterol, since there are similarities of mechanisms of steroid hydroxylations, particularly 11β-hydroxylation. It has been shown that hydroxylation of the steroid molecule at the C-11 position requires NADPH and a mixed oxidase system, comprising a flavoprotein, nonheme iron, cytochrome P450 and oxygen (MASON, 1957; OMURA et al., 1966). Indeed, this latter system alone will bring about side chain cleavage of cholesterol (HALL, 1967). Another question concerns the source of NADPH, the required cofactor for these enzymatic hydroxylations. One system suggested is that which utilizes succinate, a substrate which stimulates side chain cleavage in rat adrenal mitochondria (KORITZ, 1966) by a mechanism involving reversed electron flow for the production of NADH. It has been proposed that the NADH so produced can in turn reduce NADP via a transhydrogenation reaction, which in turn can pass electrons on to cytochrome P450 for the ultimate oxidative conversion of cholesterol to 20α-hydroxycholesterol.

More recent work has shown that there exists an NADP-dependent malate dehydrogenase (malic enzyme) within the mitochondrion. This mitochrondrial enzyme appears to favor the reaction which decarboxylates malate to form pyruvate and NADPH, whereas the cytoplasmic enzyme favors the reverse reaction of CO_2 fixation (SIMPSON et al., 1969). The NADPH produced by the decarboxylation of malate could be utilized as a cofactor for the enzymatic hydroxylation and a transhydrogenation step need not be invoked. A question still remaining relates to the possibility of compartmentalization of the different hydroxylation systems, so that one need not be concerned with the difficulty that would arise were both systems required to draw upon the same pool of NADPH. There are apparently some situations in which side chain hydroxylation and 11β-hydroxylation are independent of one another, suggesting a separation of cofactor pools. This will have to be affirmed.

It appears that the formation of pregnenolone from cholesterol is the rate limiting step for overall steroidogenesis (SULIMOVICI and BOYD, 1969). This system is dependent on gonadotropin since the activities of the enzymes are decreased after hypophysectomy and restored after the administration of gonadotropin (HALL, 1966). It is now considered that the gonadotropin effects are mediated by cyclic-3',5'-AMP, since perfusion of testis tissue with this cyclic nucleotide resulted in increased production of testicular steroids (CONNELL and EIK-NES, 1969). The stimulatory response of steroidogenesis to cyclic AMP may be prevented by inhibitors of protein synthesis, such as puromycin or chloramphenicol (MARSH and SAVARD, 1966; DORRINGTON and KIRKPATRICK, 1967). At the present time, the actual mechanism by which cyclic AMP stimulates steroidogenesis is not known.

Having formed pregnenolone, further conversion occurs, but at this point, branched pathways arise. That is, pregnenolone can be converted to progesterone by dehydrogenation and isomerization or to 17-hydroxypregnenolone by hydroxylation. Further conversions occur by separate pathways, depending on the initial substrate, and intermediates formed can potentially enter the other pathway. This is shown in Fig. 1 (SAVARD et al., 1956; NEHER and WETTSTEIN, 1960; CONNELL and EIK-NES, 1969; EIK-NES, 1970; HEFTMANN, 1970).

Thus, depending on the cellular environment in which pregnenolone may be found, it may act as a substrate for the 3β-ol dehydrogenase complex, which is composed of a 3β-hydroxy dehydrogenase and a Δ^{4-5} isomerase, and thus be converted to progesterone. Alternately, pregnenolone may act as a substrate for a 17α-hydroxylase enzyme and be converted to 17α-hydroxypregnenolone. Until purified enzymes are obtained for study, the available data do not indicate which substrate is favored by which enzyme (low K_m).

Pregnenolone is converted to 17α-hydroxypregnenolone by the action of a microsomal 17α-hydroxylase, utilizing NADPH and molecular oxygen. The next step in this pathway is the removal of the C-20 and C-21 functions by a microsomal enzyme(s), also requiring NADPH and oxygen, to form dehydroepiandrosterone.

A 17α-hydroxysteroid dehydrogenase reduces the ketone group at *C*-17 of dehydroepiandrosterone to form androstenediol. The latter compound in turn is converted to testosterone by the 3β-ol dehydrogenase enzyme complex, which is a NAD-dependent enzyme system.

The other major pathway, starting with the conversion of pregnenolone to progesterone, will produce testosterone by the formation of 17α-hydroxypro-

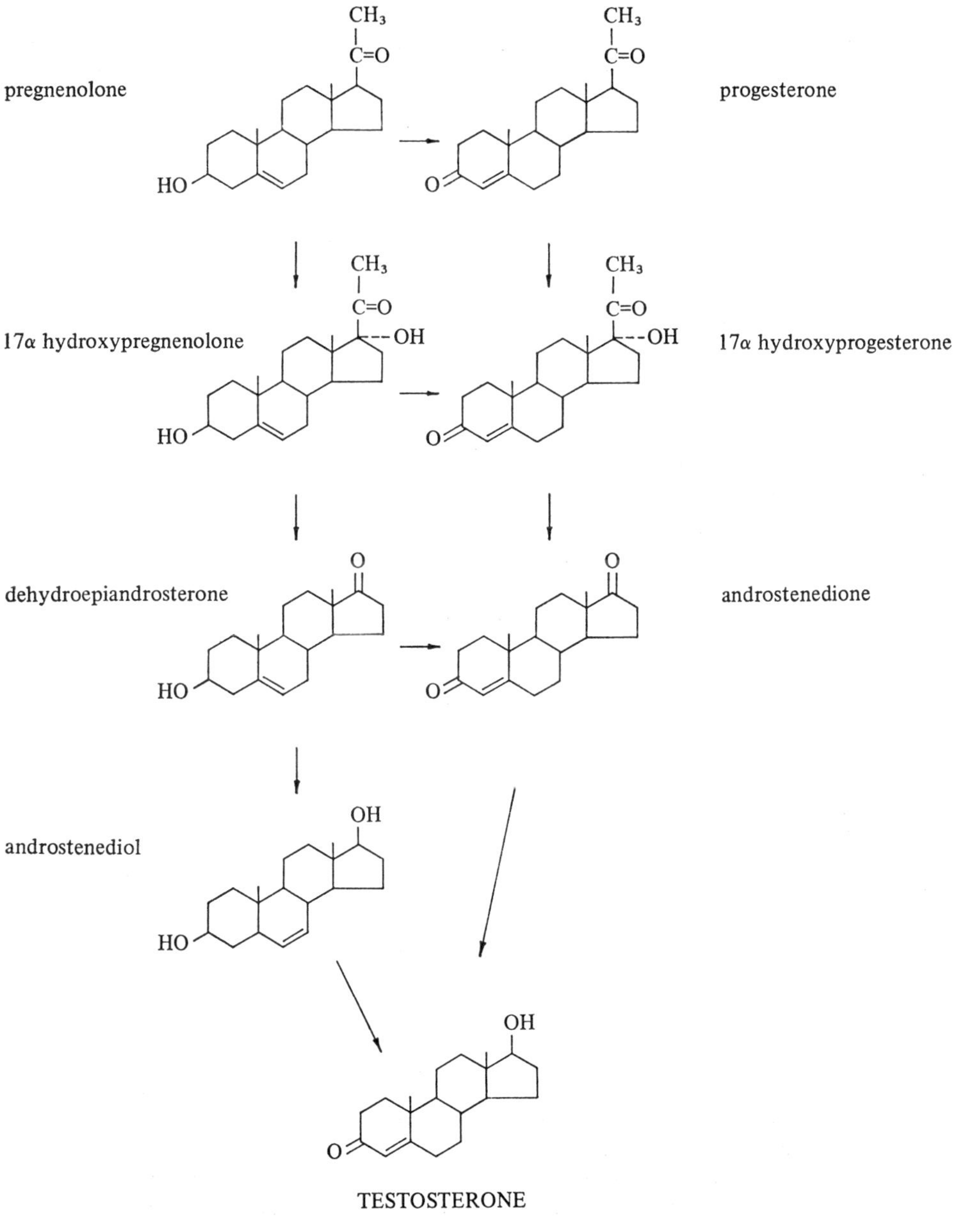

pregnenolone → progesterone

17α hydroxypregnenolone → 17α hydroxyprogesterone

dehydroepiandrosterone → androstenedione

androstenediol

TESTOSTERONE

Fig. 1. Biosynthesis of testosterone in testes

gesterone, followed by side chain cleavage (removal of C-20 and C-21) to form androstenedione, and finally, reduction of the C-17 position to yield testosterone. All of these enzymes require NADPH and, for the first two steps, molecular oxygen. All of these enzymes are localized in the microsomes.

As indicated in Fig. 1, the presence of all of these enzymes in the testis suggests the capability of interconversion from one compound to another, such that 17α-hydroxypregnenolone could be transformed to 17α-hydroxyprogesterone by the action of the 3β-ol dehydrogenase enzyme complex and dehydroepiandrosterone could be converted to androstenedione. There still remains to be established the relative flow of these intermediates through the numerous pathways available to substrates in their conversion to testosterone.

Relative Potency of Androgens

The most common assays for determination of androgenic activity are: (a) the increase in weight of seminal vesicles and prostate of immature or castrate male rats in response to administration of the test material (Dorfman and Shipley, 1956), and (b) increase in weight or area of the comb of the chick in response to injection or to inunction directly on the comb (Frank and Klempner, 1937). The relative potency of the naturally occurring androgens is as follows: testosterone, 100; 5α-dihydrotestosterone, 90; androstanediol, 60; androstenedione, 20; dehydroepiandrosterone, 10; androsterone, 10; and epitestosterone, >1. Much of the biological activity of the naturally occurring androgens must be attributed to the C-17 β-hydroxyl group, since replacement of the β-hydroxyl group with a ketone function reduces androgenic potency. It should also be noted that a 17α-hydroxyl function, as found in epitestosterone, essentially eliminates androgenic activity. Substitution of a 7α-methyl group appears to enhance androgenic potency and reduction of the A-ring to give 5α-dihydrotestosterone also increases androgenicity. The latter compound appears to be formed in androgen target tissues and may be the active cellular androgen (discussed later).

The major impetus of the organic chemist has been to synthesize compounds possessing less androgenic activity but having enhanced myotrophic (anabolic) potency. The two most commonly used anabolic agents are 4-estren-17β-ol-3-one phenylpropionate (Durabolin) and 17α-ethyl-4-estren-17β-ol-3-one (Nilevar), both of which demonstrate favorable myotrophic activities with reduced androgenicity when compared with testosterone or testosterone propionate as the standard (Herschberger et al., 1953). It should be noted that both of these compounds are 19-nor steroids.

Since testosterone is virtually inactive when administered by oral route, there are numerous synthetics in which an alkyl substitution at the 17α position has proven to enhance oral activity. It is believed that this type of substitution protects the 17β-hydroxyl group from oxidation. Some of these compounds are 9α-fluoro-17α-methyl-4-androsten-11β, 17β-diol-3-one (fluoxymesterone), 9α-fluoro-11-keto-17α-methyl testosterone, and 7α, 17-dimethyltestosterone.

Actions on Target Organs

A. Testis and Male Accessory Sex Organs

The major role of androgens is the development and maintenance of function of the male reproductive system, which includes the testis, the seminal vesicles and prostate, as well as the vas deferens and Cowpers glands. If removal of the testis is accomplished prior to puberty, the secondary sex organs, including the seminal vesicles, prostate, vas deferens, epididymis, Cowpers gland, and the preputial gland, fail to develop.

Androgens act directly on the seminiferous tubules and indirectly through the pituitary. For example, if relatively large doses of testosterone are administered to immature rats, one will obtain an increase in testis size due to stimulation of the seminiferous tubules, although there will be atrophy of the Leydig cells. This latter effect is due to inhibition of pituitary FSH. A similar situation of inhibiting pituitary FSH can be accomplished if relatively low doses of androgen are administered to young male rats (before 40 days of age), and this will result in a decrease in testis weight, arrest of spermatogenesis, and degenerative changes in the germinal epithelium (Moore and Price, 1937, 1938).

The accessory sex organs are quite sensitive to androgen for maintenance and function. Within 2 to 5 days after castration of the mature rat, the seminal vesicle shows signs of involution, changes that can be prevented by concomitant administration of testosterone (Moore and Price, 1937, 1938; Shorr et al., 1938). The response of the seminal vesicle in the castrate rat after administration of androgens is quite rapid; within 10 h one can obtain an increase in weight due to an increase in intracellular water and an increase in fructose content (Rudolph and Samuels, 1949). The response to androgen is an increase in the epithelial cells, whereas administration of estrogen will increase the fibromuscular elements of the seminal vesicles (Selye and Friedman, 1941).

Like the seminal vesicle, the prostate will undergo involution after castration (Moore et al., 1930). Androgens prevent the castration induced involution and androgens stimulate prostatic epithelium and prostatic secretions. One response to androgen administration is an increase in acid phosphatase in the prostate gland and in prostatic fluid (Huggins and Hodges, 1941). Estrogens in large doses inhibit the androgen-induced changes of the prostate.

B. Ovaries and Female Accessory Sex Organs

Androgens have been shown to induce maturation of ovarian follicles in the female rat (Noble, 1939) and administration of testosterone can lead to cyst formation in the ovary (Korenchevsky and Hall, 1940). This result is probably due to enhancement of secretion of FSH from the pituitary. However, prolonged administration of androgens will cause suppression of the ovaries (Laqueur and Fluhmann, 1942). An important action of androgens is their uterotrophic effect, producing a progesterone-like effect on the uterine endometrium (Nelson and Merckel, 1937; Selye, 1939). Like progesterone, androgens inhibit uterine motility (Robson, 1937) but unlike progesterone, androgens do not cause deciduoma (Brooksby, 1938). Although testosterone will maintain vaginal weight in ovariectomized rats, androgens antagonize the estrogen induced cornification of the vaginal mucosa (Robson, 1938). Again, this property of androgens is similar to the effects of progesterone. Finally, androgens cause enlargement of the clitoris, an undesirable response noted in women receiving androgen therapy.

C. Pituitary

Androgens, like other steroid sex hormones, are under the control of the anterior pituitary. The hormone in the male pituitary which stimulates the Leydig cells of the testis to secrete androgens is ICSH (interstitial cell stimulating hormone), whereas the germinal epithelium is apparently influenced by FSH. However, it should be noted that the two hormones show an interrelationship in their action on the testis, since androgens secreted by the Leydig cells are necessary for development and maintenance of functional germinal cells. In the castrate male, the pituitary was found to increase in weight and contained greater amounts of FSH (LEONARD, 1937). Administration of pharmacologic amounts of androgens will inhibit pituitary gonadotrophins (FSH and ICSH or LH), probably by inhibition of hypothalamic releasing factors that control the secretion of the gonadotrophins. Direct implantation of testosterone into the median eminence resulted in atrophy of the testis, seminal vesicles, and prostate and a decrease in pituitary ICSH (LH) and LH-releasing factor.

D. Breast and Breast Cancer

The administration of androgens stimulates the growth of mammary ducts and will cause development of alveoli, perhaps a response that reflects the similarity of androgens to progesterone (NELSON and GALLAGHER, 1936). It has been reported that androgens can induce a secretory state in the mammary gland epithelium of ovariectomized rhesus monkeys (VAN WAGENEN and FOLLEY, 1939). It would appear, however, that the pituitary gland is necessary for androgens to stimulate the breast. In contrast, large doses of androgen inhibit lactation and this property of androgens has been used with success to inhibit postpartum lactation (FOLLEY and KON, 1936).

Androgens have been successful in palliation of advanced metastatic cancer of the breast. Careful studies have demonstrated that objective regressions during androgen therapy are associated with increased survival. Approximately 20 % of postmenopausal women treated in this manner demonstrate objective responses, although the response rate is influenced by age of the patient, prior response to hormonal manipulation, and location of the dominant lesion. Although it had been thought that androgenicity was essential for antitumor activity, the ability of 2α-methyldihydrotestosterone propionate, which is a weaker androgen than testosterone propionate, and that of Δ'-testololactone, which possesses no inherent androgenicity, to induce approximately the same number of responses as testosterone propionate clearly indicates that virilization and antineoplastic activity are not necessarily correlated (SEGALOFF, 1966).

The mechanisms by which androgens induce regression of tumor mass are not known. The fact that the doses used inhibit pituitary gonadotrophins and/or exert an antagonism to estrogens may not be the only explanation. For example, remissions have been observed in hypophysectomized patients receiving fluoxymesterone (KENNEDY, 1958) and no reduction in urinary gonadotrophin excretion was found in patients treated with 2α-methyldihydrotestosterone propionate (BLACKBURN and ALBERT, 1959). Additional studies of the influence of androgens on growth hormone, prolactin, and TSH are necessary to determine the role that these pituitary factors may play in patients who have not been hypophysectomized.

There are several investigations of the effects of androgens on the growth and biochemistry of rodent mammary tumors. These studies have utilized transplantable autonomous hormone-responsive carcinomas as well as primary hormone-dependent carcinogen-induced mammary tumors. In general, administration of testosterone propionate resulted in inhibition of tumor growth or regression of tumor mass, accompanied by significant decreases in the activities of glucose-6-phosphate dehydrogenase, isocitrate dehydrogenase, and phosphoglucomutase in all of these experimental neoplasms (HILF et al., 1967; HILF, 1968). This effect is similar to that observed after ovariectomy of animals bearing hormone dependent tumors. It is of interest that an androgen conditioned line of the 13762 autonomous neoplasm, which required androgen for sustained growth, demonstrated an increase in the activities of the above enzymes in the presence of stimulating doses of testosterone propionate (HILF et al., 1968b). A study of the influence of androgen treatment on DMBA-induced mammary tumors revealed a decrease in aspartate transcarbamylase and phosphoglucomutase activities in those neoplasms regressing after treatment (HEISE et al., 1970). In another series of experiments, several androgens were found to be effective inhibitors of the incorporation of labeled glycine into TCA-precipitable protein of a transplantable rat fibroadenoma (ROOKS et al., 1963). In contrast, the solid Ehrlich tumor, which is a mammary cancer in origin, showed a stimulation of glycine incorporation into nucleic acids and proteins at 24 h after the administration of testosterone to tumor bearing mice (KODAMA and KODAMA, 1970).

E. Metabolic Actions

Under this category of androgen activity, target organs such as the muscle mass, kidney, and the reticulo endothelial system can be discussed together as a general anabolic response to the administration of androgens. It is well established that androgens cause nitrogen retention, an effect first demonstrated in castrate dogs (KOCHAKIAN, 1935). This effect is seen as a decrease in urinary nitrogen excretion and is probably due to a stimulation of muscle mass (myotrophic effect). This effect can be demonstrated in the absence of the testis, pituitary, pancreas, and adrenals. It is possible to enhance the nitrogen-sparing effect of androgens during periods of rapid protein anabolism, such as refeeding after a period of fasting. The effect on muscle mass of androgens has prompted investigations to find compounds possessing myotrophic activity with reduced virilizing potency. Such compounds should show an ability to increase the size of the levator ani muscle and should possess reduced potency on such end organs as the seminal vesicles and prostate.

Androgens stimulate kidney size, a result first suggested by the larger kidneys in men compared to women (MACKAY and MACKAY, 1927). Castration causes a decrease in kidney size and this decrease can be prevented by administration of androgens. Testosterone, testosterone propionate, and methyltestosterone all demonstrate strong renotrophic activity in the castrate male rat (KOCHAKIAN, 1947).

Another anabolic effect of androgens is on the blood-forming system. Androgens have been shown to increase red blood cell count in castrate or hypophysectomized rats (FINKELSTEIN et al., 1944), in castrate hamsters (STEIN and CARRIER, 1945), and in eunichoid men (MCCULLAGH and JONES, 1942). An increase in hematocrit results from androgen treatment and, in some studies, there was a suggestion of an increase in hemoglobin content in the red cells (VOLLMER et al., 1941).

F. Antiandrogens

There is a need to have available compounds that specifically inhibit the effects of androgens and that do not possess inherent hormonal activity. Such compounds would have utility in prostatic carcinoma or in virilizing syndromes, such as precocious puberty, hirsutism, etc. The most desirable antiandrogen should antagonize androgens at the target organ site, such as the prostate, but not at other sites, such as the pituitary. Finally, the antiandrogen should be effective at moderate dose levels for a reasonable length of time.

Usually, antiandrogenic activity is detected by the use of androgen bioassays, such as the chick comb or the seminal vesicles and prostate in castrate rats. By administration of a selected dose of androgen, a dose-related inhibition of the androgen effects is sought by concomitant administration of the test compound (LERNER, 1964). Two general categories of compounds have been found to possess antiandrogenic activity. In the first category are those steroids with modifications in the number of carbons in the ring system. For example, A-norprogesterone (LERNER et al., 1960), which possesses a 5-carbon A-ring, C-nor-D-homo-17α-epitestosterone acetate, containing a 5-carbon C-ring and a 6-carbon D-ring (LERNER et al., 1964), and 17α-methyl-B-nor-testosterone (SAUNDERS et al., 1964) containing a 5-carbon B-ring, all have been reported to possess antiandrogenic activity. The above compounds are relatively inactive as androgens or progestogens.

Since progesterone is itself antiandrogenic, compounds related structurally to progesterone have been found to be potent antiandrogens. Such compounds as cyproterone acetate (6-chloro-1α,2α-methylene-4,6-pregnadien-17α-ol-3,20-dione acetate) (NEUMANN et al., 1970) and chlormadinone acetate (6-chloro-1,4,6-pregnatrien-17α-ol-3,20-dione acetate) possess considerable potency as antiandrogens. These compounds antagonize testosterone-induced growth of seminal vesicles in rat, testosterone-induced growth of the chick comb, and block direct effects of testosterone on the testis. However, it should be pointed out that these agents are also potent progestational compounds.

A recent report demonstrated that antiandrogenic activity was found in 6α-bromo-17β-hydroxy-17α-methyl-4-oxa-5α-androstan-3-one, a compound which did not demonstrate androgenic, estrogenic, or progestational activity. However, the compound did inhibit pituitary gonadotrophins (BORIS et al., 1971). Thus, there may be found other substituted androgens that will inhibit the actions of strong androgens.

Mechanisms of Action

It has now become very popular to investigate the mechanism of action of hormones. With an increasing sophistication of biochemical techniques, and with an increasing accumulation of knowledge on the control of gene expression in bacterial systems, many biochemists have turned to hormone responsive target organs as models for the study of control mechanisms. The most commonly employed experimental approach to elucidate mechanisms is to use a castrate rat, to wait some period of time to allow atrophy of the seminal vesicles and prostate, to administer a dose of testosterone, and to sacrifice animals at various times after hormone perturbation to obtain tissue for analyses. The closer to the time of hormone administration that the measured response has occurred, the more confident the investigator becomes that he is examining a meaningful mechanism of action. While this may appear to be true, many effects of hormones may not be rapid or immediate, but rather, the hormone-induced events may occur at a later time in coordination with other events. Also, it should be kept in mind that the most studied responses are those that show a marked hypertrophy in the target organ and these responses may be exaggerated as a result of the considerable stimulus presented to the tissue by the use of large doses of hormones. Greater validity in hormone-induced responses may be placed on those studies that clearly demonstrate a biochemical event is related to the dose of hormone used. Several reviews on the actions of androgens have appeared recently and the reader is referred to these more thorough treatments of this subject (YOUNG, 1961; OFNER, 1969; BRIGGS and BROTHERTON, 1970; WILLIAMS-ASHMAN, 1970; WILLIAMS-ASHMAN and REDDI, 1971).

A. Effects of Androgens on Synthesis of Macromolecules

The central role that the gene plays in its control of differentiation of a cell has stimulated numerous investigations of the influence that a hormone may exert at the gene locus. Some of the earliest studies of this aspect of metabolism demonstrated that, after castration, the involution of the accessory sex organs was accompanied by decreases in the amount of RNA extracted from the cells and this decrease resulted in a decrease in the RNA/DNA ratio (DNA levels reflect an approximation of the number of cells) (WILLIAMS-ASHMAN et al., 1964; LIAO, 1965). Further, upon administration of androgen, one can demonstrate either maintenance of RNA levels and RNA/DNA ratios in the castrate rat, or, as the dose of androgen administered was elevated, a dose-related increase in RNA and RNA/DNA ratio was observed. The seminal vesicles show a more gradual, dose-related elevation than the ventral prostate in studies on castrate, immature rats; the androgen-induced increase in RNA was effectively prevented by concomitant administration of the antiandrogen, A-norprogesterone, but the antagonism of the androgen-induced effects was not found with the antiestrogen, ethamoxytriphetol (MER-25) (LERNER et al., 1968). In a like manner, the uterotrophic activity of testosterone was expressed by an increase in uterine RNA levels and RNA/DNA ratios, the response being antagonized by A-norprogesterone (LERNER et al., 1966).

The above studies measured total RNA, the majority of which is ribosomal (cytoplasmic) RNA. However, the advances in knowledge of RNA biosynthesis have led to more discrete studies on the effects of androgens at target organ sites. Studies of animal tissues have shown that ribosomal RNA's are derived from nuclear RNA precursors, a very large molecule having 45 S sedimentation characteristics. This 45 S molecule appears to be degraded in the nucleolus to one molecule of 18 S size and one molecule of 32 S to 35 S in size. This latter species undergoes another "trimming" to form a 28 S RNA, which along with the 18 S RNA, combine to form the ribosome in the cytoplasm. All of the ribosomal and pre-ribosomal species of RNA are relatively high in guanine and cytosine (GC rich) content and, as usually expressed as the ratio of adenine + uracil (A + U) divided by guanine + cytosine (G + C), demonstrate ratios of $A + U/G + C \cong 0.7$ (GEORGIEV, 1967).

With this background, studies were performed that demonstrated a dramatic decrease in cytoplasmic RNA in prostatic tissue after orchiectomy, but there was no indication that the overall base compositions were altered. Further, using DNA from castrate rat prostate as a template for bacterial RNA polymerase, the RNA produced was virtually identical to the RNA produced utilizing DNA from prostates of animals treated with androgen. Another parameter, amino acid polymerizing activity, was reduced in ribosomes from prostates of castrate rats and activity was restored after injection of testosterone to castrate rats (LIAO and WILLIAMS-ASHMAN, 1962). Initially, conclusions were reached that mRNA was deficient in ribosomes from prostate tissues of castrate rats and that testosterone appeared to increase the amount of mRNA associated with the prostatic ribosomes. However, in a careful study of early RNA synthesis after hormone stimulation, it was found that androgens stimulated 2 to 3 times the amount of rapidly labeled RNA and a heterogeneous RNA (WICKS and KENNEY, 1964). This rapidly labeled RNA had a base composition intermediate between total RNA (ribosomal) and DNA and could be confused with mRNA; hence, the investigators concluded that this represented a heterogeneous RNA and was probably a reflection of degradation of higher molecular weight RNA species (WICKS et al., 1965; GREENMAN et al., 1965).

Another series of studies showed that testosterone was capable of increasing RNA polymerase activity within 1 h after administration of the hormone (Liao et al., 1965). Hormone effects were more clear cut when the polymerase assay was conducted in a low ionic strength medium, since increasing the ionic strength of the medium narrowed the differences in polymerase activity of prostatic nuclei from androgen treated animals versus castrate control animals. These results led to the conclusion that androgen treatment enhanced polymerase activity by some mechanism which led to enhanced template activity of the DNA (Liao, 1968). This conclusion is probably too simple; more recent studies suggest that the increased template activity of RNA from androgen stimulated prostatic tissue may not be due to hormone-induced enhancement of discrete mRNA, but rather to an increase in the number of newly synthesized ribonucleoprotein particles, which are rich in mRNA. A proposal has been made that perhaps the increase in mRNA results from increased ribosomal synthesis of proteins that can protect mRNA from degradation; the decrease in ribosomal particles shortly after castration (cytoplasmic RNA decreases by 50% within 2 days after orchiectomy) suggest a relationship between the need for synthesis of numerous species of RNA and maintenance of physiologic integrity of the prostate (Liao and Fang, 1970). At this time, it is safe to conclude that a simplistic answer to the mechanism of action of testosterone on the accessory sex organs has not evolved.

Considerable work has been performed on the relationship between polyamines and androgens. Polyamines have been implicated in regulation of turnover of macromolecules, since they interact with polynucleotides and proteins and may exert an influence on the synthesis of RNA, DNA, and proteins (Tabor and Tabor, 1964; Williams-Ashman et al., 1969). The fact that the prostate has the highest quantity of spermidine and spermine may not be fortuitous; certainly, the effects that these polyamines might have on the accessory sex organ have not been elucidated. It has recently been shown that following castration, spermidine concentration decreases most rapidly, whereas putrescine and spermine decrease more gradually in the ventral prostate of the rat. Daily injections of testosterone propionate to castrate rats produced a significant increase in spermidine and putrescine levels within 24 h, whereas spermine levels did not increase until five days after initiation of hormonal treatment (Pegg et al., 1970). In the same tissues, ornithine decarboxylase, which catalyzes the formation of putrescine, was decreased soon after castration; within 6 h after administration of testosterone propionate, ornithine decarboxylase activity was increased twofold in prostates of castrate rats. In a similar manner, *S*-adenosyl-L-methionine decarboxylase was stimulated twofold in 3 h and tenfold within 48 h after androgen was administered to the castrate rat. These data demonstrate a good correlation between the enzymes responsible for biosynthesis and the accumulation of the polyamines, spermidine and putrescine. Thus, there appears to be a good temporal relationship between polyamine synthesis and an increase in RNA polymerase activity, along with a decrease in ATP levels, and these changes are the earliest ones reported to date in androgen target organs responding to the administration of testosterone. Several investigators have suggested that polyamines are interrelated with RNA synthesis, especially in situations where rapid tissue growth occurs (Raina, 1963; Tabor and Tabor, 1964; Dykstra and Herbst, 1965; Caldarera et al., 1965). However, a clear cut cause and effect relationship has not yet been established. For example, one report indicated that spermine was most effective in stimulating RNA polymerase activity of prostatic nuclei from castrate rats (Caldarera et al., 1968); yet, spermine levels showed little or no alterations for several days after treatment with androgen (Pegg et al., 1970). In addition, the very significant decrease in nuclear RNA polymerase activity after castration occurred prior to any change in the levels of spermine in prostatic tissue. Finally, the levels of polyamines are different in different lobes of the prostate (RHODES and WILLIAMS-ASHMAN, 1964), although the androgen-induced alterations in RNA content and DNA polymerase activity were similar despite the large differences in polyamine content. Therefore the discrete roles of polyamines, nucleic acid metabolism, and mechanism of action of androgens remain to be resolved.

B. Androgen Receptor Macromolecules

It would be highly desirable to define a hormone target organ by the presence of a chemical recognition mechanism, specific for that class of hormone and mechanistically accessible to or influential on the genetic apparatus of the target cell. The now classical work of JENSEN and his colleagues (JENSEN and JACOBSON, 1962) on the selected retention of labeled estradiol in estrogen target organs has led to a profusion of studies localizing steroids having very high specific radioactivity in numerous tissues of the experimental animal. Injection of labeled testosterone or androstenedione resulted in selective uptake of these steroids by the prostate and seminal vesicles. This localization was shown to occur within a few hours after injection of the hormone and appeared in the nuclei of the cells of the target organ (BRUCHOVSKY and WILSON, 1968a; ANDERSON and LIAO, 1968; MANGAN et al., 1968; TVETER, 1969). Further, uptake of labeled testosterone has been demonstrated in the hypothalamus, pituitary (RESKO et al., 1967; WHALEN and EDWARDS, 1969b), and preputial gland (BRUCHOVSKY and WILSON, 1968a), whereas this uptake was not seen in muscle, such as the levator ani. The uptake can be depressed by administration of unlabeled androgens (TVETER and AAKVAAG, 1969) or by androgen antagonists (WHALEN et al., 1969a). Thus, as with estrogens, there appear to be specific mechanisms for concentrating and/or retaining androgens in cells of target organs.

Unlike estradiol, testosterone may not be the ultimate androgen. It is now well established that there is a rapid conversion of testosterone to 5α-dihydrotestosterone (17β-hydroxy-5α-androstane-3-one) occurring in the cytoplasm of the ventral prostate (BRUCHOVSKY and WILSON, 1968a; OFNER, 1969; FANG et al., 1969; MAINWARING, 1969a) and this metabolic conversion has also been shown to occur in the androgen responsive comb, wattles, and coccygeal gland of chicks (GLOYNA and WILSON, 1969). Other investigators (GOMEZ and HSIA, 1968; WILSON and WALKER, 1969) have shown that slices of human skin, particularly from the perineal areas, actively reduce testosterone to 5α-dihydrotestosterone. Incubation of 5α-dihydrotestosterone with minces of prostatic tissue demonstrated that considerable amounts of unchanged steroid were recovered in the nuclei of these cell preparations, whereas selective retention of unchanged hormone was not demonstrated after incubation with minces of liver, diaphragm, and brain *in vitro* (FANG et al., 1969). Finally, a 5α-reductase enzyme has been identified bound to chromatin of prostatic nuclei and this enzyme catalyzes an NADPH-dependent reduction of the A-ring of testosterone (BRUCHOVSKY and WILSON 1968a; FANG et al., 1969). This finding confirms earlier work on the transformation of testosterone to 5α-dihydrotestosterone (FARNSWORTH and BROWN, 1963; SHIMAZAKI et al., 1965a, b; OFNER, 1969). Orchiectomy produced a decrease in 5α-reductase activity in the prostate; androgen administration restored enzyme activity. Cyproterone acetate, an antiandrogen, did not influence conversion of testosterone to 5α-dihydrotestosterone (BELHAM et al., 1969); its action appears to be limited to a competition with androgens for receptor substances (see below). Additional classical characterization of the 5α-reductase will be necessary and may be useful in seeking anti-androgenic compounds devoid of other hormonal properties.

Following the discovery of specific estrogen binding substances, data were reported on the existence of a macromolecular substance in prostatic nuclei from which considerable amounts of labeled 5α-dihydrotestosterone could be extracted. The binding of the steroid to the macromolecule(s) was destroyed by incubation with proteolytic enzymes, but not by treatment with RNase or DNase, strongly suggesting that proteins were the binding substances (BRUCHOVSKY and WILSON, 1968b). This has been confirmed by several other investigators (MAINWARING, 1969a; UNJHEM and TVETER, 1969a; PARSONS et al., 1970; BAULIEU and JUNG, 1970), which is in contrast with an earlier report that testosterone was associated mainly with nuclear DNA (MANGAN et al., 1968). A cytoplasmic receptor of the prostate, protein in nature and demonstrating a high affinity for 5α-dihydrotestosterone, was reported to have an 8 S sedimentation coefficient in one paper (MAINWARING, 1969b), whereas another investigator reported a receptor having a sedimentation coefficient of 9.3 S (UNHJEM et al., 1969b). FANG et al. (1969), in a very thorough investigation, reported that a cytoplasmic receptor from the prostate had a very high affinity for 5α-dihydrotestosterone and had a sedimentation coefficient of 3.5 S. Furthermore, these investigators found what appeared to be another receptor, isolated from nuclei of the prostate by extraction with 0.4 M KCl, which sedimented at 3.0 S. They found that incubation of isolated nuclei with 5α-dihydrotestosterone resulted in little or no specific binding by the 3.0 S receptor; addition of a cytoplasmic fraction to the system allowed considerable binding of the labeled steroid to the receptor isolated with solutions of high ionic strength. They postulated that the interaction of androgen with the prostate, just like that reported for the interaction of estradiol with the uterus, was a two step process: first, binding by a cytoplasmic 3.5 S receptor and second, a translocation of the steroid to the nucleus where the androgen is found associated with a 3.0 S receptor substance. Whether both receptors are one and the same protein remains to be shown. Data have been obtained demonstrating that cyproterone acetate can effectively prevent the association of the labeled androgen and these receptor substances.

WILLIAMS-ASHMAN and REDDI (1971), in a recent review, have clearly outlined the possible significance of the interaction of steroid with receptor molecules in the steroid target tissue. The most obvious postulate is that the receptor is the mechanism whereby the steroid can gain access to the nucleus and once there, interacts with the genetic machinery of the cell to stimulate transcription and the formation of RNA. Another possibility is that the receptor-steroid complex is the active form of the hormone; *in vitro* studies of the active complex would be required if one is to examine the direct effects of the "hormone" on a target tissue. It might also be mentioned that another possibility would consider that the receptor-steroid complex in the cytoplasm may be effective by stabilizing the ribosome-mRNA complex or by increasing the speed of message reading; in other words, the receptor-steroid complex could exert its effect at the level of translation. The third postulate by WILLIAMS-ASHMAN is also a most intriguing thought. It might very well be that the receptor proteins are the important substances regarding control of cell metabolism, and the steroids, by interacting with these macromolecules, cause a change in their configuration such that the receptors can now enter the nucleus and exert their effects at the gene level. One might propose that the receptors are analogous to the repressor (regulator proteins) of bacterial systems; alteration of the conformation of the repressor prevents its interaction with the regulatory sites and transcription proceeds. However, we are still in a highly speculative area at this time and many definitive experiments need to be conducted before the meaning of these interactions will be elucidated.

C. Energy Metabolism and Enzyme Changes

In the haste to ascertain mechanisms of hormone action, other aspects of cell metabolism may be overlooked while seeking to find the first event that occurs between hormone and target cell. It is obvious that a trophic response can be accomplished only as a result of energy expenditure and the limitation of this response may be a reflection of the metabolic capacity of the cell to supply the energy necessary for growth and secretion. It seems logical, then, to briefly outline the effects of androgens on various metabolic parameters in accessory sex organs and to see how these are coordinated with the morphologic changes induced by hormonal perturbation.

The early finding (BARRON and HUGGINS, 1944) that respiration in prostatic tissue decreased after castration has been confirmed several times (RUDOLPH and SAMUELS, 1949; NYDEN and WILLIAMS-ASHMAN, 1953; LEVEY and SZEGO, 1955). However, a discrepancy appeared regarding the effects of castration on succinic dehydrogenase, which in one paper was reported to decrease after castration (RUDOLPH and SAMUELS, 1949), but was shown to be unchanged in another report (LEVEY and SZEGO, 1955). A more recent report indicated that the decrease in succinate:cytochrome c dehydrogenase was a reflection of a decrease in the total number of mitochondria per unit weight of the prostate after castration; isolated mitochondria were similar in enzyme activity per mg mitochondrial nitrogen, whether obtained from castrate or intact rat prostatic tissue (EDELMAN et al., 1963).

RITTER (1966) reported that there was a rapid rise in NADH in the prostates of rats injected with testosterone, and simultaneously, a rapid decrease in ATP concentration. The levels of these substances returned to control values within 5 to 10 h. There was also reported a fourfold increase in NADPH levels at 2 to 4 h after treatment with androgen. A later report confirmed the rapid decrease in ATP following administration of androgen, but only marginal alterations in NAD and NADH levels were observed (COFFEY et al., 1968). However, nicotinamide mononucleotide adenyltransferase, which catalyzes the formation of deamido-NAD, was decreased in prostatic tissue after castration and was returned to normal levels following treatment with testosterone. The time courses of these enzyme changes were rather slow and this was interpreted as militating against the role of NAD as a primary event in androgen action (COFFEY et al., 1968). Further work seems warranted to confirm the reported change in NADPH, as this cofactor is required for the 5α-reductase and might play a role in controlling the rate of conversion of testosterone to 5α-dihydrotestosterone.

Various studies of the influence of androgens on enzyme activities in the prostate and seminal vesicles have been conducted. WILLIAMS-ASHMAN (1954) reported that at seven days after orchiectomy, a significant decrease in the activities of aconitase, fumarase, and malic dehydrogenase was produced in the prostate and these enzyme activities were returned to normal levels (intact animal) after administration of testosterone propionate for seven days. Lactate dehydrogenase activity showed an opposite pattern; it was increased after orchiectomy and returned to normal levels following treatment with androgen. In the same paper, it was reported that isocitrate dehydrogenase, glucose-6-phosphate dehydrogenase, and enolase activities were unchanged after orchiectomy or after treatment with testosterone propionate. In another report (BUTLER and SCHADE, 1958), α-glycerol-phosphate dehydrogenase in the prostate was shown to increase after castration, whereas acid phosphatase activity was unchanged. More recently, the availability of specific antiandrogens has enabled the investigator to determine the specificity of androgen-induced alterations in accessory sex organs. Lerner and his colleagues (Lerner et al., 1968) employed A-norprogesterone as a probe of androgen-induced morphologic and biochemical changes in ventral prostate and seminal vesicles of rats. Using the immature castrate rat, a dose related increase in the activities of glucose-6-phosphate dehydrogenase and NADP-malate dehydrogenase was observed in the ventral prostate, employing daily doses of testosterone propionate from 8 μg to 1.0 mg per rat for seven days. Similar results were obtained in the seminal vesicles of these animals. When a fixed dose of testosterone propionate (0.2 mg/day) was administered along with various doses of A-norprogesterone, significant antagonism of the androgen-induced enzyme changes was obtained in both the prostate and seminal vesicles. These studies were subsequently extended to demonstrate that the androgen-induced biochemical changes were not antagonized by antiestrogenic agents. In other studies, androgen-induced increases in glucose-6-phosphate dehydrogenase activity in the uterus were effectively prevented by antiandrogens, actinomycin D, or cycloheximide, suggesting that the androgen-induced trophic response in accessory sex organs is accompanied by stimulation of certain specific enzymes (Hilf et al., 1968a). These results were confirmed by Singhal and his associates (Singhal, 1967; Singhal and Valadares, 1968), who found that the androgen-induced increases in glucose-6-phosphate dehydrogenase, as well as phosphofructokinase and hexokinase, in the seminal vesicles were effectively prevented by concomitant administration of actinomycin D, cycloheximide, or ethionine. When a single dose of testosterone propionate (5 mg/100 g body weight) was administered to castrate young adult rats, the activities of glucose-6-phosphate dehydrogenase and hexokinase showed a significant elevation in the seminal vesicles at 16 h after hormone treatment. These investigators also presented data indicating that estradiol-17β, which was claimed to have no effect on the seminal vesicles, could antagonize the androgen-induced increases in enzyme activity. This is somewhat unexpected, since it is well established that estrogens stimulate the weight of the seminal vesicles, as well as the levels of RNA and glucose-6-phosphate dehydrogenase activity (Lerner et al., 1968). Additionally, the antiestrogen MER-25 can antagonize the estrogen-induced increase in seminal vesicles, but not the androgen-induced changes. Because the cytoplasmic androgen receptor of the prostate shows some affinity for estradiol-17β, if a similar situation holds for the seminal vesicles, one might anticipate a partial inhibition of androgen responses on the basis of competitive antagonism. This remains for further study.

Finally, it is rare to find any review on hormone action that does not mention or invoke cyclic-3′,5′-AMP (cAMP) as a mediator of the response of a target organ. It seems fitting, therefore, to point out that two reports appearing simultaneously discuss the role of cAMP in androgen-mediated response of the male accessory sex organs. One report (Singhal et al., 1970) indicated that administration of cAMP plus theophylline produced testosterone-like increases in the activities of hexokinase, phosphofructokinase, pyruvate kinase, and glucose-6-phosphate dehydrogenase in seminal vesicles of castrate rats. These changes were prevented by actinomycin D or cycloheximide. The other report (Rosenfeld and O'Malley, 1970) clearly demonstrated that no change in the activity of adenyl cyclase was evident in the prostate over the first 24 h after a large dose of testosterone was given to hypophysectomized rats. It is obvious that additional studies will be required to resolve this issue.

References

ANDERSON, K.M., LIAO, S.: Selective retention of dihydrotestosterone by prostatic nuclei. Nature (Lond.) **219**, 277—279 (1968).

BARRON, E.S.G., HUGGINS, C.: The metabolism of isolated prostatic tissue. J. Urol. **51**, 630—634 (1944).

BAULIEU, E.E., JUNG, I.: A prostatic cytosol receptor. Biochem. biophys. Res. Commun. **38**, 599—606 (1970).

BELHAM, J.E., NEAL, G.E., WILLIAMS, D.C.: Testosterone metabolism in the rat ventral prostate. Biochim. biophys. Acta (Amst.) **187**, 159—162 (1969).

BLACKBURN, C.M., ALBERT, A.: Effects of 2-methyl-dehydrotestosterone and of testosterone on human pituitary gonadotrophin. J. clin. Endocrinol. **19**, 603—607 (1959).

BORIS, A., DEMARTINO, L., TRMAL, T.: Some endocrine studies of a new antiandrogen, 6α-bromo-17β-hydroxy-17α-methyl-4-oxa-5α-androstan-3-one (BOMT). Endocrinology **88**, 1086—1091 (1971).

BRIGGS, M.H., BROTHERTON, J.: Steroid Biochemistry and Pharmacology. London-New York: Academic Press 1970.

BROOKSBY, J.B.: Uterine reaction to testosterone in the rat. Proc. Soc. exp. Biol. (N.Y.) **38**, 235—237 (1938).

BRUCHOVSKY, N., WILSON, J.D.: The conversion of testosterone to 5α-androstan-17β-ol-3-one by rat prostate *in vivo* and *in vitro*. J. biol. Chem. **243**, 2012—2021 (1968a).

BRUCHOVSKY, N., WILSON, J.D.: The intranuclear binding of testosterone and 5α-androstan-17β-ol-3-one by rat prostate. J. biol. Chem. **243**, 5953—5960 (1968b).

BURSTEIN, S., GUT, M.: A preliminary report on the intermediates in the conversion *in vitro* of cholesterol to pregnenolone in adrenal preparations. Steroids **14**, 207—217 (1969).

BUTLER, W.W.S., SCHADE, A.L.: The effects of castration and androgen replacement on the nucleic acid composition, metabolism, and enzymatic capacities of the rat ventral prostate. Endocrinology **63**, 271—279 (1958).

CALDARERA, C.M., BARBIROLI, B., MORUZZI, G.: Polyamines and nucleic acids during development of the chick embryo. Biochem. J. **97**, 84—88 (1965).

CALDARERA, C.M., MORUZZI, M.S., BARBIROLI, B., MORUZZI, G.: Spermine and spermidine of the prostate gland of orchiectomized rats and their effect on RNA polymerase activity. Biochem. biophys. Res. Commun. **33**, 266—271 (1968).

COFFEY, D.S., ICHINOSE, R.R., SHIMAZAKI, J., WILLIAMS-ASHMAN, H.G.: Effects of testosterone on adenosine triphosphate and nicotinamide adenine dinucleotide levels, and on nicotinamide mononucleotide adenyltransferase activity in the ventral prostate of castrated rats. Molec. Pharmacol. **4**, 580—590 (1968).

CONNELL, G.M., EIK-NES, K.B.: Metabolism leading to the formation of testosterone in the rabbit and dog testis. In: MCKERNS, K.W. (Ed.): The gonads, chapter 17. New York: Appleton-Century-Crofts 1969.

CONSTANTOPOULOS, G., CARPENTER, A., SATOH, P.S., TCHEN, T.T.: Formation of isocaproaldehyde in the enzymatic cleavage of cholesterol side chain by adrenal extract. Biochemistry **5**, 1650—1652 (1966).

CONSTANTOPOULOS, G., TCHEN, T.T.: Cleavage of cholesterol side chain by adrenal cortex. J. biol. Chem. **236**, 65—67 (1961).

DORFMAN, R.I., SHIPLEY, R.A.: Androgens. New York: John Wiley & Sons 1956.

DORRINGTON, J.H., KIRKPATRICK, R.: Effect of adenosine 3′,5′-(cyclic)-monophosphate on the synthesis of progestational steroids by rabbit ovarian tissue *in vitro*. Biochem. J. **104**, 725—730 (1967).

DYKSTRA, W.G., HERBST, E.J.: Spermidine in regenerating liver: relation to rapid synthesis of ribonucleic acid. Science **149**, 428—429 (1965).

EDELMAN, J.C., BRENDLER, H., ZORGNIOTTI, A.W., EDELMAN, P.M.: Effects of castration on mitochondria of rat ventral prostate. Endocrinology **72**, 853—858 (1963).

EIK-NES, K.B.: The androgens and the testis. New York: Marcel Dekker 1970.

FANG, S., ANDERSON, K.M., LIAO, S.: Receptor proteins for androgens. J. biol. Chem. **244**, 6584—6595 (1969).

FARNSWORTH, W.E., BROWN, J.R.: Metabolism of testosterone by the human prostate. J. Amer. med. Assoc. **183**, 436—439 (1963).

FINKELSTEIN, G., GORDON, A.S., CHARIPPER, H.A.: The effect of sex hormones on the anemia induced by hemorrhage in the rat. Endocrinology **35**, 267—277 (1944).

FOLLEY, S.J., KON, S.K.: The effect of sex hormones on lactation in the rat. Proc. roy. Soc. B **124**, 476—492 (1936).

FRANK, R.T., KLEMPNER, E.: The comb of the baby chick as a test for the male sex hormone. Proc. Soc. exp. Biol. (N.Y.) **36**, 763—765 (1937).

GEORGIEV, G. P.: The nature and biosynthesis of nuclear ribonucleic acids. Progr. nucleic acid Res. Molec. Biol. **6**, 259—351 (1967).

GLOYNA, R. E., WILSON, J. D.: A comparative study of the conversion of testosterone to 17β-hydroxy-5α-androstan-3-one (dihydrotestosterone) by prostate and epididymis. J. clin. Endocrinol. **29**, 970—977 (1969).

GOMEZ, E. C., HSIA, S. L.: *In vitro* metabolism of testosterone-4-,^{14}C and Δ^4-androstene-3,17-dione-4-^{14}C in human skin. Biochemistry **7**, 24—32 (1968).

GREENMAN, D. L., WICKS, W. D., KENNEY, F. T.: Stimulation of ribonucleic acid synthesis by steroid hormones. II. High molecular weight components. J. biol. Chem. **240**, 4420—4426 (1965).

HALKERSTON, I. D. K., EICHHORN, J., HECHTER, O.: A requirement for reduced triphosphopyridine nucleotide for cholesterol side-chain cleavage by mitochondrial fractions of bovine adrenal cortex. J. biol. Chem. **236**, 374—380 (1961).

HALL, P. F.: On the stimulation of testicular steroidogenesis in the rabbit by interstitial cell-stimulating hormone. Endocrinology **78**, 690—698 (1966).

HALL, P. F.: Electron transport in relation to steroid biosynthesis. Inhibition of side-chain cleavage of cholesterol by hyperbaric oxygen. Biochemistry **6**, 2794—2802 (1967).

HANCOCK, R. L., ZELIS, R. F., SHAW, M., WILLIAMS-ASHMAN, H. G.: Incorporation of ribonucleoside triphosphates into ribonucleic acid by nuclei of the prostate gland. Biochim. biophys. Acta (Amst.) **55**, 257—260 (1962).

HEFTMANN, E.: Steroid biochemistry. New York-London: Academic Press 1970.

HEISE, E., GORLICH, M., BACIGALUPO, G.: Biochemical studies in advancing and regressing rat mammary carcinomas induced by 7,12-dimethylbenz(a)anthracene (Huggins tumors). J. nat. Cancer Inst. **45**, 1—10 (1970).

HERSCHBERGER, L. G., SHIPLEY, E. G., MEYER, R. K.: Myotrophic activity of 19-nortestosterone and other steroids determined by modified levator ani muscle method. Proc. Soc. exp. Biol. (N.Y.) **83**, 175—180 (1953).

HILF, R.: Biochemical studies of hormone-responsive tumors. Cancer Res. **28**, 1888—1890 (1968).

HILF, R., LERNER, L. J., HARRIS, D. N.: The effect of actidione and actinomycin D on androgen-induced biochemical changes in the R3230AC mammary carcinoma and uterus of the rat. Trans. N.Y. Acad. Sci. **30**, 794—803 (1968a).

HILF, R., MICHEL, I., BELL, C.: Biochemical and morphological responses of normal and neoplastic mammary tissue to hormonal treatment. Rec. Progr. Hormone Res. **23**, 229—295 (1967).

HILF, R., SEGALOFF, A., LERNER, L. J.: Influence of hormonal treatment of Fischer rats on the biochemistry of a transplantable dimethylbenz(a)anthracene-induced mammary carcinoma and its sublines. Cancer Res. **28**, 1550—1558 (1968b).

HUGGINS, C., HODGES, C. V.: Studies on prostatic cancer. I. The effect of castration, of estrogen and of androgen injection on serum phosphatases in metastatic carcinoma of the prostate. Cancer Res. **1**, 293—297 (1941).

JENSEN, E. V., JACOBSON, H. I.: Basic guides to the mechanism of estrogen action. Rec. Progr. Hormone Res. **18**, 387—414 (1962).

KENNEDY, B. J.: Fluoxymesterone therapy in advanced breast cancer. New Eng. J. Med. **259**, 673—675 (1958).

KOCHAKIAN, C. D.: Effect of male hormone on protein metabolism of castrate dogs. Proc. Soc. exp. Biol. (N.Y.) **32**, 1064—1065 (1935).

KOCHAKIAN, C. D.: The role of hydrolytic enzymes in some of the metabolic activities of steroid hormones. Rec. Progr. Hormone Res. **1**, 177—216 (1947).

KODAMA, M., KODAMA, T.: Effect of steroid hormones on the *in vivo* incorporation of glycine-2-^{14}C into solid Ehrlich tumor, kidney and liver. Cancer Res. **30**, 228—235 (1970).

KORENCHEVSKY, V., HALL, K.: Pathological changes in the sex organs after prolonged administration of sex hormones to female rats. J. path. Bact. **50**, 295—315 (1940).

KORITZ, S, B.: The energy linked synthesis of pregnenolone in beef adrenal cortex mitochondria. Biochem. biophys. Res. Commun. **23**, 485—489 (1966).

LAQUEUR, G. L., FLUHMANN, C. F.: Effects of testosterone propionate in immature and adult female rats. Endocrinology **30**, 93—101 (1942).

LEONARD, S. L.: Changes in the relative amounts of the follicle stimulating and luteinizing hormones in the hypophysis of the female rat under varying experimental conditions. Endocrinology **21**, 330—334 (1937).

LERNER, L. J.: Hormone antagonists: Inhibitors of specific activities of estrogen and androgen. Rec. Progr. Hormone Res. **20**, 435—490 (1964).

LERNER, L. J., BIANCHI, A., BORMAN, A.: A-norprogesterone, an androgen antagonist. Proc. Soc. exp. Biol. (N.Y.) **103**, 172—175 (1960).

LERNER, L. J., BIANCHI, A., DZELZKALNS, M., BORMAN, A.: Anti-androgenic activities of A-norprogesterone and C-nor-D-homo-17α-epitestosterone acetate. Proc. Soc. exp. Biol. (N. Y.) **115**, 924—927 (1964).

LERNER, L. J., HILF, R., HARRIS, D. N.: The effect of antagonists on androgen- and estrogen-induced changes in the male accessory sex organs of the rat. Trans. N. Y. Acad. Sci. **30**, 783—793 (1968).

LERNER, L. J., HILF, R., TURKHEIMER, A. R., MICHEL, I., ENGEL, S. L.: Effects of hormone antagonists on morphological and biochemical changes induced by hormonal steroids in the immature rat uterus. Endocrinology **78**, 111—124 (1966).

LEVEY, H. A., SZEGO, C. M.: Effects of castration and androgen administration on metabolic characteristics of guinea pig seminal vesicle. Amer. J. Physiol. **183**, 371—376 (1955).

LIAO, S.: Influence of testosterone on template activity of prostatic ribonucleic acids. J. biol. Chem. **240**, 1236—1243 (1965).

LIAO, S.: Evidence for a discriminatory action of androgenic steroids on synthesis of nucleolar ribonucleic acids in prostatic nuclei. Am. Zoologist **8**, 233—242 (1968).

LIAO, S., FANG, S.: Receptor-proteins for androgens and the mode of action of androgens on gene transcription in ventral prostate. Vitam. and Hormones **27**, 17—90 (1970).

LIAO, S., LEININGER, K. R., SAGHER, D., BARTON, R. W.: Rapid effect of testosterone on ribonucleic acid polymerase activity of rat ventral prostate. Endocrinology **77**, 763—765 (1965).

LIAO, S., WILLIAMS-ASHMAN, H. G.: An effect of testosterone on amino acid incorporation by prostatic ribonucleoprotein particles. Proc. nat. Acad. Sci. (Wash.) **48**, 1956—1964 (1962).

MACKAY, L. L., MACKAY, E. M.: Factors which determine renal weight. III. Sex. Amer. J. Physiol. **83**, 196—201 (1927).

MAINWARING, W. I. P.: The binding of (1,2-^{3}H) testosterone within the nucleus of the rat prostate. J. Endocrinol. **44**, 323—333 (1969a).

MAINWARING, W. I. P.: A soluble androgen receptor in the cytoplasm of rat prostate. J. Endocrinol. **45**, 531—541 (1969b).

MANGAN, F. R., NEAL, G. E., WILLIAMS, D. C.: Subcellular distribution of testosterone in rat prostate and its possible relationship to nuclear ribonucleic acid synthesis. Arch. Biochem. Biophys. **124**, 27—40 (1968).

MARSH, J. M., SAVARD, K.: Studies on the mode of action of luteinizing hormone on steroidogenesis in the corpus luteum *in vitro*. J. Reprod. Fertil. **1**, 113—126 (1966).

MASON, H. S.: Mechanisms of oxygen metabolism. Science **125**, 1185—1188 (1957).

MCCULLAGH, E. P., JONES, R.: Effect of androgens on the blood count of men. J. Clin. Endocrinol. **2**, 243—251 (1942).

MOORE, C. R., PRICE, D.: Some effects of synthetically prepared male hormone (androsterone) in the rat. Endocrinology **21**, 313—329 (1937).

MOORE, C. R., PRICE, D.: Some effects of testosterone and testosterone propionate in the rat. Anat. Rec. **71**, 59—78 (1938).

MOORE, C. R., PRICE, D., GALLAGHER, T. F.: Rat-prostate cytology as a testis-hormone indicator and the prevention of castration changes by testis-extract injections. Amer. J. Anat. **45**, 71—108 (1930).

NEHER, R., WETTSTEIN, A.: Occurrence of Δ^5-3β-hydroxysteroids in adrenal and testicular tissue. Acta Endocrinol. **35**, 1—7 (1960).

NELSON, W. O., GALLAGHER, T. F.: Some effects of androgenic substances in the rat. A. The effect of male hormone extracts on the testes of hypophysectomized rats. Science **84**, 230—232 (1936).

NELSON, W. O., MERCKEL, C. G.: Effects of androgenic substances in the female rat. Proc. Soc. exp. Biol. (N. Y.) **36**, 823—825 (1937).

NEUMANN, F., VON BERSWORDT-WALLRABE, R., ELGER, W., STEINBECK, H., HAHN, J. D., KRAMER, M.: Aspects of androgen-dependent events as studied by antiandrogens. Rec. Progr. Hormone Res. **26**, 337—410 (1970).

NOBLE, R. L.: Direct gynaecogenic and indirect oestrogenic action of testosterone propionate in female rats. J. Endocrinol. **1**, 184—200 (1939).

NYDEN, S. I., WILLIAMS-ASHMAN, H. G.: Influence of androgen on synthetic reactions in ventral prostate tissue. Amer. J. Physiol. **172**, 588—600 (1953).

OFNER, P.: Effects and metabolism of hormones in normal and neoplastic prostate tissue. Vitam. and Hormones **26**, 237—291 (1969).

OMURA, T., SANDERS, E., ESTABROOK, R. W., COOPER, D. Y., ROSENTHAL, O.: Isolation from adrenal cortex of a nonheme iron protein and a flavoprotein as a reduced triphosphopyridine nucleotide-cytochrome P-450 reductase. Arch. Biochem. Biophys. **117**, 660—673 (1966).

PARSONS, I. C., MANGAN, F. R., NEAL, G. R.: Some effects of testosterone on the rat ventral prostate. Biochem. J. **117**, 425—430 (1970).

PEGG, A. E., LOCKWOOD, D. H., WILLIAMS-ASHMAN, H. G.: Concentrations of putrescine and polyamines and their enzymatic synthesis during androgen-induced prostatic growth. Biochem. J. **117**, 17—31 (1970).
RAINA, A.: Studies on the determination of spermidine and spermine and their metabolism in the developing chick embryo. Acta Physiol. Scand. **60**, Suppl. 218, 1—81 (1963).
RESKO, J. A., GOY, R. W., PHOENIX, C. H.: Uptake and distribution of exogenous testosterone-1,2-^{3}H in neural and genital tissues of the castrate guinea pig. Endocrinology **80**, 490—498 (1967).
RHODES, J. B., WILLIAMS-ASHMAN, H. G.: Observations on polyamines in male accessory glands of reproduction. Med. Exp. **10**, 281—285 (1964).
RITTER, C.: NAD biosynthesis as an early part of androgen action. Molec. Pharmacol. **2**, 125—133 (1966).
ROBSON, J. M.: Reactions of the uterine muscle and endometrium of the rabbit to testosterone. Quart J. Exp. Physiol. **26**, 355—359 (1937).
ROBSON, J. M.: Quantitative data on the inhibition of oestrus by testosterone, progesterone and certain other compounds. J. Physiol. **92**, 371—382 (1938).
ROOKS, W. H., HRADA, T., ABE, O., DORFMAN, R. I.: The inhibition of glycine-2-C^{14} uptake in a rat mammary fibroadenoma by steroids. Chemotherapia **7**, 61—66 (1963).
ROSEMBERG, E., PAULSEN, C. A.: The human testis. New York: Plenum Press 1970.
ROSENFELD, M. G., O'MALLEY, B. W.: Steroid hormones: effects on adenyl cyclase activity and adenosine 3',5'-monophosphate in target tissues. Science **168**, 253—255 (1970).
RUDOLPH, G. G., SAMUELS, L. T.: Early effects of testosterone propionate on the seminal vesicles of castrate rats. Endocrinology **44**, 190—196 (1949).
SATOH, P. G., CONSTANTOPOULOS, G., TCHEN, T. T.: Cleavage of cholesterol side chain by adrenal cortex. IV. Effect of phosphate and various nucleotides on a soluble enzyme system. Biochemistry **5**, 1646—1650 (1966).
SAUNDERS, H. L., HOLDEN, K., KERWIN, J. F.: The anti-androgenic activity of 17α-methyl-B-nortestosterone (SKF 7690). Steroids **3**, 687—698 (1964).
SAVARD, K., DORFMAN, R. I., BAGGETT, B., ENGEL, L. L.: Biosynthesis of androgens from progesterone by human testicular tissue *in vitro*. J. clin. Endocrinol. **16**, 1629—1630 (1956).
SEGALOFF, A.: Hormones and breast cancer. Rec. Progr. Hormone Res. **22**, 351—379 (1966).
SELYE, H.: Morphological changes in female mice receiving large doses of testosterone. J. Endocrinol. **1**, 208—215 (1939).
SELYE, H., FRIEDMAN, S.: The action of various steroid hormones on the testis. Endocrinology **28**, 129—140 (1941).
SHIMAZAKI, J., KURIHARA, H., ITO, Y., SHIDA, K.: Testosterone metabolism in prostate; formation of androstan-17β-ol-3-one and androst-4-ene-3,17-dione and the inhibitory effect of natural and synthetic estrogens. Gunma J. med. Sci. **14**, 313—325 (1965a).
SHIMAZAKI, J., KURIHARA, H., ITO, Y., SHIDA, K.: Metabolism of testosterone in prostate. Gunma J. med. Sci. **14**, 326—333 (1965b).
SHIMIZU, K., GUT, M., DORFMAN, R. I.: 20α,22ξ-Dihydroxycholesterol, an intermediate in the biosynthesis of pregnenolone (3β-hydroxypregn-5-en-20-one) from cholesterol. J. biol. Chem. **237**, 699—702 (1961a).
SHIMAZU, K., HAYANO, M., GUT, M., DORFMAN, R. I.: The transformation of 20α-hydroxycholesterol to isocaproic acid and C_{21} steroids. J. biol. Chem. **236**, 695—699 (1961b).
SHORR, E., PAPANICOLAOU, G. N., STIMMEL, B. F.: Neutralization of ovarian follicular hormone in women by simultaneous administration of male sex hormone. Proc. Soc. exp. Biol. (N. Y.) **38**, 759—762 (1938).
SIMPSON, E. R., COOPER, D. Y., ESTABROOK, R. W.: Metabolic events associated with steroid hydroxylation by the adrenal cortex. Rec. Progr. Hormone Res. **25**, 523—562 (1969).
SINGHAL, R. L.: Testosterone-induced increase in phosphofructokinase activity of rat seminal vesicle. Life Sci. **6**, 405—411 (1967).
SINGHAL, R. L., VALADARES, J. R. E.: Metabolic control mechanisms in mammalian systems. Biochem. J. **110**, 703—711 (1968).
SINGHAL, R. L., VIJAYVARGIYA, R., LING, G. M.: Cyclic adenosine monophosphate: andromimetic action on seminal vesicular enzymes. Science **168**, 261—263 (1970).
STEIN, K. F., CARRIER, E.: Changes in erythrocytes of hamsters following castration, splenectomy, and subsequent liver, iron and testosterone injections. Proc. Soc. exp. Biol. (N. Y.) **60**, 313—318 (1945).
SULIMOVICI, S. I., BOYD, G. S.: The cholesterol side-chain cleavage enzymes in steroid hormone-producing tissues. Vitam. and Hormones **27**, 199—234 (1969).
TABOR, H., TABOR, C. W.: Spermidine, spermine and related amines. Pharmacol. Rev. **16**, 245—300 (1964).
TOREN, D., MENON, K. M. J., FORCHIELLI, E., DORFMAN, R. I.: *In vitro* enzymatic cleavage of the cholesterol side chain in rat testis preparations. Steroids **3**, 381—390 (1964).

TVETER, K. J.: Subcellular localization of androgen in the rat ventral prostate *in vivo*. Endocrinology **85**, 597—600 (1969).
TVETER, K. J., AAKVAAG, A.: Uptake and metabolism *in vivo* of testosterone-1,2-^{3}H by accessory sex organs of male rats; influence of some hormonal compounds. Endocrinology **85**, 683—689 (1969).
UNHJEM, O., TVETER, K. J.: Localization of an androgen binding substance from the rat ventral prostate. Acta Endocrinol. **60**, 571—578 (1969a).
UNHJEM, O., TVETER, K. J., AAKVAAG, A.: Preliminary characterization of an androgen-macromolecular complex from the rat ventral prostate. Acta Endocrinology **62**, 153—164 (1969b).
VAN WAGENEN, G., FOLLEY, S. J.: The effect of androgens on the mammary gland of the female rhesus monkey. J. Endocrinol. **1**, 367—372 (1939).
VOLLMER, E. P., GORDON, A. S., LEVENSTEIN, I., CHARIPPER, H. A.: Effects of sex and gonadotropic hormones on red cell counts in rats. Proc. Soc. exp. Biol. (N.Y.) **46**, 409—410 (1941).
WHALEN, R. E., EDWARDS, D. A.: Effects of the anti-androgen cyproterone acetate on mating behavior and seminal vesicle tissue in male rats. Endocrinology **84**, 155—156 (1969a).
WHALEN, R. E., LUTTGE, W. G., GREEN, R.: Effects of the anti-androgen cyproterone acetate on the uptake of 1,2-^{3}H-testosterone in neural and peripheral tissues of the castrate rat. Endocrinology **84**, 217—222 (1969b).
WICKS, W. D., GREENMAN, D. L., KENNEY, F. T.: Stimulation of ribonucleic acid synthesis by steroid hormones. I. Transfer ribonucleic acid. J. biol. Chem. **240**, 4414—4419 (1965).
WICKS, W. D., KENNEY, F. T.: RNA synthesis in rat seminal vesicles: stimulation by testosterone. Science **144**, 1346—1347 (1964).
WILLIAMS-ASHMAN, H. G.: Changes in the enzymatic constitution of the ventral prostate gland induced by androgenic hormones. Endocrinology **54**, 121—129 (1954).
WILLIAMS-ASHMAN, H. G.: Androgenic control of nucleic acid and protein synthesis in male accessory genital organs. J. cell. comp. Physiol. **66**, 111—124 (1965).
WILLIAMS-ASHMAN, H. G.: Biochemistry of testicular androgen action. In: EIK-NES, K. B. (Ed.): The androgens of the testis, pp. 117—143. New York: Marcel Dekker 1970.
WILLIAMS-ASHMAN, H. G., LIAO, S., HANCOCK, R. L., JURKOWITZ, L., SILVERMAN, D. A.: Testicular hormones and the synthesis of ribonucleic acids and proteins in the prostate gland. Rec. Progr. Hormone Res. **20**, 247—301 (1964).
WILLIAMS-ASHMAN, H. G., PEGG, A. E., LOCKWOOD, D. H.: Mechanisms and regulation of polyamine and putrescine biosynthesis in male genital glands and other tissues of mammals. Adv. Enzyme Reg. **7**, 291—323 (1969).
WILLIAMS-ASHMAN, H. G., REDDI, A. H.: Actions of vertebrate sex hormones. Ann. Rev. Physiol. **33**, 31—82 (1971).
WILSON, J. D., WALKER, J. D.: The conversion of testosterone to 5α-androstan-17β-ol-3-one (dihydrotestosterone) by skin slices of man. J. clin. Invest. **48**, 371—379 (1969).
YOUNG, W. C.: Sex and Internal Secretions. Baltimore: Williams & Wilkins 1961.

Chapter 39

Mechanism of Action of Progesterone

BERT W. O'MALLEY and CHARLES A. STROTT

With 1 Figure

Biologic Responses to Progesterone

Progesterone has been established as an obligatory steroid mediator of pregnancy (CORNER, 1947; REYNOLDS, 1949; REEL et al., 1969). The primary physiologic effect of progesterone appears to be the induced transformation of uterine endometrial cells so that implantation of the developing blastocyst is facilitated. Other probable effects of this steroid hormone are grouped as follows: myometric activity is suppressed aiding in retention of the embryo during implantation and growth prior to normal parturition; this steroid is thought to support mammary development; progesterone acts as a direct antagonist to estrogen stimulation of numerous metabolic activities; certain metabolic mechanisms are altered which may have no major effect on maintenance or termination of pregnancy or reproductive processes in general. Although progesterone has been thought to be needed for alveolar development in the breast tissue of some species, this chapter will be limited to discussing progesterone action in uterus and oviduct.

The effects of progesterone on the myometrial cell have been studied by a number of investigators (CSAPO, 1969). Uterine muscle functions normally only if these cells possess, as a result of estrogen stimulation, sufficient amounts of contractile proteins. In addition, the excitable membrane of the uterine muscle cell must be capable of undergoing periodic changes between rest and activity. The spontaneous rhythmic activity of the individual cell membrane must be transferred to the contractile system of the myoplasm through an effective excitation. In the rabbit, progesterone exerts a "blocking effect" so that an excitation wave cannot spread from one region to another. This steroid has been reported to increase the membrane potential to an extent where spontaneous activity is suppressed (CSAPO, 1961) and a gradual reduction in spike discharge occurs. This "quieting" effect on uterine myometrial contractions could conceivably play a physiologic role to aid implantation and retention of the embryo. Nevertheless, this phenomenon is not a universal one for, in the guinea pig, progesterone has been shown not to be a myometrial blocking agent (PORTER, 1969). A similar role in the primates has not been adequately investigated yet. Therefore, a general concept for the role of progesterone in the regulation of gestational length and determination of the onset of labor is presently lacking.

The most important function which appears in animals in response to progesterone is the ability of the uterine endometrial cells to accept the blastocyst. Under the influence of estrogen, the endometrium proliferates and becomes dense. Progesterone inhibits further endometrial proliferation and the epithelium becomes secretory. The endometrium is now able to accept, retain, and nourish the blastocyst. This "sensitivity" for implantation must reflect a series of as yet unproven earlier intracellular biochemical events.

The deciduoma reaction has been used as a model for implantation of the blastocyst into the uterine endometrium (DEFEO, 1967). Physical or chemical irritation of the endometrial cells of a "receptive" uterus leads to a proliferative reaction which resembles the uterine reaction to the normal blastocyst as evidenced by both light and electron microscopy (DEFEO, 1967). The uterus of a pregnant (or pseudopregnant) animal is "receptive" to implantation (or decidualization) on day 4 but not day 3 or 5 of pregnancy. The decidual reaction has been found to be determined by progesterone alone since the castrate immature rat will respond with resultant decidual growth when treated only with progesterone. Progesterone also exerts a profound stimulatory influence on decidual RNA and protein synthesis in untreated or estrogen-treated castrates. Furthermore, the response is specific for progestational agents (natural or synthetic) but not androgens, glucocorticoids, or mineralocorticoids. Actinomycin D blocks the decidual reaction, suggesting that the response is dependent on new RNA synthesis (GLASSER, personal communication).

The relative lack of suitable tissue models to investigate a "positive" progesterone effect has thwarted our progress in understanding the mechanism of action of this important steroid hormone. Unfortunately, we cannot as yet specifically define the newly synthesized proteins responsible for the "uterine sensitivity" which leads to the deciduoma reaction.

Hormonal changes that occur in the chick oviduct have been characterized in terms of both the long-term developmental and the early biochemical effects caused by estrogens and progestins (O'MALLEY and MCGUIRE, 1968; O'MALLEY et al., 1969). These sex steroids are responsible for the differentiation of the cells of the epithelial mucosa of the immature chick oviduct and for the eventual synthesis of new tissue proteins. Estrogenic substances are known to stimulate oviduct growth, and after estrogen treatment three new cell types emerge from the primitive mucosa (KOHLER et al., 1969). Two of these, the goblet cells and the tubular gland cells, will subsequently synthesize tissue-specific proteins, whereas the third cell type is ciliated and concerned with motility. After a single exposure to progesterone, the goblet cells of the estrogen stimulated oviduct will synthesize the protein, avidin (KORENMAN and O'MALLEY, 1968; O'MALLEY et al., 1969).

Avidin then serves as a specific intracellular biochemical marker for the action of progesterone in reproductive target tissue of the chicken. The protein can easily be quantified and serves as a definite endpoint for progesterone action. Events prior to avidin induction can then be related in a time sequence manner. The studies performed in the chick oviduct will be summarized later in this chapter.

The Uptake and Metabolism of Progesterone

Aside from the uterus and breast, it is not clear exactly which tissues are physiologic targets for progesterone. For instance, it has been demonstrated that progesterone can alter hepatic function, e.g., increase conversion of amino acids into urea resulting in reduced concentration of plasma amino acids (LANDAU and LUGIBIHL, 1961). Progesterone can influence the renal handling of sodium leading to a natriuresis (LANDAU and LUGIBIHL, 1961). The physiologic importance of these observations to the total body economy is not understood and may simply represent pharmacologic effects of progesterone when present in large amounts.

A commonly used approach to determine "target" tissues for hormones involves the *in vivo* injection of tracer amounts of radio-labeled hormone followed by monitoring radioactivity distribution in order to study the fate of the hormone. Thus, labeled progesterone has been given to animals and the radioactivity measured in blood and various tissues during time-course experiments. Tissues demonstrating a capacity to concentrate the hormone relative to blood can then be considered as potential target tissues. Such studies have demonstrated the "target tissue" nature of the uterus in a number of species (LAUMOS and FAROOG, 1966; EDWARDS et al., 1969; WIEST, 1971; FALK and BARDIN, 1970). It has also been shown that priming animals with estrogen results in greater amounts of progesterone uptake by the uterus and longer retention times (FALK and BARDIN, 1970). This latter finding is interesting in light of evidence which reveals a specific induction of progesterone receptor protein in target tissue by estrogen (O'MALLEY et al., 1970). Similarly, progesterone uptake and retention by vaginal tissue was increased by pretreatment with estradiol (KATZMAN et al., 1971).

Large concentrations of radioactivity found in liver and kidney (LAUMOS and FAROOG, 1966) were thought to reflect the metabolic and secretory role of these organs in handling progesterone.

The potential importance of progesterone uptake by the hypothalamus and pituitary (LAUMOS and FAROOG, 1966) lies in the fact that progesterone can inhibit gonadotropin secretion (SWERDLOFF and ODELL, 1966). This presumably is part of a feed-back mechanism in the control of luteinizing hormone (LH) release during the reproductive cycle (ROSS et al., 1970). It has been reported that progesterone was not taken up into any selective region of the rat hypothalamus. It was thus concluded that in the rat, specific progesterone binding receptors do not exist in the hypothalamus and pituitary gland (SEIKI et al., 1969). However, in a subsequent study, also using rats, the results suggested the existence of limited capacity binding sites for progesterone in the mesencephalon and diencephalon, as well as in the pituitary (WHALEN and LUTTGE, 1971).

During tissue retention, steroid hormones are subject to various enzyme systems which transform them into a variety of metabolites. Once progesterone enters a "target" cell it may effect a particular response by a direct action or through the formation of a specific metabolite(s). It is not as yet clear whether progesterone metabolism is related solely to a local regulation of its concentration or if the formation of a metabolite might also act as a mediator of a specific biochemical or biological effect. It is even conceivable that different metabolites perform independent functions such as have been demonstrated for testosterone metabolites in androgen dependent tissue (ROBEL et al., 1971). Without introducing additional oxygen functions there are at least 26 different metabolites of progesterone that can be formed. The problem is thus a complex one, and it is not clear as to why a cell should form so many different metabolites. If, however, the importance in the formation of any particular metabolite is to be understood, it will be necessary to examine each metabolite, as it is identified, for some biological or biochemical activity. Such an approach has been initiated in several animal model systems. Some preliminary results are now available for the chick oviduct (KORENMAN and O'MALLEY, 1968) and the rat deciduoma reaction (DEFEO, 1967). The following discussion will be directed to these two systems.

Because it had been previously shown that in the chick oviduct there is a specific cytoplasmic receptor for progesterone which appears to function in transporting progesterone into the nucleus where it acts (O'MALLEY et al., 1970), the metabolism of progesterone associated with the cytoplasmic and nuclear receptors was examined. This was done by incubating intact oviduct tissue with ^{3}H-progesterone for varying periods of time followed by homogenization, cell fractionation, and sucrose-density-gradient analysis of the cytosol and nuclear protein preparations. This was followed by extraction and isolation of steroids from the top of the gradients (free steroids) and from the protein peaks in the gradients (bound steroids).

Several metabolites, in addition to unreacted progesterone, have been positively identified by recrystallization to constant specific activity, though the list is far from complete. These compounds include 5α-pregnane-3,20-dione; 5β-pregnane-3,20-dione; 3α-hydroxy-5β-pregnan-20-one; 3β-hydroxy-5α-pregnan-20-one; 3β-hydroxy-5β-pregnan-20-one; 20β-hydroxy-4-pregnen-3-one; and 20β-hydroxy-5α-pregnan-3-one. No radioactivity was recovered when 20α-hydroxy-4-pregnen-3-one was recrystallized suggesting that chick oviduct tissue may be lacking in 20α-hydroxysteroid dehydrogenase activity.

In terms of radioactive incorporation, 5α-pregnane-3,20-dione was the major metabolite recovered from nuclear chromatin, a finding which confirms a previous report (MORGAN and WILSON, 1970). After 30 min incubation, 5α-pregnane-3,20-dione and progesterone were present in essentially equal amounts for as long as four hours. This finding prompted the examination of avidin synthesis after giving 5α-pregnane-3,20-dione *in vivo* as previously done with progesterone (KORENMAN and O'MALLEY, 1968). Interestingly, it was found that this metabolite could induce avidin synthesis with a potency equal to, if not greater than, progesterone. This would be analogous to the conversion of testosterone to 5α-dihydrotestosterone in the rat prostate (BRUCHOVSKY and WILSON, 1968) and the finding that 5α-dihydrotestosterone has important biological activity in that system (BAULIEU et al., 1968). It was also found that 5α-pregnane-3,20-dione competed equally well with progesterone for binding to the cytoplasmic receptor (O'MALLEY et al., 1970). The question thus arises: in the chick oviduct, does progesterone induce avidin synthesis directly or through the formation of 5α-pregnane-3,20-dione, or are both compounds active? In addition, it is possible that further metabolism of 5α-pregnane-3,20-dione is important. This approach will need to be used for each metabolite as it is identified and examined for ability to bind to the cytoplasmic receptor and nuclear chromatin and induce avidin synthesis. Of course, avidin synthesis is a measurable biological response, and a metabolite of progesterone may effect some biochemical change that may or may not lead to measurable biological activity. It is also not known how the cell ultimately disposes of the progesterone molecule it originally extracted from the extracellular fluid.

The pattern of metabolites associated with the cytosol protein peak was similar to that found in the nucleus with the possible exception that there was relatively more radioactivity found in the more polar region of the chromatogram. At the end of a four hour incubation period, the greatest amount of radioactivity was found at the origin of the chromatogram. This unknown polar material accounted for approximately 30 % of the recoverable radioactivity in the bound nuclear fraction and 50 % in the bound cytosol fraction.

Examination of the unbound progesterone in both the cytosol and nuclear fractions revealed that after 5 min most of the radioactivity was found in the more polar region of the chromatogram, particularly at the origin. In fact, the polar material at the origin accounted for 70 to 80 % of the recoverable radioactivity by the end of a four hour incubation. Presumably the latter material contains additional oxygen functions. It is conceivable that this polar material is the ultimate disposal product of progesterone. It is of interest that a similar observation in an *in vivo* study has been reported for another animal species (REEL et al., 1969).

Several metabolites have been identified following incubation of deciduoma tissue with ^{3}H-progesterone. These include 5α-pregnane-3,20-dione; 5β-pregnane-3,20-dione; 3α-hydroxy-5β-pregnan-20-one; 20α-hydroxy-4-pregnen-3-one; and

20β-hydroxy-4-pregnen-3-one. In contrast to the chick oviduct, very little 5α-pregnane-3,20-dione was formed. Instead, the major metabolite in this animal model system appears to be 3α-hydroxy-5α-pregnan-20-one (tentatively identified by chromatographic behavior of the free alcohol and after derivative formation). This was also the case when highly purified nuclear preparations were extracted. Though only short-term incubations have been performed to date (15 to 60 min), all time points examined demonstrated that progesterone was at least 3 to 4 times more abundant than any possible metabolite. The control horn and the horn containing the deciduoma appeared to metabolize progesterone similarly.

Thus, an interesting species difference exists for 5α-pregnane-3,20-dione. It was the major *in vitro* metabolite in the chick oviduct and had biological activity in that system at least equivalent to progesterone. In contrast, it was a relatively minor *in vitro* metabolite in the rat uterus, and unlike progesterone was unable to support the deciduoma reaction or maintain pregnancy in the ovariectomized rat (Glasser, personal communication).

Similar experimental evidence is required which can be used to correlate tissue metabolism of progesterone with biologic activity of the individual metabolites in many different species. In this way, the complex metabolic pattern of this steroid may become more meaningful in relation to progesterone physiology.

Binding of Progesterone to Target Cells

A number of investigators have reported binding of ^{3}H-progesterone to target cells. Both mouse vagina (Podratz and Katzman, 1968) and guinea pig uterus (Falk and Bardin, 1970) have been reported to bind ^{3}H-progesterone following *in vivo* injections of the hormone. The guinea pig progesterone receptor has been subsequently isolated and shown to be a heat-labile protein with a Ka of 2×10^{-9} M for the steroid and a sedimentation value of 6.75 S on sucrose gradient analysis (Milgrom et al., 1970). The presence of specific progesterone-binding proteins has also been demonstrated in both cytosol and nuclear fractions of rabbit uteri (Wiest and Rao, 1971). In this tissue, the progesterone-binding protein is separate from transcortin (CBG), and the concentration of progesterone-binding sites in castrate rabbit uterus can be increased by prior estrogen treatment (Wiest and Rao, 1971). Finally, specific progesterone-binding sites have been shown to be present in human endometrium (Wiest and Rao, 1971; Eaton, W. L., unpublished data).

Preferential binding of progestins has also been reported for rat uterine tissue (McGuire and DeDella, 1971). However, studies in this model system have been less clear in that substantial binding of glucocorticoids is present in uterus. Both glucocorticoids and progestins bind to macromolecules sedimenting at 4 S upon sucrose gradient analysis. In fact, published studies have not as yet shown the progesterone binding capacity to be distinct from rat transcortin (Milgrom and Baulieu, 1970).

In the different species thus far studied, i.e., rat (McGuire and DeDella, 1971), guinea pig (Milgrom et al., 1970), rabbit (Wiest and Rao, 1971), chicken (O'Malley et al., 1970), and human (Wiest and Rao, 1971), these uterine and oviduct progesterone receptors have consistently demonstrated specificity for progesterone when compared to other classes of biologically active steroids. That is, cortisol, estradiol-17β, and testosterone have been shown not to compete effectively for the receptor. In addition, various kinds of steroids (precursors, metabolites, and synthetic forms) have been tested. So far only those synthetic compounds known to have progestational biological activity have been shown to bind to the receptor.

Few of the naturally occurring metabolites of progesterone have been tested, but one in particular has proven to be of some interest, i.e. 5α-pregnane-3,20-dione. This is the only metabolite thus far that has demonstrated significantly important binding to the receptor, and in this regard there is remarkable species variability. In the chicken it competes equally well with progesterone for the receptor, in the guinea pig about half as well. In the rat, rabbit, and human, however, it competes very little. In the chicken, 5α-pregnane-3,20-dione is known to have substantial biological activity, whereas in the rat it does not (the rabbit and human have not been tested). Also, in the chicken the 5β-pregnane-3,20-dione isomer has been shown to bind very little to the receptor, and likewise has been found to have little biological activity. Only a limited amount of work has been done to date on the relation of progesterone metabolites in target tissue to the progesterone receptor and biological activity. Studies of species variability in this regard will be important in order to understand the nature of progesterone metabolism in target tissue and the relationship of this process to its mechanism of action.

Sequence of Events in the Action of Progesterone

Since we have not yet elucidated the complete sequence of steps in steroid hormone action, we have tended to place major emphasis on the earliest events occurring in target cells following exposure to steroids. One of the earliest detectable intracellular events in steroid hormone action is thought to be the binding of the steroid hormone to a specific macromolecular component of the target tissue cytoplasm. Since only target cells have this macromolecular component, the distribution of these "receptor" molecules[1] might determine tissue specificity. Perhaps it is the hormone-receptor complex rather than the free hormone which participates in the regulation of RNA and protein metabolism in the target tissue.

The chick oviduct has been the subject of the bulk of the studies on molecular mechanisms of progesterone action. Following an *in vivo* injection of ^{3}H-progesterone to an estrogen pretreated chick, the labeled steroid is found distributed in both the cytoplasm and nucleus of the oviduct. The cytoplasmic radioactivity appears to exist bound to a macromolecular complex that does not dissociate on passage of the cytosol (105000 g supernatant extract) through a Sephadex G-200 column (O'Malley et al., 1969). Cytosol and nuclear extracts can be centrifuged through 5 to 20 % sucrose gradients and identified as radioactive peaks. A small amount of ^{3}H-progesterone is bound in the cytoplasm as early as one minute after injection and maximum binding occurs at 25 min; the percent of total steroid partitioned into the nucleus progressively increases during this same period. The cytosol and nuclear progesterone-binding macromolecules have sedimentation coefficients of 4 S during sucrose gradient centrifugation in the presence of 0.3 M KCl, but the cytosol-binding molecule aggregates to 5 S and 8 S forms under low salt (no KCl) conditions (Sherman et al., 1970; O'Malley et al., 1970). The oviduct-binding component shows a striking affinity for progesterone ($K_d \times 10^{-10}$ at 4 °C) and appears to comprise only 0.02 % of the cytosol protein.

Because of the high affinity displayed by transcortin for progesterone, tissue contamination by the plasma protein must be ruled out, especially since it also sediments at about 4 S in high-salt sucrose gradients. The cytosol progesterone-binding macromolecule has thus been unequivocally distinguished from plasma transcortin by agarose gel chromatography, discontinuous polyacrylamide electro-

1 At present, the steroid binding protein cannot unequivocally be defined as a receptor in the strictest pharmacologic sense of the word since the subsequent functional significance of this steroid-protein complex has not been proven.

phoresis, isoelectric gradient chromatography, and protamine sulfate precipitation (SHERMAN et al., 1970; O'MALLEY et al., 1970).

The progesterone-binding molecule can be destroyed by proteolytic enzymes, but not RNase or DNase. Thus, the active molecular-binding site for the steroid may be proteinaceous in nature. Furthermore, the receptor is a heat-sensitive, nondialyzable, and ammonium sulfate-precipitable protein with an isoelectric point of pH 4.0. Indirect physical-chemical calculations suggest that the molecule can exist in the shape of a prolate ellipsoid with a monometric molecular weight of approximately 90000 daltons.

The cytosol-binding protein of oviduct shows very little affinity for estrogens (estradiol, estrone), mineralocorticoids (aldosterone), glucocorticoids (cortisol), or progesterone precursors and inactive metabolites. However, 5α-pregnane-3,20-dione does bind to the progesterone receptor. The tissue concentration of progesterone-binding protein can be markedly increased by prior estrogen treatment (O'MALLEY et al., 1970). This estrogen mediated stimulation of progesterone-binding capacity correlates quite closely with the estrogen-induced quantitative enhancement of the oviduct-progesterone response, i.e. avidin synthesis. In addition, the progesterone-binding protein was found only in progesterone responsive target tissue (oviduct). For these reasons, the evidence can be considered as compatible with the concept that the progesterone-binding protein may be a "functional receptor" for progesterone. These receptors might thus interact initially with the steroid upon its entrance into the target cell and play a major role in the subsequent events involved in the action of the hormone.

Since progesterone is thought to act in the nucleus to influence gene transcription, it was of interest to establish whether the hormone is also bound to a receptor in the nucleus of the target cell. Purification of oviduct nuclei and extraction with salt revealed the presence of such a nuclear receptor which appeared almost identical to that which is found in the cytoplasm of the oviduct (O'MALLEY et al., 1970). No progesterone receptor could be detected in the nucleus prior to exposure to the hormone. However, upon incubation of tissue slices with ^{3}H-progesterone at 37° for short periods of time, it was possible to detect and monitor the actual transfer of the receptor-progesterone complex from the cytosol to the nucleus of the oviduct target cell (O'MALLEY et al., 1970). This same transfer process can be accomplished under more defined cell-free conditions by incubating cytosol receptor preparations labeled with ^{3}H-progesterone together with purified nuclei (O'MALLEY et al., 1970). This *in vitro* binding of receptor to oviduct nuclei showed specificity requirements for both oviduct cytosol and oviduct nuclei. Cytosol and nuclear preparations from nontarget tissues were ineffective. The intranuclear progesterone was subsequently shown to be contained on the chromatin. This series of events involving the progesterone receptor of chick oviduct is quite similar to those noted for estrogens (JENSEN, 1964; WIEST, 1971; TOFT and GORSKI, 1966; NOTEBOOM and GORSKI, 1965; JENSEN et al., 1968, 1969; TOFT et al., 1967), androgens (FANG et al., 1969; MAINWARING, 1969; BAULIEU and JUNG, 1970), aldosterone (EDELMAN and FIMOGNARI, 1968; HERMAN et al., 1968; SWANECK et al., 1970) and glucocorticoids (BEATO et al., 1969; BAXTER and TOMKINS, 1970; WIRA and MUNCK, 1970) in their respective target tissues.

Since there is a specific requirement for oviduct nuclei in the binding of the progesterone-receptor complex to chromatin, we began a search for specific "acceptor" sites on the nuclear chromatin-DNA for the receptor-hormone complex. Indeed, incubation of the cytosol receptor with purified oviduct chromatin revealed a limited number of chromatin sites capable of specifically binding the steroid-receptor complex (O'MALLEY et al., 1970). Very little binding was noted in nontarget chromatins. Determination of the nature of these chromatin sites was considerably more difficult. Experiments were performed in which a progesterone-receptor interaction with chromatin was monitored during selective removal of histones, nonhistone proteins, and chromosomal RNA. Further experiments were carried out using reconstituted "hybrid chromatins," containing the histones from one organ or species and the nonhistone acidic proteins and DNA from another organ or species (SPELSBERG et al., 1971). These rather complex experiments can be summarized by stating that the receptor-hormone complex appeared to interact with the genome at specific DNA sites which are determined by the chromatin acidic proteins (SPELSBERG et al., 1971). Histones did not appear to be involved in the interaction of the hormone-receptor complex with target cell chromatin (SPELSBERG et al., 1971). In subsequent experiments, these chromatin nonhistone "acceptor" proteins have been partially purified and characterized (SPELSBERG et al., 1972). The speculation that these DNA sites are activator sites in the genes regulating progesterone functional responses in the target cell is an attractive one, but wholly unproven at this time.

The experimental results described above are thus compatible with the following time sequence of events purported for the mechanism of action of progesterone in the chick oviduct: (1) steroid permeation of the cell membrane, (2) binding of progesterone to a specific cytoplasmic receptor, (3) transfer of the steroid-receptor complex to the nucleus, and (4) binding of the steroid-receptor complex to specific sites on the chromatin-DNA.

If the specific interaction of progesterone with the target tissue DNA is related to gene activation, it would be expected that new gene transcription products (RNA) should appear in response to progesterone. Some effort, then, has gone toward attempts to demonstrate that progesterone induces the synthesis of specific types of RNA prior to induction of avidin.

Experimental evidence from studies of progesterone induction of avidin in the presence of known inhibitors of DNA, RNA, and protein synthesis suggested that new DNA-dependent RNA synthesis and continued protein synthesis are required for induction to occur. New DNA synthesis itself is not necessary since hydroxyurea, a specific inhibitor of DNA synthesis did not affect the induction process at low concentrations (O'MALLEY et al., 1969). Further confirmation of this point came from the fact that ^{3}H-thymidine incorporation into DNA was not enhanced during induction. However, actinomycin D, which inhibits DNA-dependent RNA synthesis, caused a 90% reduction of avidin synthesis without blocking general protein synthesis, whereas cycloheximide, which blocks protein synthesis by inhibiting the transfer of activated amino acids from transfer RNA to the growing polypeptide chain, caused a complete inhibition of avidin induction (O'MALLEY et al., 1969).

In order to confirm the importance of RNA in the induction process, RNA polymerase activity was assessed at various intervals after progesterone (MCGUIRE and O'MALLEY, 1968). The activity of this enzyme increased and this increase preceded the initial rise in avidin synthesis. Similarly, the pattern of rapidly labeled nuclear RNA synthesis was altered. These results point to an effect of progesterone at the transcriptional level. In addition, analysis of RNA synthesized *in vitro* from oviduct chromatin shows that there was a qualitative change in the dinucleotide composition of nuclear RNA after progesterone administration (O'MALLEY et al., 1969).

New species of hybridizable rapidly labeled nuclear RNA (repeating sequences) were also found following administration of progesterone but prior to induction of avidin (O'MALLEY and MCGUIRE, 1968a, b; HAHN et al., 1968). That this new

RNA contains the messenger RNA for avidin is possible, but proof of such a hypothesis must await the development of a cell-free assay system that can detect a specific RNA template controlling the synthesis of this protein. Taken together, the above studies seem to indicate that progesterone exerts a primary influence at the level of transcription.

In attempting to explain how progesterone transforms the mammalian endometrium into a receptive state for the new blastocyst, we might postulate two major mechanisms. Progesterone may suppress the synthesis of an agent which inhibits implantation. More likely, the steroid may induce the synthesis of a protein molecule which facilitates implantation. We feel the latter mechanism to be more probable for the following reasons: (1) the cell structure is primarily composed of protein and all aspects of cell metabolism (i.e. carbohydrate, lipid, protein) are ultimately controlled by enzyme proteins; (2) progesterone has been shown to stimulate the synthesis of RNA and protein in the best defined model systems (deciduoma and chick oviduct); (3) finally, other steroid hormones are generally thought to exert effects in their target tissues by first stimulating production of RNA and protein.

The temporary acquisition of the capacity for the uterine endometrium to accept the new blastocyst during reproduction would then seem to be most efficiently

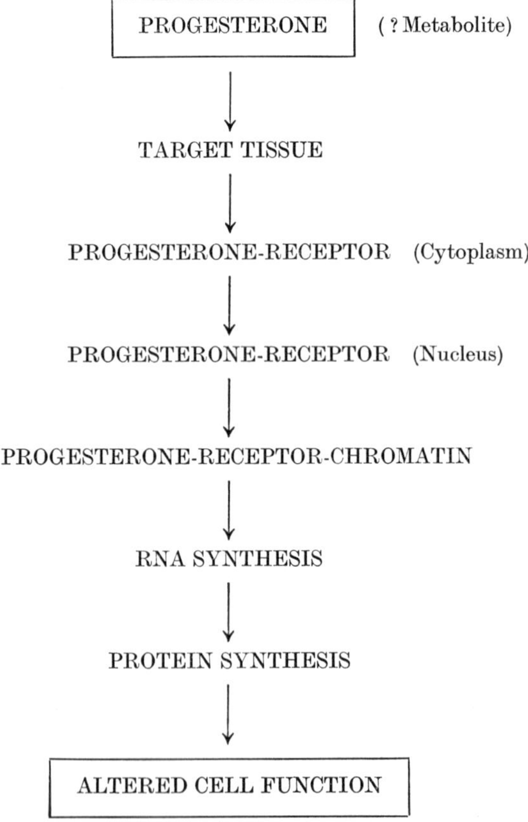

Fig. 1. Summary of the biochemical sequence of events occurring during progesterone action in the cells of target tissues

regulated by the induction of synthesis of a limited number of enzymes. A hypothetical scheme, based on current knowledge, for the series of biochemical events occurring in progesterone action in target tissue is listed in Fig. 1.

References

BAULIEU, E. E., JUNG, I.: A prostatic cytosol receptor. Biochem. biophys. Res. Commun. **38**, 599—606 (1970).

BAULIEU, E. E., LASNITZKI, I., ROBEL, P.: Metabolism of testosterone and action of metabolites on prostate glands grown in organ culture. Nature (Lond.) **219**, 1155—1156 (1968).

BAXTER, J. D., TOMKINS, G. M.: The relationship between glucocorticoid binding and tyrosine aminotransferase induction in hepatoma tissue culture cells. Proc. nat. Acad. Sci. (Wash.) **65**, 709—715 (1970).

BEATO, M., BIESEWIG, D., BRANDLE, W., SEKERIS, C. E.: Biochim. biophys. Acta (Amst.) **192**, 494 (1969).

BRUCHOVSKY, N., WILSON, J. D.: The conversion of testosterone to 5α-androstan-17β-ol-3-one by rat prostate *in vivo* and *in vitro*. J. biol. Chem. **243**, 2012—2021 (1968).

CHATTERTON, R. T., JR.: Progesterone and mammary gland development. In: MCKERNS, K. W. (Ed.): The sex steroids: molecular mechanisms. New York: Appleton-Century-Crofts 1971.

CORNER, G. W.: The hormones in human reproduction, p. 281. Princeton: Univ. Press, 1947.

CSAPO, A.: Brook Lodge Symposium on Progesterone, p. 7. Augusta, Michigan: Brook Lodge Press 1961.

DEFEO, V. J.: Decidualization. In: WYNN, R. M. (Ed.): Cellular biology of the uterus, pp. 191—290. New York: Appleton-Century-Crofts 1967.

EDELMAN, I. S., FIMOGNARI, G.: On the biochemical mechanisms of action of aldosterone. Rec. Progr. Horm. Res. **24**, 1—44 (1968).

EDWARDS, R., BRUSH, M. G., TAYLOR, R. W.: The uptake and intracellular distribution of (1,2-^{3}H) progesterone by human endometrium. J. Endocrinol. **45**, iii (1969).

FALK, R. J., BARDIN, C. W.: Uptake of tritiated progesterone by the uterus of the ovariectomized guinea pig. Endocrinology **86**, 1059—1063 (1970).

FANG, S., ANDERSON, K. M., LIAO, S.: Receptor proteins for androgens. J. biol. Chem. **244**, 6584—6595 (1969).

GLASSER, S. R.: Personal communication.

HAHN, W. E., CHURCH, R. B., GORBMAN, A., WILMOT, L.: Estrone- and progesterone-induced synthesis of new RNA species in the chick oviduct. Gen. comp. Endocrinol. **10**, 438—442 (1968).

HERMAN, T. S., FIMOGNARI, G. M., EDELMAN, I. S.: Studies on renal aldosterone-binding proteins. J. biol. Chem. **243**, 3849—3856 (1968).

JENSEN, E. V.: Proceedings of the 2nd international congress of endocrinology, p. 420. London: Amsterdam: Excerpta Medica 1964.

JENSEN, E. V., DESOMBRE, E. R., JUNGBLUT, P. W., STUMPF, W. E., ROTH, L. J.: In: ROTH, L. J., STUMPF, W. E. (Eds.): Autoradiography of diffusible substances, p. 81. New York: Academic Press 1969.

JENSEN, E. V., SUZUKI, T., KAWASHIMA, T., STUMPF, W. E., JUNGBLUT, P. W., DESOMBRE, E. R.: A two-step mechanism for the interaction of estradiol with rat uterus. Proc. nat. Acad. Sci. (Wash.) **59**, 632—638 (1968).

KATZMAN, P. A., LARSON, D. L., PODRATZ, K. C.: Effects of estradiol on metabolism of vaginal tissue. In: MCKERNS, K. W. (Ed.): The sex steroids: molecular mechanisms. New York: Appleton-Century-Crofts 1971.

KOHLER, P. O., GRIMLEY, P. M., O'MALLEY, B. W.: Estrogen-induced cytodifferentiation of the ovalbumin secreting glands of the chick oviduct. J. cell Biol. **40**, 8—27 (1969).

KORENMAN, S. G.: Comparative binding affinity of estrogens and its relation to estrogenic potency. Steroids **13**, 163—177 (1969).

KORENMAN, S. G., O'MALLEY, B. W.: Progesterone action: regulation of avidin biosynthesis by hen oviduct *in vivo* and *in vitro*. Endocrinology **83**, 11—17 (1968).

LANDAU, R. L., LUGIBIHL, K.: The catabolic and natriuretic effects of progesterone in man. Rec. Progr. Horm. Res. **17**, 249—292 (1961).

LAUMOS, K. R., FAROOG, A.: The uptake *in vivo* of (1,2-^{3}H) progesterone by the brain and genital tract of the rat. J. Endocrinol. **36**, 95—96 (1966).

MAINWARING, W. I. P.: A soluble androgen receptor in the cytoplasm of rat prostate. J. Endocrinol. **45**, 531—541 (1969).

McGuire, W. L., Dedella, C.: Endocrinology 88, 1099 (1971).
McGuire, W. L., O'Malley, B. W.: Ribonucleic acid polymerase activity of the chick oviduct during steroid-induced synthesis of a specific protein. Biochim. biophys. Acta (Amst.) **157**, 187—194 (1968).
Milgrom, E., Atger, M., Baulieu, E.: Steroids **16**, 741 (1970).
Milgrom, E., Baulieu, E.: Endocrinology **87**, 276 (1970).
Morgan, M. D., Wilson, J. D.: Intranuclear metabolism of progesterone-1,2-^{3}H in the hen oviduct. J. biol. Chem. **245**, 3781—3789 (1970).
Noteboom, W. D., Gorski, J.: Steriospecific binding of estrogens in the rat uterus. Archs. Biochem. Biophys. **111**, 559 (1965).
O'Malley, B. W., McGuire, W. L.: Progesterone-induced synthesis of a new species of nuclear RNA. Endocrinology **84**, 63—68 (1968).
O'Malley, B. W., McGuire, W. L.: Studies on the mechanisms of estrogen-mediated tissue differentiation: regulation of nuclear transcription and induction of new RNA species. Proc. nat. Acad. Sci. (Wash.) **60**, 1527—1534 (1968).
O'Malley, B. W., McGuire, W. L.: Changes in hybridizable nuclear RNA during progesterone induction of a specific oviduct protein. Biochem. biophys. Res. Commun. **32**, 595—598 (1968).
O'Malley, B. W., McGuire, W. L., Kohler, P. O., Korenman, S. G.: Studies on the mechanism of steroid hormone regulation of synthesis of specific proteins. Rec. Progr. Horm. Res. **25**, 105—160 (1969).
O'Malley, B. W., Sherman, M. R., Toft, D. O.: Progesterone "receptors" in the cytoplasm and nucleus of chick oviduct target tissue. Proc. nat. Acad. Sci. (Wash.) **67**, 501—508 (1970).
O'Malley, B. W., Sherman, M. R., Toft, D. O., Spelsberg, T. C., Schrader, W. T., Steggles, A. W.: A specific oviduct target-tissue receptor for progesterone: identification, characterization, partial purification, inter-compartmental transfer kinetics and specific interaction with the genome. In: Advances of the Biosciences: Steroid Hormone Receptors. Schering Symposium, Berlin, 1970.
Podratz, K. C., Katzman, P. A.: Fed. Proc. **27**, 497 (1968).
Porter, D. G.: Progesterone and the guinea pig myometrium. In: Wolstenholme, G. E. W., Knight, J. (Eds.): Progesterone: its regulatory effect on the myometrium, p. 79. London: J. and A. Churchill 1969.
Reel, J. R., Lee, S., Callantine, M. R.: Specific retention of an unconjugated polar metabolite in the rat uterus following labeled progesterone administration, p. 113. Fifty-first Meeting of the Endocrine Society, New York 1969.
Reynolds, S. R. M.: Physiology of the uterus, p. 611. New York: P. B. Hoeber 1949.
Robel, P., Lasnitzki, I., Baulieu, E.: Hormone metabolism and action: testosterone and metabolites in prostate organ culture. Biochimie **53**, 81 (1971).
Ross, G. T., Cargille, C. M., Lipsett, M. B., Rayford, P. L., Marshall, J. R., Strott, C. A., Rodbard, D.: Pituitary and gonadal hormones in women during spontaneous and induced ovulatory cycles. Rec. Progr. Horm. Res. **26**, 1—62 (1970).
Seiki, K., Miyamoto, M., Yamashita, A., Kotani, M.: Further studies on the uptake of labeled progesterone by the hypothalamus and pituitary of rats. J. Endocrinol. **43**, 129—130 (1969).
Sherman, M. R., Corvol, P. L., O'Malley, B. W.: Progesterone-binding components of chick oviduct: I. Preliminary characterization of cytoplasmic components. J. biol. Chem. **245**, 6085—6096 (1970).
Spelsberg, T. C., Steggles, A. W., Chytil, F., O'Malley, B. W.: Progesterone-binding components of chick oviduct. V. Exchange of progesterone binding capacity from target to non-target tissue chromatins. J. biol. Chem., **247**, 1368—1374 (1972).
Spelsberg, T. C., Steggles, A. W., O'Malley, B. W.: Progesterone-binding components of chick oviduct. III. Chromatin acceptor sites. J. biol. Chem. **246**, 4188—4197 (1971).
Swaneck, G. E., Chu, L. L. H., Edelman, I. S.: Stereo-specific binding of aldosterone to renal chromatin. J. biol. Chem. **245**, 5382—5389 (1970).
Swerdloff, R. S., Odell, W. O.: Serum luteinizing and follicle stimulating hormone levels during sequential and non-sequential contraceptive treatment of eugonadal women. J. clin. Endocr. **29**, 157—163 (1966).
Toft, D., Gorski, J.: A receptor molecule for estrogens: isolation from the rat uterus and preliminary characterization. Proc. nat. Acad. Sci. (Wash.) **55**, 1574—1581 (1966).
Toft, D. O., Shyamala, G., Gorski, J.: A receptor molecule for estrogens: studies using a cell-free system. Proc. nat. Acad. Sci. (Wash.) **57**, 1740 (1967).
Whalen, R. E., Luttge, W. G.: Differential localization of progesterone uptake in brain. Role of sex, estrogen pretreatment and adrenalectomy. Brain Res. **33**, 147—155 (1971).

WIEST, W. G.: The distribution and metabolism of progesterone in the uterus. In: MCKERNS, K.W. (Ed.): The sex steroids: molecular mechanisms. New York: Appleton-Century-Crofts, 1971.
WIEST, W. G., RAO, B. R.: Advances in the biosciences: Schering Workshop on Steroid Hormone 'Receptors' **7**, 251 (1971).
WIRA, C., MUNCK, A.: Specific glucocorticoid receptors in thymus cells. J. biol. Chem. **245**, 3436—3438 (1970).
YOKOYAMA, I.: In: Lactogenesis: the initiation of milk formation. REYNOLDS, M. (Ed.), 1969.

Chapter 40

Pharmacology and Clinical Utility of Hormones in Hormone Related Neoplasms

THOMAS L. DAO

Introduction

The isolation of estrone in 1929 independently by DOISY (1929) in the United States and by BUTENANDT (1929) in Germany made possible the classic experiment of LACASSAGNE (1932) in which mammary tumors in male mice were induced by giving injections of estrone. This experiment established a causal relationship between estrogenic hormones and mammary tumorigenesis. The proof that hormones can influence the growth of cancer was derived from experiments by HUGGINS and CLARK (1940) on tumors of the prostate of the dog.

The metabolic study of the effect of hormones on prostatic secretion in a dog with a benign prostatic tumor led to the discovery by HUGGINS (1940) that excision of the testes or the administration of estrogen resulted in a remarkable shrinkage of the canine prostatic tumor. Subsequently, HUGGINS et al. (1941) demonstrated that these same methods could induce spectacular regression of metastatic cancer of the prostate in man. This antiandrogenic control by orchiectomy or administration of estrogenic compounds (HUGGINS et al., 1941) thus ushered in the era of chemotherapy of malignant disease.

Appreciation of the results of the investigations of HUGGINS and his coworkers led to an intensive search for effective therapy with steroid hormones in many forms of cancers in humans. The control of neoplasia, either by removal of hormonal factors or by administration of hormones, represents a challenging area of research which has real clinical implications. There are at least 5 different cancers in humans that are hormone related (steroid hormones) and are amenable to control by steroid hormones.

In recent years, new steroidal agents, with greater biological activities, have been synthesized and their antitumor efficacy has been studied in human trials. The beneficial effect of hormonal therapy at best is only palliative and often limited to a few patients. The discovery of new useful agents must necessarily be dependent on the understanding of the mechanism of tumor inhibition by steroidal hormones. A broader spectrum of biological investigations must also be established for examination of compounds. It is with these goals in mind that the author considers in more detail the relationship of biological activities of steroid hormones to their antitumor activity, and the possible mechanism(s) by which hormones induce tumor regression. A brief survey is made of the clinical use of hormones in different cancers, but no attempt is made to cover the entire literature on the subject of antineoplastic steroidal agents.

Hormone-Induced Tissue Growth and Neoplasia

Hormones, directly or indirectly, can cause cellular proliferation resulting in increments in tissue mass. A large gap exists in our knowledge of the relationship between hormone stimulated tissue growth and the neoplastic process. The obvious question to be answered is whether these hormone induced tissue growths are related to the subsequent development of neoplasia. Understanding of the relationship between hormone induced tissue growth and neoplasia may provide knowledge for better use of hormonal agents in the treatment of cancer.

It has been known that alteration of the endogenous hormonal environment disturbs the homeostatic force controlling the endocrine balance between "trophic" hormone activity and target organ response. Thus, hypersecretion of pituitary trophic hormones can cause an increase in the size of the target tissue and the rate of function of that organ (increased secretion of hormones) (DAO, 1967). Hyperplasia as a result of overstimulation seems to be a prerequisite for neoplasia. The trigger mechanism of this imbalance appears to be the hypofunctioning of a target organ causing an interference with the feedback regulatory mechanism of the pituitary target relationship. Thus, thyroid tumors can be induced in a number of ways, all of which produce hypothyroidism as an initial step with subsequent stimulation of thyroid tissue by an increase in the thyrotrophic hormone (TSH) secretion from the pituitary (PURVES and GRIESBACH, 1947; MORRIS et al., 1951; AXELRAD and LEBLOND, 1955; GOLDBERG and CHIAKOFF, 1951). Neoplasia of the thyroid as a result of this endocrine imbalance can easily be prevented by administering thyroid hormones which restore the normal feedback mechanism. Similarly, ovarian tumors can be induced by methods that depress gonadal function (BISKIND and BISKIND, 1944). Again, this neoplastic transformation can be reversed if gonadal hormones are given to these animals. Neoplasms induced as a result of hormonal deficiency of the target organs apparently do not grow in normal hosts. It appears that continued stimulation by the trophic hormones is necessary to sustain the tumor growth.

The diversified biological activity of estrogens for tissue growth and the genesis of neoplasms of the mammary glands, uterus, gonads, and vagina are further examples that there are certain functional denominators between hormone induced tissue growth and neoplasms of these tissues. Disturbances of endocrine feedback regulatory mechanisms as a result of treatment with exogenous estrogens induces a state of "endocrine imbalance" in the host. The sequence of events occurring in the process of neoplastic transformation appears to resemble that following alterations in the endogenous hormonal status. In most instances, estrogens induce neoplastic growth in tissues in which non-malignant hyperplasia is stimulated by hormones. These changes are reversible and last only as long as enough estrogen is available to maintain them. These characteristics are almost identical to the normal physiological behavior of the tissue of origin. This apparent dependency on hormones for maintenance and growth of tumors that are derived from the organs and tissues normally dependent on these same hormones for physiological and metabolic activities has important clinical implications in therapy for hormone related neoplasms in humans.

Effects of hormones on normal tissue growth and the induction and growth of neoplasms, however, are not the same. Normal tissue response to endocrine stimulation is often rapid if not immediate. Induction of neoplasia by hormones requires a long period, often constituting a major portion of the life span of the species involved. It has also been well established that although normal hormone sensitive or target tissues respond to withdrawal of hormonal support by involution and atrophy, tumors of endocrine sensitive tissue may regress or remain unchanged after endocrine withdrawal. These observations suggest that neoplastic transformation in hormone sensitive tissues is a deviation from normal growth response to hormonal stimulation.

The clinical application of the principle of hormone dependency of neoplasms in hormone sensitive organs led to some remarkable therapeutic accomplishments in the management of many human cancers, particularly those of the breast and the prostate. In spite of the apparent clinical success in some patients, the overall cancer mortality has not been altered. The concept of hormone dependency is, in the true sense, only operational. We observe the regression of cancer after withdrawal of endogenous sources of hormones, but we do not understand the exact mechanism of this phenomenon. We know that some cancers are hormone responsive and others are not, and we also observe that hormone dependent cancers invariably will progress into hormone non-responsive tumors, but we are in total darkness as to the nature of this progression. These are the challenging fields of research in endocrine oncology.

Antineoplastic Property of Steroid Hormones as Related to Their Biological Activities

That steroid hormones can both induce tissue growth and inhibit endocrine related neoplasms has been well established. These seemingly paradoxical effects of hormones have been exploited, leading to the introduction of hormonal therapies in several human cancers. The lack of understanding of the exact mechanism by which steroid hormones induce regression of cancer has become the major obstacle preventing significant progress in the field of chemotherapy for endocrine related cancers.

Existing knowledge of the relation of steroid hormones to their biological activities and therapeutic effects will be considered to provide insights for designing new antineoplastic agents for cancer chemotherapy.

A. Estrogens and Antiandrogenic Effect

The therapeutic effectiveness of estrogen in the treatment of prostatic cancer is believed to be due to its "antiandrogenic effect". The classical experiments of HUGGINS et al. (1939) in which they isolated the prostate gland of dogs, thereby studying the output and biochemistry of canine prostatic secretion, led to the understanding of the androgenic control of growth and function of the prostate. Castration induces marked involution of the prostate, but this can be prevented or reversed by the administration of androgens.

During their experiments with the canine prostate, HUGGINS and CLARK (1940) also discovered that estrogenic hormones possessed an antiandrogenic effect. It was demonstrated that estrogens exert remarkable inhibition of the androgenic effect of testosterone on the growth of prostate epithelium and the prostatic secretion. In these studies it was also discovered that estrogen could inhibit the production of a prostatic enzyme, acid phosphatase, which was found to be elevated in some men with cancer of the prostate (HUGGINS and HODGES, 1941). Androgen, on the other hand, increases the concentration of acid phosphatase in the prostate. Thus, when estrogen was administered to men with advanced prostate cancer, regression of the cancer was accompanied by prompt decrease of greatly elevated serum acid phosphatase, an early biochemical alteration in the cancerous prostate.

The apparent antiandrogenic effect of estrogen has been considered to be the mechanism for the therapeutic effect of estrogen on cancer of the prostate. But what is the nature of this antiandrogenic effect? Is this antiandrogenic effect of estrogen the result of an inhibition of the response of the prostate epithelium to androgens? The antineoplastic activity of estrogen may be attributed to the suppression of pituitary gonadotrophin activity, thus reducing the production of androgens.

In human males, the interrelationship between interstitial cell stimulating hormone (ICSH) and testosterone appears to be clear. Lowering of testosterone level (Leydig cell damage, etc.) causes increase in pituitary ICSH levels. Estrogens such as estradiol or diethylstilbestrol, when administered to the male, cause inhibition of pituitary gonadotrophin secretion, thus impairing the testicular function. Inhibition of ICSH secretion causes depression of Leydig cell activity in the production of testosterone. This appears to be the mechanism of the antiandrogenic effect of estrogen in human males.

This supposition, however, is not tenable since administration of testosterone to patients with cancer of the prostate causes changes in testicular function similar to those seen with estrogens. Testosterone usually induces depression of urinary gonadotrophin to almost zero level within a period of 6 weeks. There is almost complete disappearance of Leydig cells and an "absence" of testosterone production. Unlike estrogens, testosterone, however, fails to induce regression of cancer of the prostate. It is conceivable that estrogen inhibits prostate growth by an interference with the peripheral action of androgens.

B. Androgen and its Antiestrogenic Effect

Androgen and estrogen are antagonistic. It is believed that the antineoplastic activity of androgen in mammary cancer is due to its antiestrogenic effect. Estrogen has been shown to induce mammary cancer in both mice and rats. LACASSAGNE (1937) and NATHANSON and ANDERVONT (1939) demonstrated with certainty that androgen can prevent breast cancer in mice. The major impetus in using testosterone in humans with breast cancer came after the reported successful treatment of prostatic cancer by estrogen and castration.

The antitumor activity of testosterone is not clearly understood. The antiestrogenic activity of androgen has been demonstrated by its effect on the inhibition of response of the female reproductive system to estrogen, such as the inhibition of uterine growth (VELARDO, 1959). Such an effect, however, has not been conclusively demonstrated in the response of mammary glands to estrogen in the presence of androgen. The antiestrogenic property of testosterone has been ascribed to its effect on the hypothalamic-pituitary level by inhibiting the synthesis and release of gonadotrophin. It is well recognized that testosterone and many other androgens are inhibitory to pituitary gonadotrophin production and thus bring about a temporary reduction or cessation of ovarian activity. If testosterone is continued for a long period of time, ovarian atrophy can result. Many androgenic compounds that effectively inhibit pituitary gonadotrophin have been shown to be entirely devoid of antitumor activity (DAO, unpublished data). Clinical remissions have been observed (KENNEDY, 1959; BECKETT and BRENNAN, 1959) in hypophysectomized patients receiving androgens (fluoxymestrone) and in patients who do not show reduction of pituitary gonadotrophin activity after treatment with fluoxymestrone (SEGALOFF, 1958) or with 2α-methyldihydrotestosterone (BLACKBURN and ALBERT, 1959). These observations seem to suggest that regression of breast cancer in these patients cannot be explained solely on the basis of pituitary gonadotrophin inhibition.

It is well known that testosterone is an anabolic steroid, capable of inducing nitrogen retention and stimulating the hematopoietic system. This biological activity of testosterone certainly is desirable in patients with advanced breast cancer, particularly in those with extensive bone metastases.

C. Antineoplastic Effect of Estrogen and Hypothalamic-Pituitary Regulation of Prolactin

In mammalian species, the principal early effect of estrogen on the mammary gland is ductal growth. In later life, estrogen also stimulates acinar growth. All experimental evidence suggests that the mechanism by which estrogens produce effects on the mammary epithelium is a dual process. Indirectly, estrogen exerts its effect on the anterior pituitary to secrete prolactin, an essential mammotrophic hormone, but estrogen also has a direct effect on the mammary epithelium and the connective tissue.

It has now been well established that estrogens inhibit PIF (prolactin inhibitory factor) of the hypothalamus, thus increasing the release of prolactin by the pituitary (NICOLL and MEITES, 1962). In rats, castration causes rapid decrease of plasma prolactin levels and administration of estrogen restores plasma prolactin to precastration levels. Thus, in rats bearing carcinogen induced mammary cancer, tumors rapidly regress following castration, but resume growth after injections of estrogens (STERENTAL et al., 1963). It is suggested that estrogen stimulates mammary cancer growth indirectly via the anterior pituitary. Thus, the antineoplastic effect of castration on mammary tumor growth is believed to be due to a lowering of the prolactin level. However, administration of large doses of estrogen to mammary tumor-bearing rats induces regression of cancer, while plasma prolactin levels are elevated (MEITES et al., 1971). The biphasic effect of estrogen on tumorigenesis of the mammary gland has been well established. Small doses of estrogen cause acceleration of tumor growth, whereas large doses inhibit such growth. In both situations, serum prolactin levels are elevated. This apparent paradoxical phenomenon has yet to be elucidated. Recent experiments reported by PEARSON (1972) suggest that large doses of estrogen interfere with the peripheral action of prolactin.

Progesterone in large doses suppresses plasma prolactin levels (PEARSON, 1972), but progesterone has no effect on mammary tumor growth in rats. Testosterone has little or no effect on plasma prolactin levels (PEARSON, 1972), but this steroid induces regression of carcinogen induced mammary cancer in rats. The antineoplastic activity of estrogen and androgen on mammary cancer growth cannot be explained entirely on the basis of their effect on prolactin secretion or release.

D. Effect of Progestogens on Endometrium, Mammary Gland, and Kidney, and Their Antitumor Activity

Hormonal effects upon the endometrium regulate the estrus or menstrual cycle so as to condition the endometrium for implantation. Following ovulation, the follicles are converted to corpus luteum which secretes progesterone, a hormone that transforms a proliferative endometrium into a secretory type. Protracted action of estrogen (endogenous or exogenous) if unopposed by progesterone, may play a pathogenic role in endometrial malignancy. Thus ovarian abnormalities such as the Stein-Leventhal Syndrome (JACKSON and DOCKERTY, 1957), cortical stromal hyperplasia (SOMMERS and MEISSNER, 1957), thecomas (WALL et al., 1948), and feminizing ovarian neoplasms (LARSON, 1954) have been described as coexisting with endometrial carcinoma. It seems that failure of ovulation over long periods of time predisposes endometrium to malignant changes.

In the rabbit, experimental evidence implicates estrogens as important factors in the pathogenesis of endometrial carcinoma (BURROWS and HORNING, 1952; MEISSNER et al., 1957). GRIFFITHS et al. (1963) demonstrated that induction of endometrial carcinoma in rabbits by 3-methylcholanthrene (3-MC) is estrogen dependent. They also reported that simultaneous administration of progestins can neutralize the cocarcinogenic effect of estrogens. Progesterone has been used to treat patients with metastatic endometrial carcinoma with beneficial effects.

The mammary gland responds to progestin in a manner similar to the endometrium and its effect is dependent on previous stimulation by estrogens. Like estrogen and androgen, progesterone inhibits the pituitary gonadotrophin. Based on bioassay, progesterone is both "antiestrogenic and antiandrogenic." Progestogens have been used for treatment of women with advanced breast cancer, but their results have often been inconsistent and insignificant.

Progestins have also been used in the treatment of advanced renal cell carcinoma in man. Primary carcinoma of the kidney can be induced by prolonged administration of estrogen in hamsters (MATTHEWS et al., 1947; KIRKMAN and BACON, 1952a, b; HORNING, 1952). HORNING (1956) and KIRKMAN (1959) showed that primary renal cell carcinoma induction in hamsters by estrogen can be inhibited by simultaneous administration of progesterone or testosterone. BLOOM et al. (1963) used the transplantable renal adenocarcinoma of the golden hamster as an experimental model for studies on the efficacy of certain antiestrogenic compounds and other hormonal agents in the treatment of advanced renal cell carcinoma in man.

The antitumor activity of progestogens in patients with breast cancer or endometrial or renal cell carcinoma appears to be an "antiestrogen" effect. Again, we do not understand the mechanism of this putative "antiestrogenic" effect of progestins.

E. Corticosteroids and Their Antitumor Activity

Among the adrenal corticosteroids, the glucocorticoids are the hormones which have been shown to possess antitumor activity. Of the manifold functions of glucocorticoids, the effect on lymphoid tissues has important clinical applications in the treatment of neoplastic diseases.

DOUGHERTY and WHITE (1944, 1945) were the first to describe the profound acute changes in the lymphoid tissues several hours after injections of an active glucocorticoid (e.g. cortisol) in mice, rats, and rabbits, as well as in man. These dramatic changes, as manifested by pycnosis and karyorrhexis of the lymphocyte nuclei, ultimately lead to a dissolution of lymphocytes in the thymus and lymph nodes and a peripheral lymphopenia.

Adrenal corticosteroids in large amounts were shown to induce marked regression of lymphosarcoma in mice (HEILMAN and KENDALL, 1944). Later, PEARSON et al. (1949) demonstrated profound regression of leukemia and Hodgkin's disease following cortisone acetate or ACTH treatment. These observations clearly show that hormones can indeed destroy the neoplastic counterparts of lymphocytes as well as lymphocytes themselves.

The effects of adrenal corticosteroids (e.g. cortisol) on lymphoid tissues appear to be direct since they occur both *in vivo* and *in vitro*. WHITE (1967) showed that exposure of thymocytes to cortisol *in vivo* or *in vitro* and subsequent incubation of these cells *in vitro* resulted in (a) inhibition of RNA, DNA, and protein synthesis, and (b) decreased transport of nucleic acid and protein precursors into the cells. These early changes appear to be in harmony with the early profound histological alterations in the lymphoid tissues exposed to cortisol.

Recently, KIRKPATRICK et al. (1972) have studied the specific binding components for glucocorticoids in a rat lymphosarcoma P1798. These authors showed that the glucocorticoid resistant lymphosarcoma bound significantly less ^{3}H-triamcinolone acetonide than the sensitive tumor.

Steroids with glucocorticoid activity have also been extensively studied for their effects on mammary cancer in both animals and man. Since adrenalectomy has been demonstrated to induce objective regression of breast cancer (HUGGINS and BERGENSTAL, 1951; DAO and HUGGINS, 1955), the beneficial effects of exogenous adrenocorticoid therapy seem to be the result of inhibition of the hypophyseal elaboration of ACTH, thus inducing an atrophy of the adrenal gland ("medical adrenalectomy").

Glucocorticoids have also been widely studied in the treatment of metastatic cancer of the prostate. In patients with relapsing carcinoma of the prostate after castration, urinary 17-ketosteroid often rose to above the immediate post-castration level (SCOTT and VERMEULEN, 1942). The post-castration rise of 17-ketosteroid excretion has been attributed to the increased secretion of adrenal androgens. This rationale led to the performing of adrenalectomy in patients with metastatic cancer of the prostate by HUGGINS in 1950. The beneficial effects of exogenous corticoid therapy appear to be due to an inhibition of elaboration of ACTH by the pituitary followed by atrophy of the adrenal glands.

F. Direct Effect of Steroid Hormones on Tumor Growth

Both androgens and estrogens can exert direct effects on certain target tissues. Thus, androgens have been shown experimentally to stimulate directly both the prostatic epithelium and normal mammary gland tissue (LASNITZKI, 1955; AHREN and HAMBERG, 1962). It has also been demonstrated that estrogens have a direct effect on the mammary gland epithelium (LYONS and SAKO, 1940; SPEERT, 1940), and perhaps also on the endometrium, the connective tissue, and the gonads. It is conceivable that both estrogens and androgens can produce beneficial effects in breast and prostatic cancer by virtue of their direct effect on these tumors. How a steroid hormone can induce regression of hormone-responsive tumors by its direct effect is a question that remains to be answered.

JENSEN and JACOBSON (1959) first reported the uptake of steroid estrogen in "target tissues" after administering physiological doses of tritiated estradiol of high specificity. In hormone nonresponsive tissues such as liver, kidney, muscle, diaphragm, and cerebrum, there was little incorporation of radioactivity from estrogen, whereas in uterus, vagina, and pituitary tissues, there was an extensive uptake and a prolonged retention of radioactivity. These findings led to subsequent studies on intracellular macromolecules with a great and stereospecific affinity for estrogens and revealed the existence of specific protein "receptors" in estrogen responsive tissues such as the uterus, vagina, anterior pituitary, and mammary glands (JENSEN et al., 1967). The pioneering work of JENSEN et al. (1962, 1966, 1967) has thus led to numerous investigations on the binding of other steroids in hormone sensitive tissues and tumors. Detailed descriptions are presented in other chapters in this volume.

It has been shown that estrogen is bound to specific protein components of both the cytosol and nucleus (JENSEN et al., 1967). It seems that the estrogen binding proteins may be a device to allow capture of the hormonally responsive cells and to transport estrogen into the cell nucleus. The physiological importance of binding is further supported by data showing that large concentrations of steroids are found mainly in the target tissues. It was further demonstrated that binding of estrogens can easily be impeded by a group of putative estrogen inhibitors (JENSEN et al., 1967). These observations strongly suggest that the presence or absence of specific binding sites in a target tissue may be closely related to the hormone responsiveness of this tissue.

Similar work with prostate tissues from the rat has been carried out by BRUCHOVSKY and WILSON (1968) and ANDERSON and LIAO (1968). These authors demonstrated that 5α-dihydrotestosterone can be selectively retained by prostate cell nuclei *in vivo* and by minced prostate tissue *in vitro*. LIAO et al. (1969) further demonstrated that there are at least two soluble proteins in the cytoplasm which bind 5α-dihydrotestosterone specifically, but only one complex of the androgen and protein is retained by the prostate cell nuclear acceptor (FANG and LIAO, 1971). Although there appear to be some chemical similarities in the binding of testosterone and estradiol in these tissues, no evidence has been obtained to suggest that estrogen and androgen compete for binding sites in either the breast or prostate tissues.

That there is a correlation between hormone dependence and the presence or absence of specific binding proteins in the cytosols of both human and animal breast cancers has been convincingly demonstrated (JENSEN et al., 1970, 1972; MCGUIRE and JULIAN, 1971). In these studies, data clearly show that hormone independent mammary cancers do not possess estrogen specific binding proteins, whereas hormone dependent tumors contain substantial amounts of estrogen specific binding proteins. Whether a similar mechanism exists in prostatic cancer awaits further study.

Metabolism of Steroids in Cancer

The earlier work of DOBRINER and LIBERMAN (1950) suggested that metabolism of endogenous steroid hormones may be abnormal in patients with cancer. These authors reported the presence of 11-hydroxyetiocholanolone, an adrenal corticosteroid metabolite, in the urine of many patients with malignant disease, and showed that 11-hydroxyetiocholanolone was absent or rarely found in the urine of normal individuals. Subsequent studies by many investigators, however, have been unable to confirm these earlier findings. Studies on steroid metabolism in patients with cancer have at least two apparent objectives: to find an abnormal metabolite which may be unique to cancer patients, and to determine whether metabolism of endogenous hormones in patients with cancer differs from that in a normal state. Although no evidence has been obtained as yet to indicate the presence of an abnormal metabolite in patients with cancer, results from several investigations have shown that metabolism of some steroids may be different among normal and cancerous individuals. These studies were done mainly in women with breast cancer. They are of some interest and importance and are worthy of brief discussion.

A. Metabolism of Estrogens

One of the objectives in studying endogenous metabolism of estrogen in women with breast cancer is to define the environment in which the disease evolves. These investigations, however, have often been discouraged because of our reservations about the methods employed for assaying estrogens. Recently, results from studies comparing the level of urinary estrogens in women with breast cancer with that in women with benign disease and "normal" controls revealed some interesting findings. MARMORSTON et al. (1965) measured urinary estrone, estradiol, and estriol in 133 pre- and postmenopausal women. The results showed that the pre- and postmenopausal breast cancer patients excreted a significantly higher proportion of total estrogen as estriol when compared with "normal" controls. The premenopausal women with benign disease also excreted high levels of estriol. LEMON et al. (1966) on the other hand, found in their studies with 26 breast cancer patients and 34 controls, that women with breast cancer excreted less estriol than the "normal" controls. Neither of these studies, however, has been confirmed. Recently, MACMAHON et al. (1971) studied the estrogen profile of women with breast cancer from two cities of North America where breast cancer rates are high and three areas of Asia where rates are supposed to be low. They reported that estriol levels, among the three estrogens, were considerably greater in Asian than in North American women. The data seem to agree with the earlier report of LEMON et al. (1966).

Most studies of urinary excretion of estrogens were done in women with advanced breast cancer prior to and after endocrine treatment or ablative surgery. The apparent objectives of these studies were to seek a method for predicting response to therapy, particularly the endocrine ablative procedures, and to determine the hormonal effects of endocrine treatment of the disease. Thus, estrogen excretion in premenopausal women with advanced breast cancer decreases rapidly after castration, but gradually returns to precastration levels and adrenalectomy causes a rapid decline to low levels, or in some cases, to disappearance of estrogen excretion (DAO, 1953). The postcastration elevation seems to occur in the estrone fraction, among the three estrogens (DAO, 1957 a). This data, however, is too limited to draw any conclusions.

The *in vivo* transformation of estrogens in patients with breast cancer has also been investigated. ZUMOFF et al. (1966) and GALLAGHER et al. (1967) studied the pattern of estradiol metabolism in human males and females with breast cancer. The data showed that after intravenous administration of a trace amount of labeled estradiol (either ^{14}C or tritium) to males with breast cancer, the major metabolite obtained was estriol and there were no discernable changes in this pattern even at 3 months after orchiectomy. A similar study was carried out in a group of healthy elderly men as a control, and the data disclosed a different pattern; the major metabolite after intravenous injection of labeled estradiol in these "normal" elderly men was 2-hydroxyestrone rather than estriol, as seen with men with breast cancer. These authors also reported that the metabolism of estradiol in elderly women with breast cancer closely resembled that of the "normal" elderly men (i.e. estradiol transforms mainly to 2-hydroxyestrone rather than estriol). These results may bear some relevance to the tumor-host problem. Further investigations are needed.

One of the most intriguing problems in the metabolism of estrogen in women with breast cancer lies in the persistence of this steroid in women in whom both ovaries and adrenals were removed (DAO, 1957 a; STRONG et al., 1956; BULBROOK and GREENWOOD, 1957). The challenging question is: "What is the source of estrogen in a patient supposedly devoid of steroid producing organs?" Convincing evidence has begun to evolve in recent years that the cancerous tissues contain a variety of enzyme systems that catalyze the metabolic transformation of steroid hormones (CHANG and DAO, 1962; ADAMS and WONG, 1968). Mammary cancer tissue can indeed synthesize steroid hormones (DAO et al., 1972; ADAMS et al.,

1972; GRIFFITHS et al., 1972). These studies demonstrate that breast cancer tissue can perform metabolic transformation of a variety of steroid hormones including cholesterol, pregnenolone, dehydroepiandrosterone (DHEA), testosterone, and estrone. The breast cancer tissue apparently contains the desmolase system, 16α-hydroxylating enzymes, 17β-estradiol dehydrogenase, and the aromatase system.

B. Metabolism of Androgens

Evidence of abnormal metabolism of androgen in breast cancer is lacking. Administration of androgen to women with advanced breast cancer yields metabolites similar to those obtained in normal individuals. Testosterone is converted almost completely to various hydrogenated 17-oxo-steroids. Administration of testosterone to patients with breast cancer causes an increase in urinary 17-ketosteroid excretion. This increase occurs in all patients whether they respond to the treatment or not.

Testosterone is known to be converted to estrogens *in vivo*. The biosynthesis of estrogens in women with breast cancer who have undergone oophorectomy and adrenalectomy was demonstrated earlier by WEST et al. (1956). Administration of testosterone to these patients resulted in the isolation and identification of estrone and estradiol. Subsequently, DAO and MORREAL (1968) conclusively demonstrated that testosterone, given to patients devoid of steroid producing organs (ovaries and adrenals), was metabolically converted to estriol and estrone. These findings led to the search for the site or sites of this transformation. Both testosterone and DHEA have now been shown to be converted by breast cancer tissue to physiologically active estrogens (ADAMS and WONG, 1968; DAO and VARELA, 1972).

In the last 2 decades, many investigators have been measuring urinary 17-oxosteroids in breast cancer patients before and after adrenalectomy or hypophysectomy to determine whether the level of excretion can be correlated with the response to treatment. These attempts have been largely unrewarding. However, studies of BULBROOK et al. (1960) demonstrated that the urinary excretion of testosterone metabolites and etiocholanolone was significantly greater in patients with hormone responsive as compared with nonresponsive mammary cancers. When it was measured together with 17-hydroxycorticosterone, a discriminant function was devised for predicting hormone responsive and nonresponsive cancers.

In subsequent papers these authors claimed that 35 % of patients with positive discriminants will respond to adrenalectomy or hypophysectomy, whereas 60 % of discriminant negative patients fail to respond to these endocrine ablative procedures (HAYWOOD and BULBROOK, 1968).

Clinical Use of Hormonal Steroids in the Treatment of Cancer

A. Cancer of the Prostate

The rationale for the use of hormonal steroids in the treatment of cancer of the prostate has been discussed earlier in this chapter. Estrogenic hormones administered alone or in combination with castration are beneficial to patients with cancer of the prostate.

I. Diethylstilbestrol (α,α′-diethyl-4,4′-stilbenediol)

Among the many synthetic compounds possessing estrogenic effects, diethylstilbestrol is perhaps the most widely used compound in the treatment of advanced cancer of the prostate. About 60 to 80 % of the patients with disseminated carcinoma of the prostate are benefited by diethylstilbestrol. The dosage recommended has varied from 0.1 to 500 mg three times daily. The most satisfactory dose is between 3 and 5 mg each day. In the majority of cases, the drug is administered orally, but parenteral injection has also been used.

The sodium salt of diethylstilbestrol (Na diphosphate, "Honvan") has been used for intravenous injections in these patients. The compound is guite soluble in water and can be readily transported to the prostate, causing local reactions. DRUCKREY and RAABES (1952) have reported that acid phosphatase, present abundantly in the prostatic tumor tissues, is responsible for the enzymic liberation of stilbestrol at the site of action. Honvan has not been widely used because it has not been proven to be more effective than stilbestrol in inducing regression of cancer of the prostate. The recommended dose of Honvan is 250 to 750 mg/day; it has been shown to be beneficial in 30 to 40 % of the cases.

II. Chlorotrianisene (tri-p-anisylchloroethylene, TACE)

The search for new, less toxic estrogenic compounds with antitumor activity has led to the synthesis of chlorotrianisene. This compound causes minimal effects on the adrenal and pituitary even when large doses are given. It has been used in the treatment of carcinoma of the prostate with some good results, but there is a lack of evidence that the efficacy of this compound is comparable to diethylstilbestrol. The recommended dose is 12 to 24 mg/day.

Toxicities as a result of estrogen therapy in man with advanced prostatic cancer consist of gastrointestinal disturbance, gynecomastia, and salt and water retention. Gastrointestinal symptoms are nausea and vomiting which are common and are associated with oral medication. Gynecomastia is often accompained by pain and pigmentation of the areola. These symptoms are severe, particularly after prolonged administration of the hormone. The most serious complication, perhaps, is the production of sodium retention which can be marked in men of old age. Administration of estrogen in aged patients with pre-existing cardiac or renal disease can easily trigger or lead to congestive heart failure.

III. Corticosteroid Therapy

The rationale for using adrenocorticosteroid hormones in metastatic cancer of the prostate is derived from the observation that adrenalectomy induced remission in some patients having relapse of disease following orchiectomy and estrogen therapy. It is thought that removal of the adrenals will eradicate the extragonadal source of androgen (DAO, 1957b). DAO (1957b) demonstrated that administration of cortisone at a dose of 50 mg/day to these patients induces subjective improvement comparable to the beneficial effects obtained in adrenalectomized patients. An analog of cortisone such as prednisone at a dose of 30 to 40 mg/day gives results similar to cortisone acetate. Objective regression of metastatic prostatic cancer following corticosteroid therapy has rarely been observed. The levels of acid and alkaline phosphatases do not change after corticosteroid therapy even in patients with marked symptomatic relief of bone pain. The excretion of 17-ketosteroids decreases in some patients receiving cortisone therapy (DAO, 1957b).

B. Cancer of the Breast

Hormonal steroids including androgens, estrogens, progestins, and adrenocorticosteroids have been used in the treatment of advanced breast cancer. It appears that the steroid hormones have little specificity in inducing regression of breast cancer, since nearly all of them show effectiveness even though they possess very different biological activities.

I. Androgen Therapy

1. Testosterone

Testosterone in the form of testosterone propionate (for intramuscular administration) 100 mg, three times weekly, has been used in the treatment of metastatic cancer of the breast for decades. Tumor regression occurs in from 15 to 20 % of patients so treated both in the premenopausal and postmenopausal ages. Testosterone when used in premenopausal women causes cessation of menstruation. Production of estrogen in these women declines, but does not cease completely.

The potent anabolic effect of testosterone is desirable in patients with advanced breast cancer. Patients often have improved appetite, weight gain, and recalcification of osteolytic bone metastases after testosterone therapy. This hormone also stimulates hematopoiesis, thus improving the hemogram in patients who are anemic. Testosterone therapy, however, has little if any antitumor effect on lung, liver, and central nervous system metastases.

Side effects as a result of androgen therapy are often very disturbing to the patients. Virilizing symptoms, such as hirsutism, hoarseness of voice, and acne, are most objectionable to young women. Increase in libido often occurs in older women, and amenorrhea invariably develops in premenopausal patients. Prolonged administration of testosterone may induce profound changes in electrolyte metabolism. Sodium retention may cause congestive heart failure in patients with preexisting cardiac disease. Hypercalcemia developing in women receiving androgen therapy can be fatal.

2. Dihydrotestosterone (Stanolone, Androstanolone, Androstan-17β-ol-3-one)

Reduction of the double bond of testosterone to give etiocholanolone causes a reduction in androgenicity and also clinical effectiveness in patients with advanced breast cancer. The isomer of etiocholanolone, 5α-dihydrotestosterone, however, is an effective antitumor agent in both lower animals and humans (KENNEDY, 1955; HUGGINS et al., 1959). Androstanolone possesses a degree of androgenicity about equal to testosterone. The virilizing effect produced by dihydrotestosterone therapy is no less than that from testosterone therapy. This compound induces objective regression in 20 to 24 % of patients with disseminated breast cancer. Regression occurs mostly in osseous and soft tissue lesions. Androstanolone can be given either in saline suspension or in oil at a dose of 100 mg intramuscularly three times a week.

Androstanolone causes an increase in output of urinary 17-ketosteroid and a decrease in urinary gonadotrophin (SEGALOFF et al., 1955). These changes occur in all patients irrespective of their response to the treatment. KENNEDY (1955) reported a decrease in excretion of urinary calcium and phosphorus after androstanolone therapy in patients with relief of bone pain.

Another synthetic androgen, Dromostanolone (2α-methyl-dihydrotestosterone), is markedly anabolic, but less androgenic than testosterone. Whereas testosterone has an anabolic: androgenic ratio of 1 : 1, the ratio for Dromostanolone is 5 :1. It is less androgenic than testosterone, but its antitumor effect is not different from that of testosterone (Cooperative Breast Cancer Group, 1964). The recommended dose for Dromostanolone is 100 mg, three times weekly, intramuscularly.

3. 17α-Methyltestosterone

Oxidation of the 17α-hydroxy group of testosterone to 17-oxo reduced clinical effectiveness and androgenicity. The introduction of a 17α-methyl group increases both androgenicity and antitumor effect. 17α-Methyltestosterone is given orally in doses of 10 mg, three times daily.

The therapeutic effectiveness of methyltestosterone in patients with metastatic breast cancer is about equal to that of testosterone. The virilizing effect is as severe as testosterone. Although methyltestosterone has an advantage in that it can be administered orally, it often causes cholestasis resulting in the development of jaundice. It can be mistaken as metastases to the liver by clinicians who are not familiar with this compound. The differential diagnosis, however, can easily be made by discontinuing drug administration, since jaundice regularly subsides if it is due to methyltestosterone toxicity.

4. Fluoxymestrone
(9α-fluoro-11β-hydroxy-17α-methyltestosterone, Halotestin)

It would be anticipated that the influence of the 17α-methyl group together with the 9α-fluoro group in androst-4-ene-17α-methyl-9α-fluoro-11β, 17β-diol-3-one (9α-fluoro-11β-hydroxy-17α-methyltestosterone, fluoxymestrone, Halotestin) would result in a compound in which combined electronic and steric effects enhance the biological activity. Fluoxymestrone is five times more potent an oral anabolic steroid than 17α-methyltestosterone or testosterone (KENNEDY, 1957). The antitumor effect, however, is similar to testosterone propionate or 17α-methyltestosterone.

Fluoxymestrone has now been widely used because of its therapeutic effectiveness and the ease with which it can be administered. In our own experience with a large number of cases, no jaundice has ever been observed in these patients even after one or two years of continuous administration. The side effects resulting from fluoxymestrone therapy are similar to those from testosterone.

5. 19-Nor-testosterone

19-Nor-steroids are progestational compounds, but they also possess estrogenic and androgenic activities. 19-Nor-17α-methyltestosterone is at least as androgenic as 17α-methyltestosterone, and 19-nor-17α-ethynyltestosterone (Norlutin) is slightly estrogenic (McGINTY and DJERASSI, 1958). 19-Nor-steroids are also antigonadotropic and anabolic.

Both 19-nor-17α-methyltestosterone and 19-nor-17α-ethynyltestosterone have been tried in patients with metastatic cancer of the breast. Their antitumor effect is about the same as testosterone propionate or fluoxymestrone (SEGALOFF, 1966). Both of these compounds are given at a dose of 40 mg orally per day. Remission occurs in about 20 % of the patients so treated.

6. Δ^1-Testololactone (Teslac)

Δ^1-Testololactone was synthesized by FRIED et al. (1953). This compound is devoid of androgenic activity as determined by its biological activities. It does not change the weight of the accessory sex organs in the castrated male rat, nor does it alter chick comb growth (LERNER and HILF, 1967). Bioassay shows that Δ^1-testololactone is not estrogenic or progestational. This compound possesses no antiestrogenic, antiprogestational, or antigonadotrophic activity. It appears that Δ^1-testololactone is devoid of any significant hormonal activity. It, however, can augment the androgenic effect of testosterone in castrated male rats (LERNER et al., 1960).

The antitumor effect of this agent was first reported by SEGALOFF et al. (1960). Subsequent studies, however, failed to reproduce earlier results (Cooperative Breast Cancer Group, 1964). Δ^1-Testololactone given 100 mg intramuscularly three times weekly induces remission in about 15% of patients with metastatic cancer of the breast. It is obvious that the efficacy of Δ^1-testololactone in women with advanced breast cancer is at best equal to that obtained with testosterone. The lack of disturbing side effects of testosterone in patients receiving Δ^1-testololactone is certainly desirable.

The mechanism by which Δ^1-testololactone exerts its antitumor effect is not understood. It is not likely that Δ^1-testololactone exerts its inhibitory effect via the pituitary; this compound may have a direct effect. Administered simultaneously with estrogen, Δ^1-testololactone can enhance the tumor inhibitory effect of estrogen (LERNER, 1967).

7. Other Synthetic Androgens

9α-Fluoro-11-keto-17α-methyltestosterone, 40 mg daily by mouth and 4-androstene-3β,17α-diol diacetate, given 300 mg per week intramuscularly, have shown some effects in women with advanced breast cancer (OLSON and ANSFIELD, 1960). These compounds induce regression of osseous and soft tissue metastases but are ineffective for visceral lesions. The antitumor efficacy of these compounds is again equal to that obtained with testosterone.

II. Estrogen Therapy

The use of estrogen in the treatment of breast cancer seems to be contradictory to the concept that estrogen plays an important role in the genesis of mammary cancer. In clinical observations, the growth stimulation effect of estrogen has also been demonstrated by exacerbation of breast cancer following the administration of estrogenic hormones in women who were oophorectomy responders (PEARSON et al., 1955). HADDOW et al. (1944) first found that phenolic estrogens can have ameliorative effects in human breast cancer, a paradox yet to be explained.

It has been established that estrogen has a biphasic effect on tumorigenesis of the mammary gland. Small doses of estrogen can accelerate tumor growth, whereas large doses inhibit neoplastic growth. The mechanism by which estrogen exerts this biphasic effect on tumor growth is not understood. Both small and large doses of estrogen increase pituitary secretion and release of prolactin so that levels of circulating prolactin are increased. It has also been demonstrated that both small and large doses of estrogens can inhibit the pituitary production of gonadotrophin. Recently, PEARSON et al. (1972) reported evidence suggesting that large doses of estrogen may interfere with the peripheral action of prolactin.

Because of the possible stimulatory effect of estrogen on breast cancer, it should be used in women with disseminated breast cancer with caution. In the usual clinical practice, estrogen is employed in women of older age and in those who are at least 5 or more years postmenopausal. Such criteria are arbitrary and without convincing scientific evidence. Large doses of estrogen have also been used in premenopausal women with some benefit (KENNEDY, 1962), but the wisdom of this method is questioned particularly because bilateral oophorectomy benefits 25 to 30% of premenopausal women with disseminated breast cancer.

Estrogen induces regression mainly in soft tissue metastases; less often in those with osseous and visceral metastases. Twenty to 25% of the patients with metastatic breast cancer are benefited by estrogen therapy. Remission usually is of short duration, lasting from 6 to 12 months, although occasional prolonged regression may be seen in women with soft tissue metastases.

The most economical and convenient method of administration of estrogen is the oral use of diethylstilbestrol, 5 mg three times daily, or ethinyl estradiol, 1 mg three times daily.

For parenteral administration, estradiol dipropionate or estradiol benzoate in doses of 5 mg twice weekly have been used. The drug should be continued at this dose level until either evidence of tumor progression or regression can be demonstrated.

Although toxicities as a result of estrogen therapy are less disturbing than those of androgen therapy, they can be serious, particularly in those whose diseases are augmented. Hypercalcemia in patients with osseous metastases can be fatal. The early toxic manifestations of estrogen therapy are nausea and vomiting which usually subsides in a few days without having to discontinue the medication. Omission of one or two doses during prolonged administration of estrogen often causes uterine bleeding which can easily be controlled by temporarily increasing the dose or omitting the drug until the bleeding stops. Uterine bleeding also occurs in patients when estrogen is discontinued following a period of treatment.

Urinary incontinence as a result of estrogen administration is an unusual complication probably due to the relaxation of the pelvic floor. Pigmentation of the nipple frequently occurs in patients on continuous estrogen therapy. As was discussed earlier, estrogen can induce sodium retention and result in congestive failure in older women.

III. Adrenocorticoid Therapy

The impressive clinical results of adrenalectomy in women with advanced breast cancer led to the use of adrenal corticosteroids such as cortisone and hydrocortisone in an attempt to suppress adrenocorticoid activity sufficiently to induce a similar tumor regression. Objective tumor regression in cancer of the breast following large doses of adrenal corticosteroids was reported by PEARSON et al. (1955). These remissions lasted for only 2 to 3 months despite continuous therapy. Others reported occasional remission or no tumor regression with similar treatment (SEGALOFF, 1954; DAO, 1961). DAO et al. (1961) reported the result of a study comparing cortisone therapy with adrenalectomy which demonstrated that response to adrenalectomy is not due to the effect of cortisone used for maintenance in adrenalectomized patients. It is now generally agreed that cortisone therapy does not reproduce the definitive regression observed in patients following adrenalectomy.

Cortisone (Compound E) and hydrocortisone (Compound F), both in the form of acetate, have been used in the earlier studies. Cortisone acetate has been given in the following schedule: a loading dose of as much as 200 mg per day (in 4 divided doses) is followed by a decreasing daily dose of 150, 100, and 50 mg and, thereafter, patients are placed on 50 mg daily for maintenance. This dose schedule, however, was later proven no more effective than dosage with 50 mg given initially, as well as for maintenance. Although hydrocortisone is more potent than cortisone in its physiologic effects, doses similar to those of cortisone are required to obtain antitumor effects.

The search for steroids with desirable anti-inflammatory activity but less toxicity, resulted in the synthesis of Δ^1-C^{21} compounds. The introduction of a double bond in the 1,2-positions of cortisone yields prednisone; similar treatment of hydrocortisone yields prednisolone. This alteration of chemical configuration produces remarkable changes in the biologic activity of these compounds. Prednisone and prednisolone are 3- to 5-times more potent in their glucocorticoid activity than their parent compounds. The antitumor activity of these Δ^1-compounds, however, is about the same as their parent compounds. The usual dose of prednisone for patients with advanced breast cancer is 5 mg four times daily, orally. Larger doses only increase toxicity without increasing antineoplastic potency.

Halogenated corticoids synthesized by FRIED and SABO (1957) are biologically very potent glucocorticoids. 9α-Fluoro analogs of cortisone or cortisol have greatly increased glucocorticoid and mineralocorticoid activity. The glucocorticoid activity of 9α-fluoro analogs is about 10- to 11-times greater than that of their parent compounds and the sodium retaining potency is of the order of that of aldosterone. Although these compounds are extremely potent with respect to their biological properties, the effective antitumor dose is too toxic because they cause severe water and salt retention.

Toxicity induced by adrenal corticosteroids is not entirely the same with different preparations. In the treatment of metastatic breast cancer, a daily dose of cortisone acetate exceeding 100 mg may cause disturbances in electrolyte metabolism, impairment of glucose tolerance and glycosuria. Muscle weakness may occur as a result of increased potassium excretion. Sodium and water retention cause edema. The toxic effect of Δ^1-compounds appears to be more marked. At the recommended dose of 20 mg of prednisone daily, patients may develop "Cushingoid" signs after a period of several months of continued administration. Prednisone above 30 mg daily produces symptoms of Cushing's Syndrome almost without exception.

IV. Progesterone

Progestational steroids have been used for treatment of women with advanced breast cancer, but results have been inconsistent. HUGGINS and YOUNG (1962) reported inhibition of mammary cancer in rats when progesterone was administered in combination with estrogen. Subsequently, clinical trial was carried out by LANDAU et al. (1962), who reported regression of advanced cancer of the breast after estrogen-progesterone therapy. In most studies, progestogens devoid of other hormonal activities were much less effective in inducing tumor regression when compared with androgens and corticoids.

Hydroxyprogesterone caproate (17α-hydroxyprogesterone caproate) was shown to have very little effect in patients with advanced cancer of the breast (Cooperative Breast Cancer Group, 1964). Many synthetic progestational steroids, such as 19-nor-testosterone derivatives, were shown to possess antitumor activity in man. These compounds, however, are actually androgens possessing progestational activity. It appears that their effectiveness in breast cancer is most probably due to their androgenic properties rather than to the incidental progestational activity which these compounds also possess.

Halogenated progestogens have also been studied in patients with breast cancer. 9α-Bromo-11-oxoprogesterone (bromoketoprogesterone) given in a dose of 300 mg orally daily in patients with advanced breast cancer induced a 20 % regression rate. Regression of cancer occurs mainly in soft tissue and osseous metastases.

Oxylone acetate (progesterone, 1-dehydro-9-fluoro-11β, 17-dihydroxy-6α-methyl-17-acetate, fluorometholone), another halogenated progesterone, has been studied in patients with breast cancer (Cooperative Breast Cancer Group, 1964).

This compound, given at a dose level of 50 mg per day orally, was shown to produce remission in about 20 % of the patients with advanced breast cancer.

Both of these progestational compounds possess corticoid activity, particularly oxylone acetate, which, in 50 mg doses, causes Cushingoid symptoms, hypertension, and osteoporosis. On withdrawal of the drug, vaginal bleeding occurs frequently.

Progesterone like agents with no other steroid activity may induce general metabolic effects such as sodium retention and increase of urinary nitrogen excretion. Intramuscular administration of 10 to 25 mg of progesterone for several doses may induce vaginal bleeding. Withdrawal bleeding usually occurs 2 to 3 days after the discontinuation of the therapy. Large doses of progesterone, 50 to 100 mg daily administered intramuscularly, cause marked sodium and water retention. Progesterone-like compounds with glucocorticoid activity, such as oxylone, induce severe Cushingoid symptoms such as plethora, moonface, glycosuria, marked weight gain, and hypertension, requiring discontinuation of the drug.

C. Endometrial Carcinoma

The coexistence of endometrial hyperplasia and endometrial carcinoma in humans suggests that endometrial cancer may be related to overstimulation with estrogens. The profound effect of progesterone on the endometrium suggests the possibility that these effects may similarly occur in the neoplastic endometrium. More importantly, the success in the treatment of breast and prostatic cancers by hormonal alterations has apparently prompted an investigation of the treatment of endometrial carcinoma with hormonal agents.

Progesterone or progesterone-like compounds have been used in metastatic recurrent endometrial carcinoma since 1951 (KELLEY and BAKER, 1960). Progesterone in oil, at a dose level of 50 to 200 mg daily by intramuscular injection, induced regression of metastatic endometrial cancer in 30 % of patients. Remission lasted for several months to 3 years.

17α-Hydroxyprogesterone-17-*n*-caproate (Delalutin) in a dose schedule of 250 to 500 mg twice weekly intramuscularly is effective in inducing response. Another compound, 6α-methyl-17α-acetoxyprogesterone in similar doses has been used for the treatment of metastatic cancer of the endometrium with effectiveness equal to 17α-hydroxyprogesterone caproate. It has been shown that large doses up to 5 mg weekly do not improve the remission rate (KELLEY and BAKER, 1965).

D. Carcinoma of the Kidney

The susceptibility of hamsters to renal tumorigenesis by estrogen led to the experimental trial of treatment of renal carcinoma by antiestrogenic compounds. BLOOM et al. (1963) investigated the effects of various steroids on transplanted renal tumors in hamsters and found that combinations of cortisone and Provera (6α-methyl-17α-hydroxyprogesterone acetate, medroxyprogesterone) induced striking reduction of tumor growth. The authors also reported a lack of effect of testosterone in renal cell tumors in hamsters.

Recently, BLOOM (1971) reported the results of treatment of 80 patients with advanced metastatic renal cancer with hormones. Provera, in a dose of 100 mg three times daily by mouth, was given to these patients. Regression of cancer was observed in 13 patients, more often in men (21 %) than in women (8 %). No serious toxic effects have been observed even after prolonged administration.

E. Lymphomas and Leukemia

HEILMAN and KENDALL (1944) reported that cortisone caused temporary regressions of transplantable lymphosarcomas in mice. When ACTH and cortisone became available in quantity, they were used in patients with acute leukemia and tumors of lymphoid origin.

Cortisone acetate is given in divided doses of 150 to 200 mg orally in children and 200 to 300 mg daily for adults. With the introduction of newer synthetic corticoids such as Δ^1-compounds (e.g. prednisone), cortisone has largely been replaced. Prednisone, 50 mg, is given orally in divided doses in children and 50 to 100 mg daily in the adult. Cortisone infusion I.V. with ACTH in doses of 25 mg daily in children and 50 mg daily in adults is recommended for critically ill patients. These large doses may be continued for several weeks unless marked improvement or toxic effects develop.

Toxicities are frequently observed in those patients receiving excessive doses of adrenocorticoids. Sodium and water retention, causing edema, may be controlled by low salt intake and diuretics. Metabolic disturbances, particularly increased excretion of potassium, should be corrected by administration of potassium chloride orally.

Diabetes mellitus, resulting from prednisone therapy, may increase the susceptibility to infection which is particularly undesirable in these patients. Hypertension, which may often be severe in children, can lead to fatality due to cerebral hemorrhage.

These hormones are useful in chronic lymphatic leukemia, lymphosarcoma, HODGKIN's disease, and multiple myeloma. They reduce the size of enlarged lymph nodes, liver, and spleen and produce marked relief of symptoms. They are used nearly always in combination with other chemotherapeutic agents such as 6-mercaptopurine and methotrexate.

Conclusions

The lack of significant progress in the chemotherapy of endocrine responsive neoplasms can largely be attributed to our ignorance of the mechanisms of hormone action in both hormone responsive tissues and neoplasms. We are almost completely in the dark as to how hormonal steroids induce tumor regression. It is apparent that an increase in biological activity of a hormonal steroid is not always commensurate with its antitumor activity. We speak of compounds with antiestrogenic or antiandrogenic effects, but we understand practically nothing about the mechanism by which the antagonistic effects are produced. The antieffects of steroid hormones must be studied with respect to their receptor systems. Recent progress in studies on intracellular macromolecules with a high and stereospecific affinity for estrogens has revealed the existence of specific protein "receptors" in estrogen responsive tissues. This work, pioneered by JENSEN et al. (1959, 1966), has now been extended by other investigators to androgens (LIAO et al., 1969), progestogens (SHERMAN et al., 1970), and adrenocorticoids (KIRKPATRICK et al., 1972). The better understanding of the nature of hormone receptor proteins and their binding to specific hormones may elucidate the antieffects of steroid hormones. Already, several antiestrogenic substances have been shown to have an inhibitory action on initiation and growth of mammary cancer in rats. Antiuterotrophic compounds such as ethamoxytriphetol (MER-25), and Nafoxidine (Upjohn 11,100) have been shown to block the specific incorporation of estrogen into hormone dependent tissues (JENSEN et al., 1967). Nafoxidine has been shown to be effective in inhibiting breast cancer in both experimental animals and in women with advanced breast cancer (HEUSON, personal communication). Recently, TERENIUS (1971) demonstrated the inhibitory effect of MER-25 on initiation of mammary cancer in rats. These studies present sufficient evidence to suggest that more effective antitumor compounds can be synthesized based on sound pharmaco-physiological approaches.

References

ADAMS, J. B., WONG, M. S. F.: Paraendocrine behaviour of human breast carcinoma: *in vitro* transformation of steroids to physiologically active hormones. J. Endocrinol. **41**, 41—52 (1968).

AHREN, D., HAMBERGER, L.: Direct action of testosterone propionate on the rat mammary gland. Acta Endocrinol. **40**, 265—276 (1962).

ANDERSON, K. M., LIAO, S.: Selective retention of dihydrotestosterone by prostatic nuclei. Nature (Lond.) **219**, 277—279 (1968).

AXELRAD, A. A., LEBLOND, C. P.: Induction of thyroid tumors in rats by a low iodine diet. Cancer **8**, 339—367 (1955).

BECKETT, V. L., BRENNAN, M. J.: Treatment of advanced breast cancer with fluoxymestrone (Halotestin). Surg. gynecol. Obstet. **109**, 235—239 (1959).

BISKIND, M. S., BISKIND, G. S.: Development of tumors in rat ovary after transplantation into spleen. Proc. Soc. exp. Biol. (N.Y.) **55**, 176—179 (1944).

BLACKBURN, C. M., ALBERT, A.: Effects of 2-methyldihydrotestosterone and testosterone on human pituitary gonadotrophin. J. clin. endocrinol. Metab. **19**, 603—607 (1959).

BLOOM, H. J. G.: Medroxyprogesterone acetate (Provera) in the treatment of metastatic renal cancer. Brit. J. Cancer **25**, 250—265 (1971).

BLOOM, H. J. G., DUKES, C. E., MITCHLEY, B. C. V.: Hormone-dependent tumors of kidney. I. The oestrogen-induced renal tumor of the Syrian hamster. Hormone treatment and possible relationship to carcinoma of the kidney in man. Brit. J. Cancer **17**, 611—645 (1963).

BRUCHOVSKY, N., WILSON, J. D.: The conversion of testosterone to 5α-androstan-17β-ol-3-one by rat prostate *in vivo* and *in vitro*. J. biol. Chem. **243**, 2012—2021 (1968).

BULBROOK, R. D., GREENWOOD, F. C.: Persistence of urinary oestrogen excretion after oophorectomy and adrenalectomy. Brit. med. J. **1**, 662—666 (1957).

BULBROOK, R. D., GREENWOOD, F. C., HAYWARD, J. L.: Selection of breast cancer patients for hypophysectomy by determination of urinary 17-hydroxycorticosteroids and etiocholanolone. Lancet **1**, 1154—1157 (1960).

BURROWS, H.: Tumours of the uterus. In: BURROWS, H., HORNING, E. S. (Eds.): Oestrogen and neoplasia, pp. 94—109. Springfield: Charles C. Thomas Co. 1952.

BUTENANDT, A.: Progynon, a crystalline female sexual hormone. Naturwiss. **17**, 879 (1929).

CHANG, E., DAO, T. L., MITTLEMAN, A.: Adrenal estrogens. II. Conversion of 4-^{14}C cortisone to 11β-hydroxyestrone by human breast tumor slices. In: CONNOLLY, M. (Ed.): International Congress on Hormonal Steroids, pp. 237. Amsterdam: Excerpta Medica 1962.

DAO, T. L.: A method for the separation of four phenolic estrogens in human urine by paper chromatography and an evaluation of biological assay of these compounds. Endocrinology **61**, 242—255 (1957a).

DAO, T. L.: Present status of adrenalectomy in the palliation of metastatic carcinoma of the prostate. In: Third National Cancer Conference Proceedings, pp. 292—296. Philadelphia: The J. B. Lippincott Co. 1957b.

DAO, T. L.: Endocrine environment and neoplasia. In: WISSLER, R. W., DAO, T. L., WOOD, S., JR. (Eds.): Endogenous factors influencing host-tumor balance, pp. 75—97. Chicago: University of Chicago Press 1967.

DAO, T. L., HUGGINS, C.: Bilateral adrenalectomy in treatment of cancer of the breast. Arch. Surg. **71**, 645—657 (1955).

DAO, T. L., TAN, E., BROOKS, V.: A comparative evaluation of adrenalectomy and cortisone in the treatment of advanced mammary cancer. Cancer **14**, 1259—1265 (1961).

DAO, T. L., VARELA, R., MORREAL, C.: Metabolic transformation of steroids by human breast cancer. In: DAO, T. L. (Ed.): Estrogen target tissues and neoplasia, pp. 163—179. Chicago: University of Chicago Press 1972.

DOBRINER, K., LIBERMAN, S.: The metabolism of steroid hormones in humans. In: GORDON, E. S. (Ed.): A Symposium on Steroid Hormones, pp. 46—90. Wisconsin: The University of Wisconsin Press 1950.

DOISY, E.A., VELLER, C.D., THAYER, S.A.: Folliculin from urine of pregnant women. Amer. J. Physiol. **90**, 329—330 (1929).

DOUGHERTY, T.F., WHITE, A.: Effect of prolonged stimulation of adrenal cortex and of adrenalectomy on the numbers of circulating erythrocytes and lymphocytes. Endocrinology **35**, 1—14 (1944).

DOUGHERTY, T.F., WHITE, A.: Functional alterations in lymphoid tissue induced by adrenal cortical secretion. Amer. J. Anat. **44**, 81—116 (1945).

DRUCKREY, H., RAABES, S.: Organspezifische Chemotherapie des Krebs. (Prostata-Karzionom). Klin. Wchschr. **30**, 882—884 (1952).

FANG, S., LIAO, S.: Androgen receptors: steroid and tissue-specific retention of a 17β-hydroxy-5α-androstan-3-one-protein complex by the cell nuclei of ventral prostate. J. biol. Chem. **246**, 16—24 (1971).

FRIED, J., SABO, E.F.: 9α-Fluoro derivatives of cortisone and hydrocortisone. J. Amer. chem. Soc. **76**, 1455—1456 (1954).

FRIED, J., THOMA, R.W., KLINGSBERG, A.: Oxidation of steroids by microorganisms. III. Side chain degradation, ring D-cleavage, and dehydrogenation in ring A. J. Amer. chem. Soc. **75**, 5764—5765 (1953).

GALLAGHER, T.F., FISHMAN, J., SUMOFF, B., CASSOUTO, J., HELLMAN, L.: Studies of production and metabolism of estrogens in human breast cancer. In: WISSLER, R.W., DAO, T.L., WOOD, S., JR. (Eds.): Endogenous factors influencing host-tumor balance., pp. 127—135. Chicago: University of Chicago Press 1967.

GOLDBERG, R.C., CHAIKOFF, I.L.: Development of thyroid neoplasms in rats following a single injection of radioactive iodine. Proc. Soc. exp. Biol. (N.Y.) **76**, 563—566 (1951).

GRIFFITHS, C.T., TOMIC, M., CRAIG, J.M., KISTNER, R.W.: Effect of progestins, estrogens, and castration on induced endometrial carcinoma in the rabbit. Surg. Forum **14**, 339—401 (1963).

HADDOW, A.L., WATKINSON, J.M., PATTERSON, E., KOLLER, P.C.: Influence of synthetic oestrogens upon advanced malignant disease. Brit. med. J. **2**, 393—398 (1944).

HAYWARD, J.L., BULBROOK, R.D.: Urinary steroids and prognosis in breast cancer. In: FORREST, A.P.M., KUNKLER, P.B. (Eds.): Prognostic factors in breast cancer, pp. 383—392. Baltimore: Williams and Wilkins Co. 1967.

HEILMAN, F.R., KENDALL, E.C.: The influence of 11-dehydro-17-hydroxycorticosterone (Compound E) on the growth of a malignant tumor in the mouse. Endocrinology **34**, 416—420 (1944).

HORNING, E.S.: The influence of unilateral nephrectomy on the development of stilboestrol-induced renal tumours in male hamsters. Brit. J. Cancer **8**, 627—634 (1954).

HORNING, E.S.: Observations on hormone dependent renal tumours in the golden hamster. Brit. J. Cancer **10**, 678—687 (1956).

HUGGINS, C., BERGENSTAL, D.M.: Surgery of the adrenals. J. Amer. med. Assoc. **147**, 101—106 (1951).

HUGGINS, C., BRIZIARELLI, G., SUTTON, H., JR.: Rapid induction of mammary carcinoma in the rat and the influence of hormones on the tumors. J. exp. Med. **109**, 25—42 (1959).

HUGGINS, C., CLARK, P.J.: Quantitative studies of prostate secretion. II. The effect of castration and estrogen injection on normal and on the hyperplastic prostate glands of dogs. J. exp. Med. **72**, 747—761 (1940).

HUGGINS, C., HODGES, C.V.: Studies on prostatic cancer. I. The effect of castration, of estrogen, and of androgen injection on serum phosphatases in metastatic carcinoma of the prostate. Cancer Res. **1**, 293—297 (1941).

HUGGINS, C., MASINA, M.H., EICHELBERGER, L., WARTON, J.D.: Quantitative studies of prostatic secretion. I. Characteristics of the normal secretion, the influence of thyroid, suprarenal and testis extirpation and androgen substitution on the prostatic output. J. exp. Med. **70**, 543—556 (1939).

HUGGINS, C., SCOTT, W.W., HODGES, C.V.: Studies on prostatic cancer. III. The effects of fever, of desoxycorticosterone and of estrogen on clinical patients with metastatic carcinoma of the prostate. J. Urol. **46**, 997—1006 (1941).

HUGGINS, C., STEVENS, R.E., JR., HODGES, C.V.: Studies on prostatic cancer. II. Effect of castration on advanced carcinoma of the prostate gland. Arch. Surg. **43**, 209—223 (1941).

HUGGINS, C., YANG, N.P.: Induction and extinction of mammary cancer. Science **137**, 257—262 (1962).

JACKSON, R.L., DOCKERTY, M.B.: Stein-Leventhal syndrome: analysis of 43 cases with special reference to association with endometrial carcinoma. Amer. J. obstet. Gynecol. **73**, 161—173 (1957).

Jensen, E. V., DeSombre, E. R., Jungblut, P. W.: Estrogen receptors in hormone responsive tissues and tumors. In: Wissler, R. W., Dao, T. L., Wood, S., Jr. (Eds.): Endogenous factors influencing host-tumor balance, pp. 15—30. Chicago: University of Chicago Press 1967.

Jensen, E. V., Jacobson, H.: Fate of steroid estrogens in target tissues. In: Pincus, G., Vollmer, E. P. (Eds.): Biological activities of steroids in relation to cancer, pp. 161—178. New York: Academic Press 1959.

Jensen, E. V., Jacobson, H. I.: Basic guides to the mechanism of estrogen action. In: Pincus, G. (Ed.): Recent progress in hormone research, Vol. XVIII, pp. 387—414. New York: Academic Press 1962.

Jensen, E. V., Jacobson, H. I., Flesher, J. W., Saha, N. N., Grupta, G. N., Smith, S., Volucci, V., Shiplacoff, D., Neumann, G. H., DeSombre, E. R., Jungblut, P. W.: Estrogen receptors in target tissues. In: Nakao, T., Pincus, G., Tait, J. (Eds.): Steroid dynamics, pp. 133—157. New York: Academic Press 1966.

Kelley, R., Baker, W.: Clinical observations on the effect of progesterone in the treatment of metastatic endometrial carcinoma. In: Pincus, G., Vollmer, E. P. (Eds.): Biological activities of steroids in relation to cancer, pp. 427—443. New York: Academic Press 1960.

Kelley, R. M., Baker, W. H.: The role of progesterone in human endometrial cancer. In: Meigs, J. V., Sturgin, S. H. (Eds.): Progress in gynecology, pp. 436—444. New York: Grune & Stratton 1963.

Kennedy, B. J.: The effect of stanolone in the treatment of advanced breast cancer. Cancer 8, 488—497 (1955).

Kennedy, B. J.: Fluoxymestrone in the treatment of advanced breast cancer. Cancer **10**, 813—818 (1957).

Kennedy, B. J.: Fluoxymestrone therapy in advanced breast cancer. New Eng. J. Med. **259**, 673—675 (1958).

Kennedy, B. J.: Massive estrogen administration in premenopausal women with breast cancer. Cancer **15**, 614—648 (1962).

Kennedy, B. J.: Hormone therapy for advanced breast cancer. Cancer **18**, 1551—1557 (1965).

Kirkman, H.: Estrogen-induced tumors of the kidney. III. Growth characteristics in the Syrian hamster. Nat. Cancer Inst. Monograph, No. 1, 1—57 (1959).

Kirkman, H., Bacon, R. L.: Estrogen-induced tumors of the kidney. I. Incidence of renal tumors in intact and gonadectomized male golden hamsters treated with diethylstilbestrol. J. nat. Cancer Inst. **13**, 745—756 (1952a).

Kirkman, H., Bacon, R. L.: Estrogen-induced tumors of the kidney. II. Effect of dose, administration, type of estrogen, and age on the induction of renal tumors in intact male golden hamsters. J. nat. Cancer Inst. **13**, 757—772 (1952b).

Kirkpatrick, A. F., Kaiser, N., Milholland, R. J., Rosen, F.: Glucocorticoid-binding macromolecules in normal tissues and tumors: stabilization of the specific binding component. J. biol. Chem. **247**, 70—74 (1972).

Lacassagne, A.: Apparition de cancers de la mamelle chez la souris male à des injections de folliculine. Compt. Rend. Acad. Sci. **195**, 630—632 (1932).

Lacassagne, A.: Tentative pour modifier, par la progesterone ou par la testosterone, l'apparition des adenocarcinomes mammaires provoqués par l'oestrone chez la souris. Compt. Rend. Soc. de Biol. **126**, 385—387 (1937).

Landau, R. L., Ehrlich, E. N., Huggins, C.: Estradiol benzoate and progesterone in advanced human breast cancer. J. Amer. med. Assoc. **182**, 632—636 (1962).

Larson, J. A. L.: Estrogens and endometrial carcinoma. Obstet. Gynecol. **3**, 551—572 (1954).

Lasnitzki, I.: The effect of testosterone propionate on organ cultures of the mouse prostate. J. Endocrinol. **12**, 236—240 (1955).

Lemon, H. E., Wotiz, H. H., Parsons, L., Mozden, P.: Reduced estriol excretion in patients with breast cancer prior to endocrine therapy. J. Amer. med. Assoc. **196**, 1128—1136 (1966).

Lerner, L. J., Bianchi, A., Borman, A.: Δ^1-Testololactone, a non-androgenic augmentor and inhibitor of androgens. Cancer **13**, 1201—1205 (1960).

Lerner, L. J., Hilf, R.: Biological activities of steroids and their relationship to breast cancer therapy. In: Segaloff, A., Meyer, K. K., DeBakey, S. (Eds.): Current concepts in breast cancer, pp. 80—93. Baltimore: Williams and Wilkins Co. 1967.

Liao, S., Fang, S.: Receptor-proteins for androgens and the mode of action of androgens on gene transcription in ventral prostate. Vitamins and Hormones **27**, 17—90 (1969).

Lyons, W. R., Sako, Y.: Direct action of estrone on the mammary gland. Proc. Soc. exp. Biol. (N.Y.) **44**, 398—401 (1940).

MacMahon, B., Cole, P., Brown, J. B., Aoki, K., Lin, T. M., Morgan, R. W., Woo, N. C.: Oestrogen profiles of Asian and North American women. Lancet *II*, 900—904 (1971).

MARMORSTON, J., CROWLEY, L. G., MYERS, S. M., STERNS, E., HOPKINS, C. E.: Urinary excretion of estrone, estradiol, and estriol by patients with breast cancer and benign breast disease. Amer. J. obstet. Gynecol. **92**, 460—467 (1965).

MATTHEWS, V. S., KIRKMAN, H., BACON, R. L.: Kidney damage in the golden hamster following chronic administration of diethylstilbestrol and sesame oil. Proc. Soc. exp. Biol. (N.Y.) **66**, 195—196 (1947).

McGINTY, D. A., DJERASSI, C.: Some chemical and biological properties of 19-nor-17α-ethynyltestosterone. Ann. New York Acad. Sci. **71**, 500—515 (1958).

McGUIRE, W. L., JULIAN, J. A.: Comparison of macromolecular binding of estradiol in hormone-dependent and hormone-independent rat mammary carcinoma. Cancer Res. **31**, 1440—1445 (1971).

MEISSNER, W. A., SOMMERS, S. C., SHERMAN, G.: Endometrial hyperplasia, endometrial carcinoma, and endometriosis produced experimentally by estrogen. Cancer **10**, 500—509 (1957).

MEITES, J., CASSELL, E., CLARK, J.: Estrogen inhibition of mammary tumor growth in rats; counteraction by prolactin. Proc. Soc. exp. Biol. (N.Y.) **137**, 1225—1227 (1971).

MORRIS, H. P., DALTON, A., GREEN, C.: Malignant thyroid tumors occurring in mouse after prolonged hormonal imbalance during ingestion of thiouracil. J. clin. endocrinol. Metab. **11**, 1281—1295 (1951).

NATHANSON, J. T., ANDERVONT, H. B.: Effect of testosterone propionate on development and growth of mammary carcinoma in female mice. Proc. Soc. Exp. Biol. (N.Y.) **40**, 421—422 (1939).

NICOLL, C. S., MEITES, J.: Estrogen stimulation of prolactin production by adenohypophyseal explants *in vitro*. Endocrinology **70**, 272—277 (1962).

OLSON, K. B., ANSFIELD, F. J.: Evaluation of 4-androstene-3β,17β-diol diacetate in the treatment of advanced breast cancer. In: PINCUS, G., VOLLMER, E. P. (Eds.): Biological activities of steroids in relation to cancer, pp. 385—388. New York: Academic Press 1960.

PEARSON, O. H.: ACTH- and cortisone-induced regression of lymphoid tumors in man. Cancer **2**, 943—945 (1949).

PEARSON, O. H., MOLINA, A., BUTLER, T. P., LLERENA, L., NASR, H.: Estrogen and prolactin in mammary cancer. In: DAO, T. L. (Ed.): Estrogen target tissues and neoplasia, pp. 287—305. Chicago: University of Chicago Press 1972.

PEARSON, O. H., WEST, C. D., LI, M. C., McLEAN, J. P., TRAVIS, N.: Endocrine therapy of metastatic breast cancer. Arch. Int. Med. **95**, 357—364 (1955).

PURVES, H. D., GRIESBACH, W.: Studies on experimental goitre. VIII. Thyroid tumours in rats treated with thiourea. Brit. J. exp. Path. **28**, 46—53 (1947).

Results of studies of the cooperative breast cancer group. Cancer Chemotherapy Reports, **41**, 1—24 (1964).

SCOTT, W. W., VERMEULEN, C.: Studies on prostatic cancer: excretion of 17-ketosteroids, estrogens, and gonadotrophin before and after castration. J. clin. Endocrinol. **2**, 450—456 (1942).

SEGALOFF, A.: Comparative objective regression resulting from steroid treatment in women suffering from breast cancer. In: DORFMAN, R. I. (Ed.): Methods in hormone research, Vol. 5, pp. 215—233. New York: Academic Press 1966.

SEGALOFF, A., BOWERS, C. Y., RONGONE, E. L., MURISON, P. J., SCHLOSSER, J. V.: Hormonal therapy in cancer of the breast. XIII. The effect of 9α-fluoro-17α-methyl-Δ^4-androsten-3-one-11β,17β-diol (Fluoxymesterone) therapy on clinical course and hormonal excretion. Cancer **11**, 1187—1189 (1958).

SEGALOFF, A., CARABASI, R., HORWITT, B. N., SCHLOSSER, J. V., MURISON, P. J.: Hormonal therapy in cancer of the breast. VI. Effect of ACTH and cortisone on clinical course and hormonal excretion. Cancer **7**, 331—334 (1954).

SEGALOFF, A., HORWITT, B. N., GORDON, D. L., MURISON, P. J., SCHLOSSER, J. V.: Hormonal therapy in cancer of the breast. VIII. The effect of dihydrotestosterone (Androstanolone) on clinical course and hormonal excretion. Cancer 8, 82—86 (1955).

SEGALOFF, A., WEETH, J. B., RONGONE, E. L., MURISON, P. J., BOWERS, C. Y.: Hormonal therapy in cancer of the breast. XVI. The effect of Δ^1-testololactone on chemical course and hormonal excretion. Cancer **13**, 1017—1020 (1960).

SHERMAN, M. R., CORVAL, P. L.: Progesterone-binding components of chick oviduct. J. biol. Chem. **245**, 6085—6096 (1970).

SOMMERS, S. C., MEISSNER, W. A.: Endocrine abnormalities accompanying human endometrial cancer. Cancer **10**, 516—521 (1957).

SPEERT, H.: Mode of action of estrogens on the mammary gland. Science **92**, 461—462 (1940).

STERENTAL, A., DOMINGUEZ, J. M., WEISSMAN, C., PEARSON, O. H.: Pituitary role in the estrogen dependency of experimental mammary cancer. Cancer Res. **23**, 481—484 (1963).

STRONG, J. A., BROWN, J. B., BRUCE, J., DOUGLAS, M., KLOPPER, A. I., LORAINE, J. A.: Sex-hormone excretion after bilateral adrenalectomy and oophorectomy in patients with mammary carcinoma. Lancet 1956 *II*, 955—956.

TERENIUS, L.: Effect of anti-oestrogens on initiation of mammary cancer in the female rat. Europ. J. Cancer **7**, 65—70 (1971).

VELARDO, J. T.: Steroid hormones and uterine growth. Ann. N. Y. Acad. Sci. **75**, 441—442 (1959).

WALL, E., HERTIG, A. T., SMITH, G. V. S., JOHNSON, L. C.: Ovary in endometrial carcinoma. Am. J. obstet. Gynecol. **56**, 617—633 (1948).

WHITE, A.: Mechanisms of hormone action of corticosteroids in relation to control of neoplasia. In: DAO, T. L. (Ed.): Endogenous factors influencing host-tumor balance, pp. 43—48. Chicago, University of Chicago Press 1967.

ZUMOFF, B., FISHMAN, J., CASSOUTO, J., HELLMAN, L., GALLAGHER, T. F.: Estradiol transformation in men with breast cancer. J. clin. Endocrinol. **26**, 960—966 (1966).

Chapter 41

Fluorinated Pyrimidines and Their Nucleosides

CHARLES HEIDELBERGER

With 10 Figures

Introduction

Since their introduction (HEIDELBERGER et al., 1957), the fluorinated pyrimidines and their nucleosides have been widely used as biochemical tools for the elucidation of a number of problems encountered in cell biology and molecular biology. Of more practical importance, however, has been their extensive use as drugs for the palliative treatment of patients suffering from disseminated cancer. One of the compounds is now clinically useful in the curative treatment of herpes simplex viral infections of the eye. Although these compounds have generated an enormous literature, this chapter will deal primarily with a review of the major pharmacological and biochemical effects of these compounds; the coverage of the literature, by necessity, will focus only on key references that are germane to the topics being described. Several reviews of this topic have appeared elsewhere (HEIDELBERGER and ANSFIELD, 1963; HEIDELBERGER, 1965, 1966, 1967, 1969, 1970, 1973; MANDEL, 1969; CARTER, 1970).

Rationale

The origin of the fluorinated pyrimidines represents one of the relatively rare cases in which a new series of clinically useful drugs was designed, based on a very definite rationale, which led to specific predictions of the biological and biochemical properties of the various compounds involved. The initial observation (RUTMAN et al., 1954) was that uracil was utilized for nucleic acid pyrimidine biosynthesis by a chemically induced rat hepatoma but not by normal liver. In our laboratory we confirmed that in other tumors uracil was utilized to a greater extent than was orotic acid, the major precursor of nucleic acid pyrimidines in normal tissues (HEIDELBERGER et al., 1957); there was also an enhanced incorporation of uracil into the nucleic acids of intestinal mucosa, a normal tissue with rapid cellular proliferation. It was then decided to synthesize an antimetabolite that would resemble uracil as closely as possible with only one modification in the molecule. Since a remarkable increase in toxicity had been found when fluoroacetate was compared with acetate (LÍEBECQ and PETERS, 1949), the substitution of a fluorine atom for a hydrogen atom bound to carbon seemed appropriate. We chose to do this at the 5-position and to synthesize 5-fluorouracil, which we expected to inhibit tumors because of the apparently special role of uracil in tumor metabolism. Because of the small size of the fluorine atom (for VAN DER WAAL'S radii and structures, see Fig. 1) we anticipated that the analog would be incorporated into RNA and not into DNA. Because of the stability of the C-F bond and the inductive effect that it exerts, we predicted that the increased acidity of the molecule would cause it to be bound to enzymes more tenaciously than the normal metabolite and to base-pair occasionally with guanine as if it were cytosine. Because thymidylate, an essential building block of DNA, is made biosynthetically by the attachment of a methyl group to the 5-position of deoxyuridylate, we postulated that the

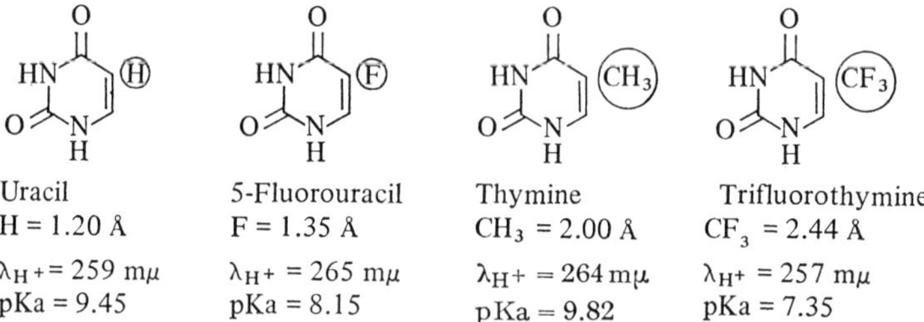

Fig. 1. The structures of two fluorinated pyrimidines and their normal counterparts

5-fluoro analog would block this reaction, leading to an inhibition of DNA biosynthesis. Finally, we predicted that because 5-fluorouracil would block DNA synthesis, it would exert some toxicity to normal tissues that have a high rate of cellular multiplication, particularly bone marrow and intestinal mucosa. All of these predictions have been fulfilled.

It then seemed appropriate to make a similar modification of thymine and to substitute the three hydrogens on the methyl group by fluorine atoms. The resulting compound, 5-trifluoromethyluracil (trifluorothymine, Fig. 1), would have a group about the same size as the methyl group. Since mammalian cells lack the enzyme to convert thymine into thymidine, we immediately proceeded to synthesize the nucleoside, trifluorothymidine (F_3TDR). We predicted that this analog should be incorporated into DNA and not into RNA, that it should consequently be mutagenic, and that it should inhibit the enzyme that methylates deoxyuridylate, as does the 5-fluoro series. Furthermore, since it was known that 5-iodo-2'-deoxyuridine inhibits the replication of DNA viruses (cf. KAUFMAN, 1965; GOZ and PRUSOFF, 1970), we expected that trifluorothymidine should also inhibit DNA viruses. All these predictions were also fulfilled. Seven compounds with clinical utility have emerged from the work thus far; four of these are currently available as drugs.

Further synthetic efforts in this field have naturally led to the synthesis of various nucleosides of FU, whose structures are shown in Fig. 2. 5-Fluorocytosine is clinically useful in the treatment of fungal infections (UTZ, 1968). FU[1], FUDR,

[1] Abbreviations: FU, 5-fluorouracil; FUR, 5-fluorouridine; FUDR, 5-fluoro-2'-deoxyuridine; FO, 5-fluoroorotate; FC, 5-fluorocytosine; FCDR, 5-fluoro-2'-deoxycytidine; ara-FCDR, 5-fluoro-β-D-arabinosylcytosine; F_3T, 5-trifluoromethyluracil, trifluorothymine; F_3TDR, 5-trifluoromethyl-2'-deoxyuridine, trifluorothymidine; 5-COOH-U, 5-carboxyuracil; FUH_2, 5,6-dihydro-5-fluorouracil; FUPA, α-fluoro-β-ureidopropionic acid; FGPA, α-fluoro-β-guanidopropionic acid; FBA, α-fluoro-β-alanine; FUMP, 5-fluorouridine-5'-monophosphate; FUDP, 5-fluorouridine-5'-diphosphate; FUTP, 5-fluorouridine-5'-triphosphate; FdUMP, 5-fluoro-2'-deoxyuridine-5'-monophosphate; FdUDP, 5-fluoro-2'-deoxyuridine-5'-diphosphate; dUMP, 2'-deoxyuridine-5'-monophosphate, deoxyuridylate; dTMP, deoxythymidylate; F_3dTMP, 5-trifluoromethyl-2'-deoxyuridine-5'-monophosphate, trifluorothymidylate; F_3dTDP, trifluorothymidine-5'-diphosphate; F_3dTTP, trifluorothymidine-5'-triphosphate; ara-C, β-D-arabinofuranosylcytosine; AP, 2-aminopurine; tRNA, transfer RNA; rRNA, ribosomal RNA; mRNA, messenger RNA.

and F_3TDR have shown clinical activity against various types of advanced cancer; FCDR and ara-FC showed some activity in a very few patients. F_3TDR is clinically useful in the treatment of herpes viral infections of the eye (WELLINGS et al., 1972).

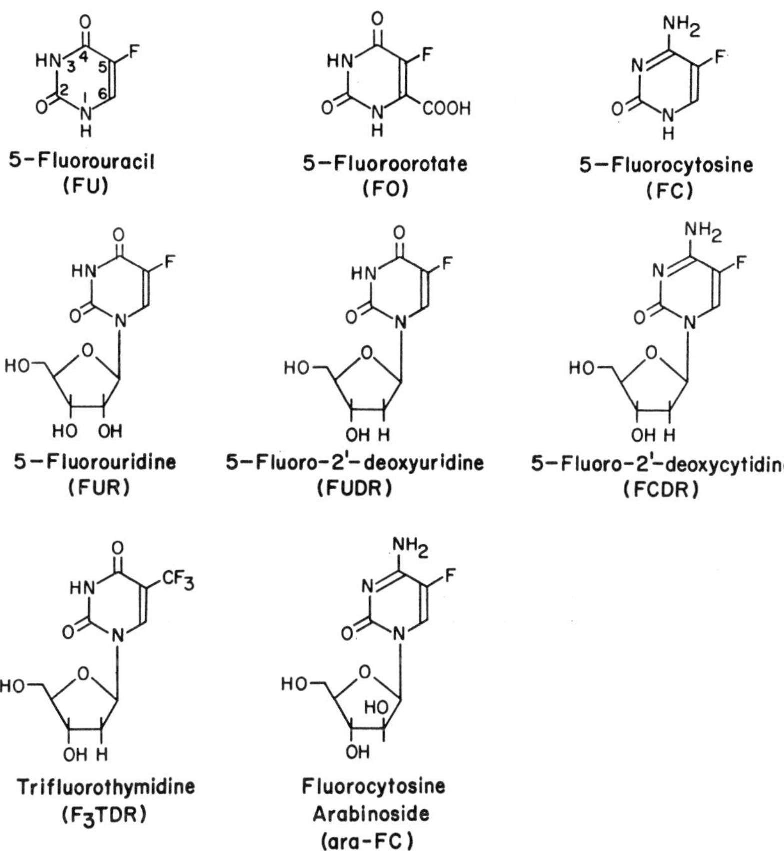

Fig. 2. The structures of fluorinated pyrimidines and their nucleosides

Synthesis

The synthesis of 5-fluorouracil was accomplished by the scheme shown in Fig. 3, in which the ring was built from acyclic precursors (DUSCHINSKY et al., 1957); the same method is still used for commercial production. By using minor variations of the same synthetic procedure, 5-fluoroorotic acid and 5-fluorocytosine were prepared. Until very recently, direct fluorination attempts had been unsuccessful. However, direct fluorination of uracil, uridine, deoxyuridine, cytosine, cytidine, and ara-C by the use of CF_3OF has been accomplished (ROBINS and NAIK, 1971, 1972). 6-Fluorouracil has also been synthesized, but it is chemically unstable and devoid of biological activity (WEMPEN and FOX, 1964a).

Originally, the ribonucleoside and deoxyribonucleoside of FU were prepared by enzymatic exchange. This method soon gave way to chemical synthesis via the mercury salt of FU and suitably blocked halo sugars (HOFFER et al., 1959; YUNG et al., 1961). FCDR was then synthesized by thiation and ammonolysis of FUDR (WEMPEN et al., 1961), and ara-FC was also synthesized (FOX et al., 1966).

A compound resembling FU, 5-fluoro-4-pyrimidinol, has been synthesized and called "fluoxidine" (BUDESINSKY et al., 1962). This compound has activity against L1210 leukemia comparable to that of FU (PUJMAN et al., 1970). It has been shown (SARTORELLI and CREASEY, 1967) that it must be oxidized to FU in order to inhibit tumors; this reaction is carried out by aldehyde oxidase and xanthine oxidase (JOHNS et al., 1966). Fluoxidine produces some tumor regressions in patients with advanced cancer and is active orally (KOLÁŘ and MECHL, 1971).

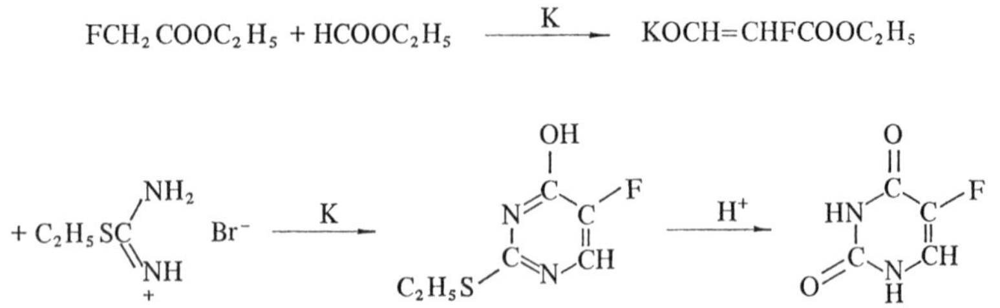

$$FCH_2COOC_2H_5 + HCOOC_2H_5 \xrightarrow{K} KOCH{=}CHFCOOC_2H_5$$

$$+ C_2H_5SC(NH_2)=NH^+ \; Br^- \xrightarrow{K} \text{2-ethylthio-4-hydroxy-5-fluoropyrimidine} \xrightarrow{H^+} \text{5-fluorouracil}$$

Fig. 3. The synthesis of 5-fluorouracil (DUSCHINSKY et al., 1957)

The initial synthesis of F_3T also involved building the pyrimidine ring from acyclic precursors; F_3T was then converted into F_3TDR by an enzymatic exchange (HEIDELBERGER et al., 1964). The synthesis was improved by the one-step conversion of the readily accessible 5-carboxyuracil to F_3T was achieved by the use of SF_4 (MERTES and SAHEB, 1963). A chemical synthesis of F_3TDR by a condensation reaction between the *bis*-trimethylsilyl derivative of F_3T and di-*p*-nitrobenzoyl-deoxyribofuranosyl chloride (RYAN et al., 1966). The 3′-deoxyribonucleosides of FU and F_3T have been synthesized recently, but are devoid of significant biological activity (NESNOW et al., 1972), as is the ribonucleoside of F_3T (KHWAJA and HEIDELBERGER, 1969). The deoxyribonucleoside of 5-fluoropyrimidine-2-one, which corresponds to FUDR lacking the keto group at *C*-4, has been prepared and is inhibitory to the growth of *E. coli* (ØYEN and LALAND, 1969).

An unsaturated nucleoside, 2′,3′-dehydro-FUDR, has been prepared and has demonstrated considerable activity against FUDR-resistant cells, as well as other tumors (KHWAJA and HEIDELBERGER, 1967); however, it was subsequently shown to exert its effects only as the result of cleavage to FU (KENT and HEIDELBERGER, 1970). In a structure-activity study, all possible mono- and dimethylated derivatives of FUDR were synthesized (KHWAJA and HEIDELBERGER, 1970), but only 3′-*O*-methyl-FUDR retained some biological and enzymatic activity (KENT et al., 1970). In an attempt to find a nucleotide derivative that might penetrate into cells, a number of esters and amides of FdUMP were prepared (REMY et al., 1961), but none of these exerted a more powerful effect on DNA synthesis in suspensions of Ehrlich ascites carcinoma cells than the parent nucleotide (MUKHERJEE and HEIDELBERGER, 1962). Two types of analogs were combined into the same molecule when 5-trifluoromethyl-6-aza-2′-deoxyuridine was synthesized; however, this compound was biologically inert, probably because its acidity was such that the compound is completely ionized at physiological pH and does not resemble the normally nonionized pyrimidine nucleosides (DIPPLE and HEIDELBERGER, 1966). A number of fatty acid mono- and diesters of FUDR were prepared, and some of these, when given orally to mice, were more tumor-inhibitory than was FUDR (NISHIZAWA et al., 1965). Finally, a bromomethoxy derivative of FUDR was synthesized (DUSCHINSKY et al., 1967), which had clinical activity in a few cancer patients about equivalent to FUDR (VAN DYK et al., 1967).

Physical, Chemical, and Conformational Properties

In general, the physical properties of the 5-fluorouracil series resemble those of the uracil series. However, the fluoro analogs are more soluble and more acidic than the corresponding uracil derivatives; F_3T and F_3TDR are even more acidic (Fig. 1). Some of the biological consequences of this increased activity will be discussed below. A thorough ultraviolet spectrophotometric study has shown clearly that the first proton in the FU series to dissociate is located on nitrogen-3 and that in the monoanion the negative charge of the resonance hybrid is localized primarily at the same atom (WEMPEN and FOX, 1964b). A comparably thorough study of the series by NMR spectroscopy has found a long-range spin coupling between the fluorine atom and the anomeric proton at *C*-1′ in FUR and FUDR (CUSHLEY et al., 1968).

In two independent studies of the x-ray crystallographic structure of FUDR it has been determined that, compared with natural deoxyribonucleosides, the *C*-2′ of the deoxyribose moiety is out of plane of the furanosyl ring on the same side as the *C*-5′ (HARRIS and MACINTYRE, 1964; SUNDARALINGAM, 1965).

Since the incorporation of fluorinated pyrimidines into both DNA and RNA produces biological effects that undoubtedly result from anomalous base-pairing (see below), some x-ray diffraction studies have been carried out on crystalline complexes of pairs of compounds in order to gain detailed structural information about base-pairing. It was found in the 1 : 1 complex of 9-ethyl-2-aminopurine and 1-methyl-5-fluorouracil that hydrogen bonds occurred between the *O*-2 of the 1-Me-FU and the amino group of 9-Et-2-AP, and between the *N*-3 of 1-Me-FU and *N*-1 of 9-Et-2-AP; this corresponds to classical WATSON-CRICK base-pairing (MAZZA et al., 1969). By contrast, it was found in the 1 : 1 complex of 9-ethyladenine and 1-methyl-5-fluorouracil that hydrogen bonds formed between the *N*-3 of 1-Me-FU and the *N*-7 of 9-Et-A and between *O*-4 of 1-Me-FU and the amino group of 9-Et-A, corresponding to "Hoogsteen" base-pairing (TOMITA et al., 1967). Moreover, a 2 : 1 intermolecular complex of 1-methyl-5-fluorouracil and 9-methyl-2,6-diaminopurine was obtained in which one of the pyrimidines forms a triple hydrogen-bonded Watson-Crick pair with the purine, while the other pyrimidine forms hydrogen bonds to the purine through the *N*-7 nitrogen; there are also purine-purine hydrogen bonds (CHANDROSS and RICH, 1971). The reason for these differences in base-pairing of very similar compounds is not clear.

Two non-Watson-Crick base-pair complexes involving fluorinated pyrimidines have also been studied. In the case of 5-fluorouracil and 1-methylcytosine, x-ray diffraction analysis of the complex showed hydrogen bonds between the *N*-1 of FU and *N*-4 of 1-Me-C, and between the *O*-2 of FU and the amino group of 1-Me-C (KIM and RICH, 1969). In the complex between FU and cytosine, hydrogen bonds were not only between the *O*-2 of FU and the amino group of C, but also between the *N*-3 of C and the *O*-4 of FU; however, no hydrogen bonds were formed when 1-methyl-FU and cytosine were mixed (VOET and RICH, 1969). It is evident that this approach is not very helpful in providing a physical basis for an understanding of the anomalous base-pairing behavior of FU.

The chemistry of the 5-fluoropyrimidines closely resembles that of the corresponding nonfluorinated compounds, and the C-F bond is stable. 6-Fluorouracil, on the other hand, is quite unstable (Wempen and Fox, 1964a). In contrast to most trifluoromethyl groups, which are stable, those of F_3T and F_3TDR are extraordinarily labile. Under very mild alkaline conditions F_3T is hydrolyzed to 5-carboxyuracil and at neutral pH reacts with glycine to give the product, $RCONHCH_2COOH$ (R = uracil) (Heidelberger et al., 1964). Careful kinetic studies of the hydrolysis of F_3T and some of its derivatives have led to the conclusion that the mechanism involves an initial nucleophilic attack on the *C*-6, followed by the elimination of HF to give the highly reactive $C{=}F_2$, which is rapidly converted by hydrolysis to COOH (Santi and Sakai, 1971). This reactivity has important repercussions in the mechanism of the interaction of F_3T derivatives with enzymes.

Ultraviolet irradiation of FU led to the isolation of an alkali-labile, acid-stable compound that was identified by synthesis as 5-fluoro-5-hydroxy-5,6-dihydrouracil; there was no indication of dimer formation (Lozeron et al., 1964). The analogous photochemical reaction also occurs with 1,3-dimethyl-FU, FUR, FUDR, FdUMP, and polyfluorouridylate (Fikus et al., 1964). The incorporation of FU into the RNA of tobacco mosaic virus sensitizes it to ultraviolet irradiation, doubtless as a consequence of the above reaction (Lozeron and Gordon, 1964).

The physical and chemical properties of polyfluorouridylic acid (poly-FU) have been carefully examined. Poly-FU exists as a random coil in solution at room temperature, but exhibits some secondary structure below 5°. It forms a double-stranded complex with poly-A, which has a lower stability than the corresponding poly-U : poly-A and poly-BrU : poly-A complexes, as indicated by a lower T_m (Szer and Shugar, 1963).

Tumor-Inhibitory Properties

Following the initial reports (Heidelberger et al., 1957, 1958a) of the marked activity of FU in inhibiting a number of transplantable tumors in rats and mice, these findings were confirmed in many other laboratories. FU was found to be superior to FO in tumor-inhibitory activity, and FC was devoid of such activity (Heidelberger et al., 1958a). When the nucleosides, FUR and FUDR, became available, it was found that the former was considerably more toxic than FU, and the latter was less so; FUDR appeared to have a considerably better therapeutic index against most tumors than either FU or FUR (Heidelberger et al., 1958b). Therefore, FU, FUR, and FUDR have all been selected for clinical evaluation. FdUMP had tumor-inhibitory activity comparable to that of FUDR (Heidelberger et al., 1960b). In a comparative study of the effects of the fluorocytosine and the fluorouracil nucleosides against transplantable mouse leukemias, it was found that FCR and FUR had approximately equivalent activities, as did FCDR and FUDR, the latter pair being more active than the former (Burchenal et al., 1959). Ara-FC was found to have somewhat more activity than ara-C against various transplanted mouse leukemias (Burchenal et al., 1966), which finding qualified it for clinical trial. F_3TDR was also very active against many transplanted tumors in mice, and on the basis of the fact that its therapeutic index against adenocarcinoma 755 was superior to that of FUDR (Heidelberger and Anderson, 1964), it was also selected for clinical trial.

A number of experiments have been carried out in experimental tumors to discover effective combinations of FU and other tumor-inhibitory compounds. The most promising of these has been the combination of FU with methotrexate (Kline et al., 1966) and with dimethyltriazenoimidazolecarboxamide (DIC) (Kline et al., 1971). A definite synergism has been observed between FU and x-irradiation in the inhibition of a transplantable mouse lymphoma (VIETTI et al., 1971).

In spite of very extensive experiments, FU has never been found to have carcinogenic activity (SCHMÄHL and OSSWALD, 1970).

Other Biological Effects

A. Inhibition of the Growth of Cultured Cells

The initial studies on the inhibition of human cells in culture by fluorinated pyrimidines established that thymidine addition prevented the toxicity exerted by FUDR, but not that of FU and FUR (RICH et al., 1958). A comprehensive comparative study of many fluorinated pyrimidines was carried out in various cell lines, including two that were resistant to FUDR. The latter cells, which lack thymidine kinase, were also resistant to F_3TDR; they were not resistant, however, to FU and FUR (UMEDA and HEIDELBERGER, 1968). Reversal studies with thymidine and uridine contributed to an understanding of the complicated alternative pathways of the metabolic activation of these compounds (see below). The inhibition produced by FUDR and its reversal by thymidine have been used as a means of synchronizing cultured cells (RUECKERT and MUELLER, 1960).

B. Antiviral Activity

The effect of FUDR on the replication of DNA viruses was first demonstrated by its inhibition of the replication of bacteriophages in *E. coli* (COHEN et al., 1958). It was found that the inhibition of replication of T-even bacteriophages produced by FUDR was reversed by thymidine (GOODMAN, 1963). T4 bacteriophage replication is also inhibited by F_3TDR (GOTTSCHLING and HEIDELBERGER, 1963). FU and its nucleosides can also cause induction of lysogenic phage, but the mechanism of this phenomenon is poorly understood (BERTANI, 1964).

The first report of inhibition of the replication of an animal DNA virus was the use of FUDR in cultures of HeLa cells in which vaccinia virus replicated (SALZMAN, 1960). It was shown that FUDR in the above system inhibits viral DNA synthesis, which occurs 2 to 3 h prior to the appearance of infectious virus; during such inhibition of viral DNA synthesis the formation of viral proteins continued. FUDR did not inhibit the replication of poliovirus, and this property was suggested as a means of distinguishing between DNA and RNA viruses (SALZMAN et al., 1963). This work was followed by many other reports of FUDR inhibition of replication of other DNA viruses in cell culture systems (reviewed by HEIDELBERGER, 1965). It is of interest, however, that FUDR has not been found to have any antiviral activity *in vivo*.

Following the discovery that 5-iodo-2'-deoxyuridine (IUDR) inhibits the replication of herpes simplex virus in rabbit and human eyes (KAUFMAN, 1965), probably as a consequence of its incorporation into viral DNA (cf. GOZ and PRUSOFF, 1970), it appeared that F_3TDR might possess similar activity. It was found to inhibit herpes simplex viral replication in rabbit eyes and cured such infections, even those of a virus strain resistant to IUDR (KAUFMAN and HEIDELBERGER, 1964). Furthermore, F_3TDR is more active on a molar basis than IUDR, FUDR, and ara-C against herpes virus in the rabbit eye system (KAUFMAN, 1965) and against the replication of vaccinia virus in HeLa cells (UMEDA and HEIDELBERGER, 1969). Finally, a clinical double blind comparison between IUDR and F_3TDR in the treatment of herpes simplex keratitis revealed that the latter drug was considerably more effective and less toxic to the normal corneal epithelium (WELLINGS et al., 1972).

Although FU and FUDR do not greatly inhibit the production of RNA viruses, FU does produce mutations in RNA viruses (see below). However, a very interesting case was found by TEMIN (1964), who showed that FUDR in the presence of uridine prevented the transformation of chick fibroblasts by the Rous Sarcoma Virus (RSV). He interpreted this and other observations to mean that the RSV, an RNA virus, had DNA as its proviral form (TEMIN, 1964). This heretical hypothesis was proven correct by his subsequent discovery of RNA-directed DNA polymerase (TEMIN and MIZUTANI, 1970). Thus, the sagacious use of specific metabolic inhibitors led to a most important discovery in the field of tumor virology and molecular biology. F_3TR has been synthesized but has no activity against either DNA or RNA viruses (KHWAJA and HEIDELBERGER, 1969).

C. Mutagenic Activity

FU and FUDR are not ordinarily incorporated into DNA. The only case in which this is not so is that of *B. subtilis* phage PBS2, which contains uracil instead of thymine in its DNA; in this phage, FUDR is incorporated into DNA in place of uracil, which enhances its ultraviolet sensitivity (LOZERON and SZYBALSKI, 1967).

F_3TDR is incorporated into DNA, and as a consequence is mutagenic to bacteriophage T4 (GOTTSCHLING and HEIDELBERGER, 1963). However, it is incorporated into mammalian cells only to a very small extent and is not mutagenic to Chinese hamster cells in culture, although in this system ara-C is highly mutagenic (HUBERMAN and HEIDELBERGER, 1972).

Since FU is incorporated into RNA, it is not surprising that it has been found to be mutagenic for various RNA viruses, including: RNA bacteriophages (DAVERN, 1964), poliovirus (COOPER, 1964), Rous Sarcoma Virus (KAWAI and HANAFUSA, 1971), and tobacco mosaic virus (KRAMER et al., 1964), where appropriate amino acid substitutions have been found in the coat proteins of the mutants (WITTMANN-LIEBOLD and WITTMANN, 1965).

D. Teratogenic Activity

FU, FUDR, and F_3TDR all exert teratogenic effects in various experimental systems (reviewed by CHAUBE and MURPHY, 1968). However, it is of interest that IUDR, when administered into the eyes of pregnant rats under the conditions required for the treatment of ocular herpes infections, is highly teratogenic; F_3TDR under the same conditions is not teratogenic (Dr. I. ITOI, private communication).

E. Effects on Chromosomes

It was found that when *Vicia faba* was treated with FUDR there was a "shattering" of the chromosomes, and the breaks could be healed by incubation with thymidine (TAYLOR et al., 1962). Chromosome breaks were also observed in Chinese hamster cells treated with FUDR; in this case, after prolonged incubation with the analog the breaks could not be joined after thymidine addition (HSU et al., 1964). When these cells were synchronized and treated with FUDR, maximum damage to the chromosomes occurred when FUDR was added early in the *S*-phase of DNA synthesis (OCKEY et al., 1968). A number of similar studies have been carried out with various cells, but the mechanism of this effect is not yet understood.

F. Effects on Bacterial Cell Walls

FU can exert a profound influence on the biosynthesis of bacterial cell walls. It inhibits cell wall mucopeptide synthesis in *Staph. aureus* by causing the accumulation of several nucleotide peptides containing FU which were partially characterized (ROGERS and PERKINS, 1960). In *E. coli* K-12, FU produced an osmotically sensitive state resulting from an alteration of cell wall synthesis in which the incorporation of diaminopimelic acid into cell walls was inhibited, accompanied by the accumulation of *N*-acetylhexosamine esters (THOMASZ and BOREK, 1962). An alteration in the structure of the cell wall of *S. aureus* in the presence of FU has been demonstrated by immunological techniques (DE REPENTIGUY et al., 1964). Since that time, little work has been done to elucidate further the nature of these effects. However, it has been found that FUDP-glucose can be oxidized to FUDP-glucuronic acid by UDP-glucose dehydrogenase, and the kinetics of the reaction showed that in order for this reaction to occur the uracil moiety of the nucleotide must be nonionized (GOLDBERG et al., 1963).

G. Antifungal Effects

All the fluorinated pyrimidines exhibit antifungal activity. However, their toxicity precludes them from being used clinically in fungus infections. 5-Fluorocytosine is a striking exception in that it is nontoxic in animals, retains antifungal activity, and is highly effective against fungal infections in mice (PITTILLO and RAY, 1969). It is also clinically effective against fungal and cryptococcal infections in patients when given orally, without exerting significant side effects (UTZ, 1968). In a thorough study, it was found that labeled FC is not metabolized in mice, dogs, and man, but is excreted unchanged in the urine. The blood level persists for a long time in humans, and, like cytosine, the fluorinated pyrimidine base is not utilized for nucleic acid biosynthesis (KOECHLIN et al., 1966). Therefore, it is clear that mammals lack the enzyme to convert FC to the active nucleosides and nucleotides, whereas fungi have the enzyme. This is a good example of species differences in enzymatic makeup which make effective chemotherapy possible.

H. Immunosuppression

FU and FUDR have both been shown to have immunosuppressive activity in animals and in man, but compared with many other drugs that have been more extensively studied, the fluorinated pyrimidines can be considered to be relatively weak immunosuppressants (MAKINODAN et al., 1970). When FU and FUDR are given a few days before the antigenic stimulus, they appear to be most effective. In one clinical study of patients undergoing cancer chemotherapy with FU, 4 of 9 patients had their secondary humoral immune response completely inhibited, whereas 8 or 10 patients failed to show a primary humoral immune response (MITCHELL and DECONTI, 1970). On the other hand, in 51 patients undergoing chemotherapy with FU and FUDR for advanced cancer, the delayed skin hypersensitivity reaction was enhanced rather than inhibited (BLOMGREN et al., 1965). It is conceivable that this apparent discrepancy could be explained on the basis of an effect of FU on the humoral immune system rather than on the cell-bound immune system.

Biochemical Summary

The present state of knowledge about the metabolism and biochemical mechanisms of action of the fluorinated pyrimidines is summarized in Fig. 4. The reactions shown are in every case analogous to those occurring with the corresponding uracil or thymine derivatives, with the exception of reaction 14. Each of the enzymatic steps will be described separately, and the first reference reporting each conversion will be listed below.

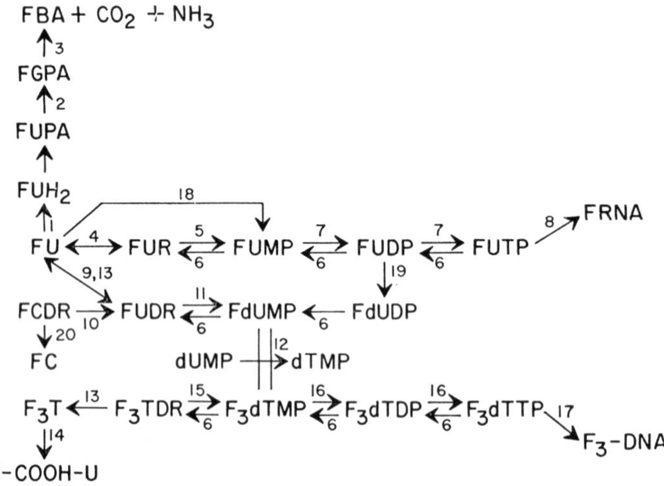

Fig. 4. A summary of the biochemistry and metabolism of the fluorinated pyrimidines

A. Metabolic Degradation of the Pyrimidine Ring

FU is converted enzymatically to dihydro-FU (1), which is then hydrolyzed nonenzymatically to α-fluoro-β-ureidopropionic acid, which is converted to α-fluoro-β-guanidopropionic acid (2), and thence to α-fluoro-β-alanine, carbon dioxide, and ammonia (3) (CHAUDHURI et al., 1959; MUKHERJEE and HEIDELBERGER, 1960). These conversions take place in all normal tissues of the mouse, including those that have rapid cell division, but do not take place in experimental tumors (MUKHERJEE and HEIDELBERGER, 1960) or in human tumors (MUKHERJEE et al., 1963b). The rings of FC (KOECHLIN et al., 1966) and F_3T are not metabolically degraded, but the latter is converted to 5-carboxyuracil (14); it is not known whether the latter reaction is enzymatic (HEIDELBERGER et al., 1965).

B. Anabolic Reactions along the Ribonucleotide Pathway

FU can react with ribose-1-phosphate to give FUR; this enzymatic reaction (4) is reversible (SKÖLD, 1958). FUR is then phosphorylated by uridine kinase to the monophosphate (CHAUDHURI et al., 1958) and by uridylate kinase to the di- and triphosphates (7) (HARBERS et al., 1959). Various phosphatases can act on the nucleotides to dephosphorylate them (6). FU can be converted directly with phosphoribosylpyrophosphate (PRPP) to FUMP by an enzyme which is present to a greater extent in tumors than in liver and which does not react appreciably with uracil (18) (REYES, 1969). The incorporation of FU into RNA, presumably via the triphosphate, has been demonstrated in many species (CHAUDHURI et al., 1958).

C. Anabolic Reactions along the Deoxyribonucleotide Pathway

FU reacts with deoxyribose-1-phosphate to give FUDR (9) (SKÖLD, 1958), which is phosphorylated to FdUMP by thymidine kinase (HARBERS et al., 1959). FdUMP was isolated after formation from FU, but FdUDP and FdUTP could not be detected in Ehrlich ascites cells (BOSCH et al., 1958). FdUMP is a powerful inhibitor of the enzyme, thymidylate synthetase (12), which methylates dUMP to dTMP (COHEN et al., 1958; HARTMANN and HEIDELBERGER, 1961).

F_3T cannot be converted in mammalian cells to F_3TDR. F_3TDR is phosphorylated by thymidine kinase (15) to F_3dTMP (BRESNICK and WILLIAMS, 1967). F_3dTMP is a powerful and irreversible inhibitor of thymidylate synthetase (12) (REYES and HEIDELBERGER, 1965). The monophosphate is phosphorylated to the di- and triphosphates by thymidylate kinase (16) (HEIDELBERGER et al., 1965). F_3TDR is incorporated into DNA, presumably as the triphosphate (17) (GOTTSCHLING and HEIDELBERGER, 1963). Very recently it was shown that FUDP is a substrate for ribonucleotide reductase (19) (KENT and HEIDELBERGER, 1972).

D. Nucleoside Catabolic Reactions

FUDR is cleaved to FU by both thymidine and deoxyuridine phosphorylases; these enzymes are present quite ubiquitously and are responsible for a decrease in the effectiveness of FUDR in whole animals and in humans (9) (BIRNIE et al., 1963). Similarly, F_3TDR is cleaved to F_3T by thymidine phosphorylase (13) (HEIDELBERGER et al., 1963). FCDR is split to FC (20) and is deaminated to FUDR (10) (HARBERS et al., 1959). Since FCDR and FUDR are equally active in most systems, FCDR probably exerts its action as a result of this deamination.

Inhibition of DNA Synthesis

A. Cellular

The incorporation of ^{14}C-formate, administered to mice, into the nucleic acids of various tissues was studied, and it was found that in mice given FU there was

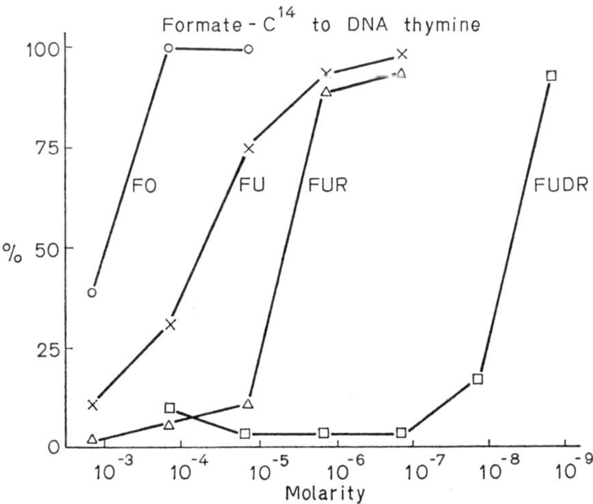

Fig. 5. The effect of fluorinated pyrimidines on the incorporation of formate-^{14}C into the DNA thymine of suspensions of Ehrlich ascites carcinoma cells (BOSCH et al., 1958)

a marked inhibition of incorporation into DNA thymine, particularly in transplanted tumors. FU had no effect on incorporation of formate into DNA or RNA purines. Since formate is a precursor of the methyl group of thymine and the 2- and 8-carbons of purines, this experiment shows that FU specifically blocks the methylation reaction leading to thymine as originally predicted, and that FU does not act as a folate antagonist (DANNEBERG et al., 1958). When suspensions of Ehrlich ascites cells were incubated with labeled formate in the presence of various concentrations of fluorinated pyrimidines and its incorporation into DNA thymine was measured, the results shown in Fig. 5 were obtained. All compounds inhibited this process in order of decreasing activity: FUDR, FUR, FU, and FO (BOSCH et al., 1958). COHEN et al. (1958) found that FU and FUDR produced thymineless death in *E. coli*, which is characterized by an increase in RNA and protein, while the DNA content remains constant; histochemical similarities to this phenomenon were found in Ehrlich ascites tumor cells obtained from FU-treated mice (LINDNER, 1959). Inhibition of DNA synthesis was also produced by FU and FUDR in HeLa cells (RUECKERT and MUELLER, 1960) and in many other cells and organisms, including human tumors (WOLBERG, 1969).

B. Enzymatic Mechanism

The enzymatic mechanism of this inhibition was elucidated when it was shown that the nucleotide, FdUMP, inhibited thymidylate synthetase (enzyme 12, Fig. 4) obtained from phage-infected *E. coli* (COHEN et al., 1958). Studies of the kinetics of inhibition of the enzyme in Ehrlich ascites cells by FdUMP showed that it is a powerful competitive inhibitor, with the $K_m/K_i = 1000$ (HARTMANN and HEIDELBERGER, 1961). The mechanism of this enzyme, in which methylenetetrahydrofolic acid functions as the coenzyme, was found by kinetic studies to be ordered and sequential. F_3dTMP also inhibits this enzyme competitively without preincubation. When this inhibitor is preincubated with the enzyme, the kinetics become noncompetitive, and a dialysis experiment showed that F_3dTMP is irreversibly bound to the enzyme. A mechanism involving an acylation of an amino group at the active site was proposed, based upon the chemical reactivity of the CF_3 group, as described above (REYES and HEIDELBERGER, 1965). As a prelude to an investigation of the chemistry of this irreversible binding, mammalian thymidylate synthetase was purified to homogeneity (FRIDLAND et al., 1971).

In an attempt to determine the importance of the contribution to cancer chemotherapy of this inhibition of DNA synthesis consequent upon the inhibition of thymidylate synthetase, an FU-resistant Ehrlich ascites tumor was developed and studied. In the resistant tumor, 1000 times the concentration of FU was required to inhibit formate incorporation into DNA thymine compared with the sensitive tumor. This established the major role of the inhibition of DNA synthesis in the inhibition of at least this tumor. Interestingly, in this resistant tumor FdUMP did not inhibit thymidylate synthetase; thus, the mechanism of resistance involved an altered enzyme (HEIDELBERGER et al., 1960). The bulk of much additional evidence in many different cells and tumors suggests that inhibition of DNA synthesis is the primary mechanism of tumor inhibition by fluorinated pyrimidines in the majority of cases. The role of tumor inhibition as a consequence of the incorporation of FU into RNA remains to be firmly established.

Incorporation into DNA

As mentioned above (Section C of other biological effects), the only known case of the incorporation of FU into DNA is in a uracil-containing DNA bacteriophage

(LOZERON and SZYBALSKI, 1967). On the other hand, F_3TDR is incorporated into DNA and is mutagenic to bacteriophage T4; the DNA containing a 10% replacement of T by F_3T has a lower T_m than the normal phage DNA (GOTTSCHLING and HEIDELBERGER, 1963). The incorporation of F_3TDR into the DNA of mammalian cells is very minimal unless forcing conditions are used, and F_3TDR produced no detectable mutations in Chinese hamster cells under conditions in which ara-C is highly mutagenic (HUBERMAN and HEIDELBERGER, 1972). When labeled F_3TDR was given at chemotherapeutic doses to tumor-bearing mice, the incorporation into the DNA of the tumor and spleen amounted to a replacement of T of only 0.1 to 0.3%, which could hardly account for the potent chemotherapeutic activity of this drug (HEIDELBERGER et al., 1965). As in the case of FU and FUDR, the cancer chemotherapeutic effect of F_3TDR can be attributed primarily to its inhibition of thymidylate synthetase.

When HeLa cells and L5178Y mouse leukemia cells in culture were blocked for 16 h with FUDR and released with thymidine, two waves of synchronous division occurred. When the block of DNA thymine synthesis was released with BUDR or IUDR, the cells underwent one synchronous division and thereafter did not divide. When the FUDR-blocked cells were treated with F_3TDR, no cell division occurred and the cells rapidly died, even though some DNA synthesis had occurred and the F_3TDR was all incorporated into the newly synthesized strand. When the DNA of such cells was analyzed by alkaline sucrose gradient sedimentation and compared with normal DNA at different times after F_3TDR addition, it was found that the assembly of the small pieces of DNA into large chains was greatly inhibited when F_3TDR was incorporated into the DNA. Such DNA evidently cannot support normal cell division (FUJIWARA et al., 1970).

Since F_3TDR is a powerful inhibitor of the replication of vaccinia virus, its incorporation into virion DNA was studied. It was found that the analog was incorporated into the virion DNA to a greater extent than into the DNA of the HeLa cells in which the virus was replicating. Even when the replacement of T by F_3T in the vaccinia virion DNA was only 5%, such virions were completely noninfective. Sucrose gradient sedimentation of the virion DNA containing such a low level of incorporation of F_3TDR revealed that the DNA was considerably smaller in size than normal (FUJIWARA and HEIDELBERGER, 1970). Furthermore, the transcription of late vaccinia messenger RNA in the presence of F_3TDR is decreased (OKI and HEIDELBERGER, 1971) and in such mRNA many of the normal sequences are missing (DEXTER and HEIDELBERGER, 1972). Thus, it appears that the incorporation of F_3TDR into vaccinia viral DNA causes the DNA to be too small, poorly replicated, and incompletely transcribed. The consequences of these effects on viral-induced and viral-structural proteins is under current investigation. Thus, it appears clear that the antiviral activity of F_3TDR is a consequence of its incorporation into viral DNA.

Effects on RNA Synthesis

A. Mammalian

In the first report on this subject, it was found that when FU and FO were administered to mice at doses somewhat above the chemotherapeutic optimum, there was an inhibition of the incorporation of labeled orotic acid and uracil into the RNA of liver, spleen, and Ehrlich ascites tumor cells. However, the extent of inhibition at the doses used was less than the inhibition produced in the incorporation of formate into DNA thymine (DANNEBERG et al., 1958). When suspensions of Ehrlich ascites cells were studied, no effect on glycolysis was found, and there was no effect of any fluorinated pyrimidine on the incorporation of uracil into mixed nucleic acid cytosine. FUDR, while completely inhibiting the incorporation of uracil into DNA thymine, did not inhibit its incorporation into RNA uracil; FO, FU, and FUR partially inhibited the latter incorporation at higher concentrations than those required to inhibit the former reaction (BOSCH et al., 1958). Thus, it is clear from these two studies that the fluorinated pyrimidines inhibit DNA synthesis to a much greater extent than RNA synthesis. FCR also inhibited DNA and RNA synthesis in suspensions of Ehrlich ascites tumor cells (HARBERS et al., 1959). When rats were treated with FU and FO, the pseudouridine content of their liver tRNA was decreased, and the incorporation of labeled orotate into the pseudouridylate was inhibited to a greater extent by FO than was its incorporation into the uridylate of tRNA (WAGNER and HEIDELBERGER, 1962). In cultures of HeLa cells, FUDR produced inhibitions in the time sequence: DNA, nuclear RNA, and cytoplasmic RNA (PAUL and HAGIWARA, 1962).

In more recent *in vivo* studies in rats, it was found that FU delayed and inhibited the incorporation of labeled cytidine into liver preribosomal RNA and greatly delayed the transport of 18 and 29 S RNA from the nucleus to the cytoplasm, whereas labeled 4 to 7 S RNA entered the cytoplasm without delay. This effect of FU was dose-dependent, but the largest effect was seen only at lethal doses (WILLEN, 1970). The inhibition of the maturation of ribosomes produced by FU, to be discussed below (Section C of effects on RNA synthesis) in bacterial systems, has also been demonstrated with FO in rat liver (WILKINSON et al., 1970).

B. Microorganisms

In an *E. coli* mutant that required uracil, FU markedly inhibited RNA synthesis as well as DNA synthesis (HOROWITZ et al., 1960). In yeast, it was found that FU inhibited the synthesis of ribosomal RNA (rRNA) without affecting the synthesis of messenger RNA (mRNA) or transfer RNA (tRNA) (DEKLOET and STRIJKERT, 1966).

C. Effects on Ribosome Biosynthesis

There have been a number of studies of this topic, mostly in bacteria. In the first publication it was reported that, when FU was added to *E. coli*, ribosomal particles smaller than normal were produced, and in low Mg^{++} medium ribosomal synthesis was inhibited (ARONSON, 1961b). It was then found that ribosomal particles made in the presence of FU had abnormal sedimentation properties and were less stable than normal ribosomes both *in vivo* and *in vitro*. These particles were not the precursors for normal ribosomes, but were degraded in the cells to furnish material for normal ribosomal synthesis. The RNA of these abnormal particles behaved differently from normal in sucrose gradient sedimentation, on MAK columns, and had a lower T_m (ANDOH and CHARGAFF, 1965). On the other hand, while agreeing with the other reports on the physical properties, KONO and OSAWA (1964) believed that these particles were normal intermediates in ribosomal biosynthesis. However, further work led the same group to the conclusion that these "FU-particles" are not normal biosynthetic intermediates because the proteins of these particles were not available for use in normal ribosomes (IWABUCHI et al., 1966). This finding was extended by the observation that in the presence of actinomycin D no "FU-particles" were converted into normal ribosomes during the recovery period (HILLS and HOROWITZ, 1966); therefore, they are not normal intermediates in ribosome synthesis. Further aspects of the ribosomal problem will be considered below (Section D of incorporation into RNA).

In *Staph. aureus* it was found that FU led to the production of altered ribosomes that were sensitive to RNase treatment, that it blocked the production of new ribosomes, and that the old ribosomes functioned normally in protein biosynthesis for one hour after FU addition to the culture (HIGNETT, 1966). In yeast, it was also found that abnormal ribosomes were produced in the presence of FU; the RNA from these particles had a composition more like DNA than normal, and upon incubation in the absence of the analog the abnormal RNA disappeared and was replaced by normal RNA (DEKLOET, 1968). Similar effects on the maturation of ribosomes have been observed in rat liver (WILKINSON et al., 1971).

Incorporation into RNA

This subject has previously been reviewed (HEIDELBERGER, 1965; MANDEL, 1969).

A. Total Cellular

In the initial report, labeled FU was given to tumor-bearing mice and incubated with suspensions of Ehrlich ascites tumor cells, and it was found that radioactivity was incorporated into the RNA, but not the DNA of various tissues. When the combined total nucleic acid fractions were hydrolyzed with strong acid to the pyrimidine bases, which were separated by ion-exchange chromatography, the results shown in the top of Fig. 6 were obtained. Peaks of ultraviolet light-absorbing material corresponding to the normal pyrimidines were obtained, which

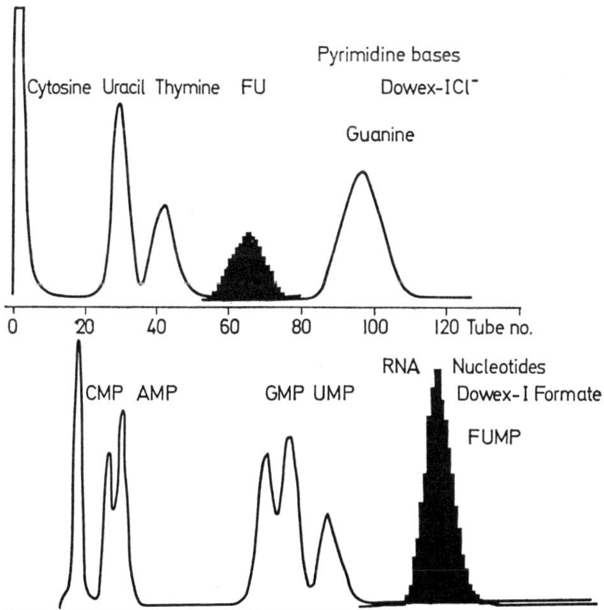

Fig. 6. The incorporation of 5-fluorouracil-2-^{14}C into RNA in suspensions of Ehrlich ascites carcinoma cells. The RNA was hydrolyzed with acid (top curve) and with alkali (lower curve), and the bases (upper curve) and nucleotides (lower curves) were separated by ion-exchange chromatography. The open peaks represent A_{260}, and the solid peaks represent radioactivity (CHAUDHURI et al., 1958)

were devoid of radioactivity; all the label was localized in a peak identified as FU. When the RNA was hydrolyzed with alkali and the nucleotides separated by ion-exchange chromatography, as shown at the bottom of Fig. 6, the normal nucleotides were devoid of radioactivity and all of the label was in a peak identified as fluorouridylate. There was no conversion of FU into nucleic acid FC and no evidence of defluorination to uracil (CHAUDHURI et al., 1958). When cell fractionations were carried out, it was found that FU was incorporated more rapidly into nuclear than into cytoplasmic RNA, and conversion into the various acid-soluble nucleotides shown in Fig. 4 was demonstrated (HARBERS et al., 1959). The incorporation of FU into total *E. coli* RNA was reported, and it was found that up to 50 % of the uracil was replaced by FU. Again, no conversion to FC and no incorporation into DNA was found (HOROWITZ and CHARGAFF, 1959). Since that time, the incorporation of FU into various types of RNA has been studied and will be described below.

Some studies have been carried out on the incorporation of FUTP into RNA catalyzed by purified *E. coli* RNA polymerase. It was found that FUTP supported the incorporation of other triphosphates, and the base ratios were normal (KAHAN and HURWITZ, 1962). When various templates were used, FUTP was incorporated to a lesser extent than UTP. When the two nucleoside triphosphates were measured in competition, the latter was incorporated in preference to the former. The Michaelis constant was larger for FUTP, and the maximum velocity was slower than for UTP (SLAPIKOFF and BERG, 1967). Because of its increased acidity as compared with U, FU might base-pair with G as if it were C to give rise to the major biological consequences described below. Such errors in copying could be introduced at the transcriptional or translational levels. We had postulated that these errors were made in transcription (HEIDELBERGER, 1965). In order to test this hypothesis, the incorporations of UTP and FUTP into RNA were compared, using purified *E. coli* RNA polymerase and several synthetic DNA templates which would force incorrect base-pairing. However, within the sensitivity of the method, no difference between FUTP and UTP in the frequency of errors could be detected (BUJARD and HEIDELBERGER, 1966). This negative experiment, taken together with others described below (Section C of consequences of incorporation into RNA), makes it almost certain that the errors of base-pairing of FU in RNA occur in translation and not in transcription.

B. Viral RNA

The first instance of incorporation of FU into RNA of a virus was the report of up to 50 % replacement of U by FU in the RNA of tobacco mosaic virus (TMV) (GORDON and STAEHELIN, 1958). The mutagenesis of RNA viruses caused by the incorporation of FU has been described above (Section C of other biological effects).

In spite of the massive incorporation of FU into the RNA of TMV and the few mutants produced, there is remarkably little biological effect upon the properties of this virus, which has normal infectivity and whose progeny have a normal base composition (GORDON and STAEHELIN, 1959). In another study of TMV containing 31 % replacement of U by FU in its RNA, there was no detectable change from normal in the quantitative amino acid analysis of the coat protein, the specific infectivity, and in the reconstitution of the virus from the RNA and protein (HOULABEK, 1962). Moreover, no antigenic differences were found between FU-containing and normal TMV (SUTIC and DJORDJEVIC, 1964).

In the case of poliovirus containing 35 % replacement, no differences from normal could be detected in quantitative amino acid composition of the coat protein, plaque morphology, host-range specificity, and neutralization by specific antibody (MUNYON and SALZMAN, 1962).

A complete study of the effects of FU on bacteriophage MS2 has been carried out. FU inhibited the production of infective phage to a greater extent when added early in the course of infection than when added later. FU is incorporated into the phage RNA with up to 80 % replacement, and this increases the buoyant density of the phage in cesium chloride; however, the T_m of this phage RNA is the same as that of the normal phage. The specific infectivity of this FU-containing phage was only slightly reduced (SHIMURA et al., 1966). It was also found that another phage particle formed in the presence of FU had a lower density than normal. This phage particle was noninfective and did not adsorb to the *E. coli* receptor. Although there was no difference from normal in the coat protein, its RNA content was only 65 % of normal. This RNA was noninfectious, but successfully directed the synthesis of some phage-specific proteins; therefore, it was suggested that the defective phage lacked a specific part of the normal phage RNA (SHIMURA et al., 1967). *In vitro* translation experiments indicated that the RNA of this defective phage represents about 2/3 of the 5′ end. It directs the synthesis of coat protein, but not that of phage RNA synthetase (SHIMURA et al., 1968). Thus, it is evident that the incorporation of FU into viral RNA can lead to a spectrum of effects ranging from none to major ones. What determines the extent of such effects is not yet understood.

C. Transfer RNA

There have been a number of studies of the incorporation of FU into tRNA of *E. coli* and the properties of the molecule containing the analog. Replacements of U by FU of up to 100 % have been reported without alterations in the base composition of the major bases (LOWRIE and BERGQUIST, 1968; KAISER, 1969a; JOHNSON et al., 1969). However, there were major alterations in the minor bases. In confirmation of our earlier work (WAGNER and HEIDELBERGER, 1962), the amount of pseudouridine was reduced from the normal level (LOWRIE and BERGQUIST, 1968; JOHNSON et al., 1969). With a high degree of FU incorporation in the RNA, there was a greatly reduced level of dihydrouridine in the tRNA, which paralleled the amount of U remaining. From this proportionality it was concluded that there is no dihydro-FU present in tRNA (KAISER et al., 1969; KAISER, 1971). The presence of FU in tRNA also decreased the amount of 4-thiouridine present; the decrease was proportional to the decrease in U-content, so it was concluded that FU cannot be thiolated because of the effect of the F atom in the molecule (KAISER, 1969b). This latter conclusion has been questioned on the basis of very indirect evidence (HIPKISS and ARNSTEIN, 1971). A diminution in the quantity of 5-methyl-U in FU-containing tRNA has also been found (LOWRIE and BERGQUIST, 1968; JOHNSON et al., 1969; BALIGA et al., 1969). A more detailed study of the methylation of tRNA obtained from a mutant of *E. coli* deficient in methyl groups has revealed that the decrease in 5-methyl-U was greater than the amount of FU substitution. This result, taken together with the fact that there is only one 5-Me-U residue in tRNA, led to the conclusion that the incorporation of FU into tRNA is a nonrandom process which probably depends on the secondary structure of the tRNA molecule (BALIGA et al., 1969).

Various systems of column chromatography have made it possible to separate the FU-containing RNA from the bulk of the normal tRNA present in *E. coli*

(LOWRIE and BERGQUIST, 1968; JOHNSON et al., 1969; KAISER, 1969a). With a purified preparation it was found that 100% replacement of U by FU produces only very minor effects on the secondary and tertiary structure of the tRNA, as shown by the techniques of gel electrophoresis, thermal denaturation, RNase digestion, cochromatography on Sephadex, and cosedimentation in sucrose gradients. From this and the foregoing, it was concluded that the minor bases are not essential for the stabilization of the three-dimensional structure of the tRNA molecule (KAISER, 1971a).

Several studies of the functional activity of FU-containing tRNA have been done. In general, FU substitution has little effect on amino acid-accepting activity; some amino acids were accepted to the same extent as normal, whereas others were accepted to a somewhat greater or lesser extent (LOWRIE and BERGQUIST, 1968; KAISER, 1969a; JOHNSON et al., 1969). In view of these facts, it would seem that the presence of the minor bases does not play an important role in aminoacyl synthetase recognition or amino acid acceptance (KAISER et al., 1969). However, there was some inhibition of the conversion of lysine to polypeptides, with use of phage R17 template and FU-containing tRNA, which was not attributed to errors in codon recognition (LOWRIE and BERGQUIST, 1968). 5 S RNA containing FU has also been isolated from *E. coli* and seems to be normally associated with the ribosomes (JOHNSON et al., 1969; KAISER, 1970).

The growth of yeast is inhibited by FC, but only FU and not FC was present in the tRNA. As in the case of *E. coli*, the yeast tRNA accepts amino acids normally. In a yeast mutant lacking in cytosine deaminase, there was no inhibition of growth produced by FC and no incorporation into tRNA. Thus, FC cannot be incorporated into RNA and can be effective in growth inhibition only if it is deaminated to FU, which is then incorporated (GEIGE and WEIL, 1970).

D. Ribosomal RNA

The effects of FU on the process of ribosome synthesis and ribosomal maturation have been described above (Section C of effects on RNA synthesis). These effects result largely from the incorporation of FU into the ribosomal RNA, which was first described in *E. coli*. Such rRNA had 70% of U replaced by FU and behaved differently from normal on MAK columns, in sucrose gradient sedimentation, and with respect to the T_m (ANDOH and CHARGAFF, 1965). The new "FU-particles" had sedimentation constants of 27, 33, and 42 S and readily broke down so that the FU which had been incorporated appeared in the acid-soluble fraction and was then reincorporated in lower amounts into normal ribosomes (HILLS and HOROWITZ, 1966; IWABUCHI et al., 1966).

The incorporation of FU into yeast tRNA was also demonstrated, and the rRNA containing the analog had a more DNA-like base composition than did the normal rRNA (DEKLOET and STRIJKERT, 1966). The incorporation of FO into rat liver RNA was studied, and it was found that the analog was selectively incorporated into nonribosomal nucleoprotein particles, which were released from polyribosomes by EDTA treatment and were quite different from normal ribosomal subunit particles. There was no incorporation of FO into 18 or 28 S rRNA for 3 hours. In the nucleus, FO was incorporated rapidly into the 45 S ribosomal precursor, but its subsequent conversion to mature 18 and 28 S rRNA was greatly inhibited (WILKINSON et al., 1971).

E. Messenger RNA

The incorporation of FU into *E. coli* mRNA was first demonstrated by GROS et al. (1961). The formation of FU-containing mRNA in *E. coli* during β-galactosidase induction and under the conditions of catabolite repression was described (NAKADA and MAGASANIK, 1964). Actinomycin D completely prevented the incorporation of both U and FU into *E. coli* mRNA; when this antibiotic was added after the labeling of the mRNA, the decay of U and FU-containing mRNA's was determined, and the $T_{1/2}$ of both was 2.0 to 2.5 minutes (YAGIL and SILBERSTEIN, 1969).

The incorporation of FO into a cytoplasmic rat liver RNA fraction with the characteristics of mRNA has also been demonstrated (WILKINSON et al., 1971).

Consequences of Incorporation into RNA

A. Mutagenesis to RNA Viruses

This topic has been discussed above (Section C of other biological effects), as has the lack of effect of massive FU incorporation on the properties of viral coat proteins (Section B of incorporation into RNA).

B. Effects on Protein Synthesis

It was initially reported that various fluorinated pyrimidines exerted no inhibition of the incorporation of labeled lysine into the total proteins of suspensions of Ehrlich ascites cells (HARBERS et al., 1959). In yeast, FU did not inhibit the incorporation of amino acids into total protein (DEKLOET and STRIJKERT, 1966), and in *Staph. aureus* the early stages of protein synthesis were normal in the presence of FU (HIGNETT, 1966). In noninfective particles of MS2 bacterophage containing heavily FU-substituted RNA, the fingerprint of coat protein hydrolysate was normal (SHIMURA et al., 1967).

In cultures of mouse fibroblasts, FUDR inhibited the incorporation of amino acids into nuclear proteins, and to a lesser extent into cytoplasmic proteins (PAUL and HAGIWARA, 1962). On the other hand, in cultures of human basal cell carcinoma, FU caused a stimulation of incorporation of amino acids into proteins (KORFSMEIER, 1970). In *E. coli*, FU produced an inhibition of leucine incorporation into total cellular proteins (HOROWITZ et al., 1960). When T_4 phage was replicated in *E. coli*, FU greatly inhibited phage production. If thymine was added to FU, phage DNA accumulated, and if uracil was added to FU, phage precursor protein accumulated; this finding indicates that FU prevented the synthesis of phage precursor proteins (ARONSON, 1961a). The effect of FU on the incorporation of amino acids into the total protein of *E. coli* was studied. Although there was no detectable change in the chromatographic properties of the soluble proteins, the incorporation of proline and tyrosine was inhibited and the incorporation of arginine increased as compared with the controls (NAONO and GROS, 1960a).

When HeLa cells were infected with poliovirus in the presence of FU, the virus-induced RNA polymerase had normal properties. However, when cells were infected with FU-containing poliovirus, the RNA polymerase had altered properties; it was concluded that the mRNA for this enzyme is transcribed from the parental viral RNA (TERSHAK, 1966). When SV40 virus (a DNA virus) was replicated in the presence of FU, although infectious viral production was inhibited, there was no inhibition of the synthesis of viral antigens, which were not, however, assembled into the viral protein capsid (MELNICK et al., 1964).

Thus, it can be seen that FU exerts different effects on protein synthesis, depending on the system and the circumstances.

C. Effects on Enzyme Induction

The induction in *E. coli* of the enzymes β-galactosidase and serine dehydratase was completely inhibited by FU, and the inhibition was partly reversed by uracil. By contrast, the synthesis of the constitutive enzymes, succinic dehydrogenase and catalase, was stimulated by the presence of FU (HOROWITZ et al., 1960). Further studies on the induction of β-galactosidase revealed that upon addition of FU an enzymatically inactive but immunologically cross-reacting protein was formed (BUSSARD et al., 1960). When the induction of alkaline phosphatase in *E. coli* occurred in the presence of FU, the enzyme had a normal affinity for the substrate but a markedly increased thermal sensitivity (NAONO and GROS, 1960b; GROS and NAONO, 1961). In contrast, although FU markedly inhibits RNA synthesis and is incorporated into RNA in yeast, it had little effect on the induction of β-galactosidase in this organism (STRIJKERT, 1969).

A thorough study of the mechanism of β-galactosidase induction in *E. coli* and its inhibition by FU has been carried out (NAKADA and MAGASANIK, 1964). When FU was added to the culture during the induction phase (3 to 4 min after addition of the inducer), it was incorporated into mRNA and led to the production of an altered protein serologically related to the enzyme. On the other hand, when FU was added after the induction period, it did not interfere with enzyme production in previously induced cells. The half-life of the β-galactosidase-forming activity after exposure to the inducer was 2.5 min at 30°; this is probably a measure of the specific mRNA. When protein synthesis was inhibited during the induction phase by chloramphenicol or elimination of an amino acid from the medium, there was no effect on enzyme formation; however, the same treatment during the phase of enzyme production prevented its synthesis. When the cells were grown under conditions of excess catabolites, the induction of the enzyme was inhibited, but such treatment did not affect enzyme production in previously induced cells. It was concluded that the inducer stimulated the production of unstable mRNA specific for β-galactosidase and that the catabolite repressor inhibited this synthesis (NAKADA and MAGASANIK, 1964).

These conclusions have been questioned as a result of experiments in which cells grown in media containing a poor source of energy and FU carried on β-galactosidase synthesis under conditions in which FU is incorporated into mRNA, which consequently must function normally. Therefore, it was suggested that FU inhibits the induction of β-galactosidase and serine dehydratase largely as the result of catabolite repression and not because of miscoding in an FU-containing mRNA (HOROWITZ and KOHLMEIER, 1967). This view is supported by the fact that four other enzymes which are not known to be inhibited by catabolite repression are synthesized by *E. coli* in the presence of FU. Furthermore, when cells were suddenly exposed to anaerobic conditions, which are known to alleviate catabolite repression, FU-inhibited *E. coli* then synthesized β-galactosidase (HOROWITZ and KOHLMEIER, 1967). Further support for this view comes from studies in a mutant of *E. coli* that is not sensitive to catabolite repression. In this situation, FU did not inhibit the induction of β-galactosidase, but did inhibit the induction of tryptophan synthetase, an enzyme whose induction is not susceptible to catabolite repression (PECK et al., 1971). If catabolite repression is the sole mechanism by which FU inhibits β-galactosidase induction, then the finding of serologically cross-reacting proteins produced in the presence of FU (BUSSARD et al., 1960; NAKADA and MAGASANIK, 1964) cannot be explained. Obviously, further work is needed to clarify this important matter.

The inhibitory effect of fluorinated pyrimidines on enzyme induction in rat liver has also been demonstrated. When fluoroorotate (which is utilized by liver more effectively than FU) was injected into rats, it prevented the dietary induction of rat liver threonine dehydratase; however, when the analog was added 6 h after dietary induction it had no effect, as shown in Fig. 7 (PITOT and PERAINO, 1964).

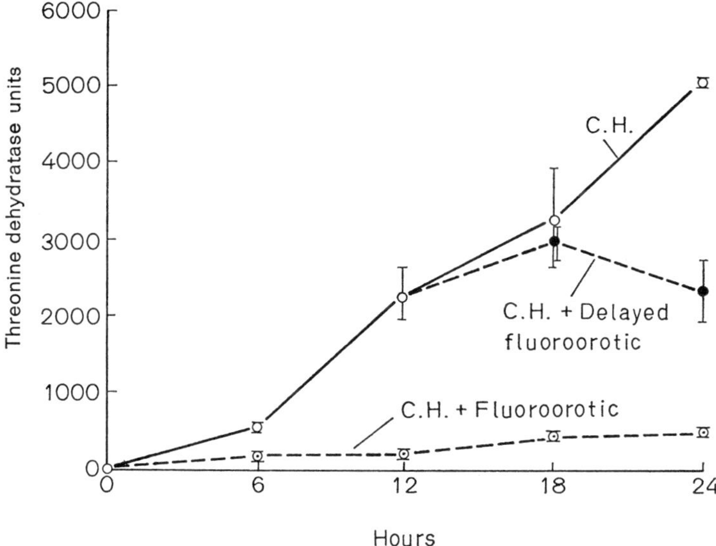

Fig. 7. The effect of 5-fluoroorotic acid administration on the dietary induction of threonine dehydratase. C. H., casein hydrolysate (PITOT and PERANO, 1964)

Similar inhibition by FO of the induction of histidase and tryptophan oxygenase in rat liver was observed, but FO caused an increase in the activity of cortisol-induced tyrosine aminotransferase (CIHAK et al., 1971). In the latter case, evidence was provided to suggest that FO inhibits the degradation of the enzyme, without interfering with its synthesis. As mentioned above (Section C of effects on RNA synthesis), when FO is administered to rats, it inhibits the maturation of liver ribosomes as a result of being incorporated into nonribosomal nucleoprotein particles (WILKINSON et al., 1971). In my opinion, the most reasonable explanation for the mechanism of the inhibition of enzyme induction in rat liver produced by FO is as follows. It seems on the basis of the above considerations that the synthesis of induced enzymes must take place on newly formed ribosomes or polyribosomes. Since FO inhibits ribosome formation for at least 3 h (WILKINSON et al., 1971), it would consequently prevent the induction of synthesis of the enzyme. However, if FO is added after 6 h, the induction of enzyme synthesis has already occurred on normal ribosomes, and the FO would be expected to be, and is (Fig. 7), without effect on the further production of the enzyme. Similarly, if new ribosomes are required for enzyme degradation, the stabilization by FO of tyrosinc aminotransferase can also be explained.

D. Coding Properties

It has been repeatedly stated that because of its increased acidity as compared with U, FU could have a tendency to base-pair incorrectly with guanine, as if it were cytosine, and thus give rise to errors in transcription or translation. Thus, the coding properties in translation were investigated. It was found that poly-FU had only a very small effect on phenylalanine incorporation stimulated by poly-U in a ribosomal system from *E. coli* (LENGYEL et al., 1961). Furthermore, poly-FU by itself stimulated little phenylalanine incorporation, but a mixed copolymer of poly-U : poly-FU gave a good stimulation of phenylalanine incorporation; no explanation was offered for this finding (WAHBA et al., 1963). In a more thorough study, it was found that poly-FU alone and in copolymers stimulated only the incorporation of phenylalanine in a ribosome system; in fact, the poly-U-directed ambiguous incorporation of leucine did not occur with poly-FU (GRUNBERG-MANAGO and MICHELSON, 1964). Thus, no translational errors could be detected in these systems which were used to establish the nature of the genetic code. Nor, as mentioned above (Section A of incorporation into RNA), could transcriptional errors be detected in a cell-free system (BUJARD and HEIDELBERGER, 1966). These findings on coding, taken together with the fact that coat proteins of RNA viruses appear to be normal, suggest that if coding errors are made by fluorinated pyrimidines in RNA they are very rare events. This concept is strengthened if one accepts the proposition that the inhibition of enzyme induction produced in bacteria and rat liver by fluorinated pyrimidines is due to catabolite repression and inhibition of the maturation of ribosomes, respectively.

E. Translational Errors

The elucidation of the mechanism by which fluorinated pyrimidines cause errors in translation has come from investigators working with systems in which rare events can be studied to the exclusion of common events. This apparently paradoxical stituation can be realized in the case of amber mutants of *E. coli* and its *T*-even bacteriophages. In amber mutants there is a "nonsense" codon, UAG, which codes for no amino acid and hence causes termination of polypeptide chains. Such amber mutants cannot grow under ordinary conditions, but can grow if the amber codon is altered to one that can code for an amino acid, thus preventing chain termination and allowing protein synthesis to proceed. It was found that a number of mutants in the r_{II} locus of bacteriophage T_4 (subsequently identified as amber), which could not grow in *E. coli* K, did grow in low frequency in the presence of FU. This phenomenon is called phenotypic revision, because phage replication occurred only in the presence of FU and progeny phage could not replicate in the absence of FU; thus, this could not be a genotypic reversion. It was concluded that this low-frequency event probably resulted from incorrect base-pairing of FU as C with G instead of as U with A in the process of translation; this mispairing caused a repair of the lesion in the original mutant mRNA (CHAMPE and BENZER, 1962). FU also produced phenotypic reversion of *E. coli* amber mutants of alkaline phosphatase (GAREN and SIDDIQI, 1962). A further study was carried out on a double mutant that was amber in the structural gene and constitutive in the regulator gene. This mutant *E. coli* synthesizes alkaline phosphatase at a very low rate in the absence of FU, but the rate increases greatly after FU addition. After purification it was found that the FU-repaired enzyme was indistinguishable from normal with respect to the following properties: specific activity, chromatographic behavior on DEAE-cellulose, kinetics of heat inactivation, stability to pronase digestion, temperature-dependent hydrolysis of *p*-nitrophenylphosphate, mobility in starch gel electophoresis, and isozyme bands. Insofar as could be determined, the FU-repaired enzyme was identical to the wild-type enzyme (ROSEN, 1965). The latter system was used for further refinement of mechanism, once the codon of the amber mutation was known. A comparison was made between fingerprints of tryptic digests of the alkaline phosphatases of the wild-type, the FU-repaired enzyme, and two other suppressed revertants (not produced by FU), which had different electrophoretic properties from the wild-type. The fingerprints of the alkaline phosphatase of wild-type and FU-repaired mutants were identical and differed from the fingerprints of the enzyme digests from the two other mutants. Amino acid analysis of the peptides established that in one of the suppressed mutants a tyrosine was substituted for a glutamine. This shows that in the suppressed mutant the amber codon, UAG, was replaced by the codon CAG (the only properly coding replacement possible with a single base alteration). Since the amino acid composition of the peptide was the same in the FU-repaired and wild-type enzymes, the insertion of glutamine in the repaired enzyme must have resulted in the mistranslation of the amber codon FUAG as CAG (ROSEN et al., 1969). This proves the coding error that had previously been postulated by many people. Other amber mutants were also reverted by FU. These results could be explained only by mispairing in translation and not in transcription, because the amber codon (UAG) contains uracil and the DNA codon (ATC) does not contain guanine; therefore, FU could not mispair in transcription with the DNA codon as if it were C (ROSEN et al., 1969).

It appears, then, that mispairing errors in translation of FU-containing RNA are very rare events which can only be detected and characterized as just described or as mutants of RNA viruses. Therefore, most of the altered biological consequences of the incorporation of FU into RNA must be explained on some basis other than that of mispairing errors.

Pathways of Activation and Resistance

The chemotherapeutically active form of the 5-fluoropyrimidines is the deoxyribonucleoside monophosphate, FdUMP. Thus, the several pathways of metabolic activation shown in Fig. 4 determine the chemotherapeutic effectiveness of the drugs, and the response of individual tumors is in part a function of the activity and amounts of the enzymes of the various pathways that metabolize whatever drug products are presented to them from the host's metabolism and tissue distribution.

A. Role of Catabolism

The effectiveness of FUDR (BIRNIE et al., 1963) and F_3TDR (HEIDELBERGER et al., 1963) is greatly diminished by the nucleoside phosphorylases that are present in tissues and in serum. In order to improve this situation, various derivatives of FUDR have been synthesized in an effort to find one that would not be cleaved to the pyrimidine base, yet retain biological activity (KHWAJA and HEIDELBERGER, 1970). One such compound was found, 3'-*O*-methyl-FUDR, which was not cleaved; but it was only about 1/100 as active as FUDR at inhibiting the growth of cells in culture (KENT et al., 1970). Various compounds have been reported in the literature to inhibit nucleoside phosphorylases, but none of these in combination with FUDR has provided increased therapeutic effectiveness. Nevertheless, work along these lines should be continued.

The pyrimidine ring of FU is cleaved by the sequence of reactions shown in Fig. 4 (CHAUDHURI et al., 1959; MUKHERJEE and HEIDELBERGER, 1960). The lack of degradation that was observed in a number of tumors, including human (MUKHERJEE and HEIDELBERGER, 1960; MUKHERJEE et al., 1963b), has been considered to be the major cause of whatever selectivity against tumors FU exerts

(HEIDELBERGER, 1965). However, this conclusion has been questioned. It has been found that 5-diazouracil irreversibly inhibits dihydrouracil dehydrogenase (enzyme 1, Fig. 4) and hence pyrimidine ring degradation. Nevertheless, when combined with FU, diazouracil caused an increase both in toxicity and in chemotherapeutic activity; consequently there was no improvement in therapeutic index (COOPER et al., 1972). In a comparative study of the incorporation of several precursors into DNA in slices of human colon cancers and normal colonic mucosa, the effect of FU was the same, from which result it was concluded that FU has no chemotherapeutic selectivity for the tumor; the lack of catabolism mentioned above was questioned (WOLBERG, 1972). Thus, the role of catabolism in the chemotherapeutic activity of FU is not fully established.

B. Activation

The various pathways of the conversion of FU into the active form of the drug, FdUMP, are shown in Fig. 4. We shall now consider studies that have related these pathways to chemotherapeutic activity. The fact that FU is effective against cells in culture that are resistant to FUDR because they lack thymidine kinase (enzyme 11, Fig. 4) (UMEDA and HEIDELBERGER, 1958) shows that the pathway of activation via ribonucleotide reduction (19, Fig. 4) is operative (KENT and HEIDELBERGER, 1972).

It was reported that in suspensions of Ehrlich ascites cells the addition of inosine increased the incorporation of FU into RNA; this suggests the importance of uridine phosphorylase (4, Fig. 4) in the conversion of FU into ribonucleotides (GOTTO et al., 1969). Although the addition of various ribose donors stimulated the conversion of FU into ribonucleotides in several mouse leukemias, they did not enhance the chemotherapeutic effectiveness of FU. From these observations it was concluded that the major determinant of effectiveness is the further conversion of ribonucleotides to FdUMP (KESSEL and HALL, 1969). When FU was given to mice bearing the L1210 leukemia, FdUMP was retained for more than 72 h as the major metabolite in the tumor cells (CHADWICK and ROGERS, 1970). In various cells in culture, it was concluded that the uridine and deoxyuridine phosphorylase pathways (4, 9, and 13, Fig. 4) are not significantly involved in FU inhibition (KENT and HEIDELBERGER, 1972). Uridine phosphorylase activities were found to be very low in a series of mouse leukemias (KESSEL et al., 1969).

Of probably greater importance in the activation of FU along the ribonucleotide pathway is its reaction with PRPP to give FUMP directly (REYES, 1969). It was found in a series of 12 transplantable mouse leukemias that there was an excellent direct correlation between the levels of this phosphoribosyltransferase activity (18, Fig. 4) and the prolongation of survival of tumor-bearing mice treated with FU (REYES and HALL, 1969). This conclusion was strengthened by the finding of high levels of enzyme 18 and the conversion of FU into FUMP in a series of susceptible mouse leukemias (KESSEL et al., 1969) and plasma cell tumors (EVERSON et al., 1970).

In 11 transplanted mouse leukemias it was observed that there was an inverse correlation between their response to FUDR and their level of thymidine kinase (11, Fig. 4), the enzyme that activates FUDR. This paradox is explained by the fact that thymidine kinase also phosphorylates any available thymidine, which would then bypass the block produced by the inhibition of thymidylate synthetase (KESSEL and WODINSKY, 1970). The high efficiency of the inhibition of the latter enzyme by the FdUMP that is formed in the tumors (HARTMANN and HEIDELBERGER, 1961) is in accord with this inverse correlation. FUR has been shown to be chemotherapeutically effective in a series of mouse leukemias only when they have low levels of the catabolic enzyme uridine phosphorylase (4, Fig. 4) (KESSEL et al., 1971).

Very extensive investigations of nucleic acid metabolism in slices of human tumors, with and without the addition of FU, have been carried out in order to obtain a method for the prognosis of the response of individuals to the drug. Great individual variations in response were found in the incorporation of both thymidine and formate into DNA and in their response to FU among various tumors (WOLBERG, 1969). Whereas there was no correlation between the *in vitro* thymidine labeling index of individual human tumors and their response to chemotherapy with FU (WOLBERG and ANSFIELD, 1971), there was a correlation with clinical response when the effect of FU on the incorporation of thymidine and uridine into DNA was determined. When neither precursor was incorporated or FU produced no effect, the patients did not respond. When FU produced an inhibition of thymidine incorporation and an inhibition of uridine incorporation, the patients showed a favorable response. When thymidine incorporation was increased and uridine decreased, the responses of the patients to chemotherapy were intermediate (WOLBERG, 1971).

C. Resistance

Because of the diversity of enzymatic reactions involved in the mechanism of action of the fluorinated pyrimidines, it is not surprising that several mechanisms of resistance have been elucidated. It has been found that the thymidylate synthetase (12, Fig. 4) of an FU-resistant Ehrlich ascites tumor was not inhibited by FdUMP (HEIDELBERGER et al., 1960), and that a line of Novikoff hepatoma cells in culture was resistant to FUDR because the cells lacked thymidine kinase (11, Fig. 4) (MORSE and POTTER, 1965) and consequently were also resistant to F_3TDR (UMEDA and HEIDELBERGER, 1968). In a series of four FU-resistant Ehrlich ascites tumors there was a marked decrease in the activity of uridine kinase (5, Fig. 4) (REICHARD et al., 1962; SKÖLD et al., 1962); this decrease was also found in some FU-resistant mouse leukemias (KESSEL et al., 1971).

In *E. coli* resistant to inhibition by FU, there was no detectable level of uracil phosphoribosyltransferase (18, Fig. 4) (BROCKMAN et al., 1960). It had been thought that this enzyme occurred only in bacteria, but in an FU-resistant Gardner lymphosarcoma it was found that there was a loss in activity of enzyme 18 (KASBEKAR and GREENBERG, 1963), which was subsequently purified and characterized (REYES, 1969). It seems very likely that other mechanisms of resistance to FU will be discovered in the future.

Effects on the Cell Cycle

The cell cycle can be defined in the following time sequence: mitosis (M), gap 1 (G_1), DNA synthesis (S), gap 2 (G_2), and M. In a study of the lethal effects of FU on mouse L cells, it was found that the drug exerted much more lethality on logarithmically growing cells than on stationary cells (MADOC-JONES and BRUCE, 1968). Thus, FU can be considered as "cycle-specific" in that it kills only cells that are proliferating in the cell cycle. The inhibition of the growth produced by FU in cells in culture is usually completely reversed by the addition of thymidine (cf. UMEDA and HEIDELBERGER, 1968), in accord with previous conclusions that the major mechanism of growth inhibition is a consequence of the blockade of thymidylate synthetase. In L cells, when thymidine was added simultaneously with FU or up to 40 h afterwards, the lethality of the drug was prevented. When the thymidine was added more than 40 h after FU, the lethality was not prevented. This was interpreted to mean that, as the result of the incorporation of FU into RNA, irreversible lethality was produced (MADOC-JONES and BRUCE, 1968). An alternative interpretation is that after a sufficient exposure to FU, thymineless death occurred as a result of an imbalance caused by continued synthesis of RNA and protein in the absence of DNA synthesis (cf. COHEN et al., 1958). This interpretation does not attach importance to the incorporation of FU into RNA in the mechanism of cell killing.

Two studies have been carried out in lines of cells synchronized by the colcemid reversal method, and contradictory results were obtained. In one, FUDR produced equal toxicity when added at all phases of the cell cycle (LOZZIO, 1969), and in the other, FUDR was considerably more lethal when added during S phase (BHUYAN et al., 1972). The reason for this difference is not explained.

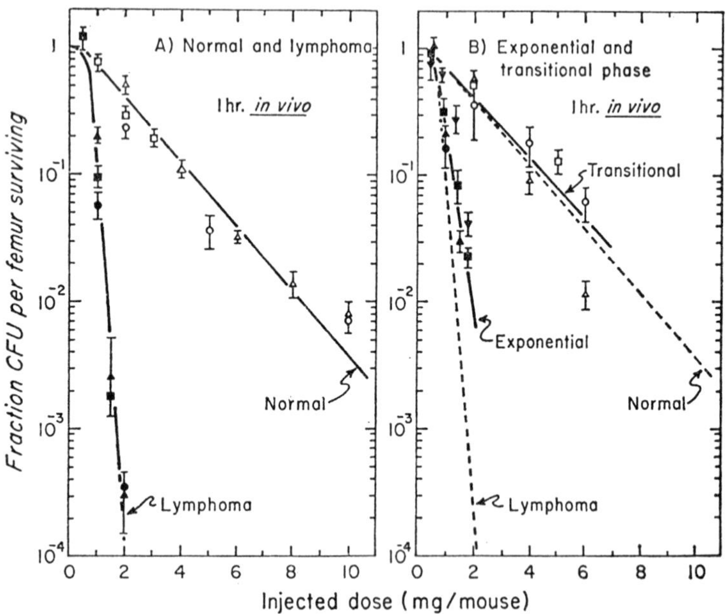

Fig. 8. The fraction of colony-forming units (CFU) surviving in the femurs of mice 1 hour after the injection of up to 10 mg of 5-fluorouracil. (A) Results for normal hematopoietic (open symbols) and lymphoma (closed symbols) CFU. (B) Results for transitional phase (open symbols) and exponential phase (closed symbols) hematopoietic CFU compared with the results for normal and lymphoma CFU (dashed lines) (BRUCE and MEEKER, 1967)

The selectivity of action of FU administered to mice, on the formation of colonies in the spleen of normal hematopoietic cells and lymphoma cells, showed (Fig. 8) that the drug was very much more lethal to the lymphoma than to the normal cells. However, normal exponentially growing hematopoietic cells (obtained from the bone marrow of lethally irradiated mice) had a sensitivity to FU equal to that of the lymphoma cells. Hence, it was concluded that FU is selectively toxic to proliferating cells, whether they be normal or lymphoma (BRUCE and MEEKER, 1967). Other aspects of drugs and the cell cycle have been reviewed (BRUCE and VALERIOTE, 1968).

Preclinical Pharmacology

Very little published material on the preclinical pharmacology of the fluorinated pyrimidines is available. Most of the work done with FU and FUDR is in the files of Hoffman-LaRoche, Inc. The preclinical pharmacology of F_3TDR is in reports of A.D. Little, Inc. The main findings are that there is toxicity to most tissues with a high rate of cellular proliferation, particularly the bone marrow and gastrointestinal mucosa. F_3TDR, although toxic to the bone marrow, exerts little toxicity on the gastrointestinal tract. Neurotoxicity, has been observed in FU-treated animals, particularly in cats, and very rarely in patients. The presence of fluorocitrate in the brains of FU-treated cats, which has been detected, indicates that fluoroacetate was present (KOENIG, 1967). It is conceivable that fluoroacetate could somehow be obtained by a reductive deamination of the catabolite, α-fluoro-β-alanine.

The tissue distribution of radioactivity in mice given FU (CHAUDHURI et al., 1958) and F_3TDR (HEIDELBERGER et al., 1965) has been studied, and no remarkable tissue localization was observed. In the case of FU-2-^{14}C, the ring is rapidly and extensively degraded in mice, as evidenced by the production of radioactive respiratory CO_2 amounting to up to 90 % of the dose in 24 h (CHAUDHURI et al., 1958). On the other hand, in mice given F_3TDR-2-^{14}C, there was no significant production of label in the respiratory CO_2; this shows that the ring was not degraded. In the urine of these mice the only compounds detectable were unchanged F_3TDR, F_3T, and 5-carboxyuracil (HEIDELBERGER et al., 1965); the results were identical for dogs and monkeys (ROGERS et al., 1969). A method for the analysis of F_3T and F_3TDR has been devised (ROGERS and WILSON, 1969) by determination of inorganic fluoride released by alkaline treatment of these compounds (HEIDELBERGER et al., 1964).

Clinical Use

The use of FU and FUDR in the treatment of patients suffering from disseminated cancer has been reviewed (HEIDELBERGER and ANSFIELD, 1963; CARTER, 1970; HEIDELBERGER, 1972). It is clearly beyond the scope of this chapter to furnish detailed clinical information, and so only the highlights will be considered. FU has been used very extensively in the treatment of patients with advanced solid cancers. FUDR has been widely but less extensively studied, partly because of its greater cost. FUR has received relatively little clinical trial because of its high toxicity. FCDR and ara-FC have produced some responses in very limited clinical trials (J.H. BURCHENAL, private communication). F_3TDR has produced an encouraging number of tumor regressions in patients with advanced breast cancer, but these regressions were difficult to maintain (ANSFIELD and RAMIREZ, 1971). Some encouraging results in the treatment with F_3TDR of children with various malignancies has also been reported (HELSON et al., 1970). F_3TDR is clinically highly effective in the treatment of herpes simplex infections of the eye (WELLINGS et al., 1972). FC is used for the treatment of human infections by fungi and cryptococci (UTZ, 1968).

In general, FU and FUDR do not seem to be effective against leukemias and lymphomas, but do produce objective regressions in advanced solid cancers, particularly breast, gastrointestinal, and gynecological. The drugs are toxic and must be given with great caution. The principal manifestations of toxicity are leukopenia, stomatitis, diarrhea, anorexia, nausea, and vomiting; toxic effects of less frequent occurrence include thrombocytopenia, hemorrhage, gastrointestinal ulceration, alopecia, dermatitis, nail changes, and, very rarely, cerebellar disturbances. In spite of the fact that FU has been widely used in the clinic for 14 years, there is still no agreement on the best mode of administration and dosage schedule. Originally, FU was given intravenously in monthly courses consisting of 5 to 7 consecutive daily treatments to moderate toxicity. Now, weekly maintenance doses appear to be as effective, and produce less toxicity and discomfort. Very recently, therapeutic effectiveness via the oral route has been reported. No cures have been reported with FU or FUDR, but they are considered useful in the palliation and prolongation of life in those patients who respond favorably.

In the initial clinical report, FU produced the toxic symptoms enumerated above, and objective regressions in some patients with various advanced malignancies (CURRERI et al., 1958). In a ten year study of FU in the treatment of 676 patients with disseminated breast cancer, it was found that there was a significant increase in the median survival of those patients who showed objective regression of their lesion and of those whose tumors stopped growing, as compared with those patients whose tumors continued to progress under treatment (Fig. 9) (ANSFIELD et al., 1969). In a direct comparison of the effectiveness of FU and FUDR in the treatment of advanced colorectal cancer, no difference was found (MOERTEL and REITEMEIER, 1967), probably because of the rapid cleavage of FUDR to FU.

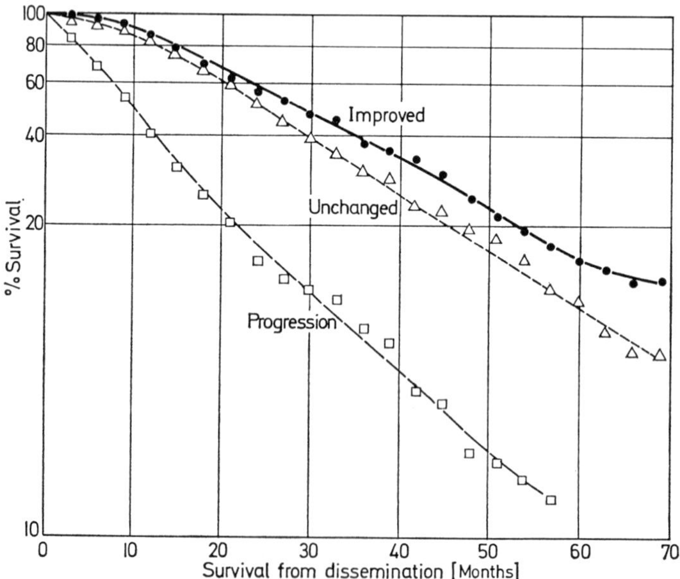

Fig. 9. The survival of human patients with disseminated breast carcinoma who had been treated with 5-fluorouracil (Ansfield et al., 1969)

Several studies on the comparison of various dosage regimens of FU have been carried out. A single weekly intravenous dose of FU produced less toxicity than multiple doses, with apparently equal therapeutic effect (JACOBS et al., 1971). Orally administered FU was shown to be effective in the treatment of advanced colorectal cancer, including liver metastases (LAHIRI et al., 1971). In a randomized comparison of equal single weekly intravenous and oral doses of FU, it was observed that there was a greater incidence of objective responses in the oral group, accompanied by less hematological and more gastrointestinal toxicity than in the intravenous group (BATEMAN et al., 1971). The administration of FU by continuous intra-arterial infusion into the hepatic artery of patients with liver metastases has been found to give minimal systemic toxicity, major tumor regressions, and increased survival in responders as compared with comparable patients receiving conventional intravenous FU therapy (ANSFIELD et al., 1971b). The use of topical administration of FU (preparation called Efudex) has given very gratifying results in the treatment of premalignant actinic keratoses, as well as multiple primary superficial basal cell and squamous cell carcinomas of the skin. However, this treatment is not recommended for use against invasive basal cell carcinomas (WILLIAMS and KLEIN, 1970; the entire issue of Dermatologica, Vol. 140, Supplement 1, 1970 is devoted to this topic).

Although the combination of FU with other cancer chemotherapeutic drugs is only in its infancy, there is preliminary evidence that FU combined with vincristine, methotrexate, cyclophosphamide, and prednisone produces considerably greater therapeutic effect against advanced breast cancer than any of those drugs given alone (ANSFIELD et al., 1971a). The combination of FU and x-irradiation has produced increased survival of patients with advanced cancer of the tonsil and of the inside of the mouth as compared with those treated with radiation alone (ANSFIELD et al., 1970). An additive effect of FU and x-irradiation has been observed in patients suffering from inoperable bronchogenic carcinoma (COHEN et al., 1971). When FU was given intraluminally at the time of surgery for carcinoma of the colon and then intravenously 1 and 2 days later, the survival of patients so treated was greater than those who had surgery alone (ROUSSELOT et al., 1968). Further studies of FU as an adjuvant to surgery are being carried out.

Clinical Pharmacology

Extensive studies of the metabolism of FU-2-^{14}C and FUDR-2-^{14}C in advanced cancer patients have been carried out with various modes of administration. Following intravenous injection, the half-times of total plasma radioactivity were about 1 hour. There was very rapid respiratory excretion of radioactive CO_2 following injection of both drugs, with approximately 90 % of the dose excreted in 12 h following oral administration, compared with approximately 70 % following intravenous injection. The total urinary excretion of radioactivity generally amounted to 5 to 10 % of the dose, and in the case of FUDR very little unchanged drug was found in the urine, while most of the label was present as FU and urea. A small amount of unchanged FU was detected in the cerebrospinal fluid following intravenous injection of FU (MUKHERJEE et al., 1963a).

The tissue distribution of radioactivity was investigated following administration of labeled FU and FUDR to patients with various cancers prior to surgical extirpation of their tumors. Although the distribution of total radioactivity between carcinoma of the colon and normal colonic mucosa varied among the patients, when the tissues were fractionated a higher percentage of the label was found as unchanged FU or as nucleotides in the tumor, and more degradation products were detected in the normal mucosa. This was taken as confirmation of the decreased degradation carried out *in situ* by the patients' tumors. Intra-arterial injection into an isolated loop of intestine containing a carcinoma was carried out with the labeled drugs, and a recovery of close to 100% was found in the tumor on the first pass (MUKHERJEE et al., 1963b).

Blood levels of FU following administration to cancer patients were measured by observing the cytotoxicity to cultured cells of serum and urine samples. The cytotoxic activity could also be determined by elution of metabolites separated by paper chromatography. This was primarily a feasibility study; too few patients were investigated to give meaningful clinical pharmacological data (SMITH et al., 1965).

A very extensive investigation of the blood levels and urinary excretion of FU and FUDR in patients has been done with the inhibition of growth of *Strep. faecalis* used as the assay system. FU and FUDR were separated chromatographically and the eluates subjected to microbiological assay. Although the plasma half-times of FU following intravenous injection were not given, they appeared to be equivalent for FU and FUDR and were approximately 15 min. When the drugs were given orally, the blood level was maintained for a longer time, but the level was much lower than that achieved during the first hour following intravenous injection. Many other findings were reported in this study, which cannot be described here because of limitations of space (CLARKSON et al., 1964).

When FU-6-^{14}C was given intravenously to patients, 60 to 97 % of the dose was recovered in the urine in the first 72 h. When the labeled FU was applied in an ointment to the skin of healthy patients, only 1 % of the label was recovered in the urine during the same period. However, in a comparable local application to patients with diseased skin (psoriasis, ulcers), 18 to 61 % of the dose was recovered in the urine. This shows that FU is not absorbed by healthy skin. But even with diseased skin the amount absorbed would in general be insufficient to cause systemic toxicity, which in fact was not seen in patients treated by topical application of Efudex (ERLANGER et al., 1970).

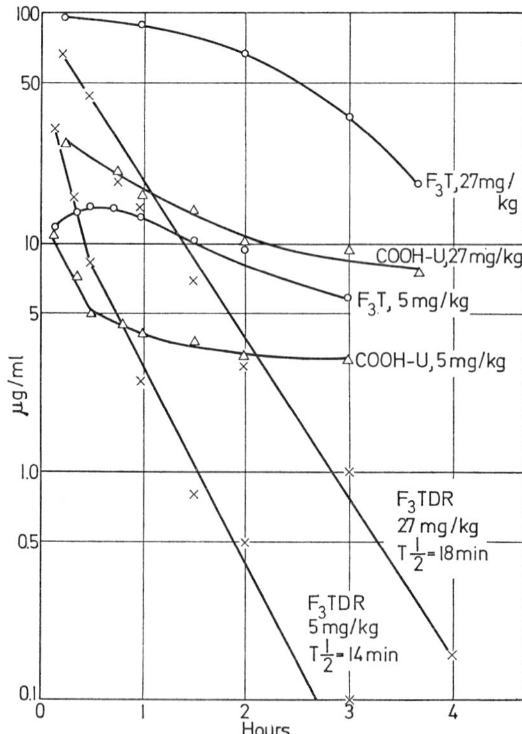

Fig. 10. The time-course of the serum levels of F_3TDR-2-^{14}C and its catabolites in two patients (DEXTER et al., 1972)

The clinical pharmacology of F_3TDR-2-^{14}C in cancer patients has been studied. As in the case of mice and monkeys, the only metabolites detectable in the urine were F_3TDR, F_3T, and 5-COOH-U, and there was no significant radioactivity in respiratory CO_2. The plasma distribution of these three compounds following intravenous injection of F_3TDR is shown in Fig. 10, where a first order disappearance of F_3TDR with a half-time of about 18 min and a precursor-product relationship between F_3T and 5-COOH-U can be seen. Children degraded the drug more slowly than adult patients, but clinical response to the drug could not be correlated with the rate of degradation. In the urine, F_3T was the major compound found, and the recovery of inorganic fluoride in the urine was about 50 % of the amount liberated in the conversion to 5-COOH-U; the remainder was presumably incorporated into the bones (DEXTER et al., 1972).

References

ANDOH, T., CHARGAFF, E.: Formation and fate of abnormal ribosomes of *E. coli* cells treated with 5-fluorouracil. Proc. nat. Acad. Sci. (Wash.) **54**, 1181—1189 (1965).

ANSFIELD, F. J., RAMIREZ, G.: Phase I and II studies of 2′-deoxy-5-(trifluoromethyl)uridine. Cancer Chemother. Rep. **55**, 205—208 (1971).

ANSFIELD, F. J., RAMIREZ, G., DAVIS, H. L., JR., KORBITZ, B. C., VERMUND, H., GOLLIN, F. F.: Treatment of advanced cancer of the head and neck. Cancer **25**, 78—82 (1970).

ANSFIELD, F. J., RAMIREZ, G., KORBITZ, B. C., DAVIS, H. L., JR.: Five-drug therapy for advanced breast cancer. A phase I study. Cancer Chemother. Rep. **55**, 183—187 (1971a).

ANSFIELD, F. J., RAMIREZ, G., MACKMAN, S., BRYAN, G. T., CURRERI, A. R.: A ten year study of 5-fluorouracil in disseminated breast cancer with clinical results and survival times. Cancer Res. **29**, 1062—1066 (1969).

ANSFIELD, F. J., RAMIREZ, G., SKIBBA, J. L., BRYAN, G. T., DAVIS, H. L., WIRTANEN, G. W.: Intrahepatic arterial infusion with 5-fluorouracil. Cancer, **28**, 1147—1151 (1971b).

ARONSON, A. I.: The inhibition of bacteriophage protein synthesis by 5-fluorouracil. Biochim. biophys. Acta (Amst.) **49**, 89—97 (1961a).

ARONSON, A. I.: The effect of 5-fluorouracil on bacterial protein and ribonucleic acid synthesis. Biochim. biophys. Acta (Amst.) **49**, 98—107 (1961b).

BALIGA, B. S., HENDER, S., SRINIVASAN, P. R.: Incorporation of 5-fluorouracil into the transfer RNA of *Escherichia coli* $K_{22}N_6$ and its effect on the methylation of uracil. Biochim. biophys. Acta (Amst.) **186**, 25—32 (1969).

BATEMAN, J. R., PUGH, R. P., CASSIDY, F. R., MARSHALL, G. J., IRWIN, L. E.: 5-Fluorouracil given once weekly: comparison of intravenous and oral administration. Cancer **28**, 907—913 (1971).

BERTANI, L. E.: Lysogenic conversion by bacteriophage P_2 resulting in an increased sensitivity of *Escherichia coli* to 5-fluorodeoxyuridine. Biochim. biophys. Acta (Amst.) **87**, 631—640 (1964).

BHUYAN, B. K., SCHEIDT, L. G., FRASER, T. J.: Cell cycle phase specificity of antitumor agents. Cancer Res. **32**, 398—407 (1972).

BIRNIE, G. D., KROEGER, H., HEIDELBERGER, C.: Studies on fluorinated pyrimidines. XVIII. The degradation of 5-fluoro-2′-deoxyuridine and related compounds by nucleoside phosphorylase. Biochemistry **2**, 566—572 (1963).

BLOMGREN, S. E., WOLBERG, W. H., KISKEN, W. A.: The effect of fluoropyrimidines on delayed cutaneous hypersensitivity. Cancer Res. **25**, 977—979 (1965).

BOSCH, L., HARBERS, E., HEIDELBERGER, C.: Studies on fluorinated pyrimidines. V. Effects on nucleic acid metabolism *in vitro*. Cancer Res. **18**, 335—343 (1958).

BRESNICK, E., WILLIAMS, S. S.: Effects of 5-trifluoromethyldeoxyuridine upon deoxythymidine kinase. Biochem. Pharmacol. **16**, 503—507 (1967).

BROCKMAN, R. W., DAVIS, J. M., STUTTS, P.: Metabolism of uracil and 5-fluorouracil by drug-sensitive and by drug-resistant bacteria. Biochim. biophys. Acta (Amst.) **40**, 22—32 (1960).

BRUCE, W. R., MEEKER, B. E.: Comparison of the sensitivity of hematopoietic colony-forming cells in different proliferative states to 5-fluorouracil. J. nat. Cancer Inst. **38**, 401—405 (1967).

BRUCE, W. R., VALERIOTE, F. A.: Normal and malignant stem cells and chemotherapy. In: 21st Symposium on Fundamental Cancer Research. M. D. Anderson Hospital, Houston, Texas, pp. 435—464, 1968.

BUDĚŠÍNSKÝ, Z., JELINEK, U., PŘIKRYL, J.: 5-Halogenpyrimidine. I. Darstellung von 4-hydroxy-5-halogenpyrimidinen. Coll. Czech. Chem. Commun. **11**, 2550—2557 (1962).

BUJARD, H., HEIDELBERGER, C.: Fluorinated pyrimidines. XXVII. Attempts to determine transcription errors during the formation of fluorouracil-containing messenger ribonucleic acid. Biochemistry **5**, 3339—3345 (1966).

BURCHENAL, J. H., ADAMS, H. H., NEWELL, N. S., FOX, J. J.: Comparative activity of 1-β-D-arabinofuranosyl-5-fluorocytosine and related compounds against transplanted mouse leukemias *in vivo* and *in vitro*. Cancer Res. **26**, 370—373 (1966).

BURCHENAL, J. H., HOLMBERG, E. A. D., FOX, J. J., HEMPHILL, S. C., REPPERT, J. A.: The effects of 5-fluorodeoxycytidine, 5-fluorodeoxyuridine and related compounds on transplanted mouse leukemias. Cancer Res. **19**, 494—500 (1959).

BUSSARD, A., NAONO, S., GROS, F., MONOD, J.: Effects d'un analogue de l'uracile sur les proprietés d'une protèine enzymatique synthetisée en sa presence. C. R. Acad. Sci. (Paris) **250**, 4049—4051 (1960).

CARTER, S. K., Ed.: Proceedings of the conference on the chemotherapy of solid tumors; appraisal of 5-fluorouracil and BCNU. Cancer Evaluation Branch, National Cancer Institute 1970.

CHADWICK, M., ROGERS, W. L.: The distribution of 5-fluoro-2'-deoxyuridine-5'-monophosphate in mice after 5-fluorouracil administration. Proc. Amer. Ass. Cancer Res. **11**, 15 (1970).

CHAMPE, S. P., BENZER, S.: Reversal of mutant phenotypes by 5-fluorouracil: an approach to nucleotide sequences in messenger-RNA. Proc. nat. Acad. Sci. (Wash.) **48**, 532—546 (1962).

CHANDROSS, R., RICH, A.: The crystal structure of the 2 : 1 intramolecular complex containing 1-methyl-5-fluorouracil and 9-ethyl-2,6-diaminopurine. Biopolymers **10**, 1795—1807 (1971).

CHAUBE, S., MURPHY, M. L.: The teratogenic effects of the recent drugs active in cancer chemotherapy. Advan. Teratol. **3**, 181—237 (1968).

CHAUDHURI, N. K., MONTAG, B. J., HEIDELBERGER, C.: Studies on fluorinated pyrimidines. III. The metabolism of 5-fluorouracil-2-^{14}C and 5-fluoroorotic acid-2-^{14}C *in vivo*. Cancer Res. **18**, 318—328 (1958).

CHAUDHURI, N. K., MUKHERJEE, K. L., HEIDELBERGER, C.: Studies on fluorinated pyrimidines VII. The degradative pathway. Biochem. Pharmacol. **1**, 328—341 (1959).

ČIHÁK, A., WILKINSON, D., PITOT, H. C.: The effect of pyrimidine analogues and tryptophan on enzyme synthesis and degradation in rat liver. Adv. Enzyme Regulation **9**, 267—289 (1971).

CLARKSON, B., O'CONNOR, A., WINSTON, L., HUTCHISON, D.: The physiologic disposition of 5-fluorouracil and 5-fluoro-2'-deoxyuridine in man. Clin. Pharmacol. Ther. **5**, 581—610 (1964).

COHEN, J. L., KRANT, M. J., SHNIDER, B. I., MATIAS, P. I., HORTON, J., BAXTER, D.: Radiation plus 5-fluorouracil (NSC-19893): clinical demonstration of an additive effect in bronchogenic carcinoma. Cancer Chemother. Rep. **55**, 253—258 (1971).

COHEN, S. S., FLAKS, J. G., BARNER, H. D., LOEB, M. R., LICHTENSTEIN, J.: The mode of action of 5-fluorouracil and its derivatives. Proc. nat. Acad. Sci. (Wash.) **44**, 1004—1012 (1958).

COOPER, G. M., DUNNING, W. F., GREER, S.: Role of catabolism in pyrimidine utilization for nucleic acid synthesis *in vivo*. Cancer Res. **32**, 390—397 (1972).

COOPER, P. D.: The mutation of poliovirus by 5-fluorouracil. Virology **22**, 186—192 (1964).

CURRERI, A. R., ANSFIELD, F. J., MCIVER, F. A., WAISMAN, H. A., HEIDELBERGER, C.: Clinical studies with 5-fluorouracil. Cancer Res. **18**, 478—484 (1958).

CUSHLEY, R., WEMPEN, I., FOX, J. J.: Nucleosides. XLIV. Long-range protein-fluorine spin-spin coupling in 5-fluoropyrimidine nucleosides. J. Amer. chem. Soc. **90**, 709—715 (1968).

DANNEBERG, P. B., MONTAG, B. J., HEIDELBERGER, C.: Studies on fluorinated pyrimidines. IV. Effects on nucleic acid metabolism *in vivo*. Cancer Res. **18**, 329—334 (1958).

DAVERN, C. I.: The inhibition and mutagenesis of an RNA bacteriophage by 5-fluorouracil. Austral. J. biol. Sci. **17**, 726—737 (1964).

DE KLOET, S. R.: Effects of 5-fluorouracil and 6-azauracil on the synthesis of ribonucleic acid and protein in *Saccharomyces carlsbergensis*. Biochem. J. **106**, 167—178 (1968).

DE KLOET, S. R., STRIJKERT, P. J.: Selective inhibition of ribosomal RNA synthesis in *Saccharomyces carlsbergensis* by 5-fluorouracil. Biochem. biophys. Res. Commun. **23**, 49—55 (1966).

DE REPENTIGNY, J., SONEA, S., FRAPPIER, A.: Differentiation by immunodiffusion and by quantitative immunofluorescence between 5-fluorouracil-treated and normal cells from a toxinogenic *Staphylococcus aureus* strain. J. Bact. **88**, 444—448 (1964).

DEXTER, D. L., HEIDELBERGER, C.: Effect of trifluorothymidine on transcription of vaccinia virus mRNA. Molec. Pharmacol. **9**, 283—296 (1973).

DEXTER, D. L., WOLBERG, W. H., ANSFIELD, F. J., HELSON, L., HEIDELBERGER, C.: The clinical pharmacology of 5-trifluoromethyl-2'-deoxyuridine. Cancer Res. **32**, 247—253 (1972).

DIPPLE, A., HEIDELBERGER, C.: Fluorinated pyrimidines. XXVIII. The synthesis of 5-trifluoromethyl-6-azauracil and 5-trifluoromethyl-6-aza-2'-deoxyuridine. J. med. Chem. **9**, 715—718 (1966).

DUSCHINSKY, R., GABRIEL, T., TAUTZ, W., NUSSBAUM, A., HOFFER, M., GRUNBERG, E., BURCHENAL, J. H., FOX, J. J.: Nucleosides. XXXVII. 5,6-Substituted 5-fluorodihydropyrimidines and their 2'-deoxyribonucleosides. J. med. Chem. **10**, 47—58 (1967).
DUSCHINSKY, R., PLEVEN, E., HEIDELBERGER, C.: The synthesis of 5-fluoropyrimidines. J. Amer. chem. Soc. **79**, 4559—4560 (1957).
ERLANGER, M., MARTZ, G., OTT, F., STORCK, H., RIEDER, J., KESSLER, S.: Cutaneous absorption and urinary excretion of 6-^{14}C-5-fluorouracil applied in an ointment to healthy and diseased skin. Dermatologica (Napol.) **140**, 7—14 (1970).
EVERSON, R., KESSEL, D., HALL, T. C.: Enzymatic determinants of responsiveness of the LPC-1 plasma cell neoplasm to fluorouracil and fluorodeoxyuridine. Biochem. Pharmacol. **19**, 2932—2934 (1970).
FIKUS, M., WIERZCHOWSKI, K. L., SHUGAR, D.: Reversible photochemical transformation of 5-fluorouracil analogues and poly-5-fluorouridylic acid. Biochem. biophys. Res. Commun. **16**, 478—483 (1964).
FOX, J. J., MILLER, N., WEMPEN, I.: Nucleosides. XXIX. 1-β-D-Arabinofuranosyl-5-fluorocytosine (FCA) and related arabinonucleosides. J. med. Chem. **9**, 101—105 (1966).
FRIDLAND, A., LANGENBACH, R. J., HEIDELBERGER, C.: Purification of thymidylate synthetase from Ehrlich ascites carcinoma cells. J. biol. Chem. **246**, 7110—7114 (1971).
FUJIWARA, Y., HEIDELBERGER, C.: Fluorinated pyrimidines. XXXVIII. The incorporation of 5-trifluoromethyl-2'-deoxyuridine into the deoxyribonucleic acid of vaccinia virus. Molec. Pharmacol. **6**, 281—291 (1970).
FUJIWARA, Y., OKI, T., HEIDELBERGER, C.: Fluorinated pyrimidines. XXXVII. Effects of 5-trifluoromethyl-2'-deoxyuridine on the synthesis of deoxyribonucleic acid of mammalian cells in culture. Molec. Pharmacol. **6**, 273—280 (1970).
GAREN, A., SIDDIQI, O.: Suppression of mutations in the alkaline phosphatase structural cistron of *E. coli*. Proc. nat. Acad. Sci. (Wash.) **48**, 1121—1127 (1962).
GIEGE, R., WEIL, J-H.: Étude des tRNA de levure avant incorporé du 5-fluorouracile provenant de la desamination *in vivo* de la 5-fluorocytosine. Bull. Soc. chim. Biol. **52**, 135—144 (1970).
GOLDBERG, N. D., DAHL, J. L., PARKS, R. E., JR.: pH Dependence of the reactions with the 5-fluorouracil and 6-azauracil analogues of uridine diphosphate glucose. J. biol. Chem. **238**, 3109—3114 (1963).
GOODMAN, F.: Nucleic acid metabolism and bacteriophage multiplication: effects of 5-fluorouracil on coliphage synthesis. Virology **21**, 249—257 (1963).
GORDON, M. P., STAEHELIN, M.: Studies on the incorporation of 5-fluorouracil into a virus nucleic acid. Biochim. biophys. Acta (Amst.) **36**, 351—361 (1959).
GOTTO, A. M., BELKHODE, M. L., TOUSTER, O.: Stimulatory effects of inosine and deoxyinosine on the incorporation of uracil-2-^{14}C, 5-fluorouracil-2-^{14}C, and 5-bromouracil-2-^{14}C into nucleic acids by Ehrlich ascites tumor cells *in vitro*. Cancer Res. **29**, 807—811 (1969).
GOTTSCHLING, H., HEIDELBERGER, C.: Fluorinated pyrimidines. XIX. Some biological effects of 5-trifluoromethyl-2'-deoxyuridine on *Escherichia coli* and bacteriophage T4B. J. mol. Biol. **7**, 541—560 (1963).
GOZ, B., PRUSOFF, W. H.: Pharmacology of viruses. Ann. Rev. Pharmacol. **10**, 143—170 (1970).
GROS, F., GILBERT, W., HIATT, H. H., ATTARDI, G., SPAHR, P. F., WATSON, J. D.: Molecular and biological characterization of messenger RNA. Cold Spr. Harb. Symp. quant. Biol. **26**, 111—126 (1961).
GROS, F., NAONO, S.: Bacterial synthesis of "modified" enzymes in the presence of a pyrimidine analog. In: HARRIS, R. J. C. (Ed.): Protein biosynthesis, pp. 195—205. London: Academic Press 1961.
GRUNBERG-MANAGO, M., MICHELSON, A. M.: Polynucleotide analogues. IV. Polyfluorouridylic and copolymers containing fluorouridylic acid. Biochim. biophys. Acta (Amst.) **87**, 593—600 (1964).
HARBERS, E., CHAUDHURI, N. K., HEIDELBERGER, C.: Studies on fluorinated pyrimidines. VIII. Further biochemical and metabolic investigations. J. biol. Chem. **234**, 1255—1262 (1959).
HARRIS, D. R., MACINTYRE, W. M.: The crystal and molecular structure of 5-fluoro-2'-deoxy-β-uridine. Biophys. J. **4**, 203—225 (1964).
HARTMANN, K-U. HEIDELBERGER, C.: Studies on fluorinated pyrimidines. VIII. Inhibition of thymidylate synthetase. J. biol. Chem. **236**, 3006—3013 (1961).
HEIDELBERGER, C.: Fluorinated pyrimidines. Progr. nucleic Acid Res. molec. Biol. **4**, 1—50 (1965).
HEIDELBERGER, C.: Fluorinated pyrimidines, biochemically and clinically useful antimetabolites. In: Molekulare Biologie des malignen Wachstums, pp. 155—176. Berlin-Heidelberg-New York: Springer 1966.
HEIDELBERGER, C.: Cancer chemotherapy with purine and pyrimidine analogues. Ann. Rev. Pharmacol. **7**, 101—124 (1967).

Heidelberger, C.: The need for additional alkylating agents and antimetabolites. Cancer Res. **29**, 2435—2442 (1969).
Heidelberger, C.: Chemical carcinogenesis, chemotherapy: cancer's continuing core challenges, G.H.A. Clowes Memorial Lecture. Cancer Res. **30**, 1549—1569 (1970).
Heidelberger, C.: Pyrimidine and pyrimidine nucleoside antimetabolites. In: Frei, E. III, Holland, J.F. (Eds.): Cancer medicine. pp. 768—791. Philadelphia: Lea and Febiger 1973.
Heidelberger, C., Anderson, S.W.: Fluorinated pyrimidines. XXI. The tumor-inhibitory activity of 5-trifluoromethyl-2′-deoxyuridine. Cancer Res. **24**, 1979—1985 (1964).
Heidelberger, C., Ansfield, F.J.: Experimental and clinical use of fluorinated pyrimidines in cancer chemotherapy. Cancer Res. **23**, 1226—1243 (1963).
Heidelberger, C., Birnie, G.D., Boohar, J., Wentland, D.: Fluorinated pyrimidines. XX. Inhibition of the nucleoside phosphorylase cleavage of 5-fluoro-2′-deoxyuridine by 5-trifluoromethyl-2′-deoxyuridine. Biochim. biophys. Acta (Amst.) **76**, 315—318 (1963).
Heidelberger, C., Boohar, J., Kampschroer, B.: Fluorinated pyrimidines. XXIV. *In vivo* metabolism of 5-trifluoromethyluracil-2-^{14}C and 5-trifluoromethyl-2′-deoxyuridine-2-^{14}C. Cancer Res. **25**, 377—381 (1965).
Heidelberger, C., Chaudhuri, N.K., Danneberg, P., Mooren, D., Griesbach, L., Duschinsky, R., Schnitzer, R.J., Pleven, E., Scheiner, T.: Fluorinated pyrimidines, a new class of tumor-inhibitory compounds. Nature (Lond.) **179**, 663—666 (1957).
Heidelberger, C., Griesbach, L., Cruz, O., Schnitzer, R.J., Grunberg, E.G.: Fluorinated pyrimidines. VI. Effect of 5-fluorouridine and 5-fluoro-2′-deoxyuridine on transplanted tumors. Proc. Soc. exp. Biol. (N.Y.) **97**, 470—475 (1958b).
Heidelberger, C., Griesbach, L., Montag, B.J., Mooren, D., Cruz, O., Schnitzer, R.J., Grunberg, E.: Studies on fluorinated pyrimidines. II. Effects on transplanted tumors. Cancer Res. **18**, 305—317 (1958a).
Heidelberger, C., Kaldor, G., Mukherjee, K.L., Danneberg, P.B.: Studies on fluorinated pyrimidines. XI. *In vitro* studies on tumor resistance. Cancer Res. **20**, 903—909 (1960a).
Heidelberger, C., Leibman, K.C., Harbers, E., Bhargava, P.M.: The comparative utilization of uracil-2-^{14}C by liver, intestinal mucosa and Flexner-Jobling carcinoma in the rat. Cancer Res. **17**, 399—404 (1957).
Heidelberger, C., Parsons, D.G., Remy, D.C.: Synthesis of 5-trifluoromethyluracil and 5-trifluoromethyl-2′-deoxyuridine. J. med. Chem. **7**, 1—5 (1964).
Heidelberger, C., Sunthankar, A.V., Griesbach, L., Randerson, S.: Fluorinated pyrimidines. XXII. Effects of simple nucleotides on transplanted tumors. Proc. Soc. exp. Biol. (N.Y.) **104**, 127—129 (1960b).
Helson, L., Yagoda, A., McCarthy, M., Murphy, M.L., Krakoff, I.H.: Clinical trials with 5-trifluoromethyl-2′-deoxyuridine (F_3TDR). Proc. Amer. Assoc. Cancer Res. **11**, 35 (1970).
Hignett, R.C.: Interference of 5-fluorouracil in the biosynthesis of ribosomes in *Staphylococcus aureus* (strain Duncan). Biochim. biophys. Acta (Amst.) **114**, 559—564 (1966).
Hills, D.C., Horowitz, J.: Ribosome synthesis in *E. coli* treated with 5-fluorouracil. Biochemistry **5**, 1625—1632 (1966).
Hipkiss, A.R., Arnstein, H.R.V., Edmunds, M.E.: Thionucleotide formation in *Escherichia coli* transfer ribonucleic acid in the presence of 5-fluorouracil. FEBS Let. **16**, 109—113 (1971).
Hoffer, M., Duschinsky, R., Fox, J.J., Yung, N.: Simple synthesis of pyrimidine-2′-deoxyribonucleosides. J. Amer. Chem. Soc. **81**, 4112—4113 (1959).
Horowitz, J., Chargaff, E.: Massive incorporation of 5-fluorouracil into a bacterial ribonucleic acid. Nature (Lond.) **184**, 1213—1215 (1959).
Horowitz, J., Kohlmeier, V.: Formation of active β-galactosidase by *E. coli* treated with 5-fluorouracil. Biochim. biophys. Acta (Amst.) **142**, 208—218 (1967).
Horowitz, J., Saukkonen, J.J., Chargaff, E.: Effect of fluoropyrimidines on the synthesis of bacterial proteins and nucleic acids. J. biol. Chem. **235**, 3266—3272 (1960).
Houlabek, V.: The composition of tobacco mosaic virus protein after the incorporation of 5-fluorouracil into the virus. J. molec. Biol. **6**, 164—166 (1963).
Hsu, T.C.. Humphrey, R.M., Somers, C.E.: Responses of Chinese hamster and L cells to 2′-deoxy-5-fluorouridine and thymidine. J. nat. Cancer Inst. **32**, 839—855 (1964).
Huberman, E., Heidelberger, C.: The mutagenicity to mammalian cells of pyrimidine nucleoside analogs. Mutation Res. **14**, 130—132 (1972).
Iwabuchi, M., Okata, E., Kono, M., Osawa, S.: The effect of 5-fluorouracil on the ribosome formation in *E. coli*. Biochim. biophys. Acta (Amst.) **114**, 83—94 (1966).
Jacobs, E.M., Reeves, W.J., Wood, D.A., Rugh, R., Braunwald, J., Bateman, J.R.: Treatment of cancer with weekly intravenous 5-fluorouracil. Cancer **27**, 1302—1305 (1971).
Johns, D.G., Sartorelli, A.C., Bertino, J.R., Iannotti, A.T., Booth, B.A., Welch, A.D.: Enzymatic hydroxylation of 5-fluoropyrimidines by aldehyde oxidase and xanthine oxidase. Biochem. Pharmacol. **15**, 400—403 (1966).

JOHNSON, J. L., YAMAMOTO, K. R., WEISLOGEL, P. O., HOROWITZ, J.: Some properties of transfer ribonucleic acids from 5-fluorouracil-treated *Escherichia coli*. Biochemistry **8**, 1901—1908 (1969).

KAHAN, F. M., HURWITZ, J.: The role of deoxyribonucleic acid in ribonucleic acid synthesis. J. biol. Chem. **237**, 3778—3785 (1962).

KAISER, I. I.: Studies on 5-fluorouracil-containing ribonucleic acid. I. Separation and partial characterization of fluorouracil-containing transfer ribonucleic acids from *Escherichia coli*. Biochemistry **8**, 231—238 (1969a).

KAISER, I. I.: Studies on 5-fluorouracil-containing RNA. II. Gross reduction of 4-thiouracil-containing tRNA from *E. coli*. Biochim. biophys. Acta (Amst.) **182**, 449—453 (1969b).

KAISER, I. I.: Isolation of 5-fluorouracil-containing 5 S ribonucleic acid from *Escherichia coli*. Biochemistry **9**, 569—573 (1970).

KAISER, I. I.: Structural properties of 5-fluorouracil-containing transfer ribonucleic acids from *Escherichia coli*. Biochemistry **10**, 1540—1545 (1971a).

KAISER, I. I.: Reduced levels of 5,6-dihydrouridine in fluorouracil-containing transfer RNA's from *Saccharomyces cerevisiae*. FEBS Let. **17**, 249—252 (1971b).

KAISER, I. I., JACOBSON, M., HEDGCOTH, C.: Studies on 5-fluorouracil-containing ribonucleic acid. III. Greatly reduced level of 5,6-dihydrouridine in fluorouracil-containing transfer RNA from *E. coli*. J. biol. Chem. **244**, 6707—6708 (1969).

KASBEKAR, D. K., GREENBERG, D. M.: Studies on tumor resistance to 5-fluorouracil. Cancer Res. **23**, 818—824 (1963).

KAUFMAN, H. E.: *In vivo* studies with antiviral agents. Ann. N.Y. Acad. Sci. **130**, 168—180 (1965).

KAUFMAN, H. E., HEIDELBERGER, C.: Therapeutic antiviral action of 5-trifluoromethyl-2'-deoxyuridine in herpes simplex keratitis. Science **145**, 585—586 (1964).

KAWAI, S., HANAFUSA, H.: The effects of reciprocal changes in temperature and the transformed state of cells infected with a Rous sarcoma virus mutant. Virology **46**, 470—479 (1971).

KENT, R. J., HEIDELBERGER, C.: Fluorinated pyrimidines. XXXV. The metabolism of 2',3'-dehydro-5-fluoro-2'-deoxyuridine in Ehrlich ascites cells. Biochem. Pharmacol. **19**, 1095—1104 (1970).

KENT, R. J., HEIDELBERGER, C.: Fluorinated pyrimidines. XL. The reduction of 5-fluorouridine-5'-diphosphate by ribonucleotide reductase. Molec. Pharmacol. **8**, 465—475 (1972).

KENT, R. J., KHWAJA, T. A., HEIDELBERGER, C.: Fluorinated pyrimidines. XXXIV. Structure-activity studies on methylated 5-fluoro-2'-deoxyuridine derivatives. J. med. Chem. **13**, 70—73 (1970).

KESSEL, D., BRUNS, R., HALL, T. C.: Determinants of responsiveness to 5-fluorouridine in transplantable murine leukemias. Molec. Pharmacol. **7**, 117—121 (1971).

KESSEL, D., HALL, T. C.: Influence of ribose donors on the action of 5 fluorouracil. Cancer Res. **29**, 1749—1754 (1969).

KESSEL, D., HALL, T. C., REYES, P.: Metabolism of uracil and 5-fluorouracil in P388 murine leukemia cells. Molec. Pharmacol. **5**, 481—486 (1969).

KESSEL, D., WODINSKY, I.: Thymidine kinase as a determinant of the response to 5-fluoro-2'-deoxyuridine in transplantable murine leukemias. Molec. Pharmacol. **6**, 251—254 (1970).

KHWAJA, T. A., HEIDELBERGER, C.: Fluorinated pyrimidines. XXIX. Synthesis of 2',3'-dehydro-5-fluoro-2'-deoxyuridine and 2',3'-dideoxy-5-fluorouridine. J. med. Chem. **10**, 1066—1070 (1967).

KHWAJA, T. A., HEIDELBERGER, C.: Fluorinated pyrimidines. XXXII. Synthesis of 2',3'-dehydro-5-trifluoromethyl-2'-deoxyuridine and 5-trifluoromethyluridine. J. med. Chem. **12**, 543—545 (1969).

KHWAJA, T. A., HEIDELBERGER, C.: Fluorinated pyrimidines. XXXIII. Synthesis of methylated 5-fluoro-2'-deoxyuridine derivatives. J. med. Chem. **13**, 64—69 (1970).

KIM, S-H., RICH, A.: A non-complementary hydrogen-bonded complex containing 5-fluorouracil and 1-methylcytosine. J. molec. Biol. **42**, 87—95 (1969).

KLINE, I., VENDITTI, J. M., MEAD, J. A. R., TYRER, D. D., GOLDIN, A.: The antileukemic effectiveness of 5-fluorouracil and methotrexate in the combination chemotherapy of advanced L-1210 in mice. Cancer Res. **26**, 848—852 (1966).

KLINE, I., WOODMAN, R. J., GANG, M., WARAVDEKAR, V. S., GOLDIN, A., VENDITTI, J. M.: Enhanced response of leukemic (L-1210) mice to combination chemotherapy with 5-(3,3-dimethyl-1-triazeno)-imidazole-4-carboxamide (NSC-45388) and 5-fluorouracil (NSC-19893). Cancer **27**, 1363—1368 (1971).

KOECHLIN, B. A., RUBIO, F., PALMER, S., GABRIEL, T., DUSCHINSKY, R.: The metabolism of 5-fluorocytosine-2-^{14}C and of cytosine-^{14}C in the rat and the disposition of 5-fluorocytosine-2-^{14}C in man. Biochem. Pharmacol. **15**, 435—446 (1966).

KOENIG, H.: Neurobiological action of some pyrimidine analogs. Int. Rev. Neurobiol. **10**, 199—230 (1967).

Kolář, V., Mechl, Z.: Fluoxidin (preliminary report on clinical evaluation). Neoplasma (Bratisl.) **18**, 485—487 (1971).

Kono, M., Osawa, S.: Intermediary steps of ribosome formation in *Escherichia coli*. Biochim. biophys. Acta (Amst.) **87**, 326—334 (1964).

Korfsmeier, K. H.: Wirkung von 5-fluorouracil auf den Protein Stoffwechsel von Tumoren und gesundem Gewebe in der Kultur. Zeit. Krebsforsch. **74**, 20—27 (1970).

Kramer, G., Wittmann, H. G., Schuster, H.: Die Erzeugung von Mutanten des Tabakmosaik Virus durch den Einbau von Fluorouracil in die Virusnucleinsäure. Z. Naturforsch. **19**b, 46—51 (1964).

Lahiri, S. R., Boileau, G., Hall, T. C.: Treatment of metastatic colorectal carcinoma with 5-fluorouracil by mouth. Cancer **28**, 902—906 (1971).

Lengyel, P., Speyer, J. F., Ochoa, S.: Synthetic polynucleotides and the amino acid code. Proc. nat. Acad. Sci. (Wash.) **47**, 1936—1942 (1961).

Líebecq, C., Peters, R. A.: The toxicity of fluoroacetate and the tricarboxylic acid cycle. Biochim. biophys. Acta (Amst.) **3**, 215—230 (1949).

Lindner, A.: Cytochemical effects of 5-fluorouracil on sensitive and resistant Ehrlich ascites tumor cells. Cancer Res. **19**, 189—194 (1959).

Lowrie, R. J., Bergquist, P. L.: Transfer ribonucleic acids from *E. coli* treated with 5-fluorouracil. Biochemistry **7**, 1761—1770 (1968).

Lozeron, H. A., Gordon, M. P.: Ultraviolet sensitization and photoreactivation of tobacco mosaic virus ribonucleic acid containing 5-fluorouracil. Biochemistry **3**, 507—510 (1964).

Lozeron, H. A., Gordon, M. P., Gabriel, T., Tautz, W., Duschinsky, R.: The photochemistry of 5-fluorouracil. Biochemistry **3**, 1844—1850 (1964).

Lozeron, H. A., Szybalski, W.: Incorporation of 5-fluorodeoxyuridine into the DNA of *B. subtilis* phage PBS2 and its radiobiological consequences. J. molec. Biol. **30**, 277—290 (1967).

Lozzio, C. B.: Lethal effects of fluorodeoxyuridine on cultured mammalian cells at various stages of the cell cycle. J. cell. Physiol. **74**, 57—62 (1969).

Madoc-Jones, H., Bruce, W. R.: On the mechanism of the lethal action of 5-fluorouracil on mouse L cells. Cancer Res. **28**, 1976—1981 (1968).

Makinodan, T., Santos, G. W., Quinn, R. P.: Immunosuppressive drugs. Pharmacol. Rev. **22**, 189—247 (1970).

Mandel, H. G.: The incorporation of 5-fluorouracil into RNA and its molecular consequences. Progr. molec. subcell. Biol. **1**, 82—135 (1969).

Mazza, F., Sobell, H. M., Kartha, G.: Base-pairing configurations between purines and pyrimidines in the solid state. IV. Crystal and molecular structure of two 1:1 hydrogen-bonded complexes, 1-methyl-5-bromouracil: 9-ethyl-2-aminopurine and 1-methyl-5-fluorouracil: 9-ethyl-2-aminopurine. J. molec. Biol. **43**, 407—422 (1969).

Melnick, J. L., Stinebaugh, S. E., Rapp, F.: Incomplete simian papovavirus SV40, formation of non-infectious viral antigen in the presence of fluorouracil. J. exp. Med. **119**, 313—326 (1964).

Mertes, M. P., Saheb, S. E.: Use of sulfur tetrafluoride in synthesis of potential anticancer agents. J. pharm. Sci. **52**, 508—509 (1963).

Mitchell, M. S., DeConti, R. C.: Immunosuppression by 5-fluorouracil. Cancer **29**, 884—889 (1970).

Moertel, C. G., Reitemeier, R. J.: Fluorouracil, floxuridine controversy. J. Amer. med. Assoc. **201**, 780 (1967).

Morse, P. A., Potter, V. R.: Pyrimidine metabolism in tissue culture cells derived from rat hepatomas. I. Suspension cell cultures derived from Novikoff hepatoma. Cancer Res. **25**, 499—508 (1965).

Mukherjee, K. L., Boohar, J., Wentland, D., Ansfield, F. J., Heidelberger, C.: Studies on fluorinated pyrimidines. XVI. Metabolism of 5-fluorouracil-2-^{14}C and 5-fluoro-2'-deoxyuridine-2-^{14}C in cancer patients. Cancer Res. **23**, 49—66 (1963a).

Mukherjee, K. L., Curreri, A. R., Javid, M., Heidelberger, C.: Studies on fluorinated pyrimidines. XVII. Tissue distribution of 5-fluorouracil-2-^{14}C and 5-fluoro-2'-deoxyuridine in cancer patients. Cancer Res. **23**, 67—77 (1963b).

Mukherjee, K. L., Heidelberger, C.: Studies on fluorinated pyrimidines. IX. The degradation of 5-fluorouracil-6-^{14}C. J. biol. Chem. **235**, 433—437 (1960).

Mukherjee, K. L., Heidelberger, C.: Studies on fluorinated pyrimidines. XV. Inhibition of the incorporation of formate-^{14}C into DNA thymine of Ehrlich ascites carcinoma cells by 5-fluoro-2'-deoxyuridine-5'-monophosphate and related compounds. Cancer Res. **22**, 815—822 (1962).

Munyon, W., Salzman, N. P.: The incorporation of 5-fluorouracil into poliovirus. Virology **18**, 95—101 (1962).

NAKADA, D., MAGASANIK, B.: The roles of inducer and catabolite repressor in the synthesis of β-galactosidase by *Escherichia coli*. J. molec. Biol. 8, 105—127 (1964).
NAONO, S., GROS, F.: Éffects d'un analogue de base nucleique sur la biosynthèse de proteines bacteriennes. Changements de la composition globale des proteins. C. R. Acad. Sci. (Paris) **250**, 3527—3529 (1960a).
NAONO, S., GROS, F.: Synthèse par *E. coli* d'une phosphatase modifiee en presence d'un analogue primidique. C. R. Acad. Sci. (Paris) **250**, 3889—3891 (1960b).
NESNOW, S., MIAN, A.M., OKI, T., DEXTER, D. L., HEIDELBERGER, C.: Fluorinated pyrimidines. XLI. Synthesis of 5-trifluoromethyl-3'-deoxyuridine and 5-fluoro-3'-deoxyuridine. J. med. Chem. **15**, 676—677 (1972).
NIZHIZAWA, Y., CASIDA, J.E., ANDERSON, S.W., HEIDELBERGER, C.: 3',5'-Diesters of 5-fluoro-2'-deoxyuridine: synthesis and biological activity. Biochem. Pharmacol. **14**, 1605—1620 (1965).
OCKEY, C.H., HSU, T.C., RICHARDSON, L.C.: Chromosome damage induced by 5-fluoro-2'-deoxyuridine in relation to the cell cycle of the Chinese hamster. J. nat. Cancer Inst. **40**, 465—475 (1968).
OKI, T., HEIDELBERGER, C.: Fluorinated pyrimidines. XXXIX. Effects of 5-trifluoromethyl-2'-deoxyuridine on the replication of vaccinia viral messenger RNA and protein. Molec. Pharmacol. **7**, 653—662 (1971).
ØYEN, T.B., LALAND, S.G.: 5-Fluoropyrimidin-2-one deoxyriboside and its growth-inhibiting properties. Biochim. biophys. Acta (Amst.) **182**, 567—569 (1969).
PAUL, J., HAGIWARA, A.: A kinetic study of the action of 5-fluoro-2'-deoxyuridine on synthetic processes in mammalian cells. Biochim. biophys. Acta (Amst.) **61**, 243—249 (1962).
PECK, R.M., MARKEY, F., YUDKIN, M.D.: Effect of 5-fluorouracil on β-galactosidase synthesis in an *Escherichia coli* mutant resistant to catabolite repression of the Lac operon. FEBS Lett. **16**, 43—44 (1971).
PITOT, H.C., PERAINO, C.: Studies on the induction and repression of enzymes in rat liver. J. biol. Chem. **239**, 1783—1788 (1964).
PITTILLO, R.F., RAY, B.J.: Chemotherapeutic activity of 5-fluorocytosine against a lethal *Candida albicans* infection in mice. Appl. Microbiol. **17**, 773—774 (1969).
PUJMAN, V., SANDBERG, J., HOWSDEN, L., GOLDIN, A.: The effect of fluoxidine on L-1210 leukemia in mice. Neoplasma (Bratisl.) **17**, 133—136 (1970).
REICHARD, P., SKÖLD, O., KLEIN, G., REVESZ, L., MAGNUSSON, P.H.: Studies on resistance against 5-fluorouracil. I. Enzymes of the uracil pathway during development of resistance. Cancer Res. **22**, 235—243 (1962).
REMY, D.C., SUNTHANKAR, A.V., HEIDELBERGER, C.: Studies on fluorinated pyrimidines. XIV. The synthesis of derivatives of 5-fluoro-2'-deoxyuridine-5'-phosphate and related compounds. J. org. Chem. **27**, 2491—2500 (1961).
REYES, P.: The synthesis of 5-fluorouridine-5'-phosphate by a pyrimidine phosphoribosyltransferase of mammalian origin. I. Some properties of the enzyme from P1534 J mouse leukemic cells. Biochemistry 8, 2057—2062 (1969).
REYES, P., HALL, T.C.: Synthesis of 5-fluorouridine-5'-phosphate by a pyrimidine phosphoribosyltransferase of mammalian origin. II. Correlation between the tumor levels of the enzyme and the 5-fluorouracil-promoted increase in survival of tumor-bearing mice. Biochem. Pharmacol. **18**, 2587—2590 (1969).
REYES, P., HEIDELBERGER, C.: Fluorinated pyrimidines. XXVI. Mammalian thymidylate synthetase: Its mechanism of action and inhibition by fluorinated nucleotides. Molec. Pharmacol. **1**, 14—30 (1965).
RICH, M.A., BOLAFFI, J.L., KNOLL, J.E., CHEONG, L., EIDINOFF, M.L.: Growth inhibition of a human cell strain by 5-fluorouracil, 5-fluorouridine, and 5-fluoro-2'-deoxyuridine-reversal studies. Cancer Res. **18**, 730—735 (1958).
ROBINS, M.J., NAIK, S.R.: Nucleic acid related compounds. III. A facile synthesis of 5-fluorouracil bases and nucleosides by direct fluorination. J. Amer. chem. Soc. **93**, 5277—5278 (1971).
ROBINS, M.J., NAIK, S.R.: A direct synthesis of 5-fluorocytosine and its nucleosides using trifluoromethyl hypofluorite. J. chem. Soc. chem. Commun., 18—19 (1972).
ROGERS, H.J., PERKINS, H.R.: 5-Fluorouracil and mucopeptide biosynthesis by *Staph. aureus*. Biochem. J. **77**, 448—459 (1960).
ROGERS, W.I., HARTMAN, A.C., PALM, P.E., OKSTEIN, C., KENSLER, C.L.: The fate of 5-trifluoromethyl-2'-deoxyuridine in monkeys, dogs, mice, and tumor-bearing mice. Cancer Res. **29**, 953—961 (1969).
ROGERS, W.I., WILSON, J.A.: Determination of labile trifluoromethyl compounds with a fluoride-ion electrode: differential analysis of 5-trifluoromethyluracil and 5-trifluoromethyl-2'-deoxyuridine. An. Biochem. **32**, 31—37 (1969).

ROSEN, B.: Characteristics of 5-fluorouracil-induced synthesis of alkaline phosphatase. J. molec. Biol. **11**, 845—850 (1965).
ROSEN, B., ROTHMAN, F., WEIGERT, M. G.: Miscoding caused by 5-fluorouracil. J. molec. Biol. **44**, 363—375 (1969).
ROUSSELOT, L. M., COLE, D. R., GROSSI, C. E., CONTE, A. J., GONZALES, E. M., PASTERNAK, B. S.: A five year progress report on the effectiveness of intraluminal chemotherapy (5-fluorouracil) adjuvant to surgery for colorectal cancer. Amer. J. Surg. **115**, 140—157 (1968).
RUECKERT, R. R., MUELLER, G. C.: Studies on unbalanced growth in tissue culture. I. Induction and consequences of thymidine deficiency. Cancer Res. **20**, 1584—1591 (1960).
RUTMAN, R. J., CANTAROW, A., PASCHKIS, K. E.: Studies in 2-acetylaminofluorene carcinogenesis. III. The utilization of uracil-2-^{14}C by preneoplastic rat liver and rat hepatoma. Cancer Res. **14**, 119—134 (1954).
RYAN, K. J., ACTON, E. M., GOODMAN, L.: Chemical synthesis of 2′-deoxy-5-(trifluoromethyl)-uridine and its α anomer. J. org. Chem. **31**, 1181—1184 (1966).
SALZMAN, N. P.: The rate of formation of vaccinia deoxyribonucleic acid and vaccinia virus. Virology **10**, 150—152 (1960).
SALZMAN, N. P., SHATKIN, A. J., SEBRING, E. D.: Viral protein and DNA synthesis in vaccinia virus-infected HeLa cell cultures. Virology **19**, 542—550 (1963).
SANTI, D. V., SAKAI, T. T.: Thymidylate synthetase. Model studies of inhibition by 5-trifluoroethyl-2′-deoxyuridylic acid. Biochemistry **10**, 3598—3607 (1971).
SARTORELLI, A. C., CREASEY, W. A.: The antineoplastic and biochemical effects of some 5-fluoropyrimidines. Cancer Res. **27**, 2201—2206 (1967).
SCHMÄHL, D., OSSWALD, H.: Experimental studies of the carcinogenic activity of antitumor and immunosuppressive agents. Arzneimittel-Forsch. **20**, 1461—1467 (1970).
SHIMURA, Y., KAIZER, H., NATHANS, D.: Fragments of MS 2 RNA as messengers for specific bacteriophage proteins: fragments from fluorouracil-containing particles. J. molec. Biol. **38**, 453—455 (1968).
SHIMURA, Y., MOSES, R. E., NATHANS, D.: Coliphage MS2 containing 5-fluorouracil. I. Preparation and physical properties. J. molec. Biol. **12**, 266—279 (1965).
SHIMURA, Y., MOSES, R. E., NATHANS, D.: Coliphage MS2 containing 5-fluorouracil. II. RNA-deficient particles formed in the presence of 5-fluorouracil. J. molec. Biol. **28**, 95—102 (1967).
SKÖLD, O.: Enzymic ribosidation and ribotidation of 5-fluorouracil by extracts of the Ehrlich ascites tumor. Biochim. biophys. Acta (Amst.) **29**, 651 (1958).
SKÖLD, O., MAGNUSSON, P-H., REVESZ, L.: Studies on resistance against 5-fluorouracil. III. Selective value of resistant uridine kinase-deficient tumor cells. Cancer Res. **22**, 1226—1229 (1962).
SLAPIKOFF, S., BERG, P.: Mechanism of ribonucleic acid polymerase action. Effect of nearest neighbors on competition between uridine triphosphate and uridine triphosphate analogs for incorporation into ribonucleic acid. Biochemistry **6**, 3654—3658 (1967).
SMITH, C. G., GRADY, J. E., KUPIECKI, F. P.: Blood and urine levels of antitumor agents determined with cell culture methods. Cancer Res. **25**, 241—245 (1965).
STRIJKERT, P. J.: The effect of 5-fluorouracil on induced enzyme synthesis in yeast. Biochim. biophys. Acta (Amst.) **182**, 262—263 (1969).
SUNDARALINGAM, M.: Conformations of the furanose ring in nucleic acids and other carbohydrate derivatives in the solid state. J. Amer. chem. Soc. **87**, 599—606 (1965).
SUTIC, D., DJORDJEVIC, B.: Effect of 5-fluorouracil on antigenic properties of tobacco mosaic virus. Nature (Lond.) **203**, 434—435 (1964).
SZER, W., SHUGAR, D.: Preparation of poly-5-fluorouridylic acid and the properties of halogenated polyuridylic acids and their complexes with polyadenylic acid. Acta biochim. pol **10**, 219—231 (1963).
TAYLOR, J. H., HAUT, W. F., TUNG, J.: Effects of fluorodeoxyuridine on DNA replication, chromosome breakage, and reunion. Proc. nat. Acad. Sci. (Wash.) **48**, 190—198 (1962).
TEMIN, H. M.: Nature of the provirus of Rous sarcoma. Nat. Cancer Inst. Monogr. **17**, 557—570 (1964).
TEMIN, H. M., MIZUTANI, S.: RNA-dependent DNA polymerase in virions of Rous sarcoma virus. Nature (Lond.) **226**, 1211—1213 (1970).
TERSHAK, D. R.: Effect of 5-fluorouracil on poliovirus-induced RNA polymerase. J. molec. Biol. **21**, 43—50 (1966).
THOMASZ, A., BOREK, E.: The mechanism of an osmotic instability induced in *E. coli* K-12 by 5-fluorouracil. Biochemistry **1**, 543—552 (1962).
TOMITA, K.I., KATZ, L., RICH, A.: Crystal structure of the intermolecular complex 9-ethyladenine: 1-methyl-5-fluorouracil. J. molec. Biol. **30**, 545—549 (1967).
UMEDA, M., HEIDELBERGER, C.: Fluorinated pyrimidines. XXX. Comparative studies of fluorinated pyrimidines with various cell lines. Cancer Res. **28**, 2529—2538 (1968).

UMEDA, M., HEIDELBERGER, C.: Fluorinated pyrimidines. XXXI. Mechanisms of inhibition of vaccinia virus replication in HeLa cells by pyrimidine nucleosides. Proc. Soc. exp. Biol. (N.Y.) **130**, 24—29 (1969).

UTZ, J.P.: Current status of the chemotherapy of systemic mycoses. Ann. intern. Med. **68**, 1177—1178 (1968).

VAN DYK, J.J., CLARKSON, B.D., DUSCHINSKY, R., KELVER, O., LA SALA, E., KRAKOFF, I.H.: Clinical evaluation of 5-bromo-5-fluoro-6-methoxy-dihydro-2′-deoxyuridine. Cancer Res. **27**, 2129—2136 (1967).

VIETTI, T., EGGERDING, F., VALERIOTE, F.: Combined effect of x-radiation and 5-fluorouracil on survival of transplanted leukemic cells. J. nat. Cancer Inst. **49**, 865—870 (1971).

VOET, D., RICH, A.: The structure of an intermolecular complex between cytosine and 5-fluorouracil. J. Amer. chem. Soc. **91**, 3069—3075 (1969).

WAGNER, N.J., HEIDELBERGER, C.: Some effects of 5-fluoroorotate and 5-fluorouracil on the soluble ribonucleic acid of rat liver. Biochim. biophys. Acta (Amst.) **61**, 373—379 (1962).

WAHBA, A.J., GARDNER, R.S., BASILIO, C., MILLER, R.S., SPEYER, J.F., LENGYEL, P.: Synthetic polynucleotides and the amino acid code. VIII. Proc. nat. Acad. Sci. (Wash.) **49**, 116—121 (1963).

WELLINGS, P.C., AWDRY, P.N., BORS, F.H., JONES, B.R., BROWN, D.C., KAUFMAN, H.E.: Double-blind clinical evaluation of trifluorothymidine in the treatment of herpes simplex ulcers of the cornea. Amer. J. Ophthamol. **73**, 932—942 (1972).

WEMPEN, I., DUSCHINSKY, R., KAPLAN, L., FOX, J.J.: Thiation of nucleosides. IV. The synthesis of 5-fluoro-2′-deoxycytidine and related compounds. J. Amer. chem. Soc. **83**, 4755—4766 (1961).

WEMPEN, I., FOX, J.J.: Pyrimidines. II. Synthesis of 6-fluorouracil. J. med. Chem. **7**, 207—209 (1964a).

WEMPEN, I., FOX, J.J.: Spectrophotometric studies of nucleic acid derivatives and related compounds. VI. On the structure of certain 5- and 6-halogenouracils and cytosines. J. Amer. chem. Soc. **86**, 2475—2477 (1964b).

WILKINSON, D.S., ČIHÁK, A., PITOT, H.C.: Inhibition of ribosomal ribonucleic acid maturation in rat liver by 5-fluoroorotic acid resulting in the selective labeling of cytoplasmic messenger ribonucleic acid. J. biol. Chem. **246**, 6418—6427 (1971).

WILLEN, R.: Polyacrylamide-agarose electrophoretic patterns of the RNA labeling in liver cytoplasm and total liver of 5-fluorouracil-treated rats. Hoppe-Seyler's Z. Physiol. Chem. **351**, 1141—1150 (1970).

WILLIAMS, A.C., KLEIN, E.: Experiences with local chemotherapy and immunotherapy in premalignant and malignant skin lesions. Cancer **25**, 450—462 (1970).

WITTMANN-LIEBOLD, B., WITTMANN, H.C.: Lokalisierung von Aminosäure-austauschen bei Spontanmutanten und nach Fluoruracileisbau isolierten Mutanten des Tabakmosaikvirus. Z. Vererbungsl. **97**, 218—225 (1965).

WOLBERG, W.H.: The effect of 5-fluorouracil on DNA thymine synthesis in human tumors. Cancer Res. **29**, 2137—2144 (1969).

WOLBERG, W.H.: Biochemical approaches to prediction of response in solid tumors. Nat. Cancer Inst. Monogr. **34**, 189—195 (1971).

WOLBERG, W.H.: Response of DNA thymine synthesis in human tumor and normal tissue to 5-fluorouracil. Cancer Res. **32**, 130—132 (1972).

WOLBERG, W.H., ANSFIELD, F.J.: The relation of thymidine labeling index in human tumors *in vitro* to the effectiveness of 5-fluorouracil chemotherapy. Cancer Res. **31**, 448—450 (1971).

YAGIL, E., SILBERSTEIN, N.: Decay of normal and 5-fluorouracil-substituted messenger ribonucleic acid of alkaline phosphatase in *Escherichia coli*. J. Bact. **100**, 1364—1370 (1969).

YUNG, N.C., BURCHENAL, J.H., FECHER, R., DUSCHINSKY, R., FOX, J.J.: Nucleosides. XI. Synthesis of 1-β-D-arabinosyl-5-fluorouracil and related nucleosides. J. Amer. chem. Soc. **83**, 4060—4065 (1961).

Chapter 42

Arabinosylcytosine

William A. Creasey

With 1 Figure

Introduction

Arabinosylcytosine (1-β-D-arabinofuranosylcytosine; cytosine arabinoside; cytosar; ara-C; cytarabine) is a member of a class of nucleosides in which D-arabinose constitutes the pentose sugar moiety. Thus, these compounds are analogs of ribonucleosides in which the hydroxyl group at the 2′-position is inverted. However, in most respects the arabinosides do not behave biologically as ribonucleoside analogs. Certain arabinosides are naturally occurring, both arabinosylthymine and arabinosyluracil (ara-U) having been isolated from the sponge *Cryptotethya crypta* (Bergman and Feeney, 1951; Bergman and Burke, 1955). Cohen (1963) has reviewed some aspects of the occurrence, isolation, and relevance to chemotherapy of the arabinosides, and suggested a possible role for these nucleosides in aging. The same author in a later review (Cohen, 1966) has outlined methods for chemical synthesis of these compounds, the metabolism of ara-C and ara-U in bacteria, and some effects of the arabinosides on mammalian cells. Much of the pharmacological information regarding ara-C that was available through 1968 may be found briefly reviewed in an article on cancer chemotherapy by Sartorelli and Creasey (1969). Clinical brochures that include some information about the chemistry, antitumor activity in experimental systems, and preliminary data obtained in man, have been prepared by Livingston and Carter (1968) and the Upjohn Company (1970). Notari et al. (1972) have defined the stability of the drug under various storage conditions and found that at neutral pH the drug retains 90 % of its potency after 6 months at room temperature.

In this chapter the intent is to present an outline of studies carried out on the mechanisms of action, metabolism, biological interactions, and cell-kinetic relationships of ara-C. The major emphasis throughout will be on the enzymatic factors that are involved in the action of this important therapeutic agent. Some of the chemical and biological aspects of the agent will also be discussed. Clinical aspects of ara-C form the topic of Chapter 43 of this volume.

Synthesis and Structure-Activity Relationships of the Arabinosides

A variety of synthetic routes have been utilized to obtain the arabinosides and their derivatives; Cohen (1966) has reviewed some of these. Fox et al. (1957) described the synthesis of arabinosylthymine (spongothymidine) starting from the trityl derivative of ribofuranosylthymine. This was treated with methanesulfonyl chloride to give the *O*-mesyl derivative, cyclized by reaction with aqueous methanol and ammonia, and finally subjected to acid hydrolysis. A convenient procedure for the synthesis of arabinoside diphosphates involves phosphorylation of ribonucleosides with polyphosphoric acid and then hydrolysis of the cyclized product (WALWICK et al., 1959; ROBERTS and DEKKER, 1967). HUNTER (1965) started from 1-β-D-xylofuranosyl uracil nucleosides, which were first blocked at the 3'- and 5'-positions and then had a 2'-O-alkyl sulfonyl group introduced; the products underwent transformation to arabinosides via the 2',3'-epoxy derivatives. Apart from ara-C and ara-U, the 5-halogenated and 5-methyl substituted compounds were also prepared by this method. SMRT (1967) obtained arabinoside monophosphates by phosphorylating the 2',3'-di-O-benzoyl derivatives of the nucleosides with cyanoethyl phosphate in the presence of dicyclohexylcarbodiimide. The cytosine derivatives required protection of the N_4-position with dimethylaminomethylene or acetyl groups. A number of N_4-substituted cytosine and 5-fluorocytosine arabinosides were prepared by thiation with phosphorus pentasulfide, alkylation, and reaction with nucleophiles (WEMPEN et al., 1968). FALCO and FOX (1968) first converted 5'-deoxyuridine to a 2,2'-anhydro compound by reaction with thiocarbonyldiimidazole, and then, by successive benzoylation, thiation, and hydrolysis with alcoholic ammonia, obtained 5'-deoxyarabinosylcytosine. The 3-N-oxide of ara-C was prepared by heating the parent compound with m-chlorobenzoic acid (PANZICA et al., 1971). Reaction with partially hydrolyzed phosphorus oxychloride has been employed to synthesize both 2,2'-O-cyclocytidine from cytidine (KANAI et al., 1970), and 5'-O-methyl derivatives of both ara-C and ara-U from 5'-O-methylcytidine (GIZIEWICZ et al., 1972). An alternative method for obtaining O-methyl derivatives of ara-C involved direct methylation with dimethylsulfate (DARZYNKIEWICZ et al., 1972). Acylation of ara-C with acid anhydrides was used to prepare the butyryl, benzoyl, palmitoyl, and steroyl-O-esters which may be of value as depot forms of ara-C (MONTGOMERY and THOMAS, 1972; WARNER et al., 1972). Finally, the L-enantiomer of ara-C was synthesized from the aminooxazoline derivative of L-arabinose by initial reaction with cyanoacetylene to bring about ring closure, followed by acid hydrolysis of the resulting cyclonucleoside (GISH et al., 1971; TOLMAN and ROBINS, 1971).

Changes in the base or sugar moieties profoundly affect the activity of the arabinosides as tumor inhibitors or as antiviral or immunosuppressive agents. The L-enantiomer of ara-C has no significant activity against mouse leukemia L1210 or Ridgeway osteogenic sarcoma (TOLMAN and ROBINS, 1971), both of which respond to therapy with ara-C, nor is it a substrate for the pyrimidine nucleoside deaminase from *Escherichia coli*. In contrast, conversion of ara C to the 5' ada mantoate ester did not lead to any marked loss in activity against leukemia L1210. However, the schedule dependence so characteristic of ara-C was lost, together with the reversal of activity by deoxycytidine (NEIL et al., 1970). In view of the retention of antitumor activity by this and other esters, including the octanoate, benzoate, palmitate, butyrate, and stearate, compounds of this type might have some application as depot forms of ara-C. Deamination to ara-U produces a compound that is virtually completely inactive (CHU and FISCHER, 1962); induction of a megaloblastic marrow that has been described during administration of ara-U probably resulted from amination of this material at the nucleotide level (CREASEY et al., 1968). Substitution of fluorine at the 5 position of the cytosine ring to give arabinosyl-5-fluorocytosine did not cause loss of inhibitory potency against DNA synthesis and cellular proliferation of normal mouse tissues (LENAZ et al., 1969) and HeLa cell cultures (KIM et al., 1966). The N_4-hydroxy derivatives of both ara-C and arabinosyl-5-fluorocytosine displayed growth inhibitory activity against L1210 leukemia and, to a much lesser extent, a BURKITT's tumor culture (BURCHENAL et al., 1967; DOLLINGER et al., 1967). This is in marked contrast to the loss of activity that accompanies N_4-butyrylation of the 3′,5-di-*O*-butyryl-ester of ara-C; 2′,3′-di-*O*-ester formation also leads to loss of activity (Montgomery and Thomas, 1972). The N_4-methyl and hydrazino derivatives of ara-C and its 5-fluorinated analog were also inactive as tumor inhibitors (Dollinger et al., 1967). However, this class of N_4-substituted derivatives is of interest because the compounds are not subject to deamination by either the mouse kidney or the human liver deaminase systems.

Thioarabinosylcytosine appeared to have similar effects to ara-C in terms of reducing the mitotic index and producing giant cells in L cell cultures (Bremerskov et al., 1970). Kimball et al. (1966) showed that arabinosyl-6-mercaptopurine exerted both antitumor and inhibitory biochemical effects on the Ehrlich ascites carcinoma. Cyclocytidine, a compound found to be active against leukemia L1210, indeed to have a better therapeutic index than ara-C itself (Hoshi et al., 1971), apparently is slowly converted to ara-C; furthermore, it is resistant to enzymatic deamination. Another derivative that may be resistant to deamination, and which displays considerable activity against the L1210 leukemia, is the 3-*N*-oxide of ara-C (Panzica et al., 1971). Arabinosyladenine, arabinosylguanine, arabinosylhypoxanthine, and arabinosyl-5-fluorouracil exhibit varied activity as growth inhibitors for bacteria or mammalian tumors (Cohen, 1963, 1966). The antitumor effect of ara-C-5′-monophosphate on L1210 leukemia apparently requires an initial dephosphorylation to the free nucleoside which then enters the cells (Schrecker and Goldin, 1968).

Assay Methods for Arabinosylcytosine

Many pharmacological studies on the distribution and metabolism of ara-C have utilized tritium labeled drug. Basically, all of these procedures involve preliminary determination of the levels of radioactivity in body fluids, followed by chromatographic separation of ara-C from its metabolite ara-U. Blood and plasma are usually deproteinized before chromatography, which is commonly performed on paper. An example of such a study is that of Creasey et al. (1966), one of the earliest clinical investigations of this drug.

As a second alternative approach, and one that is in many ways more convenient since it obviates the use of radioisotopes, is to carry out a bioassay using sensitive cell lines or microorganisms. Pitillo and Hunt (1967) and Hunt and Pitillo (1968) have described the use of actinobolin-resistant strains of *Streptococcus faecalis* as an assay system for ara-C. In this case, the authors used the method to follow the plasma clearance of ara-C in mice. More recently, Hanka et al. (1970) used the same actinobolin-resistant strain (ATCC 8043), but included in the assay system tetrahydrouridine to inhibit the deamination of ara-C by the organism, a process that would lead to falsely low estimates of drug concentrations. With this modified method, levels of ara-C as low as 0.1 mg/ml could be measured. Borsa et al. (1969) employed L cells in tissue culture to assay for methotrexate and ara-C in mouse serum.

A third approach to the assay of ara-C is to use a biochemical system. In one such procedure described by Baguley and Falkenhaug (1971), the incorporation of tritium labeled thymidine into DNA by suspensions of L cells or mouse spleen cells was employed as the test parameter. This process was so sensitive to ara-C that human plasma concentrations as low as 0.04 µg/ml could be detected. Momparler et al. (1972) determined ara-C by phosphorylating the drug with deoxyuridine kinase and ATP-γ-^{32}P in the presence of magnesium ions. The 5′-ara

CMP was isolated by thin-layer chromatography on DEAE cellulose. This method could detect concentrations of ara-C down to 2.5 mM (0.6 μg/ml).

Biological Actions

A. Antitumor Effects in Experimental Systems

The first example of growth inhibition by ara-C was reported by SLECHTA (1961) who found that both this compound and ara-U inhibited the growth of *Escherichia coli*; this action was reversed by a number of purine and pyrimidine nucleosides. EVANS et al. (1961, 1964a) were the first to report the effect of ara-C on a spectrum of mouse tumors including leukemia L1210, Sarcoma 180, Ehrlich ascites carcinoma, L5178Y lymphoma, and T_4 lymphoma. This inhibition could be reversed or prevented by the administration of deoxycytidine (EVANS and MENGEL, 1964). In studies by DIXON and ADAMSON (1965), ara-C was found to be active as an inhibitor of the growth of the L1210, P288, P388, and K1964 mouse tumors, but to have little or no effect on mast cell tumor P815 or plasma cell tumor YPC. A large spectrum of mouse tumors was tested and 38 were found to be sensitive to ara-C; only one subline of the L1210 leukemia was resistant. Both the Walker 256 ascites tumor and the Novikoff hepatoma of rats were sensitive, but the Dunning leukemia and the Walker 256 solid carcinosarcoma were not (WODINSKY and KENSLER, 1965).

The growth of L5178Y cells in culture was inhibited by ara-C, and in this system deoxycytidine acted as an antagonist (CHU and FISCHER, 1962). Similar effects in terms both of inhibition by ara-C and of protection by deoxycytidine were reported for HeLa S-3 cells (KIM and EIDINOFF, 1965) and Don C cells (YOUNG and FISCHER, 1968). These studies, carried out *in vitro*, provided evidence for imbalanced growth of the treated cells, with formation of giant cells, accumulation of RNA and protein, and some degree of partial synchronization after recovery. This latter phenomenon has also been reported to occur *in vivo* in the LIEBERKÜHN's crypt cells of rats treated with ara-C (VERBIN et al., 1972). The resemblance of some of these findings to "thymineless death" is close, and it is relevant that in several strains of *Escherichia coli* the kinetics of "thymineless death" and lethality from ara-C are identical (ATKINSON and STACEY, 1968; CUMMINGS, 1969). WILKOFF et al. (1967) have found that in cultured L1210 mouse leukemia cells, the kinetics of cell killing are first-order, with the rate of reduction dependent at least in part on the heterogeneity of the cell population.

Ara-C is effective against established as well as newly implanted tumors, but its efficacy does decline with the age of the neoplasms (KLINE et al., 1966; GRISWOLD et al., 1970), probably reflecting the diminished population of actively dividing cells. Much attention has been paid to scheduling of ara-C therapy to take advantage of its cell-cycle dependence. This dependence presumably results from its specificity as an inhibitor of DNA synthesis, which, except for unscheduled repair, is of course restricted to S-phase. It should be borne in mind, however, that the data of KARON and SHIRAKAWA (1969) do not rule out the possibility of an effect late in the G_1 phase of Don C cells, while TOBEY (1972) found in Chinese hamster cell cultures evidence for an effect on transition of cells from G_1 into S, as well as the inhibition of DNA synthesis. Nevertheless, the predominant S-phase activity of ara-C has led to the development of experimental treatment schedules by SKIPPER et al. (1967, 1970) that take account of this relative specificity. Clinical implications of cycle dependence are discussed in Chapter 43.

Many reports have appeared claiming that synergism, or greater than additive antitumor effects, occurred when ara-C was administered in combination with other agents. Thus, when mice bearing L5178Y lymphoma were treated with ara-C and 6-mercaptopurine, greater than additive responses were seen (EVANS et al., 1964a). In this same tumor and the L1210 leukemia, EVANS et al. (1964b) demonstrated that there was synergism between ara-C and mitomycin C or porfiromycin (methyl mitomycin C), provided that the arabinoside was administered at its optimal dosage level. SCHABEL (1968) found that in combination with nitrosourea or cyclophosphamide, ara-C was able to produce a high cure rate in mice with advanced L1210 leukemia which cannot be cured by ara-C alone. In another study, 1,3-*bis*-(2-chloroethyl)-1-nitrosourea (BCNU), also produced a markedly greater suppression of the growth of leukemia L1210 when given in combination with ara-C (TYRER et al., 1968). Consideration of the topic of the place of ara-C in clinical combination chemotherapy may be found in the article by SARTORELLI and CREASEY (1973), and in greater detail in Chapter 43 of this volume.

B. Other Biological Effects

Antitumor action is but one aspect of the generalized growth inhibition produced by ara-C. Effects on cellular proliferation in normal host tissues are also noted. This is particularly true of the bone marrow, where arrest of mitosis occurs together with a megaloblastosis that primarily affects the erythroid precursors (TALLEY and VAITKEVICIUS, 1963; BLOCK et al., 1965). In a system in which marrow recolonization by donor cells occurred after lethal irradiation of mice, ara-C prevented this process from taking place. Its action could be reversed in time and dose-dependent fashion by deoxycytidine (PAPAC et al., 1965a). As was mentioned earlier, the Lieberkühn's crypt cells of rats are sensitive to ara-C (VERBIN et al., 1972). Embryonic development also is susceptible to ara-C, and examples of this are available from species as diverse as the chick (KARNOFSKY and LACON, 1966) and the sea urchin, *Sphaerochinus granularis* (FLICKINGER, 1967). Whereas in the chick, delay in development was associated with the appearance of growth abnormalities, in the sea urchin these were not seen, growth continuing normally once the drug was removed.

The appearance of various morphologic abnormalities during treatment with ara-C has been widely reported, both for man and for experimental animals. This class of lesions has been especially intensively studied in human bone marrow cells in which, apart from megaloblastosis, nuclear bleb formation (AHEARN et al., 1967), chromatid breaks, despiralization, and other abnormalities primarily of the erythroid elements (BELL et al., 1966) are seen. Formation of nucleolar vacuoles, elongation of the nuclei, and decreased retention of stain have been described in human diploid cells (WI-38) treated with ara-C (HENEEN and NICHOLS, 1967). Chromosomal breaks and aberrations are prominent in cultures of human leukocytes exposed to ara-C (KIHLMAN et al., 1963; BREWEN, 1965; BREWEN and CHRISTIE, 1967). The kinetics of production of such breaks in relation to the cell cycle have been examined by BENEDICT et al. (1970) in Don C hamster fibroblasts. Ara-C produced chromatid breaks in all phases of the cell cycle except M, but maximum sensitivity occurred during late S and early G_2 phases. Deoxycytidine prevented breaks from developing in any phase when present simultaneously with ara-C, but when it was added after the antimetabolite, the number of breaks was reduced only during S phase. Interestingly, exposure of these cells to ultraviolet light reduced the frequency of chromatid breaks induced by ara-C in S and G_2 phases in a manner that could be correlated temporally with the decreased uptake of tritiated thymidine into DNA produced by the radiation (BENEDICT and KARON, 1971). Thus, there would appear to be a relation between the genesis of such breaks and DNA synthesis, including nonscheduled repair.

Chromosomal abnormalities would be expected to lead to developmental effects. Thus, teratogenesis has been observed in rat embryos in a number of different laboratories. CHAUBE et al. (1968) described the types of lesions produced, including cleft palate and lip, encephalocele, and deformed appendages and tail, and defined the critical time for teratogenic effects as days 10 to 12 of gestation. Deoxycytidine acted as an antagonist unless more than 10 min elapsed between injection of the two compounds. A similar sensitive period during gestation was noted by RITTER et al. (1971), who further determined that significant, prolonged reduction in DNA synthesis in the fetus had little correlation with the morphological effects produced by ara-C. In *Drosophila melanogaster*, ara-C produced no point mutations but only small chromosome deletions, notably in the spermatocytes and spermatogonia, similar in incidence and degree to those induced by halogenated pyrimidine deoxynucleosides, azauridine, and azacytidine (FAHMY et al., 1966).

As an inhibitor of DNA synthesis, ara-C is effective in suppressing replication of DNA viruses, and indeed was shown to have utility in treating herpes simplex keratitis as early as 1962 (UNDERWOOD). Among the viruses found to be sensitive to ara-C are adenoviruses 2, 7, and 12 (FELDMAN and RAPP, 1966), vaccinia virus (RENIS and JOHNSON, 1962), herpes simplex, vaccinia, pseudorabies, swine pox, fowl pox, and B viruses (BUTHALA, 1964), and Rauscher and Maloney murine leukemia viruses (HIRSCHMAN et al., 1969). Ara-C, when present at appropriate times, can inhibit the replication of Rous sarcoma (BADER, 1966) and avian sarcoma (TEMIN, 1966) viruses although they are RNA viruses, presumably by preventing the formation of the DNA provirus within the infected cells. Among the viruses (mainly RNA type) not inhibited are Newcastle virus, influenza A (PR8), vesicular stomatitis virus, Coe virus, adenoviruses 3, 6, 8, and 10, and hemadsorption type I virus.

Ara-C, both in experimental systems and at the clinical level, has proved to be a very effective agent in suppressing both primary and secondary immune responses (BUSKIRK et al., 1965; FISCHER et al., 1966; MITCHELL et al., 1969). Indeed there is a real possibility that the immunosuppressive activity of the drug may interfere with its antitumor effect (BALDINI et al., 1968). It has been shown, for example, that the dose requirements for suppression of formation of blocking antibodies and of the cell-mediated immune response, may determine whether inhibition of tumor growth can be attained (HEPPNER and CALABRESI, 1972). Immunosuppressive action is retained by the 5′-acylates of ara-C (GRAY et al., 1972).

Metabolic Fate of Arabinosylcytosine

The metabolic fate of ara-C has been investigated rather intensively because of the importance of pharmacodynamic factors in determining the effectiveness of this schedule-dependent drug. Although in aqueous buffered solutions ara-C undergoes deamination to ara-U in a reaction that is catalyzed by anions such as bisulfite, lactate, and phosphate (NOTARI, 1967), this spontaneous conversion does not appear to be significant *in vivo*. Rather, the predominant process is an enzyme catalyzed deamination which was first reported to occur in *Escherichia coli* (PIZER and COHEN, 1960; SLECHTA, 1961; TONO and COHEN, 1962). All the strains of this organism tested deaminated ara-C, and in addition, strains W, B, and 9637 cleaved the glycosyl linkage of ara-U to form free uracil. The first demonstration that mammalian cells in culture were able to deaminate ara-C was made by SMITH et al. (1965) who studied a PPLO-contaminated strain of KB cells. Interestingly, the PPLO strain from these cells could deaminate ara-C in the absence of the KB cells. Ara-U was able to inhibit the deamination. Conversion of ara-C to ara-U *in vivo* was a prominent finding in the earliest clinical pharmacologic studies with this agent (PAPAC et al., 1965b; CREASEY et al., 1966), and was not unexpected in view of the very rapid deamination of 5-iodo-2′-deoxycytidine in man (CALABRESI et al., 1963). Between 86 and 96% of the radioactivity recovered in the urine after administration of tritiated ara-C was present in the form of ara-U; urinary excretion was very rapid and complete. Levels of ara-C in the plasma declined rapidly, becoming undetectable by chromatographic techniques after 20 min (CREASEY et al., 1966). TALLEY et al. (1967), using a biological assay, also found that ara-C became undetectable in human serum within 15 min; only a very limited amount of unchanged drug appeared in the urine. Rates of urinary excretion of radioactivity were compared after administration of labeled ara-C by various routes to a group of children with leukemia. Recovery of radioactivity in the 24 hour urine was similar for all routes, (i.e., 68 to 81%) except intravenous injection (87 to 91%) (TALLEY et al., 1966). When administered into the lateral ventricles of patients through an Ommaya reservoir, ara-C was metabolized very slowly with a half-life of 5.4 to 11.4 h in the spinal fluid (CREASEY et al., 1968). In another study in which different routes were used, the half-life of the tritium body load varied from 3 h (intravenous) to 8.5 h (intrathecal), and the rate of conversion to ara-U was not much affected by the route of administration (FINKELSTEIN et al., 1970). The data obtained by GOLDENBERG (1971) in hamsters would suggest that in this species absorption and/or metabolism of ara-C must be different after oral administration, however, since larger doses were needed to inhibit the A. melanoma number 3 when oral rather than parenteral therapy was used. More recent clinical studies have confirmed these earlier reports of rapid disappearance of ara-C from human plasma, and provided a more complete description, due in many cases to more sensitive assay systems that were employed. In general, a biphasic plasma clearance pattern has been described with values for the initial half-life variously reported as 3 to 9 min (BAGULEY and FALKENHAUG, 1971), 12 min (MULLIGAN and MELLET, 1968; HO and FREI, 1971), and 15 min (MOMPARLER et al., 1972). The secondary phase has a significantly longer half-life, HO and FREI (1971) estimating it to be 111 min.

Although in both mice and dogs the urinary excretion of tritium after administration of labeled ara-C is rapid as in humans (DIXON and ADAMSON, 1965), there are considerable species differences in the rate and extent of metabolism of the drug. In mice the half-life of free drug in the serum has been estimated as 16 (BAGULEY and FALKENHAUG, 1971) and 20 min (BORSA et al., 1969), values close to, although slightly higher than in man. MULLIGAN and MELLETT (1968) described a whole range of half-lives varying from 95 min in dogs, through 43 min in rats and 35 min in hamsters, to no measurable value in monkeys, where no serum ara-C could be detected. Thus, deamination of ara-C proceeded rather slowly in dogs and rats. In no mammals has cleavage of the arabinose moiety been seen.

The enzyme responsible for deamination of ara-C is a pyrimidine nucleoside deaminase. Activity of this type, capable of deaminating cytidine, was described long ago in dog liver (SCHMIDT, 1932) and mouse kidney (GREENSTEIN et al., 1947). Such activity has since been reported in a wide range of animal and human tissues (CREASEY, 1963; HALL and LEVINE, 1967; CAMIENER and SMITH, 1965). The mouse kidney system is one of the two tissues that has been studied most intensively.

CREASEY (1963) found that the 107 fold purified deaminase from this tissue was active against a wide range of substrates. Deoxyribonucleosides were deaminated less rapidly than ribonucleosides, and ara-C even more poorly. Free bases were not substrates in general, except for a small degree of activity against 5-hydroxymethyl and 5-methyl-cytosine. Substitution at the 5-position of the pyrimidine ring increased the rate of deamination by the enzyme. The human liver deaminase was studied by CAMIENER (1967a, b) and a Km value for ara-C established as 1.2 to 1.6×10^{-4} M. Like the mouse kidney enzyme, the human liver deaminase was sulfhydryl dependent. Groups necessary for activity were a 2-keto group, an unsubstituted ring N_3, pentofuranose at position 1′, free 3′-α-OH groups, and a nonphosphorylated 5′-OH. Substitution by chlorine or bromine at the 5-position increased the rate of deamination. Inhibitory activity was increased by N_4 substitution in the order: methylamino, keto, hydrazino, thio, amino, hydroxyamino. The most effective enzyme inhibitor was N_4-hydroxymethyl-2′-deoxycytidine, when ara-C was used as the substrate. DOLLINGER et al. (1967) extended these studies with the human liver and mouse kidney deaminases to a variety of derivatives of ara-C. Both ara-C and its 5-fluorinated derivate were deaminated at the same rate. Replacement of the amino group at the 4 position by hydroxylamino, methylamino, hydrazino, or acetylamino functions led to loss of ability to serve as a substrate. The N_4 hydroxyl derivatives of 2′-deoxycytidine, 5-methyl-2′-deoxycytidine, and 5-fluoro-2′-deoxycytidine were not deaminated, but they functioned as potent inhibitors of the deaminases.

Although many compounds have been found to inhibit the deamination of ara-C, the most effective compound is tetrahydrouridine, synthesized by catalytic reduction of cytidine in the presence of rhodium, followed by hydrolysis of the intermediate (HANZE, 1967). Tetrahydrouridine is a potent inhibitor of the partial or regulatory type, with the reduced rate of ara-U formation dependent on preincubation (CAMIENER and SMITH, 1968). In both dogs and monkeys, pretreatment with tetrahydrouridine produced a marked increase in both the plasma half-life of ara-C and the excretion of unchanged drug in the urine (MULLIGAN and MELLETT, 1968).

Biochemical Studies with Arabinosylcytosine

Biochemical studies with ara-C have focused on five major areas: uptake and phosphorylation of the drug, inhibition of DNA synthesis in general, interaction with the ribonucleoside diphosphate reductase system, inhibition of DNA polymerase, and incorporation of the analog into nucleic acids. These areas of study will be reviewed, and in addition, the approaches that have been made toward elucidating the mechanisms of resistance to ara-C will be examined.

A. Uptake and Phosphorylation of Ara-C

The earliest work of CHU and FISCHER (1962) showed that metabolic phosphorylation was a necessary prerequisite for ara-C to inhibit cellular proliferation. Indeed, there appears to be a relationship between the ability of human and mouse leukemic cells to take up and retain ara-C in phosphorylated form, and the response of the cells to drug (KESSEL, 1967; KESSEL and HALL, 1967; KESSEL et al., 1967). As with other studies undertaken by KESSEL and his coworkers, the intracellular label derived from tritiated ara-C that is retained by the cells after thorough washing, is assumed to be in the form of nucleotides. This affords a rapid and convenient form of assay. The transport of ara-C into mammalian cells is a rapid process, and of the intracellular material, 70 % or more is in the form of nucleotides, with the 5′-triphosphate as the major component. Deoxycytidine profoundly inhibits both uptake and phosphorylation of ara-C, but since the nucleoside itself is not concentrated by cells, it is most probable that the reduced uptake is merely a reflection of the failure to accumulate the phosphate esters (Chu and Fischer, 1965; Creasey et al., 1968; Schrecker and Urshel, 1968; Uchida et al., 1968). This inhibition by deoxycytidine of the phosphorylation of ara-C undoubtedly represents a major factor in prevention of the antitumor and antiviral effects of the analog, both *in vitro* (Chu and Fischer, 1962, 1965; Renis and Johnson, 1962) and *in vivo* (Evans and Mengel, 1964). Furthermore, the implication clearly is that the same kinase is responsible for the phosphorylation of both deoxycytidine and ara-C. Kozai and Sugino (1971) studied the system which phosphorylates pyrimidine nucleosides, including ara-C, in calf thymus. Kinetic study of fairly crude preparations was the technique primarily employed. Cytidine kinase and deoxycytidine kinase activities were separable, the former enzyme being apparently unable to phosphorylate deoxycytidine and ara-C. Further phosphorylation to the diphosphate esters also was catalyzed by two different enzymes, one for dCMP and ara-CMP, the other for CMP; this was concluded on the basis of the differential effects of glutathione. Formation of triphosphates appeared to occur by a common enzymatic mechanism. As a critical agent in the activation of ara-C, deoxycytidine kinase has been given much attention. The enzyme occurs at highest levels in lymphoid tissues, and calf thymus afforded a very useful source for studies by Durham and Ives (1967, 1969). The partially purified kinase had little phosphate donor specificity, ATP, GTP, UTP, and dATP showing some activity. Although deoxycytidine was the preferred substrate, ara-C, deoxyguanosine, and deoxyadenosine could all be phosphorylated, and each functioned as a competitive inhibitor for the other substrates. The enzyme was markedly inhibited by dCTP, and less efficiently by dCDP and dCMP; dTTP was able to reverse the inhibition produced by dCTP. Momparler and Fischer (1968) purified deoxycytidine kinase about 100 fold from calf thymus cells. They determined the Km values for the enzyme as 4.0×10^{-5} M for ara-C compared with 1.4×10^{-5} M for deoxycytidine, thus explaining the efficacy of deoxycytidine reversal. It is of interest that phosphorylation of ara-C was more sensitive to the effects of inhibitors such as dCTP than was the corresponding reaction with deoxycytidine. Inhibition by dCTP was competitive with ATP and noncompetitive with ara-C or deoxycytidine.

The deoxycytidine kinase system of L1210 cells has been especially targeted for study by Kessel and his colleagues (Kessel, 1968a, b; Kessel and Shurin, 1968). Uptake of ara-C by these cells was very rapid, a cell/medium concentration ratio of 1 being achieved in 1 min. Loss of label from the cells was biphasic with the initial fast phase being inhibited by UO_2^{2+}; at 0° this rapid exit phase was inhibited. Phosphorylation of deoxycytidine by the partially purified enzyme (150 fold) was competitively inhibited by ara-C, dCMP, dCDP, and dCTP. The K_i for deoxycytidine was forty times smaller than the Km for ara-C. Thus, in these cells too the effectiveness of deoxycytidine reversal rests on relative affinities for the enzyme. The leukemia L1210 deoxycytidine kinase was estimated to have a molecular weight of about 60000, it exhibited a dependence on divalent cations, notably Mg^{2+} or Mn^{2+}, and was relatively insensitive to sulfhydryl inhibitors and surface active agents. Grindey et al. (1967, 1968) found that administration of uridine to mice bearing L1210 leukemia prior to a suboptimal dose of ara-C greatly increased the antitumor effect of the analog. Experiments performed with a supernatant derived from mouse spleen showed that the rate of phosphorylation of ara-C with UTP as the phosphate donor was twice that obtained with ATP, whereas in contrast, the phosphorylation of deoxycytidine was only slightly increased with

UTP. Thus, formation of UTP from administered uridine, with resultant stimulation of the anabolism of ara-C to its nucleotides, affords a reasonable explanation of the increased antitumor efficacy.

The subject of deoxycytidine kinase will be returned to later, when the problem of resistance to ara-C is considered, which appears in many cases to involve changes with respect to the kinase.

B. Inhibition of DNA Biosynthesis

The volume of literature testifying to an inhibitory effect of ara-C on the biosynthesis of DNA is very extensive, so that it is impossible to document every reported instance of such activity. Thus, this chapter will be confined to giving some idea of the variety of situations in which this inhibitory effect has been described, and to pointing out some of the findings that are particularly suggestive of the type of mechanisms involved.

One aspect of this area of study that has caused controversy, as to the underlying biochemical mechanism, is the selectivity of the inhibitory effect. Incorporation of labeled thymidine, of radioactivity derived from ribonucleosides such as cytidine and uridine, and of inorganic phosphate labeled with ^{32}P, has been observed fairly generally to be inhibited in the presence of ara-C. On the other hand, the incorporation of deoxycytidine has been found to be frequently unaffected, or even enhanced. This type of finding is suggestive of interference with nucleotide interconversions.

Uptake of precursors into both the ribonucleotide pools and RNA has not been significantly affected in most of the systems studied. This lack of effect of ara-C ties in both with the picture akin to "thymineless death" that has been reported in *Escherichia coli* (Atkinson and Stacey, 1968; Cummings, 1969), and with the failure of the drug to inhibit steroid-mediated enzyme induction in hepatoma cell cultures (Peterkofsky and Tomkins, 1967).

The earliest reports of inhibition of DNA synthesis described the effects of ara-C on cells in tissue culture, including L5178Y lymphoma (Chu and Fischer, 1962, 1968), HeLa cells (Young and Hodas, 1965; Kim and Eidinoff, 1965), and L cells (Silagi, 1965). In these systems, the incorporation of thymidine was depressed by ara-C, while in some cases uptake of deoxycytidine was unaffected. Subsequently, this type of study, using thymidine, cytidine, or uridine as precursors of DNA pyrimidines, was extended to KB spinner cultures (Karon et al., 1966), rabbit kidney cells (Kaplan et al., 1968), human leukemic leukocytes, and normal bone marrow cells (Creasey et al., 1968), and mammalian cells infected with reovirus (Loh and Soergel, 1967). Treatment of animals with ara-C, followed by administration of labeled thymidine showed that the drug could exert a profound inhibition of DNA synthesis in growing rat embryos (Ritter et al., 1971). Some inhibition of the incorporation of tritiated cytidine into the DNA of leukemic leukocytes *in vitro* was noted when the activity of such suspensions was measured in samples obtained prior to, and during, therapy of patients with ara-C (Creasey et al., 1968). Apart from ara-C, various other arabinosides also inhibit DNA synthesis. These include arabinosyladenine (Furth and Cohen, 1967), arabinosyl-6-mercaptopurine (Kimball et al., 1966), arabinosyl-5-fluorocytosine (Kim et al., 1966; Lenaz et al., 1969), and thioarabinosylcytosine (Bremerskov et al., 1970).

In all such studies, nuclear DNA would be the major component, and the data would primarily reflect the effect of ara-C on this fraction. Something is known about the relative sensitivity of different DNA compartments to the analog. Synthesis of nonmitochondrial cytoplasmic DNA, a fraction considered to be informational DNA, is less sensitive to ara-C than is the fabrication of nuclear DNA in chick breast muscle cells (BELL, 1971). The repair of ultraviolet-induced lesions in HeLa cells containing DNA substituted with 5-bromouracil in one strand was not inhibited by ara-C (CLEAVER, 1968). This finding is compatible with the relative insensitivity to ara-C of polymerase I, the enzyme that catalyzes repair in *Escherichia coli* (RAMA REDDY et al., 1971). In rabbit kidney cells infected with herpes virus, BEN-PORAT et al. (1968) found that DNA synthesis was less sensitive to ara-C than it was in uninfected cells. Although this could have been due to a lower sensitivity of the viral DNA synthesizing system, it is probable that the finding resulted from the failure of ara-C to induce deoxycytidine kinase, a process that occurred in the normal cells.

This body of evidence for DNA synthesis being a target area for the action of ara-C requires explanation at a more fundamental level. Three lines of investigation have been pursued to approach this. First, study of the ribonucleoside diphosphate reductase system is the oldest approach. Second are kinetic studies with polymerase preparations and phosphate esters of ara-C. Third are studies of the incorporation of ara-C into nucleic acids.

C. Ribonucleoside Diphosphate Reductase

Early biochemical studies, notably those of CHU and FISCHER (1962, 1965), were suggestive of inhibition of the ribonucleoside diphosphate reductase system by some phosphorylated form of ara-C. This conclusion was based on both nutritional data, including the reversal or protection by deoxycytidine, and experiments in which the amount of label derived from tritiated uridine was reduced in both the DNA and deoxycytidine nucleotides, but unchanged in RNA, and uridine and thymidine nucleotides of L5178Y cells exposed to ara-C. Such evidence suggested that the protection afforded by deoxycytidine resulted both from inhibition of the activation of ara-C, and from a bypass of the metabolic blockade of the conversion of CDP to dCDP, by supplying the needed end product. Inhibition by ara-C of the uptake of precursors such as cytidine or thymidine into DNA, without any effect on the incorporation of deoxycytidine, has been a consistent finding. Reports of this have come from experiments with mammalian cells as diverse as L cells (SILAGI, 1965), HeLa cells (KIM and EIDINOFF, 1965), human leukemic leukocytes (CREASEY et al., 1966, 1968; ROBERTS et al., 1968), L5178Y cells (CHU and FISCHER, 1968a), and rabbit kidney cell cultures (KAPLAN et al., 1968). Several problems exist, however, in regarding inhibition of the production of dCDP as the major, or even as a significant factor in the cytotoxic action of ara-C. Firstly, there is clearly an irreversible component to the damage produced by the drug, one that is manifested after prolonged exposure (SILAGI, 1965; CHU and FISCHER, 1968b). This irreversible damage is unlikely to arise from any competitive inhibition of one specific enzyme. Secondly, data have been obtained recently concerning the magnitude of intracellular pools of deoxyribonucleotides, by enzymatic approaches such as those of NORDENSKJÖLD et al. (1970), or by radiochromatographic techniques (COLBY and EDLIN, 1970). When applied to ara-C, it was found that the drug caused only a transient decrease in the dCTP pool of mouse embryo cells, with increases in the levels of dATP, dGTP, and dTTP (SKOOG and NORDENSKJÖLD, 1971), while in human leukemic leukocytes, ara-C had no effect on the pools of cytidine and deoxycytidine phosphates (INAGAKI et al., 1969). KAPLAN et al. (1968) found indications that only when some deoxycytidine was present in the medium did inhibition of ribonucleoside diphosphate reductase occur. This was probably the result of feedback inhibition resulting from elevated dCTP levels; it has been known since 1961 that this enzyme is inhibited by deoxyribonucleoside triphosphates (REICHARD et al., 1961). Thirdly, MOORE and COHEN (1967) have shown that the di- and triphosphate esters of ara-C exert only a moderate degree of inhibition of the partially purified ribonucleoside diphosphate reductase from the Novikoff ascites tumor. This inhibition was certainly no greater than that produced by dCTP, in contrast to ara-ATP whose much more potent inhibitory effect resembled in type the action of dATP, which is believed to be an allosteric effector, stabilizing an inactive state of the enzyme (LARSSON and REICHARD, 1966).

Thus, while it is reasonable to conclude that the nucleotides of ara-C may reach, under appropriate conditions, intracellular levels sufficient to exert some pseudo-feedback inhibition of ribonucleoside diphosphate reductase, this process is almost certainly not a major factor in the cytotoxic action of ara-C. For this reason attention has switched to two other sites, inhibition of DNA polymerase enzyme systems and incorporation of analog into nucleic acids.

D. DNA Polymerase

At a time when the mechanism of action of ara-C was widely assumed to be inhibition of ribonucleoside diphosphate reductase, CARDEILHAC and COHEN (1964) prepared the 5′-nucleotides of ara-C and tested them as both substrates and inhibitors of polynucleotide biosynthesis. Ara-CDP produced greater than 95% inhibition of the polymerization of ADP and CDP catalyzed by polynucleotide phosphorylase. However, ara-CTP was inert when tested as an inhibitor of DNA and RNA polymerases from *Escherichia coli*. Crude DNA polymerase preparations from Ehrlich ascites carcinoma (KIMBALL and WILSON, 1968) and human leukemic leukocytes (INAGAKI et al., 1969) were both inhibited by ara-CTP, competitively with dCTP. FURTH and COHEN (1968a, b) examined in some detail the DNA and RNA polymerase enzymes from calf thymus and bovine lymphosarcoma. For the calf thymus enzyme, ara-CTP acted as a competitive inhibitor (versus dCTP) with a K_i value of 1 μM, the same as for ara-ATP, compared with Km values of 3 μM for dCTP and 2.5 μM for dATP. These levels of arabinonucleotides would be readily achievable intracellularly. In L cells, GRAHAM and WHITMORE (1970a) demonstrated that ara-CTP was a competitive inhibitor of DNA polymerase with a K_i of 8.7 ± 5.2 μM compared with a Km of 9.0 ± 4.3 μM for dCTP. Thus, it would appear that mammalian polymerases have generally proved more sensitive to ara-CTP than the bacterial enzymes.

Recent studies with mammalian and Rauscher murine leukemia virus polymerases have extended knowledge regarding the specificity of the inhibition by ara-CTP (TUOMINEN and KENNEY, 1972; MÜLLER et al., 1972). The most surprising aspect of these findings was that the RNA-dependent DNA polymerase, the virally induced reverse transcriptase, was 200 times as sensitive to ara-CTP as the DNA-dependent enzyme, although the kinetics of the inhibition was competitive for both enzymes. This presumably forms the basis for the ability of ara-C to interfere with replication and transformation by oncogenic RNA viruses. That the inhibitory effect of ara-CTP depends on competition with dCTP, as indicated by the studies described above, is confirmed by the failure of the nucleotide analog to inhibit the synthesis of poly (dA-dT) (FURLONG and GRESHAM, 1971; MOMPARLER, 1972). Reexamination of the *Escherichia coli* enzyme by RAMA REDDY et al. (1971) has shown that polymerase II, the presumed replicase, is sensitive to ara-CTP, whereas the repair enzyme I, and the polymerase III of undefined function, are much more resistant.

Although inhibition of DNA polymerase is undoubtedly a major site of action of ara-C, the existence of irreversible damage resulting from exposure to drug (Silagi, 1965; Chu and Fischer, 1968b) and the ability of mouse L cells to maintain their viability despite a 97 % reduction in DNA synthesis over a 14 hour period (Graham and Whitmore, 1970b) suggest that competitive inhibition of this type cannot be the only factor that determines cytotoxicity. For this reason attention has been turned to one of the most controversial areas of research on ara-C, the question of its incorporation into nucleic acids.

E. Incorporation of Ara-C into Nucleic Acids

Many purine and pyrimidine antimetabolites that are activated by phosphorylation are known to be incorporated into nucleic acids. Since ara-C is rapidly phosphorylated up to the level of its 5′-triphosphate, incorporation of the agent into polynucleotides would be expected. The first efforts to find such incorporated arabinosides were made in *Escherichia coli* by Cohen and his coworkers (Tono and Cohen, 1962; Cardeilhac and Cohen, 1964). In this organism, ara-U was not incorporated into the nucleic acids, although some of the carbon atoms of the arabinose moiety found their way into the ribose of RNA. Ara-CDP and ara-CTP did not appear to be substrates for polynucleotide phosphorylase and DNA polymerase, respectively; with RNA polymerase, ara-C was less than 1 % as effective as CTP. Later studies carried out in the same laboratory with partially purified polymerases from calf thymus and bovine lymphosarcoma also failed to demonstrate that ara-CTP and ara-ATP could function to any significant extent as substrates for either DNA or RNA polymerase (Furth and Cohen, 1968a, b).

Meanwhile, many other investigators were studying the metabolism of tritiated ara-C by suspensions of various cell lines. It was reported consistently that radioactivity was found in the nucleic acid fractions, but the amounts involved were very small. In his comments on this situation, Cohen (1966) was correct in his insistence that rigorous identification of the incorporated label was necessary, since contamination by metabolites of ara-C from the acid-soluble fraction could easily be responsible for the tritium associated with nucleic acids. Chu and Fischer (1965, 1968a) found that when L5178Y cells were incubated with tritiated ara-C, radioactivity was found in the RNA and DNA. Later the same authors (1968b) degraded the nucleic acids and were able to isolate ara-CMP. Other systems in which incorporation of ara-C into nucleic acids was observed include L cells (Silagi, 1965), human leukemic leukocytes (Creasey et al., 1966, 1968), rat embryos (Chaube et al., 1968), herpes simplex virus growing in human and rat kidney cells (Nutter and Rapp, 1973), and mouse lymphoma cells (Zahn et al., 1972). In some of these reports (Creasey et al., 1966; Zahn et al., 1972), degradation of the nucleic acids was carried out to confirm that the incorporated radioactivity was indeed ara-C.

At the enzymatic level, incorporation has been demonstrated with a variety of mammalian enzymes. Furlong and Gresham (1971), using a partially purified Walker 256 carcinosarcoma DNA polymerase, found evidence for some substitution of ara-CTP for dCTP in DNA biosynthesis, but no evidence that this incorporated analog brought about chain termination, confirming the earlier conclusions of Doering et al. (1966) regarding mouse fibroblasts. Graham and Whitmore (1970a) used both whole L cells and DNA polymerase preparations to establish inhibition of the latter enzyme by ara-CTP, and incorporation of the analog into DNA. The labeled DNA was degraded with micrococcal nuclease and spleen phosphodiesterase, and once again there was no evidence for concentration of ara-C in a terminal position. In whole cells, ara-C was initially present in the small Okazaki fragments, but shifted into longer strands when the cells were washed and incubated without labeled ara-C. MOMPARLER (1972) found that although the Km values for ara-CTP and dCTP in a mammalian polymerase system were similar, the value for the maximum velocity with dCTP was eight times greater than for ara-CTP. Ara-CTP was incorporated also into poly (dC-dG), but not into poly (dA-dT). The data for enzymatic digestion of DNA labeled with ara-CMP-^{32}P were suggestive of some activity of ara-CTP in causing termination of chain growth.

Despite such evidence that ara-C is incorporated into DNA, the problem remains as to how this uptake relates to cell death. Terminal incorporation with cessation of chain growth could be a serious lesion, but there is as yet no conclusive evidence that this is always a significant process. Furthermore, GRAHAM and WHITMORE (1970a) could find no correlation between lethality and the incorporation of ara-C into DNA. CHU and FISCHER (1968a, b) performed some experiments with L5178Y cells to attempt to resolve this problem. Acute cell death, which was not amenable to reversal by deoxycytidine, occurred at higher drug levels; it correlated, not with the incorporation of ara-C into DNA, but rather with uptake of the analog into RNA. Pretreatment with methotrexate reduced the incorporation of ara-C into nucleic acids, but sensitized the cells to the lethal effects of the drug. This phenomenon was later examined in more detail by CHU (1971). She incubated L5178Y cells with tritiated ara-C for up to 4 h and showed that uptake of drug into the DNA fraction ceased in one hour, although cell lethality continued to increase. On the other hand, incorporation into RNA continued with a linear rate of increase that could be correlated with the increments in cell death. When the cells were pretreated with 5-fluoro-2′-deoxyuridine or methotrexate, the incorporation of labeled ara-C into DNA was greatly reduced, although the pretreatment caused a four fold increase in the cell kill produced by the arabinoside. When the radioactive RNA was subjected to gradient centrifugation, it was found that the label was concentrated in the 2 to 16 S RNA, appearing first in 1 to 2 S RNA, then in 2 to 4 S material, and finally in heavier fractions.

Thus, while it is evident that ara-C is incorporated into all polynucleotides, the available evidence suggests that only the antimetabolite that is present in lower molecular weight RNA fractions is truly crucial in terms of acute cell kill. Messenger RNA for histone synthesis is of a 7 to 9 S particle size, and it is perhaps significant that treatment with ara-C inhibits histone synthesis in HeLa cells and causes disappearance of the messenger from the polyribosomes (BORUN et al., 1967). Should incorporation of ara-C occur in the 7 to 9 S messenger RNA, which has a short half-life, interference with its function and resultant inhibition of histone synthesis might occur. Whether the analog that is incorporated into DNA is able to bring about any long-term effects as a result of miscoding is as yet unresolved. Nevertheless, the fact that chromosome damage and teratogenesis occur with this drug suggests that such delayed effects are probable.

F. Miscellaneous Biochemical Effects

Relatively few studies of the effects of ara-C on other biochemical processes have been reported, and most of these are processes involved in nucleotide metabolism. ROBERTS et al. (1968) followed a number of leukocyte enzymes in a group of patients undergoing therapy with ara-C. The leukemic leukocytes showed a good correlation between the incorporation of deoxyuridine and that of thymidine into DNA *in vitro*, processes that were generally inhibited but occasionally stimulated. The levels of thymidylate synthetase, uridine kinase, and thymidine kinase showed no consistent pattern of change after exposure to ara-C, but were highly correlated together, whereas the changes in dihydrofolate reductase did not relate to the other parameters. In a recent study with the human lymphoblastic cell line CCRF-CEM, Roberts and Loehr (1971) found that ara-C lowered the thymidylate synthetase activity, whereas methotrexate increased it. Changes in the rate of enzyme turnover were postulated to account for the findings. Kit et al. (1966) reported that in monkey kidney and LM cell cultures, exposure to ara-C led to a significant increase in thymidine kinase and a smaller elevation of thymidylate kinase. These changes were not produced by ara-U, arabinosylthymine, deoxyuridine, cytidine, or thymidine. Cycloheximide prevented the increase in thymidine kinase, indicating that synthesis of new enzyme was required. In contrast to such findings of increased formation of some proteins, Smith and Chu (1972) described differential inhibition of protein synthesis in Chinese hamster cell cultures; histones were the proteins most affected. Histone and histone messenger RNA synthesis in L cells is also inhibited by ara-C (Schochetman and Perry, 1972). However, induction of dihydrofolate reductase by viral infection of mouse kidney cell cultures is not affected by ara-C (Pearson et al., 1966). Finally, Russell (1972) has suggested that the ability of ara-C to decrease the synthesis and accumulation of polyamines in mouse spleen and to prevent the increase in the ratio of spermidine to spermine that accompanies the growth of leukemia L1210 may be an index of drug antitumor efficacy. Methotrexate was superior to ara-C on this basis.

G. Resistance to Arabinosylcytosine

There are two forms of drug resistance, one that is innate, the natural resistance of a tissue, and the other which develops during therapy and presents a major problem for cancer chemotherapy. Natural resistance will of course be encountered among any group of neoplasms. Here the pharmacological problem is not to determine the mechanism of resistance with a view to circumventing it, but rather to find methods of identifying the intractable tumor and thus to avoid subjecting the patient to needless ineffectual therapy. Cline (1967) has suggested that the leukemic leukocytes that are sensitive to ara-C may be recognized by incubating them with the drug and tritiated thymidine or uridine for 24 h, and measuring the amount of incorporation of these precursors into nucleic acids. Thymidine incorporation appeared to be the more sensitive index (Cline, 1967; Cline and Rosenbaum, 1968). On the other hand, a very close relationship between the rate of conversion of ara-C to its nucleotides and the response to therapy of a group of murine and human leukemias has been found (Kessel, 1967; Kessel et al., 1969).

Turning to acquired resistance, several mechanisms have been proposed. Of these, the first and most plausible, involves changes in the enzymes that convert ara-C to active inhibitory nucleotides. As early as 1965, Chu and Fischer isolated an ara-C-resistant mutant of L5178Y lymphoma that had an impaired capacity to phosphorylate both ara-C and deoxycytidine to their 5′-phosphate esters. Subsequently, mutants of the L1210 tumor resistant to ara-C were isolated and studied; in these cells the ability to phosphorylate ara-C or deoxycytidine was also reduced by as much as 97% (Kessel, 1967; Schrecker and Urschel, 1967, 1968). In addition to changes in the ability to phosphorylate the two previous nucleosides, Schrecker (1970) found that the ara-C-resistant L1210 tumor also was severely depleted in deoxyguanosine kinase activity, with only minor decreases in the levels of deoxyadenosine and thymidine kinases. Extracts of the resistant tumor did not inhibit deoxycytidine kinase and the level of 5′-nucleotidase was not different from that of the sensitive tumor. BACH (1969) also reported a reduced deoxycytidine kinase in another mutant of L1210 leukemia resistant to ara-C. In this case, the decrease in the level of enzyme was less profound, and there seemed to be additional changes with respect to DNA polymerase and to an increased dependence on exogenous thymidine. The P815 tumor has also provided mutants resistant to ara-C, and in these, reduced levels of deoxycytidine kinase have been reported consistently (UCHIDA et al., 1968; DRAHOVSKY and KREIS, 1970; KREIS et al., 1972). It is interesting that in this tumor (DRAHOVSKY and KREIS, 1970) as in the resistant L1210 leukemia (SCHRECKER, 1970), the deletion is primarily at the level of the nucleoside kinase, nucleotide kinase activities being retained. In the studies of KREIS et al. (1972), which made use of electrophoretic and immunological procedures, the resistant P815 cells were found to contain a protein with similar migration and antigenic reaction to the kinase of sensitive cells, but which lacked enzymatic activity. DNA hybridization studies failed to show any difference between the sensitive and resistant lines. Finally, phosphorylation of ara-C has also been found to take place at a very low rate in leukemic cells from patients resistant to therapy with ara-C (KESSEL et al., 1969).

Another type of mutant was isolated from L5178Y cultures by MOMPARLER et al. (1968). This strain, which was approximately 5 times more resistant to ara-C than the parent, showed little or no difference in the conversion of nucleosides, including ara-C, to the corresponding nucleotides. However, there was a pattern of increased incorporation of labeled uridine and cytidine into the acid-soluble deoxycytidine nucleotide pool, coupled with little change in the incorporation of these precursors into nucleic acids. The authors considered that the mutant possessed elevated synthesis and a larger pool of deoxycytidine nucleotides, perhaps through an enhanced nucleoside diphosphate reductase system. SMITH and CHU (1972) have also claimed that the latter enzyme may be involved in resistance to ara-C in cultured Chinese hamster cells.

The L1210 mutant resistant to ara-C studied by BACH (1969) deserves further mention. Examination of the DNA polymerase prepared from this cell line disclosed that its affinity for dCTP was unchanged from that seen in the parent strain, but ara-CTP was very much less inhibitory with a 3 or 4 fold change in the K_i. In addition to this change in affinity, and the relatively small reduction in kinase activity mentioned earlier, there was also a low level nonspecific change in cell permeability to nucleosides.

While changes in the system for activation of ara-C, or in the target enzymes, are logical sites for resistance to develop, one other mechanism is available to the cell that on the surface appears very suitable. This is an elevation in nucleoside deaminase activity. STEUART and his colleagues (STEUART and BURKE, 1971; STEUART et al., 1971) have studied the bone marrow and peripheral leukocytes of leukemic patients treated with ara-C. The ratio of the relative rates of phosphorylation to deamination correlated with the clinical response to ara-C. However, it could be argued that of the two components of this ratio, the rate of phosphorylation is by far the more critical. There was evidence for an increased level of deaminase during sequential courses of therapy, and this was associated with diminished duration of remission.

Thus, in summary, it can be said that there is one major mechanism of resistance to ara-C encountered in both experimental tumors and human leukemias, and that is a diminished deoxycytidine kinase activity, leading to reduced formation of ara-CTP. Increased deamination of ara-C within human leukemia cells may be involved in the resistance of these cells to ara-C, but is clearly an accompaniment to changed kinase activity. Since the levels of deoxycytidine nucleotides may be relatively unaffected by ara-C in most cells, elevation of the intracellular concentrations of these nucleotides is unlikely to be a major factor in acquisition of resistance, unless these elevated levels exert significant feedback inhibition of deoxycytidine kinase. Finally, changes in affinity of DNA polymerase, while of great biochemical interest, have not yet been demonstrated to represent a widely distributed mechanism.

Conclusions

In this review it has been made amply clear that ara-C is a drug possessing multiple sites of action (Fig. 1). As such, it is probably not meaningful to speculate

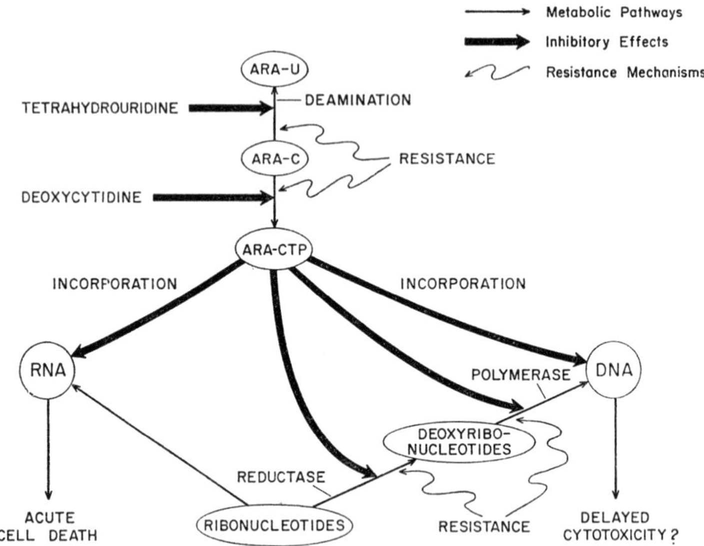

Fig. 1. Metabolism, possible sites of action, and known mechanisms of resistance of arabinosylcytosine

on which is the more critical mechanism for expression of cytotoxicity. Presumably the various possible mechanisms (i.e., inhibition of DNA polymerase, incorporation into DNA, uptake into RNA, interference with histone biosynthesis, and inhibition of ribonucleoside diphosphate reductase) will occur to different degrees among individual tumor types. Some may only be manifest under special conditions, and suppression of ribonucleoside diphosphate reductase activity in a pseudofeedback fashion clearly comes in this category. Again, just what role incorporation into RNA plays in the antitumor activity of ara-C in man is currently unclear. In tissue culture systems, the acute cell kill so closely associated with this incorporation requires relatively prolonged exposure to relatively large drug levels, whereas in the therapeutic situation, plasma levels of ara-C are very transient. Thus, at the present time the metabolic lesion that is most clearly defined in terms of its implication for antitumor action is inhibition of DNA polymerase.

As regards the mechanisms for acquired resistance, it is evident that deletion or a change in the level of deoxycytidine kinase activity is the one that occurs most frequently. If the data of KREIS et al. (1972) reflect the status in neoplasms apart from the P815 tumor, it would appear that the kinase protein is still present, but has undergone changes that make it essentially inactive. In human leukemic cells there is evidence that increased levels of nucleoside deaminase may form a further element which, combined with reduced kinase levels, raises the resistance of the cells to drug.

A final word should be mentioned about the concept of scheduling of therapy with ara-C. Since, of the possible mechanisms of action, most relate directly or indirectly to DNA and its biosynthesis, ara-C is classed as an S-phase-dependent drug (SKIPPER et al., 1967). Thus, the use of this agent in combination with other drugs should be devised, ideally, so as to take advantage of this fact. For example, a degree of synchrony could be induced with one of several other agents so as to present to the administered ara-C a tumor population containing a larger percentage of cells in the sensitive *S*-phase. A converse aspect to this is that it is also possible to take advantage of the differences in cell cycle characteristics of the host and the tumor. A particularly elegant demonstration of this was reported recently by HAUS et al. (1972). By tailoring the doses of ara-C in sinusoidal fashion to the circadian rhythm of mice bearing leukemia L1210, significantly improved tumor response was achieved with less toxicity. Such approaches, made with the overall biology of both the host and tumor in mind, offer hope for greatly improved therapeutic efficacy.

References

AHEARN, M.J., LEWIS, C.W., CAMPBELL, L.A., LUCE, J.K.: Nuclear bleb formation in human bone marrow cells during cytosine arabinoside therapy. Nature (Lond.) **215**, 196—197 (1967).

ATKINSON, C., STACEY, K.A.: Thymineless death induced by cytosine arabinoside. Biochim. biophys. Acta (Amst.) **166**, 705—707 (1968).

BACH, M.K.: Biochemical and genetic studies of a mutant strain of mouse leukemia L1210 resistant to 1-β-D-arabinofuranosylcytosine (cytarabine) hydrochloride. Cancer Res. **29**, 1036—1044 (1969).

BADER, J.P.: Metabolic requirements for infection by Rous sarcoma virus. I. The transient requirement for DNA synthesis. Virology **29**, 444—451 (1966).

BAGULEY, B.C., FALKENHAUG, E.M.: Plasma half-life of cytosine arabinoside (NSC-63878) in patients treated for acute myeloblastic leukemia. Cancer Chemother. Rep. **55**, 291—298 (1971).

BALDINI, L., BRAMBILLA, G., CAVANNA, M., PARODI, S.: Immunosuppressive activity of methotrexate and arabinosylcytosine in mice bearing L1210 leukemia. Brit. J. Pharmacol. **34**, 674P-676P (1968).

BELL, E.: Informational DNA synthesis distinguished from that of nuclear DNA by inhibitors of DNA synthesis. Science **174**, 603—606 (1971).

BELL, W.R., WHANG, J.J., CARBONE, P.P., BRECHER, G., BLOCK, J.B.: Cytogenetic and morphologic abnormalities in human bone marrow cells during cytosine arabinoside therapy. Blood **27**, 771—781 (1966).

BENEDICT, W.F., HARRIS, N., KARON, M.: Kinetics of 1-β-D-arabinofuranosylcytosine-induced chromosome breaks. Cancer Res. **30**, 2477—2483 (1970).

BENEDICT, W.F., KARON, M.: Chromatid breakage: cytosine arabinoside-induced lesions inhibited by UV irradiation. Science **171**, 680—682 (1971).

BEN-PORAT, T., BROWN, MCK., KAPLAN, A.S.: Effect of 1-β-D-arabinofuranosylcytosine on DNA synthesis. II. In rabbit kidney cells infected with herpes viruses. Molec. Pharmacol. **4**, 139—146 (1968).

BERGMANN, W., BURKE, D.C.: Contributions to the study of marine products. XXXIX. The nucleosides of sponges. III. Spongothymidine and spongouridine. J. org. Chem. **20**, 1501—1507 (1955).

BERGMANN, W., FEENEY, R.J.: Contributions to the study of marine products. XXXII. The nucleosides of sponges. I. J. org. Chem. **16**, 981—987 (1951).

BLOCK, J.B., BELL, W., WHANG, J., CARBONE, P.P.: Hematologic and cytogenetic abnormalities during cytosine arabinoside (CA) therapy. Proc. Amer. Ass. Cancer Res. **6**, 6 (1965).

Borsa, J., Whitmore, G. F., Valeriote, F. A., Collins, D., Bruce, W. R.: Studies on the persistence of methotrexate, cytosine arabinoside and leukovorin in the serum of mice. J. nat. Cancer Institute **42**, 235—242 (1969).

Borun, T. W., Scharff, M. D., Robbins, E.: Rapidly labeled, polyribosome-associated RNA having the properties of histone messenger. Proc. nat. Acad. Sci. (Wash.) **58**, 1977—1983 (1967).

Bremerskov, V., Kaden, P., Mittermayer, C.: DNA synthesis during the life cycle of L cells: morphological, histochemical and biochemical investigations with arabinosylcytosine and thioarabinosylcytosine. Europ. J. Cancer **6**, 379—392 (1970).

Brewen, J. G.: The induction of chromatid lesions by cytosine arabinoside in post-DNA synthetic human leukocytes. Cytogenetics **4**, 28—36 (1965).

Brewen, J. G., Christie, N. T.: Studies on the induction of chromosomal aberrations in human leukocytes by cytosine arabinoside. Exp. Cell Res. **46**, 276—291 (1967).

Burchenal, J. H., Wiggins, R., Butterbaugh, J.: Activity of *N*4-hydroxyl derivatives of 1-β-D-arabinofuranosylcytosine (ara-C) in Burkitt cell culture and mouse leukemia. Proc. Amer. Ass. Cancer Res. **8**, 8 (1967).

Buskirk, H. H., Crim, J. A., Petering, H. G., Merritt, K., Johnson, A. G.: Effect of uracil mustard and several antitumor drugs on the primary antibody response in rats and mice. J. nat. Cancer Inst. **34**, 747—758 (1965).

Buthala, D. A.: Cell culture studies on antiviral agents: 1-Action of cytosine arabinoside and some comparisons with 5-iodo-2′-deoxyuridine. Proc. Soc. Exp. Biol. (N.Y.) **115**, 69—77 (1964).

Calabresi, P., Creasey, W. A., Prusoff, W. H., Welch, A. D.: Clinical and pharmacological studies with 5-iodo-2′-deoxycytidine. Cancer Res. **23**, 583—592 (1963).

Camiener, G. W.: Studies of the enzymatic deamination of cytosine arabinoside. II. Properties of the deaminase of human liver. Biochem. Pharmacol. **16**, 1681—1689 (1967a).

Camiener, G. W.: Studies of the enzymatic deamination of cytosine arabinoside. III. Substrate requirements and inhibitors of the deaminase of human liver. Biochem. Pharmacol. **16**, 1691—1702 (1967b).

Camiener, G. W., Smith, C. G.: Studies of the enzymatic deamination of cytosine arabinoside. I. Enzyme distribution and species specificity. Biochem. Pharmacol. **14**, 1405—1416 (1965).

Camiener, G. W., Smith, C. G.: Studies of the enzymatic deamination of ara-cytidine. V. Inhibition *in vitro* and *in vivo* by tetrahydrouridine and other reduced pyrimidine nucleosides. Biochem. Pharmacol. **17**, 1981—1991 (1968).

Cardeilhac, P. T., Cohen, S. S.: Some metabolic properties of nucleotides of 1-β-D-arabinofuranosylcytosine. Cancer Res. **24**, 1595—1603 (1964).

Chaube, S., Kreis, W., Uchida, K., Murphy, M. L.: The teratogenic effect of 1-β-D-arabinofuranosylcytosine in the rat. Protection by deoxycytidine. Biochem. Pharmacol. **17**, 1213—1226 (1968).

Chu, M. Y.: Incorporation of arabinosylcytosine into 2—7 S ribonucleic acid and cell death. Biochem. Pharmacol. **20**, 2057—2063 (1971).

Chu, M. Y., Fischer, G. A.: A proposed mechanism of action of 1-β-D-arabinofuranosylcytosine as an inhibitor of the growth of leukemic cells. Biochem. Pharmacol. **11**, 423—430 (1962).

Chu, M. Y., Fischer, G. A.: Comparative studies of leukemic cells sensitive and resistant to cytosine arabinoside. Biochem. Pharmacol. **14**, 333—341 (1965).

Chu, M. Y., Fischer, G. A.: Effects of cytosine arabinoside on the cell viability and uptake of deoxypyrimidine nucleosides in L5178Y cells. Biochem. Pharmacol. **17**, 741—751 (1968a).

Chu, M. Y., Fischer, G. A.: The incorporation of ^{3}H-cytosine arabinoside and its effect on murine leukemic cells (L5178Y). Biochem. Pharmacol. **17**, 753—767 (1968b).

Cleaver, J. E.: Repair replication and degradation of bromouracil-substituted DNA in mammalian cells after irradiation with ultraviolet light. Biophys. J. **8**, 775—791 (1968).

Cline, M. J.: Prediction of *in vivo* cytotoxicity of chemotherapeutic agents by their effect on malignant leukocytes *in vitro*. Blood **30**, 176—188 (1967).

Cline, M. J., Rosenbaum, E.: Prediction of *in vivo* cytotoxicity of chemotherapeutic agents by their *in vitro* effect on leukocytes from patients with acute leukemia. Cancer Res. **28**, 2516—2521 (1968).

Cohen, S. S.: Sponges, cancer chemotherapy and cellular aging. Perspect. biol. Med. **6**, 215—227 (1963).

Cohen, S. S.: Introduction to the biochemistry of D-arabinosyl nucleotides. Progr. nucleic Acid Res. **5**, 1—88 (1966).

Colby, C., Edlin, G.: Nucleotide pool levels in growing, inhibited, and transformed chick fibroblast cells. Biochemistry **9**, 917—920 (1970).

Creasey, W. A.: Studies on the metabolism of 5-iodo-2′-deoxycytidine *in vitro*. J. biol. Chem. **238**, 1772—1776 (1963).

CREASEY, W. A., DECONTI, R. C., KAPLAN, S. R.: Biochemical studies with 1-β-D-arabinofuranosylcytosine in human leukemic leukocytes and normal bone marrow cells. Cancer Res. **28**, 1074—1081 (1968).

CREASEY, W. A., FLANIGAN, S., MCCOLLUM, R. W., CALABRESI, P.: Intraventricular administration of antimetabolites in patients with neoplasms and infections of the CNS. Proc. Amer. Ass. Cancer Res. **9**, 16 (1968).

CREASEY, W. A., PAPAC, R. J., MARKIW, M. E., CALABRESI, P., WELCH, A. D.: Biochemical and pharmacological studies with 1-β-D-arabinofuranosylcytosine in man. Biochem. Pharmacol. **15**, 1417—1428 (1966).

CUMMINGS, D. J.: Comments on "thymineless death induced by cytosine arabinoside". Biochim. biophys. Acta (Amst.) **179**, 237—238 (1969).

DARŻYNKIEWICZ, E., KUŚMIEREK, J. T., SHUGAR, D.: o'-Methyl derivatives of arabinosylcytosine. Biochem. biophys. Res. Commun. **46**, 1734—1741 (1972).

DIXON, R. L., ADAMSON, R. H.: Antitumor activity and pharmacologic disposition of cytosine arabinoside (NSC 63878). Cancer Chemother. Rep. **48**, 11—16 (1965).

DOERING, A., KELLER, J., COHEN, S. S.: Some effects of D-arabinosylnucleosides on polymer synthesis in mouse fibroblasts. Cancer Res. **26**, 2444—2450 (1966).

DOLLINGER, M. R., BURCHENAL, J. H., KREIS, W., FOX, J. J.: Analogs of 1-β-D-arabinofuranosylcytosine. Studies on mechanisms of action in BURKITT's cell culture and mouse leukemia, and *in vitro* deamination studies. Biochem. Pharmacol. **16**, 689—706 (1967).

DOLLINGER, M., KREIS, W., STOLL, D., FOX, J., BURCHENAL, J. H.: Deamination of cytosine arabinoside and its analogs. Proc. Amer. Ass. Cancer Res. **8**, 14 (1967).

DRAHOVSKY, D., KREIS, W.: Studies on drug resistance-II. Kinase patterns in P815 neoplasms sensitive and resistant to 1-β-D-arabinofuranosylcytosine. Biochem. Pharmacol. **19**, 940—944 (1970).

DURHAM, J. F., IVES, D. H.: Feedback control of calf thymus deoxycytidine kinase. Fed. Proc. **26**, 808 (1967).

DURHAM, J. P., IVES, D. H.: Deoxycytidine kinase. 1. Distribution in normal and neoplastic tissues and inter-relationships of deoxycytidine and 1-β-D-arabinofuranosylcytosine phosphorylation. Molec. Pharmacol. **5**, 358—375 (1969).

EVANS, J. S., BOSTWICK, L., MENGEL, G. D.: Synergism of the antineoplastic activity of cytosine arabinoside by porfiromycin. Biochem. Pharmacol. **13**, 983—988 (1964).

EVANS, J. S., MENGEL, G. D.: The reversal of cytosine arabinoside activity *in vivo* by deoxycytidine. Biochem. Pharmacol. **13**, 989—994 (1964).

EVANS, J. S., MUSSER, E. A., BOSTWICK, L., MENGEL, G. D.: The effect of 1-β-D-arabinofuranosylcytosine hydrochloride on murine neoplasms. Cancer Res. **24**, 1285—1293 (1964).

EVANS, J. S., MUSSER, E. A., MENGEL, G. D., FORSBLAD, K. R., HUNTER, J. H.: Antitumor activity of 1-β-D-arabinofuranosylcytosine hydrochloride. Proc. Soc. exp. Biol. (N.Y.) **106**, 350—353 (1961).

FAHMY, O. G., FAHMY, M. J., DE VRYE, C. E.: The mutagenic properties of the nucleosides of pyrimidine analogues in *Drosophilia melanogaster*. Biochem. Pharmacol. **15**, 299—316 (1966).

FALCO, E. A., FOX, J. J.: Nucleosides XLVIII. Synthesis of 1-(5-deoxy-β-D-arabinosyl) cytosine and related compounds. J. med. Chem. **11**, 148—151 (1968).

FELDMAN, L. A., RAPP, F.: Inhibition of adenovirus replication by 1-β-D-arabinofuranosylcytosine. Proc. Soc. exp. Biol. (N.Y.) **122**, 243—247 (1966).

FINKELSTEIN, J. Z., SCHER, J., KARON, M.: Pharmacologic studies of tritiated cytosine arabinoside (NSC-63878) in children. Cancer Chemother. Rep. **54**, 35—39 (1970).

FISCHER, D. S., CASSIDY, E. P., WELCH, A. D.: Immunosuppression by pyrimidine nucleoside analogs. Biochem. Pharmacol. **15**, 1013—1022 (1966).

FLICKINGER, R. A.: Delay of normal development of sea urchin embryos by cytosine arabinoside. Experientia (Basel) **23**, 136 (1967).

FOX, J. J., YUNG, N., BENDICH, A.: Pyrimidine nucleosides. II. The synthesis of 1-β-D-arabinofuranosylthymine (spongothymidine). J. Amer. chem. Soc. **79**, 2775—2778 (1957).

FURLONG, N. B., GRESHAM, C.: Inhibition of DNA synthesis but not of poly-dAT synthesis by the arabinose analogue of cytidine *in vitro*. Nature (Lond.) **233**, 212—214 (1971).

FURTH, J. J., COHEN, S. S.: Inhibition of mammalian DNA polymerase by the 5'-triphosphate of 9-β-D-arabinofuranosyladenine. Cancer Res. **27**, 1528—1533 (1967).

FURTH, J. J., COHEN, S. S.: Effect of the 5'-triphosphates of 1-β-D-arabinofuranosylcytosine and 9-β-D-arabinofuranosyladenine on the enzymatic synthesis of nucleic acid in mammalian tissues. Proc. Amer. Ass. Cancer Res. **9**, 23 (1968a).

FURTH, J. J., COHEN, S. S.: Inhibition of mammalian DNA polymerase by the 5'-triphosphate of 1-β-D-arabinofuranosylcytosine and the 5'-triphosphate of 9-β-D-arabinofuranosyladenine. Cancer Res. **28**, 2061—2067 (1968b).

GISH, D. T., NEIL, G. L., WECHTER, W. J.: Nucleic acids. 12. Synthesis of the L-enantiomer of 1-β-D-arabinofuranosylcytosine and of O^2, $O^{2'}$-anhydro-1-β-D-arabinofuranosylcytosine. J. med. Chem. **14**, 882—883 (1971).

GIZIEWICZ, J., KUŚMIEREK, J. T., SHUGAR, D.: 5′-o-Methyl derivatives of 1-β-D-arabinofuranosylcytosine and 1-β-D-arabinofuranosyluracil. J. med. Chem. **15**, 839—840 (1972).

GOLDENBERG, D. M.: Oral activity of 1-β-D-arabinofuranosylcytosine in a transplantable hamster melanoma. Chemotherapy **16**. 294—299 (1971).

GRAHAM, F. L., WHITMORE, G. F.: Studies in mouse L-cells on the incorporation of 1-β-D-arabinofuranosylcytosine into DNA and on inhibition of DNA polymerase by 1-β-D-arabinofuranosylcytosine-5′-triphosphate. Cancer Res. **30**, 2636—2644 (1970a).

GRAHAM, F. L., WHITMORE, G. F.: The effect of 1-β-D-arabinofuranosylcytosine on growth, viability and DNA synthesis of mouse L-cells. Cancer Res. **30**, 2627—2635 (1970b).

GRAY, G. D., NICHOL. R., MICKELSON, M. M., CAMIENER, G. W., GISH, D. T., KELLY, R. C., WECHTER, W. J., MOXLEY, T. E., NEIL, G. L.: Immunosuppressive, antiviral and antitumor activities of cytarabine derivatives. Biochem. Pharmacol. **21**, 465—475 (1972).

GREENSTEIN, J. P., CARTER, C. E., CHALKLEY, H. W.: Enzymatic degradation of ribose-nucleic and desoxyribosenucleic acids with an addendum on the effect of nucleates on the heat stability of proteins. Cold Spr. Harb. Symp. Quant. Biol., **12**, 64 (1947).

GRINDEY, G. B., SASLAW, L. D., WARAVDEKAR, V. S.: Relationship of uracil derivatives to the metabolism of arabinosylcytosine (ara-C). Proc. Amer. Ass. Cancer Res. **8**, 24 (1967).

GRINDEY, G. B., SASLAW, L. D., WARAVDEKAR, V. S.: Effects of uracil derivatives on phosphorylation of arabinosylcytosine. Molec. Pharmacol. **4**, 96—103 (1968).

GRISWOLD, D. P., JR., SIMPSON-HERREN, L., SCHABEL, F. M., JR.: Altered sensitivity of a hamster plasmacytoma to cytosine arabinoside (NSC-63878). Cancer Chemother. Rep. **54**, 337—346 (1970).

HALL, T. C., LEVINE, R.: Deamination of cytosine arabinoside by normal and malignant tissues. Proc. Amer. Ass. Cancer Res. **8**, 24 (1967).

HANKA, L. J., KUENTZEL, S. L., NEIL, G. L.: Improved microbiological assay for cytosine arabinoside (NSC-63878). Cancer Chemother. Rep. **54**, 393—397 (1970).

HANZE, A. R.: Nucleic acids. IV. The catalytic reduction of pyrimidine nucleosides (human liver deaminase inhibitors). J. Amer. chem. Soc. **89**, 6720—6725 (1967).

HAUS, E., HALBERG, F., SCHEVING, L. E., PAULY, J. E., CARDOSO, S., KÜHL, J. F. W., SOTHERN, R. B., SHIOTSUKA, R. N., HWANG, D. S.: Increased tolerance of leukemic mice to arabinosylcytosine with schedule adjusted to circadian system. Science **177**, 80—82 (1972).

HENEEN, W. K., NICHOLS, W. W.: Cell morphology of a human diploid cell strain (WI-38) after treatment with arabinosylcytosine. Cancer Res. **27**, 242—250 (1967).

HEPPNER, G. H., CALABRESI, P.: Suppression by cytosine arabinoside of serum-blocking factors of cell-mediated immunity to syngeneic transplants of mouse mammary tumors. J. nat. Cancer Inst. **48**, 1161—1167 (1972).

HIRSCHMAN, S. Z., FISCHINGER, P. J., O'CONNOR, T. E.: The inhibition by cytosine arabinoside of the replication of murine leukemia and sarcoma viruses in mouse embryo cultures. J. Cancer **4**, 671—677 (1969).

HO, D. H. W., FREI, E., III: Clinical pharmacology of 1-β-D-arabinofuranosylcytosine. Clin. Pharmacol. Therap. **12**, 944—954 (1971).

HO, D. H. W., FREIREICH, E. J.: Clinical pharmacology of arabinosylcytosine. In: SARTORELLI, A. C., JOHNS, D. J. (Eds.): Handbook of experimental pharmacology, Vol. 38. Antineoplastic and immunosuppressive agents. Berlin-Heidelberg-New York: Springer 1975.

HOSHI, A., KANZAWA, F., KURETANI, K., SANEYOSHI, M., ARAI, Y.: 2,2′-o-Cyclocytidine, antitumor cytidine analog resistant to cytidine deaminase. Gann **62**, 145—146 (1971).

HUNT, D. E., PITTILLO, R. F.: Determination of certain antitumor agents in mouse blood by microbiologic assay. Cancer Res. **28**, 1095—1109 (1968).

HUNTER, J. H.: Transforming 1-β-D-xylofuranosyluracil nucleosides into 1-β-D-arabinofuranosyluracil nucleosides. U.S. Patent 3,183,226, May 11, 1965, in Chem. Abstr. **63**, 16446g (1965).

INAGAKI, A., NAKAMURA, T., WAKISAKA, G.: Studies on the mechanism of action of 1-β-D-arabinofuranosylcytosine as an inhibitor of DNA synthesis in human leukemic leukocytes. Cancer Res. **29**, 2169—2176 (1969).

KANAI, T., KOJIMA, T., MARUYAMA, O., ICHINO, M.: Pyrimidine nucleosides. III. Reaction of cytidine or N-4-acetylcytidine with partially hydrolyzed phosphorous oxychloride. Chem. pharm. Bull. (Tokyo) **18**, 2569—2570 (1970).

KAPLAN, A. S., BROWN, MCK., BEN-PORAT, T.: Effect of 1-β-D-arabinofuranosylcytosine on DNA synthesis I. In normal rabbit kidney cell cultures. Molec. Pharmacol. **4**, 131—138 (1968).

KARNOFSKY, D. A., LACON, C. R.: The effects of 1-β-D-arabinofuranosylcytosine on the developing chick embryo. Biochem. Pharmacol. **15**, 1435—1442 (1966).

KARON, M., HENRY, P., WEISSMAN, S., MEYER, C.: The effect of 1-β-D-arabinofuranosylcytosine on macromolecular synthesis in KB spinner cultures. Cancer Res. **26**, 166—171 (1966).
KARON, M., SHIRAKAWA, S.: The locus of action of 1-β-D-arabinofuranosylcytosine in the cell cycle. Cancer Res. **29**, 687—696 (1969).
KESSEL, D.: Transport and phosphorylation of cytosine arabinoside by normal and leukemic cells. Proc. Amer. Ass. Cancer Res. **8**, 36 (1967).
KESSEL, D.: Some observations on the phosphorylation of cytosine arabinoside. Molec. Pharmacol. **4**, 402—410 (1968a).
KESSEL, D.: Properties of deoxycytidine kinase partially purified from L1210 cells. J. biol. Chem. **243**, 4739—4744 (1968b).
KESSEL, D., HALL, T. C.: Transport and phosphorylation as factors in the antitumor action of cytosine arabinoside. Science **156**, 1240—1241 (1967).
KESSEL, D., HALL, T. C., ROSENTHAL, P.: Uptake and phosphorylation of cytosine arabinoside by normal and leukemic blood cells *in vitro*. Cancer Res. **29**, 459—463 (1969).
KESSEL, D., HALL, T. C., WODINSKY, I.: Transport and phosphorylation as factors in the antitumor action of cytosine arabinoside. Science **156**, 1240—1241 (1967).
KESSEL, D., SHURIN, S. B.: Transport of two non-metabolized nucleosides, deoxycytidine and cytosine arabinoside, in a sub-line of the L1210 murine leukemia. Biochim. biophys. Acta (Amst.) **163**, 179—187 (1968).
KIHLMAN, B. A., NICHOLS, W. W., LEVAN, A.: The effect of deoxyadenosine and cytosine arabinoside on the chromosomes of human leukocytes *in vitro*. Hereditas **50**, 139—143 (1963).
KIM, J. H., EIDINOFF, M. L.: Action of 1-β-D-arabinofuranosylcytosine on the nucleic acid metabolism and viability of HeLa cells. Cancer Res. **25**, 698—702 (1965).
KIM, J. H., EIDINOFF, M. L., FOX, J. J.: Action of 1-β-D-arabinofuranosyl-5-fluorocytosine on the nucleic acid metabolism and viability of HeLa cells. Cancer Res. **26**, 1661—1664 (1966).
KIMBALL, A. P., BOWMAN, B., BUSH, P. S., HERRIOT, J., LEPAGE, G. A.: Inhibitory effects of the arabinosides of 6-mercaptopurine and cytosine on purine and pyrimidine metabolism. Cancer Res. **26**, 1337—1343 (1966).
KIMBALL, A. P., WILSON, M. J.: Inhibition of DNA polymerase by 1-β-D-arabinosylcytosine and reversal of inhibition by deoxycytidine-5'-triphosphate. Proc. Soc. exptl. Biol. (N.Y.) **127**, 429—432 (1968).
KIT, S., DETORRES, R. A., DUBBS, D. R.: Arabinofuranosylcytosine-induced stimulation of thymidine kinase and deoxycytidylic deaminase activities of mammalian cultures. Cancer Res. **26**, 1859—1866 (1966).
KLINE, I., VENDITTI, J. M., TYRER, D. D., GOLDIN, A.: Chemotherapy of leukemia L1210 in mice with 1-β-D-arabinofuranosylcytosine hydrochloride I. Influence of treatment schedules. Cancer Res. **26**, 853—859 (1966).
KOZAI, Y., SUGINO, Y.: Enzymatic phosphorylation of 1-β-D-arabinofuranosylcytosine. Cancer Res. **31**, 1376—1382 (1971).
KREIS, W., DRAHOVSKY, D., BORBERG, H.: Characterization of protein and DNA in P815 cells sensitive and resistant to 1-β-D-arabinofuranosylcytosine. Cancer Res. **32**, 696—701 (1972).
LARSSON, A., REICHARD, P.: Enzymatic synthesis of deoxyribonucleotides X. Reduction of purine ribonucleotides; allosteric behavior and substrate specificity of the enzyme system from *Escherichia coli* B. J. biol. Chem. **241**, 2540—2549 (1966).
LENAZ, L., STERNBERG, S. S., PHILIPS, F. S.: Cytotoxic effects of 1-β-D-arabinofuranosyl-5-fluorocytosine and of 1-β-D-arabinofuranosylcytosine in proliferating tissues in mice. Cancer Res. **29**, 1790—1798 (1969).
LIVINGSTON, R. B., CARTER, S. K.: Cytosine arabinoside (NSC-63878)-clinical brochure. Cancer Chemother. Rep. **1**, 179—205 (1968).
LOH, P. C., SOERGEL, M.: Macromolecular synthesis in cells infected with reovirus type 2 and the effect of ara-C. Nature (Lond.) **214**, 622—623 (1967).
MITCHELL, M. S., WADE, M. E., DECONTI, R. C., BERTINO, J. R., CALABRESI, P.: Immunosuppressive effects of cytosine arabinoside and methotrexate in man. Ann. intern. Med. **70**, 535—547 (1969).
MOMPARLER, R. L.: Kinetic and template studies with 1-β-D-arabinofuranosylcytosine 5'-triphosphate and mammalian deoxyribonucleic acid polymerase. Molec. Pharmacol. **8**, 362—370 (1972).
MOMPARLER, R. L., CHU, M. Y., FISCHER, G. A.: Studies on a new mechanism of resistance of L5178Y murine leukemia cells to cytosine arabinoside. Biochim. biophys. Acta (Amst.) **161**, 481—493 (1968).
MOMPARLER, R. L., FISCHER, G. A.: Mammalian deoxynucleoside kinases I. Deoxycytidine kinase: purification, properties, and kinetic studies with cytosine arabinoside. J. biol. Chem. **243**, 4298—4304 (1968).
MOMPARLER, R. L., LABITAN, A., ROSSI, M.: Enzymatic estimation and metabolism of 1-β-D-arabinofuranosylcytosine in man. Cancer Res. **32**, 408—412 (1972).

Montgomery, J.A., Thomas, H.J.: Acyl derivatives of 1-β-D-arabinofuranosylcytosine. J. med. Chem. **15**, 116—118 (1972).
Moore, E.C., Cohen, S.S.: Effects of arabinonucleotides on ribonucleotide reduction by an enzyme system from rat tumor. J. biol. Chem. **242**, 2116—2118 (1967).
Müller, W.E.G., Yamazak, Z.I., Sögtrop, H.H., Zahn, R.K.: Action of 1-β-D-arabinofuranosylcytosine on mammalian tumor cells-2. Inhibition of mammalian and oncogenic viral polymerases. Europ. J. Cancer **8**, 421—428 (1972).
Mulligan, L.T., Jr., Mellett, L.B.: Comparative metabolism of cytosine arabinoside and inhibition of deamination by tetrahydrouridine. Pharmacologist **10**, 167 (1968).
Neil, G.L., Wiley, P.F., Manak, R.C., Moxley, T.E.: Antitumor effect of 1-β-D-arabinofuranosylcytosine 5′-adamantoate (NSC-117614) in leukemic mice. Cancer Res. **30**, 1047—1054 (1970).
Nordenskjöld, B.A., Skoog, L., Brown, N.C., Reichard, P.: Deoxyribonucleotide pools and deoxyribonucleic acid synthesis in cultured mouse embryo cells. J. biol. Chem. **245**, 5360—5368 (1970).
Notari, R.E.: A mechanism for the hydrolytic deamination of cytosine arabinoside in aqueous buffer. J. pharm. Sci. **56**, 804—809 (1967).
Notari, R.E., Chin, M.L., Wittebort, R.: Arabinosylcytosine stability in aqueous solutions: pH profile and shelflife predictions. J. pharm. Sci. **61**, 1189—1196 (1972).
Nutter, R.L., Rapp, F.: The effect of cytosine arabinoside on virus production in various cells infected with herpes simplex virus types 1 and 2. Cancer Res. **33**, 166—170 (1973).
Panzica, R.P., Robins, R.K., Townsend, L.B.: Synthesis and anticancer activity of cytosine arabinoside 3-N-oxide (ara-C 3-*N*-oxide). J. med. Chem. **14**, 259 (1971).
Papac, R.J., Calabresi, P., Hollingsworth, J.W., Welch, A.D.: Effects of 1-β-D-arabinofuranosylcytosine hydrochloride on regenerating bone marrow. Cancer Res. **25**, 1459—1462 (1965).
Papac, R.J., Creasey, W.A., Calabresi, P., Welch, A.D.: Clinical and pharmacological studies with 1-β-D-arabinofuranosylcytosine (cytosine arabinoside). Proc. Amer. Ass. Cancer Res. **6**, 50 (1965).
Pearson, P.M., Kit, S., Dubbs, D.R.: Induction of dihydrofolate reductase by SV^{40} and polyoma virus. Cancer Res. **26**, 1653—1660 (1966).
Peterkofsky, B., Tomkins, G.M.: Effect of inhibitors of nucleic acid synthesis on steroid-mediated induction of tyrosine aminotransferase in hepatoma cell cultures. J. molec. Biol. **30**, 49—61 (1967).
Pitillo, R.F., Hunt, D.E.: Cytosine arabinoside sensitivity in actinobolin-resistant *Streptococcus fecalis:* the basis of a utilitarian microbiological assay. Proc. Soc. exp. Biol. (N.Y.) **124**, 636—640 (1967).
Pizer, L.I., Cohen, S.S.: Metabolism of pyrimidine arabinonucleotides and cyclonucleosides in *Escherichia coli.* J. biol. Chem. **235**, 2387—2392 (1960).
Rama Reddy, G.V., Goulian, M., Hendler, S.S.: Inhibition of *E. coli* DNA polymerase II by ara CTP. Nature (Lond.) **234**, 286—288 (1971).
Reichard, P., Cannalakis, Z.N., Cannalakis, E.S.: Studies on a possible regulatory mechanism for the biosynthesis of deoxyribonucleic acid. J. biol. Chem. **236**, 2514—2519 (1961).
Renis, H.E., Johnson, H.G.: Inhibition of plaque formation of vaccinia virus by cytosine arabinoside hydrochloride. Bacteriol. Proc. 140 (1962).
Ritter, E.J., Scott, W.J., Wilson, J.G.: Teratogenesis and inhibition of DNA synthesis induced in rat embryos by cytosine arabinoside. Teratology **4**, 7—14 (1971).
Roberts, D.W., Hall, T.C., Rosenthal, D.: Sequential changes in biochemical parameters following cytosine arabinoside administration. Proc. Amer. Ass. Cancer Res. **9**, 60 (1968).
Roberts, D.W., Loehr, E.V.: Methotrexate and cytosine arabinoside modulation of thymidylate synthetase activity in CCRF-CEM cells. Cancer Res. **31**, 457—462 (1971).
Roberts, W.K., Dekker, C.A.: A convenient synthesis of arabinosylcytosine (cytosine arabinoside). J. org. Chem. **32**, 816—817 (1967).
Russell, D.H.: Effects of methotrexate and cytosine arabinoside on polyamine metabolism in a mouse L1210 leukemia. Cancer Res. **32**, 2459—2462 (1972).
Sartorelli, A.C., Creasey, W.A.: Cancer Chemotherapy. Ann. Rev. Pharmacol. **9**, 51—72 (1969).
Sartorelli, A.C., Creasey, W.A.: Combination chemotherapy. In: Holland, J.F., Frei, E. III (Eds.): Cancer medicine, pp. 707—717. Philadelphia: Lea and Febiger 1973.
Schabel, F.M., Jr.: *In vivo* leukemia cell kill kinetics and "curability" in experimental systems. In: The proliferation and spread of neoplastic cells, pp. 379—408. Baltimore: Williams and Wilkins 1968.
Schmidt, G.: Über den fermentativen Abbau der Guanylsäure in der Kaninchenleber. Hoppe-Seyler Z. physiol. Chem. **208**, 185—224 (1932).

SCHOCHETMAN, G., PERRY, R. P.: Early appearance of histone messenger RNA in polyribosomes of cultured L cells. J. molec. Biol. **63**, 591—596 (1972).
SCHRECKER, A. W.: Metabolism of 1-β-D-arabinofuranosylcytosine in leukemia L1210: nucleoside and nucleotide kinases in cell-free extracts. Cancer Res. **30**, 632—641 (1970).
SCHRECKER, A. W., GOLDIN, A.: Antitumor effect and mode of action of 1-β-D-arabinofuranosylcytosine 5′-phosphate in leukemia L1210. Cancer Res. **28**, 802—803 (1968).
SCHRECKER, A. W., URSHEL, M. J.: Nucleoside kinases in leukemia L1210 and a subline resistant to arabinosylcytosine. Proc. Amer. Ass. Cancer Res. **8**, 58 (1967).
SCHRECKER, A. W., URSHEL, M. J.: Metabolism of 1-β-D-arabinofuranosylcytosine in leukemia L1210: studies with intact cells. Cancer Res. **28**, 793—801 (1968).
SILAGI, S.: Metabolism of 1-β-D-arabinofuranosylcytosine in L cells. Cancer Res. **25**, 1446—1453 (1965).
SKIPPER, H. E., SCHABEL, F. M., JR., MELLETT, L. B., MONTGOMERY, J. A., WILKOFF, L. J., LLOYD, H. H., BROCKMAN, R. W.: Implications of biochemical, cytokinetic, pharmacologic, and toxicologic relationships in the design of optimal therapeutic studies. Cancer Chemother. Rep. **54**, 431—449 (1970).
SKIPPER, H. E., SCHABEL, F. M., JR., WILCOX, W. S.: Experimental evaluation of potential anticancer agents. XXI. Scheduling of arabinosylcytosine to take advantage of its *S*-phase specificity against leukemia cells. Cancer Chemother. Rep. **51**, 125—165 (1967).
SKOOG, L., NORDENSKJÖLD, B.: Effects of hydroxyurea and 1-β-D-arabinofuranosylcytosine on deoxyribonucleotide pools in mouse embryo cells. Europ. J. Biochem. **19**, 81—89 (1971).
SLECHTA, L.: Effect of arabonucleosides on growth and metabolism of *E. coli*. Fed. Proc. **20**, 357 (1961).
SMITH, C. G., BUSKIRK, H. H., LUMMIS, W. L.: Effect of arabinofuranosyluracil on the cytotoxicity of arabinofuranosylcytosine in PPLO-contaminated cell cultures. Proc. Amer. Ass. Cancer Res. **6**, 60 (1965).
SMITH, D. B., CHU, E. H. Y.: A genetic approach to the study of cytotoxicity and resistance of cultured Chinese hamster cells in the presence of cytosine arabinoside. Cancer Res. **32**, 1651—1657 (1972).
SMRT, J.: Nucleic acid components and their analogues. C. Arabinofuranosyluracil and arabinofuranosylcytosine phosphates. Coll. Czech. Chem. Commun. **32**, 3958—3965 (1967).
STEUART, C. D., BURKE, P. J.: Cytidine deaminase and the development of resistance to arabinosylcytosine. Nature (Lond.) **233**, 109—110 (1971).
STEUART, C. D., BURKE, P. J., OWENS, A. H., JR.: Correlation of ara-C metabolism and clinical response in adult acute leukemia. Proc. Amer. Ass. Cancer Res. **12**, 89 (1971).
TALLEY, R. W., O'BRYAN, R. M., TUCKER, W. G., LOO, R. V.: Clinical pharmacology and human antitumor activity of cytosine arabinoside. Cancer **20**, 809—816 (1967).
TALLEY, R., VAITKEVICIUS, V.: Megaloblastosis produced by a cytosine antagonist, 1-β-D-arabinofuranosylcytosine, Blood **21**, 352—362 (1963).
TEMIN, H. M.: Studies on carcinogenesis by avian sarcoma viruses. V. Requirement for new DNA synthesis and for cell division. J. Cell Physiol. **69**, 53—64 (1967).
TOBEY, R. A.: Effects of cytosine arabinoside, daunomycin, mithramycin, azacytidine, adriamycin, and camptothecin on mammalian cell cycle traverse. Cancer Res. **32**, 2720—2725 (1972).
TOLMAN, R. L., ROBINS, R. K.: Synthesis of 1-β-L-arabinofuranosylcytosine, the enantiomer of cytosine arabinoside. J. med. Chem. **14**, 1112 (1971).
TONO, H., COHEN, S. S.: The activity of nucleoside phosphorylase on 1-β-D-arabinosyluracil within *Escherichia coli*. J. biol. Chem. **237**, 1271—1282 (1962).
TUOMINEN, F. W., KENNEY, F. T.: Inhibition of RNA-directed DNA polymerase from Rauscher leukemia virus by the 5′-triphosphate of cytosine arabinoside. Biochem. biophys. Res. Commun. **48**, 1469—1475 (1972).
TYRER, D. D., KLINE, I., VENDITTI, J. M., GOLDIN, A.: Separate and sequential chemotherapy of mouse leukemia L1210 with 1-β-D-arabinofuranosylcytosine hydrochloride and 1,3-*bis*-(2-chloroethyl)nitrosourea. Cancer Res. **27**, 873—879 (1967).
UCHIDA, K., KREIS, W., HUTCHISON, D. J.: Distribution of 1-β-D-arabinofuranosylcytosine (ara-C) and enzyme profiles of mice carrying ara-C-sensitive and -resistant P815 neoplasms. Proc. Amer. Ass. Cancer Res. **9**, 72 (1968).
UNDERWOOD, G. E.: Activity of 1-β-D-arabinofuranosylcytosine hydrochloride against herpes simplex keratitis. Proc. Soc. exp. Biol. (N.Y.) **111**, 660—664 (1962).
UPJOHN COMPANY: Cytarabine (Cytosar). Clin. Pharmacol. Therap. **11**, 155—160 (1970).
VERBIN, R. S., DILUISO, G., LIANG, H., FARBER, E.: Synchronization of cell division *in vivo* through the combined use of cytosine arabinoside and colcemid. Cancer Res. **32**, 1489—1495 (1972).

WALWICK, E. R., ROBERTS, W. K., DEKKER, C. A.: Cyclization during the phosphorylation of uridine and cytidine by polyphosphoric acid; a new route to the O^2,2'-cyclonucleosides. Proc. chem. Soc. 84 (1959).
WARNER, D. T., NEIL, G. L., TAYLOR, A. J., WECHTER, W. J.: Nucleic acids. 13. 3'-*O*- and 2'-*O*-esters of 1-β-D-arabinofuranosylcytosine as antileukemic and immunosuppressive agents. J. med. Chem. **15**, 790—792 (1972).
WEMPEN, I., MILLER, N., FALCO, E. A., FOX, J. J.: Nucleosides XLVII. Synthesis of some N_4-substituted derivatives of 1-β-D-arabinofuranosyl-cytosine and -5-fluorocytosine. J. med. Chem. **11**, 144—148 (1968).
WILKOFF, L. J., WILCOX, W. S., BURDESHAW, J. A., DIXON, G. J., DULMADGE, E. A.: Effect of antimetabolites on kinetic behavior of proliferating cultured L1210 leukemia cells. J. nat. Cancer Inst. **39**, 965—975 (1967).
WODINSKY, I., KENSLER, C. J.: Activity of cytosine arabinoside (NSC-63878) in a spectrum of rodent tumors. Cancer Chemother. Rep. **47**, 65—68 (1965).
YOUNG, C. W., HODAS, S.: Acute effects of cytotoxic compounds on incorporation of precursors into DNA, RNA, and protein of HeLa cell monolayers. Biochem. Pharmacol. **14**, 205—214 (1965).
YOUNG, R. S. K., FISCHER, G. A.: The action of arabinosylcytosine on synchronously growing populations of mammalian cells. Biochem. biophys. Res. Commun. **32**, 23—29 (1968).
ZAHN, R. K., MÜLLER, W. E. G., FORSTER, W., MAIDHOF, A., BEYER, R.: Action of 1-β-D-arabinofuranosylcytosine on mammalian tumor cells-1. Incorporation into DNA. Europ. J. Cancer 8, 391—396 (1972).

Chapter 43

Clinical Pharmacology of Arabinosylcytosine

D. H. W. Ho and E. J Freireich

With 1 Figure

Introduction

The drug, 1-β-D-arabinofuranosylcytosine (ara-C), is of importance because of its effectiveness against the acute myeloblastic form of leukemia in man. Its antineoplastic activity is profoundly affected by pharmacological parameters such as dosage, route, and schedule of administration. Furthermore, ara-C has proven to have synergistic activity in combination with a number of different classes of therapeutically active anticancer drugs. Thus, an understanding of the pharmacology of ara-C profoundly influences the strategy of its use and its effectiveness.

Effect of Route of Administration

A. Intravenous Administration — Single Dose

I. Volume of Distribution

As indicated in Table 1, the apparent volume of distribution of ara-C is inversely proportional to the dose of drug administered. At doses of 67 mg/M^2 or less, the volume of distribution is greater than the volume of total body water (> 1000 ml/kg). This probably reflects the rapid metabolism and localization of the drug in cells and is consistent with the observation that the influx of ara-C from the plasma to the peripheral compartment (tissues) is 6 times greater than

Table 1. *Volume of distribution in patients after receiving various doses of ara-C*

Patient	Dose mg/M^2	Apparent volume of distribution ml/kg of ara-C
L. D. (1st dose)[a]	47	1500
L. D. (15th dose)[a]	47	1237
V. M. (1st dose)[a]	67	2892
V. M. (15th dose)[a]	67	1511
E. L.	200	778
L. S.	200	598
E. J.	1500	370
S. W.	3000	433

[a] Patients L. D. and V. M. received 15 doses of ara-C and pharmacologic studies were performed on the 1st and 15th doses.

its efflux (Loo and Ho, unpublished data). At larger doses, the influx of ara-C to the tissues is saturated, and a greater fraction of the drug is, therefore, present in plasma. Because the total ara-C deaminase activity in human plasma is less than 1 % of that in liver, this results in a much smaller apparent volume of distribution at large doses.

II. Half-life

After administration of a single intravenous injection of tritiated ara-C (ara-C-^{3}H) to patients, the levels of total radioactivity in the blood, determined in the acid-soluble fraction, fell rapidly, with a half-life of 30 to 60 min. Examination by paper chromatography of the acid extracts from whole blood of patients failed to reveal unchanged ara-C 5 to 20 min after drug injections (Creasey et al., 1966). Microbiological assay of ara-C from the blood of patients who received the drug showed disappearance of ara-C from the blood within 15 min (Talley et al., 1967).

It has also been reported that blood radioactivity decreased rapidly in 1 of 2 children receiving tritiated ara-C i.v., and that the half-life was less than 30 min. The levels of radioactivity were too low to permit separation into unchanged drug and metabolites by paper chromatography (Finkelstein et al., 1970). Recently, however, clinical pharmacologic studies of ara-C have been further extended (Ho and Frei, 1971). In these investigations, most of the plasma radioactivity was in 1-β-D-arabinofuranosyluracil (ara-U), and all of the radioactivity could be accounted for as ara-C and ara-U. The plasma disappearance curve of

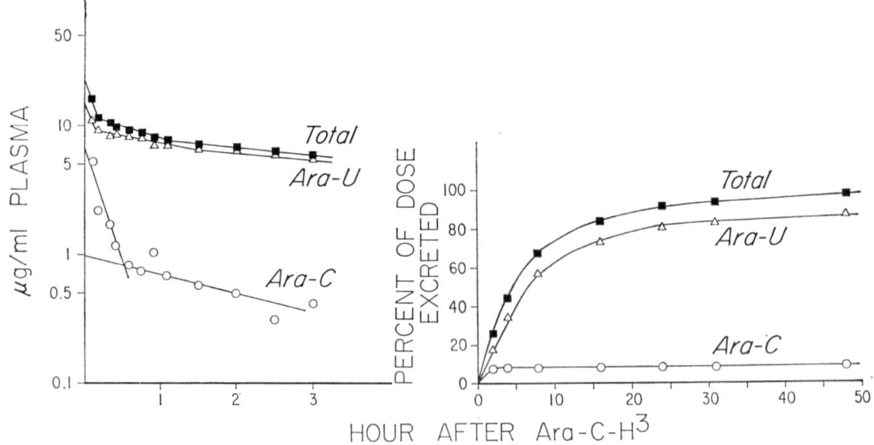

Fig. 1. The distribution of total radioactivity, ara-C, and ara-U in patients' plasma and urine after receiving a single dose of ara-C-^{3}H (200 mg/M^2). (With permission of the C.V. Mosby Company, copyright 1971)

ara-C, when plotted on a semilog scale, was biphasic, with an initial fast phase (mean half-time 12 min) and a slower second phase (mean half-time 111 min) (Fig. 1) (Ho and Frei, 1971). The half-time of ara-C in plasma was independent of the dose, and a linear correlation between the dose and plasma concentration of ara-C was found. Using enzyme kinetic data obtained *in vitro* together with a suitable pharmacokinetic model, plasma concentration of ara-C can be predicted in adult patients after i.v. injections of ara-C (Dedrick et al., 1972).

III. Metabolism

Ara-C is converted to ara-U by an ara-C deaminase (i.e., pyrimidine nucleoside deaminase), and is phosphorylated to its triphosphate level by various kinase enzymes.

1. Plasma

CREASEY et al. (1966) were first to identify ara-U as the only metabolite present in the plasma of patients who received ara-C. Recent studies corroborated these findings and showed that essentially all of the radioactivity in plasma was accounted for by ara-C and ara-U (HO and FREI, 1972). The initial plasma ara-U to ara-C ratio was lower at the larger doses of ara-C, suggesting saturation of ara-C deaminase activity (HO and FREI, 1971).

2. Leukemic Cells

Ara-C-^{3}H has been shown to enter leukemic lymphocytes rapidly when the drug was incubated with cells *in vitro* (CREASEY et al., 1966). The capacity for ara-C phosphorylation was greatest in mature lymphocytes, lymphoblasts, and in some cases, myeloblasts. A patient with chronic myelogenous leukemia in blast crisis received continuous i.v. infusion of ara-C; a steady level of ara-C was maintained after a 3-hour infusion. Ninety-six percent of the radioactivity of white blood cells was present as ara-C nucleotides, this concentration being twenty-two fold greater than plasma ara-C levels (HO and FREI, 1971).

IV. Excretion

Ara-C is converted to ara-U, which is rapidly excreted in the urine. This rapid conversion to ara-U largely accounts for the extremely short half-life of ara-C. Most of the drug (85 %) is recovered in urine by 24 h, 8 % as ara-C and the remainder as ara-U (Fig. 1) (HO and FREI, 1971).

B. Oral Administration

I. Absorption

The activity of orally administered ara-C in experimental systems is well documented (EVANS et al., 1964b; GOLDENBERG et al., 1968; KLINE et al., 1968); the oral dose required to exert an effect is three- to ten-fold greater than the parenteral dose. All of 7 cancer patients treated daily with oral ara-C showed megaloblastic bone marrow changes (GOLDENBERG et al., 1968). Patients receiving ara-C-^{3}H orally excreted only 14 % of the dose in the urine with less than 3 % of the dose being ara-C, and the remainder ara-U (HO and FREI, 1971). Radioactivity increased steadily in the plasma, reaching a plateau after 6 h. Approximately 70 % of the radioactivity was ara-U and 30 % was ara-C (HO and FREI, 1971). The relatively poor absorption (i.e., less than 20 %) of ara-C from the gastrointestinal tract in man and monkeys (HO and FREI, 1971; MELLETT et al., 1971) is consistent with the fact that ara-C is less effective when given orally.

II. Effect of 1-(β-D-ribofuranosyl)-4-hydroxy-3,4,5,6-tetrahydropyrimidine-2-(1H)-one (Tetrahydrouridine, THU)

THU is an effective inhibitor of pyrimidine nucleoside deaminase *in vitro* and *in vivo* (CAMIENER and SMITH, 1968; HANZE, 1967; MULLIGAN and MELLETT, 1968). THU markedly enhances the therapeutic effect of ara-C administered orally to mice bearing L1210 leukemia (Neil et al., 1970a). The effect exceeds that achieved with intraperitoneally administered ara-C alone, presumably by greatly prolonging the half-life of ara-C. Since studies with ara-C in man, as well as in experimental systems, have shown that frequent i.v. injections or continuous i.v. infusion for 5 days is a better regimen than 5 daily single injections (Burke et al., 1968; Carey and Ellison, 1965; Ellison et al., 1968; Frei et al., 1969; Freireich et al., 1970; Kline et al., 1966a; Skipper et al., 1967), it would be advantageous to have an orally active form of ara-C which is capable of maintaining a constant blood level over these time periods.

C. Intrathecal Administration

Ara-C is moderately effective when given systemically against intracranially transplanted L1210 leukemic cells (Kline et al., 1966b). This would suggest that ara-C passes the blood brain barrier. A single cerebrospinal fluid (CSF) sample taken after a pulse dose of ara-C in man revealed a very low concentration of the drug (Ho and Frei, 1971). However, when ara-C was given by continuous i.v. infusion over a 2 h period, the level of ara-C in the spinal fluid was 50 % that of simultaneous plasma samples (Ho and Frei, 1971). The ratio of ara-C to ara-U in the spinal fluid was much larger than in the plasma (Ho and Frei, 1971). The intrathecal administration of ara-C (50 mg/M^2) results in large concentrations of ara-C and a half-time of 2 h. The ratio of ara-C to ara-U, even after 7 h, is 6:1 (Ho and Frei, 1971); this is probably because of very low ara-C deaminase levels in the CSF and brain. The concentration of radioactivity in the plasma following intrathecal injection is small, and by 24 h, 70 % of the radioactivity appears in the urine. At 7 h, the concentration of ara-C in the CSF is still 40 μg/ml; assuming a continued exponential decrease in ara-C concentration, levels greater than 0.1 μg/ml would persist for approximately 24 h. Studies in cell culture have shown that exposure to low concentrations of ara-C (0.1 μg/ml) for long periods of time may be as lethal to cells as larger concentrations for shorter periods (Graham and Whitmore, 1970; Wilkoff et al., 1967). Thus, daily intrathecal therapy at doses of about 50 mg/M^2 or continuous i.v. infusion should provide continuous levels of ara-C greater than 0.1 μg/ml, and should be a useful regimen for meningeal leukemia.

D. Intramuscular and Subcutaneous Administration

Finkelstein et al. (1970) have performed pharmacological studies in man with intramuscularly and subcutaneously injected ara-C-^{3}H, which are indistinguishable from intravenously injected ara-C. The administered radioactivity was almost completely excreted within the first 24 h and the conversion of ara-C to ara-U approached 90% within 4 h of administration. The levels of radioactivity in plasma were too low to permit the separation of ara-C from ara-U. This study led to the suggestion that ara-C should have similar therapeutic effect in man regardless of the route of administration (Finkelstein et al., 1970). However, the ara-C levels in human plasma achieved by different routes of administration should be defined before any clinical applications can be inferred.

Toxicity

A. Myelosuppression

It is well documented that the major toxic manifestations of ara-C are leukopenia and thrombocytopenia (Bernard et al., 1966; Bodey et al., 1969; Burke et al., 1968; CAREY and ELLISON, 1965; HENDERSON and BURKE, 1965; HOWARD et al., 1966; LIVINGSTON and CARTER, 1968; LOO et al., 1965; TALLEY and FREI, 1968), and that the leukocyte depression is largely attributable to granulocyte depression with little lymphocyte involvement (TALLEY and FREI, 1968). Reticulocytopenia was more consistently observed with 48- and 96-hour continuous infusion and with the larger dose levels employed with 24-hour infusion (TALLEY and FREI, 1968).

B. Megaloblastosis and Unbalanced Growth

TALLEY and VAITKEVICIUS (1963) were the first to report that ara-C produced megaloblastosis; this has been confirmed by other investigators (BELL et al., 1966; BLOCK et al., 1965; CAREY and ELLISON, 1965; CARTER and LIVINGSTON, 1969; LIVINGSTON and CARTER, 1968; LOO et al., 1965; TALLEY and FREI, 1968). However, megaloblastosis was rapidly reversed after the cessation of treatment.

Ara-C is a specific inhibitor of DNA synthesis (CHU and FISCHER, 1962; FURTH and COHEN, 1968; INAGAKI et al., 1969; KIM and EIDENOFF, 1965; KIMBALL and WILSON, 1968). Thus, cells prevented from making DNA cannot divide, even though active RNA and protein synthesis can still proceed, leading to imbalanced growth and eventually to permanent loss of proliferative capacity (SKINNER et al., 1967). Therefore, if an effective blood concentration of ara-C can be maintained for long enough in patients with nonsynchronous leukemic cell populations, all of the cells will be arrested in *S*-phase, and this will eventually be followed by cell death (SKIPPER et al., 1967). The effect of ara-C on KB cells is a partial inhibition of DNA synthesis, leading to a cessation of mitosis and cell proliferation. The synthesis of RNA continues normally as the cells undergo marked enlargement (KARON et al., 1966). This pattern is similar to that observed in megaloblastosis (KARON et al., 1966; REISNER, 1958).

C. Chromosomal Aberrations and Teratogenesis

Ara-C has been shown to be potent in inducing chromosome breakage (BELL et al., 1966; BENEDICT et al., 1970; BENEDICT and KARON, 1971; BREWER, 1965; BREWER and CHRISTIE, 1967; CHU, 1965; KIHLMAN et al., 1963). These chromosome breaks resulted from the inhibition of DNA synthesis (BENEDICT et al., 1970; KIHLMAN et al., 1963). Ara-C has been shown to produce teratogenic effects in lower animals (CHAUBE et al., 1968; DIXON and ADAMSON, 1965; KARNOFSKY and LACON, 1966; RITTER et al., 1971).

D. Other Toxic Effects

Nausea, vomiting, anemia, and mild hepatic and gastrointestinal toxicity are also seen, but are not dose-limiting factors (BODEY et al., 1969; CARTER and LIVINGSTON, 1969).

Effect of Schedule, Dose, and Strategy of Treatment

A. Effect of Duration of Continuous Infusion on Clinical Toxicity

With single doses of up to 4200 mg/M², no significant toxicity to the bone marrow is detectable, as measured by changes in circulating blood cells. This lack of toxicity of a single injection is presumably caused by the short biological half-life of ara-C, resulting in a minimal effect on cells in cycle. When the drug is administered by continuous infusion for a 24-hour period, however, there is moderate but reversible toxicity observed with doses of 600 to 800 mg/M^2, although a further increase of dose by a factor of two is not associated with any increase in toxicity. The plateau observed after 24-hour infusion presumably reflects that the fraction of cells which was exposed during *S*-phase is maximally suppressed and that cells not in cycle are not suppressed. Thus, no further enhancement of toxicity was observed with increasing doses. However, when the infusion period is prolonged to 48 h or longer, there is a progressive increase in myelosuppression with doses increasing up to 1000 mg/M^2 (Burke et al., 1968; Frei et al., 1969). This is presumably caused by the fact that in 48 h a major fraction of the proliferating marrow cells has gone through the cell cycle.

B. Effect of Dose and Schedule on Pharmacological Findings

I. Dose

Pharmacological studies have been performed in patients receiving varying doses of ara-C from 47 to 3000 mg/M^2 intravenously; ara-C and ara-U are the only products found. The half-life of ara-C in plasma is independent of the dose, and a linear correlation between the dose and plasma levels of ara-C was found (Ho and Frei, 1971). The ratios of plasma concentrations of ara-U to ara-C at 5 min are inversely proportional to the dose; the larger the dose, the lower the ratio (Ho and Frei, 1971). This suggests the saturation of ara-C deaminase activity (Ho and Frei, 1971), which has been extensively studied (Camiener, 1967a, b; Camiener and Smith, 1965). A wide tissue and species variation in the enzyme activity was reported, with high activity in human liver (Camiener, 1967a). The enzyme activity of human tissues was determined on the basis of units per gram of tissue. The liver deaminase activity converts 1.9 mg of ara-C to ara-U per gram of liver per hour or 31 μg of ara-C to ara-U per minute. A patient who received 4.5 g of ara-C (3.0 g/M^2) had a body weight of 52 kg and an estimated liver weight of 1430 g; thus, a total liver deaminase activity of 45 mg of ara-C per minute. The injected 4.5 g of ara-C would take approximately 100 min to be deaminated (Ho, unpublished data). Therefore, it appears that with large doses, the deaminase activity is initially saturated with ara-C.

II. Schedule

The therapeutic effect of ara-C is profoundly affected by the schedule of administration. In the mouse, administration every 3 h for 8 doses twice weekly has proved to be superior to daily treatment (Kline et al., 1966a; Skipper et al., 1967). This reflects the short cell cycle time of the experimental tumors being investigated, and the administration every 3 to 4 days permits recovery of normal organ function between courses of treatment. In man, a schedule of administration utilizing continuous infusion for 5 days or i.v. injections every 8 h for 15 doses over 120 h gave comparable results, which were better than the results from 5 daily single injections (Frei et al., 1969; Freireich et al., 1971; Wang et al., 1970). Pharmacological studies were performed at the first and fifteenth doses in patients receiving injections every 8 h, and it was found that the plasma half-time of ara-C, as well as the excretion of both ara-C and ara-U, were similar for both doses (Ho and Frei, 1971). Thus, the pharmacological disposition is not affected by prior exposure to ara-C over the 120-hour period. Recent studies have shown that there is a significant correlation between the half-life of ara-C *in vivo* and the response to ara-C treatment in man (Baguley and Faikenhaug, 1971). Thus, patients with a short half-life for ara-C have a poor response. This emphasizes the importance of pharmacology to the therapeutic results.

Clinical pharmacological studies of ara-C administered by constant intravenous infusion have been performed after a loading dose, the purpose of the latter being to reach a steady state of ara-C promptly. Constant infusion of ara-C in the therapeutic dose range (112 mg/M²/day) resulted in a constant plasma level of ara-C of 0.07 μg/ml (Ho and Frei, 1971). There was a correlation between the dose and ara-C plasma level; an infusion rate of 400 mg/M²/day produced a constant plasma level of ara-C of 0.4 μg/ml (Ho and Frei, 1971). The best present schedule of continuous infusion therapy for acute myelogenous leukemia is 200 mg/M²/day for 5 days (Bodey et al., 1969). This results in a constant plasma level of ara-C of approximately 0.15 μg/ml. This concentration is effective in decreasing substantially the synthesis of DNA; the decrease presumably results from arrest of cells at the G_1-S interphase or from progression delay during the S period (Wilkoff et al., 1967).

C. Clinical Results for Acute Leukemia and the Relationship of Schedule to Effectiveness

Ara-C has its primary clinical activity against the acute myeloblastic form of leukemia that occurs primarily in adults. While activity has been reported in the childhood or lymphoblastic variety, the striking activity is in myeloblastic leukemia. Considering the virtually specific myelosuppressive effect on normal bone marrow, the specificity for myeloblastic leukemia is relevant. The most effective regimen reported to date for ara-C administered alone is continuous intravenous infusion over 120 h, with rest periods of 9 or more days between courses of treatment to allow for recovery of normal myeloid tissue (Bodey et al., 1969). Comparable results have been obtained with a schedule of i.v. injections every 8 h for 15 doses over 120 h using a similar strategy. Moreover, this drug can be continued at roughly 3- to 4-week intervals in maintenance therapy for long periods of time. This regimen has resulted in remissions with median durations of over 60 weeks and, in a small fraction of patients, in excess of 2 years.

Combination Chemotherapy

The first report of the synergism between ara-C and other agents was reported by Evans et al. (1964a), who used the drug in combination with porfiromycin. This was soon followed by the observations of synergism between ara-C and either nitrosoureas or thiopurines in experimental animals (Schabel, 1968).

A. Ara-C and Cyclophosphamide

Ara-C alone will prolong life, but will not cure mice bearing L1210 leukemia when given in the advanced stage of disease (Hoffman et al., 1969; Schabel, 1968). In combination with nitrosourea or cyclophosphamide, ara-C is synergistic against L1210 leukemia and produces a high cure rate (Schabel et al., 1968). These results suggested that similar combination therapy could be effective in acute leukemia. Cyclophosphamide was chosen rather than a nitrosourea because it is able to induce remission when used alone in human leukemia (Fernbach et al., 1962). Initial studies of a combination of ara-C and cyclophosphamide gave promising results in adults with acute myeloblastic leukemia (Bodey et al., 1970). This was followed by a report of better response when the 4 drug combination of vincristine, prednisone, ara-C, and cyclophosphamide (COAP) was given to 50 consecutive patients (Whitecar et al., 1972). The COAP regimen was established as superior to ara-C alone in a prospective randomized study (Bodey et al., 1972). This has led to a comparative evaluation of COAP against a 3 drug combination of ara-C, vincristine, and prednisone (Southwest Cancer Chemotherapy Study Group protocol 560/561). Thus, while improved results with cyclophosphamide have been reported, the synergism observed in experimental animals has not been solidly and comparatively established in man.

B. Ara-C and 1,3-*bis*-(2-Chloroethyl)-1-Nitrosourea (BCNU)

There is some biochemical evidence that ara-C and BCNU act at two different sites in nucleic acid synthesis (Groth et al., 1972; Wheeler and Bowdon, 1965), and that they are synergistic against L1210 mouse leukemia (Tyrer et al., 1968). This combination was tried and well tolerated in patients with metastatic cancer and acute leukemia (Vogler et al., 1971). Remissions were achieved, but the results were not significantly better than those seen using ara-C alone; the major problem was early death caused by infections (Hersh et al., 1965). Another study of ara-C and BCNU in a different schedule achieved a better remission rate with little toxicity (Hayes and Ellison, 1969). However, further studies are necessary to explore the usefulness of this combination in man.

C. Ara-C and 6-Thioguanine (TG)

Following the report of synergistic activity between ara-C and 6-mercaptopurine in the mouse (Burchenal and Dollinger, 1967), Gee et al. (1969) reported that remissions averaging 6 months were achieved in 21 of 38 patients treated with a combination of ara-C and TG. This observation has subsequently been confirmed in a larger series of patients. Simultaneous treatment with ara-C and TG protects mice from TG toxicity (Schmidt et al., 1970). When given simultaneously, the administration of ara-C inhibits TG incorporation into DNA, but the incorporation is augmented when TG is given 12 to 18 h after ara-C (LePage and White, 1972). Thus, studies in man of the temporal relationship between ara-C and TG are of great importance, and such studies in patients with acute leukemia using the 2 drugs at 12-hour intervals or other time schedules may prove to be highly informative.

D. Ara-C and Methyl Mitomycin (Porfiromycin)

The possible effectiveness of combination therapy with ara-C and porfiromycin in man was indicated by studies of the synergistic effects of these two drugs on median survival time in experimental animals (Evans et al., 1964a). Studies of this combination in children with acute leukemia showed no advantage over the use of ara-C alone (Kaplan et al., 1966). Information should be obtained on modification of dose and schedule of administration of these two drugs.

Resistance to Ara-C as Related to Kinase: Deaminase Ratios and to Intracellular Ribonucleotide Concentrations

Phosphorylation of ara-C to nucleotides by ara-C kinase is required for the action of the drug, and impaired kinase activity has been correlated with the development of drug resistance by P5178Y leukemic cells in culture (Chu and Fischer, 1965). Survival of mice bearing different transplantable leukemias treated with ara-C was compared with uptake and subsequent phosphorylation of ara-C *in vitro*.

The degree of drug phosphorylation was correlated with response, and is an important determinant of drug sensitivity (KESSEL et al., 1967). The kinase activity of cell extracts was decreased in L1210 leukemic cells resistant to ara-C (SCHRECKER, 1970). The same mechanism was reported in the P815 tumor resistant to ara-C *in vivo* (UCHIDA and KREIS, 1969). It has been demonstrated that the lack of ara-C-5'-diphosphate (ara-CDP) and ara-C-5'-triphosphate (ara-CTP) in the resistant cells is the result of a very low ara-C kinase activity (DRAHOVSKY and KREIS, 1970; UCHIDA and KREIS, 1969). Leukemic cells from patients who responded to ara-C treatment demonstrated a rapid conversion of ara-C to nucleotides, and the capacity of ara-C phosphorylation was lowest in circulating lymphoblasts and myeloblasts from patients resistant to ara-C (HALL et al., 1968; KESSEL et al., 1969). The deamination of ara-C did not appear to be an important factor in ara-C resistance (HALL et al., 1968; KESSEL et al., 1967; UCHIDA and KREIS, 1969). However, the difference in phosphorylation of ara-C is not a general finding in all of the strains reported resistant to ara-C (BACH, 1969; MOMPARLER et al., 1968). Deoxycytidylic deaminase activity increased in mammalian cells exposed to ara-C *in vitro* (KIT et al., 1966). It was reported that the response to ara-C in 34 patients correlated with the ratio of kinase and deaminase activity in bone marrow and peripheral leukemic cells (STEUART et al., 1971b). In a later report by the same group, responses in human leukemia to ara-C are correlated with lower intracellular concentrations of deaminase than those present in nonresponders (STEUART and BURKE, 1971a). Furthermore, in sequential treatment schedules, increasing deaminase activities are associated with markedly reduced susceptibility of the tumor cell to ara-C (STEUART and BURKE, 1971a).

Ara-C-5'-phosphate was found to have an antitumor effect similar to ara-C in L1210 leukemia; the dephosphorylation could take place by phosphohydrolases on the cell membrane or within the cell (SCHRECKER and GOLDIN, 1968; SCHRECKER and MEAD, 1966). Thus, the rate of hydrolysis of ara-C nucleotides could also be a factor in determining the response to ara-C. However, 5'-nucleotidase was found in about equal amounts in experimental tumors sensitive or resistant to ara-C (DRAHOVSKY and KREIS, 1970; SCHRECKER, 1970).

Large ara-C kinase activities have been demonstrated in peripheral white blood cells of patients with chronic lymphocytic leukemia and acute myelocytic and lymphocytic leukemia (KESSEL et al., 1969). Further studies with peripheral leukemic and bone marrow cells have shown that cells of patients with acute myelogenous leukemia (AML) and chronic lymphocytic leukemia (CLL) have high kinase and low deaminase activities (HO, unpublished data). Since AML patients treated with ara-C showed a response rate of about 40 % (FREIREICH et al., 1971), the high kinase and deaminase activities in CLL cells are suggestive that patients with CLL may likewise respond to ara-C. In fact, remission has been induced in patients with CLL treated with ara-C and cyclophosphamide (GUTTERMAN et al., 1972). However, further studies with either drug alone in CLL patients are necessary before a positive correlation between kinase and deaminase ratios and responsiveness to ara-C therapy can be established unequivocally. Studies of kinase and deaminase activities of solid tumors are quite preliminary. However, in a study of patients with malignant melanoma, two patients were found to have relatively high kinase activities and both patients showed objective response to ara-C treatment. Another 12 patients were found to have relatively lower kinase activities and failed to respond to ara-C treatment (HART et al., 1972). If further investigation of melanoma and other solid tumors support these preliminary findings, the determination of kinase and deaminase ratios may be of great predictive value for determining responsiveness to ara-C therapy.

Perspectives

The therapeutic effectiveness of ara-C could be substantially improved if the biological half-life of the drug could be prolonged by protecting it from rapid deamination. However, modification of the chemical formulation of ara-C, resulting in either delayed release or improved oral absorption of the drug, could also be considered as a potential approach.

A. Tetrahydrouridine (THU)

THU is a potent inhibitor of ara-C deaminase *in vitro* and *in vivo* (Camiener and Smith, 1968; Hanze, 1967; Mulligan and Mellett, 1968). It has also been demonstrated that THU inhibits human liver ara-C kinase activity (Ho, 1972). In experimental animals, THU has no toxicity or intrinsic antitumor activity, but markedly enhances the therapeutic effect of ara-C administered orally (Neil et al., 1970a). Therapeutic results obtained with combinations of THU and ara-C administered orally are comparable to those achieved with intraperitoneal ara-C alone (Neil et al., 1970a). However, ara-C has not been adequately studied with oral regimens, and it has not been shown to have antitumor activity in limited studies. It would be advantageous to have an orally active form of ara-C to eliminate the clinical need for frequent i.v. injections or continuous i.v. infusion.

In addition to its ability to improve oral administration, THU may be useful for converting tumors from resistance to sensitivity. If the basis for resistance is high deaminase activity, then the administration of significant concentrations of THU may result in increased susceptibility of these tumors to ara-C.

B. 1-β-D-Arabinofuranosylcytosine 5′-Adamantoate (AdO-Ara-C)

Therapy with a single dose of AdO-ara-C was almost as effective as ara-C on an optimum schedule with injections every 3 h for L1210 leukemia in mice (Neil et al., 1970b). The agent is active even when administered as early as 48 h prior to tumor inoculation. These studies suggest that esters of ara-C might be useful as depot forms of the drug, permitting infrequent dosages with sustained release of ara-C to maintain constant blood levels over extended periods. This would obviate the need for continuous i.v. infusion for 5 days, and would greatly extend the therapeutic range of this drug clinically.

Preliminary pharmacological studies of patients after a single intramuscular injection of ara-C-5′-palmitate-^{14}C (palmo-ara-C-^{14}C) revealed a slow absorption of the drug. In 7 days, only 40 % of the given drug was excreted, of which less than 2 % was ara-C (Ho and Frei, unpublished data). This study confirmed the lack of myelosuppression in patients receiving palmo-ara-C in a phase I study (Frei, unpublished data). It is therefore desirable to have depot forms of ara-C that are more soluble and better absorbed than palmo-ara-C. Ara-C-5′-benzoate and 5′-octanoate may prove to be more useful agents (Gray et al., 1972).

C. Other Ara-C Analogs

Attempts have been made to find ara-C analogs which are less easily deaminated and therefore possibly more effective.

I. 2,2′-*O*-Cyclocytidine (Cyclocytidine)

Cyclocytidine was synthesized from cytidine (Kanai et al., 1970; Kikugawa and Ichino, 1970) and was active against L1210 leukemia (Hoshi et al., 1971).

It appeared that the drug was less toxic, but more effective than ara-C administered once daily for 5 days for treatment of mice bearing L1210 leukemia. Four of six mice survived for over 45 days after treatment with cyclocytidine, whereas none were cured with ara-C therapy (HOSHI et al., 1971). At a larger dose than ara-C, cyclocytidine inhibits DNA, but not RNA or protein synthesis of human marrow cells and peripheral leukemic cells *in vitro*, and is not deaminated during incubation with human liver extracts at 37° for 2 h, whereas ara-C is completely deaminated within 20 min under the same conditions (Ho, unpublished data). If cyclocytidine is slowly hydrolyzed and serves as a reservoir of ara-C, this may obviate the current clinical practice of continuous i.v. infusion or injections every 8 h for 5 days.

II. Arabinosyl Cytosine 3-N-Oxide (Ara-C-3-*N*-Oxide)

This compound was synthesized to protect ara-C from rapid deamination (PANZICA et al., 1971). Preliminary studies indicated that ara-C-3-*N*-oxide is a potent inhibitor of L1210 leukemia, and long-term survivors were observed in L1210 leukemia-bearing mice treated with ara-C-3-*N*-oxide (PANZICA et al., 1971). This derivative certainly may have clinical application in those situations in which the deaminase activity is very high in human tissues.

D. Sparing Action by Uridine

Uridine administered in conjunction with a suboptimal dose of ara-C produced an increase in the life span of mice bearing leukemia L1210 (SASLAW et al., 1968). It is noteworthy that this synergism was achieved with a naturally occurring compound with ara-C rather than with another antileukemic agent. Enzymatic studies demonstrated that a dialyzed spleen supernatant from L1210 leukemia-bearing mice phosphorylated ara-C with uridine triphosphate (UTP) at twice the initial rate, as compared to a molar equivalent level of adenosine triphosphate (ATP) (GRINDEY et al., 1968). Thus, the potentiating effect of uridine on ara-C was suggested to be a consequence of increased phosphorylation of ara-C in the presence of UTP. Preliminary studies with the ara-C kinase of human spleen and leukemic cells from patients with acute or chronic lymphocytic and myelocytic leukemia showed that ATP is a better phosphate donor than UTP (Ho, unpublished data). However, it was shown in L1210 cells that UTP was the better phosphate donor only if the level of the substrate, ara-C, was low (KESSEL, 1968). In other words, the effect of UTP is strictly a concentration dependent phenomenon.

References

BACH, M.K.: Biochemical and genetic studies of a mutant strain of mouse leukemia L1210 resistant to 1-β-D-arabinofuranosyl cytosine (cytarabine) hydrochloride. Cancer Res. **29**, 1036—1044 (1969).

BAGULEY, B.C., FAIKENHAUG, E.M.: Plasma half-life of cytosine arabinoside in patients treated for acute myeloblastic leukemia. Cancer Chemother. Rep. **55**, 291—298 (1971).

BELL, W.R., WHANG, J.J., CARBONE, P.P., BRECHER, G., BLOCK, J.B.: Cytogenetic and morphologic abnormalities in human bone marrow cells during cytosine arabinoside therapy. Blood **27**, 771—781 (1966).

BENEDICT, W.R., HARRIS, N., KARON, M.: Kinetics of 1-β-D-arabinofuranosylcytosine-induced chromosome breaks. Cancer Res. **30**, 2477—2483 (1970).

BENEDICT, W.F., KARON, M.: Chromatid breakage: ara-C induced lesions inhibited by UV irradiation. Science **171**, 680—682 (1971).

BERNARD, J., BOIRON, M., JACQUILLAT, C., LORTHOLARY, P., WEIL, M.: Les leucemies aiguës granulocytaires. Bull. Soc. med. Hop. (Paris) **117**, 699—709 (1966).

BLOCK, J.B., BELL, W., WHANG, J., CARBONE, P.P.: Hematologic and cytogenic abnormalities during cytosine arabinoside therapy. Proc. Amer. Ass. Cancer Res. **6**, 6 (1965).

BODEY, G.P., COLTMAN, C.A., FREIREICH, E.J, BONNET, J.D., GEHAN, E.A., HAUT, A.B., HEWLETT, J.S., McCREDIE, K.B., SAIKI, J.H., WILSON, H.E.: Arabinosyl cytosine (ara-C) versus combination chemotherapy (COAP) for adult acute leukemia. Proc. Amer. Ass. Cancer Res. **13**, 107 (1972).

BODEY, G.P., FREIREICH, E.J, MONTO, R.W., HEWLETT, J.S.: Cytosine arabinoside (NSC 63878) therapy for acute leukemia in adults. Cancer Chemother. Rep. **53**, 59—66 (1969).

BODEY, G.P., RODRIGUEZ, V., HART, J.S., FREIREICH, E.J: Therapy of acute leukemia with the combination of cytosine arabinoside (NSC 63878) and cyclophosphamide (NSC 26271). Cancer Chemother. Rep. **54**, 255—262 (1970).

BREWER, J.G.: The induction of chromatid lesions by cytosine arabinoside in post-DNA-synthetic human leukocytes. Cytogenetics **4**, 28—36 (1965).

BREWER, J.G., CHRISTIE, N.T.: Studies on the induction of chromosomal aberrations in human leukocytes by cytosine arabinoside. Exp. Cell Res. **46**, 276—291 (1967).

BURCHENAL, J.H., DOLLINGER, M.R.: Cytosine arabinoside in combination with 6-mercaptopurine, methotrexate or fluorouracil in L1210 mouse leukemia. Cancer Chemother. Rep. **51**, 435—438 (1967).

BURKE, P.J., SERPICK, A.A., CARBONE, P.P., TARR, N.A.: Clinical evaluation of dose and schedule of administration of cytosine arabinoside (NSC 63878). Cancer Res. **28**, 274—279 (1968).

CAMIENER, G.W.: Studies of the enzymatic deamination of cytosine arabinoside. II. Properties of the deaminase of human liver. Biochem. Pharmacol. **16**, 1681—1689 (1967a).

CAMIENER, G.W.: Studies of the enzymatic deamination of cytosine arabinoside. III. Substrate requirements and inhibitors of the deaminase of human liver. Biochem. Pharmacol. **16**, 1691—1702 (1967b).

CAMIENER, G.W., SMITH, C.G.: Studies of the enzymatic deamination of cytosine arabinoside. I. Enzyme deamination and species specificity. Biochem. Pharmacol. **14**, 1405—1416 (1965).

CAMIENER, G.W., SMITH, C.G.: Studies of the enzymatic deamination of ara-cytidine. V. Inhibition *in vitro* and *in vivo* by tetrahydrouridine and other reduced pyrimidine nucleosides. Biochem. Pharmacol. **17**, 1981—1991 (1968).

CAREY, R.W., ELLISON, R.R.: Continuous cytosine arabinoside infusions in patients with neoplastic disease. Clin. Res. **13**, 337 (1965).

CARTER, S.K., LIVINGSTON, R.B.: Ara-C: development and application. Proceedings of the Chemotherapy Conference, National Cancer Institute, October (1969).

CHAUBE, S., KREIS, W., UCHIDA, K., MURPHY, M.L.: The teratogenic effect of 1-β-D-arabinofuranosylcytosine in the rat. Biochem. Pharmacol. **17**, 1213—1226 (1968).

CHU, E.H.Y.: Effects of ultraviolet radiation on mammalian cells. I. Induction of chromosome aberrations. Mutat. Res. **2**, 75—94 (1965).

CHU, M.Y., FISCHER, G.A.: A proposed mechanism of action of 1-β-D-arabinofuranosylcytosine as an inhibitor of the growth of leukemic cells. Biochem. Pharmacol. **11**, 423—430 (1962).

CHU, M.Y., FISCHER, G.A.: Comparative studies of leukemic cells sensitive and resistant to cytosine arabinoside. Biochem. Pharmacol. **14**, 333—341 (1965).

CREASEY, W.A., PAPAC, R.J., MARKIW, M.E., CALABRESI, P., WELCH, A.D.: Biochemical and pharmacological studies with 1-β-D-arabinofuranosylcytosine in man. Biochem. Pharmacol. **15**, 1417—1428 (1966).

DEDRICK, R.L., FORRESTER, D.D., HO, D.H.W.: *In vitro-in vivo* correlation of drug metabolism — 1-β-D-arabinofuranosyl cytosine. Biochem. Pharmacol. **21**, 1—16 (1972).

DIXON, R.L., ADAMSON, R.H.: Antitumor activity and pharmacologic disposition of cytosine arabinoside (NSC 63878). Cancer Chemother. Rep. **48**, 11—16 (1965).

DRAHOVSKY, D., KREIS, W.: Studies on drug resistance — II. Kinase patterns in P815 neoplasms sensitive and resistant to 1-β-D-arabinofuranosyl cytosine. Biochem. Pharmacol. **19**, 940—944 (1970).

ELLISON, R.R., HOLLAND, J.F., WEIL, M., JACQUILLAT, C., BOIRON, M., BERNARD, J., SAWITSKY, A., ROSNER, F., GUSSOFF, B., SILVER, R.T., KARANAS, A., CUTTNER, J., SPURR, C.L., HAYES, D.M., BLOM, J., LEONE, L.A., HAURANI, F., KYLE, R., HUTCHISON, J.L., FORCIER, R.J., MOON, J.H.: Arabinosyl cytosine: a useful agent in the treatment of acute leukemia in adults. Blood **32**, 507—523 (1968).

EVANS, J., BOSTWICK, L., MENGEL, G.D.: Synergism of the antineoplastic activity of cytosine arabinoside by porfiromycin. Biochem. Pharmacol. **13**, 983—988 (1964a).

EVANS, J.S., MUSSER, E.A., BOSTWICK, L., MENGEL, G.D.: The effect of 1-β-D-arabinofuranosyl cytosine hydrochloride on murine neoplasms. Cancer Res. **24**, 1285—1293 (1964b).

FERNBACH, D.J., SUTOW, W.W., THURMAN, W.G., VIETTI, T.S.: Clinical evaluation of cyclophosphamide. A new agent for the treatment of children with acute leukemia. J. Amer. med. Ass. **182**, 30—37 (1962).

FINKELSTEIN, J.Z., SCHER, J., KARON, M.: Pharmacologic studies of tritiated cytosine arabinoside. Cancer Chemother. Rep. **54**, 35—39 (1970).

FREI, E., III, BICKERS, J.N., HEWLETT, J.S., LANE, M., LEARY, W.V., TALLEY, R.W.: Dose schedule and antitumor studies of arabinosyl cytosine (NSC 63878). Cancer Res. **29**, 1325—1332 (1969).

FREIREICH, E.J, BODEY, G.P., HART, J.S., RODRIGUEZ, V., WHITECAR, J.P., FREI, E., III: Remission induction in adults with acute myelogenous leukemia. In: RENTCHNICK, P. (Ed.): Recent results in cancer research, Vol. 30, pp. 85—91. Berlin-Heidelberg-New York: Springer 1970.

FREIREICH, E.J, BODEY, G.P., HART, J.S., WHITECAR, J.P., JR., MCCREDIE, K.B.: Current status of therapy for acute leukemia. In: Recent results in cancer research, Vol. 36. Current concepts in the management of leukemia and lymphoma, pp. 119—125. Berlin-Heidelberg-New York: Springer 1971.

FURTH, J.J., COHEN, S.S.: Inhibition of mammalian DNA polymerase by the 5′-triphosphate of 1-β-D-arabinofuranosyl cytosine and the 5′-triphosphate 1-β-D-arabinofuranosyl adenine. Cancer Res. **28**, 2061—2067 (1968).

GEE, T.S., YU, K.P., CLARKSON, B.D.: Treatment of adult acute leukemia with arabinosyl cytosine and thioguanine. Cancer **23**, 1019—1032 (1969).

GOLDENBERG, D.M., SCHRICKER, K.T., VON DER EMDES, J., SOGTROP, H.H.: Peroral therapy with cytosine arabinoside. Preliminary laboratory and clinical findings. Arzneimittelforschung **18**, 712—714 (1968).

GRAHAM, F.L., WHITMORE, G.F.: The effect of 1-β-D-arabinofuranosyl cytosine on growth viability and DNA synthesis of mouse L-cells. Cancer Res. **30**, 2627—2635 (1970).

GRAY, G.D., NICHOL, R., MICKELSON, M.M., CAMIENER, G.W., GISH, D.T., KELLY, R.C., WECHTER, W.J., MOXLEY, T.E., NEIL, G.L.: Immunosuppressive antiviral and antitumor activities of cytarabine derivatives. Biochem. Pharmacol. **21**, 465—475 (1972).

GRINDEY, G.B., SASLAW, L.D., WARAVDEKAR, V.S.: Effects of uracil derivatives on phosphorylation of arabinosylcytosine. Molec. Pharmacol. **4**, 96—103 (1968).

GROTH, D.P., D'ANGELO, J.M., VOGLER, W.R., MINGIOLI, E.S., BETZ, B.: Selective metabolic effects of 1,3-*bis* (2-chloroethyl)-1-nitrosourea upon *de novo* purine biosynthesis. Proc. Int. Cancer Congress 1972.

GUTTERMAN, J.U., CURTIS, J.E., FREIREICH, E.J: Combination therapy with cytosine arabinoside (ara-C) and cyclophosphamide (Ctx) of chronic lymphocytic leukemia (CLL). American Society of Clin. Oncology, May 1972.

HALL, T.C., KESSEL, D., LEVINE, R., ROBERTS, D.: In: WITTE, S., ZAHN, R.K. (Eds.): Studies on the cellular pharmacology of cytosine arabinoside. Cytosin-Arabinosid Symposium. Arzneimittelforschung 20—30 (1968).

HANZE, A.R.: Nucleic acids. IV. The catalytic reduction of pyrimidine nucleosides (human liver deaminase inhibitors). J. Amer. chem. Soc. **89**, 6720—6725 (1967).

HART, J.S., HO, D.H.W., SALEM, P., FREI, E., III: Clinical and kinetic evaluation of continuous 5-day arabinosyl cytosine (ara-C) on melanoma. Proc. Amer. Ass. Cancer Res. **13**, 101 (1972).

HAYES, D.M., ELLISON, R.R.: Production of remissions in blastic phase of chronic myelocytic leukemia (CML) and acute myelocytic leukemia (AML) by arabinosyl cytosine (ara-C) plus 1,3-*bis*-β(2-chloroethyl)-1-nitrosourea (BCNU). Blood **34**, 840 (1969).

HENDERSON, E.S., BURKE, P.J.: Clinical experience with cytosine arabinoside. Proc. Amer. Ass. Cancer Res. **6**, 102 (1965).

HERSH, E.M., BODEY, G.P., NIES, B.A., FREIREICH, E.J: Cause of death in acute leukemia. J. Amer. med. Ass. **193**, 105—109 (1965).

HO, D.H.W.: Inhibition of 1-β-D-arabinofuranosyl cytosine phosphorylation in human livers by tetrahydrouridine. Biochem. Pharmacol. **21**, 2936 (1972).

HO, D.H.W., FREI, E., III: Clinical pharmacology of 1-β-D-arabinofuranosyl cytosine. Clin. Pharmacol. Ther. **12**, 944—954 (1971).

HOFFMAN, G.S., KLINE, I., GANG, M., TYRER, D.D., GOLDIN, A., MANTEL, N., VENDITTI, J.M.: Sequential chemotherapy with cyclophosphamide (NSC 26271) and cytosine arabinoside (NSC 63878) in mice with advanced leukemia L1210. Cancer Chemother. Rep. **53**, 265—271 (1969).

HOSHI, A., KANZAWA, F., KURETANI, K., SANEYOSHI, M., ARAI, Y.: 2,2′-*O*-Cyclocytidine, antitumor cytidine analog resistant to cytidine deaminase. Gann **62**, 145—146 (1971).

HOWARD, J.P., CEVIK, W., MURPHY, L.M.: Cytosine arabinoside (NSC 63878) in acute leukemia in children. Cancer Chemother. Rep. **50**, 287—291 (1966).

INAGAKI, A., NAKAMURA, T., WAKISAWA, G.: Studies on the mechanism of action of 1-β-D-arabinofuranosyl cytosine as an inhibitor of DNA synthesis in human leukemic leukocytes. Cancer Res. **29**, 2169—2176 (1969).

KANAI, T., KOJIMA, T., MARUYAMA, O., ICHINO, M.: Pyrimidine nucleosides. III. Reaction of cytidine or *N*-4-acetyl cytidine with partially hydrolyzed phosphorousoxychloride. Chem. pharm. Bull. **18**, 2569—2570 (1970).

Kaplan, S., Wade, M., Clement, D., DeConti, R., Calabresi, P.: Enhancement of the cytotoxic activity of cytosine arabinoside by porfiromycin. Proc. Amer. Ass. Cancer Res. **7**, 35 (1966).
Karnofsky, D., Lacon, C.: The effect of 1-β-D-arabinofuranosyl cytosine on the developing chick embryo. Biochem. Pharmacol. **15**, 1435—1442 (1966).
Karon, M., Henry, P., Weissman, S., Meyer, C.: The effect of 1-β-D-arabinofuranosyl cytosine on macromolecular synthesis in KB spinner cultures. Cancer Res. **26**, 166—171 (1966).
Kessel, D.: Some observations on the phosphorylation of cytosine arabinoside. Molec. Pharmacol. **4**, 402—404 (1968).
Kessel, D., Hall, T. C., Rosenthal, D.: Uptake and phosphorylation of cytosine arabinoside by normal and leukemic human blood cells *in vitro*. Cancer Res. **29**, 459—463 (1969).
Kessel, D., Hall, T. C., Wodinsky, I.: Transport and phosphorylation as factors in the antitumor action of cytosine arabinoside. Science **156**, 1240—1241 (1967).
Kihlman, B. A., Nichols, W. W., Levan, A.: The effect of deoxyadenosine and cytosine arabinoside on the chromosomes of human leukocytes *in vitro*. Hereditas **50**, 139—143 (1963).
Kikugawa, K., Ichino, M.: On the reaction of Vilsmeier-Haack reagents with nucleoside: a convenient synthesis of 2,2′-cyclocytidine. Tetrahedron Let. **11**, 867—870 (1970).
Kim, J. H., Eidenoff, M. L.: Action of 1-β-D-arabinofuranosylcytosine and nucleic acid metabolism and viability of HeLa cells. Cancer Res. **25**, 698—702 (1965).
Kimball, A. P., Wilson, M. J.: Inhibition of DNA polymerase by 1-β-D-arabinosylcytosine and reversal of inhibition of deoxycytidine-5′-triphosphate. Proc. Soc. exp. Biol. (N.Y.) **127**, 429—432 (1968).
Kit, S., Detorres, R. A., Dubbs, D. R.: Arabinofuranosyl cytosine-induced stimulation of thymidine kinase and deoxycytidylic deaminase activities of mammalian cultures. Cancer Res. **26**, 1859—1866 (1966).
Kline, I., Tyrer, D. D., Gang, M., Venditti, J. M., Goldin, A.: Influence of route of administration on antileukemic activity of cytosine arabinoside (NSC 63878) in advanced leukemia L1210 in mice. Cancer Chemother. Rep. **52**, 399—404 (1968).
Kline, I., Venditti, J. M., Tyrer, D. D., Goldin, A.: Chemotherapy of leukemia L1210 in mice with 1-β-D-arabinofuranosyl cytosine hydrochloride. I. Influence of treatment schedules. Cancer Res. **26**, 853—859 (1966a).
Kline, I., Venditti, J. M., Tyrer, D. D., Mantel, N., Goldin, A.: Chemotherapy of leukemia L1210 in mice with 1-β-D-arabinofuranosyl cytosine hydrochloride. II. Effectiveness against intracerebrally and subcutaneously inoculated leukemic cells. Cancer Res. **26**, 1930—1937 (1966b).
LePage, G. A., White, S. C.: Scheduling of arabinosylcytosine (ara-C) and 6-thioguanine (TG) therapy. Proc. Amer. Ass. Cancer Res. **13**, 11 (1972).
Livingston, R. B., Carter, S. K.: Cytosine arabinoside (NSC 63878) — clinical brochure. Cancer Chemother. Rep. **1**, 179—205 (1968).
Loo, R. V., Brennan, M. J., Talley, R. W.: Clinical pharmacology of cytosine arabinoside. Proc. Amer. Ass. Cancer Res. **6**, 161 (1965).
Mellett, L. B., Eldareer, S. M., Chen, F. P.: Anomalous metabolism of 5-^{3}H-1-β-D-arabinofuranosyl cytosine (ara-C) in the rhesus monkey after oral administration. Proc. Amer. Ass. Cancer Res. **12**, 68 (1971).
Momparler, R. L., Chu, M. Y., Fischer, G. A.: Studies on a new mechanism of resistance of L5178Y murine leukemia cells to cytosine arabinoside. Biochim. biophys. Acta (Amst.) **161**, 481—493 (1968).
Mulligan, L. T., Jr., Mellett, L. B.: Comparative metabolism of cytosine arabinoside and inhibition of deamination by tetrahydrouridine. Pharmacologist **10**, 167 (1968).
Neil, G. L., Moxley, T. E., Manak, R. C.: Enhancement by tetrahydrouridine of 1-β-D-arabinofuranosyl cytosine (cytarabine) oral activity in L1210 leukemic mice. Cancer Res. **30**, 2166—2172 (1970a).
Neil, G. L., Wiley, P. F., Manak, R. C., Moxley, T. E.: Antitumor effect of 1-β-D-arabinofuranosyl cytosine 5′-adamantoate (NSC 117614) in L1210 leukemic mice. Cancer Res. **30**, 1047—1054 (1970b).
Panzica, R. P., Robins, R. K., Townsend, L. B.: Synthesis and antitumor activity of cytosine arabinoside 3-*N*-oxide. J. med. Chem. **14**, 259 (1971).
Reisner, E. H., Jr.: The nature and significance of megaloblastic blood cell formation. Blood **13**, 313—338 (1958).
Ritter, E. J., Scott, W. J., Wilson, J. G.: Teratogenesis and inhibition of DNA synthesis induced in rat embryos by cytosine arabinoside. Teratology **4**, 7—14 (1971).
Saslaw, L. D., Grindey, G. B., Kline, I., Waravdekar, V. S.: Sparing action of uridine on the antileukemic activity of cytosine arabinoside. Cancer Res. **28**, 11—20 (1968).

SCHABEL, F. M., JR.: *In vivo* leukemic cell kill kinetics and curability in experimental systems. In: The proliferation and spread of neoplastic cells, p. 379. Baltimore: Williams and Wilkins 1968.

SCHMIDT, L. H., MONTGOMERY, J. A., LASTER, W. R., JR., SCHABEL, F. M.: Combination therapy with arabinosyl cytosine and thioguanine. Proc. Amer. Ass. Cancer Res. **11**, 70 (1970).

SCHRECKER, A. W.: Metabolism of 1-β-D-arabinofuranosyl cytosine in leukemia L1210: nucleoside and nucleotide kinases in cell-free extracts. Cancer Res. **30**, 632—641 (1970).

SCHRECKER, A. W., GOLDIN, A.: Antitumor effect and mode of action of 1-β-D-arabinofuranosyl cytosine 5′-phosphate in leukemia L1210. Cancer Res. **28**, 802—803 (1968).

SCHRECKER, A. W., MEAD, J. A. R.: Isolation and antileukemic activity in mice of 1-β-D-arabinofuranosyl cytosine 5′-phosphate present in synthetic 5′-cytidylic acid. Biochem. Pharmacol. **15**, 1443—1452 (1966).

SKIPPER, H. E., SCHABEL, F. M., JR., WILCOX, W. S.: Experimental evaluation of potential anticancer agents: XXI. Scheduling of arabinosyl cytosine to take advantage of its *S*-phase specificity against leukemic cells. Cancer Chemother. Rep. **51**, 125—141 (1967).

STEUART, C. D., BURKE, P. J.: Cytidine deaminase and the development of resistance to arabinosyl cytosine. Nature (Lond.) **233**, 109—110 (1971a).

STEUART, C. D., BURKE, P. J., OWENS, A. H.: Correlation of ara-C metabolism and clinical response in adult acute leukemia. Proc. Amer. Ass. Cancer Res. **12**, 353 (1971b).

TALLEY, R. W., FREI, E., III: Summary of clinical experience with cytosine arabinoside. Arzneimittelforschung **18**, 93—105 (1968).

TALLEY, R. W., O'BRYAN, R. M., TUCKER, W. G., LOO, R. V.: Clinical pharmacology and human antitumor activity of cytosine arabinoside. Cancer **20**, 809—816 (1967).

TALLEY, R. W., VAITKEVICIUS, V. K.: Megaloblastosis produced by a cytosine antagonist 1-β-D-arabinofuranosyl cytosine. Blood **21**, 352—362 (1963).

TYRER, D. D., KLINE, I., VENDITTI, J. M., GOLDIN, A.: Separate and sequential chemotherapy of mouse leukemia L1210 with 1-β-D-arabinofuranosyl cytosine hydrochloride and 1,3-*bis*-(2-chloroethyl)-1-nitrosourea. Cancer Res. **27**, 873—879 (1968).

UCHIDA, K., KREIS, W.: Studies on drug resistance. I. Distribution of 1-β-D-arabinofuranosyl cytosine, cytidine and deoxycytidine in mice bearing ara-C sensitive and resistant P815 neoplasms. Biochem. Pharmacol. **18**, 1115—1128 (1969).

VOGLER, W. R.: Clinical trials of 1-β-D-arabinofuranosyl cytosine and 1,3-*bis*-(2-chloroethyl)-1-nitrosourea combination in metastatic cancer and acute leukemia. Cancer **27**, 1081—1088 (1971).

WANG, J. J., SELAWRY, O. S., VIETTI, T. J., BODEY, G. P.: Prolonged infusion of arabinosyl cytosine in childhood leukemia. Cancer **25**, 1—6 (1970).

WHEELER, G. P., BOWDON, B. J.: Some effects of 1,3-*bis*-(2-chloroethyl)-1-nitrosourea upon the synthesis of protein and nucleic acids *in vivo* and *in vitro*. Cancer Res. **25**, 1770—1778 (1965).

WHITECAR, J. P., JR., BODEY, G. P., FREIREICH, E. J, MCCREDIE, K. B., HART, J. S.: Cyclophosphamide, vincristine, arabinosyl cytosine and prednisone (COAP) combination chemotherapy for adult acute leukemia. Cancer Chemother. Rep. **54**, 543—550 (1972).

WILKOFF, L. J., WILCOX, W. S., BURDESHAW, J. A., DIXON, G. J., DULMADGE, E. A.: Effect of antimetabolites on kinetic behavior of proliferating cultured L1210 leukemia cells. J. nat. Cancer Inst. **39**, 965—975 (1967).

Chapter 44

Halogenated Pyrimidine Deoxyribonucleosides

William H. Prusoff and Barry Goz

With 4 Figures

Introduction

The halogenated uracil derivatives are not only powerful tools for elucidation of many intricate biochemical events of importance to molecular biology but also they have valuable clinical utility. This review is directed to an understanding of why these compounds function as they do, and in addition to indicate the many uses that they have.

Chemistry

Aknowledge of the chemical and physical properties of 5-iodo-2′-deoxyuridine (IdUrd, IUdR, IUDR, IDU) is germane to understanding the basis of the biological effects observed.

A. Synthesis

I. Synthesis of Nucleosides Halogenated in the Pyrimidine Moiety

Johnson and Johns (1905) replaced the hydrogen on carbon-5 of the pyrimidine ring by an iodine atom in an alkaline reaction mixture. This synthetic procedure is applicable to the iodination of uridine and deoxyuridine; however, iodination in dilute nitric acid results in the direct formation of crystals of 5-iodouracil ribonucleoside (Prusoff et al., 1953) or 5-iodouracil-2′-deoxyribonucleoside, respectively (Prusoff, 1959). This latter procedure affords efficient, as well as facile preparation of large amounts of these compounds.

Prior to the availability of these synthetic approaches to the preparation of the halogenated nucleosides, IdUrd was isolated by Zamenhof et al. (1956a) and by Dunn and Smith (1954, 1957) from the DNA of microorganisms grown in media supplemented with 5-iodouracil. Friedkin and Roberts (1954) presented evidence for the *in vitro* enzyme catalyzed formation of IdUrd by incubation of 5-iodouracil, deoxyribose-1-phosphate, and a mammalian source of thymidine phosphorylase.

The 5-chloro and 5-bromo derivatives of the ribo- and deoxyribonucleosides of uracil and cytosine have been prepared (Fukuhara et al., 1955; Frisch and Visser, 1959) by a photocatalytic procedure, and 5-bromo-2′-deoxyuridine (BrdUrd) by direct bromination of deoxyuridine by Beltz and Visser (1955). Various other methods have been used for halogenation of nucleosides by Hilbert and Johnson (1930), Hoffer et al. (1959), Cheong et al. (1960), Chang and Welch (1961), Yung et al. (1961), Michelson et al. (1962), Chang and Welch

(1963), LIPKIN et al. (1963), HORWITZ et al. (1964), PRYSTAS and ŠORM (1964), CHANG (1965), YOSHIDA et al. (1968), SRIVASTAVA and NAGPAL (1970).

Several conditions have been used for the synthesis of IdUrd: (1) by treatment of deoxyuridine with excess iodine under oxidizing conditions in dilute HNO_3 (PRUSOFF, 1959; CHEONG et al., 1960); (2) with iodic acid (CHANG and WELCH, 1963); (3) in alkaline solution (PRUSOFF, 1959); (4) with iodine monochloride (BUI et al., 1965; BROWNSTONE, 1963).

II. Synthesis of Radioactive Halogenated Nucleosides and Nucleotides

A modification of the method of PRUSOFF (1959) has been used for the synthesis of IdUrd of high specific activity labeled with radioactive ^{125}I, ^{131}I, or ^{132}I (SILVESTER and WHITE, 1963), as well as that of radioactive 5-iodo-2'-deoxyuridylic acid (HAMPTON and EIDENOFF, 1961). BROWNSTONE (1963) and BUI et al. (1965) prepared ^{131}I-5-IdUrd using ICl.

2-^{14}C-5-BrdUrd was synthesized enzymically from 2-^{14}C-5-bromouracil by FUCIK and KARA (1964) with *trans-N*-deoxyribosylase isolated from *Lactobacillus helveticus*. FRIEDKIN and ROBERTS (1954), using a mammalian enzyme, synthesized radioactive thymidine by a method that is directly applicable for the formation of radioactive IdUrd. FILIP and NEJEDLY (1969) prepared various radioactive deoxyribonucleosides labeled in the base moiety by incubation of the labeled base, the dicyclohexylammonium salt of 2-deoxy-α-D-ribose-1-phosphate and an *E. coli* enzyme preparation.

A precaution in the measurement of ^{125}I used as the label in radioactive IdUrd was reported by BAKHLE et al. (1964). They observed that some solvents or electrolytes absorb the soft gamma radiation from ^{125}I ($E = 0.035$ Mev) to a markedly greater extent than that from ^{131}I ($E = 0.36$ Mev).

III. Synthesis of Nucleosides Halogenated in the Sugar Moiety

The substitution of halogens in the sugar moiety of nucleosides has been described. The biological activity of several of these compounds indicates a potential in the chemotherapy of viral and neoplastic diseases, as well as in elucidating biochemical mechanisms. LEVINE and TIPSON (1934) described the preparation of 2',3'-dimethyl-5'-iodouridine and 2',3'-ditosyl-5'-iodouridine, and MICHELSON and TODD (1955) described the preparation of 3'-iodo-3'-deoxythymidine, 5'-iodo-5'-deoxythymidine, and 5'-bromo-5'-deoxythymidine. 5'-Iodo-5'-deoxyuridine was subsequently shown to form a cyclo derivative (BROWN et al., 1957).

Replacement of the 5'-OH of thymidine with a hydrogen or halogen has resulted in compounds that are unique, in that they inhibit thymidylate kinase. The synthesis of 5'-fluorothymidine was described by LANGEN and KOWOLLIK (1968), and the synthesis of the 5'-fluoro derivative of thymidine, deoxyuridine, 5-fluoro-2'-deoxyuridine, as well as of the 5'-fluoro derivative of IdUrd was described by LANGEN et al. (1969a). LANGEN et al. (1969a) also reported the synthesis of 5'-deoxy, 5'-bromo, and 5'-iodothymidine by the procedure of MICHELSON and TODD (1955), and of 5'-chlorothymidine. KARA and DUSCHINSKY (1969) reported the isolation of 5'-deoxy-5'-iodothymidine as an intermediate in the formation of 5'-deoxythymidine. DUSCHINSKY et al. (1969) also described the synthesis of 5'-deoxy, 5'-chloro, 5'-bromo, and 5'-iodothymidine. The preparation of 3'-deoxy-3'-fluorothymidine, an inhibitor of DNA biosynthesis, was reported by LANGEN et al. (1969b).

IV. Synthesis of Nucleotides Halogenated in the Pyrimidine Moiety

The synthesis of the nucleotide corresponding to IdUrd, 5-iodo-2′-deoxyuridine-5′-phosphate, has been accomplished by iodination in dilute nitric acid by HAMPTON et al. (1962). The 5′-mono and diphosphate derivatives of 5-iodouridine have been synthesized by MICHELSON et al. (1962) in high yield from uridylic acid.

LIPKIN et al. (1963) synthesized 5-iodouridine triphosphate by N-iodosuccinimide iodination of the tetraethylammonium salt of UTP in a solution of anhydrous dimethyl sulfoxide containing the catalyst *n*-butyl disulfide. PRUSOFF and CHANG (1968) reported the synthesis of 5-iodo-2′-deoxyuridine triphosphate from 5-iodo-2′-deoxycytidine 5′-phosphate in good yield.

CANELLAKIS et al. (1960) described the enzymic synthesis of radioactive pyrimidine and purine nucleoside-5′-triphosphates in yields of 85 to 95 %. Other methods include CANELLAKIS (1957), HURLBERT (1957), STONE and POTTER (1957), CANELLAKIS and MANTSAVINOS (1958), LEHMAN et al. (1958), and MALEY and OCHOA (1958).

V. Synthesis of Halogenated Nucleic Acid

The biosynthesis of DNA in which a halogenated uracil is present in place of the normal thymine moiety was achieved by WEYGAND et al. (1952a), ZAMENHOF and GRIBOFF (1954), WACKER et al. (1954), and DUNN and SMITH (1954, 1957) by growth of a microorganism in a medium supplemented with the appropriate halogenated uracil analog. Similarly, incorporation of IdUrd or BrdUrd into the DNA of mammalian cells, plant cells, and viruses has been demonstrated. The synthetic incorporation of halogens into preformed polynucleotides has also been accomplished.

COMMERFORD (1971) incorporated iodine into the 5-position of cytosine of DNA and RNA by heating the polymer in an aqueous solution of either iodine or of the oxidizing agent thallic trichloride plus iodide at pH 5. Incorporation into single stranded DNA occurred more readily than into double stranded DNA. With single stranded DNA, over 95 % of the DNA-cytosine could be iodinated. The thymine and adenine moieties of DNA were not iodinated, and the guanine little, if at all. Cytosine in RNA was preferentially iodinated in relation to the uracil moiety; however, small amounts of 5-iodouracil and large amounts of uracil hydrate were observed.

ASCOLI and KAHAN (1966) used ^{131}I-iodine monochloride to halogenate RNA and DNA in an organic solvent. The uracil and cytosine moieties of RNA were labeled in the 5-position and guanine in the 8-position. DNA-guanine and -cytosine were labeled 1.4 and 14 %, respectively. DUVAL and EBEL (1964, 1965) brominated RNA in dimethyl formamide in the 8-position of guanine and the 5-position of cytosine and uracil. As the extent of bromination of sRNA increased, an alteration of secondary structure was observed, and with ribosomal RNA, a decrease in sedimentation constant occurred.

BRAMMER (1963) iodinated infectious tobacco mosaic virus (TMV)-RNA with *N*-iodosuccinimide, with the cytosine moiety being the most readily iodinated base, and found that 2 to 3 atoms of iodine per infectious RNA molecule were lethal. Loss of infectivity was also observed during bromination of TMV-RNA with *N*-bromosuccinimide, during which uracil reacted less readily than guanine or cytosine, and adenine not at all.

MICHELSON et al. (1962) prepared enzymically polyhalogen uridylic acid by incubation of 5-bromo, 5-chloro, or 5-iodouridine 5′-diphosphate with polynucleotide phosphorylase, and found that the presence of the halogen in the uracil moiety did not interfere with the enzymic activity of ribonuclease, venom phosphodiesterase, 5′-nucleotidase, and semen phosphomonoesterase.

B. Stability of Nucleosides

Although BrdUrd and IdUrd are stable substances when stored in the dry state, they are susceptible to degradation in solution. The reaction products and their rate of formation in solution are markedly dependent upon pH, temperature, and exposure to radiation.

GREER and ZAMENHOF (1962) and BERENS and SHUGAR (1963) reported that 5-BrdUrd has a greater lability in phosphate buffer (pH 6.8) relative to thymidine. WACKER and TRÄEGER (1963) studied the acid hydrolysis of various 5-halogen substituted deoxyuridines and found them to be 3 to 4 times more readily cleaved than thymidine or deoxyuridine, and under these conditions deoxycytidine was cleaved 16 times more rapidly. PFITZNER and MOFFATT (1964) reported that deoxyuridine was more readily hydrolyzed at low pH than uridine. The greater stability of the ribonucleoside relative to the deoxyribonucleoside was observed by BERENS and SHUGAR (1963) who found that the deoxyribonucleoside, but not the ribonucleoside of 5-bromouracil undergoes cleavage of the glycoside bond on heating at 100° at neutral pH.

RAVIN et al. (1964b) studied the hydrolytic degradation of IdUrd in aqueous solution at 60° from pH 1.3 to 12.0 and found the rate of disappearance to be a first-order reaction. The rate of degradation was independent of pH between pH 1.3 and 6.3. Between pH 6.3 and 9.0 a sharp increase was observed in the reaction rate, which coincided with the appearance of the ionized form of IdUrd ($pK_a =$ 8.25). Above pH 11.0 the reaction rate increased markedly and changed from first order to pseudo first order.

RAVIN et al. (1964a) found the main products formed during acid hydrolysis were 5-iodouracil and 2′-deoxyribose; no significant amount of uracil was formed. Product formation in alkaline solution is complex, with the formation of deoxyuridine and a non-UV absorbing compound that has the deoxyribose moiety attached.

GARRETT et al. (1964) found that under acidic conditions the final products from IdUrd were iodide, uracil, and degraded deoxyribose; however, in agreement with RAVIN et al. (1964a), deoxyribose and iodouracil were identified as the initial products.

GARRETT et al. (1965) described two routes of degradation of IdUrd during alkaline hydrolysis at 80° (Fig. 1). The rate of appearance of iodine ion as measured polarographically closely paralleled the degradation of IdUrd as measured spectrophotometrically. Based on chromatographic and spectral analysis 5-hydroxy-2′-deoxyuridine was identified as a product of the major route of IdUrd alkaline hydrolysis. 5-Hydroxy-dUrd, being unstable in alkali, is rapidly degraded and does not accumulate. 5-Hydroxy-dUrd could be formed by either an SN-2 displacement reaction with direct formation of iodide ion, or by hydration of the 5—6 double bond with the hydroxyl on position 5 and subsequent elimination of HI. The formation of deoxyuridine during alkaline hydrolysis via the minor route is postulated to be by hydration of the 5—6 double bond with the hydroxyl in the 6 position, and subsequent elimination of hypoiodous acid (IOH). The hypoiodous acid may rearrange to form iodate which subsequently reacts with decomposition products of 5-hydroxy-dUrd to form iodide ion.

SHAPIRO and KANG (1969) studied the stability of the *N*-glycosyl bond of deoxyuridine, thymidine, and 5-BrdUrd and found a slow uncatalyzed hydrolysis in aqueous solution between pH 3 to 7 at 75°, 85.5°, and 95°. The rate constant for hydrolysis at 85.5° in H_2O is about 20-fold greater for BrdUrd (15.7×10^6 K/sec) in comparison to deoxyuridine, and the latter is hydrolyzed 2-fold faster than thymidine. The rate of hydrolysis increased below pH 3, and decreased above pH 8.

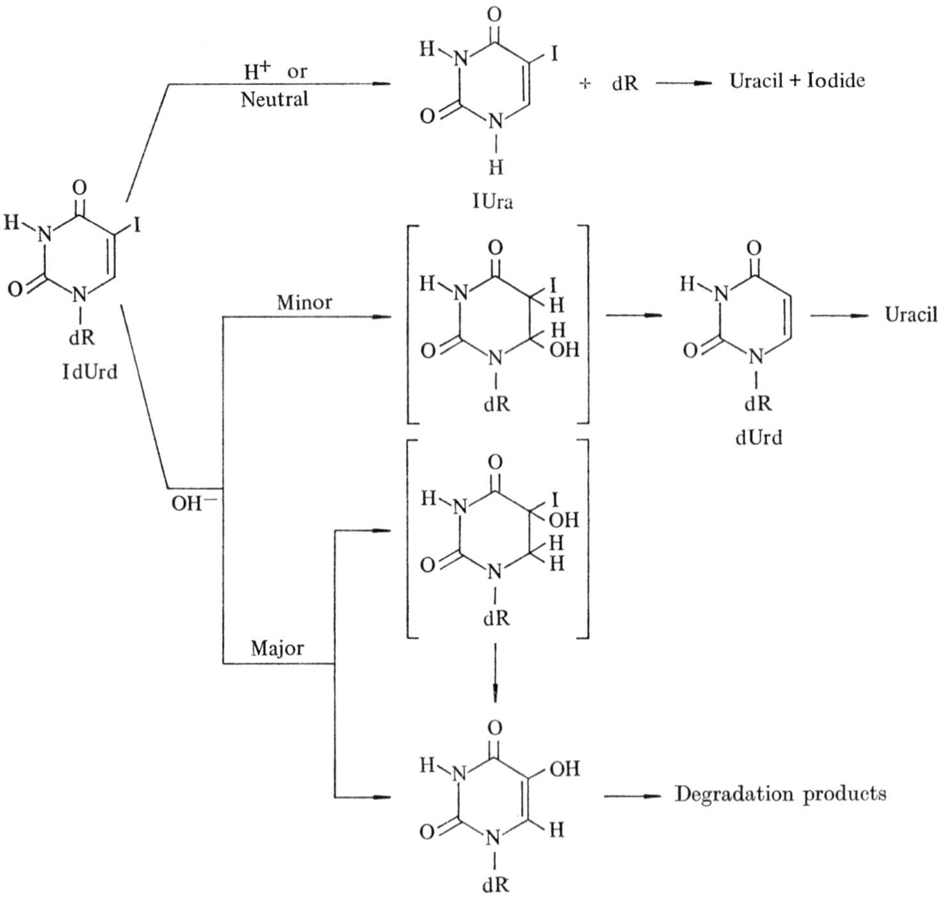

Fig. 1. Pathways for the acid, neutral, and alkaline degradation of 5-iodo-2′-deoxyuridine (GARRETT et al., 1965)

GARRETT and YAKATAN (1968) studied the kinetics and possible mechanisms of solvolysis of several derivatives of uridine substituted in the 5-position with I, Br, Cl, and CH_3 at both neutral and alkaline pH and at high temperature (i.e., 80°). The order of reactivity to alkaline solvolysis is IUrd > BrUrd > ClUrd > Urd, and hence is in agreement with the relative susceptibility of the halogenated deoxyribonucleosides relative to thymidine and dUrd. Several pathways for the alkaline hydrolysis of these compounds have been described by GARRETT and YAKATAN (1968). Hydroxyl addition to the 6 position results in the formation of a 5-6 saturated bond, and subsequent elimination of HX results in the formation of the unstable ribosylbarbituric acid. The more labile the carbon halogen bond, the greater the ease of solvolysis (i.e., HX elimination). Although the 6-hydroxy uracil nucleoside is postulated to form during alkaline hydrolysis of both IdUrd and IUrd, it is difficult to reconcile the different subsequent reactions, that is, the formation of dUrd versus "degradation product".

A second pathway for solvolysis of halouridines is via direct hydration of the 5-6 bond of the pyrimidine moiety to form 5-halo, 5-hydroxy, 6-dihydrouridine and then subsequent elimination of HX to form 5-hydroxyuridine, a rapidly degradable substance in alkali (WANG, 1959; GARRETT and YAKATAN, 1968).

Another reaction sequence was reported by LIPKIN et al. (1964) who observed that treatment of 5-iodouridine in alkali resulted in the formation of 6,5'-anhydro-ribosyl barbituric acid presumably by attack on the 6-position by the anion produced in the 5'-position by alkali.

C. Steric Effects

The incorporation of iodine in place of the methyl group of thymidine results in an increase in the bulk volume, since the methyl group has a van der Waals atomic radius of 2.00, whereas that of the iodine atom is 2.15. Although the size of the halogen substituent is greater than the methyl group, any hindrance by the halogenated deoxyribonucleoside to its capacity to substitute for the thymidine component of the double helix of DNA appears to be small. Indeed, consideration of the composition of this double helix, as proposed by Watson and Crick, clearly indicates that there should not be any problem for incorporation of IdUrd into DNA because of steric hindrance. The iodine atom is well removed from the groups required for hydrogen bonding with the adenine moiety of the complementary DNA strand of the double helix. Thus, the increased volume of the substituent on the 5-position of the pyrimidine ring does not appear seriously to affect the structure of the resultant DNA, nor seriously to affect the Km of IdUrd or its phosphorylated derivatives as substrates for various enzymes. The biological consequence of incorporation of IdUrd into DNA, as well as the effect of IdUrd and its phosphorylated derivatives on enzyme function will be discussed in a later section.

The van der Waals radii of halogen atoms vary from 1.35 Å for fluorine to 2.15 Å for iodine. In systems that can incorporate free pyrimidines into nucleic acids, 5-fluorouracil enters only RNA, while 5-bromouracil and 5-iodouracil enter DNA, and the 5-chloroderivative (chlorine has a van der Waals radius intermediate between that of fluorine and bromine) may enter both RNA and DNA. The failure to find uracil in DNA, is not because deoxyuridine triphosphate is not a substrate for DNA polymerase instead of deoxythymidine triphosphate, but because accumulation of deoxyuridine triphosphate fails to occur, as it undergoes rapid enzymic breakdown (GREENBERG and SOMMERVILLE, 1962; BERTANI et al., 1963). OKAZAKI, T. and KORNBERG (1964) have shown that deoxyuridine triphosphate, and to a lesser extent 5-fluoro-2'-deoxyuridine triphosphate, can substitute partially for deoxythymidine triphosphate in the reaction catalyzed by DNA polymerase. Thus, the failure of incorporation of 5-fluoro-2'-deoxyuridine into DNA is related to the failure of incorporation of deoxyuridine.

D. Ionization Effects

The effect of pH on the ionization of the halogenated nucleosides and their phosphorylated derivatives (i.e., nucleotides and nucleic acid) is a very important parameter in understanding their biological activities. In halogenated pyrimidines, the electronic configuration of the ring is altered because of the inductive effect of the halogen, and this results in more acidic dissociation constants. Titration of IdUrd revealed that the molecule has a lower pK_a, 8.25, than that of thymidine, 9.8. Thus, at pH 7.4, the proportion of the enolic form of IdUrd is greater than that of thymidine by a factor of 34. This has obvious implications not only in the forces binding the two strands of DNA together, but also in the potential problem of incorrect genetic coding. The genetic aspect will be discussed in more detail later.

BERENS and SHUGAR (1963) provided evidence that below pH 6 all of the 5-halogenated uracil derivatives exist in the diketo form, as do uracil and thymine. They tabulated the UV spectra of the various halogenated uracils, their ribonucleosides and deoxyribonucleosides as a function of pH, and their dissociation constants. The pK_a values of the halogenated deoxyuridine derivatives shown in Table 1 are derived in part from their publication. A number of ionic and nonionic species of IdUrd that may exist in solution at various pH values are depicted in Fig. 2.

Table 1. *The pK_a of thymidine, deoxyuridine, and their halogenated derivatives*

Compound	pK_a^a
Thymidine	9.80
Deoxyuridine	9.30
5-Iodo-2′-deoxyuridine	8.20; 8.25 (PRUSOFF, 1963)
5-Bromo-2′-deoxyuridine	7.90; 8.1 (LAWLY and BROOKE, 1962)
5-Chloro-2′-deoxyuridine	7.90
5-Fluoro-2′-deoxyuridine	7.80; 7.66 (WEMPEN et al., 1961)

[a] (BERENS and SHUGAR, 1963).

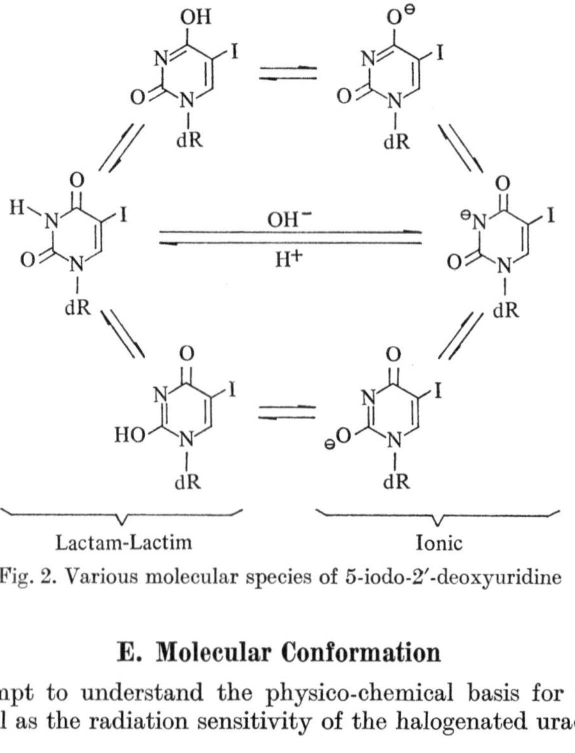

Fig. 2. Various molecular species of 5-iodo-2′-deoxyuridine

E. Molecular Conformation

In an attempt to understand the physico-chemical basis for the biological activity, as well as the radiation sensitivity of the halogenated uracil derivatives subsequent to incorporation into the nucleic acids, several investigators have examined the molecular conformation, as well as the crystal structure of these analogs, either alone or in complex with normal purine components (VOET and RICH, 1970). To facilitate these studies, alkylated halogenated bases on occasion have been used as model compounds.

CAMERMAN and TROTTER (1964) examined the crystal and molecular structure of IdUrd by x-ray diffraction and proposed that the antiviral activity may be related to the unusually short intermolecular distance of 2.96 Å between the iodine atom and the oxygen of a carbonyl group, whereas the calculated sum of their van der Waals radii is 3.55 Å. They postulated that the ability of iodine to form charge transfer bonds may cause the increased interchain attraction that could either prevent or delay the synthesis of virus DNA, thereby permitting normal host defense mechanisms to operate. Perhaps a charge transfer complex may form between the iodine of IdUrd and an adjacent base in the same strand, and such a distortion could conceivably affect transcription.

RAHMAN and WILSON (1970) in a similar study of the crystal and molecular structure of 5-iodouridine did not find such a close approach of the iodine atoms; that is, there was not a shortening, so that the interatomic distances were smaller than the sum of normal van der Waals radii. Two forms of 5-iodouridine, molecule I and II, are described by RAHMAN and WILSON (1970). The pyrimidine base is less planar in molecule I than in molecule II. These results are in agreement with the pyrimidine base described by CAMERMAN and TROTTER (1965). RAHMAN and WILSON (1970) report 5-iodouridine to be in the *anti* conformation with the pucker in the sugar ring being C3′ *endo* in molecule I and C2′ *endo* in molecule II. In molecule I the C5′-O5′ bond is *gauche* with respect to both the C4′-O1′ bond and the C4′-C3′ bond, and hence in a *gauche-gauche* conformation, whereas the conformation of molecule II is *trans-gauche* (RAHMAN and WILSON, 1970). When the environment of the crystalline nucleosides is altered, changes occur in conformation similar to those observed when DNA changes from the B or A form (WILSON, 1970). IBALL et al. (1966) similarly investigated by x-ray analysis the structure of 5-bromouracil-2′-deoxyribonucleoside and 5-bromouracil ribonucleoside.

Mutation caused by incorporation of halogenated uracil derivatives into DNA has been attributed to 5-iodouracil or 5-bromouracil base pairing with guanine rather than with adenine, and comparison has, therefore, been made of the hydrogen bonding between halogenated uracil derivatives and various purine derivatives. The high electronegativity of the bromine or iodine atom results in a marked alteration of the electron distribution in the pyrimidine base which affects the mode of hydrogen bonding. MIZUNO et al. (1970) observed bromine substitution in 1-ethyl-5-bromouracil to cause two types of hydrogen bonding: (1) between O4 and H of N3 and (2) between O2 and H of N3. Similar studies have been made by TAVALE et al. (1969) on the base-pairing configuration of 9-ethyl-8-bromoadenine and 1-methyl-5-bromouracil in the solid crystalline state.

The presence of a halogen on the 5-carbon of the pyrimidine moiety of a polynucleotide exerts a stability on the ordered form as evidenced by the resultant Tm (i.e., $X > Me > H$). This effect in ribopolymers has been explored and reviewed by RILEY and PAUL (1970) and MAUSSOULI et al. (1966).

Metabolism

A. Anabolism

The close structural and chemical similarities between thymidine and IdUrd or BrdUrd allow the utilization of these compounds and their phosphorylated derivatives as substrates for the various enzymes concerned with the biosynthesis of DNA. Thus, IdUrd and BrdUrd are incorporated into the DNA, but not RNA or protein of mammalian cells, plant cells, bacterial cells, as well as phage and animal viruses.

Mathias et al. (1959) isolated the DNA from murine L5178Y leukemia cells grown in culture containing ^{131}I-IdUrd. After removal of protein and RNA, the DNA was enzymically hydrolyzed and the formed deoxyribonucleotides separated by ion-exchange chromatography. Quantitative analysis unequivocally showed that IdUMP had substituted for dTMP, since the molar content of IdUMP plus dTMP was essentially equivalent to the molar concentration of dAMP. Of the newly synthesized DNA, about 66% of the DNA-thymine had been replaced by IdUrd.

The free halogenated pyrimidine bases, 5-chloro, 5-bromo, and 5-iodouracil are incorporated into the DNA of bacteria (Weygand and Wacker, 1952; Weygand et al., 1952; Dunn and Smith, 1954; Zamenhof and Griboff, 1954; Zamenhof et al., 1956a).

A pronounced selectivity for thymine relative to 5-bromouracil was observed in a thymine-requiring strain of *E. coli* by Hackett and Hanawalt (1966) and Kanner and Hanawalt (1968). Similarly, Laird and Bodner (1967) found *Bacillus subtilis thy*$^-$ to preferentially utilize thymine or thymidine relative to bromouracil or BrdUrd for the biosynthesis of DNA. What the limiting factor is for such preferential utilization was not investigated.

In mammalian systems, 5-iodo or 5-bromouracil are not readily utilized for the biosynthesis of DNA relative to their deoxyribonucleosides. This is in accord with thymine being a very poor precursor of DNA-thymine in mammalian systems. This may be related, however, to the limited availability of a source of deoxyribose-1-phosphate as shown by Breitman et al. (1966) and Gotto et al. (1969).

Comparison of the relative uptake of IdUrd and thymidine into mammalian DNA revealed a marked preference for the normal metabolite thymidine (Prusoff, 1960; Hughes et al., 1964; Fox and Prusoff, 1965; Baugnet-Makiew and Goutier, 1968). Five to ten percent of injected IdUrd has been shown by Hughes et al. (1964) to be retained by the mouse; 40 to 50 percent of thymidine injected is utilized by the rat (Potter, 1959). A similar pattern has been reported by Rubini et al. (1960) for man. Furthermore, IdUrd has been claimed to be preferentially incorporated into mitochondrial DNA relative to nuclear DNA in normal and certain malignant tissues of mice (Georgatsos et al., 1970) and rats (Neubert et al., 1968). Localized pool sizes could affect such interpretation.

Prusoff (1960) compared the relative uptake of equimolar amounts of ^{14}C-2-thymidine and ^{131}I-IdUrd into the DNA of Ehrlich ascites cells *in vivo* and found a 40-fold greater utilization of thymidine. The uptake of IdUrd into DNA was increased to that of thymidine when the total amount of IdUrd was increased 12-fold and the frequency of administration doubled. The preferential utilization of thymidine relative to IdUrd was attributed to a variety of possible circumstances that include differences in: (a) the rate of transport into the cell, (b) the rate of formation of the mono-, di-, and triphosphate derivatives, (c) the rate of utilization of IdUTP relative to dTTP by DNA polymerase, (d) the rate of catabolism of the nucleosides or their phosphorylated derivatives, and (e) the rate of egress from the abdominal cavity.

Baugnet-Makiew and Goutier (1968) found the uptake of thymidine relative to IdUrd into DNA varied from tissue to tissue by a factor of two in bone marrow, thymus, and normal liver, by a factor of 3.8 in spleen, and by a factor of 5 to 6 in regenerating rat liver. The difference in utilization may be related to their findings that, whereas *in vitro* phosphorylation of thymidine in the various tissue extracts resulted in the formation of significant amounts of di- and triphosphate derivatives in addition to the monophosphate, phosphorylation of IdUrd appeared to stop at the monophosphate level with essentially no pool of the di- and triphosphates of IdUrd. Since IdUrd is indeed incorporated into DNA and hence must form the di- and triphosphates, one must be concerned with the relative susceptibility to catabolism of the di- and triphosphate derivatives of thymidine and IdUrd as a limiting factor for utilization of the nucleoside for the biosynthesis of DNA.

Thus, in comparing the relative utilization of thymidine and IdUrd in a particular tissue or cell type it is of interest to determine the K_m of IdUrd and thymidine for thymidine kinase, the K_m of IdUMP and TMP for thymidylate kinase, the K_m of IdUDP and TDP for thymidine diphosphokinase, the K_m of IdUTP and TTP for DNA polymerase, and the K_m of these compounds for the appropriate catabolic enzymes. The question is whether the pool sizes of the intermediate nucleotides are controlled by catabolic or anabolic limitations, or both.

DETHLEFSEN (1969a, b) showed a direct correlation between the amount of IdUrd administered to a tumor-bearing mouse and the amount incorporated into the tumor DNA. Thymidine affects the incorporation of IdUrd into DNA (HUGHES et al., 1964; DETHLEFSEN, 1969a,b, 1971). HUGHES et al. (1964) observed that thymidine (0.05 μmole), when injected simultaneously with trace amounts of IdUrd of very high specific activity into mice, depressed incorporation of IdUrd into intestinal DNA by 50%. Thymidine in larger amounts (10 μmoles) completely prevented the utilization of IdUrd for DNA biosynthesis. DETHLEFSEN (1971) observed that thymidine, when administered i.p. to mice in 40-fold excess of ^{131}I-IdUrd, either 10 min prior to or simultaneously with the labeled analog, decreased the incorporation of IdUrd into DNA by 2 and 15% of controls, respectively. However, DETHLEFSEN (1971) observed no thymidine effect when given 30 min before or after IdUrd, but did find a 44% decrease when thymidine was given 15 min after IdUrd.

A comparison of the relative utilization of IdUrd, thymidine, and their phosphorylated derivatives has been explored in a cell-free system by BAKHLE and PRUSOFF (1969). In two murine leukemic cell lines they found a 5.8-fold greater utilization of thymidine than of IdUrd and a 5.0-fold greater utilization of TMP than of IdUMP as substrates for thymidine kinase and thymidylate kinase, respectively. Since purified enzymes were not studied, it is difficult to determine whether these observations were indicative of differences in K_m values between the normal metabolite and its analog, or whether they represent a five-fold greater susceptibility of the halogenated analog to catabolic enzymes.

MAK and TILL (1963) measured the rate of DNA biosynthesis with ^{125}I-IdUrd in mammalian cells *in vitro* and observed the apparent K_m for IdUrd to be 4 times greater than that for thymidine, as measured by competition studies for DNA biosynthesis. CYSYK and PRUSOFF (1972) found the K_m for IdUrd (1.2×10^{-5} M) to be essentially equivalent to that for thymidine (1.67×10^{-5} M) for a highly purified preparation of *E. coli* thymidine kinase. BRESNICK and THOMPSON (1965), using a partially purified thymidine kinase from the rat Walker tumor, found the K_i for 5-bromo, 5-chloro, and 5-iododeoxyuridine to be of the same order of magnitude as the apparent K_m for thymidine (3.7 μM). A Lineweaver-Burk plot indicated the nature of the inhibition to be competitive both with mammalian (BRESNICK and THOMPSON, 1965) and bacterial (VOYTEK et al., 1972) thymidine kinase.

BAKHLE and PRUSOFF (1969) observed equimolar utilization of dTTP and IdUTP for the biosynthesis of DNA by a preparation of DNA polymerase derived from L5178Y cells. BESSMAN et al. (1958) demonstrated that there is no preferential utilization of BrdUTP over dTTP by *E. coli* DNA polymerase. KAROL and SIMPSON (1968) used BrdUTP as a marker to prove that DNA biosynthesis by isolated mitochondria occurred by a replicative rather than a repair process.

It has been proposed by SPEYER et al. (1965, 1966) that DNA polymerase may play a critical role in selection of the correct nucleoside triphosphate for incorporation into DNA either by selective interaction with the nucleotide prior to the base hydrogen bonding with the template DNA, or by failure to form the phosphodiester bond subsequent to base pairing by the free nucleoside triphosphate with the DNA template. If there were selective interaction between the nucleotide and the enzyme, then the electronic alterations induced in the pyrimidine moiety by the halogen in the 5-position does not influence this interaction. This would be rather surprising! For example, in all situations where the feedback or allosteric inhibition of IdUTP relative to dTTP has been compared, a more marked effect has been exerted by IdUTP (DIWAN and PRUSOFF, 1968; PRUSOFF and CHANG, 1968). SEKELY and PRUSOFF (1969) found that a 2-fold excess of IdUTP was required to observe a 50% inhibition of dTTP utilization by DNA polymerase derived from either noninfected African green monkey kidney cells or from cells infected with herpes simplex virus. However, since crude extracts were used it is difficult to evaluate the influence of triphosphatase activity, if present, on the relative availability to DNA polymerase of dTTP and IdUTP.

B. Catabolism

The effective use of BrdUrd or IdUrd *in vivo* has been limited in part by its rapid catabolism to the free base and subsequent dehalogenation of the free halogenated base (BARRETT and WEST, 1956; PAHL et al., 1959; WELCH and PRUSOFF, 1960; PRUSOFF et al., 1960; HAMPTON and EIDINOFF, 1961; KRISS and REVESZ, 1962; KRISS et al., 1963; OPPELT et al., 1971). PRUSOFF et al. (1960) studied the metabolism of labeled IdUrd in mice and proposed the sequence of events depicted in Fig. 3. Direct dehalogenation of IdUrd does not occur.

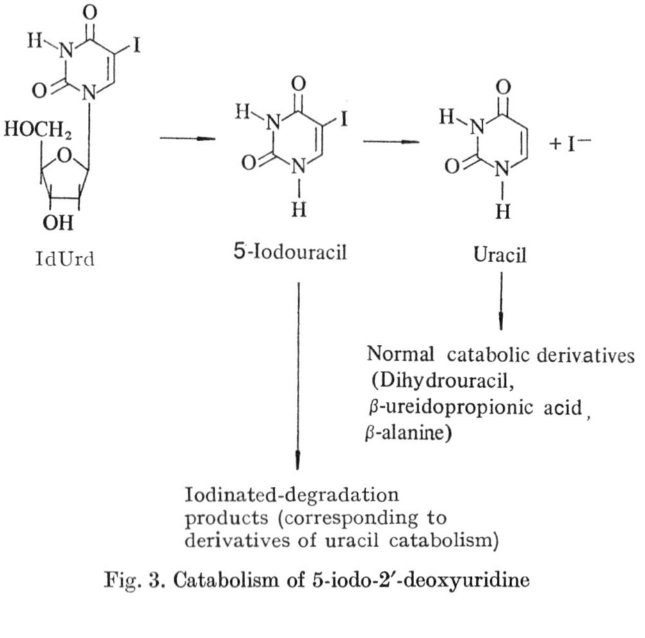

IdUrd → 5-Iodouracil → Uracil + I^-

Uracil → Normal catabolic derivatives (Dihydrouracil, β-ureidopropionic acid, β-alanine)

5-Iodouracil → Iodinated-degradation products (corresponding to derivatives of uracil catabolism)

Fig. 3. Catabolism of 5-iodo-2′-deoxyuridine

The free pyrimidine, thymine, is utilized poorly relative to thymidine for the biosynthesis of DNA-thymine by mammalian cells, and 5-bromo or 5-iodouracil are utilized even less efficiently because the latter are preferentially catabolized (FRIEDKIN and ROBERTS, 1954; BAUEROVA and SORMOVA, 1961; SEBESTA et al., 1961). Similarly, IdUrd is more rapidly catabolized than thymidine (HUGHES et al., 1964; CLARKSON et al., 1967; O'FARRELL and DUNAWAY, 1967).

5-Bromouracil was reported by BARRETT and WEST (1956) and SCHOLLER et al. (1965) to be dehalogenated metabolically in the rat. This analog was postulated to be reduced enzymically to the dihydro derivative (WALLACH and GRISOLIA, 1957; GRISOLIA and CARDOSO, 1957), a form that readily loses HBr to form uracil (BARRETT and WEST, 1956). PAHL et al. (1959) administered radioactive 5-bromouracil to a leukemic patient orally and 16% of the radioactivity appeared in the urine. Evidence was presented for conversion to uracil, as well as subsequent extensive reduction and cleavage of the pyrimidine ring.

5-Substituted halogenated derivatives of uracil are degraded in a manner (BARRETT and WEST, 1956; CHAUDHURI et al., 1958; PAHL et al., 1959; PRUSOFF et al., 1960) similar to that of thymine and uracil (RUTMAN et al., 1954; CANELLAKIS, 1956; FINK et al., 1956; FRITZSON, 1957). Thus, it is not unexpected that 5-halogenated uracils will affect the catabolism of thymine or uracil (SEBESTA et al., 1961; AGRAWAL et al., 1969).

BARRETT et al. (1964) studied the ability of a number of pyrimidine derivatives (5-F, Cl, Br, and I-uracil) to inhibit the degradation by rat tissue of radiolabeled uracil and thymine and observed inhibition of the initial reduction of the 5—6 double bond due to substrate competition for the active site of the enzyme dihydrouracil dehydrogenase (4,5-dihydrouracil:NADP oxidoreductase, EC 1.3.1.2). Only liver, of the various tissues studied, had significant degrading activity. Partially purified dihydrouracil dehydrogenase with NADPH has been shown by NEWMARK et al. (1962) to catalyze the reduction of 5-halogenated uracils.

IdUrd and BrdUrd are rapidly degraded in the animal body (EIDINOFF et al., 1959b; CALABRESI et al., 1961; WELCH and PRUSOFF, 1960; PRUSOFF, 1960; PRUSOFF et al., 1960; HAMPTON and EIDINOFF, 1961; KRISS and REVESZ, 1962; KRISS et al., 1962, 1963). BrdUrd and thymidine are rapidly degraded by liver (GERBER and REMY-DEFRAIGNE, 1963; KRISS and REVESZ, 1962), and this tissue is probably the site of IdUrd degradation also (WELCH and PRUSOFF, 1960; CALABRESI et al., 1961; KRISS et al., 1962). HUGHES et al. (1964) reported that the liver is the primary site of IdUrd catabolism.

IdUrd incorporated into DNA is stable and deiodination of the labeled DNA does not occur *in vivo* (PRUSOFF, 1960; HUGHES et al., 1964). The IdUrd used for DNA biosynthesis must be trapped fairly rapidly by the cell, presumably by phosphorylation. Thus, KRUEGER et al. (1960) showed that utilization of ^{131}I-IdUrd for DNA biosynthesis occurs within the hour, and HUGHES et al. (1964) reported a half-life for incorporation of IdUrd into DNA of about 5 min.

Radioiodine derived from iodouracil or IdUrd is rapidly excreted in the urine (PRUSOFF et al., 1960; WELCH and PRUSOFF, 1960; COMMERFORD et al., 1960). PRUSOFF et al. (1960) showed that ^{131}I-IdUrd is catabolized initially to iodouracil, which in turn is reduced to iodide and uracil.

FEINENDEGEN et al. (1966b) and HOFER and HUGHES (1970) found that incorporation of IdUrd into DNA, like thymidine, proceeded in the mouse with a half-time of 5 min, whereas the rate of degradation had a half-time of 3 min. However, the half-life of intracellular phosphorylated IdUrd is probably considerably longer. The main site of IdUrd catabolism, analogous to thymidine (GERBER and

REMY-DEFRAIGNE, 1963), appears to be the liver, where more than one-half of IdUrd injected into the portal vein is broken down with a 95 % conversion to iodide (HUGHES et al., 1964).

Part of the explanation for the more efficient use of thymidine relative to IdUrd for DNA biosynthesis is the preferential degradation of IdUrd relative to thymidine (HUGHES et al., 1964). ZIMMERMAN (1962) has observed IdUrd to be cleaved phosphorylytically more rapidly than thymidine.

O'FARRELL and DUNAWAY (1967) studied the incorporation and tissue distribution of labeled IdUrd in the cotton rat and found over 95 % to be eliminated 48 h post injection. The majority of the retained radioactivity was associated with the intestine. Of the radioiodine released metabolically from ^{131}I-IdUrd, about 99 % was excreted and the rest was associated with skin and hair, where it was retained with a long biological half-life, and with the prostate and seminal vesicle-coagulation glands.

CLARKSON et al. (1967) have studied the fate of IdUrd when injected into the brain of the dog. ^{125}I-IdUrd administered i.v. disappeared from plasma with a half-time of about 3.5 h, whereas that in cerebrospinal fluid (CSF) increased, reaching a maximum after about 2.5 h. About 80 % of the radioactivity that entered the CSF was in the form of ^{125}I-iodide. Thus, IdUrd or iodouracil either do not cross the blood-brain barrier or are rapidly degraded after entrance. However, such a barrier may not exist when brain tumors or viral encephalitis are present. Intracarotid infusion of BrdUrd or IdUrd has been reported to be efficacious in these conditions.

Intracisternally administered labeled IdUrd is rapidly degraded so that within 20 min at least 50 % of the nucleoside is cleaved to iodouracil. However, incubation of ^{125}I-IdUrd in CSF *in vitro* for 8 h produced no degradation; hence, enzymes responsible for the catabolism of IdUrd must be present in the cellular components of the brain, as well as in the liver. Such considerations are important in the establishment of an effective regimen in therapy of viral encephalitis or brain tumors.

MERITS and CAIN (1970) studied the incorporation of low levels of high specific activity labeled ^{131}I-IdUrd and ^{82}Br-BrdUrd into rat brain and observed a rapid disappearance of the labeled DNA with a half-life of about 6 h. The hypothesis was offered that the labeled DNA was specifically degraded due to the radiations emanating from the label. The specific activity of the ^{131}I-IdUrd was reported to be 100 to 1000 Ci/mmole.

The metabolism of IdUrd has been studied in man following intravenous infusion during 2 h periods, in dosages of 17 to 120 mg/kg daily, usually for 5 successive days (WELCH and PRUSOFF, 1960; CALABRESI et al., 1961). The level of radioactivity following infusions of ^{131}I-IdUrd progressively fell, reaching 50 % of the 5 min level in 7 to 10 h. Four hours following cessation of the infusion, the urine already contained about 44 % of the injected radioactivity; the values at 24 and 48 h were approximately 88 and 94 %, respectively. Five minutes following the termination of an infusion lasting for about 2 h, the total blood of the individual contained only about 9 % of the injected radioactivity. Two hours after the injection, the radioactivity excreted in the urine was primarily in the form of iodouracil and iodide, with very little IdUrd.

The extreme physiological lability of IdUrd limits in part its clinical use, and practicable means have been sought to inhibit its catabolism (see below). The ease with which IdUrd is degraded by intestinal enzymes would appear to preclude its oral use.

C. Enzyme Inhibition

DELAMORE and PRUSOFF (1962) observed with cells of both the Ehrlich ascites carcinoma and the L5178Y lymphoma that the specific metabolic site affected primarily by IdUrd was characteristic of the individual tissue. Thus, a marked accumulation of dTTP was produced by IdUrd in Ehrlich ascites carcinoma cells, implying inhibition of DNA polymerase, whereas in L5178Y lymphoma cells, primary inhibition of the phosphorylation of dTMP was indicated, implying blockage of thymidylate kinase. Furthermore, at concentrations of IdUrd that exerted no inhibition of the formation of thymidylate *de novo* in Ehrlich ascites cells, a significant inhibition was observed in L5178Y cells, suggesting inhibition of thymidylate synthetase in this cell line presumably by pseudoproduct inhibition by IdUMP formed by phosphorylation of IdUrd. BAKHLE and PRUSOFF (1969) studied the effects of IdUrd and its mono- and triphosphate derivatives on those enzymes involved in the formation of thymidine and its phosphorylated derivatives, as well as on the biosynthesis of DNA in cell-free extracts of these two murine neoplasms. The differences previously found with whole cells by DELAMORE and PRUSOFF (1962) were not observed. The natural substrate was utilized preferentially to the corresponding iodinated analog by thymidine kinase and thymidylate kinase, but DNA polymerase used either dTTP or IdUTP equally well. Inhibition of the conversion of thymidine to thymidylate, of thymidylate to dTTP, and of dTTP to DNA-thymine by the appropriate derivative of IdUrd was reversible and presumably competitive. The differences between the experiments of DELAMORE and PRUSOFF (1962) and BAKHLE and PRUSOFF (1969) were attributed to the complexities of the intact cell where problems of cell transport, rates of phosphorylation, and size and stability of metabolite pools must be considered. The cell-free studies were performed with crude extracts in an attempt to mimic the intact cell, but yet devoid of membrane effects. Although a 5-fold excess of IdUrd to thymidine and of IdUMP to TMP was required to achieve 50 % inhibition of thymidine kinase and thymidylate kinase, respectively, one cannot assume that a corresponding difference in K_m for these substrates exists, since these are crude extracts that contain nucleosidase and nucleotidase activities for which the halogenated substrate may be preferentially utilized. Thus, for example, in purified enzyme systems the K_m for IdUrd and thymidine have been reported to be essentially identical (BRESNICK and THOMPSON, 1965), however, the rate of catabolism of IdUrd is greater than that of thymidine (see references in section on Anabolism).

Deoxythymidine kinase, purified from extracts of *Escherichia coli* B cells (OKAZAKI, R. and KORNBERG, 1964a, b), as well as the enzyme present in animal tumors (IVES et al., 1962; BRESNICK and THOMPSON, 1965) is subject to allosteric or feedback inhibition by not only dTTP, but also with the *E. coli* enzyme, by the corresponding halogenated analog BrdUTP. The bacterial enzyme was activated by dCDP and dCTP, however, the mammalian enzyme was inhibited by dCTP. The K_m for thymidine was increased by dTTP, whereas the activator, dCDP, caused a decrease in K_m and an increase in V_{max} (IWATSUKI and OKAZAKI, 1967). Those nucleotides that exert either an inhibitory or an activating effect caused an increase in sedimentation coefficient of the *E. coli* enzyme, with a doubling of the molecular weight of the enzyme. The allosteric nature of thymidine kinase derived from either *E. coli* or mammalian cells has been well established.

VOYTEK et al. (1971) examined the effect of various halogenated nucleoside triphosphates on a highly purified preparation of deoxythymidine kinase from *E. coli*. They observed that 5-iodo-2'-deoxycytidine 5'-triphosphate and 5-bromo-

2′-deoxycytidine 5′-triphosphate were more potent allosteric activators of deoxythymidine kinase than the naturally occurring effector 2′-deoxycytidine 5′-triphosphate throughout the pH range of 5.2 to 9.3. 5-Iodo-2′-deoxyuridine 5′-triphosphate (IdUTP) activated the enzymes at basic pH values; however, it exerted an inhibitory effect in a manner comparable to 2′-deoxythymidine 5′-triphosphate below pH 6.5. Whereas the inhibitory effect produced by IdUTP at pH 5.4 could not be prevented by up to a 12-fold excess of dCTP, the activation caused by IdUTP at pH 7.8 was completely prevented by dTTP.

The influence of various allosteric effectors on the sedimentation rate of deoxythymidine kinase was investigated by VOYTEK et al. (1971). Zone sedimentation studies in sucrose gradients showed that the sedimentation coefficient of deoxythymidine kinase (pH 5.6 = 3.5; pH 7.8 = 3.5) is increased at pH 7.8 by 5-bromo-2′-deoxycytidine 5′-triphosphate (5.6) and 5-iodo-2′-deoxycytidine 5′-triphosphate (5.6) to a greater extent than that produced by dCTP (5.3). IdUTP caused an even more marked increase in the sedimentation coefficient at both pH 5.6 (6.0) and 7.8 (5.9), and was similar to that produced by dTTP (5.9).

Kinetic analysis of the effect of the various allosteric effectors on the rate of thymidine phosphorylation was performed by VOYTEK et al. (1971). Linear double reciprocal plots were obtained of initial velocity against varying concentrations of deoxythymidine in the presence and absence of the halogenated effectors at both pH 5.4 and 7.8. The K_m is reduced by dCTP, and the halogenated derivatives of dCTP produce a similar effect.

OKAZAKI, R. and KORNBERG (1964a, b) reported that BrdUTP was equivalent to dTTP in its inhibitory action, but 5-fluoro-2′-deoxyuridine triphosphate had marginal activity. In the study of VOYTEK et al. (1971), IdUTP was an inhibitor or an activator, and these contrasting effects were dependent on the pH of the incubation mixture. IWATSUKI and OKAZAKI (1967) showed at pH values above 8.7 that dTTP exerted little or no inhibitory effect on deoxythymidine kinase activity, but rather a small activation. Similarly, VOYTEK et al. (1971) found that the inhibitory potency of dTTP is diminished at basic pH values. Since the pK_a of dTTP is 9.8, it is conceiveable that as dTTP becomes more ionized its inhibitory action is decreased and activation increases. However, OKAZAKI, T. and KORNBERG (1964) reported that at pH 7.8, BrdUTP, which has a pK_a of 8.05 and, hence, is more ionized than dTTP at pH 7.8, is equivalent to dTTP in inhibiting deoxythymidine kinase. IdUTP has a pK_a of 8.25 and, therefore, in the study of VOYTEK et al. (1971) was expected to exert an inhibitory effect at a different pH in a manner similar to BrdUTP as reported by OKAZAKI, T. and KORNBERG (1964); however, they observed IdUTP to be a potent activator above pH 6.5 and an inhibitor at more acidic pH values. Therefore, the pK_a parameters of these effectors may not be the critical factor in determining whether the effector molecule will be an activator or an inhibitor. CAMERMAN and TROTTER (1964) have shown by x-ray diffraction methods that fairly strong charge transfer bonding between oxygen and iodine exists in crystals of 5-iodo-2′-deoxyuridine, and HASSEL and ROMMING (1962) have reported that the stability of the charge transfer bonds is proportional to the atomic weight of the halogen; hence, the bonds formed should be stronger when iodine rather than bromine atoms are the electron acceptors. It is conceivable that a charge transfer bond, which is pH dependent, forms between some electron donor group in deoxythymidine kinase and the iodine atom in IdUTP, and that this interaction may produce a subtle change in the conformation of the enzyme, which distinguishes it as an activator rather than an inhibitor such as dTTP or BrdUTP.

Prusoff and Chang (1969/70) have reported that deoxythymidine kinase from Ehrlich ascites carcinoma cells is inhibited by dTTP and IdUTP at both pH 5.0 and 7.5. The kinetic studies of this mammalian enzyme indicated that dTTP and IdUTP acted as competitive inhibitors with deoxythymidine at pH 7.5, but that the inhibition caused by both nucleotides was more complex at pH 5.0 and 6.5, giving parabolic double reciprocal plots. In contrast, Voytek et al. (1971) reported that the activation kinetics of the *E. coli* enzyme show normal Lineweaver-Burk relationships with dCTP, BrdCTP, IdCTP, and IdUTP at pH 7.5, as well as at pH 5.4. IdUTP and dTTP act as competitive inhibitors of thymidine at pH 5.4. The explanation for the difference in the inhibition kinetics between thymidine kinase derived from *E. coli* and that from Ehrlich ascites carcinoma cells is not known. Furthermore, whereas IdUTP was about 3 times more inhibitory than dTTP in the inhibition of deoxythymidine kinase derived from Ehrlich ascites cells, IdUTP is, if anything, slightly less inhibitory than dTTP to the *E. coli* enzyme.

dCTP has been shown to be a specific activator of deoxycytidylate deaminase derived from several sources. dTTP, regardless of the source of deoxycytidylate deaminase, is the most effective naturally occurring inhibitor. IdUTP has been shown by Prusoff and Chang (1968), not only to mimic dTTP in the exertion of a feedback inhibition of dCMP deaminase, but also to cause a greater inhibitory effect than that of dTTP. The relationship between dCTP and dTTP is one of reversible inhibition or activation dependent upon the molar ratio of the activator and inhibitor (Scarano et al., 1967). Similarly, with extracts derived from Ehrlich ascites carcinoma and L5178Y lymphoma cells, IdUTP behaved qualitatively in a manner similar to dTTP, and in addition IdUTP qualitatively mimicked dTTP at all levels of pH investigated (Prusoff and Chang, 1968).

Diwan and Prusoff (1968) observed an increase in deoxycytidylate deaminase activity after infection of African green monkey kidney cells with herpes simplex virus. They made a comparison of the relative susceptibility to inhibition by IdUTP of this enzyme present in the uninfected and infected cells. No alteration in the susceptibility of the "induced" enzyme to inhibition by either IdUTP or dTTP was observed. IdUTP, however, was about 2.5 times more potent an inhibitor than dTTP of this enzymic reaction.

Since relatively small amounts of IdUTP are required for feedback inhibition of deoxycytidylate deaminase, relative to those derivatives of IdUrd required for competitive inhibition of the anabolic reactions of thymidine and its phosphorylated derivatives (Bakhle and Prusoff, 1969), it would appear that this site of inhibition may be of importance in the IdUrd inhibition of cellular reproduction. Whether inhibition of this enzyme occurs *in vivo* is dependent upon a number of factors that include, for example, the pool size of dCMP, dCTP, and dTTP, which presumably varies from cell to cell depending on the phase of growth of the individual cell. Accumulation of an inhibitory level of IdUTP is related to a complex series of reactions that vary not only with the species of cell, but also with the phase of growth. The rate of transport of IdUrd into the cell may be critical if the cell contains an active pyrimidine deoxyribonucleosidase, an enzyme that converts IdUrd into innocuous 5-iodouracil. If the rate of transport of IdUrd into the cell were slower than the rate of cleavage of IdUrd, the amount of IdUrd available for subsequent phosphorylation would be limiting. Thus, the activity of the three kinases required for the conversion of IdUrd to its triphosphate is critical to the formation of the pool of IdUTP. The formed pool of IdUTP is not stagnant, but is subjected to depletion by either incorporation into DNA or to dephosphorylation by nucleoside triphosphatase. Thus, critical evaluation of the contributory role of

IdUTP as an allosteric inhibitor *in vivo* of either deoxycytidylate deaminase or of other enzymes that are affected similarly is a complex problem. The various sites of inhibition by IdUrd and its anabolically derived phosphorylated derivatives are depicted in Fig. 4.

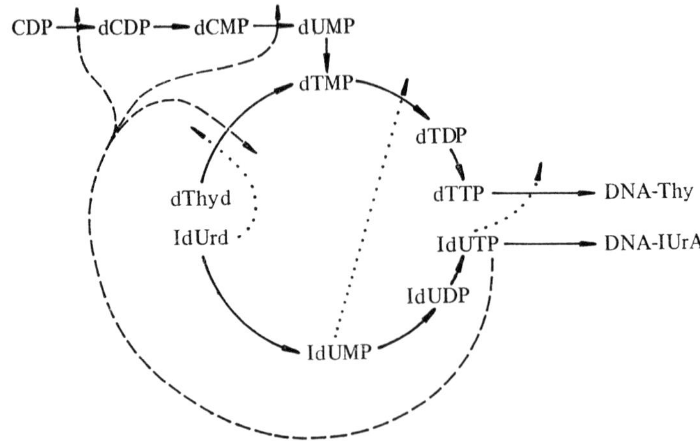

Fig. 4. Sites of inhibition by 5-iodo-2′-deoxyuridine and its phosphorylated derivatives

D. Augmentation of Utilization of Halogenated Deoxyribonucleosides

One of the major problems in the use of IdUrd or BrUrd is their very rapid metabolic degradation, and hence many laboratories have made a variaty of approaches to provide means that would enhance halogen analog incorporation into DNA. Although IdUrd and its phosphorylated derivatives exert an inhibitory effect on the various enzymes concerned with the incorporation of thymidine and its phosphorylated derivatives into DNA, the type of inhibition exerted appears to be the competitive type. Hence, a decrease in the pool size of the halogenated analog or an increase in the pool size of the appropriate derivative of thymidine readily overcome such an impermanent inhibition. The major site to be affected in order to obtain the desired biological effect (i.e., tumor inhibition, radiosensitization, antiviral activity, marker for study of cell kinetics, detection of malignant tissue, etc.) is incorporation into DNA, an irreversible event.

I. Inhibition of Thymidylate Synthetase

Phosphorylated derivatives of thymidine compete with phosphorylated derivatives of IdUrd along the pathway of DNA biosynthesis (Fig. 4). The phosphorylated derivatives of thymidine are derived from two major sources: (1) exogenous thymidine from metabolic degradation of DNA present either in ingested food or from dead cells within the organism and (2) endogenous thymidylate formed *de novo* by thymidylate synthetase, which uses methylene tetrahydrofolate as the coenzyme.

HAKALA (1959, 1962) found BrdUrd could replace completely the thymidine requirement of a mammalian cell when methotrexate, an inhibitor of thymidylate synthetase, was present in the medium. HAKALA (1962) replaced with BrdUrd 93 to 100 % of DNA-thymine in human uterine fibroblasts and mouse fibroblasts when the *de novo* formation of thymidylate was prevented with methotrexate. HAMPTON and EIDINOFF (1961) augmented by 3-fold the uptake of IdUrd into rat tumor DNA similarly by the coadministration of methotrexate.

Thymidylate synthetase may also be inhibited by the monophosphate of FdUrd (COHEN et al., 1958; HARTMANN and HEIDELBERGER, 1961; HEIDELBERGER, 1965). Thus, FdUrd has been used to increase the uptake of BrdUrd or IdUrd into DNA of bacterial DNA (LORKIWCZ and SZYBALSKI, 1960) and mammalian DNA (DJORDJEVIC and SZYBALSKI, 1960; ROTENBERG et al., 1962; KRISS et al., 1962; CLIFTON et al., 1963). For example, KRISS et al. (1962) increased the uptake of labeled IdUrd into tissues of the rat by a factor of 2 to 5 by the concurrent injection of FdUrd.

II. Inhibition of Nucleoside Phosphorylase

The availability of a greater amount of IdUrd for the biosynthesis of DNA in mammalian cells should be obtained by a reduction in the activity of the catabolic enzymes responsible for the cleavage of IdUrd to iodouracil. Preliminary studies by PERKINS and PRUSOFF (cited in PRUSOFF, 1963) and by FOX and PRUSOFF (1966) had shown that thymine ribonucleoside is an effective inhibitor of the nucleoside phosphorylase responsible for the cleavage of IdUrd. The kinetics of this inhibition have been investigated by FOX et al. (1969/70).

KRISS and BOND (1964) found a variety of natural and unnatural pyrimidines and pyrimidine nucleosides, when present in 3-fold excess, inhibited the phosphorolysis of IdUrd by a crude mouse liver extract.

The effect of thymine ribonucleoside on the metabolism of ^{125}I-IdUrd in mice was studied by FOX and PRUSOFF (1966). Although thymine ribonucleoside is indeed an effective inhibitor of catabolism *in vitro*, the results in mice were disappointing, since a high molar ratio of thymine ribonucleoside to ^{125}I-IdUrd increased the rate of urinary excretion of total radioactivity, which was composed mainly of iodouracil and unchanged IdUrd. This may be due to either a block in cell transport, a block in catabolism, or a diuretic effect of thymine ribonucleoside. The distribution of radioactivity among various tissues indicates a 2.5- to 3-fold greater uptake of radioactivity into the liver, heart, kidney, and muscle, than into tissues that show a normal high rate of division such as small intestine, spleen, and bone marrow. There was no increase in the utilization of IdUrd for the biosynthesis of DNA, but thymine ribonucleoside merely altered the amount of ^{125}I-IdUrd present in the intracellular fluids.

LANGEN and ETZOLD (1963) observed that deoxyglucosylthymine inhibits the cleavage of pyrimidine nucleosides by extracts of Ehrlich ascites tumor cells, partially by extracts of rat liver and not at all by extracts of horse liver. The inhibition was of the competitive type with the affinity of deoxyglucosylthymine for the enzyme being 5 times that of uridine, 20-times that of thymidine and 80-times that of deoxyuridine. Similar results were obtained by ZIMMERMAN and SEIDENBERG (1964).

Two enzymes possessing deoxyribonucleosidase activity have been reported to be present in mammalian tissues, of which only one is inhibited by thymine deoxyglucoside (KRENITSKY et al., 1964, 1965). Thymidine phosphorylase (EC 2.4.2.4) catalyzes the phosphorolysis of thymidine and deoxyuridine and is not sensitive to inhibition by thymine deoxyglucoside, whereas uridine-deoxyuridine phosphorylase (EC 2.4.2.3) is inhibited (ZIMMERMAN, 1964; LANGEN and ETZOLD, 1966a, b; ETZOLD et al., 1968). LANGEN et al. (1967), ETZOLD et al. (1968), PREUSSEL et al. (1969), BAKER (1967), and BAKER and BZESTOTARSKI

(1964, 1968), have developed a variety of compounds as potential inhibitors of the phosphorylytic cleavage of compounds such as IdUrd, BrdUrd, and FdUrd.

LANGEN and ETZOLD (1966a, b) have shown that administration of 1-(2′-deoxy-β-D-glucopyranosyl)thymine to cats will augment the incorporation of IdUrd into the DNA of intestine, spleen, and bone marrow. Unfortunately, these compounds inhibit only uridine-deoxyuridine phosphorylase, but not thymidine phosphorylase, the enzyme responsible for cleavage of FdUrd and IdUrd in human tissues (ETZOLD et al., 1968).

HAMPTON and EIDINOFF (1961) used 5-iodouridine in an attempt to increase the utilization of IdUrd for the biosynthesis of DNA. A 60-fold molar excess of 5-iodouridine did not influence the uptake of labeled IdUrd into tumor or intestinal tissue, although the radioactivity taken up by the liver was increased 5-fold. DETHLEFSEN (1971) observed a 2-fold increase in the utilization of a tracer dose of ^{125}I-IdUrd when 5-iodouridine was given 30 min prior to administration of the labeled compounds, but not when given simultaneously or 30 min afterwards.

Since pyrimidine nucleoside phosphorylase cleaves thymidine, IdUrd, or BrdUrd to the free base plus deoxyribose-1-phosphate, it is theoretically possible to reutilize the free pyrimidine base by supplying a large pool of deoxyribose-1-phosphate. In this manner, deoxyadenosine has been used to supply a source of deoxyribose-1-phosphate to shift the reaction towards pyrimidine nucleoside anabolism (BOYCE and SETLOW, 1962; BUDMAN and PARDEE, 1967; KAMMEN, 1967).

LANGEN and VENKER (1963) studied the utilization of 5-bromouracil for the synthesis of DNA of tumor-bearing mice, and under conditions where no incorporation of 5-bromouracil occurred, they found that the administration of very large doses of bromouracil (i.e., 20 mg) plus deoxyguanosine (20 mg) three times per day subcutaneously, with or without 5-fluorouracil, resulted in marked uptake of the halogenated uracil (25 % substitution) into tumor, intestine, spleen, and liver.

GOTTO et al. (1969) found that deoxyinosine, by serving as a supply of deoxyribose-1-phosphate, can stimulate the incorporation of 5-bromouracil into the DNA of Ehrlich ascites tumor cells *in vitro*. The reason why thymine or halogenated uracil derivatives are poor precursors relative to their corresponding nucleosides for DNA biosynthesis may be because of an inadequate pool of the phosphorylated sugar moiety. The obvious therapeutic implication is to determine whether deoxyinosine does indeed afford a therapeutic advantage when combined with IdUrd or even iodouracil.

ROSNER and YAGIL (1970) successfully have combined two approaches in an attempt to augment incorporation of BrdUrd into *E. coli* DNA by not only the coadministration of FdUrd to inhibit thymidylate synthetase after conversion to FdUMP but also by the inclusion of deoxyadenosine to supply a large pool of deoxyribose-1-phosphate.

III. Inhibition of Pyrimidine Degradation

COOPER and GREER (1970) have approached the problem of augmentation of IdUrd incorporation into tumor DNA by inhibition of the degradation of the cleaved pyrimidine moiety. They observed both 5-cyanouracil, an inhibitor of dihydrouracil dehydrogenase (DORSETT et al., 1969), and 5-diazouracil, to inhibit the dehalogenation of iodouracil. 5-Diazouracil exerted an irreversible inhibition and 5-cyanouracil a reversible inhibition of the dehalogenation of 5-iodouracil by an enzyme present in the 105000 × g rat liver supernatant fluid. The potential of 5-diazouracil under *in vivo* conditions was investigated; it was found that 3 h after administration of 5-diazouracil the enzyme present in the rat liver supernatant fluid responsible for dehalogenation was inhibited by over 90%. Unfortunately, the IdUrd cleavage is not impaired and hence the authors suggest that inclusion of a source of deoxyribose-1-phosphate by supplying deoxyinosine (GOTTO et al., 1969) should stimulate incorporation into DNA. COOPER et al. (1972) reported a combination of 5-diazouracil with deoxyguanosine, to serve as a source of deoxyribose-1-phosphate, increased the uptake of iodouracil and thymine into DNA by twenty-fold in tissues of tumor-bearing rats.

IV. Complex Formation

WOODMAN (1966, 1968) augmented the uptake of IdUrd into DNA of several murine and hamster tumors, but not into spleen and intestinal mucosa, by forming a salt complex between IdCMP or IdUrd and a variety of polycations. Thus, the protamine-IdCMP complex relative to IdCMP alone produced a tumor to normal tissue ratio of DNA-iodine content 3 fold higher in mice and 6 fold higher in hamsters. Since the surface of the tumor cell has been reported to be more acidic than that of normal cells, the polycation, by interacting with the tumor cell surface to a greater extent than the normal cell, may produce in this manner a higher localized concentration of IdCMP and hence greater absorption. However, other possible mechanisms have been presented by WOODMAN (1968).

V. Alteration of Structure

Because the rapid metabolism of IdUrd *in vivo* limits in part the potential clinical effectiveness of this compound, and since cytosine nucleosides are resistant to nucleosidase cleavage (DEVERDIER and POTTER, 1960), it was suggested by WELCH (1961) that 5-iodo-2′-deoxycytidine could serve as a stable reservoir of IdUrd. The synthesis of 5-iodo-2′-deoxycytidine was reported by CHANG and WELCH (1961). However, studies in mice (CRAMER et al., 1962; KRISS et al., 1962) and in man (CALABRESI et al., 1963b) have shown that the cytosine analog is in fact rapidly and extensively degraded. CREASEY (1963) studied the metabolism of 5-iododeoxycytidine in various tissues of the mouse and found the first step in this degradation is deamination to IdUrd.

5-Iodo-2′-deoxyuridine-5′-phosphate, although less susceptible to the degradative enzymes that cleave IdUrd, nevertheless was not taken up to any greater extent than IdUrd (HAMPTON and EIDINOFF, 1961).

VI. Improved Regimens

PRUSOFF (1960) reported markedly increased uptake of IdUrd into the DNA of Ehrlich ascites cells *in vivo* when the total amount of IdUrd was increased by 12-fold and the frequency of administration doubled.

IdUrd was administered as an oil emulsion by HAMPTON and EIDINOFF (1961) to provide a depot; however, these investigators, as well as CLIFTON et al. (1963), found that injected IdUrd was used more efficiently for DNA biosynthesis than when given in depot form.

Since the liver has been implicated as the primary site of metabolic degradation of IdUrd or BrdUrd, attempts have been made to either circumvent or minimize this parameter by the administration of the halogenated nucleoside directly into the tumor site by intraarterial infusion (BAGSHAW et al., 1967; SANO et al., 1965; SANO et al., 1968).

HOFER and HUGHES (1970) found that the total amount of labeled IdUrd retained by leukemic mice, as well as the tissue distribution, was dependent upon the route of administration. Thus, intraperitoneal injection of IdUrd into mice bearing a peritoneal tumor produced a 3-fold greater retention of label than when the drug was given by intravenous or subcutaneous injection; however, in the nonleukemic mouse no difference was observed with respect to the mode of administration.

Physical Effects of Incorporation of Halogenated Uracil Derivatives into DNA

Incorporation of IdUrd or BrdUrd into DNA exerts a marked effect on the replication of mammalian cells, bacteria, and viruses. The biochemical and physical effects that result from incorporation of halogenated uracils into nucleic acids have been reviewed by KIT (1962), SZYBALSKI (1962), BROCKMAN and ANDERSON (1963), ELION and HITCHINGS (1965), PRUSOFF et al. (1965), and PRUSOFF (1967).

A. Increased Lability to Stress

DNA substituted with halogenated deoxyuridine is more sensitive to hydrodynamic shearing forces (SZYBALSKI, 1962); this finding may explain the lower intrinsic viscosity of substituted DNA relative to normal DNA. MCCREA and LIPMAN (1967) found IdUrd-substituted DNA liberated by osmotic shock to be extensively fragmented, in contrast to the normal DNA that was consistently relatively long and continuous. These investigators proposed that the decreased pock-forming ability of the IdUrd-substituted virus particles may be attributed, at least in part, to the increased fragility of the DNA when released within the host cell by the "uncoating enzyme". Whether the procedure used for isolation of the halogenated DNA resulted in the increased fragility or whether this condition exists within the intact virus particle must still be elucidated.

EASTERBROOK and DAVERN (1963) suggested, that BrdUrd substituted vaccinia DNA may be fragmented within the viral particle; this was corroborated by later observations of MCCREA and LIPMAN (1967). A related observation was made by FUJIWARA et al. (1970) that 5-(trifluoromethyl)-2′-deoxyuridine, an analog of thymidine, is incorporated into DNA and the substituted DNA polymer is smaller than the normal unsubstituted DNA. This decreased size of the DNA polymer was attributed to an inhibition by the fluorinated analog of the rate of formation of the DNA chains.

B. Increased Density

Centrifugation of DNA in a CsCl gradient results in a migration of the polymer that is dependent upon its density. Incorporation of a bromine (atomic weight: 80) or of iodine (atomic weight: 127) in place of the methyl group (atomic weight: 15) of DNA-thymine results in a marked increase in the buoyant density of the halogenated DNA (MESELSON et al. 1957; ERIKSON and SZYBALSKI, 1963b).

C. Increased Temperature (Tm) for DNA Denaturation

Heating a solution of nucleic acid results in a transition of the native nucleic acid to denatured DNA, as evidenced by an increase in ultraviolet absorbancy as the structure of DNA changes from a helical to a random coil (DOTY et al., 1959). The T_m or melting temperature is the temperature at which 50 % of the maximal increase in optical density occurs as the temperature of the solution is raised.

Replacement of DNA-thymine by bromouracil during replication results in enhanced stability of the polymer, as measured by an increase in T_m (KIT and HSU, 1961; SZYBALSKI and MENNIGMAN, 1962). PIETRZYKOWSKA and SHUGAR (1967) compared the T_m of phage T_3 normal DNA and of DNA in which 60 % of thymine residues had been replaced by 5-bromouracil and found about a 3° increase in the substituted DNA ($T_m = 74.4°$). This difference decreased as the salt concentration of the DNA solution increased, in agreement with the finding of INMAN and BALDWIN (1962).

LORKIEWICZ and SZYBALSKI (1960) and SZYBALSKI (1962) found that at equivalent degrees of incorporation, IdUrd causes a greater increase in T_m than BrdUrd.

MICHELSON et al. (1967) have presented an excellent review of the physical properties of synthetic polynucleotides, as well as of the 5-fluoro, 5-chloro, 5-bromo, 5-iodo, and 5-hydroxyuracil analogs of polyuridylate (SZER and SHUGAR, 1963; MASSOULI et al., 1966). Both 5-bromo and 5-iodouridylate increase the stability of the secondary structure of the homopolynucleotide, as well as the stability of hetero complexes, the latter effect being manifest by about a 30° increase in the T_m of poly (I) · poly (IC) relative to the nonhalogenated polymer poly [I] · poly (C) (MASSOULI et al., 1966). Studies by MASSOULI et al. (1966) of the temperature-UV absorption profiles of substituted homopolymers found that bromo or iodouracil increased stability, whereas chlorouracil substitution decreased the stability of the structure from (T_m: I > Br > U > Cl > F). Since the pK_a values of the various halogenated uracils are not markedly different from each other, they attributed the increased stability not to an effect on the hydrogen bonds responsible for base pairing but rather to interplane interactions (i.e., stacking energy).

A similar stabilizing effect by halogens is observed with synthetic polydeoxyribonucleotides. DAVIES and BALDWIN (1963) observed poly (dA-dBrU) to have an 8° larger T_m than poly (dA-dU), and INMAN and BALDWIN (1964) found poly d(I) · poly (dBrC) to have a T_m 26° greater than poly d(I) · poly (dC).

RILEY and ANIKO (1971) compared the T_m of synthetic polydeoxyribonucleotide complexes containing adenine and bromouracil and found that base sequence affected the thermal stability of both d(A-BrU) polymers and d(A-T) polymers. The thermal stabilities (i.e., T_m values) of the polymers d(A-T) and d(A-BrU) were about 7° more than the copolymers d(A-T) · d(A-T) and d(A-BrU) · d(A-BrU), respectively. The thermal stabilities as a function of pH were investigated and both the halogen substituted and unsubstituted homo- and copolymers showed decreased stability at high pH levels, with both the halogen-substituted homo- and copolymers being less stable at the high pH than the unsubstituted polymer. In agreement with previous investigators, they found that both bromine and the methyl group substituents in the 5-position of the pyrimidine moiety of these polymers confer stability to thermal denaturation with BrU > T > U. Although bromine or iodine in the 5-position of the pyrimidine moiety has been stated to increase the strength of the hydrogen bond, MICHELSON et al. (1967) believe other factors such as the increased interplanar interactions (i.e., free energy of stacking of base pairs), as well as solvent-polymer organization may be more important in imparting increased thermal stability. HOWARD et al. (1969) have studied by spectrophotometric methods the interaction of poly (BrC) with poly (I). They found evidence that the dependence of T_m upon bromocytosine content is linear and that the stabilizing effect of bromine is probably not due to solvent effects or to increased hydrogen bonding between the hypoxanthine-cytosine base pair, but rather to the increased polarizability (i.e., induced dipole and dispersion interactions) of bromine acting upon adjacent cytosine residues in the same strand.

PULLMAN and PULLMAN (1969), in their excellent review of the electronic structure of nucleic acids, addressed themselves to the problem of forces responsible for the stability of the double-helical structure of DNA and gave equal weight to the in-plane interactions between the hydrogen-bonded bases, the vertical interactions between the stacked bases, and the contribution of solvation effects.

D. Decreased pH for DNA Denaturation

When a solution of DNA is exposed to either an increase or a decrease in pH, an increase in absorbancy is observed as the structure of DNA changes from a helical to a random coil.

INMAN and BALDWIN (1962) and BALDWIN and SHOOTER (1963) observed a decreased helical stability (i.e. helix-coil transition) to alkali of the alternating copolymer d(ABrU) · (dABrU) compared to the polymer (dAT) · (dAT) with the pH of the melt being 9.42 and 10.95, respectively. The pH transitions were followed by the increase in buoyant densities during denaturation. BALDWIN and SHOOTER (1963) found *E. coli* DNA with 88% bromouracil substitution melts at pH 10.66, whereas the unsubstituted DNA melts at pH 11.42.

Confirmation of A · BrU rich regions of DNA melting at a lower pH than A-T rich regions was provided by INMAN and SCHNOS (1970) using electron microscopy of partially denatured DNA solutions at high pH. The extent of denaturation of BrU-DNA derived from phage, after 10 min at pH 10.45, was similar to that found for unsubstituted phage DNA after 48 to 90 min at pH 11.29. RILEY and ANIKO (1971) prepared the homopolymers (dBrU, rBrU) and copolymers d(A-BrU), r(A-BrU) and studied by alkaline titration the pH_m, which they define as "the pH at the midpoint of an absorbancy transition". Comparison of the pH_m of the following homopolymers and copolymer complexes was made: d(A-T) · d(A-T) (11.06); dA · dT (11.13); d(A-BrU) · d(A-BrU) (9.57); dA · dBrU (9.70); r(A-U) · r(A-U) (10.9); rA · rU (10.4); r(A-BrU) · r(A-BrU) (10.1); rA · rBrU (9.7). The order of effectiveness of the substituent on the 5-carbon of the pyrimidine moiety, with regard to the resultant sensitivity to alkali denaturation, is Br > T > U. Comparison of the ribose and deoxyribose polymers shows that the effect of the bromine substituent is more marked in the deoxyribose polymers. They suggest that runs of BrU in DNA, in substitution for runs of thymine, may have unique properties that cause the altered biological properties that result from such incorporation of halogenated uracils into DNA.

E. Increased Sensitivity to Heat Degradation

GREER (1960) has reported that *E. coli* $15T^-$ which contained 5-bromouracil in its DNA in place of thymine is hypersensitive to heat. This is supported by the findings of SZYBALSKI (1962) that halogenated DNA is more sensitive to heat degradation than unsubstituted DNA.

WESTRA and DEWEY (1971) found that mammalian cells during mitosis or in S phase were more sensitive to heat-induced mortality than cells heated during G_1 or G_2. BrdUrd, however, did not sensitize to heat either P-815 cells (SCHINDLER et al., 1966) or Chinese hamster cells (DEWEY et al., 1971). The lethal effect of heat was attributed by DEWEY et al. (1971) to a prime effect on chromosomal protein which interacts subsequently with the DNA. Thus a major difference appears to exist between bacterial and mammalian cells with regard to the influence of BrdUrd on heat sensitization.

Biological Consequences of Incorporation of Halogenated Uracil Derivatives into DNA

A. Mutagenic Effects

The initial observations of the incorporation of 5-bromo or 5-iodouracil into nucleic acid were made in the 1950's. WEYGAND et al. (1952) detected the incorporation of bromouracil labeled with ^{82}Br into the nucleic acid of *Streptococcus faecalis*. They did not determine whether the incorporation was specific for DNA or RNA. In 1954, three groups reported that 5-bromouracil was incorporated into the DNA of various microorganisms in place of thymine (DUNN and SMITH, 1954; ZAMENHOF and GRIBOFF, 1954; WACKER et al., 1954). Additionally, DUNN and SMITH (1954) reported that 5-iodouracil was similarly incorporated and that both analogs were incorporated into the DNA of phages T_2 and T_5. A more complete study was described later by DUNN and SMITH (1957). ZAMENHOF et al. (1956a, b) reported that 5-chlorouracil is incorporated into *E. coli* DNA, in addition to 5-bromo and 5-iodouracil, and KOZINSKI and SZYBALSKI (1959) reported that BrdUrd is incorporated into the single stranded DNA of ΦX174.

The incorporation of halogenated uracils into mammalian DNA was established in 1959 to 1960. HAKALA (1958, 1959) demonstrated BrdUrd incorporation into HeLa cell DNA. EIDINOFF et al. (1959a, b) showed incorporation of BrdUrd and IdUrd into the DNA of H.Ep. 1 cells in culture, and incorporation of IdUrd into human leukemic leucocytes *in vivo* (EIDENOFF et al., 1959b). IdUrd was shown to be incorporated into the DNA of both Ehrlich ascites cells (PRUSOFF, 1959a, b, 1960) and L5178Y mouse leukemia cells (MATHIAS et al., 1959). Incorporation of BrdUrd (EASTERBROOK and DAVERN, 1963) and IdUrd (PRUSOFF et al., 1963) into the DNA of vaccinia virus and incorporation of BrdUrd into pseudorabies virus DNA (KAPLAN and BEN-PORAT, 1964) was subsequently demonstrated. More recently, KAROL and SIMPSON (1968) showed that isolated rat liver mitochondria incubated with BrdUTP yield DNA with about 33% bromouracil substitution.

Thus, the incorporation of IdUrd and BrdUrd into DNA is well substantiated in a variety of organisms. The physico-chemical consequences of such incorporation are treated elsewhere in this chapter. The following discussion deals with the biological effects of BrdUrd and IdUrd incorporation into DNA. The most thoroughly studied effect, that of increased mutation frequency, will be discussed first.

Of the many studies of the mutagenic action of the halogenated pyrimidine analogs that have been performed, mainly with bromouracil, perhaps the most decisive has been done with the phages ΦX174, S13, and T_4. At about the same time that 5-bromo and 5-iodouracil were shown to be incorporated into DNA, various studies were published establishing the mutagenicity of these compounds. Thus, LITMAN and PARDEE (1956) reported that chloro, bromo, and iodouracil were all mutagenic relative to phage T_2, as indicated by reversion to the r^+ plaque type.

In 1958, the first of a series of papers appeared by BENZER and FREESE (1958) comparing spontaneous and bromouracil induced mutations in the rII system of T_4 by genetic fine structure analysis. These workers extended the finding of LITMAN and PARDEE (1956) with T_2 and bromouracil to the T_4 rII system; bromouracil raised the total frequency of occurrence of all rII mutants several hundred fold above the spontaneous rate. Furthermore, and most importantly, they found that the loci of the bromouracil induced mutations within the A and B cistrons of the rII region were markedly different from those that arose spontaneously. Only three sites, of 132 spontaneous mutants and 67 induced mutants, were found in common. The "hot spots" (i.e., map sites where mutations occur with high probability) for the spontaneous mutants differed from those induced by bromouracil. Parenthetically, the origin of "hot spots" is still at present a matter for conjecture. A model for "hot spots", together with a review of other hypotheses, has recently been published (YAMAGATA and SAKAMOTO, 1971).

FREESE (1959) proposed the mispairing of bases, engendered by bromouracil during DNA replication, as the mechanism of bromouracil induced mutagenesis. Mispairing was proposed to occur either during or after bromouracil incorporation into DNA. In the former case, bromouracil mispairs with a guanine rather than an adenine moiety in the DNA template, and subsequently correctly pairs with adenine in later replication of DNA. This results in the transition from a G:C base pair to an A:T base pair. In the latter type of mispairing, bromouracil (BU) in the DNA pairs with a guanine rather than the correct base adenine, thereby leading to the transition from a BU:A (T:A) base pair to a C:G base pair. Similar reasoning exists in the case of iodouracil.

The most commonly given explanations for the increased mispairing by bromo or iodouracil relate to their ability to undergo keto-enol isomerization, and to ionization properties related to differences in the pK_a values of thymine, bromouracil and iodouracil. The pK_a of thymine is 9.8 (SHUGAR and FOX, 1952), while that of bromouracil is 8.0 (BERENS and SHUGAR, 1963); the decrease is due to the electrophilic activity of the bromine atom. Therefore, with thymine at pH 7.0 the ionized anionic species occurs with about 0.1 % frequency, whereas the frequency of the ionized form for bromouracil is 6.6 %. Similar reasoning suggests that the electrophilic bromine or iodine should also increase the frequency of occurrence of the ionized or enol tautomer. The possible configurations of IdUrd are depicted in Fig. 2.

The fact that mispairing during incorporation permits the transition of G:C to A:T, whereas mispairing after incorporation allows an A:T to G:C transition, leads to the so-called "dirty-growth" and "clean-growth" experiments. In "dirty-growth," the appearance of mutations in an organism is monitored during replication in the presence of the mutagen, in this case the halogenated analogs. In contrast, for "clean-growth" the induction of mutations is followed after the analog has been incorporated into DNA and in the absence of the analog in the medium. Assumedly, it is also absent from the cell except for that incorporated into DNA. It is presumed that during "dirty-growth", incorporation mutations should be detected (i.e., G:C to A:T), and in "clean-growth," replication errors should be detected, i.e., errors produced by previously incorporated analog (A:T to G:C). Furthermore, the two should then be specific in not inducing a mutation at the same site or, as is usually the case, causing reversion of the same mutant.

"Clean-growth" mutagenesis was first shown by LITMAN and PARDEE (1960a, b) with T_2 phage and bromouracil. STRELZOFF (1961, 1962) demonstrated that bromouracil could induce "dirty-growth" and "clean-growth" reversions in *E. coli*, and that some of the mutants were only reverted in the presence of bromouracil. The reversion of lysozyme deficient mutants was studied by TERZAGHI et al. (1962) with T_4 and bromouracil. These investigators were able to show that of the lysozyme mutants studied, two gave reversion during "clean-growth" while four other mutants showed only "dirty-growth" reversion. However, these results of TERZAGHI et al. (1962) were somewhat mitigated by the finding that hydroxylamine, which only mutates cytosine to thymine (TESSMAN et al., 1964), caused reversion of one of the mutants found to revert during "clean-growth" and which was therefore presumed to contain an A:T pair at the site of mutation. Moreover, hydroxylamine caused no reversion of the four mutants found to revert only during "dirty-growth" with bromouracil. These mutants were presumed to have had, prior to reversion, a G:C pair at the mutation site which should have also responded to hydroxylamine.

An interesting approach to proving the existence of a mispaired G:BU was reported by PRATT and STENT (1959) with rII mutants of T_2 and T_4. These investigators found that if cells infected with a particular rII mutant were exposed to BrdUrd for only 4.5 min and lysed, as much as 81 % of the revertants to the r^+ wild type were heterozygotes, whereas a 50-minute BrdUrd exposure followed by lysis resulted in only 26 % of the revertants being heterozygotes. It may be argued that this result is in agreement with the existence of a G:BU base pair which causes reversion to the r^+ type. With a short pulse of BrdUrd and a short period of infection the G:BU remains in the same molecule of DNA and is coated. Such a phage on plating analysis would be a heterozygote. However, consistent with the data, further replication of the heterozygote molecule would separate the guanine and bromouracil containing strands into two daughter molecules with the resultant formation of one mutant and one nonmutant, thus decreasing the proportion of heterozygotes.

The work of TESSMAN et al. (1964) and HOWARD and TESSMAN (1964) with phage S13 more firmly established that BrdUrd preferentially induced the transition of thymine to cytosine and of adenine to guanine. This conclusion rests upon the genetic and chemical evidence that with the single-stranded DNA phages S13 and ΦX174, hydroxylamine only mutates cytosine to thymine (TESSMAN et al., 1964). The study of halogenated uracil induced mutagenesis in phage S13 eliminates the problem in determining the actual base transition involved, since this phage has a single stranded DNA and thus there is no question as to which base of a base pair is the primary target. The transitions A to G and T to C induced by BrdUrd were suppressed by thymidine while the reverse of these transitions was unaffected by thymidine but was suppressed by deoxycytidine. This is again consistent with the idea that the G:C to A:T transition is induced by bromouracil replacing cytosine, while in an A:T to G:C transition, bromouracil replaces thymine (HOWARD and TESSMAN, 1964).

The mutagenicity of halogenated analogs has also been tested in *Drosophila* (FAHMY et al., 1966; RIZKI and RIZKI, 1969). The mechanism of mutagenesis by halogenated uracils has been most thoroughly analyzed and established. The incorporation of these halogenated uracils into DNA leads not only to possible mutagenesis but also to many other interesting biological consequences. A question which must always be asked in each instance is whether the mutagenic activity of these compounds can account for the observed effects.

B. Inhibition of Cellular Division

I. Cell Culture

BrdUrd or IdUrd in sufficiently high concentration will inhibit mammalian cell division. HeLa cells treated with 30 µM BrdUrd in combination with methotrexate will undergo one division in the normal time before cellular replication ceases. Giant cells develop which eventually disintegrate, and under these conditions, BrdUrd substitutes for about 50 % of DNA-thymine. The effect is irreversible (HAKALA, 1958, 1959). On the other hand, Sarcoma 180, L cells, and human uterine fibroblasts can undergo at least 2 to 3 divisions at these drug concentrations, and in the case of L cells 94 to 100 % of the DNA-thymine was substituted by BrdUrd (HAKALA, 1962). LITTLEFIELD and GOULD (1960) reported similar inhibition for HeLa, as well as rabbit KD cells, with BrdUrd alone at concentrations of 3.3 to 326 μM, although unlike the 94 to 100% substitution of DNA-thymine reported by HAKALA (1962) for L cells, they obtained only 49 and 62% maximal substitution in HeLa and KD cells, respectively. Inclusion of fluorouracil in the culture medium did not increase BrdUrd substitution.

A human cell line from bone marrow (DJORDJEVIC and SZYBALSKI, 1960) can grow indefinitely in 33 μM BrdUrd, which at this concentration produces 14% substitution. At 163 μM, cell viability is impaired, although BrdUrd substitution of DNA-thymine is only increased to 39%. In this same cell line, exposure to as little as 14 μM IdUrd for 7 days markedly reduced viability on replating in IdUrd-free medium (DJORDJEVIC and SZYBALSKI, 1960). MATHIAS et al. (1959) and MATHIAS and FISCHER (1962) examined the effect of IdUrd on the murine leukemic cell line L5178Y and found that concentrations of 10 to 100 μM allowed only one division and cell death invariably commenced. In 1 mM IdUrd no division occurred, and the effect of 30 μM was preventable by 8 μM thymidine. The DNA synthesized by L5178Y cells, when grown in media supplemented with 30 μM IdUrd, had two-thirds of the DNA-thymine replaced by the analog (MATHIAS et al., 1959).

HEp No. 1 cells similarly will divide on the average only once subsequent to addition of 75 μM BrdUrd or IdUrd. Replication of cells in media containing 140 μM IdUrd resulted in approximately 25% substitution of DNA thymidine (EIDINOFF and RICH, 1959; EIDINOFF et al., 1959a; CHEONG et al., 1960).

MORRIS and CRAMER (1966) similarly found that cells of the P815Y murine mast cell tumor completed only one doubling of both cell number and DNA with IdUrd concentrations of 100 to 200 μM.

WILKOF et al. (1970) studied the kinetics of inhibition of IdUrd on replicating L1210 cells in culture and observed not only that first order kinetics did not apply, but also that the kinetic parameters were independent of concentration. Thus, they observed that the kinetics of population reduction by IdUrd could be described by the Gompertz function, whereas that due to hydroxyurea followed the first-order rate equation.

On the other hand, LANGEN and LISS (1962) studied fluorouracil inhibition of DNA synthesis in ascites tumor cells *in vitro* and found that both thymidine and BrdUrd were equally effective in reversing the inhibition. In the newly synthesized DNA, 85 to 90% of the thymine was replaced by bromouracil. The free bases thymine, bromouracil, and iodouracil are equally effective if given simultaneously with a donor of deoxyribose-1-phosphate such as deoxyguanosine or deoxyadenosine, but not deoxycytidine. Bromouracil and iodouracil both replaced 85% of the thymine residues in newly synthesized DNA. KIHLMAN (1966) had previously observed that many of the effects of FdUrd were reversed by thymidine and its analogs. Although IdUrd (10^{-4} M), BrdUrd (10^{-4} M), and thymidine (10^{-3} M) cause a decline in the mitotic index of root tips of *Vicia faba* during cell division, with the effect of IdUrd being most potent, both IdUrd and BrdUrd can substitute for thymidine in reversing an FdUrd-induced mitotic inhibition (HOFFMAN, 1970).

Other studies demonstrating the ability of BrdUrd or IdUrd to inhibit cellular replication include those of ERIKSON and SZYBALSKI (1961), SIMON (1961), MOHLER and ELKIND (1963), EYE et al. (1964), GEERAETS, et al. (1965), COGGIN et al. (1967), FUJIWARA et al. (1970).

Cells that do not possess thymidine kinase activity are resistant to BrdUrd and IdUrd, as the analogs must be phosphorylated by this enzyme and subsequent catalysts in order to be incorporated into DNA and cause inhibition (KIT et al., 1963; KIT et al., 1966; DUBBS et al., 1967; LITTLEFIELD, 1965). In addition to such resistant cells, BrdUrd tolerant cells have been described by DJORDJEVIC and SZYBALSKI (1960) and SIMON (1963). These cells incorporate BrdUrd into their DNA, but continue to replicate.

SIMON and coworkers have extensively studied the phenomenon of BrdUrd tolerance in HeLa cells. SIMON (1963) reported that the inclusion of 66 μM BrdUrd in the medium of cultured cells allows a single division with no delay, but only a small portion of the cells divides more than twice. Eventually, however, a population of slow growing cells evolves which tolerates 66 μM BrdUrd in its environment. The appearance of such cells is blocked if FdUrd or methotrexate is added with the BrdUrd. In the tolerant cells approximatelx 30 % of the DNA-thymine is replaced by BrdUrd. The DNA from cells which divided only once had 75 % DNA-thymine replaced in the replicated strand. Determination of thymidine kinase activity in the tolerant and control HeLa cells showed enzyme activity of the same order of magnitude, so that the difference in DNA substitution is not attributable to decreased thymidine kinase activity (TOLIVER and SIMON, 1967). A prominent feature of the tolerant cells is their increased generation time which TOLIVER and SIMON (1967) reported was due to a three-fold increase in the duration of the *S* phase of the cell cycle. Returning the tolerant cells to normal medium restored the normal generation time after 60 h. In a later communication TOLIVER et al. (1968) explored the difference between HeLa cells grown in the presence of BrdUrd alone, from which BrdUrd tolerant cells evolve, and cells grown in BrdUrd plus FdUrd which divide only once and produce no tolerant cells. Analysis of the pyrimidine oligonucleotides from cells grown in the presence of BrdUrd with and without FdUrd revealed an unknown peak. This "unique" peak is found in the enzymically hydrolyzed DNA derived from cells either grown in the presence of BrdUrd and FdUrd or from BrdUrd tolerant cells, but not from control cells. The significance of the unknown peak has not been resolved to date; however, it may represent an oligonucleotide that contains bromouracil, which would indeed alter chromatographic properties.

KAJIWARA and MUELLER (1964) tested whether the time of BrdUrd addition to synchronized HeLa cells affected the inhibition of division. Interestingly, the first 3 h of the 6-hour DNA synthetic period was very sensitive to BrdUrd, *vis-a-vis* inhibition of cloning efficiency which was 22 % of control efficiency, whereas the second 3-hour portion of the period was virtually insensitive (i.e. 95 % of control cloning efficiency). During the first 3 h 34 % of BrdUrd-substituted DNA is synthesized, while during the second 3 h 65 % of the substituted DNA is made. The authors speculate that either a special species of DNA is synthesized in the early period or that the DNA synthesized initially codes for protein essential to cell viability. KIM et al. (1967) do not confirm these findings. Although they too find maximal inhibition of synchronized HeLa cells during the DNA synthetic period, such inhibition was coincident with maximum DNA synthesis in the middle of the period rather than in the beginning as found in KAJIWARA and MUELLER (1964). KIM et al. (1967) opine that the discrepancy in results is due to the difference employed in the method of synchronization; theirs involved collecting cells in mitosis, whereas KAJIWARA and MUELLER (1964) used methotrexate. These results deserve reconciliation of the discrepancy.

Another provocative but unresolved series of studies is that of Morris and Cramer (MORRIS and CRAMER, 1966, 1968; CRAMER and MORRIS, 1966) with IdUrd and the murine mastocytoma P815Y. As previously cited, 100 to 200 μM IdUrd allows one doubling of the cell number and DNA. Although the amount of DNA remains constant, the synthesis of DNA occurs in only about one-half of the cells. MORRIS and CRAMER hypothesize that substitution of IdUrd in one strand blocks

DNA replication, whereas substitution in the complementary strand has no effect. RNA synthesis is decreased in the treated cells, but the inhibition is similar whether cells are synthesizing or not synthesizing DNA (MORRIS, personal communication of the work of CRAMER, MORRIS, and MILTON).

A perhaps related finding of KASAMAKI et al. (1968) demonstrates that primary mouse embryo cells in which the synthesis of DNA is inhibited by IdUrd will resume cellular DNA synthesis upon infection with polyoma virus. Two possible explanations given are that a new polyoma-coded DNA polymerase is able to use IdUrd-substituted DNA as a template or that the polyoma genome specifies a regulatory protein required for DNA synthesis which cannot be transcribed from substituted DNA.

There have been several reports of cytologically observable chromosomal aberrations induced by BrdUrd principally in mouse cells (HSU et al., 1961; HSU and SOMERS, 1961, 1962; HUMPHREY and HSU, 1965). For example, treatment of L cells with 83 μM BrdUrd for 5 days results in lengthening of centromeric regions, secondary constrictions, and chromatid breaks (HSU and SOMERS, 1961). PALMER (1970) made a similar observation with cultures of human peripheral leukocytes exposed to 245 μM BrdUrd for 5 to 7 h, and moreover found a reproducible pattern of BrdUrd-induced constrictions in the D and sex chromosomes. She concurs with HSU and SOMERS (1961) in that the constriction regions in reaction to BrdUrd may be composed of heterochromatin rich in A-T base pairs. Lastly, BrdUrd affects mitosis in HeLa cells causing cytoplasmic as well as chromosomal abnormalities after 20 h. Furthermore, multiple chromosomal fragmentation and many akinetic fragments were observed just outside the metaphase spindle. Polar chromosomes were also found and subsequent chromosome separation was irregular with formation of many bridges. Cytokinesis was also irregular (IZUTSU and BIESELE, 1966).

In nonmammalian systems bromouracil alters the sequence of chromosome replication in *E. coli* K12 (ABE and TOMIZAWA, 1967) and in T_4-infected *E. coli* causes a 40% decrease in the rate of movement of growing points of phage DNA (WERNER, 1968).

II. Animals

The potential of IdUrd as an inhibitor of neoplastic growth has been explored in a number of animal systems.

IdUrd, when injected into mice in amounts of 100 or 150 mg/kg daily for 6 days, inhibited significantly the growth of Sarcoma 180 and lymphoma L1210 and L5178Y without evidence of host toxicity (JAFFE and PRUSOFF, 1960). When the drug was administered to mice in combination with azaserine, 6-azathymine, 6-azauridine, 5-fluorodeoxyuridine, or methotrexate, only additive inhibitory effects on the growth of lymphoma L 1210 were seen (JAFFE and PRUSOFF, 1960). Other investigators have observed, however, that IdUrd can potentiate the activity of 5-fluorodeoxyuridine in mice or rats bearing various neoplasms (BURCHENAL et al., 1960; HEIDELBERGER et al., 1960). Similarly, in mice bearing the neoplasm P815, the effects of combinations of IdUrd and 2-chloro-terephthalanilide-4′,4′-*bis* (imidazolin-2-yl), as well as of the latter with 5-iodouridine, 5-bromouridine, or 5-bromodeoxyuridine, were more than additive (BURCHENAL et al., 1962). The results obtained by JAFFE and PRUSOFF (1960) were not significantly different whether the drug was administered daily in a single dose or in divided parenteral doses; oral administration of IdUrd in amounts equivalent to those administered parenterally was much less effective. In no instance was a "cure" obtained, but marked inhibition of tumor growth was observed. Tumor viability was retained even under conditions that resulted in over 95% inhibition of tumor growth, accompanied by marked host toxicity. GOLDIN et al. (1961) evaluated several antileukemic agents in advanced leukemia L1210 in mice and found that IdUrd is only 20 % as effective as methotrexate.

Thus, on the basis of experiments in mice, eradication or "cure" of a neoplasm does not appear feasible by the administration of IdUrd alone. In this respect, however, it is pertinent to cite the following two encouraging experiments. BOOTH and SARTORELLI (1963) have observed that IdUrd in combination with uracil mustard [5-*bis*-2-(chloroethyl)aminouracil] resulted in a potentiation of the antitumor activity in mice bearing the transplanted neoplasm, Sarcoma 180. This combination of an alkylating agent with IdUrd is in contrast to the additive effects seen when IdUrd was combined with known antimetabolites (JAFFE and PRUSOFF, 1960). The desirability of extending these studies to man is obvious. Other encouraging experiments are those of BERRY and ANDREWS (1962a, b), who demonstrated a marked potentiating effect on the growth of the ascitic P-388 lymphocytic leukemia in mice by combinations of IdUrd and x-irradiation, as compared with either type of therapy alone. The capacity of halogenated uracil derivatives to reduce the threshold of cells to the damaging effects of radiation had been described previously for bacteria by GREER (1960) and GREER and ZAMENHOF (1957) and for mammalian cells in culture by DJORDJEVIC and SZYBALSKI (1960) and CRAMER et al. (1963).

Biochemical studies with mammalian cells, either *in vitro* or *in vivo*, have also been performed that show that IdUrd inhibits competitively the utilization of radioactive thymidine for the biosynthesis of DNA-thymine, and under these conditions is utilized in lieu of thymidine for the formation of the DNA polymer. The appearance of radioactivity in the thymidylate of the DNA of Ehrlich ascites tumor cells *in vitro* from such precursors as radioactive orotic acid, formate, or thymidine is inhibited by IdUrd, but, as might be expected, the utilization of orotic acid for the biosynthesis of DNA-cytosine or of RNA-pyrimidines is not affected (PRUSOFF, 1960). Thus, both the exogenous and the *de novo* pathways concerned with the formation of phosphorylated derivatives of thymidine were affected by IdUrd or its derivatives. Studies by DELAMORE and PRUSOFF (1962) of the specific enzymic reaction affected by IdUrd in various normal and neoplastic murine tissues revealed that the decreased incorporation, in the presence of IdUrd, of ^{14}C-formate or of ^{3}H-thymidine into DNA-thymine is a reflection of an inhibition of the utilization of thymidine, thymidylic acid, or thymidine triphosphate, presumably by IdUrd acting in the form of the corresponding phosphorylated derivative of IdUrd. The specific metabolic site primarily affected in the various tissues studied is a characteristic of the individual tissue; thus, DNA polymerase was preferentially inhibited in the Ehrlich ascites carcinoma and in human chronic granulocytic and acute monocytic leukemia, whereas studies with L5178Y leukemia cells, with ^{3}H-thymidine and ^{14}C-formate, indicated a primary inhibition of thymidine kinase and thymidylic acid kinase, respectively. At concentrations of IdUrd that exerted no inhibition of the formation of thymidylate from ^{14}C-formate by Ehrlich ascites cells, a significant degree of inhibition was observed in L5178Y leukemia cells; the former finding is in agreement with that of HARTMAN and HEIDELBERGER (1961) with Ehrlich ascites cells, in which IdUrd, under conditions in which IdUMP would be formed, caused no inhibition of thymidylate synthetase. Studies by BAKHLE and PRUSOFF (1969) with cell-free extracts of these cells disclosed no such differences and a possible explanation for the divergence in the results obtained from cell-free and whole cell experiments was presented.

Biochemical studies with BrdUrd showed similar results. Thus, BrdUrd inhibits the incorporation of labeled formaldehyde (KIT et al., 1958), formate, orotic acid and thymidine (HAKALA, 1958) into DNA-thymine of mammalian tissues *in vitro* and of labeled formaldehyde into DNA-thymine of spleen and tumor tissues *in vivo* (KIT et al., 1958).

C. Inhibition of Viral Replication

Several communications have cited the antiviral activity of BrdUrd and IdUrd. Most of them have indicated that these analogs are most efficacious when present at the initiation of infection, with delay in exposure to analog resulting in less inhibition and finally no inhibition. It was originally observed by THOMPSON et al. (1949) that bromouracil significantly inhibited vaccinia replication. Inhibition of polyoma virus production by BrdUrd was observed by SMITH et al. (1960).

HERRMANN (1961) observed that both IdUrd and BrdUrd inhibited the replication of several DNA containing viruses in cell culture, particularly vaccinia and herpes simplex. Since then, there have been numerous reports concerned with the inhibitory effect of these analogs on a variety of viruses as indicated below:

(1) Herpes simplex virus: KAUFMAN (1962); KAUFMAN et al. (1962a, b); PERKINS et al. (1962); CRAMER et al. (1963); KAUFMAN and MALONEY (1963); ROIZMAN et al. (1963); SMITH (1963b); DUBBS and KIT (1964b); RAPP (1964); SIMINOFF (1964); SMITH and DUKES (1964); NEMES and HILLMAN (1965), PRUSOFF et al. (1965); SCHNEWEISS (1965a, b); KUCERA and HERRMANN (1966); SHEN et al. (1966); SIMINOFF and MENEFEE (1966); HERRMANN (1968); SCHIEK and SCHIEK (1969); PERSON et al. (1970); RENIS (1970).

(2) Pseudorabies virus: KAPLAN et al. (1965); KAPLAN and BEN-PORAT (1967); GREIG and BIRARD (1969); RENIS (1970).

(3) H-1 (hamster osteolytic virus): LEDINKO (1967).

(4) Equine herpes 3: KARPAS (1967).

(5) Malignant catarrhal fever virus (a group B herpes): PLOWRIGHT et al. (1963).

(6) Varicella Zoster virus: RAPP and VANDERSLICE (1964); RAWLS et al. (1964).

(7) Herpes virus simiae (B virus): MILLER (1967).

(8) Cytomegalovirus virus (a herpes virus): HENSEN et al. (1966); SIDWELL et al. (1970).

(9) Vaccinia virus: THOMPSON et al. (1949); HERRMANN (1961); SIMON (1961); KIT and DUBBS (1962a, b); CALABRESI et al. (1963a); PRUSOFF et al. (1963); EASTERBROOK and DAVERN (1963); KAUFMANN (1963); SHEN et al. (1966); LODDO et al. (1963b); SCHNEWEISS (1965b); KUCERA and HERRMANN (1966); RADA and BLASKOVIC (1966); HERMANN (1968); NEUFAHRT et al. (1969); RENIS (1970).

(10) Polyoma virus: SMITH et al. (1960); MUNYON et al. (1964); BOWEN et al. (1964); MORI and KIMURA (1965); WEIL et al. (1965); BOWEN et al. (1966); HIRT (1966); KIMURA and MORI (1966).

(11) SV40 virus: HAAS and MAASS (1964); TODARO and GREEN (1964); ASHKENAZI (1965); MAAS et al. (1965); MELNICK and RAPP (1965); RAPP et al. (1965a, b).

(12) SV15 virus: OMELCHENKOV et al. (1969).

(13) Adenovirus: KJELLEN (1962); SCHNEWEISS (1965b); KEJLLEN et al. (1963); MUNTONI and LODDO (1963); FURUSAWA et al. (1964); SHEN et al. (1966).

(14) Aujeszky virus: RUSSEFF et al. (1969).

(15) Bovine Rhinotracheitis virus: PERSECHINO and ORFEI (1965); LILLIE and MOHANTY (1968).

(16) African Swine virus: MOULTON and COGGINS (1968).

(17) Porcine Picodna virus: MAYR et al. (1968).

(18) Visna virus: THOMAS (1965).

(19) Columbia SK virus: FORCE and STEWART (1964b).
(20) Encephalomyocarditis virus: FEELY (1965).
(21) Rabbit pox virus: APPLEYARD and WESTWOOD (1964).

In a series of papers cited elsewhere in this chapter PRUSOFF and his associates have examined the effect of IdUrd and its phosphorylated derivatives on various pertinent enzymes in infected and noninfected cells. Although IdUrd and its derivatives interacted with the various enzymes studied, no differential effect was found which could account for the magnitude of the antiviral activity of the compound. Attention, therefore, has been directed toward the role of IdUrd (or BrdUrd) substituted viral DNA to antiviral activity (DUNN and SMITH, 1954, 1957; PRUSOFF et al., 1963; EASTERBROOK and DAVERN, 1963; KAPLAN and BEN-PORAT, 1964). Also reinforcing the logic of this approach is the finding that mutants of vaccinia (DUBBS and KIT, 1964a) and herpes simplex virus (DUBBS and KIT, 1964b), which are resistant to BrdUrd, also lack the ability to induce thymidine kinase activity which is necessary for analog incorporation into DNA. LODO et al. (1963a) and FERRARI et al. (1965) also isolated an IdUrd-resistant vaccinia virus, but did not verify that it lacked thymidine kinase.

Studies by SMITH (1963) and SMITH and DUKES (1964) support the view that IdUrd does not prevent adsorption of herpes virus to cells. SCHNEWEISS (1965b) observed that noninfectious herpes virus formed in the presence of BrdUrd lost its capacity to be adsorbed by the host cell. The virus particles formed in the presence of IdUrd which are noninfectious appear ragged and often empty, as shown for vaccinia virus (PRUSOFF et al., 1963), herpes zoster virus (RAPP and VANDERSLICE, 1964), herpes simplex virus (SMITH and DIKES, 1964), and SV40 virus (RAPP et al., 1965b).

SCHIEK and SCHIEK (1969) observed that herpes virus hominis grown in HeLa cells in the presence of BrdUrd had an increased buoyant density and a faster sedimentation velocity in a CsCl density gradient. The marked decrease in infectivity of the virus is presumed to be due to the formation of faulty coat proteins. WATSON et al. (1964) showed that IdUrd permits the partial assembly of the virion.

KJELLEN et al. (1963) found that structural adenovirus proteins are synthesized in the presence of BrdUrd even though the virions formed are noninfectious. SIMINOFF and MENEFEE (1966) examined with the electron microscope normal and BrdUrd-inhibited herpes infected cells at various stages of viral growth and noted that BrdUrd prevents virus maturation at the step involved in the formation of immature (i.e., naked) virus particles. Viral antigen is made and may be specified by the parental genome. Thus, BrdUrd allows the formation of at least certain viral structural units, but prevents their assembly.

ROIZMAN et al. (1963) studied extensively the effect of IdUrd on the reproduction of herpes simplex virus, and found that this analog had no inhibitory effect during the first two hours after infection. Three to four hours after infection, multiplication of the virus was inhibited, and after four hours the inhibition could not be reversed. These investigators (ROIZMAN et al., 1963) observed that the simultaneous addition of a 17 or 83 molar excess of thymidine reversed the inhibition by IdUrd to approximately 20 and 55 %, respectively, of the noninhibited control. ROIZMAN et al. (1963) did not find incorporation of ^{3}H-IdUrd into the DNA of herpes simplex virus; however, based on an uncertain plating efficiency of their virus, they placed an upper limit of DNA-thymine replacement of not more than 1.5 or 15 %. CRAMER et al. (1963) also apparently did not find incorporation of ^{14}C-IdUrd into herpes simplex when the analog was given in a subinhibitory concentration six hours after infection. KAPLAN et al. (1965) and KAPLAN and BEN-PORAT (1967), however, have reported that IdUrd and BrdUrd are incorporated into the DNA of pseudorabies virus, a member of the herpes group. Studies with vaccinia virus have demonstrated an incorporation of IdUrd (PRUSOFF et al., 1963) or BrdUrd (EASTERBROOK and DAVERN, 1963) into the viral DNA. EASTERBROOK and DAVERN (1963) have shown that vaccinia virus had a 140-fold decrease in infectivity when grown under conditions that resulted in 13 % replacement of DNA-thymine by bromouracil.

Although these analogs inhibit the formation of infectious virus, the synthesis of specific viral antigen is not prevented (EASTERBROOK and DAVERN, 1963; SIMINOFF, 1964; MAAS et al., 1965; RAPP et al., 1965a, b; SCHNEWEISS, 1965a, b; SIMINOFF and MENEFEE, 1966; KARPAS, 1967); however, MAASS and HAAS (1966) investigated the effect of IdUrd on the formation of virus specific SV40 antigen and found a marked decrease when the virus replicates in the presence of 280 μM IdUrd. Haemagglutinin synthesis by SV15 virus (OMELCHENKOV et al., 1969) and H-1 virus (LEDENKO, 1967) was markedly inhibited by FdUrd (OMELCHENKOV et al., 1969) and by cytosine arabinoside (LEDINKO, 1967), but not by IdUrd.

BrdUrd and IdUrd, although inhibiting the formation of infectious virus, do not prevent the cytopathic effect exerted on infected cells (SMITH, 1963; MUNYON et al., 1964; RAPP and VANDERSLICE, 1964; SMITH and DUKES, 1964; SCHNEWEISS, 1965b; HENSEN et al., 1966). RAPP and VANDERSLICE (1964) reported that the spread of zoster virus from cell to cell was inhibited by IdUrd; however, in agreement with the studies of SMITH (1963) and SMITH and DUKES (1964) with herpes virus, IdUrd, although preventing replication, did not inactivate intracellular infectious virus nor prevent or reverse cytopathic changes caused by the virus. Thus, although spread of the virus was prevented by IdUrd some distribution of zoster antigens to neighboring cells occurred either by direct transfer of protein or of viral DNA capable of forming viral specific proteins but not infectious virions.

EASTERBROOK and DAVERN (1963) did a comprehensive study of the effect of BrdUrd on vaccinia virus multiplication. With their virus-cell system 2 μM BrdUrd was sufficient to completely inhibit infectious virus production. In the presence of BrdUrd, vaccinia DNA with a mean bromouracil substitution of DNA-thymine of 13 % was formed, and on the basis of buoyant density gradient profiles the authors proposed that the substituted DNA was smaller in molecular weight than unsubstituted DNA and heterogeneous in density. The former proposal is in agreement with a later finding of MCCREA and LIPMAN (1967) that IdUrd-substituted vaccinia virus DNA is also more fragile and hence in small molecular weight pieces. EASTERBROOK and DAVERN (1963) also reported that in cells exposed to BrdUrd there are large numbers of abnormal viral particles that are noninfectious and which cannot be reactivated. JOKLIK (1964) also investigated the effect of BrdUrd on vaccinia virus and found that when infection was carried out with virus in which 13 % of the thymidine of the DNA was replaced by BrdUrd, the DNA appeared to be prematurely broken down as soon as it was uncoated in the vesicles within which the virus particles were taken up into the cells.

SMITH (1963) and SMITH and DUKES (1964) performed studies similar to those of EASTERBROOK and DAVERN (1963) but with IdUrd and herpes simplex infected cells. As with BrdUrd-treated infected cells, abnormal particles were formed. These workers interpreted their results to indicate that assembly of viral components rather than their production was inhibited by IdUrd.

KAPLAN and coworkers (KAMIYA et al., 1965; KAPLAN et al., 1965; KAPLAN and BEN-PORAT, 1966) examined the mechanism of the antiviral activity of BrdUrd and IdUrd in the pseudorabies virus-rabbit kidney cell system. Neither BrdUrd nor IdUrd inhibited the synthesis of viral DNA or viral antigens. To the contrary, both DNA and antigen synthesis were greater in drug-treated infected cells, and such synthesis continued beyond the time when in untreated infected cells there was no further synthesis of DNA and antigen. When the infected cells were tested for the formation of DNase insensitive DNA (assumed to indicate at least coated DNA if not fully assembled mature virions) in the presence or absence of drug, the BrdUrd-treated cells yielded levels of DNase insensitive DNA similar to control, whereas IdUrd-treated cells failed to form significant amounts of DNase insensitive DNA. Since in both BrdUrd- and IdUrd-treated infected cells, the yield of infectious virus formed is greatly reduced, it follows that BrdUrd treatment results in formation of noninfectious virus particles, which is in accord with the results of EASTERBROOK and DAVERN (1963) with vaccinia virus, and that IdUrd treatment results in a failure to form significant amounts of either normal or abnormal appearing viral particles. This result with IdUrd is in contradistinction to the results of SMITH (1963), SMITH and DUKES (1964), and PRUSOFF et al. (1963) with vaccinia virus, where significant although abnormal appearing viral particles were found when IdUrd was used. This probably reflects a difference in the properties of the two viruses, although in the vaccinia experiments DNase insensitive DNA was not measured. KAPLAN et al. (1965) and KAPLAN and BEN-PORAT (1966), however, could obtain DNase insensitive, IdUrd substituted DNA if after a 7-hour incubation IdUrd containing medium was replaced with thymidine containing medium or if after 4-hours incubation in thymidine containing medium IdUrd containing medium was substituted. With the latter protocol the virus titer was 9 % of control as compared to 0.37 % of control when IdUrd was present throughout infection. KAPLAN and BEN-PORAT (1966) found that the infectivity of the virus formed when IdUrd was added 4 h postinfection was as sensitive to γ-ray inactivation as the virus formed when IdUrd was present throughout infection, and both preparations were about twice as sensitive as normal virus. From this they concluded that the virus formed under the former conditions contained IdUrd-DNA and that, therefore, such virus can initiate infection and yield normal DNA. Although not explicitly stated, such substituted virus should also yield normal progeny.

A somewhat different approach to the mechanism of the antiviral activity of IdUrd was undertaken by GOZ and PRUSOFF (1968, 1970a). These investigators studied the effect of IdUrd on phage T_4 and took advantage of the great knowledge of T_4 replication processes and the fact that this virus could be grown in large chemically measureable quantities. In their first study, GOZ and PRUSOFF (1968) found that a normal yield of viral particles was obtained when cells were infected in the presence of IdUrd. These viruses appeared morphologically normal (GOZ et al., unpublished observations) and, contrary to the findings of LITMAN and PARDEE (1960), were capable of killing host bacteria upon reinfection. This discrepancy may be due to a difference in experimental conditions. LITMAN and PARDEE (1960a, b) employed a medium with sulfanilamide to promote analog incorporation, whereas GOZ and PRUSOFF (1968, 1970a) made use of thymine requiring mutants of *E. coli* and T_4, obviating the need for addition of a second drug which may produce unobserved effects of its own. In addition, the IdUrd substituted T_4 were inactivated by antiserum prepared to normal phage, thus indicating normal tail protein in substituted phage (GOZ and PRUSOFF, 1970a). In the 1968 study, it was found that infection with IdUrd substituted T_4 resulted in induction of markedly decreased levels of viral enzymes such as deoxycytidylate hydroxymethylase, dihydrofolate reductase, and lysozyme. A companion study by AAMODT and GOZ (1970) with antibody made against purified deoxycytidylate hydroxymethylase of T_4 indicated that the reduced levels of activity of this enzyme after infection by IdUrd substituted virus was apparently due to reduced synthesis of enzyme molecules rather than to a normal rate of synthesis of enzyme molecules which were inactive.

GOZ and PRUSOFF (1970a) extended their study of the range of viral products synthesized by IdUrd substituted virus with the use of T_4 amber mutants in genotypic and phenotypic rescue experiments. By this method also, IdUrd substituted T_4 appeared to induce reduced quantities of various proteins including enzymes, structural proteins, and products related to virus maturation or morphogenesis. Moreover, different gene products were affected to different extents and for several gene products a direct relationship between the degree of IdUrd substitution and decrease in viral protein was demonstrated. Thus, in contrast to the general findings with animal viruses, the antiviral activity of IdUrd was manifested upon reinfection of substituted virus and at that time all viral synthesis was affected, albeit to different extents relative to the protein made.

The question of specificity of antiviral action of IdUrd has been raised by SMITH (1963), DEINHARDT (1965), HANNA and WILKENSON (1965), and KAUFMAN (1965). The problem of whether IdUrd is a specific antiviral agent or exerts its effect by producing cell toxicity was investigated by CRAMER et al. (1963). They found inhibition of herpes simplex virus at a concentration of 0.1 of that required to inhibit cell reproduction. Similarly RADA and BLASKOVIC (1966) observed that a 2.8 μM concentration of IdUrd, which produced 95 % inhibition of vaccinia virus, had no effect when noninfected HeLa cells were exposed to this concentration for 24 h. However, a 10-fold increase in IdUrd concentration exerted about 10 % cell damage. Furthermore, MUNYON et al. (1964) found that in mouse embryo cells that had been exposed to 28 μM IdUrd for as long as 69 h before infection with polyoma virus, and then transferred to a medium free of drug, infectious virus was formed in normal or even greater than normal amounts. This concentration of IdUrd inhibited irreversibly the replication of the mouse embryo cells and resulted in enlarged cells which permitted the formation of increased amounts of virus. DUNNEBACKE and REAUME (1958) had observed that the yield of polio virus particles is directly related to the size of cells.

SIMON (1961) reported that HeLa cells pretreated with BrdUrd for 5 days supported vaccinia virus replication; however, when BrdUrd was present at the time of infection there was a marked inhibition of viral replication. Similar experiments with IdUrd have been performed with pseudorabies virus (KAPLAN and BEN-PORAT, 1967), and SV40 virus (HAAS and MAASS, 1964).

Another approach to support specificity of action of IdUrd or BrdUrd was the demonstration that concentrations of these analogs which inhibit replication of DNA viruses had no effect on the replication of RNA viruses, such as Bittner virus (LYONS et al., 1966), H-1 virus (LEDINKO, 1967), and influenza virus (BADER, 1965).

Additional support for specificity of the antiviral action of BrdUrd was provided by BADER (1964) who found that cells pretreated with BrdUrd for 3 or 4 days would support the replication of the virus as satisfactorily as did untreated cells if Rous sarcoma virus was added after removal of the analog.

LEONTIEVA and FADUVA (1969) made the interesting observation that low concentrations of BrdUrd enhanced the reproduction of Gheta and O'Nyong-Nyong virus in cell culture.

The method of assay may be important with regard to the effect these analogs have on viral replication. KUCERA and HERRMANN (1966) applied the gradient plate technique to the study of the effect of various antiviral substances, and, in general, agreement was found with results obtained by the disc plate method. Vaccinia virus was found to be more susceptible to inhibition by BrdUrd than was herpes simplex virus. Thymidine, as expected, prevented the inhibitory effect of

IdUrd. The authors submit this procedure as another useful technique for bioassay of IdUrd and other agents, as well as for the detection and isolation of IdUrd resistant strains of virus.

HERRMANN (1968) studied, by the plaque suppression test, the effect of various halogenated deoxyribonucleosides on the replication of herpes simplex virus, vaccinia virus, and adenovirus types 1,2,5, and 7. The various strains of adenovirus were not inhibited by concentrations of BrdUrd and IdUrd that were inhibitory to vaccinia and herpes simplex virus. IdUrd and BrdUrd had been reported previously to inhibit adenovirus type 5 (MUNTONI and LODDO, 1963; KJELLEN, 1962) and adenovirus type 12 (FURUSAWA et al., 1964).

PERSON et al. (1970) found herpes simplex virus I, responsible for cutaneous and oral herpes infection, to be more sensitive than herpes virus II, responsible for genital herpes infection. Differences in sensitivity to IdUrd and adenine arabinoside varied depending on the cell culture system used, as well as on the prior passage history of the virus. Thus, with chick embryo fibroblasts, herpes virus I was more sensitive than herpes virus II to inhibition, whereas with HeLa cells, depending on the strain, either a slight or no difference was observed.

IdUrd and other halogenated deoxyuridine derivatives have been used to determine whether a virus contains RNA or DNA (SALZMAN, 1960; HAMPARIAN et al., 1963). Although this approach has been used by many investigators there is a hazard in identifying a virus as containing DNA by virtue of its being inhibited by IdUrd or BrdUrd, since it has clearly been established that RNA oncogenic virus are dependent on DNA biosynthesis. That DNA may be required for RNA viruses replication has been reported by TEMIN (1963, 1964) for Rous sarcoma virus, by BERRY et al. (1962) for influenza virus, and by THOMAS (1965) for visna virus.

D. Effect on Oncogenic Viruses

BrdUrd and IdUrd have a number of interesting interactions with oncogenic viruses. First, the formation of infectious progeny of several oncogenic viruses is inhibited by these drugs. BrdUrd inhibits infectious virus formation of polyoma (SMITH et al., 1960), SV40 (DIDERHOLM, 1963), and adenovirus types 3 (SCHNEWEIS, 1965b) and 5 (KJELLEN, 1962; KJELLEN et al., 1963). IdUrd likewise inhibits polyoma (BOWEN et al., 1962; MUNYON et al., 1964; MORI and KUMURA, 1965), SV40 (HAAS and MAASS, 1964; MELNICK and RAPP, 1965; RAPP and MELNICK, 1965) and SV15 adenovirus (OMELCHENKO et al., 1969). Polyoma virus will replicate in the presence of 141 μM IdUrd if IdUrd-resistant mouse cells are used (KIMURU and MORI, 1966). Replication of Rous sarcoma virus, an RNA virus, is also inhibited by BrdUrd when added within 12 h post infection (BADER, 1964; LEVINSON et al., 1970) and by IdUrd (FORCE and STEWART, 1964a; BADER, 1965). In addition, BrdUrd inhibits visna virus replication which also contains RNA (THOMAS, 1965). IdUrd, however, does not prevent induction of deoxycytidylate deaminase or uridine kinase by Rous sarcoma virus (KARA, 1968). These latter experiments were executed to demonstrate the requirement for DNA synthesis in replication of the RNA Rous sarcoma virus and are in agreement with the now generally accepted hypothesis of a DNA provirus intermediate conceived and reviewed recently by TEMIN (1971).

BrdUrd, as reviewed in another section, is incorporated into mammalian DNA. WEIL et al. (1965) have also shown that BrdUrd may be incorporated into the cellular DNA that is formed when synthesis is stimulated by polyoma infection.

IdUrd, although preventing formation of infectious SV40 progeny, does not block formation of viral or tumor antigens (MELNICK and RAPP, 1965; RAPP et al.,

1965a). BrdUrd, similarly, does not prevent polyoma hemagglutinin (capsid proteins) synthesis or cytopathic effects, although no infectious virus is formed. However, BrdUrd plus FdUrd will block polyoma-induced cytopathic effects (WEIL et al., 1965), so that the type of inhibition may depend upon the relative incorporation of the analog into DNA. It is also possible that the block of cytopathic development is attributable directly to FdUrd. HIRT (1966) reports that BrdUrd and FdUrd, under conditions yielding fully substituted DNA, results in 1 % infectivity and 10 % hemagglutination titer relative to normal.

Studies of tumor induction in whole animals indicate that IdUrd will suppress the development of adenovirus 12 induced tumors (HUEBNER et al., 1963), as well as polyoma virus induced tumors in newborn hamsters (FISCHER et al., 1965). Suppression of tumor formation occurred even if the IdUrd was injected at a site distant from the point of viral inoculation. COGGIN et al. (1967), however, reported that "inoculation of 1 ml solution containing 100 mg of IdUrd into newborn hamsters infected with SV40 virus" did not prevent neoplastic development.

TODARO and GREEN (1964) made the observation that BrdUrd and IdUrd can markedly (up to nine-fold) increase the frequency of 3T3 cell transformation by SV40. Such enhancement occurs even if the cells are exposed to the drugs only prior to addition of virus. The authors imply that the analogs may be increasing transformation by SV40 by causing some sort of chromosomal aberrations (reviewed in another section). ASHKENAZI (1965) made similar observations.

A very interesting effect of BrdUrd and IdUrd recently has been published. LOWY et al. (1971) found that exposure of growing cultures of cells from embryos of the high leukemic mouse strain AKR to BrdUrd (66 to 326 μM) or IdUrd (56 to 282 μM) for 24 to 48 h induced synthesis of murine leukemia virus in as many as 0.5% of the cells. These cells prior to treatment had shown no evidence of viral particles, antigens, or RNA-directed DNA polymerase. In a similar fashion BrdUrd induced C-type virus in clonal lines of virus-free BALB/3T3, BALB/3T12-1, and BALB/3T12-4 cells (AARONSON et al., 1971). Under similar conditions, BrdUrd rescues mouse sarcoma virus from rat cells transformed by this virus (KLEMENT et al., 1971). As might be anticipated, studies have also begun to appear at this writing reporting activation of latent viruses in human tumors. This has been seen with particles resembling C-type virus (STEWART et al., 1972a, b) and also with Epstein-Barr virus, a DNA virus (HAMPAR et al., 1972; GERBER, 1972). No evidence is available as to how BrdUrd or IdUrd can activate RNA or DNA tumor viruses in virus negative cells.

E. Effects on Transformation, Conjugation and Transduction

It might be expected that incorporation of 5-bromo or 5-iodouracil into transforming DNA would exert a significant effect. This appears not to be the case. In an early report, EPHRATI-ELIZUR and ZAMENHOF (1959) did find a reduction in three of four genetic markers monitored in bromouracil substituted transforming DNA of *B. subtilis*. However, the following year SZYBALSKI et al. (1960) stated that in the same transforming system BrdUrd substitution of one or both strands of the DNA did not alter significantly the transforming activity of all of the markers tested. LITMAN and SZYBALSKI (1963) in a later paper observed that DNA synthesized *in vitro* from a BrdUrd labeled primer functioned normally in transformation. GIMLIN et al. (1963, 1966) also found that bromouracil substituted transforming DNA of *B. subtilis* was only slightly decreased in effectiveness relative to the indole marker, but further observed that there was a decrease in the number of viable cells grown on control medium after treatment with bromouracil-substituted transforming DNA. Unsubstituted transforming DNA also produced this latter effect, but to a significantly lesser extent. No explanation of this action is as yet known.

In retrospect, the failure of bromouracil substituted DNA to differ in transforming capability from unsubstituted DNA may not be surprising. The experimental design of the reported studies was such that one marker at a time was monitored and a small decrease would hardly be detected. It is suggested that changes induced by substitution with bromouracil would be of a mutagenic nature and thus occur at the relatively low frequency associated with mutagenic alterations, rather than in the more pronounced fashion associated with, for example, the proposed inhibition of the initiation of mRNA synthesis. A system geared to observe smaller changes might show a significant difference between normal and substituted transforming DNA, for example, transformation of indole$^-$ cells using normal and substituted DNA also from indole$^-$ cells, and in this case looking for increased reversion in the bromouracil substituted indole$^-$ transforming DNA to the indole$^+$ state.

BrdUrd and IdUrd appear to have an effect on conjugation and recombination in *E. coli* K12. FOLSOME (1960) observed that BrdUrd reduced both the transfer and integration of DNA when the males contained the substituted DNA. COOPER et al. (1971) obtained similar results with IdUrd. Although incorporation of IdUrd into the DNA of the female strains decreased viability, there was little effect on their ability to receive DNA and carry out recombination after conjugation. In contrast, and as with BrdUrd substitution of male DNA, IdUrd interfered with both transfer and genetic linkage. The authors speculate that these effects are attributable to an IdUrd-induced instability of the male chromosome.

WILKINS (1968) has examined the effect of bromouracil containing DNA on recombination in *Salmonella typhimurium* via transduction with phage PLT-22. The thymine of the DNA was 70% substituted by bromouracil. In this instance, substitution of donor DNA had no effect on genetic linkage. Bromouracil substitution of the recipient DNA had a slight effect. The frequency of transductants was 40% reduced and the linkage of cotransduced markers decreased about 5%.

It appears, therefore, from the above, that the only bacterial genetic system in which recombination is affected is conjugation in *E. coli* K-12 when the donor DNA is substituted by bromouracil or iodouracil.

F. Inhibition of Antibody Production

Another specialized cell function that is inhibited by BrdUrd and IdUrd is antibody production. BIEBER et al. (1962) found that 4 successive intraperitoneal doses of 7.5 mg/kg of BrdUrd significantly suppressed the immune response in mice. FISCHER et al. (1966) failed to find immunosuppression in mice with up to 300 mg/kg/day of IdUrd, and BrdUrd was only slightly effective at a dosage of 100 mg/kg/day. GULATI and PATEL (1971) reported that injecting guinea pigs with bromouracil (50 mg/kg intraperitoneally) daily for 5 days starting 15 days after the third monthly injection of insulin antigen reduced the serum antibody titer for insulin measured after the drug treatment. These are perhaps exceptional findings, for as GABRIELSEN and GOOD (1967) state, neither BrdUrd nor IdUrd are effective immunosuppressive agents *in vivo*. There are, however, examples in which BrdUrd or IdUrd were efficacious as immunosuppressants when *in vitro* systems were employed. DUTTON et al. (1960) first reported this effect in detail. In their study rabbits were first immunized *in vivo* with ovalbumin. The spleen was then removed and cultured *in vitro*, at which time antibody was measured and

BrdUrd tested. In these cells antibody was produced for about 48 h. BrdUrd (20 μM) caused a marked inhibition of synthesis, although increasing the concentration of BrdUrd to 2.5 mM did not appreciably inhibit further antibody production. Thymidine partially prevents this effect of BrdUrd, implying that BrdUrd is acting through incorporation into DNA or on DNA synthesis. Indeed DNA synthesis was inhibited by this agent by about 30%, while there was no effect on RNA synthesis or on incorporation of amino acids into protein. DUTTON and PEARCE (1962) enlarged upon these findings and also reported that IdUrd was active in this regard, although slightly less effective.

O'BRIEN (1961, 1963) also found BrdUrd to be immunosuppressive *in vitro* when tested in a system of cultured fragments of popliteal lymph nodes excised from rabbits immunized with bovine serum albumin and diphtheria toxoid. Administration of BrdUrd (6 μg/ml) during the second to fourth day of culturing, a time associated with cell division, caused a substantial reduction in antibody titer.

G. Effects on Embryonic Development and Differentiation

A considerable body of literature has accrued on the effects of BrdUrd and IdUrd on embryonic development and cellular differentiation. As these effects for the most part have been prevented by coadministration of thymidine and correlated with analog incorporation in DNA, they will be discussed in this section.

Early experiments demonstrated that IdUrd or BrdUrd had a teratogenic and lethal effect on developing embryos. The teratogenic effect is well documented. BrdUrd is teratogenic in rats where a dose of 800 mg/kg intraperitoneally on the 12th day of pregnancy produces abnormalities (MURPHY, 1965), in pregnant hamsters where 400 mg/kg iv on the seventh and eighth days caused malformations (RUFFOLO and FERM, 1965), and in mice by either small daily doses of 60 to 124 mg/kg intraperitoneally throughout gestation (DI PAOLO, 1964) or by single doses intraperitoneally of 300 to 500 mg/kg during days 7 to 11 (SKALKO et al., 1971). 5-Chloro-2′-deoxyuridine is teratogenic in rats (125 to 1000 mg/kg on the twelvth day of pregnancy) and the effect is completely prevented by coadministration of thymidine (CHAUBE and MURPHY, 1964).

KARNOFSKY and BASCH (1960) first reported that BrdUrd (0.33 μM) will cause embryonic death beginning at the blastula stage of the sand dollar embryo. Coadministration of thymine or thymidine will protect against the lethal effect of BrdUrd, but not entirely. The block of development through the cleavage stage and early blastula stage by FdUrd was prevented by BrdUrd. NEMER (1962) reported similar results for IdUrd and the *Paracentrotus lividus* embryo. IdUrd blocked development at the blastula stage and reversed the inhibition of development by FdUrd, allowing division to the blastula stage. Labeled IdUrd was incorporated into total acid-precipitable material and this incoporation was reduced to about one-third by an equimolar concentration of thymidine. WHEELER et al. (1963) also report incorporation of labeled IdUrd into the embryo of *Arbacia punctalata* and the prevention of this incorporation by thymidine. ZAMENHOF et al. (1971) have reported that BrdUrd injected into the albumin of developing chick eggs decreased hatchability, body and brain weight, and brain DNA (equated to cell number) when measured at hatching. The effect was demonstrable with small doses at 3 days, but increased dosage was required at later times in development until at the 12th and 16th day even a 100-fold increment over the 3-day dose produced no effect on the parameters measured. Examination of the chromosomes in early cleavage mitosis of the sand dollar and sea urchin embryos (MAZIA and GONTCHAROFF, 1964; GONTCHAROFF and MAZIA, 1967) revealed that incorporation of bromouracil into DNA caused difficulty in anaphase separation of chromosomes. In the sand dollar this resulted in prevention of further development, but in the sea urchin the chromosomes did separate allowing early development to continue to the blastula stage. For this type of effect on chromosomes in the sea urchin embryo relatively large concentrations of BrdUrd were used (33 to 652 μM), although in the sand dollar *Dendraster excentricus* 1 μM BrdUrd added shortly after fertilization resulted in an abnormal cleavage pattern.

It is perhaps not surprising that usually no observable effect of BrdUrd or IdUrd occurs until late blastula or gastrula stage. In the sea urchin, *Arbacia*, actinomycin D does not interfere with protein synthesis to the blastula stage, and enucleated eggs can carry on protein synthesis (reviewed by GROSS, 1967). Thus, if the halogenated uracils produce lethality after incorporation into DNA by introducing lethal errors into proteins via the transcriptional-translational processes, such effect would not occur in a system apparently independent of DNA-directed RNA synthesis. However, at gastrulation newly synthesized RNA may be important and the effect of bromouracil or iodouracil in DNA is observed.

Investigators have also reported effects of BrdUrd (IdUrd has similar activity but has not been investigated as thoroughly) on differentiation and specific functions of cells in culture. Such data were first reported by STOCKDALE et al. (1964) and OKAZAKI and HOLTZER (1965) who observed that presumptive chick embryo myoblasts in culture with low levels of BrdUrd continue to grow and replicate, but do not fuse to form characteristic multinucleated myotubes. In addition, striated myofibrils did not appear and the synthesis of myosin and tropomyosin was not detected. These results have since been elaborated on for myogenesis [COLEMAN et al., 1969; BISCHOFF and HOLTZER, 1970 (IdUrd and CldUrd have similar activity), COLEMAN et al., 1970; SANGER and HOLTZER, 1970].

Similar effects with BrdUrd have been found in other systems. Thus, BrdUrd prevents matrix accumulation around chick embryo chondrocytes in culture (ABBOT and HOLTZER, 1968; LASHER and CAHN, 1969; HOLTHAUSEN et al., 1969; CHACKO et al., 1969). In most of these studies, the synthesis of chondrocyte specific molecules such as chondroitin sulfate was also impeded by BrdUrd. Chick embryo amnion cells exposed to BrdUrd failed in the synthesis of mucopolysaccharides (BISCHOFF and HOLTZER, 1968; MAYNER et al., 1971). The study of ANDERSON et al. (1970) is a fine structure analysis of chick embryo chondrocytes cultured in the presence of BrdUrd. The cells which lost their polygonal form and assumed a flattened fibroblast-like structure showed a decrease in rough endoplasmic reticulum with less prominent Golgi apparatus and more free ribosomes, microtubules, and cytoplasmic filaments. Matrix granules were smaller in size and number, or absent. Finally, KOYAMA and ONO (1971) reported that BrdUrd reduced hyaluronic acid synthesis in a clonal hybrid line which had this synthetic ability and which was derived from a mouse mammary carcinoma and a cell from new born Chinese hamster tissue.

COLEMAN et al. (1970), who also studied muscle cells and cartilage cells, reported that chick embryo pigmented retina cells in culture media supplemented with BrdUrd (10 to 100 μM) lost melanoma granules. SILAGI and BRUCE (1970) also reported loss of pigmentation in a mouse melanoma by BrdUrd treatment and, of even greater interest, this treatment reduced or eliminated the tumorigenicity of these cells when injected into mice.

BrdUrd inhibits terminal differentiation of pancreatic epithelial rudiments (WESSELS, 1964; RUTTER et al., 1968). It also inhibits detectable hemoglobin synthesis and erythropoietic foci in chick embryos (WILT, 1965; MIURA and WILT, 1971). In mammary organ cultures of pregnant mice, BrdUrd, as well as IdUrd, inhibited the prolactin induced increase in the milk proteins, casein and α-lacttalbumin, while there was no effect on induction of galactosyl transferase (TURKINGTON et al., 1971). Induction of tyrosine aminotransferase by dexamethasone in the HTC line of rat hepatoma is also blocked by BrdUrd (STELLWAGEN and TOMKINS, 1971a, b). Lastly, SCHUBERT and JACOB (1970) reported that rather than blocking differentiation, BrdUrd induces the differentiation of a mouse neuroblastoma into cells that morphologically resemble mature neurons.

Several explanations have been advanced for this effect of BrdUrd and IdUrd. Incorporation of the analog into DNA is a prerequisite for the effect, which does not occur if DNA synthesis is blocked or sufficient thymidine is added with the BrdUrd. An important exception to this, which on further study may prove the rule, is reported by SCHUBERT and JACOB (1970). When cytosine arabinoside or mitomycin C was added to block DNA synthesis, BrdUrd still induced mouse neuroblastoma cells to differentiate into cells morphologically resembling mature neurons. SCHUBERT and JACOB (1970) propose that BrdUrd increases the affinity between the cells and the culture dish surface, which, on the basis of experiments to be published, is responsible for the induced differentiation of the neuroblastoma cells. Thus, BrdUrd causes an unspecified metabolic change in the cells which indirectly induces the differentiation of the neuroblast, probably by increasing the affinity between the limiting membrane of the cell and the culture dish surface. To support their contention, the authors cite the findings of others that in the systems in which BrdUrd affects differentiation, there is a flattening of the cells, suggesting an increased affinity between the cells and the culture dish surface. Needless to say, further experimentation on this point is warranted.

If the SCHUBERT and JACOB (1970) report is set aside, other explanations centering upon analog incorporation into DNA may be entertained. Mutagenesis is obviously not responsible, as this would mean that almost 100 percent of the cells would show the mutation, which is not very likely. Also the effect is readily reversible. Furthermore, since in several studies single cell derived clones could be shown to be affected by BrdUrd, selection of an aberrant cell type in the treated cells can be ruled out.

BISCHOFF and HOLTZER (1970) suggest three explanations: (1) the genes coding for the products affected by BrdUrd have pyrimidine-rich initiator sites and are thus sensitive, while the nonsensitive genes making essential products for cell viability and growth are always active and do not have an initiator region; (2) genes coding for essential nonBrdUrd functions are highly redundant, thus requiring greater BrdUrd incorporation to block them entirely — this idea is deemed less likely as cells can grow for many generations in BrdUrd without loss of viability; and (3) certain regions of the DNA molecule are less prone to bromouracil substitution for thymine.

MIURA and WILT (1971) propose that the physical presence of BrdUrd affects chromosomal organization or reorganization at mitosis or S phase, such organization being essential for regulatory events in the differentiation process. Although the authors cite evidence for chromosomal abnormalities associated with BrdUrd incorporation into DNA, they present no hypothesis as to how a specific effect on differentiative or specialized processes might occur.

STELLWAGEN and TOMKINS (1971a, b) also invoke the idea of a selective inhibition by BrdUrd of translation, possibly related to the base composition of the initiator sites. In addition, a model is derived (STELLWAGEN and TOMKINS, 1971b) to explain, at least in part, the differential effect based on differential labilities of certain messengers and their proteins. Thus, a stable molecule would show little immediate decrease in concentration even though its mRNA synthesis was decreased by BrdUrd, while a labile component would more quickly reflect inhibition of transcription by BrdUrd.

H. Toxicity

Biochemical studies in bacteria and cell cultures clearly indicate a competitive relationship between thymidine and IdUrd. Such a relationship has been observed in a number of mammalian systems *in vivo*. The successful prevention of the toxic effects of an otherwise lethal sequence of daily doses (18 μmoles; about 250 mg/kg) of IdUrd, when administered intraperitoneally to mice repeatedly, was obtained by the prior administration of thymidine (100 μmoles) (PRUSOFF et al., 1960). The amount of IdUrd required to produce a toxic effect in the absence of thymidine appeared to be critical, since a decrease in the quantity of administered IdUrd to one-half of the dose that produced 100 % lethality, caused no discernable toxic effects. Thymidine may have saturated either the transport mechanism involved in the penetration of IdUrd into cells or the pyrimidine deoxyribonucleoside kinase within the cells for a sufficiently long period of time such that catabolism and excretion of IdUrd resulted in a diminution of the size of the pool of IdUrd to a nontoxic level. In any case, a toxic intracellular concentration of IdUrd, or more probably of phosphorylated derivatives of IdUrd, can be prevented by thymidine.

One of the limitations in therapy of cancer with many agents is the toxicity exerted on normal actively replicating tissues such as the bone marrow and intestinal epithelium. HOFFMAN and POST (1966) studied the replication of a breast tumor and the coexistent normal ileal epithelium in the female rat *in vivo* and found that the ileal cells replicate 4 times more rapidly than the tumor cells. Thus, they also observed IdUrd to be incorporated more rapidly into the ileal cells than into tumor cells, a finding that implies ensured toxicity if IdUrd therapy is extended for a period of time, at least in those situations where the generation time of the tumor is considerably less than normal tissue. Of relevance, of course, is the ability of a normal tissue to replace those cells that are damaged by the drug under consideration.

POST and HOFFMAN (1969) examined the effect *in vivo* of IdUrd on the replication of ileal and spleen cells in rats as tissues representative of replicating normal cells of the gastrointestinal and hematopoietic systems, respectively. IdUrd was found to cause a delay in DNA synthesis, as well as in G_2 of the cell cycle. Spleen lymphocytes were more susceptible to IdUrd than were ileal cells. Whether these effects constitute a trivial or a major concern in therapy is not known.

OEHLERT and MAGNUSSEN (1965) studied by radioautography the uptake of ^{3}H-IdUrd into Yoshida hepatoma cells in the rat. After 48 h, they observed nuclear enlargement and cytoplasmic changes.

The ability of thymidine to protect an animal from the lethal effects of IdUrd was extended to man by CALABRESI (1962) and MARK and CALABRESI (1962). These workers prevented some of the toxic manifestations of IdUrd in man, such as alopecia and stomatitis, by infusion of a very small amount of thymidine into the external carotid artery while IdUrd was administered intravenously; however, the effects of IdUrd on bone marrow and on neoplastic tissues were not abolished by this regimen. This inability to control the toxicity of IdUrd to the bone marrow in man by the regional administration of thymidine has prevented any increase in the amount of IdUrd administered to patients. This is a major clinical problem that must be solved before any significant increase in the amount of IdUrd administered can be accomplished. Of pertinence, is the observation by JAFFE and PRUSOFF (1960) that the coadministration of a 10 to 30 molar excess of thymidine with IdUrd reduced the inhibition of the growth of leukemia L1210 by IdUrd by only one-half. The toxicity in man is concentration dependent (CALABRESI et al., 1961). The major toxic effects with doses of 100 to 120 mg of IdUrd per kg, infused intravenously for periods of 2 to 3 h daily for 5 or 6 days, are stomatitis, leukopenia, and alopecia (CALABRESI et al., 1961).

Marker Function

Since thymidine uniquely is incorporated into the DNA polymer, it affords the opportunity for use as a marker for the study of cell kinetics (i.e. rate of turnover, metastasis, etc.). The ideal DNA marker is one that not only specifically enters DNA, but in addition is metabolically stable once incorporated, is not toxic, and most important, is not reutilized after cell death. Unfortunately, no ideal DNA marker exists. Many reports substantiate the reutilization of thymidine derived from DNA, and in some instances this has been as great as 60 % (POTTER, 1959; RUBINI, 1960; BRYANT, 1962; DIDERHOLM et al., 1962; RICKE, 1962; ROBINSON and BRECHER, 1963; FEINENDEGEN et al., 1964, 1966b; MARUYAMA, 1964; COMMERFORD, 1965; TANNACH, 1965; STEEL, 1966; DETHLEFSEN et al., 1969; DETHLEFSEN, 1970; HEINIGER et al., 1971a, b). The pool sizes of thymidine, TMP, TDP, and TTP must be relatively small (POTTER and NYGAARD, 1963) to permit as much as 50 % of a tracer dose of injected thymidine to be utilized by rats and mice (POTTER, 1959; FEINENDEGEN and BOND, 1962).

Incorporation of radio-labeled IdUrd occurs exclusively into cellular DNA (EIDINOFF et al., 1959a, b; PRUSOFF, 1959a, b; HUGHES et al., 1964; COMMERFORD, 1965; FOX and PRUSOFF, 1965), hence, this analog has been shown to be an index of the rate of cell replication in tissues (KRUEGER et al., 1960; GITLIN et al., 1962; DETHLEFSEN and MENDELSOHN, 1964; HUGHES et al., 1964; CUMMERFORD, 1965; DETHLEFSEN, 1967, 1969a, b; HOFER et al., 1968, 1969a, b; CLIFTON and YATVIN, 1970), as well as of the localization of human tumors (DJORDJEVIC and SZYBALSKI, 1960; WELCH and PRUSOFF, 1960). ROTENBERG et al. (1962) concluded from a study of mice bearing spontaneous mammary tumors, in reference to the kinetics of labeling and retention of ^{131}I-IdUrd in tumors and tissues, that a clinical trial of ^{131}I-IdUrd for localization of human tumors was merited. Similar studies were performed by HAMPTON and EIDINOFF (1961) with transplanted tumors in mice.

IdUrd as a marker in lieu of thymidine affords the opportunity of not only labeling with ^{3}H or ^{14}C, but in addition with radioactive iodine (^{125}I or ^{131}I). The greater energy of the iodine isotopes permits more facile monitoring. The 10 fold decrease in energy of the γ-radiation emitted by ^{125}I, as well as the Auger and internal conversion electron induced by ^{125}I electron emission, permits more effective use of ^{125}I (compared to ^{131}I) in some biological studies (MYERS and VANDERLEEDEN, 1960; DANIEL et al., 1962; GITLIN et al., 1962; MAK and TILL, 1963; SMITH et al., 1963; CUDKOWICZ et al., 1964). The advantages (MYERS and VANDERLEEDEN, 1960; DANIEL et al., 1962; HOFER and HUGHES, 1971) and disadvantages (BAKHLE et al., 1964; AHNSTRÖM et al., 1970; FIDLER, 1970; HOFER and HUGHES, 1971; KRISCH, 1972) of the use of iodine-125 as a label have been reported. Care must be exercised in regard to choice of isotope, as well as its specific activity, because of the potential lethal damage that may result from radio-decay.

ERTL et al. (1970) report that toxicity to mammalian cells by DNA labeled with ^{125}IdUrd can exceed that from ^{3}H-IdUrd by a factor of about ten. They reviewed the physical properties and basis for the biological effects of iodine-125. The biological (i.e., genetic) damage caused by ^{125}I exceeds that produced by its primary radiation effects (i.e., Auger and conversion electrons) and they attribute the increased damage to charge transfer as a consequence of the Auger effect. Intramolecular charge transfer may occur also when the formed positively charged tellurium atom is bound to the uracil moiety, leading to molecular distortion and bond disruption. Thus, radioactive decay of ^{125}I involves electron capture, transition to metastable ^{125}Te, and finally to a multiple ionized ion with charges ranging from $+1$ to $+18$. This multiply ionized tellurium can produce considerable damage to the immediate environment due to its extremely great oxidizing power.

HOFER and HUGHES (1971) have made a critical analysis of the relative radiotoxicity of tritium labeled thymidine and ^{125}I- and ^{131}I-labeled IdUrd. They found ^{125}I was more toxic than either ^{3}H or ^{131}I-labels by a factor of 4 to 5 and concluded "the excessive toxicity of intranuclear ^{125}I results from the high electron flux associated with the Auger cascade which leads to concentrated energy deposition within a radiosensitive volume considerably smaller than the cell nucleus". Calculation of the number of internal disintegrations per cell per hour required to cause 50 percent lethality of L1210 cells is 4 for ^{125}I, 47 for ^{131}I, and 62 for ^{3}H.

FIDLER (1970) found cell cultures exposed to ^{125}I-IdUrd for 24 h at a concentration of 0.5 μc/ml had no alteration of biological behavior; however, a concentration of greater than 2 μc/ml produced toxicity.

A disadvantage of IdUrd relative to thymidine is the 2- to 40-fold greater utilization of the latter for the biosynthesis of DNA (PRUSOFF, 1960; HUGHES et al., 1964; FOX and PRUSOFF, 1965; BAUGNET-MAKIEW and GOUTIER, 1968). The preferential uptake of thymidine over IdUrd has been attributed to a predilection by thymidine kinase for thymidine relative to IdUrd (PONTIS et al., 1961; BIRNIE et al., 1963; BAUGNET-MAKIEW and GOUTIER, 1968; BAKHLE and PRUSOFF, 1969), as well as an enhanced enzymic degradation of IdUrd (HUGHES et al., 1964). FOX et al. (1969/70), however, have reported that although the apparent K_m of the mouse liver enzyme for IdUrd is not significantly different from that for thymidine, the maximum velocity of cleavage of thymidine is about 5 times less. This greater rate of catabolism of IdUrd in the presence of thymidine would therefore account, at least in part, for the more rapid removal of IdUrd from the mixture present in the cell pool. This mechanism would explain the recognized advantage of isotopically labeled IdUrd as a "pulse" label for DNA *in vivo*, since its presence as a nucleoside within the cell would be of much shorter duration than that of the naturally occurring nucleoside. Thus, a significant advantage of IdUrd over thymidine as a marker of DNA is the relatively low rate of reutilization of IdUrd, being on the order of at most a few percent (KRUEGER et al., 1960; FEINENDEGEN et al., 1964, 1966a, b; HUGHES et al., 1964; COMMERFORD, 1965; HOFER et al., 1969a, b; PORSCHEN and FEINENDEGEN, 1969; DETHLEFSEN, 1970, 1971). Although the reutilization of IdUrd may be minimal in an area far removed from the site of cell death, it could be appreciable if cell death occurs in or near a tumor or tissue that is undergoing rapid cellular reproduction.

DETHLEFSEN (1970), in discussing various investigations (HUGHES et al., 1964; FEINENDEGEN et al., 1966a, b; MENDELSOHN and DETHLEFSEN, 1968; DETHLEFSEN et al., 1969; HOFER et al., 1969a, b) concerned with the relative reutilization of thymidine (22 to 52 %) and of IdUrd (0 to 21 %), suggested that the efficiency of reutilization of thymidine and IdUrd is related to their relative original utilization. An attempt was made to decrease the reutilization of ^{131}I-IdUrd by inclusion of nonradioactive thymidine (20 mM) in the drinking water; however, no striking effect was observed and furthermore this amount of thymidine intake may produce some cytotoxicity.

That IdUrd is a stable label after incorporation into DNA until cell death has been demonstrated (HUGHES et al., 1964; COMMERFORD, 1965; FEINENDEGEN et al., 1966a; HOFER et al., 1968, 1969a, b; CLIFTON and YATVIN, 1970). The stability of ^{131}I-IdUrd in DNA is attested to by the observation that in "resting" cells in the mouse the label declined by less than 10% in more than 100 days (COMMERFORD, 1965).

Originally, concern existed as to the specificity of iodine labeled IdUrd as a marker for DNA because of the presence of radioactivity in tissue components other than DNA (PRUSOFF et al., 1960; DETHLEFSEN, 1969b) and this was attributed to interaction of the catabolically released iodine from IdUrd with proteins and lipids (WELCH and PRUSOFF, 1960). However, HUGHES et al. (1964) correctly attributed this apparent nonspecific labeling to incomplete extraction of labeled DNA. This interpretation was confirmed by FOX and PRUSOFF (1965) and by DETHLEFSEN (1969a).

A disadvantage of IdUrd relative to thymidine is its pharmacological effects, such as inhibition of cellular replication or prolongation of the cell cycle, which are related to the extent of uptake into DNA (see section on biological consequences of incorporation of halogenated uracil derivatives into DNA).

DETHLEFSEN (1971) has evaluated the use of ^{125}I-labeled IdUrd as a tracer for measuring cell loss from solid tumors due to metastasis and cell lysis, and alerted investigators to the problem of highly variable radio-iodine contamination in the skin above the tumor, as well as in the acid-soluble fractions of the tumor. Thus, he proposes that the tumor DNA must be extracted prior to determination of the radioactive content.

The use of radioactive iodine as a label imposes a problem due to radiation effects (HOFER et al., 1969b); however, use of radio-labeled IdUrd with high specific activity may minimize this effect (DUBBS and KIT, 1964c; FEINENDEGEN et al., 1966a; FOX and LAJTHA, 1967; HOFER et al., 1969b). Nevertheless, DETHLEFSEN (1971) cautions that the use of iodine labeled IdUrd may be particularly toxic for sensitive, rapidly proliferating tissues such as duodenum, spleen, and murine lymphoma (HOFER et al., 1969b; POST and HOFFMAN, 1969; DETHLEFSEN, 1971).

The technique of prelabeling ascites cells with ^{125}I-IdUrd (HOFER et al., 1969b) has been used to evaluate the effect of various antitumor drugs (HOFER, 1969; HOFER et al., 1969a) and radiation (HOFER, 1970) on cell death and migration. HOFER and HOFER (1971) used ^{125}I-IdUrd to label the DNA of L1210 leukemia cells for a study of their kinetics of proliferation, migration, and death. The rate of cell death was determined by measuring the rate of excretion of ^{125}I from mice injected with ^{125}I-IdUrd labeled cells. Of relevance to their interpretation, is the accumulation of catabolically formed radioiodine in the thyroid, a factor that would be interpreted as a decreased rate of cell death. This factor was minimized by the inclusion of NaI in the drinking water 1 to 2 days prior to inoculation with the labeled cells (HOFER et al., 1969b). Metastases or cell migrations were measured, at various intervals of time after injection of the labeled cells, by determination of the radio-iodine content of various organs. Again, a concern may be the reutilization of ^{125}I-IdUrd from dead cells which occurs, albeit to a small degree, as well as the question of the viability of the migrated radioactive cells. Of interest is their finding that 79% of the L1210 ascites cells injected i.p. into mice migrated from the peritoneal cavity during the first 24 h. HOFER and HOFER (1971) indicated that when ^{125}I-IdUrd is administered in low concentration over a protracted period of time to mice bearing the L1210 ascites tumor and the cells used subsequently as an inoculum, the following ideal situation exists: "(a) the ^{125}I in the inoculum is associated exclusively with the DNA of the tumor cells and is not released from the DNA of the labeled cells while they are alive; (b) the radioactive label is distributed uniformly throughout the initial cell population; (c) the incorporated radioisotope does not affect the rate of division or death of labeled cells; and (d) radioactively labeled compounds are rapidly excreted following the death of labeled cells".

FIDLER (1970) has raised the objection to the technique described by HOFER et al. (1969b), in which cells are labeled *in vivo* with ^{125}I-IdUrd for study of the kinetics of cell death and metastases in nonlabeled mice, that small numbers of tumor cells would not be detected because of low incorporation of label. As discussed elsewhere in this chapter, one must limit the amount of radioactivity per cell to avoid cell destruction from internal radiation (HOFER and HUGHES, 1971). FIDLER (1970) labeled cells in culture with ^{125}I-IdUrd, administered these cells i.v. to mice, and at various times analyzed the distribution of radioactivity in the various organs. The criteria that FIDLER set for use of a labeled cell for a study of metastasis include: (1) the label is not removed from the cell until it dies; (2) once the label is released it must not be reutilized, but rather rapidly excreted; (3) the label should not alter the normal sequence of biological events of the cell; (4) the label should be present in sufficient amount to readily detect few cells; and (5) the label should be homogenous in concentration per cell.

A precaution in the use of ^{125}I as a radioactive label arises from the toxicity produced from the emanating radiations (HOFER et al., 1969b, 1970). However, HOFER et al. (1969b) were able to minimize this factor if the incorporation of ^{125}I into the L1210 ascites cells was kept below 0.03 μCi per million labeled cells. Such a situation may be achieved if the dose of ^{125}I-IdUrd administered to label the cells is not in excess of 2 μCi per mouse (HOFER et al., 1969).

Although ^{3}H-thymidine has been used generally as a tool for investigations of the biosynthesis of DNA, serious limitations exist in the measurement of the tritium. The very low energy of the β-emanations limits the usefulness of measurement in a Geiger-Müller counter. Liquid scintillation counting occasionally requires large corrections for quenching, and sample size for counting is limited, hence, quantitative work with this precursor is tedious. On the other hand, the γ-radiations of ^{131}I or ^{125}I are readily counted using a sodium iodide (Tl) crystal, not only with high efficiency (60%), but also the sample size relative to liquid scintillation counting may be at least 30-fold greater. Therefore, although the amount of radioactivity (dpm) in DNA derived from ^{3}H-thymidine or ^{125}I-IdUrd may be about the same, the factors discussed result in more efficient counting of the iodine isotope. Thus, MAK and TILL (1963) had previously indicated that an advantage of iodine labeled IdUrd over tritium labeled thymidine is the greater ability of measuring low levels of radioiodine relative to the tritium.

FOX and PRUSOFF (1965) made a comparison of the rate of metabolic decay of the radioactive low molecular weight metabolites derived from ^{125}I-IdUrd and ^{3}H-thymidine, and a striking decrease in the size of the ^{125}I-labeled cold acid-soluble fraction was observed relative to the ^{3}H-labeled fraction. This indicates that a marked difference in the metabolism of IdUrd and thymidine exists in the mouse which may have an important bearing on the relative merits of these two compounds as potential labels of DNA. The preferential utilization of thymidine compared to IdUrd for the biosynthesis of DNA may be related to possible differences in the rates of transport out of the abdominal cavity, transport into the cell, phosphorylation, catabolism, and excretion from the organism.

FOX and PRUSOFF (1965) observed the ratio of tritium labeled derivatives to those labeled with ^{125}I, 17.5 h following the last administration of ^{3}H-thymidine or ^{125}I-IdUrd, in the cold acid-soluble fractions derived from four tissues; the ratio ranged from 10 to 35. This finding is in agreement with the greater incorporation of thymidine into DNA relative to IdUrd. DETHLEFSEN (1971) compared the metabolism of tritium versus iodine labeled IdUrd and also found a marked difference in the rate of loss of the two labels from the acid-soluble fractions.

Although IdUrd and thymidine are each substrates for thymidine kinase and nucleoside phosphorylase, the relative enzyme activities that lead to the formation of nucleotides or of the cleavage of the nucleoside to the free pyrimidine base may vary with the particular tissue. Free thymidine per se is found in some tissues, notably spleen and thymus, to a greater extent than previously appreciated, although cellular thymidine is considered to be only partially available for equilibration with added thymidine (POTTER and NYGAARD, 1963). Phosphorylated derivatives of thymidine (i.e., the mono-, di-, and triphosphate) also exist in these and other tissues. Hence, catabolism of DNA labeled with radioactive thymidine results in the formation of thymidine monophosphate which equilibrates with these pools of phosphorylated derivatives of thymidine. Thus, the labeled thymidine may be trapped as the nucleoside or as phosphorylated derivatives, during both the formation and the degradation of DNA. Although the nucleoside is subject to the action of the competing kinase and phosphorylase, it is usually considered lost as a precursor of DNA once it is catabolized to free thymine. However, mechanisms do exist in mammalian systems for the conversion of thymine to the ribonucleoside and, to a lesser extent, to its deoxyribonucleoside (DEVERDIER and POTTER, 1960; GAITO and PRUSOFF, 1962). This latter conversion permits the reutilization of the thymine moiety for the biosynthesis of DNA (REICHARD and ESTBORN, 1951; BROWN et al., 1952; HAMPTON et al., 1962). In contrast, radioactive IdUrd is more vulnerable to catabolism, since preformed pools of nonradioactive IdUrd or its phosphorylated derivatives do not exist. Thus, a larger percentage of ^{125}I-IdUrd, in comparison to ^{3}H-thymidine, is susceptible to catabolism. It has been demonstrated that IdUrd, in comparison to thymidine, is preferentially attacked by nucleoside phosphorylase (PONTIS et al., 1961; ZIMMERMAN, 1962; BIRNIE et al., 1963; FOX et al., 1969/70), and hence IdUrd would presumably be removed from the cold acid-soluble fraction at a greater rate. Similarly, an additional increase in the rate of loss of ^{125}I-labeled compounds would result if the affinities of the mono-, di-, and triphosphates of IdUrd and thymidine were different for the other catabolic and anabolic enzymes. Thus, a combination of these catabolic and anabolic events may be the explanation for the unequal rate of loss of the ^{125}I- and ^{3}H-labels from the acid-soluble fraction. Such differences between the two precursors of DNA are responsible for the preferential use of IdUrd as a marker relative to thymidine.

In addition to the above references to the marker use of IdUrd, the following uses should be mentioned: (1) to study the effects of ionizing radiation (COMMERFORD et al., 1960; GITLIN et al., 1961; MAK and TILL, 1963; O'FARREL and DUNAWAY, 1967a); (2) to study cell population growth and cell loss in normal and neoplastic tissues (DAVIS et al., 1968; CLIFTON and YATVIN, 1970; HOFER et al., 1970), and in tumor metastases (HOFER and HUGHES, 1970), the fate of lymphoblasts and immunoblasts injected into rat lymph (HALL and SMITH, 1970), and cell proliferation in regenerating rat liver (BÜRKI et al., 1969); (3) to study the extent and kinetics of asparaginase destruction of murine leukemic cells *in vivo* (HOFER et al., 1970), of heterologous antilymphocytic serum on lymphoid cells (TAUB, 1970), and of phytohaemagglutinin on human lymphocytes (CRAIG et al., 1969).

Radiosensitization

A very important property of the halogenated derivatives of uracil is their capacity after incorporation into DNA to increase the sensitivity of mammalian cells, bacteria, and viruses to the lethal effects of UV and ionizing radiations. For appropriate references see ELKIND and WHITMORE (1967), SZYBALSKI (1967), and KAPLAN (1970). Since radiation sensitization will be discussed in detail elsewhere in this book, there will be no attempt to cover this area extensively. Discussion will be limited to possible mechanisms of action, as well as to studies in progress that are relevant.

The sensitization phenomenon was first observed in bacteria by GREER and ZAMENHOF (1957) and reported in detail by GREER (1960). This observation was extended to include mammalian cells *in vitro* by DJORDEVIC and SZYBALSKI (1960) and *in vivo* by BERRY and ANDREWS (1962a, b).

The potential of chemotherapeutic agents to enhance radiation therapy has been reviewed by BAGSHAW and DOGGETT (1969) and by KAPLAN (1970). The therapeutic potential of BrdUrd and IdUrd as radiosensitizers has received minimal study (WELCH and PRUSOFF, 1960; CALABRESI et al., 1961; BAGSHAW et al., 1967; SANO et al., 1968; HOSHINO and SANO, 1969; LANDOLT, 1971). The studies with IdUrd were encouraging but limited in scope. Although BAGSHAW and coworkers did obtain evidence for clinical radiosensitization by BrdUrd, differential radiosensitization between neoplastic and normal tissue was not achieved. The studies by SANO et al. (1968) concern the use of BrdUrd in the radiosensitization of malignant brain tumors in man and these workers have expressed cautious optimism; however, LANDOLT (1971) treated 10 patients with glioblastoma similarly and the reported apparent effectiveness was attributed to patient selection. The recent reports of successful use of halogenated nucleosides to sensitize neoplastic tissues relative to normal tissue in animals (BROWN et al., 1971; GOFFINET, 1972) would imply that problems of pharmacology in man may have to be solved before more effective use is attained (see SUIT, 1966). Among the halogenated deoxyribonucleosides, the iodinated analogs are the most potent sensitizers to x-rays. The increase in sensitivity has been attributed to their incorporation into DNA by replacement of thymidine. ERIKSON and SZYBALSKI (1963) have hypothesized that the radiosensitizing effect may be related to the greater photoelectric absorption of the halogen atoms. Whether the effect is manifest by an inhibition of post-irradiation repair or by an increased fragility of the DNA molecule is still under consideration (for discussion see LETT et al., 1970).

Mechanistically, WACKER (1963) and SMITH (1964) reported that UV and ionizing radiations caused the loss of bromine from bromouracil substituted DNA with the formation of uracil; LION (1970) observed the formation of an alkali labile bond in irradiated bromouracil labeled DNA. HOTZ and REUSCHL (1967) found that bromouracil in DNA increased the amount of the sugar deoxyribose destroyed by UV irradiation, and electron spin data obtained by KOEHLEIN and HUTCHINSON (1969) was consistent with the appearance of a free radical in the sugar moiety of BU-DNA. ZIMBRICK (1969a, b) also supports the formation of a uracil free radical during radiolysis of bromouracil substituted DNA and abstraction of a hydrogen from a neighboring deoxyribose. The bromine radical (Br·) has been observed during flash photolysis of bromouracil derivatives by DANZIGER et al. (1968). Recent studies by HUTCHINSON and HALES (1970) support previous observations of an increase in the induction of breaks in bromouracil-DNA compared to normal DNA. These observations are readily explained by the experiments of RUPP and PRUSOFF (1964, 1965a, b) which proposed and provided evidence that radiation causes the release of the halogen at the 5-position of the uracil moiety with the formation of a uracil free radical. Presumably this uracil free radical when present in DNA can abstract a hydrogen from the deoxyribose of DNA, thereby labilizing the DNA backbone; hence, one observes an increase in the number of breaks in the bromouracil-substituted DNA.

Previous studies in our laboratory on the photochemistry of iodouracil (RUPP and PRUSOFF, 1964, 1965a, b) indicated that when iodouracil is exposed to ultraviolet light a dehalogenation occurs with the formation of a uracil free radical which subsequently undergoes several possible reactions dependent upon the specific environmental conditions. Irradiation of iodouracil in an aqueous environment results in the formation of a rearranged molecule, alloxanic acid. Irradiation in the presence of a compound from which a hydrogen can be abstracted results in the formation of uracil, whereas irradiation of iodouracil in the presence of the disulfide, cystamine, results in the cleavage of cystamine by the formed uracil free radical with the formation of the thioether, *S*-(5-uracilyl)cysteamine. It is this latter observation that prompted our present investigations described below.

Evidence has been obtained that irradiation of 5-iodo-2′-deoxyuridine, when present in a substrate-enzyme complex, will produce a photochemical reaction that results in the conversion of the analog to the deoxyuridine free radical when at the active site of the enzyme. The free radical produced may then interact with an amino acid at or adjacent to the catalytic site, producing a covalent linkage that prevents subsequent enzyme activity. Thus, what is accomplished is the novel conversion of a competitive inhibitor into an irreversible inhibitor. Since there is preferential interaction of a substrate with a specific protein, it is conceivable that preferential inactivation of specific enzymes may be achieved by this approach.

Supporting evidence has been obtained for these concepts in our laboratory using extensively purified thymidine kinase prepared from *E. coli* (VOYTEK et al., 1971) by a modification of the procedure described by OKAZAKI, T. and KORNBERG (1964). Irradiation of the enzyme in the presence of the normal substrate, thymidine, resulted in a decreased rate of inactivation by UV-irradiation, whereas the presence of IdUrd increased the rate of inactivation of this enzyme (CYSYK and PRUSOFF, 1972). All studies with tritium-labeled IdUrd showed a straight line relationship between the irradiation dose and the amount of radioactivity that became irreversibly associated with the protein. Similar studies with radioiodine-labeled IdUrd revealed no attachment of radioiodine to the enzyme. These results support a covalent interaction between the radiation-formed deoxyuridine free radical and the enzyme. That the photolytic reaction is an active site interaction is supported by the following evidence. (1) An enzyme-IdUrd complex forms because IdUrd is a substrate for thymidine kinase (i.e., K_m for IdUrd is identical to that for thymidine). (2) IdUrd sensitizes only, or preferentially, the catalytic activity (the regulatory activity of those enzyme molecules not so inactivated are not affected). (3) The IdUrd effect is increased by the activator, dCDP, which increases the affinity for the substrate, and is decreased by the allosteric inhibitor, dTTP, which decreases the affinity for substrate. (4) The IdUrd-sensitizing effect is decreased and eventually is abolished by increasing prior to radiation the concentrations of thymidine. (5) The enhancement is a hyperbolic function of the IdUrd concentration and a maximum sensitizing effect is attained, closely resembling the substrate saturation curve for thymidine kinase activity. In contrast, the UV-sensitization of thymidine kinase by 5-iodo-2′-deoxycytidine (a nonsubstrate) or NaI is a linear function of the concentration of these sensitizers.

Whereas both BrdUrd and IdUrd undergo photochemical reaction when incorporated into DNA, these nucleosides in solution behave very differently. The photosensitivity of the various halogenated pyrimidine and deoxyribonucleoside derivatives is dependent upon many factors which include pH, frozen or nonfrozen state, the presence of organic substances, and the presence or absence of oxygen

(PRUSOFF, 1962; RUPP and PRUSOFF, 1964, 1965a,b). Thus, bromouracil and 5-bromo-2′-deoxyuridine were unaffected when irradiated in water or in the frozen state (WACKER, 1961; WACKER et al., 1961; SMITH, 1962), but when irradiated in the presence of other pyrimidine derivatives or at high pH a marked photolability of bromouracil was observed (SMITH, 1962, 1963).

Bromouracil or iodouracil, when incorporated into DNA, not only is in a highly structured environment, but also is in intimate proximity to other organic components of DNA. Hence, as observed, 5-bromouracil in DNA is very sensitive to photochemical alteration, with uracil being a major photoproduct (WACKER et al., 1961). When bromouracil-substituted DNA is irradiated, energy absorbed randomly by other purine and pyrimidine components may be transferred in sufficient amount to the carbon-bromine bond of bromouracil to result in dehalogenation. A discussion of the excited states and energy transfer in bromouracil substituted DNA has been presented by FIELDEN and LILLICARP (1970–72) in which it was stated that absorbed radiation energy may migrate a distance of about 200 base pairs. The bromouracil acts as an energy sink for the excited system as a whole. Similarly, the IdUrd in the enzyme-substrate complex form is more sensitive than IdUrd in solution to photoactivation because of the transfer of the energy absorbed by the protein, thymidine kinase, to the complexed substrate. The mechanism for the formation of DNA-uracil from DNA-bromouracil is similar to that observed during photolysis of 5-iodouracil in solution (WACKER et al., 1961; HOTZ and REUSCHL, 1967; KOEHLIN and HUTCHINSON, 1969; HUTCHINSON and HALES, 1970).

Recent studies of the photochemistry of 5-bromouracil (ISHIHARA and WANG, (1966) and of 5-fluorouracil (FIKUS et al., 1964, 1965; LOZERON et al., 1964) confirm that dehalogenation results from photolysis; however, the primary photoproduct of fluorouracil and its nucleosides is the hydrate which is subsequently dehalogenated to barbituric acid by elimination of HF (FIKUS et al., 1965). The photochemistry of 5-chlorouracil has not been as thoroughly studied as that of 5-fluoro, 5-bromo, or 5-iodouracil. However, in view of the bond-dissociation energy of the carbon-chlorine bond (66.5 kcal per mole) in relation to that of the corresponding fluoro (107.0 kcal per mole), bromo (54.0 kcal per mole), and iodo (45.5 kcal per mole) carbon bonds (PAULING, 1960), it would not be surprising if dehalogenation of 5-chlorouracil were also involved as either a primary or a secondary event during photolysis. KAZIMIERCZUK and SHUGAR (1971) refer to unpublished observations of FIKUS and SHUGAR that 5 chlorouracil is radiation resistant with a quantum yield of less than 10^{-4}, however, 6-chlorouracil in the monoionic form, but not the neutral form, undergoes photohydration of the 5,6-bond with subsequent halogen elimination to yield barbituric acid. When the photosensitivities of the deoxyribonucleosides of 5-fluorouracil, 5-chlorouracil, 5-bromouracil, and 5-iodouracil were compared in phosphate buffer, 0.01 M, pH 7.1 at room temperature, the 5-chloro and 5-bromo-2′-deoxyuridines were inert, whereas 5-fluoro and 5-iodo-2′-deoxyuridine were appreciably photoreactive, as measured by a decrease in absorbance (PRUSOFF, 1962). Thus the greater photochemical reactivity of IdUrd relative to BrdUrd and CldUrd is related to the strength of the carbon-halogen bond, which is related to the electronegativity of the halogen substituent. Therefore, less energy is required to break the C-I bond than the C-Br bond (PAULING, 1960).

The strength of the carbon-halogen bond of uracil, its nucleosides, and oligonucleotides was studied by WRONA and CZOCHRALSKA (1970) by classical polarography, and they observed that the ease of electroreduction of the carbon-halogen bond increases in the order F < Cl < Br < I. The electroreduction mechanism of

5-iodo, 5-bromo, and 5-chlorouracil involves a two electron carbon-halogen bond fission with the formation of uracil or its glycoside and a halogen ion, whereas that of 5-fluorouracil is a four-electron process with the formation of 5,6-dihydrofluorouracil and the fluoride ion.

Elkind and Whitmore (1967) commented that although it is reasonable to associate increased sensitivity of cells to irradiation with the incorporation of 5-chloro, 5-bromo, and 5-iodo-2′-deoxyuridine into cellular DNA, unequivocal evidence has not been presented that the DNA is the principal or sole target molecule. The various other biochemical sites of inhibition exerted by 5-iodo-2′-deoxyuridine and its phosphorylated derivatives have been reviewed (Goz and Prusoff, 1970b, see Fig. 4).

Although 5-iodo-, 5-bromo-, 5-chloro-, and 5-fluoro-2′-deoxyuridine are each substrates for thymidine kinase and all undergo photolysis with UV light under appropriate circumstances, only IdUrd increases the sensitization of the enzyme to photoinactivation (Voytek et al., 1972; Cysyk and Prusoff, 1972). This observation presumably is related to the difference in the bond energy of the C-I bond as compared to the C-Br bond, as well as to the amount of energy absorbed by the protein during irradiation that can be transported to the halogenated substrate. Apparently the amount of energy that can be funneled to the C-Br bond is much greater when BrdUrd is a component of DNA relative to the enzyme-substrate complex. The clinical implications of this reaction are discussed in the section on clinical use.

Clinical Use

Two major areas in which the clinical potential of IdUrd has been investigated in man are the therapy of neoplasia and therapy of viral infections. As of today, IdUrd has found a major role as an antiviral agent. The antiviral activity of IdUrd and BrdUrd has been established in cell culture, in animals and in man. After the report of Herrmann (1961) that IdUrd and BrdUrd inhibit the replication of several DNA-containing viruses *in vitro*, particularly vaccinia and herpes simplex, Kaufman and associates (Kaufman, 1962; Kaufman et al., 1962a, b), found that solutions of either IdUrd or BrdUrd applied frequently to the cornea, suppressed the keratitis caused by these two viruses in rabbits and, more importantly, suppressed herpes simplex of the corneal epithelium in man. The studies in rabbits were confirmed and extended to other derivatives of IdUrd (Perkins et al., 1962). Kaufman (1965b) has presented the results of five independent double-blind studies that confirm the efficacy of IdUrd in acute dendritic keratitis in man.

Thus, today, among the various halogenated derivatives, IdUrd has achieved the status of a drug permitted by the Food and Drug Administration to be sold in the United States for the therapy of herpetic keratitis in man. The clinical antiviral use of IdUrd and related agents has been extensively reviewed (Prusoff, 1967; Goz and Prusoff, 1970b; Schabel and Montgomery, 1971). A tabulation of the various viral diseases that have been treated with IdUrd, and in a few instances with BrdUrd, are listed in Table 2.

Table 2. *Disease entities in which therapy with IdUrd or BrdUrd have been investigated*

1. Herpes simplex keratitis	6. Smallpox
2. Cutaneous herpes	7. Herpes encephalitis
3. Herpes zoster	8. Congenital cytomegalovirus infection
4. Herpes genitalis	9. Subacute sclerosing panencephalitis
5. Vaccinia gangrenosum	10. Cancer

Although the efficacy of IdUrd in the topical therapy of herpes simplex infection of the corneal epithelium in man has been confirmed, its effectiveness in deep stromal infections is doubtful. Cutaneous herpes infections have been treated with IdUrd. The results of such topical therapy are controversial, the problem being one of insuring penetration of the drug into the infected cells. MacCallum and Juel-Jensen (1966) successfully treated herpes simplex lesions of the skin in man by application of a 5% solution of IdUrd in dimethylsulfoxide. This solvent enables about a ten-fold greater solubility of the drug relative to water and may also result in more effective penetration of the drug into cells.

Herpes varicella virus is responsible for varicella (i.e. chicken pox) and herpes zoster (i.e. shingles). Although the replication of herpes varicella virus and the zoster virus were markedly affected by IdUrd in culture, therapy of herpes zoster by topical application in man was not effective. The suggestion was made that since the virus resides in the posterior root ganglia, the drug may not have reached the site of viral replication. Juel-Jensen et al. (1970), however, using a very concentrated solution of IdUrd (i.e. 40% in dimethyl sulfoxide), reported accelerated healing and a reduction in the duration of pain from an average of over a month to that of less than 3 days. Waltuch and Sachs (1968) treated disseminated herpes zoster, which developed in a patient with Hodgkin's disease, with systemically administered IdUrd and reported an excellent response.

Herpes genitalis has been treated with a 0.5% ointment and beneficial effects have been reported.

Conchie et al. (1968) reported cytomegalovirus to be favorably affected by IdUrd in that the urinary excretion of the virus was reduced; however, further study by Barton and Tobin (1970) indicated that clinical improvement had not been achieved.

Success in the treatment of various localized infections with IdUrd is based on the ability to achieve an adequate concentration in a restricted area. The logical extension is the determination of whether systemic infections could also be suppressed. The extensive experience of Calabresi et al. (1961) in the treatment of neoplasms of man by systemic administration of IdUrd led to the experiments of Calabresi et al. (1963a), who showed that vaccinia infections, both in rabbits and in patients with advanced neoplastic disease, could be suppressed by the intravenous administration of well tolerated amounts of IdUrd. Although the acute toxicity (i.e. stomatitis, alopecia, and hematopoietic depression) observed was reversible (Calabresi et al., 1963a), it has been recommended by Welch (1965) that the use of this compound be restricted to patients with severe or potentially lethal DNA-viral infections, because incorporation of IdUrd into the genome of the host cell conceivably could express itself by genetic damage, infertility, or even neoplastic change. Although FdUrd, BrdUrd, and IdUrd inhibit antibody formation *in vitro*, BrdUrd, not IdUrd, inhibited the immune response in animal systems (Fischer et al., 1966). This may be an advantage in the use of IdUrd for systemic antiviral therapy because a possible host defense mechanism is apparently not impaired by this drug. The teratogenic potential of these halogenated deoxyribonucleosides, including IdUrd, has also been reviewed (see Prusoff, 1967 and the section on embryonic development and differentiation).

A potentially exciting use of IdUrd is in the systemic therapy of herpes encephalitis. The initial report by Breeden et al. (1966) described the successful treatment of a patient with encephalitis caused by herpes simplex virus by administering an intravenous injection of IdUrd (total dose 39 g) during a 7-day period after surgical decompression. This provocative finding has stimulated numerous investigators to use this drug in the therapy of viral encephalitis. However, only a few case reports have been presented. Although not uniformly enthusiastic, reports clearly indicate the need for a properly controlled study of IdUrd efficacy to evaluate its true potential in the treatment of herpetic encephalitis. It is obviously essential to establish that the disease entity under study is caused by a herpes virus or other DNA virus. Some investigators have assumed that this disease is uniformly fatal or disabling, but fortunately for the patient, this is not so. Thus, interpretation of reports that describe treatment of relatively few cases are subject to question. Nevertheless, the majority of these reports indicate that IdUrd merits continued evaluation in the therapy of this dread disease. Of particular importance is the study of RAPPEL and BRIHAYE (1969), who observed favorable response in 9 of 11 cases treated with IdUrd.

A number of other purine and pyrimidine derivatives have demonstrated marked antiviral activity *in vivo*, and these have been tabulated by SCHABEL and MONTGOMERY (1971). Several of these agents have been reviewed recently (GOZ and PRUSOFF, 1970b).

Whereas the aim in the chemotherapy of neoplasms is the total destruction of the neoplastic cell, it is not essential to have complete eradication of a virus to achieve successful therapy. For example, it has been reported that if a patient with smallpox has a virus blood level of 10^4 per milliliter infecting doses (chorioallantoic membrane assay) or greater in the second day of illness, the patient will probably die; however, if the titer is 10^2 infecting doses per milliliter or less, the viremia will disappear and the patient will recover. Thus, the body is able to recover from at least certain virus infections by utilization of host defense mechanisms, provided the intensity of the infection is not above a critical level.

The potential role of IdUrd in neoplasm therapy in man, for which it was originally prepared (PRUSOFF, 1959), is still under investigation, particularly in combination with irradiation. Initial studies of the antineoplastic potential of IdUrd have been reported by WELCH and PRUSOFF (1960) and CALABRESI et al. (1961). Objective improvement was reported in one patient with malignant melanoma, one with abdominal fibrosarcoma, and one with epidermal cancer of the tongue. Although some objective evidence of moderately favorable effects was observed in other patients, in none was the general picture improved significantly. Several reviews of the antineoplastic potential of IdUrd have appeared (CALABRESI, 1963; CALABRESI and WELCH, 1962).

Clinical and pharmacological studies in man with a closely related analog, 5-iodo-2′-deoxycytidine, were reported by CALABRESI et al. (1963b), and a close parallelism exists between the biological activity and the rate of deamination to form IdUrd.

The ability of IdUrd or BrdUrd to sensitize mammalian cells *in vitro* and *in vivo* to radiation afforded the opportunity to investigate its potential in man. The administration intra-arterially of BrdUrd plus methotrexate to patients with advanced head and neck tumors led to extensive tumor regression in all patients upon x-irradiation, however, extensive radiosensitization occurred in normal skin and mucous membranes (BAGSHAW et al., 1967; DOGGETT et al., 1967; BAGSHAW and DOGGETT, 1969). The improvement observed in 36 % of patients from the combined therapy of BrdUrd, methotrexate, and radiation was not significantly different from conventional irradiation alone.

SANO et al. (1968) and HOSHINO and SANO (1969) obtained encouraging results in the therapy of patients with malignant brain tumors by irradiation after a continuous arterial infusion of BrdUrd, methotrexate, and 5-fluorouracil or FdUrd. However, long-term follow up is required before the efficacy of this mixture can be unequivocally established.

Initial experiments of VOYTEK et al. (1972) and CYSYK and PRUSOFF (1972) have demonstrated that IdUrd or N-methyl IdUrd, analogs of thymidine which specifically interact with the enzyme thymidine kinase, can be converted by UV-irradiation into irreversible inhibitors when associated with the enzyme at the active site. Thus, if a similar sequence of reactions were to occur with ionizing radiation, then an opportunity is afforded for a more effective utilization of IdUrd and possibly other compounds in the therapy of neoplasms. In a preliminary study, performed to determine the effect of x-rays on thymidine kinase in the presence and absence of IdUrd, an augmentation of the rate of inactivation in the presence of IdUrd was indeed observed. What is envisioned is a two-pronged attack that involves initially an incorporation of a maximal amount of IdUrd into the DNA of neoplastic tissue, to be followed by irradiation at a time subsequent to administration of an additional dose of IdUrd when the pools of phosphorylated derivatives of IdUrd are at a maximum. Thus, not only will one observe an effect on DNA, but also on those enzymes concerned with the biosynthesis of DNA. This should result in marked enhancement of the lethal effects of radiation, because the processes concerned with DNA function, DNA biosynthesis, and DNA repair will be adversely affected. Hitherto, the clinical approach to the use of IdUrd or BrdUrd as potential sensitizers of x-irradiation has been concerned with attainment of maximal incorporation into DNA only.

Mode of Inhibition

The studies reviewed above document the different effects engendered by incorporation of BrdUrd or IdUrd into DNA. It is the purpose of this section to review mechanisms postulated in the studies already cited, as well as others bearing on this topic.

The basis for the mutagenic action of BrdUrd or IdUrd is base pairing errors, either in the replication or transcription of substituted DNA. Therefore, analysis of DNA or RNA made from substituted DNA might reveal these errors. TRAUTNER et al. (1962) have done such a study. Unfortunately, their results are anomalous and, as it appears, the wrong enzyme was studied [the arguments for this latter conclusion are reviewed by GOULIAN (1971)].

Other evidence in cell-free systems for the ability of halogenated uracil to cause miscoding has been provided by GRUNBERG-MANAGO and MICHELSON (1964) and MICHELSON (1965) who studied the coding ability of poly 5-chloro, bromo, and iodouridylic acid relative to polyuridylic acid. With regard to stimulation of phenylalanine incorporation, the iodo analog was as effective as polyuridylic acid, but the bromo analog was about 30 % less effective and the chloro derivative about 67 % less effective. On the other hand, polyuridylic acid stimulation of isoleucine incorporation was negligible, while the halogenated analogs stimulated considerable incorporation, with the bromo derivative being most efficacious. The pH effect on incorporation was also investigated and thus, for example, polybromouridylic acid stimulation of isoleucine incorporation was three-fold greater at pH 7.43 than at pH 7.97.

Many investigators have ascribed the various effects of IdUrd and BrdUrd, such as differential inhibition of syntheses of certain proteins (STELLWAGEN and TOMKINS, 1971a, b; GOZ and PRUSOFF, 1968, 1970a), to A-T rich clusters in DNA as described by SZYBALSKI et al. (1966). In this regard, INMAN and SCHNOS (1970) have shown, with electron microscopic observation of DNA, that the A-BU rich regions are located at similar positions along the molecule as the A-T rich regions. SZYBALSKI et al. (1966) had postulated that RNA polymerase may bind at A-T rich regions and in supporting evidence recently published it was found that *E. coli* RNA polymerase was bound more by thymine-rich fragments of phage F1 DNA than by the mean or nonthymine-rich fragments. In addition, RNA synthesis was twice as fast on the thymine-rich fragments (SHISHIDO and IKEDA, 1970). Of course, it is a large step from such *in vitro* results to RNA synthesis in the intact cells; however, PAINTER et al. (1970) found RNA synthesis in ultraviolet irradiated cells with bromouracil substituted DNA decreased by 95% relative to irradiated normal cells which had only a 30% decrease. More recently, JONES and DOVE (1972), in studies with BrdUrd substituted bacteria and phage, found that BrdUrd substitution reduces DNA-directed RNA production about seven-fold and sensitizes transcription to near visible light irradiation.

Work with synthetic polymers has also been interesting in this area. JONES and BERG (1966) observed that poly dT inhibited the binding of RNA polymerase to T_7 DNA, and that the inhibition was greater than that with poly A or heat-denatured T_7 DNA. The intriguing finding has also been made (LINN and RIGGS, 1971) that poly d(A-BU) competes about 40 times more effectively for *E. coli* lac repressor than poly d(A-T) which in turn is 20 times more effective than poly d(A-U).

Another explanation for differential effects of BrdUrd or IdUrd, often invoked, and companion to the idea of A-T rich regions, is the concept of the critical thymidine site or sites. Such ideas generally take the form of the critical sites only being substituted at large analog concentrations thus accounting for the apparent ability of cells to grow in the presence of the analogs at lower concentration.

The relation of mutation to the effects of BrdUrd and IdUrd as described in the preceding sections has been considered by many investigators. In general, the effects of BrdUrd and IdUrd cannot be explained by increased mutation rate. The principal argument against this is that many of the effects are relatively rapidly reversed when the analog is removed, a feature not expected if a mutational event has occurred.

In this regard, BYRD (1971) has shown by several approaches that the lethal effect of iodouracil is not due to mutagenic alterations in phage T_4. First, after demonstrating that iodouracil-substituted T_4*td*8, a thymine-requiring mutant, can be multiplicity reactivated, he used this procedure to study the mutation frequency of the viable and nonviable portions of a population of iodouracil-substituted T_4*td*8rII, a double mutant. The rII reversion frequency in the multiplicity reactivated, nonviable, substituted phage was not significantly different from the viable substituted phage. If mutagenesis were the cause of lethality, the nonviable phage would be expected to have a higher reversion frequency than the viable phage. Second, BYRD (1971) compared reversion frequency and lethality at various degrees of iodouracil substitution and found that the reversion frequency increases most markedly at lower levels of substitution, while lethality is apparent only when greater substitution is achieved. Third, the order of efficacy of producing lethality by chloro, bromo, and iodouracil is different from that for producing mutagenesis. Lastly, while rII reversion frequency increases linearly with time in cells infected in the presence of iodouracil, the degree of lethality remains constant throughout infection.

Conclusions

It is obvious from the above that a great deal of further work is needed to understand the mechanism(s) of action of the sundry effects of BrdUrd and IdUrd. The answer to the question of how these analogs inhibit cell division, viral replication, and specialized cell functions, while also being capable of inducing oncogenic viruses in cells previously lacking such viruses, should be of great value. As greater understanding of these halogenated deoxyribonucleosides is acquired, it is to be hoped that more sophisticated use may ensue, as well as synthesis of related compounds with greater selectivity of action. Clinically one can readily envision advances in at least two important areas, radiosensitization of neoplasms and antiviral chemotherapy.

References

AAMODT, L., GOZ, B.: An immunological study of an enzyme made by phage containing 5-iodo-2′-deoxyuridine-substituted deoxyribonucleic acid. Biochem. Pharmacol. **19**, 2400—2403 (1970).

AARONSON, S.A., TODARO, G.T., SCOLNICK, E.M.: Induction of murine C-type viruses from clonal lines of virus-free BALB/3T3 cells. Science **174**, 157—159 (1971).

ABBOTT, J., HOLTZER, H.: The loss of phenotypic traits by differentiated cells. V. The effect of 5-bromodeoxyuridine on cloned chondrocytes. Proc. nat. Acad. Sci. (Wash.) **59**, 1144—1151 (1968).

ABE, M., TOMIZAWA, J.I.: Replication of the *Escherichia coli* K12 chromosome. Proc. nat. Acad. Sci. (Wash.) **58**, 1911—1918 (1967).

AGARWAL, D.P., EICKHOFF, K., GOEDDE, H.W.: A note on *in vitro* inhibition of thymine degradation by some pyrimidine analogues and related products. Z. Natur. Forsch. (b) **24**, 469—470 (1969).

AHNSTROM, G., EHRENBERG, L., HUSSAIN, S., NATARAJAN, A.T.: On the killing and mutagenic actions in *E. coli* associated with Auger effect during ^{125}I decay. Mutation Res. **10**, 247—250 (1970).

ANDERSON, H.C., CHACKO, S., ABBOTT, J., HOLTZER, H.: The loss of phenotypic traits by differentiated cells *in vitro*. VII. Effect of 5-bromodeoxyuridine and prolonged culturing on fine structure of chondrocytes. Amer. J. Pathol. **60**, 289—311 (1970).

APPLEYARD, G., WESTWOOD, J.C.N.: The growth of rabbitpox virus in tissue culture. J. gen. Microbiol. **37**, 391—401 (1964).

ASCOLI, F., KAHAN, F.M.: Iodination of nucleic acids in organic solvents with iodine monochloride. J. biol. Chem. **241**, 428—431 (1966).

ASHKENAZI, A.: Action of 5-iodo-2′-deoxyuridine (IUdR) on *in vitro* transformation of hamster kidney cells by SV40 virus. Israel J. med. Sci. **1**, 1012—1014 (1965).

BADER, J.P.: The role of deoxyribonucleic acid in the synthesis of Rous Sarcoma Virus. Virology **22**, 462—468 (1964).

BADER, J.P.: The requirements for DNA synthesis in the growth of Rous Sarcoma and Rous Associated viruses. Virology **26**, 253—261 (1965).

BAGSHAW, M.A., DOGGETT, R.L.S.: A clinical study of chemical radiosensitization. Front. Radiat. Ther. Oncol. **4**, 164—173 (1969).

BAGSHAW, M.A., DOGGETT, R.L.S., SMITH, K.C., KAPLAN, H.S., NELSON, T.S.: Intra-arterial 5-bromodeoxyuridine and x-ray therapy. Amer. J. Roetgenol. Radium. Therapy Nucl. Med., **99**, 886—894 (1967).

BAKER, B.R.: Irreversible enzyme inhibitors. LXXV. Inhibitors of thymidine phosphorylase. I. Mode of ribofuranose binding. J. med. Chem. **10**, 297—301 (1967).

BAKER, B.R., BZESZOTARSKI, W.: Irreversible enzyme inhibitors. CIV. Inhibitors of thymidine phosphorylase. VIII. Further studies on hydrophobic bonding with 6-substituted uracils. J. med. Chem. **10**, 1109—1113 (1967).

BAKER, B.R., BZESZOTARSKI, W.: Irreversible enzyme inhibitors. CXXI. Thymidine phosphorylase. IX. On the nature and dimensions of the hydrophobic bonding region. J. med. Chem. **11**, 639—644 (1968).

BAKHLE, Y.S., PRUSOFF, W.H.: The effect of 5-iodo-2′-deoxyuridine and its mono- and triphosphates on some enzymes concerned with the biosynthesis of DNA in cell-free extracts of murine neoplastic cells. Biochim. biophys. Acta (Amst.) **174**, 302—308 (1969).

BAKHLE, Y.S., PRUSOFF, W.H., MCCREA, J.F.: Precaution in the use of iodine-125 as a radioactive tracer. Science **143**, 799—800 (1964).

BALDWIN, R.L., SHOOTER, E.M.: The alkaline transition of BU-containing DNA and its bearing on the replication of DNA. J. molec. Biol. **7**, 511—526 (1963).

BARRETT, H.W., MUNAVALLI, S.N., NEWMARK, P.: Synthetic pyrimidines as inhibitors of uracil and thymine degradation by rat-liver supernatant. Biochim. biophys. Acta (Amst.) **91**, 199—204 (1964).

BARRETT, H.W., WEST, R.A.: Dehalogenation of substituted pyrimidines *in vivo*. J. amer. Chem. Soc. **78**, 1612—1615 (1956).

BARRY, R. D., IVES, D. R., CRUICKSHANK, J. G.: Participation of deoxyribonucleic acid in the mutiplication of influenza virus. Nature (Lond.) **194**, 1139—1140 (1962).
BARTON, B. W., TOBIN, J. O. H.: The effect of idoxuridine on the excretion of cytomegalovirus in congenital infection. Ann. N. Y. Acad. Sci. **173**, 90—95 (1970).
BAUEROVA, J., SEBESTA, K., ŠORM, F., ŠORMOVA, Z.: Effect of uracil analogs on the metabolism of pyrimidines in cucumber seedlings. Coll. Czech. Chem. Commun. **25**, 2906—2911 (1960).
BAUGNET-MANIEU, GOUTIER, R.: Mechanisms responsible for the low incorporation into DNA of the thymidine analogue, 5-iodo-2′-deoxyuridine. Biochem. Pharmacol. **17**, 1017—1023 (1968).
BELTZ, R. E., VISSER, D. W.: Growth inhibition of *Esherichia coli* by new thymidine analogs. J. Amer. chem. Soc. **77**, 736—738 (1955).
BENZER, S., FREESE, E.: Induction of specific mutations with 5-bromouracil. Proc. nat. Acad. Sci. (Wash.) **44**, 112—119 (1958).
BERENS, K., SHUGAR, D.: Ultraviolet absorption spectra and structure of halogenated uracils and their glycosides. Acta biochim. polon. **10**, 25—47 (1963).
BERRY, R. J., ANDREWS, J. R.: Modification of radiation effect on mammalian tumor cells by pharmacological agents. Nature (Lond.) **196**, 185—186 (1962a).
BERRY, R. J., ANDREWS, J. R.: Modification of the radiation effect on the reproductive capacity of tumor cells *in vivo* with pharmacological agents. Radiol. Res. **16**, 82—88 (1962b).
BERRY, R. J., ANDREWS, J. R.: Quantitative relationships between radiation dose and the reproductive capacity of tumor cells in a mammalian system *in vivo*. Radiology **77**, 824—830 (1962c).
BERTANI, L. E., HAGGMARK, A., REICHARD, P.: Enzymatic synthesis of deoxyribonucleotides. J. biol. Chem. **238**, 3407—3413 (1963).
BESSMAN, J. J., LEHMAN, I. R., SIMMS, E. S., KORNBERG, A.: Enzymatic synthesis of deoxyribonucleic acid. II. General properties of the reaction. J. biol. Chem. **233**, 171—177 (1958).
BIEBER, S., ELION, G. B., HITCHINGS, G. H., HOOPER, D. C., NATHAN, H. C.: Suppression of the immune response by drugs in combinations. Proc. Soc. exp. Biol. (N. Y.) **111**, 334—337 (1962).
BIRNIE, G. D., KROEGER, H., HEIDELBERGER, C.: Studies of fluorinated pyrimidines. XVIII. The degradation of 5-fluoro-2′-deoxyuridine and related compounds by nucleoside phosphorylase. Biochemistry **2**, 566—572 (1963).
BISCHOFF, R., HOLTZER, H.: Inhibition of hyaluronic acid synthesis by BUdR in cultures of chick amnion cells. Anat. Rec. **160**, 317 (1968).
BISCHOFF, R., HOLTZER, H.: Inhibition of myoblast fusion after one round of DNA synthesis in 5-bromodeoxyuridine. J. Cell Biol. **44**, 134—150 (1970).
BOOTH, B. A., SARTORELLI, A. C.: Growth inhibition of a spectrum of transplanted mouse tumors by combinations of inhibitors of nucleic acid biosynthesis and alkylating agents. Cancer Res. **23**, 1762—1768 (1963).
BOWEN, J. M., ELLIOTT, A. Y., SYKES, J. A., DMOCHOWSKI, L. L.: Effect of halogenated pyrimidines on polyoma virus multiplication *in vitro*. Proc. Amer. Assoc. Cancer Res. **3**, 306 (1962).
BOWEN, J. M., ELLIOTT, A. Y., SYKES, J. A., DMOCHOWSKI, L. L.: Fluorescent microscopy of polyoma-infected cells treated with halogenated pyrimidine analogues. Acta. un. int. contra cancrum. **20**, 1062—1063 (1964).
BOWEN, J. M., HUGHES, R. G., DMOCHOWSKI, L. L.: Studies on the inhibition of polyoma virus replication *in vitro:* comparison of the effects of phenethyl alcohol, 5-iodo-2′-deoxyuridine, puromycin, and actinomycin D. Texas Rep. biol. Med. **24**, 143—157 (1966).
BOYCE, R. P., SETLOW, R. B.: A simple method of increasing the incorporation of thymidine into the deoxyribonucleic acid of *Escherichia coli*. Biochim. biophys. Acta (Amst.) **61**, 618—620 (1962).
BRAMMER, K. W.: Chemical modification of viral ribonucleic acid. II. Bromination and iodination. Biochim. biophys. Acta (Amst.) **72**, 217—229 (1963).
BREEDEN, C. J., HALL, T. C., TYLER, H. R.: Herpes simplex encephalitis treated with systemic 5-iodo-2′-deoxyuridine. Ann. intern. Med. **65**, 1050—1056 (1966).
BREITMAN, T. R., PERRY, S., COOPER, R. A.: Pyrimidine metabolism in human leukocytes. III. The utilization of thymine for DNA-thymine synthesis by leukemic leukocytes. Cancer Res. **26**, 2282—2285 (1966).
BRESNICK, E., THOMPSON, U. B.: Properties of deoxythymidine kinase partially purified from animal tumors. J. biol. Chem. **240**, 3967—3974 (1965).
BROCKMAN, R. W., ANDERSON, E. P.: Biochemistry of cancer (metabolic aspects). Ann. Rev. Biochem. **32**, 463—512 (1963).
BROWN, D. M., TODD, A. R., VARADARAJAN, S.: Nucleotides. Part XL. O^2: 5′-cyclouridine and a synthesis of isocytidine. J. chem. Soc., 868—872 (1957).
BROWN, G. B., WEINFELD, H., ROLL, P. M.: In: MCELROY, W. D., GLASS, B. (Eds.): Phosphorus metabolism, p. 388. Baltimore: Johns Hopkins Press 1952.

BROWN, J. M., GOFFINET, D. R., CLEAVER, J. E., KALLMAN, R. F.: Preferential radiosensitization of mouse sarcoma relative to normal skin by chronic intra-arterial infusion of halogenated pyrimidine analogs. J. nat. Cancer Inst. **47**, 75—89 (1971).
BROWNSTONE, A. D.: A simple preparation of 5-iodo-2′-deoxyuridine labelled with iodine-131 using iodine monochloride. Nature (Lond.) **199**, 1285 (1963).
BRYANT, B. J.: Reutilization of leukocyte DNA by cells of regenerating liver. Exp. Cell Res. **27**, 70—79 (1962).
BUDMAN, D. R., PARDEE, A. B.: Thymidine and thymine incorporation into deoxyribonucleic acid: inhibition and repression by uridine of thymidine phosphorylase of *Escherichia coli*. J. Bact. **94**, 1546—1550 (1967).
BUI, N. M., GILLETT, R., DUMONT, P.: An improved synthesis of 5-iodo-2′-deoxyuridine-I^{131} and 5-iodouracil-I^{131}. Int. J. Appl. Rad. Isotopes **16**, 337—339 (1965).
BURCHENAL, J. H., OETTGEN, H. F., REPPERT, J. A., COLEY, V.: Studies on the synergism of fluorinated pyrimidines and certain pyrimidine and purine derivatives against transplanted mouse leukemia. Cancer Chemother. Rep. **6**, 1—5 (1960).
BURKI, K., SHAER, J. C., SCHINDLER, R.: Die Verwendung von Jod-desoxyuridin ^{131}I zur Messung der Zellproliferation in der regenerierenden Rattenleber. Schweiz. med. Wochen. **99**, 1163—1164 (1969).
BYRD, D. M.: On the lethal effect of 5-iodouracil on bacteriophage T4. Ph. D. Dissertation. New Haven: Yale University (1971).
CALABRESI, P.: Regional protection in cancer chemotherapy. I. Infusions of thymidine into external cartotid artery of patients receiving systemic 5-iodo-2′-deoxyuridine. J. clin. Invest. **41**, 1484—1491 (1962).
CALABRESI, P.: Current status of clinical investigations with 6-azauridine, 5-iodo-2′-deoxyuridine, and related compounds. Cancer Res. **23**, 1260—1267 (1963).
CALABRESI, P., CARDOSO, S. C., FINCH, S. C., KLIGERMAN, M. M., VON ESSEN, C. F., CHU, M. Y., WELCH, A. D.: Initial clinical studies with 5-iodo-2′-deoxyuridine. Cancer Res. **21**, 550—559 (1961).
CALABRESI, P., CREASEY, W. A., PRUSOFF, W. H., WELCH, A. D.: Clinical and pharmacological studies with 5-iodo-2′-deoxycytidine. Cancer Res. **23**, 583—592 (1963a).
CALABRESI, P., MCCOLLUM, R. W., WELCH, A. D.: Suppression of infections resulting from a deoxyribonucleic acid virus (vaccinia) by systemic administration of 5-iodo-2′-deoxyuridine. Nature (Lond.) **197**, 767—769 (1963b).
CALABRESI, P., WELCH, A. D.: Chemotherapy of neoplastic diseases. Ann. Rev. Med. **13**, 147—202 (1962).
CAMERMAN, N., TROTTER, J.: 5-Iodo-2′-deoxyuridine: relation of structure to its antiviral activity. Science **144**, 1348—1350 (1964).
CAMERMAN, N., TROTTER, J.: The crystal and molecular structure of 5-iodo-2′-deoxyuridine. Acta crystalog. **18**, 203—211 (1965).
CANELLAKIS, E. S.: Pyrimidine metabolism. I. Enzymatic pathways of uracil and thymine degradation. J. biol. Chem. **221**, 315—322 (1956).
CANELLAKIS, E. S.: Pyrimidine metabolism. II. Enzymatic pathways of uracil anabolism. J. biol. Chem. **227**, 329—338 (1957).
CANELLAKIS, E. S., GOTTESMAN, M. E., KAMMEN, H. O.: A method for the synthesis of ribonucleoside and deoxyribonucleoside-5′-triphosphate. Biochim. biophys. Acta (Amst.) **39**, 82—87 (1960).
CANELLAKIS, E. S., MANTSAVINOS, R.: The conversion of ^{14}C-deoxynucleoside 5′-monophosphates to the corresponding di- and triphosphates by soluble mammalian enzymes. Biochim. biophys. Acta (Amst.) **27**, 643—645 (1958).
CHACKO, S., HOLTZER, S., HOLTZER, H.: Suppression of chondrogenic expression in mixtures of normal chondrocytes and BUdR-altered chondrocytes grown *in vitro*. Biochem. biophys. Res. Commun. **34**, 183—189 (1969).
CHANG, P. K.: Iodination of 2′-deoxycytidine and related substances. A reinvestigation of the structures of the by-product, $C_9H_{10}I_2N_2O_5$ and its derivatives. J. org. Chem. **30**, 3913—3915 (1965).
CHANG, P. K., WELCH, A. D.: Preparation of 5-iodo-2′-deoxycytidine. Biochem. Pharmacol. **8**, 327—328 (1961).
CHANG, P. K., WELCH, A. D.: Iodination of 2′-deoxycytidine and related substances. J. med. Chem. **6**, 428—430 (1963).
CHAUBE, S., MURPHY, M. L.: Teratogenic effects of 5-chlorodeoxyuridine on the rat fetus; protection by physiological pyrimidines. Cancer Res. **24**, 1986—1990 (1964).
CHAUDHURI, N. K., MUKHERJEE, K. L., HEIDELBERGER, C.: Studies on fluorinated pyrimidines. VII. The degradative pathway. Biochem. Pharmacol. **1**, 328—341 (1958).
CHEONG, L., RICH, M. A., EIDINOFF, M. L.: Introduction of the 5-halogenated uracil moiety into deoxyribonucleic acid of mammalian cells in culture. J. biol. Chem. **235**, 1441—1447 (1960).

CLARKSON, D. R., OPPELT, W. W., BYVOET, P.: The fate of 5-iodo-2′-deoxyuridine (IUdR) in plasma and cerebrospinal fluid of dogs. J. Pharmacol. exp. Ther. **157**, 581—588 (1967).
CLIFTON, K. H., SZYBALSKI, W., HEIDELBERGER, C., GOLLIN, F. F., ANSFIELD, F. J., VERMUND, H.: Incorporation of I^{125} labeled iododeoxyuridine into the deoxyribonucleic acid of murine and human tissues following therapeutic doses. Cancer. Res. **23**, 1715—1723 (1963).
CLIFTON, K. H., YATVIN, M. B.: Cell population growth and cell loss in the MTG-B mouse mammary carcinoma. Cancer. Res. **30**, 658—664 (1970).
COGGIN, J. H., LARSON, V. M., HILLEMAN, M. R.: Prevention of SV_{40} virus tumorigenesis by irradiated, disrupted and iododeoxyuridine treated tumor cell antigens. Proc. Soc. exp. Biol. (N.Y.) **124**, 774—784 (1967).
COHEN, S. S.: The biochemistry of viruses. Ann. Rev. Biochem. **32**, 83—154 (1963).
COHEN, S. S., FLAKS, J. G., BARNER, H. D., LOEB, M. R., LICHTENSTEIN, J.: The mode of action of 5-fluorouracil and its derivatives. Proc. nat. Acad. Sci. **44**, 1004—1012 (1958).
COLEMAN, J. R., COLEMAN, A. W., HARTLINE, E. J. H.: A clonal study of the reversible inhibition of muscle differentiation by the halogenated thymidine analog 5-bromodeoxyuridine. Dev. Biol. **19**, 527—548 (1969).
COLEMAN, A. W., COLEMAN, J. R., KANKEL, D., WERNER, I.: The reversible control of animal cell differentiation by the thymidine analog 5-bromodeoxyuridine. Exp. Cell Res. **59**, 319—328 (1970).
COMMERFORD, S. L.: Biological stability of IUdR labeled with ^{125}I after incorporation into the DNA of the mouse. Nature (Lond.) **206**, 949—950 (1965).
COMMERFORD, S. L.: Iodination of nucleic acids *in vitro*. Biochemistry **10**, 1993—1999 (1971).
COMMERFORD, S. L., GITLIN, D., HUGHES, W. L.: Inhibitory effect of small doses of x-radiation on incorporation of iododeoxyuridine (IDU) into DNA. Fed. Proc. **19**, 359 (1960).
CONCHIE, A. F., BARTON, B. W., TOBIN, J. O'H.: Congenital cytomegalovirus infection treated with idoxuridine. Brit. med. J. **4**, 162—163 (1968).
COOPER, A. D., BURGEN, M. W., WHITE, C. W., HERRMANN, R. L.: Effect of iododeoxyuridine upon conjugation and the fate of transferred deoxyribonucleic acid in *Escherichia coli*. K12. J. Bact. **107**, 433—441 (1971).
COOPER, G. M., DUNNING, W. F., GREER, S.: Role of catabolism in pyrimidine utilization for nucleic acid synthesis *in vivo*. Cancer Res. **32**, 390—397 (1972).
COOPER, G. M., GREER, S.: Irreversible inhibition of dehalogenation of 5-iodouracil by 5-diazouracil and reversible inhibition by 5-cyanouracil. Cancer Res. **30**, 2937—2941 (1970).
CRAIG, A. W., GARRETT, J. V., JACKSON, S. M.: Quantitation of lymphocyte transformation using radioactive iododeoxyuridine. J. clin. Path. **22**, 558—559 (1969).
CRAMER, J. W., MORRIS, N. R.: Absence of DNA synthesis in one-half of a population of mammalian tumor cells inhibited in culture by 5-iodo-2′-deoxyuridine. Molec. Pharmacol. **2**, 363—367 (1966).
CRAMER, J. W., PRUSOFF, W. H., WELCH, A. D., SARTORELLI, A. C., DELAMORE, I. W., VON ESSEN, C. F., CHANG, P. K.: Studies on the biochemical pharmacology of 5-iodo-2′-deoxycytidine *in vitro* and *in vivo*. Biochem. Pharmacol. **11**, 761—768 (1962).
CRAMER, J. W., WACKER, A., WELCH, A. D.: Biochemical studies of the effect of 5-iodo-2′-deoxyuridine (IUdR) on herpes simplex virus (HSV) infection of HeLa cells. Biochem. J. **87**, 26P (1963).
CREASY, W. H.: Studies on the metabolism of 5-iodo-2′-deoxycytidine *in vitro*. Purification of nucleoside deaminase from mouse kidney. J. biol. Chem. **238**, 1772—1776 (1963).
CUDKOWICZ, G., UPTON, A. C., SMITH, L. H., GOSSLEE, D. G., HUGHES, W. L.: An approach to the characterization of stem cells in mouse bone marrow. Ann. N.Y. Acad. Sci. **117**, 571—582 (1964).
CYSYK, R., PRUSOFF, W. H.: Alteration of ultraviolet sensitivity of thymidine kinase by allosteric regulators, normal substrates, and a photoaffinity label, 5-iodo-2′-deoxyuridine, a metabolic analog of thymidine. J. biol. Chem. **247**, 2522—2532 (1972).
DANIEL, P. M., GALE, M. M., PRATT, O. E.: Advantages of iodine-125 for studying thyroid function in experimental animals. Nature (Lond.) **196**, 1065—1066 (1962).
DANZIGER, R. M., HAYON, E., LANGMUIR, M. E.: Pulse radiolysis and flash photolysis study of aqueous solutions of simple pyrimidines. Uracil and bromouracil. J. phys. Chem. **72**, 3842—3849 (1968).
DAVIS, D. R., BALDWIN, R. L.: x-Ray studies of two synthetic DNA copolymers. J. molec. Biol. **6**, 251—255 (1963).
DAVIS, W. E., SCHOFIELD, R., COLE, L. J.: Deficient Fe^{59} and I^{125} deoxyuridine uptake by lympho-hemopoietic cell transplants engaged in homograft reactions. J. Cell Physiol. **71**, 185—196 (1968).
DEINHARDT, F.: In discussion in symposium on antiviral substances. Ann. N.Y. Acad. Sci. **130**, 218—219 (1965).

DELAMORE, I. W., PRUSOFF, W. H.: Effect of 5-iodo-2′-deoxyuridine on the biosynthesis of phosphorylated derivatives of thymidine. Biochem. Pharmacol. **11**, 101—112 (1962).
DETHLEFSEN, L. A.: Tumor radioactivity from ^{125}I or ^{3}H-labeled IUdR. Cancer. Res. **29**, 1717—1720 (1969a).
DETHLEFSEN, L. A.: Incorporation of ^{125}I-labeled 5-iodo-2′-deoxyuridine into the DNA of mouse mammary tumors. In: FRY, R. J. M., GRIEM, M. L., KIRSTEN, W. H. (Eds.): Normal and malignant cell growth, p. 186—201. Berlin-Heidelberg-New York: Springer 1969b.
DETHLEFSEN, L. A.: Reutilization of ^{131}I-5-iodo-2′-deoxyuridine as compared to ^{3}H-thymidine in mouse duodenum and mammary tumor. J. nat. Cancer Inst. **44**, 827—840 (1970).
DETHLEFSEN, L. A.: An evaluation of radioiodine-labeled 5-iodo-2′-deoxyuridine as a tracer for measuring cell loss from solid tumors. Cell Tissue Kinet. **4**, 123—138 (1971).
DETHLEFSEN, L. A., CUNNINGHAM, J., POWELL, E.: Reutilization of ^{131}I-5-iodo-2′-deoxyuridine as compared to ^{3}H-thymidine in mouse duodenum and mammary tumor. Proc. Amer. Assoc. Cancer. Res. **10**, 19 (1969).
DETHLEFSEN, L. A., MENDELSOHN, M. L.: Uptake of labeled 5-iodo-2′-deoxyuridine (I^{125}IUDR) as an index of tumor growth. Radiat. Res. **22**, 182 (1964).
DEVERDIER, C. H., POTTER, V. R.: Alternative pathways of thymine and uracil metabolism in the liver and hepatoma. J. nat. Cancer Inst. **24**, 13—29 (1960).
DEWEY, W. C., WESTRA, A., MILLER, H. H., NAGASAWA, H.: Heat-induced lethality and chromosomal damage in synchronized Chinese hamster cells with 5-bromodeoxyuridine. Inst. J. Radiat. Biol. **20**, 505—520 (1971).
DIDERHOLM, H., FICHTELIUS, O., LINDER, O.: Availability time of ^{3}H-label after administration of ^{3}H-thymidine *in vivo*. Exp. Cell Res. **27**, 431—435 (1962).
DIPAOLO, J. A.: Polydactylism in the offspring of mice injected with 5-bromodeoxyuridine. Science **145**, 501—503 (1964).
DIWAN, A., PRUSOFF, W. H.: The effect of 5-iodo-2′-deoxyuridine-5′-triphosphate, an allosteric inhibitor, on deoxycytidylate deaminase "induced" by herpes simplex virus. Virology **34**, 184—186 (1968).
DJORDJEVIC, B., SZYBALSKI, W.: Genetics of human cell lines. III. Incorporation of 5-bromo- and 5-iododeoxyuridine into the deoxyribonucleic acid of human cells and its effect on radiation sensitivity. J. exp. Med. **112**, 509—531 (1960).
DOGGETT, R. L. S., BAGSHAW, M. A., KAPLAN, H. S.: Combined therapy using chemotherapeutic agents and radiotherapy. In: DEELY, T. J., WOOD, C. A. P. (Eds.): Modern trends in radiotherapy, pp. 107—131. London: Butterworth's 1967.
DORSETT, M. T., MORSE, P. A., GENTRY, G. A.: Inhibition of rat dihydropyrimidine dehydrogenase by 5-cyanouracil *in vitro*. Cancer. Res. **29**, 79—82 (1969).
DOTY, P., BOEDTKER, H., FRESCO, J. R., HASELKORN, R., LITT, M.: Secondary structure in ribonucleic acids. Proc. nat. Acad. Sci. **45**, 482—499 (1959).
DUBBS, D. R., KIT, S.: Isolation and properties of vaccinia mutants deficient in thymidine kinase-inducing activity. Virology **22**, 214—225 (1964a).
DUBBS, D. R., KIT, S.: Mutant strains of herpes simplex virus deficient in thymidine kinase-inducing activity. Virology **22**, 493—502 (1964b).
DUBBS, D. R., KIT, S.: Effect of halogenated pyrimidine and thymidine on growth of L-cells and a subline lacking thymidine kinase. Exp. Cell Res. **33**, 19—28 (1964c).
DUBBS, D. R., KIT, S.: Effect of temperature on deoxythymidine kinase activity by herpes simplex mutants. Virology **25**, 256—270 (1965).
DUBBS, D. R., KIT, S., DE TORRES, R. A., ANKEN, M.: Virogenic properties of bromodeoxyuridine-sensitive and bromodeoxyuridine-resistant simian virus 40-transformed mouse kidney cells. J. Virol. **1**, 968—979 (1967).
DUNN, D. B., SMITH, J. D.: Incorporation of halogenated pyrimidines into the deoxyribonucleic acids of *Bacterium coli* and its bacteriophages. Nature (Lond.) **174**, 305—306 (1954).
DUNN, D. B., SMITH, J. D.: The occurrence of 6-methyl aminopurine in deoxyribonucleic acids. Biochem. J. **68**, 627—636 (1956).
DUNN, D. B., SMITH, J. D.: Effects of 5-halogenated uracils on the growth of *E. coli* and their incorporation into deoxyribonucleic acids. Biochem. J. **67**, 494—506 (1957).
DUNNEBACKE, T. H., REAUME, M. G.: Correlation of the yield of poliovirus with the size of isolated tissue culture cells. Virology **6**, 8—13 (1958).
DUSCHINSKY, R., WALKER, H., KARA, J.: Synthesis of 5′-deoxy and 5′-deoxy-5′-halonucleosides as inhibitors of thymidylate kinase. Abstr. 158th meeting Amer. Chem. Soc., New York Sept. 8—12, (1969).
DUTTON, R. W., DUTTON, A. H., VAUGHN, J. H.: The effect of 5-bromouracil deoxyribonucleoside on the synthesis of antibody *in vitro*. Biochem. J. **75**, 230—235 (1960).
DUTTON, R. W., PEARCE, J. D.: A survey of the effects of metabolic antagonists on the synthesis of antibody in an *in vitro* system. Immunology **5**, 414—423 (1962).

DUVAL, J., EBEL, J.P.: Halogénation des acides nucléiques. I. Action du brome sur les bases et les nucleosides en milieu diméthylformamide. Bull. Soc. chim. Biol. **46**, 1059—1071 (1964).
DUVAL, J., EBEL, J.P.: Halogénation des acides nucléiques. II. bromuration des acides ribonucléiques de levure en milieu diméthylformamide. Bull. Soc. chim. Biol. **47**, 787—806 (1965).
EASTERBROOK, K.B., DAVERN, C.I.: The effect of 5-bromodeoxyuridine on the multiplication of vaccinia virus. Virology **19**, 509—520 (1963).
EIDINOFF, M.L., CHEONG, L., GAMBETTA, G.E., BENUA, S., ELLISON, R.R.: Incorporation of 5-iodouracil labeled with iodine-131 into the deoxyribonucleic acid of human leukemic leucocytes following *in vivo* administration of 5-iododeoxyuridine labeled with iodine 131. Nature (Lond.) **183**, 1686—1687 (1959b).
EIDINOFF, M.L., CHEONG, L., RICH, M.A.: Incorporation of unnatural pyrimidine bases into the DNA of mammalian cells. Fed. Proc. **18**, 220 (1959a).
EIDINOFF, M.L., RICH, M.A.: Incorporation of unnatural pyrimidine bases into deoxyribonucleic acid of mammalian cells. Science **129**, 1550—1551 (1959).
ELION, G.B., HITCHINGS, G.H.: Metabolic basis for the actions of analogs of purines and pyrimidines. Advanc. Chemother. **2**, 91—177 (1965).
ELKIND, M.M., WHITMORE, G.F.: In: Radiobiology of cultured mammalian cells, p. 155—183. New York: Gordon and Breach 1967.
EPHRATI-ELIZUR, E., ZAMENHOF, S.: Incorporation of 5-bromouracil into transforming principle of *Bacillus subtilis* and its biological effects. Nature (Lond.) **184**, 472—473 (1959).
ERIKSON, R.L., SZYBALSKI, W.: Molecular radiobiology of human cell lines. I. Comparative sensitivity to x-rays and ultraviolet light of cells containing halogen-substituted DNA. Biochem. biophys. Res. Commun. **4**, 258—261 (1961).
ERIKSON, R.L., SZYBALSKI, W.: Molecular radiobiology of human cell lines. V. Comparative radiosensitizing properties of 5-halodeoxycytidines and 5-halodeoxyuridines. Radiat. Res. **20**, 252—262 (1963a).
ERIKSON, R.L., SZYBALSKI, W.: Molecular radiobiology of human cell lines. III. Radiation-sensitizing properties of 5-iododeoxyuridine. Cancer Res. **23**, 122—130 (1963b).
ERTL, H.H., FEINENDEGEN, L.E., HEINIGER, H.J.: Iodine 125, a tracer in cell biology; physical properties and biological aspects. Phys. med. Biol. **15**, 447—456 (1970).
ETZOLD, G., PREUSSEL, B., HINTSCHE, R., LANGEN, P.: Thymin-2′-desoxypentopyranoside als Hemmstoffe der Uridin-desoxyuridin-phosphorylase Konfigurations-Wirkungs-Beziehungen. Acta biol. med. germ. **20**, 437—442 (1968a).
ETZOLD, G., PREUSSEL, B., LANGEN, P.: Structural requirements for the inhibition of uridine-deoxyuridine phosphorylase by thymine nucleosides containing an unnatural carbohydrate moiety. Molec. Pharmacol. **4**, 20—24 (1968b).
EY, R.C., HUGHES, W.F., HOLMES, A.W.: Clinical and laboratory evaluation of idoxuridine (IDU) therapy in herpes simplex keratitis. Arch. Ophthalmal. **71**, 325—331 (1964).
FAHMY, O.G., FAHMY, M.J., DE VRYE, C.E.: The mutagenic properties of the nucleosides of pyrimidine analogues in *drosophila melanogaster*. Biochem. Pharmacol. **15**, 299—316 (1966).
FEELEY, E.J.: Effect of iododeoxyuridine on encephalomyocarditis virus. Antimicrob. Agent Chemother. 574—577 (1965).
FEINENDEGEN, L.E., BOND, V.P.: Differential uptake of ^{3}H-thymidine into the soluble fraction of single bone marrow cells, determined by autoradiography. Exp. Cell Res. **27**, 474—484 (1962).
FEINENDEGEN, L.E., BOND, V.P., CRONKITE, E.P., HUGHES, W.L.: RNA turnover in normal rat bone marrow. Ann. N.Y. Acad. Sci. **113**, 727—741 (1964).
FEINENDEGEN, L.E., BOND, V.P., HUGHES, W.L.: 125-IDU (5-iodo-2′-deoxyuridine) in autoradiographic studies of cell proliferation. Exp. Cell Res. **43**, 107—119 (1966a).
FEINENDEGEN, L.E., BOND, V.P., HUGHES, W.L.: Physiological thymidine reutilization in rat bone marrow. Proc. Soc. exp. Biol. (N.Y.) **122**, 448—455 (1966b).
FERRARI, W., GESSA, G.L., LODDO, B., SCHIVO, M.C.: Decreased pathogenicity for rabbit skin of IDU-resistant vaccinia virus. Virology **26**, 154—155 (1965).
FIDLER, I.J.: Metastasis: quantitative analysis of distribution and fate of tumor emboli labeled with ^{125}I-5-iodo-2′-deoxyuridine. J. nat. Cancer Inst. **45**, 773—782 (1970).
FIELDEN, E.M., LILLICARP, S.C.: Excited states and energy transfer in biomolecular systems. Curr. Topics Radiat. Res. Quart. **7**, 133—180 (1970—72).
FIKUS, M., WIERZCHOWSKI, K., SHUGAR, D.: Reversible photochemical transformation of 5-fluorouracil analogues and poly-5-fluorouridylic acid. Biochem. biophys. Res. Commun. **16**, 478—483 (1964).
FIKUS, M., WIERZCHOWSKI, K., SHUGAR, D.: Photochemistry of 5-fluorouracil analogues, glycosides and polyFU. Photochem. Photobiol. **4**, 521—536 (1965).

FILIP, J., NEJEDLY, Z.: Preparation of 5-halogeno derivatives of deoxyuridine labelled in base with ^{14}C. J. labelled Compounds **5**, 241—249 (1969).
FINK, K., CLINE, R. E., HENDERSON, R. B., FINK, R. M.: Metabolism of thymine (methyl-C^{14} or -2-C^{14}) by rat liver *in vitro*. J. biol. Chem. **221**, 425—433 (1956).
FISCHER, D. S., BLACK, F. L., WELCH, A. D.: Inhibition by nucleoside analogues of tumor formation by polyoma virus. Nature (Lond.) **206**, 839—840 (1965).
FISCHER, D. S., CASSIDY, E. P., WELCH, A. D.: Immunosuppression by pyrimidine nucleoside analogs. Biochem. Pharmacol. **15**, 1013—1022 (1966).
FOLSOME, C. E.: Effects of 5-bromodeoxyuridine upon gene recombination in *Escherichia coli* K12. Genetics **45**, 1111—1122 (1960).
FORCE, E. E., STEWART, R. C.: Effect of 5-iodo-2'-deoxyuridine on multiplication of Rous sarcoma virus *in vitro*. Proc. Soc. exp. Biol. Med. (N.Y.) **116**, 803—806 (1964a).
FORCE, E. E., STEWART, R. C.: Effect of 5-iodo-2'-deoxyuridine on the pathogenesis of Columbia-SK virus in mice. J. Immunol. **93**, 872—878 (1964b).
FOX, B. W., PERKINS, J. P., PRUSOFF, W. H.: Inhibitory action of thymine ribonucleoside and other pyrimidine derivatives on the cleavage of 5-iodo-2'-deoxyuridine by mouse-liver extract. Chem. biol. Interact. **1**, 331—340 (1969—70).
FOX, B. W., PRUSOFF, W. H.: The comparative uptake of I^{125} labeled 5-iodo-2'-deoxyuridine and thymidine-H^3 into tissues of mice bearing hepatoma-129. Cancer Res. **25**, 234—240 (1965).
FOX, B. W., PRUSOFF, W. H.: Effect of thymine ribonucleoside on the metabolism of ^{125}I-5-iodo-2'-deoxyuridine. Biochem. Pharmacol. **15**, 1317—1324 (1966).
FOX, E., MESELSON, M.: Unequal photosensitivity of the two strands of DNA in bacteriophage λ. J. molec. Biol. **7**, 583—589 (1963).
FOX, M., LAJTHA, L.: Continuous irradiation of P388F lymphoma *in vitro* sensitization by 5-iodo-2'-deoxyuridine. Int. J. Radiat. Biol. **12**, 251—264 (1967).
FREESE, E.: The specific mutagenic effect of base analogues on phage T4. J. molec. Biol. **1**, 87—105 (1959).
FRIEDKIN, M., ROBERTS, D.: The enzymatic synthesis of nucleosides. II. Thymidine and related pyrimidine nucleosides. J. biol. Chem. **207**, 257—266 (1954).
FRISCH, D. M., VISSER, D. W.: 5-Bromodeoxycytidine and 5-chlorodeoxycytidine. J. Amer. chem. Soc. **81**, 1756—1758 (1959).
FRITZON, P.: The catabolism of C^{14} labeled uracil, dihydrouracil and β-ureidopropionic acid in rat liver slices. J. biol. Chem. **226**, 223—228 (1957).
FUČÍK, V., KARA, J.: Enzymatic synthesis of 5-bromo-2'-deoxyuridine-2-^{14}C and 5-iodo-2'-deoxyuridine-2-^{14}C and their incorporation into deoxyribonucleic acid *(Allium cepa)*. Biol. Plant Acad. Sci. Bohemoslav **6**, 232—235 (1964).
FUJIWARA, Y., OKI, T., HEIDELBERGER, C.: Fluorinated pyrimidines. XXXVII. Effect of 5-trifluoromethyl-2'-deoxyuridine on the synthesis of deoxyribonucleic acid of mammalian cells in culture. Molec. Pharmacol. **6**, 273—280 (1970).
FUKUHARA, T. K., VISSER, D. W.: Cytidine derivatives. J. Amer. chem. Soc. **77**, 2393—2395 (1955).
FURUSAWA, E., CUTTING, W., BUCKLEY, P., FURUSAWA, S.: Complete cure of DNA virus infection in cultured cells by drug combinations. Proc. Soc. exp. Biol. (N.Y.) **116**, 938—944 (1964).
GABRIELSEN, A. E., GOOD, R. A.: Chemical suppression of adaptive immunity. Advanc. Immunol. **6**, 91—229 (1967).
GAITO, R. A., PRUSOFF, W. H.: Studies on the metabolism of thymine and 6-azathymine. Biochem. Pharmacol. **11**, 323—336 (1962).
GARRETT, E. R., CHERMBURKAR, P. B., SUZUKI, T.: Prediction of stability in pharmaceutical preparations. XIV. The complete pH dependent solvolytic degradations of an iodinated nucleoside, the antiviral 5-iodo-2'-deoxyuridine. Chem. pharm. Bull **13**, 1113—1130 (1965).
GARRETT, E. R., SUZUKI, T., WEBER, D. J.: The acidic solvolytic transformation of an iodinated nucleoside, the antiviral 5-iodo-2'-deoxyuridine. J. Amer. chem. Soc. **86**, 4460—4468 (1964).
GARRETT, E. R., YAKATAN, G. J.: Solvolysis of 5-halouridines and related nucleosides. J. pharm. Sci. **57**, 1478—1487 (1968).
GEERAETS, W. J., WONG, G., GUERRY, D. III: The effect of idoxuridine (IDU) on corneal stromal cells in tissue culture. Med. College Virginia Quart. 30—33 (1965).
GEORGATOS, J. G., ANTONOGLOU, O., GABRIELDER, C.: Incorporation of 5-iodo-2'-deoxyuridine-I^{131} into nuclear and mitochondrial DNA of normal and malignant mouse tissues. Arch. biochem. Biophys. **136**, 219—222 (1970).
GERBER, P.: Activation of Epstein-Barr virus by 5-bromodeoxyuridine in "virus-free" human cells. Proc. nat. Acad. Sci. (Wash.) **69**, 83—85 (1972).
GERBER, G. B., REMY-DEFRAIGNE, J.: Synthese der Desoxyribonucleinsäure in der isolierten perfundierten Rattenleber. Z. Naturforsch. **186**, 216—218 (1963).

Gimlin, D. M., Farquharson, E., Leach, F. R.: Effect of bromouracil-labelled transforming deoxyribonucleic acid of *Bacillus subtilis* on cell growth. Nature (Lond.) **197**, 407—408 (1963).

Gimlin, D. M., Hardman, S. D., Kelley, B. N., Butler, G. C., Leach, F. R.: Effect of bromouracil-containing deoxyribonucleic acid on *Bacillus subtilis*. J. Bact. **92**, 366—374 (1966).

Gitlin, D., Commerford, S. L., Amsterdam, E., Hughes, W.: x-Rays affect the incorporation of 5-iododeoxyuridine into deoxyribonucleic acid. Science **133**, 1074—1075 (1962).

Goffinet, D. R., Brown, J. M., Bagshaw, M. A., Kaplan, H. S.: Prolonged carotid arterial radiosensitizer infusion and radiation therapy of mouse gliomas. Amer. J. Roentgenol. Radium **114**, 7—15 (1972).

Goldin, A., Venditti, J. M., Kline, I., Mantel, N.: Evaluation of antileukemic agents employing advanced leukemia L1210 in mice IV. Cancer Res. **21**, CS 27 (1961).

Gontcharoff, M., Mazia, D.: Developmental consequences of introduction of bromouracil into the DNA of sea urchin embryos during early division stages. Exp. Cell Res. **46**, 315—327 (1967).

Gotto, A. M., Belkhode, M. L., Touster, O.: Stimulatory effects of inosine and deoxyinosine on the incorporations of uracil-2-^{14}C, 5-fluorouracil-2-^{14}C, and 5-bromouracil-2-^{14}C into nucleic acids of Ehrlich ascites tumor cells *in vitro*. Cancer Res. **29**, 807—811 (1969).

Goulian, M.: Biosynthesis of DNA. Ann. Rev. Biochem. **40**, 855—898 (1971).

Goz, B., McCrea, J. F., Prusoff, W. H.: Unpublished observations.

Goz, B., Prusoff, W. H.: The ability of phage containing 5-iodo-2′-deoxyuridine-substituted deoxyribonucleic acid to induce enzymes. J. biol. Chem. **243**, 4750—4756 (1968).

Goz, B., Prusoff, W. H.: The relation of antiviral activity of IUdR to gene function in phage. Ann. N. Y. Acad. Sci. **173**, 379—389 (1970a).

Goz, B., Prusoff, W. H.: Pharmacology of viruses. Ann. Rev. Pharmacol. **10**, 143—170 (1970b).

Green, M., Pina, M.: Stimulation of the DNA synthesizing enzymes of cultured human cells by vaccinia virus infection. Virology **17**, 603—604 (1962).

Green, M., Pina, M., Chagoya, V.: Biochemical studies on adenovirus multiplication. V. Enzymes of deoxyribonucleic acid synthesis in cells infected by adenovirus and vaccinia virus. J. biol. Chem. **239**, 1188—1197 (1964).

Greenberg, G., Sommerville, R. L.: Deoxyuridylate kinase activity and deoxyuridine triphosphatase in *Escherichia coli*. Proc. nat. Acad. Sci. (Wash.) **48**, 247—257 (1962).

Greer, S.: Studies on ultraviolet irradiation of *Escherichia coli* containing 5-bromouracil in its DNA. J. gen. Micro. Biol. **22**, 618—634 (1960).

Greer, S., Zamenhof, S.: Effect of 5-bromouracil in deoxyribonucleic acid of *E. coli* on sensitivity to ultraviolet radiation. Abstr. papers 131st meeting. Amer. chem. Soc. 3C. 1957,

Greer, S., Zamenhof, S.: Studies of depurination of DNA by heat. J. molec. Biol. **4**, 123—141 (1962).

Grisolia, S., Cardoso, S. S.: The purification and properties of hydropyrimidine dehydrogenase. Biochim. biophys. Acta (Amst.) **25**, 430—431 (1957).

Gross, P. R.: The control of protein synthesis in embryonic development and differentiation. In: Moscona, A. A., Monroy, A. (Eds.): Current topics in developmental biology. New York: Academic Press 1967.

Grunberg-Manago, M., Michelson, A. M.: Polynucleotide analogues. II. Stimulation of amino acid incorporation by polynucleotide analogues. Biochim. biophys. Acta (Amst.) **80**, 431—440 (1964).

Gulati, O. D., Patel, D. G.: Effects of various drugs on insulin antibodies. Brit. J. Pharmac. **42**, 66—77 (1971).

Haas, R., Maass, G.: Die Wirkung von 5-jod-2′-desoxyuridine auf die Vermehrung von SV-40 in Gewebekulturen. Arch. Ges. Virusforsch. **14**, 567—582 (1964).

Hackett, P., Hanawalt, P.: Selectivity for thymine over 5-bromouracil by a thymine-requiring bacterium. Biochim. Biophys. Acta (Amst.) **123**, 356—363 (1966).

Hakala, M. T.: Tissue culture studies on mechanisms of action of some purine and thymine analogs. Fed. Proc. **17**, 236 (1958).

Hakala, M. T.: Mode of action of 5-bromodeoxyuridine on mammalian cells in culture. J. biol. Chem. **234**, 3072—3076 (1959).

Hakala, M.: Effect of 5-bromodeoxyuridine incorporation on survival of cultured mammalian cells. Biochim. biophys. Acta (Amst.) **61**, 815—823 (1962).

Hall, J. G., Smith, M. E.: Homing of lymph-borne immunoblasts to the gut. Nature (Lond.) **226**, 262—263 (1970).

Hampar, B., Derge, J. G., Martos, L. M., Walker, J. L.: Synthesis of Epstein-Barr virus after activation of the viral genome in a "virus-negative" human lymphoblastoid cell (Ragi) made resistant to 5-bromodeoxyuridine. Proc. nat. Acad. Sci. (Wash.) **69**, 78—82 (1972).

HAMPARIAN, V. V., HILLEMAN, M. R., KETLER, A.: Contributions to characterization and classification of animal viruses. Proc. Soc. exp. Biol. (N.Y.) **112**, 1040—1050 (1963).

HAMPTON, A., HAMPTON, E. G., EIDINOFF, M. L.: Nucleotides. III. Synthesis and effects with cells in culture of ^{131}I-labeled 5-iodo-2'-deoxyuridine-5'-phosphate. Biochem. Pharmacol. **11**, 155—159 (1962).

HAMPTON, E. G., EIDINOFF, M. L.: Administration of 5-iododeoxyuridine-I^{131} in the mouse and rat. Cancer Res. **21**, 345—352 (1961).

HAMPTON, E. G., RICH, M. A., EIDINOFF, M. L.: Introduction of the 5-iodouracil moiety into deoxyribonucleic acid of mammalian cells. J. biol. Chem. **235**, 3562—3566 (1960).

HANNA, C.: Effect of several analogs of idoxuridine on the uptake of tritium labeled thymidine in the rabbit cornea infected with herpes simplex. Exp. Eye Res. **5**, 164—167 (1966).

HANNA, C., WILKINSON, K. P.: Effect of idoxuridine on the uptake of tritium-labeled thymidine in the rabbit cornea infected with herpes simplex. Exp. Eye Res. **4**, 31—35 (1965).

HARTMAN, K., HEIDELBERGER, C.: Studies on fluorinated pyrimidines. XIII. Inhibition of thymidylate synthetase. J. Biol. Chem. **236**, 3006—3013 (1961).

HASSEL, O., ROMMING, C.: Direct structural evidence for weak charge transfer bonds in solids containing chemically saturated molecules. Quart. Rev. (Lond.) **16**, 1—18 (1962).

HEIDELBERGER, C.: Fluorinated pyrimidines. Prog. nucl. Acid. Res. **4**, 1—50 (1965).

HEIDELBERGER, C., GRIESBACH, L., GHOBAR, A.: The potentiation by 5-iodo-2'-deoxyuridine (IDUR) of the tumor-inhibitory activity of 5-fluoro-2'-deoxyuridine (FUDR). Cancer Chemother. Rept. **6**, 37—38 (1960).

HEINIGER, H. J., FEINENDEGEN, L. E., BURKE, K.: Reutilization of thymidine in various groups of rat bone marrow cells. Blood **37**, 340—348 (1971a).

HEINIGER, H. J., FRIEDRICH, G. D., FEINENDEGEN, L. E., CANTELMO, F.: Reutilization of 5 ^{125}I-iodo-2'-deoxyuridine and ^{3}H-thymidine in regenerating liver of mice. Proc. Soc. exp. Biol. (N.Y.) **137**, 1381—1384 (1971b).

HENSEN, D., SMITH, R. P., GEHRKE, J.: Murine cytomegalovirus: observations on growth *in vitro*, cytopathic effect, and inhibition with iododeoxyuridine. Arch ges. Virusforsch. **18**, 433—444 (1966).

HERRMANN, E. C., JR.: Plaque inhibition test for detection of specific inhibitors of DNA containing viruses. Proc. Soc. exp. Biol. (N.Y.) **107**, 142—145 (1961).

HERRMANN, E. C.: Sensitivity of herpes simplex virus, vaccinia virus, and adenoviruses to deoxyribonucleic acid inhibitors and thiosemicarbazones in a plaque suppression test. Appl. Microbiol. **16**, 1151—1155 (1968).

HILBERT, G. E., JOHNSON, T. B.: Researches on pyrimidines. CXVII. A method for the synthesis of nucleosides. J. Amer. chem. Soc. **52**, 4489—4499 (1930).

HIRT, B.: Evidence for semiconservative replication of circular polyoma DNA. Proc. nat. Acad. Sci. (Wash.) **55**, 997—1004 (1966).

HOFER, K. G.: Tumor cell death *in vivo* after administration of chemotherapeutic agents. Cancer Chemother. Rept. **53**, 273—281 (1969).

HOFER, K. G.: Radiation effects on death and migration of tumor cell in mice. Radiat. Res. **43**, 663—678 (1970).

HOFER, K. G., DIBENEDETTO, J., HUGHES, W. L.: Natural and asparaginase induced death of L5178Y leukemia cells *in vitro*. Z. Krebsforsch. **75**, 34—44 (1970).

HOFER, K. G., HOFER, M.: Kinetics of proliferation, migration and death of L1210 ascites cells. Cancer. Res. **31**, 402—408 (1971).

HOFER, K. G., HUGHES, W. L.: Incorporation of iododeoxyuridine-^{125}I into the DNA of L1210 leukemia cells during tumor development. Cancer Res. **30**, 236—243 (1970).

HOFER, K. G., HUGHES, W. L.: Radiotoxicity of intranuclear tritium, ^{125}iodine and ^{131}iodine. Radiat. Res. **47**, 94—109 (1971).

HOFER, K. G., PRENSKY, W., HUGHES, W. L.: The measurement of tumor cell death *in vivo* with iodine-125 labelled iododeoxyuridine. J. Cell. Biol. **39**, 62a (1968).

HOFER, K. G., PRENSKY, W., HUGHES, W. L.: Death and metastatic distribution of tumor cells in mice monitored with ^{125}I-iododeoxyuridine. J. nat. Cancer Inst. **43**, 763—773 (1969a).

HOFER, K. G., ROSENOFF, S., PRENSKY, W., HUGHES, W. L.: Spontaneous and amethopterin induced death of L1210 leukemia cells *in vivo*. Nature (Lond.) **221**, 576—577 (1969b).

HOFFER, M., DUSCHINSKY, R., FOX, J. J., YUNG, N.: Simple synthesis of pyrimidine-2'-deoxyribonucleosides. J. Amer. chem. Soc. **81**, 4112—4113 (1959).

HOFFMAN, J., POST, J.: Replication and 5-iodo-2'-deoxyuridine-^{3}H incorporation by tumor and normal cells. Cancer. Res. **26**, 1313—1318 (1966).

HOFFMANN, G. R.: Studies on the reversal of 5-fluorodeoxyuridine-induced mitotic inhibition by thymidine and thymidine analogs. Canad. J. Genet. Cytol. **12**, 230—240 (1970).

HOLTHAUSEN, H. S., CHACKO, S., DAVIDSON, E. A., HOLTZER, H.: Effect of 5-bromodeoxyuridine on expression of cultured chondrocytes grown *in vitro*. Proc. nat. Acad. Sci. (Wash.) **63**, 864—870 (1969).

Horwitz, J. P., Chua, J., Noel, M., DaRooge, M. A.: Nucleosides. IV. 1-(2-Deoxy-β-D-lyxofuranosyl) 5-iodouracil. J. med. Chem. **7**, 385—386 (1964).
Hoshino, T., Sano, K.: Radiosensitization of malignant brain tumors with bromouridine (thymidine analogue). Acta radiologica **8**, 15—26 (1969).
Hotz, G., Reuschl, H.: Damage to deoxyribose molecules and to U-gene reactivation in UV-irradiated 5-bromouracil-DNA of phage T4 Bor as influenced by cysteamine. Molec. Gen. Genet. **99**, 5—11 (1967).
Howard, B. D., Tessman, I.: Identification of the altered bases in mutated single-stranded DNA. J. molec. Biol. **9**, 364—371 (1964).
Howard, F. B., Frazier, J., Miles, H. T.: Interaction of poly-5-bromocytidylic acid with polyinosinic acid. A study of helix stability and spectroscopic properties. J. biol. Chem. **244**, 1291—1302 (1969).
Hsu, T. C., Billen, D., Levan, A.: Mammalian chromosomes *in vitro*. XV. Patterns of transformation. J. nat. Cancer Inst. **27**, 515—541 (1961).
Hsu, T. C., Somers, C. E.: Effect of 5-bromodeoxyuridine on mammalian chromosomes. Proc. nat. Acad. Sci. (Wash.) **47**, 396—403 (1961).
Hsu, T. C., Somers, C. E.: Properties of L cells resistant to 5-bromodeoxyuridine. Exp. cell. Res. **26**, 404—410 (1962).
Huebner, R. J., Lane, W. T., Welch, A. D., Calabresi, P., McCollum, R. W., Prusoff, W. H.: Inhibition by 5-iododeoxyuridine of the oncogenic effects of adenovirus type 12 in hamsters. Science **142**, 488—490 (1963).
Hughes, W. L., Commerford, S. L., Gitlin, D., Krueger, R. C., Schultze, B., Shah, V., Reilly, P.: Deoxyribonucleic acid metabolism *in vivo*. I. Cell proliferation and death as measured by incorporation and elimination of iododeoxyuridine. Fed. Proc. **23**, 640—648 (1964).
Humphrey, R. M., Hsu, T. C.: Further studies on biological properties of mammalian cell lines resistant to 5-bromodeoxyuridine. Texas Rep. Biol. Med. **23**, 321—336 (1965).
Hurlbert, R. P.: Preparation of nucleoside diphosphates and triphosphates. Meth. Enzymol. **3**, 785—805 (1957).
Hutchinson, F., Hales, H. B.: Mechanism of the sensitization of bacterial transforming DNA to ultraviolet light by the incorporation of 5-bromouracil. J. molec. Biol. **50**, 59—69 (1970).
Iball, J., Morgan, C. H., Wilson, H. R.: Structures of 5-bromodeoxyuridine and 5-bromouridine. Nature (Lond.) **209**, 1230—1232 (1966).
Inman, R. B., Baldwin, R. L.: Helix-random coil transition in synthetic DNA's of alternating sequence. J. molec. Biol. **5**, 172—184 (1962).
Inman, R. B., Baldwin, R. L.: Helix-random coil transitions in DNA homopolymer pair. J. molec. Biol. **8**, 452—469 (1964).
Inman, R. B., Schnos, M.: Partial denaturation of thymine and 5-bromouracil-containing DNA in alkali. J. molec. Biol. **49**, 93—98 (1970).
Ishihara, H., Wang, S. Y.: Photochemistry of 5-bromo-1,3-dimethyluracil in aqueous solution. Biochemistry **5**, 2302—2307 (1966).
Ives, D. H., Morse, P. A., Potter, V. R.: Feedback inhibition of thymidine kinase by thymidine triphosphate. Fed. Proc. **21**, 383 (1962).
Iwatsuki, N., Okazaki, R.: Mechanism of regulation of deoxythymidine kinase of *Escherichia coli*. I. Effect of regulatory deoxynucleotides on the state of aggregation of the enzyme. J. molec. Biol. **29**, 139—154 (1967).
Izutsu, K., Biesele, J. J.: Effects on HeLa cell division of physiologic deoxyribonucleosides and deoxyribonucleotides. Cancer Res. **26**, 910—928 (1966).
Jaffe, J. J., Prusoff, W. H.: The effect of 5-iododeoxyuridine upon the growth of some transplantable rodent tumors. Cancer Res. **20**, 1383—1388 (1960).
Johnson, T. B., Johns, C. O.: Researches on pyrimidines; some 5-iodo pyrimidine derivatives; 5-iodocytosine. J. biol. Chem. **1**, 305—318 (1905—06).
Joklik, W. K.: The intracellular fate of rabbitpox virus rendered noninfectious by various reagents. Virology **22**, 620—633 (1964).
Jones, O. W., Berg, P.: Studies on the binding of RNA polymerase to polynucleotides. J. molec. Biol. **22**, 199—209 (1966).
Jones, T. C., Dove, W. F.: Photosensitization of transcription by bromodeoxyuridine substitution. J. molec. Biol. **64**, 409—416 (1972).
Juel-Jensen, B. E.: Results of the treatment of zoster with idoxuridine in dimethylsulphoxide. Ann. N.Y. Acad. Sci. **173**, 74—82 (1970).
Kajiwara, K., Mueller, G. C.: Molecular events in the reproduction of animal cells. III. Fractional synthesis of DNA with BUdR and its effect on cloning efficiency. Biochim. biophys. Acta (Amst.) **91**, 486—493 (1964).
Kamiya, T., Ben-Porat, T., Kaplan, A. S.: Control of certain aspects of the infective process by progeny viral DNA. Virology **26**, 577—589 (1965).

KAMMEN, H. O.: Thymine metabolism in *Escherichia coli*. I. Factors involved in utilization of exogenous thymine. Biochim. biophys. Acta (Amst.) **134**, 301—311 (1967).
KANNER, L., HANAWALT, P.: Efficiency of utilization of thymine and 5-bromouracil for normal and repair DNA synthesis in bacteria. Biochim. biophys. Acta (Amst.) **157**, 532—545 (1968).
KAPLAN, A. S., BEN-PORAT, T.: Mode of replication of pseudorabies virus DNA. Virology **23**, 90—95 (1964).
KAPLAN, A. S., BEN-PORAT, T.: Mode of antiviral action of 5-iodouracil deoxyriboside. J. molec. Biol. **19**, 320—332 (1966).
KAPLAN, A. S., BEN-PORAT, T.: Differential incorporation of iododeoxyuridine into DNA of pseudorabies virus-infected and noninfected cells. Virology **31**, 734—736 (1967).
KAPLAN, A. S., BEN-PORAT, T., KAMIYA, T.: Incorporation of 5-bromodeoxyuridine and 5-iododeoxyuridine into viral DNA and its effect on the infective process. Ann. N.Y. Acad. Sci. **130**, 226—239 (1965).
KAPLAN, H. S.: Radiosensitization by the halogenated pyrimidine analogues: Laboratory and clinical investigations. In: MOROSON, H. L., QUINTILIANI, M. (Eds.): Radiation protection and sensitization. New York: Barnes and Noble 1970.
KARA, J.: Induction of deoxycytidylate deaminase and uridine kinase and activation of cellular DNA synthesis in the course of transformation of chicken embryo cells infected by Rous sarcoma virus *in vitro*. Folio Biolog. (Praha) **14**, 249—265 (1968).
KARA, J., DUSCHINSKY, R.: Inhibition of thymidylate kinase and DNA synthesis in HeLa cells by 5′-deoxythymidine. Biochim. biophys. Acta (Amst.) **186**, 223—225 (1969).
KARNOFSKY, D. A., BASCH, R. S.: Effect of 5-fluorodeoxyuridine and related halogenated pyrimidines on the sand-dollar embryo. J. biophys. biochem. Cytol. **7**, 61—71 (1960).
KAROL, M. H., SIMPSON, M. V.: DNA biosynthesis by isolated mitochondria: a replicative rather than repair process. Science **162**, 470—473 (1968).
KARPAS, A.: The effect of 5-bromo-2′-deoxyuridine on the multiplication of equine herpes 3 virus in rabbit kidney cells. Ann. Inst. Past. **112**, 308—315 (1967).
KASAMAKI, A., BEN-PORAT, T., KAPLAN, A. S.: Polyoma virus-induced release of inhibition of cellular DNA synthesis caused by iododeoxyuridine. Nature (Lond.) **217**, 756—758 (1968).
KAUFMAN, H. E.: Clinical cure of herpes simplex keratitis by 5-iodo-2′-deoxyuridine. Proc. Soc. exp. Biol. (N.Y.) **109**, 251—252 (1962).
KAUFMAN, H. E.: Treatment of herpes simplex and vaccinia keratitis by 5-iodo- and 5-bromo-2′-deoxyuridine, pp. 90—107. In: POLLARD, E. C. (Ed.): Perspectives in virology III. New York: Paul B. Hoeber 1963.
KAUFMAN, H. E.: *In vivo* studies with antiviral agents. Ann. N.Y. Acad. Sci. **130**, 168—180 (1965a).
KAUFMAN, H. E.: Problems in virus chemotherapy. Progr. med. Virol. **7**, 116—159 (1965b).
KAUFMAN, H. E., MALONEY, E. D.: Therapeutic antiviral activity in tissue culture. Proc. Soc. exp. Biol. (N.Y.) **112**, 4—7 (1963).
KAUFMAN, H. E., MARTOLA, E., DOHLMAN, C.: Use of 5-iodo-2′-deoxyuridine (IDU) in treatment of herpes simplex keratitis. Arch. Opthalmol **68**, 235—239 (1962a).
KAUFMAN, H. E., NESBURN, A. B., MALONEY, D. E.: IDU therapy of herpes simplex. Arch. Opthalmol. **67**, 583—591 (1962b).
KAZIMIERCZUK, Z., SHUGAR, D.: Photochemical transformation of 6-chlorouracil and some alkylated analogues. Biochim. biophys. Acta (Amst.) **254**, 157—166 (1971).
KIHLMAN, B. A.: Actions of chemicals on dividing cells. Englewood Cliffs N.J.: Prentice-Hall 1966.
KIM, J. H., GELBARD, A. S., PEREZ, A. G., EIDINOFF, M. L.: Effect of 5-bromodeoxyuridine on nucleic acid and protein synthesis and viability in HeLa cells. Biochim. biophys. Acta (Amst.) **134**, 388—394 (1967).
KIMURA, G., MORI, R.: Multiplication of polyoma virus in iododeoxyuridine (IUdR) — resistant mouse cells in the presence of IUdR. Life Sci. **5**, 1707—1714 (1966).
KIMURA, G., MORI, R., AMALEO, K.: Further studies on the effect of 5-iodouridine on polyoma virus multiplication in mouse cells. Japanese J. Microbiol. **10**, 211—219 (1966).
KIT, S.: Physicochemical studies on the deoxyribonucleic acids of mouse tissues. In: The molecular basis of neoplasia, pp. 133—146. Austin: Univ. of Texas Press 1962.
KIT, S., BECK, C., GRAHAM, O. L., GROSS, A.: Effect of 5-bromodeoxyuridine on deoxyribonucleic acid thymine synthesis and cell metabolism of lymphatic tissues and tumors. Cancer Res. **18**, 598—602 (1958).
KIT, S., DUBBS, D. R.: Biochemistry of vaccinia infected mouse fibroblasts (strain L-M). I. Effects on nucleic acid and protein synthesis. Virology **18**, 274—285 (1962a).
KIT, S., DUBBS, D. R.: Biochemistry of vaccinia-infected mouse fibroblasts (strain L-M). II. Properties of the chromosomal DNA of infected cells. Virology **18**, 286—293 (1962b).

KIT, S., DUBBS, D. R., FREARSON, P. M.: HeLa cells resistant to bromodeoxyuridine and deficient in thymidine kinase activity. Int. J. Cancer 1, 19—30 (1966).
KIT, S., DUBBS, D. R., PIERKARSKI, L. J., HSU, T. C.: Deletion of thymidine kinase activity from L cells resistant to bromodeoxyuridine. Exp. Cell Res. 31, 297—312 (1963).
KIT, S., HSU, T. C.: Relative stability to thermal denaturation of deoxyribonucleic acid (DNA) preparations containing bromodeoxyuridine. Biochem. biophys. Res. Commun. 5, 120—124 (1961).
KJELLEN, L.: Effect of 5-halogenated pyrimidines on cell proliferation and adenovirus multiplication. Virology 18, 64—70 (1962).
KJELLEN, L., PERIERA, H. G., VALENTINE, R. C., ARMSTRONG, J. A.: An analysis of adenovirus particles and soluble antigens produced in the presence of 5-bromodeoxyuridine. Nature (Lond.) 199, 1210—1211 (1963).
KLEMENT, V., NICOLSON, M. O., HUEBNER, R. J.: Rescue of the genome of focus forming virus from rat non-productive lines by 5-bromodeoxyuridine. Nature — New Biol. 234, 12—14 (1971).
KLEMPERER, H. G., HAYNES, G. R., SHEDDEN, W. I. H., WATSON, D. K.: A virus-specific thymidine kinase in BHK21 cells infected with herpes simplex virus. Virology 31, 120—128 (1967).
KLIGERMAN, M. M.: The roll of combination radiation and chemotherapy. Proc. Conference Research Radiotherapy Cancer, pp. 147—157. New York: Amer. Cancer Soc. 1961.
KNIGHT, V., GERONE, P. J., GRIFFITH, W. R., CAUDI, R. B., CATE, T. R., JOHNSON, K. M., LONG, D. J., EVANS, H. E., SPICHARD, A., KASEL, J. A.: Studies in volunteers with respiratory viral agents: small particle aerosol; heterotypic protections; viral chemotherapy; bovine reovirus. Amer. Rev. Respirat. Dis. 88, 135—147 (1963).
KOHNELEIN, W., HUTCHINSON, F.: ESR-studies of normal and 5-bromouracil substituted DNA of *Bacillis subtilis* after irradiation with ultraviolet light. Radiat. Res. 39, 745—757 (1969).
KOYAMA, H., ONO, T.: Effect of 5-bromodeoxyuridine on hyaluronic acid synthesis of a clonal hybrid line of mouse and chinese hamster in culture. J. cell. Physiol. 78, 265—272 (1971).
KOZINSKI, A. W., SZYBALSKI, W.: Dispersive transfer of the parental DNA molecule to the progeny of phage Φ X174. Virology 9, 260—274 (1959).
KRENITSKY, T. A., BARCLAY, M., JACQUEZ, J. A.: Specificity of mouse uridine phosphorylase chromotography, purification and properties. J. biol. Chem. 239, 805—812 (1964).
KRENITSKY, T. A., MELLORS, J. W., BARCLAY, R. K.: Pyrimidine nucleosidases: their classification and relationship to uric acid ribonucleoside phosphorylase. J. biol. Chem. 240, 1281—1286 (1965).
KRISCH, R. E.: Lethal effects of iodine-125 decay by electron capture in *Escherichia coli* and in bacteriophage T1. Int. J. Radiat. Biol. 21, 167—189 (1972).
KRISS, J. P., BOND, S. B.: The effect of natural and unnatural pyrimidines and pyrimidine nucleosides on the phosphorolysis of 5-iododeoxyuridine by mouse liver extract. Biochem. Pharmacol. 13, 365—370 (1964).
KRISS, J. P., MARUYAMA, Y., TUNG, L. A., BOND, S. B., REVESZ, L.: The fate of 5-bromodeoxyuridine, 5-bromodeoxycytidine, and 5-iododeoxycytidine in man. Cancer Res. 23, 260—268 (1963).
KRISS, J. P., REVESZ, L.: The distribution and fate of bromodeoxyuridine and bromodeoxycytidine in the mouse and rat. Cancer Res. 22, 254—265 (1962).
KRISS, J. P., TUNG, L., BOND, S.: The distribution and fate of iododeoxycytidine in the mouse and rat. Cancer Research 22, 1257—1264 (1962).
KRUEGER, R. C., GITLIN, D., COMMERFORD, S. L., STEIN, J., HUGHES, W. L.: Iododeoxyuridine (IDU) as a tracer of DNA metabolism *in vivo*. Fed. Proc. 19, 307 (1960).
KUCERA, L. S., HERRMANN, E. C.: Gradient plate technique applied to the study of antiviral substances. Proc. Soc. exp. Biol. (N.Y.) 122, 258—262 (1966).
LAIRD, C. D., BODMER, W. F.: 5-Bromouracil utilization by *Bacillis subtilis*. J. Bact. 94, 1277—1278 (1967).
LANDOLT, A. M.: Resultate der postoperativen Behandlung des Glioblastoma Multiforme mit einer strahlensensibilisierenden Substanz (5-bromo 2′-deoxyuridine). Acta Neurochirurgica 24, 263—268 (1971).
LANGEN, P., ETZOLD, G.: Desoxyglucosyl-thymin als Hemmstoff einer Pyrimidin Nucleosid-Phosphorylase aus Ascites-Tumorzellen. Bio. Zeitschrift 339, 190—197 (1963).
LANGEN, P., ETZOLD, G.: Enhancement of 5-iododeoxyuridine incorporation into DNA of cat tissues *in vivo* by inhibition of uridine-deoxyuridine phosphorylase. Molec. Pharmacol. 2, 89—92 (1966a).
LANGEN, P., ETZOLD, G.: Enhancement by deoxyglucosyl-thymine of the 5-iododeoxyuridine incorporation into DNA *in vivo* at high doses of 5-iododeoxyuridine. Acta biol. med. germ. 17, Kl-K3 (1966b).

LANGEN, P., ETZOLD, G., BARWOLFF, D., PREUSSEL, B.: Inhibition of thymidine phosphorylase by 6-aminothymine and derivatives of 6-aminouracil. Biochem. Pharmacol. **16**, 1833—1837 (1967).
LANGEN, P., ETZOLD, G., HINTSCHE, R., KOWOLLIK, G.: 3′-Deoxy-3′-fluorothymidine, a new selective inhibitor of DNA-synthesis. Acta biol. med. germ. **23**, 759—766 (1969a).
LANGEN, P., KOWOLLIK, G.: 5′-Deoxy-5′-fluorothymidine, a biochemical analogue of thymidine 5′-monophosphate selectively inhibiting DNA synthesis. Eur. J. Biochem. **6**, 344 (1968).
LANGEN, P., KOWOLLIK, G., SCHUTT, M., ETZOLD, G.: Thymidylate kinase as a target enzyme for 5′-deoxythymidine and various 5′-deoxy-5′-halogeno pyrimidine nucleosides. Acta. biol. med. germ. **23**, K19 (1969a).
LANGEN, P., LISS, E.: Die Verwertung von Thymidin, Bromdesoxyuridin und den freien Pyrimidenbasen Thymin, Bromouracil und Joduracil zur Desoxyribonucleinsäure-Synthese durch Ascites-Tumorzellen *in vitro*. Biochem. Zeit. **336**, 139—153 (1962).
LANGEN, P., VENKER, P.: Über die Einführung von Bromuracil in die Desoxyribonucleinsäure tumortragender Mäuse durch Gabe von Bromuracil und Desoxyguanosin. Acta biol. med. germ. **11**, 799—805 (1963).
LASHER, R., CAHN, R. D.: The effects of 5-bromodeoxyuridine on the differentiation of chondrocytes *in vitro*. Dev. Biol. **19**, 415—435 (1969).
LAWLEY, P. D., BROOKES, P.: Ionization of DNA bases or base analogues as a possible explanation of mutagenesis, with special reference to 5-bromodeoxyuridine. J. molec. Biol. **4**, 216—219 (1962).
LEDINKO, N.: Plaque assay of the effects of cytosine arabinoside and 5-iodo-2′-deoxyuridine on the synthesis of H-1 virus particles. Nature (Lond.) **214**, 1346—1347 (1967).
LEHMAN, I. R., BESSMAN, M. J., SIMMS, E. S., KORNBERG, A.: Enzymatic synthesis of deoxyribonucleic acid. I. Preparation of substrates and partial purification of enzyme from *Escherichia coli*. J. biol. Chem. **233**, 163—170 (1958).
LEONTIEVA, N. A., FADEEVA, L. L.: Investigation of biological and hemogglutinating properties of Ghetah arbovirus. Voprosy Virusologii **14**, 464—468 (1969).
LETT, J. T., CALDWELL, I., LITTLE, J. G.: Repair of x-ray damage to the DNA in *Micrococcus radiodurans*: the effect of 5-bromodeoxyuridine. J. molec. Biol. **48**, 395—408 (1970).
LEVENE, P. A., TIPSON, S.: The structure of monotrityl uridine. J. biol. Chem. **105**, 419—430 (1934).
LEVINSON, W. E., BISHOP, J. M., QUINTRELL, N., JACKSON, J., FANSHIER, L.: Synthesis of RNA in normal and Rous sarcoma virus-infected cells. Effect of bromodeoxyuridine. Virology **42**, 221—224 (1970).
LILLIE, M. G., MOHANTY, S. B.: The effect of 5-iodo-2′-deoxyuridine on the multiplication of infectious bovine Rhinotracheitis virus. Cornell Veterinarian **58**, 278—288 (1968).
LIN, S. Y., RIGGS, A. D.: Lac repressor binding to operator analogues. Comparison of poly (dA-T), poly (dA-BrU) and poly (dA-U). Biochem. biophys. Res. Commun. **45**, 1542—1547 (1971).
LION, M. B.: UV photoproducts in 5-bromouracil substituted DNA of *Escherichia coli* 15T. Third Inst. Cong. Radiation Res. Abstr. **25**, 211 (1965).
LION, M. B.: Search for a mechanism for the increased sensitivity of 5-bromouracil-substituted DNA to ultraviolet radiation. II. Single strand breaks in the DNA of irradiated 5-bromouracil-substituted T3 coliphage. Biochim. biophys. Acta (Amst.) **209**, 24—33 (1970).
LIPKIN, D., HOWARD, F. B., NOWOTNY, D., SANO, M.: The iodination of nucleosides and nucleotides. J. biol. Chem. **238**, 2249—2251 (1963).
LITMAN, R. M., PARDEE, A. B.: Production of bacteriophage mutants by a disturbance of deoxyribonucleic acid metabolism. Nature (Lond.) **178**, 529—531 (1956).
LITMAN, R. M., PARDEE, A. B.: The induction of mutants of bacteriophage T2 by 5-bromouracil. III. Nutritional and structural evidence regarding mutagenic action. Biochim. biophys. Acta (Amst.) **42**, 117—130 (1960a).
LITMAN, R. M., PARDEE, A. B.: The induction of mutants of bacteriophage T2 by 5-bromouracil. IV. Kinetics of bromouracil-induced mutagenesis. Biochim. biophys. Acta (Amst.) **42**, 131—140 (1960b).
LITMAN, R. M., SZYBALSKI, W.: Enzymatic synthesis of transforming DNA. Biochem. biophys. Res. Commun. **10**, 473—481 (1963).
LITTLEFIELD, J. W.: Studies on thymidine kinase in cultured mouse fibroblasts. Biochim. biophys. Acta (Amst.) **95**, 14—22 (1965).
LITTLEFIELD, J. W., GOULD, E. A.: The toxic effect of 5-bromodeoxyuridine on cultured epithelial cells. J. biol. Chem. **235**, 1129—1133 (1960).
LODDO, B., SCHIVO, M. L., FERRARI, W.: Development of vaccinia virus resistant to 5-iodo-2′-deoxyuridine. Lancet **2**, 914—915 (1963).

Lorkiewicz, Z., Szybalski, W.: Genetic effects of halogenated thymidine analogs incorporated during thymidylate synthetase inhibition. Biochem. biophys. Res. Commun. **2**, 413—418 (1960).

Lowy, D. R., Rowe, W. P., Teich, N., Hartley, J. W.: Murine leukemia virus; high-frequency activation *in vitro* by 5-iododeoxyuridine and 5-bromodeoxyuridine. Science **174**, 155—156 (1971).

Lozeron, H. A., Gordon, M. P., Gabriel, T., Tautz, W., Duschinsky, R.: The photochemistry of 5-fluorouracil. Biochemistry **3**, 1844—1850 (1964).

Lyons, M. J., Lasfargues, E. Y., Came, P.: Effect of actinomycin D and halogenated deoxyuridine on the replication of Bittner virus *in vitro*. Nature (Lond.) **212**, 100—101 (1966).

Maass, G., Haas, R.: Über die Bildung von virusspezifischem SV-40 Antigen in Gegenwart von 5-Jod-2'-Desoxyuridin. Arch. ges. Virusforsch. **18**, 253—256 (1966).

Maass, G., Müller, J., Nakanoin, K., Vogt, A., Haas, R.: Die Bildung inkompletter SV-40 Viren in Gegenwart von 5-Jod-2'-Desoxyuridin. Arch. ges. Virusforsch. **15**, 549—564 (1965).

MacCallum, F. O., Juel-Jensen, B. E.: Herpes simplex virus skin infection in man treated with idoxuridine in dimethylsulphoxide. Results of double blind controlled trial. Brit. med. J. **2**, 805—807 (1966).

Mak, S., Till, J. E.: Use of I^{125} labeled 5-iodo-2'-deoxyuridine for the measurment of DNA synthesis in mammalian cells *in vitro*. Canad. J. Biochem. **41**, 2343—2351 (1963).

Maley, F., Ochoa, S.: Enzymatic phosphorylation of deoxycytidylic acid. J. biol. Chem. **233**, 1538—1543 (1958).

Mark, J. B. D., Calabresi, P.: Regional protection in cancer chemotherapy. II. Preliminary studies with hypogastric artery infusion of thymidine during treatment with 5-iodo-2'-deoxyuridine. Cancer Chemother. Rep. **16**, 545—549 (1962).

Maruyama, Y.: Re-utilization of thymidine during death of a cell. Nature (Lond.) **201**, 93—94 (1964).

Massoulie, J. A., Michelson, A. M., Pochon, F.: Polynucleotide analogues. VI. Physical studies on 5-substituted pyrimidine polynucleotides. Biochim. biophys. Acta (Amst.) **114**, 16—26 (1966).

Mathias, A. P., Fischer, G. A.: The metabolism of thymidine by murine leukemic lymphoblasts (L5178Y). Biochem. Pharmacol. **11**, 57—68 (1962).

Mathias, A. P., Fischer, G. A., Prusoff, W. H.: Inhibition of the growth of mouse leukemia cells in culture by 5-iodo-deoxyuridine. Biochim. biophys. Acta (Amst.) **36**, 560—561 (1959).

Mayne, R., Sanger, J. W., Holtzer, H.: Inhibition of mucopolysaccharide synthesis by 5-bromodeoxyuridine in cultures of chick amnion cells. Dev. Biol. **25**, 547—567 (1971).

Mazia, D., Gontcharoff, M.: The mitotic behavior of chromosomes in echinoderm eggs following incorporation of bromodeoxyuridine. Exp. Cell Res. **35**, 14—25 (1964).

McAuslan, B. R., Joklik, W. K.: Stimulation of the thymidine phosphorylase system in HeLa cells on infection with poxvirus. Biochem. biophys. Res. Commun. **8**, 486—491 (1962).

McCrea, J. R., Lipman, M. B.: Strand-length measurements of normal and 5-iodo-2'-deoxyuridine treated vaccinia virus deoxyribonucleic acid released by the Kleinschmidt method. J. Virol. **1**, 1037—1044 (1967).

Melnick, J. L., Rapp, F.: The use of antiviral compounds in analyzing the sequential steps in the replication of SV40 papovavirus. Ann. N. Y. Acad. Sci. **130**, 291—309 (1965).

Mendelsohn, M. L., Dethlefsen, L. A.: Tumor growth and cellular kinetics. In: The proliferation and spread of neoplastic cells, pp. 197—212. Baltimore: William and Wilkins 1968.

Merits, I., Cain, J. C.: Loss of labeled DNA from rat brain following injections of precursors with high specific radioactivity. II. DNA labeled with 5-(^{131}I)iodo-2'-deoxyuridine and 5-(^{82}Br) bromo-2'-deoxyuridine. Biochim. biophys. Acta (Amst.) **209**, 327—338 (1970).

Meselson, M., Stahl, F. W., Vinograd, J.: Equilibrium sedimentation of macromolecules in density gradient. Proc. nat. Acad. Sci. **43**, 581—588 (1957).

Michelson, A. M.: Polynucleotides forme d'analogues de bases. Bull. Soc. chim. Biol. **47**, 1553—1562 (1965).

Michelson, A. M., Dondon, J., Grunberg-Manago, M.: The action of polynucleotide phosphorylase on 5-halogenouridine-5'-pyrophosphates. Biochim. biophys. Acta (Amst.) **55**, 529—540 (1962).

Michelson, A. M., Massoulie, J., Guschlbauer, W.: Synthetic polynucleotides. Progr. nucl. Acid. Res. **6**, 83—141 (1967).

Michelson, A. M., Todd, A. R.: Deoxyribonucleosides and related compounds. Part V. Cyclothymidines and other thymidine derivatives. The configuration at the glycosidic centre in thymidine. J. chem. Soc. 816—823 (1955).

Miller, F. A.: Inhibition of B virus in cell culture by 5-iodo-2'-deoxyuridine. Appl. Microbiol. **15**, 733—735 (1967).

MIURA, Y., WILT, F. H.: The effects of 5-bromodeoxyuridine on yolk sac erythropoiesis in the chick embryo. J. Cell Biol. **48**, 523—532 (1971).

MIZUNO, H., NAKANISHI, N., FUJIWARA, T., TOMITA, K., TSUKIHARA, T., ASHIDA, T., KAKUDO, M.: The crystal structure of two forms of 1-ethyl-5-bromouracil. Biochem. biophys. Res. Commun. **41**, 1161—1165 (1970).

MOHLER, W. C., ELKIND, M. M.: Radiation response of mammalian cells grown in culture. III. Modification of x-ray survival of Chinese hamster cells by 5-bromodeoxyuridine. Exp. Cell. Res. **30**, 481—491 (1963).

MONTONI, S., LODDO, B.: Attivita inhibente *in vitro* della 5-iododesossiuridin verso l'adenvirus 5. Boll. Soc. Ital. Biol. Sper. **39**, 4—6 (1963).

MORI, R., KIMURA, G.: Inhibitory effect of 5-Iododeoxyuridine on polyoma virus multiplication in mouse embryo cells. Life Sci. **4**, 1503—1507 (1965).

MORRIS, N. R., CRAMER, J. W.: DNA synthesis by mammalian cells inhibited in culture by 5-iodo-2'-deoxyuridine. Molec. Pharmacol. **2**, 1—9 (1966).

MORRIS, N. R., CRAMER, J. W.: 5-iodo-2'-deoxyuridine and DNA synthesis in mammalian cells. Exp. Cell Res. **51**, 555—563 (1968).

MOULTON, J., COGGIN, L.: Synthesis and cytopathogenesis of African swine fever virus in porcine cell cultures. Amer. J. Vet. Res. **29**, 219—232 (1968).

MUNYON, W., HUGHES, R., ANGERMANN, J., BERECZKY, E., DMOCHOWSKI, L.: Studies on the effect of 5-iododeoxyuridine and *p*-fluorophenylalanine on polyoma virus formation *in vitro*. Cancer Res. **24**, 1880—1886 (1964).

MURPHY, M. L.: Dose-response relationships in growth inhibitory drugs in the rat: time of treatment as a teratological determinant. In: WILSON, J. G., WARKANY, J. (Eds.): Teratology: Principles and techniques, pp. 161—184. Chicago: University of Chicago Press 1965.

MYERS, W. G., VANDERLEEDEN, J. C.: Radioiodine-125. J. nucl. Med. **1**, 149—164 (1960).

NEMER, M.: Characteristics of the utilization of nucleosides by embryos of *Paraentrotus lividus*. J. biol. Chem. **237**, 143—149 (1962).

NEMES, M., HILLEMAN, M. R.: Effective treatment of experimental herpes simplex keratitis with new derivative, 5-methylamino-2'-deoxyuridine (MADU). Proc. Soc. exp. Biol. (N.Y.) **119**, 515—520 (1965).

NEUBERT, D., OBERDISSE, E., BASS, R.: Biosynthesis and degradation of mitochondrial DNA. In: SLATER, E. C. (Ed.): Biochemical aspects of biogenesis of mitochondria, Proc. round table discuss. 1967, pp. 103—131. Bari: Italy 1968.

NEUFAHRT, A., ROLLY, H., SCHUTZ, E.: Einfluß von Mykoplasmen auf die antivirale Wirkung von 5-Joduracil-Desoxyribosid (JUdR). Zeit. Balk. Parasit. Inif. Hyg. **209**, 470—477 (1969).

NEWMARK, P., STEPHENS, J. D., BARRETT, H. W.: Substrate specificity of the dihydrouracil dehydrogenase and uridine phosphorylase of rat liver. Biochim. biophys. Acta (Amst.) **62**, 414—416 (1962).

O'BRIEN, T. F.: The effect of 5-bromodeoxyuridine on entirely *in vitro* secondary antibody response. Fed. Proc. **20**, 27 (1961).

O'BRIEN, T. F., COONS, A. H.: Studies on antibody production. VII. The effect of 5-bromodeoxyuridine on the *in vitro* anamnestic antibody response. J. exp. Med. **117**, 1063—1074 (1963).

OEHLERT, W., MAGNUSSEN, B.: Autoradiographic studies and the incorporation of 5-iodo-2'-deoxyuridine (IUdR) into the DNA of cells of Yoshida hepatoma AH130. Z. Krebsforsch. **66**, 455—459 (1965).

O'FARREL, T. P., DUNAWAY, P. B.: Effect of acute ionizing radiation on incorporation of ^{131}IUDR by cotton rats, *Sigmodon hispidus*. Radiat. Res. **38**, 109—124 (1967).

OKAZAKI, K., HOLTZER, H.: An analysis of myogenesis using fluorescein-labeled antimyosin. J. Histochem. Cytochem. **13**, 726—739 (1965).

OKAZAKI, R., KORNBERG, A.: Deoxythymidine kinase of *Escherichia coli*. I. Purification and some properties of the enzyme. J. biol. Chem. **239**, 269—274 (1964a).

OKAZAKI, R., KORNBERG, A.: Deoxythymidine kinase of *Escherichia coli*. II. Kinetics and feedback control. J. biol. Chem. **239**, 275—284 (1964b).

OKAZAKI, T., KORNBERG, A.: Enzymatic synthesis of deoxyribonucleic acid. XV. Purification and properties of a polymerase from *Bacillus subtilis*. J. biol. Chem. **239**, 259—268 (1964).

OMELCHENKOV, T. N., CIAMPOR, F., NADOCHEY, G. A., AVAKYAN, A. A., ALTSHTEIN, A. D.: Effects of inhibitors of DNA synthesis on heamagglutinin and infectious SV 15 virus formation in green monkey kidney cells. Acta. virol. **13**, 461—468 (1969).

OPPELT, W. W., CLARKSON, D. R., MELVIN, S. L.: Metabolism of 5-iodo-2'-deoxyuridine (IUdR) in brain and liver of dogs. Res. Commun. Clin. Pathol. Pharmacol. **2**, 553—566 (1971).

PAHL, H. B., GORDON, M. P., ELLISON, R. R.: Some aspects of the metabolism of 5-bromouracil. Arch. Biochem. Biophys. **79**, 245—251 (1959).

Painter, R. B., Goodman, M. G., Reisner, B. L.: The effect of ultraviolet light on RNA metabolism in bromouracil deoxyriboside-grown HeLa cells. Photochem. Photobiol. **12**, 49—55 (1970).
Palmer, C. G.: 5-Bromodeoxyuridine-induced constrictions in human chromosomes. Canad. J. Genet. Cytol. **12**, 816—830 (1970).
Pauling, L.: The nature of the chemical bond, 3rd ed. Ithaca, New York: Cornell University Press 1960.
Perkins, E. S., Wood, R. M., Sears, M. L., Prusoff, W. H., Welch, A. D.: Anti-viral activities of several iodinated pyrimidine deoxyribonucleosides. Nature (Lond.) **194**, 985—986 (1962).
Person, D. A., Sheridan, P. J., Herrmann, E. C.: Sensitivity of types 1 and 2 herpes simplex virus to 5-iodo-2′-deoxyuridine and 9-β-D-arabinofuranosyladenine. Infect. Immunol. **2**, 815—820 (1970).
Pfitzmer, K. E., Moffatt, J. G.: The synthesis and hydrolysis of 2′,3′-dideoxyuridine. J. org. Chem. **29**, 1508—1511 (1964).
Pietrzykowska, I., Shugar, D.: Replacement of thymine by 5-ethyluracil in bacteriophage DNA. Biochem. biophys. Res. Commun. **25**, 567—572 (1967).
Plowright, W., MacAdam, R. F., Armstrong, J. A.: Growth and characterization of the virus of bovine malignant catarrhal fever in East Africa. J. gen. Microbiol. **39**, 253—266 (1963).
Pontis, H., Degerstedt, G., Reichard, P.: Uridine and deoxyuridine phosphorylases from Ehrlich ascites tumor. Biochim. biophys. Acta (Amst.) **51**, 138—147 (1961).
Porschen, W., Feinendegen, L.: *In vivo*-Bestimmung der Zellverlustrate bei Experimentaltumoren mit markiertem Joddeoxyuridin. Strahlentherap. **137**, 718—723 (1969).
Post, J., Hoffman, J.: The effects of 5-iodo-2′-deoxyuridine upon the replication of ileal and spleen cells *in vivo*. Cancer Res. **29**, 1859—1865 (1969).
Potter, R. L., Nygaard, O. F.: The conversion of thymidine to thymine nucleotides and deoxyribonucleic acid *in vivo*. J. biol. Chem. **238**, 2150—2155 (1963).
Potter, V. R.: Metabolic products formed from thymidine. In: Stohlman, F., Jr. (Ed.): The kinetics of cellular proliferation, pp. 104—110. New York-London: Grune and Stratton 1959.
Pratt, D., Stent, G. S.: Mutational heterozygotes in bacteriophages. Proc. nat. Acad. Sci. (Wash.) **45**, 1507—1515 (1959).
Preussel, B., Etzold, G., Barwolf, D., Langen, P.: Differential inhibitor sensitivities of thymidine phosphorylases from *E. coli* and mammalian tissues. Biochem. Pharmacol. **18**, 2035—2037 (1969).
Prusoff, W. H.: Synthesis and biological activities of iododeoxyuridine, an analog of thymidine. Biochim. biophys. Acta (Amst.) **32**, 295—296 (1959a).
Prusoff, W. H.: Incorporation of iododeoxyuridine, an analog of thymidine, into mammalian deoxyribonucleic acid. Fed. Proc. **18**, 305 (1959b).
Prusoff, W. H.: Incorporation of iododeoxyuridine into the deoxyribonucleic acid of mouse Ehrlich-ascites-tumor cells *in vivo*. Biochim. biophys. Acta (Amst.) **39**, 327—331 (1960).
Prusoff, W. H.: Studies on the mechanism of cellular sensitization to ultraviolet radiation by halogenated pyrimidines. I., Biochem. biophys. Acta (Amst.) **58**, 588—590 (1962).
Prusoff, W. H.: A review of some aspects of 5-iododeoxyuridine and azauridine. Cancer. Res. **23**, 1246—1259 (1963).
Prusoff, W. H.: Recent advances in chemotherapy of viral diseases. Pharmacol. Rev. **19**, 209—250 (1967).
Prusoff, W. H., Bakhle, Y. S., McCrea, J. F.: Incorporation of 5-iodo-2′-deoxyuridine into the deoxyribonucleic acid of vaccinia virus. Nature (Lond.) **199**, 1310—1311 (1963).
Prusoff, W. H., Bahkle, Y. S., Sekely, L.: Cellular and antiviral effects of halogenated deoxyribonucleosides. Ann. N. Y. Acad. Sci. **130**, 135—150 (1965).
Prusoff, W. H., Chang, P. K.: 5-Iodo-2′-deoxyuridine 5′-triphosphate, an allosteric inhibitor of deoxycytidylate deaminase. J. biol. Chem. **243**, 223—230 (1968).
Prusoff, W. H., Chang, P. K.: Regulation of thymidine kinase activity by 5-iodo-2′-deoxyuridine 5′-triphosphate and deoxythymidine 5′-triphosphate. Chemico. biol. Int. **1**, 285—299 (1969—70).
Prusoff, W. H., Holmes, W. L., Welch, A. D.: Nonutilization of radioactive iodinated uracil, uridine, and orotic acid by animal tissues *in vivo*. Cancer. Res. **13**, 221—225 (1953).
Prusoff, W. H., Jaffe, J. J., Gunther, H.: Studies in the mouse of the pharmacology of 5-iododeoxyuridine, an analog of thymidine. Biochem. Pharmacol. **3**, 110—121 (1960).
Prystaš, M., Šorm, F.: Nucleic acid components and their analogues. XLIII. Synthesis of anomeric 5-iodo-2′-deoxyuridines. Collection Czech. Chem. Commun. **29**, 121—142 (1964).
Pullman, B., Pullman, A.: Quantum-mechanical investigations of the electronic structure of nucleic acids and their constituents. Progr. nucl. Acid. Res. **9**, 327—402 (1969).
Rada, B., Blaskovic, D.: Some characteristics of the effects of 6-azauridine on vaccinia virus multiplication, in comparison with those of 5-iododeoxyuridine. Acta virol. **10**, 1—9 (1966).

RAHMAN, A., WILSON, H. R.: The crystal and molecular structure of 5-iodouridine. Acta cryst. B **26**, 1765—1775 (1970).
RAPP, F.: Inhibition by metabolic analogues of plaque formation by herpes zoster and herpes simplex viruses. J. Immunol. **93**, 643—648 (1964).
RAPP, F., BUTEL, J. S., FELDMAN, L. A., KITAHARA, T., MELNICK, J. L.: Differential effects of inhibitors on the steps leading to the formation of SV40 tumor and virus antigens. J. exp. Med. **121**, 935—944 (1965b).
RAPP, F., MELNICK, J. L., KITAHARA, T.: Tumor and virus antigens of simian virus 40: differential inhibition of synthesis by cytosine arabinoside. Science **147**, 625—627 (1965a).
RAPP, F., VANDERSLICE, D.: Spread of zoster virus in human embryonic lung cells and the inhibitory effect of iododeoxyuridine. Virology **22**, 321—330 (1964).
RAPPEL, M., BRIHAYE, J.: Traitement de l'encéphalite necrosante herpetique par l'idoxuridine. Rev. Neurol. (Paris) **121**, 93—98 (1969).
RAVIN, L. S., SIMPSON, C. A., ZAPPALA, A. F.: Idoxuridine — a preliminary report. J. pharm. Sci. **53**, 976 (1964a).
RAVIN, L. J., SIMPSON, C. A., ZAPPALA, A. F., GULESICH, J. J.: Hydrolysis of idoxuridine. J. Pharm. Sci. **53**, 1064—1066 (1964b).
RAWLS, W. F., COHEN, R. A., HERRMANN, E. C.: Inhibition of varicella virus by 5-iodo-2'-deoxyuridine. Proc. Soc. exp. Biol. (N.Y.) **115**, 123—127 (1964).
REICHARD, P., ESTBORN, B.: Utilization of desoxyribosides in the synthesis of polynucleotides. J. biol. Chem. **188**, 839—846 (1951).
RENIS, H. E.: Comparison of cytotoxicity and antiviral activity of 1-β-D-arabinofuranosyl-5-iodocytosine with related compounds. Cancer Res. **30**, 189—194 (1970).
RICKE, W. O.: The *in vivo* reutilization of lymphocytic and sarcoma DNA by cells growing in the peritoneal cavity. J. Cell Biol. **13**, 205—216 (1962).
RILEY, M., PAUL, A.: Properties of synthetic polydeoxyribonucleotide complexes containing adenine and bromouracil. Biochemistry **10**, 3819—3825 (1971).
RIZKI, R. M., RIZKI, T. M.: Somatic cell lesions induced by the base analog 5-bromodeoxyuridine. Cancer Res. **29**, 201—208 (1969).
ROIZMAN, B., AURELIAN, L., ROANE, P. R., JR.: The multiplication of herpes simplex virus. I. The programming of viral DNA duplication in HEp-2 cells. Virology **21**, 482—498 (1963).
ROSNER, A., YAGIL, E.: Incorporation of 5-bromodeoxyuridine into DNA of wild type *Escherichia coli* and its use for enrichment of auxtrophic mutants. Molec. gen. Genet. **106**, 254—262 (1970).
ROTENBERG, A. D., BRUCE, W. R., BAKER, R. G.: Incorporation of 5-iododeoxyuridine-^{131}I in spontaneous C3H mouse mammary tumors. Brit. J. Radiol. **35**, 337—342 (1962).
RUBINI, J. R., CRONKITE, E. P., BOND, V. P., FLIEDNER, T. M.: The metabolism and fate of tritiated thymidine in man. J. clin. Invest. **39**, 909—918 (1960).
RUFFOLO, P. R., FERM, V. H.: The embryocidal and teratogenic effects of 5-bromodeoxyuridine in the pregnant hamster. Lab. Inv. **14**, 1547—1553 (1965).
RUPP, W. D., PRUSOFF, W. H.: Incorporation of 5-iodo-2'-deoxyuridine into bacteriophage T1 as related to ultraviolet sensitization or protection. Nature (Lond.) **202**, 1288—1290 (1964).
RUPP, W. D., PRUSOFF, W. H.: Photochemistry of iodouracil. I. Photoproducts obtained in water. Biochem. biophys. Res. Commun. **18**, 145—151 (1965a).
RUPP, W. D., PRUSOFF, W. H.: Photochemistry of iodouracil. II. Effects of sulfur compounds, ethanol and oxygen. Biochem. biophys. Res. Commun. **18**, 158—164 (1965b).
RUSSEFF, C., WASSELEWA, L., MATEWA, V.: Der Einfluß einiger Antimetaboliten auf die Vermehrung des Aujeszkyvirus. I. Untersuchungen mit 5-Jod-2'-Desoxyuridin (JUDR). Zbl. Vet. Med. B. **16**, 702—708 (1969).
RUTMAN, R. J., CANTAROW, A., PASCHKIS, K. E.: The catabolism of uracil *in vivo* and *in vitro*. J. biol. Chem. **210**, 321—329 (1954).
RUTTER, W. J., KEMP, J. D., BRADSHAW, W. S., CLARK, W. R., RONZIO, R. A., SANDERS, T. G.: Regulation of specific protein synthesis in cytodifferentiation. J. Cell Physiol. **72** (Suppl. 1), 1—18 (1968).
SALZMAN, N. P.: The rate of formation of vaccinia deoxyribonucleic acid and vaccinia virus. Virology **10**, 150—152 (1960).
SANGER, J. W., HOLTZER, H.: "Nuclear complementation" in 5-bromodeoxyuridine and cytochalasin B-treated myogenic cells. J. Cell Biol. **47**, 178a (1970).
SANO, K., HOSINO, T., NAGAI, M.: Radiosensitization of brain tumor cells with a thymidine analogue (bromouridine). J. Neurosurg. **28**, 530—538 (1968).
SANO, K., SATO, F., HOSHINO, T., NAGAI, M.: Experimental and clinical studies of radiosensitizers in brain tumors, with special reference to BUdR-antimetabolite continous regional infusion-radiation therapy (BAR Therapy). Neurol. Med. Chir. **7**, 51—72 (1965).

SCARANO, E., GERACI, G., ROSSI, M.: Deoxycytidylate aminohydrolase. II. Kinetic properties. The activatory effect of deoxycytidine triphosphate and the inhibitory effect of deoxythymidine triphosphate. Biochemistry **6**, 192—201 (1967).

SCHABEL, F. M., MONTGOMERY, J. A.: Antiviral agents-purines and pyrimidines. In: BAUER, D. J. (Ed.): The international encylopedia of pharmacology and therapeutics, Section 61. The chemotherapy of virus disease. Oxford-New York: Pergamon Press 1972.

SCHALLER, J., GORDON, M., STERNBERG, S. S.: Studies with 5-bromouracil in rodents and dogs. Proc. Soc. exp. Biol. (N.Y.) **93**, 124—128 (1965).

SCHIEK, W., SCHIEK, E.: Untersuchung über infektiöses bromdesoxyuridin-haltiges Herpes virus hominis, Bestimmung der Dichte und der Sedimentationskonstanten im CsCl-H_2O-Dichtegradienten. Arch. Ges. Virusforsch. **28**, 229—238 (1969).

SCHINDLER, R., RAMSIER, L., GRIEDER, A.: Increased sensitivity of mammalian cell culture to radiomimetic alkylating agents following incorporation of 5-bromodeoxyuridine into cellular DNA. Biochem. Pharmacol. **15**, 2013—2023 (1966).

SCHNEWEIS, K. E.: Das Verhalten von DNA-Viren in 5-Bromdesoxyuridin-behandelten Zellkulturen. I. Untersuchungen am Herpesvirus zur antigenen Eigenschaft und zur Adsorptionsfähigkeit des infektionsuntüchtigen Virus. Arch. Ges. Virusforsch. **15**, 565—582 (1965a).

SCHNEWEIS, K. E.: Das Verhalten von DNA-Viren in 5-Bromodesoxyuridin-behandelten Zellkulturen. II. Die Virusproduktion in Abhängigkeit von der infizierenden Virusdosis und vom Zeitpunkt des Zusatzes von 5-Bromodesoxyuridin. Archiv. Ges. Virusforsch. **15**, 583—597 (1965b).

SCHUBERT, D., JACOB, F.: 5-Bromodeoxyuridine-induced differentiation of a neuroblastoma. Proc. nat. Acad. Sci. (Wash.) **67**, 247—254 (1970).

SEBESTA, K., BAUEROVA, J., SORMOVA, Z.: Inhibitions of uracil and thymine degradation by some 5-substituted uracil analogues. Biochim. biophys. Acta (Amst.) **50**, 393—394 (1961).

SEKELY, L., PRUSOFF, W. H.: The effect of 5-iodo-2′-deoxyuridine-5′-triphosphate on DNA polymerase of uninfected and herpes simplex infected cells. Pharmacol. Res. Commun. **1**, 3—6 (1969).

SHAPIRO, R., KANG, S.: Uncatalyzed hydrolysis of deoxyuridine, thymidine, and 5-bromodeoxyuridine. Biochemistry **8**, 1806—1810 (1969).

SHEN, T. Y., MCPHERSON, J. F., LINN, B. O.: Nucleosides. III. Studies on 5-methylamino-2′-deoxyuridine as a specific antiherpes agent. J. med. Chem. **9**, 366—369 (1966).

SHISHIDO, K., IKEDA, Y.: Preferential binding of RNA polymerase to the thymidylic acid-rich fragments obtained from bacteriophage F1 DNA. J. Biochem. **68**, 881—884 (1970).

SHUGAR, D., FOX, J. J.: Spectrophotometric studies of nucleic acid derivatives and related compounds as a function of pH. Biochim. biophys. Acta (Amst.) **9**, 199—218 (1952).

SIDWELL, R. W., ARNETT, G., BROCKMAN, R. W.: Comparison of the anticytomegalovirus activity of a group of pyrimidine analogs. Ann. N.Y. Acad. Sci. **173**, 592—602 (1970).

SILAGI, S., BRUCE, S. A.: Suppression of malignancy and differentiation in melanotic melanoma cells. Proc. nat. Acad. Sci. (Wash.) **66**, 72—78 (1970).

SILVESTER, D. J., WHITE, W. D.: Preparation of very high specific activity IUdR, IUR and iodouracil labelled with iodine 125, 131, 132. Nature (Lond.) **200**, 65—67 (1963).

SIMINOFF, P.: The effect of 5-bromodeoxyuridine on herpes simplex infection of HeLa cells. Virology **24**, 1—12 (1964).

SIMINOFF, P., MENEFEE, M. G.: Normal and 5-bromodeoxyuridine inhibited development of herpes simplex virus. Exp. cell. Res. **44**, 241—255 (1966).

SIMON, E. H.: Evidence for the nonparticipation of DNA in viral RNA synthesis. Virology **13**, 105—118 (1961).

SIMON, E. H.: Effect of 5-bromodeoxyuridine on cell division and DNA replication in HeLa cells. Exp. cell. Res. **9**, 263—269 (1963).

SKALKO, R. G., PACKARD, D. S., JR., SCHWENDIMANN, R. N., RAGGIO, J. R.: The teratogenic response of mouse embryos to 5-bromodeoxyuridine. Teratology **4**, 87—93 (1971).

SMITH, H. H., KUGELMAN, B. H.: Incorporation of tritiated base analogues in plant chromosomes. Radiat. Res. **14**, 504 (1961).

SMITH, H. H., KUGELMAN, B. H., COMMERFORD, S. L., SZYBALSKI, W.: Incorporation of 5-iododeoxyuridine into DNA of plant cells. Proc. nat. Acad. Sci. (Wash.) **49**, 451—457 (1963).

SMITH, J. D., FREEMAN, G., VOGT, M., DULBECCO, R.: The nucleic acid of polyoma virus. Virology **12**, 185—196 (1960).

SMITH, K. C.: A chemical basis for the sensitization of bacteria to ultraviolet light. Biochem. biophys. Res. Commun. **6**, 458—463 (1962).

SMITH, K. C.: Photochemical reactions of thymine, uracil, uridine, cytosine, and bromouracil, in frozen solution and in dried films. Photochem. Photobiol. **2**, 503—517 (1963).

SMITH, K. C.: The photochemistry of thymine and bromouracil *in vivo*. Photochem. Photobiol. **3**, 1—10 (1964).

SMITH, K. O.: Some biological aspects of herpes virus-cell interactions in the presence of 5-iodo-2′-deoxyuridine (IDU); demonstrations of a cytotoxic effect by herpes virus. J. Immunol. **91**, 582—590 (1963).
SMITH, K. O., DUKES, C. D.: Effect of 5-iodo-2′-deoxyuridine (IDU) on herpes virus synthesis and survival in infected cells. J. Immunol. **92**, 550—554 (1964).
SPEYER, J. F.: Mutagenic DNA polymerase. Biochem. biophys. Res. Commun. **21**, 6—8 (1965).
SPEYER, J. F., KARAM, J. D., LENNY, A. B.: On the role of DNA polymerase in base selection. Cold Spr. Harb. Symp. Quant. Biol. **31**, 693—697 (1966).
SRIVASTAVA, P. C., NAGPAL, K. L.: Bromination of nucleosides. Experientia (Basel) **26**, 220 (1970).
STELLWAGEN, R. H., TOMKINS, G. M.: Preferential inhibition by 5-bromodeoxyuridine of the synthesis of tyrosine aminotransferase in hepatoma cell cultures. J. molec. Biol. **56**, 167—182 (1971a).
STELLWAGEN, R. H., TOMPKINS, G. M.: Differential effect of 5-bromodeoxyuridine on the concentrations of specific enzymes in hepatoma cells in culture. Proc. nat. Acad. Sci. (Wash.) **68**, 1147—1150 (1971b).
STEWART, S. E., KASNIC, G., JR., BEN, T.: Activation of viruses in human tumors by 5-iododeoxyuridine and dimethyl sulfoxide. Science **175**, 198—199 (1972b).
STEWART, S. E., KASNIC, G., JR., DRAYCOTT, C., FELLER, W., GOLDEN, A., MITCHELL, E., BEN, T.: Activation *in vitro*, by 5-iododeoxyuridine, of a latent virus resembling C-type virus in a human sarcoma cell line. J. nat. Cancer. Inst. **48**, 273—277 (1972a).
STOCKDALE, F., OKAZAKI, K., MAMEROFF, M., HOLTZER, H.: 5-Bromodeoxyuridine: effect on myogenesis *in vitro*. Science **146**, 533—535 (1964).
STONE, J. E., POTTER, V. R.: Biochemical screening of pyrimidine antimetabolites. II. The development of a system with a nonoxidative energy source. Cancer. Res. **17**, 794—799 (1957).
STRELZOFF, E.: Identification of base pairs involved in mutations induced by base analogues. Biochem. biophys. Res. Commun. **5**, 384—388 (1961).
STRELZOFF, E.: DNA synthesis and induced mutations in the presence of 5-bromouracil. 2. Induction of mutations. Z. Vererbungslehre **93**, 301—318 (1962).
SUIT, H. D.: Theoretical evaluation of a limitation in the use of pyrimidine analogs in radiation therapy. Radiology **87**, 1065—1068 (1966).
SZER, W., SHUGAR, D.: Preparation of poly-5-fluorouridylic acid and the properties of halogenated poly-uridylic acids and their complexes with poly-adenylic acid. Acta biochim. polon. **10**, 219—231 (1963).
SZYBALSKI, W.: Properties and applications of halogenated deoxyribonucleic acids. In: The molecular basis of neoplasia, pp. 147—171. Austin Texas: University of Texas Press 1962.
SZYBALSKI, W.: Molecular events resulting in radiation injury, repair and sensitization of DNA. Radiat. Res. **7**, 147—159 (1967).
SZYBALSKI, W., KUBINSKI, H., SHELDRICK, P.: Pyrimidine clusters on the transcribing strand of DNA and their possible role in the initiation of RNA synthesis. Cold Spr. Harb. Symp. Quant. Biol. **31**, 123—127 (1966).
SZYBALSKI, W., MENNIGMANN, H.: The recording thermospectrophotometer, an automatic device for determining the thermal stability of nucleic acids. Anal. Biochem. **3**, 267—275 (1962).
SZYBALSKI, W., OPARA-KUBINSKA, Z., LORKIEWICZ, L., EPHRATI-ELIZUR, E., ZAMENHOF, S.: Transforming activity of deoxyribonucleic acid labelled with 5-bromouracil. Nature (Lond.) **188**, 743—745 (1960).
TAUB, R. N.: Effects of heterologous antilymphocyte serum on lymphoid cells labeled with 5-iodo-2′-deoxyuridine-^{125}I. Fed. Proc. **29**, 142—144 (1970).
TAVALE, S. S., SAKORE, T. D., SOBELL, H. M.: Base-pairing configurations between purines and pyrimidines in the solid state. II. Crystal and molecular structure of 9-ethyl-8-bromoadenine-1-methyl-5-bromouracil. J. molec. Biol. **43**, 375—384 (1969).
TEMIN, H. M.: The effects of actinomycin D on growth of Rous sarcoma virus *in vitro*. Virology **20**, 577—582 (1963).
TEMIN, H. M.: The participation of DNA in Rous sarcoma virus production. Virology **23**, 486—494 (1964).
TEMIN, H. M.: Mechanism of cell transformation by RNA tumor viruses. Ann. Rev. Microbiol. **25**, 609—648 (1971).
TERZAGHI, B. E., STREISINGER, G., STAHL, F. W.: The mechanism of 5-bromouracil mutagenesis in the bacteriophage T4. Proc. nat. Acad. Sci. (Wash.) **48**, 1519—1524 (1962).
TESSMAN, I., PODDAR, R. K., KUMAR, S.: Identification of the altered bases in mutated single-stranded DNA. 1. *In vitro* mutagenesis by hydroxylamine, ethyl methanesulfonate and nitrous acid. J. molec. Biol. **9**, 352—363 (1964).

THOMAS, H.: Effect of 5-bromodeoxyuridine and actinomycin D on the growth of Visna virus in cell cultures. Virology **26**, 36—43 (1965).
THOMPSON, R. L., WILKIN, M. L., HITCHINGS, G. H., ELION, G. B., FALCO, E. A., RUSSELL, P. B.: The effects of antagonists on the multiplication of vaccinia virus *in vitro*. Science **110**, 454—455 (1949).
TODARO, G. J., GREEN, H.: Enhancement by thymidine analogs of susceptibility of cells to transformation by SV40. Virology **24**, 393—400 (1964).
TOLIVER, A., SIMON, E. H.: DNA synthesis in 5-bromouracil tolerant HeLa cells. An autoradiographic study. Exp. cell. Res. **45**, 603—617 (1967).
TOLIVER, A., SIMON, E. H., GILHAM, T. P.: On the mechanism of 5-bromouracil inhibition of DNA synthesis and cell division. Exp. cell. Res. **53**, 506—518 (1968).
TRAUTNER, T. A., SWARTZ, M. N., KORNBERG, A.: Enzymatic synthesis of deoxyribonucleic acid. X. Influence of bromouracil substitutions on replication. Proc. nat. Acad. Sci. (Wash.) **48**, 449—455 (1962).
TURKINGTON, R. W., MAJUMDER, G. C., RIDDLE, M.: Inhibition of mammary gland differentiation *in vitro* by 5 bromo-2′-deoxyuridine. J. biol. Chem. **246**, 1814—1819 (1971).
VOET, D., RICH, A.: The crystal structures of purine, pyrimidines and their intermolecular complexes. Progr. nucl. Acid. Res. **10**, 183—265 (1970).
VOYTEK, P., CHANG, P., PRUSOFF, W. H.: Purification of deoxythymidine kinase by preparative disc gel electrophoresis and the effects of various halogenated nucleoside triphosphates on its enzymatic activity. J. biol. Chem. **246**, 1432—1438 (1971).
VOYTEK, P., CHANG, P., PRUSOFF, W. H.: Kinetic and photochemical studies of 3-*N*-methyl-5-iodo-2′-deoxyuridine. J. biol. Chem. **247**, 567—572 (1972).
WACKER, A.: Alteration of pyrimidines by radiation *in vivo* and *in vitro*. J. chim. Phys. **58**, 1041—1045 (1961).
WACKER, A.: Molecular mechanisms of radiation effects. Progr. nucl. Acid. Res. **1**, 369—399 (1963).
WACKER, A., DELLWEG, H., WEINBLUM, D.: Über die strahlensensibilisierende Wirkung des 5-Bromouracils. J. molec. Biol. **3**, 787—789 (1961).
WACKER, A., TRAEGER, L.: Über die Säurehydrolyse der Desoxyriboside und Riboside. Zeit. Naturforsch. **18**b, 13—16 (1963).
WACKER, A., TREBST, A., JACHERTS, D., WEYGAND, F.: Über den Einbau von 5-Bromouracil-(2-^{14}C) in die Desoxyribonucleinsäure verschiedener Bakterien. Z. Naturforsch. **9**b, 616—617 (1954).
WALLACH, D. P., GRISOLIA, S.: The purification and properties of hydropyrimidine hydrase. J. biol. Chem. **226**, 277—288 (1957).
WALTUCK, G., SACHS, F.: Herpes zoster in a patient with Hodgkins disease. Arch. Intern. Med. **121**, 458—462 (1968).
WANG, S. Y.: Chemistry of pyrimidines. II. The conversion of 5-bromo to 5-hydroxyuracils. J. Amer. chem. Soc. **81**, 3786—3789 (1959).
WATSON, D. H., WILDY, P., RUSSELL, W. C.: Quantitative electron microscope studies on the growth of herpes virus using the technique of negative staining and ultramicrotomy. Virology **24**, 523—538 (1964).
WEIL, R., MICHEL, M. R., RUSCHMANN, G.: Induction of cellular DNA synthesis by polyoma virus. Proc. nat. Acad. Sci. (Wash.) **53**, 1468—1475 (1968).
WELCH, A. D.: Some metabolic approaches to cancer chemotherapy. Cancer Res. **21**, 1475—1490 (1961).
WELCH, A. D.: Some mechanisms involved in selective chemotherapy. Ann. N. Y. Acad. Sci. **123**, 19—41 (1965).
WELCH, A. D., PRUSOFF, W. H.: A synopsis of recent investigations of 5-iodo-2′-deoxyuridine. Cancer Chemother. Rept. **6**, 29—36 (1960).
WEMPEN, I., DUSCHINSKY, R., KAPLAN, L., FOX, J. J.: Thiation of nucleosides. IV. The synthesis of 5-fluoro-2′-deoxycytidine and related compounds. J. Amer. chem. Soc. **83**, 4755—4766 (1961).
WERNER, R.: Distribution of growing points in DNA of bacteriophage T4. J. molec. Biol. **33**, 679—692 (1968).
WESSELLS, N. K.: DNA synthesis, mitosis and differentiation in pancreatic acinar cells *in vitro*. J. Cell Biol. **20**, 415—433 (1964).
WESTRA, A., DEWEY, W. C.: Variation in sensitivity to heat shock during the cell-cycle of Chinese hamster cells *in vitro*. Int. J. Radiat. Biol. **19**, 467—477 (1971).
WEYGAND, F., WACKER, A.: Stoffwechseluntersuchungen bei Mikroorganismen mit Hilfe radioaktiver Isotope. III. Z. Naturforsch. **7**b, 26—28 (1952).
WEYGAND, F., WACKER, A., DELLWEG, H.: Stoffwechseluntersuchungen bei Mikroorganismen mit Hilfe radioaktiver Isotope. II. Z. Naturforsch. **7**b, 19—25 (1952).

WILKINS, B. M.: The recombination of bromouracil-containing deoxyribonucleic acid in *Salmonella typhimurium* transduction. J. gen. Microbiol. **51**, 107—114 (1968).
WILKOFF, L. J., LLOYD, H. H., DULMADGE, E. A., DIXON, G. J.: Kinetic evaluation of the effect of hydroxyurea on viability of replicating cultured leukemia L1210 cells. J. nat. Cancer Inst. **44**, 201—209 (1970).
WILSON, H. R.: Changes in nucleoside conformation. Nature (Lond.) **225**, 545 (1970).
WILT, F. H.: Regulation of initiation of chick embryo hemoglobin synthesis. J. molec. Biol. **12**, 331—341 (1965).
WOODMAN, R. J.: Increased localization and incorporation of iododeoxyuridine into tumor DNA *in vivo* when coupled to polycation. Nature (Lond.) **209**, 1362—1363 (1966).
WOODMAN, R. J.: Localized incorporation of iododeoxyuridine from polycation-complexed iododeoxycytidylic acid into DNA of several murine and hamster tumors. Cancer. Res. **28**, 2007—2016 (1968).
WRONA, M., CZOCHRALSKA, B.: Electroreduction of halogeno-pyrimidines. Electrochemical reduction of 5-halogenoderivatives of uracil, its nucleosides and oligonucleotides. Acta. biochim. polon. **17**, 351—360 (1970).
YAMAGATA, Y., SAKAMOTO, M.: Possible origin of the hot spot. J. theor. Biol. **30**, 215—217 (1971).
YOSHIDA, H., DUVAL, J., EBEL, J. P.: Halogenation des acides nucleiques. VI. Ioduration des nucleosides en milieu dimethylformamide. Biochim. Biophys. Acta (Amst.) **161**, 13—22 (1968).
YUNG, N. C., BURCHENAL, J. H., FECHER, R., DUSCHINSKY, R., FOX, J. J.: Nucleosides. XI. Synthesis of 1-β-arabinofuranosyl-5-fluorouracil and related nucleosides. J. Amer. chem. Soc. **83**, 4060—4065 (1961).
ZAMENHOF, S., DEGIOVANNI, R., RICH, K.: *Escherichia coli* containing unnatural pyrimidines in its deoxyribonucleic acid. J. Bact. **71**, 60—69 (1956a).
ZAMENHOF, S., GRAUEL, L., VAN MARTHEN, E.: The effect of thymidine and 5-bromodeoxyuridine on developing chick embryo brain. Res. Commun. Chem. Pathol. Pharmacol. **2**, 261—270 (1971).
ZAMENHOF, S., GRIBOFF, G.: *E. coli* containing 5-bromouracil in its deoxyribonucleic acid. Nature (Lond.) **174**, 307—308 (1954).
ZAMENHOF, S., REINER, B., DEGIOVANNI, R., RICH, K.: Introduction of unnatural pyrimidines into deoxyribonucleic acid of *E. coli*. J. biol. Chem. **219**, 165—173 (1965b).
ZIMBRICK, J. D., WARD, J. F., MYERS, L. S.: Studies on the chemical basis of cellular radiosensitization by 5-bromouracil substitution in DNA. I. Pulse and steady state radiolysis of 5-bromouracil and thymine. Int. J. Radiat. Biol. **16**, 505—523 (1969a).
ZIMBRICK, J. D., WARD, J. F., MYERS, L. S.: Studies on the chemical basis of cellular radiosensitization by 5-bromouracil substitution in DNA. II. Pulse and steady state radiolysis of bromouracil substituted and unsubstituted DNA. Int. J. Radiat. Biol. **16**, 525—534 (1969b).
ZIMMERMAN, M.: The possible identity of thymidine phosphorylase and pyrimidine deoxyribosyl transferase of rat liver. Biochem. biophys. Res. Commun. **8**, 169—174 (1962).
ZIMMERMAN, M.: Selective inhibition by deoxyglucosyl thymine of thymidine phosphorylases not catalyzing deoxyribosyl transfer. Biochem. biophys. Res. Commun. **16**, 600—603 (1904).
ZIMMERMAN, M., SEIDENBERG, J.: Deoxyribosyl transfer. I. Thymidine phosphorylase and nucleoside deoxyribosyltransferase in normal and malignant tissues. J. biol. Chem. **239**, 2618 (1964).

Chapter 45

Azapyrimidine Nucleosides

J. Škoda

With 3 Figures

Introduction

Azapyrimidine analogs are derived from pyrimidine compounds through the replacement of one of the methine groups with an atom of nitrogen. The replacement may be effected in position 5 or 6 of the pyrimidine ring so that the numerous azapyrimidine bases, nucleosides and their derivatives fall into two categories:

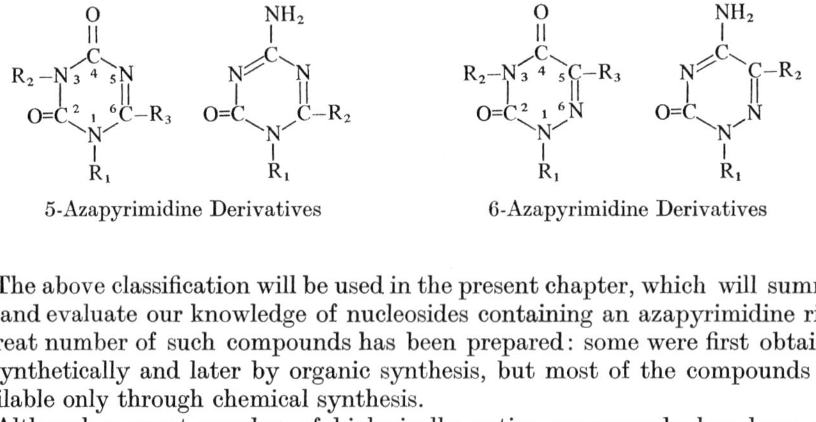

5-Azapyrimidine Derivatives

6-Azapyrimidine Derivatives

The above classification will be used in the present chapter, which will summarize and evaluate our knowledge of nucleosides containing an azapyrimidine ring. A great number of such compounds has been prepared: some were first obtained biosynthetically and later by organic synthesis, but most of the compounds are available only through chemical synthesis.

Although a great number of biologically active compounds has been discovered among the azapyrimidine nucleosides, only two of the analogs have attained practical importance, having passed pharmacological and clinical tests, and are now serving as drugs or tools for biochemical and pharmacological research. The older of the two is 6-azauridine, obtained by an industrial microbial process. The newer is 5-azacytidine, which was first prepared synthetically and only later discovered as an antibiotic produced by the microorganism *Streptoverticillium lakadanus*. Special sections will be devoted to these two azapyrimidine nucleosides.

Review of Existing Azapyrimidine Nucleosides

A. 6-Azapyrimidine Nucleosides

The history of 6-azapyrimidine nucleosides began in 1955 with the discovery of 6-azathymidine. The formation of this anomalous deoxyribonucleoside from 6-azathymine by a transdeoxyribosylation mechanism was observed in a bacterial subcellular system (PRUSOFF, 1955). It was then shown that the biosynthesis of 6-azathymidine was involved in the mechanism of the inhibitory action of 6-azathymine; thus, the metabolically formed 6-azathymidine displayed markedly greater inhibitory effects than the parent compound, 6-azathymine.

Shortly afterward, the most important member of the azapyrimidine nucleosides, 6-azauridine, was described. The compound was discovered as an extracellular anabolite of 6-azauracil in *Escherichia coli* (ŠKODA et al., 1957) and as an intracellular anabolite in *Streptococcus faecalis* (HANDSCHUMACHER, 1957); in the *Escherichia coli* culture the ribosylation of 6-azauracil was so efficient that it was employed for the production of 6-azauridine by industrial fermentation (ŠKODA and ŠORM, 1958a). 6-Azauridine was also prepared synthetically (HANDSCHUMACHER, 1960a; PRYSTAŠ and ŠORM, 1962; CRISTESCU, 1968). The mechanism of the inhibitory action of 6-azauridine and its applications in different biological systems are dealt with in detail in a later section of this chapter.

Several derivatives of 6-azauridine were also prepared synthetically; these included 3-methyl-6-azauridine (PRYSTAŠ et al., 1962), 5-methyl-6-azauridine (PRYSTAŠ and ŠORM, 1962), and the rather curious compound 6-azapseudouridine (BOBEK et al., 1969).

6-Aza-2′-deoxyuridine, obtained synthetically (PLIML et al., 1963), as well as by enzymic transdeoxyribosylation (KÁRA and ŠORM, 1963), does not show significant biological activity; extracts from animal tissues, including some tumor tissues, possess only a minimal capacity to phosphorylate 6-aza-2′-deoxyuridine (KÁRA and ŠORM, 1963). 6-Aza-3′-deoxyuridine (BERÁNEK and ŠORM, 1968a) and 5-hydroxymethyl-6-aza-2′-deoxyuridine (BOBEK et al., 1967) have also been prepared.

6-Azacytidine and some of its derivatives have been synthesized from 6-azauridine obtained by fermentation (ŠORM et al., 1961; ŽEMLIČKA and ŠORM, 1965; ČERNĚCKIJ et al., 1962; BERÁNEK et al., 1964). In addition, a nitrogen mustard derivative of 6-azacytidine was described (ŽEMLIČKA et al., 1964). The carcinostatic effect of 6-azacytidine on the Ehrlich tumor is slight, but in combination with the alkylating agent 5-*bis*-(2-chloroethyl)aminomethyluracil, a synergistic inhibition of this tumor was observed (ŠORM and VESELÝ, 1961). However, no extensive investigations of the carcinostatic effects of 6-azacytidine have been carried out. The metabolism of this compound was studied in detail *in vivo* and *in vitro* using mice bearing the Ehrlich ascites carcinoma. It was shown that 6-azacytidine is phosphorylated to the 5′-phosphate both in ascitic cells and in liver and that the anomalous nucleotide that was formed interferes with the *de novo* biosynthesis of pyrimidine nucleotides by inhibiting orotidine 5′-phosphate decarboxylase; simultaneously, deamination of 6-azacytidine to 6-azauridine takes place (HANDSCHUMACHER et al., 1963). The degree of deamination of 6-azacytidine is tissue-specific (HANDSCHUMACHER et al., 1963), as well as species-specific (NOVOTNÝ et al., 1965). Similarly, a subcellular extract of *Escherichia coli* deaminates 6-azacytidine, but at a much slower rate than cytidine (LISÝ and ŠKODA, 1966). 6-Azacytidine inhibits the incorporation of cytidine into the RNA of fowl leukemic cells and normal myeloblasts (VESELÝ, 1964). The acute toxicity of 6-azacytidine in mice is very low, but after repeated daily administration a leukopenia and hemorrhagic diarrhea develop which result in death (JIŘIČKA et al., 1965). Large intraperitoneal doses of 6-azacytidine do not affect the exploratory activity of rats; however, the same activity is decreased in mice. In addition, large doses of 6-azacytidine antagonize the lethal effect of nicotine. Administration of 6-azacytidine into cerebral ventricles produces ataxia and loss of postural reflexes (JANKŮ et al., 1965a) and 6-azacytidine interrupts pregnancy in mice if administered before the 15th day after fertilization (Elis and Rašková, 1964; Čerey et al., 1965). Polyribonucleotides containing 6-azacytidine in place of cytidine or uridine (Škoda and Šorm, 1964) are not active in the translation process (Škoda et al., 1966; Lisý et al., 1968). Another analog prepared in this group was 6-azaisocytidine (Žemlička and Šorm, 1967).

The deoxy analog of 6-azacytidine, 6-aza-2′-deoxycytidine, was prepared synthetically (Pliml and Šorm, 1962; Tong et al., 1966). This analog inhibits the growth of *Thermobacterium acidophilus*, shows a partial inhibitory effect in leukemic mice, and is partly deaminated by cells of the Ehrlich ascites tumor (quoted from Pliml and Šorm, 1962). It was also found that 6-aza-2′-deoxycytidine activates in Ehrlich ascites tumor cells the biosynthesis of deoxyribonucleic acids (Kára, 1964). 6-Aza-2′-deoxycytidine 5′-phosphate activates the deoxycytidylate deaminase of embryonic and tumor tissues; this effect is species-specific (Kára and Šorm, 1964; Sagar and Kára, 1966). The synthesis of the 5-methyl derivative of 6-aza-2′-deoxycytidine has also been reported (Pryštaš and Šorm, 1963).

Finally, a series of 6-azapyrimidine nucleosides with an "anomalous" sugar moiety has been prepared. However, 6-azacytosine arabinoside (Farkaš et al., 1966), the aza analog of the cytostatically effective cytosine arabinoside, did not display any inhibitory effects (Škoda and Veselý, unpublished results).

Other compounds prepared in this series are 1-β-D-xylofuranosyl-6-azauracil (Tkaczynski et al., 1964), 1-β-D-arabinofuranosyl-6-azauracil (Farkaš et al., 1966), 1-β-D-arabinofuranosyl-6-azaisocytosine (Beránek and Šorm, 1968b), 1-(2′,3′-epoxy-β-D-lyxofuranosyl)-6-azaisocytosine (Wierczorkowski et al., 1968) and 1-β-D-lyxofuranosyl-6-azauracil (Beránek, 1969); none of these derivatives possessed pronounced biological activity. Recently, the group was enlarged by the 6-azauracil and 6-azathymine nucleosides of 2-deoxy-D-arabinohexapyranose (Durr et al., 1967) and by 1-(2-deoxy-D-arabinohexapyranosyl)-5-bromo-6-azauracil (Durr and Hammond, 1970).

B. 5-Azapyrimidine Nucleosides

5-Azapyrimidine nucleosides, unlike 6-azapyrimidine derivatives, are unstable in aqueous media, being liable to hydrolytic cleavage of the triazine ring.

When studying the mechanism of the antibacterial effects of 5-azauracil (allantoxaidine), 5-azauridine was discovered (Škoda et al., 1962). This compound is decomposed to ribosyl biuret (Škoda et al., 1962) via ribosyl 1-formylbiuret (Čihák et al., 1964):

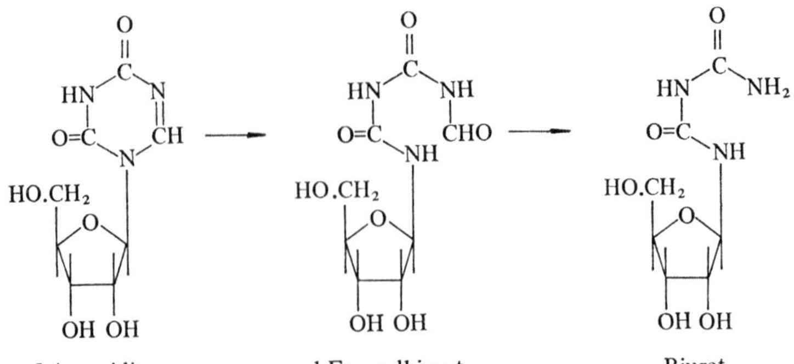

5-Azauridine → 1-Formylbiuret Ribonucleoside → Biuret Ribonucleoside

The discovery of 5-azauridine as a metabolite of 5-azauracil stimulated its synthetic preparation, in the course of which 5-azacytidine was also prepared (PÍSKALA and ŠORM, 1964).

5-Azauridine completely inhibits growth and protein synthesis in *Escherichia coli* (DOSKOČIL and ŠORM, 1970a, b).

5-Aza-2′-deoxyuridine has not yet been synthesized, but it is formed by the enzymic deamination of 5-aza-2′-deoxycytidine (DOSKOČIL and ŠORM, 1970c).

The most important member of the group of 5-azapyrimidine nucleosides is 5-azacytidine. Its inhibitory effects were first described with the synthetically obtained preparation (ŠORM et al., 1964); two years later 5-azacytidine was isolated as an antibiotic (HAŇKA et al., 1966). 5-Azacytidine is treated in greater detail later in this chapter.

The corresponding deoxyribo analog, 5-aza-2′-deoxycytidine, was prepared synthetically (PLIML and ŠORM, 1964); it shows potent antibacterial effects (ČIHÁK and ŠORM, 1965) and displays antileukemic properties in AKR mice (ŠORM and VESELÝ, 1968). In the latter system it inhibits extensively the incorporation of 2′-deoxyuridine and 2′-deoxycytidine into nucleic acids (VESELÝ et al., 1969). Resistance to this agent is attained rapidly; leukemic cells resistant to 5-aza-2′-deoxycytidine retain their sensitivity toward 5-azacytidine (VESELÝ et al., 1968a). 5-Aza-2′-deoxycytidine-resistant cells contain a reduced level of deoxycytidine kinase, thereby minimizing activation of this drug (VESELÝ et al., 1969a).

The distribution of 5-aza-2′-deoxycytidine in mouse organs has been studied; a greater retention was found in lymphatic tissues after intraperitoneal application, than in other organs (RAŠKA et al., 1965), apparently associated with the selective ability of the spleen and of the thymus (as well as of leukemic tissues) to phosphorylate 5-aza-2′-deoxycytidine (ŠORM et al., 1966).

5-Aza-2′-deoxycytidine inhibits the phosphorolysis of thymidine *in vivo* and is a donor of the deoxyribosyl group for deoxyribosylation of thymine in *Escherichia coli* (DOSKOČIL and PAČES, 1968; DOSKOČIL, 1970). This transdeoxyribosylation is preceded by a deamination of 5-aza-2′-deoxycytidine. In deaminase-less mutants of *Escherichia coli*, 5-aza-2′-deoxycytidine shows practically no inhibitory activity. However, in wild-type cells of *Escherichia coli*, 5-aza-2′-deoxycytidine inhibits protein synthesis and the replication of phage f2 as effectively as 5-azacytidine, but has a much weaker effect on the replication of phage T4 (DOSKOČIL and ŠORM, 1970c).

5-Azacytosine derivatives of 1-β-ribopyranose and of glucopyranose have been prepared (PÍSKALA and ŠORM, 1964) and have been found to be noninhibitory to the growth of *Escherichia coli* (ČIHÁK and ŠORM, 1965).

C. 6-Azauridine[1]

I. Molecular Mechanism of Inhibitory Effects

The mechanism of the inhibitory effects of most anomalous nucleosides is thought to be the process known as lethal synthesis. This is involved in the action of 6-azauridine, which is phosphorylated in the presence of adenosine 5′-triphosphate to the final inhibitor, 6-azauridine 5′-monophosphate [6-azauridine itself is an intermediate in the mechanism of action of 6-azauracil (ŠKODA et al.,

1 2-β-D-Ribofuranosyl-*as*-triazine-3,5(2*H*,4*H*)-dione.

1957a, b; Handschumacher, 1957)]. 6-Azauridine is phosphorylated both in microorganisms (Škoda and Šorm, 1959), and in animal tissues (Handschumacher and Pasternak, 1958; Habermann and Šorm, 1958; Pasternak and Handschumacher, 1959). The phosphorylation is catalyzed by uridine kinase (Sköld, 1960) and uridine competes with 6-azauridine[2] for this enzyme. The 6-azauridine 5′-phosphate formed inhibits orotidine 5′-phosphate decarboxylase (Handschumacher and Pasternak, 1958; Habermann and Šorm, 1958; Handschumacher, 1960b). Due to the blockade of the utilization of orotidine 5′-phosphate, this intermediate is accumulated and degraded to orotidine and orotic acid. The above degradation products then accumulate in bacterial culture media (Škoda and Šorm, 1959b), in the urine (Habermann and Šorm, 1958), and in experimental tumors (Pasternak and Handschumacher, 1959) of mice, as well as in human urine (Fallon et al., 1961; Buttoo et al., 1965). In animal systems, 6-azauridine 5′-phosphate is not further phosphorylated; the biosynthesis of 6-azauridine 5′-di- and triphosphates was observed only in the protozoan *Trypanosoma equiperdum* (Rubin et al., 1962). Synthetically prepared higher phosphates of 6-azauridine were found to inhibit the biological synthesis of polyribonucleotides and ribonucleic acids: 6-azauridine 5′-diphosphate is an inhibitor of polynucleotide phosphorylase (Škoda et al., 1959a, b) and 6-azauridine 5′-triphosphate inhibits RNA polymerase (Goldberg and Rabinowitz, 1963). Since these inhibitory effects require relatively large concentrations of the anomalous nucleotides, 6-azauridine 5′-di- and triphosphates apparently play no significant role in the mechanism of action of 6-azauridine in animal systems; the main site of action of 6-azauridine thus remains the inhibition of orotidine 5′-phosphate decarboxylase by 6-azauridine 5′-phosphate. A general scheme of the mechanism of the inhibitory effects of 6-azauridine is presented in Fig. 1.

The interaction of 6-azauridine with animal systems, however, must be viewed in a more complex way. Pyrimidine starvation, induced by 6-azauridine in Sarcoma 180 cells growing in culture, produced a three- to four-fold increase in the level of aspartate transcarbamylase (Ennis and Lubin, 1963), and human diploid cell lines grown in a medium containing 6-azauridine developed augmented levels of orotidine 5′-phosphate pyrophosphorylase and orotidine 5′-phosphate decarboxylase (Pinsky and Krooth, 1967a, b). Studies of the utilization of orotic acid-6-^{14}C in patients with chronic myelogenous leukemia in the presence and absence of 6-azauridine have been interpreted as indicating that 6-azauridine may cause an increase in the biosynthesis of uridylic acid (Bono and Weissman, 1964). 6-Azauridine can thus regulate, whether directly or indirectly, the metabolism of pyrimidine nucleotide precursors.

No incorporation of 6-azauridine into the nucleic acids of animal tissues has been observed thus far following intraperitoneal or intravenous administration. Only after intracerebral injection of 6-azauridine in the cat were brain ribonucleic acids shown to contain 6-azauridine 2′(3′)-phosphate and 6-azacytidine 2′(3′)-phosphate following hydrolysis (Wells et al., 1963). Therefore, special attention has been devoted to the molecular and genetic consequences of a *potential* incorporation of 6-azauridine into nucleic acids. To this end, use has been made of modern techniques of studying code triplets (Nirenberg and Leder, 1964). The principle of the technique lies in estimating the ability of trinucleoside diphosphates (i.e. triplets) to form a bond between the corresponding ^{14}C-aminoacyl-tRNA and ribosomes. The results obtained with the aid of this method indicated un-

2 At the same time, 6-azauridine is relatively resistant to enzymes attacking pyrimidine nucleosides (Pontis et al., 1961). One may thus use with advantage 6-azauridine-^{14}C as a substrate for determining uridine kinase activity (Winkler et al., 1962).

equivocally that introduction of 6-azauridine into the codon triplet gives rise to dead codon triplets, which are unable to stimulate the binding of aminoacyl-tRNA to ribosomes (LISÝ et al., 1968). It may therefore be concluded that if incorporation

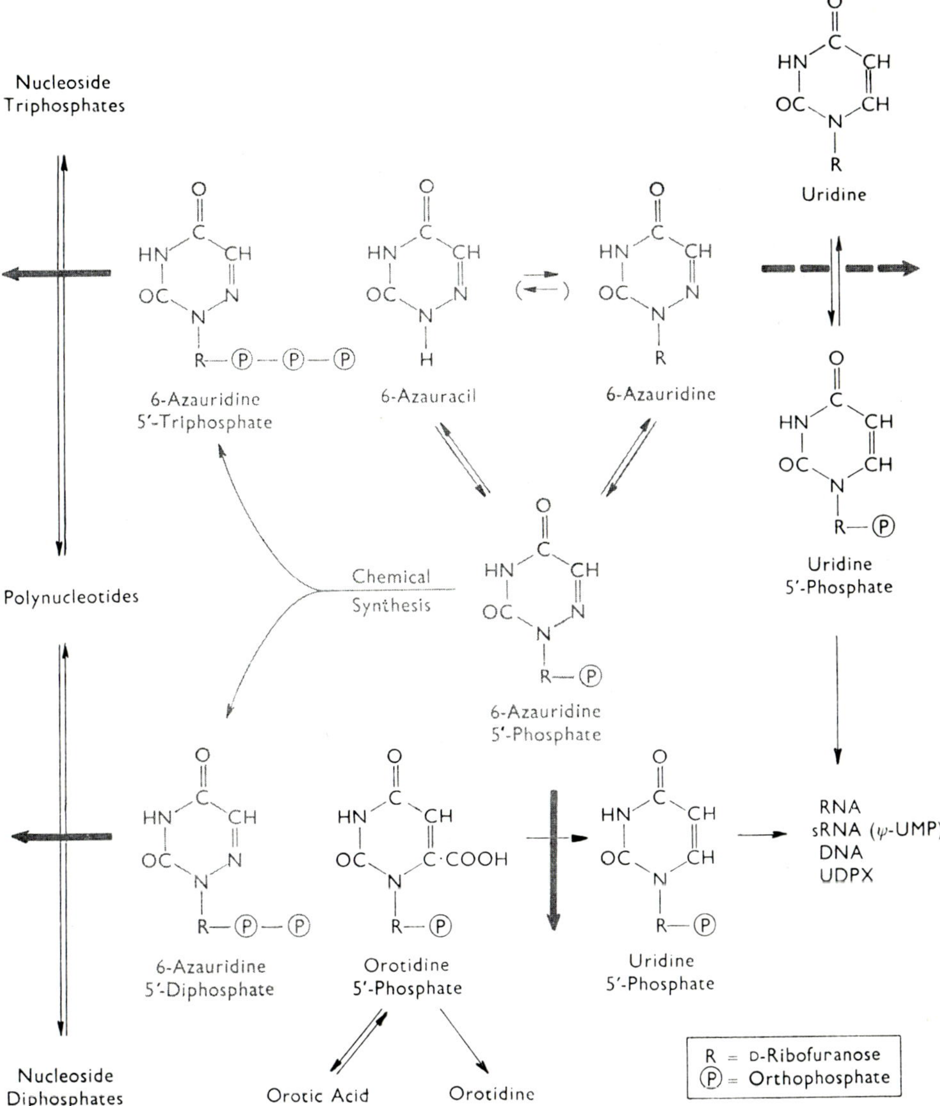

Fig. 1. Schematic representation of the inhibitory effects of 6-azauridine and its phosphates. The heavy arrows indicate inhibition, the heavy broken arrow a competition with substrate

of 6-azauridine (even in the form of 6-azacytidine) into informational macromolecules takes place, none of the codons and anticodons containing 6-azapyrimidine nucleosides would possess any coding activity and they would hence be unable to cause errors in the translation process.

II. Biological Effects

1. Virostatic Activity

The virostatic effects of 6-azauridine were first observed with vaccinia virus in a tissue culture of chicken fibroblasts (Rada et al., 1960), and later with the same virus in chorioallantoic membrane cultures (Rada and Blaškovič, 1961) and in HeLa cells (Loh, 1964; Rada and Blaškovič, 1966). 6-Azauridine also delayed the mortality rate of mice inoculated with the IHD variant of vaccinia virus (Jasińska et al., 1962); similarly, 6-azauridine inhibited vaccinia virus in rabbits (Šmejkal and Šorm, 1962).

A selective activity is displayed by 6-azauridine toward Rous sarcoma virus *in vitro* (Rada and Závada, 1962), as well as *in vivo* (Rada et al., 1964). It inhibits the formation of malignant centers by this virus on the chick embryo chorioallantoic membrane (Vrba, 1964).

6-Azauridine inhibits markedly the multiplication of type 5 adenovirus in a monolayer culture of HeLa cells (Flanagan and Ginsberg, 1964); at the same time, the biosynthesis of virus-specific antigens is inhibited. The following viruses were found to be sensitive to 6-azauridine: dengue virus (Stollar et al., 1966), polyoma virus (Gershon and Sachs, 1966), reovirus (Rada and Shatkin, 1967), Venezuelan equine encephalitis virus (Kaverin and Emeliyanov, 1967), para-influenza 3 virus (Korbecki et al., 1968), Newcastle disease virus (Schäfer et al., 1967; Bukrinskaya and Asadullaev, 1968), herpes simplex virus (Galegov et al., 1968), myxovirus (Bukrinskaya and Asadullaev, 1968), ornithosis virus (Terskikh et al., 1968), lymphocytic choriomeningitis virus (Buck and Pfau, 1969), cytomegalovirus (Demidova et al., 1969), herpes-virus hominis (Falke and Rada, 1970), and measles virus (Leonard et al., 1971).

In the meningovirus, 6-azauridine inhibited the incorporation of labeled uridine into viral specific ribonucleic acids and into mature virus without affecting viral yield (Korbecki et al., 1969); in Newcastle disease virus-infected cells it inhibited the synthesis of ribonucleic acids (Wilson and LoGerfo, 1964).

During a viral eye infection in rabbits caused by herpes simplex virus, 6-aza-uridine showed a clear therapeutic effect (Galegov et al., 1970). The inhibitory action of 6-azauridine in viral eye infections of man is dealt with elsewhere in this chapter.

The existing studies of the antiviral effects of 6-azauridine permit the following conclusions. 6-Azauridine shows pronounced antiviral effect against a number of viruses; however, it inhibits others very little or not at all. The sensitivity of viruses to 6-azauridine is rather different not only among viruses of different groups, but also within the same group or subgroup of viruses.

6-Azauridine inhibits also the reproduction of the T2 bacteriophage (Pravdina et al., 1969).

An important role in the mechanism of the antiviral effect of 6-azauridine is ascribed to an increase in the level of uridine kinase in infected cells evoked by the virus infection. An increased level of uridine kinase was observed in chorioallantoic membranes infected with vaccinia virus and in embryonic cells and muscles of chicks infected with Rous sarcoma virus (Rada and Gregušová, 1964; Gelbard et al., 1966). In infected cells an increase in the biosynthesis of 6-azauridine 5′-phosphate, the final inhibitor, is observed. The important role of uridine kinase in the antiviral activity of 6-azauridine is borne out by studies in which inhibition of virus by 6-azauridine was significantly increased by the addition of cell-free extracts containing uridine kinase (RADA and ALTANEROVÁ, 1970; RADA and HANUŠOVSKÁ, 1970; RADA, 1970).

6-Azauridine did not show any ability to activate murine leukemia virus in AKR cell lines (LOWY et al., 1971).

2. Antineoplastic Effects

The cancerostatic effects of 6-azauridine were described for the first time in a tissue culture of Sarcoma 180 (SCHINDLER and WELCH, 1957); the inhibitory effect of 6-azauridine in this system was relieved by uridine. Somewhat later, the antineoplastic effects of 6-azauridine were described in a series of experimental neoplasms (JAFFE et al., 1957; ŠORM and KEILOVÁ, 1958; CONN et al., 1967). The effects of 6-azauridine on the Rous sarcoma were mentioned previously.

A more exact comparison of the results attained is complicated by the fact that the antineoplastic effects of this compound are significantly dependent on the maintenance of an adequate concentration of 6-azauridine in the tissues (Table 1).

Table 1. *Dependence of the degree of inhibition of leukemia L 1210 by 6-azauridine on the frequency of dosage* (HANDSCHUMACHER et al., 1962)

μMoles/dose	Time intervals between administration (h)	Total dose per day (μmoles)	Change in body weight (g)	Inhibition of tumor growth (%)
2	8	6	0	50
3	12	6	+1.0	17
6	24	6	+1.5	8
12	48	6	+2.0	0

Of the experimental neoplasms studied, 6-azauridine inhibits pronouncedly the L 5178 Y lymphoma in mice and the H lymphoma of rats (HANDSCHUMACHER et al., 1962). The antitumor effect of 6-azauridine in these cancers is associated with an inhibition of the formation of pyrimidine nucleotides *de novo* (HANDSCHUMACHER and PASTERNAK, 1958).

The antitumor effect of 6-azauridine toward the Ehrlich ascitic tumor may be potentiated by an alkylating agent [5-*bis*-(2-chloroethyl)-aminomethyluracil] (ŠORM and VESELÝ, 1961). Using the same tumor, it was possible to observe an antagonism between the therapeutic effect of irradiation and 6-azauridine if the antimetabolite was administered shortly before the irradiation (GROZDANOVIČ et al. 1968). However, if 6-azauridine was administered 24 h before irradiation, it potentiated the cancerostatic effect of the ionizing radiation (MAGDON and KONOPATZKY, 1967). 6-Azauridine applied before irradiation prevented an increase in the diameter of the cell nuclei of Ehrlich ascites carcinoma cells (GROZDANOVIČ et al., 1970).

As with other antimetabolites of the nucleic acid components, resistance appeared against 6-azauridine. Thus, e.g., using a serial subculture, a strain of experimental leukemia developed a 1500 times greater resistance toward 6-azauridine. It was found that the cells of the resistant strain lost their ability to phosphorylate 6-azauridine to the active inhibitory nucleotide form (PASTERNAK et al., 1961).

The antineoplastic effects of 6-azauridine in man are treated elsewhere in this chapter.

3. Immunosuppressive Activity

The immunosuppressive activity of 6-azauridine is not particularly strong, but in view of the large doses of 6-azauridine employed in the treatment of malignant diseases, as well as in nonlethal conditions, one must consider this activity.

The formation of antibodies in young rabbits is inhibited only at relatively high doses of 6-azauridine; complete inhibition can be achieved at a dose of 5 g/kg body weight, and significant inhibition can be attained in some animals at a dose of 0.5 g/kg body weight (ŠTERZL, 1961). By combining 6-azauridine with chloramphenicol it was possible to suppress the primary immune response to an intraperitoneal injection of sheep erythrocytes in mice. Combination therapy using both 6-azauridine and chloramphenicol at a lower dose level did not result in potentiation; however, admixture of either drug in a low dose with the other in a larger dose led to a significant potentiation, which was more marked when 6-azauridine was used at the larger dose (FISCHER et al., 1966).

In large doses, 6-azauridine displayed an immunosuppressive effect in the allotransplantation reaction in mice (NOUZA, 1966). The immunosuppressive effects of 6-azauridine, or rather of 6-azauridine 2′,3′,5′-triacetate[3] were studied in greater detail with a number of cell-mediated responses in mice (transplantation reaction, graft-versus-host reaction, and experimental autoimmune aspermatogenesis). In all of the cases studied 6-azauridine displayed a low to medium immunosuppressive activity, but only when certain conditions of dose and timing were maintained (NOUZA et al., 1970). Small doses of 6-azauridine or its short-term application may lead to a paradoxical enhancement of antibody synthesis *in vitro* (STEJSKALOVÁ et al., 1970), as well as *in vivo* (NOUZA et al., 1970).

4. Cholesterol and Lipid Changes Induced by 6-Azauridine

Protracted administration of 6-azauridine (intravenous drip) or its acetyl derivative (orally) to leukemic (BUTTOO et al., 1965) and psoriatic (SLAVÍK et al., 1970) patients led to a decrease in serum cholesterol levels. This hypocholesterolemia was observed also with rats following an oral application of 6-azauridine triacetate (BUTTOO et al., 1965). Repeated application of 6-azauridine to rats was shown to decrease not only plasma cholesterol levels, but also the concentrations of free fatty acids, phospholipids, and esterified fatty acids; plasma glucose and total protein concentration were not affected (GRAFNETTER and GRAFNETTEROVÁ, 1967). In experiments with liver slices and epididymal fat pads of rats injected for two weeks with 6-azauridine, a pronounced decrease was produced in the incorporation of labeled acetate into lipids (GRAFNETTEROVÁ et al., 1968a).

5. Embryotoxic Effects

In tests with a screening system for substances capable of interrupting pregnancy, 6-azauridine was described as a compound which closely approached the goal of finding an agent which might control human pregnancy, with minimal toxic effects (SANDERS et al., 1961). Single doses of 1 mg/g interrupted every pregnancy in mice; one-half of this dose level interrupted, under the same conditions, about 50% of the pregnancies. The antifertility activity of 6-azauridine was less effective in the very earliest and during the later stages of pregnancy. The following important facts were observed by the above authors: (a) young animals born to mothers exposed to 6-azauridine during early pregnancy survived

3 The 6-azauridine preparation used orally: 2-β-D-ribofuranosyl-*as*-triazine-3,5($2H$,$4H$)-dione 2′,3′,5′-triacetate, or Triazure.

and were apparently quite normal, (b) litters born to mothers dosed late in pregnancy were smaller in number and most of the young died within two days of birth, and (c) in doses capable of interrupting pregnancy, 6-azauridine has no pronounced effect on the unfertilized ovum or on the mother, and the young, which were exposed to the effects of 6-azauridine during their intrauterine life, were themselves capable in due course of producing and rearing normal offspring.

At a dose of 2 to 4 g/kg of mouse body weight and at a dose of 4 to 6 g/kg of rat body weight the drug showed marked embryotoxic effects between the 5th and 10th days of pregnancy. The necrotic embryos and placentas were resorbed *in utero*. If 6-azauridine was applied before the 4th day it showed no embryotoxicity. If applied after the 10th day it resulted in premature delivery of either sick or dead progeny. In mice exposed to massive doses of 6-azauridine, no trophoblastic proliferation resembling the hydatiform mole was observed (VORHERR and WELCH, 1970). Further, the teratogenic effect of 6-azauridine in rats was shown to depend upon (a) the stage of embryonic development and (b) the antimetabolite dose (GUTOVÁ et al., 1971).

6-Azauridine triacetate also caused an inhibition of pregnancy in successfully mated female rabbits (SAKSENA and CHAUDHURY, 1970). While young mice born to mothers inadequately dosed appeared to be perfectly healthy, it was observed that when 500 mg of 6-azauridine/kg was given from day 13 to 17 to 1 female rabbit there appeared to be a reduction in litter size and 1 fetus showed an abnormality in the development of the nostrils (MORRIS et al., 1967).

The abortifacient effect of 6-azauridine triacetate was studied also in the macaque monkey. Of 14 pregnancies examined, 13 were terminated by spontaneous abortion without any correlation between dosage, weight of animals, and time of abortion. One pregnancy (with a low dose of 6-azauridine triacetate) carried to term, when fetal dystocia required a hysterotomy, and a teratogenic infant was delivered (VAN WAGENEN et al., 1970).

The effect of 6-azauridine given intravenously in single doses of 7.5 to 15.0 g was examined in 15 pregnant women preceding curettage. In three of the women with advanced pregnancy, which was interrupted 24 h after application of 6-azauridine, no changes in trophoblast could be detected. In the other women, changes of the chorionic villi were observed during the interval of 1 to 8 days after application of the antimetabolite, which represents incontestable proof of damage to the ovum. 6-Azauridine thus shows definite deleterious effects in early human pregnancy (VOJTA and JIRÁSEK, 1966).

In chick embryos, 6-azauridine was also embryotoxic, particularly during the first phases of incubation; the occurrence of malformations and even of fetal death was observed (GRAFNETTEROVÁ et al., 1966).

Several attempts have been made to elucidate the basis of the embryotoxic effect of 6-azauridine. The degree of inhibition of the incorporation of ^{14}C-orotic acid *in vivo*, as well as the effect of the drug on the formation of $^{14}CO_2$ from ^{14}C-carboxylorotic acid *in vitro*, is practically the same both at the time of high sensitivity (6-day embryos) and during the period of relative insensitivity (15-day fetuses) in mice (RAŠKA et al., 1966). In chick embryos, 6-azauridine not only produced an inhibition of orotic acid incorporation, but also a remarkable decrease in the rate of incorporation of uridine into embryonal RNA (WELCH, ŠKODA and GUTOVÁ, 1965, unpublished results). In the brain of chick embryos exposed to 6-azauridine, a relatively large concentration of this antimetabolite was found (GRAFNETTEROVÁ and GRAFNETTER, 1968). It was further shown that the brain of chick embryos, exposed to 6-azauridine during the first developmental phases, possessed a relatively larger content of total steroids and a slightly increased content of desmosterol (Grafnetterová et al., 1966). During embryonic development of chicks, 6-azauridine causes a decrease in the calcium level of plasma and an increase of bone dry weight and ash, as well as of the calcium content (Grafnetterová et al., 1968b).

In the studies on the effect of 6-azauridine on chick, mouse, and rat embryos and fetuses, a direct interference by the analog with morphogenetic systems of the embryo was observed during the period of formation of organ systems (Jelínek et al., 1970), organs (Jelínek et al., 1971), and organ components, e.g., of the coronary system of the heart (Rychter et al., 1972; Rychter and Jelínek, 1973). 6-Azauridine apparently is active throughout morphogeny; the final effect is determined by the developmental stage of the embryo at the time of exposure to 6-azauridine. According to the latest observations, the embryotoxic effects of 6-azauridine in the mouse are directed especially against the developing fetal brain (Seifertová et al., 1973).

III. Pharmacological Studies

The toxicity of 6-azauridine is highly species specific. In man, 6-azauridine may be employed over long periods for therapeutic purposes in extremely large doses of 600 mg/kg/24 h; doses of 24 mg/kg/24 h cause leukopenia and death in the dog (Handschumacher et al., 1962). Acute toxicity for mice after intraperitoneal injection is very low ($LD_{50} = 11.25$ g/kg); however, if it is given to mice in repeated daily doses, leukopenia and hemorrhagic diarrhea occur and lead to the death of the animals. A linear relationship exists between the logarithm of the daily dose of 6-azauridine and the logarithm of the mean lethal time (Jiřička et al., 1965). Small doses of 6-azauridine (50 mg/kg/24 h) cause a stimulation of lymphopoiesis in the spleen and the lymph nodes; larger doses (500 mg/kg/24 h) lead to a progressive depression of lymphopoiesis and to proliferation of reticulum cells. Following large doses of 6-azauridine, necrobiotic changes of the intestinal epithelium, morphological changes in the kidney, and fatty degeneration of the liver were observed.

Acute and chronic toxicity of 6-azauridine 2′,3′,5′-triacetate correspond in rats to the toxicity of 6-azauridine (compared on a molar base); in mice the triacetate is more toxic. In rats, repeated oral administration caused serious side effects; however, under these conditions it did not lead to any undesirable changes in pigs (Plevová et al., 1970a).

Injected 6-azauridine is apparently generally distributed throughout body water and is relatively rapidly excreted unchanged in the urine; 75% of a dose is excreted within 4 h, and over 95% within 8 h (Handschumacher et al., 1962). 6-Azauridine is excreted by the kidney through glomerular filtration and tubular excretion, with glomerular filtration playing a more important role. No significant difference was found in excretion following intravenous or intramuscular administration (Šmahel et al., 1967).

6-Azauridine administered orally is very poorly absorbed and the blood levels attained are short lived. 6-Azauracil is formed in the process and this pyrimidine produces highly undesirable central nervous system toxicity.

The effect of 6-azauridine on the central nervous system was studied in mice and in rats. The most sensitive indicator of its action was found to be depression of exploratory activity. Conditioned avoidance behavior remained unchanged even at very large doses. Following injection of 6-azauridine into the cerebral ventricles of mice, the effect on motor behavior is raised 50 to 100 times when compared with intraperitoneal application. An antagonism between 6-azauridine and some convulsants has also been described (JANKŮ et al., 1965b). Studies were undertaken on the effect of 6-azauridine on the peripheral nervous system (BAUER and ČAPEK, 1969a, b) and on the contractile responses of the isolated ileum to drugs and to coaxial stimulation (ŠEFERNA et al., 1966). 6-Azauridine (500 mg/kg) injected intraperitoneally into rats inhibited some types of experimental inflammation (TRNAVSKÝ and LAPÁROVÁ, 1967).

Parenteral application of large doses of 6-azauridine, however, produced no serious side effects in humans. In the course of treatment of patients with nonterminal malignant disease with 6-azauridine, orotic aciduria (Fig. 2) and uricosuria (FALLON et al., 1961) were observed. These may lead to crystalluria (HANDSCHUMACHER et al., 1962). Prolonged administration of 6-azauridine or its triacetate in massive oral doses interferes with the formation of erythrocytes, but a slowly developing anemia promptly disappears on temporary withdrawal of the drug.

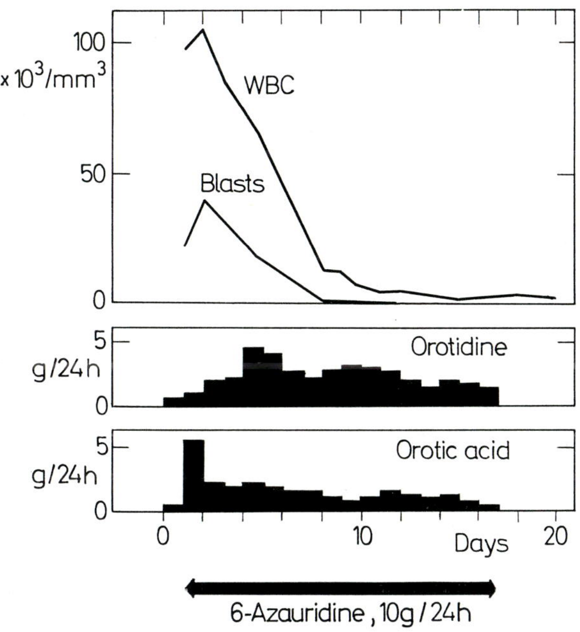

Fig. 2. Leukocytes and urinary excretion of orotidine and orotic acid during the therapy of monocytic leukemia with 6-azauridine (BUTTOO et al., 1965)

In contrast to 6-azauridine, its triacetate is rapidly absorbed from the gastrointestinal tract. Free 6-azauridine appears in the blood stream together with a smaller amount of 6-azauridine 5′-monoacetate (Fig. 3) (HANDSCHUMACHER et al., 1962). Deacetylation of 6-azauridine triacetate takes place during its incubation with blood serum (CREASEY et al., 1963). A rapid deacetylation is observed in rodents, while slower deacetylation occurs in the serum of nonrodent species (PLEVOVÁ et al., 1970b). Following oral administration of 6-azauridine 2′, 3′,5′-triacetate to man, most of the compound was excreted in the form of 6-azauridine and a portion as 6-azauridine monoacetate; in one patient, the urine was found to contain 6-azauridine diacetate. In none of the patients, however, was unchanged triacetate excreted in the urine (GRAFNETTEROVÁ et al., 1966b).

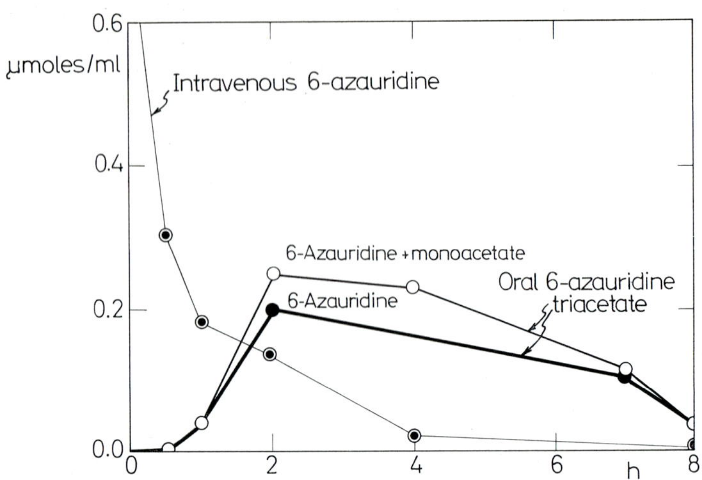

Fig. 3. Blood levels of 6-azauridine after equimolar dosage of 6-azauridine (intravenously) or its triacetyl derivative (orally) (Handschumacher et al., 1962)

IV. Clinical Application

1. Virostatic Effects

6-Azauridine was administered orally for 2 to 3 weeks up to a total dose of about 100 g to patients with a viral eye infection in which the herpes simplex virus was found or the clinical course pointed strongly to this etiology (Myška et al., 1967). The healing was rapid, especially in patients with dendritic ulcers combined with iridocyclitis. All patients selected for this study suffered from considerable stromal involvement for which other therapy, including topical 5-iodo-2′-deoxyuridine, is practically ineffective.

In a controlled clinical experiment with nonvaccinated patients suffering from smallpox of the so-called ordinary type, 6-azauridine was found to reduce mortality by 50% (Elis and Rašková, 1971).

2. Antineoplastic and Antihyperplastic Effects

The first clinical application of 6-azauridine was in patients with cancer. 6-Azauridine does not affect solid tumors (Elis and Rašková, 1971; Erukhimov and Vermel, 1969). Only in the gynecological area was tumor regression described after massive doses of 6-azauridine (Kafka et al., 1961). More significant application of 6-azauridine lies in the treatment of leukemia. According to American (Handschumacher et al., 1962) and Czechoslovak (Elis and Misařová, 1964; Elis and Rašková, 1966) studies, the results obtained may be summarized as follows: In infant leukemia, 6-azauridine produces complete remissions less frequently than 6-mercaptopurine, but it induces more frequent partial remissions. The duration of complete as well as partial remissions is shorter following administration of 6-azauridine than 6-mercaptopurine. In adult patients with leukemia no complete remissions were observed, but partial remissions were achieved. Here, too, the duration of the remission was shorter than with other therapeutic modalities. In several cases of acute leukemia of children and adults, which were resistant to conventional cytostatics, the administration of 6-azauridine resulted in a complete or partial remission. A relatively rapid effect is achieved with patients suffering from chronic granulocytic leukemia in blastic crisis where in 3 to 5 days a practically normal white blood cell count is achieved (HANDSCHUMACHER et al., 1962). The most striking results of treating leukemia with 6-azauridine are the preferential effects on the blast cells which were diminished dramatically in all 13 acute leukemias studied[4] (WILKINSON, 1963). 6-Azauridine may thus be useful in producing a rapid depression of the leukemic cell population before resorting to further treatment.

Promising results were achieved in the treatment of mycosis fungoides (ZÁRUBA et al., 1963; CALABRESI and TURNER, 1966). In addition, 6-azauridine is highly effective in all kinds of trophoblast proliferation (malignant chorionepithelioma, destructive and hydatiform mole) where a normalization of chorionic gonadotropins is also achieved (ŠMAHEL et al., 1965).

Following administration of 6-azauridine or of its triacetate to patients with polycythemia vera, amelioration of symptoms was observed, together with a decrease in splenomegaly and a reduction of the hematocrit; this effect of 6-azauridine is apparently due to suppression of erythropoiesis (DECONTI and CALABRESI, 1970).

3. Effect on Psoriasis

6-Azauridine displays a selective inhibitory effect on psoriatic epidermis. Of the first series of ten patients with severe, disabling psoriasis, all showed clinical improvement of their skin lesions following oral administration of 6-azauridine triacetate. The most rapid improvement was seen in the patients with exfoliative erythroderma. The doses applied at the onset of treatment were 270 mg/kg/24 h and later were gradually decreased to one-half this level. No case of oral, gastrointestinal, or skin ulceration was observed and hair loss did not occur (TURNER and CALABRESI, 1964). The usefulness of 6-azauridine in the treatment of psoriasis was demonstrated in further work (CALABRESI and TURNER, 1966) carried out by a double-blind test method (RAŠKOVÁ et al., 1967; VOGLER and OLANSKY, 1970). Here, too, no toxic side effects were observed; a mild depression of the bone marrow was the only toxicity observed. 6-Azauridine triacetate is not recommended for pregnant women during the period of growth of the fetus (RAŠKOVÁ et al., 1967) or for patients with rheumatoid arthritis[5] (ELIS et al., 1970). Patients suffering from psoriasis and treated with 6-azauridine triacetate displayed a typical hyperaminoaciduria (SLAVÍK et al., 1969).

D. 5-Azacytidine[6]

I. Molecular Mechanism of Inhibitory Action

The inhibitory effects of 5-azacytidine are polyvalent. They involve 5-azauridine which is formed by deamination, as well as other decomposition products. Pronounced growth-inhibition is produced by 5-azacytidine in bacteria; this inhibition may be relieved by pyrimidine nucleosides added together with the antimetabolite (ČIHÁK and ŠORM, 1964). 5-Azacytidine in *Escherichia coli* inhibits the induction of β-galactosidase, as well as general protein synthesis, while the synthesis of total RNA is inhibited only slightly (DOSKOČIL et al., 1967). 5-Aza-

4 In the course of treatment of acute myeloblastic leukemia, chromosome changes in peripheral leukocytes were described (ELVES et al., 1963).

5 In smaller doses (50 mg/kg/24 h) applied over long periods, 6-azauridine triacetate reportedly had an ameliorative effect on rheumatoid arthritis (HAVELKA et al., 1969).

6 1-β-D-Ribofuranosyl-4-amino-*s*-triazine-2(1*H*)-one.

cytidine is incorporated into bacterial RNA and DNA. The inhibition of β-galactosidase induction is apparently due to the formation of fraudulent mRNA (Pačes et al., 1968a). With *Escherichia coli* deficient in cytidine deaminase, the incorporation of leucine into proteins is inhibited by 5-azacytidine only slightly, while in the wild strain the inhibition is complete. However, sensitivity toward 5-azauridine is retained even in the deaminase-deficient strain (Doskočil and Šorm, 1970b). 5-Azauridine apparently plays an important role in the mechanism of the inhibitory effects of 5-azacytidine. In the presence of 5-azacytidine one may observe disturbances in the formation of bacterial ribosomes: both 23S and 16S ribosomal RNAs are formed, but are not incorporated into the ribosomes (Pačes et al., 1968b).

After the intraperitoneal administration of 5-azacytidine to mice, the urine was found to contain orotidine and orotic acid (Raška et al., 1965), and in leukemic mice, the incorporation of orotic acid into liver RNA was markedly inhibited after 5-azacytidine (Veselý et al., 1968b); these findings point to an inhibition of orotidine 5′-phosphate decarboxylase by 5-azacytidine 5′-phosphate. In addition, 2 to 8 h following an intraperitoneal injection of 5-azacytidine to rats, cell-free extracts of their livers contained a lower level of orotidine 5′-phosphate decarboxylase. The activity of this enzyme returned to normal after 30 to 36 h. The decreased utilization of orotic acid was observed for only a few hours after the administration of the analog, and after 18 to 24 h a pronounced increase in the incorporation of orotic acid was noted (Čihák and Brouček, 1972).

The mechanism of the inhibitory effects of 5-azacytidine is characterized by the incorporation of the analog into nucleic acids (Čihák et al., 1965; Jurovčík et al., 1965). In a culture of L 1210 leukemia cells, inhibition of DNA synthesis occurred to a greater extent than that of RNA synthesis. 5-Azacytidine is phosphorylated to the 5′-triphosphate, the formed nucleotides are reduced to the corresponding deoxyribonucleotides and the analog is incorporated into both RNA and DNA. Incorporation into polynucleotides is thought to be the main cause of the marked antileukemic effects of 5-azacytidine (Li et al., 1970a).

Interference with the synthesis of pyrimidine nucleotides *de novo* on the one hand and the formation of fraudulent nucleic acids due to incorporation of 5-azacytidine, on the other, represent, according to present knowledge, the main molecular consequences of exposure to 5-azacytidine.

II. Biological Effects in Animal Systems

Larger doses of 5-azacytidine bring about depression of the bone marrow in mice and a hypoplastic involution of the lymphatic system (LD_{50} is about 150 mg/kg). In therapeutic doses, 5-azacytidine is a potent inhibitor of lymphoid leukemia in mice (Šorm et al., 1964); a single dose of 100 mg/kg produced, in 50% of the treated animals, a complete or considerable eradication of leukemic cells given in a supralethal dose (Šorm and Veselý, 1964). Using proper dosage regimens, a threefold increase in survival was achieved in mice with leukemia L 1210 (Evans and Haňka, 1968). The antileukemic effect and immunosuppressive activity (Fischer et al., 1966) of 5-azacytidine in mice are depressed by concurrent treatment with either 6-azauridine (Šorm and Veselý, 1965), or uridine (Vadlamudi et al., 1970).

Due to incorporation of 5-azacytidine into DNA (Li et al., 1970a) the L 1210 leukemia cells in culture display considerable chromosome damage[7] (Li et al., 1970b). 5-Azacytidine was also used for the preparation of mutants of arboviruses

[7] Chromosomal mutations are caused by 5-azacytidine in the root meristem of *Vicia faba* (Fučík et al., 1965, 1970).

(HALLE, 1968) and for obtaining conditional lethal mutants of vesicular stomatitis virus (PRINGLE, 1970).

The acquisition of resistance toward 5-azacytidine[8] by mouse leukemia cells is accompanied by (a) a decrease in uridine and deoxycytidine kinase activities, (b) a decrease in the incorporation of cytidine and 5-azacytidine into nucleic acids, (c) an increase in triphosphatase activity (VESELÝ et al., 1968c), and (d) an increase in RNA and DNA polymerase activities (VESELÝ et al., 1970). Leukemic cells resistant to 5-aza-2′-deoxycytidine are sensitive to 5-azacytidine, but cells resistant to 5-azacytidine are also insensitive to 5-aza-2′-deoxycytidine (VESELÝ et al., 1968a).

Incorporation of 5-azacytidine into ribonucleic acids is the most likely cause of inhibition of hormonal induction of tryptophan pyrrolase observed after administration of 5-azacytidine to rats (ČIHÁK et al., 1967), as well as of the inhibition of thymidine kinase synthesis in rat liver after partial hepatectomy (ČIHÁK et al., 1968). On the other hand, the levels of tyrosine aminotransferase (ČIHÁK et al., 1971) and of uridine kinase (ČIHÁK et al., 1972) in regenerating rat liver, as well as in the liver of intact rats, are increased after 5-azacytidine. This antimetabolite causes a destruction of liver polyribosomes to inactive monomers and dimers in rats (ČIHÁK et al., 1968; LEVITAN and WEBB, 1969).

5-Azacytidine interrupts pregnancy in mice during the first week (with an optimum effect between the 4th and the 6th day), while it has no discernible effect during the last 10 days of pregnancy (SVATÁ et al., 1966); 4- to 6-day-old embryos are completely resorbed. With 11- to 13-day-old fetuses damage to liver and nerve tissue was observed (SEIFERTOVÁ et al., 1968). In developing sea urchin embryos, 5-azacytidine inhibited the synthesis of RNA, as well as of DNA, but not the formation of proteins; morphological development was not affected up to the 8-cell stage, but thereafter a retardation of development occurred (CRKVENJAKOV et al., 1970).

5-Azacytidine, administered for three days before a supralethal dose of x-irradiation, markedly reduced the mortality of mice (VESELÝ et al., 1969b).

Recently, a high frequency induction of mouse leukemia in the AKR strain by 5-azacytidine was described; 5-azacytidine was a more potent inducer than 5-iodo-2′-deoxyuridine (VESELÝ and ČIHÁK, 1973). 5-Azacytidine also induced virus production in a virogenic hamster cell line transformed by Rous sarcoma virus (ALTANEROVÁ, 1972).

III. Clinical Studies

Successful therapeutic application of 5-azacytidine in experimental leukemias was followed by clinical administration of the antimetabolite to 20 children with acute leukemia and to one child with chronic myeloid leukemia (HRODEK and VESELÝ, 1971). 5-Azacytidine (1 to 2 mg/kg/24 h) produced a considerable depression of leukocyte count in 90% of the children and a decrease or disappearance of blasts in the blood. The improvement of the bone marrow was either partial or insignificant. If, however, prednisone was employed together with 5-azacytidine, complete remission was achieved in a large percentage of the patients. The duration of remission was between 2 and 16 months. During the later stages of the disease the effect of 5-azacytidine by itself, as well as in combination with prednisone, was generally unsatisfactory.

8 In *Bacillus subtilis*, the acquisition of resistance to 5-azacytidine is accompanied by a loss in the ability of the bacteria to incorporate the antimetabolite into nucleic acids (JUROVČÍK et al., 1972). The transfer of resistance to a sensitive strain was achieved by a transformation process (FUČÍK et al., 1972).

Tolerance to 5-azacytidine is relatively high. In only 2 out of 21 cases was vomiting observed following an intramuscular injection; however, intramuscular injection of children was accompanied by considerable thrombocytopenia which resulted in hematomas.

5-Azacytidine also showed an impressive activity in children with acute myelogenous leukemia resistant to cytosine arabinoside (KARON et al., 1973).

References

ALTANEROVÁ, V.: Virus production induced by various chemical carcinogens in a virogenic hamster cell line transformed by Rous sarcoma virus. J. Natl. Cancer Inst. **49**, 1375—1380 (1972).

BAUER, V., ČAPEK, R.: The effects of 6-azauridine on the peripheral nervous system. I. The action on ganglionic transmission. Int. J. Neuropharmacol. **8**, 263—269 (1969a).

BAUER, V., ČAPEK, R.: The effects of 6-azauridine on the peripheral nervous system. II. The action on neuromuscular transmission and on striated muscle. Int. J. Neuropharmacol. **8**, 721—727 (1969b).

BERÁNEK, J.: Nucleic acid components and their analogues. CXIX. Synthesis of 1-β-D-lyxofuranosyl-6-azauracil. Coll. Czech. Chem. Commun. **34**, 618—629 (1969).

BERÁNEK, J., PIŤHA, J.: Nucleic acid components and their analogues. XLVI. Some derivatives of 6-azacytidine and 6-azauridine. Coll. Czech. Chem. Commun. **29**, 625—634 (1964).

BERÁNEK, J., ŠORM, F.: Nucleic acid components and their analogues. CVIII. Synthesis of 3′-deoxy-6-azauridine. Coll. Czechoslov. Chem. Commun. **33**, 901—912 (1968a).

BERÁNEK, J., ŠORM, F.: Nucleic acid components and their analogues. CIX. Synthesis of 1-β-D-arabinofuranosyl-6-azaisocytosine. Coll. Czech. Chem. Commun. **33**, 913—923 (1968b).

BOBEK, M., FARKAŠ, J., ŠORM, F.: Nucleic acid components and their analogues. XCVII. Synthesis of 5-hydroxymethyl-6-aza-2′-deoxyuridine and 5-hydroxymethyl-6-aza-2′-deoxycytidine. Coll. Czech. Chem. Commun. **32**, 3581—3586 (1967).

BOBEK, M., FARKAŠ, J., ŠORM, F.: Nucleic acid components and their analogues. CXXIV. Synthesis of 5-β-D-ribofuranosyl-6-azauracil (6-azapseudouridine). Coll. Czech. Chem. Commun. **34**, 1690—1695 (1969).

BONO, V. H., WEISSMAN, S. M., FREI, E. III.: The effect of 6-azauridine administration on *de novo* pyrimidine production in chronic myelogenous leukemia. J. clin. Invest. **43**, 1486—1494 (1964).

BUCK, L. L., PFAU, C. J.: Inhibition of lymphocytic choriomeningitis virus replication by actinomycin D and 6-azauridine. Virology **37**, 698—701 (1969).

BUKRINSKAYA, A. G., ASADULLAEV, T. A.: Comparative effect of histon and 6-azauridine on myxovirus reproduction. Vop. virus. **13**, 549—554 (1968) (in Russian).

BUTTOO, A. S., ISRAËLS, M. C. G., WILKINSON, J. F.: Hypocholesterolaemia and orotic aciduria during treatment with 6-azauridine. Brit. med. J. **1**, 552—554 (1965).

CALABRESI, P., TURNER, R. W.: Beneficial effects of triacetyl azauridine in psoriasis and mycosis fungoides. Ann. intern. Med. **64**, 352—371 (1966).

ČEREY, K., ELIS, J., RAŠKOVÁ, H.: Studies on 6-azauridine and 6-azacytidine. V. Influence of 6-azacytidine on prenatal development in mice. Biochem. Pharmacol. **14**, 1549—1556 (1965).

ČERNĚCKIJ, V., CHLÁDEK, S., ŠORM, F., SMRT, J.: Nucleic acid components and their analogues. XIV. 6-Azacytidine and some of its N_4-derivatives. Coll. Czech. Chem. Commun. **27**, 87—93 (1962).

ČIHÁK, A., BROUČEK, J.: Dual effect of 5-azacytidine on the synthesis of liver ribonucleic acids. Lack of the relationship between metabolic transformation of orotic acid *in vitro* and its incorporation *in vivo*. Biochem. Pharmacol. **21**, 2497—2507 (1972).

ČIHÁK, A., SEIFERTOVÁ, M., VESELÝ, J.: Enhanced uridine kinase and RNA synthesis in regenerating rat liver after 5-azacytidine administration. Arch. Biochem. Biophys. **148**, 400—406 (1972).

ČIHÁK, A., ŠKODA, J., ŠORM, F.: Formation of 5-azauridine, ribosyl N-formylbiuret, ribosyl biuret, and their 5′-phosphates in *Escherichia coli* culture from 5-azauracil. Coll. Czech. Chem. Commun. **29**, 300—308 (1964).

ČIHÁK, A., ŠORM, F.: Biochemical effects and metabolic transformations of 5-azacytidine in *Escherichia coli*. Coll. Czech. Chem. Commun. **30**, 2091—2102 (1965).

ČIHÁK, A., VESELÝ, J., INOUE, H., PITOT, H. C.: Effect of 5-azacytidine on dietary and hormone induction of serine dehydratase and tyrosine aminotransferase in rat liver. Biochem. Pharmacol. **21**, 2545—2553 (1972).

ČIHÁK, A., VESELÝ, J., ŠORM, F.: Incorporation of 5-azacytidine into liver ribonucleic acids of leukemic mice sensitive and resistant to 5-azacytidine. Biochim. biophys. Acta (Amst.) **108**, 516—518 (1965).

ČIHÁK, A., VESELÝ, J., ŠORM, F.: Complete inhibition by 5-azacytidine of hormonal induction of tryptophan pyrrolase. Biochim. biophys. Acta (Amst.) **134**, 486—489 (1967).

ČIHÁK, A., VESELÝ, J., ŠORM, F.: Thymidine kinase and polyribosome distribution in regenerating rat liver following 5-azacytidine. Biochim. biophys. Acta (Amst.) **166**, 277—279 (1968).

CONN, H. O., CREASEY, W. A., CALABRESI, P.: Effect of 6-azauridine on plasma cell tumors of mice: correlation of antitumor effect with inhibition of orotic acid metabolism. Cancer Res. **27**, 618—625 (1967).

CREASEY, W. A., FINK, M. E., HANDSCHUMACHER, R. E., CALABRESI, P.: Clinical and pharmacological studies with 2′,3′,5′-triacetyl-6-azauridine. Cancer Res. **23**, 444—453 (1963).

CRISTESCU, C.: 6-Azauracil derivatives with potential cytostatic activity. VI. An improved synthesis of 2-β-D-ribofuranosyl-*as*-triazine-3,5(2*H*,4*H*)dione (6-azauridine). Rev. Roumaine Chim. **12**, 365—369 (1968).

CRKVENJAKOV, R., BAJKOVIČ, N., GLIŠIN, V.: The effect of 5-azacytidine on development, nucleic acid and protein metabolism in sea urchin embryos. Biochem. biophys. Res. Commun. **39**, 655—660 (1970).

DECONTI, R. C., CALABRESI, P.: Treatment of polycythemia vera with azauridine and azaribine. Ann. intern. Med. **73**, 575—579 (1970).

DEMIDOVA, S. A., AZADOVA, N. B., MARTYNOVA, V. N., GALEGOV, G. A., ZHDANOV, V. M.: The injurious effect of 6-azauridine on the multiplication of cytomegalovirus in man. Dokl. Akad. Nauk SSSR **186**, 709—710 (1969) (in Russian).

DOSKOČIL, J.: The kinetics of metabolic transformations of nucleosides by whole cells of *Escherichia coli*. Coll. Czech. Chem. Commun. **35**, 2656—2672 (1970).

DOSKOČIL, J., PAČES, V.: The effect of azapyrimidine nucleosides and deoxynucleosides on the metabolism of thymidine and thymine in cultures of *Escherichia coli*. Coll. Czech. Chem. Commun. **33**, 4369—4378 (1968).

DOSKOČIL, J., PAČES, V., ŠORM, F.: Inhibition of protein synthesis by 5-azacytidine in *Escherichia coli*. Biochim. biophys. Acta (Amst.) **145**, 771—779 (1967).

DOSKOČIL, J., ŠORM, F.: The effects of 5-azacytidine and 5-azauridine on protein synthesis in *Escherichia coli*. Biochem. biophys. Res. Commun. **38**, 569—574 (1970a).

DOSKOČIL, J., ŠORM, F.: The inhibitory effects of 5-azacytidine and 5-azauridine in *Escherichia coli*. Coll. Czech. Chem. Commun. **35**, 1880—1891 (1970b).

DOSKOČIL, J., ŠORM, F.: The mode of action of 5-aza-2′-deoxycytidine in *Escherichia coli*. Europ. J. Biochem. **13**, 180—187 (1970c).

DURR, G. J., HAMMOND, S.: The synthesis of 1-(2-deoxy-D-arabinohexopyranosyl)-5-bromo-6-azauracil(1). J. heterocycl. Chem. **7**, 743—745 (1970).

DURR, G. J., KEISER, J. F., IERARDI, P. A.: The 6-azauracil and 6-azathymine nucleosides of 2-deoxy-D-arabinohexopyranose(1). J. heterocycl. Chem. **4**, 291—294 (1967).

ELIS, J., RAŠKOVÁ, H.: La toxicité foetale de l'azacytidine. J. Physiol. (Paris) **56**, 559—560 (1964).

ELIS, J., RAŠKOVÁ, H.: Controlled clinical trials with new cytostatic preparations produced in Czechoslovakia. Rev. Czech. Med. **12**, 9—19 (1966).

ELIS, J., RAŠKOVÁ, H.: New indications for 6-azauridine treatment in man. A review. Europ. J. Clin. Pharm. **4**, 77—81 (1971).

ELIS, J., SLAVÍK, M., RAŠKOVÁ, H.: Side effects of 6-azauridine triacetate in rheumatoid arthritis. Clin. Pharmacol. Ther. **11**, 404—407 (1970).

ELVES, M. W., BUTTOO, A. S., ISRAËLS, M. C. G., WILKINSON, J. F.: Chromosome changes caused by 6-azauridine during treatment of acute myeloblastic leukemia. Brit. med. J. **1**, 156—159 (1963).

ENNIS, H. L., LUBIN, M.: Capacity for synthesis of a pyrimidine biosynthetic enzyme in mammalian cells. Biochem. biophys. Acta (Amst.) **68**, 78—83 (1963).

ERUKHIMOV, L. S., VERMEL, E. M.: The use of azauridine in cancer of the bladder. Vop. onkol. **15**, 91 (1969) (in Russian).

EVANS, J. S., HAŇKA, L. J.: The *in vivo* activity of combinations of 5-azacytidine and cytidine on leukemia L-1210. Experientia (Basel) **24**, 922—923 (1968).

FALKE, D., RADA, B.: 6-Azauridine as an inhibitor of the synthesis of herpesvirus hominis. Acta virol. **14**, 115—123 (1970).

FALLON, H. J., FREI, E., III, BLOCK, J., SEEGMILLER, J. E.: The uricosuria and orotic aciduria induced by 6-azauridine. J. clin. Invest. **40**, 1906—1914 (1961).

Farkaš, J., Beránek, J., Šorm, F.: Nucleic acid components and their analogues. LXXXVI. Synthesis of 1-β-D-arabinofuranosyl-6-azacytosine. Coll. Czech. Chem. Commun. **31**, 4002—4008 (1966).
Fischer, D.S., Cassidy, E.P., Welch, A.D.: Immunosuppression by pyrimidine nucleoside analogs. Biochem. Pharmacol. **15**, 1013—1022 (1966).
Flanagan, J.F., Ginsberg, H.S.: Role of ribonucleic acid biosynthesis in multiplication of type 5 adenovirus. J. Bact. **87**, 977—987 (1964).
Fučík, V., Michaelis, A., Rieger, R.: On the induction of segment extension and chromatid structural changes in *Vicia faba* chromosomes after treatment with 5-azacytidine and 5-aza-deoxycytidine. Mutation Res. **9**, 599—606 (1970).
Fučík, V., Šormová, Z., Šorm, F.: The effect of 5-azacytidine on the root meristem of *Vicia faba*. Biol. plant. (Prague) **7**, 58—64 (1965).
Fučík, V., Zadražil, S., Jurovčík, M., Šormová, Z.: Mechanism of resistance to 5-azacytidine in *Bacillus subtilis*. I. Isolation and properties of mutants resistant to 5-azacytidine and 5-aza-2′-deoxycytidine. Folia Microbiol. (Prague) **17**, 517—521 (1972).
Galegov, G.A., Bikbulatova, T.M., Vanag, K.A., Shen, R.M.: Inhibiting effect of 6-aza-uridine upon reproduction of herpes simplex virus. Vop. Virus. **13**, 18—21 (1968) (in Russian).
Galegov, G.A., Kukhar, E.E., Bikbulatov, R.M.: Treatment of keratitis in rabbits due to herpes simplex virus with 6-azauridine. Vop. Virus. **15**, 351—354 (1970) (in Russian).
Gelbard, A.S., Kim, S.H., Eidinoff, M.L.: Nucleoside kinase activities in tissue infected with Rous sarcoma virus. Cancer Res. **26**, 748—751 (1966).
Gershon, D., Sachs, L.: The early synthesis of RNA in polyoma virus (PV) development. Virology **29**, 44—48 (1966).
Goldberg, I.H., Rabinowitz, M.: Inhibition of RNA nucleotidyltransferase by 6-azauridine triphosphate. Biochim. biophys. Acta (Amst.) **72**, 116—119 (1963).
Grafnetter, D., Grafnetterová, J.: Effect of 6-azauridine on lipid metabolism in the rat. Neoplasma (Bratisl.) **14**, 145—153 (1967).
Grafnetterová, J., Beránek, J., König, J., Šmahel, O., Šorm, F.: Catabolism of 2′,3′,5′-tri-*O*-acetyl-6-azauridine in human organism. Neoplasma (Bratisl.) **13**, 241—249 (1966b).
Grafnetterová, J., Grafnetter, D.: 6-Azauridine in brain tissue during chick embryonal development. Experientia (Basel) **24**, 53 (1968).
Grafnetterová, J., Grafnetter, D., Poledne, R.: Lipid changes induced by 6-azauridine. Estratto dal Volume degli Atti del Congresso Internazionale su "Clinical evaluation of testing methods of vasoactive drug effects". Roma, 1—4 maggio 1968a.
Grafnetterová, J., Grossi, E., Fumagalli, R., Morganti, P., Grafnetter, D.: Effects of 6-azauridine on the developing chick embryo. Neoplasma (Bratisl.) **13**, 251—258 (1966a).
Grafnetterová, J., Jedlička, V., Šmahel, O.: Influence of 6-azauridine on the calcium content of plasma and bones in new-born chicks. Experientia (Basel) **24**, 1144—1145 (1968b).
Grozdanovič, J., Vích, Z., Truxová, G.: The combined effect of 6-azauridine and irradiation *in vivo* and *in vitro*. I. The acute effect on the mouse Ehrlich ascites carcinoma. Neoplasma (Bratisl.) **15**, 247—249 (1968).
Grozdanovič, J., Vích, Z., Truxová, G., Kratochvíl, J.: Combined effect of 6-azauridine and irradiation *in vivo* and *in vitro*. VI. Nuclear diameters of Ehrlich ascites carcinoma cells after repeated irradiation and 6-AzUR application. Neoplasma (Bratisl.) **17**, 601—606 (1970).
Gutová, M., Elis, J., Rašková, H.: Teratogenic effect of 6-azauridine in rats. Teratology **4**, 287—292 (1971).
Habermann, V., Šorm, F.: Mechanism of the cancerostatic action of 6-azauracil and its riboside. Coll. Czech. Chem. Commun. **23**, 2201—2206 (1958).
Halle, S.: 5-Azacytidine as a mutagen for arboviruses. J. Virol. **2**, 1228—1229 (1968).
Handschumacher, R.E.: Studies of bacterial resistance to 6-azauracil and its riboside. Biochim. biophys. Acta (Amst.) **23**, 428—430 (1957).
Handschumacher, R.E.: Bacterial preparation of orotidine-5′-phosphate and uridine-5′-phosphate. Nature (Lond.) **182**, 1090—1091 (1958).
Handschumacher, R.E.: Azauracil ribonucleoside and ribonucleotides: isolation and chemical synthesis. J. biol. Chem. **235**, 764—768 (1960a).
Handschumacher, R.E.: Orotidylic acid decarboxylase: inhibition studies with azauridine 5′-phosphate. J. biol. Chem. **235**, 2917—2919 (1960b).
Handschumacher, R.E., Calabresi, P., Welch, A.D., Bono, V.H. Jr., Fallon, H.J., Frei, E. III: Summary of current information on 6-azauridine. Cancer Chemother. Rep. **21**, 1—18 (1962).
Handschumacher, R.E., Pasternak, C.A.: Inhibition of orotidylic acid decarboxylase, a primary site of carcinostasis by 6-azauracil. Biochim. biophys. Acta. (Amst.) **30**, 451—452 (1958).

HANDSCHUMACHER, R. E., ŠKODA, J., ŠORM, F.: Metabolic and biochemical effects of 6-azacytidine in mice with Ehrlich ascites carcinoma. Coll. Czech. Chem. Commun. **28**, 2983—2990 (1963).

HAŇKA, L. J., EVANS, J. S., MASON, D. J., DIETZ, A.: Microbiological production of 5-azacytidine. I. Production and biological activity. Antimicrob. Agents Chemother. 619—624 (1966).

HAVELKA, S., PĚGŘIMOVÁ, E., TRNAVSKÝ, K., SLAVÍK, M., ELIS, J.: 6-Azauridin-Triacetat in der Therapie der chronischen Polyarthritis. Z. f. Rheumaforsch. **28**, 29—35 (1969).

HRODEK, O., VESELÝ, J.: 5-Azacytidine in childhood leukemia. Neoplasma (Bratisl.) **18**, 493—503 (1971).

JAFFE, J. J., HANDSCHUMACHER, R. E., WELCH, A. D.: Studies on the carcinostatic activity in mice of 6-azauracil riboside (6-azauridine), in comparison with that of 6-azauracil. Yale J. biol. Med. **30**, 168—175 (1957).

JANKŮ, I., KRŠIAK, M., NOVOTNÝ, J., VOLICER, L., ČAPEK, R.: Studies on 6-azauridine and 6-azacytidine. IV. Correlations between metabolism and central nervous effects of 6-azacytidine. Biochem. Pharmacol. **14**, 1545—1548 (1965a).

JANKŮ, I., KRŠIAK, M., VOLICER, L., ČAPEK, R., SMETANA, R., NOVOTNÝ, J.: Studies on 6-azauridine and 6-azacytidine. II. The effects of 6-azauridine on the central nervous system. Biochem. Pharmacol. **14**, 1526—1535 (1965b).

JASIŃSKA, S., LINK, F., BLAŠKOVIČ, D., RADA, B.: Studies on the effect of antiviral substances on experimental virus infections. III. The effect of 6-azauracil riboside and urethane on vaccina virus infection in mice. Acta virol. (Bratisl.) **6**, 17—23 (1962).

JELÍNEK, R., RYCHTER, Z., KLIKA, E.: Syndrome of caudal regression and dystrophic malformations of the spinal cord. Folia morphol. (Prague) **19**, 58—70 (1971).

JELÍNEK, R., RYCHTER, Z., SEICHERT, V.: Syndrome of caudal regression in the chick embryo. Folia Morphol. (Prague) **18**, 125—137 (1970).

JIŘIČKA, Z., SMETANA, K., JANKŮ, I., ELIS, J., NOVOTNÝ, J.: Studies on 6-azauridine and 6-azacytidine. I. Toxicity studies of 6-azauridine and 6-azacytidine. Biochem. Pharmacol. **14**, 1517—1523 (1965).

JUROVČÍK, M., RAŠKA, K., ŠORMOVÁ, Z., ŠORM, F.: Anabolic transformation of a novel antimetabolite, 5-azacytidine, and evidence for its incorporation into ribonucleic acid. Coll. Czech. Chem. Commun. **30**, 3370—3376 (1965).

JUROVČÍK, M., ZADRAŽIL, S., FUČÍK, V., ŠORMOVÁ, Z.: Mechanism of resistance to 5-azacytidine in *Bacillus subtilis*. II. Utilization of 5-azacytidine and of natural pyrimidines. Coll. Czech. Chem. Commun. **37**, 299—308 (1972).

KAFKA, V., MUSIL, J., PADOVEC, J., ŠORM, F.: Chemotherapie maligner Tumoren in der Gynäkologie. Bericht über eine Therapie mit Azauridin (6-Azauracilribosid). Gynaecologia **152**, 191—197 (1971).

KÁRA, J.: Activation of DNA biosynthesis in Ehrlich ascites cells *in vivo* following application of 6-aza-2′-deoxycytidine. Biochem. biophys. Res. Commun. **17**, 377—382 (1964).

KÁRA, J., ŠORM, F.: Study of the substrate specificity of deoxynucleoside phosphokinases. Phosphorylation of ^{3}H-thymidine, 6-azathymidine, deoxyuridine, 6-azadeoxyuridine and 5-hydroxymethyldeoxyuridine labelled with ^{14}C, by enzymes from normal and malignant mammalian tissues *in vitro*. Coll. Czech. Chem. Commun. **28**, 1441—1448 (1963).

KÁRA, J., ŠORM, F.: Activation of deoxycytidylate deaminase from Ehrlich ascites-tumor cells by 6-aza-2′-deoxycytidine 5′-phosphate. Biochim. biophys. Acta (Amst.) **80**, 154—157 (1964).

KARON, M., SIEGER, L., LEIMBROCK, S., FINKELSTEIN, J. Z., NESBIT, M. E., SWANEY, J. J.: 5-Azacytidine: a new active agent for the treatment of acute leukemia. Blood **42**, 359—365 (1973).

KAVERIN, N. V., EMELIYANOV, B. A.: The effect of 6-azauridine on the course of latent period in RNA viruses. Vop. Virus. **12**, 51—54 (1967) (in Russian).

KORBECKI, M., ŁUCZAK, M., KLIMOWITZ, Z.: Influence of 6-azauridine on the multiplication of the parainfluenza 3 virus. Bull. Acad. Polonaise Sci. **16**, 539—543 (1968).

KORBECKI, M., PLAGEMANN, P. G. W.: Competitive inhibition of uridine incorporation by 6-azauridine in uninfected and mengovirus-infected Novikoff hepatoma cells. Proc. Soc. exp. Biol. (N.Y.) **132**, 587—595 (1969).

LEONARD, L. L., MEULEN, V. TER, FREEMAN, J. M.: *In vitro* sensitivity of measles virus to 6-azauridine. Proc. Soc. exp. Biol. (N.Y.) **136**, 857—862 (1971).

LEVITAN, I. B., WEBB, T. E.: Effect of 5-azacytidine on polyribosomes and on the controls of tyrosine transaminase in rat liver. Biochim. biophys. Acta (Amst.) **182**, 491—500 (1969).

LI, L. H., OLIN, E. J., BUSKIRK, H. H., REINEKE, L. M.: Cytotoxicity and mode of action of 5-azacytidine on L 1210 leukemia. Cancer Res. **30**, 2760—2769 (1970a).

LI, L. H., OLIN, E. J., FRASER, T. J., BHUYAN, B. K.: Phase specificity of 5-azacytidine against mammalian cells in tissue culture. Cancer Res. **30**, 2770—2775 (1970b).

Lisý, V., Škoda, J.: Deamination of some cytosine and cytidine analogues by an *Escherichia coli* extract. Coll. Czech. Chem. Commun. **31**, 3020—3022 (1966).
Lisý, V., Škoda, J., Rychlík, I., Smrt, J., Holý, A., Šorm, F.: Changes in coding properties of poly- and oligonucleotides containing 6-azapyrimidine ribonucleosides. Coll. Czech. Chem. Commun. **33**, 4111—4119 (1968).
Loh, P. C.: The role of RNA in the synthesis of vaccinia virus. Proc. Soc. exp. Biol. (N. Y.) **116**, 789—792 (1964).
Lowy, D. R., Rowe, W. P., Teich, N., Hartley, J. W.: Murine leukemia virus: high-frequency activation in vitro by 5-iododeoxyuridine and 5-bromodeoxyuridine. Science **174**, 155—156 (1971).
Magdon, E., Konopatzky, R.: Untersuchungen zur Wirkung von 6-Azaurazilribosid bei der Bestrahlung von experimentellen Tiertumoren. Arch. Geschwulstforsch. **29**, 259—245 (1967).
Misařová, Z., Elis, J.: Azauracilriboside and azauracilribosidetriacetate in the therapy of leukemia in children. Čs. Pediat. **19**, 161—165 (1964) (in Czech).
Morris, J. M., van Wagenen, G., Hurteau, G. D., Johnston, D. W., Carlsen, R. A.: Compounds interfering with ovum implantation and development. Fertil. Steril. **18**, 7—17 (1967).
Myška, V., Elis, J., Plevová, J., Rašková, H.: Azauridine in viral eye infections. Lancet **I**, 1230—1231 (1967).
Nirenberg, M., Leder, P.: RNA codewords and protein synthesis. The effect of trinucleotides upon the binding of sRNA to ribosomes. Science **145**, 1399—1407 (1964).
Nouza, K.: Screening of immunosuppressive drugs in the allotransplantation reaction between mice differing at the H-3 locus. Folia Biol. (Prague) **12**, 266—277 (1966).
Nouza, K., Pokorná, Z., Slavík, M., Gottwaldová, A.: The immunosuppressive effects of 6-azauridine. Folia Biol. (Prague) **16**, 188—195 (1970).
Novotný, J., Smetana, R., Rašková, H.: Studies on 6-azauridine and 6-azacytidine. III. The fate of 6-azacytidine in various animal species. Biochem. Pharmacol. **14**, 1537—1544 (1965).
Pačes, V., Doskočil, J., Šorm, F.: Incorporation of 5-azacytidine into nucleic acids of *Escherichia coli*. Biochim. biophys. Acta (Amst.) **161**, 352—360 (1968a).
Pačes, V., Doskočil, J., Šorm, F.: The effect of 5-azacytidine on the synthesis of ribosomes in *Escherichia coli*. FEBS Let. **1**, 55—58 (1968b).
Pasternak, C. A., Fischer, G. A., Handschumacher, R. E.: Alteration in pyrimidine metabolism in L 5178 Y leukemia cells resistant to 6-azauridine. Cancer Res. **21**, 110—117 (1961).
Pasternak, C. A., Handschumacher, R. E.: The biochemical activity of 6-azauridine: interference with pyrimidine metabolism in transplantable mouse tumors. J. biol. Chem. **234**, 2992—2997 (1959).
Pinsky, L., Krooth, R. S.: Studies on the control of pyrimidine biosynthesis in human diploid cell strains. I. Effect of 6-azauridine on cellular phenotype. Proc. nat. Acad. Sci. (Wash.) **57**, 925—932 (1967a).
Pinsky, L., Krooth, R. S.: Studies on the control of pyrimidine biosynthesis in human diploid cell strains. II. Effects of 5-azaorotic acid, barbituric acid, and pyrimidine precursors on cellular phenotype. Proc. nat. Acad. Sci. (Wash.) **57**, 1267—1274 (1967b).
Pískala, A., Šorm, F.: Nucleic acid components and their analogues. LI. Synthesis of l-glycosyl derivatives of 5-azauracil and 5-azacytosine. Coll. Czech. Chem. Commun. **29**, 2060—2076 (1964).
Plevová, J., Janků, I., Šeda, M.: Toxicity of 6-azauridine triacetate. Toxicol. Appl. Pharmacol. **17**, 511—518 (1970a).
Plevová, J., Šeda, M., Janků, I.: The deacetylation of 6-azauridine-triacetate in the plasma of various species correlated with toxicity. Proc. Europ. Soc. Study Drug Toxicity. **11**, 240—241 (1970b).
Pliml, J., Prystaš, M., Šorm, F.: Nucleic acid components and their analogues. XXXIX. Synthesis of anomeric 2′-deoxy-6-azauridines and of 6-azathymidine. Coll. Czech. Chem. Commun. **28**, 2588—2597 (1963).
Pliml, J., Šorm, F.: Nucleic acid components and their analogues. XXVIII. Synthesis of 6-aza-2′-deoxycytidine. Coll. Czech. Chem. Commun. **28**, 546—550 (1963).
Pliml, J., Šorm, F.: Synthesis of a 2-deoxy-*D*-ribofuranosyl-5-azacytosine. Coll. Czech. Chem. Commun. **29**, 2576—2578 (1964).
Pontis, H., Degerstedt, G., Reichard, P.: Uridine and deoxyuridine phosphorylase from Ehrlich ascites tumor. Biochim. biophys. Acta (Amst.) **51**, 138—147 (1961).
Pravdina, N. F., Lysenko, A. M., Linevich, Yu. G., Galegov, G. A.: The action of 6-azauridine on reproduction of T2 phage. Mikrobiologija **38**, 295—298 (1969) (in Russian).
Pringle, C. R.: Genetic characteristics of conditional lethal mutants of vesicular stomatitis virus induced by 5-fluorouracil, 5-azacytidine, and ethyl methane sulfonate. J. Virol. **5**, 559—567 (1970).

PRUSOFF, W. H.: Studies on mechanism of action of 6-azathymine. I. Biosynthesis of the deoxyriboside. J. biol. Chem. **215**, 809—821 (1955).
PRYSTAŠ, M., GUT, J., ŠORM, F.: Nucleic acid components and their analogues. XXI. Synthesis of 3-methyl-6-azauridine. Structure proof and general approach to the synthesis of 6-azauridines. Coll. Czech. Chem. Commun. **27**, 1572—1577 (1962).
PRYSTAŠ, M., ŠORM, F.: Nucleic acid components and their analogues. XXII. Synthesis of 6-azauridine and 5-methyl-6-azauridine. Coll. Czech. Chem. Commun. **27**, 1578—1584 (1962).
PRYSTAŠ, M., ŠORM, F.: Nucleic acid components and their analogues. XL. Synthesis of 5-methyl-2'-deoxy-6-azacytidine. Coll. Czech. Chem. Commun. **28**, 2598—2604 (1963).
RADA, B.: The effect of cell-free extracts on the inhibition of virus multiplication by 6-azauridine. Ann. N.Y. Acad. Sci. **173**, 176—184 (1970).
RADA, B., ALTANEROVÁ, V.: Virus-inhibitory activity of 6-azauridine dependent on cell-free extracts containing uridine kinase. I. Inhibition of plaque-formation. Acta virol. (Bratisl.) **14**, 425—434 (1970).
RADA, B., BLAŠKOVIČ, D.: Inhibition of vaccinia virus multiplication *in vitro* by 6-azauracil riboside. Acta virol. (Bratisl.) **5**, 308—316 (1961).
RADA, B., BLAŠKOVIČ, D.: Some characteristics of the effects of 6-azauridine on vaccinia virus multiplication in comparison with those of 5-iododeoxyuridine. Acta virol. (Bratisl.) **10**, 1—9 (1966).
RADA, B., BLAŠKOVIČ, D., ŠORM, F., ŠKODA, J.: The inhibitory effect of 6-azauracil riboside on the multiplication of vaccinia virus. Experientia (Basel) **16**, 487—488 (1960).
RADA, B., GREGUŠOVÁ, V.: Increase of uridine kinase activity after infection of cells with vaccinia and Rous sarcoma viruses. Biochem. biophys. Res. Commun. **15**, 324—328 (1964).
RADA, B., HANUŠOVSKÁ, T.: Virus-inhibitory activity of 6-azauridine dependent on cell-free extracts containing uridine kinase. II. Quantitative aspects, efficacy of pretreatment. Acta virol. (Bratisl.) **14**, 435—444 (1970).
RADA, B., SHATKIN, A. J.: The inhibitory effect of 6-azauridine on reovirus multiplication. Acta virol. (Bratisl.) **11**, 551—553 (1967).
RADA, B., SMIDOVÁ, V., ZÁVADA, J.: The inhibitory effect of some antimetabolites and antibiotics on Rous sarcoma growth. Neoplasma (Bratisl.) **11**, 553—559 (1964).
RADA, B., ZÁVADA, J.: Screening-test for cytostatic and virostatic substances. Neoplasma (Bratisl.) **9**, 57—65 (1962).
RAŠKA, K., JUROVČÍK, M., ŠORMOVÁ, Z., ŠORM, F.: On the metabolism of 5-azacytidine and 5-aza-2'-deoxycytidine in mice. Coll. Czech. Chem. Commun. **30**, 3001—3006 (1965).
RAŠKA, K., ZEDECK, M. S., WELCH, A. D.: Relationship between the metabolic effects and the pregnancy interrupting property of 6-azauridine in mice. Biochem. Pharmacol. **15**, 2136—2138 (1966).
RAŠKOVÁ, H., ELIS, J., GUTOVÁ, M., NIŽŇANSKÁ, J., MIKULECKÝ, Z., KUBÍČKOVÁ, V., BORČ, K., PŘIBÍKOVÁ, V, HULÍNSKÝ, K., KANTNER, V., BELSAN, I., KŮTA, A., ERBERTOVÁ, B., KLEIBEL, K., SEYČEK, V., DUCHKOVÁ, H.: Indications for 6-azauridine triacetate — psoriasis. Čs. lék. čes. **106**, 870—873 (1967) (in Czech.).
RAŠKOVÁ, H., ELIS, J., PERLÍK, F., POLANSKÝ, F., SLAVÍK, M.: Unexpected sideeffects of 6-azauridine in rheumatoid arthritis and feedback in animal experiments. Proc. Europ. Soc. Study Drug Toxicity **12**, 191—198 (1971).
RUBIN, R. J., JAFFE, J. J., HANDSCHUMACHER, R. E.: Qualitative differences in the pyrimidine metabolism of *Trypanosoma equiperdum* and mammals as characterized by 6-azauracil and 6-azauridine. Biochem. Pharmacol. **11**, 563—572 (1962).
RYCHTER, Z., JELÍNEK, R.: Change in shape and location of non-vascularized area of ventricular myocardium in chick embryo during terminal phase of heart vascularization after administration of 6-azauridine in different doses. Folia morphologica (Prague) **21**, 1—11 (1973).
RYCHTER, Z., OŠŤÁDAL, B., JELÍNEK, R.: Weight analysis of development of the chick embryo myocardium during the terminal phase of its vascularization after administration of 6-azauridine. Physiologia Bohemoslovaca **21**, 569—580 (1972).
SAGAR, P., KÁRA, J.: Activation of deoxycytidylate deaminase from certain embryonal and tumor tissues by 6-aza-2'-deoxycytidine-5'-monophosphate and 2'-deoxycytidine-5'-triphosphate. Folia biol. (Prague) **12**, 75—79 (1966).
SAKSENA, S. K., CHAUDHURY, R. R.: The antifertility effect of 2',3',5'-tri-*O*-acetyl-6-azauridine. Part II. In rabbits. Indian J. med. Res. **58**, 374—376 (1970).
SANDERS, M. A., WIESNER, B. P., YUDKIN, J.: Control of fertility by 6-azauridine. Nature (Lond.) **189**, 1015—1016 (1961).
SCHÄFER, W., PISTER, L., SCHNEIDER, R.: Analyse des Vermehrungsmechanismus des Newcastle disease Virus (NDV) mit Hilfe verschiedener Inhibitoren. Z. Naturforsch. **22b**, 1319—1330 (1967).

Schindler, R., Welch, A. D.: Ribosidation as a means of activating 6-azauracil as an inhibitor of cell reproduction. Science **125**, 548—549 (1957).
Šeferna, I., Loukomskaya, N., Kadlec, O., Janků, I.: The effect of 6-azauridine on the contractile responses of the isolated ileum of the guinea-pig to drugs and to coaxial stimulation. J. pharm. Pharmacol. **18**, 501—506 (1966).
Seifertová, M., Čihák, A., Veselý, J.: Effect of 5-azacytidine and 6-azauridine on the synthesis of DNA in embryonic mouse brain, mitotic activity and migration of ventricular cells. Neoplasma (Bratisl.) **20**, 243—249 (1973).
Seifertová, M., Veselý, J., Šorm, F.: Effect of 5-azacytidine on developing mouse embryo. Experientia (Basel) **24**, 487—488 (1968).
Škoda, J., Hess, V. F., Šorm, F.: The biosynthesis of 6-azauracil riboside by *Escherichia coli* growing in the presence of 6-azauracil. Experientia (Basel) **13**, 150—151 (1957a).
Škoda, J., Hess, V. F., Šorm, F.: Production of 6-azauracil riboside by *Escherichia coli* growing in the presence of 6-azauracil. Coll. Czech. Chem. Commun. **22**, 1330—1333 (1957b).
Škoda, J., Kára, J., Čihák, A., Šorm, F.: Formation of the ribonucleoside of 5-azauracil by *Escherichia coli* and isolation of ribosyl biuret as the main decomposition product of 5-azauridine. Coll. Czech. Chem. Commun. **27**, 1692—1694 (1962).
Škoda, J., Kára, J., Šormová, Z.: Interaction of 6-azauridine-5′-diphosphate with *Escherichia coli* polynucleotide phosphorylase. Coll. Czech. Chem. Commun. **24**, 3783—3789 (1959b).
Škoda, J., Kára, J., Šormová, Z., Šorm, F.: Inhibition of *Escherichia coli* polynucleotide phosphorylase by 6-azauridine diphosphate. Biochim. biophys. Acta (Amst.) **33**, 579—580 (1959a).
Škoda, J., Lisý, V., Smrt, J., Holý, A., Šorm, F.: Formation of a dead code triplet through replacement of the terminal ribonucleoside in guanylyl-uridylyl-uridine and guanylyl-uridylyl-cytidine by 6-azacytidine. Molec. Pharmacol. **2**, 608—610 (1966).
Škoda, J., Šorm, F.: Czechoslovak patent No. 88063 (1958a) (in Czech).
Škoda, J., Šorm, F.: Accumulation of nucleic acid metabolites in *Escherichia coli* exposed to the action of 6-azauracil. Biochim. biophys. Acta (Amst.) **28**, 659—660 (1958b).
Škoda, J., Šorm, F.: The accumulation of orotic acid, uracil and hypoxanthine by *Escherichia coli* in the presence of 6-azauracil and the biosynthesis of 6-azauridylic acid. Coll. Czech. Chem. Commun. **24**, 1331—1337 (1959).
Škoda, J., Šorm, F.: Biosynthesis of co-polymers of uridylic and cytidylic acids with 6-azacytidylic acid. Biochim. biophys. Acta (Amst.) **91**, 352—354 (1964).
Sköld, O.: Uridine kinase from Ehrlich ascites tumor: purification and properties. J. biol. Chem. **235**, 3273—3279 (1960).
Slavík, M., Elis, J., Rašková, H., Gutová, M., Duchková, M., Kubíková, M., Seyček, V.: Therapeutic effects of 6-azauridine triacetate in psoriasis. Pharm. Clin. **2**, 120—125 (1970).
Slavík, M., Hyánek, J., Elis, J., Homolka, J.: Typical hyperaminoaciduria after high doses of 6-azauridine triacetate. Biochem. Pharmacol. **18**, 1782—1784 (1969).
Šmahel, O., Černoch, A., Šorm, F., König, J., Valenta, O., Švehla, C., Švorc, J., Bláha, V., Uher, V., Gerberová, J.: An attempt to treat chorionepithelioma with 6-azauridine. Čs. lék. čes. **104**, 1085—1087 (1965) (In Czech.).
Šmahel, O., Grafnetterová, J., König, K., Schück, O.: Der Blutspiegel und die renale Ausscheidung von 6-Azauridin bei verschiedenem Applikations- und Dosierungsmodus. Internationale Zeitschrift für Klinische Pharmakologie. Therap. Toxikol. **2**, 101—105 (1967).
Šmejkal, F., Šorm, F.: The effect of 6-azauracil riboside against vaccinia virus in rabbits. Acta virol. (Bratisl.) **6**, 282 (1962).
Šorm, F., Keilová, H.: The anti-tumor activity of 6-azauracil riboside. Experientia (Basel) **14**, 215 (1958).
Šorm, F., Pískala, A., Čihák, A., Veselý, J.: 5-Azacytidine, a new, highly effective cancerostatic. Experientia (Basel) **20**, 202—203 (1964).
Šorm, F., Smrt, J., Černěckij, V.: 6-Azacytidine — a new antimetabolite. Experientia (Basel) **17**, 64—65 (1961).
Šorm, F., Šormová, Z., Raška, K., Jurovčík, M.: Comparison of the metabolism and inhibitory effects of 5-azacytidine and 5-aza-2′-deoxycytidine in mammalian tissues. Rev. Roumaine Biochim. **3**, 139—147 (1966).
Šorm, F., Veselý, J.: Potentiation of the cancerostatic effect of 6-azauridine and 6-azacytidine with 5-*bis*-(2-chloroethyl)-aminomethyluracil. Experientia (Basel) **17**, 355 (1961).
Šorm, F., Veselý, J.: The activity of a new antimetabolite, 5-azacytidine, against lymphoid leukemia in AK mice. Neoplasma (Bratisl.) **11**, 123—130 (1964).
Šorm, F., Veselý, J.: Partial reversal of toxic effects of 5-azacytidine by 6-azauridine in normal mice. Experientia (Basel) **21**, 581—582 (1965).
Šorm, J., Veselý, J.: Effect of 5-aza-2′-deoxycytidine against leukemic and hemopoietic tissues in AKR mice. Neoplasma (Bratisl.) **15**, 339—343 (1968).

STOLLAR, V., STEVENS, T. M., SCHLESINGER, R. W.: Studies on the nature of dengue viruses. II. Characterization of viral RNA and effects of inhibitors of RNA synthesis. Virology **30**, 303—312 (1966).

STEJSKALOVÁ, V., IVÁNYI, J., KÁRA, J.: Enhancement of antibody synthesis *in vitro* by 6-azauridine, uridine and actinomycin D. Folia Biol. (Prague) **16**, 250—258 (1970).

ŠTERZL, J.: Effect of some metabolic inhibitors on antibody formation. Nature (Lond.) **189**, 1022—1023 (1961).

SVATÁ, M., RAŠKA, K., ŠORM, F.: Interruption of pregnancy by 5-azacytidine. Experientia (Basel) **22**, 53 (1966).

TERSKIKH, I. I., GALEGOV, G. A., CHUTKOV, N. A., BEKLESHOVA, A. IU.: The inhibitory effect produced by 5-bromo-2′-deoxyuridine and 6-azauridine on the reproduction of the causative organism of ornithosis. Dokl. Akad. Nauk SSSR **180**, 480—481 (1968) (in Russian).

TKACZYNSKI, T., ŠMEJKAL, J., ŠORM, F.: Nucleic acid components and their analogues. L. Synthesis of 1-β-D-xylofuranosyl-6-azauracil. Coll. Czech. Chem. Commun. **29**, 1736—1738 (1964).

TONG, G. L., LEE, W. L., GOODMAN, L.: A convenient synthesis of 6-aza-2′-deoxycytidine (1). J. Heterocycl. Chem. **3**, 226—227 (1966).

TRNAVSKÝ, K., LAPÁROVÁ, V.: Anti-inflammatory activity of 6-azauridine. Med. Pharmacol. Exp. **16**, 171—177 (1967).

TURNER, R. W., CALABRESI, P.: The effect of triacetyl azauridine on psoriasis. J. Invest. Derm. **43**, 551—557 (1964).

VADLAMUDI, S., PADARATHSINGH, M., BONMASSAR, E., GOLDIN, A.: Reduction of antileukemic and imunosuppressive activities of 5-azacytidine in mice by concurrent treatment with uridine. Proc. Soc. exptl. Biol. (N. Y.) **133**, 1232—1238 (1970).

VAN WAGENEN, G., DECONTI, R. C., HANDSCHUMACHER, R. E., WADE, M. E.: Abortifacient and teratogenic effects of triacetyl-6-azauridine in the monkey. Am. J. Obstet. Gynec. **108**, 272—281 (1970).

VESELÝ, J.: The effect of 6-azauridine and 6-azacytidine on the intracellular synthesis of RNA in fowl leukemic and normal myeloblasts *in vitro*. Acta biol. med. german. **12**, 60—64 (1964).

VESELÝ, J., ČIHÁK, A.: High-frequency induction in vivo of mouse leukemia in AKR strain by 5-azacytidine and 5-iodo-2′-deoxyuridine. Experientia (Basel) **29**, 1132—1133 (1973).

VESELÝ, J., ČIHÁK, A., ŠORM, F.: Characteristics of mouse leukemic cells resistant to 5-azacytidine and 5-aza-2′-deoxycytidine. Cancer Res. **28**, 1995—2000 (1968a).

VESELÝ, J., ČIHÁK, A., ŠORM, F.: Biochemical mechanism of drug resistance. VII. Inhibition of orotic acid metabolism by 5-azacytidine in leukemic mice sensitive and resistant to 5-azacytidine. Biochem. Pharmacol. **17**, 519—524 (1968b).

VESELÝ, J., ČIHÁK, A., ŠORM, F.: Enhanced triphosphatase activity of mouse leukemic cells resistant to 5-azacytidine. Coll. Czech. Chem. Commun. **33**, 341—345 (1968c).

VESELÝ, J., ČIHÁK, A., ŠORM, F.: Biochemical mechanisms of drug resistance. IX. Metabolic alterations in leukemic mouse cells following 5-aza-2′-deoxycytidine. Coll. Czech. Chem. Commun. **34**, 901—909 (1969a).

VESELÝ, J., ČIHÁK, A., ŠORM, F.: Association of decreased uridine and deoxycytidine kinase with enhanced RNA and DNA polymerase in mouse leukemic cells resistant to 5-azacytidine and 5-aza-2′-deoxycytidine. Cancer Res. **30**, 2180—2186 (1970).

VESELÝ, J., GOSTOF, R., ČIHÁK, A., ŠORM, F.: Radioprotective effect of 5-azacytidine in AKR mice. Z. Naturforsch. **24**b, 318—320 (1969b).

VOGLER, W. R., OLANSKY, S.: A double-blind study of azaribine in the treatment of psoriasis. Ann. intern. Med. **73**, 951—956 (1970).

VOJTA, M., JIRÁSEK, J.: 6-Azauridine-induced changes of the trophoblast in early human pregnancy. Clin. Pharmacol. Ther. **7**, 162—165 (1966).

VORHERR, H., WELCH, A. D.: The mode of interruption of pregnancy by 6-azauridine in mice and rats. Biochem. Pharmacol. **19**, 1001—1006 (1970).

VRBA, M.: Titration of Rous sarcoma virus on the chick embryo chorioallantoic membrane. Acta virol. (Bratisl.) **7**, 525—533 (1964).

WELLS, W., GAINES, D., KOENIG, H.: Studies of pyrimidine nucleotide metabolism in the central nervous system. I. Metabolic effects and metabolism of 6-azauridine. J. Neurochem. **10**, 709—723 (1963).

WIECZORKOWSKI, J., ŠORM, F., BERÁNEK, J.: Nucleic acid components and their analogues. CX. Synthesis of 1-(2′,3′-epoxy-β-D-lyxofuranosyl)-6-azaisocytosine. Coll. Czech. Chem. Commun. **33**, 924—930 (1968).

WILKINSON, J. F.: Treatment of leukemias. Proc. roy. Soc. Med. **56**, 644—648 (1963).

WILSON, D. E., LOGERFO, P.: Inhibition of ribonucleic acid synthesis in Newcastle disease virus-infected cells by puromycin and 6-azauridine. J. Bact. 88, 1550—1555 (1964).

WINKLER, A., DRAHOVSKÝ, D., GREGUŠOVÁ, V., THURZO, V., KÁRA, J., ŠKODA, J., ŠORM, F.: Determination of uridine kinase activity in some tumours and in leukaemic cells using 4,5-^{14}C-azauridine as substrate. Neoplasma (Bratisl.) **9**, 101—103 (1962).
ZÁRUBA, F., KŮTA, A., ELIS, J.: Treatment of mycosis fungoides with 6-azauracilriboside. Lancet **II**, 275 (1963).
ŽEMLIČKA, J., SMRT, J., ŠORM, F.: Nucleic acid components and their analogues. XLVIII. Synthesis and structure of nitrogen mustard derivatives of cytidine and 6-azacytidine. Coll. Czech. Chem. Commun. **29**, 635—644 (1964).
ŽEMLIČKA, J., ŠORM, F.: Nucleic acid components and their analogues. LXIII. The reaction of dimethylchloromethylenammonium chloride with 2′,3′,5′-tri-O-acyl derivatives of uridine and 6-azauridine; a new synthesis of 6-azacytidine. Coll. Czech. Chem. Commun. **30**, 2052—2067 (1965).
ŽEMLIČKA, J., ŠORM, F.: Nucleic acid components and their analogues. LXXXIX. Synthesis of 2′,3′-O-isopropylidene-O^2,5′-cyclo-6-azauridine and 2-(β-D-ribofuranosyl)-3-amino-4,5-dihydro-1,2,4-triazine-3-one (6-azaisocytidine). Coll. Czech. Chem. Commun. **32**, 576—590 (1967).

Chapter 46

Showdomycin, 5-Hydroxyuridine, and 5-Aminouridine

D. W. VISSER

With 1 Figure

Introduction

The antibiotic, showdomycin, has a structural similarity to N-ethylmaleimide, a thiol binding reagent, and also to the nucleosides, uridine and pseudouridine. Its reactivity toward sulfhydryl-groups of susceptible proteins results from its maleimide-like structure and accounts for its cytotoxic effects. However, its nucleoside like structure is also related to its function as evidenced by the capacity of nucleosides to reverse its inhibitory effects on growth and on the transport of sugars and amino acids in *Escherichia coli*. This interesting specificity, as well as the remarkable changes which occur in showdomycin-resistant mutants of *E. coli*, are the basis for continued interest in this antibiotic.

The 5-substituted nucleosides, 5-aminouridine and 5-hydroxyuridine, are synthetic products which, unlike showdomycin, exert their primary inhibitory effects only after conversion to phosphorylated derivatives. Both 5-substituted nucleoside analogs inhibit RNA synthesis and the function of pyrimidine containing cofactors, and are incorporated to a minor extent into RNA. These nucleoside analogs inhibit tumor growth in experimental animals, but neither has been tested clinically.

Chemistry of Showdomycin

Showdomycin was isolated from a filtrate of *Streptomyces showdoensis* by NISHIMURA et al. (1964). Its chemical structure was shown to be 3-β-D-ribofuranosylmaleimide (DARNALL et al., 1967; NAKAGAWA et al., 1967). It bears a structural similarity to uridine and can be visualized as pseudouridine which has lost an NH group in the contraction to a five-membered ring. Other chemical and physical properties of the antibiotic have been described by NISHIMURA et al. (1964) and DARNALL et al. (1967).

A chemical property of the antibiotic which explains most of its inhibitory effects in biological systems is the alkylating action of its maleimide moiety. Another chemical property worthy of special note is the instability of its maleimide structure under alkaline conditions (NISHIMURA et al., 1964).

Metabolism of Showdomycin

In contrast to most other nucleoside analogs, showdomycin exerts its inhibitory effects as the unmetabolized nucleoside (ROY-BURMAN, S. et al., 1968). The antibiotic is not phosphorylated by enzyme preparations from Ehrlich ascites cells which actively convert uridine to UTP. These results do not exclude the possibility of a very small degree of conversion to the nucleotide level; however, in context with several reports which relate the inhibitory effects of showdomycin to its alkylating ability, it seems unlikely that phosphorylation is essential for its action. As might be predicted from the chemical stability of its carbon-linked glycosyl bond, showdomycin is not a substrate for nucleoside phosphorylase (ROY-BURMAN, S. et al., 1968).

Inhibitory Effects of Showdomycin

The antibiotic is a moderately active antibacterial agent against gram-positive and gram-negative bacteria, and is particularly active toward *Streptococcus haemolyticus* and *Streptococcus pyogenes* (NISHIMURA et al., 1964). Showdomycin is also active against cultured HeLa cells (MATSUURA et al., 1964) and inhibits Ehrlich ascites cell proliferation *in vitro* and *in vivo* (MATSUURA et al., 1964; NISHIMURA et al., 1964).

Experimental evidence that showdomycin exerts its inhibitory effect by alkylation was provided independently by ROY-BURMAN, S. et al. (1968) and NISHIMURA and KOMATSU (1968), confirming the earlier suggestion of DARNALL et al. (1967). An investigation of the effects of showdomycin on uridine and orotic acid metabolism in a cell-free preparation from Ehrlich ascites cells showed that the antibiotic inhibits uridine 5'-monophosphokinase, uridine phosphorylase, and possibly orotidylic acid pyrophosphorylase, but has no effect on the activity of uridine kinase (ROY-BURMAN, S. et al., 1968). The demonstration that showdomycin is not phosphorylated to the nucleotide level and is not a substrate for nucleoside phosphorylase suggested to these authors that the inhibitory effects on specific enzymes of orotic acid and uridine metabolism might not be related to the nucleoside structure of the antibiotic, but rather, result from its reaction in a nonspecific manner with accessible sulfhydryl groups of enzymes involved in pyrimidine metabolism. This concept of showdomycin action was supported by the noncompetitive inhibition of liver uridine 5'-diphosphate-α-D-glucose dehydrogenase by showdomycin, by the protective effect of cysteine, and by the rapid and almost quantitative conversion of the antibiotic to a ninhydrin-positive derivative in the presence of cysteine.

NISHIMURA and KOMATSU (1968) reached similar conclusions on the mode of action of showdomycin *in vivo*. They found that mercaptoethanol, cysteine, and glutathione are equally effective in reversing the inhibitory effect of the antibiotic on the growth of *E. coli*, and none of the other amino acids tested is effective. The alkylating action of showdomycin *in vivo* and *in vitro* has been confirmed as a major effect of the antibiotic by several subsequent reports as mentioned below.

HADLER et al. (1968) measured the mitochondrial volume change induced by showdomycin and interpreted their data to implicate a mitochondrial thiol group in oxidative phosphorylation (HADLER and MOREAU, 1969). Their data do not point out unique differences in action between showdomycin and other sulfhydryl reagents, but are consistent with the concept that the antibiotic acts primarily as an alkylating agent.

N-Ethylmaleimide and showdomycin act similarly to increase the radiosensitization of *Escherichia coli* (TITANI and KATSUBE, 1969). Non-toxic levels of the nucleoside also enhance the lethal effects of the alkylating agents 2,2'-dichlorodiethylamine and methyl methanesulfonate (TITANI and KATSUBE, 1970), which are believed to exert their primary effect by altering DNA structure. These authors proposed two possible explanations: (1) a decrease in reactive SH-groups which normally detoxify the alkylating agent before it can attack the target molecules, (2) an inhibition of DNA repair enzymes.

Recently, BERMEK et al. (1970) reported that showdomycin inhibits polyphenylalanine synthesis in a human cell-free system. Two specific effects of the antibiotic are its inactivation of the elongation factor and of the enzymatic and non-enzymatic binding of phenylalanyl-tRNA to ribosomes. Both of these effects are produced by other sulfhydryl reagents.

An interesting finding which relates the nucleoside structure of the antibiotic to its biological activity has been reported by NISHIMURA and KOMATSU (1968). These authors found that the inhibitory action of showdomycin on the proliferation of *E. coli* is specifically reversed by most nucleosides, whereas purines, pyrimidines, ribose, deoxyribose, nucleotides, and phosphate derivatives of ribose are inactive as reversing agents. Ribosyl- and deoxyribosyl-derivatives of all common purines or pyrimidines are almost equally effective as reversing agents, indicating a general requirement for the nucleoside structure for protection against the inhibitory action of the antibiotic.

KOMATSU and TANAKA (1968) extended these studies by showing that *N*-ethylmaleimide and showdomycin each inhibit in a similar manner the incorporation of amino acids and purine and pyrimidine bases into macromolecules of *E. coli*. However, nucleosides, with the notable exception of pseudouridine, reverse the inhibitory effects of showdomycin, but not those of *N*-ethylmaleimide. The authors concluded that the *N*-glycosyl linkage of the common nucleosides may be a structural requirement for their ability to reverse the inhibitory action of showdomycin.

These indications that showdomycin has structural specificity related to its function, and the well established fact that the transport of amino acids and sugars is inhibited by sulfhydryl reagents, led to investigations on the effects of showdomycin on sugar and amino acid uptake in *E. coli* (ROY-BURMAN et al., 1971). These studies showed that showdomycin inhibits uptake of glucose, α-methyl-D-glucoside, and leucine into whole cells. The inhibitory effects are reversed completely by preincubation of the cells with cysteine or with the common nucleosides excepting guanosine, deoxyguanosine, and pseudouridine. Both showdomycin and *N*-ethylmaleimide inhibit glucose uptake at similar concentration levels. However, nucleosides are ineffective in reversing *N*-ethylmaleimide inhibition of transport, but restore the showdomycin inhibited transport of glucose completely. Concentration levels of the antibiotic which inhibit transport processes are similar to those which inhibit growth and protein and nucleic acid synthesis. These data suggest that inhibition of transport may be a primary effect of showdomycin action.

The mechanism of the protective action of nucleosides on the transport processes is not clear. Presumably, nucleosides interact at sites on the cell surface, thereby preventing transport of the structurally related antibiotic and its reaction with susceptible sulfhydryl groups. It appears that the nucleoside itself is required, rather than the phosphorylated derivative or a product of nucleoside catabolism. This conclusion is apparent from the protective effect of 5-hydroxydeoxyuridine, which is not phosphorylated by *E. coli*, and from the ineffectiveness of nucleotides, purines, pyrimidines, ribose, or deoxyribose (ROY-BURMAN et al., 1971). Furthermore, guanine-containing nucleosides which do not prevent inhibition by showdomycin are susceptible to nucleoside phosphorylase. Thus, the products of nucleoside phosphorylase, ribose-1-phosphate or deoxyribose-1-phosphate, are apparently not directly involved in the protective effect.

Several reports regarding the remarkable ability of showdomycin to induce an extensive alteration in the base composition of ribosomal RNA and rapidly-labeled RNA have appeared recently. BELJANSKI and BELJANSKI (1968) found that the composition of DNA from bacteria grown in the presence of showdomycin is not altered, whereas the purine to pyrimidine ratio of rapidly-labeled RNA is doubled and the nucleotide composition of ribosomal RNA is changed drastically. Mutants of *E. coli* resistant to both small (1 to 10 μg/ml) and large (20 to 500 μg/ml) concentrations of showdomycin have been developed (BELJANSKI et al., 1969, 1971). These mutants exhibit similar drastic changes in both rapidly labeled and ribosomal RNA when they are grown on synthetic medium in the absence of showdomycin (BELJANSKI et al., 1969, 1971). Lack of complementarity between the altered, rapidly labeled RNA and either the mutant or wild-type DNA was demonstrated, and a similar lack of complementarity has been shown for ribosomal RNA (BELJANSKI et al., 1970, 1971). Ribosomes from a mutant of *E. coli* which is resistant to 500 μg showdomycin/ml contain RNA species in which the purine concentrations greatly exceed those of pyrimidines, and both the 50 S and 30 S ribosomal subunits have a highly altered protein pattern after electrophoretic separation on polyacrylamide gel. Surprisingly, these "mutant" ribosomes are as active as wild-type ribosomes for protein synthesis in cell-free systems.

Rationalization of these data with current concepts of molecular biology is difficult. As pointed out by BELJANSKI et al. (1971), "one would expect that a mutation of almost all of the RNAs of *E. coli* and of ribosomal proteins, as is the case with one of the mutants, would be lethal". A possible partial explanation for the existence of abnormal RNA is provided by the finding that polynucleotide phosphorylase from one of the resistant mutants exhibits new properties. This enzyme from the mutant has a pronounced preference for ADP and GDP as substrates, and synthesizes poly-AGUC *in vitro* in which the amount of purine bases is doubled as compared to normal (BELJANSKI et al., 1970). In addition, DNA dependent RNA polymerase from this mutant exhibits a markedly reduced specific activity when compared to the wild-type enzyme. These findings, however, are still inadequate to explain the tolerance of the mutant to the gross changes in the RNA and protein composition. We have verified the facile development of showdomycin resistant *E. coli* mutants (VISSER and ROY-BURMAN, 1971) and, in addition, have shown that one of the mutants is resistant to inhibition of glucose transport by concentrations of showdomycin which inhibit by 90% or more in wild-type *E. coli*.

While all of the effects of showdomycin reported thus far may be explained by the reactivity of its maleimide moiety with sulfhydryl groups, it is apparent that showdomycin is not simply an alkylating agent. It possesses interesting specificities relating to its nucleoside structure which enhance its potential for applications in transport studies and provide a model for the synthesis of related analogs.

Chemistry and Metabolism of 5-Hydroxyuridine

The nucleoside analog, 5-hydroxyuridine, synthesized by LEVENE and LA FORGE (1912), is one of the first synthetic pyrimidine nucleoside derivatives reported. Corresponding 5-hydroxy derivatives of deoxyuridine (BELTZ and VISSER, 1955) and cytidine (FUKUHARA and VISSER, 1962) have also been synthesized, but their activity in biological systems has not been studied extensively. Preparation of 5-hydroxyuridine from uridine has been improved (ROBERTS and VISSER, 1952; UEDA, 1960) and conditions have been developed which are sufficiently mild to allow chemical synthesis of 5-hydroxy-UDP and 5-hydroxy-UTP from the corresponding uridine nucleotides (ROY-BURMAN et al., 1966). Synthetic procedures and physical characteristics of these nucleoside (VISSER, 1968) and nucleotide analogs (VISSER and ROY-BURMAN, 1968) have been reviewed. The 5-hydroxy derivatives of UDP-glucose, UDP-glucuronate (Roy-Burman, P., et al., 1968) and UDP-xylose (Huang et al., 1971) were prepared enzymatically from 5-hydroxy-UTP.

The introduction of a hydroxyl group at the 5-position of uridine induces chemical changes which are related to some of the inhibitory effects of the analog. In addition to the potential steric hindrance resulting from replacement of a hydrogen by the relatively bulky (0.96 Å radius) hydroxyl group and its contribution of a new hydrogen-bonding center, the electro-negative hydroxyl group induces a change in pK_a from 9.2 to 7.8 (Roy-Burman et al., 1966). Thus, at physiological pH values, a significant fraction of the nucleoside analog may exist in its ionized form, which could alter its enzyme binding properties and formation of hydrogen-bonded base-pairs.

Inhibitory Effects of 5-Hydroxyuridine

The inhibitory effects of 5-hydroxyuridine in biological systems were initially reported by Roberts and Visser (1952). 5-Hydroxyuridine and 5-aminouridine were of interest since they inhibit growth of wild type Neurospora, whereas other pyrimidine nucleoside analogs studied inhibit growth of a pyrimidine-requiring mutant only. It was concluded from these early "inhibition analysis" studies that uridine and cytidine are not intermediates in the synthesis *de novo* of pyrimidine nucleotides, and that 5-hydroxyuridine and 5-aminouridine inhibit reactions involved in the pathway of pyrimidine nucleotide biosynthesis. Subsequently, the analog has been reported to inhibit the growth of bacteria (Slotnick et al., 1953), viruses (Visser et al., 1952), and animal tumors (Sugiura and Creech, 1956).

The temporary nature of the inhibitory effect of 5-hydroxyuridine on the growth of *E. coli* and Neurospora was explained by its degradation to the inert pyrimidine analog, 5-hydroxyuracil (Slotnick et al., 1954). Nonproliferating cell suspensions of *E. coli* degrade 5-hydroxyuridine at approximately the same rate as uridine and cytidine.

The induction of β-galactosidase in *E. coli* is prevented completely by low concentrations of 5-hydroxyuridine which have no effect on protein synthesis (Spiegelman et al., 1955). At higher concentrations of the analog both RNA and protein synthesis are inhibited in *E. coli* 15 T^- (Ben-Ishai and Volcani, 1956). The precise mechanism of these inhibitory effects and the metabolism of the analog were studied by Smith and Visser (1965) in Ehrlich ascites cells and cell-free extracts. RNA and protein syntheses are inhibited by 5-hydroxyuridine in whole cells, but in contrast to the results with *E. coli* 15 T^-, the effect of the analog on RNA synthesis is much more pronounced than the effect on protein synthesis. These studies indicated that 5-hydroxyuridine inhibits primarily nucleic acid synthesis and only secondarily the formation of protein. The analog is metabolized by Ehrlich ascites cells or cell-free extracts to the 5-hydroxy derivatives of UMP, UDP, UTP, UDP-glucose, and is incorporated into RNA. A comparison of the amounts of uridine and 5-hydroxyuridine which are metabolized to corresponding nucleotides and incorporated into RNA by whole cells revealed that the amounts of the respective acid-soluble nucleotides are not grossly different, while the amount of uridine incorporated into nucleic acids is 27 times that of 5-hydroxyuridine. These data imply a marked difference in the utilization of UTP and 5-hydroxy-UTP as substrates for DNA-dependent RNA polymerase. This difference may be attributed to impairment of the hydrogen bonding efficiency between 5-hydroxyuracil and adenine due to the negative inductive effect of the 5-hydroxyl group. This conclusion was substantiated by the subsequent finding that 5-hydroxy-UTP is an inefficient, but specific, substitute for UTP in the *E. coli* RNA polymerase reaction *in vitro* (Roy-Burman et al., 1966).

A partial explanation for the inhibitory effect of 5-hydroxyuridine on RNA synthesis is the strong inhibition of orotidylic acid decarboxylase by 5-hydroxy-UMP, one of the products of 5-hydroxyuridine metabolism (Smith and Visser, 1965). This explanation is based on the finding that synthetically prepared 5-hydroxy-UMP does not inhibit appreciably the conversion of UMP to UTP in a cell-free preparation from Ehrlich ascites cells, whereas conversion of orotic acid to UTP is inhibited completely at a molar ratio of inhibitor to orotic acid of 5:1, and the inhibition is accompanied by an accumulation of orotidylic acid.

Poly-5-hydroxyuridylate has been isolated as a product of polynucleotide phosphorylase using synthetically prepared 5-hydroxy-UDP as substrate. The polynucleotide analog was shown to be an inefficient (Grunberg-Manago and Michelson, 1964) or completely ineffective (Smith and Visser, 1965) polynucleotide in its ability to direct phenylalanine polymerization. These results substantiated the prior evidence that the 5-hydroxyl group impairs base-pairing of uracil with adenine. Furthermore, it has been reported that poly-5-hydroxyuridylate stimulates incorporation of amino acids other than phenylalanine into polypeptides, implying aberrant base-pairing of the uracil analog (Grunberg-Manago and Michelson, 1964).

The cellular conversion of 5-hydroxyuridine to 5-hydroxy-UTP and 5-hydroxy-UDP-sugars led to investigations of the possible consequence of these nucleotide analogs on, respectively, DNA dependent RNA polymerase (Roy-Burman et al., 1966) and UDPG dehydrogenase (Roy-Burman, P. et al., 1968). Synthetically prepared 5-hydroxy-UTP is incorporated into RNA to a very low extent by RNA polymerase from *E. coli* and acts as a competitive inhibitor of UTP in the polymerase reaction. The ability of 5-hydroxy-UTP to replace UTP in RNA synthesis decreases markedly at pH values above 7. The inhibitory effect of 5-hydroxy-UTP on the polymerase reaction is least at pH 7.0 and increases with increasing pH values to a maximum at pH 9.0. These effects are related to the relatively low pK_a of 5-hydroxyuridine as compared to uridine, the analog serving as a more efficient substrate in unionized form and a more efficient inhibitor in ionized form. The data are consistent with the conclusion that 5-hydroxy-UTP inhibits RNA synthesis because it has a strong affinity for a DNA-polymerase complex but does not participate readily in polynucleotide synthesis. It is of interest in this connection that 5-hydroxy-dUTP is incorporated into DNA and acts as a competitive inhibitor of dTTP in the DNA-dependent DNA polymerase reaction; but, in contrast to the behavior of 5-hydroxy-UTP in RNA synthesis, the ionized form is ineffective as either substrate or inhibitor (Roy-Burman et al., 1970).

A crude preparation of UDP-glucose pyrophosphorylase from yeast was used to prepare 5-hydroxy-UDP-glucose from 5-hydroxy-UTP and glucose-1-phosphate (Roy-Burman, P. et al., 1968). The cofactor analog is oxidized at a slower rate than UDP-glucose by the dehydrogenase and produces non-competitive inhibition with respect to UDP-glucose and a mixed-type inhibition with respect to NAD^+. The nonionized form of the cofactor analog is the more effective inhibitor of UDP-glucose oxidation. Rate constants indicate that the analog inhibits binding of NAD^+ to the enzyme to a greater extent than binding of UDP-glucose, thus accounting for the noncompetitive kinetics with respect to UDP-glucose. The cofactor analog, 5-hydroxy-UDP-xylose, prepared from 5-hydroxy-UTP and xylose-1-phosphate with a crude yeast extract, inhibits UDP-glucose dehydrogenase, but to a lesser extent than does UDP-xylose, the naturally occurring allosteric effector of this reaction (Huang et al., 1971).

A summary of the present knowledge of the metabolism of 5-hydroxyuridine and the known inhibitory effects of phosphorylated derivatives are given in Fig. 1. The metabolic lesion which is largely responsible for the observed inhibitory effects on cell growth and RNA synthesis has not been ascertained. Although 5-hydroxy-UMP strongly inhibits orotidylate decarboxylase, the concentration of 5-hydroxy-UMP in Ehrlich ascites cells is low as compared to 5-hydroxy-UTP. Thus, inhibition of either the polymerase or the decarboxylase reaction may conceivably predominate, depending upon cell type and environmental conditions. Similarly, although incorporation of the analog into RNA is low as compared with certain other analogs, a very small degree of incorporation of 5-hydroxyuracil into RNA may be assumed to cause its malfunction due to the inability of the analog to form appropriate base pairs. It is probable that the sequence of inhibitory effects which limits RNA synthesis or its function, namely, the inhibition of UTP synthesis *de novo*, the inhibition of UTP utilization for RNA synthesis, and the incorporation of the analog to form nonfunctional RNA is a more likely explanation for its overall cytotoxic effects than any one of the metabolic lesions alone.

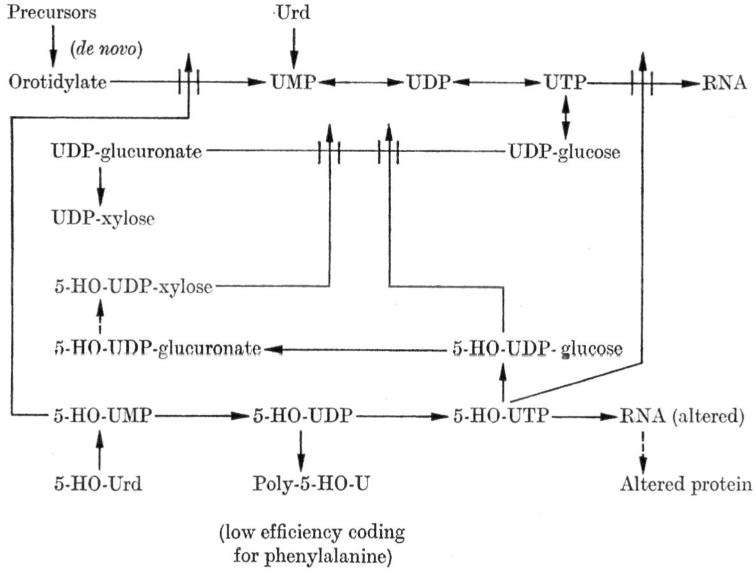

Fig. 1. Metabolism of 5-hydroxyuridine and known enzymatic sites of inhibition. Inhibition is indicated by —‡—. Reactions which have not been established are indicated by dashed lines

Chemistry, Metabolism, and Inhibitory Effects of 5-Aminouridine

Procedures for the synthesis of 5-aminouridine (Roberts and Visser, 1952) and the related analogs, 5-aminouracil and 5-aminodeoxyuridine, have been described (Beltz and Visser, 1957). The chemistry, metabolism, and inhibitory actions of 5-aminouridine have been reviewed (Visser, 1968a; Roy-Burman, 1970).

5-Aminouridine, 5-aminouracil, and 5-aminodeoxyuridine produce a wide range of biological effects. These analogs inhibit growth of bacteria (Theil and Zamenhof, 1963; Dunn and Smith, 1958; Beltz and Visser, 1957), fungi (Roberts and Visser, 1952), viruses (Visser et al., 1952), protozoa (Kidder and Dewey, 1949), tumors (Stock and Suguira, reported by Visser, 1955), and plant root meristems (Smith et al., 1963). The 6-methylamino purine content of DNA is increased up to nine fold in a thymine-requiring mutant of *E. coli* by 5-aminouracil (Dunn and Smith, 1958; Thiel and Zamenhof, 1963), and this analog has been used to produce partial synchronization of nuclear divisions in plant root meristems (Smith et al., 1963).

Thymidylate synthetase is inhibited by 5-aminodeoxyuridine, but the analog does not inhibit incorporation of the hydroxymethyl group of serine into adenine of *E. coli* (Friedland and Visser, 1961). 5-Aminodeoxyuridine (Wacker et al., 1960; Kabat and Visser, 1964) and 5-aminouracil (Wacker et al., 1960) are incorporated into bacterial DNA, whereas 5-aminouridine is metabolized like uridine and is incorporated into RNA (Smith et al., 1966). In this regard, the 5-amino-substituted nucleosides act in a manner similar to that of corresponding 5-chloro-substituted nucleosides, since both types of analogs may be directed into either RNA or DNA.

Preliminary evidence that 5-aminouridine interferes with pyrimidine nucleotide synthesis *de novo* was provided by the observations that the analog inhibits carbamylphosphate incorporation into nucleic acid pyrimidines (Werkheiser and Visser, 1955), and phosphate incorporation into nucleotides and phospholipids of rat liver slices and hepatoma (Werkheiser et al., 1955). The mechanism of these inhibitory effects was elucidated by Smith et al. (1966) using Ehrlich ascites cells and cell-free preparations. The analog is metabolized by whole cells to the 5-amino derivatives of UMP, UDP, UTP, and UDP-sugars, and is incorporated into RNA. Under identical conditions, the amount of uridine incorporated into RNA is 6.7 times greater than that of 5-aminouridine. These results are explained in part by the relatively slow rate of phosphorylation of the nucleoside 5′-phosphate analogs as compared to UMP, and in part by the inefficient utilization of the nucleoside triphosphate analogs as compared to UTP in the DNA-dependent RNA polymerase reaction (Smith et al., 1966; Roy-Burman et al., 1970). The presence of 5-amino-UMP inhibits formation of uridine nucleotides in cell-free preparations of Ehrlich ascites cells, due to its strong inhibition of orotidylic acid decarboxylase (Smith et al., 1966). As previously indicated for 5-hydroxyuridine, the importance *in vivo* of the inhibition of orotidylic acid decarboxylase cannot be assessed accurately.

The cofactor analog, 5-amino-UDP-glucose, has been prepared from 5-amino-UTP using UDP-glucose pyrophosphorylase of yeast (Roy-Burman et al., 1970). The analog is oxidized by UDP-glucose dehydrogenase at a rate one-half that of UDP-glucose. 5-Amino-UDP-xylose, prepared from 5-amino-UTP and xylose-1-phosphate by a yeast extract, inhibits UDP-glucose dehydrogenase with respect to UDP-glucose (Huang et al., 1971). It is conceivable that the inhibitory effects of these amino-substituted cofactors may contribute to the cytotoxic effects of 5-aminouridine. However, in general, the cofactor analogs appear to serve primarily as alternate substrates for the natural cofactors and may be predicted to be of lesser consequence than inhibitory effects of the analog of RNA synthesis and function.

The nucleotide analog, 5-amino-UTP, substitutes specifically for UTP with an efficiency of about 40% in the DNA-dependent RNA polymerase reaction of *E. coli* (Roy-Burman et al., 1970). In contrast to 5-hydroxy-UTP, 5-amino-UTP does not inhibit RNA synthesis significantly, and apparently serves primarily as an alternate substrate for UTP in RNA synthesis. It is of interest in this regard that certain viruses grown in the presence of 5-aminouridine are hypersensitive to nitrous acid (THIRY, 1966), presumably becauseof the substitution of the nitrous acid susceptible analog for nonreactive uridine.

In summary, 5-aminouridine limits UTP synthesis *de novo* and is metabolized to 5-amino-UTP which serves as an alternate substrate for UTP in the RNA polymerase reaction. This sequence accounts for the substantial incorporation of 5-amino-UMP into RNA, but the consequence of the altered RNA is not known. As compared to 5-hydroxyuridine, the 5-amino-derivative is a more acceptable alternate substrate for several enzymes involved in uridine metabolism and is less effective as a nonsubstrate inhibitor. In other aspects of their metabolism and inhibitory effects the two analogs are similar.

References

BELJANSKI, M., BELJANSKI, M.: Synthèse dans *Escherichia coli* des ARN dont la structure primaire diffère totalement de celle de l' ADN. C. R. Acid. Sc. Paris, D **267**, 1058—1060 (1968).

BELJANSKI, M., BELJANSKI, M., BOURGAREL, P., CHASSAGNE, J.: Synthèse chez les bactéries d'ARN nouveaux n'étant pas la copie de l'ADN. C. R. Acad. Sc. Paris, D **269**, 240—243 (1969).

BELJANSKI, M., BOURGAREL, P., BELJANSKI, M.: Showdomycene et biosynthese d'ARN non-complementaires de l'ADN. Ann. Inst. Pasteur. **118**, 253—276 (1970).

BELJANSKI, M., BOURGAREL, P., BELJANSKI, M.: Drastic alteration of ribosomal RNA and ribosomal proteins in showdomycin-resistant *Escherichia coli*. Proc. nat. Acad. Sci. (Wash.) **68**, 491—495 (1971).

BELTZ, R. E., VISSER, D. W.: Growth inhibitiou of *Escherichia coli* by new thymidine analogs. J. Amer. chem. Soc. **77**, 736—738 (1955).

BELTZ, R. E., VISSER, D. W.: Studies on the action of thymidine analogues. J. biol. Chem. **226**, 1035—1045 (1957).

BEN-ISHAI, R., VOLCANI, B. E.: Dependence of protein synthesis on ribonucleic acid formation in a thymine-requiring mutant of *Escherichia coli*. Biochim. biophys. Acta (Amst.) **21**, 265—270 (1956).

BERMEK, E., KRAMER, W., MONKEMEYER, H., MATTHAEI, H.: Mechanisms in protein synthesis XII. Sites of action of showdomycin in a cell-free polyphenylalanine synthesizing system from human lymphatic tissue: ribosomes and elongation factor TF II. Biochem. biophys. Res. Comm. **40**, 1311—1318 (1970).

DARNALL, K. R., TOWNSEND, L. B., ROBINS, R. K.: The structure of showdomycin, a novel carbon-linked nucleoside antibiotic related to uridine. Proc. nat. Acad. Sci. (Wash.) **57**, 548—553 (1967).

DUNN, D. B., SMITH, J. D.: The occurrence of 6-methylaminopurine in deoxyribonucleic acids. Biochem. J. **68**, 627—635 (1958).

FRIEDLAND, M., VISSER, D.W.: Studies on 5-aminodeoxyuridine. Biochim. biophys. Acta (Amst.) **51**, 148—152 (1961).

FUKUHARA, T. K., VISSER, D. W.: Uridine, cytidine, and deoxyuridine derivatives. Biochemistry **1**, 563—568 (1962).

GRUNBERG-MANAGO, M., MICHELSON, A. M.: Polynucleotide analogues. II. Stimulation of amino acid incorporation by polynucleotide analogues. Biochim. biophys. Acta (Amst.) **80**, 431—440 (1964).

HADLER, H. I., CLAYBOURN, B. E., TSCHANG, T. P.: Mitochondrial volume changes induced by the antibiotic showdomycin. Biochem. biophys. Res. Comm. **31**, 25—31 (1968).

HADLER, H. I., MOREAU, T. L.: The induction of ATP energized mitochondrial volume changes by the combination of the two antitumor agents showdomycin and lapachol. J. Antibiot. **22**, 513—520 (1969).

HUANG, Y. H. J., ROY-BURMAN, D., VISSER, D.W.: Uridine diphosphate glucose dehydrogenase of calf liver. Properties and inhibition characteristics with uridine diphosphate xylose analogues. Biochem. Pharmacol. **20**, 2447—2453 (1971).

KABAT, S., VISSER, D. W.: The incorporation of aminodeoxyuridine into deoxyribonucleic acid of *Escherichia coli* 15 T^-. Biochim. biophys. Acta (Amst.) **82**, 680—681 (1964).

KIDDER, G. W., DEWEY, V. C.: The biological activity of substituted pyrimidines. J. biol. Chem. **178**, 383—387 (1949).

KOMATSU, Y., TANAKA, K.: Mechanism of action of showdomycin. Part I. Effect of showdomycin on the syntheses of nucleic acids and proteins in *Escherichia coli* K-12. Agr. biol. Chem. **32**, 1021—1027 (1968).

Levene, P. A., La Forge, F. B.: Über die Hefe — Nucleinsäure. V. Die Struktur der Pyrimidin-Nucleoside Berichte der Deutschen Chemischen Gesellschaft **45**, 608—620 (1912).

Matsuura, S., Shiratori, O., Katagiri, K.: Antitumor activity of showdomycin. J. Antibiot. **17**, 234—237 (1964).

Nakagawa, Y., Kano, H., Tsuda, T., Koyama, H.: Structure of a new class of C-nucleoside antibiotic showdomycin. Tetrahedron Lett. **42**, 4105—4109 (1967).

Nishimura, H., Komatsu, Y.: Reversal of inhibiting action of showdomycin on the proliferation of *Escherichia coli* by nucleosides and thiol compounds. J. Antibiot. **21**, 250—254 (1968).

Nishimura, H., Mayama, M., Komatsu, Y., Kato, H., Shimaoka, N., Tanaka, Y.: Showdomycin, a new antibiotic from a streptomyces sp. J. Antibiot. **17**, 148—155 (1964).

Roberts, M., Visser, D. W.: Antimetabolite activity of uridine and cytidine derivatives. J. biol. Chem. **194**, 695—701 (1952).

Roy-Burman, P.: Analogues of nucleic acid components. In: Rentchnick, P. (Ed.): Recent results in cancer research, p. 64—66. New York-Heidelberg-Berlin: Springer 1970.

Roy-Burman, P., Roy-Burman, S., Visser, D. W.: Uridine diphosphate glucose dehydrogenase. Studies with 5-hydroxyuridine diphosphate glucose and 5,6-dihydrouridine diphosphate glucose. J. biol. Chem. **243**, 1692—1697 (1968).

Roy-Burman, S., Huang, Y. H. J., Visser, D. W.: Inhibition of amino acid and sugar transport by showdomycin. Biochem. biophys. Res. Comm. **42**, 445—453 (1971).

Roy-Burman, S., Roy-Burman, P., Visser, D. W.: Inhibition of ribonucleic acid polymerase by 5-hydroxyuridine 5′-triphosphate. J. biol. Chem. **241**, 781—786 (1966).

Roy-Burman, S., Roy-Burman, P., Visser, D. W.: Showdomycin, a new nucleoside antibiotic. Cancer Res. **28**, 1605—1610 (1968).

Roy-Burman, S., Roy-Burman, P., Visser, D. W.: Studies on the effect of triphosphates of 5-aminouridine and 5-hydroxydeoxyuridine on ribonucleic acid and deoxyribonucleic acid polymerases. Biochem. Pharmacol. **19**, 2745—2756 (1970).

Slotnick, I. J., Visser, D. W., Rittenberg, S. C.: Growth inhibition of purine-requiring mutants of *Escherichia coli* by 5-hydroxyuridine. J. biol. Chem. **203**, 647—652 (1953).

Slotnick, I. J., Visser, D. W., Rittenberg, S. C.: Degradation of substituted pyrimidine nucleosides by *Escherichia coli* and *Bacillus subtilis*. J. biol. Chem. **208**, 217—223 (1954).

Smith, D. A., Roy-Burman, P., Visser, D. W.: Studies on 5-aminouridine. Biochim. biophys. Acta (Amst.) **119**, 221—228 (1966).

Smith, D. A., Visser, D. W.: Studies on 5-hydroxyuridine. J. biol. Chem. **240**, 446—453 (1965).

Smith, H. H., Fussel, C. P., Kugelman, B. H.: Partial synchronization of nuclear divisions in root meristems with 5-aminouracil. Science **142**, 595 (1963).

Spiegelman, S., Halvorson, H. O., Ben-Ishai, R.: Free amino acids and the enzyme-forming mechanism. In: McElroy, W. D., Glass, B. (Eds.): A symposium on amino acid metabolism, p. 124—169. Baltimore: Johns Hopkins Press 1955.

Sugiura, K., Creech, H. J.: Merits of ascites tumors for chemotherapeutic screening. Ann. N. Y. Acad. Sci. **63**, 962—982 (1956).

Theil, E., Zamenhof, S.: Studies on 6-methylaminopurine (6-methyladenine) in bacterial deoxyribonucleic acid. J. biol. Chem. **238**, 3058—3064 (1963).

Thiry, L.: Viruses grown in the presence of base analogs: specific alteration of susceptibility to inactivation by radiations, mutagens, and protodyes. Virology **28**, 543—554 (1966).

Titani, Y., Katsube, Y.: Radiosensitization of *Escherichia coli* B/r by showdomycin. Biochim. biophys. Acta (Amst.) **192**, 367—369 (1969).

Titani, Y., Katsube, Y.: Enhancement of the lethal effect of alkylation to *Escherichia coli* B/r by showdomycin. J. Antibiot. **23**, 43—44 (1970).

Ueda, T.: Studies on coenzyme analogs. III. Syntheses of 5-substituted uridine 5′-phosphates. Chem. pharm. Bull. 8, 455—458 (1960).

Visser, D. W.: Antimetabolites of nucleic acid precursors. In: Rhoads, C. P. (Ed.): Antimetabolites and cancer, pp. 47—62. Am. Soc. Adv. Sci. 1955.

Visser, D. W.: 5-Hydroxyuridine. In: Zorbach, W. W., Tipson, R. S. (Eds.): Synthetic procedures in nucleic acid chemistry, Vol. 1, pp. 428—430. New York: John Wiley & Sons 1968.

Visser, D. W.: 5-Aminouridine. In: Zorbach, W. W., Tipson, R. S. (Eds.): Synthetic procedures in nucleic acid chemistry, Vol. 1, p. 407—408. New York: John Wiley & Sons 1968a.

Visser, D. W., Lagerborg, D. L., Pearson, H. E.: Inhibition of mouse encephalomyelitis virus, *in vitro*, by certain nucleoprotein derivatives. Proc. Soc. exp. Biol. (N. Y.) **79**, 571—573 (1952).

Visser, D. W., Roy-Burman, P.: 5-Hydroxyuridine 5′-phosphate derivatives. In: Zorbach, W. W., Tipson, R. S. (Eds.): Synthetic procedures in nucleic acid chemistry, Vol. 1, p. 493 to 496. New York: John Wiley & Sons 1968.

VISSER, D. W., ROY-BURMAN, S.: Unpublished data, 1971.

WACKER, A., KIRSCHFIELD, S., HARTMANN, D., WEINBLUM, U. D.: Über den Einbau von 5-nitrouracil, 5-aminouracil und 2-thiothymin in die bakteriendeoxyribonukleinsäure. J. mol. Biol. **2**, 69—71 (1960).

WERKHEISER, W. C., VISSER, D. W.: Metabolic inhibitors and nucleotide turnover. II. Inhibition of uptake of C^{14}-precursors in rat liver and hepatoma slices. Cancer Research **15**, 644—649 (1955).

WERKHEISER, W. C., WINZLER, R. J., VISSER, D. W.: Metabolic inhibitors and nucleotide turnover. I. Inhibition of uptake of radiophosphate in rat liver and hepatoma slices. Cancer Res. **15**, 641—643 (1955).

Chapter 47

6-Thiopurines

A. R. P. PATERSON and D. M. TIDD

With 1 Figure

Introduction

It was recognized through early studies with 2,6-diaminopurine, 8-azaguanine, and 6-mercaptopurine that chemotherapy with analogs of nucleic acid bases might afford control of some aspects of neoplastic disease (ELION and HITCHINGS, 1965). The inhibitory activity of thiopurines toward rodent tumors, and the value of 6-mercaptopurine in the treatment of human leukemias (the latter was first reported by BURCHENAL et al., 1953), focused a great deal of attention on the thiopurines; the immunosuppressive and anti-inflammatory properties of the thiopurines were subsequently recognized (thiopurine immunosuppressive effects have been reviewed by SCHWARTZ and ANDRÉ, 1962; HITCHINGS and ELION, 1963, 1969; BERENBAUM, 1967; ASHTON et al., 1970; anti-inflammatory effects have been discussed by PAGE et al., 1962a, b; HERSH et al., 1966; BERENBAUM, 1967; FURTH, 1970). A great effort has been made to synthesize related analogs and to understand the metabolism and metabolic effects of thiopurines in a variety of cell systems. It has become apparent that 6-mercaptopurine and its homolog, 6-thioguanine, produce cytotoxic effects which are manifested in rapidly proliferating cell populations *in vivo* and *in vitro*. Despite an extensive research effort, the biochemical bases of the cytotoxic effects of 6-mercaptopurine and 6-thioguanine are only dimly perceived at present.

The metabolism and metabolic effects of the 6-thiopurines have been reviewed frequently; see for examples BROCKMAN (1963a), BROCKMAN and ANDERSON (1963), ELION et al. (1963), HENDERSON and MANDEL (1963), HUTCHISON (1963), ELION and HITCHINGS (1965), STOCK (1966), ELION (1967), BALIS (1968), MONTGOMERY (1970), and ROY-BURMAN (1970).

The metabolism of 6-mercaptopurine, 6-thioguanine, and 6-methylthioinosine is summarized in Fig. 1, which refers to transformations that take place in animal cells. Abbreviations used in this diagram are explained in the text. Figure 1 presents findings from a variety of mammalian cell types; particular cells may be unable to effect some of the conversions indicated. The concept that analogs of the natural purine bases become active as antimetabolites after conversion to ribosyl 5′-phosphate derivatives appears to have originated in the suggestion by KIDDER and DEWEY (1949) that 8-azaguanine acted in this way. It has since been established that this process is the first essential step in the anabolism and mechanism of action of the three major thiopurines considered in this chapter.

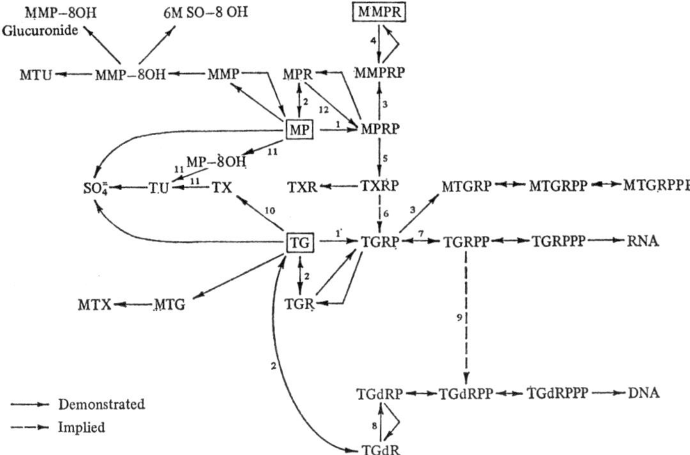

Fig. 1. Thiopurine metabolism: enzymes. (1) Hypoxanthine-guanine phosphoribosyltransferase. (2) Purine nucleoside phosphorylase. (3) Methyltransferase. (4) Adenosine kinase. (5) Inosinate (IMP) dehydrogenase. (6) Xanthylate (XMP) aminase. (7) Guanylate (GMP) kinase. (8) Deoxynucleoside kinase. (9) Ribonucleotide reductase. (10) Guanase. (11) Xanthine oxidase. (12) Inosine kinase.

Key to abbreviations: MP, 6-Mercaptopurine. TG, 6-Thioguanine. MMPR, 6-Methylthioinosine. TX, 6-Thioxanthine. MP-8 OH, 8-Hydroxy-6-mercaptopurine. TU, 6-Thiouric acid. 6MSO-8OH, 6-Methylsulfinyl-8-hydroxypurine. $SO_4^{=}$, Inorganic sulfate. R, Ribosyl group at purine 9-position. dR, Deoxyribosyl group at purine 9-position. M, Methyl group on 6-thiol of 6-thiopurine. P, Monophosphate group at pentosyl 5′-position. PP, Diphosphate group at pentosyl 5′-position. PPP, Triphosphate group at pentosyl 5′-position.

Metabolism of 6-Mercaptopurine and 6-Methylthioinosine

A. Anabolism

I. 6-Thioinosinate

The initial reaction in the anabolism of 6-mercaptopurine (MP) is conversion to 6-thioinosinate (MPRP) (see Fig. 1) by hypoxanthine-guanine phosphoribosyltransferase (LUKENS and HERRINGTON, 1957; BROCKMAN et al., 1959). This step was recognized as essential to the inhibitory action of MP in experiments which showed that certain MP-resistant sublines of rodent neoplasms were devoid of this particular enzyme activity (see review by BROCKMAN, 1963a).

The term "activation" has been used to describe this step; however, with hindsight, it now appears that earlier reference to 6-thioinosinate as the "active" form of the drug may have been misleading because, in addition to enzymatic inhibitions directly attributable to 6-thioinosinate, further metabolites of this compound are probably involved in MP cytotoxicity. The di- and triphosphate derivatives of 6-thioinosine have not been identified as MP metabolites; however, it is possible that these may be among the uncharacterized minor metabolites of MP detected by CALDWELL (1969).

II. 6-Methylthioinosinate

MP and other 6-thiopurine derivatives are substrates for an *S*-adenosylmethionine — requiring methyltransferase activity in animal cells (REMY, 1963,

1965). 6-Methylthioinosinate (MMPRP) is formed by methylation of 6-thioinosinate and is evidently responsible for certain metabolic effects of MP (see below). This compound is a major metabolite of MP in several cell types (ALLAN et al., 1966; CALDWELL, 1969; PATERSON and WANG, 1970a; BENNETT and ALLAN, 1971).

6-Methylthioinosinate is the principle metabolite of 6-methylthioinosine (MMPR) in several cell types, including the human erythrocyte (LOO et al., 1969). This compound is a substrate for adenosine kinase (see Fig. 1) and is converted thereby to the 5′-monophosphate ester (BENNETT et al., 1965; CALDWELL et al., 1966; see also references 5 to 11, HENDERSON et al., 1972).

6-Methylthioinosinate does not appear to be a substrate for nucleoside monophosphate kinases because the di- and triphosphate derivatives have not been detected in several cell types where formation of the monophosphate has been demonstrated. Accordingly, incorporation of 6-methylthioinosinate into nucleic acids would not be expected. Intracellular 6-methylthioinosinate persists for long periods in Ehrlich ascites carcinoma cells and in human erythrocytes (LOO et al., 1968; PATERSON and WANG, 1970a), but in cultured L5178Y cells, this compound has a half-time of less than one hour (WARNICK, C.T., PATERSON, A.R.P., unpublished results).

III. 6-Thioxanthylate

6-Thioinosinate is a substrate for IMP dehydrogenase from *Aerobacter aerogenes* (HAMPTON, 1963); the product of this reaction, 6-thioxanthylate (TXRP) (see Fig. 1), is a major metabolite of MP in 2 mouse neoplasms, the Ehrlich ascites carcinoma and leukemia L1210 (ATKINSON et al., 1965; CALDWELL, 1969; MELONI and ROGERS, 1969).

IV. Other Anabolites of 6-Mercaptopurine

By anion exchange chromatography on columns of DEAE Sephadex, CALDWELL (1969) showed that MP-treated Ehrlich ascites carcinoma cells contain a number of MP metabolites (perhaps 8) other than those mentioned above. A clue to the identity of some of these uncharacterized compounds may be found in the work of SCANNELL and HITCHINGS (1966), who demonstrated that DNA from an MP-treated tumor contained deoxythioguanosine (TGdR), evidently incorporated in nucleotide linkage in the isolated DNA. It is implicit in this finding that nucleotide derivatives of 6-thioguanine (TG) are formed from MP. Although this has not been studied directly, it may be presumed that amination of 6-thioxanthylate is a step in the formation of the 6-thioguanosine phosphates from MP and that deoxythioguanosine phosphates are derived therefrom. These compounds have not been demonstrated as metabolites of MP; however, their implied existence is likely because TG is also anabolized by these sequences (see Fig. 1 and below). The implied existence of thioguanosine phosphates as MP anabolites suggests that MP would be incorporated into RNA as well as into DNA. The incorporation of TG into RNA nucleotides in mouse tumor cells has been demonstrated by LEPAGE (1968). Incorporation of MP into RNA has been reported (BIEBER et al., 1961); however, characterization of this material was not rigorous. HANSEN and coworkers presented evidence to suggest that MP may be bound firmly to RNA by forming metal mercaptides with divalent ions associated with the nucleic acid (HANSEN and NADLER, 1961; HANSEN et al., 1962). The amount of MP bound to RNA was of the order of magnitude of that reported as "incorporated" by BIEBER et al. (1961).

V. 6-Thioinosine

6-Thioinosine (MPR) (see Fig. 1) is a substrate for purine nucleoside phosphorylase (KRENITSKY, 1967); Ehrlich ascites carcinoma cells cleave this compound phosphorolytically, with liberation of the free base (PATERSON and SUTHERLAND, 1964). However, direct phosphorylation of 6-thioinosine has been demonstrated in extracts of a thiopurine-resistant subline of the Ehrlich ascites carcinoma, which lacked hypoxanthine-guanine phosphoribosyltransferase (PIERRE et al., 1967). The enzyme responsible has been identified as "inosine kinase" (PIERRE and LEPAGE, 1968); previously, the existence of this enzyme activity had been doubted (BROCKMAN and ANDERSON, 1963). This activity may not be significant in the intact cell since thiopurine-resistant tumors, which lack hypoxanthine-guanine phosphoribosyltransferase, are cross resistant to 6-thioinosine.

B. Catabolism

The urinary excretion products of the 6-thiopurines are derived by oxidation and methylation processes. In the mouse, MP is converted to 6-thiouric acid (TU) by xanthine oxidase (see Fig. 1), probably by way of the intermediate 6-thio-8-hydroxypurine (MP-8OH). In the mouse, both MP and 6-thiouric acid are excreted in the urine; a portion of the 6-thiouric acid may be further degraded by uricase, with the ultimate formation of sulfate (ELION et al., 1959, 1963; ELION, 1967). In man, MP, 6-thiouric acid, and sulfate are also MP excretion products; the route of sulfate formation is unknown, but does not involve uricase since this enzyme is absent in man. 6-Methylsulfinyl-8-hydroxypurine and several other methylated oxidation products have also been identified as urinary excretion products of MP in man (ELION, 1967). 6-Methylthiopurine (MMP) occurs in rat urine after administration of MP (SARCIONE and STUTZMAN, 1959), but has not been found in mouse or human urine (ELION, 1967).

The xanthine oxidase inhibitor, allopurinol (4-hydroxypyrazolo[3,4-*d*]pyrimidine), inhibits the oxidation of purines and of MP *in vivo* and *in vitro* in both mouse and man; the toxicity of MP, and its potency as an antineoplastic agent, are increased several-fold in the presence of allopurinol in both mouse and man (ELION et al., 1963; HITCHINGS, 1963; ANONYMOUS, 1968). Very little oxidative catabolism of MP occurs within tumor tissue; however, in leukemia L1210 cells there is a small amount of direct dethiolation of MP, presumably with the production of hypoxanthine (MELONI and ROGERS, 1969).

Metabolism of 6-Thioguanine

A. Anabolism

I. 6-Thioguanosine Phosphates

The initial step in the anabolism of TG is conversion to the ribonucleoside monophosphate derivative, 6-thioguanylate (TGRP) (see Fig. 1). As with MP, this reaction is catalyzed by hypoxanthine-guanine phosphoribosyltransferase. This became apparent when particular mouse tumors, which were resistant to MP through deletion of this enzyme, were found to be cross resistant to TG and also to lack the ability to convert TG to 6-thioguanylate (LAW, 1958; ELLIS and LEPAGE, 1963; STUTTS and BROCKMAN, 1963). As with MP, the formation of the ribonucleoside monophosphate derivative is essential to the cytotoxic action of TG, but metabolites beyond 6-thioguanylate are involved in cytotoxicity. 6-Thioguanylate is a prominent metabolite of TG in mouse tumor cells; metabolites tentatively identified as thioguanosine di- and triphosphates (TGRPP and TGRPPP) have also been detected (MOORE and LEPAGE, 1958; MIECH et al., 1967; LEPAGE, 1968). This is in accordance with the demonstration by MIECH et al. (1967) that 6-thioguanylate is a substrate for the highly specific guanylate kinase of Sarcoma 180 cells; 6-thioguanylate behaves as an alternative substrate for this enzyme, but the reaction has a low maximum velocity relative to that with GMP. That TG becomes incorporated into RNA (see Fig. 1) is apparent in the recovery of TG nucleotides from RNA isolated from TG treated mouse tumor cells (LEPAGE, 1968).

II. Deoxythioguanosine Phosphates

Although free deoxyribonucleoside phosphate derivatives of TG have not been isolated, they are evidently formed in cells because TG is incorporated into DNA in nucleotide linkage (LEPAGE, 1960; LEPAGE et al., 1964; LEPAGE and WHITECAR, 1971). In demonstrating the latter, DNA was degraded with deoxyribonuclease and phosphodiesterase and the incorporated analog was recovered in the form of a mononucleotide; this has been demonstrated in several mouse tumors and in normal mouse tissues (LEPAGE et al., 1964). The incorporation of TG into DNA nucleotides has also been demonstrated with bone marrow from normal and leukemic patients (LEPAGE and WHITECAR, 1971).

III. Other Anabolites of 6-Thioguanine

ALLAN and BENNETT (1971) have demonstrated that 6-methylthioguanylate (MTGMP) (see Fig. 1) is an anabolite of TG in H.Ep.No.2 cells grown in culture, and is apparently formed by the methylation of 6-thioguanylate involving the previously mentioned methyltransferase (REMY, 1965). The di- and triphosphates of 6-methylthioguanosine were also tentatively identified.

IV. 6-Thioguanosine and β-2'-Deoxythioguanosine

One route by which β-2'-deoxythioguanosine (TGdR) is anabolized in normal and neoplastic cells is by way of a kinase-catalyzed phosphorylation (see Fig. 1) with eventual incorporation into DNA (IWAMOTO et al., 1963; LEPAGE et al., 1964; PEERY and LEPAGE, 1969). A kinase activity present in Ehrlich ascites carcinoma cells also catalyzes the phosphorylation of 6-thioguanosine (PIERRE et al., 1967). The corresponding di- and triphosphate derivatives of both 6-thioguanosine and its deoxyribosyl homolog (see Fig. 1) have been demonstrated in acid extracts of tumor cells which were treated *in vivo* with the analog nucleosides (LEPAGE, 1968). α-2'-Deoxythioguanosine is also converted to mono-, di-, and triphosphate derivatives, and incorporation into the terminal nucleoside positions of RNA and DNA in a mouse tumor has been shown. In contrast, β-2'-deoxythioguanosine is incorporated into internal nucleotide positions in DNA (LEPAGE, 1968).

In an alternate anabolic route, the ribosyl and deoxyribosyl derivatives of TG are cleaved by phosphorolysis (see Fig. 1) with release of the base which is then available for conversion to the nucleotide by hypoxanthine-guanine phosphoribosyltransferase. Phosphorolysis of the ribosyl and β-2'-deoxyribosyl derivatives o TG has been demonstrated in tumor cell extracts, but α-2'-deoxythioguanosine is not cleaved by purine nucleoside phosphorylase (LEPAGE, 1968).

B. Catabolism

TG is a substrate for guanase and the deamination product is 6-thioxanthine (TX) (see Fig. 1) (CURRIE et al., 1967). The latter is oxidized by xanthine oxidase and the reaction product is 6-thiouric acid. 6-Thioxanthine and 6-thiouric acid have been identified as catabolites of TG in mouse tissues (MOORE and LEPAGE, 1958). 6-Thioxanthine and 6-thiouric acid are major catabolites of TG in patients with tumors of the head and neck (LEFKOWITZ et al., 1965). However, degradation of TG by this route occurs only to a small extent during therapy of human leukemias (ELION, 1967). Methylated excretion products of TG are more abundant in these patients, and 2-amino-6-methylthiopurine (MTG) (see Fig. 1) is a prominent urinary constituent (ELION et al., 1962). LEFKOWITZ et al. (1965) suggested that these differences in man may be related to the type of disease. Sulfate is a major end product in the catabolism of TG. Small amounts of TG undergo direct dethiolation in tumor tissue and the products have been detected as nucleic acid purines, principally as guanine (SARTORELLI et al., 1958).

Metabolic Effects of 6-Mercaptopurine and 6-Methylthioinosine

HIRSCHBERG (1963) noted that since its synthesis (ELION et al., 1952) MP had been tested against 120 different experimental neoplasms and, of these, 75 were sensitive to the drug. Rapidly multiplying cells are more susceptible to MP than stationary cell populations (BERENBAUM, 1967; AOKI and MOORE, 1969; LASTER et al., 1969; SCHABEL, 1969; MONTGOMERY, 1970), and this is reflected in the toxicity of MP toward the proliferating elements of bone marrow and intestinal epithelium (BURCHENAL et al., 1953, 1954; PHILIPS et al., 1954a). Thus, SCHABEL et al. (1965) found that "resting" cultures of L1210 mouse leukemia cells were insensitive to MP in contrast to the response of proliferating L1210 cells *in vivo*. However, it is unlikely that the rate of cell proliferation is the only determinant of the selectivity of MP cytotoxicity toward tumor tissue. MP has had extensive use in the treatment of human acute leukemia (see reviews by HENDERSON, 1969, and GOLDIN et al., 1971). In the treatment of acute lymphocytic leukemia (GOLDIN et al., 1971), MP has been used in combination with prednisone, or with other agents in 3- and 4-drug combinations, in very effective remission-inducing therapy. Singly, and in combination with other drugs, MP is effective in remission maintenance in this disease. The frequency of remission induction in the chemotherapy of acute myelogenous leukemia is much lower than that of acute lymphocytic leukemia; however, singly, and in combination with other drugs, MP does have activity in remission induction and maintenance.

Efforts to elucidate the biochemical mechanisms of MP cytotoxicity have involved searching for biochemical disturbances produced by the drug and its metabolites which could account for the drug's biological effects. ELION and HITCHINGS (1965) have summarized some of the metabolic effects of MP anabolites; the present discussion of these effects does not attempt to be comprehensive and is admittedly selective.

A. The Free Base, 6-Mercaptopurine

The free base, MP, has been shown to inhibit hypoxanthine-guanine phosphoribosyltransferase (ATKINSON and MURRAY, 1965) and xanthine oxidase (SILBERMAN and WYNGAARDEN, 1961); in both inhibitions the analog is a competitive substrate. Since conversion to 6-thioinosinate is the first step essential to the cytotoxic activity of MP (see review by BROCKMAN, 1963a), inhibitory effects of the free base are of doubtful chemotherapeutic significance.

B. Nucleotide Anabolites

Studies of MP "mechanism of action" have concentrated upon metabolic effects of the anabolites, 6-thioinosinate and 6-methylthioinosinate (see Fig. 1); enzymatic inhibitory effects of possible importance in the present context are not known for 6-thioxanthylate, the other major anabolite of MP. The isolation of deoxythioguanosine from DNA of MP-treated cells (SCANNELL and HITCHINGS, 1966) revealed that TG nucleotides are formed in the metabolism of MP. TG nucleotides would appear to be derived by way of 6-thioinosinate conversion to 6-thioguanylate, presumably via 6-thioxanthylate. It is at least theoretically possible that MP-treated cells will express the superimposed metabolic effects of several MP anabolites, including TG nucleotides. The nature of the MP effect would depend upon the relative proportion of the MP anabolites. The following discussion will be concerned mainly with the metabolic effects of 6-thioinosinate and 6-methylthioinosinate.

I. Inhibition of Purine Ribonucleotide Synthesis *de novo*

It was originally demonstrated that MP inhibited the incorporation of ^{14}C-labeled formate or glycine into acid-soluble purines (FERNANDES et al., 1956) and nucleic acid purines of experimental neoplasms (SKIPPER, 1954; HEIDELBERGER and KELLER, 1955; LEPAGE and GREENLEES, 1955; GREENLEES and LEPAGE, 1956). The inhibition by MP of incorporation of phosphate into nucleic acids (DAVIDSON and FREEMAN, 1955) could be interpreted in terms of these observations, which suggested that MP inhibited either purine ribonucleotide synthesis *de novo* or purine ribonucleotide interconversions, or both of these processes.

It was demonstrated that MP inhibited the accumulation of α-N-formylglycineamide ribonucleotide (FGAR) in azaserine-treated tumor cells, either *in vivo* or *in vitro* (LEPAGE and JONES, 1961; BROCKMAN, 1963b; BROCKMAN and CHUMLEY, 1965). Azaserine, a glutamine analog, inhibits the glutamine-requiring amidation of FGAR; flux through the preceding steps of purine synthesis continues and FGAR accumulates in azaserine-treated cells. Thus, the inhibition by MP of FGAR accumulation indicated that MP inhibited an early step in purine ribonucleotide synthesis *de novo*. BROCKMAN (1963b) showed that MP did not inhibit the accumulation of FGAR in thiopurine-resistant cells that lacked the capacity to form 6-thioinosinate, in agreement with earlier results of LEPAGE and JONES (1961) which suggested that a nucleotide metabolite of the drug was responsible for the inhibition of the purine nucleotide biosynthetic pathway. Natural purines also inhibited accumulation of FGAR (HENDERSON, 1962), and it then became apparent that mammalian cells were similar to *E. coli* in that purine ribonucleotide synthesis *de novo* was subject to feedback regulation and thiopurine metabolites evidently mimicked natural purine nucleotides as feedback inhibitors of an early enzyme step (GOTS and GOLLUB, 1959). On the basis of similar experiments with intact tumor cells, 6-methylthioinosine (as the 5′-monophosphate) was shown to be a very potent inhibitor of the *de novo* pathway of purine nucleotide synthesis (HENDERSON and KHOO, 1965).

6-Thioinosinate and 6-methylthioinosinate have been reported to inhibit various preparations of glutamine-5-phosphoribosylpyrophosphate (PRPP) amidotransferase, the first enzyme unique to the pathway of purine ribonucleotide synthesis *de novo* (MCCOLLISTER et al., 1962, 1964; CASKEY et al., 1964; HILL and BENNETT, 1969; TAY et al., 1969). In this action, the thiopurine nucleotides mimicked the effect of natural purine nucleotides and the concept that these analog ribonucleotides act as pseudofeedback inhibitors of *de novo* purine nucleotide synthesis became synthesized. 6-Methylthioinosinate is the most potent of the reported nucleotide inhibitors of the amidotransferase (HILL and BENNETT, 1969; TAY et al., 1969), and it has been suggested that intracellular 6-methylthioinosinate, formed as a metabolite of MP (see Fig. 1), is responsible for most, if not all, of the inhibition of purine nucleotide synthesis *de novo* observed in MP-treated cells (BENNETT and ALLAN, 1971).

BENNETT et al. (1963) concluded that for three mouse neoplasms treated *in vivo* with MP, interference with an early step in purine nucleotide synthesis *de novo* was of greater significance in inhibition of purine nucleotide synthesis than was interference with purine ribonucleotide interconversions. In these experiments, MP markedly inhibited the incorporation of ^{14}C-formate or ^{14}C-glycine into nucleic acid purines, but had little or no effect on the incorporation of ^{14}C-aminoimidazole carboxamide (AIC).

Similarly, BROCKMAN and CHUMLEY (1965) found that incorporation of AIC into purine ribonucleotides in drug-sensitive cells was not inhibited at concentrations of MP which strongly inhibited the azaserine-induced accumulation of FGAR. HAKALA and NICHOL (1964) reported that AIC partially prevented MP inhibition of tumor cell growth in culture. They suggested that a metabolic block prior to the formation of AIC ribonucleotide on the *de novo* purine nucleotide pathway was at least partially responsible for growth inhibition in this system in which cell proliferation was totally dependent upon endogenous formation of purine nucleotides. In contrast, LEPAGE and coworkers found no correlation between tumor growth inhibition and feedback inhibition of purine ribonucleotide synthesis *de novo* by MP (GREENLEES and LEPAGE, 1956; LEPAGE and JONES, 1961). Also, HITCHINGS and ELION (1967) reported that MP elicited feedback inhibition of purine nucleotide synthesis *de novo* to the same extent in lines of Adenocarcinoma 755 which were MP-sensitive and MP-resistant. Thus, inhibition of purine nucleotide synthesis *de novo* by a metabolite of MP is an important biochemical effect of the drug; however, a relationship between this effect and cytotoxicity has not been established.

An argument against the idea that MP cytotoxicity derives from inhibition of purine nucleotide synthesis *de novo* may be found in the fact that therapeutic effects are enhanced synergistically when MP and several inhibitors of purine nucleotide synthesis *de novo* are used in combination chemotherapy of various rodent tumors. The glutamine analogs, azaserine and 6-diazo-5-oxo-L-norleucine, inhibit *de novo* purine nucleotide synthesis, and both synergize with MP (HITCHINGS, 1955; CLARKE et al., 1957; TARNOWSKI and STOCK, 1957). In addition, it has been demonstrated that 6-methylthioinosine potentiates the cytotoxic activity of MP, apparently by increasing the availability of PRPP for phosphoribosyltransferase catalyzed reactions; in this way, the anabolism of MP is enhanced (SCHABEL et al., 1967; WANG et al., 1967; PATERSON and MORIWAKI, 1969; PATERSON and WANG, 1970a, b; SCHOLAR et al., 1972). It is difficult to imagine how combinations of these agents with MP would result in synergistic enhancement of cytotoxic effects, if MP toxicity were due solely to inhibition of PRPP-amidotransferase. However, inhibition of purine nucleotide synthesis *de novo* would appear to be the basis of the "self-enhancement" effect of MP, in which the ability of cells to convert MP to 6-thioinosinate is enhanced by prior exposure to MP (PATERSON, 1959, 1964; MELONI and ROGERS, 1969).

HITCHINGS and ELION (1967) concluded that potentiation of azaserine by MP was inconsistent with the concept that the purine analog acts primarily on *de novo* purine nucleotide synthesis. They suggested that effects on purine ribonucleotide interconversions may play an important role in tumor inhibition.

II. Inhibition of Purine Ribonucleotide Interconversions

Experiments with microorganisms provided the first evidence that thiopurines inhibited purine ribonucleotide interconversions (see reviews by ELION and HITCHINGS, 1957; SKIPPER and BENNETT, 1958; BROCKMAN, 1963a; BROCKMAN and ANDERSON, 1963; BALIS, 1968). HAKALA and NICHOL (1959) and DAVIDSON (1960) found that MP, presumably as the nucleotide, inhibited the conversion of IMP to AMP in intact tumor cells, and SIMPSON et al. (1962) reported that formation of GMP from IMP by Ehrlich ascites cells *in vivo* was also inhibited by MP and was apparently more susceptible to inhibition by MP than was the formation of AMP. Cell-free preparations of Sarcoma 180 exhibited reduced capacity to convert IMP to AMP and XMP when the tumor was obtained from animals which had been treated with MP (SALSER and BALIS, 1965). In contrast, BAKER and BENNETT (1964) concluded that the concentration of 6-thioinosinate required to inhibit the conversion of IMP to AMP in a cell-free system from Adenocarcinoma 755 was sufficiently great that this inhibition was not likely to be of primary significance *in vivo*. However, IMP concentrations in cells are low and ELION (1967) has suggested that the 6-thioinosinate levels achieved in MP-treated cells would probably inhibit IMP metabolism, despite the fact that 6-thioinosinate has a lower affinity than IMP for IMP dehydrogenase and adenylosuccinate synthetase. Whether or not these metabolic effects of 6-thioinosinate contribute to the therapeutic result is still an open question because intracellular pools of 6-thioinosinate have only a transient existence (PATERSON, 1959; BALIS, 1968).

IMP dehydrogenase catalyzes conversion of IMP to XMP; preparations of this enzyme from pigeon liver (SALSER et al., 1960) and from Ehrlich ascites tumor cells (ATKINSON et al., 1963) were inhibited by 6-thioinosinate. Adenylosuccinate synthetase catalyzes conversion of IMP to adenylosuccinate, and adenylosuccinate lyase is responsible for the conversion of adenylosuccinate into AMP. ATKINSON et al. (1964) reported that both enzymes (partially purified from Ehrlich ascites tumor cells) were inhibited by 6-thioinosinate and concluded from a comparison of the activities and kinetic parameters of IMP dehydrogenase, adenylosuccinate sythetase, and adenylosuccinate lyase that the first of these enzyme activities was probably most sensitive to inhibition by 6-thioinosinate in intact Ehrlich ascites tumor cells. SALSER and BALIS (1965) demonstrated that the intrinsic capacity for synthesis of AMP and XMP was lower in Sarcoma 180 than in normal mouse liver and suggested that the lower enzyme activities in tumors might account for the selective cytotoxic action of MP toward neoplastic tissue. In spite of these observations, a causal relationship between inhibition of purine nucleotide interconversions and MP cytotoxicity has not been established. Further, it has not been established that temporary constriction of the production of purine nucleotides is necessarily lethal to the cell.

III. Incorporation into DNA

SCANNELL and HITCHINGS (1966) demonstrated that deoxythioguanosine was present within the internucleotide linkages of DNA of an MP resistant subline of Adenocarcinoma 755 after treatment with MP. The amount of deoxythioguanosine associated with the DNA of the resistant tumor was twice that found in the sensitive parent line and was of the same order of magnitude as that reported for incorporation of TG into DNA under comparable conditions (LEPAGE, 1963). Although it appears that incorporation of TG into DNA is centrally involved in the cytotoxic activity of TG (see below), the mechanism by which the incorporated analog exerts its toxic effect is not evident. It would seem that in some resistant mutants toxic effects of the DNA-incorporated analog are suppressed in some manner.

IV. Resistance to 6-Mercaptopurine

In a number of instances, MP resistance in experimental tumors has been associated with loss of the ability to convert MP to 6-thioinosinate (see review by BROCKMAN, 1963a). This has usually involved reduced activity of or deletion of hypoxanthine-guanine phosphoribosyltransferase. However, it is clear that resistance to MP may be acquired by other means, as will be apparent in the following examples. A subline of the Ehrlich ascites carcinoma selected for MP resistance (PATERSON and HORI, 1962) possessed MP phosphoribosyltransferase activity comparable to that of the MP-sensitive parent line. WOLPERT et al. (1971) suggested that enhanced breakdown of thiopurine nucleotides by alkaline phosphohydrolase may be at least partially responsible for the insensitivity of a subline of Sarcoma 180 to these agents.

BIEBER et al. (1961) have described an MP-resistant line of Adenocarcinoma 755 which apparently incorporated at least as much MP into acid-soluble nucleotides and into the nucleic acids as the MP-sensitive line. It was this resistant tumor in which SCANNELL and HITCHINGS (1966) demonstrated that deoxythioguanosine was present within the internucleotide linkages of DNA after treatment with MP.

What little is known about thiopurine resistance in human neoplastic disease also indicates that mechanisms other than phosphoribosyltransferase deletion are operative; for example, assay of phosphoribosyltransferase activities of leukocytes from leukemic patients who had become resistant to therapy with MP after initially responding, revealed a deficiency of hypoxanthine phosphoribosyltransferase in cells of only one of the fifteen subjects tested (DAVIDSON and WINTER, 1964).

V. Conclusions

The intracellular presence of the MP anabolites, 6-methylthioinosinate and 6-thioinosinate, results in inhibition of purine ribonucleotide synthesis and interconversions. The specific enzymatic sites are inhibition of glutamine-PRPP amidotransferase by 6-thioinosinate and 6-methylthioinosinate, and inhibitions by 6-thioinosinate of IMP dehydrogenase, adenylosuccinate synthetase, and adenylosuccinate lyase. Conversion of MP to TG nucleotides introduces the possibility of still further loci of action for MP. 6-Methylthioinosinate is the only major metabolite of 6-methylthioinosine (see Fig. 1) and the only known action of this compound, inhibition of purine ribonucleotide synthesis *de novo*, would appear to account for its growth inhibitory effects. Intracellular 6-methylthioinosinate persists for long periods, at least in some cell types, suggesting that inhibition of purine nucleotide synthesis might be maintained for a period sufficient for the accumulation of lethal cell damage. Differences in the effects of MP in various experimental systems may reflect differences in the proportions of MP anabolites, as well as differences in the intrinsic sensitivities of their sites of action.

At present, there is not sufficient evidence to attribute the lethal effects of MP exposure to the enzymatic inhibitions discussed above.

Metabolic Effects of 6-Thioguanine

TG inhibits the growth of a number of transplantable rodent tumors, including adenocarcinoma 755, leukemia L1210, Ehrlich ascites carcinoma, and others (SARTORELLI and LEPAGE, 1958a; VENDITTI et al., 1960; SCHABEL et al., 1961;

WHITE, 1961). Useful therapeutic responses were obtained in clinical trials of TG in treatment of acute lymphocytic leukemia and chronic myelogenous leukemia (MURPHY et al., 1955; FARBER et al., 1956; HALES et al., 1957; ELLISON and BURCHENAL, 1960). TG and MP appear to have the same therapeutic spectrum, and TG was not effective in leukemias resistant to MP (HALES et al., 1957). TG alone, and in combination with azaserine, was ineffective against multiple myeloma (CARBONE et al., 1964; HAYES et al., 1967); the latter combination was of limited value in the treatment of other solid neoplasms (SCHROEDER et al., 1964). It has been a general opinion among clinical investigators that TG and MP were similar in action and that therapeutic responses to each were similar, although TG was more toxic on a molar basis. Of the two, MP has been the most studied.

On a molar basis, TG is about 25 times more toxic to the mouse than MP (SKIPPER and SCHMIDT, 1962). The principal feature of TG toxicity in mammals is the highly selective action against bone marrow (PHILIPS et al., 1954a, 1956). In man, toxic effects include leukopenia and thrombocytopenia with some gastrointestinal disturbances (PHILIPS et al., 1954b). Marrow depression is also the principal toxicity associated with the combination of TG and arabinosylcytosine (GEE et al., 1969).

A. The Free Base, 6-Thioguanine

TG was shown to inhibit the incorporation of guanine into nucleic acids of ascites tumor cells, and it was suggested that this effect might be partly attributable to competition between TG and guanine for hypoxanthine-guanine phosphoribosyltransferase (SARTORELLI and LEPAGE, 1958b).

B. Nucleotide Anabolites

6-Thioguanylate (TGRP) (see Fig. 1) is a major metabolite of TG in normal tissues of the mouse, guinea pig bone marrow, and in several ascitic tumors of the mouse (MOORE and LEPAGE, 1958; MIECH et al., 1967; LEPAGE, 1968). 6-Thioguanosine di- and triphosphates have also been tentatively identified as TG metabolites in mouse ascites tumors. In Ehrlich ascites carcinoma cells which were treated *in vivo* with TG, intracellular 6-thioguanylate persisted for substantial periods [after 24 h thioguanylate concentrations were about 20% of those at 1 h (MOORE and LEPAGE, 1958)], suggesting that this metabolite may turn over more slowly than 6-thioinosinate (PATERSON, 1959).

It was established that formation of 6-thioguanylate is necessary for the cytotoxic action of TG in experiments with thiopurine-resistant sublines of mouse tumors which were devoid of hypoxanthine-guanine phosphoribosyltransferase activity and were therefore unable to anabolize TG (BROCKMAN, 1963a). This finding focussed attention on the effects of 6-thioguanylate on the intermediary metabolism of purine nucleotides. However, it was also apparent that the involvement of 6-thioguanylate in TG cytotoxicity did not preclude the involvement of metabolites other than 6-thioguanylate. In attempts to relate TG cytotoxicity to the biochemical effects of TG metabolites, three areas have been investigated: (a) purine nucleotide synthesis *de novo*, (b) interconversions of purine nucleotides, and (c) incorporation of TG into DNA. Studies on the first two areas have attempted to identify inhibitory actions of 6-thioguanylate and to relate these to growth inhibition.

I. Inhibition of Purine Ribonucleotide Synthesis *de novo*

The presence of 6-thioguanylate in cells has a number of direct consequences. The first enzyme in the reaction sequence by which purine nucleotides are synthesized *de novo*, glutamine-PRPP amidotransferase, is subject to allosteric regulation by purine nucleotides, and is inhibited by several nucleotide derivatives of thiopurines (McCollister et al., 1964). Allan and Bennett (1971) have compared the abilities of 6-thiopurine ribonucleotides to inhibit partly purified glutamine-PRPP amidotransferase from mouse tumor cells; the results [expressed in terms of the concentration (mM) required for 50 % inhibition of amidotransferase activity] are as follows: 6-thioinosinate (1.11), 6-thioguanylate (0.27), 6-methylthioinosinate (0.09), and 6-methylthioguanylate (1.15). From the concentrations of 6-thioguanylate achievable in tumor cells [about 0.1 to 0.2 mM (Moore and LePage, 1958; Miech et al., 1967)], it would appear that this metabolic effect of 6-thioguanylate may be operative in TG-treated tumor cells. Consistent with these facts are the demonstrations that TG blocks (a) the first portion of the *de novo* pathway of purine nucleotide synthesis and (b) the incorporation of glycine-^{14}C into the purine bases of the nucleic acids of tumor cells (LePage, 1961). The formation of 6-methylthio derivatives of the thioguanosine phosphates (see Fig. 1) probably does not contribute to the inhibition by TG of purine nucleotide synthesis *de novo* (Allan and Bennett, 1971).

II. Inhibition of Purine Ribonucleotide Interconversions

IMP dehydrogenase is inhibited by 6-thioinosinate and 6-thioguanylate, apparently because the analogs form disulfide bonds with an enzymic sulfhydryl group at the IMP reaction site (Atkinson et al., 1963; Hampton, 1963). The inactivation by thiopurine nucleotides of the IMP dehydrogenase activities of *Aerobacter aerogenes* and of Sarcoma 180 cells is reversible by sulfhydryl reagents (Hampton, 1963; Miech et al., 1967). 6-Thioguanylate is an inhibitor of guanylate kinase from Sarcoma 180 cells and from hog brain. The analog behaves as a competitive inhibitor of the substrate guanylate with a K_i of about 6×10^{-5} M and is itself a substrate for the enzyme, although the maximum velocity of the reaction is low (Miech et al., 1969).

Miech et al. (1967, 1969) have proposed that the presence of 6-thioguanylate in tumor cells should impair the synthesis of guanylate through inhibition at the 2 sites noted above, glutamine-PRPP amidotransferase and IMP dehydrogenase. The authors suggest that these inhibitions, together with that of guanylate kinase, might result in a general lowering of intracellular concentrations of guanine nucleotides, a situation which might have serious consequences for the cell. It remains in the realm of speculation whether a temporary constriction in the synthesis of guanosine phosphates would have lethal consequences for cells.

III. Incorporation into DNA

On the basis of investigations into the metabolic effects of TG, LePage concluded that TG incorporation into DNA consistently correlated with tumor inhibition and was therefore a likely basis for TG cytotoxicity (Sartorelli and LePage, 1958b; LePage, 1960, 1963, LePage and Jones, 1961; LePage and Junga, 1967). A number of TG-sensitive mouse tumors incorporated TG in DNA, whereas such incorporation was much less in the TG-insensitive C3HED and Mecca lymphosarcomas (LePage and Jones, 1961; LePage, 1963). In contrast, inhibition of the *de novo* pathway of purine synthesis by 6-thioguanylate did not correlate with tumor sensitivity to TG; this effect of TG was operative in the TG-insensitive lymphomas, as well as in sensitive neoplasms (LePage and Jones, 1961). The postulate that TG cytotoxicity was due to entry into DNA structure suggested that β-2′-deoxythioguanosine might be an effective antitumor agent with some advantage over TG in that fewer metabolic steps would be required for its incorporation into DNA. The α- and β-anomers of 2'-deoxythioguanosine were found to have antitumor activity and were inhibitory to TG-resistant tumor sublines and to the naturally insensitive Mecca lymphosarcoma (LEPAGE et al., 1964). Mecca cells incorporated the β-anomer into DNA at a much greater rate than TG; the α-anomer also entered DNA, partly in the form of chain termini (LEPAGE and JUNGA, 1967).

LEPAGE and WHITECAR (1971) have shown that bone marrow of patients with acute leukemia responded rapidly to TG treatment with the disappearance of a large fraction of the original cells. A course of 5 daily treatments projected the surviving cells into a proliferative state, and in those cells, one-half to essentially all DNA guanine was replaced by TG. The specific toxicity of TG for bone marrow may be attributable to the ability of other rapidly proliferating tissues to deaminate the analog.

IV. Delayed Cytotoxicity

Consistent with the idea that TG incorporation into DNA has lethal consequences are the experiments of BARRANCO and HUMPHREY (1971) which show that cultured Chinese hamster ovary cells are sensitive to β-2'-deoxythioguanosine during the early and middle portions of the *S* phase of the mitotic cycle. In these experiments, synchronized cells were exposed to β-2'-deoxythioguanosine for 1 h intervals at various times in the cell cycle; cells treated in this way were assayed for viability by a cloning method, and it was found that progression through the cell cycle was not affected by a β-2'-deoxythioguanosine exposure which was ultimately lethal to 90 % of the cells. In other words, the lethality of the treatment was not expressed immediately and cells completed the cycle during which they were exposed to β-2'-deoxythioguanosine. Delayed manifestations of MP cytotoxicity have been described in which MP-treated cells in culture underwent further proliferation in the absence of MP before lysis occurred (BASES, 1959; TOMIZAWA and ARONOW, 1960; TIDD et al., 1972). This type of cell death could possibly explain why MP gave a negative result (on the borderline of scoring as a potential cancer chemotherapeutic agent) in early screening against sarcoma 180 (HITCHINGS and ELION, 1954). CLARKE et al. (1953) subsequently demonstrated that the majority of Sarcoma 180 transplants from MP-treated animals failed to grow in their new hosts despite poor apparent responses to therapy with MP. The appearance of large cells was a characteristic feature of the delayed cytotoxic effect of MP *in vitro* (BASES, 1959; TIDD et al., 1972) and this was also described for MP-treated Sarcoma 180 (CLARKE et al., 1953). TG and β-2'-deoxythioguanosine produced delayed cytotoxic effects similar to those of MP in cultures of L5178Y cells; the concentration of TG or β-2'-deoxythioguanosine was 0.01 times that of MP required for a comparable effect (TIDD and KIM, 1972). It remains to be determined whether the delayed response of MP is due to metabolically derived TG nucleotides. It is conceivable that the delayed cytotoxic effects are a consequence of incorporation of thiopurine into genetic material and that lethal effects appear when transcription or translation of these impaired genes is undertaken. BERENBAUM (1967) has discussed such effects of MP in terms of the concept of "reproductive death".

V. Conclusions

6-Thioguanylate inhibits the *de novo* pathway of purine nucleotide synthesis and purine nucleotide interconversions; the enzymes inhibited by the analog nucleotide are glutamine-PRPP amidotransferase, IMP dehydrogenase, and guanylate kinase. However, there is reasonable doubt that the cytotoxic effects of TG can be attributed to these inhibitions. Incorporation of TG into DNA correlates with drug lethality, but the mechanism by which the incorporated analog exerts its effect is not apparent. Delayed cytotoxic effects of MP and TG may share a common biochemical mechanism.

Combination Chemotherapy

The effects of combining thiopurines with other agents in the chemotherapy of cancer will be treated here only briefly; the reader is referred to reviews by VENDITTI and GOLDIN (1964) and SARTORELLI (1965). Combination chemotherapy is considered elsewhere in these volumes. Combinations of MP or TG with the glutamine antagonists, azaserine or 6-diazo-5-oxo-L-norleucine, are synergistic in the chemotherapy of various experimental tumors. However, in clinical trials, MP in combination with either glutamine analog failed to afford advantage in the treatment of acute lymphocytic leukemia (HEYN et al., 1960; SULLIVAN et al., 1962). The TG-azaserine combination has had very limited clinical testing; some improvement was seen in a small group of breast tumor patients, but thrombocytopenia and toxicity to epithelia were serious (SCHROEDER et al., 1964; HAYES et al., 1967). The biochemical basis for the therapeutic potentiation which results from combining the 6-thiopurines with the glutamine antagonists is uncertain; however, a prominent consequence of this combination is that anabolism of the thiopurines is markedly enhanced (for example, SARTORELLI et al., 1958; PATERSON, 1964). Undoubtedly involved in these effects is the fact that the glutamine antagonists are potent inhibitors of the *de novo* pathway of purine nucleotide synthesis.

Treatment with a combination of MP and 6-methylthioinosine induced complete remissions in 7 out of 29 patients with acute myelogenous leukemia (FREIREICH et al., 1967); 6-methylthioinosine alone was found to be inactive in the treatment of patients with MP-resistant acute leukemia (LUCE et al., 1967). The combination of arabinosylcytosine and TG has been employed in the treatment of acute myelogenous leukemia in adults producing the relatively high remission rate of 45 % (GEE et al., 1969).

References

ALLAN, P. W., BENNETT, L. L., JR.: 6-Methylthioguanylic acid, a metabolite of 6-thioguanine. Biochem. Pharmacol. **20**, 847—852 (1971).

ALLAN, P. W., SCHNEBLI, H. P., BENNETT, L. L., JR.: Conversion of 6-mercaptopurine and 6-mercaptopurine ribonucleoside to 6-methylmercaptopurine ribonucleotide in human epidermoid carcinoma No. 2 cells in culture. Biochim. biophys. Acta (Amst.) **114**, 647—650 (1966).

ANONYMOUS: Allopurinol and the control of hyperuricemia in neoplastic disease. Med. Let. Drugs Therap. **10**, 103—104 (1968).

AOKI, Y., MOORE, G. E.: Comparative sensitivity to various antimetabolites of several established cell lines derived from the buffy coat of normal humans and patients with neoplastic diseases. Cancer Res. **29**, 1307—1312 (1969).

ASHTON, H., BEVERIDGE, G. W., STEVENSON, C. J.: Therapeutics. XI. Immunosuppressive drugs. Brit. J. Derm. **83**, 326—330 (1970).

ATKINSON, M. R., ECKERMANN, G., STEPHENSON, J.: Formation of 6-thioxanthosine 5′-phosphate from 6-mercaptopurine and from 6-thioxanthine in Ehrlich ascites tumor cells. Biochim. biophys. Acta (Amst.) **108**, 320—322 (1965).

ATKINSON, M. R., MORTON, R. K., MURRAY, A. W.: Inhibition of inosine 5′-phosphate dehydrogenase from Ehrlich ascites-tumour cells by 6-thioinosine 5′-phosphate. Biochem. J. **89**, 167—172 (1963).

ATKINSON, M. R., MORTON, R. K., MURRAY, A. W.: Inhibition of adenylosuccinate synthetase and adenylosuccinate lyase from Ehrlich ascites-tumour cells by 6-thioinosine 5′-phosphate. Biochem. J. **92**, 398—404 (1964).

ATKINSON, M. R., MURRAY, A. W.: Inhibition of purine phosphoribosyltransferases of Ehrlich ascites-tumour cells by 6-mercaptopurine. Biochem. J. **94**, 64—74 (1965).

BAKER, H. T., BENNETT, L. L., JR.: Inhibition by 6-mercaptopurine ribonucleotide of the conversion of inosinic acid to adenylic acid in cell-free systems from mercaptopurine sensitive and mercaptopurine-resistant mammalian cells. Biochim. biophys. Acta (Amst.) **80**, 497—499 (1964).

BALIS, M. E.: Antagonists and nucleic acids. In: Frontiers of biology, Vol. 10. Amsterdam: North Holland Publishing Co. 1968.

BARRANCO, S. C., HUMPHREY, R. M.: The effects of β-2'-deoxythioguanosine on survival and progression in mammalian cells. Cancer Res. **31**, 583—586 (1971).

BASES, R. E.: Some applications of tissue culture methods to radiation research. Cancer Res. **19**, 311—315 (1959).

BENNETT, L. L., JR., ALLAN, P. W.: Formation and significance of 6-methylthiopurine ribonucleotide as a metabolite of 6-mercaptopurine. Cancer Res. **31**, 152—158 (1971).

BENNETT, L. L., JR., BROCKMAN, R. W., SCHNEBLI, H. P., CHUMLEY, S., DIXON, G. J., SCHABEL, F. M., JR., DULMADGE, E. A., SKIPPER, H. E., MONTGOMERY, J. A., THOMAS, H. J.: Activity and mechanism of action of 6-methylthiopurine ribonucleoside in cancer cells resistant to 6-mercaptopurine. Nature (Lond.) **205**, 1276—1279 (1965).

BENNETT, L. L., JR., SIMPSON, L., GOLDEN, J., BARKER, T. L.: The primary site of inhibition by 6-mercaptopurine on the purine biosynthetic pathway in some tumors *in vivo*. Cancer Res. **23**, 1574—1580 (1963).

BERENBAUM, M. C.: Immunosuppressive agents and allogeneic transplantation. J. clin. Pathol. **20**, 471—498 (1967).

BIEBER, S., DIETRICH, L. S., ELION, G. B., HITCHINGS, G. H., MARTIN, D. S.: The incorporation of 6-mercaptopurine-S^{35} into the nucleic acids of sensitive and nonsensitive transplantable mouse tumors. Cancer Res. **21**, 228—231 (1961).

BROCKMAN, R. W.: Mechanisms of resistance to anticancer agents. Advanc. Cancer Res. **7**, 129—234 (1963a).

BROCKMAN, R. W.: Biochemical aspects of mercaptopurine inhibition and resistance. Cancer Res. **23**, 1191—1201 (1963b).

BROCKMAN, R. W., ANDERSON, E. P.: Biochemistry of cancer. Ann. Rev. Biochem. **32**, 463—512 (1963).

BROCKMAN, R. W., BENNETT, L. L., JR., SIMPSON, M. S., WILSON, A. R., THOMPSON, J. R., SKIPPER, H. E.: A mechanism of resistance to 8-azaguanine. II. Studies with experimental neoplasms. Cancer Res. **19**, 856—869 (1959).

BROCKMAN, R. W., CHUMLEY, S.: Inhibition of formylglycinamide ribonucleotide synthesis in neoplastic cells by purines and analogs. Biochim. biophys. Acta (Amst.) **95**, 365—379 (1965).

BURCHENAL, J. H., ELLISON, R. R., MURPHY, M. L., KARNOFSKY, D. A., SYKES, M. P., TAN, T. C., MERMANN, A. C., YUCEOGLU, M., MYERS, W. P. L., KRAKOFF, I., ALBERSTADT, N.: Clinical studies on 6-mercaptopurine. Ann. N. Y. Acad. Sci. **60**, 359—368 (1954).

BURCHENAL, J. H., MURPHY, M. L., ELLISON, R. R., SYKES, M. P., TAN, T. C., LEONE, L. A., KARNOFSKY, D. A., CRAVER, L. F., DARGEON, H. W., RHOADS, C. P.: Clinical evaluation of a new antimetabolite, 6-mercaptopurine, in the treatment of leukemia and allied diseases. Blood **8**, 965—999 (1953).

CALDWELL, I. C.: Ion exchange chromatography of tissue nucleotides. J. Chromat. **44**, 331—341 (1969).

CALDWELL, I. C., HENDERSON, J. F., PATERSON, A. R. P.: The enzymic formation of 6-(methylmercapto)-purine ribonucleoside 5'-phosphate. Canad. J. Biochem. **44**, 229—245 (1966).

CARBONE, P. P., FREI, E., III, OWENS, A. H., JR., OLSON, K. B., MILLER, S. P.: 6-Thioguanine (NSC-752) therapy in patients with multiple myeloma. Cancer Chemother. Rep. **36**, 59—62 (1964).

CASKEY, C. T., ASHTON, D. M., WYNGAARDEN, J. B.: The enzymology of feedback inhibition of glutamine phosphoribosylpyrophosphate amidotransferase by purine ribonucleotides. J. biol. Chem. **239**, 2570—2579 (1964).

CLARKE, D. A., PHILIPS, F. S., STERNBERG, S. S., STOCK, C. C., ELION, G. B., HITCHINGS, G. H.: 6-Mercaptopurine: effects in mouse sarcoma 180 and in normal animals. Cancer Res. **13**, 593—605 (1953).

CLARKE, D. A., REILLY, H. C., STOCK, C. C.: A comparative study of 6-diazo-5-oxo-L-norleucine and *O*-diazoacetyl-L-serine on sarcoma 180. Antibiot. and Chemother. **7**, 653—671 (1957).

CURRIE, R., BERGEL, F., BRAY, R. C.: Enzymes and cancer. Preparation and some properties of guanase from rabbit liver. Biochem. J. **104**, 634—638 (1967).

DAVIDSON, J. D.: Studies on the mechanism of action of 6-mercaptopurine in sensitive and resistant L1210 leukemia *in vitro*. Cancer Res. **20**, 225—232 (1960).

Davidson, J. D., Freeman, B. B.: The effects of antitumor drugs upon P^{32} incorporation into nucleic acids of mouse tumors. Cancer Res. **15**, 31—37 (1955).

Davidson, J. D., Winter, T. S.: Purine nucleotide pyrophosphorylases in 6-mercaptopurine sensitive and resistant human leukemias. Cancer Res. **24**, 261—267 (1964).

Elion, G. B.: Biochemistry and pharmacology of purine analogs. Fed. Proc. **26**, 898—903 (1967).

Elion, G. B., Burgi, E., Hitchings, G. H.: Studies on condensed pyrimidine systems. IX. The synthesis of some 6-substituted purines. J. Amer. chem. Soc. **74**, 411—414 (1952).

Elion, G. B., Callahan, S. W., Hitchings, G. H., Rundles, R. W., Laszlo, J.: Experimental, clinical, and metabolic studies of thiopurines. Cancer Chemother. Rep. **16**, 197—202 (1962).

Elion, G. B., Callahan, S. W., Rundles, R. W., Hitchings, G. H.: Relationship between metabolic fates and antitumor activities of thiopurines. Cancer Res. **23**, 1207—1217 (1963).

Elion, G. B., Hitchings, G. H.: Biochemical effects of 6-mercaptopurine. In: CIBA foundation symposium on the chemistry and biology of purines. London: J. and A. Churchill, Ltd. 1957.

Elion, G. B., Hitchings, G. H.: Metabolic basis for the actions of analogs of purines and pyrimidines. In: Advances in chemotherapy., Vol. 2. New York-London: Academic Press 1965.

Elion, G. B., Mueller, S., Hitchings, G. H.: Studies on condensed pyrimidine systems. XXI. The isolation and synthesis of 6-mercapto-2,8-purinediol(6-thiouric acid). J. Amer. chem. Soc. **81**, 3042—3045 (1959).

Ellis, D. B., LePage, G. A.: Biochemical studies of resistance to 6-thioguanine. Cancer Res. **23**, 436—443 (1963).

Ellison, R. R., Burchenal, J. H.: Treatment of chronic granulocytic leukemia with the 6-substituted purines 6-mercaptopurine, thioguanine, and 6-chloropurine. Clin. Pharmacol. Ther. **1**, 631—644 (1960).

Farber, S., Toch, R., Sears, E. M., Pinkel, D.: Advances in the chemotherapy of cancer in man. In: Advances in cancer research, Vol. IV. New York-London: Academic Press 1956.

Fernandes, J. F., LePage, G. A., Lindner, A.: The influence of azaserine and 6-mercaptopurine on the *in vivo* metabolism of ascites tumor cells. Cancer Res. **16**, 154—161 (1956).

Freireich, E. J., Bodey, G. P., Harris, J. E., Hart, J. S.: Therapy for acute granulocytic leukemia. Cancer Res. **27**, 2573—2577 (1967).

Furth, R., van: Origin and kinetics of monocytes and macrophages. Semin. Hemat. **7**, 125—141 (1970).

Gee, T. S., Yu, K. P., Clarkson, B. D.: Treatment of adult acute leukemia with arabinosylcytosine and thioguanine. Cancer **23**, 1019—1032 (1969).

Goldin, A., Sandberg, J. S., Henderson, E. S., Newman, J. W., Frei, E., III, Holland, J. F.: The chemotherapy of human and animal acute leukemia. Cancer Chemother. Rep. **55**, 309—507 (1971).

Gots, J. S., Gollub, E. G.: Purine analogs as feedback inhibitors. Proc. Soc. exp. Biol. (N.Y.) **101**, 641—643 (1959).

Greenlees, J., LePage, G. A.: Purine biosynthesis and inhibitors in ascites cell tumors. Cancer Res. **16**, 808—813 (1956).

Hakala, M. T., Nichol, C. A.: Studies on the mode of action of 6-mercaptopurine and its ribonucleoside on mammalian cells in culture. J. biol. Chem. **234**, 3224—3228 (1959).

Hakala, M. T., Nichol, C. A.: Prevention of the growth-inhibitory effect of 6-mercaptopurine by 4-aminoimidazole-5-carboxamide. Biochim. biophys. Acta (Amst.) **80**, 665—668 (1964).

Hales, D. R., Jerner, R. W., Hall, B. E., Willet, F. M., Franco, J., Feichtmeir, T. V.: Comparison of therapeutic effects of 6-methylmercaptopurine, 6-chloropurine, 6-thioguanine and 6-mercaptopurine in human acute leukemia. Clin. Res. Proc. **5**, 32 (1957).

Hampton, A.: Reactions of ribonucleotide derivatives of purine analogs at the catalytic site of inosine 5'-phosphate dehydrogenase. J. biol. Chem. **238**, 3068—3074 (1963).

Hansen, H. J., Bennett, S. J., Nadler, S. B.: Studies on the binding of 6-mercaptopurine by ribonucleic acids in the presence of metals. Arch. Biochem. **98**, 379—383 (1962).

Hansen, H. J., Nadler, S. B.: Chemical interaction of S^{35}-6-mercaptopurine and ribonucleic acids. Proc. Soc. exp. Biol. (N.Y.) **107**, 324—326 (1961).

Hayes, D. M., Costa, J., Moon, J. H., Hoogstraten, B., Harley, J. B.: Combination therapy with thioguanine (NSC-752) and azaserine (NSC-742) for multiple myeloma. Cancer Chemother. Rep. **51**, 235—238 (1967).

Heidelberger, C., Keller, R. A.: The effects of twenty-nine compounds on nucleic acid and protein biosynthesis in slices of Flexner-Jobling carcinoma and rat spleen. Cancer Res. **15**, 106—112 (1955).

Henderson, E. S.: Treatment of acute leukemia. Semin. Hemat. **6**, 271—319 (1969).

Henderson, J. F.: Feedback inhibition of purine biosynthesis in ascites tumor cells. J. biol. Chem. **237**, 2631—2635 (1962).

Henderson, J. F., Khoo, M. K. Y.: On the mechanism of feedback inhibition of purine biosynthesis *de novo* in Ehrlich ascites tumor cells *in vitro*. J. biol. Chem. **240**, 3104—3109 (1965).
Henderson, J. F., Mandel, H. G.: Purine and pyrimidine antimetabolites in cancer chemotherapy. Advanc. clin. Pharmacol. **2**, 297—343 (1963).
Henderson, J. F., Mikoshiba, A., Chu, S. Y., Caldwell, I. C.: Kinetic studies of adenosine kinase from Ehrlich ascites tumor cells. J. biol. Chem. **247**, 1972—1975 (1972).
Hersh, E. M., Wong, V. G., Freireich, E. J.: Inhibition of the local inflammatory response in man by antimetabolites. Blood **27**, 38—48 (1966).
Heyn, R. M., Brubaker, C. A., Burchenal, J. H., Cramblett, H. G., Wolff, J. A.: Comparison of 6-mercaptopurine with the combination of 6-mercaptopurine and azaserine in the treatment of acute leukemia in children: results of a cooperative study. Blood **15**, 350—359 (1960).
Hill, D. L., Bennett, L. L., Jr.: Purification and properties of 5-phosphoribosylpyrophosphate amidotransferase from Adenocarcinoma 755 cells. Biochemistry **8**, 122—130 (1969).
Hirschberg, E.: Patterns of response of animal tumors to anticancer agents. Cancer chemother. screening data XXI, Cancer Res. **23**, 521—980 (1963).
Hitchings, G. H.: Purine and pyrimidine antagonists. Amer. J. clin. Nutr. **3**, 321—327 (1955).
Hitchings, G. H.: Summary of informal discussion on the role of purine antagonists. Cancer Res. **23**, 1218—1225 (1963).
Hitchings, G. H., Elion, G. B.: The chemistry and biochemistry of purine analogs. Ann. N.Y. Acad. Sci. **60**, 195—199 (1954).
Hitchings, G. H., Elion, G. B.: Chemical suppression of the immune response. Pharmacol. Rev. **15**, 365—405 (1963).
Hitchings, G. H., Elion, G. B.: Mechanisms of action of purine and pyrimidine analogs. In: Cancer Chemotherapy, Basic and Clinical Applications. New York: Grune and Stratton 1967.
Hitchings, G. H., Elion, G. B.: The role of antimetabolites in immunosuppression and transplantation. Accounts chem. Res. **2**, 202—209 (1969).
Hurd, E. R.: Effect of 6-mercaptopurine on enzymes of the polymorphonuclear leucocyte. Proc. Soc. exp. Biol. (N.Y.) **129**, 882—885 (1968).
Hutchison, D. J.: Cross resistance and collateral sensitivity studies in cancer chemotherapy. In: Advances in Cancer Research, Vol. 7. New York-London: Academic Press 1963.
Iwamoto, R. H., Acton, E. M., Goodman, L.: 2′-Deoxythioguanosine and related nucleosides. J. med. Chem. **6**, 684—688 (1963).
Kidder, G. W., Dewey, V. C.: The biological activity of substituted purines. J. biol. Chem. **179**, 181—187 (1949).
Krenitsky, T. A.: Purine nucleoside phosphorylase: kinetics, mechanism, and specificity. Molec. Pharmacol. **3**, 526—536 (1967).
Laster, W. R., Jr., Mayo, J. G., Simpson-Herren, L., Griswold, D. P., Jr., Lloyd, H. H., Schabel, F. M., Jr., Skipper, H. E.: Success and failure in the treatment of solid tumors. II. Kinetic parameters and "cell cure" of moderately advanced Carcinoma 755. Cancer Chemother. Rep. **53**, 169—188 (1969).
Law, L. W.: Some aspects of drug resistance in neoplasms. Ann. N.Y. Acad. Sci. **71**, 976—992 (1958).
Lefkowitz, E. R., Creasey, W. A., Calabresi, P., Sartorelli, A. C.: Clinical and pharmacologic effects of combinations of 6-thioguanine and Duazomycin A in patients with neoplastic disease. Cancer Res. **25**, 1207—1212 (1965).
LePage, G. A.: Incorporation of 6-thioguanine into nucleic acids. Cancer Res. **20**, 403—408 (1960).
LePage, G. A.: Symposium on the experimental pharmacology and clinical use of antimetabolites. Part V. Use of combinations of antimetabolites for chemotherapy of cancer. Clin. Pharmacol. Ther. **2**, 121—129 (1961).
LePage, G. A.: Basic biochemical effects and mechanism of action of 6-thioguanine. Cancer Res. **23**, 1202—1206 (1963).
LePage, G. A.: The metabolism of α-2′-deoxythioguanosine in murine tumor cells. Canad. J. Biochem. **46**, 655—661 (1968).
LePage, G. A., Greenlees, J. L.: Incorporation of glycine-2-C^{14} into ascites tumor cell purines as a biological test system. Cancer Res. **15**, 102—105 (1955).
LePage, G. A., Jones, M.: Purinethiols as feedback inhibitors of purine synthesis in ascites tumor cells. Cancer Res. **21**, 642—649 (1961).
LePage, G. A., Junga, I. G.: The utilization of α-2′-deoxythioguanosine by murine tumor cells. Molec. Pharmacol. **3**, 37—43 (1967).
LePage, G. A., Junga, I. G., Bowman, B.: Biochemical and carcinostatic effects of 2′-deoxythioguanosine. Cancer Res. **24**, 835—840 (1964).

LePage, G. A., Whitecar, J. P., Jr.: Pharmacology of 6-thioguanine in man. Cancer Res. **31**, 1627—1631 (1971).
Loo, T. L., Ho, D. H. W., Blossom, D. R., Shepard, B. J., Frei, E., III: Cellular uptake of purine antimetabolites *in vitro*. I. Uptake of 6-methylthiopurine ribonucleoside by human erythrocytes. Biochem. Pharmacol. **18**, 1711—1725 (1969).
Loo, T. L., Luce, J. K., Sullivan, M. P., Frei, E., III: Clinical pharmacologic observations on 6-mercaptopurine and 6-methylthiopurine ribonucleoside. Clin. Pharmacol. Ther. **9**, 180—194 (1968).
Luce, J. K., Frenkel, E. P., Vietti, T. J., Isassi, A. A., Hernandez, K. W., Howard, J. P.: Clinical studies of 6-methylmercaptopurine riboside (NSC-40774) in acute leukemia. Cancer Chemother. Rep. **51**, 535—546 (1967).
Lukens, L. N., Herrington, K. A.: Enzymic formation of 6-mercaptopurine ribotide. Biochim. biophys. Acta (Amst.) **24**, 432—433 (1957).
McCollister, R. J., Gilbert, W. R., Jr., Ashton, D. M., Wyngaarden, J. B.: Pseudofeedback inhibition of purine synthesis by 6-mercaptopurine ribonucleotide and other purine analogues. J. biol. Chem. **239**, 1560—1563 (1964).
McCollister, R. J., Gilbert, W. R., Jr., Wyngaarden, J. B.: Pseudofeedback inhibition of purine synthesis by 6-mercaptopurine and other purine analogues. J. clin. Invest. **41**, 1383 (1962).
Meloni, M. L., Rogers, W. I.: Enhancement of 6-thioinosine-5'-monophosphate synthesis in solid L1210 lymphocytic leukemia cells by prior exposure to 6-mercaptopurine. Biochem. Pharmacol. **18**, 413—417 (1969).
Miech, R. P., Parks, R. E., Jr., Anderson, J. H., Jr., Sartorelli, A. C.: An hypothesis on the mechanism of action of 6-thioguanine. Biochem. Pharmacol. **16**, 2222—2227 (1967).
Miech, R. P., York, R., Parks, R. E., Jr.: Adenosine triphosphate-guanosine 5'-phosphate phosphotransferase. II. Inhibition by 6-thioguanosine 5'-phosphate of the enzyme isolated from hog brain and Sarcoma 180 ascites cells. Molec. Pharmacol. **5**, 30—37 (1969).
Montgomery, J. A.: The biochemical basis for the drug actions of purines. Prog . med. Chem. **7**, 69—123 (1970).
Moore, E. C., LePage, G. A.: The metabolism of 6-thioguanine in normal and neoplastic tissues. Cancer Res. **18**, 1075—1083 (1958).
Murphy, M. L., Tan, T. C., Ellison, R. R., Karnofsky, D. A., Burchenal, J. H.: Clinical evaluation of chloropurine and thioguanine. Proc. Amer. Ass. Cancer Res. **2**, 36 (1955).
Page, A. R., Condie, R. M., Good, R. A.: Effect of 6-mercaptopurine on inflammation. Amer. J. Path. **40**, 519—530 (1962a).
Page, A. R., Condie, R. M., Good, R. A.: Clinical studies on the anti-inflammatory activity of 6-mercaptopurine. Blood **20**, 118—119 (1962b).
Paterson, A. R. P.: The formation of 6-mercaptopurine riboside phosphate in ascites tumor cells. Canad. J. Biochem. **37**, 1011—1023 (1959).
Paterson, A. R. P.: Enhancement of thioinosinate synthesis in the Ehrlich ascites carcinoma by prior treatment with 6-mercaptopurine or azaserine. Acta Un. int. Cancr. **20**, 1033—1036 (1964).
Paterson, A. R. P., Hori, A.: Resistance to 6-mercaptopurine. I. Biochemical differences between the Ehrlich ascites carcinoma and a 6-mercaptopurine-resistant subline. Canad. J. Biochem. **40**, 181—194 (1962).
Paterson, A. R. P., Moriwaki, A.: Combination chemotherapy: synergistic inhibition of lymphoma L5178Y cells in culture and *in vivo* with 6-mercaptopurine and 6-(methylmercapto) purine ribonucleoside. Cancer Res. **29**, 681—686 (1969).
Paterson, A. R. P., Sutherland, A.: Metabolism of 6-mercaptopurine ribonucleoside by Ehrlich ascites carcinoma cells. Canad. J. Biochem. **42**, 1415—1423 (1964).
Paterson, A. R. P., Wang, M. C.: Mechanism of the growth inhibition potentiation arising from combination of 6-mercaptopurine with 6-(methylmercapto)-purine ribonucleoside. Cancer Res. **30**, 2379—2387 (1970a).
Paterson, A. R. P., Wang, M. C.: Combination chemotherapy: treatment of the Ehrlich ascites carcinoma and several drug resistant sublines with combinations of 6-mercaptopurine and 6-(methylmercapto)-purine ribonucleoside. Canad. J. Biochem. **48**, 79—83 (1970b).
Peery, A., LePage, G. A.: Nucleotide formation from α- and β-2'-deoxythioguanosine in extracts of murine and human tissues. Cancer Res. **29**, 617—623 (1969).
Philips, F. S., Sternberg, S. S., Hamilton, L. D., Clarke, D. A.: The toxic effects of 6-mercaptopurine and related compounds. Ann. N.Y. Acad. Sci. **60**, 283—296 (1954a).
Philips, F. S., Sternberg, S. S., Hamilton, L. D., Clarke, D. A.: The effects of thioguanine in mammals. Proc. Amer. Ass. Cancer Res. **1**, 37—38 (1954b).
Philips, F. S., Sternberg, S. S., Hamilton, L. D., Clarke, D. A.: Effects of thioguanine in mammals. Cancer **9**, 1092—1101 (1956).

PIERRE, K. J., KIMBALL, A. P., LEPAGE, G. A.: The effect of structure on nucleoside kinase activity. Canad. J. Biochem. **45**, 1619—1632 (1967).
PIERRE, K. J., LEPAGE, G. A.: Formation of inosine-5'-monophosphate by a kinase in cell-free extracts of Ehrlich ascites cells *in vitro*. Proc. Soc. exp. Biol. (N.Y.) **127**, 432—440 (1968).
REMY, C. N.: Metabolism of thiopyrimidines and thiopurines. *S*-Methylation with *s*-adenosylmethionine transmethylase and catabolism in mammalian tissues. J. biol. Chem. **238**, 1078—1084 (1963).
REMY, C. N.: Methylation of synthetic and normal purines, pyrimidines and ribonucleosides. In: Transmethylation and methionine biosynthesis. Chicago: University of Chicago Press 1965.
ROY-BURMAN, P.: Analogs of nucleic acid components. In: Recent results in cancer research, Vol. 25. New York-Heidelberg-Berlin: Springer 1970.
SALSER, J. S., BALIS, M. E.: The mechanism of action of 6-mercaptopurine. II. Basis for specificity. Cancer Res. **25**, 544—551 (1965).
SALSER, J. S., HUTCHISON, D. J., BALIS, M. E.: Studies on the mechanism of action of 6-mercaptopurine in cell free preparations. J. biol. Chem. **235**, 429—432 (1960).
SARCIONE, E. J., STUTZMAN, L.: 6-Methylmercaptopurine: identification as metabolite of 6-mercaptopurine *in vivo* and its activity *in vitro*. Proc. Soc. exp. Biol. (N.Y.) **101**, 766—769 (1959).
SARTORELLI, A. C.: Approaches to the combination chemotherapy of transplantable neoplasms. In: Progress in experimental tumor research, Vol. 6. New York: Hafner Publishing Co. Inc. 1965.
SARTORELLI, A. C., LEPAGE, G. A.: Inhibition of ascites cell growth by combinations of 6-thioguanine and azaserine. Cancer Res. **18**, 938—942 (1958a).
SARTORELLI, A. C., LEPAGE, G. A.: Metabolic effects of 6-thioguanine. II. Biosynthesis of nucleic acid purines *in vivo* and *in vitro*. Cancer Res. **18**, 1329—1335 (1958b).
SARTORELLI, A. C., LEPAGE, G. A., MOORE, E. C.: Metabolic effects of 6-thioguanine. I. Studies on thioguanine-resistant and -sensitive Ehrlich ascites cells. Cancer Res. **18**, 1232—1239 (1958).
SCANNELL, J. P., HITCHINGS, G. H.: Thioguanine in deoxyribonucleic acid from tumors of 6-mercaptopurine-treated mice. Proc. Soc. exp. Biol. (N.Y.) **122**, 627—629 (1966).
SCHABEL, F. M., JR.: The use of tumor growth kinetics in planning "curative" chemotherapy of advanced solid tumors. Cancer Res. **29**, 2384—2389 (1969).
SCHABEL, F. M., JR., LASTER, W. R., JR., SKIPPER, H. E.: Chemotherapy of leukemia L1210 by 6-mercaptopurine (NSC 755) in combination with 6-methylthiopurine ribonucleoside (NSC 40774). Cancer Chemother. Rep. **51**, 111—124 (1967).
SCHABEL, F. M., JR., MONTGOMERY, J. A., SKIPPER, H. E., LASTER, W. R., JR., THOMSON, J. R.: Experimental evaluation of potential anticancer agents. I. Quantitative therapeutic evaluation of certain purine analogs. Cancer Res. **21**, 690—699 (1961).
SCHABEL, F. M., JR., SKIPPER, H. E., TRADER, M. W., WILCOX, W. S.: Experimental evaluation of potential anticancer agents: XIX. Sensitivity of non-dividing leukemic cell populations to certain classes of drugs *in vivo*. Cancer Chemother. Rep. **48**, 17—30 (1965).
SCHOLAR, E. M., BROWN, P. R., PARKS, R. E., JR.: Synergistic effect of 6-mercaptopurine and 6-methyl-mercaptopurine ribonucleoside on the levels of adenine nucleotides of Sarcoma 180 cells. Cancer Res. **32**, 259—269 (1972).
SCHROEDER, J. M., ANSFIELD, F. J., CURRERI, A. R., LEPAGE, G. A.: Toxicity and clinical trial of azaserine and 6-thioguanine in advanced solid malignant neoplasms. Brit. J. Cancer **18**, 449—458 (1964).
SCHWARTZ, R. S., ANDRÉ, J.: The chemical suppression of immunity. In: Immunopathology 2nd International Symposium, 1961. Basel: Benno Schwabe 1962.
SILBERMAN, H. R., WYNGAARDEN, J. B.: 6-Mercaptopurine as substrate and inhibitor of xanthine oxidase. Biochim. biophys. Acta (Amst.) **47**, 178—180 (1961).
SIMPSON, L., BENNETT, L. L., JR., GOLDEN, J.: Effects of 6-mercaptopurine (MP) on the synthesis of purines in ascites tumor cells. Proc. Amer. Ass. Cancer Res. **3**, 361 (1962).
SKIPPER, H. E.: On the mechanisms of action of 6-mercaptopurine. Ann. N.Y. Acad. Sci. **60**, 315—321 (1954).
SKIPPER, H. E., BENNETT, L. L., JR.: Biochemistry of cancer. Ann. Rev. Biochem. **27**, 137—166 (1958).
SKIPPER, H. E., SCHMIDT, L. H.: A manual on quantitative drug evaluation in experimental tumor systems. Part 1. Background, description of criteria, and presentation of quantitative therapeutic data on various classes of drugs obtained in diverse experimental tumor systems. Cancer Chemother. Rep. **17**, 1—143 (1962).
STOCK, J. A.: Antimetabolites. In: Experimental Chemotherapy, vol. IV. New York-London: Academic Press 1966.

STUTTS, P., BROCKMAN, R.W.: A biochemical basis for resistance of L1210 mouse leukemia to 6-thioguanine. Biochem. Pharmacol. **12**, 97—104 (1963).

SULLIVAN, M.P., BEATTY, E.C., JR., HYMAN, C.B., MURPHY, M.L., PIERCE, M.I., SEVERO, N.C.: A comparison of the effectiveness of standard dose 6-mercaptopurine, combination 6-mercaptopurine and DON, high-loading 6-mercaptopurine therapies in the treatment of acute leukemia in children: results of a cooperative study. Cancer Chemother. Rep. **16**, 161—164 (1962).

TARNOWSKI, G.S., STOCK, C.C.: Effects of combinations of azaserine and of 6-diazo-5-oxo-L-norleucine with purine analogs and other antimetabolites on the growth of two mouse mammary carcinomas. Cancer Res. **17**, 1033—1039 (1957).

TAY, B.S., LILLEY, R.McC., MURRAY, A.W., ATKINSON, M.R.: Inhibition of phosphoribosylpyrophosphate amidotransferase from Ehrlich ascites-tumour cells by thiopurine nucleotides. Biochem. Pharmacol. **18**, 936—938 (1969).

TIDD, D.M., KIM, S.C.: A delayed cytotoxic effect of 6MP. Proc. Amer. Ass. Cancer Res. **13**, 52 (1972).

TIDD, D.M., KIM, S.C., HORAKOVA, K., MORIWAKI, A., PATERSON, A.R.P.: A delayed cytotoxic reaction for 6-mercaptopurine. Cancer Res. **32**, 317—322 (1972).

TOMIZAWA, S., ARONOW, L.: Studies on drug resistance in mammalian cells. II. 6-Mercaptopurine resistance in mouse fibroblasts. J. Pharmacol. exp. Therap. **128**, 107—114 (1960).

VENDITTI, J.M., FREI, E., III, GOLDIN, A.: The effectiveness of 2-amino-6-[(1-methyl-4-nitro-5-imidazolyl)thio]purine against transplantable mouse leukemia. Cancer Chemother. Rep. **8**, 44—46 (1960).

VENDITTI, J.M., GOLDIN, A.: Drug synergism in antineoplastic chemotherapy. In: Advances in Chemotherapy, Vol. 1. New York-London: Academic Press 1964.

WANG, M.C., SIMPSON, A.I., PATERSON, A.R.P.: Combinations of 6-mercaptopurine (NSC 755) and 6-(methylmercapto)purine ribonucleoside (NSC 40774) in the therapy of Ehrlich ascites carcinoma. Cancer Chemother. Rep. **51**, 101—109 (1967).

WHITE, F.R.: Data summaries of selected purine antagonists. Thioguanine and thioguanosine. Cancer Chemother. Rep. **11**, 202—213 (1961).

WOLPERT, M.K., DAMLE, S.P., BROWN, J.E., SZNYCER, E., AGRAWAL, K.C., SARTORELLI, A.C.: The role of phosphohydrolases in the mechanism of resistance of neoplastic cells to 6-thiopurines. Cancer Res. **31**, 1620—1626 (1971).

Chapter 48

Azathioprine

Gertrude B. Elion and George H. Hitchings

Introduction (Basic Aspects)

Azathioprine ("Imuran") is an *S*-substituted 6-mercaptopurine:

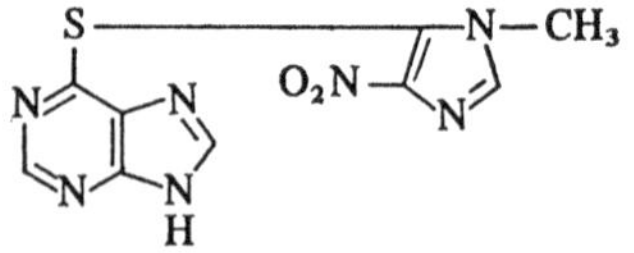

S—N—CH_3 O_2N N N N N H

In vitro it reacts almost quantitatively with sulfhydryl ion with formation of 6-mercaptopurine (6-MP) and 5-mercapto-1-methyl-4-nitroimidazole. This reflects a nucleophilic attack of -SH on the imidazole-5 position, since ^{35}S-labeled azathioprine yields ^{35}S-6-mercaptopurine almost quantitatively on reaction with H_2S or glutathione (Bresnick, 1959; Elion et al., 1961). Azathioprine is likewise split readily by hydroxyl ions, and is converted rapidly to 6-MP in 0.1 *N* sodium hydroxide, especially on warming (Elion et al., 1961).

Biochemical Effects

Many, but not all, of the biological and biochemical effects of azathioprine are attributable to its cleavage to 6-MP and the subsequent anabolic transformation of the free purine to its ribonucleotide, thioinosinic acid, and other thioanalogs of purine derivatives. These reactions have been more fully discussed elsewhere (Hitchings and Elion, 1963a, 1972; Elion and Hitchings, 1965; Elion, 1967).

6-MP is a competitive inhibitor of and a substrate for hypoxanthine-guanine phosphoribosyltransferase (HGPRT). 6-Thioinosinic acid is an inhibitor of succinoadenylate synthetase and lyase, and of inosinate dehydrogenase. Since ^{35}S-6-mercaptopurine was traced to ^{35}S-thioguanine deoxyriboside derived from a tumor-DNA, a series of as yet unstudied further anabolic reactions must have occurred. These would involve thioinosinate or thioguanylate, or both, as substrates for kinases, ribonucleoside diphosphate reductase, polymerases, etc. It has been shown, further, that thioinosinate is *S*-methylated, and that methylthiopurine ribonucleotide is a stronger feed-back inhibitor than thioinosinate of glutamine-phosphoribosylpyrophosphate amidotransferase, the first step in purine nucleotide biosynthesis. The consequences of incorporation of foreign base residues into nucleic acids have not been fully evaluated. Any attempt to pin-point the locus of action of 6-MP in a given tissue at a given time, therefore, is confronted with complexities of impressive proportions.

With azathioprine the complications are compounded. *In vivo*, as dealt with below, the cleavage of the molecule is by no means the unilateral reaction found *in vitro*. Attack by reactive molecules can be on either side of the S-atom, since ^{35}S-labeled imidazole metabolites are found among the metabolites of ^{35}S-azathioprine. One must consider not only potentially biologically active metabolites, but also the reaction of the methylnitroimidazole moiety with active metabolites or even with reactive groups (e.g. ,protein-SH and -NH_2) as possible contributors to the biological activities of azathioprine. This multiplicity of potential *loci* affects the evaluation of biological responses in several ways. One must be wary of accepting as meaningful an effect that occurs only at a high concentration that exceeds the therapeutic range (high range ca. 2 μg/ml = 7 μM by a significant factor. Direct comparisons of 6-MP and azathioprine are notable for their scarcity, which adds to the problem of interpretation of the role of the imidazole moiety in the responses of azathioprine (cf. the section on Biological effects, part E).

Biological Effects

A. Classes of Lymphocytes and Their Interactions

Recent developments dealing with the classification of lymphocytes and their cooperativity in the production of immune responses have provided considerable insight into the cellular mechanisms of the immune response. In brief, lymphocytes are classified as T (thymus-derived) or B (bursa or bone marrow-derived) and considerable progress has been made in allocating specialized functions to each. Cooperativity between the two types generally is required for maximal immune responses of all types. In a broad way, T-cells mediate cellular responses and B-cells humoral responses. Memory and tolerance have been more clearly demonstrated for T-cells, and T-cells apparently are more easily made tolerant. Nevertheless, tolerance of B-cells for antigens with repetitive sequences (e.g., pneumococcal polysaccharide, polyvinylpyrrolidone) has been shown (HOWARD, 1972). Such substances are poor inducers of delayed hypersensitivity reactions, and it may be that responses to them do not involve T-cells (MILLER et al., 1971).

Very little has been done in the way of testing the effects of drugs in the types of systems in which the activities of T and B-cells have been separated. However, evidence appears to be accumulating that azathioprine has a selective effect on T-cells. In particular, there are: its effect on rosette formation in nonimmunized mice, its inhibition of the mixed lymphocyte reaction, and its ability to selectively inhibit the migration of labeled lymph-node cells to the lymph nodes of syngeneic recipients (FOURNIER et al., 1972).

B. Effects on Cells *in Vitro*

The levels at which azathioprine exhibits definite cytotoxicity in cell systems *in vitro* are of the order of 5 (BOLL et al., 1971) to 10 (WILSON, 1965) μg/ml for bone marrow and lymph node cells, respectively. However, the mitotic rate of bone marrow cells was reduced significantly at 1 μg/ml, and transitory effects on regeneration were observed at 0.5 μg/ml (BOLL et al., 1971). Much higher levels of azathioprine are tolerated for short periods. For example, CHAN and STONE (1970) found that mouse spleen cells survived (ca. 75 %) 2 mg/ml for 2 h, while over the same period survival was as great as with controls (ca. 85 %) when the concentration was 0.2 mg/ml. These concentrations strikingly reduced the incorporations of thymidine, uridine, and leucine into macromolecules as early as 30 min after the addition of the drug. It is difficult to assess the importance of effects that are observed only at elevated concentrations. Thus, protein synthesis (i.e., leucine incorporation) by human lymphocytes is inhibited at 6.8×10^{-5} M (19 μg/ml) and larger concentrations (SCHWARTZ et al., 1969). DUTTON and PEARCE (1962) studied the effects of a variety of agents on antibody synthesis by spleen cell suspensions from sensitized rabbits and concluded that inhibition was a secondary manifestation of cytotoxicity. SMITH and FORBES (1967, 1970) also found inhibition of the capacity of human lymphocytes to synthesize proteins, and found azathioprine to be more active than 6-MP, however, at azathioprine concentrations of 60 μg/ml and upward. LEUNG and VAS (1968), using lymph node fragment cultures from hyperimmunized rabbits, found a selective inhibition of antibody synthesis, as compared with nonspecific protein synthesis, by both azathioprine and 6-MP at the respective lower concentration levels, whereas chloramphenicol inhibited nonspecific protein synthesis more than antibody synthesis. In these studies, azathioprine was strikingly more active than 6-MP (10 to 20 μg/ml vs 177 to 250 μg/ml respectively), but possibly only at concentrations greater than those attainable *in vivo*. UYEKI and LLACER (1970) found 6-MP highly active in inhibiting hemolysin plaque-forming spleen cells from sensitized mice. The concentration causing 50 % inhibition ($I.C._{50}$) was 0.06 μM, but the dose-response curve had a shallow slope. Azathioprine was not tested.

A number of biological and biochemical responses have been found to occur at or below toxic levels. These, in the main, are responses that have significance for immunosuppression. Thus, WILSON (1965) found the attack of sensitized lymph node cells on target cells was inhibited at 1 to 5 μg/ml (dose-dependent), with cytotoxicity not evident below 10 μg/ml. The mixed lymphocyte reaction was inhibited in the range 1 to 10 μg/ml, although it was abolished only at 100 μg/ml (VAS and LOWENSTEIN, 1965). Similarly, BACH and BACH (1972) found the viability of lymphocytes unaffected by the presence of azathioprine at 10 μg/ml or less over a 7-day period. At this concentration thymidine incorporation into DNA was strongly suppressed in the mixed human lymphocyte culture. At smaller doses the response was variable, in over one-half of the trials the minimum effective concentration was 0.1 μg/ml or less, in one-third ,0.01 μg/ml or less. Mixed cultures, even from the same pair of subjects, gave variable results. In contrast to methotrexate, the effectiveness of azathioprine fell off sharply with 1 or 2 days' delay in its addition.

Azathioprine did not protect the target cell from humorally mediated, complement-dependent immune damage in a cytolytic system employing fibroblast Chinese hamster lung cells and rabbit hyperimmune serum (SHIPLEY, 1972).

BACH and coworkers have been very active in studies of the rosette inhibition test (BACH et al., 1969; BACH and DARDENNE, 1971a). Sheep erythrocytes adhere to an occasional mouse spleen cell to form a "rosette" when the two cell populations are incubated together. The incidence of rosette-forming cells (RFC) in nonimmunized mice is 1 or 2 per 1000, depending on the strain of mouse involved (BACH, 1971a). Azathioprine inhibits rosette formation at 1 μg/ml, however, its potency is markedly increased in sera from azathioprine-treated patients, or after an "activation" step. This is discussed below in connection with the clinical pharmacology of azathioprine. Rosette forming cells are also found in bone marrow, but the sensitivity of such cells to azathioprine is now believed to be in some way thymus-dependent. Neonatal thymectomy suppresses the sensitivity of RFC to azathioprine (BACH et al., 1971a); thymosin endows sensitivity to bone marrow RFC, and to spleen cells from adult thymectomized mice (BACH and DARDENNE, 1972a; BACH et al., 1971). Azathioprine-sensitive RFC are believed to be antigen-recognizing T-cells since their depletion is associated with immuno-incompetence, and injection of thymus cells causes them to reappear along with immune responsiveness.

C. Effects on the Immune Response

The effects of 6-MP and azathioprine on immune responses have been reviewed previously (Hitchings and Elion, 1963, 1969, 1969a; Hitchings, 1963; Schwartz and André, 1962).

I. Antibody Formation

The earliest observations of the immunosuppressive activity of 6-MP were those of Schwartz et al. (1958, 1959) on the response of rabbits to bovine serum albumen. These studies brought out the importance of timing. In contrast to other agents, 6-MP was most effective when given during the induction period of the response, with or shortly after antigen. It was relatively ineffective during the phase of antibody production. The action could be shown to be similar to immune paralysis or tolerance. Rabbits whose reaction to an antigen was suppressed by 6-MP were unreactive when challenged later with the same antigen (Schwartz and Dameshek, 1959). This tolerance did not, however, reduce the response to another antigen, and tolerance to one and reactivity to another antigen could be demonstrated to exist simultaneously. Subsequently, it was shown with azathioprine (Meyer zum Büschenfelde et al., 1969; Hitchings and Elion, 1969a) and with 6-MP (Nathan et al., 1961; Schwartz and Dameshek, 1963; Brooke, 1966) that the induction of nonresponsiveness or tolerance depends on the intensity of the antigenic stimulus, as well as the drug; tolerance was induced best with the greatest level of antigen and the greatest level of drug.

With many antigens the first antibody produced is the macroglobulin, IgM, 19 S. As antibody production continues, IgG, 7 S antibody begins to appear and IgM production declines rapidly. There may be some kind of feedback control of IgG upon IgM production. Persistent IgM production has been observed in a number of experiments where the induction of tolerance was incomplete due to inadequate drug dosage (Sahiar and Schwartz, 1964; Borel et al., 1965). The alternate, inadequate antigen dosage, has not been demonstrated clearly, but can be inferred in some instances. This splitting of the two phases of response is of particular interest, because production of IgG is associated with immunological memory. Where IgM, but not IgG is formed, a subsequent challenge with the same antigen produces a repetition of the primary response (i.e., IgM appears and only after a normal delay is IgG formed), in contrast to a true secondary response where IgG appears rapidly (cf. the section on Clinical pharmacology, part E I).

Although patients treated with azathioprine for autoimmune disease have not shown a consistent fall in serum IgG or IgM levels (Swanson and Schwartz, 1967; Levy et al., 1972), turnover studies with radioiodinated gamma globulins have revealed that the rate of synthesis of both IgG and IgM has been significantly reduced in a number of such patients at therapeutic doses (Levy et al., 1972).

II. Cell-Borne Immunity

6-MP and azathioprine clearly suppress cell-borne immunity, as shown by their effects in prolonging the survival of renal allografts (Starzl, 1964; Calne, 1967; Merrill, 1968; Hamburger et al., 1972). Their effects on cellular immunity, however, are limited and difficult to interpret. Although skin graft prolongation has been reported in rabbits with azathioprine (Patkowski, 1968), the extensions of skin graft survival that have been observed are generally unimpressive (Alexandre et al., 1963; Murray et al., 1964; Gelfand et al., 1971). If skin rejection is primarily a T-cell phenomenon, one would conclude that azathioprine's effects on T-cells are not great. On the other hand, significant suppression of induced thyroiditis and accompanying delayed hypersensitivity reactions were observed in guinea pigs with 6-MP (SPIEGELBERG and MIESCHER, 1963), with only minor effects on antithyroglobulin antibody.

In another experimental animal model for autoimmune disease, experimental allergic encephalomyelitis (EAE), azathioprine has also shown suppressive activity (ROSENTHALE et al., 1969; BABINGTON and WEDEKING, 1971), as it has against adjuvant arthritis in rats (PERPER et al., 1971; VINEGAR et al., 1968), a cutaneous graft-versus-host reaction in chickens (FLOERSHEIM and SEILER, 1967), and delayed skin reactions in guinea pigs (ARINOVICHE and LOEWI, 1970). It did not, however, suppress secondary disease in monkeys with bone marrow grafts (ELTRINGHAM, 1966). SCHWARTZ and BELDOTTI (1965) had reported a similar lack of effect of 6-MP in chronic homologous disease in mice. Despite its inability to prolong first set skin graft survival in mice, azathioprine did succeed in preventing sensitization of the host by the intraperitoneal injection of allogeneic spleen cells (SKOPINSKA et al., 1969; KENNEALEY et al., 1971). Thus, many cell-mediated responses are inhibited by azathioprine, and the reasons for the failures in some systems are still obscure.

There have been several suggestions that 6-MP and azathioprine have anti-inflammatory effects (HITCHINGS and ELION, 1963; BOREL and SCHWARTZ, 1964; STEVENS and WILLOUGHBY, 1969; ARINOVICHE and LOEWI, 1970). For example, azathioprine suppressed both the appearance of mononuclear exudate cells in skin windows and the granuloma formation caused by polyvinyl sponge implantation in rats (ARINOVICHE and LOEWI, 1970). On the other hand, in adjuvant arthritis in rats, azathioprine behaved like an immunosuppressive agent rather than an anti-inflammatory agent, as judged by its suppression of nonestablished arthritis but its inactivity on established arthritis (PERPER et al., 1971). The insensitivity of immunologically committed cells to azathioprine was also seen when immune lymphoid cells were passively transferred to normal mice which were then challenged with *Listeria monocytogenes* (TRIPATHY and MACKANESS, 1969). The resistance of long-lived lymphocytes and plasma cells in rat lymph nodes to treatment with 6-MP (MILLER and COLE, 1967) is in agreement with this lack of effect. To add to the apparent contradictions, the compound had no effect on delayed hypersensitivity responses to PPD (tuberculin purified protein derivative) in immunized rats, but did affect the response to BGG (bovine γ-globulin) or PPD in immunized guinea pigs (ARINOVICHE and LOEWI, 1970).

D. Antitumor Effects

I. In Rodents

Azathioprine has shown activity against a wide variety of transplantable rodent tumors (ELION et al., 1961). In mice bearing adenocarcinoma 755 it showed a much better chemotherapeutic index (maximum tolerated dose/minimum effective dose) when given orally than when given intraperitoneally; with 6-MP the chemotherapeutic index was superior when the drug was given intraperitoneally. This superiority of the oral route for azathioprine is due to a lower toxicity, without equivalent loss of antitumor activity.

II. In Man

In man, the responsiveness of acute leukemia and chronic granulocytic leukemia to treatment with azathioprine appears to be similar to that obtained with 6-MP (RUNDLES et al., 1961). However, STORTI et al. (1968) have reported unusually good remissions with large intermittent doses of azathioprine in acute leukemia.

E. Comparison of 6-Mercaptopurine and Azathioprine

The question as to whether azathioprine is superior to 6-MP as an immunosuppressive agent has been raised often. In the *in vitro* systems discussed above (e.g., rosette inhibition and inhibition of protein synthesis in peripheral lymphocytes or immunized lymph node cultures) azathioprine is clearly active at smaller absolute concentrations than 6-MP. *In vivo* the situation is more complex. The route and frequency of administration of drug, as well as the nature and size of the antigenic challenge, can determine whether 6-MP or azathioprine is more effective at the same fraction of the toxic dose. BERENBAUM (1971), using large single doses of drug in mice and measuring the effect on hemolysin plaque-forming cells, found 6-MP to be better than azathioprine by the intraperitoneal route, but azathioprine was somewhat better by the subcutaneous route. However, azathioprine has shown equal activity on circulating antibody and on hemolysin plaques at doses 50 to 65 % of the molecular equivalent dose of 6-MP when the drugs were given orally or intraperitoneally for four consecutive days following antigenic stimulation (NATHAN et al., 1961; BLANCUZZI and ELION, unpublished).

In a number of systems, the superiority of azathioprine appears to lie not in greater absolute activity, but in lower toxicity at the active dose. Thus, in skin grafts from AKR to CBA mice, no prolongation of graft survival could be obtained with 6-MP at doses below an LD_{90}, whereas azathioprine gave 10 days' prolongation at 20 mg/kg, with only a 10 % mortality (BLANCUZZI and ELION, unpublished). In adjuvant arthritis in rats, VINEGAR (unpublished) found azathioprine and 6-MP to be equally effective at equimolar doses when the drugs were given in the diet, but the 6-MP was significantly more toxic. On the other hand, if the rats were dosed orally only three times per week, 6-MP was superior. In general, the better chemotherapeutic index of azathioprine appears to exist when the drugs are given orally on a chronic basis.

The superior results with azathioprine in dog kidney allografts (CALNE et al., 1962; ALEXANDRE et al., 1963), which were also felt to be due to its lower toxicity at active doses, led to its choice for initial experiments in human renal transplantation.

Thus, either 6-MP or azathioprine may show superiority in a specific model system, by a specific regimen of administration. Azathioprine, however, on balance, does seem to have the better safety-efficacy ratio in the uses to which it is usually put: oral administration to patients with an organ transplant or autoimmune disease.

Clinical Pharmacology

A. Toxicity

The maximum tolerated doses (MTD) for a variety of species and the LD_{50} values for rodents are given in Table 1. Single doses of the drug are relatively nontoxic, but repeated doses show a greatly enhanced toxicity. Even at toxic doses, however, deaths are delayed, rather than being acute. Guinea pigs are much less sensitive to the toxic effects of azathioprine or 6-MP than other animals. This probably reflects a different metabolic disposition of the drug in this species.

The principal toxic effect of azathioprine is bone marrow depression (ELION et al., 1961; HUNSTEIN et al., 1967). Lymphoid tissue (e.g., spleen, thymus) also has shown depletion on chronic administration (ELION et al., 1961; GABOR and SCOTT, 1968; GOTJAMANOS, 1971). Consequently, animals on relatively large doses for a prolonged period often develop infections. Germ-free mice tolerate larger doses than normal mice (SILAS and NANCE, 1968). There is no effect by azathioprine on the phagocytic activity of liver and spleen macrophages (GOTJAMANOS, 1971).

Table 1. *Toxicity of azathioprine in different species*

Animal	Acute LD_{50} (mg/kg)	Maximum tolerated dose (mg/kg × days)	Ref.
Mouse	650 i.p.	100 × 5 i.p.	ELION et al. (1961)
		200 × 4 i.p.	QUINN and ELION (unpublished)
	2500 p.o.	200 × 5 p.o.	ELION et al. (1961)
		20 p.o. chronically	WALFORD (1966, 1969)
Rat	310 i.p.	50 × 10 i.p.	ELION et al. (1961)
	400 p.o.		
		15 p.o. chronically	FRANKEL et al. (1970)
Dog		7.5 × 10 p.o.	ELION et al. (1961)
		2 p.o. chronically	
Rabbit		20 × 4 i.m.	LEIBOWITZ and ELLIOTT (1966)
		25 × 4 p.o.	
		10 i.p. p.o. chronically	SCHWARTZ and ANDRÉ (1962)
Guinea Pig		175 × 5 i.p.	PAINE (personal communication)
Patas Monkey		3 p.o. × 28	SKARPA and UDALL (personal communication)
		1 p.o., chronically	
Man		2—3, p.o. chronically	CALNE (1967)

Dogs are more sensitive to the toxic effects of azathioprine than are rodents (ELION et al., 1961). At 10 mg/kg for 10 days, deaths were due to agranulocytosis of the marrow and spleen; acute ulcers of the rectal region were also seen. Dogs are particularly susceptible to liver function changes with azathioprine (STARZL et al., 1965; HAXHE et al., 1967; ARONSEN et al., 1969), although hepatotoxicity has not been a consistent finding in dogs (WORTH, 1968). Biliary stasis is probably responsible for the observed changes in liver enzymes, since liver function can return to normal even on continued treatment (ARONSEN et al., 1969). Azathioprine has been reported to accentuate the liver toxicity of carbon tetrachloride in rats (REUBER, 1970).

Azathioprine inhibited DNA synthesis in regenerating rat liver (GONZALEZ et al., 1970; MALAMUD et al., 1972). However, when the drug was stopped, there was a rebound in DNA synthesis (VAN VROONHOVEN and MALT, 1971).

In rhesus monkeys, azathioprine produced a specific nephrotoxic effect at doses which had only a moderate effect on lymphoid tissue (HUSER and MURPHY, 1966).

In man, as in other species, the principal toxic effect of azathioprine is bone marrow depression (CALNE, 1967; BACH and DARDENNE, 1971). Patients who have been on immunosuppressive therapy for prolonged periods with azathioprine have shown no effects on jejunal mucosa (EGGER and ACKMAN, 1971), and growth in children has not been affected (SUNDERMAN and PEARSON, 1969). Hepatotoxicity, in the form of liver enzyme changes or cholestatic jaundice, has been reported occasionally (STARZL, 1964; MERRILL, 1968) but is generally reversible when drug is withheld. Epidemiologic studies and the detection of Australia antigen suggest that a large percentage of the hepatitis in transplant patients is of viral origin (HAMBURGER et al., 1972).

B. Tissue Distribution

Tissue levels of ^{35}S following intraperitoneal administration of ^{35}S-azathioprine to mice showed no unusually large concentration in any particular tissue (ELION, unpublished). During the first two hours, levels of ^{35}S in liver and intestine were 1.5 to 2 times the plasma levels; by 4 h the concentration of ^{35}S was greatest in intestine (i.e., 3.5 times plasma level). The concentrations of ^{35}S in kidney, spleen, lung, and muscle were equal to or lower than plasma levels; there was very little ^{35}S found in brain. Because of the rapidity with which azathioprine is split *in vivo*, and the multiplicity of its metabolites, these ^{35}S concentrations cannot be assumed to be due to azathioprine or "active" metabolites.

C. Metabolism of Azathioprine

I. Introduction

The conversion of azathioprine to 6-MP *in vivo* is chemical, rather than enzymatic, and results principally from nucleophilic attack on the 5-position of the nitroimidazole ring. It occurs in blood, but not in plasma, suggesting that the red cells, which contain glutathione as well as other sulfhydryl-containing compounds, play an important part in the splitting *in vivo*. In man, the splitting appears to be much more complete than in the mouse or dog (ELION et al., 1961, 1962, 1963), and very little azathioprine is excreted in human urine at the usual therapeutic dose levels (ELION et al., 1962, 1963; ELION, 1968, 1972).

The anabolism of 6-MP to its biologically active form, thioinosinic acid, occurs inside the cells through the action of hypoxanthine-guanine phosphoribosyltransferase. Thioinosinic acid is then transformed into other biologically active nucleotides (e.g., methylthioinosinic acid and thioguanylic acid). Since the nucleotides do not transverse cell membranes without dephosphorylation, they do not circulate in the plasma, nor are they excreted in the urine. Consequently, the determination of the plasma levels of 6-MP or azathioprine has no prognostic value with respect to the therapeutic effectiveness or toxicity of these two compounds. The toxic effects of thioinosinic acid and related nucleotides upon cell division are manifest long after the drug and its metabolites have disappeared from the circulation. To date, it has not been possible to devise methods sufficiently sensitive to measure the nucleotides in the tissues of patients under treatment.

II. Urinary Metabolites

1. ^{35}S-Azathioprine

Early investigations determined the urinary metabolites of azathioprine in man after administration of nonradioactive drug (ELION et al., 1961, 1963). Little or no unchanged azathioprine was found; a few percent of the dose was excreted as free 6-MP and 13 to 21 % as 6-thiouric acid in 24 h. CHALMERS et al. (1967) reported a 24-h urinary excretion of thiouric acid equivalent to 38 % of the dose of azathioprine in one individual. However, the precipitation method used by CHALMERS gives high values for thiouric acid compared with the isotope dilution technique (ELION, unpublished observations), probably because 6-methylthiouric acid precipitates along with the thiouric acid.

The use of ^{35}S-azathioprine revealed that its absorption from the gastrointestinal tract was good; over 50 % of the radioactive dose was excreted in the urine in 24 h, and only 12.6 % was found in the 48-h stool specimen (ELION, 1968, 1972). There were individual variations in the amount of thiouric acid excreted (i.e., 10 to 25 % of the dose) and in the amount of inorganic sulfate derived from ^{35}S in the first 24 h (i.e., 10 to 20 % of the dose) (ELION, 1972). Because of the variations, a quantitative comparison of the metabolic fate of azathioprine and 6-MP can be valid only in the same individual. Such a direct comparison, made in one individual (ELION, 1968, 1969, 1972), indicated somewhat better absorption of azathioprine from the gastrointestinal tract, lower excretion of free 6-MP and thiouric acid, but a larger excretion of ^{35}S-sulfate when azathioprine was given. Other oxidized and methylated products of 6-MP catabolism (e.g., 6-methylthiouric acid, 6-thioxanthine, 6-methylsulfinyl-8-hydroxypurine) were present in the urine after azathioprine administration. Less than 2 % of the ^{35}S-azathioprine was excreted in the urine unchanged and approximately 10 % of the ^{35}S appeared in the urine as 1-methyl-4-nitro-5-thioimidazole (ELION, 1969). This intensely yellow compound, $\lambda_{max} = 415$ nm at pH 1, was known to be a urinary metabolite of azathioprine, as well as a reaction product of azathioprine with hydrogen sulfide or with glutathione *in vitro* (BRESNICK, 1959; CHALMERS et al., 1967; ELION, 1968). The fact that it contained ^{35}S indicated that splitting of azathioprine was not exclusively by nucleophilic attack at the 5-position of the nitroimidazole ring, and that, therefore, a molecule of azathioprine would not necessarily yield one molecular equivalent of 6-MP. Another detoxication mechanism for azathioprine is its oxidation to 8-hydroxyazathioprine by aldehyde oxidase (CHALMERS et al., 1969). Animals possessing high levels of aldehyde oxidase (e.g., rabbit, guinea pig) may detoxify azathioprine more readily than 6-MP. Subsequent reaction of 8-hydroxyazathioprine *in vivo* with glutathione or other nucleophilic reagents would release 8-hydroxy-6-thiopurine, which would then be oxidized by xanthine oxidase to thiouric acid. That the aldehyde oxidase route to thiouric acid is not an important one in man is indicated by two facts: (1) in the comparative metabolic study in the same individual, less thiouric acid was produced from azathioprine than from 6-MP (ELION, 1972) and (2) the molecular equivalence of the tolerated doses of the two drugs in man (RUNDLES et al., 1961).

2. ^{14}C-Azathioprine

Investigations using azathioprine labeled with ^{14}C in the 4 and 5 carbons of the methyl-nitroimidazole ring showed that azathioprine was subject to attack *in vivo* by nucleophiles other than sulfhydryl compounds (ELION et al., 1970; DEMIRANDA and CHU, 1970; DEMIRANDA et al., 1972). A considerable portion of the ^{14}C was retained in the body longer than the ^{35}S had been; only 20 % was excreted in 24 h and 37 % in 48 h. Over 11 different ^{14}C-containing metabolites were excreted in the urine. Among these were 1-methyl-4-nitro-5-thioimidazole, a very small amount of 8-hydroxyazathioprine, and at least four metabolites with the ultraviolet absorption characteristics of 5-substituted amino-1-methyl-4-nitroimidazole (ELION et al., 1970). One of these amino derivatives, 1-methyl-4-nitro-5-carboxymethylaminoimidazole, was shown to be derived from azathioprine *in vivo* in the rat (DEMIRANDA and CHU, 1970). The other amino compounds are undoubtedly derived from other amino acids. Recently, another urinary metabolite of azathioprine in the rat has been identified as 1-methyl-4-nitro-5-*N*-acetyl-*S*-cysteinylimidazole (DEMIRANDA et al., 1972). This is believed to be the biotransformation product of 1-methyl-4-nitro-5-*S*-glutathionylimidazole, formed in the blood.

III. Blood Levels

1. ^{35}S-Azathioprine

Following an oral dose of 100 mg of ^{35}S-azathioprine, the peak of radioactivity in the plasma (equivalent to approximately 2 μg of azathioprine per ml) occurred at 2 h, with a half-life for the radioactivity of 4.5 to 5 h (ELION, 1969, 1972). After 10 h, when the ^{35}S was essentially all in the form of inorganic sulfate, clearance of the ^{35}S was much slower. BACH and DARDENNE (1972) obtained similar results when giving ^{35}S-azathioprine, 3 mg/kg orally, to patients with normal renal function, except that the peak of radioactivity in the serum occurred at 40 to 60 min. Because of the rapidity with which azathioprine is metabolized *in vivo*, the radioactivity, even after the first hour, comprises a mixture of ^{35}S-containing metabolites. The rapidity with which azathioprine itself disappears from the plasma is reflected in the fact that little or no azathioprine is excreted in the urine. Methods are not yet available for measuring the multiple sulfur-containing metabolites in the serum quantitatively.

2. ^{14}C-Azathioprine

The peak radioactivity in the plasma following oral administration of 90 mg of ^{14}C-azathioprine (labeled at *C*-4 and 5 of the methyl-nitroimidazole ring) occurred after 6 h and was equivalent to 0.4 μg of azathioprine per ml. Six hours later, the ^{14}C level dropped to 50 % of the peak radioactivity and remained at that approximate level for the next 24 h. The clearance of the ^{14}C is undoubtedly slowed by the binding of the methyl-nitroimidazole moiety to a variety of nucleophilic groups in proteins, since the level of azathioprine per se falls rapidly (ELION et al., 1970, unpublished).

3. Rosette Inhibitory Activity (RIA)

The ability of azathioprine to inhibit rosette formation of sheep red blood cells on nonimmunized mouse spleen cells has been used as a measure of immunosuppressive activity present in the serum following azathioprine administration (BACH and DARDENNE, 1970, 1971, 1972). This rosette inhibitory activity (RIA) appears in the serum 30 min after an oral dose of azathioprine and reaches its maximum 30 to 60 min after the peak of radioactivity with ^{35}S-azathioprine. Thereafter, the RIA decreases rapidly; 50 % disappears within 4 h and 80 % within 12 h. The appearance and decay of RIA in the serum after intravenous administration of azathioprine is not significantly different from that after oral administration. The level of serum RIA is dose-dependent (BACH and DARDENNE, 1972).

The level of RIA is greater than can be accounted for by the concentration of azathioprine itself. Thus, some activation of azathioprine to one or more compounds with greater RIA is indicated (BACH and DARDENNE, 1970; BACH, 1971). This action seems to require the presence of hypoxanthine-guanine phosphoribosyltransferase, since no serum RIA was found in a patient deficient in this enzyme (BACH and DARDENNE, 1970). In normal subjects, the serum RIA after a dose of 6-MP of 1.5 mg/kg is similar to that obtained with azathioprine at 3 mg/kg.

Concurrent measurement of RIA and ^{35}S in serum following ^{35}S-azathioprine administration has revealed that the two are not necessarily related. Thus, patients with severe liver dysfunction have shown little or no RIA in the serum following either oral or intravenous azathioprine (MITCHELL et al., 1970; BACH and DARDENNE, 1972), although no abnormality in azathioprine metabolism was apparent from the curve showing the disappearance of ^{35}S in the serum (BACH and DARDENNE, 1972) or from urinary metabolites (ELION, unpublished). Moreover, patients with abnormally long ^{35}S retention in the serum, such as those with kidney failure, have generally shown normal RIA curves (BACH and DARDENNE, 1971).

IV. Effect of Disease Conditions

1. Renal Insufficiency

It has been the clinical impression of a number of groups (STARZL, 1964; CALNE, 1967, SIMMONS et al., 1971) that the dose of azathioprine should be reduced when temporary renal insufficiency occurs. Since renal clearance plays a minor role in the disposal of the drug as compared with metabolic inactivation, the reason for such a reduction in dose has not been apparent. BACH and DARDENNE (1971), in 59 patients treated continually with azathioprine for long periods, showed no correlation between renal failure and the incidence, severity, or duration of leucopenia. Nevertheless, two of their patients with renal failure showed severe bone marrow aplasia and abnormally prolonged RIA titers within 15 days of treatment with azathioprine at 3 mg/kg (BACH and DARDENNE, 1970, 1972). Since it is not known how frequently this pattern of abnormally prolonged RIA titers and toxicity may occur in patients with renal failure, discretion dictates that the dose of azathioprine in such individuals should be individualized.

2. Gout

Gouty overproducers of uric acid have shown a reduction in the incorporation of glycine-^{14}C into uric acid and reduction of serum and urinary uric acid when treated with azathioprine (SORENSEN, 1966; KELLEY et al., 1967); the same has been true in 3 out of 4 gout patients with normal uric production (KELLEY et al., 1967). In normal individuals azathioprine does not show this type of suppression (SORENSEN, 1966). Since all of these patients appeared to be capable of converting azathioprine to 6-MP and then to thioinosinic acid, the reason for their differences in sensitivity to feedback inhibition of *de novo* purine nucleotide biosynthesis is not clear.

3. Lesch-Nyhan Syndrome

Children with the Lesch-Nyhan syndrome lack the enzyme hypoxanthine-guanine phosphoribosyltransferase (HGPRT) and are, therefore, unable to convert 6-MP to thioinosinic acid. Azathioprine produces no hematological toxicity in these patients nor does it have any effect on uric acid production (NYHAN et al., 1966). An individual lacking HGPRT failed to show any RIA titer after the administration of azathioprine (BACH and DARDENNE, 1972).

4. Liver Disease

In patients with severe liver disease, or in those with liver transplants in whom liver function is failing, the administration of azathioprine results in little or no RIA in the serum (BACH and DARDENNE, 1969, 1972; MITCHELL et al., 1970). In several such patients, an improvement in liver function resulted in a return of the immunosuppressive titer to the serum. The reason for the absence of RIA in azathioprine-treated patients with severe liver dysfunction is difficult to explain. Since splitting of azathioprine to 6-MP does not require the liver, it may be inferred that, in severe liver disease, the action of HGPRT is impaired or that there is excessive catabolism of 6-MP or thioinosinic acid. The data in the literature are not adequate to correlate immunosuppressive activity and bone marrow depression in patients with liver disease.

D. Teratology

I. Chromosome Studies

Azathioprine produced chromosomal aberrations in leucocytes *in vitro*, but only at concentrations (50 μg/ml) much greater than those attainable *in vivo* (OBE, 1971). In another *in vitro* study, azathioprine induced chromosomal mutations at 7 μg/ml only when it was added in a particular solvent, "oximazon," not when dissolved in water (HAMPEL et al., 1971).

In pregnant rabbits, a single i.p. dose of azathioprine on day 11 of gestation produced chromatid breaks and abnormal metaphase figures in both the fetuses and the dams during the 72 h post treatment period. Thereafter, the incidence of aberrations declined to control levels (MOORE and KOZMA, unpublished).

Although chromosomal aberrations have been found in patients receiving azathioprine (JENSEN, 1967; EBERLE et al., 1968; FRIEDRICH and ZEUTHEN, 1970), there is considerable question as to whether these are attributable to drug or to the autoimmune conditions or uremia existing in the treated patients.

II. Teratogenesis in Laboratory Animals

Unlike 6-MP, which is teratogenic in mice, rats, and rabbits, azathioprine showed teratogenic activity only in rabbits under comparable dosage regimens (TUCHMANN-DUPLESSIS and MERCIER-PAROT, 1964, 1964a, 1966). However, considerable teratogenicity with azathioprine in mice has been reported with certain dosage and timing schedules (GITHENS et al., 1965; ROSENKRANTZ et al., 1967). Azathioprine was embryocidal in rats at doses which did not produce gross malformation (THIERSCH, 1962; CONNON, 1969) and had a harmful effect on the nidation phase of the ovum in several rodent species without producing fetal abnormalities (LAURO et al., 1969). A single dose did not produce any dominant lethal mutations in male Swiss-Webster mice (MOORE and KOZMA, unpublished).

A suppression of fertility in male mice for two weeks followed a single dose of azathioprine in one study (MOORE and KOZMA, unpublished), but ROSENKRANTZ et al. (1967) found no effect on male or female fertility in mice, and CONNON (1969) found no effect on conception rates in rats.

III. Clinical Experience

Although azathioprine must be considered potentially teratogenic on the basis of animal studies, a number of normal healthy infants have been delivered to kidney homograft recipients. PENN et al. (1971a) reviewed the experience with parenthood in 19 male recipients and 8 female recipients of renal homografts. Eighteen of the 19 infants whose fathers had renal homografts were normal; one infant was born with a myelomeningocele and other anomalies. Two of the pregnancies in female homograft recipients were terminated by therapeutic abortion; the other six resulted in live births. One of these infants was premature and died shortly after birth; the other five survived, two with a completely uncomplicated course, the others after some neonatal complications.

In 10 pregnancies among female kidney recipients reported by others, 9 have led to normal infants and one to a spontaneous abortion (MURRAY et al., 1963; BOARD et al., 1967; KAUFMAN et al., 1967; CAPLAN et al., 1970; MERKARTZ et al.,

1971). One patient with systemic lupus erythematosus (GILLIBRAND, 1966) and one with active chronic hepatitis (POWELL, 1969) treated with azathioprine have also had normal infants.

E. Effects on Immunological Status

I. Tests for Immunological Reactivity

Patients who are under immunosuppressive treatment with azathioprine after renal transplantation or for autoimmune disease are generally also receiving corticosteroids. It is, therefore, difficult to divorce the effects of the two drugs when studying the ability of such individuals to respond to various antigenic stimuli. Nevertheless, some studies have been instructive in delineating the selectivity of the immunosuppression produced by such treatment, particularly in the few experiments in which azathioprine alone has been used.

In vitro tests employing the lymphocytes of azathioprine-treated patients showed no decrease in responsiveness to phytohemagglutinin (HEINE et al., 1969; DENMAN et al., 1970; ZWEIMAN and SILBERBERG, 1971; PAGÉ et al., 1971), Streptolysin O (HEINE et al., 1969), or naturally encountered antigens such as streptokinase or endotoxin (DENMAN et al., 1970). This is in contrast to the inhibition of *in vitro* lymphocyte transformation observed by HERSH and OPPENHEIM (1967) in patients with malignant disease receiving intensive chemotherapy with cytotoxic drugs.

Lymphocytes from recipients of renal allografts were able to inhibit colony formation of donor fibroblasts *in vitro*. However, the sera from most of these patients were able to specifically block this effect (QUADRACCI et al., 1970). This suggests that immunosuppression did not prevent either the sensitization of the lymphocytes or the formation of "enhancing" antibodies capable of blocking the cell-mediated reaction.

Patients receiving azathioprine have shown a normal antibody response to primary antigenic stimulation by flagellin (ROWLEY et al., 1969; LEE et al., 1971), influenza vaccine, tetanus toxoid, and brucella antigen. However, treated patients did not produce IgG antibody after an early secondary stimulation with flagellin, indicating an interference with immunological memory (ROWLEY et al., 1969). SWANSON and SCHWARTZ (1967) found some abnormal antibody responses to keyhole limpet hemocyanin (KLH) in patients with autoimmune disease being treated with azathioprine; in particular, IgG antibody synthesis was absent or delayed, even when the IgM response was normal.

Delayed skin reactions were not inhibited by treatment with azathioprine in patients previously sensitized to PPD or streptokinase (DENMAN et al., 1970). However, delayed hypersensitivity reactions were inhibited when treatment was given during immunization with KLH (SWANSON and SCHWARTZ, 1967).

The phagocytic activity of the reticuloendothelial system in renal transplant patients was found to be slower during the early phase of phagocytosis (PALMER et al., 1971).

II. Infections

Infections may be a serious problem in patients under immunosuppressive therapy following renal or cardiac transplantation. The responsible organisms are often species which do not ordinarily produce clinical disease: *Candida*, *Aspergillus*, *Pneumocystis*, and cytomegalovirus (HILL et al., 1964; RIFKIND et al., 1964; STINSON et al., 1971). A study by FOLB and TROUNCE (1970) suggests that the depression of cellular immunity rather than humoral immunity is responsible for the *Candida* infections in immunosuppressed patients.

Viral infections (e.g., with herpes zoster) also appear to be activated in transplant patients (RIFKIND, 1966; MERIGAN and STEVENS, 1971). Azathioprine does not interfere with interferon production or release, but does decrease and delay neutralizing antibody (GLASGOW, 1971). Whether viral infection in transplant recipients is the result of immunosuppression or of the immunological stimulation created by the allograft, or both, is difficult to say. Herpes virus infections are common in a variety of clinical conditions having in common the sustained proliferation of lymphocytes [e.g., systemic lupus erythematosus (DALLDORF et al., 1969), infectious mononucleosis, and Burkitt's lymphoma (KLEIN, 1971)]. Moreover, transformed lymphocytes have been found to support the replication of viruses (BLOOM et al., 1970). The relationship between viral activation and immunoregulation is discussed below in relation to carcinogenesis.

III. Carcinogenesis

Long-term studies in mice with azathioprine in the diet showed no evidence of carcinogenicity (WALFORD, 1966, 1969; UDALL, unpublished). A few squamous cell ear duct tumors have been reported in Fischer strain rats fed an azathioprine-containing diet for one year (FRANKEL et al., 1970), but not in Sprague-Dawley rats.

Azathioprine did not increase the incidence of plasma cell tumors in mice treated with Bayol F (MANDEL and DECOSSE, 1970), or of liver tumors in rats fed a liver carcinogen (FRANKEL et al., 1970). When hamster cheek pouches were painted with a carcinogen (dimethylbenzanthracene), azathioprine-treated animals had smaller tumors than the controls at 14 weeks and were free of tumor at 17 weeks (SHEEHAN et al., 1971), suggesting an antitumor effect of azathioprine.

A greater than normal incidence of lymphomas and other neoplasms has been reported in kidney transplant patients, in whom graft rejection is suppressed by azathioprine and prednisone, with the addition in many instances of antilymphocyte globulin, actinomycin C, and x-irradiation (PENN et al., 1971). This has raised the question as to whether the suppression of "immunological surveillance" is responsible for the increased incidence of neoplasia, or whether it is the combination of persistent immunological stimulation coupled with immunosuppression which is responsible. Attempts have been made to answer this question by animal experiments. The studies of KRUEGER et al. (1971) and KRUEGER and HEINE (1972) in mice treated with azathioprine alone, compared with those given azathioprine + persistent antigenic stimulation (e.g., by vaccinia virus, HeLa cells, Freund's adjuvant) support the thesis that lymphoma development is the result of the combination of antigenic stimulation and immunosuppression, rather than either one alone.

Immunosuppression with azathioprine has been shown to potentiate the expression of a virally-induced leukemia in Balb/c mice; the combination of azathioprine + antilymphocyte serum was much more active in this system than azathioprine alone (REID et al., 1972). On the other hand, VREDEVOE and HAYS (1969) found no potentiation by azathioprine of the Gross leukemia virus in C3H/HeJ mice or of the normal incidence of leukemia in AKR mice. It has been suggested that the induction of lymphomas in NZB or (NZB $\times$ NZW) F_1 mice by azathioprine (CASEY, 1968a, b; MELLORS, 1969) may be due to the activation of a latent virus (MELLORS, 1969). Since these strains have a very high incidence of spontaneous autoimmune disease, it is conceivable that their immunological reactivity may also be responsible for activation of oncogenic viruses.

SCHWARTZ (1972) has suggested that the transformation of lymphocytes to lymphoblasts by an immunological stimulus results in the activation of oncogenic virogenes. This theory is supported by facts such as the activation of leukemia viruses by graft-versus-host disease(GLEICHMANN et al., 1972; HIRSCH et al., 1970) and by mixed lymphocyte reactions *in vitro* (HIRSCH et al., 1972). He also postulates that feedback loops (e.g., with IgG antibody) control the immune response and prevent activation of oncogenic viruses in transformed lymphocytes. Faulty immunoregulation would lead to sustained lymphocyte proliferation and would favor the activation of such viruses. In transplant patients, the continuously circulating lymphocytes are constantly exposed to the cell-surface antigens of the graft, and threatened rejection is accompanied by an outpouring of transformed lymphocytes.

In patients with autoimmune disease, in whom the incidence of lymphomas would be expected to be greater than normal, treatment with azathioprine and corticosteroids has not led to a high incidence of malignancies; only 3 have been reported in a group of 4000 treated patients (MCEWAN and PETTY, 1972), as compared with 3 in a smaller group of placebo controls. This suggests that diminished surveillance through immunosuppression is not the predominating cause of the increased incidence of malignancies in transplant patients.

Conclusions

A satisfactory rationalization of the immunosuppressive effects of azathioprine is at present beyond reach. One can reject, as insufficient, the hypothesis that it acts simply as a cytotoxic agent with selective effects on rapidly multiplying cells. Cell division and DNA synthesis are integral events in the primary immune response. Cellular multiplication is significantly greater in the secondary response, however, and the secondary is much less sensitive than the primary response to treatment with azathioprine.

The key to the eventual understanding of the mechanism of action of azathioprine appears to lie in its effects on cellular differentiation. In some way it sensitizes the antigen recognition mechanism so that the induction of tolerance can be achieved at lower doses of antigen. When the effect falls short of tolerance, a suppression of the development of immunological memory can still be observed. In these circumstances IgG is not produced, IgM persists, and a later challenge with the same antigen results in the repetition of the primary type response. This could result from inhibition of lymphoblastic transformation, selective destruction of lymphoblasts, or inhibition of further differentiation of the lymphoblasts induced by antigen.

In biochemical terms, many of the actions of azathioprine are attributable to the ultimate formation of thioinosinic acid, but many indicators suggest that the initial splitting of the molecule and the imidazole moiety play some role in its actions, more or less important depending on the system under study.

The immunosuppressive effects of azathioprine in allograft retention clearly fall short of the induction of true tolerance. But the presence of the drug seems to become less important with the passage of time, either because of an ultimate exhaustion of the host versus graft mechanism, or more likely, because partial suppression permits the gradual accumulation of enhancing antibody that protects the graft from attack by sensitized lymphocytes, and a sort of pseudotolerance is achieved.

The thiopurine derivatives have attained some practical success in immunology in the role they play in renal transplantation. They have also, through the separation of IgM and IgG responses, and through some selective effects on T- versus B-lymphocytes, helped to identify some critical targets for further studies, both immunological and biochemical.

References

ALEXANDRE, G. P. J., MURRAY, J. E., DAMMIN, G. J, NOLAN, B.: Immunosuppressive drug therapy in canine renal and skin homografts. Transplantation **1**, 432—461 (1963).

ARINOVICHE, R., LOEWI, G.: Comparison of the effects of two cytotoxic drugs and of anti-lymphocytic serum, on immune and non-immune inflammation in experimental animals. Ann. rheum. Dis. **29**, 32—39 (1970).

ARONSEN, K. F., HUSBERG, B., PIHL, B.: Immunosuppressive treatment in non-transplanted dogs. Azathioprine versus azathioprine-antilymphocyteimmunoglobulin-G. Acta chir. scand. **135**, 475—481 (1969).

BABINGTON, R. G., WEDEKING, P. W.: The influence of cinanserin and selected pharmacologic agents on experimental allergic encephalomyelitis (EAE). J. Pharmacol. exp. Ther. **177**, 454—460 (1971).

BACH, J. F.: Immunosuppression by chemical agents. Transplant. Proc. **3**, 27—33 (1971).

BACH, J. F.: Antigen-binding cells. In: Cell-mediated immunity. In vitro correlates, pp. 51—74. Basel: Karger 1971a.

BACH, J. F., DARDENNE, M.: Études sur le métabolisme de l'azathioprine. C. R. Acad. Sci. (Paris) **271**, 453—456 (1970).

BACH, J. F., DARDENNE, M.: The metabolism of azathioprine in renal failure. Transplantation **12**, 253—259 (1971).

BACH, J. F., DARDENNE, M.: Activities of immunosuppressive agents *in vitro*. I. Rosette inhibition by azathioprine. Rev. Europ. études clin. et biol. **16**, 770—777 (1971a).

BACH, J. F., DARDENNE, M.: Serum immunosuppressive activity of azathioprine in normal subjects and patients with liver diseases. Proc. roy. Soc. Med. **65**, 260—263 (1972).

BACH, J. F., DARDENNE, M.: Antigen recognition by T lymphocytes. II. Similar effects of azathioprine, antilymphocyte serum and anti-theta serum on rosette-forming lymphocytes in normal and neonatally thymectomized mice. Cell. Immunol. **3**, 11—21 (1972a).

BACH, J. F., DARDENNE, M., CROSNIER, J.: Bone marrow-reactivity to azathioprine due to metabolism abnormality. Ann. intern. Med.

BACH, J. F., DARDENNE, M., DAVIES, A. J. S.: Early effect of adult thymectomy. Nature (Lond.) **231**, 110—111 (1971a).

BACH, J. F., DARDENNE, M., FOURNIER, C.: *In vitro* evaluation of immunosuppressive drugs. Nature (Lond.) **222**, 998—999 (1969).

BACH, J. F., DARDENNE, M., GOLDSTEIN, A. L., GUHA, A., WHITE, A.: Appearance of T-cell markers in bone marrow rosette-forming cells after incubation with thymosin, a thymic hormone. Proc. nat. Acad. Sci. (Wash.) **68**, 2734—2738 (1971).

BACH, M. A., BACH, J. F.: Activities of immunosuppressive agents *in vitro*. II. Different timing of azathioprine and methotrexate in inhibition and stimulation of mixed lymphocyte reaction. Clin. exp. Immunol. **11**, 89—98 (1972).

BERENBAUM, M. C.: Is azathioprine a better immunosuppressive than 6-mercaptopurine? Clin. exp. Immunol. **8**, 1—8 (1971).

BLANCUZZI, V., ELION, G. B.: Unpublished.

BLOOM, B. R., JIMENEZ, L., MARCUS, P. I.: A plaque assay for enumerating antigen-sensitive cells in delayed-type hypersensitivity. J. exp. Med. **132**, 16—30 (1970).

BOARD, J. A., LEE, H. M., DRAPER, D. A., HUME, D. M.: Pregnancy following kidney homotransplantation from a non-twin: Report of a case with concurrent administration of azathioprine and prednisone. Obstet. Gynec. **29**, 318—323 (1967).

BOLL, I., KLIMAS, J., WILLIGERODT, B.: Die Wirkung von 6-Mercaptopurin und Azathioprin auf menschliches Knochenmark *in vitro*. Arzneimittel-Forsch. **21**, 502—504 (1971).

BOREL, Y., FAUCONNET, M., MIESCHER, P. A.: Effect of 6-mercaptopurine (6-MP) on different classes of antibody. J. exp. Med. **122**, 263—275 (1965).

BOREL, Y., SCHWARTZ, R. S.: Inhibition of immediate and delayed hypersensitivity in the rabbit by 6-mercaptopurine. J. Immunol. **92**, 754—761 (1964).

BRESNICK, E.: The metabolism *in vitro* of antitumor imidazolyl derivatives of mercaptopurines. Fed. Proc. **18**, 371 (1959).

BROOKE, M. S.: Immunological paralysis in mice exposed to sublethal irradiation or treated with 6-mercaptopurine. Transplantation **4**, 1—7 (1966).

CALNE, R. Y.: Renal transplantation, 2nd Ed. London: Edward Arnold, Ltd. 1967.

CALNE, R. Y., ALEXANDRE, G. P. J., MURRAY, J. E.: A study of the effects of drugs in prolonging survival of homologous renal transplants in dogs. Ann. N. Y. Acad. Sci. **99**, 743—761 (1962).
CAPLAN, R. M., DOSSETOR, J. B., MAUGHAN, G. B.: Pregnancy following cadaver kidney transplantation. Amer. J. Obstet. Gynec. **106**, 644—648 (1970).
CASEY, T. P.: The development of lymphomas in mice with autoimmune disorders treated with azathioprine. Blood **31**, 396—399 (1968a).
CASEY, T. P.: Azathioprine (Imuran) administration and development of malignant lymphomas in NZB mice. Clin. exp. Immunol. **3**, 305—312 (1968b).
CHALMERS, A. H., KNIGHT, P. R., ATKINSON, M. R.: Conversion of azathioprine into mercaptopurine and mercaptoimidazole derivatives *in vitro* and during immunosuppressive therapy. Aust. J. exp. Biol. med. Sci. **45**, 681—691 (1967).
CHALMERS, A. H., KNIGHT, P. R., ATKINSON, M. R.: 6-Thiopurines as substrates and inhibitors of purine oxidases: a pathway for conversion of azathioprine into 6-thiouric acid without release of 6-mercaptopurine. Aust. J. exp. Biol. med. Sci. **47**, 263—273 (1969).
CHAN, G. Y., STONE, R. L.: Inhibition of nucleic acid and protein synthesis in mouse spleen cells *in vitro* by azathioprine. Appl. Microbiol. **20**, 910—912 (1970).
CONNON, A. F.: Effects of azathioprine on reproduction in rats. J. Reprod. Fertil. **18**, 165—166 (1969).
DALLDORF, G., CARVALHO, R. P. S., JAMARA, M., FROST, P., EHRLICH, D., MARIGO, C.: The lymphomas of Brazilian children. J. Amer. med. Ass. **208**, 1365—1368 (1969).
DEMIRANDA, P., BEACHAM, L. M., III, CREAGH, T., ELION, G. B.: Metabolic fate of the imidazole moiety of azathioprine (Imuran). Abstract, Fifth International Congress on Pharmacology 55 (1972).
DEMIRANDA, P., CHU, L. C.: Reaction of azathioprine (Imuran) with ^{14}C-glycine in the rat. Fed. Proc. **29**, 608 (1970).
DENMAN, E. J., DENMAN, A. M., GREENWOOD, B. M., GALL, D., HEATH, R. B.: Failure of cytotoxic drugs to suppress immune responses of patients with rheumatoid arthritis. Ann. rheum. Dis. **29**, 220—231 (1970).
DUTTON, R. W., PEARCE, J. D.: A survey of the effect of metabolic antagonists on the synthesis of antibody in an *in vitro* system. Immunology **5**, 414—423 (1962).
EBERLE, P., HUNSTEIN, W., PERINGS, E.: Chromosomes in patients treated with Imuran. Hum. Genet. **6**, 69—73 (1968).
EGGER, G., ACKMAN, D.: Light microscopic examination of the jejunum after long-standing azathioprine treatment. Experientia (Basel) **27**, 326 (1971).
ELION, G. B.: Unpublished.
ELION, G. B.: Biochemistry and pharmacology of purine analogues. Fed. Proc. **26**, 898—904 (1967).
ELION, G. B.: Discussion. In: MIESCHER, P. A., GRABOR, P. (Eds.): International symposium on immunopathology, Fifth, Italy, June 1967, pp. 399—401. New York: Grune and Stratton 1968.
ELION, G. B.: The comparative metabolism of "Imuran" and 6-mercaptopurine (6-MP) in man. Proc. Amer. Ass. Cancer Res. **10**, 21 (1969).
ELION, G. B.: The significance of azathioprine metabolites. Proc. roy. Soc. Med. **65**, 257—260 (1972).
ELION, G. B., BENEZRA, F. M., CARRINGTON, L. O., STRELITZ, R. A.: Metabolic fate of ^{14}C-azathioprine. Fed. Proc. **29**, 607 (1970).
ELION, G. B., CALLAHAN, S. W., BIEBER, S., HITCHINGS, G. H., RUNDLES, R. W.: A summary of investigations with 6-[(1′-methyl-4′nitro-5′-imidazolyl)] thiopurine. Cancer Chemother. Rep. **14**, 93—98 (1961).
ELION, G. B., CALLAHAN, S. W., HITCHINGS, G. H., RUNDLES, R. W., LASZLO, J.: Experimental, clinical and metabolic studies of thiopurines. Cancer Chemother. Rep. **16**, 197—202 (1962).
ELION, G. B., CALLAHAN, S. W., RUNDLES, R. W., HITCHINGS, G. H.: Relationship between metabolic fates and antitumor activities of thiopurines. Cancer Res. **23**, 1207—1217 (1963).
ELION, G. B., HITCHINGS, G. H.: Metabolic basis for the actions of analogs of purines and pyrimidines. In: Advances in chemotherapy, Vol. 2, pp. 91—177. New York: Academic Press 1965.
ELTRINGHAM, J. R.: Effect of azathioprine and amethopterin on secondary disease in the rhesus monkey. Exp. Hematol. **10**, 12—13 (1966).
FLOERSHEIM, G. L., SEILER, K.: Differential effects of immunosuppressive drugs on a cutaneous graft-versus-host reaction in chickens. Transplantation **5**, 1355—1370 (1967).
FOLB, R. I., TROUNCE, J. R.: Immunological aspects of candida infection complicating steroid and immunosuppressive drug therapy. Lancet **II**, 1112—1114 (1970).
FOURNIER, C., BACH, M. A., DARDENNE, M., BACH, J. F.: Selective action of azathioprine on T cells. Transplant. Proc. **5**, 523—526 (1973).

FRANKEL, H. H., YAMAMOTO, R. S., WEISBURGER, E. K., WEISBURGER, J. H.: Chronic toxicity of azathioprine and the effect of this immunosuppressant on liver tumor induction by the carcinogen *N*-hydroxy-*N*-2-fluorenylacetamide. Toxicol. appl. Pharmacol. **17**, 462—480 (1970).

FRIEDRICH, U., ZEUTHEN, E.: Chromosomenabnormitäten und Behandlung mit Imuran (Azathioprin) nach Nierentransplantationen. Hum. Genet. **8**, 289—294 (1970).

GABOR, E. P., SCOTT, J. L.: Effect of thiopurines on rat lymphoid tissues. Clin. Res. **16**, 154 (1968).

GELFAND, M. C., NOWAKOWSKI, A., FRIEDMAN, E. A., KNEPSHIELD, J. H.: Synergism in immunosuppression. III. Allograft rejection and humoral antibody production in intact and splenectomized mice. Transplantation **12**, 377—383 (1971).

GILLIBRAND, P. N.: Systemic lupus erythematosus in pregnancy treated with azathioprine. Proc. roy. Soc. Med. **59**, 834 (1966).

GITHENS, J. H., ROSENKRANTZ, J. G., TUNNOCK, S. M.: Teratogenic effects of azathioprine (Imuran). J. Pediat. **66**, 959—961 (1965).

GLASGOW, L. A.: Immunosuppression, interferon, and viral infections. Fed. Proc. **30**, 1846—1851 (1971).

GLEICHMANN, E., GLEICHMANN, H., SCHWARTZ, R. S.: Immunologic induction of malignant lymphoma: genetic factors in the graft-versus-host model. J. nat. Cancer Inst. **49**, 793—801 (1972).

GONZALEZ, E. M., KREJCZY, K., MALT, R. A.: Modification of nucleic acid synthesis in regenerating liver by azathioprine. Surgery **68**, 254—259 (1970).

GOTJAMANOS, T.: The effect of azathioprine on phagocytic activity and morphology of reticulo-endothelial organs in mice. Pathology **3**, 171—179 (1971).

HAMBURGER, J., CROSNIER, J., DORMONT, J., BACH, J. F.: Renal transplantation. Theory and practice. Baltimore: Williams and Wilkins 1972.

HAMPEL, K. E., LACKNER, A., SCHULZ, G., BUSSE, V.: Chromosomal mutations by azathioprine in human leukocytes *in vitro*. Z. Gastroent. **9**, 47—51 (1971).

HAXHE, J. J., ALEXANDRE, G. P. J., KESTENS, P. J.: The effect of Imuran and azaserine on liver function tests in the dog. Its relation to the detection of graft rejection following liver transplantation. Arch. int. Pharmacodyn. **168**, 366—372 (1967).

HEINE, K. M., STOBBE, H., KLATT, R., APOSTOLOFF, E., DUTZ, W.: Lymphocyte transformation tests in patients under treatment with immunosuppressive drugs. Helv. med. Acta **35**, 140—145 (1969/70).

HERSH, E. M., OPPENHEIM, J. J.: Inhibition of *in vitro* lymphocyte transformation during chemotherapy in man. Cancer Res. **27**, 98—105 (1967).

HILL, R. H., JR., ROWLANDS, D. T., JR., RIFKIND, D.: Infectious pulmonary disease in patients receiving immunosuppressive therapy for organ transplantation. New Engl. J. Med. **271**, 1021—1027 (1964).

HIRSCH, M. S., BLACK, P. H., TRACY, G. S., LEIBOWITZ, S., SCHWARTZ, R. S.: Leukemia virus activation in chronic allogeneic disease. Proc. nat. Acad. Sci. (Wash.) **67**, 1914—1917 (1970).

HIRSCH, M. S., PHILLIPS, S. M., SOLNIK, C., BLACK, P. H., SCHWARTZ, R. S., CARPENTER, C. B.: Activation of leukemia viruses by graft-versus-host and mixed lymphocyte reactions *in vitro*. Proc. nat. Acad. Sci. (Wash.) **69**, 1069—1072 (1972).

HITCHINGS, G. H.: Summary of informal discussion on the role of purine antagonists. Cancer Res. **23**, 1218—1225 (1963).

HITCHINGS, G. H., ELION, G. B.: Chemical suppression of the immune response. Pharmacol. Rev. **15**, 365—405 (1963).

HITCHINGS, G. H., ELION, G. B.: Purine analogues. In: HOCHSTER, R. M., QUASTEL, J. H. (Eds.): Metabolic inhibitors, Vol. 1, pp. 215—237. New York: Academic Press 1963a.

HITCHINGS, G. H., ELION, G. B.: Thiopurines as inhibitors of the immune response. In: SHUGAR, D. (Ed.): FEBS Symposium, Biochemical aspects of antimetabolites and of drug hydroxylation, Vol. 16, pp. 1—10. London and New York: Academic Press 1969.

HITCHINGS, G. H., ELION, G. B.: The role of antimetabolites in immunosuppression and transplantation. Accounts chem. Res. **2**, 202—209 (1969a).

HITCHINGS, G. H., ELION, G. B.: Mechanisms of action of purine and pyrimidine analogues. In: BRODSKY, I., KAHN, S. B., MOYER, J. H. (Eds.): Cancer chemotherapy II, 22nd Hahnemann Symposium, pp. 23—32. New York: Grune and Stratton 1972.

HOWARD, J. G.: Cellular events in the induction and loss of tolerance to pneumococcal polysaccharides. Transplant. Rev. **8**, 50—75 (1972).

HUNSTEIN, W., PERINGS, E., KLOSE, U.: Long-term animal experiments with azathioprine (Imuran) to test its myelotoxic effect. Vehr. dtsch. Ges. inn. Med. **73**, 450—453 (1967).

HUSER, H. J., MURPHY, G. P.: The renal and hematologic effects of immunosuppression in the rhesus monkey. Survival of autotransplants following azathioprine. Amer. Surg. **32**, 243—248 (1966).

JENSEN, M. K.: Chromosome studies in patients treated with azathioprine and amethopterin. Acta med. scand. **182**, 445—455 (1967).
KAUFMAN, J. J., DIGNAM, W., GOODWIN, W. E., MARTIN, D. C., GOLDMAN, R., MAXWELL, M. H.: Successful normal childbirth after kidney homotransplantation. J. Amer. med. Ass. **200**, 338—341 (1967).
KELLEY, W. N., ROSENBLOOM, F. M., SEEGMILLER, J. E.: The effects of azathioprine (Imuran) on purine synthesis in clinical disorders of purine metabolism. J. clin. Invest. **46**, 1518—1529 (1967).
KENNEALEY, G. T., LYTTON, B., RUDDLE, N., MITCHELL, M. S.: Modification of response to histocompatibility antigens with chemotherapeutic agents. Transplantation **12**, 522—523 (1971).
KLEIN, G.: Immunological aspects of Burkitt's lymphoma. Advanc. Immunol. **14**, 187—243 (1971).
KRUEGER, G. R. F., HEINE, U. I.: Morphogenesis of two immunologically induced mouse lymphomas. Cancer Res. **32**, 573—582 (1972).
KRUEGER, G. R. F., MALMGREN, R. A., BERARD, C. W.: Malignant lymphomas and plasmacytosis in mice under prolonged immunosuppression and persistent antigenic stimulation. Transplantation **11**, 138—144 (1971).
LAURO, V., SANTILLI GIORNELLI, F. E., DOMINICI, C., FANELLI, A., CUCCHIA, G.: Effetti della 6-mercaptopurina e dell'azathioprina sulla fase di annidamento dell'uovo: indagine comparativa in alcune specie di roditori. Arch. Ginec. Obstet. **74**, 164—177 (1969).
LEE, A. K. Y., MACKAY, I. R., ROWLEY, M. J., YAP, C. Y.: Measurement of antibody-producing capacity of flagellin in man. IV. Studies in autoimmune disease, allergy, and after azathioprine treatment. Clin. exp. Immunol. **9**, 507—518 (1971).
LEIBOWITZ, H. M., ELLIOTT, J. H.: Chemotherapeutic immunosuppression of the corneal graft reaction. II. Combined systemic antimetabolite and topical corticosteroid therapy. Arch. Ophthal. **76**, 338—344 (1966).
LEUNG, F. C., VAS, S. I.: Effects of immunosuppressive drugs on secondary antibody response *in vitro*. Canad. J. Microbiol. **14**, 7—11 (1968).
LEVY, J., BARNETT, E. V., MACDONALD, N. S., KLINENBERG, J. R., PEARSON, C. M.: The effect of azathioprine on gammaglobulin synthesis in man. J. clin. Invest. **51**, 2233—2238 (1972).
MALAMUD, D., GONZALEZ, E. M., CHIU, H., MALT, R. A.: Inhibition of cell proliferation by azathioprine. Cancer Res. **32**, 1226—1229 (1972).
MANDEL, M. A., DECOSSE, J. J.: Enhancement of tumor induction in mice by long term immunosuppression. Surg. Forum **21**, 129—131 (1970).
MCEWAN, A., PETTY, L. G.: Oncogenicity of immunosuppressive drugs. Lancet **I**, 326—327 (1972).
MELLORS, R. C.: Murine leukemialike virus and the immunopathological disorders of New Zealand Black mice. J. infect. Dis. **120**, 480—487 (1969).
MERIGAN, T. C., STEVENS, D. A.: Viral infections in man associated with acquired immunological deficiency states. Fed. Proc. **30**, 1858—1864 (1971).
MERKATZ, I. R., SCHWARTZ, G. H., DAVID, D. S., STENZEL, K. H., RIGGIO, R. R., WHITSELL, J. C.: Resumption of female reproductive function following renal transplantation. J. Amer. med. Ass. **216**, 1749—1754 (1971).
MERRILL, J. P.: Medical management of the transplant patient. In: RAPAPORT, F. T., DAUSSET, J. (Eds.): Human transplantation, pp. 66—79. New York: Grune and Stratton 1968.
MEYER ZUM BÜSCHENFELDE, K. H., FREUDENBERG, J.: Tierexperimentelle Untersuchungen über die Wirkung von Azathioprin auf die Bildung zirkulierender Antikörper. Klin. Wschr. **47**, 379—482 (1969).
MILLER, J. F. A. P., BASTEN, A., SPRENT, J., CHEERS, C.: Interaction between lymphocytes in immune responses. Cell. Immunol. **2**, 469—495 (1971).
MILLER, J. J., COLE, L. J.: Resistance of long-lived lymphocytes and plasma cells in rat lymph nodes to treatment with prednisone, cyclophosphamide, 6-mercaptopurine, and actinomycin D. J. exp. Med. **126**, 109—125 (1967).
MITCHELL, C. G., EDDLESTON, A. L. W. F., SMITH, M. G. M., WILLIAMS, R.: Serum immunosuppressive activity due to azathioprine and its relation to hepatic function after liver transplantation. Lancet **I**, 1196—1199 (1970).
MOORE, H. L., JR., KOZMA, C.: Unpublished.
MURRAY, J. E., REID, D. E., HARRISON, J. H., MERRILL, J. P.: Successful pregnancies after human renal transplantation. New Engl. J. Med. **269**, 341—343 (1963).
MURRAY, J. E., SCHEIL, A. G. R., MOSELEY, R., KNIGHT, P. R., MCGAVIC, J. D., DAMMIN, G. J.: Analysis of mechanism of immunosuppressive drugs in renal homotransplantation. Ann. Surg. **160**, 449—473 (1964).
NATHAN, H. C., BIEBER, S., ELION, G. B., HITCHINGS, G. H.: Detection of agents which interfere with the immune response. Proc. Soc. exp. Biol. (N.Y.) **107**, 796—799 (1961).

NYHAN, W. L., SWEETMAN, L., CARPENTER, D. G., CARTER, C. H., HOEFNAGEL, D.: Effects of azathioprine in a disorder of uric acid metabolism and cerebral function. J. Pediat. **72**, 111—118 (1968).
OBE, G.: Die Wirkung von 6-Mercaptopurin und Azathioprin auf menschliche Chromosomen *in vitro*. Arzneimittel-Forsch. **21**, 504—505 (1971).
PAGÉ, D., POSEN, G., STEWART, T., HARRIS, J.: Immunological detection of renal allograft rejection in man. Increased deoxynucleic acid synthesis by peripheral lymphoid cells. Transplantation **12**, 341—347 (1971).
PAINE, K. W. E.: Personal communication.
PALMER, D. L., RIFKIND, D., BROWN, D. W.: ^{131}I-Labeled colloidal human serum albumin in the study of reticuloendothelial system function. III. Phagocytosis and catabolism compared in normal, leukemic, and immunosuppressed human subjects. J. infect. Dis. **123**, 465—469 (1971).
PATKOWSKI, J.: On the mode of action of some immunosuppressant drugs. J. Pharm. Pharmacol. **20**, 957—959 (1968).
PENN, I., HALGRIMSON, C. G., STARZL, T. E.: *De novo* malignant tumors in organ transplant recipients. Transplant. Proc. **3**, 773—778 (1971).
PENN, I., MAKOWSKI, E., DROEGEMUELLER, W., HALGRIMSON, C. G., STARZL, T. E.: Parenthood in renal homograft recipients. J. Amer. med. Ass. **216**, 1755—1761 (1971 a).
PERPER, R. J., ALVAREZ, B., COLOMBO, C., SCHRODER, H.: The use of a standardized adjuvant arthritis assay to differentiate between antiinflammatory and immunosuppressive agents. Proc. Soc. exp. Biol. (N.Y.) **137**, 506—512 (1971).
POWELL, D.: Pregnancy in active chronic hepatitis on immunosuppressive therapy. Postgrad. med. J. **45**, 292—294 (1969).
QUADRACCI, L. J., HELLSTRÖM, I. E., STRIKER, G. E., MARCHIORO, T. L., HELLSTRÖM, K. E.: Immune mechanisms in human recipients of renal allografts. Cell. Immunol. **1**, 561—566 (1970).
QUINN, R. P., ELION, G. B.: Unpublished.
REID, R. H., PIROFSKY, B., DAWSON, P. J.: The influence of immunosuppression on virus-induced lymphatic leukemia in mice. Transplantation **13**, 61—65 (1972).
REUBER, M. D.: Accentuation of carbon tetrachloride-induced cirrhosis by azathioprine in the rat. Arch. Path. **90**, 567—571 (1970).
RIFKIND, D.: The activation of varicella-zoster virus infections by immunosuppressive therapy. J. Lab. clin. Med. **68**, 463—474 (1966).
RIFKIND, D., MARCHIORO, T. L., WADDELL, W. R., STARZL, T. E.: Infectious diseases associated with renal homotransplantation. I. Incidence, types and predisposing factors. J. Amer. med. Ass. **189**, 397—407 (1964).
ROSENKRANTZ, J. G., GITHENS, J. H., COX, S. M., KELLUM, D. L.: Azathioprine (Imuran) and pregnancy. Amer. J. Obstet. Gynec. **97**, 387—394 (1967).
ROSENTHALE, M. E., DATKO, L. J., KASSARICH, J., SCHNEIDER, F.: Chemotherapy of experimental allergic encephalomyelitis (EAE). Arch. int. Pharmacodyn. **179**, 251—275 (1969).
ROWLEY, M. J., MACKAY, I. R., MCKENZIE, I. F. C.: Antibody production in immunosuppressed recipients of renal allografts. Lancet **II**, 708—710 (1969).
RUNDLES, R. W., LASZLO, J., ITOGA, T., HOBSON, J. B., GARRISON, F. E., JR.: Clinical and hematologic study of 6-[(1-methyl-4-nitro 5 imidazolyl)thio]-purine and related compounds. Cancer Chemother. Rep. **14**, 99—115 (1961).
SAHIAR, K., SCHWARTZ, R. S.: Inhibition of 19 S antibody synthesis by 7 S antibody. Science **145**, 395—397 (1964).
SCHWARTZ, G. H., STENZEL, K. H., RUBIN, A. L.: Depression of lymphocyte transformation by drugs *in vitro*. Effects of a new immunosuppressant, Cinanserin. Transplantation **8**, 704—711 (1969).
SCHWARTZ, R. S.: Immunoregulation, oncogenic viruses, and malignant lymphomas. Lancet **I**, 1266—1269 (1972).
SCHWARTZ, R. S., ANDRÉ, J.: The chemical suppression of immunity. Mechanism of cell and tissue damage produced by immune reactions. 2nd International symposium on immunopathology 1961, pp. 385—409. Basel: Benno Schwabe & Co. 1962.
SCHWARTZ, R. S., BELDOTTI, L.: The treatment of chronic murine homologous disease: a comparative study of four "immunosuppressive" agents. Transplantation **3**, 79—97 (1965).
SCHWARTZ, R. S., DAMESHEK, W.: Drug-induced immunological tolerance. Nature (Lond.) **183**, 1682—1683 (1959).
SCHWARTZ, R. S., DAMESHEK, W.: The role of antigen dosage in drug-induced immunologic tolerance. J. Immunol. **90**, 703—710 (1963).
SCHWARTZ, R. S., EISNER, A., DAMESHEK, W.: The effect of 6-mercaptopurine on primary and secondary immune responses. J. clin. Invest. **38**, 1394—1403 (1959).

SCHWARTZ, R. S., STACK, J., DAMESHEK, W.: Effect of 6-mercaptopurine on antibody production. Proc. Soc. exp. Biol. (N.Y.) **99**, 164—167 (1958).

SHEEHAN, R., SHKLAR, G., TENNEBAUM, R.: Azathioprine effects on the development of hamster pouch carcinomas. Arch. Path. **21**, 264—270 (1971).

SHIPLEY, W. U.: Immunosuppressive agents and immune cytolysis *in vitro*. The effect of azathioprine, hydrocortisone, and radiation on antiserum and complement-mediated lysis of cultured mammalian cells. Transplantation **14**, 392—395 (1972).

SILAS, D. E., NANCE, F. C.: Increased tolerance to high doses of azathioprine by germfree animals. Clin. Res. **16**, 84 (1968).

SIMMONS, R. L., KJELLSTRAND, C. M., BUSELMEIER, T. J., NAJARIAN, J. S.: Current practice of renal transplantation at the University of Minnesota. Minn. Med. **54**, 115—120 (1971).

SKARPA, M., UDALL, V.: Unpublished.

SKOPIŃSKA, E., SANKOWSKI, A., NOUZA, K.: Effect of azathioprine on the development of allograft sensitivity in mice. Bull. Acad. pol. Sci. Cl. 6 **17**, 85—88 (1969).

SMITH, J. L., FORBES, I. J.: Use of human lymphocytes in studies of drug action. Nature (Lond.) **215**, 538—539 (1967).

SMITH, J. L., FORBES, I. J.: Inhibition of protein synthesis in human lymphocytes by thiopurines. Aust. J. exp. Biol. med. Sci. **48**, 267—276 (1970).

SORENSEN, L. B.: Suppression of the shunt pathway in primary gout with azathioprine. Proc. nat. Acad. Sci. (Wash.) **55**, 571—575 (1966).

SPIEGELBERG, H. L., MIESCHER, P. A.: The effect of 6-mercaptopurine and aminopterin on experimental immune thyroiditis in guinea pigs. J. exp. Med. **118**, 869—890 (1963).

STARZL, T. E.: Experience in renal transplantation. Philadelphia: W. B. Saunders (1964).

STARZL, T. E., MARCHIORO, T. L., PORTER, K. A., TAYLOR, P. D., FARIS, T. D., HERMANN, T. J., HLAD, C. L., WADDELL, W. R.: Factors determining short- and long-term survival after orthotopic liver homotransplantation in the dog. Surgery **58**, 131—155 (1965).

STEVENS, J. E., WILLOUGHBY, D. A.: The anti-inflammatory effect of some immunosuppressive agents. J. Path. **97**, 367—373 (1969).

STINSON, E. B., BIEBER, C. P., GRIEPP, R. B., CLARK, D. A., SHUMWAY, N. E., REMINGTON, J. S.: Infectious complications after cardiac transplantation in man. Ann. intern. Med. **74**, 22—36 (1971).

STORTI, E., TRALDI, A., QUAGLINO, D.: Clinical studies on the effect of Imuran and vincristine in the treatment of leukemia. Acta Genet. med. (Roma) **17**, 220—231 (1968).

SUNDERMAN, C. R., PEARSON, H. A.: Growth effects of long-term antileukemic therapy. J. Pediat. **75**, 1058—1062 (1969).

SWANSON, M. A., SCHWARTZ, R. S.: Immunosuppressive therapy: the relation between clinical response and immunological competence. New Eng. J. Med. **277**, 163—170 (1967).

THIERSCH, J. B.: Effect of 6-(1′-methyl-4′-nitro-5′-imidazolyl)mercaptopurine and 2-amino-6-(1′-methyl-4′-nitro-5′-imidazolyl)mercaptopurine on the rat litter *in utero*. J. Reprod. Fertil. **4**, 297—302 (1962).

TRIPATHY, S. P., MACKANESS, G. B.: The effect of cytotoxic agents on the passive transfer of cell-mediated immunity. J. exp. Med. **130**, 17—30 (1969).

TUCHMANN-DUPLESSIS, H., MERCIER-PAROT, L.: Production de malformations des membres chez le Lapin par administration d'un antimétabolite: l'azathioprine. C. R. Acad. Sci. (Paris) **259**, 3648—3651 (1964).

TUCHMANN-DUPLESSIS, H., MERCIER-PAROT, L.: Considérations sur les tests tératogènes. Différences de réaction de trois espèces animales à l'égard d'un antitumoral. C. R. Soc. Biol. (Paris) **158**, 1984—1990 (1964a).

TUCHMANN-DUPLESSIS, H., MERCIER-PAROT, L.: Réactions provoquées chez l'embryon par deux antimétabolites chimiquement voisins. Bull. schweiz. Akad. med. Wiss. **22**, 153—165 (1966).

UDALL, V.: Unpublished.

UYEKI, E. M., LLACER, V.: Anti-tumour agents on antibody-forming cells *in vitro*. Biochem. Pharmacol. **19**, 2419—2424 (1970).

VAN VROONHOVEN, T. J., MALT, R. A.: Rebound hyperplasia of regenerating liver after cessation of azathioprine. Surg. Forum **22**, 339—340 (1971).

VAS, M., LOWENSTEIN, L.: The effect of prednisone and azathioprine in mixed leucocyte culture. In: Conference and workshop on histocompatibility testing, pp. 213—215. Baltimore: Williams and Wilkins 1965.

VINEGAR, R.: Unpublished.

VINEGAR, R., SCHREIBER, W., HUGO, R.: Inhibitory effects of immunosuppressive agents on adjuvant arthritis (AA) and delayed skin reactions (DSR). Pharmacologist **10**, 184 (1968).

VREDEVOE, D. L., HAYES, E. F.: Effect of antilymphocytic and antithymocytic sera on the development of mouse lymphoma. Cancer Res. **29**, 1685—1690 (1969).
WALFORD, R. L.: Generalizing biologic hypotheses and aging: an immunological approach. In: KROHN, P. L. (Ed.): Topics in biology of aging, pp. 163—169. New York: John Wiley and Sons 1966.
WALFORD, R. L.: Immunologische Aspekte des Alterns. Klin. Wschr. **47**, 599—605 (1969).
WILSON, D. B.: Quantitative studies on the behavior of sensitized lymphocytes *in vitro*. II. Inhibitory influence of the immune suppressor, Imuran, on the destructive reaction of sensitized lymphoid cells against homologous target cells. J. exp. Med. **122**, 167—172 (1965).
WORTH, W. S.: Azathioprine effect on normal canine liver and kidney function. Toxicol. appl. Pharmacol. **12**, 1—6 (1968).
ZWEIMAN, B., SILBERBERG, D. H.: *In vitro* lymphocyte responsiveness of human subjects receiving azathioprine. Int. Arch. Allergy **41**, 428—433 (1971).

Chapter 49

Purine Arabinosides, Xylosides, and Lyxosides

G. A. LePage

With 1 Figure

Introduction

Arabinosyluracil and arabinosylthymine were identified in extracts of the sponge, *Crytotethya crypta* (Bergmann and Burke, 1955), but arabinosylpurines were first obtained by chemical synthesis (Lee et al., 1960; Reist et al., 1962). Eventually one of these, arabinosyladenine, was found as an antibiotic in cultures of *Streptomyces antibioticus* (Parke-Davis and Company, 1967). A considerable number of arabinosylpurines have now been obtained, some with interesting biological properties. Their chemistry and a range of biological tests have received detailed discussion (Cohen, 1966; Suhadolnik, 1970). This discussion will be limited to those having most relevance to tumor and virus studies, and particularly to those on which an appreciable volume of data has accumulated. The structures of relevant arabinosylpurines are shown in Fig. 1.

9-β-D-ribofuranosyladenine (adenosine)

9-β-D-arabinofuranosyladenine (ara-A)

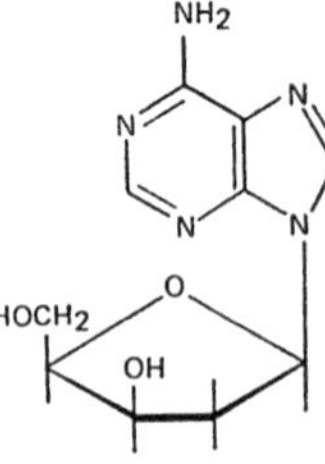

9-β-D-xylofuranosyladenine (xyl-A)

9-β-D-lyxofuranosyladenine (lyx-A)

9-β-D-arabinofuranosyl-6-mercaptopurine (ara-6-MP)

9-β-D-arabinofuranosylthioguanine (ara-TG)

Fig. 1

9-β-D-Arabinofuranosyladenine (Ara-A)

Synthesis of ara-A has been achieved by several approaches, the conversion of a xylonucleoside to ara-A (LEE et al., 1960; REIST et al., 1962), the condensation of tri-o-benzyl-D-arabinofuranosyl chloride with benzoyladenine (GLAUDEMANS and FLETCHER, 1968), and fermentation with *Streptomyces antibioticus* (PARKE-DAVIS and Company, 1967). All yield a β-nucleoside, and the fermentation procedure is probably now the most economical.

The biological effects of ara-A were first studied in a bacterial system (HUBERT-HABART and COHEN, 1961). Ara-A was deaminated to arabinosylhypoxanthine (ara-H) or converted to the nucleotide level. It killed bacterial cells, and the observed biochemical effects were the inhibition of DNA synthesis and incorporation of ara-A into terminal nucleosides of RNA.

Ara-A was found to be an inhibitor of several experimental tumors in mice (BRINK and LEPAGE, 1964a, b, 1965). Murine tissues also either converted ara-A to nucleotide forms, predominantly the 5'-triphosphate, or rapidly deaminated it. It was excreted in the urine as ara-H to the extent of 75 to 87 % of a therapeutic dose in 4 h. There appeared to be little or no cleavage to the free base by nucleoside phosphorylase. When ara-A labeled with ^{14}C was used, small amounts of ^{14}C appeared in the RNA-adenine and RNA-guanine. A later study showed that some cleavage and efficient reutilization of the base can explain this incorporation into RNA (LEPAGE, 1970). A study with crude extracts of a susceptible murine tumor indicated that the nucleotide, not ara-A as such, was the active form and that growth inhibition could be explained by the inhibition of DNA polymerase by ara-ATP (YORK and LEPAGE, 1966). A species difference appeared involved here, since ara-ATP did not inhibit the DNA polymerase obtained from *E. coli*. However, confirmation of the effect on mammalian DNA polymerase was obtained in a comparison of purified DNA polymerases from *E. coli*, calf thymus, and bovine lymphosarcoma (FURTH and COHEN, 1967). The mammalian DNA polymerases were inhibited, but that from *E. coli* was not, and the inhibition of DNA polymerase was demonstrated to be of the competitive type (FURTH and COHEN, 1968). In view of recent findings of several DNA polymerases of *E. coli*, this should perhaps be reexamined. Ara-A nucleotides were also shown to inhibit ribonucleoside diphosphate reductase from mammalian cells (FURTH and COHEN, 1968).

Since the active form of ara-A is ara-ATP, and ara-A can be converted in tissues either to ara-H by adenosine deaminase or to nucleotides by kinases, the relative amounts of these enzymes in a tissue would seem likely to govern the extent to which DNA synthesis, and therefore growth, would be inhibited. The mouse has a relatively high level of adenosine deaminase in red blood cells, higher than is the case for human erythrocytes. Inhibitors of this deamination were sought with some limited success (KOSHIURA and LEPAGE, 1968). It is not known which kinases are involved in the phosphorylation of ara-A to nucleotides. It has been established that deoxycytidine kinase phosphorylates arabinosylcytidine (MOMPARLER and FISCHER, 1968). By analogy, one might expect that deoxyadenosine kinase would phosphorylate ara-A; however, a purified deoxyadenosine kinase (KRYGIER and MOMPARLER, 1971) did not phosphorylate ara-A.[1] Nevertheless, crude extracts of calf thymus, the tissue used as the source of the purified deoxyadenosine kinase, showed a considerable capacity to phosphorylate ara-A.[2]

The earlier studies on murine ascites tumors indicated that those neoplasms with high levels of deaminase were resistant to ara-A. Tumors that had low or

1 Personal communication from Dr. R. L. MOMPARLER.
2 LEPAGE, G. A., SATO, J.: Unpublished results.

moderate levels of deaminase were responsive (Brink and LePage, 1964a, b). Some recent experiments[2] were conducted on mice bearing the 6C3HED lymphosarcoma (very low deaminase), Ehrlich carcinoma (moderate deaminase), and L1210 leukemia (very high deaminase), respectively. Groups of mice were injected i.p. with ara-A at 25 mg/kg and pulsed with tritiated thymidine for 30 min at intervals thereafter. DNA was isolated from each tumor sample and incorporation of tritium measured as an assay of DNA synthesis. All three tumors showed profound inhibition initially, but the L1210 cells recovered in 6 h, the Ehrlich cells in 8 h, and the 6C3HED cells had not recovered by 24 h. Thus, a sufficient level of ara-ATP for inhibition was achieved in all three, but decline to ineffective concentrations was more rapid in those cells with higher levels of activity of the degradative deaminase enzyme.

The utility of ara-A as an anticancer agent might be expected to derive from the situation in which normal cells are protected because of relatively high deaminase: kinase ratios and certain tumors with relatively low ratios would suffer a differential toxicity. Some data indicating wide variations in the deaminase: kinase ratios of human tumor cells have been obtained (LePage, 1969). Ratios of deamiase: kinase varied from 3.1 to 154. In a series of assays on peripheral leucocytes from leukemia patients[2], the ratios have varied from 7 to 2975. Such variations should surely result in considerable differences in susceptibility to ara-A.

Ara-A has shown considerable potential as an antiviral agent. Quite striking responses were obtained in the treatment of DNA virus infections in cell cultures, hamsters, and mice. The viruses showing responses included intracerebral infections with Herpes simplex and vaccinia. No such response was obtained in cell cultures infected with various RNA viruses (Miller et al., 1968a, b; Sidwell et al., 1968, 1969; Schardein and Sidwell, 1968; Sloan et al., 1968; Dixon et al., 1968).

Some toxicity tests have been conducted in mice and rabbits (Kurz et al., 1968). The LD_{50} for mice given a single i.p. dose of ara-A was 4677 mg/kg. No mortality occurred, however, at a dose of 7950 mg/kg given orally. When mice were given the drug orally at daily doses of 177 to 1532 mg/kg for 28 days, the most significant effect was a generalized weight loss. This effect was also seen when i.p. doses of 240 mg/kg/day were given mice for 6 days (Brink and LePage, 1964b). In this study a 25 % loss of body weight occurred and was regained by day 23. No repressive effect on the hemopoietic system was observed, in contrast to the action of other purine antimetabolites (Brink and LePage, 1964b). This was corroborated by the finding that immunity to viruses was developed normally in animals that received ara-A therapy and recovered (Sloan et al., 1968).

Ara-A has also shown some antimalarial activity (Ilan et al., 1970).

A preliminary study has been made on the distribution and excretion of ara-A in man. The half-time in blood was relatively short and reasonably comparable to that of ara-C (Ch'ien et al., 1971). There is every indication that clinical trials of ara-A as an antiviral and antitumor agent should be conducted.

9-β-D-Arabinofuranosylguanine (Ara-G)

This nucleoside was synthesized by a fusion of 2,6-dichloropurine with xylofuranose tetraacetate and inversion of the hydroxyls to yield the ara-G derivative (Reist and Goodman, 1964). A small sample was used for studies in an ascites tumor line (Brink and LePage, 1964a). At doses comparable to levels of ara-A that were effective as an antitumor agent, ara-G was less effective. The difficulty of obtaining a quantity of this nucleoside, and these discouraging preliminary results, have prevented a more detailed examination of its biological effects. A better synthesis has apparently now been obtained (LEE et al., 1971). It may, therefore, become possible to test ara-G at more adequate dosage levels.

9-β-D-Arabinofuranosylhypoxanthine (Ara-H)

This nucleoside is the product of metabolism of ara-A in bacteria (HUBERT-HABART and COHEN, 1962), in mice (BRINK and LEPAGE, 1964a, b), and in man (KOSHIURA and LEPAGE, 1968). A relatively low activity was ascribed to it in antiviral chemotherapy studies (SCHABEL, 1968). It seems likely that this activity results from a small amount of metabolic conversion to ara-A (LEPAGE, 1969).

9-β-D-Arabinofuranosyl-6-Mercaptopurine (Ara-6-MP)

Ara-6-MP was obtained by chemical synthesis (REIST et al., 1962). Although it is a purine nucleoside analog, the initial biological tests indicated that its only metabolic effect was on the incorporation of pyrimidine precursors into DNA-cytosine (KIMBALL et al., 1964). It was equally effective against 6-mercaptopurine (6-MP) sensitive and resistant lines of the Ehrlich carcinoma. Use of the radio-sulfur-labeled drug permitted the demonstration that it was rapidly excreted in the urine by mice (i.e., 75 % in 6 h). The material excreted was largely (88 %) unchanged ara-6-MP. Two minor metabolites were observed; however, no cleavage to 6-MP or conversion to nucleotide could be detected. Several murine tumors were completely eradicated by combining ara-6-MP with a low dose of the glutamine antagonists azaserine or diazonorleucine. Further studies (KIMBALL et al., 1966, 1967a) indicated that synergistic responses with these combinations were due to a "sequential block" of deoxypyrimidine nucleotide synthesis. The glutamine antagonists inhibited the conversion of uridylate to cytidylate, reducing the pools of cytidylate, and ara-6-MP inhibited the conversion of cytidylate to deoxycytidylate. There was no effect of ara-GMP on reduction of adenylate or guanylate by ribonucleoside diphosphate reductase. Relatively large and frequent dosages were required to inhibit the bone marrow of mice. A very large dose level (500 mg/kg) given to mice during the 9th to 11th day of pregnancy caused malformations of the fetuses, but smaller doses (250 mg/kg) did not. A correlation was obtained, in extracts of a limited spectrum of mouse tumor lines, between inhibition of the enzyme ribonucleoside diphosphate reductase and carcinostatic effects (LEPAGE, 1971). It was also shown that the ribonucleoside diphosphate reductase in extracts of 5 to 16 human tumor biopsies was significantly inhibited. It may, therefore, be speculated that ara-6-MP acts as an allosteric inhibitor of cytidylate reductase, and, thereby, produces an imbalance in the synthesis of precursors for DNA.

Ara-6-MP is unusual in that it is active as the nucleoside and is not converted to the nucleotide level (LEPAGE et al., 1969). In mice it is rapidly distributed and equilibrated in body water, even in the necrotic areas of tumors.[3] It was excreted in the urine at the same rate in mice, in dogs (LOO et al., 1970), and in man.[4] Some toxicological studies were conducted in dogs (HENRY, 1970) and the only toxic effects observed were a few instances of liver damage which apparently were not dose-dependent. Since ara-6-MP is immunosuppressive, these animals may have had activation of latent hepatitis. Phase I testing in man has involved doses as

3 LEPAGE, G. A.: Unpublished results.
4 Personal communication from Dr. T. L. LOO.

large as 6700 mg/M^2. This level, about 100 mg/kg, approximates carcinostatic doses in mice and produced no apparent toxicity in man.[5]

Ara-6-MP has been shown to have some unusual immunosuppressive effects. While it had no influence on the production of humoral antibodies in mice, it did prolong the survival of skin homografts, the latter assumed to be an effect upon the cellular immune response (Kimball et al., 1965, 1967b; Gisler and Bell, 1969a, b). Ara-6-MP also showed a protective effect against general anaphylaxis. A study of human lymphocytes in culture showed that ara-6-MP inhibited DNA synthesis in lymphocytes stimulated with mitogens, but did not influence the morphological events of blastogenesis (Hersh and LePage, 1971).

9-β-D-Arabinofuranosyl-6-Thioguanine (Ara-TG)

Ara-TG was obtained by chemical synthesis (Lee et al., 1971) and has been reported to have activity against the murine L1210 leukemia. Until this recent report, it was very difficult to synthesize, and investigations have apparently not yet proceeded any further.

9-β-D-Xylofuranosyladenine (Xyl-A)

Xyl-A has been synthesized chemically (Lee et al., 1963). It exhibited carcinostatic properties in the same experimental tumors as ara-A and was, like ara-A, deaminated by adenosine deaminase. The activity and catabolism of these two agents were, therefore, similar (Koshiura and LePage, 1968). However, unlike ara-A, xyl-A was inhibitory to both RNA and DNA synthesis. Xyl-A was readily converted to xyl-ATP and in this form was an inhibitor of the formation of 5-phosphoribosyl-1-pyrophosphate (PRPP). Since PRPP is required for the synthesis of purine and pyrimidine nucleotides, inhibition of its synthesis seems to explain the metabolic effects of xyl-A (Ellis and LePage, 1965a, b). Xyl-A was labeled in the base with radiocarbon for studies of its metabolism and distribution (Ellis and LePage, 1966). Murine tissues converted it to ara-H and this catabolite was rapidly excreted in the urine by mice. No indication was obtained for conversion of xyl-A to the free base. Like ara-A, it was not immunosuppressive, probably because the relatively high levels of adenosine deaminase present in the thymus, spleen, and bone marrow cells protect these tissues. Toxicity of xyl-A observed in mice was, as with ara-A, a general weight loss.

A report has appeared indicating that xyl-A may have antiviral effects. A saline solution or a cream containing xyl-A showed activity against experimental herpes virus infections in the eye and against herpes virus replication in cell cultures (Bossier et al., 1966).

It is conceivable that xyl-A might have utility against tumors having low levels of adenosine deaminase, as was suggested for ara-A. In addition, since it influences both RNA and DNA synthesis, it might, unlike ara-A, be capable of affecting tumor cells not in rapid growth. Preclinical toxicology and clinical testing have apparently not yet been initiated.

9-β-D-Xylofuranosyl-6-Mercaptopurine (Xyl-6-MP)

The chemical synthesis of xyl-6-MP has been described (Reist et al., 1971). Antitumor effects were observed in three experimental murine tumors, Sarcoma 180, the Ehrlich carcinoma, and the TA 3 adenocarcinoma (Sato et al., 1966).

5 Personal communication from Dr. E. Frei, III.

An additive antineoplastic response was observed in experimental tumors with combinations of xyl-6-MP and azaserine. Use of the radiosulfur labeled nucleoside showed that there was little or no cleavage of the nucleoside to 6-MP and little or no nucleotide formation was observed. Only traces of radioactivity were detected in nucleic acid or protein fractions. Excretion of xyl-6-MP in the urine was rapid, about 50 % in 3 h. Unchanged nucleoside and three minor metabolites were found on chromatography of the urine. Xyl-6-MP inhibited the utilization of guanine for nucleic acid synthesis, but did not interfere with guanine nucleotide formation *de novo* or with other reactions of nucleic acid or protein metabolism. No further reports have appeared on studies of xyl-6-MP.

9-β-D-Xylofuranosyl-6-Thioguanine (Xyl-TG)

Xyl-TG has been obtained by chemical synthesis (LEE et al., 1971). One limited report has appeared concerning its activity against experimental murine tumors (KANEKO and LEPAGE, 1970). In this study it appeared to have immunosuppressive effects and it prolonged the survival of tumor-bearing mice only when combined with azaserine. Xyl-TG was very rapidly excreted in the urine (88 % in 4 h), without any indication of metabolite formation. In addition, no nucleotide formation was detected in mouse tissues. Since its antineoplastic effects appeared marginal, studies were not pursued in any further depth.

9-β-D-Lyxofuranosyladenine (Lyx-A)

The chemical synthesis of lyx-A has been described (REIST et al., 1967). It was tested against the murine L1210 leukemia and showed only marginal effects. Murine tissues deaminated and phosphorylated it.[6] No further studies with this agent appear to have been reported.

9-β-D-Lyxofuranosyl-6-Mercaptopurine (Lyx-6-MP)

Lyx-6-MP has been chemically synthesized (REIST et al., 1967). A limited study with this agent was carried out in mice[7], including an investigation of distribution and excretion conducted with radiosulfur-labeled lyx-6-MP. Mice excreted lyx-6-MP in the urine very rapidly. Excretion was almost complete (95 %) in 3 h and almost all of the radioactivity was recovered as unchanged drug. The only tissue showing an appreciable accumulation was the kidney, and this might be expected because of the rapid excretion. Mice bearing the Ehrlich ascites carcinoma treated with lyx-6-MP at a dosage level of 40 mg/kg twice daily for 6 consecutive days showed a 56 % increase in survival time over untreated tumor-bearing controls. Groups of mice bearing the Ehrlich carcinoma treated simultaneously with azaserine and lyx-6-MP showed a synergistic response with some tumor-free survivors. No consistent effect could be detected upon the utilization of precursors of purines, pyrimidines, or proteins in Ehrlich tumor cells treated with lyx-6-MP. In view of the marginal effects and difficulties in synthesis, studies of lyx-6-MP have not been pursued further.

References

BERGMANN, W., BURKE, D. C.: Marine products. XXXIX. The nucleosides of sponges. III. Spongothymidine and spongouridine. J. org. Chem. **20**, 1501—1507 (1955).

6 LEPAGE, G. A.: Unpublished results.
7 MILTON, J. D., LEPAGE, G. A.: Unpublished results.

Boissier, J. R., Levine, P., DeRudder, J., Privat de Garilke, M.: Antiviral 9-β-D-xylofuranosyladenine. Societe Insturielle pour la Fabrication des Antibiotiques. Fr. M. 6164 (Cl A 61k, C 07D) 14 Aug. (1968). Appli. 13 Oct. 1966.
Brink, J. J., LePage, G. A.: Metabolic effects of 9-arabinosylpurines in ascites tumor cells. Cancer Res. **24**, 312—318 (1964a).
Brink, J. J., LePage, G. A.: Metabolism and distribution of 9-β-D-arabinosyladenine in mouse tissues. Cancer Res. **24**, 1042—1049 (1964b).
Brink, J. J., LePage, G. A.: 9-β-D-Arabinofuranosyladenine as an inhibitor of metabolism in normal and neoplastic cells. Canad. J. biochem. **43**, 1—15 (1965).
Ch'ien, L. T., Glazko, A. J., Buchanan, R. A., Alford, C. A.: Human metabolic disposition of 9-β-D-arabinofuranosyladenine (Ara-A). XI. Interscience Conf. on Antimicrob. Agents and Chemother. New York 1971.
Cohen, S. S.: Introduction to the biochemistry of D-arabinosyl nucleosides. In: Davidson, J. N., Cohn, W. E. (Eds.): Progress in nucleic acid research and molecular biology, pp. 1—83. New York: Academic Press 1966.
Dixon, G. J., Sidwell, R. W., Miller, F. A., Sloan, B. J.: Antiviral activity of 9-β-D-arabinofuranosyladenine. V. Activity against intracerebral vaccinia virus infections in mice. Antimicrob. Ag. Chemother. 172—179 (1968).
Ellis, D. B., LePage, G. A.: The effect of β-xylosyladenine on the formation of 5-phosphoribosyl-1-pyrophosphate by cell-free extracts of TA3 cells. Canad. J. Biochem. **43**, 617—619 (1965a).
Ellis, D. B., LePage, G. A.: Some inhibiting effects of 9-β-D-xylofuranosyladenine, an adenosine analog, on nucleotide metabolism in ascites tumor cells. Molec. Pharmacol. **1**, 231—238 (1965b).
Ellis, D. B., LePage, G. A.: Metabolic fate of 9-β-D-xylofuranosyladenine in mice bearing susceptible tumor cells. Cancer Res. **26**, 893—897 (1966).
Furth, J. J., Cohen, S. S.: Inhibition of mammalian DNA polymerase by the 5'-triphosphate of 9-β-D-arabinofuranosyladenine. Cancer Res. **27**, 1528—1533 (1967).
Furth, J. J., Cohen, S. S.: Inhibition of mammalian DNA polymerase by the 5'-triphosphate of 9-β-D-arabinofuranosylcytosine and the 5'-triphosphate of 9-β-D-arabinofuranosyladenine. Cancer Res. **28**, 2061—2067 (1968).
Gisler, R. H., Bell, J. P.: Studies on immunosuppression by purine nucleoside analogues. I. Effects on the immune response to sheep red blood cells in mice. Biochem. Pharmacol. **18**, 2115—2122 (1969a).
Gisler, R. H., Bell, J. P.: Studies on immunosuppression by purine nucleoside analogues. II. Effects on skin-graft rejection and immediate hypersensitivity in mice. Biochem. Pharmacol. **18**, 2123—2136 (1969b).
Glaudemans, C. P. J., Fletcher, H. J., Jr.: 9-β-D-Arabinofuranosyladenine (spongoadenosine). Direct synthesis of a *cis* nucleoside. In: Zorbach, W. W., Tipson, R. S. (Eds.): Synthetic procedures in nucleic acid chemistry, pp. 126—131. New York: Interscience Publishers 1968.
Henry, M. C.: Preclinical toxicology of NSC 406021 (Ara-6 MP). U. S. Gov't Res. Develop. Rep. **70**, 63—68 (1970).
Hersh, E. M., LePage, G. A.: The effect of arabinosyl-6-mercaptopurine on the *in vitro* blastogenic responses of human lymphocytes to mitogenic agents. Biochem. Pharmacol. **20**, 2459—2468 (1971).
Hubert-Habart, M., Cohen, S. S.: The toxicity of 9-β-D-arabinofuranosyladenine to purine-requiring *Escherichia coli*. Biochim. biophys. Acta. (Amst.) **59**, 468—471 (1962).
Ilan, Joseph, Tokuyasu, K., Ilan, Judith: Phosphorylation of D-arabinosyladenine by *Plasmodium berghei* and its partial protection of mice against malaria. Nature (Lond.) **228**, 1300—1301 (1970).
Kaneko, T., LePage, G. A.: Studies on β-D-xylofuranosyl-6-thioguanine in mice. Cancer Res. **30**, 699—701 (1970).
Kimball, A. P., Bowman, B., Bush, P. S., Herriot, J., LePage, G. A.: Inhibiting effects of the arabinosides of 6-mercaptopurine and cytosine on purine and pyrimidine metabolism. Cancer Res. **26**, 1327—1343 (1966).
Kimball, A. P., Herriot, S. J., Allinson, P. S.: Studies on immune suppressive drugs. Proc. Soc. exp. Biol. (N.Y.) **126**, 181—184 (1967b).
Kimball, A. P., LePage, G. A., Allinson, P. S.: Further studies on the metabolic effects of 9-β-D-arabinofuranosyl-9-H-purine-6-thiol. Cancer Res. **27**, 106—116 (1967a).
Kimball, A. P., LePage, G. A., Bowman, B.: The metabolism of 9-arabinosyl-6-mercaptopurine in normal and neoplastic tissues. Canad. J. Biochem. **42**, 1753—1768 (1964).
Kimball, A. P., LePage, G. A., Bowman, B., Herriot, S. J.: Suppression of the homograft response by purinethiol nucleosides. Proc. Soc. exp. Biol. (N.Y.) **119**, 248—252 (1965).

KOSHIURA, R., LEPAGE, G. A.: Some inhibitors of deamination of 9-β-D-arabinofuranosyladenine and 9-β-D-xylofuranosyladenine by blood and neoplasms of experimental animals and humans. Cancer Res. **28**, 1014—1020 (1968).
KRYGIER, V., MOMPARLER, R. L.: Mammalian deoxynucleoside kinases: II. Deoxyadenosine kinase: purification and properties. J. biol. Chem. **246**, 2745—2751 (1971).
KURTZ, S. M., FISKEN, R. A., KAUMP, D. H., SCHARDEIN, J. L.: Toxicity of 9-β-D-arabinofuranosyladenine in mice and rabbits. Antimicrob. Ag. Chemother. 180—189 (1968).
LEE, W. W., BENITEZ, A., GOODMAN, L., BAKER, B. R.: Potential anticancer agents. XL. Synthesis of the β-anomer of 9-(D-arabinofuranosyl)adenine. J. Amer. chem. Soc. **82**, 2648—2649 (1960).
LEE, W. W., MARTINEZ, A. P., BLACKFORD, R. W., BARTUSKA, V. J., REIST, E. J., GOODMAN, L.: Xylo- and arabinofuranosylthioguanine and related nucleosides derived from 2-acetamido-6-chloropurine. J. med. Chem. **14**, 819—823 (1971).
LEE, W. W., MARTINEZ, A. P., TONG, G. L., GOODMAN, L.: Simultaneous formation of both α- and β-nucleosides by the fusion method. Chem. Ind. (Lond.) **52**, 2007—2008 (1963).
LEPAGE, G. A.: Alterations in enzyme activity in tumors and the implications for chemotherapy. Adv. Enz. Regul. **8**, 323—332 (1969).
LEPAGE, G. A.: Arabinosyladenine and arabinosylhypoxanthine metabolism in murine tumor cells. Canad. J. Biochem. **48**, 75—78 (1970).
LEPAGE, G. A.: Studies with analogues of purine nucleosides. Prediction of response to cancer therapy. Nat. Cancer Inst. Monograph **34**, 184—187 (1971).
LEPAGE, G. A., BELL, J. P., WILSON, M. J.: Arabinosyl-6-mercaptopurine and arabinosyl-6-mercaptopurine-5'-phosphate: comparison of their metabolic effects. Proc. Soc. exp. Biol. (N. Y.) **131**, 1038—1041 (1969).
LOO, T. L., LU, K., RICHARDS, M. B., LEPAGE, G. A.: Pharmacologic disposition of arabinosyl-6-mercaptopurine and β-deoxythioguanosine in the dog. Pharmacologist **12**, 302 (1970).
MILLER, F. A., DIXON, G. J., EHRLICH, J., SLOAN, B. J., MCLEAN, J. W., JR.: Antiviral activity of 9-β-D-arabinofuranosyladenine. I. Cell culture studies. Antimicrob. Ag. Chemother. 136—147 (1968a).
MILLER, F. A., SLOAN, B. J., SILVERMAN, C. A.: Antiviral activity of 9-β-D-arabinofuranosyladenine. VI. Effects of delayed treatment on herpes simplex virus in mice. Antimicrob. Ag. Chemother. 192—195 (1968b).
MOMPARLER, R. L., FISCHER, G. A.: Mammalian deoxynucleoside kinases. I. Deoxycytidine kinase: purification, properties and kinetic studies with cytosine arabinoside. J. biol. Chem. **243**, 4298—4304 (1968).
Parke-Davis and Company, Belgian Pat. No. 671557 (1967).
REIST, E. J., BARTUSKA, V. J., GOODMAN, L.: Xylosyl-6-mercaptopurine. In preparation.
REIST, E. J., BENITEZ, A., GOODMAN, L., BAKER, B. R., LEE, W. W.: Potential anticancer agents. LXXVI. Synthesis of purine nucleosides of β-D-arabinofuranose. J. org. Chem. **27**, 3274—3279 (1962).
REIST, E. J., CALKINS, D. F., GOODMAN, L.: Purine nucleosides of β-D-lyxofuranose. J. org. Chem. **32**, 169—173 (1967).
REIST, E. J., GOODMAN, L.: Synthesis of 9-β-D-arabinofuranosylguanine. Biochemistry **3**, 15—18 (1964).
SATO, K., LEPAGE, G. A., KIMBALL, A. P.: The metabolism of 9-β-D-xylofuranosyl-6-mercaptopurine in normal and neoplastic tissues. Cancer Res. **26**, 741—747 (1966).
SCHABEL, F. M., JR.: The antiviral activity of 9-β-D-arabinofuranosyladenine. Chemotherapy **13**, 321—338 (1968).
SCHAREIN, J. L., SIDWELL, R. W.: Antiviral activity of 9-β-D-arabinofuranosyladenine. III. Reduction in evidence of encephalitis in treated herpes simplex-infected hamsters. Antimicrob. Ag. Chemother. 155—160 (1968).
SIDWELL, R. W., ARNETT, G., SCHABEL, F. M., JR.: Effects of 9-β-D-arabinofuranosyladenine on myxoma and pseudorabies viruses. Progr. Antimicrob. Anticancer Chemother., Proc. Int. Congr. Chemother. **2**, 44—48 (1969).
SIDWELL, R. W., DIXON, G. J., SCHABEL, F. M., JR., KAUMP, D. H.: Antiviral activity of 9-β-D-arabinofuranosyladenine. II. Activity against herpes simplex keratitis in hamsters. Antimicrob. Ag. Chemother. 148—154 (1968).
SLOAN, B. J., MILLER, F. A., EHRLICH, J., MCLEAN, W. J., JR.: Antiviral activity of 9-β-D-arabinofuranosyladenine. IV. Activity against intracerebral herpes simplex virus infections in mice. Antimicrob. Ag. Chemother. 161—171 (1968).
SUHADOLNIK, R. J.: Nucleoside antibiotics. 1st Ed. New York: Wiley-Interscience 1970.
YORK, J. L., LEPAGE, G. A.: A proposed mechanism for the action of 9-β-D-arabinofuranosyladenine as an inhibitor of the growth of some ascites cells. Canad. J. Biochem. **44**, 19—26 (1966).

Chapter 50

Antibiotics Resembling Adenosine: Tubercidin, Toyocamycin, Sangivamycin, Formycin, Psicofuranine, and Decoyinine

CHARLES A. NICHOL

With 3 Figures

Introduction

The antibiotics which resemble adenosine comprise a growing family of nucleosides with unique structures and diverse actions. Only selected members can be considered here, with emphasis on the relation of structure to metabolism and locus of action. As analogs of adenosine, these cytotoxic agents have useful application to studies exploring binding sites of adenine nucleotides and structural features of polynucleotide polymers. As more information emerges it will be feasible to classify these nucleosides, along with synthetic relatives, according to their sites of action. In this regard, a broad distinction can be made separating this family of adenosine related nucleosides from other nucleoside antibiotics, which bind at ribosomal sites to inhibit protein synthesis and which, like puromycin, bear substituents that classify them as analogs of aminoacyl-tRNA.

The nucleosides discussed in this chapter further illustrate that single modifications in either the base or the sugar confer remarkable changes in biological activity. Some of these are among the most potent cytotoxic agents known. Tubercidin preferentially enters anabolic pathways of adenosine and is compared with related pyrrolopyrimidine nucleosides, toyocamycin, and sangivamycin. Formycin represents an unusual C-C linkage of the base to the sugar. Comparison of formycin and tubercidin with the corresponding analogs of inosine indicates the importance of the amino group for cytotoxicity. Psicofuranine illustrates unusual specificity of binding as a nucleoside. Its action as an inhibitor of guanylic acid biosynthesis is shared by a closely related nucleoside, decoyinine, and an antibiotic of unrelated structure, mycophenolic acid.

Other members of this family of nucleoside antibiotics, which are not included in this chapter, have interesting structural features. Nucleocidin, 9-(4′-fluoro-5′-O-sulfamoylpentofuranosyl)adenosine, is the only antibiotic known to contain a fluoro sugar (MORTON et al., 1969). Its 5′-sulfamyloxy group confers resemblance to a nucleotide. Nucleocidin is the most potent trypanocidal agent known, but unfortunately has a small chemotherapeutic index (FLORINI et al., 1966; FLORINI, 1967). Aristeromycin is a unique analog of adenosine in which the oxygen bridge of ribose is replaced by a methylene group (KUSAKA et al., 1967; SHEALY and CLAYTON, 1969). Nebularine, 9-β-D-ribofuranosylpurine, is a cytotoxic antibiotic which is also found in certain mushrooms (FOX et al., 1966). Although lacking the 6-amino substituent, it is still a substrate for adenosine kinase. Several related antibiotics isolated from culture filtrates of *Cordyceps militaris* are analogs or derivatives of adenosine, i.e.l 3'-deoxyadenosine (cordycepin), 3'-amino-3'-deoxyadenosine, homocitrullyladenosine, and lysylaminoadenosine (SUHADOLNIK, 1970). The extensive work on the antiviral activity and mode of action of arabinosyladenine is included in a separate chapter in this volume (LEPAGE, Chapter 49). Characterization of naturally occurring analogs of adenosine such as spongosine (9-β-D-ribofuranosyl-2-methoxyadenine) isolated from sponges (BERGMAN and STEMPIEN, 1957; SCHAEFFER and THOMAS, 1958) and isopentenyladenosine which is found as a component of sRNA (ROBINS et al., 1967; LEONARD et al., 1968), has stimulated similar study of their metabolic actions and has led to synthesis of related compounds.

The capacity to synthesize an antibiotic is thought to confer some survival advantage, allowing the organism to maintain its ecological niche. Presumably, synthesis of a particular antibiotic persists because of its capacity to inhibit some vulnerable metabolic site. It is curious, therefore, that among these nucleoside antibiotics so many are structural and functional analogs of adenosine, whereas the corresponding analogs of guanosine are lacking. Since screening for antibiotics discloses agents of such diverse structure, the biological basis for this circumstance is open to speculation.

Most of these nucleoside antibiotics have shown pronounced anticancer activity in experimental studies; yet, for reasons of limited availability or because of technical problems, few have received adequate clinical evaluation. Among those that have entered clinical trials, some limiting toxicity was encountered with each, and none has emerged so far as a useful anticancer drug. Studies on their activity against bacteria, viruses, and parasitic organisms have encouraged further exploratory studies, but toxicity at low doses in experimental animals indicates limitations for any prolonged administration. Interest continues to grow in the synthesis of compounds containing some of their unique structural features. Indeed, the close interplay between the structural elucidation of antibiotics and synthesis of related nucleosides is indicated by awareness that arabinosyladenine, 3'-deoxyadenosine, and aristeromycin were synthesized and studied before they were characterized as antibiotics. Certainly, separate consideration of naturally occurring and synthetic nucleosides is an artificial distinction with regard to biochemical and chemotherapeutic studies. Work in each of these areas will continue to reinforce work in the other.

The literature concerning the discovery and structural elucidation of these compounds has also been covered in a comprehensive monograph by SUHADOLNIK (1970) and a review by FOX et al. (1966). No attempt is made in this brief presentation to list the full range of activities in biological and biochemical systems. Instead, the examples selected are discussed with regard to their potential for chemotherapy and their use as biochemical probes to disclose sites of action deserving further exploration.

Pyrrolopyrimidine Nucleosides: Tubercidin, Toyocamycin, and Sangivamycin

A. Common Pathway of Biosynthesis

The similar structure of these antibiotics suggests the likelihood that they share a common biosynthetic pathway (Fig. 1). By comparing the incorporation of adenine-2-^{14}C and adenine-8-^{14}C into toyocamycin produced by *S. rimosus*, UEMATSU and SUHADOLNIK (1970) obtained evidence that the pyrimidine ring, but not the 8-carbon, can serve as a precursor. When adenosine containing C^{14} in the ribose moiety was used, carbon atoms of the ribose contributed to the formation of the pyrrole ring of toyocamycin (SUHADOLNIK and UEMATSU, 1970). Experiments on the incorporation of precursors into tubercidin by *S. tubercidicus* gave evidence of a similar pathway (SMULSON and SUHADOLNIK, 1967). Thus, a mechanism involving opening of the imidazole ring followed by rearrangement of the ribose, in a manner similar to the synthesis of a pteridine from GTP (BROWN, 1972), seems feasible if both *N* 7 and *C* 8 of the purine nucleotide precursor can be removed (SUHADOLNIK, 1970). The enzymes involved in such cleavage and in the formation of the nitrile have not been studied. Evidence is available, however, that sangivamycin and toyocamycin are present in the same culture filtrates (SUHADOLNIK and UEMATSU, 1969) and rapid conversion of toyocamycin to sangivamycin occurs in cell-free extracts of *Streptomyces* (SUHADOLNIK, 1970).

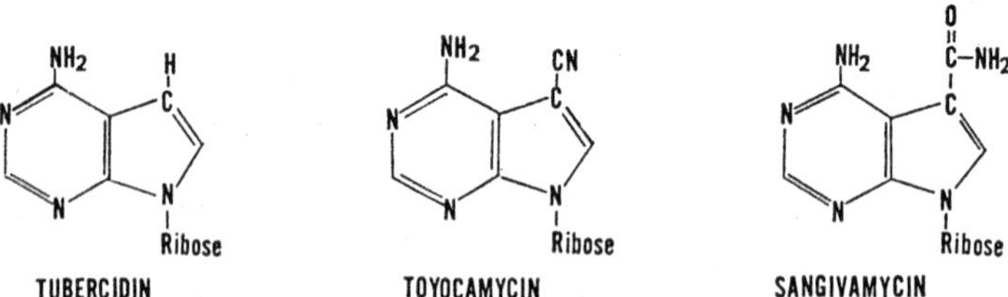

Fig. 1. 7-Deaza analogs of adenosine: tubercidin, 4-amino-7-(D-ribofuranosyl)-7*H*-pyrrolo-[2,3-*d*] pyrimidine; toyocamycin, 4-amino-5-cyano-7-(D-ribofuranosyl)-7*H*-pyrrolo-[2,3-*d*] pyrimidine; sangivamycin, 4-amino-5-carboxamide-7-(D-ribofuranosyl)-7*H*-pyrrolo-[2,3-*d*] pyrimidine

B. Tubercidin: An Anabolic Analog of Adenosine

The design of a compound able to enter anabolic pathways of adenosine and at the same time remain inert to degradative enzymes would be an arduous task by synthetic molecular manipulation alone. Yet these are the properties of this naturally occurring compound (BLOCH and NICHOL, 1964). Awareness that the aglycone of tubercidin, 4-aminopyrrolo[2,3-d]-pyrimidine, is biologically inactive causes one to question what heterocyclic bases among the many already synthesized for chemotherapeutic tests may have similar potential for activity if converted to the nucleoside form. The aglycone of tubercidin does not inhibit cultures of mammalian or bacterial cells. This can be attributed to lack of any activity as a substrate for AMP pyrophosphorylase or any metabolic conversion to a nucleotide (ACS et al., 1964; BLOCH et al., 1967).

The presence of a carbon atom replacing the 7-nitrogen of adenosine has marked effects on the stability of the glycosidic bond and on the properties of the amino group (FOX et al., 1966). Tubercidin is inert as a substrate for purified adenosine deaminase from intestinal mucosa. Also, adenosine phosphorylase in cell-free extracts of Sarcoma 180 has little or no effect on tubercidin under conditions that cleave adenosine completely within a few minutes (BLOCH et al., 1967). Replacement of the imidazole ring with a pyrrole ring still allows good substrate activity for adenosine kinase (SCHNEBLI et al., 1967; BLOCH et al., 1967). Conversion to the nucleotide is apparently essential for activity since tubercidin did not inhibit a line of mammalian cells that lacked adenosine kinase (BENNETT et al., 1966).

The evidence that tubercidin is incorporated into both RNA and DNA of mammalian and bacterial cells (ACS et al., 1964; BLOCK et al., 1967) indicates that this antibiotic can mimic adenosine as a substrate for many anabolic enzymes. Tubercidin readily enters erythrocytes and is rapidly converted to the triphosphate (SMITH et al., 1967; 1970). The conversion of adenosine to ATP by cell-free extracts of Sarcoma 180 is suppressed by the presence of tubercidin primarily by substrate competition for nucleoside diphosphokinase (BLOCH et al., 1967). When incubated under suitable conditions in the presence of nicotinamide mononucleotide and ATP, tubercidin monophosphate is incorporated into a diphosphopyridine nucleotide (BLOCH et al., 1967). Tubercidin triphosphate serves as a substrate for ribonucleotide reductase (SUHADOLNIK et al., 1968); this finding is consistent with the isolation of the deoxynucleotide of 7-deaza-adenosine from DNA (ACS et al., 1964; BLOCH et al., 1967). A dinucleoside monophosphate synthesized from tubercidin was readily cleaved by a nonspecific ribonuclease, but not by a ribonuclease which preferentially splits internucleotide bonds adjacent to the 3′-phosphate of adenosine residues (HASHIMOTO et al., 1970). A tubercidin polymer containing at least 100 nucleotide units was formed from tubercidin diphosphate by polynucleotide phosphorylase (IKEHARA and FUKUI, 1968). Tubercidin triphosphate and certain other nucleotide analogs can replace ATP as substrates for the DNA dependent RNA polymerase of Mengo virus infected cells (KAPULER et al., 1969). Polymers formed from this and related nucleotides have been examined with regard to structural and functional differences (URETSKY et al., 1968; WARD and REICH, 1969).

C. Biochemical Basis for the Cytotoxicity of Tubercidin

The critical metabolic site vulnerable to inhibition when cells are exposed to tubercidin is still an enigma. Attempting evaluation of available data discloses the dilemma that occurs when any antimetabolite enters anabolic pathways and is incorporated into macromolecules. In this case, tubercidin and its nucleotide metabolites are such good substitute substrates for enzymes involved in the anabolism of adenosine that it is difficult to relate the kinetics of reactions studied in cell-free systems to peculiar characteristics that might account for cytotoxicity. The various possibilities for which there is some experimental evidence include the following.

I. Feedback Inhibition of Purine Nucleotide Biosynthesis by Tubercidin Monophosphate

HENDERSON and KHOO (1965) presented evidence that the exposure of Ehrlich ascites tumor cells to tubercidin resulted in inhibition of PRPP biosynthesis. HILL and BENNETT (1969) extended previous studies of tubercidin as an inhibitor of purine nucleotide biosynthesis (BENNETT and SMITHERS, 1964) by using a partially purified phosphoribosyl pyrophosphate (PRPP) amidotransferase from adenocarcinoma 755 and found that tubercidin monophosphate was as active as AMP.

II. Impairment of Some Vital Function of ATP

As an energy source for the formation of aminoacyl-tRNA, tubercidin triphosphate could not replace ATP, whereas it could readily replace ATP as a substrate for the terminal tRNA pyrophosphorylase (URETSKY et al., 1968). The utilization of glucose by a bacterial suspension was impaired by tubercidin (BLOCH et al., 1967), but interference with glycolysis was not found in *S. mansoni* (ROSS and JAFFE, 1972). The possibility that tubercidin triphosphate interferes with some reaction critical for energy metabolism remains open for further exploration.

III. Formation of an Analog of Cyclic AMP

Tubercidin 3′,5′-cyclic phosphate was synthesized by DRUMMOND and POWELL (1970) and found to be slightly more active than cyclic AMP as an activator of phosphorylase b. It was also more active than cyclic AMP as a substrate for cyclic 3′,5′-nucleotide phosphodiesterase. By analogy with other enzymes, it is likely that tubercidin cyclic phosphate is formed in tissues following administration of the antibiotic, but direct evidence for this reaction is lacking at present. In view of the multiple binding sites for cyclic AMP in different tissues, the possibility that some of the hormonally mediated functions may be adversely affected by the analog deserves consideration.

IV. Impairment of Some Reaction Depending on NAD Cofactors

Following the observation that an NAD analog containing 7-deaza-adenine could be formed enzymatically (BLOCH et al., 1967), the chemical synthesis of this NAD analog was carried out using tubercidin monophosphate and nicotinamide mononucleotide. Instead of acting as an inhibitor, this dinucleotide replaced NAD as a cofactor for alcohol dehydrogenase (NICHOL, 1968). In this regard, other analogs of NAD derived from formycin and 2,6-diaminopurine were active as cofactors for several dehydrogenase enzymes (WARD et al., 1972). From the few enzymes studied so far, substitution rather than inhibition appears to be the pattern. Before concluding that interference in this manner is unlikely, however, biosynthetic reactions requiring NADP need to be examined.

V. Formation of Fraudulent Macromolecules that can Impede Protein or Nucleic Acid Synthesis

The incorporation of tubercidin and related nucleosides into tRNA, anticodon trinucleotides, mono and mixed polymers, as well as cellular and viral RNA and DNA, has enabled study of the structure and function of those macromolecules by sophisticated techniques, which can be mentioned only briefly here, with regard to potential sites of action. The objective is to explain the rapid inhibition of protein, RNA, and DNA synthesis following exposure of mammalian cells to tubercidin observed by ACS et al. (1964).

tRNA containing tubercidin phosphate in place of the terminal adenylate was synthesized by URETSKY et al. (1968) using a preparation of tRNA pyrophosphorylase. This analog of tRNA was able to esterify amino acids, and the aminoacyl-tRNA could function in the formation of peptide bonds although at a somewhat reduced rate. IKEHARA and OHTSUKA (1965) synthesized trinucleoside diphosphates containing tubercidin and observed that these served as templates for the binding of aminoacyl-tRNA to ribosomes. Polymers corresponding to poly-A and poly U-A containing 7-deaza-adenine in place of adenine functioned as templates for the enzymatic formation of polylysine (URETSKY et al., 1968). These observations make it doubtful that the incorporation of tubercidin would impair coding or peptide bond formation sufficiently to account for impaired protein synthesis *in vivo*.

The incorporation of an analog into DNA or some form of RNA with consequent impairment of some vital function could be related to the irreversible nature of tubercidin inhibition of mammalian cells. One observation that casts some doubt on the relation of such incorporation to cytotoxicity is the ability of bacterial cells, unlike mammalian cells, to continue growing, while incorporating substantial amounts of tubercidin into RNA and DNA (BLOCH et al., 1967). In a medium containing pyruvate, *S. faecalis* is insensitive to the presence of tubercidin, with the consequence that growth continues despite the continuing incorporation.

VI. Different Action of Tubercidin in Cells of Different Origin

Obtaining evidence concerning a metabolic site of action which might account for the cytotoxicity of tubercidin is rendered more difficult than in the case of psicofuranine, since supplementation of the culture medium for mammalian cells with any precursors, metabolites, or vitamin nutrients does not counteract its inhibition. Furthermore, renewal of growth does not occur upon transfer to drug-free medium of cells once exposed to the antibiotic (OWEN and SMITH, 1964; ACS et al., 1964).

In contrast, adenosine competitively prevents the inhibitory action of tubercidin on the growth of *S. faecalis* (BLOCH et al., 1967). Pursuing an explanation for this observation led to the finding that this is not a specific effect, but is shared by other nucleosides including uridine. This directed attention to the ribose moiety and pathways of carbohydrate utilization. Fermentative pathways present in microbial, but not in mammalian cells, allow the utilization of ribose-5-phosphate and pyruvate as an alternative to glycolysis for the generation of ATP. The preferential utilization of pyruvate rather than glucose in the presence of tubercidin implied that interference with glycolysis or some ATP-dependent reaction in energy metabolism may occur in bacteria (BLOCH et al., 1967). In studies of glucose consumption and lactate production by the parasite *Schistosoma mansoni*, the adverse effects of tubercidin could not be accounted for on the basis of inhibition of glucose uptake, phosphorylative glycolysis, or glycogen depletion (ROSS and JAFFE, 1972).

D. Comparison of Toyocamycin and Sangivamycin with Tubercidin

The cytotoxic potency of these pyrrolopyrimidine nucleosides against mammalian cells in culture is measured in the nanogram rather than the microgram concentration range. Both toyocamycin and sangivamycin are more active *in vitro* than tubercidin. The concentration in the medium producing 50 % inhibition of growth of murine and human cells was 6 ng per ml for tubercidin, 2 ng per ml for sangivamycin, and 0.5 ng per ml for toyocamycin. Inhibition of the growth of tumors in rodents was observed with daily doses in the range of 0.1 to 0.5 mg per kg of body weight. Based on the subacute LD_{50} doses, however, the chemotherapeutic index is small in each case (OWEN and SMITH, 1964; RAO, 1968).

Biochemical studies of each of these antibiotics indicate substantial similarity as anabolic analogs of adenosine. Comparison in many cases is difficult since reports concern individual antibiotics available to different investigators. Sangivamycin has been studied in only a few laboratories and toyocamycin was available to investigators who did not compare it to tubercidin. For instance, the observation that toyocamycin abolished the maturation of nucleolar ribosomal RNA into 28 and 18 S cytoplasmic ribosomal RNA, but allowed the synthesis of other RNA species, may represent the closest approach to the biochemical basis for cytotoxicity, which may be common to the other pyrrolopyrimidine antibiotics (TAVITIAN et al., 1969; MANTEUIL et al., 1970). Such selective inhibition could be attributed to some alteration in the structure of the nucleolar precursors. This area of study is of continuing interest since inhibition of RNA synthesis occurs to a greater extent than inhibition of protein or DNA synthesis. Also, such selective inhibition of RNA synthesis may have particular application in probing steps in the synthesis of RNA viruses. Treatment of chick embryo cultures with actinomycin D did not reveal any actinomycin-resistant RNA synthesis related to infection with avian leukosis virus; whereas, after treatment with toyocamycin, RNA synthesis in infected cells differed notably from that in noninfected cells (Riman et al., 1969). Also of interest in this regard is the report by Ehrman (1968) that in *Drosophila*, toyocamycin retards the formation of a cytoplasmic factor (virus or rickettsia), which causes maternally transmitted sterility of hybrid males.

The diphosphates and triphosphates of tubercidin, toyocamycin, and sangivamycin were used to study the substrate specificity and chemical requirements for binding at the regulatory site of ribonucleotide reductase from *L. leichmannii* and *E. coli* (Suhadolnik et al., 1968; Chassy and Suhadolnik, 1968). The triphosphate analogs served as substrates for the *L. leichmannii* enzyme, but the cyano group of toyocamycin triphosphate markedly decreased activity both as a substrate and as an allosteric activator. For the *E. coli* enzyme, which reduces the diphosphate nucleotides, replacement of the cyano group with the carboxamide group eliminated activity as a substrate. A number of analogs of 5′-AMP were used to characterize the allosteric AMP binding site of threonine dehydrase (Rabinowitz et al., 1968). The monophosphate forms of tubercidin, toyocamycin, and sangivamycin had essentially the same allosteric activity as AMP, indicating by these alterations in the imidazole ring that there is little binding function or steric restriction in that portion of the adenine. Thus, these analogs have proven to be useful in probing the dimensions of nucleotide binding sites.

E. Potential for Chemotherapy

The anticancer activity of each of these antibiotics against experimental tumors in rodents was sufficient to encourage clinical trials. In a Phase I study of sangivamycin, the major side effects of hypotension and flushing were reduced by slow infusion. The severe local reaction encountered with toyocamycin and tubercidin were not a problem with sangivamycin. The small number of cases and restricted range of tumor types prevented evaluation of antitumor effects of sangivamycin and no responses to treatment with total doses in the range of 0.1 to 2.8 mg/kg were observed among the 47 patients studied (Cavins et al., 1967). Although a Phase II study with larger doses was proposed, other agents with more favorable properties apparently displaced such trials. A Phase I study of toyocamycin disclosed side effects of hypotension and nephrotoxicity, and intravenous administration was restricted by severe local reaction and phlebitis. In a similar trial of tubercidin in 93 patients, nephrotoxicity was observed in 18 cases and venous thromboses proximal to sites of injection occurred in 12 cases (Bisel et al., 1970). Although this study was primarily for evaluation of dose range and side effects it is of interest that the 3 instances of a favorable effect were all on cases of primary pancreatic carcinoma among only 6 patients in this series with this type of tumor.

An unusual mode of administration was devised to circumvent the distressing problem of venous thrombosis and necrosis at the site of injection of tubercidin. Studies on the disposition in the body showed that tubercidin is rapidly taken up by the blood cells of different species. When tubercidin is added to animal or human blood *in vitro* it rapidly enters erythrocytes and is maintained there in nucleotide form, primarily as the triphosphate (Smith et al., 1970). Human blood cells are saturated with tubercidin at a concentration of 200 to 400 μg per ml of whole blood. Tubercidin is released from this reservoir over a long period of time and the half-life of the antibiotic loaded erythrocytes is not altered. When administered by rapid i.v. injection, 25 % of the dose appeared in dog urine within 24 h. When tubercidin was administered to the dog inside its own blood cells, 18 % of the dose was excreted in the urine in 21 days (SMITH et al., 1970).

The administration of tubercidin following its uptake into each patient's own erythrocytes *in vitro* proved to be quite feasible for a Phase I study. Whole blood, withdrawn by phlebotomy into sterile plastic bags containing EDTA, was incubated at 37° for 1 h with the appropriate amount of tubercidin introduced in sterile saline. The blood was then retransfused into the patient from the same vacutainer. The severe local reactions associated with direct intravenous injection were avoided. Drug toxicity in 45 patients (hematological depression in 6 patients and renal toxicity in 5 cases) receiving 200 to 1500 µg/kg at weekly intervals for two doses was infrequent, mild, and reversible (GRAGE et al., 1970).

This experience in the area of cancer chemotherapy may have important clinical application in the area of parasitic infections. Certain parasites apparently lack the metabolic capacity to synthesize purines *de novo* and are true parasites depending upon their hosts for preformed purines. *Schistosoma mansoni* feeds on red blood cells beginning about two weeks after the cercariae invade the host. Since tubercidin was found to be the most active purine analog tested *in vitro*, JAFFE et al. (1971) used the technique of absorption into red cells to test the activity of tubercidin on *S. mansoni* infected mice. The marked effect on viability and egg-laying capacity of schistosomes in all of the treated mice encouraged further evaluation of the efficacy of tubercidin. This selective administration based on the eating habits of schistosomes may exploit their metabolic dependence on preformed purines. These studies illustrate productive liaison between two different areas in the field of chemotherapy.

Formycin

The detection and isolation of formycin was based on screening for activity against Yoshida rat sarcoma cells (HORI et al., 1964). This highly cytoxic nucleoside was subsequently found to inhibit viruses, fungi, bacteria, and experimental tumors. Formycin appeared in culture broths at early stages of fermentation, but was replaced gradually by another antibiotic, laurusin, which was found to be identical with formycin B (AIZAWA et al., 1965; OTAKE et al., 1965). Both formycin and formycin B were very effective inhibitors of *Xanthomonas oryzae* which infects the rice plant and therefore are of economic importance in Japan (KOYAMA and UMEZAWA, 1965), but formycin B was less effective or inactive in most biological tests (ISHIZUKA et al., 1968).

Formycin can be viewed as an analog of adenosine in which the *C* 8 and *N* 9 have been interchanged (Fig. 2). Although this change retains close structural similarity, the increased length of the C-C glycosyl bond in formycin compared with the C-N bond in adenosine seems to facilitate freedom of rotation. The interaction between atoms of the furanose ring with the hydrogen of *C* 8 of adenosine, which provides one of the major rotational barriers for purine nucleosides (HASCHEMEYER and RICH, 1967), is absent in formycin. Thus, the conformational transitions, which can occur in polynucleotide polymers containing formycin residues, are of particular interest (WARD and REICH, 1968; WARD et al., 1969a, b). The occurrence of other carbon linked nucleosides as natural products is illustrated by the structure of showdomycin (3-β-D-ribofuranosylmaleimide) which can be considered to be a structural relative of pseudouridine (TOWNSEND and ROBINS, 1969).

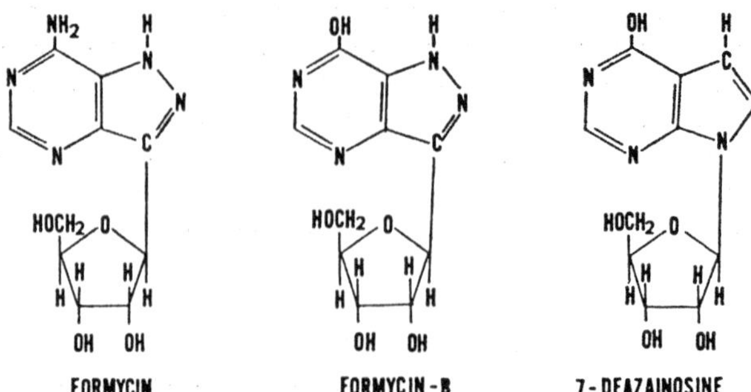

Fig. 2. Formycin, a *C*-glycoside analog of adenosine and two analogs of inosine; formycin, 7-amino-3-(β-D-ribofuranosyl)-pyrazolo [4,3-*d*] pyrimidine; formycin B, 7-hydroxy-3-(β-D-ribofuranosyl)-pyrazolo [4,3-*d*] pyrimidine; 7-deazainosine, 4-hydroxy-7-(β-D-ribofuranosyl)-7*H*-pyrrolo [2,3-*d*] pyrimidine

A. Enzymatic Studies

Formycin is another anabolic analog of adenosine and its nucleotides are readily accepted in place of adenine nucleotides by most enzymes studied so far. As in the case of tubercidin, the diverse enzymatic studies provide no clear understanding of the cytotoxicity or antiviral action of formycin. Thus, to explain the remarkable activity of this antibiotic is still a challenging problem.

Formycin is rapidly converted to phosphorylated derivatives by tumor cells *in vitro* in concentrations approaching those of adenosine phosphates. In the presence of an adequate energy supply, the 5'-triphosphate is the major metabolite (CALDWELL et al., 1969). Conversion to the nucleotide is necessary for the expression of antitumor effects, since a tumor subline known to be deficient in adenosine kinase was not inhibited by formycin (CALDWELL et al., 1969) and feedback inhibition of purine nucleotide biosynthesis did not occur in cells unable to phosphorylate formycin (HENDERSON et al., 1967). Formycin-5'-phosphate is readily formed in the presence of partially purified preparations of mammalian adenosine kinase (SCHNEBLI et al., 1967; LINDBERG, 1969). As with other active nucleotides, some inhibition of nucleotide synthesis from guanine and hypoxanthine, interference with conversion to adenine nucleotides, and inhibition of nucleic acid synthesis occurs in intact cells exposed to formycin (HENDERSON et al., 1967). ATP concentrations are the same in control and formycin-treated cells (CALDWELL et al., 1969) and formycin does not inhibit glycolysis in tumor cells (HORI et al., 1964). Consequently, it is unlikely that the cytotoxicity of formycin can be associated with any impairment of energy metabolism.

In a comprehensive biochemical study, WARD et al. (1969c) observed that formycin and its derivatives substituted effectively for the corresponding adenosine substrates of various enzymes of nucleotide metabolism including hexokinase, myokinase, and phosphoenolpyruvate kinase. With RNA polymerase, aminoacyl-tRNA synthetase, and polynucleotide phosphorylase, the affinities of the formycin nucleotides closely approximated those of the adenine nucleotides. tRNA molecules bearing formycin nucleoside termini are readily aminoacylated and efficiently transfer amino acids into polypeptides. Formycin triphosphate is the first nucleotide analog containing an abnormal base that can substitute for ATP with aminoacyl-tRNA synthetase. For two reactions, however, differences were observed.

Formycin triphosphate could not substitute for ATP in NAD synthetase from yeast, and formycin triphosphate did not serve efficiently as a substrate for homopolymer synthesis by RNA polymerase (WARD et al., 1969c). Formycin triphosphate was used as a substrate by DNA dependent RNA polymerase and could replace ATP when DNA from calf thymus, salmon sperm, or *E. coli* was used as a template. The rate of synthesis of formycin-containing RNA, however, was 47 to 68 % of that for the formation of RNA from natural nucleoside triphosphates (IKEHARA et al., 1968).

B. Biopolymers Containing Formycin

Certain properties of formycin facilitate study of polymers containing this nucleoside. Its ultraviolet absorption maximum is appreciably different from those of the normal nucleic acid constituents, thus allowing absorption and optical rotatory dispersion measurements even in the presence of a large excess of the normal bases (WARD and REICH, 1968). Also, formycin and its derivatives fluoresce at neutral pH, thus providing a parameter useful for measurement of physical properties and enzyme substrate interactions (WARD et al., 1969). In addition to obtaining information basic to understanding the relation between structure and function of macromolecules, the study of polymers containing formycin may shed some light on the role of another *C*-ribosyl nucleoside, pseudouridine.

In an extensive study of the relationship between nucleoside conformation and biological activity, formycin polymers were particularly useful (WARD and REICH, 1968, 1969; WARD et al., 1969a, b, c). Attention was directed to several paradoxical characteristics of formycin polynucleotides that are related to the presence of repeating sequences of formycin residues in polymers. (1) The synthesis of the homopolymer, poly F, proceeds poorly and the efficient utilization of formycin nucleotides by RNA polymerase and polynucleotide phosphorylase is dependent on the concurrent polymerization of other nucleotides. (2) Random copolymers containing a mixture of formycin and normal nucleotides code quite efficiently for polypeptide synthesis *in vitro* and their coding properties are indistinguishable from the corresponding polymers that contain adenosine, yet, in contrast to poly A, poly F fails to direct the synthesis *in vitro* of polylysine. (3) Poly F is readily degraded by pancreatic ribonuclease, but is highly resistant to degradation by nonspecific nucleases such as micrococcal nuclease and the phosphodiesterases of spleen and rattlesnake venom, whereas the converse is true for poly-A.

A variety of different techniques was used to study these polymers containing formycin. The thermal denaturation profile and the ultraviolet absorption and fluorescence spectra indicated that poly F is single-stranded at neutral pH and suggested that formycin residues can exist in different conformations depending on the proportion of formycin residues, the base sequence, and the degree of strandedness of the polymers. The biochemical anomalies were related to repeating sequences of formycin residues in the single stranded state, which can exist in an abnormal conformation because of the glycosyl bond. By drawing together considerations based on structural studies, substrate specificity of pancreatic ribonuclease, and model building, WARD and REICH (1968, 1969) and WARD et al. (1969b) concluded that formycin residues in polynucleotides are *anti* in ordered double-stranded structures of the Watson-Crick type, *syn* in neutral poly-F, and probably a mixture of *syn* and *anti* in single stranded copolymers. Thus, the extent of incorporation of formycin into nucleic acids may be a factor in the expression of its biological activity. Incorporation of other analogs into polynucleotides conferred properties related to their existence in the *syn* conformation.

The template activities of ribopolynucleotides containing formycin for the binding of tRNA to ribosomes and for polypeptide synthesizing systems were studied by IKEHARA et al. (1969). The nature of RNA as the messenger did not change greatly and the polypeptides formed had the exact amino acid sequences as expected from the regular codon.

C. Potential for Chemotherapy

As an anticancer agent, the potential of formycin is limited by its extensive deamination *in vivo*. As an immunosuppressive agent, formycin is active in contrast to formycin B (OKADA et al., 1969). As an antiviral agent, formycin has displayed substantial activity against vaccinia, polio, and influenza viruses *in vitro* in cultures of HeLa and chick embryo cells (ISHIDA et al., 1967a, b). In particular, the equal activity of formycin and formycin B against influenza A_1 virus grown on chorioallantoic membrane is noteworthy in relation to the lower toxicity of formycin B in animals (TAKEUCHI et al., 1967). Since both antibiotics inhibited viral multiplication, an important question is whether they act in a similar manner to inhibit viruses, yet differ so markedly in cytotoxic activity.

Inosine Analogs: Formycin B and 7-Deazainosine

Two analogs of inosine (Fig. 2) can be obtained by deamination of formycin (UMEZAWA et al., 1965; TOWNSEND and ROBINS, 1969) and tubercidin (MIZUNO et al., 1963; BLOCH et al., 1969). Their availability permits comparison of biochemical and biological activities related to the functional amino group of the adenosine analogs. Metabolic deamination of formycin occurs readily. In contrast, 7-deazainosine is not a direct metabolic product of tubercidin. Deazainosinate may be derived, however, from tubercidin-5′-phosphate by the action of adenylate deaminase (BLOCH et al., 1967) which apparently differs considerably from adenosine deaminase with regard to the structural requirements of the base. The extent to which metabolic amination of both inosine analogs can occur, however, presumably via the adenylosuccinase pathway, is of considerable importance. The occurrence of this amination in different organisms and tissues infers potential for selective cytotoxicity.

A. Formycin B

Formycin is rapidly deaminated to the corresponding inosine analog, formycin B, when incubated with microorganisms (SAWA et al., 1967b) or with tumor cells (CALDWELL et al., 1969). Hepatic aldehyde oxidase oxidizes formycin B to the corresponding xanthine analog, oxoformycin B (ISHIZUKA et al., 1968a, b; TSUKADA et al., 1969; SHEEN et al., 1970). In the presence of coformycin, a compound isolated from culture filtrates along with formycin, the activity of formycin as an inhibitor of *E. coli* and mammalian cells *in vitro* was greatly increased (SAWA et al., 1967a, b). This effect is attributed to the inhibition of adenosine deaminase by coformycin ($K_i = 6.5 \times 10^{-8}$ M) (UMEZAWA et al., 1967). Thus, deamination can be considered an inactivation reaction. Although the inosine analog retains activity against *X. oryzae* (AIZAWA et al., 1965) and has some antiviral activity against influenza virus (TAKEUCHI et al., 1967; KUNIMOTO et al., 1968), it has little cytotoxicity for bacteria, fungi, or mammalian cells (UMEZAWA et al., 1965).

Only few microorganisms have the capacity to aminate formycin B. SAWA et al. (1968) reported that cells of *Nocardia interforma* can convert formycin B to formycin and found that the monophosphate form of each antibiotic was present in these cells. In other studies, however, factors other than amination seemed to account for the inhibition of *X. oryzae* by formycin B. Formycin B interferes with the entry of exogenous nucleosides into these cells and the inhibitory action can be prevented by adding purine and pyrimidine nucleosides to the medium (HORI et al., 1968). The report by TAKEUCHI et al. (1967) that formycin B is as active as formycin against influenza A_1 virus *in vitro* is also of particular interest, since formycin B does not inhibit the growth of mammalian cells. The biochemical basis for this selectivity of action has not been disclosed. Formycin also inhibits multiplication of tobacco mosaic virus, and its effect on leaf lesions was prevented by adenine, but not by hypoxanthine (TEZUKA and TOKUZO, 1969).

In contrast to the potency of formycin as an inhibitor of purine nucleotide biosynthesis by tumor cells, formycin B was inactive (HENDERSON et al., 1967). This may be related to its lack of activity as a substrate for inosine kinase in mammalian cells (SHEEN et al., 1970). Formycin B is a competitive inhibitor ($K_i = 1 \times 10^{-4}$ M) of purified erythrocyte purine nucleoside phosphorylase (SHEEN et al., 1968). These authors suggested that formycin B might be used to increase the antitumor activity of other nucleoside analogs which may be inactivated by phosphorolysis.

B. 7-Deazainosine

A striking difference between deazainosine and tubercidin was observed by SMITH et al. (1970) when these compounds were incubated with whole human blood. Their data suggest that tubercidin will be present in the body primarily inside the blood cells, whereas deazainosine will be distributed primarily in the plasma. In dogs, only 0.25 % of the tubercidin injected i.v. is excreted in the urine within 24 h in contrast to 25 % of a similar dose of deazainosine within the same period (SMITH et al., 1967). Differences between the toxicological effects of tubercidin and deazainosine implied that conversion of the latter compound into anabolites of tubercidin was required to exert biological effects (NICHOL et al., 1967; MIHICH et al., 1969). Severe local and renal toxicity occurred in dogs treated with tubercidin, but not with deazainosine. On the other hand, liver toxicity was a major toxic effect of deazainosine treatment. Thus, there is the likelihood that metabolic activation contributed to the localization of toxicity. In this regard it is noteworthy that tubercidin was 6- to 20-fold more toxic than deazainosine in rodents and dogs (MIHICH et al., 1969).

Experimental tumors not inhibited by tubercidin were not affected by deazainosine and the difference in relative potency against responsive tumors was consistently 1:16 (BLOCH et al., 1969). The relatively weak activity of deazainosine as a competitive inhibitor of inosine phosphorylase does not appear to be sufficient to account for its cytotoxicity (BLOCH et al., 1969). Tubercidin is a potent inhibitor of bacterial *(S. faecalis)* and mammalian (Sarcoma 180) cells. In contrast, deazainosine is inert as an inhibitor of *S. faecalis*, but is only slightly less active than tubercidin as an inhibitor of Sarcoma 180 cells *in vitro*. This differential inhibition is correlated with the observation that deazainosinate and tubercidin nucleotides were formed from deazainosine by the mammalian cells, but not by these bacterial cells (BLOCH et al., 1969). Thus, there is the prospect that deazainosine may be inactive *per se* and represent a latent drug which can be activated selectively in cells containing inosine kinase (PIERRE and LEPAGE, 1968) and the capacity to aminate this nucleotide.

Psicofuranine, Decoyinine, and Mycophenolic Acid

In contrast to the other nucleoside analogs discussed in this chapter, the locus of action of these antibiotics is relatively well-defined. They share ability to inhibit the biosynthesis of guanylic acid from inosinic acid. Psicofuranine and decoyinine are active as nucleosides and are not dependent on metabolic conversion to the corresponding nucleotides. Substantial evidence now indicates that the cellular pools of guanylate nucleotides are considerably smaller than those of the other nucleotides and the amount of dGTP is sufficient to sustain DNA synthesis for only a brief period unless the supply is renewed (SKOOG, 1970; REICHARD, 1972). Thus, it is likely that impairment of guanylate synthesis to even a slight extent by these antibiotics may adversely affect growth and survival of cells with limited ability to supply this essential precursor by the salvage pathway.

Mycophenolic acid is included in this section because of its function rather than its structure. Lacking either nitrogen or any sugar moiety, it bears little resemblance to a nucleoside. When a space-filling molecular model of mycophenolic acid is oriented so that the plane of the ring corresponds to the purine ring of inosine or guanosine, then it can be readily seen that the unsaturated side chain can occupy positions where contact points or sites of potential binding closely duplicate those of the nucleoside ribose. Consideration of the structure and action of mycophenolic acid infers that our concept of inhibitors capable of binding at nucleotide substrate or allosteric sites need not be restricted to structures closely analogous to natural nucleotides. Further study of this antibiotic may yield more precise information concerning the interatomic distances between functional groups on the enzyme receptor essential for binding of nucleotides.

A. Rediscovered Antibiotics

It is not uncommon for an antibiotic to be isolated from the medium of a new organism and then to find that it has the same structure as one already described. A phenolic antibiotic was first observed in a *Penicillium* corn mold in 1896, and although named mycophenolic acid in 1913, it was not characterized until 1952 (BIRKINSHAW et al., 1952) as a product of *Penicillium brevi-compactum*. This compound was of less interest than other antibiotics when its antibacterial and antifungal activities were studied during the 1940's. The antiviral activity of beers of *P. stoloniferum* renewed interest in mycophenolic acid (WILLIAMS et al., 1968a). Also, the evaluation of the anticancer activity of mycophenolic acid proceeded independently at the same time in laboratories in the United States and England (WILLIAMS et al., 1968b; CARTER et al., 1969). Of particular interest was the spectrum of its anticancer activity against several solid experimental tumors, but not against murine leukemias (WILLIAMS et al., 1968; SWEENEY et al., 1972). Mycophenolic acid and numerous derivatives have been synthesized (BIRCH and WRIGHT, 1969). Although sixty-five analogs were obtained by modifying all positions of the molecule except *C*-1, none were as effective as mycophenolic acid in suppressing cell division of mouse fibroblast cultures (JONES and MILLS, 1971). Thus, chemical modification of the parent structure has not so far improved on the natural selection of this highly active unique compound.

Psicofuranine and decoyinine were isolated and named in this country in 1959 (SCHROEDER and HOEKSEMA, 1959) and 1964 (HOEKSEMA et al., 1964), respectively. When characterized, it became clear that they were the same as two antibiotics isolated in Japan in 1954 (YUNSTEN et al., 1954) and 1956 (YUNSTEN et al., 1956) called Angustmycin C (psicofuranine) and Angustmycin A (decoyinine). The more recent names are used here to be consistent with the nomenclature applied in many of the reported biological and biochemical studies. The names of these antibiotics are derived from the sugar, psicose, and from the name of the variety of streptomycin used for the fermentation, *decoyicus* in the United States and *angustmyceticus* in Japan (Fig. 3).

Psicofuranine and decoyinine occur together in the fermentation broth of *S. hygroscopicus* var. *decoyicus* and their close structural similarity indicated the probability that one could serve as the precursor of the other. During fermentation the interconversion of psicofuranine and decoyinine can occur (HOEKSEMA et al., 1964; CHASSY et al., 1966). Also, as part of the total chemical synthesis of decoyinine, psicofuranine was converted to decoyinine (McCARTHY et al., 1968).

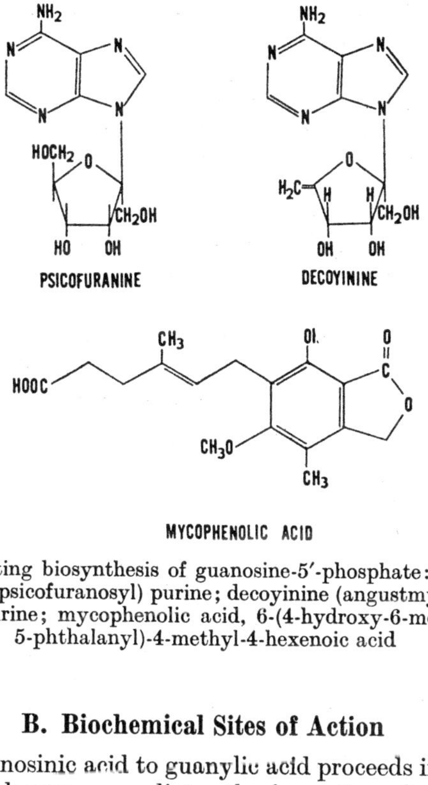

PSICOFURANINE

DECOYININE

MYCOPHENOLIC ACID

Fig. 3. Antibiotics inhibiting biosynthesis of guanosine-5′-phosphate: psicofuranine (angustmycin C) 6-amino-9-(β-D-psicofuranosyl) purine; decoyinine (angustmycin A) 6-amino-9-(β-D-5,6-psicofuranoseenyl) purine; mycophenolic acid, 6-(4-hydroxy-6-methoxy-7-methyl-3-oxo-5-phthalanyl)-4-methyl-4-hexenoic acid

B. Biochemical Sites of Action

The conversion of inosinic acid to guanylic acid proceeds in a two step process. (1) Inosinic acid dehydrogenase mediates the formation of xanthylic acid by an oxidation reaction requiring NAD as a cofactor. (2) The conversion of xanthylic acid to guanylic acid by xanthosine 5′-phosphate aminase proceeds by an ATP dependent amination reaction in which either glutamine or ammonia will serve as amine donor depending upon the species. The kinetics of the reaction and the affinity of the cofactor are influenced by the concentration and sequence of binding of the components.

The identification of the similar site of metabolic inhibition of psicofuranine, decoyinine, and mycophenolic acid was facilitated by identifying guanine and guanosine as metabolites which prevented their growth inhibitory effects on cultures of bacterial or mammalian cells. This does not infer that they occupy the same binding site. The evidence supports the interpretation, however, that impairment of guanylic acid synthesis is the locus of action involved in inhibition of growth since the availability of products of this metabolic pathway allows growth to proceed in the presence of these antibiotics.

I. Psicofuranine

The presence of a hydroxymethyl group on the ribose C-1 of adenosine is tolerated with regard to cleavage of the adjoining glycosidic bond, but markedly affects deamination at the 6 position of the purine and the addition of phosphate at the C-5 of the ribose. Nucleoside phosphorylase from Ehrlich ascites mouse tumor cells can cleave psicofuranine (LEPAGE and JUNGA, 1965) and D-psicose was identified in the urine of patients receiving psicofuranine (STRECKER et al., 1965). Psicofuranine is inactive as a substrate for adenosine deaminase from intestinal mucosa (BLOCH and NICHOL, 1964; CORY and SUHADOLNIK, 1965). Also, it is not a substrate for adenosine kinase from rat liver or mouse tumor cells (LINDBERG et al., 1967; SHIGEURA and SAMPSON, 1967).

Based on microbial inhibition of *S. aureus* by psicofuranine in the presence of natural purines, pyrimidines, and nucleosides, HANKA (1960) concluded that psicofuranine interfered primarily with the biosynthesis of GMP from XMP. The same interpretation was made by SLECHTA (1960a) using *E. coli*. In addition, xanthosine accumulated in the culture filtrates of *E. coli* grown in the presence of psicofuranine, and SLECHTA (1960b) found that xanthosine aminase was inhibited by psicofuranine in cell-free preparations.

Psicofuranine has proven to be quite useful in studies of the reaction mechanism and regulation of XMP aminase which is described by the equation:

$$\begin{gathered}\text{Xanthylic acid} + \text{ATP} + \text{glutamine} (NH_3) + H_2O \\ \rightarrow \text{Guanylic acid} + \text{AMP} + \text{PPi} + \text{glutamate}\end{gathered}$$

Most of the biochemical studies have been done using the ammonia requiring enzyme of *E. coli*, and there is relatively little information concerning the glutamine requiring reaction in mammalian tissues. MOYED and coworkers, in particular, have conducted extensive biochemical studies of changes in the behavior of this enzyme which might account for resistance to psicofuranine acquired by *E. coli*. The synthesis of both IMP dehydrogenase and XMP aminase is controlled by a feedback mechanism related to the supply of GMP (MOYED, 1961). Unlike the usual regulatory enzyme, this aminase is at the end rather than the beginning of a biosynthetic sequence, and its kinetic properties differ from those of typical end-product sensitive enzymes. Mutations decreasing XMP aminase sensitivity to adenine glycosides are frequently accompanied by decreased levels of aminase activity (DONOVAN et al., 1967). There is evidence that adenosine takes part in the regulation of XMP aminase and that psicofuranine binds at this regulatory site. The activity of XMP aminase from an adenosine sensitive mutant of *Bacillus subtilis* was strongly inhibited by either psicofuranine or adenosine, while the enzymes from the resistant and parent strains were little affected by either of these adenine glycosides (KIDA et al., 1969).

The catalytic properties of XMP aminase and its sensitivity to inhibition could be altered by chemical modification of the adenine glycoside site (KURAMITSU and MOYED, 1966). Photooxidation in the presence of methylene blue reduces the binding of psicofuranine without causing corresponding reduction in the binding of the substrates. Also, the binding of psicofuranine to a mercaptoethanol-treated aminase is undiminished, yet the enzyme is much less sensitive to its inhibitory effects. Thus, the adenine glycoside binding site is separate from the active center of the enzyme, which is in keeping with the kinetic description of the primary interaction of psicofuranine with the aminase as a noncompetitive process (UDAKA and MOYED, 1963; FUKUYAMA and MOYED, 1964). The inhibition of XMP aminase by psicofuranine depended upon the presence of the substrate, XMP, and one of the products, inorganic pyrophosphate. The interpretation of the nature of the inhibition as irreversible has been modified by the observation that a reversible change in the conformation of the enzyme is associated with the binding of XMP and that this response is greatly enhanced by the presence of PPi and magnesium ions (ZYK et al., 1969). The change in conformation is indicated by resistance to inactivation by heat or hydrolysis by proteolytic enzymes. This normal change in conformation was found to be essential for the reversible interaction of the enzyme with adenosine. The susceptibility to inhibition by adenine glycosides is determined by the extent of the response of the enzyme to the modifying effect of PPi. Such modification can be eliminated by mild treatment with urea or guanidine-HCl or by genetic alteration with consequent loss of sensitivity to the irreversible inhibition by the adenine glycosides, but without appreciable effect upon catalytic activity (ZYK et al., 1970). Thus, the recognition of the inhibitor depends upon a specific conformational state of the aminase molecule and transition to that conformation is induced by XMP and PPi.

These observations are of particular interest as an additional biochemical mechanism of drug resistance. The only mechanism observed so far that confers resistance to psicofuranine via modification of the aminase depends upon breaking the sequence of conformational transition, which is required for recognition of the inhibitor. Presumably, mutational events resulting in replacement of one or more amino acid residues can impair the flexibility of the enzyme (ZYK et al., 1970). That this is not an isolated instance of this type of drug resistance is indicated by studies on the nature of resistance to methicillin. The side chain of methicillin normally modifies the change in conformation of penicillin-β-lactamase in a way that prevents its activity. When this side chain induced modification is eliminated in resistant mutants, then inactivation of the antibiotic by the enzyme can occur (ZYK and CITRI, 1968). Thus, a mechanism of resistance, which may be applicable to other drugs, involves some constraint on a conformational change of the enzyme normally required for drug binding or drug inactivation.

II. Decoyinine

The biological activity and biochemical effects of decoyinine closely parallel those of psicofuranine (TANAKA et al., 1960, 1961). The same pattern of reversal of bacterial inhibition occurs in the presence of guanine and guanosine. Decoyinine also acts as a noncompetitive inhibitor of XMP aminase and presumably can occupy the same binding site as psicofuranine (BLOCH and NICHOL, 1964; KURAMITSU and MOYED, 1965). Decoyinine and, to a lesser extent, psicofuranine interfered with the formation of PRPP. When cell-free extracts of *S. faecalis* were incubated with ribose-5-phosphate, ATP, and radioactive guanine, GMP was readily formed, but this reaction could not proceed in the presence of decoyinine. When PRPP replaced ribose-5-phosphate and ATP, GMP was formed even in the presence of decoyinine (BLOCH and NICHOL, 1964). In this system there was no indication of conversion of decoyinine to its nucleotide and the conversion of guanine to its nucleotides via nucleoside kinase or phosphorylase was excluded. Since the reaction mechanism of pyrophosphokinase and XMP aminase each involve the pyrophosphate cleavage of ATP, the possibility was considered that decoyinine could occupy the ATP site in such reactions.

III. Mycophenolic Acid (MPA)

The structural specificity of mycophenolic acid is of particular interest in relation to the suggestion of JONES and MILLS (1971) that at least some of the polar groups in MPA may closely simulate those in purine derivatives which bind to the catalytic site or allosteric site of inosinic acid dehydrogenase. Replacing the methoxy of the parent molecule by an ethoxy group resulted in an eight-fold decrease in biological activity (the most active analog) and replacement of methoxy by propoxy, acetoxy, or hydroxy reduced activity still further. Substitution of H for the 4-methyl of MPA also resulted in a decrease in the antimitotic activity, possibly because of an increase in the susceptibility of the phthalide system to ring opening. Modification of the unsubstituted lactone ring or of the chain length of the terpenoid substituent of MPA was detrimental to antimitotic activity. Increasing the degree of unsaturation or elimination of the olefinic double bond reduced the antimitotic activity. None of the 65 compounds was as effective as MPA in suppressing cell division in mouse fibroblasts cultured *in vitro* (Jones and Mills, 1971). Despite the lack of activity on cell growth *in vitro*, the carboxamide derivative and mycophenolic acid glucuronide inhibited XMP aminase to the same degree as MPA (Sweeney et al., 1972b).

Franklin and Cook (1969) found that MPA strongly inhibited DNA synthesis in the L strain of fibroblasts *in vitro*. The extent of the inhibition of DNA synthesis was markedly increased by preincubation of the cells with MPA before the addition of ^{14}C-thymidine and was reversed by guanine in a noncompetitive manner, but not by hypoxanthine, xanthine, or adenine. They also found the reversal of inhibition by guanine can be suppressed by hypoxanthine, 6-mercaptopurine, and adenine. Carter et al. (1969) showed that MPA effectively prevented the incorporation of labeled hypoxanthine into xanthine and guanine nucleotides, but not into adenine nucleotides. Inosinic acid dehydrogenase was strongly inhibited by MPA, and the analysis showed mixed type kinetics with a K_i value of approximately 4×10^{-8} M. It was suggested that this action could account for the antimitotic and anticancer properties. Some cells may be able to bypass the block imposed by MPA by converting guanine to guanylic acid via hypoxanthine-guanine phosphoribosyltransferase. The sensitivity of a cell may therefore depend on its ability to use this salvage pathway (Carter et al., 1969; Sweeney et al., 1972b).

The different metabolic reactions inhibited by MPA all involve nucleoside or nucleotide receptors. Using a purified preparation of IMP dehydrogenase from different sources, Sweeney et al. (1972b) observed a similar degree of inhibition regardless of whether sensitive or resistant experimental tumors were the source. However, the enzyme from human adenocarcinoma of the colon was considerably more sensitive than that from adenocarcinoma 755 of the mouse (1.7×10^{-8} M vs 6.5×10^{-4} M MPA for 50% inhibition). Such differences are related more to tissue source than to species variation since the enzyme from Landschutz ascites cells of the mouse was more sensitive than that from murine Ridgeway osteogenic sarcoma (2.5×10^{-8} M vs 5.5×10^{-4} M MPA for 50% inhibition). XMP aminase was also prepared from seven rodent tumors and the concentration of MPA giving 50% inhibition ranged from 7.0 to 8.8×10^{-4} M (Sweeney et al., 1972b). Based on computation of apparent rates of enzymatic reactions in intact Ehrlich ascites cells related to the distribution of radioactive precursors into nucleotide products, Snyder et al. (1972) confirmed the inhibition of IMP dehydrogenase and in addition noted that inhibition of GDP kinase was considerably greater than that of XMP aminase. Under conditions that gave apparent inhibition of GDP kinase by 47.6%, IMP dehydrogenase was inhibited by 87.7% and XMP aminase by 14.6%.

One of the properties of a number of nucleoside 5′-monophosphates is their ability to simulate the normal feedback inhibition of purine nucleotide biosynthesis. Thus, the observation that partial inhibition of the accumulation of formylglycinamide ribonucleotide occurred in mammalian cell suspensions exposed to mycophenolic acid is of particular interest (FRANKLIN and COOK, 1969). Although the involvement of a nucleotide binding site is inferred, other sites or an effect due to indirect inhibition were not excluded. It is curious, however, that a molecule so different from a nucleoside impinges on so many reactions involving nucleotide functions.

C. Potential for Chemotherapy

Recognition of biochemical pathways that circumvent the reactions inhibited by psicofuranine, decoyinine, and mycophenolic acid support the impression that their chemotherapeutic potential depends upon combination with other drugs. In each case, their growth-inhibitory action is prevented by supplying bacterial or mammalian cells with guanine or guanosine. Consequently, cells endowed with high capacity to convert guanine to its nucleotide by hypoxanthine-guanine phosphoribosyltransferase can by-pass inhibition of inosinate dehydrogenase or xanthylate aminase (guanylate synthetase). Similarly, guanosine kinase would contribute to the same by-pass effect under circumstances in which guanosine might be available. SWEENEY et al. (1972b) measured the phosphoribosyltransferase activity of a number of rodent tumors; in general, high levels of this enzyme were associated with natural resistance to mycophenolic acid. CARTER et al. (1969) selected 6-mercaptopurine to use in combination with mycophenolic acid because of its inhibitory action on phosphoribosyltransferase. These authors interpreted the effect of the combination against Ehrlich ascites tumor as potentiation. The same rationale remains to be explored by combining each of these antibiotics with inhibitors of this transferase enzyme.

Mycophenolic acid is rapidly converted in the body to the glucuronide metabolite. The glucuronide form of the drug, however, is unable to enter cells and the intracellular concentration of mycophenolic acid depends upon the rate of hydrolysis of the metabolite by β-glucuronidase. Consequently, there is a biochemical basis for a selective cytotoxic effect on those cells or tissues that have high levels of β-glucuronidase. The level of this enzyme is related to the unusual spectrum of activity against many solid tumors, but not against ascitic cells. SWEENEY et al. (1972) found that mycophenolic acid was most effective against experimental tumors having high levels of β-glucuronidase. The rapid conversion of mycophenolic acid to its glucuronide is apparently related to the relatively low toxicity of the antibiotic in experimental animals and to the limitation of its use clinically. Large doses are required since the drug is excreted rapidly in the glucuronide form.

Psicofuranine was rated as highly active against many experimental tumors and had a relatively good chemotherapeutic index. Early studies in patients with cancer, however, disclosed a type of toxicity that could not have been anticipated on the basis of toxicity evaluation in animals. In several patients, treatment with psicofuranine was associated with pericarditis (YATES and OLSON, 1961; COSTA et al., 1961; TALLEY and CARLSON, 1963). Because of the serious implications of this type of toxicity further evaluation was discontinued and because of its similar biological and biochemical effects, clinical evaluation of decoyinine was deferred.

Concluding Comments

Within the past ten years, work on the structural elucidation and biological evaluation of nucleoside antibiotics has disclosed compounds with remarkable potency. The fact that many compounds arising through some process of natural selection resemble adenosine seems to reflect the many sites where interference with the metabolic functions of adenine derivatives can give rise to cytotoxicity.

Potency must be combined with selectivity to achieve chemotherapy. When inhibitory activity is observed *in vitro* at very low concentrations then the next question is whether there is some selective action against cells or tissues of different origin. There is no way of predicting from biochemical systems whether the potential to relieve human diseases will be related to selective action against bacteria, parasites, viruses, or malignant cells. When new compounds display such cytotoxicity, however, then an opportunity is presented to discover which metabolic sites are particularly vulnerable to inhibition by such metabolic antagonists.

Knowledge of specialized biochemical techniques combined with skill and some intuition underlie the best use of these cytotoxic nucleosides as metabolic probes. The contributions to fundamental knowledge may be the most important aspect of current work in this field. For instance, the selective action of a pyrrolopyrimidine nucleoside in preventing the formation of certain species of sRNA may provide a means of understanding better the process of viral replication. The detailed study of the regulation of xanthylate aminase has disclosed a different mechanism of drug resistance related to loss of capacity for conformational flexibility. Study of the metabolic activation of these nucleoside analogs has led to recognition that the distribution of activating enzymes in different cells can be a predominant factor determining selectivity.

The potency of these nucleoside antibiotics in contrast to the lack of activity of their corresponding free bases has stimulated interest in the synthesis of nucleoside analogs. Many purine and pyrimidine analogs were synthesized as potential anticancer agents and then used up by lengthy expensive administration to animals bearing experimental tumors without ever determining whether they displayed any activity as substrates for enzymes necessary for their activation. Consequently, the logic of testing new synthetic nucleoside analogs as substrates for activating, as well as inactivating enzymes, is all the more apparent. Indeed, by analogy it is likely that some of these, inactive as kinase substrates, will be active in biochemical systems in the nucleotide form. The limited entry of the nucleotides into cells, however, remains as a barrier to their use *in vivo* unless some means is found to circumvent this limitation.

There is already a substantial body of literature covering the structure and biological activity of synthetic relatives of these naturally occurring nucleosides, which could not be cited here. This brief survey, however, illustrates the type of new information that can be derived by curiosity about the biochemical basis for the cytotoxicity of such potent compounds. Looking ahead, the marriage between synthetic and natural products chemistry will certainly give rise to new relatives of the adenosine-related antibiotics. In addition to serving as new biochemical probes, some of these may have sufficient selectivity of action to become useful drugs to alleviate human diseases.

References

ACS, G., REICH, E., MORI, M.: Biological and biochemical properties of the analogue antibiotic tubercidin. Proc. nat. Acad. Sci. (Wash.) **52**, 493—501 (1964).

AIZAWA, S., HAIDAKA, T., OTAKE, N., YONEHARA, H., ISONO, K., IGARASHI, N., SUZUKI, S.: Studies on a new antibiotic, laurusin. Agr. biol. Chem. **29**, 375—376 (1965).

BENNETT, L. L., JR., SCHNEBLI, H. P., VAIL, M. H., ALLAN, P. W., MONTGOMERY, J. A.: Purine ribonucleoside kinase activity and resistance to some analogs of adenosine. Molec. Pharmacol. **2**, 432—443 (1966).

BENNETT, L. L., JR., SMITHERS, D.: Feedback inhibition of purine biosynthesis in H.Ep. 2 cells by adenine analogs. Biochem. Pharmacol. **13**, 1331—1339 (1964).

BERGMAN, W., STEMPIEN, M. F., JR.: Contributions to the study of marine products. XLIII. The nucleosides of sponges. V. The synthesis of spongosine. J. org. Chem. **22**, 1575—1577 (1957).

BIRCH, A. J., WRIGHT, J. J.: A total synthesis of mycophenolic acid. Aust. J. Chem. **22**, 2635—2644 (1969).

BIRKINSHAW, J. H., RAISTRICK, H., ROSS, D. J.: Studies in the biochemistry of microorganisms. The molecular constitution of mycophenolic acid, a metabolic product of *Penicillium brevicompactum Dierckx*. II. Further observations on the structural formula for mycophenolic acid. Biochem. J. **50**, 630—634 (1952).

BISEL, H. F., ANSFIELD, F. J., MASON, J. H., WILSON, W. L.: Clinical studies with tubercidin administered by direct intravenous injection. Cancer Res. **30**, 76—78 (1970).

BLOCH, A.: Nucleoside antibiotics related to adenosine. Antimicrob. Ag. Chemother. **1964**, 530—539 (1965).

BLOCH, A., LEONARD, R. J., NICHOL, C. A.: On the mode of action of 7-deaza-adenosine (tubercidin). Biochim. biophys. Acta (Amst.) **138**, 10—25 (1967).

BLOCH, A., MIHICH, E., LEONARD, R. J., NICHOL, C. A.: Studies on the biologic activity and mode of action of 7-deazainosine. Cancer Res. **29**, 110—115 (1969).

BLOCH, A., NICHOL, C. A.: Inhibition of ribosephosphate pyrophosphokinase activity by decoyinine, an adenine nucleoside. Biochem. biophys. Res. Comm. **16**, 400—403 (1964).

BROWN, G. M.: The biosynthesis of pteridines. Advanc. Enzymol. **35**, 35—77 (1971).

CALDWELL, I. C., HENDERSON, J. F., PATERSON, A. R. P.: The metabolism of formycin, an adenosine analogue. Canad. J. Biochem. **47**, 901—908 (1969).

CARTER, S. B., FRANKLIN, T. J., JONES, D. F., LEONARD, B. J., MILLS, S. D., TURNER, R. W., TURNER, W. B.: Mycophenolic acid: an anti-cancer compound with unusual properties. Nature (Lond.) **223**, 848—850 (1969).

CAVINS, J. A., HALL, T. C., OLSON, K. B., KHUNG, C. L., HORTON, J., COLSKY, J., SHADDUCK, R. K.: Initial toxicity study of sangivamycin. Cancer Chemother. Rep. **51**, 197—203 (1967).

CHASSY, B. M., SUGIMORI, T., SUHADOLNIK, R. J.: The biosynthesis of the 6-deoxy-D-erythro-2,5-hexodiulose sugar of decoyinine. Biochim. biophys. Acta (Amst.) **130**, 12—18 (1966).

CHASSY, B. M., SUHADOLNIK, R. J.: Nucleoside antibiotics. II. Biochemical tools for studying the structural requirements for interaction at the catalytic and regulatory sites of ribonucleotide reductase from *Eschericia coli*. J. biol. Chem. **243**, 3538—3541 (1968).

CORY, J. G., SUHADOLNIK, R. J.: Structural requirements of nucleosides for binding by adenosine deaminase. Biochemistry **4**, 1729—1732 (1965).

COSTA, G., HOLLAND, J. F., PICKREN, J. W.: Acute pericarditis produced by psicofuranine, a nucleoside analogue. New Eng. J. Med. **265**, 1143—1146 (1961).

DONOVAN, K. L., ROWE, J. A., MOYED, H. S.: Adenine glycoside site of xanthosine-5′-phosphate aminase. Antimicrob. Ag. Chemother. **1964**, 289—296 (1968).

DRUMMOND, G. I., POWELL, C. A.: Analogs of adenosine 3′,5′-cyclic phosphate as activators of phosphorylase *b* kinase and as substrates for cyclic 3′,5′-nucleotide phosphodiesterase. Molec. Pharmacol. **6**, 24—30 (1970).

EHRMAN, L.: Antibiotics and infectious hybrid sterility in *Drosophila paulistorum*. Molec. gen. Genet. **103**, 218—222 (1968).

FLORINI, J. R.: Nucleocidin. In: GOTTLICH, I. D., SHAW, P. D. (Eds.): Antibiotics, pp. 428—433. New York: Springer 1967.

FLORINI, J. R., BIRD, H. H., BELL, P. H.: Inhibition of protein synthesis *in vitro* and *in vivo* by nucleocidin, an antitrypanosomal antibiotic. J. biol. Chem. **241**, 1091—1098 (1966).

FOX, J. J., WATANABE, K. A., BLOCH, A.: Nucleoside antibiotics. Progr. nucleic Acid Res. **5**, 251—313 (1966).

FRANKLIN, T. J., COOK, J. M.: The inhibition of nucleic acid synthesis by mycophenolic acid. Biochemistry **113**, 515—524 (1969).

FRANKLIN, T. J., COOK, J. M.: Inhibition of guanine nucleotide biosynthesis by mycophenolic acid in Yoshida ascites cells. Biochem. Pharmacol. **20**, 1334—1338 (1971).

FUKUYAMA, T. T., MOYED, H. S.: A separate antibiotic-binding site in xanthosine-5′-phosphate aminase: inhibitor- and substrate-binding studies. Biochemistry **3**, 1488—1492 (1964).

GRAGE, T. B., ROCHLIN, D. B., WEISS, A. J., WILSON, W. L.: Clinical studies with tubercidin administered after absorption into human erythrocytes. Cancer Res. **30**, 79—81 (1970).

HANKA, L. J.: Mechanism of action of psicofuranine. J. Bact. **80**, 30—36 (1960).

HASCHENMEYER, A. E. V., RICH, A.: Nucleoside conformations: an analysis of steric barriers to rotation about the glycosidic bond. J. molec. Biol. **27**, 369—384 (1967).

HASHIMOTO, J., UCHIDA, T., EGAMI, F.: Action of ribonucleases T_1, T_2, and U_2 on dinucleoside monophosphates containing 7-deazapurine base. Biochim. biophys. Acta (Amst.) **199**, 535—536 (1970).

HENDERSON, J. F., KHOO, M. K. Y.: On the mechanism of feedback inhibition of purine biosynthesis *de novo* in Ehrlich ascites tumor cells *in vitro*. J. biol. Chem. **240**, 3104—3109 (1965).

HENDERSON, J. F., PATTERSON, A. R. P., CALDWELL, I. C., HORI, M.: Biochemical effects of formycin, an adenosine analog. Cancer Res. **27**, 715—719 (1967).

HILL, D. L., BENNETT, L. L., JR.: Purification and properties of 5-phosphoribosyl pyrophosphate amidotransferase from adenocarcinoma 755 cells. Biochemistry 8, 122—130 (1969).

HOEKSEMA, H., SLOMP, G., VAN TAMELEN, E. E.: Angustmycin A and decoyinine. Tetrahedron Let. 1787—1795 (1964).

HORI, M., ITO, E., TAKITA, T., KOYAMA, G., TAKEUCHI, T., UMEZAWA, H.: A new antibiotic, formycin. J. Antibiot. 61, 96—99 (1964).

HORI, M., WAKASHIRO, T., ITO, E., SAWA, T., TAKEUCHI, T., UMEZAWA, H.: Biochemical effects of formycin B on *Xanthomonas oryzae*. J. Antibiot. 21, 264—271 (1968).

IKEHARA, M., FUKUI, T.: Some physical properties of poly 7-deazaadenylic acid (polytubercidin phosphoric acid). J. molec. Biol. 38, 437—441 (1968).

IKEHARA, M., MAURAO, K., HARADA, F., NISHIMURA, S.: Synthesis of formycin triphosphate and its incorporation into ribopolynucleotide by DNA-dependent RNA polymerase. Biochim. biophys. Acta (Amst.) 155, 82—90 (1968).

IKEHARA, M., MAURAO, K., HARADA, F., NISHIMURA, S.: Protein synthesis directed by ribopolynucleotide containing formycin. Biochim. biophys. Acta (Amst.) 174, 696—703 (1969).

IKEHARA, M., OHTSUKA, E.: Stimulation of the binding of aminoacyl-sRNA to ribosomes by tubercidin (7-deazaadenosine) and N^6-dimethyladenosine containing trinucleoside diphosphate analogs. Biochem. biophys. Res. Comm. 21, 257—264 (1965).

ISHIDA, N., HOMMA, M., KUMAGAI, K., SCHIMIZU, Y., MATSUMOTO, S., IZAWA, A.: Studies on the antiviral activity of formycin. J. Antibiot. A 20, 49—52 (1967a).

ISHIDA, N., IZAWA, A., HOMMA, M., KUMAGAI, K., SHIMIZU, Y.: Anti-myxovirus activity of formycin B. J. Antibiot. A 20, 129—131 (1967b).

ISHIZUKA, M., SAWA, T., KOYAMA, G., TAKEUCHI, T., UMEZAWA, H.: Metabolism of formycin and formycin B *in vivo*. J. Antibiot. 21, 1—4 (1968a).

ISHIZUKA, M., SAWA, T., HORI, S., TAKAYAMA, H.: Biological studies on formycin and formycin B. J. Antibiot. 21, 5—12 (1968b).

JAFFE, J. J., MEYMARIAN, E., DOREMUS, H. M.: Antischistosomal action of tubercidin administered after absorption into red cells. Nature (Lond.) 230, 408—409 (1971).

JONES, F. F., MILLS, S. D.: Preparation and antitumor properties of analogs and derivatives of mycophenolic acid. J. med. Chem. 14, 305—311 (1971).

KAPULER, A. M., WARD, D. C., MENDELSOHN, N., KLETT, H., ACS, G.: Utilization of substrate analogs by mengovirus-induced RNA polymerase. Virology 37, 701—706 (1969).

KIDA, M., KAWASHIMA, F., IMADA, A., NOGAMI, I., SUHARA, I., YONEDA, M.: Studies on the purine-sensitive mutants of *Bacillus subtilis*. I. Properties of an adenosine-sensitive mutant. J. Biochem. 66, 487—492 (1969).

KOYAMA, G., UMEZAWA, H.: Formycin B and its relation to formycin. J. Antibiot. A 18, 175—177 (1965).

KUNIMOTO, T., WAKASHIRO, T., OKAMURA, I., ASAJIMA, T., HORI, M.: Structural requirements for formycin activity. J. Antibiot. 21, 468—470 (1968).

KURAMITSU, H. K., MOYED, H. S.: A separate antibiotic binding site of xanthosine-5'-phosphate aminase. Differential alteration of catalytic properties and sensitivity to inhibition. J. biol. Chem. 241, 1596—1601 (1966).

KUSAKA, T., YAMAMOTO, H., SHIBATA, M., MUROI, M., KISHI, T., MIZUMO, K.: *Streptomyces citricolor* nov. sp. and a new antibiotic, aristeromycin. J. Antibiot. 21, 255—263 (1968).

LEONARD, N. J., HECHT, S. M., SKOOG, F., SCHMITZ, R. Y.: Cytokinins: synthesis of 6-(3-methyl-3-butenylamino)-9-β-D-ribofuranosylpurine (3IPA) and the effect of side-chain unsaturation on the biological activity of isopentylaminopurines and their ribosides. Proc. nat. Acad. Sci. (Wash.) 59, 15—21 (1968).

LEPAGE, G. A.: Purine arabinosides, xylosides and lyxosides. This volume, Chapter 49.

LEPAGE, G. A., JUNGA, I. G.: Labeling of nucleosides with tritium. Canad. J. Chem. 43, 1279—1281 (1965).

LINDBERG, B.: Some additional properties of partially purified mammalian adenosine kinase. Biochim. biophys. Acta (Amst.) 185, 245—247 (1969).

LINDBERG, B., KLENOW, H., HANSEN, K.: Some properties of partially purified mammalian adenosine kinase. J. biol. Chem. 242, 350—356 (1967).

MANTEUIL, S., TAVITIAN, A., BOIRON, M.: Comparative study of the action of two antibiotics, actinomycin D and toyocamycin, on the synthesis of ribosomal proteins in L cells. C. R. Acad. Sci. (Paris) D 270, 543—546 (1970).

MCCARTHY, J. R., JR., ROBINS, R., ROBINS, M.: Purine nucleosides. XXII. The synthesis of angustmycin A (decoyinine) and related unsaturated nucleosides. J. Amer. chem. Soc. 90, 4993—4999 (1968).

MIHICH, E., SIMPSON, L., MULHERN, A. I.: Comparative study of the toxicologic effects of 7-deazaadenosine (tubercidin) and 7-deazainosine. Cancer Res. 29, 116—122 (1969).

MIZUNO, Y., IKEHARA, M., WATANABE, K. A., SUZAKI, S.: X. Synthesis of 4-hydroxy-7-β-D-ribofuranosyl-7-*H*-pyrrolo[2,3-*d*] pyrimidine, a tubercidin analog. J. org. Chem. 28, 3331—3336 (1963).
MORTON, G. O., LANCASTER, J. E., VAN LEAR, G. E., FULMOR, W., MEYER, W. E.: The structure of nucleocidin. III (a new structure). J. Amer. chem. Soc. **91**, 1535—1537 (1969).
MOYED, H. S.: Interference with feedback control of enzyme activity. Cold Spring Harbor Symp. Quant. Biol. **26**, 323—329 (1961).
NICHOL, C. A.: The mode of action of nucleoside antibiotics and other compounds related to adenosine. Proc. Fed. Europ. Biochem. Soc. **5**, 116 (1968).
NICHOL, C. A., BLOCH, A., MIHICH, E.: Studies on the biological and biochemical activities of tubercidin and related nucleosides. In: Cancer Chemotherapy Proceedings, Takeda International Conference, Osaka, 1966, p. 185—195 (1967).
ODAKA, T., TAKIZAWA, K., YAMAURA, K., YAMAMOTO, T.: Immunosuppressive effect of formycins. Jap. J. exp. Med. **39**, 327—329 (1969).
OTAKE, N., AIZAWA, S., HIDAKA, T., SETO, H., YONEHARA, H.: Biological and chemical transformations of formycin to laurusin. Agr. biol. Chem. **29**, 377—378 (1965).
OWEN, S. P., SMITH, C. G.: Cytotoxicity and antitumor properties of the abnormal nucleoside tubercidin. Cancer Chemother. Rep. **36**, 19—23 (1964).
PIERRE, K. J., LEPAGE, G. A.: Formation of inosine-5'-monophosphate by a kinase in cell-free extracts of Ehrlich ascites cells *in vitro*. Proc. Soc. exp. Biol. (N.Y.) **127**, 432—440 (1968).
RABINOWITZ, K. W., SHADA, J. D., WOOD, W. A.: The mechanism of action of 5'-adenylic acid-activated threonine dehydrase. III. Structural requirements for nucleotide allosteric activation. J. biol. Chem. **243**, 3214—3217 (1968).
RAO, K. V.: Structure of sangivamycin. J. med. Chem. **11**, 939—941 (1968).
REICHARD, P.: Control of deoxyribonucleotide synthesis *in vitro* and *in vivo*. Advanc. Enzyme Reg. **10**, 3—16 (1972).
RIMAN, J., SVERAK, L., LANGLOIS, A. J., BONAR, A., BEARD, J. W.: Influence of toyocamycin on RNA synthesis in chick embryo cells noninfected and infected with strain MC29 avian leukosis virus. Cancer Res. **29**, 1707—1716 (1969).
ROBINS, M. J., HALL, R. H., THEDFORD, R.: A component of the transfer ribonucleic acid of yeast and of mammalian tissue, methods of isolation, and characterization. Biochemistry 6, 1837—1848 (1967).
ROSS, A. F., JAFFE, J. J.: Effects of tubercidin and its ribonucleotides on various metabolic pathways in *Schistosoma mansoni*. Biochem. Pharmacol. **21**, 3059—3069 (1972).
SAWA, T., FUKAGAWA, Y., HOMMA, I., TAKEUCHI, T., UMEZAWA, H.: Mode of inhibition of coformycin on adenosine deaminase. J. Antibiot. A **20**, 227—231 (1967a).
SAWA, T., FUKAGAWA, Y., HOMMA, I., TAKEUCHI, T., UMEZAWA, H.: Formycin-deaminating activity of microorganisms. J. Antibiot. A **20**, 317—321 (1967b).
SAWA, T., FUKAGAWA, Y., HOMMA, I., WAKASHIRO, T., TAKEUCHI, T., HORI, M., KOMAI, T.: Metabolic conversion of formycin B to formycin A and to oxoformycin B in *Nocardia interforma*. J. Antibiot. **21**, 334—339 (1968).
SCHAEFFER, H., THOMAS, H. J.: Synthesis of potential anticancer agents. XIV. Ribosides of 2,6-disubstituted purines. J. Amer. chem. Soc. **80**, 3738—3742 (1958).
SCHNEBLI, H. P., HILL, D. L., BENNETT, L. L., JR.: Purification and properties of adenosine kinase from human tumor cells of type H. Ep. No. 2. J. biol. Chem. **242**, 1997—2004 (1967).
SCHROEDER, W., HOEKSEMA, H.: A new antibiotic, 6-amino-9-D-psicofuranosylpurine. J. Amer. chem. Soc. **81**, 1767—1768 (1959).
SHEALY, Y. F., CLAYTON, J. D.: Synthesis of carbocyclic analogs of purine ribonucleosides. J. Amer. chem. Soc. **91**, 3075—3083 (1969).
SHEEN, M. R., KIM, B. K., PARKS, R. E., JR.: Purine nucleoside phosphorylase from human erythrocytes. III. Inhibition by the inosine analog formycin B of the isolated enzyme and of nucleoside metabolism in intact erythrocytes and sarcoma 180 cells. Molec. Pharmacol. **4**, 293—299 (1968).
SHEEN, M. R., MARTIN, H. F., PARKS, R. E., JR.: The interaction of the nucleoside analogues, formycins A and B with xanthine oxidase and hepatic aldehyde oxidase. Molec. Pharmacol. **6**, 255—265 (1970).
SHIGEURA, H. T., SAMPSON, S. D.: Structural basis for phosphorylation of adenosine congeners. Nature (Lond.) **25**, 419—420 (1967).
SKOOG, L.: An enzymatic method for the determination of dCTP and dGTP in picomole amounts. Europ. J. Biochem. **17**, 202—208 (1970).
SLECHTA, L.: Studies on the mode of action of psicofuranine. Biochem. Pharmacol. **5**, 96—107 (1960a).
SLECHTA, L.: Inhibition of xanthosine-5'-phosphate aminase by psicofuranine. Biochem. biophys. Res. Commun. **3**, 596—598 (1960b).

Smith, C. G., Gray, G. D,; Carlson, R. G., Hanze, A. R.: Biochemical and biological studies with tubercidin (7-deaza-adenosine), 7-Deazainosine and certain nucleotide derivatives of tubercidin. Advanc. Enzyme Reg. **5**, 121—151 (1967).

Smith, C. G., Reineke, L. M., Harpootlian, H., Burch, M. R., Shefner, A. M., Muirhead, E. C.: Studies on the uptake of tubercidin (7-deazaadenosine) by blood cells and its distribution in animals. Cancer Res. **30**, 69—75 (1970).

Smulson, M. E., Suhadolnik, R. J.: The biosynthesis of the 7-deazaadenine ribonucleoside, tubercidin, by *Streptomyces tubercidicus*. J. biol. Chem. **242**, 2872—2876 (1967).

Strecker, G., Goubet, B., Montreuil, J.: Les cétoses de l'urine humaine. Identification du D(+)-allulose. C. R. Acad. Sci. (Paris) **260**, 999—1002 (1965).

Suhadolnik, R. J.: Nucleoside antibiotics. New York-London-Sidney-Toronto: Wiley-Interscience 1970.

Suhadolnik, R. J., Finkel, S. I., Chassy, B. M.: Nucleoside antibiotics. I. Biochemical tools for studying the structural requirements for interaction at the catalytic and regulatory sites of ribonucleotide reductase from *Lactobacillus leichmannii*. J. biol. Chem. **243**, 3532—3537 (1968).

Suhadolnik, R. J., Uematsu, T.: Biosynthesis of the pyrrolopyrimidine nucleoside antibiotic, toyocamycin. VII. Origin of the pyrrole carbons and the cyano carbon. J. biol. Chem. **245**, 4365—4371 (1970).

Sweeney, M. J., Gerzon, K., Harris, P. N., Holmes, R. E., Poore, G. A., Williams, R. H.: Experimental antitumor activity and preclinical toxicology of mycophenolic acid. Cancer Res. **32**, 1795—1802 (1972).

Sweeney, M. J., Hoffman, D. H., Esterman, M. A.: Metabolism and biochemistry of mycophenolic acid. Cancer Res. **32**, 1803—1809 (1972).

Takeuchi, T., Iwanaga, J., Aoyagi, T., Murase, M., Sawa, T., Umezawa, H.: Antiviral effects of formycin derivatives. J. Antibiot. A **20**, 297—298 (1967).

Takeuchi, T., Iwanaga, J., Aoyagi, T., Umezawa, H.: Antiviral effect of formycin and formycin B. J. Antibiot. A **19**, 286—287 (1966).

Talley, R. W., Carlson, R. G.: Polyserositis induced by psicofuranine in man and comparative toxicity in the rat, mouse, dog, chicken, and monkey. Toxicol. appl. Pharmacol. **5**, 235—246 (1963).

Tanaka, N., Miyairi, N., Umezawa, H.: Studies on antagonists to angustmycins. J. Antibiot. A **13**, 265—269 (1960).

Tanaka, N., Nishimura, T., Yamaguchi, H., Umezawa, H.: Activity of angustmycins against experimental infections and transplantable tumors. J. Antibiot. A **15**, 98—102 (1961).

Tavitian, A., Uretsky, S. C., Acs, G.: The effect of toyocamycin on cellular RNA synthesis. Biochem. biophys. Acta (Amst.) **179**, 50—57 (1969).

Tezuka, N., Hirai, T.: Effects of formycin B on tobacco mosaic virus multiplication. Jap. J. Microbiol. **13**, 367—374 (1969).

Townsend, L. B., Robins, R. K.: The mass spectra of formycin, formycin B, and showdomycin carbon linked nucleoside antibiotics. J. heterocycl. Chem. **6**, 459—464 (1969).

Tsukada, I., Kunimoto, T., Hori, M., Komai, T.: Isolation and properties of the enzyme which catalyzes the oxidation of formycin B. J. Antibiot. **22**, 36—38 (1969).

Udaka, S., Moyed, H. S.: Inhibition of parental and mutant xanthosine 5'-phosphate aminases by psicofuranine. J. biol. Chem. **238**, 2797—2803 (1963).

Umezawa, H., Sawa, T., Fukagawa, Y., Homma, I., Ishizuka, M., Takeuchi, T.: Studies on formycin and formycin B in cells of Ehrlich carcinoma and *E. coli*. J. Antibiot. A **20**, 308—316 (1967).

Umezawa, H., Sawa, T., Fukagawa, Y., Koyama, G., Murase, M., Hamada, M., Takeuchi, T.: Transformation of formycin to formycin B and their biological activities. J. Antibiot. A **18**, 178—181 (1965).

Uematsu, T., Suhadolnik, R. J.: Nucleoside antibiotics. VI. Biosynthesis of the pyrrolopyrimidine nucleoside antibiotic toyocamycin by *Streptomyces rimosus*. Biochemistry **9**, 1260—1266 (1970).

Uretsky, S. C., Acs, G., Reich, E., Mori, M., Altwerger, L.: Pyrrolopyrimidine nucleotides and protein synthesis. J. biol. Chem. **243**, 306—312 (1968).

Ward, D. C., Cerami, A., Reich, E.: Biochemical studies of the nucleoside analogue, formycin. J. biol. Chem. **244**, 3243—3250 (1969c).

Ward, D. C., Fuller, W., Reich, E.: Stereochemical analysis of the specificity of pancreatic RNase and polyformycin as substrate: differentiation of the transphosphorylation and hydrolysis reactions. Proc. nat. Acad. Sci. (Wash.) **62**, 581—588 (1969b).

Ward, D. C., Horn, T., Reich, E.: Fluorescence studies of nucleotides and polynucleotides. III. Diphosphopyridine nucleotide analogues which contain fluorescent purines. J. biol. Chem. **247**, 4014—4020 (1972).

WARD, D. C., REICH, E.: Conformational properties of polyformycin. Proc. nat. Acad. Sci. (Wash.) **61**, 1494—1501 (1968).
WARD, D. C., REICH, E.: Relationship between nucleoside conformation and biological activity. In: Annual Reports in Medicinal Chemistry, 1969, pp. 272—284. New York-London: Academic Press 1970.
WARD, D. C., REICH, E., STRYER, L.: Fluorescence studies of nucleotides and polynucleotides. I. Formycin, 2-aminopurine riboside, 2,6-diaminopurine riboside, and their derivatives. J. biol. Chem. **244**, 1228—1237 (1969a).
WILLIAMS, R. H., BOECK, L. D., CLINE, J. C., DELONG, D. C., GERZON, K., GORDEE, R. S., GORMAN, M., HOLMES, R. E., LARSEN, S. H., LIVELY, D. H., MATTHEWS, T. R., NELSON, J. D., POORE, G. A., STARK, W. M., SWEENEY, M. J.: Mycophenolic acid: fermentation, isolation, and biological properties. Antimicrob. Ag. Chemother. 229—233 (1968).
WILLIAMS, R. H., LIVELY, D. H., DELONG, D. C., CLINE, J. C., SWEENEY, M. J., POORE, G. A., LARSEN, S. H.: Mycophenolic acid: antiviral and antitumor properties. J. Antibiot. **21**, 463—464 (1968).
YATES, R. C., OLSON, K. B.: Drug-induced pericarditis. Report of three cases due to 6-amino-9-D-psicofuranosylpurine. New Engl. J. Med. **265**, 274—277 (1961).
YÜNTSEN, H., OHKUMA, K., ISHII, Y., YONEHARA, H.: Studies on angustmycin. III. J. Antibiot. A **19**, 195—201 (1956).
YÜNTSEN, H., YONEHARA, H., UI, H.: Studies on a new antibiotic, angustmycin. I. J. Antibiot. A **7**, 113—115 (1954).
ZYK, N., CITRI, N.: The interaction of penicillinase with penicillins. VI. Comparison of free and antibody-bound enzyme. Biochim. biophys. Acta (Amst.) **159**, 317—326 (1968).
ZYK, N., CITRI, N., MOYED, H. S.: Conformative response of xanthosine 5'-phosphate aminase. Biochemistry 8, 2787—2794 (1969).
ZYK, N., CITRI, N., MOYED, H. S.: Alteration of the conformative response and inhibition of xanthosine 5'-phosphate aminase by adenine glycosides. Biochemistry **9**, 677—683 (1970).

Chapter 51

8-Azaguanine

R. E. Parks, Jr. and K. C. Agarwal

Introduction

The base analog 8-azaguanine (8-azaG; guanazolo; 5-amino-7-hydroxy-1 H-v-triazolo(d)pyrimidine) holds a special place in the field of cancer chemotherapy, since it was the first purine analog to display marked carcinostatic effects against murine malignancies. This base analog, which contains a nitrogen atom in place of the carbon in position 8 of the purine ring, has not proved useful for the treatment of human cancer. However, 8-azaG has provided a valuable tool for the molecular biologist, since the molecule is readily incorporated into the ribonucleic acids and appears to exert its cytotoxic action at that level.

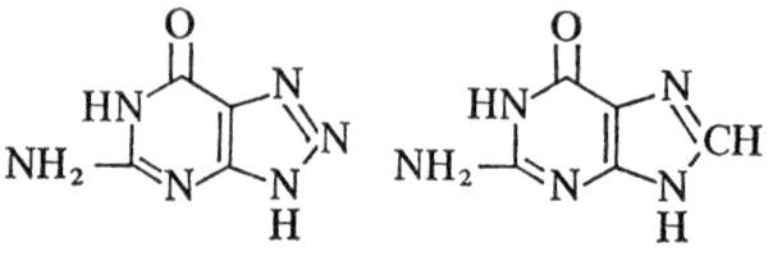

8-Azaguanine   Guanine

A number of reviews have appeared that document in detail the numerous investigations that have been performed with this compound over the past twenty-five years (Mandel, 1955, 1959; Parks, 1955, 1962, 1963; Mathews, 1958; Skipper and Bennett, 1958; Anderson and Law, 1960; Handschumacher and Welch, 1960; Brockman and Anderson, 1963; Karnofsky and Clarkson, 1963; Emmelot, 1965; Montgomery, 1965; Stock, 1966; Roy-Burman, 1970).

Early Investigations

8-Azaguanine was first synthesized in 1945 by Roblin and his associates (Roblin et al., 1945), who observed inhibition of the growth of *E. coli* competitive with guanine, with an inhibition index of 128. This guanine analog first came into prominence in 1949 through studies in the laboratory of G. W. Kidder with the ciliate protozoon, *Tetrahymena geleii* (Kidder and Dewey, 1949). This organism has an absolute nutritional requirement for guanine, guanosine, or guanylic acid and is strongly, but competitively, inhibited by 8-azaG (inhibition index 0.02) (Kidder et al., 1949). Although later experiments with ^{14}C-labeled guanine showed that it may be incorporated into the nucleic acids of a number of animal tissues, such as bone marrow, the evidence available at that time from less sensitive methods that employed ^{15}N-labeled guanine indicated little or no incorporation of preformed guanine into animal cells (Brown et al., 1948). Therefore, 8-azaG was considered as a possible chemotherapeutic agent against tumors, parasites, viruses, or other invading cells that might differ in their degree of guanine utilization from the tissues of the host. It was soon learned that 8-azaG caused marked inhibition of the growth of several murine adenocarcinomas (KIDDER et al., 1949, 1951). Other tumors, such as Sarcoma 180 and the Harding-Passey melanoma, however, did not respond (SUGIURA et al., 1950). In addition, there was evidence that the antitumor action of 8-azaG could be reversed by treatment with guanine (GOLDIN et al., 1950; KIDDER et al., 1951). That 8-azaG has carcinostatic rather than carcinolytic effects was demonstrated when it was shown that tumor growth was inhibited during treatment, but resumed promptly when therapy was stopped (KIDDER et al., 1949, 1951). For listings of 8-azaG sensitive and resistant tumors, the reader is referred to KIDDER et al. (1951) and STOCK (1966).

8-AzaG has not proved useful in the treatment of human malignancies for several reasons. First, the drug must be given by a parenteral route because its effectiveness is markedly diminished when it is administered orally. This is probably the result of deamination to the inactive compound, 8-azaxanthine, by the enzyme guanine deaminase in the intestinal mucosa and liver. Second, 8-azaguanine is only poorly soluble; therefore, on the basis of the dosage required for tumor inhibition in the mouse (about 60 mg/kg of body weight), greater than one gram per day would be required for the treatment of adult human subjects. When administered to patients by intravenous injection, 8-azaG caused skin rashes, and intramuscular injections were extremely painful (GELLHORN, 1953; HALL et al., 1962). Since other purine analogs that did not have these disadvantages, such as 6-thioguanine and 6-mercaptopurine, were soon developed (ELION et al., 1952; ELION and HITCHINGS, 1955), further intensive studies of possible clinical applications of 8-azaG were abandoned. However, HALL et al. (1962) have reported positive effects in the treatment of tumors of the head and neck with local infusions of 8-azaG.

Pharmacological Behavior

The LD_{50} for 8-azaG in adult mice administered in five intraperitoneal doses at 12-h intervals is about 120 mg per kilo per injection (CARLO and MANDEL, 1954). Other investigations indicate that 8-azaG is considerably more toxic to young, immature animals than to adult animals and that doses tolerated readily by pregnant female rats usually cause fetal death, abortions, or fetal resorptions (PARKS, 1955). Studies with ^{14}C-labeled 8-azaG in mice, rabbits, and man (MANDEL et al., 1951; GELLHORN et al., 1951; GELLHORN, 1953) showed that the drug is excreted rapidly in the urine, mostly in the form of the metabolite 8-azaxanthine, undoubtedly produced by an enzymatic reaction with guanine deaminase. In experiments with mice only about 3 % of the administered 8-azaG remained in the animals 12 h after injection (MANDEL et al., 1951). As discussed elsewhere, much of this retained 8-azaG is incorporated into the ribonucleic acids of the tissues.

Effect of 8-Azaguanine and Its Derivatives on Enzymes

A. Degradative Enzymes

8-Azaguanine interacts as a substrate with guanine deaminase (guanase) and purine nucleoside phosphorylase, and as an inhibitor with adenosine deaminase and xanthine oxidase. Deamination of 8-azaG by guanase was first reported by ROUSH and NORRIS (1950). Because the product of the deamination, 8-azaxanthine, has little biological effect, it was suggested that tumors with high guanase activity would be resistant to inhibition by 8-azaG and initial studies with several mouse neoplasms seemed to support this hypothesis (HIRSCHBERG et al., 1952). Since fetal brain tissue grown in culture is less susceptible to inhibition by 8-azaG than cultured brain tumor cells with lower guanase activity, and the human brain tumor, glioblastoma multiforme, is devoid of measurable guanase activity (HIRSCHBERG et al., 1953), it was anticipated that 8-azaG might find use in the treatment of human brain tumors. However, the hypothesis that high guanase activity is the primary factor that renders tumors and other tissues resistant to inhibition by 8-azaG was soon made untenable when a number of neoplasms were found in which this relationship did not occur (HIRSCHBERG et al., 1952). For example, the rat ascites Takeda sarcoma is more susceptible than the Yoshida sarcoma to 8-azaG, although the guanase activity of the former is much greater (KONDO and MARUYAMA, 1955), and a number of mouse leukemias with similar guanase levels varied widely in their response to 8-azaG (SCHACTER and LAW, 1957). Several laboratories have found that the treatment of tumor-bearing animals with guanine reversed the inhibition of tumors caused by 8-azaG (GOLDIN et al., 1950; KIDDER et al., 1951). It is possible that this is the result of the induction of guanase activity in normal tissues, such as liver or intestinal mucosa, rather than a direct antagonism in the tumor. This interesting possibility has not been tested. The fact that in rabbits, mice, monkeys, and man, 8-azaG is excreted in the urine principally as the deamination product 8-azaxanthine, demonstrates the importance of guanase in the pharmacological behavior of 8-azaG (GELLHORN et al., 1951; MANDEL et al., 1951; GELLHORN, 1953). Using a guanase preparation from rat liver, ROUSH and NORRIS (1950) found a K_m for guanine of 5×10^{-6} M and of 7×10^{-4} M with 8-azaG. Similarly, studies by ROSS and PARKS (1971) with a preparation of guanase from Sarcoma 180 ascites cells revealed K_m values of about 4×10^{-6} M with guanine and about 1×10^{-4} M with 8-azaG. Guanase from Sarcoma 180 was totally inactive with 6-thioguanine and 6-selenoguanine, either as inhibitors or substrates. In view of the fact that isozymes of guanase have now been reported (KRISHNAN et al., 1970), the question of the activity of guanine analogs with guanase deserves further examination.

8-AzaG has been reported to inhibit both adenosine deaminase and xanthine oxidase (FEIGELSON and DAVIDSON, 1956; ULTMANN and FEIGELSON, 1958). However, there is little evidence that these inhibitions play a role in the cytotoxic mechanism of action of the drug. Also, purine nucleoside phosphorylase reacts with 8-azaG and either ribose-1-phosphate or deoxyribose-1-phosphate to form reversibly 8-azaguanosine or 8-azadeoxyguanosine (FRIEDKIN, 1954).

B. Anabolic Enzymes

8-AzaG and its nucleoside and nucleotide derivatives react with various enzymes of purine and purine nucleotide anabolism, and the formation of 8-azaGMP, 8-azaGDP, and 8-azaGTP have been demonstrated, as well as the incorporation of 8-azaG into ribonucleic acids.

8-AzaG was first shown to serve as a substrate for hypoxanthine-guanine phosphoribosyltransferase (HGPRT) by WAY and PARKS (1958).

$$\text{8-azaG} + \text{PRPP} \xrightarrow{\text{HGPRT}} \text{8-azaGMP} + \text{PP}_i$$

This reaction is necessary for antitumor activity, since cells that lose this enzyme through genetic mutation become resistant to growth inhibition by 8-azaG (BROCKMAN et al., 1957, 1959a, b). In the cases that have been reported, when mammalian cells lose HGPRT activity they also become resistant to other purine analogs related to hypoxanthine or guanine, such as 6-mercaptopurine and

6-thioguanine, which indicates that the same enzyme catalyzes 5′-mononucleotide formation from guanine and hypoxanthine and their analogs. However, studies with *Salmonella typhimurium* showed that separate enzymes are involved in this organism and the guanine activity alone may be lost by genetic mutation (KALLE and GOTS, 1961). Different HGPRT-like enzymes were found in 8-azaG-sensitive and -resistant cells (ADYE and GOTS, 1966). Although detailed kinetic analyses have not yet been reported, striking differences in the pH optima for 8-azaG and guanine with hog liver HGPRT were observed (WAY and PARKS, 1958), perhaps due to the markedly lower pK_a of 8-azaG (pK_a of 6.5 for 8-azaG vs 9.2 for guanine). In recent studies with HGPRT from Sarcoma 180 cells, K_m values for guanine, 6-thioguanine, and 6-selenoguanine were about 5×10^{-6} M, whereas the K_m for 8-azaG was about 60-fold greater (i.e., 3×10^{-4} M) (AGRAWAL et al., 1971; ROSS and PARKS, 1971). This greater K_m value may explain the relative insensitivity of Sarcoma 180 to 8-azaG.

The formation of 8-azaGTP from 8-azaGMP was first shown in coupled enzymatic reactions of guanylate kinase and nucleoside diphosphokinase with pyruvate kinase (WAY et al., 1959), and ^{14}C-labeled 8-azaGTP was isolated. In contrast to the 5′-monophosphate nucleotides of other guanine analogs, such as 6-thioguanine, 8-azaGMP serves as a substrate for the enzyme, guanylate kinase, from hog brain, Sarcoma 180 cells, and human erythrocytes (MIECH and PARKS, 1965; MIECH et al., 1969; AGRAWAL et al., 1971). The fact that 6-thioGMP does not react with this enzyme accounts for the substantial accumulation of this analog nucleotide in tumor cells treated with 6-thioguanine. The triphosphate nucleotide, 8-azaGTP, serves as a substrate for nucleoside diphosphokinase from human erythrocytes (MOURAD and PARKS, 1966) and succinic thiokinase from pig heart (CHA and PARKS, 1964), both enzymes that normally convert GDP to GTP.

C. Metabolic Enzymes

GTP serves as the specific cofactor for a number of important enzymes in metabolism. For example, succinic thiokinase, a key enzyme in the citric acid cycle, phosphoenolpyruvate carboxykinase, the enzyme that links the citric acid cycle with glycolysis in gluconeogenesis, and adenylosuccinate synthetase, a critical enzyme in the synthesis of AMP, are enzymes that require guanosine rather than adenosine polyphosphate nucleotides as cofactors. Therefore, an attractive explanation of the action of 8-azaguanine and other guanine analogs might be that fraudulent coenzymes, such as 8-azaGTP, are formed in cells and cause blockade of one or more key enzymic reactions (PARKS, 1962). However, little evidence has been uncovered to support this hypothesis. In the above reactions, 8-azaGTP replaces GTP as the coenzyme rather than causing inhibition (PARKS, 1962; COHEN and PARKS, 1963; CHA and PARKS, 1964). In addition, the accumulation of substantial quantities of 8-azaGDP or 8-azaGTP in inhibited tissues has not been observed.

A potentially significant study was performed with adenylosuccinate synthetase (COHEN and PARKS, 1963):

$$\text{IMP} + \text{Aspartate} + \text{GTP} \rightleftharpoons \text{Adenylosuccinate} + \text{GDP} + \text{Pi}$$

8-AzaGTP replaces GTP as the essential coenzyme in this reaction; however, kinetic analysis revealed that the Michaelis constants (K_m) for 8-azaGTP and GTP are 5.4×10^{-6} M and 4.3×10^{-5} M, respectively, and the V_{max} values are 14.4 nmoles per hour and 34 nmoles per hour, respectively. Thus the K_m for 8-azaGTP is only 1/8 that of GTP, while the maximum velocity is only 42 % of that for GTP. This suggests that 8-azaGTP might serve as a partial substrate for adenylosuccinate synthetase and resemble in its behavior the partial antagonist described by ARIËNS et al. (1956). Thus, 8-azaGTP, which has a significantly greater affinity for the enzyme when it occupies the reactive site, permits a reaction velocity only 42 % of the optimal rate. It is possible that such a phenomenon could be involved in cellular inhibitions, and it is likely that careful kinetic analyses would reveal similar effects with other analog nucleotides and other enzymes. However, although these nucleotide-level effects are of considerable biochemical interest, there is no evidence that they play a significant role in the cellular inhibitions caused by 8-azaG.

D. RNA Polymerase, DNA Polymerase, and Ribonuclease (RNAase)

Studies with DNA-directed RNA polymerase isolated from *E. coli* (KAHAN and HURWITZ, 1962) showed that the ribonucleoside triphosphates of several analogs, including 8-azaG, can replace the natural ribonucleoside triphosphates. The rate of this reaction when 8-azaGTP replaced GTP with calf thymus DNA as the primer, was about 24 % of the control value, whereas negligible velocities were observed when 8-azaGTP replaced ATP, UTP, or CTP. These observations indicated that, not only can 8-azaGTP interact with the enzyme, but that the 8-azaG residue is capable of forming the proper complementary base pairs with a DNA primer, although with lowered efficiency.

In recent studies with RNA polymerase from *E. coli*, of the steps involved in the transcription of DNA (i.e., chain initiation, chain elongation, and chain release), DARLIX et al. (1971) have confirmed the observations of KAHAN and HURWITZ (1962) that the replacement of GTP by 8-azaGTP reduced the rate of RNA synthesis to 20 to 25 % of normal. In experiments with β,γ-^{32}P 8-azaGTP, it was observed that chain initiation was decreased to about 15 % of the chains initiated by GTP. Furthermore, if both ATP and GTP were replaced simultaneously by the two analog nucleotides, 8-azaGTP and formycin triphosphate (an ATP analog), very little chain initiation occurred and RNA synthesis was thereby almost completely suppressed. The analog, 8-azaGTP, functions normally in chain elongation, but an abnormal pattern of chain termination and release occurred when the RNA product contained 8-azaG. Significantly, RNA chains that contain 8-azaGMP were not released from ternary complexes, even after prolonged incubation and the formation of chains longer than 3000 nucleotide units. Under the same conditions, chains that contained normal bases were released when the length reached about 3000 nucleotide units. If such events occur in intact cells, marked interference with DNA transcription would occur and the newly synthesized 8-azaG-containing RNA molecules would be retained in the nucleus. Such an event would drastically interfere with protein synthesis. These findings might very well explain many of the observations made by a number of laboratories on the behavior of 8-azaG.

In experiments with chemically synthesized 2′-deoxy-8-azaguanosine 5′-triphosphate, it was found that this analog nucleotide does not serve as a substrate for DNA polymerase from *E. coli* (REICH, personal communication). This finding may explain the failure of significant amounts of 8-azaG to be incorporated into the DNA of most tissues studied.

Residues of 8-azaG in the polyribonucleotide, poly-8-azaG, are found predominantly in the *syn* conformation under conditions in which natural nucleotides occur in the *anti* conformation. The fact that poly-8-azaG is in the *syn* conformation permits it to serve as a substrate for bovine pancreatic RNAase, while polyguanine is resistant (LEVIN, 1962; WARD et al., 1969). However, although the transphosphorylation component of the RNAase reaction can occur with poly-8-azaG, the hydrolytic reaction is defective. Therefore, the product released is 8-azaguanosine cyclic 2′,3′-phosphate rather than 8-azaguanosine 3′-phosphate (WARD et al., 1969).

Effects of 8-Azaguanine on Protein Synthesis

Investigations to date point to effects on the protein synthesizing machinery of the cell as a major site of action of 8-azaG. Early evidence for inhibition of protein synthesis came from the laboratory of CREASER (1956) who demonstrated the inhibition by 8-azaG of induced enzyme production in bacteria. Other workers showed inhibition of hemoglobin synthesis by de-embryonated chick blastoderm (O'BRIEN, 1959), and a differential effect on the synthesis of bacterial cell wall as opposed to cellular protein (MANDEL, 1958; MANDEL and ALTMAN, 1960; ROODYN and MANDEL, 1960).

In a study of the effect of 8-azaG on induced enzyme synthesis in the liver of the adrenalectomized rat following administration of tryptophan (tryptophan pyrrolase) or hydrocortisone (glucose-6-phosphatase and fructose-1-6-diphosphatase), significant decreases in enzymatic activities were observed and the decreases were dose-related (KVAM and PARKS, 1960). Since GTP is required for protein synthesis, 8-azaGTP was tested as a cofactor in an *in vitro* system employing rat liver microsomes for the study of protein synthesis. 8-AzaGTP was found to be a partially effective replacement for GTP. Furthermore, when the microsomal system was incubated with both GTP and 8-azaGTP, additive rather than competitive effects were seen (ROY et al., 1961). These observations suggest that the effect of 8-azaguanine on protein synthesis does not occur at the level of GTP. As discussed below, marked effects occur when 8-azaG is incorporated into tRNA or mRNA that probably explain the inhibitions of protein synthesis caused by 8-azaG.

Incorporation of 8-Azaguanine into Nucleic Acids

The incorporation of 8-azaG into the ribonucleic acids of both tumor and normal tissues was first shown by BENNETT et al. (1950). 8-AzaG also enters the RNA of *Tetrahymena geleii*, and a relationship was seen between growth inhibition and amount of 8-azaG incorporated (HEINRICH et al., 1952; KIDDER et al., 1952). As in experiments with higher animals, only negligible incorporation of 8-azaG into DNA was observed. It was reported by LASNITZKI et al. (1954) that 8-azaG in bacterial, viral, and mammalian RNA may replace as much as 5 % of the guanine residues. An extremely interesting and provocative observation first made by SMITH and MATHEWS (1957) was that *B. cereus* can replace as much as 40 % of its RNA guanine by 8-azaguanine. Furthermore, the distribution of the analog was not random, with the smaller RNA molecules containing greater amounts of 8-azaG than the larger RNA's. These early results have been amply confirmed in more recent investigations by a number of laboratories that demonstrate preferential labeling of tRNA and mRNA in comparison with ribosomal RNA (MANDEL and MARKHAM, 1958; LEVIN, 1963; KARON et al., 1965). Also, in *B. cereus*, the RNA formed during partial growth inhibition by 8-azaG is somewhat less stable than normal RNA (CHANTRENNE and DEVREUX, 1960; MANDEL, 1961; LEVIN, 1963).

Several laboratories have offered evidence for the incorporation of 8-azaG into messenger RNA (LEVIN, 1965a; ZIMMERMAN and GREENBERG, 1965; WEBB, 1967; KWAN and WEBB, 1967, 1970; ZIMMERMAN, 1968). Since there is considerable evidence that 8-azaG inhibits protein synthesis, an attractive working hypothesis is that defective mRNA's are formed causing disruption and breakdown of polyribosomes or otherwise modifying the function of mRNA. Studies with regenerating liver have shown that administration of 8-azaG causes an increase in the numbers of monomers and dimers of ribosomes, and pulse-labeling experiments with radioactive amino acids indicated that the monomers and dimers of the ribosomes are inactive in protein synthesis (KWAN and WEBB, 1967). Similar conclusions were drawn from experiments with *B. cereus* in which the addition of polyribonucleotides to extracts of *B. cereus* grown in the presence of 8-azaG caused marked increases in amino acid incorporation. This suggests that a significant number of the ribosomes are dissociated from mRNA in the treated cells (ZIMMERMAN et al., 1967).

Of considerable interest is that 8-azaG is incorporated primarily into RNA, with little or no uptake into DNA. Several laboratories have reported that in the presence of 8-azaG, the synthesis of protein and DNA may be strongly inhibited while RNA synthesis proceeds. A definite explanation for the failure to incorporate significant amounts of 8-azaG into DNA has not been offered. It seems possible that the substrate activity of 8-azaGDP with the enzyme ribonucleoside diphosphate reductase may be defective, or that 2′-deoxy-8-azaGTP may be a poor substrate for the DNA polymerases. Recent studies with *E. coli* DNA polymerase indicate that 2′-deoxy-8-azaGTP does not serve as a substrate (REICH, personal communication).

A question of considerable interest is whether miscoding is caused when 8-azaG residues replace guanine in tRNA or mRNA. Since the pK_a of 8-azaG ($pK_a = 6.5$) (AGRAWAL and PARKS, 1971) is considerably lower than that of guanine ($pK_a = 9.2$), it appears that at physiological pH, 8-azaG incorporated into nucleotide forms or into nucleic acids exists predominantly in the ionized state and might be expected to cause errors in translation. This question has been subjected to careful study (LEVIN, 1965b; GRUNBERGER et al., 1966, 1967, 1968). With *B. cereus* it was found that 8-azaG replaces only guanine residues in the tRNA (LEVIN, 1963). The isolated tRNA that contained 8-azaG accepted amino acids to the same extent as normal RNA. However, although miscoding has not been observed, codons that contain 8-azaG instead of guanine perform with lowered efficiency. For example, 8-azaG can replace guanine in the codons for valine, alanine, and asparate, as well as in the second position of codons for arginine (GRUNBERGER et al., 1968). However, the template activity of the 8-azaG-containing codons was markedly decreased. The GpUpG codon activity of *E. coli* tRNA was decreased with 8-azaGpUpG or GpUp8-azaG, and was almost completely lost when both residues were replaced in 8-azaGpUp8-azaG.

References

ADYE, J. C., GOTS, J. S.: Further studies on genetically altered purine nucleotide pyrophosphorylases of Salmonella. Biochim. biophys. Acta (Amst.) **118**, 344—350 (1966).

AGARWAL, K. C., CHU, S. H., ROSS, A. F., GORSKE, A. F., PARKS, R. E., JR.: Antitumor action of 6-selenoguanine and 6-selenoguanosine. Pharmacologist **13**, 105 (1971).

AGARWAL, K. C., PARKS, R. E., JR.: Unpublished observation (1971).

AGARWAL, R. P., SCHOLAR, E. M., AGRAWAL, K. C., PARKS, R. E., JR.: Identification and isolation on a large scale of guanylate kinase from human erythrocytes (effects of monophosphate nucleotides of purine analogs). Biochem. Pharmacol. **20**, 1341—1354 (1970).

ANDERSON, E. P., LAW, L. W.: Biochemistry of cancer. Ann. Rev. Biochem. **29**, 577—608 (1960).

ARIËNS, E. J., VAN ROSSUM, J. M., SIMONIS, A. M.: Theoretical basis of molecular pharmacology; interactions of one or two compounds with one receptor system. Arzneimittel-Forsch. **6**, 282—293 (1956).

BENNETT, L. L., JR., SKIPPER, H. E., MITCHELL, J. H., SUGIURA, K.: Studies on the distribution of radioactive 8-azaguanine (guanazolo) in mice with Eo 771 tumors. Cancer Res. **10**, 644—646 (1950).

BROCKMAN, R. W., ANDERSON, E. P.: Biochemistry of cancer (metabolic aspects). Ann. Rev. Biochem. **32**, 463—512 (1963).
BROCKMAN, R. W., BENNETT, L. L., JR., SIMPSON, M. S., WILSON, A. R., THOMSON, J. R., SKIPPER, H. E.: A mechanism of resistance to 8-azaguanine. II. Studies with experimental neoplasms. Cancer Res. **19**, 856—869 (1959b).
BROCKMAN, R. W., SPARKS, M. C., HUTCHISON, D. J., SKIPPER, H. E.: A mechanism of resistance to 8-azaguanine. I. Microbiological studies on the metabolism of purines and 8-azapurines. Cancer Res. **19**, 177—188 (1959a).
BROCKMAN, R. W., SPARKS, M. C., SIMPSON, M. S.: A comparison of the metabolism of purines and purine analogs by susceptible and drug-resistant bacterial and neoplastic cells. Biochim. biophys. Acta (Amst.) **26**, 671—672 (1957).
BROWN, G. B., ROLL, P. M., PLENTL, A. A., CAVALIERI, L. F.: The utilization of adenine for nucleic acid synthesis and as a precursor of guanine. J. biol. Chem. **172**, 469 (1948).
CARLO, P. E., MANDEL, H. G.: The effect of 4-amino-5-imidazole carboxamide on the toxicity of 8-azaguanine. Cancer Res. **14**, 459—462 (1954).
CHA, S., PARKS, R. E., JR.: Succinic thiokinase. I. Purification of the enzyme from pig heart. J. biol. Chem. **239**, 1961—1967 (1964).
CHANTRENNE, H., DEVREUX, S.: Action de la 8-azaguanine sur la synthèse des protéines et des acides nucléiques chez *Bacillus cereus*. Biochim. biophys. Acta (Amst.) **39**, 486—499 (1960).
COHEN, L. H., PARKS, R. E., JR.: Inhibition and activation of adenylosuccinic synthetase by 8-azaguanosine triphosphate. Canad. J. Biochem. **41**, 1495—1501 (1963).
CREASER, E. H.: The assimilation of amino acids by bacteria. 22. The effect of 8-azaguanine upon enzyme formation in *Staphylococcus aureus*. Biochem. J. **64**, 539 (1956).
DARLIX, J. L., FROMAGEOT, P., REICH, E.: Analysis of transcription *in vitro* using purine nucleotide analogs. Biochemistry **10**, 1525—1531 (1971).
ELION, G. B., BURGI, E., HITCHINGS, G. H.: Studies on condensed pyrimidine systems. IX. The synthesis of some 6-substituted purines. J. Amer. chem. Soc. **74**, 411—414 (1952).
ELION, G. B., HITCHINGS, G. H.: The synthesis of 6-thioguanine. J. Amer. chem. Soc. **77**, 1676 (1955).
EMMELOT, P.: The molecular basis of cancer chemotherapy. In: ARIËNS, E. J. (Ed.): Molecular pharmacology, Vol. 2. New York: Academic Press. 1965.
FEIGELSON, P., DAVIDSON, J. D.: The inhibition of adenosine deaminase by 8-azaguanine *in vitro*. J. biol. Chem. **223**, 65—73 (1956).
FRIEDKIN, M.: Enzymatic synthesis of azaguanine riboside and azaguanine deoxyriboside. J. biol. Chem. **209**, 295—301 (1954).
GELLHORN, A.: Laboratory and clinical studies on 8-azaguanine. Cancer **6**, 1030—1033 (1953).
GELLHORN, A., KREAM, J., HIRSCHBERG, E.: Metabolism of 8-azaguanine in rabbits. Fed. Proc. **10**, 297—298 (1951).
GOLDIN, A., GREENSPAN, E. M., GOLDBERG, B., SCHOENBACH, E. B.: Studies on the mechanism of action of chemotherapeutic agents in cancer. IV. Relationship of guanine and guanylic acid to the action of guanazolo on lymphoid tumors in mice and rats. J. nat. Cancer Inst. **11**, 319—338 (1950).
GRÜNBERGER, D., HOLY, A., ŠORM, F.: Synthesis and coding properties of 8-azaguanosine containing triribonucleoside diphosphates. Biochim. biophys. Acta (Amst.) **161**, 147—155 (1968).
GRUNBERGER, D., MEISSNER, L., HOLY, A., ŠORM, F.: The coding properties of polymers and trinucleoside diphosphates containing 8-azaguanosine. Coll. Czech. Chem. Commun. **32**, 2625—2633 (1967).
GRÜNBERGER, D., O'NEAL, C., NIRENBERG, M.: Stimulation of amino acid incorporation into protein by polyuridylic-8-azaguanylic acid. Biochim. biophys. Acta (Amst.) **119**, 581—585 (1966).
HALL, T. C., KRANT, M. J., LLOYD, J. B., PATTERSON, W. B., ISHIBARA, A., POTEE, K. G., LOVINA, T. O., MULLEN, J. M.: Treatment of localized inoperable neoplasms with intra-arterial infusions of 8-azaguanine. Cancer **15**, 1156—1164 (1962).
HANDSCHUMACHER, R. E., WELCH, A. D.: Agents which influence nucleic acid metabolism. In: CHARGAFF, E., DAVIDSON, J. N. (Eds.): The nucleic acids, Vol. 3, pp. 453—526. New York: Academic Press 1960.
HEINRICH, M. R., DEWEY, V. C., PARKS, R. E., JR., KIDDER, G. W.: The incorporation of 8-azaguanine into the nucleic acid of *Tetrahymena geleii*. J. biol. Chem. **197**, 199—204 (1952).
HIRSCHBERG, E., KREAM, J., GELLHORN, A.: Enzymatic deamination of 8-azaguanine in normal and neoplastic tissues. Cancer Res. **12**, 524—528 (1952).
HIRSCHBERG, E., MURRAY, M. R., PETERSON, E. R., KREAM, J., SCHAFRANEK, R., POOL, J. L.: Enzymatic deamination of 8-azaguanine in normal human brain and in glioblastoma multiforme. Cancer Res. **13**, 153—157 (1953).

Kahan, F. M., Hurwitz, J.: The role of deoxyribonucleic acid in ribonucleic acid synthesis. IV. The incorporation of pyrimidine and purine analogues into ribonucleic acid. J. biol. Chem. **237**, 3778—3785 (1962).

Kalle, G. P., Gots, J. S.: Alterations in purine nucleotide pyrophosphorylases and resistance to purine analogues. Biochim. biophys. Acta (Amst.) **53**, 166—173 (1961).

Karnofsky, D. A., Clarkson, B. D.: Cellular effects of anticancer drugs. Ann. Rev. Pharmacol. **3**, 357—428 (1963).

Karon, M., Weissman, S., Meyer, C., Henry, P.: Studies of DNA, RNA, and protein synthesis in cultured human cells exposed to 8-azaguanine. Cancer Res. **25**, 185—192 (1965).

Kidder, G. W., Dewey, V. C.: The biological activity of substituted purines. J. biol. Chem. **179**, 181—187 (1949).

Kidder, G. W., Dewey, V. C., Parks, R. E., Jr.: Effect of lowered essential metabolites on 8-azaguanine inhibition. J. biol. Chem. **197**, 193—198 (1952).

Kidder, G. W., Dewey, V. C., Parks, R. E., Jr., Woodside, G. L.: Purine metabolism in *Tetrahymena* and its relation to malignant cells in mice. Science **109**, 511—514 (1949).

Kidder, G. W., Dewey, V. C., Parks, R. E., Jr., Woodside, G. L.: Further evidence on the mode of action of 8-azaguanine (guanazolo) in tumor inhibition. Cancer Res. **11**, 204—211 (1951).

Kondo, T., Maruyama, T.: The influence of 8-azaguanine on tumors and its enhancement. Gann **42**, 503—506 (1955).

Krishnan, P. S., Sitaramayya, A., Kumar, K. S.: Differential induction of cytoplasmic guanine deaminase isozymes under guanine stress in rat liver and brain. Biochem. biophys. Res. Commun. **40**, 1002—1007 (1970).

Kvam, D. C., Parks, R. E., Jr.: Inhibition of hepatic-induced enzyme formation by 8-azaguanine. J. biol. Chem. **235**, 2893—2896 (1960).

Kwan, S. W., Webb, T. E.: A study of the mechanism of polyribosome breakdown induced in regenerating liver by 8-azaguanine. J. biol. Chem. **242**, 5542—5548 (1967).

Kwan, S. W., Webb, T. E.: Differential sensitivity of the protein-synthesizing system of rat liver to 8-azaguanine. Life Sci. **9**, 975—983 (1970).

Lasnitzki, I., Mathews, R. E. F., Smith, J. D.: Incorporation of 8-azaguanine into nucleic acids. Nature (Lond.) **173**, 346 (1954).

Levin, D. H.: The polymerization of 8-azaguanosine 5′-diphosphate by polynucleotide phosphorylase. Biochim. biophys. Acta (Amst.) **61**, 75—81 (1962).

Levin, D. H.: The incorporation of 8-azaguanine into soluble ribonucleic acid of *Bacillus cereus*. J. biol. Chem. **238**, 1098—1104 (1963).

Levin, D. H.: Evidence for an active messenger ribonucleic acid containing 8-azaguanine. Biochemistry **5**, 1618—1624 (1965a).

Levin, D. H.: Amino acid acceptor and transfer functions of sRNA containing 8-azaguanine. Biochem. biophys. Res. Commun. **19**, 654—660 (1965b).

Mandel, H. G.: Some aspects of the metabolism of 8-azaguanine. In: Rhoads, C. P. (Ed.): Antimetabolites and cancer, pp. 199—218. Washington, D. C.: Am. Ass. Advance. Sci. 1955.

Mandel, H. G.: The effect of 8-azaguanine on utilization of methionine by *Bacillus cereus*. Arch. Biochem. Biophys. **76**, 230—232 (1958).

Mandel, H. G.: The physiological disposition of some anticancer agents. Pharmacol. Rev. **11**, 743—838 (1959).

Mandel, H. G.: Further studies on the modification of nucleic acid synthesis of *B. cereus* by 8-azaguanine. J. Pharmacol. exp. Ther. **133**, 141—150 (1961).

Mandel, H. G., Alpen, E. L., Winters, W. D., Smith, P. K.: The urinary metabolites of 8-azaguanine in the mouse and the monkey. J. biol. Chem. **193**, 63—71 (1951).

Mandel, H. G., Altman, R. L.: The depression of the incorporation of sulfur amino acids into *Bacillus cereus* by 8-azaguanine. J. biol. Chem. **235**, 2029—2035 (1960).

Mandel, H. G., Markham, R.: The effect of 8-azaguanine on the biosynthesis of ribonucleic acid in *Bacillus cereus*. Biochem. J. **69**, 297—306 (1958).

Mathews, R. E. F.: Biosynthetic incorporation of metabolite analogues. Pharmacol. Rev. **10**, 359—406 (1958).

Miech, R. P., Parks, R. E., Jr.: Adenosine triphosphate: guanosine monophosphate phosphotransferase (partial purification and substrate specificity). J. biol. Chem. **240**, 351—357 (1965).

Miech, R. P., York, R., Parks, R. E., Jr.: Adenosine triphosphate-guanosine 5′-phosphate phosphotransferase. II. Inhibition by 6-thioguanosine 5′-phosphate of the enzyme isolated from hog brain and sarcoma 180 ascites cells. Molec. Pharmacol. **5**, 30—37 (1969).

Montgomery, J. A.: On the chemotherapy of cancer. Progr. Drug Res. **8**, 431—507 (1965).

Mourad, N., Parks, R. E., Jr.: Erythrocytic nucleoside diphosphokinase. II. Isolation and kinetics. J. biol. Chem. **241**, 271—278 (1966).

O'BRIEN, B. R. A.: 8-Azaguanine inhibition of haemoglobin synthesis in de-embryonated chick blastoderm. Nature (Lond.) **184**, 376—377 (1959).
PARKS, R. E., JR.: Antimetabolite studies in *Tetrahymena* and tumors. In: RHOADS, C. P. (Ed.): Antimetabolites and cancer, pp. 175—197. Washington, D.C.: Am. Assoc. Advance. Sci. 1955.
PARKS, R. E., JR.: Studies with 8-azaguanine and other purine antimetabolites. Il Farmaco, **17**, 627—646 (1962).
PARKS, R. E., JR.: Cancer chemotherapy with purine antimetabolites. In: BUSCH, H. (Ed.): Biochemical frontiers in medicine, pp. 245—273.: Little, Brown and Company 1963.
ROBLIN, R. O., JR., LAMPEN, J. O., ENGLISH, J. P., COLE, Q. P., VAUGHAN, J. R.: Studies in chemotherapy. VIII. Methionine and purine antagonists and their relation to the sulfonamides. J. Am. chem. Soc. **67**, 290—294 (1945).
ROODYN, D. B., MANDEL, H. G.: The differential effect of 8-azaguanine on cell wall and protoplasmic protein synthesis in *Bacillus cereus*. J. biol. Chem. **235**, 2036—2044 (1960).
ROSS, A. F., PARKS, R. E., JR.: Unpublished observation (1971).
ROUSH, A., NORRIS, E. R.: Deamination of 8-azaguanine by guanase. Arch. Biochem. Biophys. **29**, 124—129 (1950).
ROY, J. K., KVAM, D. C., DAHL, J. L., PARKS, R. E., JR.: Effect of triphosphate nucleosides of 8-azaguanine, 6-thioguanine, and 6-mercaptopurine on amino acid incorporation *in vitro* into microsomal protein. J. biol. Chem. **236**, 1158—1162 (1961).
ROY-BURMAN, P.: Analogues of nucleic acid components. In: RENTCHNICK, P. (Ed.): Recent results in cancer research, pp. 28—32. New York: Springer 1970.
SCHACTER, B., LAW, L. W.: Azaguanine-deaminase activity of several lymphocytic leukemias of mice. J. nat. Cancer Inst. **18**, 77—81 (1957).
SKIPPER, H. E., BENNETT, L. L., JR.: Biochemistry of cancer. Ann. Rev. Biochemistry **27**, 157—166 (1958).
SMITH, J. D., MATHEWS, R. E. F.: The metabolism of 8-azapurines. Biochem. J. **66**, 323—333 (1957).
STOCK, J. A.: Antimetabolites. In: SCHNITZER, R. J., HAWKING, F. (Eds.): Experimental chemotherapy, Vol. 4, pp. 80—196. New York: Academic Press 1966.
SUGIURA, K., HITCHINGS, G. H., CAVALIERI, L. F., STOCK, C. C.: The effect of 8-azaguanine on the growth of carcinoma, sarcoma, osteogenic sarcoma, lymphosarcoma and melanoma in animals. Cancer Res. **10**, 178—185 (1950).
ULTMANN, J. E., FEIGELSON, P.: The effects of 8-azaguanine and 6-mercaptopurine on purine catabolism in the rat. Cancer Res. **18**, 1319—1323 (1958).
WARD, D. C., FULLER, W., REICH, E.: Stereochemical analysis of the specificity of pancreatic RNAase with polyformycin as substrate: differentiation of the transphosphorylation and hydrolysis reactions. Proc. nat. Acad. Sciences **62**, 581—588 (1969).
WAY, J. L., DAHL, J. L., PARKS, R. E., JR.: Polyphosphate nucleosides of purine analogues. J. biol. Chem. **234**, 1241—1243 (1959).
WAY, J. L., PARKS, R. E., JR.: Enzymatic synthesis of 5'-phosphate nucleotides of purine analogues. J. biol. Chem. **231**, 467—480 (1958).
WEBB, T. E.: Polyribosome breakdown in rat liver following administration of 8-azaguanine. Biochim. biophys. Acta (Amst.) **138**, 307—315 (1967).
ZIMMERMAN, E. F.: Azaguanine inhibition of protein synthesis. III. Sito of action in HeLa cells. Biochim. biophys. Acta (Amst.) **157**, 378—391 (1968).
ZIMMERMAN, E. F., GREENBERG, S. A.: Inhibition of protein synthesis by 8-azaguanine. I. Effects on polyribosomes in HeLa cells. Molec. Pharmacol. **1**, 113—125 (1965).
ZIMMERMAN, E. F., HOLLER, B. W., PEARSON, G. D.: Azaguanine inhibition of protein synthesis. II. Effects of poly (U) in *Bacillus cereus*. Biochim. Biophys. Acta (Amst.) **134**, 402—410 (1967).

Chapter 52

Folate Antagonists

JOSEPH R. BERTINO

With 2 Figures

Basic Considerations

A. Structure and Mechanism of Action of Folate Antagonists

The three most widely studied and clinically useful folate antagonists are aminopterin, methotrexate (MTX, amethopterin), and 3′,5′-dichloro-MTX (Fig. 1). These compounds are all 4-amino analogs of folic acid and are powerful inhibitors of the enzyme dihydrofolate reductase (DHFR) (Fig. 2). The folate antagonists have extremely low inhibition constants (ca. 10^{-10} M) and they bind in a stoichiometric manner to dihydrofolate reductase at pH 6.0 (WERKHEISER, 1961; BERTINO et al., 1964). At a more alkaline pH, they bind less tightly and the binding is competitive with the substrate, dihydrofolate. This enzyme-inhibitor complex can be dissociated with regeneration of the enzyme and inhibitor by chromatography on DEAE-cellulose or hydroxylapatite, or by gel filtration at pH 9.0 in the presence of 0.15 M KCl (MATHEWS and HUENNEKENS, 1963; BERTINO et al., 1964, 1965).

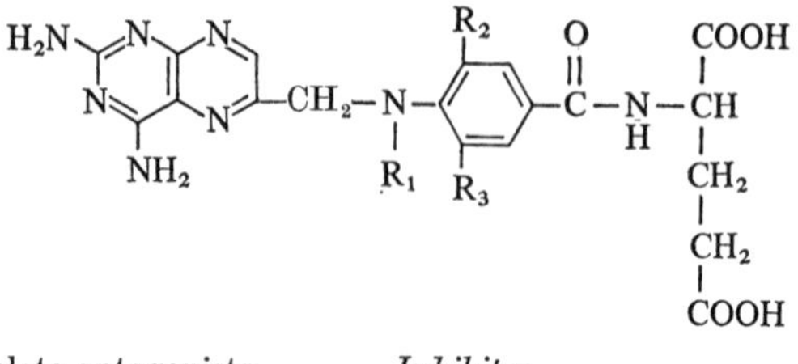

Fig. 1. Structure of folate antagonists

Inhibitor	R_1	R_2	R_3
Aminopterin	H	H	H
Methotrexate	CH_3	H	H
Dichloromethotrexate	CH_3	Cl	Cl

MTX has similar binding affinities for dihydrofolate reductase from normal mammalian tissues and from neoplastic tissues; thus, selectivity of these agents against tumors depends upon other considerations, such as differences between normal and neoplastic cells in growth rates, folate coenzyme pools, levels of dihydrofolate reductase, transport, the presence of salvage pathway enzymes for the formation of purine nucleotides and thymidylate and the rate of synthesis of the enzyme dihydrofolate reductase (BERTINO, 1963; WERKHEISER, 1971). WERK-

HEISER (1971) has described a model that attempts to take these factors into consideration to predict MTX effectiveness as a consequence of drug dosage and schedule.

In contrast, attempts to obtain selectivity with folate antagonists on the basis of differential inhibition of dihydrofolate reductases have been very successful in bacterial and protozoal chemotherapy (HITCHINGS, 1971). "Nonclassical" folate antagonists have been synthesized that exploit the species differences in dihydrofolate reductases at the hydrophobic binding regions located outside of the enzyme active site (BAKER, 1964; BURCHALL and HITCHINGS, 1965; BURCHALL, 1971). Differences among mammalian dihydrofolate reductase enzymes, in particular between neoplastic and nonneoplastic enzymes, appear to be small or nonexistent, and clinically useful compounds based on this rationale have not yet been developed (BAKER, 1971). However, the availability of affinity chromatographic procedures, in particular utilizing MTX bound to sepharose, has provided a great stimulus to this field, since highly purified dihydrofolate reductases from a number of mammalian sources are now available for careful analysis and study (KAUFMAN and PIERCE, 1971; HUENNEKENS et al., 1971; CHELLO et al., 1972; GOLDIE and HILLCOAT, 1972). The availability of antibody to mammalian dihydrofolate reductases and of a variety of nonclassical inhibitors should also facilitate the documentation of potentially exploitable differences in dihydrofolate reductase proteins in normal and neoplastic tissues. At least two forms of dihydrofolate reductase have been detected in mammalian tissues; one form appears to contain bound NADPH, while the other does not have any bound nucleotide (PERKINS et al., 1967; HUENNEKENS et al., 1971). The significance of these two forms *in vivo* is not clear, but it has been suggested that they play a role in the development of drug resistance (HUENNEKENS et al., 1971).

Although the enzyme dihydrofolate reductase has received a great deal of attention because of its inhibition by low concentrations of MTX, additional sites of action of MTX have been proposed. BORSA and WHITMORE (1969) have demonstrated that thymidylate synthetase from cultured L-cells is inhibited weakly by MTX, in a competitive manner with N^5–N^{10}-methylene tetrahydrofolate (FH_4), the folate coenzyme involved in this reaction (Fig. 2). Inhibition of dihydrofolate reductase, which leads to a depletion of N^5–N^{10}-methylene FH_4 in cells actively synthesizing DNA, thus could intensify the inhibition of thymidylate synthetase by MTX. It is of interest that one strain of *Lactobacillus casei* resistant to MTX has elevated levels of thymidylate synthetase, as well as of dihydrofolate reductase (LEARY and KISLIUK, 1971). An increase in thymidylate synthetase activity has also been observed after MTX treatment of human leukemia cells in culture (ROBERTS and LOEHR, 1971), in regenerating liver (LABOW et al., 1969), and in cells from patients with acute leukemia treated with MTX (ROBERTS et al., 1969). The mechanism of this rise in the latter circumstances is not entirely clear, but appears to result from some form of cell synchronization and a decrease in the rate of degradation of the enzyme.

B. Mechanism of Cell Death

The folate antagonists are essentially inhibitors of DNA synthesis and therefore kill cells if the drug is present during the S phase of the cell cycle (HRYNIUK et al., 1969; BRUCE, 1970). As might be expected, MTX kills cells most effectively when the cell population is in logarithmic growth; it is much less effective against plateau phase cells (HRYNIUK et al., 1969). In addition, these studies indicate that cells in the S phase during log growth are more sensitive to MTX than cells in

S phase in plateau growth. The biochemical reason for this difference in sensitivity has not been elucidated, but one factor involved may relate to MTX transport (NAHAS et al., unpublished observations).

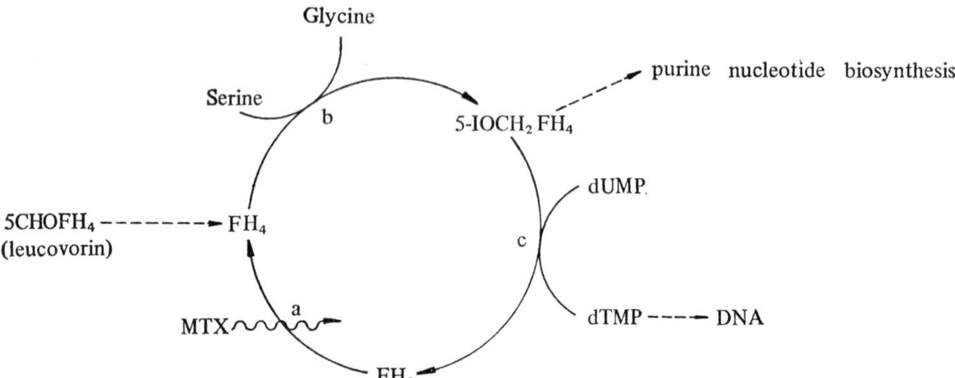

Fig. 2. Inhibition of dihydrofolate reductase by methotrexate (MTX). Abbreviations used are: FH_4, tetrahydrofolate; FH_2, dihydrofolate; dUMP, deoxyuridylate; dTMP, thymidylate. The three enzymes involved in the methylation of deoxyuridylate are: (a) dihydrofolate reductase, (b) serine transhydroxymethylase, and (c) thymidylate synthetase

As a result of inhibition of DNA synthesis by MTX, under certain conditions cells are unable to synthesize sufficient DNA for subsequent division, and "megaloblast" formation occurs, since RNA and protein synthesis continue, while the formation of DNA does not. At a critical point, cell death ensues, but the exact reasons for death are not known. This type of cell death has been referred to as unbalanced growth or "thymineless" death and is also seen with other potent inhibitors of DNA synthesis such as 5-fluorodeoxyuridine and cytosine arabinoside (COHEN, 1971).

Since MTX may also inhibit RNA synthesis via inhibition of *de novo* purine nucleotide synthesis, as well as protein synthesis, it has been suggested that MTX, unlike cytosine arabinoside or 5-fluorodeoxyuridine, is a "self-limiting" inhibitor of cell growth, since by stopping RNA and protein synthesis, metabolic imbalances caused by interference with the formation of DNA are corrected. This appears to be true of at least one mammalian cell type, the L cell grown in tissue culture (BORSA and WHITMORE, 1969a). Thus, exposure of these cells to deoxyadenosine in the presence of MTX enhanced the rate of cell kill, as compared to a purine free medium. The implications of this finding are of great importance if human tumors behave similarly. Combination chemotherapy with MTX and inhibitors of either protein or RNA synthesis may result in antagonism of MTX action. An example of this phenomenon, shown by a recent study, demonstrates that asparaginase, an inhibitor of protein synthesis, can prevent the action of MTX under certain circumstances (CAPIZZI et al., 1971). These considerations may or may not apply to normal replicating cells, and the net therapeutic effect achieved will depend upon a differential effect on normal versus neoplastic tissues. Furthermore, in other cell lines, purines partially relieved the MTX block on DNA synthesis and decreased cell kill, indicating that at least in this line "purineless" death was a major concomitant of MTX action (HRYNIUK and BERTINO, 1971). Clearly, further studies of the combination of MTX and inhibitors of protein synthesis are warranted, and conditions of dosage and scheduling may be found that lead to an improved therapeutic index of MTX for certain tumors, as well as to an antagonism (CAPIZZI, 1972).

Pharmacology of Folate Antagonists

A. Absorption

Oral doses of MTX in the usual therapeutic range (i.e., 2.5 to 10 mg) are absorbed rapidly and completely from the gastrointestinal tract (FREEMAN, 1958; HENDERSON et al., 1965). However, large oral doses (i.e., 10 mg/kg) were found to be less well absorbed, and absorption was prolonged (HENDERSON et al., 1965). Aminopterin in therapeutic doses is also absorbed quantitatively and rapidly after oral administration, but dichloro-MTX was found to be absorbed poorly and erratically, and systemic administration of this latter drug is necessary to obtain reproducible blood concentrations (DAVIDSON and OLIVERIO, 1965). The reasons for the poor absorption of dichloro-MTX are not clear, but may relate to metabolism by intestinal flora.

B. Transport

As might be expected, since MTX is a large polar lipid-insoluble molecule, transport across cell membranes depends upon specific transport mechanisms. Thus, tumor cell penetration and organ distribution may reflect the presence or absence of these transport processes, as well as the level of the enzyme DHFR in the cells. An active transport process for MTX that appears also to be utilized by the reduced folates, N^5-formyl FH_4 and N^5-methyl-FH_4, has been found in both L5178 and L1210 cells (GOLDMAN, 1971; NAHAS et al., 1972). In contrast, the vitamin, folic acid, is only poorly transported by these cells, and presumably does not employ the same carrier system utilized by MTX and the reduced folates (NAHAS et al., 1972; NIETHAMMER and HUENNEKENS, 1972). In Sarcoma 180 cells, HAKALA (1965) observed a slow influx of MTX, proportional to the extracellular MTX concentration over a wide range. Since a slight deviation was observed at large MTX concentrations and MTX uptake was inhibited by N^5-formyl-FH_4, the process may not be one of simple diffusion, but a process of facilitated diffusion with a low affinity constant.

A good correlation was obtained with a series of transplantable murine leukemias between uptake of MTX and natural sensitivity to the drug (KESSEL et al., 1965). Not surprisingly, one mechanism of acquired resistance to MTX observed in several murine neoplasms has been impaired MTX transport (FISCHER, 1962; HAKALA, 1965). In man, impaired transport of MTX may, in certain instances of acute leukemia, play a role in natural or acquired resistance (FISCHER et al., 1963; KESSEL et al., 1968), although further studies are required to establish the role of altered transport in drug resistance.

In a study of N^5-formyltetrahydrofolate (leucovorin) transport in L1210 cells, MTX competitively inhibited the uptake of this reduced folate ($K_i = 7.7$ µM) (NAHAS et al., 1972), a finding anticipated in view of the ability of leucovorin to inhibit MTX uptake competitively (GOLDMAN, 1971). Efflux of leucovorin was accelerated by MTX, while folic acid had little or no effect on the influx or efflux of MTX. Thus, leucovorin "rescue" of cells from MTX action may be due not only to the repletion of reduced folate coenzymes by leucovorin, but also to the ability of leucovorin to inhibit MTX uptake and to accelerate the efflux of some intracellular MTX. These studies also provide an explanation for the observation that the administration of either MTX or aminopterin results in a transient increase in the urinary excretion of leucovorin in both experimental animals and man (Li et al., 1958).

C. Distribution of Folate Antagonists

Organ distribution of folate antagonists appears to reflect the presence or absence of specific transport mechanisms, as well as the levels of DHFR present in cells. Thus, in liver, kidney, and the intestinal mucosa, penetration of MTX appears to be rapid, and appreciable levels are achieved. In tissues such as muscle, fat, and brain, penetration is poor (Bischoff et al., 1970). Only slight penetration of MTX from plasma into the cerebrospinal fluid occurs, as in the situation with folic acid (but not with reduced folates), therefore intrathecal administration of MTX is necessary to achieve high levels in the central nervous system (Rubin et al., 1966). MTX is found in skin after parenteral administration, perhaps bearing on its activity in patients with psoriasis, and also on its ability to cause skin rashes (Grignani et al., 1967; Anderson et al., 1970). Transport of this drug through normal or damaged skin or through mucous membranes into the parenteral circulation upon topical administration has not been adequately studied in man.

The long term tissue retention of the 2,4-diaminopteroylglutamate compounds appears to be determined by the levels of the target enzyme DHFR, and the turnover of the cells in that tissue. Thus, in liver and kidney, organs with a slow cellular turnover rate, MTX appears to be retained for months (Charache and Condit, 1960). Indeed, Werkheiser (1962) has suggested that the rate of tissue disappearance of this tightly bound MTX can be used to estimate the rate of cell turnover. Using tritium labeled MTX, Johns et al. (1964) found in man that tritium labeled MTX could be readily displaced weeks after MTX administration by dihydrofolate and unlabeled MTX, compounds with relatively great affinity for DHFR. These findings indicate that the binding of MTX to DHFR, although tight, is reversible, as might be expected from the enzyme studies previously noted (Bertino et al., 1964). The use of I^{131} labeled iodoaminopterin has also allowed the measurement, via external scintillation scanning, of the organ distribution of this folate antagonist in human subjects; in addition to the anticipated high concentration of the drug in liver and kidney, considerable drug activity was detected over the sternal bone marrow, and some excretion of the drug in the stomach was detected (Johns et al., 1968).

D. Metabolism

Marked species differences exist in the metabolism of the folate antagonists, explaining at least in part the wide range of LD_{50} values obtained with these compounds in animals. In addition, the susceptibility to metabolic alteration differs between antagonists; in general, the halogenated compounds are more extensively metabolized than the nonhalogenated derivatives (Davidson and Oliverio, 1965).

In man, metabolism of aminopterin or MTX does not appear to be quantitatively significant. Studies with ^{3}H-labeled MTX have shown that most of the drug is excreted unchanged in the first 24 h after oral or parenteral administration (Johns et al., 1964; Henderson et al., 1965). Urinary excretion of MTX during a 48 h time period varied from 56 % of the administered dose when 2.5 μg/kg was administered, to 83 % of the dose when 10 mg/kg was given (Henderson et al., 1965). This initial excretion represents drug not bound to tissue DHFR. Subsequent slow excretion (1 to 2 %/day) may represent slow release from tissue

DHFR with kidney clearance. Chromatography of this urinary material has shown small amounts of non-MTX radioactivity (JOHNS et al., 1964). HENDERSON et al. (1965) suggested that these derivatives arise from bacterial cleavage of MTX during enterohepatic circulation of the drug. Recent studies of ZAHARKO et al. (1969, 1970) support the concept of bacterial cleavage of the drug to a pteroate and glutamate during enterohepatic circulation, a catabolic pathway of considerable quantitative importance in mice and rats.

Certain species, especially the rabbit and guinea pig are capable of rapidly oxidizing MTX to 7-hydroxyMTX by liver aldehyde oxidase (JOHNS et al., 1965). 7-HydroxyMTX is less than one one-hundredth as active as MTX, accounting apparently for the tremendous tolerance of these animal species to MTX (JOHNS, 1971). In man, liver aldehyde oxidase lacks the ability to utilize MTX as a substrate, although it does hydroxylate the MTX analog, dichloroMTX.

E. Excretion

Biliary excretion of MTX in man appears to be a minor route of excretion, with only 2 to 6 % of the drug found in the feces after parenteral administration (HENDERSON et al., 1965). Again, important species differences exist; biliary excretion of this drug in the rat is quantitatively greater than in man. With dichloroMTX, as much as one-half of the drug may appear in the feces of the rat after parenteral administration (DAVIDSON and OLIVERIO, 1965).

The major route of MTX excretion is via the kidney. This process appears to be a combination of glomerular filtration and active tubular excretion. Of potential clinical importance are the findings that other compounds utilizing the same renal tubular mechanism, e.g. salicylate and *p*-aminohippurate, inhibit this process (LIEGLER et al., 1969). MTX itself, in large doses, may be toxic to the kidney, resulting in impaired tubular transport, thus increasing its own retention and toxicity (CONDIT et al., 1969).

F. Mechanisms of Drug Resistance

Three mechanisms of acquired drug resistance to MTX have been described in experimental tumor systems: an increased level of DHFR, impaired transport, and an altered DHFR with decreased affinity for MTX (reviewed by BERTINO and SKEEL, 1973). The biochemical explanation for acquired MTX resistance in patients with acute lymphatic leukemia has been difficult to document, but one instance of an altered enzyme has been detected as a possible explanation (BERTINO and SKEEL, 1973). Utilizing a simple *in vitro* test, in which incorporation of ^{3}H-deoxyuridine into DNA is measured in the absence and presence of MTX, biochemical resistance may be detected (HRYNIUK and BERTINO, 1969; BERTINO and SKEEL, 1973). Clearly, additional work is needed in this important area, since development of drug resistance may offer opportunities for alternative chemotherapeutic approaches.

In one animal study, natural resistance of a series of transplanted rodent tumors correlated relatively well with impaired transport (KESSEL et al., 1965). In man, natural resistance of patients with acute myelocytic leukemia appears to result from the ability of these cells to synthesize DHFR at a relatively faster rate than lymphoid leukemia cells (HRYNIUK and BERTINO, 1969). This rapid rate of synthesis may be detected because of the ability of MTX to stabilize the enzyme and protect it from degradation (BERTINO et al., 1965).

Clinical Application

A. General Considerations

MTX is available for both parenteral and oral administration. When large doses of drugs are to be used, or when absorption may be impaired, parenteral use is recommended (Henderson et al., 1965). DichloroMTX and aminopterin are not available for general use and must be considered experimental drugs, especially the former compound, which is under investigation as an intra-arterial agent (Cleveland et al., 1969). Toxicity to the folate antagonists, once a significant concentration is reached, is almost a direct function of the duration of drug concentration in the plasma, and probably only a log function of the dose of the drug (Bruce et al., 1966). Thus, huge amounts of drug may be administered if the duration of drug exposure is limited to 48 h or less by leucovorin administration; when exposure to high concentrations of drug exceeds 48 h, severe toxicity occurs, presumably due to the killing of significant numbers of normal stem cells that are recruited from a "G_0" state to enter the cell cycle (Schwarzenberg et al., 1969). Thus, the acute effects of MTX administration are primarily related to normal renewal systems, e.g., the gastrointestinal mucosa, the bone marrow, and the skin (Bertino and Johns, 1967; Condit, 1971).

B. Toxic Effects

After a single large dose of MTX (i.e., 1 to 5 mg/kg), leukopenia may be produced, reaching a nadir at day 9 to 10 after drug administration. Thrombocytopenia and reticulocytopenia may also be produced, the nadir of the platelet count depression being observed also on day 10 (Condit et al., 1962). All replicating forms in the bone marrow are affected, but not mature blood cell elements. Recovery then occurs within the next several days, but may be prolonged in patients in poor general condition, in particular if a clinical or subclinical folate deficient state is present, or if patients have impaired marrow function due to infection, tumor cell involvement, previous radiation therapy, or chemotherapy. Toxicity may also be enhanced in patients with impaired renal function, and a creatinine clearance test is advisable in all patients before treatment with large doses of MTX (Condit, 1969). Since MTX itself can lead to renal toxicity, repeat kidney function tests should be carried out during therapy with MTX. If MTX is to be used in patients with impaired kidney function, facilities should be available to monitor blood levels of the drug, and leucovorin "rescue" should be utilized appropriately if drug clearance is delayed significantly (Mitchell and Bertino, unpublished observations).

With minimal to moderately toxic doses of MTX, mucositis may be observed two to seven days after MTX administration. The degree of mucositis produced is a function of both the drug dose and the duration of drug administration, and may range from minimal erythema of the buccal mucosa and lower inner lip to severe ulceration of the oral mucosa, also involving the nasal epithelium. It is usually good practice to stop therapy at the first sign of mucositis, since severe toxicity may be produced with continued drug administration. Nausea and anorexia, and less commonly, vomiting, may also be noted during or after MTX administration, especially with large doses. Diarrhea is also occasionally seen. With toxic doses of MTX more severe gastrointestinal signs and symptoms, progressing to gastrointestinal ulceration and bleeding, may be produced. Fever has also been reported to accompany the use of large dose MTX with leucovorin rescue (Gottlieb et al., 1970).

Skin rash has been noted in 10 to 20 % of patients treated with MTX. Severity of the rash is often related to other signs and symptoms of severe toxicity, but occasionally skin toxicity is seen without other evidence of toxicity. The rash usually occurs one to three days after MTX administration, is maculopapular in type, occurs in the upper trunk and neck region, and may be pruritic and spread to other parts of the trunk. Occasionally, especially when associated with severe systemic MTX toxicity, the rash may be more severe, and is characterized by vasculitis and widespread herpetiform skin eruption. Hair loss after MTX administration occurs in 5 to 10 % of patients, especially in older individuals.

Two types of liver damage appear to be associated with MTX administration: a reversible transient toxicity noted with large doses of the drug, such as are employed in the treatment of choriocarcinoma (HERTZ et al., 1961) and less commonly, hepatic fibrosis associated with long term use of the drug (ROENIGK et al., 1971). Although the potential for hepatic fibrosis and cirrhosis related to chronic MTX administration does not appear to be a significant contraindication to the use of this drug in the treatment of neoplastic disease, these effects are of great significance when this drug is utilized to treat nonneoplastic disease, in particular psoriasis, and patients should be carefully followed and the drug discontinued if evidence of chronic liver disease is noted.

Left upper quadrant pain, probably due to splenic capsule inflammation, perhaps secondary to leukemia cell destruction, has been reported to occur in leukemic patients treated with large doses of MTX (HRYNIUK and BERTINO, 1969). Pulmonary infiltrates have been reported to occur with chronic MTX administration. The relationship of these effects to infection processes, especially *Pneumocystis carinii* pneumonia, is not clear, although the infiltrate is presumed to be an allergic reaction.

MTX is known to be a potent abortifacient, especially if administered during the first trimester of pregnancy. In a recent study it also has been reported to impair spermatogenesis, and may be mutagenic (CAPIZZI, unpublished observations).

C. Treatment of Neoplastic Disease: General Principles

MTX is a cell cycle specific inhibitor and kills cells only in the *S* phase of growth; thus, for significant antitumor effect, it must be present for a sufficient length of time and at an effective concentration. Since few if any biochemical differences have been noted between normal replicating tissues and tumor tissue with regard to MTX action, it is obvious that unless kinetic or pharmacologic differences exist between the tumor cells and normal replicating cells, this drug may not have any selectivity. Tumors with large growth fractions and short generation times may benefit from large dose intermittent treatment with this agent; if the treatment interval is kept short, normal cell toxicity will be manageable. The use of large doses of drug has the additional advantage that the occurrence of mutations to drug resistant forms may be less frequent. Except for the treatment of choriocarcinoma, and perhaps for Burkitt's lymphoma, where MTX treatment may be curative, this drug has limited antitumor effects, and the use of other modalities such as x-ray therapy and surgery to decrease tumor mass, as well as of other drugs in combination with MTX, appears to be necessary to obtain more significant antitumor effects and prevention of drug resistance.

It follows that neoplasms composed of cells with long generation times and with small growth fractions (e.g., chronic lymphocytic leukemia and multiple myeloma) will not benefit from MTX therapy. Conceivably, low dose continuous therapy might be effective, but since there is no differential effect on normal replicating cells, toxicity to normal tissues and possible development of drug resistance limits this approach.

In a discussion of specific diseases benefited by MTX therapy the above principles should be kept in mind. It should also be noted that optimum dosage schedules using MTX have not been ascertained in every disease, and some improvement in results might be expected with improved drug scheduling. An important limitation to MTX therapy is central nervous system (CNS) disease. Meningeal leukemia and lymphoma may be successfully treated with intrathecal MTX, but disease invariably recurs. The use of MTX intrathecally together with whole brain radiation as prophylaxis against this occurrence has led to a decreased rate of CNS involvement and an increase in survival in patients with acute lymphocytic leukemia (SULLIVAN et al., 1969).

D. Treatment of Specific Tumors

I. Choriocarcinoma

This rapidly fatal malignancy has the distinction of being the first human neoplasm cured by a chemotherapeutic agent. HERTZ et al. (1961) demonstrated that 50% of patients with choriocarcinoma may be cured by large dose aggressive therapy with MTX. Higher cure rates are achieved in patients with a shorter duration of disease and urinary chorio-gonadotrophin titers of less than 10^6 units/24 h. Attempts to utilize aggressive chemotherapy in other human tumors have not resulted in comparable improvement in tumor response, except perhaps for a smaller percentage of patients with Burkitt's lymphoma (BURKITT, 1965). Several authors have suggested that host immune responses contribute to the cure of these two tumors by MTX, although the evidence for this is only fragmentary. Certain other drugs, most notably actinomycin D, also have significant antitumor effects against choriocarcinoma and combinations of drugs have been used in late stage treatment of patients with choriocarcinoma with some success (HERTZ et al., 1964). Patients with choriocarcinoma should be treated at centers equipped to deal with the severe toxicity encountered, and the response followed by frequent determination of chorio-gonadotrophin in urine or blood.

II. Acute Leukemia

Aminopterin, the first antimetabolite of demonstrable value in the treatment of neoplastic disease, was reported to cause complete remissions in children with acute leukemia in 1947 (FARBER et al., 1947). Since this time, MTX has supplanted aminopterin in the clinic, presumably because of its improved therapeutic index, demonstrable in mice bearing the L1210 leukemia (GOLDIN et al., 1955), but not unequivocally proven in man. During the past decade it has also become clear that MTX is not an optimum drug to use by itself in "remission induction" of acute leukemia, presumably because patients appearing for treatment with acute leukemia have far advanced disease, and thus the tumor cell population is more apt to be in plateau phase growth rather than in logarithmic growth, and thus less susceptible to the effects of this drug. As might be anticipated, MTX is a highly effective drug in the treatment of patients with acute lymphatic leukemia in remission; large intermitent doses of drug every 4 days have proven to be more effective than daily low dose continuous administration (SELAWRY, 1965). Five day courses of MTX administered in a schedule similar to that used in the treatment of choriocarcinoma also have proved to be effective remission therapy. In one study, patients with far advanced acute lymphoblastic leukemia were treated with large doses of MTX given over 24 h followed by leucovorin rescue; complete or partial remissions were obtained in seven of the eleven patients treated (HRYNIUK and BERTINO, 1969). The use of leucovorin rescue appeared to decrease the gastrointestinal toxicity of MTX without decreasing its antileukemia effects. Pulses of large doses at biweekly intervals with or without leucovorin rescue also have proven to be highly effective dosage schedules in the treatment of acute lymphatic leukemia (CONDIT and ELIEL, 1960; PERRIN and MAUER, 1963; DJERASSI, 1967). The optimum dose schedule for the treatment of acute lymphocytic leukemia has not been definitely established, but it seems clear that some form of large dose intermittent treatment is preferable over low dose daily administration. Our preference for remission therapy of acute lymphocytic leukemia is MTX in large dosage, followed by leucovorin rescue at 36 h, used in combination with cytosine arabinoside and cyclophosphamide (SKEEL et al., 1973).

MTX has not been as effective in the treatment of acute myelocytic leukemia (AML) either in remission induction or in remission maintenance (VOGLER et al., 1967). Remission induction rates with this drug in AML range from 5 to 15%, when used in conventional schedules. Attempts to improve remission rates by the use of large dose infusions followed by leucovorin rescue have not proven successful, since AML cells, as well as normal stem cells, appeared to be rescued by leucovorin (HRYNIUK and BERTINO, 1969). However, despite these limitations, MTX has definite antileukemia effects in AML and has been utilized in several combination chemotherapy programs with improved remission induction rates (HENDERSON, 1968; SKEEL et al., 1973).

III. Head and Neck Cancer

MTX is probably the single most effective drug in the treatment of advanced epidermoid carcinoma of the head and neck (LEONE et al., 1968; LANE et al., 1968; CAPIZZI et al., 1970). Approximately 30 to 50% of patients may expect clinical benefit from large dose intermittent therapy with this drug, although the responses have only lasted 3 to 4 months (BERTINO et al., 1973). Leucovorin rescue, as in acute lymphatic leukemia, has been shown to improve the therapeutic index of MTX in this disease by decreasing the severe toxic effects of the drug, especially in this susceptible patient population, which often presents with subclinical folate deficiency and poor general condition (HELLMAN et al., 1964).

IV. Breast Cancer

MTX is one of the most effective drugs available for the treatment of breast cancer; most series report that about 30% of patients with advanced disease obtain an objective tumor response with MTX (LIVINGSTON and CARTER, 1970). Again, neither have optimum dose schedules been established nor does it appear that the most effective drug combination utilizing MTX has been found. Leucovorin rescue following MTX administration has also been utilized in this disease; encouraging antitumor results have been reported with minimum toxicity (VOGLER et al., 1971).

V. Lung Cancer

MTX has been demonstrated to cause objective antitumor effects in carcinoma of the lung in several reports; however, improvement in survival has only been minimal (LIVINGSTON and CARTER, 1970). In a recent small series, extremely large doses of MTX, followed by leucovorin rescue 6 h later, produced very substantial tumor regression of long duration (DJERASSI, 1972). Further studies with larger series of patients will be necessary to establish the value of this approach.

VI. Lymphoma

MTX has limited value in the treatment of lymphoma. In general, the more undifferentiated the lymphoma the more effective is MTX. In childhood lymphosarcoma, the use of MTX with leucovorin rescue has produced a large percentage of tumor regressions (DJERASSI et al., 1968), and in histiocytic and undifferentiated lymphocytic lymphoma MTX may be of value. In one program, the use of MTX as part of a combination has produced complete and partial remissions in 100 % of patients, with some individuals being free of disease for over 2 years (LEVITT et al., 1971).

MTX has also caused complete regressions and some cures in Burkitt's lymphoma, but cyclophosphamide remains the drug of choice in this disease (BURKITT, 1965).

VII. Brain Tumors

Intrathecal administration of MTX has been reported to be of value in the treatment of some brain tumors, especially of the childhood variety (NEWTON et al., 1968; WILSON and NORELL, 1969). Intrathecal administration, together with systemic leucovorin rescue either given concomitantly or following MTX administration, has also been explored recently (WILSON, 1971).

VIII. Primary or Metastatic Liver Tumors

Intra-arterial use of MTX has been attempted for primary liver cancer, as well as for metastatic disease to the liver, usually from the gastrointestinal tract. While most chemotherapists prefer the use of fluorinated pyrimidines intra-arterially, MTX has also been used successfully for this purpose. Response rates of the order of 50 % have been recorded, lasting for several months (BURROWS et al., 1967; NERVI et al., 1970).

Following the successful use of dichloroMTX in a small series of patients with head and neck cancer (CLEVELAND et al., 1969), this drug was recently used to treat patients in Africa with malignant hepatoma (VOGEL et al., 1972). While the systemic use of this drug proved disappointing, hepatic artery infusion produced substantial tumor regression for several months in the few patients studied. This drug, unlike MTX, is metabolized by normal liver and, therefore, is theoretically superior to MTX for intra-arterial use, since by using appropriate doses systemic toxicity should be minimal, while local antitumor effects should be maximum. Further studies with this drug used by intra-arterial injection are clearly indicated.

IX. Mycosis Fungoides

Remissions of several months duration have been reported following the use of MTX without (WRIGHT et al., 1960) and with leucovorin rescue (McDONALD and BERTINO, unpublished observations).

X. Miscellaneous Solid Tumors

MTX has been reported to be of some value in the treatment of various other solid tumors including carcinoma of the bladder (ELLIOT, 1962) and cervix (ROY, 1967), testicular tumors (WYATT and McANINCH, 1967), and soft tissue sarcomas (WILTSHAW, 1967). Usually, the response rates have been low and the duration of response not long, but further work is required with various dosage schedules before the maximal value of MTX in these diseases can be assessed. In a recent report, large dose MTX with leucovorin rescue was shown to cause impressive tumor regressions (both complete and partial) in several patients with osteogenic sarcoma, a tumor refractory to most chemotherapeutic agents (JAFFE, 1972).

XI. Nonneoplastic Diseases

MTX has been used to treat severe generalized psoriasis, a benign disease of the skin characterized by rapid proliferation (VAN SCOTT et al., 1964; McDONALD and BERTINO, 1969; WEINSTEIN, 1971), so-called diseases of "autoimmunity" such as Wegener's granulomatosis (CAPIZZI and BERTINO, 1970), systemic lupus erythematous, and rheumatoid arthritis (STEINBERG, 1972) and as an immunosuppressive agent, especially to treat graft versus host disease as seen after marrow transplantion (THOMAS et al., 1971). The use of MTX to treat severe psoriasis and chronic diseases such as rheumatoid arthritis is controversial, in view of the potentially serious hazards of drug therapy (BERTINO, 1973). When this drug and other potent chemotherapeutic agents are used in these diseases, the patients should be under the supervision of physicians skilled in the use of these drugs and informed consent should be obtained.

References

ANDERSON, L. L., COLLINS, G. J., OJIMA, Y., SULLIVAN, R. D.: A study of the distribution of methotrexate in human tissues and tumors. Cancer Res. **30**, 1344—1348 (1970).

BAKER, B. R.: Active-site directed irreversible inhibitors of dihydrofolate reductase. Ann. N.Y. Acad. Sci. **186**, 214—226 (1971).

BAKER, B. R., HO, B. T.: Differential inhibition of dihydrofolate reductase from different species. J. pharm. Sci. **53**, 1137—1138 (1964).

BERTINO, J. R.: The mechanism of action of the folate antagonists in man. Cancer Res. **23**, 1286—1306 (1963).

BERTINO, J. R.: Chemical action and pharmacology of methotrexate, azathioprine, and cyclophosphamide in man. Arthritis Rheum. **16**, 79—83 (1973).

BERTINO, J. R., BOOTH, B. A., CASHMORE, A. R., BIEBER, A. L., SARTORELLI, A. C.: Studies of the inhibition of dihydrofolate reductase by the folate antagonists. J. biol. Chem. **239**, 479—485 (1964).

BERTINO, J. R., CASHMORE, A. R., FINK, M., CALABRESI, P., LEFKOWITZ, E.: The induction of leukocyte and erythrocyte dihydrofolate reductase by methotrexate. Clin. Pharm. Therap. **6**, 763—770 (1965).

BERTINO, J. R., DECONTI, R. C., MOSHER, M.: Chemotherapy of head and neck cancer. Cancer **31**, 1141—1149 (1973).

BERTINO, J. R., JOHNS, D. G.: Folate antagonists. Ann. Rev. Med. **18**, 27—34 (1967).

BERTINO, J. R., SKEEL, R. T.: Resistance to chemotherapeutic agents: clinical aspects. Proc. 5th int. Congr. Pharmacol. **3**, 376—392 (1973).

BISCHOFF, K. B., DEDRICK, R. L., ZAHARKO, D. S.: Preliminary model for methotrexate pharmacokinetics. J. pharm. Sci. **59**, 149—153 (1970).

BORSA, J., WHITMORE, G. F.: Studies relating to the mode of action of methotrexate. III. Inhibition of thymidylate synthetase in tissue culture cells and in cell-free systems. Molec. Pharmacol. **5**, 318—332 (1969).

BORSA, J., WHITMORE, G. F.: Cell killing studies on the mode of action of methotrexate (MTX) on L-cells *in vitro*. Cancer Res. **29**, 737—744 (1969a).

BRUCE, W. R.: The action of chemotherapeutic agents at the cellular level and the effects of these agents on hematopoietic and lymphomatous tissue. In: Canadian cancer conference, Proc. 7th Canad. Cancer Res. Conf., Honey Harbour, Ontario **7**, 53—64 (1967).

BRUCE, W. R., MEEKER, B. E., VALERIOTE, F. A.: Comparison of the sensitivity of normal hematopoietic and transplanted lymphoma colony forming cells to chemotherapeutic agents administered *in vivo*. J. nat. Cancer Inst. **37**, 233 (1966).

BURCHALL, J. J.: Comparative biochemistry of dihydrofolate reductase. Ann. N.Y. Acad. Sci. **186**, 143—152 (1971).

BURCHALL, J. J., HITCHINGS, G. H.: Inhibitor binding analysis of dihydrofolate reductases from various species. Molec. Pharmacol. **1**, 126—132 (1965).
BURKITT, D. P.: In: BURKITT, D. P., BURCHENAL, J. H. (Eds.): Treatment of Burkitt's tumor. New York: Springer 1966.
BURROWS, J. H., TALLEY, R. W., DRAKE, E. H., SAN DIEGO, F. J., TUCKER, W. G.: Infusion of fluorinated pyrimidines into hepatic artery for treatment of metastatic carcinoma of liver. Cancer **21**, 1886—1892 (1967).
CAPIZZI, R. L.: Schedule-dependent eradication of murine leukemia with methotrexate and asparaginase. Fifteenth Ann. Meeting, Amer. Soc. Hematol. **43** (Abstr.) (1972).
CAPIZZI, R. L., BERTINO, J. R.: Methotrexate therapy of Wegener's granulomatosis. Ann. int. Med. **74**, 74—79 (1971a).
CAPIZZI, R. L., DECONTI, R. C., MARSH, J. C., BERTINO, J. R.: Methotrexate therapy of head and neck cancer: improvement in therapeutic index by the use of leucovorin "rescue". Cancer Res. **30**, 1782—1788 (1970).
CAPIZZI, R. L., SUMMERS, W. P., BERTINO, J. R.: L-Asparaginase induced alteration of amethopterin (methotrexate) activity in mouse leukemia L5178Y. Ann. N. Y. Acad. Sci. **186**, 302—311 (1971).
CHARACHE, S., CONDIT, P. T., HUMPHREYS, S. R.: Studies of the folic acid vitamins. IV. The persistence of amethopterin in mammalian tissues. Cancer **13**, 236—240 (1960).
CHELLO, P., CASHMORE, A. R., JACOBS, S. A., BERTINO, J. R.: Improved purification of tetrahydrofolate dehydrogenase from L1210 leukemia by affinity chromatography. Biochim. biophys. Acta (Amst.) **268**, 30—34 (1972).
CLARYSSE, A. M., CATHEY, W. J., CARTWRIGHT, G. E., WINTROBE, M. N.: Pulmonary disease complicating intermittent therapy with methotrexate. J. Amer. med. Ass. **209**, 1861—1864 (1969).
CLEVELAND, J. C., JOHNS, D. G., FARNHAM, G., BERTINO, J. R.: Arterial infusion of dichloromethotrexate in cancer of the head and neck: a clinical-pharmacologic study. Curr. Topics surg. Res. **1**, 113—120 (1969).
COE, R. O., BULL, F. E.: Cirrhosis associated with methotrexate treatment of psoriasis. J. Amer. med. Ass. **206**, 1514—1520 (1968).
COHEN, S.: On the nature of thymineless death. Ann. N. Y. Acad. Sci. **186**, 292—301 (1971).
CONDIT, P. T.: Chemotherapy of neoplastic disease with folate antagonists. Ann. N. Y. Acad. Sci. **186**, 475—485 (1971).
CONDIT, P. T., CHANES, R. E., JOEL, W.: The renal toxicity of methotrexate. Cancer **23**, 126—131 (1969).
CONDIT, P. T., ELIEL, L.: Effects of large infrequent doses of amethopterin on acute leukemia in children. J. Amer. med. Ass. **172**, 451—453 (1960).
CONDIT, P., SHNIDER, B. I., OWENS, A. H., JR.: Studies in the folic acid vitamins. VII. The effects of large doses of amethopterin in patients with cancer. Cancer Res. **22**, 706—712 (1962).
CRUSBERG, T. C., LEARY, R., KISLIUK, R. L.: Properties of thymidylate synthetase from dichloromethotrexate-resistant *Lactobacillus casei*. J. biol. Chem. **245**, 5292—5296 (1970).
DAVIDSON, J. O., OLIVERIO, V. T.: The physiologic disposition of dichloromethotrexate-Cl^{36} in man. Clin. Pharmacol. Ther. **6**, 325—327 (1965).
DJERASSI, I.: Methotrexate infusions and intensive supportive care in the management of children with acute lymphocytic leukemia: follow-up report. Cancer Res. **27**, 2561—2564 (1967).
DJERASSI, I., ROMINGER, C. J., KIM, J. S., TURCHI, J., SUVANSRI, U., HUGHES, D.: Phase I study of high doses of methotrexate with citrovorum factor in patients with lung cancer. Cancer **30**, 22—30 (1972).
DJERASSI, I., ROYER, G., TREAT, C., CARIM, H.: Management of childhood lymphosarcoma and reticulum cell sarcoma with high dose intermittent methotrexate and citrovorum factor. Proc. Amer. Ass. Cancer Res. **9**, 18 (1968).
ELLIOT, J.: Treatment of bladder cancer with amethopterin. Cancer Chemother. Rep. **20**, 147 (1962).
FARBER, S. L. H., DIAMOND, R. D., MERCER, R. F., SYLVESTER, J. R., WOLFF, J. O.: Temporary remissions in acute leukemia in children produced by folic acid antagonists, 4-aminopteroylglutamic acid (aminopterin). New Engl. J. Med. **238**, 787—793 (1948).
FISCHER, G. A., BERTINO, J. R., WELCH, A. D.: Uptake of tritium labeled MTX by human leukemia leukocytes. Blood **22**, 819 (1963).
FREEMAN, M. V.: The fluorometric measurement of the absorption, distribution and excretion of single doses of 4-amino-10-methylpteroylglutamic acid (amethopterin) in man. J. Pharmacol. exp. Ther. **122**, 154—162 (1958).

GOLDIN, A., VENDETTI, J. M., HUMPHREYS, S. R., DENNIS, D., MANTEL, N., GREENHOUSE, S. W.: A quantitative comparison of the antileukemic effectiveness of two folic antagonists in mice. J. nat. Cancer Inst. **15**, 1657—1664 (1955).

GOLDIE, J., HILLCOAT, B. L.: Purification of tetrahydrofolate dehydrogenase by affinity chromatography. Biochim. biophys. Acta (Amst.) **268**, 35—40 (1972).

GOLDMAN, I. D.: The characteristics of the membrane transport of amethopterin and the naturally occurring folates. Ann. N. Y. Acad. Sci. **186**, 400—422 (1971).

GOTTLIEB, J. A., SERPICK, A. A.: Prolonged intravenous methotrexate therapy in the treatment of acute leukemia and solid tumors. Cancer Res. **30**, 2132—2138 (1970).

GRIGNANI, F., MARTINELLI, M. F., TONATO, M., FINZI, A. F.: Folate dependent enzymes in human epidermis. Arch. Derm. **96**, 577—585 (1967).

HAKALA, M. T.: On the role of drug penetration in amethopterin resistance of sarcoma — 180 cells *in vitro*. Biochim. biophys. Acta (Amst.) **102**, 198—209 (1965).

HELLMAN, S., IANNOTTI, A., BERTINO, J. R.: Determinations of the levels of serum folate in patients with carcinoma of the head and neck treated with methotrexate. Cancer Res. **24**, 105—113 (1964).

HENDERSON, E. S.: Treatment of acute leukemia. Ann. int. Med. **69**, 628—632 (1968).

HENDERSON, E. S., ADAMSON, R. H., OLIVERIO, V. T.: The metabolic fate of tritiated methotrexate. II. Absorption and excretion in man. Cancer Res. **25**, 1018—1024 (1965).

HERTZ, R., LEWIS, J., JR., LIPPSETT, M. B.: 5 Years experience with the Chemotherapy of metastatic choriocarcinoma and related trophoblastic tumors in women. Amer. J. obstet. and Gynec. **82**, 631—640 (1961).

HERTZ, R., ROSS, G. T., LIPSETT, M. B.: Chemotherapy in women with trophoblastic disease; choriocarcinoma, chorioadenoma destruens, and complicated hydatidiform mole. Ann. N. Y. Acad. Sci. **114**, 881—885 (1964).

HITCHINGS, G. H.: Folate antagonists as antibacterial and antiprotozoal agents. Ann. N. Y. Acad. Sci. **186**, 444—451 (1971).

HRYNIUK, W. M., BERTINO, J. R.: The treatment of leukemia with large doses of methotrexate and folinic acid: clinical-biochemical correlates. J. clin. Invest. **48**, 2140—2155 (1969).

HRYNIUK, W. M., BERTINO, J. R.: Growth rate and cell kill. Ann. N. Y. Acad. Sci. **186**, 330—342 (1971).

HRYNIUK, W. M., FISCHER, G. A., BERTINO, J. R.: *S*-Phase cells of rapidly growing and resting populations. Differences in response to methotrexate. Molec. Pharmacol. **5**, 557—564 (1969).

HUENNEKENS, F. M., DUNLAP, R. B., FREISHEIM, J. H., GUNDERSEN, L. E., HARDING, N. G. L., LEVISON, S. A., MELL, G. P.: Dihydrofolate reductases: structural and mechanistic aspects. Ann. N. Y. Acad. Sci. **186**, 85—99 (1971).

JAFFE, N., FARBER, S., TRAGGIS, D., GEISER, C., DAS, L., KIM, B., FRANENBERGER, G., DJERASSI, I.: Favorable response of metastatic osteogenic sarcoma to pulse high dose methotrexate-citrovorum-administration. Proc. Amer. Ass. Cancer Res. **13**, 27 (1972).

JOHNS, D. G., HOLLINGSWORTH, J. W., CASHMORE, A. R., PLENDERLEITH, I. H., BERTINO, J. R.: Methotrexate displacement in man. J. clin. Invest. **43**, 621—629 (1964).

JOHNS, D. G., IANNOTTI, A. T., SARTORELLI, A. C., BOOTH, B. A., BERTINO, J. R.: The identity of rabbit liver methotrexate oxidase. Biochim. biophys. Acta (Amst.) **105**, 380—382 (1965).

JOHNS, D. G., SPENCER, R. P., CHANG, P. K., BERTINO, J. R.: I^{131} I-3′-Iodoaminopterin: a gamma-labeled active-site-directed enzyme inhibitor. J. nuclear Med. **9**, 530—536 (1968).

JOHNS, D. G., VALERINO, D. M.: Metabolism of folate antagonists. Ann. N. Y. Acad. Sci. **186**, 378—386 (1971).

KAUFMAN, B. T., PIERCE, J. V.: Purification of dihydrofolic reductase from chicken liver by affinity chromatography. Biochem. biophys. Res. Comm. **44**, 608—613 (1971).

KESSEL, D., HALL, T. C., ROBERTS, D.: Modes of uptake of methotrexate by normal and leukemic human leukocytes *in vitro* and their relation to drug response. Cancer Res. **28**, 564—570 (1968).

KESSEL, D., HALL, T. C., ROBERTS, D., WODINSKY, I.: Uptake as a determinant of methotrexate response in mouse leukemias. Science **150**, 752—754 (1965).

LABOW, R., MALEY, G. F., MALEY, F.: The effect of methotrexate on enzymes following partial hepatectomy. Cancer Res. **29**, 366—372 (1969).

LANE, M., MOORE, J. E., III., LEVIN, H., SMITH, F. E.: Methotrexate therapy for squamous cell carcinoma of the head and neck. J. Amer. med. Ass. **204**, 561—564 (1968).

LEARY, R., KISLIUK, R. L.: Crystalline thymidylate synthetase from dichlormethotrexate resistant *Lactobacillus casei*. Prep. Biochem. **1**, 47—54 (1971).

LEONE, L. A., ALBALA, M. M., REGE, V. B.: Treatment of carcinoma of the head and neck with intravenous methotrexate. Cancer **21**, 828—837 (1968).

LEVITT, M., MARSH, J. C., DECONTI, R. C., MITCHELL, M. S., SKEEL, R. T., FARBER, L. R., BERTINO, J. R.: Combination sequential chemotherapy in advanced reticulum cell sarcoma. Cancer **29**, 630—636 (1972).

LI, M. C., NIXON, N. E., FREEMAN, M. V.: Increase of urinary citrovorum factor activity in patients receiving methotrexate (amethopterin). Proc. Soc. exp. Biol. (N.Y.) **97**, 29—32 (1958).

LIEGLER, D. G., HENDERSON, E. S., HAHN, M. A., OLIVERIO, V. T.: The effect of organic acids on renal clearance of methotrexate in man. Clin. Pharmacol. Ther. **10**, 849—857 (1969).

LIVINGSTON, R. B., CARTER, S. K.: Single agents in cancer chemotherapy. London: Plenum Press 1970.

MATHEWS, C. K., HUENNEKENS, F. M.: Further studies on dihydrofolic reductase. J. biol. Chem. **238**, 3436—3442 (1963).

McDONALD, C. J., BERTINO, J. R.: Parenteral methotrexate for psoriasis. Arch. Derm. **100**, 655—668 (1969).

McDONALD, C. J., BERTINO, J. R.: unpublished observations.

NAHAS, A., CAPIZZI, R. L., BERTINO, J. R.: Methotrexate transport in logarithmic and plateau phase cells. Submitted for publication.

NAHAS, A., NIXON, P. F., BERTINO, J. R.: Uptake and metabolism of N^5-formyltetrahydrofolate by L1210 leukemia cells. Cancer Res. **32**, 1416—1421 (1972).

NERVI, C., ARCANGELI, G., CASALE, C., CARRESE, M., GUADAGNI, A., LEPERA, V.: A reappraisal of intra-arterial chemotherapy. Cancer **26**, 577—582 (1970).

NEWTON, W., SAYERS, M., SAMUELS, L.: Intrathecal methotrexate (NSC 740) therapy for brain tumors in children. Cancer Chemother. Rep. **52**, 257—261 (1968).

NIETHAMMER, D., HUENNEKENS, F. M.: Transport of folic acid, 5-methyltetrahydrofolic acid and methotrexate through the membrane of lymphocytes. 2nd International Symposium on Metabolism and Membrane Permeability of Erythrocytes, Thrombocytes and Leukocytes, p. 81, Vienna, June 14—16, 1972.

PERKINS, J. P., HILLCOAT, B. L., BERTINO, J. R.: Dihydrofolate reductase from a resistant subline of the L1210 lymphoma. J. biol. Chem. **242**, 4771—4776 (1967).

PERRIN, J., MAUER, A.: Evaluation of intravenous amethopterin therapy in acute leukemia. J. Pediat. **61**, 283—284 (1963).

ROBERTS, D. W., HALL, T. C., ROSENTHAL, D.: Coordinated changes in biochemical patterns: the effects of cytosine arabinoside and methotrexate on leukocytes from patients with acute granulocytic leukemia. Cancer Res. **29**, 571—578 (1969).

ROBERTS, D. W., LOEHR, E. V.: Elevation of thymidylate synthetase activity in CCRF—CEM cells. Cancer Res. **31**, 1181—1187 (1971).

ROENIGK, H. H., BERGFELD, W. F., ST. JACQUES, R., OWENS, F. J., HAWK, W. A.: Hepatotoxicity of methotrexate in treatment of psoriasis. Arch. Derm. **103**, 250—261 (1971).

ROY, D.: Treatment of advanced or recurrent carcinoma of the cervix by cytotoxic drugs. Indian J. Cancer **4**, 32 (1967).

RUBIN, R. C., OMMAYA, A. K., HENDERSON, E. S., BERING, E. A., RALL, D. P.: Cerebrospinal fluid perfusion for central nervous system neoplasms. Neurology **16**, 680—692 (1966).

SCHWARZENBERG, L., MATHÉ, G., HAYAT, M., DEVASSAL, F., AMIEL, J. L., CATTAN, A., SCHNEIDER, M., SCHLUMBERGER, J. R., ROSENFELD, C., JASMIN, C., NGO/MINH/MAH: Une nouvelle combinaison de methotrexate et d'acide folinique pour le traitment des cancers. La Presse Med. **77**, 385—388 (1969).

SELAWRY, O.: New treatment schedule with improved survival in childhood leukemia. Intermittent parenteral vs. daily oral administration of methotrexate for maintenance of induced remission. J. Amer. med. Ass. **194**, 75—81 (1965).

SKEEL, R. T., MARSH, J. C., DECONTI, R. C., MITCHELL, M. S., HUBBARD, S. P., BERTINO, J. R.: Development of a combination chemotherapy program for adults with acute leukemia: CAM and CAM-L. Cancer **32**, 76—81 (1973).

STEINBERG, A. D.: Efficacy of immunosuppressive drugs in rheumatic diseases. Arthr. and Rheum. (in press).

SULLIVAN, M. P., VIETTI, T. J., FERNBACH, D. J., GRIFFITH, K. M., HADDY, T. B., WATKINS, W. L.: Clinical investigations in the treatment of meningeal leukemia: radiation therapy regimens vs. conventional intrathecal methotrexate. Blood **34**, 301—319 (1969).

THIERSCH, J. B.: Therapeutic abortion with folic acid antagonist, 4-amino pteroylglutamic acid, administered by the oral route. Amer. J. Obst. Gynec. **63**, 1298 (1962).

THOMAS, E. D., STORB, R.: The effect of amethopterin on the immune response. Ann. N.Y. Acad. Sci. **186**, 467—474 (1971).

VANSCOTT, E. S., AUERBACH, R., WEINSTEIN, G. D.: Parenteral methotrexate in psoriasis. Arch. Derm. **89**, 550—556 (1964).

VOGEL, C. L., ADAMSON, R. H., DEVITA, V. T., JOHNS, D. G., KYALWAZI, S. K.: Preliminary clinical trials of dichloromethotrexate (NSC-29630) in hepatocellular carcinoma. Cancer Chemother. Rep. **56**, 249—258 (1972).

VOGLER, W. R., HUGULEY, C., RUNDLES, R.: Comparison of methotrexate with 6-mercaptopurineprednisone in treatment of acute leukemia in adults. Cancer **20**, 1221—1226 (1967).

VOGLER, W. R., JACOBS, J.: Toxic and therapeutic effects of methotrexate-folinic acid (leucovorin) in advanced cancer and leukemia. Cancer **28**, 894—901 (1971).
WEINSTEIN, G. D.: Biochemical and pathophysiological rationale for amethopterin in psoriasis. Ann. N.Y. Acad. Sci. **186**, 452—466 (1971).
WERKHEISER, W. C.: Specific binding of 4-amino folic acid analogues by folic acid reductase. J. biol. Chem. **236**, 888—893 (1961).
WERKHEISER, W. C.: The relation of folic acid reductase to aminopterin toxicity. J. Pharmacol. exp. Therap. **137**, 167—172 (1962).
WERKHEISER, W. C.: Mathematical simulation in chemotherapy. Ann. N.Y. Acad. Sci. **186**, 343—358 (1971).
WILMANNS, W.: Effects of amethopterin treatment on thymidylate synthesis in human leucocytes and bone marrow cells. Ann. N.Y. Acad. Sci. **186**, 365—371 (1971).
WILSON, C. B.: Medulloblastoma. Current views regarding the tumor and its treatment. Oncology **24**, 273—290 (1970).
WILSON, C. B., NORRELL, H.: Brain tumor chemotherapy with intrathecal methotrexate. Cancer **23**, 1038—1045 (1969).
WILTSHAW, E.: Methotrexate in treatment of sarcomata. Brit. Med. J. **2**, 142—145 (1967).
WRIGHT, J. C., GUMPORT, S. L., GOLOMB, F. M.: Remissions produced with the use of methotrexate in patients with mycosis fungoides. Cancer Chemother. Rep. **9**, 11—20 (1960).
WYATT, J., MCANINCH, L.: A chemotherapeutic approach to advanced testicular carcinoma. Canad. J. Surg. **10**, 421—426 (1967).
ZAHARKO, D. S., BRUCKNER, H., OLIVERIO, V. T.: Antibiotics alter methotrexate metabolism and excretion. Science **166**, 887—888 (1969).
ZAHARKO, D. S., OLIVERIO, V. T.: Reinvestigation of methotrexate metabolism in rodents. Biochem. Pharmacol. **19**, 2923—2925 (1970).

Chapter 53

Glutamine Antagonists

L. L. BENNETT, JR.

Introduction

This chapter deals primarily with compounds whose biological activity may be ascribed to interference with functions of glutamine. Some consideration is also given to molecules that decrease the cellular pools of glutamine either by preventing its synthesis or by metabolically altering it once it is formed.

Glutamine occurs widely in animal cells both in free form and as a constituent of protein. In the free form it is the principal free amino acid of blood plasma and a major amino acid in brain cells. Glutamine synthetase, the enzyme converting glutamic acid to glutamine, occurs widely in animal cells, and glutamine is therefore not an essential amino acid. Aside from its role as a constituent of proteins, glutamine participates in the synthesis of a number of other compounds. Its amide group is the donor of one or more nitrogen atoms to a variety of molecules essential for mammalian cells; the conversions involved are the following:

PRPP[1] → 5-phosphoribosylamine
FGARP → FGAmRP
XMP → GMP
UTP → CTP
CO_2 → Carbamylphosphate
Deamido-NAD → NAD
Fructose-6-phosphate → Glucosamine-6-phosphate
Aspartate → Asparagine

In addition, glutamine is the donor of the nitrogen atom for the following conversions important only in microbial metabolism:

Shikimic acid → *p*-Aminobenzoic acid
Chorismic acid → Anthranilic acid
1-Phosphoribosyl-AMP → Imidazoleglycerol phosphate → histidine

For documentation of these general statements the reader is referred to the text of MEISTER (1965). Each of the glutamine-requiring conversions listed will be considered in more detail below.

Although glutamine is not an essential amino acid for normal nutrition, many tumors are dependent upon exogenous glutamine. This dependence is evident in the high requirement for glutamine when the cells are placed in culture (EAGLE et al., 1956; NEUMAN and McCOY, 1956), and is associated with a low intracellular

[1] Abbreviations: RP, 5-phosphoribosyl-; PRPP, 5-phosphoribosyl-1-pyrophosphate; FGARP, 2-formamido-*N*-ribosyl acetamide 5′-phosphate (formylglycinamide ribonucleotide); FGAmRP; 2-formamido-*N*-ribosylacetamidine 5′-phosphate (formylglycinamidine ribonucleotide); XMP, xanthosine 5′-phosphate; GMP, guanosine 5′-phosphate; AMP, adenosine 5′-phosphate; ATP, adenosine 5′-triphosphate; UTP, uridine 5′-triphosphate; CTP, cytidine 5′-triphosphate; NAD, nicotinamide adenine dinucleotide; PRA, 5-phosphoribosylamine.

content of glutamine and a low activity of glutamine synthetase (Roberts and Frankel, 1949; Levintow, 1954; Roberts and Borges, 1955; Rabinovitz et al., 1956, 1957, 1959; Pasieka and Morgan, 1959; Smulson and Neal, 1965; El-Asmar et al., 1966). These metabolic characteristics provide a rationale for a selective action on tumors of agents that interfere with the uptake, synthesis, or functions of glutamine.

The structures of all of the glutamine analogs to be considered are given below in order that similarities and differences may be noted. Each of these analogs may be regarded as glutamine in which modifications have been made on *C*-4 or *C*-5 or in the amide group, while the first three carbon atoms and the 2-amino group are unchanged. Thus albizziin, *O*-carbamylserine, and *S*-carbamylcysteine may be regarded as glutamine in which *C*-4 has been replaced respectively by -NH-, -O-, or -S-.

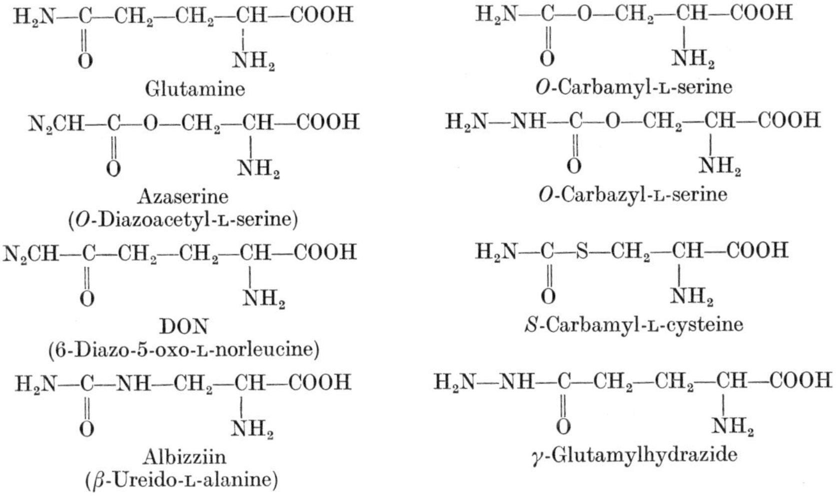

$$H_2N{-}\underset{\|}{\overset{}{C}}{-}CH_2{-}CH_2{-}CH(NH_2){-}COOH \quad (C{=}O)$$

Glutamine

$$H_2N{-}C({=}O){-}O{-}CH_2{-}CH(NH_2){-}COOH$$

O-Carbamyl-L-serine

$$N_2CH{-}C({=}O){-}O{-}CH_2{-}CH(NH_2){-}COOH$$

Azaserine
(*O*-Diazoacetyl-L-serine)

$$H_2N{-}NH{-}C({=}O){-}O{-}CH_2{-}CH(NH_2){-}COOH$$

O-Carbazyl-L-serine

$$N_2CH{-}C({=}O){-}CH_2{-}CH_2{-}CH(NH_2){-}COOH$$

DON
(6-Diazo-5-oxo-L-norleucine)

$$H_2N{-}C({=}O){-}S{-}CH_2{-}CH(NH_2){-}COOH$$

S-Carbamyl-L-cysteine

$$H_2N{-}C({=}O){-}NH{-}CH_2{-}CH(NH_2){-}COOH$$

Albizziin
(β-Ureido-L-alanine)

$$H_2N{-}NH{-}C({=}O){-}CH_2{-}CH_2{-}CH(NH_2){-}COOH$$

γ-Glutamylhydrazide

Numerous reviews have appeared in which some or all of these analogs have been discussed (Duvall, 1960a, b; Brockman and Anderson, 1963; Shive and Skinner, 1963; Pittillo and Hunt, 1967; Livingston et al., 1970). A full coverage of all of the literature on these agents is beyond the scope of the present review, which is intended to present a summary of the status of glutamine analogs with particular emphasis on mechanisms of action. For a full coverage of the earlier literature the reader is referred to the reviews named above, and for full coverage of the antitumor activities particularly to those of Duvall and Livingston et al.

Metabolic Effects of Glutamine Analogs

A. Azaserine and DON

I. Isolation and General Biological Activity

Azaserine and DON are considered together because they are both diazo compounds that act in a generally similar manner. Azaserine, isolated in 1954 from a *Streptomyces* (Bartz et al., 1954; Fusari et al., 1954a, b) was the first diazo compound found to occur naturally. DON was isolated shortly thereafter by the same group of workers (Dion et al., 1956). Both compounds have been synthesized chemically (Moore et al., 1954; Nicolaides et al., 1954; DeWald and Moore, 1956; Westland et al., 1956; Weygand et al., 1958). DON also occurs in conjugated form in three other antibiotics: duazomycin A (RAO, 1961), alazopeptin (DEVOE et al., 1957), and azotomycin (once designated duazomycin B) (RAO et al., 1960). Duazomycin A is simply *N*-acetyl-DON. Alazopeptin and azotomycin are tripeptides consisting of two molecules of DON and one of another amino acid. These antibiotics apparently exert their biological effects only after cleavage to DON, and hence will not be considered separately from DON in discussion of loci of action.

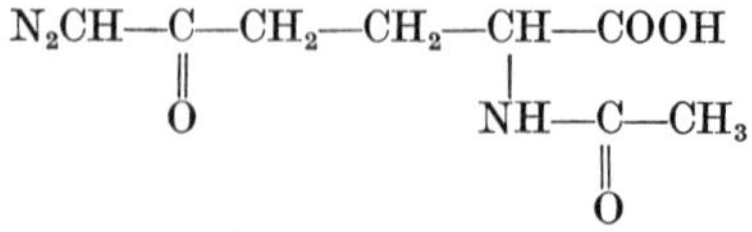

```
N2CH—C—CH2—CH2—CH—COOH
     ‖          |
     O          NH—C—CH3
                   ‖
                   O
```

Duazomycin A

```
   O                                        O
   ‖                                        ‖
   C—CH—CH3                                 C—CH2—CH2—CH—COOH
   |  |                                     |            |
   |  NH2                                   |            NH2
  HN                                       HN
   |                                        |
   CH—CH2—CH2—C—CHN2                        CH—CH2—CH2—C—CHN2
   |          ‖                             |          ‖
 O=C          O                           O=C          O
   |                                        |
  HN—CH—CH2—CH2—C—CHN2                     HN—CH—CH2—CH2—C—CHN2
     |          ‖                             |          ‖
     COOH       O                             COOH       O
```

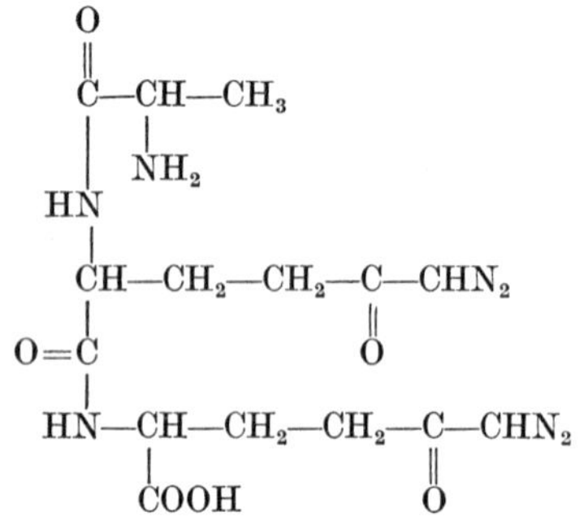

Alazopeptin 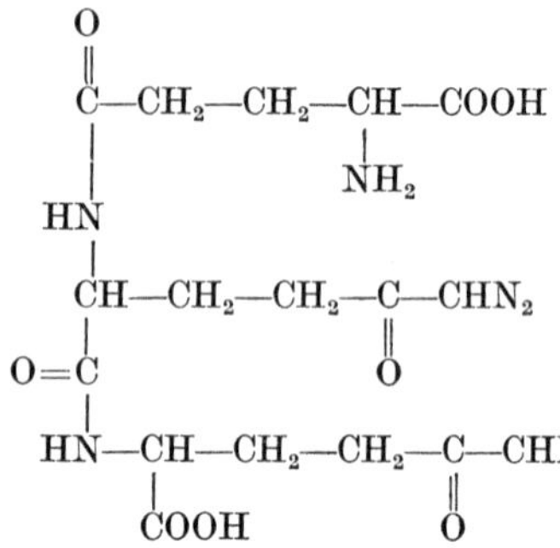 Azotomycin

Azaserine and DON have fairly broad biological activity. Both agents inhibit the growth of certain bacteria, fungi, and protozoa, though many strains are insensitive or are inhibited only by high concentrations. Both agents have been evaluated against a wide spectrum of animal tumors and have shown considerable activity against some of them (DUVALL, 1960a, b). Antitumor activity is discussed further in a later section. DON is more toxic than azaserine and is generally more potent than azaserine as a glutamine antagonist (see below). The superiority of DON to azaserine may be due to the fact that DON retains a chain of six carbon atoms and therefore is a closer structural analog of glutamine than is azaserine. The D-isomer of azaserine was inactive in a number of systems (DUVALL, 1960a). The D-isomer of DON has not been studied extensively, but has been reported to be less effective than the L-isomer in inhibiting the growth of Sarcoma 180 (DUVALL, 1960b).

II. Inhibition of Purine Biosynthesis

The amide group of glutamine is the donor of the 3- and 9-nitrogen atoms of the purine ring and of the amino N-atom of GMP (HARTMAN, 1970). Glutamine is thus involved at three separate points on the pathways leading to purine nucleotides, as shown in the condensed scheme below, and these three reactions are potential sites of action of glutamine antagonists.

The earliest observed metabolic effect of azaserine was a profound inhibition of purine nucleotide biosynthesis in mammalian cells (SKIPPER et al., 1954) at a step before the formation of the ribonucleotide of 5-amino-4-imidazole-carboxamide (BENNETT et al., 1956). This inhibition was shown to be associated with an accumulation of FGARP in avian cells (HARTMAN et al., 1956) and in *E. coli* (TOMISEK et al., 1956). Blockade of the amidination of FGARP was also observed with DON in pigeon liver (LEVENBERG et al., 1957). Following these initial observations, inhibition of the amidination of FGARP by azaserine or DON was found in a great variety of systems – mammalian cells including tumors (GREENLEES and LEPAGE, 1956; MOORE and LEPAGE, 1957; SARTORELLI and LEPAGE, 1958a; HENDERSON, 1962; ANDERSON and BROCKMAN, 1963), bacteria (TOMISEK and REID, 1962), and algae (VAN DER MEULEN et al., 1959) – and is presumably the blockade responsible for the inhibition of *de novo* synthesis of purine nucleotides observed by many other authors (DUVALL, 1960a, b; BARCLAY et al., 1962; SARTORELLI et al., 1964; HELD et al., 1969). The specificity of this blockade has made azaserine a useful agent in the study of the first few steps of purine nucleotide biosynthesis: cells treated with azaserine and ^{14}C-labeled formate or glycine accumulate ^{14}C–FGARP, and agents inhibiting one of the early steps of this pathway produce a decrease in the accumulation of FGARP (SARTORELLI and LEPAGE, 1958b; LEPAGE and JONES, 1961; HENDERSON, 1962, 1963; BENNETT and SMITHERS, 1964; BROCKMAN and CHUMLEY, 1965).

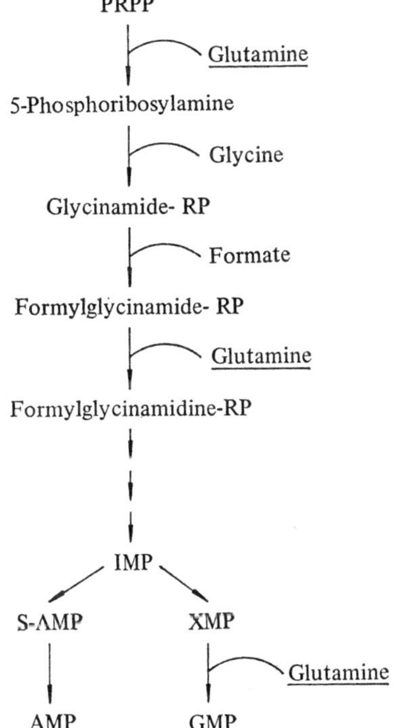

Pathway for biosynthesis of purine ribonucleotides

The accumulation of FGARP in cells inhibited by azaserine or DON indicates that, of the three glutamine-requiring enzymes involved in synthesis of purines, the one catalyzing the amidination of FGARP is the most sensitive. Inhibition of this enzyme by glutamine analogs has been studied extensively, particularly by Buchanan and his coworkers (HARTMAN et al., 1956; LEVENBERG et al., 1957; FRENCH et al., 1963; DAWID et al., 1963). Inhibition of the enzyme by azaserine or DON is at first reversible, but upon incubation with the inhibitor in the absence of glutamine, becomes irreversible (LEVENBERG et al., 1957). The inactivation of the enzyme is the result of initial reversible concentration of the inhibitor at the glutamine-binding site, after which it alkylates a sulfhydryl group on the enzyme surface. After incubation of the enzyme with ^{14}C-azaserine, digestion with proteolytic enzymes followed by acid hydrolysis yielded *S*-carboxymethylcysteine (DAWID et al., 1963); the reactions involved are shown below. The reaction of a diazoalkane with a sulfhydryl group normally proceeds at a very slow rate. The inactivation of the enzyme therefore presumably results from the binding of azaserine to the active site in such a manner that the diazomethyl group is positioned near the sulfhydryl group of the cysteine residue (see BAKER, 1967, for a discussion of this type of inhibition).

$$\cdots\cdots \underset{\displaystyle \|\atop \displaystyle O}{C}-NH-\underset{\displaystyle |\atop \displaystyle CH_2-SH}{CH}-\overset{\displaystyle O\atop \displaystyle \|}{C}-NH\cdots\cdots + N_2{}^{*}CH-\underset{\displaystyle \|\atop \displaystyle O}{C}-O-CH_2-\underset{\displaystyle |\atop \displaystyle NH_2}{CH}-COOH$$

$$\downarrow$$

$$\cdots\cdots \underset{\displaystyle \|\atop \displaystyle O}{C}-NH-\overset{\displaystyle O\atop \displaystyle \|}{CH-C}-NH\cdots\cdots \quad \text{with } CH\text{: } CH_2-S-{}^{*}CH_2-\underset{\displaystyle \|\atop \displaystyle O}{C}-O-CH_2-\underset{\displaystyle |\atop \displaystyle NH_2}{CH}-COOH$$

$$\downarrow$$

$$H_2N-\underset{\displaystyle |\atop \displaystyle CH_2-S-{}^{*}CH_2-COOH}{CH}-COOH$$

Since DON also inhibits the enzyme irreversibly, it presumably acts in a similar manner, but the product has not been isolated.

This enzyme is considerably more sensitive to DON than to azaserine. Thus, for the enzyme from pigeon liver, the K_i for reversible binding of azaserine was 3.4×10^{-5} M and that for DON was 1.1×10^{-6} M (LEVENBERG et al., 1957). For the enzyme from *Salmonella typhimurium*, the difference in sensitivity to the two inhibitors was not as marked; only three times as much azaserine as DON was required for equivalent inhibition (FRENCH et al., 1963).

Although the amidination of FGARP is the site on the purine nucleotide biosynthetic pathway most sensitive to inhibition by these analogs, it would be expected that one of the other sites might also be inhibited if the concentration of inhibitor were raised. Several observations have been made which indicate that DON, at concentrations somewhat higher than those required for inhibition of the FGARP–FGAmRP conversion, inhibits PRPP amidotransferase, the enzyme catalyzing the synthesis of phosphoribosylamine. Thus, in a mouse plasma cell neoplasm, administration of DON at 0.005 mg/kg produced a large accumulation of FGARP which decreased progressively as the dose of DON was increased, until at 0.5 mg/kg essentially no FGARP accumulated (ANDERSON and BROCKMAN, 1963). Similar effects of DON were noted in other animal systems (MOORE and LEPAGE, 1957), in *E. coli* (TOMISEK and REID, 1962), and in pigeon liver extracts (BARG et al., 1957). Inhibition of the isolated enzyme by DON has been studied in detail (HARTMAN, 1963), and the mechanism seems to be similar to that by which azaserine inactivates the enzyme catalyzing the FGARP–FGAmRP conversion. Inhibition is at first reversible, and then becomes irreversible as DON forms a covalent bond with a sulfhydryl group on the enzyme.

Although both azaserine and DON inhibit PRPP amidotransferase (GOLDTHWAIT, 1956; HARTMAN, 1963), the enzyme is much more sensitive to DON than to azaserine; for inhibition competitive with glutamine, the K_i for DON was

1.9×10^{-5} M and for azaserine 4.2×10^{-3} M (HARTMAN, 1963). In intact cells also, DON is much more effective than azaserine; in the mouse plasma cell neoplasm cited above, 0.125 mg/kg of azaserine was required to produce as much accumulation of FGARP as 0.005 mg/kg of DON, and the amount accumulating did not decrease when the dose of azaserine was raised to 150 mg/kg (ANDERSON and BROCKMAN, 1963). Thus, even at this high concentration, azaserine did not inhibit the synthesis of PRA. In an enzyme preparation from *E. coli*, DON (1 mM) produced a 53 % inhibition of the amidotransferase while azaserine at the same concentration was without effect (LEGAL et al., 1967).

Glutamine is also the source of the amino group of guanine, which is introduced by the amination of XMP.

$$\text{XMP} + \text{Glutamine} \xrightarrow{\text{ATP}} \text{GMP} + \text{Glutamate}$$

XMP aminases from both mammalian (ABRAMS and BENTLEY, 1959; LOWY and WILLIAMS, 1960) and bacterial (YAROVAYA et al., 1967) cells are inhibited by azaserine or DON. Like the other amido transferases discussed above, XMP aminase is also much more sensitive to DON than to azaserine. In a preparation of the aminase from calf thymus the K_i for azaserine was 6.7×10^{-3} M, about 15 times greater than that for DON (ABRAMS and BENTLEY, 1959). In the rabbit erythrocyte, which does not carry out the early steps of the *de novo* purine biosynthetic pathway, DON inhibited the conversion of aminoimidazole carboxamide ribonucleotide to GMP at a concentration 1/180th of that of azaserine (LOWY and WILLIAMS, 1960). This enzyme is much less sensitive to inhibition by azaserine and DON than are those catalyzing the synthesis of PRA and FGAmRP. Thus, 200 times more azaserine was required to inhibit the aminase from calf thymus than was required to inhibit the amidination of FGARP by the enzyme from pigeon liver (ABRAMS and BENTLEY, 1959). The results of *in vivo* studies also indicate that the aminase is less sensitive than the other two enzymes (BARCLAY et al., 1962; ANDERSON and BROCKMAN, 1963). In contrast to inhibition of the other two enzymes, inhibition of the aminase is not irreversible (ABRAMS and BENTLEY, 1959). This observation may mean (a) that there is not a sulfhydryl group properly positioned for alkylation by the bound inhibitor, or (b) that the binding of the inhibitor is so weak that the enzyme-inhibitor complex is not present in sufficient concentration for the alkylation to take place at a biologically significant rate (see BAKER, 1967 for a discussion of this type of inhibition). The inhibition of XMP aminase would not be expected to be a significant locus of action for azaserine and DON in those cells in which the *de novo* pathway to purine nucleotides is operative, but it could be important in those cells (such as erythrocytes, bone marrow, and certain protozoa) which do not carry out *de novo* purine synthesis.

III. Inhibition of Pyrimidine Biosynthesis

The amide nitrogen of glutamine is the source of the 3-N atom of the pyrimidine ring and of the amino group of cytosine. The steps at which these atoms are introduced are shown below.

Only a few observations have been made on the inhibition of carbamylphosphate synthetase by glutamine analogs. HAGER and JONES (1965) found that Ehrlich ascites cells incorporated ^{14}C-bicarbonate into carbon atom 2 of the uridine nucleotides and that this process was inhibited by glutamine analogs. Under conditions of reversible inhibition, DON was more effective than azaserine, but even more effective was *O*-carbamylserine. This relative order of effectiveness of inhibitors was also observed with a cell free preparation from *E. coli* and thus appears to be characteristic of this enzyme. By contrast both DON and azaserine were more effective than *O*-carbamylserine in inhibiting the amidination of FGARP (LEVENBERG et al., 1957). However, when the *E. coli* enzyme was preincubated with the inhibitors, azaserine and DON irreversibly inhibited carbamyl phosphate synthetase and were more effective than *O*-carbamylserine. DON has also been found to inhibit carbamyl phosphate synthetase in rat tumors (YIP and KNOX, 1970). Since carbamyl phosphate is utilized in other conversions, inhibition of its synthesis would have metabolic consequences in areas other than pyrimidine synthesis.

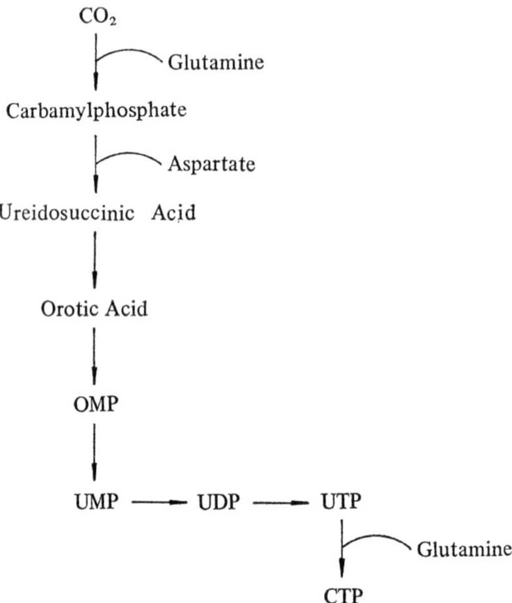

Pathway for biosynthesis of pyrimidine ribonucleotides

Inhibition of the synthesis of cytosine by a glutamine analog was first noted by EIDINOFF and coworkers (1958) in a study of the utilization of orotic acid and ureidosuccinic acid by rats; DON inhibited the conversion of these precursors to cytidine derivatives but not to derivatives of uridine or thymidine. The inhibition of the conversion of uridine nucleotides to cytidine nucleotides was studied in detail by HURLBERT and his associates (KAMMEN and HURLBERT, 1959; HURLBERT and KAMMEN, 1960; CHAKRABORTY and HURLBERT, 1961). In enzyme systems from mammalian cells, uridine nucleotides were converted to cytidine nucleotides in the presence of ATP and glutamine and the conversion was inhibited by DON irreversibly (HURLBERT and KAMMEN, 1960). In tissue suspension DON was more active (by a factor >175 times) than azaserine in inhibiting this conversion (KAMMEN and HURLBERT, 1959). In a study with a mouse plasma cell neoplasm *in vivo*, DON at 0.5 mg/kg was found to block completely the conversion of uridine to CMP (ANDERSON and BROCKMAN, 1963). This site of action may be sufficiently sensitive to DON to be of some significance for the biological activity of this agent.

IV. Inhibition of Synthesis of NAD

Two pathways exist for the synthesis of NAD, one involving the direct reaction of nicotinamide and ATP and the other the reaction of nicotinic acid and ATP to form deamido-NAD, which is then aminated (for references see PREISS and HANDLER, 1958; NARROD et al., 1961). The amidating enzyme from some sources utilizes glutamine and that from others utilizes ammonia. The yeast and mammalian enzymes utilize glutamine and are inhibited by glutamine analogs, whereas that from *E. coli* utilizes ammonia and is insensitive to DON (PREISS and HANDLER, 1958; SPENCER and PREISS, 1967). The K_i for azaserine for the yeast enzyme was 1.3×10^{-3} M; and, upon incubation, azaserine was eventually bound irreversibly to the enzyme (PREISS and HANDLER, 1958). In spite of this relatively high K_i, this inhibition apparently may take place *in vivo* since the administration of azaserine or DON to animals resulted in the marked lowering of NAD levels in liver, tumor, and brain (NARROD et al., 1959, 1961; BONASERA et al., 1963; BARCLAY and PHILLIPPS, 1966; SLATER and SAWYER, 1966). (However, an alternative explanation is that the lower level of NAD results in part from a deficiency of ATP produced by the inhibition of the purine nucleotide biosynthetic pathway.) The level of NAD in mouse liver is decreased to about 1/4 of normal value two hours after administration of azaserine (NARROD et al., 1961). This lowering was associated with an accumulation of deamido-NAD in DON treated animals and apparently results in part from the prevention of new NAD synthesis (since these analogs blocked increased synthesis of NAD induced by nicotinamide) and in part from an analog-induced increase in the turnover of NAD. For this conversion also, DON was a better inhibitor than azaserine (NARROD et al., 1961; BARCLAY and PHILLIPPS, 1966).

V. Inhibition of Synthesis of Glucosamine

Glutamine is the donor of the nitrogen atom in the conversion of fructose-6-phosphate to glucosamine-6-phosphate catalyzed by enzymes from both microbial and mammalian cells. DON inhibited the conversion and was much more effective than azaserine (GHOSH et al., 1960). Kinetic constants have not been reported and therefore this enzyme cannot be compared, with respect to sensitivity, to the other glutamine-requiring conversions already discussed. The possible importance of this site of inhibition in some cells is shown by the observation that inhibition of *E. coli* by DON could not be reversed by inosine or glucosamine alone but could be reversed completely by a mixture of these two metabolites (COGGIN and MARTIN, 1965).

VI. Inhibition of Synthesis of Asparagine

Asparagine is synthesized from aspartate in mammalian cells as shown below (PATTERSON and ORR, 1968).

$$\text{Aspartate} + \text{Glutamine} + \text{ATP} \longrightarrow \text{Asparagine} + \text{Glutamate} + \text{AMP} + \text{PP}_i$$

The enzyme is inhibited by azaserine or DON and DON is the more effective inhibitor. The enzyme from KB cells was inhibited by DON and azotomycin but not by duazomycin A or azaserine (PATTERSON and ORR, 1968; HASKELL and CANELLOS, 1970). Aside from these reports there is no information on the effects of glutamine analogs on this enzyme, but there are a number of reports of therapeutic potentiation with combinations of asparaginase and glutamine analogs which will be discussed later.

VII. Inhibition of Synthesis of Anthranilic Acid and *p*-Aminobenzoic Acid

In microbial systems the amide N-atom of glutamine may serve as the source of the amino N-atom of both anthranilic acid (SRINIVASAN and RIVERA, 1963) and *p*-aminobenzoic acid (SRINIVASAN and WEISS, 1961). The conversion of shikimate or chorismate to anthranilate was inhibited by azaserine or DON in enzymes obtained from *E. coli* (SRINIVASAN and RIVERA, 1963; GIBSON et al., 1967) and *S. typhimurium* (TAMIR and SRINIVASAN, 1969; NAGANO et al., 1970). In the enzyme system from *E. coli* DON was 200 times more effective than azaserine; γ-glutamylhydrazide and *O*-carbazylserine were without effect (SRINIVASAN and RIVERA, 1963).

NAGANO et al. (1970) have analyzed in detail the effects of DON on anthranilate synthesis by an enzyme aggregate from *S. typhimurium*. This aggregate consists of two enzymes, anthranilate synthetase and 5-phosphoribosylpyrophosphate phosphoribosyltransferase, which catalyze the following reactions.

$$\text{Chorismate} + \text{Glutamine} \xrightarrow{Mg^{++}} \text{Anthranilate} + \text{Pyruvate} + \text{Glutamate}$$

$$\text{Anthranilate} + \text{PRPP} \xrightarrow{Mg^{++}} \text{N-(5'-phosphoribosyl)anthranilate} + PP_i .$$

The isolated anthranilate synthetase can utilize NH_3 but not glutamine, whereas the synthetase moiety of the aggregate can utilize glutamine or NH_3. DON does not inactivate the unaggregated synthetase but does inactivate the aggregate; the inactivation results from the alkylation by DON of cysteine residues in the phosphoribosyltransferase moiety of the enzyme.

That inhibition of anthranilate synthesis may be of importance in the antimicrobial action of DON is shown by the observation that in a tryptophan auxotroph of *S. cerevisae* DON caused a buildup of chorismic acid (LINGENS et al., 1966).

Azaserine and DON also inhibit the conversion of shikimate to *p*-aminobenzoic acid (SRINIVASAN and WEISS, 1961). In this reaction, as contrasted to anthranilate synthetase, DON was only 40 $\times$ as effective as azaserine. When both enzymes were present, the anthranilate synthetase effectively competed with the *p*-aminobenzoic acid synthetase for DON.

VIII. Synthesis of Histidine

In the synthesis of histidine in bacteria, glutamine contributes one of the ring nitrogen atoms which is introduced in the formation of the imidazole ring from 1-(5'-phosphoribosyl)-AMP (for references see MEISTER, 1965). Direct evidence for inhibition of this conversion by glutamine analogs has not been reported. That it may be of some importance is suggested by observations of the reversal by histidine of inhibition by azaserine in certain strains of *E. coli* and of the effectiveness of histidine in increasing the degree of reversal by aromatic amino acids of azaserine-induced inhibition of bacteria (KAPLAN et al., 1959; HEDEGAARD et al., 1959a, b; PITTILLO, 1961; PITTILLO and QUINNELLY, 1962). In some microbial systems, however, histidine had little or no activity in reversing the effect of azaserine (HALVORSON, 1954; GOTS and GOLLUB, 1956).

IX. Effects on Glutaminase and Glutamine Synthetase

The reactions considered above have been those in which glutamine served as a donor of an N-atom in the synthesis of a molecule of biological importance. It might also be expected that glutamine analogs would interfere with the control of the cellular pools of glutamine, either by action on glutamine synthetase or on

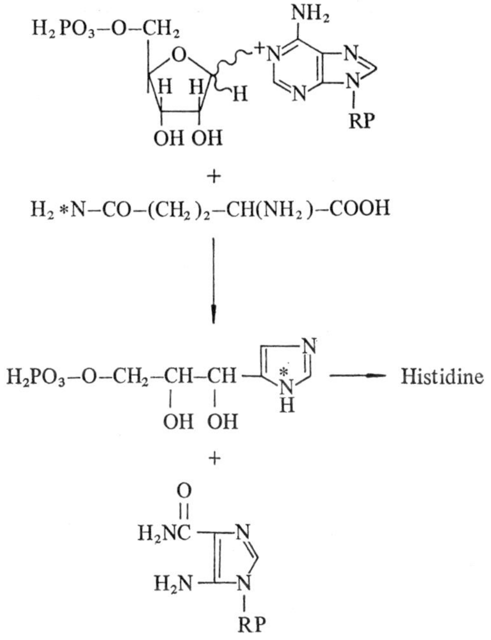

$H_2PO_3{-}O{-}CH_2$ ... NH_2 ... RP

OH OH

+

$H_2{*}N{-}CO{-}(CH_2)_2{-}CH(NH_2){-}COOH$

↓

$H_2PO_3{-}O{-}CH_2{-}CH{-}CH{-}$ ... → Histidine

OH OH

+

$H_2NC(=O)$, H_2N ... RP

Participation of glutamine in the biosynthesis of histidine

glutaminase. Both azaserine and DON have been found to inhibit glutaminase, the enzyme catalyzing the conversion of glutamine to glutamate (Klingman and Handler, 1958; Ghosh et al., 1960; Miller and Balis, 1969). DON was much more potent (by >100 times) as an inhibitor of the enzyme from *E. coli* than was azaserine (Ghosh et al., 1960). The asparaginase of *E. coli* has activity for both asparagine and glutamine; neither DON nor azaserine inhibited the activity of this enzyme, whereas DON was a potent inhibitor of *E. coli* glutaminase used in the same study (Miller and Balis, 1969).

In the only reported study of the effect of these analogs on glutamine synthetase, Wu and Yuan (1968) reasoned that subinhibitory concentrations of glutamine antagonists might induce cells to synthesize more glutamine, and found that in the presence of low concentrations of azaserine or DON, activity of glutamine synthetase in *E. coli* was increased by 25 to 30%.

X. Other Actions

There are other actions of azaserine or DON that are not obviously related directly to any one of the inhibitions discussed above. In photosynthesizing *Scenedesmus*, azaserine produced effects that were interpreted as resulting from interference with transamination (Barker et al., 1956; Van der Meulen and Bassham, 1959). However, in *Azotobacter agilis* effects of azaserine on transamination could not be detected (Delhumeau-Arrecillas and Burris, 1959). Both azaserine and DON are potent teratogens (Dagg and Karnofsky, 1955; Murphy and Karnofsky, 1956; Thiersch, 1957a, b; Blattner et al., 1958). DON was about 10 times more active than azaserine and had a greater margin between doses toxic to the mother and to the litter. The fact that adenine gave only partial protection against the effect of DON (THIERSCH, 1957b) suggests that DON acts at multiple sites in embryonic tissue, but that purine nucleotide biosynthesis is one of the significant sites of action.

Both inhibition of transaminations and teratogenicity conceivably can be related directly or indirectly to interference with the metabolism or function of glutamine. There are, however, other effects of azaserine or DON that cannot be explained readily in this manner. Azaserine is a potent mutagen (HEMMERLY and DEMEREC, 1955; GOTS et al., 1955; SZYBALSKI, 1958; IYER and SZYBALSKI, 1958, 1959; STEINMAN et al., 1958), and is also lysogenic (GOTS et al., 1955). An interesting effect of azaserine in *E. coli* is the production of filaments (MAXWELL and NICKEL, 1954; KAPLAN et al., 1959; KILGORE and GREENBERG, 1961; CURRY and GREENBERG, 1962), an effect also produced by ionizing radiation and by alkylating agents. Similarity in action of azaserine to radiation and alkylating agents is also shown by the observations that (a) radiation-resistant mutants of *E. coli* were resistant to azaserine and to a group of radiomimetic agents (GREENBERG et al., 1961; WOODY-KARRER and GREENBERG, 1963); (b) azaserine inactivated a *B. subtilis* transforming factor (TERAWAKI and GREENBERG, 1965); and (c) a spectrum of microorganisms responded similarly to azaserine and ionizing radiation (PITTILLO et al., 1965). Other effects of these agents have been observed that are also indicative, though less directly than those cited above, of similarity to effects of alkylating agents. Azaserine inhibited resting cells of *E. coli* (NARKATES and PITTILLO, 1964) and also inhibited nonproliferating leukemia L1210 cells in an exponential manner (SCHABEL et al., 1965). When proliferating leukemia L1210 cells were treated with azaserine, the kinetics of cell kill suggested that azaserine killed cells in all phases of the cycle (WILKOFF et al., 1967); however, in another study with mammalian cells, azaserine was classed among phase-specific agents (BRUCE et al., 1966). SIMARD and BERNHARD (1966) found that at high concentration azaserine caused morphological changes in the nucleolus characteristic of the action of agents known to bind with DNA.

These observations point to general similarities of the action of azaserine and classical alkylating agents, and suggest that, in addition to interference with glutamine-requiring reactions, azaserine may also react directly with DNA. The diazo group of azaserine is sufficiently reactive for such alkylation to occur, but as yet no alkylated product has been isolated from DNA, nor has any direct evidence been reported for the existence of DNA alkylated by azaserine.

The studies discussed above have also revealed some interesting differences in the actions of azaserine and DON. Despite its close structural similarity to azaserine, and despite the fact that it is generally more potent than azaserine as a growth inhibitor and as an antagonist of glutamine, DON did not induce filament formation in bacteria (MAXWELL and NICKEL, 1957; KILGORE and GREENBERG, 1961) and was not mutagenic (SZYBALSKI, 1958; STEINMAN et al., 1958). Furthermore, radiation-resistant mutants that were resistant to azaserine were not resistant to DON (WOODY et al., 1961). These differences between the two agents have not been rationalized.

XI. Mechanism of Growth Inhibition by Azaserine and DON

The results discussed above show clearly that azaserine and DON function, though perhaps not exclusively, as antagonists of glutamine, and that they not only compete with glutamine for the active sites of the enzymes but in most instances irreversibly inactivate the enzymes. Which of the enzymes will be most inhibited will of course depend on the particular cell type under study. There has been no reported study in which the glutamine-requiring enzymes have been isolated from the same source and compared with respect to sensitivity to the antagonist. However, a great deal of evidence indicates that, in cells in which the purine nucleotide synthetic pathway is operative, the FGARP–FGAmRP conversion is the site that is most sensitive to these analogs. In addition to the studies already cited in which a buildup of FGARP was noted in many cell types treated with azaserine or DON, other lines of evidence also indicate purine nucleotide synthesis as a primary site of action. The results are more clearcut with DON than with azaserine. Thus, purines reversed inhibition of *E. coli* by DON (MAXWELL and NICKEL, 1957), whereas inhibition by azaserine was reversed by purines or AIC but over a narrow range (BENNETT et al., 1956; GOTS and GOLLUB, 1956). Adenine partially protected litters against the teratogenic effects of DON but not against those of azaserine (THIERSCH, 1957 a, b), whereas in the sand dollar, purines prevented inhibition by both azaserine and DON (KARNOFSKY and BEVELANDER, 1958).

On the other hand, there are also observations that indicate that even in cells that are making purine nucleotides, this pathway may not be the critical, or only, site of inhibition. Thus, purines or AIC did not prevent azaserine-induced inhibition of growth of leukemic cells in culture (VANDEVOORDE et al., 1964). *Gaffkya homari* can grow equally well on purines or on *p*-aminobenzoic acid, and azaserine was equally inhibitory in both media (AARONSON, 1959). In one strain of *E. coli*, synthesis of purines and of glucosamine appear to be about equally sensitive to azaserine since protection was afforded by a mixture of inosine and glucosamine but not by either alone (COGGIN and MARTIN, 1965).

Certain protozoa either lack the *de novo* purine nucleotide biosynthetic pathway or have a limited capacity for *de novo* synthesis; therefore, if azaserine or DON inhibit these organisms it must be at some site other than the synthesis of PRA or FGAmRP. In *Trypanosoma equiperdum*, for example, growth inhibition by azaserine apparently results from interference with the production of cytidine nucleotides (MOMPARLER and JAFFE, 1965). Sites other than purine nucleotide synthesis must also be responsible for any effects of these analogs on other cells, such as mature erythrocytes and bone marrow, that are known to be unable to synthesize purine nucleotides *de novo*.

In microbial systems aromatic amino acids are the most effective agents in reversing or preventing inhibition by azaserine (HALVORSON, 1954; BENNETT et al., 1956; GOTS and GOLLUB, 1956; KAPLAN et al., 1959; BROCK and BROCK, 1961; LEE and YUZURIHA, 1964), and it has been suggested that these reversals result from interference by the amino acids with the uptake or binding of the inhibitors (KAPLAN et al., 1959; BROCK and BROCK, 1961). In lymphocytes (PINE, 1958), Ehrlich ascites cells (JACQUEZ, 1957, 1961), a plasma cell neoplasm (PINE, 1958; ANDERSON and JACQUEZ, 1962), and Sarcoma 180 (JACQUEZ, 1958), azaserine or DON have, in fact, been shown to be actively concentrated by an amino acid transport system. In the hamster intestine *in vitro*, both azaserine and DON were rapidly transported but did not interfere with the transport of other amino acids (SPENCER et al., 1963). It would thus appear reasonable that reversal by aromatic amino acids may result from competition for the transport system. In this respect, interesting differences are again apparent in the actions of azaserine and DON. Inhibition of growth of bacteria by DON was reversed by purines but not by aromatic amino acids (MAXWELL and NICKEL, 1957). Nevertheless DON was transported by the mammalian transport systems. It may be that the bacterial transport system can concentrate azaserine but not DON, as is suggested by the observation of FERROLUZZI-AMES (quoted in BROCKMAN and ANDERSON, 1963) that azaserine but not DON inhibited tryptophan transport in a system from *S. typhimurium*. However, competition for a transport system may not explain completely the effects of aromatic amino acids, as shown by the observation that in a cell-free system from *E. coli*, phenylalanine reversed or prevented azaserine-induced inhibition of the synthesis of the ribonucleotide of 5-amino-4-imidazole carboxamide (TOMISEK et al., 1959).

The production of a deficiency of purine nucleotides by a block of *de novo* synthesis would be expected to have wide and diverse metabolic effects because of the large number of reactions in which these nucleotides are involved either as cofactors or substrates. One of the consequences of administration of azaserine is an inhibition of DNA synthesis. SARTORELLI and coworkers (SARTORELLI and BOOTH, 1967; CRAMER and SARTORELLI, 1969) have rationalized this inhibition by showing that in azaserine-treated cells the activities of both thymidine kinase and TMP kinase decreased markedly. It was hypothesized that ATP, as a substrate for both enzymes, stabilizes the enzymes, and that, in the presence of the lowered ATP pool induced by azaserine, the activities of these enzymes decay. One might expect that similar effects would be noted for other enzymes for which purine nucleotides are substrates or effectors.

B. Conjugates of DON

Of the three conjugates of DON (i.e., alazopeptin, duazomycin, and azotomycin) only the last two have been studied to any extent. All three inhibit the growth of microorganisms and of certain experimental tumors (DEVOE et al., 1957; RAO et al., 1960; OLESON et al., 1960; PRICE et al., 1962; CARTER, 1968). These conjugates apparently act only after cleavage to DON, therefore, they would be expected to have the same metabolic effects as DON, but might differ from DON in their transport and physiological disposition. Duazomycin was readily deacetylated by mammalian acylase (ANDERSON and BROCKMAN, 1963) and azotomycin was degraded to glutamate and DON by pronase and by cell-free preparations from bacteria and tumor cells (BROCKMAN et al., 1970). Since alazopeptin differs from azotomycin only in the replacement of a glutamyl moiety by an alanyl moiety, its activity and activation would be expected to be similar. However, aside from reports on its teratogenicity (THIERSCH, 1958), and its similarity to DON in inhibiting NAD synthesis (BARCLAY and PHILLIPPS, 1966), no detailed study has been made of alazopeptin.

C. Amide Derivatives of Glutamine: γ-Glutamylhydrazide and γ-*N*-Benzylglutamine

γ-Glutamylhydrazide, a simple derivative of glutamine in which a hydrazide group replaces the amide group, was first prepared by ROPER and MCILWAIN (1948) and found to inhibit the growth of bacteria. Inhibition of *L. arabinosus* by the hydrazide was reversed by glutamine (AYENGAR and ROBERTS, 1953) and, from the limited number of studies reported, the hydrazide appears to function as a weak antagonist of glutamine. It inhibited the two-step conversion of FGARP to aminoimidazole ribonucleotide, but the principal site of inhibition was difficult to determine because it also inhibited the second reaction in this sequence (LEVENBERG et al., 1957; SCHROEDER et al., 1969). The hydrazide also slightly inhibited the nicotinamide-induced synthesis of NAD (BARCLAY and PHILLIPPS, 1966), but did not inhibit the synthesis of anthranilate (SRINIVASAN and RIVERA, 1963) or the conversion of XMP to GMP (ABRAMS and BENTLEY, 1959). The analog stimulated protein synthesis both in bacteria (NEAL et al., 1968) and in mammalian cells (RABINOVITZ et al., 1959; SMULSON and NEAL, 1965). In both systems, the hydrazide was incorporated as such into the primary structure of protein, and in the bacterial cells some was also incorporated as glutamate. This stimulation apparently is related to the capacity of the hydrazide to substitute for glutamine in protein synthesis in cells that have low levels of glutamine synthetase.

In the mouse brain, glutamylhydrazide apparently inhibited the conversion of glutamate to γ-aminobutyrate (TAPIA and AWAPARA, 1967). Of a series of γ-*N*-substituted glutamines only *N*-benzylglutamine showed biological activity; it inhibited *S. lactis*, and inhibition was reversed by glutamine (EDELSON et al., 1959).

D. *O*-Carbamyl-L-Serine and *O*-Carbazyl-L-Serine

O-Carbamyl-L-serine was synthesized as a glutamine analog similar to azaserine in being an *O*-derivative of serine, but resembling glutamine more closely than does azaserine (SKINNER et al., 1956). Inhibition of bacteria by this analog was reversed competitively by glutamine (SKINNER et al., 1956; RAVEL et al., 1958). Like γ-glutamylhydrazide, it increased protein synthesis in certain tumor cells, possibly by competing with glutamine for some reactions and thus making more glutamine available for protein synthesis (RABINOVITZ et al., 1959). In a cell-free system it inhibited the amidination of FGARP (LEVENBERG et al., 1957) and, as has already been noted, was more effective than azaserine or DON as a competitive inhibitor of carbamyl phosphate synthetase (HAGER and JONES, 1965). *Streptococcus lactis* grown in the presence of *O*-carbamylserine, azaserine, or *S*-carbamylcysteine contained decreased amounts of the enzyme converting ornithine to citrulline; the effects of *O*-carbamylserine, but not those of the other two analogs, were reversed competitively by glutamine (RAVEL et al., 1958). Of a series of derivatives of *O*-carbamylserine containing various substituents on the amide N-atom, only the methyl derivative was active against bacteria, and its effects were reversible by glutamine (MCCORD et al., 1958a).

O-Carbazylserine, a simple derivative of *O*-carbamylserine, also functions as a glutamine antagonist in inhibiting bacterial growth (MCCORD et al., 1958b).

It is noteworthy that *O*-carbamyl-D-serine is produced by a *Streptomyces* (HAGEMANN et al., 1955; OKAMI et al., 1962) and functions, not as an antagonist of glutamine, but as an antagonist of D-alanine in the synthesis of bacterial cell walls (for references see TANAKA et al., 1963; REITZ et al., 1967).

E. *S*-Carbamyl-L-Cysteine

S-Carbamyl-L-cysteine was designed as an analog of glutamine which, like azaserine, contains a chemically reactive group, and which might therefore inactivate one of the glutamine-requiring enzymes. Since the *S*-carbamyl group is more active than the *O*-carbamyl group, this compound might be expected to form a covalent bond with the enzyme whereas *O*-carbamylserine would not. A comparison of these two analogs and azaserine on the growth of bacteria and on the synthesis of the enzyme catalyzing the ornithine-citrulline conversion provided some evidence that this was the case; the effects of *O*-carbamylserine were reversed competitively by glutamine, whereas those of azaserine and *S*-carbamylcysteine were not (RAVEL et al., 1958). *S*-Carbamylcysteine and *S*-methylcarbamylcysteine inhibited GMP synthetase of *E. coli*, and the inhibition by the latter compound was irreversible (YAROVAYA et al., 1967). These irreversible inhibitions probably indicate formation of a covalent bond with groups on the enzymes, but no direct evidence was obtained for formation of such a bond. *S*-Carbamyl-L-cysteine has also been found to inhibit glutaminase from both mammalian and microbial sources (MARDASHEV and KOVALENKO, 1968) and to inhibit protein synthesis in Ehrlich ascites cells (RABINOVITZ and FISHER, 1962). A series of derivatives was prepared by ROSS et al. (1961); of these only the methyl derivative was inhibitory to bacteria and its effects were reversed by glutamine.

F. Albizziin

Albizziin, or β-ureido-L-alanine, was isolated initially from *Albizziia julibrissin Durazz.* (GMELIN et al., 1958) and later synthesized (KJAER and LARSEN, 1959). Its activity as a glutamine antagonist was first noted in studies of inhibition of glutaminase by MARDASHEV and SOKOVNINA (quoted by LINGENS et al., 1966) and later reported more fully by MARDASHEV and KOVALENKO (1968). In a tryptophan auxotroph of *S. cerevisiae*, albizziin inhibited the synthesis of anthranilate and produced a buildup of chorismic acid (LINGENS et al., 1966). BUCHANAN and his associates (SCHROEDER et al., 1969) have studied in detail the effects of albizziin on FGARP amidotransferase. Their investigations indicate that this enzyme has a glutamine binding site and an ammonia binding site. Glutamine is bound, then forms a covalent bond (a γ-glutamyl thioester) with a sulfhydryl group on the enzyme; at the same time the amide N-atom is transferred as ammonia to the ammonia binding site. Albizziin was found to inactivate the enzyme irreversibly and to bind to it covalently in a ratio of one mole of inhibitor to one mole of enzyme. This inactivation is similar to, but mechanistically distinct from, that produced by azaserine. The latter compound inactivates the enzyme by means of a highly reactive chemical group, whereas, in inactivation by albizziin, the inactivating reaction is the same enzymatic reaction by which glutamine is normally bound to the enzyme. Other studies with this analog have not been reported.

Agents Affecting Synthesis and Degradation of Glutamine

A. Inhibitors of Glutamine Synthetase

Agents that decrease the intracellular pool of glutamine by preventing its synthesis or by causing its degradation would produce metabolic effects generally similar to those produced by glutamine analogs. If the concentration of glutamine were sufficiently lowered, the rate of all of the glutamine-requiring reactions would be effectively decreased, but, under conditions of limiting concentrations, one would expect that glutamine would be used preferentially by those enzymes to which it was most tightly bound.

Glutamine synthetase, an enzyme occurring widely in animal tissues, as well as in microbial cells and in plants (MEISTER, 1965), catalyzes the synthesis of glutamine by the reaction shown below.

$$\text{Glutamate} + NH_3 + \text{ATP} \longrightarrow \text{Glutamine} + \text{ADP} + P_i$$

Two inhibitors of this enzyme are known that are of some chemotherapeutic interest: methionine sulfoximine (MSO) and δ-hydroxylysine.

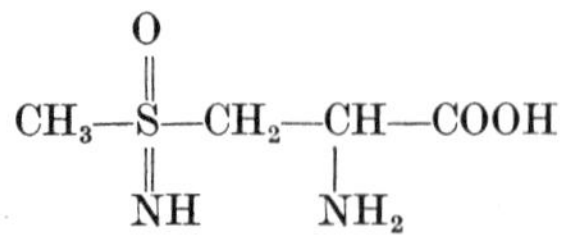

$$CH_3{-}\overset{\overset{\displaystyle O}{\|}}{\underset{\underset{\displaystyle NH}{\|}}{S}}{-}CH_2{-}\underset{\underset{\displaystyle NH_2}{|}}{CH}{-}COOH \qquad H_2N{-}CH_2{-}\underset{\underset{\displaystyle OH}{|}}{CH}{-}CH_2{-}CH_2{-}\underset{\underset{\displaystyle NH_2}{|}}{CH}{-}COOH$$

Methionine sulfoximine 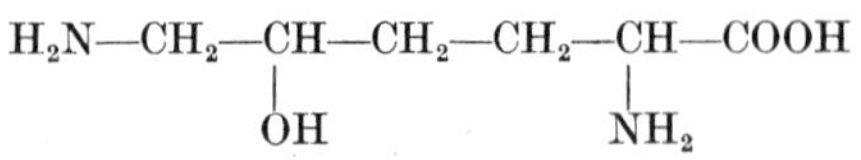 $\qquad$ δ-Hydroxylysine

Interest in MSO began with its identification as the agent responsible for the convulsant activity of flour that had been treated with nitrogen trichloride (for references see SHORT and THOMPSON, 1951; RONZIO et al., 1969). There is an extensive literature on its epileptogenic properties and it has been widely used as an agent for inducing experimental convulsions in a variety of mammals (for references see SELLINGER et al., 1968). Inhibition of microorganisms by MSO was reversed by glutamine (HEATHCOTE and PACE, 1950; NEWELL and CARMAN, 1950). MSO was early shown to inhibit cerebral glutamine synthetase (PACE and Mc DERMOTT, 1952), and a number of later studies have been concerned with inhibition of this enzyme both *in vivo* and *in vitro* (PETERS and TOWER, 1959; GERSHENOVICH et al., 1963; FOLBERGROVA, 1963; SELLINGER and WEILER, 1963; TEWS and STONE, 1964; LAMAR and SELLINGER, 1965; DE ROBERTIS et al., 1967; LAMAR, 1968; VAN DEN BERG and VAN DEN VELDEN, 1970). SELLINGER and coworkers (1968) showed that the convulsant activity of this agent was independent of its effects on glutamine synthetase, but it is as an inhibitor of this enzyme that this analog is of interest here. Although the bulk of the literature on MSO is concerned with its effects on glutamine synthetase of the brain, MSO has also been found to inhibit protein synthesis in the liver (ROTH, 1952) and in Ehrlich ascites cells (RABINOVITZ et al., 1956, 1959), apparently in the latter case by interference with the synthesis of glutamine. Analogs of MSO in which the methyl group was replaced by ethyl, propyl, or butyl groups were less active than MSO as inhibitors of the synthetase (SELLINGER and GARAZA, 1966).

In inhibiting glutamine synthetase, MSO apparently acts as an analog of glutamate. *In vitro* it inhibits the enzyme competitively with glutamate (SELLINGER and WEILER, 1963), and *in vivo* its inhibition is irreversible (LAMAR and SELLINGER, 1965). The mechanism of this inhibition was investigated by MEISTER and his associates (RONZIO and MEISTER, 1968; RONZIO et al., 1969; ROWE et al., 1969) who found that glutamine synthetase in the presence of ATP and Mg^{++} or Mn^{++} ions, converts MSO to a phosphate (in which the phosphate group is on the sulfoximine N-atom). The phosphate was tightly bound to the enzyme and apparently was responsible for its inhibition, since chemically synthesized MSO phosphate inhibited the synthetase (ROWE et al., 1969).

L-Methionine sulfoxide also inhibits glutamine synthetase (BOREK et al., 1946; ELLIOTT and GALE, 1948; SPECK, 1949; FRY, 1955; RONZIO et al., 1969), but has attracted much less attention than has MSO. L-Methionine sulfone was about as potent as MSO in inhibiting the enzyme, but the inhibition was reversible (RONZIO et al., 1969).

δ-Hydroxylysine, a relatively nontoxic analog, inhibited the incorporation of amino acids into protein of Ehrlich cells; since this inhibition was reversed by glutamine it is inferred that the analog inhibits the synthesis of glutamine (RABINOVITZ et al., 1957, 1959).

B. Glutaminase

The activity of the enzyme, glutaminase, which hydrolyses the amido group of glutamine, would be a factor controlling the cellular pools of glutamine. Use of this enzyme in therapy is discussed below.

Glutamine Analogs as Antitumor Agents

The low levels of free glutamine and the low activity of glutamine synthetase in certain tumors (see above) provide a rational basis for the selective action of glutamine analogs on tumors, and one might expect that some glutamine analogs would be ranked among the better antitumor agents. However, no glutamine analog has taken a permanent place as a clinically useful agent. In fact, of these analogs, only azaserine, DON, and the conjugates of DON, have good activity against experimental tumors. Among the other glutamine analogs, only *S*-carbamylcysteine and *S*-methylcarbamylcysteine have been reported to have any significant antitumor activity, and their activity was at best minimal (SKINNER et al., 1958, 1961). Some analogs other than azaserine and DON, however, may be of use in combination chemotherapy, and some examples are discussed below.

Azaserine and DON have been evaluated extensively as antitumor agents and a wide variety of experimental neoplasms respond to them, some to a marked degree. The responses of tumors to these agents have been tabulated in detail elsewhere (DUVALL, 1960a, b; LIVINGSTON et al., 1970) and will not be duplicated here. Despite encouraging responses in animal tumors, DON and azaserine have not proven generally satisfactory in the clinic. Extensive clinical trials, made shortly after their discovery, showed that beneficial effects of these agents were at best transient, and toxicity was a severe limitation (ELLISON et al., 1954; MAGILL et al., 1957). Although the effects of azaserine and DON were generally similar, some differences were noted. Azaserine, but not DON, was associated with hepatic toxicity in some patients and, as in animals, DON was much more toxic than azaserine (MAGILL et al., 1957). The difference in toxicity may be related to the fact that azaserine, but not DON, is degraded by liver enzymes in the rat (REILLY, 1958; JACQUEZ and SHERMAN, 1962). One clinical success, however, was obtained with DON. KARNOFSKY and coworkers (1964) noted that in the rat DON caused fetal resorption at a dose only 1/500th of that toxic to the mother, and for this reason used it to treat patients with choriocarcinoma. Five out of six patients responded and 3 to 4 months later showed no evidence of the disease.

Duazomycin (COLSKY et al., 1966; FOLEY et al., 1966) and azotomycin (ANSFIELD, 1965; WEISS et al., 1968) have also undergone extensive clinical trials and have shown no marked activity.

A large number of trials both in animals and in the clinic have been made with combinations of glutamine analogs and other agents. The definition of purine nucleotide biosynthesis as the primary site of action of azaserine and DON suggested to many workers that the combination of one of these agents with purine analogs might synergistically inhibit tumor growth by either or both of the following mechanisms: (a) inhibition of the purine nucleotide biosynthetic pathway at two points, or (b) simultaneous inhibition of *de novo* synthesis of purine nucleotides and their synthesis from preformed purines (SKIPPER, 1954; SARTORELLI and LEPAGE, 1958a; SARTORELLI and BOOTH, 1960, 1963). Potentiation of antitumor activity has been reported in experimental tumors for combinations of azaserine or DON with 6-mercaptopurine (SKIPPER, 1954; TARNOWSKI and STOCK, 1957; CLARKE et al., 1957; GOLDIN et al., 1958; SARTORELLI et al., 1964), 9-alkyl derivatives of 6-mercaptopurine (HANSEN et al., 1964); 6-thioguanine (TARNOWSKI and STOCK, 1957; SARTORELLI and LEPAGE, 1958a; SARTORELLI et al., 1964), 6-chloropurine (TARNOWSKI and STOCK, 1957; SARTORELLI and BOOTH, 1960, 1963; SARTORELLI et al., 1964), 8-azaguanine (SKIPPER, 1954), and 4-aminopyrazolo (3,4-*d*)pyrimidine and its 1-methyl derivative (HENDERSON and JUNGA, 1960). Clinical trials have been made with some of these combinations and have not been particularly successful. Some improvement in response was obtained with combinations of azaserine and 6-thioguanine in breast cancer (SCHROEDER et al., 1964) and of duazomycin and 6-thioguanine in head and neck cancer (LEFKOWITZ et al., 1965), whereas azaserine plus 6-mercaptopurine gave no enhanced effect against leukemia in children (HEYN et al., 1960), and the combination of azaserine and 6-thioguanine was relatively ineffective against multiple myeloma (HAYES et al., 1967).

Potentiation of the antitumor effects of glutamine analogs has also been noted with agents other than purine analogs. On the basis of their observation that ethidium bromide inhibited the utilization of preformed purines, KANDASWAMY and HENDERSON (1962) studied combinations of this agent with azaserine and found potentiation against Ehrlich ascites cells. Inhibition of Sarcoma 180 by the combination of azaserine and 6-chloropurine was further enhanced by glyceraldehyde (SARTORELLI et al., 1960). The activity of γ-glutamylhydrazide against Sarcoma 180 was increased by the administration of deoxypyridoxine (MICKELSON and FLIPPIN, 1958).

Potentiation might be expected from the combination of a glutamine analog with an agent that inhibits the synthesis of glutamine. The only reported observation of such potentiation is that of CLARKE et al. (1957), who found that MSO, which was without activity itself, enhanced the effects of azaserine and DON against Sarcoma 180.

The antitumor activity of asparaginase presumably is due to the low activity of asparagine synthetase in certain neoplasms (COONEY and HANDSCHUMACHER, 1970). Since glutamine is utilized in the synthesis of asparagine, it would be logical to treat tumors with a combination of asparaginase and a glutamine antagonist, with the rationale that asparaginase would destroy the free asparagine being supplied via the blood and that the glutamine analog would inhibit the synthesis of asparagine within the tumor cell. Because of the great current interest in asparaginase, a considerable literature is developing on combination therapy of this type. Combinations of asparaginase with azaserine were more effective than either agent alone against leukemia L5178Y in mice (JACOBS et al., 1969) and P1798 lymphoma (MASHBURN, 1968), and combinations of asparaginase and DON were similarly more effective against Ehrlich ascites cells, the B16 melanoma, and the Walker 256 tumor (TARNOWSKI et al., 1970). Similarly, azotomycin potentiated the action of asparaginase against L5178Y leukemia (JACOBS et al., 1969), and azaserine added slightly to the effectiveness of asparaginase against the Walker 256 tumor (SUGIURA, 1969). The combination of γ-glutamylhydrazide with asparaginase was relatively ineffective against the Ehrlich ascites tumor (TARNOWSKI et al., 1970). A clinical trial of asparaginase in combination with azaserine in patients with acute lymphatic leukemia showed no effects beyond those expected of asparaginase alone (LEVENTHAL et al., 1970).

TARNOWSKI et al. (1970) have also studied the effectiveness of a combination of asparaginase and MSO. This combination was potentiating against the Ehrlich ascites carcinoma, but only with increased toxicity.

As has already been noted, many tumors have low levels of glutamine and low activities of glutamine synthetase. Therefore, the same rationale that applies to therapy of tumors with asparaginase should also be applicable to therapy with glutaminase. GREENBERG and coworkers found that a glutaminase-asparaginase preparation from a *Pseudomonas* decreased the growth rate of Ehrlich cells, but without increasing the number of survivors, and that this activity was enhanced by azaserine or 8-azaguanine (GREENBERG et al., 1964; EL-ASMAR et al., 1966). Since asparaginase alone has antitumor activity, it was not possible to ascribe the inhibition of the tumor cells to glutaminase. However, ROBERTS and coworkers (1970) have obtained more highly purified glutaminases and shown that a preparation having only glutaminase activity was active against Ehrlich cells. It was, however, less active than a preparation that also had asparaginase activity. More recently these same workers (ROBERTS et al., 1971) have studied the antitumor activity of a homogeneous glutaminase purified from a *Diplobacillus* soil organism.

This enzyme deaminated asparagine as well as glutamine, but was highly active against a line of Ehrlich ascites carcinoma resistant to asparaginase.

Another method of lowering the cellular pools of glutamine is the use of diets deficient in glutamine or glutamine precursors. SKIPPER and THOMSON (1958) made an extensive study of the activity of a series of antitumor agents in animals on diets deficient in various amino acids. A diet deficient in glutamate and aspartate potentiated moderately the activity of azaserine against Sarcoma 180. The most marked potentiation of the action of azaserine was observed in animals on a diet deficient in isoleucine; this observation has not been rationalized.

Although the glutamine analogs have no place at present among the clinically useful antitumor agents, it is still conceivable that they may find some specialized uses, either alone against certain tumors [see, for example, their use against trophoblastic tumors (KARNOFSKY et al., 1964)], or in combination with other agents. The well documented glutamine requirement of certain tumors, which is associated with low glutamine synthetase activity, would appear to provide such a sound basis for selective action that attempts to exploit it should still be made, even though such attempts have not so far been encouraging.

Glutamine Analogs as Immunosuppressive Agents

After the initial observation of the marked activity of 6-mercaptopurine and its derivatives as immunosuppressive agents (for references see SCHWARTZ, 1967), many other antimetabolites, including glutamine analogs, were investigated for this activity. Azaserine and DON have been evaluated both alone and in combination with other drugs, notably azathioprine (Imuran), for their effectiveness in dogs with kidney or skin transplants (SHEIL et al., 1964, 1968; MURRAY et al., 1969; ALEXANDRE et al., 1963; FOUCHER et al., 1967) and in humans with kidney transplants (ALEXANDRE et al., 1964; MURRAY et al., 1963, 1968). Although, when used alone, azaserine gave increased morbidity and for this reason has been abandoned for single agent therapy (MURRAY et al., 1968), in combination with azathioprine it has been highly effective. In extensive studies in dogs, the combination of azathioprine and azaserine was the most effective of a number of drugs and drug combinations in providing for both survival and function of the transplant (ALEXANDRE et al., 1963; MURRAY et al., 1969). However, the combination of azaserine and azathioprine is synergistic in producing liver toxicity and leucopenia in dogs (HAXHE et al., 1967) and has a low margin for use (FOUCHER et al., 1967). Azaserine combined with azathioprine (MURRAY et al., 1963), or with azathioprine, actinomycin, radiation, and prednisone (ALEXANDRE et al., 1964) has been used with some success in human kidney transplants.

Glutamine analogs alone or in combination with 6-mercaptopurine have also been reported to have immunosuppressive activity in other systems. The combination of duazomycin and 6-mercaptopurine suppressed experimental allergic encephalomyelitis in rats, whereas duazomycin alone was ineffective (VOGEL and CALABRESI, 1969). This same combination was effective in suppressing the secondary immune response to diphtheria toxoid in rabbits (ROSENBERG and CALABRESI, 1963), and in autoimmune disease in humans (KAPLAN et al., 1968). In rats, challenged with tetanus or with Sarcoma 180 heterografts, azaserine inhibited antibody synthesis and enhanced the effects of azathioprine, which was not effective alone (HANSEN et al., 1964).

The only report in which a glutamine analog has been found to be a highly potent immunosuppressive agent when used alone is a recent study of the blastogenic response of human lymphocytes to phytohemagglutinin, streptolysin O, or allogenic leukocytes (HERSH and BROWN, 1971). Azotomycin produced marked inhibition in this system and its effects were enhanced by asparaginase. In the same system, glutaminase also had potent immunosuppressive activity (HERSH, 1971).

The mechanism by which antimetabolites, including the glutamine analogs, inhibit the immune response is not understood. The drugs which are effective immunosuppressive agents usually also have growth-inhibitory and antitumor activity, and therefore may act by inhibiting the reproduction of antibody-producing cells.

References

AARONSON, S.: Mode of action of azaserine on *Gaffkya homari*. J. Bact. **77**, 548—551 (1959).

ABRAMS, R., BENTLEY, M.: Biosynthesis of nucleic acid purines. III. Guanosine 5′-phosphate formation from xanthosine 5′-phosphate and L-glutamine. Arch. Biochem. Biophys. **79**, 91—110 (1959).

ALEXANDRE, G.P.J., MORELLE, J., HAXHE, J.J., MICHELSEN, P., YPERSELE, C. v., MICHAUX, M., KESTENS, P.: Considerations a propos de quatre cas d'homogreffes renales. Acta Chirurgica Belgica **63**, 367—385 (1964).

ALEXANDRE, G.P.J., MURRAY, J.E., DAMMIN, G.J., NOLAN, B.: Immunosuppressive drug therapy in canine renal and skin homografts. Transplantation **1**, 432—461 (1963).

ANDERSON, E.P., BROCKMAN, R.W.: Biochemical effects of duazomycin A in the mouse plasma cell neoplasm 70429. Biochem. Pharmacol. **12**, 1335—1354 (1963).

ANDERSON, E.P., JACQUEZ, J.A.: Azaserine resistance in a plasma-cell neoplasm without change in active transport of the inhibitor. Cancer Res. **22**, 27—37 (1962).

ANSFIELD, F.J.: Phase I study of azotomycin (NSC-56654). Cancer Chemother. Rep. **46**, 37—40 (1965).

AYENGAR, P., ROBERTS, E.: Inhibition of the utilization of glutamine by *Lactobacillus arabinosus*. Growth **17**, 201—214 (1953).

BAKER, B.R.: Design of active-site directed irreversible enzyme inhibitors. New York: John Wiley and Sons 1967.

BARCLAY, R.K., GARFINKEL, E., PHILLIPPS, M.A.: Effects of 6-diazo-5-oxo-L-norleucine on the incorporation of precursors into nucleic acids. Cancer Res. **22**, 809—814 (1962).

BARCLAY, R.K., PHILLIPPS, M.A.: Effects of 6-diazo-5-oxo-L-norleucine and other tumor inhibitors on the biosynthesis of nicotinamide adenine dinucleotide in mice. Cancer Res. **26**, 282—286 (1966).

BARG, W., BOGGIANO, E., SLOAN, N., DE RENZO, E.C.: Inhibitors of *de novo* formylglycinamide ribotide synthesis in pigeon liver extracts. Fed. Proc. **16**, 150 (1957).

BARKER, S.A., BASSHAM, J.A., CALVIN, M., QUARCK, U.C.: Sites of azaserine inhibition during photosynthesis by *scenedesmus*. J. Amer. chem. Soc. **78**, 4632—4635 (1956).

BARTZ, Q.R., ELDER, C.C., FROHARDT, R.P., FUSARI, S.A., HASKELL, T.H., JOHANNESSEN, D.W., RYDER, A.: Isolation and characterization of azaserine. Nature (Lond.) **173**, 72—73 (1954).

BENNETT, L.L., JR., SCHABEL, F.M., JR., SKIPPER, H.E.: Studies on the mode of action of azaserine. Arch. Biochem. Biophys. **64**, 423—436 (1956).

BENNETT, L.L., JR., SMITHERS, D.: Feedback inhibition of purine biosynthesis in H. Ep. 2 cells by adenine analogs. Biochem. Pharmacol. **13**, 1331—1339 (1964).

BLATTNER, R.J., WILLIAMSON, A.P., SIMONSEN, L.: Teratogenic changes in early chick embryos following administration of antitumor agent (azaserine). Proc. Soc. exp. Biol. (N.Y.) **97**, 560—564 (1958).

BONASERA, N., MANGIONE, G., BONAVITA, V.: Diphosphopyridine nucleotide synthesis in brain following injection of various compounds. Biochem. Pharmacol. **12**, 633—636 (1963).

BOREK, E., MILLER, H.K., SHEINESS, P., WAELSCH, H.: The effect of the sulfoxide from DL-methionine on glutamic acid and glutamine metabolism. J. biol. Chem. **163**, 347 (1946).

BROCK, T.D., BROCK, M.L.: Reversal of azaserine by phenylalanine. J. Bact. **81**, 212—217 (1961).

BROCKMAN, R.W., ANDERSON, E.P.: Biochemistry of cancer (metabolic aspects). Ann. Rev. Biochem. **32**, 463—512 (1963).

BROCKMAN, R.W., CHUMLEY, S.: Inhibition of formylglycinamide ribonucleotide synthesis in neoplastic cells by purines and analogs. Biochim. biophys. Acta (Amst.) **95**, 365—379 (1965).

BROCKMAN, R.W., PITTILLO, R.F., SHADDIX, S., HILL, D.L.: Mode of action of azotomycin. Antimicrobial Agents and Chemotherapy 1969, 56—62 (1970).

BRUCE, W. R., MEEKER, B. E., VALERIOTE, F. A.: Comparison of the sensitivity of normal hematopoietic and transplanted lymphoma colony-forming cells to chemotherapeutic agents administered *in vivo*. J. nat. Cancer Inst. **37**, 233—245 (1966).

CARTER, S. K.: Azotomycin (NSC-56654)-clinical brochure. Cancer Chemother. Rep. **1**, part 3, 207—217 (1968).

CHAKRABORTY, K. P., HURLBERT, R. B.: Role of glutamine in the biosynthesis of cytidine nucleotides in *Escherichia coli*. Biochim. biophys. Acta (Amst.) **47**, 607—609 (1961).

CLARKE, D. A., REILLY, H. C., STOCK, C. C.: A comparative study of 6-diazo-5-oxo-L-norleucine and *O*-diazocetyl-L-serine on Sarcoma 180. Antibiot. and Chemother. **7**, 653—671 (1957).

COGGIN, J. H., JR., MARTIN, W. R.: 6-Diazo-5-oxo-L-norleucine inhibition of *Escherichia coli*. J. Bact. **89**, 1348—1353 (1965).

COLSKY, J., SHNIDER, B. I., FRANZINO, A., PEREZ, J.: Observations in patients with metastatic malignancy treated with duazomycin A. Clin. Pharmacol. and Ther. **7**, 352—358 (1966).

COONEY, D. A., HANDSCHUMACHER, R. E.: L-Asparaginase and L-asparagine metabolism. Ann. Rev. Pharmacol. **10**, 421—440 (1970).

CRAMER, G. T., SARTORELLI, A. C.: Studies on the mechanism of the azaserine-induced decrease in the activity of thymidine kinase. Biochem. Pharmacol. **18**, 1355—1362 (1969).

CURRY, J., GREENBERG, J.: Filament formation in radioresistant mutants of *Escherichia coli S* after treatment with ultraviolet light and radiomimetic agents. J. Bact. **83**, 38—42 (1962).

DAGG, C. P., KARNOFSKY, D. A.: Teratogenic effects of azaserine on the chick embryo. J. exp. Zool. **130**, 555—572 (1955).

DAWID, I. B., FRENCH, T. C., BUCHANAN, J. M.: Azaserine-reactive sulfhydryl group of 2-formamido-*N*-ribosylacetamide 5′-phosphate: L-glutamine amido-ligase (adenosine diphosphate) II. Degradation of azaserine-C-^{14}-labeled enzyme. J. biol. Chem. **238**, 2178—2185 (1963).

DELHUMEAU-ARRECILLAS, G., BURRIS, R. H.: Effects of azaserine on *Azotobacter agilis*. J. Bact. **78**, 740—741 (1959).

DE ROBERTIS, E., SELLINGER, O. Z., DE L. ARNAIZ, G. R., ALBERICI, M., ZIEHER, L. M.: Nerve endings in methionine sulphoximine convulsant rats, a neurochemical and ultrastructural study. J. Neurochem. **14**, 81—89 (1967).

DE VOE, S. E., RIGLER, N. E., SHAY, A. J., MARTIN, J. H., BOYD, T. C., BACKUS, E. J., MOWAT, J. H., BOHONOS, N.: Alazopeptin: production, isolation and chemical characteristics. Antibiot. Ann. 1956—1957, 730—735 (1957).

DEWALD, H. A., MOORE, A. M.: 6-Diazo-5-oxo-L-norleucine, a new tumor-inhibitory substance. Preparation of L (D and L)-forms. Amer. chem. Soc. 129th Meeting Abstr. 13—14 M (1956).

DION, H. W., FUSARI, S. A., JAKUBOWSKI, Z. L., ZORA, J. G., BARTZ, Q. R.: 6-Diazo-5-oxo-L-norleucine, a new tumor-inhibitory substance. II. Isolation and characterization. J. Amer. chem. Soc. **78**, 3075—3077 (1956).

DUVALL, L. R.: New agent data summaries: azaserine. Cancer Chemother. Rep. **7**, 65—86 (1960a).

DUVALL, L. R.: New agent data summaries: 6-diazo-5-oxo-L-norleucine. Cancer Chemother. Rep. **7**, 86—98 (1960b).

EAGLE, H., OYAMA, V. I., LEVY, M., HORTON, C. L., FLEISCHMAN, R.: The growth response of mammalian cells in tissue culture to L-glutamine and L-glutamic acid. J. biol. Chem. **218**, 607—616 (1956).

EDELSON, J., SKINNER, C. G., SHIVE, W.: Synthesis and biological activity of some *N*-(substituted) glutamines. J. med. pharm. Chem. **1**, 165—170 (1959).

EIDINOFF, M. L., KNOLL, J. E., MARANO, B., CHEONG, L.: Pyrimidine studies. I. Effect of DON (6-diazo-5-oxo-L-norleucine) on incorporation of precursors into nucleic acid pyrimidines. Cancer Res. **18**, 105—109 (1958).

EL-ASMAR, F. A., GREENBERG, D. M.: Studies on the mechanism of inhibition of tumor growth by the enzyme glutaminase. Cancer Res. **26**, 116—122 (1966).

ELLIOTT, H. W., GALE, E. F.: Glutamine-synthesizing system of *Staphylococcus aureus:* its inhibition by crystal violet and methionine sulfoxide. Nature (Lond.) **161**, 129—130 (1948).

ELLISON, R. R., KARNOFSKY, D. A., STERNBERG, S. S., MURPHY, M. L., BURCHENAL, J. H.: Clinical trials of *O*-diazoacetyl-L-serine (azaserine) in neoplastic disease. Cancer (Philad.) **7**, 801—814 (1954).

FOLBERGROVA, J.: The effect of methionine sulphoximine on the protein metabolism of brain cortex slices. J. Neurochem. **10**, 775—782 (1963).

FOLEY, H. T., SHNIDER, B. I., GOLD, G. L., RIUS, J.: A pilot study of methotrexate, duazomycin A, and radiation therapy in carcinoma of the lung. J. new Drugs **6**, 105—110 (1966).

FOUCHER, G., WUYTS, J. L., MACK, G., GEISERT, J., FONTAINE, J. L.: Influence du traitement combiné azasérine/imuran sur la survie de l'allotransplant renal primaire chez le chien. Compt. Rend. Séances Soc. Biol. (Paris) **161**, 1404—1406 (1967).

French, T. C., Dawid, I. B., Day, R. A., Buchanan, J. M.: Azaserine-reactive sulfhydryl group of 2-formamido-*N*-ribosylacetamide 5′-phosphate: L-glutamine amido-ligase (adenosine diphosphate). I. The purification and properties of the enzyme from *Salmonella typhimurium* and the synthesis of L-azaserine-C^{14}. J. biol. Chem. **238**, 2171—2177 (1963).
Fry, B. A.: Glutamine synthesis by *Micrococcus pyogenes var. aureus*. Biochem. J. **59**, 579—589 (1955).
Fusari, S. A., Frohardt, R. P., Ryder, A., Haskell, T. H., Johannessen, D. W., Elder, C. C., Bartz, Q. R.: Azaserine, a new tumor-inhibitory substance. Isolation and characterization. J. Amer. chem. Soc. **76**, 2878—2881 (1954a).
Fusari, S. A., Haskell, T. H., Frohardt, R. P., Bartz, Q. R.: Azaserine, a new tumor-inhibitory substance. Structural studies. J. Amer. chem. Soc. **76**, 2881—2883 (1954b).
Gershenovich, Z. S., Krichevskaya, A. A., Kaloušek, J.: The effect of raised oxygen pressure and of methionine sulphoximine on the glutamine synthetase activity of rat brain. J. Neurochem. **10**, 79—82 (1963).
Ghosh, S., Blumenthal, H. J., Davidson, E., Roseman, S.: Glucosamine metabolism. V. Enzymatic synthesis of glucosamine 6-phosphate. J. biol. Chem. **235**, 1265—1273 (1960).
Gibson, F., Pittard, J., Reich, E.: Ammonium ions as the source of nitrogen for tryptophan biosynthesis in whole cells of *Escherichia coli*. Biochim. biophys. Acta (Amst.) **136**, 573—576 (1967).
Gmelin, R., Strauss, G., Hassenmaier, G.: Isolierung von 2 neuen pflanzlichen Aminosäuren: *S*(β-carboxyäthyl)-L-cystein und Albizziin aus den Samen von *Albizzia julibrissin Durazz. (Mimosaceae)*. Z. Naturforsch. **13** B, 252—256 (1958).
Goldin, A., Humphreys, S. R., Venditti, J. M., Mantel, N.: Factors influencing antitumor synergism: relation to screening methodology. Ann. N. Y. Acad. Sci. **76**, 932—938 (1958).
Goldthwait, D. A.: 5-Phosphoribosylamine, a precursor of glycinamide ribotide. J. biol. Chem. **222**, 1051—1068 (1956).
Gots, J. S., Bird, T. J., Mudd, S.: L-Azaserine as an inducing agent for the development of phage in the lysogenic *Escherichia coli*, K-12. Biochim. biophys. Acta (Amst.) **17**, 449—450 (1955).
Gots, J. S., Gollub, E. G.: Purine metabolism in bacteria. IV. L-Azaserine as an inhibitor. J. Bact. **72**, 858—864 (1956).
Greenberg, D. M., Blumenthal, G., Ramadan, M. A.: Effect of administration of the enzyme glutaminase on the growth of cancer cells. Cancer Res. **24**, 957—963 (1964).
Greenberg, J., Mandell, J. D., Woody, P. L.: A preliminary report-resistance and cross-resistance of *Escherichia coli* mutants to radiomimetic agents. Cancer Chemother. Rep. **11**, 51—56 (1961).
Greenlees, J., LePage, G. A.: Purine biosynthesis and inhibitors in ascites cell tumors. Cancer Res. **16**, 808—813 (1956).
Hagemann, G., Pénasse, L., Teillon, J.: Sur un dérivé de la sérine, la *O*-carbamyl-D-sérine, produit par un *streptomyces*. Biochim. biophys. Acta (Amst.) **17**, 240—243 (1955).
Hager, S. E., Jones, M. E.: Initial steps in pyrimidine synthesis in Ehrlich ascites carcinoma *in vitro*. I. Factors affecting the incorporation of ^{14}C-bicarbonate into carbon 2 of the uracil ring of the acid-soluble nucleotides of intact cells. J. biol. Chem. **240**, 4556—4563 (1965).
Halvorson, H.: Some effects of azaserine on yeast metabolism. Antibiot. and Chemother. **4**, 948—961 (1954).
Hansen, H. J., Vandevoorde, J. P., Bennett, K. J., Giles, W. G.: Azaserine and thiopurines: I. Inhibition of S-180 mouse tumor and antibody synthesis. J. lab. clin. Med. **63**, 801—818 (1964).
Hartman, S. C.: The interaction of 6-diazo-5-oxo-L-norleucine with phosphoribosyl pyrophosphate amidotransferase. J. biol. Chem. **238**, 3036—3047 (1963).
Hartman, S. C.: Purines and pyrimidines. In: Greenberg, D. M. (Ed.): Metabolic pathways, Vol. IV, pp. 1—68. 3 rd ed. New York: Academic Press 1970.
Hartman, S. C., Levenberg, B., Buchanan, J. M.: Biosynthesis of the purines. XI. Structure, enzymatic synthesis, and metabolism of glycinamide ribotide and (α-*N*-formyl)-glycinamide ribotide. J. biol. Chem. **221**, 1057—1070 (1956).
Haskell, C. M., Canellos, G. P.: Asparagine biosynthesis in KB tumor cells: inhibitor studies with asparagine and glutamine antagonists. Cancer Res. **30**, 1081—1083 (1970).
Hayes, D. M., Costa, J., Moon, J. H., Hoogstraten, B., Harley, J. B.: Combination therapy with thioguanine (NSC 752) and azaserine (NSC 742) for multiple myeloma. Cancer Chemother. Rep. **51**, 235—238 (1967).
Haxhe, J. J., Alexandre, G. P. J., Kestens, P. J.: The effect of imuran and azaserine on liver function tests in the dog. Arch. int. Pharmacodyn. **168**, 366—372 (1967).
Heathcote, J. G., Pace, J.: Inhibition of the growth of *Leuconostoc mesenteroides* by the toxic factor from "agenized" zein: reversal by L-glutamine. Nature (Lond.) **166**, 353—354 (1950).

Hedegaard, J., Maspero-Segre, S., Thoai, N.-V., Roche, J.: Influence de l'histidine et de ses métabolites sur la biosynthèse des purines par *Escherichia coli B*. IV. Action sur des cultures inhibées par l'azasérine. Comp. Rend. Seances Soc. Biol. (Paris) **153**, 767—771 (1959a).

Hedegaard, J., Maspero-Segre, S., Thoai, N.-V., Roche, J.: Influence de l'histidine et de ses métabolites sur la biosynthèse des purines par *Escherichia coli B*. V. Mode d'action dans des cultures inhibées par l'azasérine. Comp. Rend. Seances Soc. Biol. (Paris) **153**, 954—959 (1959b).

Held, I., Wells, W., Koenig, H.: Metabolic effects of azaserine in rat brain. J. Neurochem. **16**, 537—542 (1969).

Hemmerly, J., Demerec, M.: Tests of chemicals for mutagenecity. Cancer Res., Suppl. **3**, 69—75 (1955).

Henderson, J. F.: Feedback inhibition of purine biosynthesis in ascites tumor cells. J. biol. Chem. **237**, 2631—2635 (1962).

Henderson, J. F.: Feedback inhibition of purine biosynthesis in ascites tumor cells by purine analogs. Biochem. Pharmacol. **12**, 551—556 (1963).

Henderson, J. F., Junga, I. G.: Inhibition of ascites tumor growth by 4-aminopyrazolo(3,4-*d*) pyrimidine in combination with azaserine, 6-mercaptopurine, and thioguanine. Cancer Res. **20**, 1618—1624 (1960).

Hersh, E. M.: Immunosuppression by L-glutaminase *in vitro*. Proc. Amer. Ass. Cancer Res. **12**, 39 (1971).

Hersh, E. M., Brown, B. W.: Inhibition of immune response by glutamine antagonism: effect of azotomycin on lymphocyte blastogenesis. Cancer Res. **31**, 834—840 (1971).

Heyn, R. M., Brubaker, C. A., Burchenal, J. H., Cramblett, H. G., Wolff, J. A.: The comparison of 6-mercaptopurine with the combination of 6-mercaptopurine and azaserine in the treatment of acute leukemia in children: results of a cooperative study. Blood **15**, 350—359 (1960).

Hurlbert, R. B., Kammen, H. O.: Formation of cytidine nucleotides from uridine nucleotides by soluble mammalian enzymes: requirements for glutamine and guanosine nucleotides. J. biol. Chem. **235**, 443—449 (1960).

Iyer, V. N., Szybalski, W.: The mechanism of chemical mutagenesis. I. Kinetic studies on the action of triethylene melamine (TEM) and azaserine. Proc. nat. Acad. Sci. (Wash.) **44**, 446—456 (1958).

Iyer, V. N., Szybalski, W.: Mutagenic effect of azaserine in relation to azaserine resistance in *Escherichia coli*. Science **129**, 839—840 (1959).

Jacobs, S. P., Wodinsky, I., Kensler, C. J., Venditti, J.: Therapy of experimental leukemias with combinations of L-asparaginase and glutamine antagonists. Proc. Amer. Ass. Cancer Res. **10**, 43 (1969).

Jacquez, J. A.: Active transport of *O*-diazoacetyl-L-serine and 6-diazo-5-oxo-L-norleucine in Ehrlich ascites carcinoma. Cancer Res. **17**, 890—896 (1957).

Jacquez, J. A.: Concentrative uptake of 6-diazo-5-oxo-L-norleucine by Sarcoma 180, liver and muscle *in vivo*. Proc. Soc. exp. Biol. (N.Y.) **99**, 611—613 (1958).

Jacquez, J. A.: Transport and exchange diffusion of L-tryptophan in Ehrlich cells. Amer. J. Physiol. **200**, 1063—1068 (1961).

Jacquez, J. A., Sherman, J. H.: Enzymatic degradation of azaserine. Cancer Res. **22**, 56—61 (1962).

Kammen, H. O., Hurlbert, R. B.: The formation of cytidine nucleotides and RNA cytosine from orotic acid by the Novikoff tumor *in vitro*. Cancer Res. **19**, 654—663 (1959).

Kandaswamy, T. S., Henderson, J. F.: Inhibition of ascites tumor growth by the trypanocide, ethidium bromide, in combination with azaserine. Nature (Lond.) **195**, 85 (1962).

Kaplan, L. H., Reilly, H. C., Stock, C. C.: Action of azaserine on *Escherichia coli*. J. Bact. **78**, 511—519 (1959).

Kaplan, S. R., Hayslett, J. P., Calabresi, P.: Treatment of advanced Wegener's granulomatosis with azathioprine and duazomycin A. New Eng. J. Med. **278**, 239—244 (1968).

Karnofsky, D. A., Bevelander, G.: Effects of DON (6-diazo-5-oxo-L-norleucine) and azaserine on the sand-dollar embryo. Proc. Soc. exp. Biol. (N.Y.) **97**, 32—37 (1958).

Karnofsky, D. A., Golbey, R. B., Li, M. C.: Remissions induced in trophoblastic tumors by 6-diazo-5-oxo-L-norleucine (DON). Proc. Amer. Ass. Cancer Res. **5**, 33 (1964).

Kilgore, W. W., Greenberg, J.: Filament formation and resistance to 1-methyl-3-nitro-1-nitrosoguanidine and other radiomimetic compounds in *Escherichia coli*. J. Bact. **81**, 258—266 (1961).

Kjaer, A., Larsen, P. O.: Amino acid studies. Part II. Structure and synthesis of Albizziine (L-2-amino-3-ureidopropionic acid), an amino acid from higher plants. Acta chem. Scand. **13**, 1565—1574 (1959).

KLINGMAN, J. D., HANDLER, P.: Partial purification and properties of renal glutaminase. J. biol. Chem. **232**, 369—380 (1958).
LAMAR, C., JR.: The duration of the inhibition of glutamine synthetase by methionine sulfoximine. Biochem. Pharmacol. **17**, 636—640 (1968).
LAMAR, C., JR., SELLINGER, O. Z.: The inhibition *in vivo* of cerebral glutamine synthetase and glutamine transferase by the convulsant methionine sulfoximine. Biochem. Pharmacol. **14**, 489—506 (1965).
LEE, K.-H., YUZURIHA, Y.: Studies on growth and cell division. III. Action of azaserine on cell division. J. pharm. Sci. **53**, 290—293 (1964).
LEFKOWITZ, E. R., CREASEY, W. A., CALABRESI, P., SARTORELLI, A. C.: Clinical and pharmacologic effects of combinations of 6-thioguanine and duazomycin A in patients with neoplastic disease. Cancer Res. **25**, 1207—1212 (1965).
LE GAL, M.-L., LE GAL, Y., ROCHE, J., HEDEGAARD, J.: Purine biosynthesis: enzymatic formation of ribosylamine-5-phosphate from ribose-5-phosphate and ammonia. Biochem. biophys. Res. Commun. **27**, 618—624 (1967).
LE PAGE, G. A., JONES, M.: Purinethiols as feedback inhibitors of purine synthesis in ascites tumor cells. Cancer Res. **21**, 642—649 (1961).
LEVENBERG, B., MELNICK, I., BUCHANAN, J. M.: Biosynthesis of the purines. XV. The effect of aza-L-serine and 6-diazo-5-oxo-L-norleucine on inosinic acid biosynthesis *de novo*. J. biol. Chem. **225**, 163—176 (1957).
LEVENTHAL, B. G., SKEEL, R. T., YANKEE, R. A., HENDERSON, E. S.: L-Asparaginase (NSC 109229) plus azaserine (NSC 742) in acute lymphatic leukemia. Cancer Chemother. Rep. **54**, 47—51 (1970).
LEVINTOW, L.: The glutamyltransferase activity of normal and neoplastic tissues. J. nat. Cancer Inst. **15**, 347—352 (1954).
LINGENS, F., LÜCK, W., MÜLLER, G.: Über die Wirkung von 5-oxo-6-diazo-norleucin und Albizziin auf die Biosynthese der Anthranilsäure in *Saccharomyces cerevisiae*. Hoppe-Seylers Z. physiol. Chem. **343**, 282—289 (1966).
LIVINGSTON, R. B., VENDITTI, J. M., COONEY, D. A., CARTER, S. K.: Glutamine analogs in chemotherapy. Advanc. Pharmacol. and Chemother. **8**, 57—120 (1970).
LOWY, B., WILLIAMS, M. K.: The presence of a limited portion of the pathway *de novo* of purine nucleotide biosynthesis in the rabbit erythrocyte *in vitro*. J. biol. Chem. **235**, 2924—2927 (1960).
MAGILL, G. B., MEYERS, W. P. L., REILLY, H. C., PUTNAM, R. C., MAGILL, J. W., SYKES, M. P., ESCHER, G. C., KARNOFSKY, D. A., BURCHENAL, J. H.: Pharmacological and initial therapeutic observations on 6-diazo-5-oxo-L-norleucine (DON) in human neoplastic disease. Cancer (Philad.) **10**, 1138—1150 (1957).
MARDASHEV, S. R., KOVALENKO, N. A.: Effect of some glutamine analogs on glutaminase activity in rat kidney. *Clostridium welchii SR*-12 and *Mycobacterium* sp.n. Vop. med. Khim. **14**, 319—323 (1968); Biol. Abstr. **51**, 82403 (1970).
MASHBURN, L. T.: The effect of combined therapy with L-asparaginase on P1798 lymphosarcoma. Proc. Amer. Ass. Cancer Res. **9**, 45 (1968).
MAXWELL, R. E., NICKEL, V. S.: Filament formation in *E. coli* induced by azaserine and other antineoplastic agents. Science **120**, 270—271 (1954).
MAXWELL, R. E., NICKEL, V. S.: 6-Diazo-5-oxo-L-norleucine, a new tumor-inhibitory substance. V. Microbiologic studies of mode of action. Antibiot. and Chemother. **7**, 81—89 (1957).
MCCORD, T. J., SKINNER, C. G., SHIVE, W.: Some O-(substituted carbamyl) serines. J. org. Chem. **23**, 1963—1965 (1958a).
MCCORD, T. J., RAVEL, J. M., SKINNER, C. G., SHIVE, W.: *O*-Carbazyl-DL-serine, an inhibitory analog of glutamine. J. Amer. chem. Soc. **80**, 3762—3764 (1958b).
MEISTER, A.: Biochemistry of the amino acids, Vols. I and II, 2nd ed. New York: Academic Press 1965.
MICKELSON, M. N., FLIPPIN, R. S.: Effects of certain amino acid derivatives on microorganisms and Sarcoma 180. J. nat. Cancer Inst. **20**, 495—512 (1958).
MILLER, H. K., BALIS, M. E.: Glutaminase activity of L-asparagine amidohydrolase. Biochem. Pharmacol. **18**, 2225—2232 (1969).
MOMPARLER, R. L., JAFFE, J. J.: Effect of azaserine on the incorporation of ^{14}C-labeled purines and pyrimidines into the acid-soluble and nucleic acid fractions of *Trypanosoma equiperdum*. Biochem. Pharmacol. **14**, 255—262 (1965).
MOORE, E. C., LE PAGE, G. A.: *In vivo* sensitivity of normal and neoplastic mouse tissues to azaserine. Cancer Res. **17**, 804—808 (1957).
MOORE, J. A., DICE, J. R., NICOLAIDES, E. D., WESTLAND, R. D., WHITTLE, E. L.: Azaserine, synthetic studies. I. J. Amer. chem. Soc. **76**, 2884—2887 (1954).
MURPHY, M. L., KARNOFSKY, D. A.: Effect of azaserine and other growth-inhibiting agents on fetal development of the rat. Cancer (Philad.) **9**, 955—962 (1956).

MURRAY, J. E., MERRILL, J. P., HARRISON, J. H., WILSON, R. E., DAMMIN, G. J.: Prolonged survival of human kidney homografts by immunosuppressive drug therapy. New Eng. J. Med. **268**, 1315—1323 (1963).

MURRAY, J. E., SHEIL, A. G. R., MOSELEY, R., KNIGHT, P., MCGAVIC, J. D., DAMMIN, G. J.: Analysis of mechanism of immunosuppressive drugs in renal homotransplantation. Ann. Surg. **160**, 449—473 (1969).

MURRAY, J. E., WILSON, R. E., TILNEY, N. L., MERRILL, J. R., COOPER, W. C., BIRTCH, A. G., CARPENTER, C. B., HAGER, E. B., DAMMIN, G. J., HARRISON, J. H.: Five years experience in renal transplantation with immunosuppressive drugs: survival, function complications, and the role of lymphocyte depletion by thoracic duct fistula. Ann. Surg. **168**, 416—435 (1968).

NAGANO, H., ZALKIN, H., HENDERSON, E. J.: The anthranilate synthetase-anthranilate-5-phosphoribosylpyrophosphate phosphoribosyl-transferase aggregate. J. biol. Chem. **245**, 3810—3820 (1970).

NARKATES, A. J., PITTILLO, R. F.: Inhibition of nonproliferating *Escherichia coli* by azaserine. Antimicrobial Agents and Chemotherapy — 1963, 439—446 (1964).

NARROD, S. A., BONAVITA, V., EHRENFELD, E. R., KAPLAN, N. O.: Effect of azaserine on the biosynthesis of diphosphopyridine nucleotide in mouse. J. biol. Chem. **236**, 931—935 (1961).

NARROD, S. A., LANGAN, T. A., JR., KAPLAN, N. O., GOLDIN, A.: Effect of azaserine (*O*-diazoacetyl-L-serine) on the pyridine nucleotide levels of mouse liver. Nature (Lond.) **183**, 1674—1675 (1959).

NEAL, A. L., LIBMAN, L., SMULSON, M. E.: Influence of γ-glutamyl-hydrazide on protein synthesis of *Pseudomonas aeruginosa*. Arch. Biochem. Biophys. **127**, 426—428 (1968).

NEUMAN, R. E., MCCOY, T. A.: Dual requirement of Walker Carcinosarcoma 256 *in vitro* for asparagine and glutamine. Science **124**, 124—125 (1956).

NEWELL, G. W., CARMAN, W. W.: Effect of methionine on toxicity of crystalline "agene factor" against *Leuconostoc mesenteroides*. Fed. Proc. **9**, 209 (1950).

NICOLAIDES, E. D., WESTLAND, R. D., WITTLE, E. L.: Azaserine, synthetic studies. II. J. Amer. chem. Soc. **76**, 2887—2891 (1954).

OKAMI, Y., MAEDA, K., KONDO, H., TANAKA, T., UMEZAWA, H.: A streptomyces producing *O*-carbamyl-D-serine. J. Antibiot. (Tokyo) **15**, 147—151 (1962).

OLESON, J. J., REITH, A. R., THIE, R. S., MJOS, K. J., CALDERELLA, L. A.: The comparative antitumor activity of the diazomycins. Fed. Proc. **19**, 394 (1960).

PACE, J., MCDERMOTT, E. E.: Methionine sulfoximine and some enzyme systems involving glutamine. Nature (Lond.) **169**, 415—416 (1952).

PASIEKA, A. E., MORGAN, J. F.: Glutamine metabolism of normal and malignant cells cultivated in synthetic media. Nature (Lond.) **183**, 1201—1202 (1959).

PATTERSON, M. K., JR., ORR, G. R.: Asparagine biosynthesis by the Novikoff hepatoma. Isolation, purification, and mechanism studies of the enzyme system. J. biol. Chem. **243**, 376—380 (1968).

PETERS, E. L., TOWER, D. B.: Glutamic acid and glutamine metabolism in cerebral cortex after seizures induced by methionine sulphoximine. J. Neurochem. **5**, 80—90 (1959).

PINE, E. K.: Concentrative uptake of azaserine by neoplastic plasma cells and lymphocytes. J. nat. Cancer Inst. **21**, 973—984 (1958).

PITTILLO, R. F.: Studies on the antimicrobial nature of action of azaserine. Antimicrobial Agents Annual — 1960, 276—287 (1961).

PITTILLO, R. F., HUNT, D. E.: Azaserine and 6-diazo-5-oxo-L-norleucine (DON). In: GOTTLIEB, D., SHAW, P. D. (Eds.): Antibiotics, Vol. I, Mechanism of action, pp. 481—493. New York: Springer 1967.

PITTILLO, R. F., NARKATES, A. J., BURNS, J.: Comparison of the effects of some radiation modifiers on selected radiomimetic agents in microorganisms. Radiat. Res. **25**, 401—409 (1965).

PITTILLO, R. F., QUINNELLY, B. G.: Further studies on the antimicrobial nature of action of azaserine. Antimicrobial Agents and Chemotherapy — 1961, 245—253 (1962).

PREISS, J., HANDLER, P.: Biosynthesis of diphosphopyridine nucleotide. J. biol. Chem. **233**, 493—500 (1958).

PRICE, K. E., BUCK, R. E., SCHLEIN, A., SIMINOFF, P.: A comparison of the *in vitro* susceptibility of HeLa and protozoan cells to antitumor antibiotics. Cancer Res. **22**, 885—891 (1962).

RABINOVITZ, M., FISHER, J. M.: *S*-Carbamylcysteine inhibition of protein synthesis by Ehrlich ascites tumor cells. J. nat. Cancer Inst. **28**, 1165—1171 (1962).

RABINOVITZ, M., OLSON, M. E., GREENBERG, D. M.: Role of glutamine in protein synthesis by the Ehrlich ascites carcinoma. J. biol. Chem. **222**, 879—893 (1956).

RABINOVITZ, M., OLSON, M. E., GREENBERG, D. M.: δ Hydroxylysine — an inhibitor of glutamine and protein synthesis by the Ehrlich ascites carcinoma cell. Cancer Res. **17**, 885—889 (1957).

RABINOVITZ, M., OLSON, M.E., GREENBERG, D.M.: Effect of glutamine analogs on amino acid incorporation into protein of some normal and neoplastic cells *in vitro*. Cancer Res. **19**, 388—392 (1959).

RAO, K.V.: Chemistry of the duazomycins. I. Duazomycins A. Antimicrobial Agents and Chemotherapy — 1961, 178—183 (1962).

RAO, K.V., BROOKS, S.C., KUGELMAN, M., ROMANO, A.A.: Duazomycins A, B, and C, three antitumor substances. I. Isolation and characterization. Antibiotics Ann. 1959-60, 943—949 (1960).

RAVEL, J.M., MCCORD, T.J., SKINNER, C.G., SHIVE, W.: *S*-Carbamyl-L-cysteine, an inhibitory amino acid analogue. J. biol. Chem. **232**, 159—168 (1958).

REILLY, H.C.: Some aspects of azaserine, 6-diazo-5-oxo-L-norleucine, and β-2-thienylalanine. In: WOLSTENHOLME, G.E.W., O'CONNOR, C.M. (Eds.): Ciba Foundation Symposium: Amino acids and peptides with antimetabolic activity, pp. 62—74. Boston: Little, Brown and Co. 1958.

REITZ, R.H., SLADE, H.D., NEUHAUS, F.C.: The biochemical mechanisms of resistance by *Streptococci* to the antibiotics D-cycloserine and *O*-carbamyl-D-serine. Biochemistry **6**, 2561—2570 (1967).

ROBERTS, E., BORGES, P.R.F.: Patterns of free amino acids in growing and regressing tumors. Cancer Res. **15**, 697—699 (1955).

ROBERTS, E., FRANKEL, S.: Free amino acids in normal and neoplastic tissues of mice as studied by paper chromatography. Cancer Res. **9**, 645—648 (1949).

ROBERTS, J., HOLCENBERG, J.S., DOLOWY, W.C.: Antineoplastic activity of highly purified bacterial glutaminases. Nature (Lond.) **227**, 1136—1137 (1970).

ROBERTS, J., HOLCENBERG, J.S., DOLOWY, W.C.: Physico-chemical and kinetic properties of an antitumor glutaminase and its crystallization. Proc. Amer. Ass. Cancer Res. **12**, 13 (1971).

RONZIO, R.A., MEISTER, A.: Phosphorylation of methionine sulfoximine by glutamine synthetase. Proc. nat. Acad. Sci. (Wash.) **59**, 164—170 (1968).

RONZIO, R.A., ROWE, W.B., MEISTER, A.: Studies on the mechanism of inhibition of glutamine synthetase by methionine sulfoximine. Biochemistry 8, 1066—1075 (1969).

ROPER, J.A., MCILWAIN, H.: Preparation and antibacterial action of some compounds structurally related to glutamic acid. Their application in microbiological determination of small quantities of glutamine. Biochem. J. **42**, 485—492 (1948).

ROSENBERG, S., CALABRESI, P.: Enhanced suppression of the secondary immune response by combination of 6-mercaptopurine "duazomycin A." Nature (Lond.) **199**, 1101—1102 (1963).

ROSS, D.L., SKINNER, C.G., SHIVE, W.: *S*-(alkyl- and arylcarbamoyl)-L-cysteines. J. med. pharm. Chem. **3**, 519—524 (1961).

ROTH, J.S., WASE, A., REINER, L.: The distribution of S^{35}-labeled L-methionine sulfoximine in the rat. Science **115**, 236—238 (1952).

ROWE, W.B., RONZIO, R.A., MEISTER, A.: Inhibition of glutamine synthetase by methionine sulfoximine. Studies on methionine sulfoximine phosphate. Biochemistry 8, 2674—2680 (1969).

SARTORELLI, A.C., BOOTH, B.A.: Antineoplastic activity of combinations of 6-chloropurine and azaserine. Cancer Res. **20**, 198—203 (1960).

SARTORELLI, A.C., BOOTH, B.A.: Some factors affecting the tumor-inhibitory properties of combinations of azaserine and 6-chloropurine. Biochem. Pharmacol. **12**, 847—853 (1963).

SARTORELLI, A.C., BOOTH, B.A.: Inhibition of the synthesis of thymine nucleotides by azaserine. Molec. Pharmacol. **3**, 71—80 (1967).

SARTORELLI, A.C., LEPAGE, G.A.: Inhibition of ascites cell growth by combinations of 6-thioguanine and azaserine. Cancer Res. **18**, 938—942 (1958a).

SARTORELLI, A.C., LEPAGE, G.A.: Metabolic effects of 6-thioguanine. II. Biosynthesis of nucleic acid purines *in vivo* and *in vitro*. Cancer Res. **18**, 1329—1335 (1958b).

SARTORELLI, A.C., SCHOOLAR, E.J., JR., KRUSE, P.F., JR.: Chemotherapy of Sarcoma 180 by combinations of DL-glyceraldehyde with 6-thioguanine or with azaserine and 6-chloropurine. Proc. Soc. exp. Biol. (N.Y.) **104**, 266—268 (1960).

SARTORELLI, A.C., UPCHURCH, H.F., BIEBER, A.L., BOOTH, B.A.: Some metabolic effects exerted by azaserine and purine analogs *in vivo*. Cancer Res. **24**, 1202—1209 (1964).

SCHABEL, F.M., JR., SKIPPER, H.E., TRADER, M.W., WILCOX, W.S.: Experimental evaluation of potential anticancer agents. XIX. Sensitivity of nondividing leukemic cell populations to certain classes of drugs *in vivo*. Cancer Chemother. Rep. **48**, 17—30 (1965).

SCHROEDER, D.D., ALLISON, A.J., BUCHANAN, J.M.: Biosynthesis of the purines. XXXII. Effect of Albizziin and other reagents on the activity of formylglycinamide ribonucleotide amidotransferase. J. biol. Chem. **244**, 5856—5865 (1969).

SCHROEDER, J. M., ANSFIELD, F. J., CURRERI, A. R., LEPAGE, G. A.: Toxicity and clinical trial of azaserine and 6-thioguanine in advanced solid malignant neoplasms. Brit. J. Cancer **18**, 449—458 (1964).
SCHWARTZ, R. S. (Ed.): Proceedings of the symposium on immunosuppressive drugs. Fed. Proc. **26**, 879—960 (1967).
SELLINGER, O. Z., AZCURRA, J. M., OHLSSON, W. G.: Methionine sulfoximine seizures. VIII. The dissociation of the convulsant and glutamine synthetase inhibitory effects. J. Pharmacol. exp. Ther. **164**, 212—222 (1968).
SELLINGER, O. Z., GARAZA, A.: The inhibition of cerebral glutamine synthetase by structural analogs of the convulsant DL-methionine sulfoximine. Biochem. Pharmacol. **15**, 396—399 (1966).
SELLINGER, O. Z., WEILER, P., JR.: The nature of the inhibition *in vitro* of cerebral glutamine synthetase by the convulsant, methionine sulfoximine. Biochem. Pharmacol. **12**, 989—1000 (1963).
SHEIL, A. G. R., DAMMIN, G. J., MITCHELL, R. M., MOSELEY, R. V., MURRAY, J. E.: The management, function, and histology of long functioning renal allografts in dogs on immunosuppressive drug therapy. Ann. Surg. **167**, 467—485 (1968).
SHEIL, A. G. R., MOSELEY, R. V., MURRAY, J. E.: Differential skin and renal homograft survival in dogs on immunosuppressive therapy. Surg. Forum **15**, 166—168 (1964).
SHIVE, W., SKINNER, C. G.: Amino acid analogs. In: HOCHSTER, R. M., QUASTEL, J. H. (Eds.): Metabolic inhibitors, Vol. I, pp. 1—73. New York: Academic Press 1963.
SHORT, L. N., THOMPSON, H. W.: Toxic factor from agenized proteins: infra-red measurements. J. chem. Soc. 1746—1749 (1951).
SIMARD, R., BERNHARD, W.: Le phénomène de la ségrégation nucléolaire: spécificité d'action de certains antimétabolites. Int. J. Cancer **1**, 463—479 (1966).
SKINNER, C. G., MCCORD, T. J., RAVEL, J. M., SHIVE, W.: *O*-Carbamyl-L-serine, an inhibitory analog of L-glutamine. J. Amer. chem. Soc. **78**, 2412—2414 (1956).
SKINNER, C. G., MCKENNA, G. F., MCCORD, T. J., SHIVE, W.: Antitumor activity of some amino acid analogs. I. *S*-carbamylcysteine and *O*-carbazylserine. Texas Repts. Biol. Med. **16**, 493—499 (1958).
SKINNER, C. G., MCKENNA, G. F., ROSS, D. L., SHIVE, W.: Antitumor activity of amino acid analogs. II. *S*-methylcarbamoyl-L-cysteine. Texas Rep. biol. Med. **19**, 860—865 (1961).
SKIPPER, H. E.: Effects of 6-mercaptopurine on experimental tumors. Ann. N. Y. Acad. Sci. **60**, 267—272 (1954).
SKIPPER, H. E., BENNETT, L. L., JR., SCHABEL, F. M., JR.: Mechanism of action of azaserine. Fed. Proc. **13**, 298—299 (1954).
SKIPPER, H. E., THOMSON, J. R.: A preliminary study of the influence of amino acid deficiencies on experimental cancer chemotherapy. In: WOLSTENHOLME, G. E. W., O'CONNOR, C. M. (Eds.): Ciba Foundation Symposium: Amino acids and peptides with antimetabolic activity, pp. 38—58. Boston: Little, Brown and Co. 1958.
SLATER, T. F., SAWYER, B. C.: Nicotinamide adenine dinucleotides in acute liver injury: effects of azaserine and puromycin in the rat. Biochem. Pharmacol. **15**, 1267—1271 (1966).
SMULSON, M. E., NEAL, A. L.: Comparative effects of glutamine analogues on protein metabolism of 6C3H-ED and Ehrlich ascites carcinoma. Arch. Biochem. Biophys. **112**, 25—31 (1965).
SPECK, J. F.: The enzymatic synthesis of glutamine, a reaction utilizing adenosine triphosphate. J. biol. Chem. **179**, 1405—1426 (1949).
SPENCER, R. P., BOW, T. M., MARKULIS, M. A.: Intestinal transport of azaserine and NDO. Biochem. Pharmacol. **12**, 599 (1963).
SPENCER, R. L., PREISS, J.: Biosynthesis of diphosphopyridine nucleotide. The purification and the properties of diphosphopyridine nucleotide synthetase from *Escherichia coli B*. J. biol. Chem. **242**, 385—392 (1967).
SRINIVASAN, P. R., RIVERA, A, JR.: The enzymatic synthesis of anthranilate from shikimate 5-phosphate and L-glutamine. Biochemistry **2**, 1059—1062 (1963).
SRINIVASAN, P. R., WEISS, B.: The biosynthesis of *p*-aminobenzoic acid: studies on the origin of the amino group. Biochim. biophys. Acta (Amst.) **51**, 597—599 (1961).
STEINMAN, I. D., IYER, V. N., SZYBALSKI, W.: The mechanism of chemical mutagenesis. II. Interactions of selected compounds with manganous chloride. Archives Biochem. Biophys. **76**, 78—86 (1958).
SUGIURA, K.: Effect of L-asparaginase (NSC-109, 229) on transplantable and spontaneous tumors from mice and rats. Cancer Chemother. Rep. **53**, 189—194 (1969).
SZYBALSKI, W.: Special microbiological systems. II. Observations on chemical mutagenesis in microorganisms. Ann. N. Y. Acad. Sci. **76**, 475—489 (1958).
TAMIR, H., SRINIVASAN, P. R.: Purification and properties of anthranilate synthetase from *Salmonella typhimurium*. J. biol. Chem. **244**, 6507—6513 (1969).

TANAKA, N., SASHIKATA, K., WADA, T., SUGAWARA, S., UMEZAWA, H.: Mechanism of action of *O*-carbamyl-D-serine. J. Antibiot. (Tokyo) **16**, 217—221 (1963).
TAPIA, R., AWAPARA, J.: Formation of γ-aminobutyric acid (GABA) in brain of mice treated with L-glutamic acid-γ-hydrazide and pyridoxal phosphate-γ-glutamyl hydrazone. Proc. Soc. exp. Biol. (N.Y.) **126**, 218—221 (1967).
TARNOWSKI, G.S., MOUNTAIN, I.M., STOCK, C.C.: Combination therapy of animal tumors with L-asparaginase and antagonists of glutamine or glutamic acid. Cancer Res. **30**, 1118—1122 (1970).
TARNOWSKI, G.S., STOCK, C.C.: Effects of combinations of azaserine and of 6-diazo-5-oxo-L-norleucine with purine analogs and other antimetabolites on the growth of two mouse mammary carcinomas. Cancer Res. **17**, 1033—1039 (1957).
TERAWAKI, A., GREENBERG, J.: Effect of some radiomimetic agents on deoxyribonucleic acid synthesis in *Escherichia coli* and transformation in *Bacillus subtilis*. Biochim. biophys. Acta (Amst.) **95**, 170—173 (1965).
TEWS, J.K., STONE, W.E.: Effects of methionine sulfoximine on levels of free amino acids and related substances in brain. Biochem. Pharmacol. **13**, 543—545 (1964).
THIERSCH, J.B.: Effect of *O*-diazoacetyl-L-serine on rat litter. Proc. Soc. exp. Biol. (N.Y.) **94**, 27—32 (1957a).
THIERSCH, J.B.: Effect of 6-diazo-5-oxo-L-norleucine (DON) on the rat litter *in utero*. Proc. Soc. exp. Biol. (N.Y.) **94**, 33—35 (1957b).
THIERSCH, J.B.: Effect of alazopeptin (A) on litter and fetus of the rat *in utero*. Proc. Soc. exp. Biol. (N.Y.) **97**, 888—889 (1958).
TOMISEK, A.J., KELLY, H.J., SKIPPER, H.E.: Chromatographic studies of purine metabolism. I. The effect of azaserine on purine biosynthesis in *E. coli* using various C^{14}-labeled precursors. Arch. Biochem. Biophys. **64**, 437—455 (1956).
TOMISEK, A.J., REID, M.R.: Chromatographic studies of purine metabolism. V. Inhibition mechanism of diazo-oxo-norleucine in wild type and in diazo-oxo-norleucine-resistant *Escherichia coli*. J. biol. Chem. **237**, 807—811 (1962).
TOMISEK, A.J., REID, M.R., SKIPPER, H.E.: Chromatographic studies of purine metabolism. IV. Reversal of azaserine-induced inhibition by phenylalanine and tryptophan. Cancer Res. **19**, 489—493 (1959).
VAN DEN BERG, C.J., VAN DEN VELDEN, J.: The effect of methionine sulphoximine on the incorporation of labelled glucose, acetate, phenylalanine and proline into glutamate and related amino acids in the brains of mice. J. Neurochem. **17**, 985—991 (1970).
VAN DER MEULEN, P.Y.F., BASSHAM, J.A.: Study of inhibition of azaserine and diazo-oxo-norleucine (DON) on the algae *Scenedesmus* and *Chlorella*. J. Amer. chem. Soc. **81**, 2233—2239 (1959).
VANDEVOORDE, J.P., HANSEN, H.J., NADLER, S.B.: Metabolism of leukemic cells in culture; azaserine inhibition of J-128 (Osgood). Proc. Soc. exp. Biol. (N.Y.) **115**, 55—57 (1964).
VOGEL, C.L., CALABRESI, P.: Enhanced suppression of experimental allergic encephalomyelitis by combination chemotherapy with duazomycin-A and 6-mercaptopurine. Proc. Soc. exp. Biol. (N.Y.) **131**, 251—256 (1969).
WEISS, A.J., RAMIREZ, G., GRAGE, T., STRAWITZ, D., GOLDMAN, L., DOWNING, V.: Phase II study of azotomycin (NSC 56654). Cancer Chemother. Repts. **52**, 611—614 (1968).
WESTLAND, R.D., FUSARI, S.A., CROOKS, H.M., JR.: 6-Diazo-5-oxo-L-norleucine, a new tumor-inhibitory substance. Synthetic studies. Amer. chem. Soc. 129th Meeting Abstr. 14M (1956).
WEYGAND, F., BESTMANN, H.J., KLIEGER, E.: *N*-Trifluoracetyl-aminosäuren. XI. Synthese des 6-diazo-5-oxo-L-norleucins und der 7-diazo-6-oxo-2-L-amino-önanthsäure. Chem. Ber. **91**, 1037—1040 (1958).
WILKOFF, L.J., WILCOX, W.S., BURDESHAW, J.A., DIXON, G.J., DULMADGE, E.A.: Effect of antimetabolites on kinetic behavior of proliferating cultured L1210 leukemia cells. J. nat. Cancer Inst. **39**, 965—975 (1967).
WOODY, P.L., MANDELL, J.D., GREENBERG, J.: Resistance and cross-resistance of *Escherichia coli* mutants to anticancer agents. Radiat. Res. **15**, 290—297 (1961).
WOODY-KARRER, P., GREENBERG, J.: Resistance and cross resistance of *Escherichia coli S* mutants to the radiomimetic agent nitrofurazone. J. Bact. **85**, 1208—1216 (1963).
WU, C., YUAN, L.H.: Regulation of synthesis of glutamine synthetase in *Escherichia coli*. J. gen. Microbiol. **51**, 57—65 (1968).
YAROVAYA, L.M., MARDASHEV, S.R., DEBOV, S.S.: Effect of some glutamine antimetabolites on the guanine monophosphate synthetase of *Escherichia coli*. Vop. med. Khim. **13**, 176 to 180 (1967); Biol. Abstr. **49**, 25139 (1969).
YIP, M.C.M., KNOX, W.E.: Glutamine-dependent carbamyl phosphate synthetase. J. biol. Chem. **245**, 2199—2204 (1970).

Chapter 54

Cytotoxic Amino Acid Analogs

PAUL F. KRUSE, JR.

Introduction

Much of the impetus for working with antimetabolites can be traced to several key reports. One was the demonstration by WOODS (1940) of competition between sulfanilamide and *p*-aminobenzoic acid. Another was the use of a folic acid antagonist, aminopterin, by FARBER et al. (1948) against leukemia, and a third was the concept of inhibition analysis (cf. SHIVE, 1950).

Except for the recent advent of the enzyme L-asparaginase as an effective antitumor agent, the formulary of the cancer chemotherapist has been composed almost entirely of alkylating agents, purine analogs, folic acid antagonists, halogenated pyrimidines, vinca alkaloids, antibiotics, and corticosteroids (cf. KARNOFSKY and CLIFFORD, 1966; SCHWARTZ, 1968; KRAKOFF, 1971). A few other compounds such as hydroxyurea and quinacrine, which are not included in any of the preceding classifications, have also been found of benefit. Cytotoxic amino acids are a part of the present day armamentarium primarily in the sense that some amino acid moieties serve as "carriers," e.g., as in the phenylalanyl portion of the alkylating agent sarcolysin, or that a compound such as azaserine is both an antibiotic and an amino acid antagonist (of glutamine). L-Asparaginase[1], alkylating agents, and glutamine antagonists are each the subject of other chapters in this book. Thus, reference to them herein is made only occasionally when pertinent to discussion of other substances.

Even with deletion from this discussion of these three types of amino acid related agents, there is, nevertheless, considerable evidence of the potential usefulness of other types of these compounds at the clinical level of neoplasia. For example, the uses of *p*-chlorophenylalanine in carcinoid syndrome patients, of α-methyltyrosine in cases of pheochromocytoma, of penicillamine (3-mercaptovaline) in malignant melanoma, as well as the antitumor activities of other compounds will be summarized. The study of amino acid analogs has led to new findings in areas such as transport across cell membranes, metabolic pathways, pharmacodynamics, and pathogen-host interrelationships (cf. reviews by DITTMER, 1950; MATTHEWS, 1958; RICHMOND, 1962; SHIVE and SKINNER, 1963; FOWDEN et al., 1967; MILNE, 1968). This basic knowledge is of considerable importance to applied practice; in addition, several recent developments concerning amino acid depletion have stimulated renewed interest in amino acid analogs with respect to neoplasia.

The possible role of cytotoxic amino acid analogs in immunosuppression remains speculative. These substances have so far been relatively little studied in immunosuppression, unless one considers position-isomers of α-amino acids such

1 L-Asparaginase is included here as an antiamino acid substance because of its amino acid amide depletion effects.

as ε-aminocaproic acid. This compound displays marked immunosuppressive activity as described later in this chapter. However, some α-amino acid analogs have been observed to affect the immune response also, and these activities are summarized below.

In discussing cytotoxic amino acids, it is well to consider briefly at the outset several of the principal means by which these substances may act on a living system. An amino acid analog might act as a competitive inhibitor of the structurally related metabolite. In this case the degree of inhibition is proportional to the ratio of concentrations of inhibitor to metabolite, and the effect on an isolated appropriate enzyme system would be to change the slope but not the intercept of the line on a Lineweaver-Burk plot of reaction rate. If the test substance is a noncompetitive inhibitor, i.e., the corresponding metabolite does not overcome the inhibition, both the slope and the intercept of such a plot are changed. Such a compound can be shown to be an antagonist of a particular substrate only by its effect upon an enzymic reaction known to involve the specific metabolite. Another mode of action of amino acid analogs can be to alter amino acid transport. Individual amino acids are concentrated into cells by specific energy-requiring mechanisms, and they can be competitively displaced by analogs (e.g., BRITTEN et al., 1955). As might be expected, amino acid analogs can also inhibit enzyme synthesis normally induced by free amino acids (e.g., HALVORSON and SPIEGELMAN, 1952), nucleic acid synthesis (e.g., PARDEE and PRESTIDGE, 1956a), antibody response (LA VIA et al., 1960), and differentiation (e.g., WILDE, 1955). Further, they often are incorporated into protein in place of their respective metabolites (e.g., KRUSE et al., 1959). In all, it is apparent that these substances can alter the course of a wide variety of events in living systems.

Along with the reservations mentioned previously (exclusion of alkylating agents, glutamine antagonists, and amino acid depletion agents such as L-asparaginase), this discussion is confined mainly to work that has been done with cytotoxic amino acids as it pertains to neoplasia and to immunosuppression in animal systems. The terms cytotoxic amino acids and amino acid analogs are used herein interchangeably.

Amino Acid Analogs and Anticancer Properties

A. Aspartic Acid and Asparagine

Aspartic acid is a key substance in intermediary metabolism, participating in the syntheses of protein, pyrimidine nucleotides, and purine nucleotides. It can contribute nitrogen directly to the urea cycle and, by transamination, form oxaloacetic acid, a key substance in gluconeogenesis as well as in terminal oxidations. This amino acid has also been a principal target for attack via antimetabolites.

Analogs such as 3-hydroxy-, 2- and 3-methyl-, and 3-aminocysteic acid, and related compounds, such as (+)-*S*-methyl-L-cysteine sulfoxide (the lower homolog of methionine sulfoxide, an antagonist of glutamic acid) and 2-thiohydantoin-5-acetic acid, have been studied in various biological systems — some of them intensively so with microorganisms. In general, they have all proved to be effective inhibitors of aspartic acid utilization. 3-Methylaspartic acid, for example, was shown to be a potent antimetabolite of aspartic acid in growth of *E. coli* strain B (WOOLLEY, 1960) and was the subject of a recent review article (GALEGOV, 1963). To this author's knowledge, none of these compounds has proved to be an effective anticancer agent in experimental tumor systems.

Since aspartic acid is involved in a diversity of anabolic pathways, perhaps it is not surprising that diets supplemented with aspartic acid promote tumor growth, as shown in two recent reports. SZENDE and TYIHÁK (1968) fed 200 mg per kg body weight per day of L-aspartic acid to rats bearing Yoshida sarcoma and Guerin carcinoma tumors, and observed a 30 to 53 % promotion of growth compared to tumor animals on unsupplemented diets. It is known, however, that some commercial sources of aspartic acid contain significant quantities of L-asparagine (PATTERSON et al., 1969b) and caution must be used in interpretation of results of aspartic acid feeding experiments if this factor is not taken into account. SCHMIDT (1970) also observed promotion of tumor growth in animals given additional L-aspartic acid. The feature of SZENDE and TYIHÁK's (1968) report salient to this discussion was that analogous feeding experiments with 1000 mg per kg body weight per day of D-aspartic acid depressed tumor growth by 36 to 88 % of that in control animals. Reasons for the inhibitory effect of the D-isomer were not investigated, but an indication may be cited from an interesting earlier report by EISENSTADT et al. (1959). These authors found that D-aspartic acid inhibited protein synthesis, and from an analysis of metabolite reversal tests concluded that D-aspartate interfered in purine nucleotide synthesis at the reaction sequence: IMP + L-aspartate + GTP $\rightleftharpoons$ AMP + fumaric acid + GDP + P_i. Further tests with cell-free extracts showed the effectiveness of inhibition of AMP formation by D-aspartate, and the hypothesis was developed that protein synthesis inhibition was effected indirectly because of impairment with the energetics (ATP) of the system. Recently, MIURA et al. (1970a) found that D-aspartic acid had antitumor activity against asparaginase-sensitive 6C3HED cells, but not against 6C3HED asparaginase-resistant cells.

While the more common analogs of aspartic acid have not been effective tumor inhibitors, it was reported recently that the carbobenzoxy derivative of L-aspartate (disodium salt) was markedly inhibitory to the growth of SJKL/J lymphosarcoma in mice, but was relatively ineffective against two other types of tumors (SCHLESINGER et al., 1971). However, the analogous derivative of L-asparagine was active against all three tumors (SCHLESINGER et al., 1969, 1971).

In recent years considerable interest has been shown in L-asparagine analogs. This has been a research activity complementary to the development of L-asparaginase as an antitumor agent (cf. chapters 68 and 69) and to the asparagine requirement of certain tumor cell types (NEUMAN and McCOY, 1956; McCOY et al., 1959; HALEY et al., 1961). Curtailment of L-asparagine supply to certain tumors via enzyme injections or amino acid antagonists would logically be of benefit to the host. The efficacy of L-asparaginase treatment has been observed repeatedly, with evidence that depletion of asparagine in the circulatory system is a contributory factor (e.g., OHNUMA et al., 1970), but no comparable progress of a practical nature has been achieved with monomolecular L-asparagine analogs. Even though asparaginase is effective in clearing blood asparagine, other aspects of particular concern clinically are (a) pre-existent cells in the tumor population that are able to synthesize asparagine, and (b) asparagine supply from host cells via asparagine synthetase activity (cf. PATTERSON et al., 1969a; COONEY et al., 1970). Thus, combination of asparaginase with inhibitors effective against aspects (a) and (b) above has been the goal of a number of studies. Progress has been made, for example, with the enzyme plus the glutamine antagonist, 6-diazo-5-oxo-L-norleucine and azotomycin (TARNOWSKI et al., 1969, 1970; HASKELL and CANELLOS, 1970) which interfere with asparagine synthesis by preventing acquisition of the amido group from glutamine via asparagine synthetase.

Several asparagine analogs have been studied in detail; these are aspartic acid-β-hydrazide (AAH), β-aspartylhydroxamic acid (BAH), and 5-diazo-4-oxo-L-norvaline (DONV). MICKELSON and FLIPPIN (1956) found that when AAH was injected daily into mice bearing sarcoma 180 at 150 mg per kg body weight from day 3 to 10 after tumor implantation there was a 30 to 40 % reduction in tumor weight. In combination with 4-deoxypyridoxine (DOP), tumor growth was inhibited 70 to 80 %. This sort of additive effect of DOP with an amino acid analog was also to be seen later by HRUBAN and WISSLER (1960) (see B. III, this chapter). OHNUMA et al. (1967) used AAH alone in comparable doses against the 6C3HED tumor in mice and found a similar degree of inhibition, approximately 35 %; results in the two studies differed in that severe body weight loss of 25 % was observed in the former, but a slight gain of 4 % occurred in the latter. In contrast to these observations, MIURA et al. (1970a) found no prolongation of survival time in mice with asparaginase-sensitive 6C3HED cells when treated with AAH.

Among 21 aspartic acid and asparagine related compounds, MIURA et al. (1970a) found that D-aspartic acid, D-glutamic acid, hydantoin-5-acetic acid, and BAH possessed antitumor activity, with the last substance effective against both asparaginase-sensitive and -resistant 6C3HED tumors. From the work of NORTON and CHEN (1969), BAH could be effective against both because it acts not only as an L-asparagine antagonist, but also as a repressor of L-asparagine synthetase. In the presence of L-asparaginase, however, BAH is hydrolyzed as readily as is L-asparagine (SCHWARTZ et al., 1970).

To assess the anti-asparagine activity of DONV, which is the next lower homolog of the effective glutamine antagonist 6-diazo-5-oxo-L-norleucine, HANDSCHUMACHER et al. (1968) determined its effect on L-asparaginase and on asparagine-dependent and -independent cell lines *in vitro*. The enzyme was inhibited irreversibly (cf. JACKSON and HANDSCHUMACHER, 1970), while 80 % of the L-asparagine-requiring L5178Y leukemia cells in culture were killed at a concentration of DONV of 6×10^{-4} moles per liter (cf. SUMMERS and HANDSCHUMACHER, 1971), compared to a 25 % kill in P815Y mast cells that do not have an asparagine requirement. Asparagine-dependent and -independent lines of the Jensen sarcoma react to DONV in a similar manner[2].

The β-sulfonamide analog of L-asparagine, L-2-amino-2-carboxyethane-sulfonamide, was an effective inhibitor of serum asparaginase and of an asparagine-requiring mutant of *N. crassa*. It also reduced the growth of *Eremothecium ashbyii* (HEYMANN et al., 1959) and inhibited the development of sea urchin eggs (LALLIER, 1968), but was apparently without effect on the survival time of mice with 6C3HED tumors (MIURA et al., 1970a). Various α-N-alkyl derivatives of asparagine were also found to be asparaginase inhibitors (HALPERN and GROSSOWICZ, 1957; DE GROOT and LICHTENSTEIN, 1960).

B. Basic Amino Acids

I. Arginine

One of the most intensively studied amino acid analogs has been L-canavanine (2-amino-4-guanidinoxybutyric acid), a potent antimetabolite of arginine in numerous biological systems (cf. SHIVE and SKINNER, 1963), including replication of viruses (e.g., PILCHER et al., 1955; RANKI and KÄÄRIÄINEN, 1969); this analog occurs naturally in relatively high concentration, about 2 %, in jack beans. Regarding animal cell systems, L-canavanine was shown to limit growth of Walker 256 carcinosarcoma cells *in vitro* by 50 % at a 1:1 M concentration ratio with L-arginine (KRUSE and McCOY, 1958), and it was incorporated in significant amounts into the tumor cell protein (KRUSE et al., 1959). In other *in vitro* tests

2 Personal communication. Dr. M.K. PATTERSON, JR., December 1971.

it strongly inhibited survival of chick embryo fibroblasts (MORGAN et al., 1958), growth of green monkey kidney cells (TYTELL and NEUMAN, 1960), and three lines derived from human tissues, WISH, FL (amnion), and HEp-2 (carcinoma) (MIEDEMA and KRUSE, 1966). However, in *in vivo* tests against Sarcoma 180 in mice, L-canavanine exhibited only a slight antitumor activity (prolongation of survival time) either alone or in various combinations with 6-thioguaninine, azaserine, chloropurine, and several other amino acid antagonists (SARTORELLI et al., 1960). Several attempts in this author's laboratory to prepare the nitrogen analog of canavanine, 5-azaarginine (2-amino-4-guanidinaminobutyric acid), failed because of cyclization of the product (the cyclic compound was ineffective as a mammalian cell growth inhibitor *in vitro*).

Like arginine, canavanine is split by arginase but at a slower rate. The product L-canaline, 2-amino-4-aminooxybutyric acid, proved to be 4-fold more toxic to tumor cells *in vitro* than was L-canavanine (WHITE et al., 1963). The inhibition was not reversed by L-ornithine, but it was prevented by either pyridoxal phosphate or glutamic acid semialdehyde. Thus, the toxicity was possibly due to the potent "carbonyl-trapping" properties of the substituted hydroxylamine structure (WHITE et al., 1963). In this regard, one of the histidine analogs (α-hydrazino) has been found to inhibit pyridoxal phosphate-requiring enzymes (discussed later). Like canavanine, however, L-canaline had no appreciable effect on survival time of mice bearing Sarcoma 180[3]. Recently L-canaline was found to interfere with ornithine utilization in rat liver and it was estimated to be more than 100 times as effective as cycloserine in inhibiting transaminase activity (KEKOMÄKI et al., 1969). In its "open" form, cycloserine is the next lower homolog of canaline.

The distance between the 2- and 5-nitrogen substituents in arginine is not necessarily a requirement to be retained in antagonist structures, as it appears to be for the 2-, 6-substituents in lysine (discussed later). For instance, L-homoarginine was an effective inhibitor of the growth of several microorganisms, and was reversible by arginine (cf. SHIVE and SKINNER, 1963). Further, an interesting observation was made recently by FISHMAN and SIE (1970), who found that L-homoarginine is a strong, uncompetitive inhibitor of human bone and liver alkaline phosphatase while it has virtually no effect on intestinal and placental alkaline phosphatases. These four tissues are the major contributors to the serum alkaline phosphatase. The analog was found to be ineffective, however, against Jensen sarcoma cells *in vitro*, as were two lower homologs of arginine, L-2-amino-3-guanidinopropionic acid and L-2-amino-4-guanidinobutyric acid, and three corresponding homologs of ornithine and citrulline, neither of which, themselves, could spare the arginine requirement for these tumor cells *in vitro* (WHITE et al., 1963). Other compounds related to arginine that neither inhibited growth nor spared the arginine requirement for growth were the 2-hydroxy and 2-keto analogs, L-arginine amide, L-arginine methyl ester · HCl, benzoyl-L-arginine, nitro-L-arginine, agmatine, DL-2-amino-6-guanidinaminocaproic acid, and L-octopine. In contrast to these results, the tripeptide, L-prolyl-L-phenylalnyl-L-arginine supplanted arginine in the culture medium, and moreover, stimulated proliferation. Several other arginine peptides also replaced arginine in the growth medium (WHITE et al., 1963).

A nitrogen mustard derivative of arginine, N^2-*bis*(2-chloroethyl)carbamoyl-L-arginine, was said to have possible activity as an anticancer drug (DONGOROZI, 1960).

3 Unpublished results, KRUSE, P. F., JR., NASH, J., SMITH, C. W.; the L-canaline did produce signs of chronic allergic reactions with much itching and some edema in the animals.

II. Histidine

Certain analogs of histidine have been shown to be effective inhibitors of bacterial growth, including 2-thiazolealanine, 1,2,4-triazole-3-alanine, and 2-hydrazino-3-(4-imidazolyl)propionic acid (e.g., MOYED, 1961; LEVIN and HARTMAN, 1963; SHIFRIN et al., 1966). Unlike most other amino acids, no true natural products are known that act as histidine analogs; however, treatment of plants with the herbicide, 3-amino-1,2,4-triazole (amitrole), does cause production of β-3-amino-1,2,4-triazole-1-ylalanine, which proved to be (a) growth inhibitory to bacterial cultures and (b) incorporated into protein (WILLIAMS et al., 1965). Amitrole itself, while not a structural analog of an amino acid per se, is a growth inhibitor reversible by histidine (e.g., KLOPOTOWSKI and WIATER, 1965). It is of interest here to cite another heterocyclic compound, 3,4-dimethylpyrazolo(3,2-*c*)-as-triazine (DMPT); this compound and certain of its derivatives markedly inhibit several tumors in rats (BALDWIN et al., 1966); it apparently does not act as an antagonist of purines, whose structure it resembles closely, but interferes with either the metabolism or an essential function of histidine. Only histidine, among a range of amino acids and imidazole derivatives, could offset the toxicity of this antagonist. Of further interest is that it strongly inhibited histidine ammonia-lyase, being noncompetitive with histidine; furthermore, the enzyme had much higher affinity for DMPT than for histidine. Thus, the inhibitor effectively reduced the amount of active enzyme (ARDEN et al., 1970). Since histidine is part of the catalytic site of several enzymes (cf. WIELAND and DETERMANN, 1966), SCHLESINGER and SCHLESINGER (1967) studied the effect of replacement of histidine in alkaline phosphatase with the analog 1,2,4-triazole-3-alanine. The antagonist caused immediate cessation of the production of the enzyme in *E. coli* K-12, but protein synthesis continued for at least 40 min. This, and other results, indicated that the analog yielded subunits of the enzyme that were incapable of normal association.

Two interesting correlations of biological activity with analog structure were observed (SHIFRIN et al., 1966) in studies with a single analog of histidine, 2 hydrazino-3-(4-imidazoyl)propionic acid (HIPA). The structural similarity with histidine permitted the inhibitor to enter *S. typhimurium* cells via the histidine-specific transport system. HIPA inactivated several pyridoxal phosphate-containing enzymes, particularly acetylornithine transaminase in which the coenzyme is apparently relatively accessible (cf. SHIFRIN et al., 1966). These and other effects of the analog explain why not only histidine but also arginine, and to some extent aspartate, could reverse the toxicity of HIPA. Another interesting property of HIPA is its beneficial effect on survival of skin homografts (see Section on Amino Acid Analogs and Immunosuppression).

The design of analogs, which takes into account structural features, first to permit entry into the cell and second to cause specific intracellular lesions, is still an intriguing aspect of the study of antimetabolites; it was, for example, the underlying concept in design of the effective antitumor agent, sarcolysine.

Unlike D-aspartic acid, D-histidine (25 mg), given subcutaneously 4 times daily on days 5 to 10 following transplantation of the RD3 sarcoma in rats (period of rapid tumor growth), caused no appreciable effect on the rate of tumor growth compared with saline-injected tumor-bearing control animals (WISEMAN and GHADIALLY, 1957).

A nitrogen mustard derivative of histidine, *p*-[bis(2-chloroethyl)amino]-phenylacetylhistidine methyl ester · 2 HCl, appeared to be (a) particularly effective against bone tumors and (b) of low toxicity (ABARTIENE, 1967).

III. Lysine

Much has been learned regarding structural features contributory to effective lysine antagonists. For example, it appears that the distance between the two nitrogen atoms must be essentially the same as in lysine, and a *trans*-like configuration of the 2- and 6-carbons has been found of importance in certain bacterial systems (cf. Shive and Skinner, 1963). Thus, 6-*C*-methyllysine is a strong antagonist of lysine, but ornithine and homolysine are not (McLaren and Knight, 1951, 1953). Also, 3-amino-methylcyclohexaneglycine is a lysine antagonist, but the 4-amino analog is not, probably because it cannot readily assume a *trans*-like configuration (Davis et al., 1960). *trans*-4,5-Dehydrolysine, but not the *cis*-isomer, is an effective competitive inhibitor of the utilization of lysine in bacterial systems (Davis et al., 1961).

Predictably, sulphur, oxygen, and nitrogen have been substituted for a methylene group in the lysine chain, all at the 4-position, and the resultant analogs tested as growth inhibitors. The *S*-analog, *S*-(β-aminoethyl) cysteine (4-thiolysine), was a potent inhibitor of lysine incorporation into rat bone marrow *in vitro*, while 6-*C*-methyllysine, 5-hydroxylysine, and 2-amino-6-hydroxycaproic acid were moderately active, of low activity, and inactive, respectively (Rabinovitz and Tuve, 1959). 4-Thiolysine was also found by Rabinovitz and Fisher (1962) to block hemoglobin formation by rabbit reticulocytes, in which case an accumulation of ribosome-associated protein occurred. DL-4-Oxalysine (McCord et al., 1957) was a potent inhibitor of bacterial growth and also of adenocarcinoma growth in embryonated eggs (McCord, 1959); it could not protect mice with lethal infections of either *Salmonella schottmuelleri* or *Staphylococcus aureus* (Stapley et al., 1967). DL-4-Azalysine (McCord et al., 1964) also proved to be an inhibitor of lysine utilization to about the same degree as the 4-oxa analog; the aza-isostere is more difficult to make, is very hygroscopic, and so far as is known at present, has not been tested for antitumor properties[4]. Kolc (1969) described syntheses of L-, D-, and DL-4-azalysine-6-^{14}C, but the biological activity of these compounds does not appear to have been reported.

N^6-Puryl-substituted lysines were reported to have a selective toxicity to cancer cells and to affect synthesis of tumor macromolecules (Hidvegi et al., 1964), but the data are not fully documented and do not appear to have been confirmed by other workers.

Earlier in this discussion, 6-*C*-methyllysine was cited as a potent lysine antagonist. It should be mentioned here that N^6-methyl-substituted lysines have been isolated from histones obtained from various sources (Murray, 1964) and from human urine (Kakimoto and Akazawa, 1970), and 6-*N*-trimethyllysine, which has also been isolated from Ehrlich ascites tumor cells (Hempel et al., 1968), was found to promote growth of three transplantable tumors in mice by 20 to 60% on a weight basis compared with tumor-bearing control animals (Szende et al., 1970). The role of these methylated amino acids in either normal or pathological states is not clear.

Nitrogen mustard derivatives of lysine ["lysepsin", a mixture of 2-, and 6-*bis* (2-chloroethyl)-substituents] were shown to have pronounced antitumor effects, but whether or not these were as effective as or less effective than phenylalanine mustard is not clear (Larionov and Spasskaya, 1961; Novikova, 1963; Spasskaya and Larionov, 1966).

---

4 Personal communication, Dr. T.J. McCord, December 1971.

C. Aromatic Amino Acids

Analogs of phenylalanine have been prepared in greater number than of any other amino acid. Analogs of tyrosine and tryptophan have been prepared and studied relatively extensively also. The number of these aromatic amino acid analogs exceeds several dozen, including halogen, hydroxy, and alkyl substituents; ring replacement with *O*, *N*, or *S*; cycloalkenyl and alkenyl substituents, etc. (cf. SHIVE and SKINNER, 1963; FOWDEN et al., 1967). All of these compounds exhibit some degree of biological activity. The reader is reminded that discussions of alkylating agents such as sarcolysine, in which phenylalanine serves as the "carrier" moiety, are to be found elsewhere in this volume.

I. Phenylalanine

The carcinoid syndrome in man is characterized by frequent, brief episodes of cutaneous flushing and respiratory distress. Usually, functioning malignant carcinoid develops in the ileum, and metastasis often precedes the development of symptoms. Whereas the gastrointestinal mucosa is normally the major depot of serotonin in the body, in patients with malignant carcinoid, the tumor is the major site of serotonin biosynthesis. Serotonin blood levels in this disease are 5 to 10 times normal levels, and urinary excretion of 5-hydroxyindoleacetic acid (5-HIAA) is often increased over 25-fold. As much as 60 % of dietary tryptophan may be diverted to the serotonin pathway by the tumor, while normally about 1 % is metabolized in this way. The pathway from tryptophan to 5-HIAA is via tryptophan hydroxylase to 5-hydroxytryptophan, then decarboxylation to 5-hydroxytryptamine (serotonin), followed by conversion to 5-HIAA by monoamine oxidase and aldehyde dehydrogenase. It was determined in one study (GRAHAME-SMITH, 1964) that liver metastases in malignant carcinoid had an active tryptophan hydroxylating system which was not present in the surrounding liver tissue. *p*-Chlorophenylalanine is an effective inhibitor of tryptophan hydroxylase, and it has been found to be of significant value in treatment of some carcinoid patients (cf. SHANI and SHEBA, 1970; SJOERDSMA, 1971). This analog was first found by KOE and WEISSMAN (1966) to deplete brain serotonin in the rat, and since then has been the subject of a number of basic investigations (cf. GUROFF, 1969). Aside from its effects in carcinoid disease, this analog was also reported to cause hypersexuality in the rat (TAGLIAMONTE et al., 1969), but no evidence of this effect was observed in clinical studies in man (cf. SJOERDSMA, 1971).

One of the most intensively studied of all amino acid analogs has been 4-fluorophenylalanine. Most of these investigations have centered about (a) its relatively great propensity for incorporation into protein, at the expense of phenylalanine incorporation but not incorporation of tyrosine or any other amino acid (cf. RICHMOND, 1962), and (b) its antiviral activities (e.g., LEVINTOW et al., 1962; DYM and BECKER, 1969). As an antitumor agent, however, 4-fluorophenylalanine does not have an appreciable selective activity against cancer cells *in vitro* (JACQUEZ and MOTTRAM, 1953) or a significant effect on survival time of tumor-bearing mice (SARTORELLI et al., 1960). However, the combination of 4-fluorophenylalanine and phenylalanine-restricted diet did produce marked inhibition of two transplantable tumors in mice (RYAN and ELLIOTT, 1968). Another widely studied analog of phenylalanine, β-3-thienylalanine, has exhibited appreciable antitumor properties (JACQUEZ et al., 1952, 1953; BRISTOW and WISSLER, 1961), particularly in combination with administration of deoxypyridoxine (DOP) (HRUBAN and WISSLER, 1960; HRUBAN et al., 1962). Another example of the additive effect of an amino acid analog and DOP against tumors was cited previously in the Section on Aspartic Acid and Asparagine. The oncostatic effect of the β-3-isomer could not be explained on the basis of selective uptake by tumor tissue, since its uptake into Murphy-Sturm lymphosarcoma tissue in rats was negligible compared to its uptake in the kidneys, liver, jejunal mucosa, and pancreas (Samal et al., 1963).

Tumor inhibition by carbobenzoxy-L-asparagine was mentioned in the Section on Aspartic Acid and Asparagine. In related studies, Mor and Lichtenstein (1969) found that carbobenzoxy-L-phenylalanine was a strong inhibitor of rat liver asparaginase; this analog (injected as the sodium salt) was a strong inhibitor of Ehrlich ascites tumor in mice, but only slightly effective against SJL/J lymphosarcoma (Schlesinger et al., 1971).

Aminoxy and hydroxylamino analogs of phenylalanine were found to influence pyridoxal phosphate-dependent activities (Bonomi and Tenconi, 1964); the aminoxy derivative, 2-aminoxy-3-phenylpropionic acid, was a strong inhibitor of the tyrosine-oxidizing system of the liver, glutamic-oxalacetate transaminase of the liver, and 3,4-dihydroxyphenylalanine (DOPA) decarboxylase of the kidney. The inhibitions by this analog are similar in nature to effects of aminoxy and hydrazino analogs mentioned previously. The efficacy of N-haloacetylamino acids as anticancer compounds was indicated over two decades ago by Friedman and Rutenburg (1950), who observed that N-iodoacetylphenylalanine had some retarding action on growth of Sarcoma 37 in mice.

II. Tyrosine

Pheochromocytoma is a catecholamine-producing tumor arising from chromaffin cells of the sympatho-adrenal system. The first step in production of catecholamines is conversion of tyrosine to DOPA, catalyzed by tyrosine hydroxylase. The most potent inhibitor of this enzyme which has been studied in man is α- methyltyrosine, and this analog has been of value in the medical management of pheochromocytoma (e.g., Jones et al., 1968). Daily doses of 2.0 to 4.0 g produced from 50 to 80 % inhibition of catecholamine biosynthesis (cf. Sjoerdsma, 1971). In the latter studies with pheochromocytoma patients, α-methylphenylalanine was not an effective drug. Recently, an extensive study of the structural requirements of phenylalanine analogs for inhibition of tyrosine hydroxylase was made by Weinhold and Rethy (1969). The most potent compound was α-methyl-3-iodophenylalanine, but it was not as effective as the corresponding tyrosine analog (Udenfriend et al., 1965). Whereas α-methyltyrosine has been of value in pheochromocytoma, it was ineffective in reducing urine DOPA levels in two patients with metastatic melanoma, and failed to retard clinical deterioration (Greer et al., 1969).

In melanin-producing cells, tyrosinase catalyzes the conversion of tyrosine to DOPA and DOPA to DOPA quinone. Nonenzymatic polymerization of the latter then forms melanin. Inhibition of tyrosinase activity has been achieved with phenyllactic acid and L-cysteine, a combination which proved effective against S-91 mouse melanoma both *in vitro* (Duke et al., 1967) and *in vivo* (Duke and Demopoulos, 1967). Tyrosinase activity has also been inhibited by penicillamine (a valine analog) as described in the Section on Leucine, Isoleucine, Valine, and other Amino Acids.

A multifunctional compound related to tyrosine, ethyl α-acetamido-α-cyano-β-(3,5-dimethyl-4-methoxyphenyl)propionate, was found to cause 18 % and 35 % inhibition of Ehrlich carcinoma and L4946(C1) leukemia, respectively, in mice, but was inactive against Gardner lymphosarcoma (Jorgensen and Wiley, 1963).

Recently, another tyrosine analog, L-3-nitrotyrosine, was found to have activity against Taper liver tumor cells in mice (MACLEAN and HUBER, 1971).

III. Tryptophan

A number of tryptophan analogs have been studied with respect to their effect on protein synthesis. Analogs such as 2-azatryptophan (tryptazan), 7-azatryptophan, 5-, and 6-fluorotryptophan are all activated for protein synthesis, and their effects on microorganism and animal growth and metabolism are considered mostly due to incorporation into protein. A number of other analogs, including methyl-substituted, hydroxy-, and hydroxamic derivatives are not activated in protein synthesis, but in most cases inhibit tryptophan activation (e.g., PARDEE and PRESTIDGE, 1956b; SHARON and LIPMANN, 1957; BERECZ and GODIN, 1962).

Evidence that certain hydroxy- and methyl-tryptophans cannot be transported across intestinal sacs was cited by SPENCER et al. (1964). Such studies are of obvious importance to the chemotherapist, because for amino acids to be used as carriers to bring various cytoactive groups into cells, the added groups must not interfere with the transport process.

Much information about the inhibition of tryptophan synthesis and utilization has been gained in microbiological systems with the aid of tryptophan analogs (cf. SHIVE and SKINNER, 1963; FOWDEN et al., 1967). Comparable studies in animal systems are relatively few, particularly with respect to tumor-host relationships. Mustard derivatives of tryptophan have, however, been examined rather intensively, both in experimental animals and clinically in man (e.g., FISHBEIN et al., 1964; SCHMID et al., 1965; LAMPERT et al., 1966; KUNG et al., 1968).

Recently L-tryptophan itself was found to inhibit growth of Walker 256 intramuscular carcinoma in rats (GOLD, 1970). Doses of 8, 4, and 2 mmoles per kg body weight inhibited the tumor 55 %, 50 %, and 35 %, respectively. Other L-amino acids such as histidine, proline, leucine, and glutamic acid had no such effect. The primary mechanism of action of L-tryptophan was thought to be due to its capacity to inhibit the enzyme phosphoenolpyruvate carboxykinase (PEP carboxykinase) (cf. RAY et al., 1966; GOLD, 1968), a pivotal enzyme in gluconeogenesis. Inhibitors of PEP carboxykinase such as L-tryptophan and hydrazine sulfate (RAY and HANSON, 1969) are therefore possibly of value in cancer chemotherapy (GOLD, 1970). Whether or not any of the tryptophan analogs might be more effective inhibitors of this particular enzyme remains to be ascertained. Somewhat in contrast to the results of GOLD (1970), CUTTS (1964) found that tryptophan reversed the antitumor effect of vinblastine in tumor-bearing animals.

D. Sulfur-Containing Amino Acids

I. Methionine

Like aspartic acid, methionine has a complex role to play in the cell, as summarized by FOWDEN et al. (1967). Much of the interest regarding methionine antagonists has centered about ethionine; this homolog can replace methionine residues in protein while concomitantly interfering with methyl-group transfer reactions by facilitating the anomalous ethylation of substrates. Ethionine has the distinction of being the first amino acid analog found capable of incorporation into protein (LEVINE and TARVER, 1951); it was one of the first such compounds to be studied in animal systems (LEVY et al., 1953). In addition, ethionine's spectrum of activities includes tumor inhibition in some systems (e.g., LEVY et al., 1953; GUALANDI and BERGAMINI, 1954; ELY and BATT, 1955) but not in others (e.g.,

WHITE and SHIMKIN, 1954), as well as carcinogenesis (POPPER et al., 1953; FARBER, 1956). Although ethionine was ineffective alone when tested against adenocarcinoma 755 in C57BL mice, in combination with a folic acid antagonist there was a pronounced tumor inhibition (SHAPIRO and FUGMANN, 1957). This was an interesting example of the concept of sequential blockade, as defined by POTTER (1951). While neither compound alone was effective, the hypothesis was that the folic acid antagonist would inhibit 1-carbon transfer and, therefore, would interfere with homocysteine conversion to methionine. The addition of a methionine antagonist should then provide a sequential blockade effect, and the results seem to be in accord with this premise. A similar synergism was observed by SKIPPER et al. (1954) and by MORRISON and HIGGINS (1956).

Other interesting properties of this versatile amino acid analog are its rather specific action against liver urocanase activity in the rat (SPOLTER and BALDRIDGE, 1963), and its organotropy to the pancreas (GUALANDI and BERGAMINI, 1954).

Some evidence that higher homologs of ethionine also have growth inhibitory properties, presumably due to interference with protein synthesis and not methyl group transfer, was provided by RIZZOLI et al. (1962) and CESTARI et al. (1963). The ethyl ester of ethionine was not an effective agent against growth of fibroblast cultures (FEHER et al., 1961).

The proliferation of HeLa carcinoma cells *in vitro* was inhibited by oxa-analogs of methionine and ethionine (RIZZOLI et al., 1961), and several derivatives of methionine such as *N*-chloroacetyl-, *N*-dichloroacetyl-, *p*-[*bis*(2-chloropropyl) amino] phenylacetyl-DL-methionine ethyl ester, and *p*-[*bis*(2-chloroethyl)amino] phenacetyl-DL-phenylmethionine were found to have considerable anticancer activity in experimental animal systems (ABE et al., 1960; DAMARACKIS, 1963; KEBLAS, 1966).

II. Cysteine and Cystine

Much of the interest in these two amino acids with respect to chemotherapy of neoplasia resides in their capacity to modify the severe leukopenia often encountered in treatments with nitrogen mustard. This protective effect is specific, since a number of compounds with structures closely related to L-cysteine failed to prevent the leukotoxic effect of nitrogen mustard (cf. WEISBERGER and LEVINE, 1954). It is commonly assumed that L-cysteine protects cells from the radiomimetic action of alkylating agents, although in a recent study with *E. coli*, ROSENKRANZ et al. (1970) observed a synergism between L-cysteine and alkylating agents, i.e., the antibacterial action of the agents was actually enhanced by L-cysteine.

Two compounds, L-selenocysteine and phenylselenocysteine, were effective inhibitors of the incorporation of radioactive L-cystine by leukemic leukocytes (WEISBERGER et al., 1956); and selenocystine exhibited growth inhibitory properties against Murphy lymphosarcoma tumors in rats (WEISBERGER and SUHRLAND, 1956a) and caused a rapid decrease in total leukocyte count and in spleen size in human leukemia patients (WEISBERGER and SUHRLAND, 1955, 1956b).

Over a dozen compounds related to cysteine were tested as potential tumor inhibitors, and the results have been summarized by STOCK (1958). Such compounds as 2-methyl-DL-cysteine, *S*-benzyl-2-methyl-DL-cysteine, and 2- and 3-methyl-methionine actually promoted transplantable tumor growth, whereas *S*-ethyl-L-cysteine, *S*-(2-chloroethyl)-L-cysteine, and djenkolic acid (the cysteine thioacetal of formaldehyde) were partially tumor inhibitory.

Interest in derivatives of these sulfur-containing amino acids as possible tumor-inhibitory agents continues, as evidenced by recent reports of the antileukemia effects of *S*-trityl-L-cysteine and several structural modifications (e.g., TYRER et al., 1969; ZEE-CHENG and CHENG, 1970; COFFEY et al., 1971).

A matter of vital importance in oral administration of drugs is the intestinal transport process, as mentioned previously in the discussion on tryptophan analogs. Nine analogs of cystine were employed to furnish evidence that the disulfide linkage in cystine is a necessary component of the latter for transport to occur (SPENCER et al., 1965).

E. Leucine, Isoleucine, Valine, and Other Amino Acids

I. Leucine, Isoleucine, and Valine

Compounds with significant anticancer effects have sometimes been found through screening programs, but they have also been developed on a more rational basis through prior knowledge of the activities of related structures or of potentially exploitable nutritional and/or metabolic differences between tumor and host. Occasionally a promising drug emerges as a result of two or more of these approaches. For example, 1-aminocyclopentanecarboxylic acid (ACPC) was included solely by chance in a spectrum of compounds submitted for anticancer evaluation (cf. ROSS et al., 1961), while simultaneously it was being synthesized at the Chester Beatty Research Institute because of the known ability of several α-substituted amino acids to inhibit growth (CONNORS et al., 1960). Among more than six dozen α-substituted amino acids with structures related to ACPC, mostly with 3- to 8-carbon ring moieties, only ACPC and several derivatives, such as 1-hydroxylaminocyclopentanecarboxylic acid (HACPC) possessed appreciable antitumor activity. Actually, HACPC had earlier been found to be a rather potent inhibitor of Ehrlich ascites carcinoma (WILSON et al., 1959), and an indication previously of the antitumor effect of ACPC was given by MARTEL and BERLINGUET (1959). The compound ACPC is a nonmetabolizable amino acid, lacking an α-hydrogen atom, and remains essentially unchanged within the cell (e.g., CHRISTENSEN and JONES, 1962). Evidently its biological effects are due mostly to interference with valine (e.g., GREGORY et al., 1969; LINDENAUER et al., 1970). It possessed marked antitumor activity in rodents (e.g., CONNORS et al., 1960; ROSS et al., 1961), as did several ester derivatives (GOLDIN et al., 1961). In tests with human cancer patients ACPC had been found of essentially no value (cf. ROSS et al., 1961), or possibly of some benefit in multiple myeloma (e.g., KRANT et al., 1962) and leiomyosarcoma (cf. BROWN, 1967). It may possibly be useful in various immunological diseases (cf. ROSENTHALE and GLUCKMAN, 1968). It is of interest that 1-amino-3-methylcyclopentanecarboxylic acid was found to be about 1000 times more toxic to *E. coli* 9723 than ACPC but apparently much less toxic to mice (ABSHIRE, 1968).

Another branched chain amino acid analog which is an effective inhibitor of *E. coli* 9723 (APOSHIAN et al., 1959) and which has also shown promise as an antitumor agent is L-penicillamine (LITTMAN et al., 1963). Although L-, D-, and DL-forms were all active as Sarcoma 180 retardants, the L-form was the most active, being as effective against Sarcoma 180 as 5-fluorouracil and less toxic (LITTMAN et al., 1963). The simplest method of administering the drug was to dissolve it in the drinking water; at levels of 25 to 200 mg per kg per day tumor growth was inhibited 26 to 46 % (LITTMAN et al., 1964). While the toxicity of penicillamine to bacteria can be reversed to some extent by branched chain amino acids (cf. APOSHIAN et al., 1959), there is good evidence that its tumor inhibitory properties in animal systems reside not so much in anti-amino acid effects as they do in antagonism to B_6 metabolism (LITTMAN et al., 1963) and in chelating the copper cofactor for tyrosinase, an active enzyme in malignant melanocytes (HOURANI and DEMOPOULOS, 1969). The latter investigators found that subcutaneous administration of D-penicillamine to DBA/2 mice bearing already established *S*-91 malignant melanoma resulted in inhibition of tumor growth and metastases. This agent shows some promise in treatment of human melanoma by itself or possibly in combination with diets restricted in phenylalanine and/or tyrosine (cf. DEMOPOULOS, 1966a, b), but the results of clinical trials to date are inconclusive[5].

Two fluorinated compounds, DL-5,5,5-trifluoroleucine and DL-4,4,4,4',4',4'-hexafluorovaline, have shown antitumor properties. The former had a significant effect on survival time of mice bearing a spectrum of leukemias (RENNERT and ANKER, 1964), and the latter inhibited growth and killed HeLa cells *in vitro* (GALEGOV and BENYUMOVICH, 1965). A considerable number of interesting analogs of the branched chain amino acids have been prepared and studied in some detail in various life systems, including 3-cyclohexene-1-glycine and 3-cyclohexene-1-DL-alanine (EDELSON et al., 1958, 1959), α-amino-β-chlorobutyric acid (RABINOVITZ and MCGRATH, 1959), and various aza- and thia-analogs (SMITH et al., 1963; MCCORD et al., 1965, 1967, 1968). However, some of these compounds have apparently not been investigated in tumor-host systems, nor studied with regard to immunosuppressive effects.

An isostere of isoleucine, *O*-methyl-L-threonine, was an effective inhibitor of bacterial growth (SMULSON et al., 1967) and of protein synthesis in carcinoma cells (RABINOVITZ et al., 1955), but was ineffective as a growth inhibitor of Jensen rat sarcoma cells *in vitro* even at 50 μg/ml concentration[6]. Work has been done recently with the higher homolog, *O*-ethyl-L-threonine; it is also an isoleucine antagonist (cf. HIREMATH et al., 1971) and is reported to decrease the incidence of mortality of chickens with MAREK's disease, a neoplastic-like lymphoproliferative malady (cf. SHIGUERA et al., 1969).

II. Other Amino Acids

Several diazo derivatives of glycine were found to have anticancer effects, but similar derivatives of alanine were considerably less effective (BALDINI and BRAMBILLA, 1965, 1966a, b). Two compounds, diazoacetylglycinamide and diazoacetylglycine hydrazide, at levels of 180 to 300 mg per kg per day, potentiated the effect of 5-fluorouracil against the ascites form of Sarcoma 180 in mice, but not of corresponding solid tumors.

Good evidence that mustard derivatives of the various amino acids vary significantly in their effects on different tumors was observed by SCHMID et al. (1965). Glycine, alanine, and tryptophan mustards were effective against Ehrlich ascites carcinoma, but caused only slight inhibition of Ridgway osteogenic sarcoma, while phenylalanine mustard activity was the reverse.

A derivative of serine, *N*-dichloroacetyl-DL-serine, has potent anticancer properties. For example, when it was administered as the sodium salt to mice bearing Sarcoma 37, complete tumor regression was observed; further, the compound was markedly nontoxic to rats and mice even in doses of 4 g per kg body weight (LEVI et al., 1960). Other tests showed that it was effective alone against several rodent tumors, and in combination with cyclophosphamide or radiation it showed beneficial effects in a few cases of human cancer (BLONDAL et al., 1961). Another derivative of serine, the *bis*(2-chloropropyl)carbamate ester, was reported to have

5 Personal communication, Dr. H.B. DEMOPOULOS, December 1971.
6 Unpublished results, KRUSE, P.F., JR., WHITTLE, W., NASH, J.

a favorable response in 9 of 17 patients with stage IV breast cancer and in 1 of 5 patients with prostatic cancer (FALKSON and FALKSON, 1965).

Two recent papers describe some interesting properties of L-serine hydroxamate. First, it was by far the most potent growth inhibitor of *E. coli* K-12 among 8 amino acid hydroxamates tested (TOSA and PIZER, 1971a), and secondly, it was a competitive inhibitor of seryl-transfer ribonucleic acid (tRNA) synthetase (TOSA and PIZER, 1971b). In view of the apparent high demand for serine by certain tumor cell systems, i.e., neoplastic mast cells (SCHINDLER, 1963), Jensen sarcoma cells (KRUSE et al., 1967), and leukemic cells (REGAN et al., 1969), it should be of interest to test the hydroxamate analog for anticancer effects.

Amino Acid Analogs and Immunosuppression

As noted in the Introduction, amino acid analogs have received little study as immunosuppressive agents. Substances which suppress the immune response can be classified as antiproliferative agents and "others" (BERENBAUM, 1970). Because some of the amino acid analogs are potent inhibitors of proliferation, one can speculate that they might significantly affect the immune response, particularly at the level of proliferation of precursor cells. In several of the following studies, this effect was apparently observed; interference with either the antigen-reactive or precursor cells of the antibody response is probably the major goal in developing immunosuppressive agents (MAKINODAN et al., 1970). Thus, the activity of amino acid analogs in immunosuppression would seem to warrant investigation.

Most anticancer compounds are known now to be immunosuppressants also, and it has been only an accident of priorities that they have been considered anticancer drugs rather than immunosuppressants (SCHWARTZ, 1968)[7]. The unfortunate situation here is that immunosuppression often favors tumor progression (cf. REIS, 1971), so that many of the present day anticancer drugs might be said to be self-defeating because of their dual role as immunosuppressants (SCHWARTZ, 1968). On the other hand, the use of drugs having the capacity to destroy cells, impede their replication, or perhaps irreversibly bind to a specific key enzyme — as might be true for cytotoxic amino acids — is certainly sound logic in attacks against either neoplasia or the immune response. There is, therefore, little basis according to WATSON and JOHNSON (1969) for questioning the use of either cytotoxic or immunosuppressive drugs for these purposes.

Interference with antibody synthesis by amino acid analogs is not predicated on depletion of amino acids necessary for gamma-globulin synthesis. At this level of humoral antibody response, relatively small quantities of amino acids are required for these syntheses, and these can likely be obtained even in an undernourished animal from breakdown of labile liver and muscle protein (cf. CANNON, 1945). Of course, a cytotoxic amino acid substance conceivably might specifically inhibit production of globulin protein or its transport across cell membranes, but no such substance is known. Presumably, the best possibility then is an effective amino acid analog that interferes with the immune response at a point before the buildup of antibody-producing cells. There have been several observations in this regard.

Evidence for acute suppression of antibody formation in adult male albino rats by 3-thiophenealanine was reported 15 years ago by WISSLER et al. (1956). This

7 Not every antitumor compound, however, has been found to be immunosuppressive; uracil mustard did not inhibit antibody synthesis in the rat when given in doses sufficient to inhibit growth of Walker 256 tumor (BUSKIRK et al., 1965). The polysaccharide, statolon, is reported to stimulate the immune system, and it also exhibits antileukemia activity (cf. *Chem. Eng. News*, Nov. 15, 1971, p. 79).

observation was made in the course of a comprehensive study of the influence of this antimetabolite on body weight, nitrogen balance, the synthesis of specific antibody globulin, and neoplastic growth within a few days after its addition to the diet. Rations were given by stomach tube twice daily, about 12 hours apart. Antibody determinations were made by use of the hemolysin method of Cannon et al. (1944). Under the experimental conditions employed, neither a protein-free ration nor fasting had much effect on antibody formation compared with that in rats fed a control (and maintenance) diet. In three separate experiments, however, diets supplemented with 25 to 100 mg per rat of 3-thiophenealanine consistently caused pronounced depression of anti-sheep erythrocyte hemolysins, particularly at 4 days after antigen injection. The effect was abolished when additional phenylalanine was added to the diet, and in antagonist-free diets variation of the level of phenylalanine had no definite effect on humoral antibody concentration under the conditions employed. The conclusion was that metabolite-antimetabolite competition was the contributory factor in the lessened antibody response, and this was borne out in an additional experiment. Tissues were removed from the animals for histological examination 4 days after antigen injection. Whereas the antimetabolite produced no appreciable effect on the histology of the bone marrow, lymph nodes, testis, gastrointestinal tract, or the Malpighian corpuscles of the spleen, it did cause a marked depression of pyroninophilic cell response in the red pulp of the spleen. This organ is apparently responsible in the rat for most of the subsequent antibody formation in response to a single intravenous injection of particulate antigen. Why cellular proliferation was decreased in the spleen but not in some of the other tissues, such as the gastrointestinal tract, was not evident.

In view of this interesting study by Wissler et al. (1956), the immunosuppressive property of 3-thiophenealanine was also investigated by La Via et al. (1960). Again, the compound was found to inhibit antibody response in rats; however, when the antimetabolite was added to an antibody-synthesizing tissue culture system it gave no inhibition of antibody synthesis.

Thus, it appeared that the analog was effective in inhibiting precursor cell production of the antibody-forming mechanism, but was not demonstratively effective in inhibiting the production of humoral antibody *per se*.

Another amino acid analog was found recently to have immunosuppressive effects apparently similar to those observed for 3-thiophenealanine. When ACPC was given to mice 3 days before the administration of sheep erythrocytes, it prevented the synthesis of hemagglutinins and hemolysins by reducing the number of plaque-forming cells in the splenic pulp (Frisch, 1969). However, the analog did not inhibit secondary antibody response, nor did it increase graft survival. Immunosuppressive properties of ACPC were reported by Rosenthale and Gluckman (1968) who observed that it could suppress experimental allergic encephalomyelitis in animals in a dose-related manner. Their results indicated that ACPC acts by inhibiting the proliferation of immunologically active cellular lymphoid elements.

There has been considerable interest in recent years in the antitumor properties of L-asparaginase (cf. Chapter 68). Being protein, this substance is immunogenic, but because of its enzymatic activity it is also potentially immunosuppressive. For example, Astaldi et al. (1969) have shown that L-asparaginase could intensively inhibit blastic transformation of human peripheral lymphocytes exposed to phytohemagglutinin *in vitro*. This was also found to be evident in experiments by Miura et al. (1970b) who found that the L-asparagine analog, L-β-aspartohydroxamic acid exerted a similar effect. It was concluded that interference with the blastic transformation in both cases was due to an amino acid depletion (L-asparagine) effect. Suppression of blastogenesis by the glutamine antagonist, azotomycin, was observed recently by HERSH and BROWN (1971).

An interesting study of the effect of six amino acid analogs on the survival of scale homografts in fish *(Fundulus heteroclitus)* was done by Goss (1961). After grafting, circulation in the substitute scales was re-established the next day, and in control fish, foreign melanophore breakdown was invariably complete on the third day. The reliability of this sequence was such that the survival of pigment cells only one day beyond this time was said to constitute an unequivocal and statistically significant indication of the efficacy of the treatment being used. The amino acid analogs used were β-2-thienylserine, DL-β-phenylserine, DL-α-methylphenylalanine, β-2-thienylalanine, DL-β-phenyllactic acid, and ethionine. In general, all of these proved to be rather toxic and not very effective in protecting the foreign scale grafts from destruction by the host. Ethionine was the best of the six, prolonging graft survival by 1 to 2 days but at toxic levels of either 1 or 3.3 mg per fish per day. An apparently nonlethal dose of 5 mg per fish per day of β-2-thienylalanine also prolonged graft survival by 1 day. For comparative purposes, immunosuppressants such as 6-mercaptopurine and 5-fluorodeoxyuridine at doses of 2 mg per fish per day caused prolongations of 2 to 5 days.

One of the host reactions to challenge by certain antigens is an increase in proteolytic activity of the serum (e.g., MCKAY and SHAPIRO, 1958). Enzymes such as cathepsin or chymotrypsin are implicated in the rise of tissue proteases that occurs during anaphylaxis and anaphylactoid conditions (UNGAR et al., 1961). A position isomer of norleucine, ε-aminocaproic acid (EACA), has been found to be a potent suppressor of the chymotrypsin-type proteolytic enzymes (ABLONDI et al., 1959) and an inhibitor of certain hypersensitivity reactions (ZWEIFACH et al., 1962). Subsequently, this compound has received much attention as an agent which suppresses homograft rejection, complement fixation, and immunity to tumor transplantation (e.g., GILLETTE et al., 1963; TAYLOR and FUDENBERG, 1964; BONMASSAR et al., 1968). While EACA is not an amino acid analog in the usual sense of the term, it is interesting that in a study of inhibition of the C'_1 component of complement by amino acids (TAYLOR and FUDENBERG, 1964), norleucine, β-alanine, ω-aminocaprylic acid, and valeric acid were ineffective compared with EACA. Therefore, the length of the chain and the presence and position of the amino group were structural features relative to the anticomplementary effect.

Work by LINN and GOLLAN (1966) indicated that a regime of nontoxic doses of EACA and prednisolone had value in prolongation of survival of renal allografts in greyhound dogs. However, insofar as clinical use of EACA is concerned, ROWINSKI and HAGER (1966) and SMOLIN and KEATES (1967) concluded that its use in graft reactions would seem to be impractical for several reasons, including the probability of large required dosages and toxic effects.

Like EACA, another compound which has been shown to allow growth of transplanted tumors in immunized animals is *N*-diazoacetylglycine (BRAMBILLA et al., 1970). This substance was first found to have antitumor activity (BALDINI and BRAMBILLA, 1966), and in subsequent work it prolonged median survival time of skin grafts in mice as effectively as azathioprine and methotrexate. Skin grafting has been accompanied by significant increases in histamine excretion. The possibility, therefore, that histamine formation from histidine decarboxylase activity might be involved in the mechanics of homograft rejection led MOORE (1967) to test the effect of histidine decarboxylase inhibitors on rat skin homograft survival. The amino acid analog, 2-hydrazino-3(4-imidazolyl)propionic acid (α-hydrazinohistidine), more than doubled graft survival, and appeared to be more effective than 4-bromo-3-hydroxybenzyloxyamine, a compound which has been used in humans to lower histamine levels (LEVIN, 1966).

Amino acid analogs have been found to be of some value as anti-inflammatory agents. NAGAI (1969) has shown that 4-amino-3-hydroxybutyric acid, a position isomer of homoserine and an ω-amino acid like EACA, has pronounced anti-inflammatory activity both experimentally in rats and clinically in humans. Substituted lysine esters, such as N^6-benzyloxycarbonyllysine methyl ester, are considered useful (GEIGY, 1969) for treatment of inflammatory and allergic diseases.

Immunosuppression by such agents as sarcolysine and folate antagonists, compounds which contain an amino acid moiety but are not classified specifically as amino acid analogs, is well known (e.g., BERTINO et al., 1967; BONMASSAR et al., 1968a, b).

These studies re-emphasize the dual role of many cytotoxic agents, i.e., they are deleterious both to tumor growth and to the immune response.

Future Considerations

Underlying much of the rationale for investigating amino acid analogs as antitumor agents is the hypothesis that tumors may be more dependent than other tissues on exogenous amino acid supply (e.g., WISEMAN and GHADIALLY, 1958; DEBARBIERI et al., 1970), and the fact that protein synthesis is an essential preliminary event before DNA replication can begin (e.g., MAALØE and HANAWALT, 1961). Fundamentally, cancer is a problem of uncontrolled growth, and inhibition of growth by curtailing nutrient supplies has for many years been an obvious and popular approach, as exemplified in the dietary experiments early in modern cancer research by TANNENBAUM and colleagues (cf. TANNENBAUM, 1947). Because DNA synthesis is dependent upon prior protein synthesis, it depends on the availability of an adequate supply of amino acids. Logically, suppression of amino acid supply coupled with one or more types of specific amino acid and/or nucleic acid antagonism should favor the host rather than the tumor.

In a study of the effect of amino acid deficiencies on experimental cancer chemotherapy, SKIPPER and THOMSON (1958) found that the antitumor activity of certain analogs such as azaserine or DON was significantly increased by maintenance of the tumor-bearing host on diets deficient in certain amino acids. An especially interesting result in the comprehensive study by these investigators was that the most pronounced tumor inhibition occurred when mice were held on a diet deficient in isoleucine. Subsequently, Walker tumor growth was found to be retarded in rats maintained on diets deficient in isoleucine (SUGIMURA et al., 1959), and treatment of chickens with MAREK'S disease by an isoleucine antagonist resulted in a decreased incidence of mortality (SHIGUERA et al., 1969). A possible explanation of these antitumor effects of isoleucine depletion was given recently in a series of interesting papers (cf., TOBEY and LEY, 1970, 1971; LEY and TOBEY, 1970). These suggest an isoleucine-mediation of genome replication in mammalian cells. If so, exploitation of this phenomenon in the chemotherapy of neoplasia might involve one or more of the following possibilities: (a) reduction in amount of available isoleucine could retard tumor growth as indicated in several studies cited previously, (b) if the numbers of neoplastic cells traversing the cell cycle could be increased by elevating the level of isoleucine, radiotherapy, or chemotherapy might be potentiated (TOBEY and LEY, 1971), or (c) combination of isoleucine restriction and metabolic antagonists other than azaserine or DON (SKIPPER and THOMSON, 1958) might potentiate inhibition of tumor growth. Regarding (c) it is of interest to recall that the combination of phenylalanine restriction and antagonism (4-fluorophenylalanine) had a marked effect on tumor growth (RYAN and ELLIOTT, 1968).

Amino acid supplementation or restriction to control malignancy has been used in several other recent studies, for example, in childhood leukemia (ALLAN et al., 1965), in several other types of human malignancies (LORINCZ and KUTTNER, 1966), in melanoma in mice (DEMOPOULOUS, 1966a), in Burkitt's lymphoblasts *in vitro* (WEINBERG and BECKER, 1970), in adenocarcinoma in mice (THEUER, 1971), and most prominently in the treatment of leukemia in humans and animals with L-asparaginase (cf. Chapters 68 and 69). OHNUMA et al. (1971) suggest on the basis of *in vitro* studies with leukemic cells that depression of cysteine, glutamine, histidine, or tyrosine by means of an enzyme or amino acid analog could be explored as a chemotherapeutic approach with reasonable basis to anticipate success in some acute leukemias. It is conceivable, too, that amino acid restriction and drug therapy can be made more efficacious by dose schedules correlated with circadian periodicity of blood amino acids (e.g., FEIGIN et al., 1967).

From a number of unrelated studies, it is clear that several amino acid analogs function as inhibitors of certain pyridoxal phosphate-dependent enzymes. Included among these are 2-aminoxy-3-phenylpropionic acid (BONOMI and TENCONI, 1964), 2-hydrazino-3(4-imidazolyl) propionic acid (SHIFRIN et al., 1966), β-*N*-(3-hydroxy-4-pyridone)alanine (FOWDEN et al., 1967), and perhaps canaline (WHITE et al., 1963). Other reports show that amino acid analogs which are potent inhibitors of specific enzymes, such as *p*-chlorophenylalanine inhibition of tryptophan hydroxylase and α-methyltyrosine inhibition of tyrosine hydroxylase, have pronounced antitumor effects.

One must conclude from all of these developments that manipulation of amino acid supply by amino acid restrictions, imbalances, and/or antagonists can be of substantial benefit in the management of neoplasia. As more knowledge is obtained concerning the nature of the reactions to be inhibited and the type of control essential for effective treatment of particular diseases, the role of cytotoxic amino acids is likely to be enhanced in the future, with respect to both neoplasia and immunocompetence.

References

ABARTIENE, D.: Changes in blood glutathione levels after the administration of alkylating agents. Nauji laimejimai Biol. Biochem., Liet TSR Jaunuju Mokslininku-Biol. Biochem. Moksline Konf. 1967, 351—354. Chem. Abstr. **72**, 2030v (1970).

ABE, M., CHIBATA, I., HIROKAWA, H., KAMEDA, Y., MIZUNO, D.: Antitumor effect of amino acid analogs. Yakugaku Zasshi **80**, 1309—1311 (1960). Chem. Abstr. **55**, 2900h (1961).

ABLONDI, F. B., HAGEN, J. J., PHILLIPS, M., DERENZO, E. C.: Inhibition of plasmin, trypsin, and the streptokinase-activated fibrinolytic system by ε-aminocaproic acid. Arch. Biochem. Biophys. **82**, 153—160 (1959).

ABSHIRE, C. J.: A study of the toxicity of several cyclopentylamino acid analogs. J. med. Chem. **11**, 598—599 (1968).

ALLAN, J. D., IRELAND, J. T., MILNER, J., MOSS, A. D.: Treatment of leukaemia by amino acid imbalance. Lancet I, 302—303 (1965).

APOSHIAN, H. V., BLAIR, R. M., MORRIS, M., SMITHSON, C. H.: The reversal of the inhibitory activity of L-penicillamine by branched chain amino acids. Biochim. biophys. Acta **36**, 93—101 (1959).

ARDEN, G. M., GRANT, D. J. W., PARTRIDGE, M. W.: Action of tumour inhibitory pyrazolotriazines on *Klebsiella aerogenes*. I. Inhibition by 3,4-dimethylpyrazolo(3,2-*c*)-as-triazine and its antagonism by histidine. Biochem. Pharmacol. **19**, 57—69 (1970).

ASTALDI, C., BURGIO, G. R., KRČ, J., GENOVA, R., ASTALDI, A. A.: L-Asparaginase and blastogenesis. Lancet I, 423 (1969).

BALDINI, L., BRAMBILLA, G.: Antineoplastic activity of diazoacetylglycine derivatives. Cancer Res. **26**, 1754—1758 (1966a).

BALDINI, L., BRAMBILLA, G.: Antineoplastic activity of 5-fluorouracil in association with two diazoacetyl derivatives of glycine. Arch. Ital. Sci. Farmacol. **15**, 31—32 (1965). Chem. Abstr. **66**, 9735b (1967).

BALDINI, L., BRAMBILLA, G.: Amino acid and peptide diazoderivatives as possible antitumor agents. X. Experimental antineoplastic activity of N-diazoacetyl-DL-alanine ethyl ester and of *N*-diazoacetyl-DL-alanine hydrazide. Boll. Soc. Ital. Biol. Sper. **42**, 1669—1672 (1966b); — Chem. Abstr. **67**, 10115p (1967).

BALDWIN, R. W., PARTRIDGE, M. W., STEVENS, M. F. G.: Pyrazolotriazines; a new class of tumor-inhibitory agents. J. pharm. Pharmacol. suppl. **18**, 1—4 (1966).

BERECZ, A., GODIN, C.: The incorporation of tryptophan analogues into rat plasma proteins. Can. J. biochem. Physiol. **40**, 153—157 (1962).

BERENBAUM, M. C.: The complications of immunosuppression. Proc. roy. Soc. Med. **63**, 23—26 (1970).

BERTINO, J. R., HILLCOAT, B. L., JOHNS, D. G.: Folate antagonists: some biochemical and pharmacological considerations. Fed. Proc. **26**, 893—897 (1967).

BLONDAL, H., LEVI, I., LATOUR, J. P. A., FRASER, W. D.: Antitumor effect of *N*-dichloroacetyl-DL-serine (FT-9045). Radiology **76**, 945—960 (1961). Chem. Abstr. **55**, 20181f (1961).

BONMASSAR, E., CASTAGNONE, D., CELI, M. L., MELAN, F.: Interference of immunologic factors on the antitumor activity of sarcolysin. Arch. Ital. Pathol. Clin. Tumori **11**, 215—228 (1968b); — Biol. Abst. **50**, No. 31035 (1969).

BONMASSAR, E., CELI, M. L., MELAN, F., TESTORELLI, C.: Influence of epsilon-amino-caproic acid on the takes of tumor cells in immunized mice. Arch. Ital. Pathol. Clin. Tumori **11**, 187—194 (1968); — Biol. Abstr. **50**, No. 31036 (1969).

BONMASSAR, E., MELAN, F., TESTORELLI, C.: Sensitivity to sarcolysin of Ehrlich ascites tumors in mice "vaccinated" with tumor cells obtained from animals treated with sarcolysin or other antitumor drugs (thioguanine, actinomycin D). Arch. Ital. Pathol. **11**, 229—234 (1968a); — Biol. Abstr. **50**, No. 31037 (1969).

BONOMI, U., TENCONI, L. T.: Activity of aminoxy and hydroxylamino analogs of phenylalanine and glycine in some pyridoxal phosphate-dependent enzymic reactions. Acta Vitaminol. **18**, 7—12 (1964); — Chem. Abstr. **61**, 8785 (1964).

BRAMBILLA, G., PARODI, S., CAVANNA, M., BALDINI, L.: The immunodepressive activity of *N*-diazoacetylglycine amide in some transplantation systems. Transplantation **10**, 100—105 (1970).

BRISTOW, E. C., WISSLER, R. W.: Acute effects of β-3-thienylalanine on neoplastic growth in the male albino rat. Lab. Invest. **10**, 31—38 (1961).

BRITTEN, R. J., ROBERTS, R. B., FRENCH, E. F.: Amino acid adsorption and protein synthesis in *Escherichia coli*. Proc. nat. Acad. Sci. (Wash.) **41**, 863—870 (1955).

BROWN, R. R.: Aminoaciduria resulting from cycloleucine administration in man. Science **157**, 432—434 (1967).

BUSKIRK, H. H., CRIM, J. A., PETERING, H. G., MERRITT, K., JOHNSON, A. G.: Effect of uracil mustard and several antitumor drugs on the primary antibody response in rats and mice. J. nat. Cancer Inst. **34**, 747—758 (1965).

CANNON, P. R.: Relationship of protein metabolism to antibody production and resistance to infection. Advanc. Protein Chem. **2**, 135 (1945).

CANNON, P. R., WISSLER, R. W., WOOLRIDGE, R. L., BENDITT, E. P.: Relationship of protein deficiency to surgical infection. Ann. Surg. **120**, 514—524 (1944).

CESTARI, A., CONCILIO, C., DESSI, P., RIZZOLI, C.: A study of the action of methionine homologues at cellular level and in the systems of organized growth. Proc. First Intern. Pharmacol. Meeting **5**, 233—245 (1963).

CHRISTENSEN, H. N., JONES, J. C.: Amino acid transport models: renal resorption and resistance to metabolic attack. J. biol. Chem. **237**, 1203—1206 (1962).

COFFEY, J. J., PALM, P. E., DENINE, E. P., BARONOWSKY, P. E., KENSLER, C. J.: Species differences in the physiological disposition of 3-tritylthio-L-alanine (NSC 83265). Cancer Res. **31**, 1908—1914 (1971).

CONNORS, T. A., ELSON, L. A., HADDOW, A., ROSS, W. C. J.: The pharmacology and tumour growth inhibitory activity of 1-aminocyclopentane-1-carboxylic acid and related compounds. Biochem. Pharmacol. **5**, 108—129 (1960).

COONEY, D. A., CAPIZZI, R. L., HANDSCHUMACHER, R. E.: Evaluation of L-asparagine metabolism in animals and man. Cancer Res. **30**, 929—935 (1970).

CUTTS, J. H.: Effects of other agents on the biologic responses to vincaleukoblastine. Biochem. Pharmacol. **13**, 421—431 (1964).

DAMARACKIS, B.: Toxicity and anticancer properties of dichloropropylaminophenylacetic acid derivatives of phenylalanine and methionine. Onkol. Inst. Darbai Lietovos TSR **2**, 29—41 (1961). Chem. Abstr. **59**, 15798 (1963).

DAVIS, A. L., SKINNER, C. G., SHIVE, W.: 3-Aminomethylcyclohexaneglycine, a lysine analog. Arch. Biochem. Biophys. **87**, 88—92 (1960).
DAVIS, A. L., SKINNER, C. G., SHIVE, W.: The conformation of lysine on its site of biological utilization. J. Amer. chem. Soc. **83**, 2279 (1961).
DE BARBIERI, A., DI VITTORIO, P., MAUGERI, M., MISTRETTA, A. P., PERRONE, F., TASSI, G. C., TEMELCOU, O., ZAPELLI, P.: Investigations with synthetic antitumor peptides. Progr. Antimicrobial Anticancer Chemother. **2**, 146—152 (1970).
DE GROOT, N., LICHTENSTEIN, N.: The action of mammalian liver enzyme preparations on asparagine and asparagine derivatives. Biochim. biophys. Acta **40**, 92—98 (1960).
DEMOPOULOS, H. B.: Effects of low phenylalanine-tyrosine diets on S-91 mouse melanomas. J. nat. Cancer Inst. **37**, 185—190 (1966a).
DEMOPOULOS, H. B.: Effects of reducing the phenylalanine-tyrosine intake of patients with advanced malignant melanoma. Cancer **19**, 657—664 (1966b).
DITTMER, K.: The structural bases of some amino acid antagonists and their microbiological properties. Ann. N. Y. Acad. Sci. **52**, 1274—1301 (1950).
DONGOROZI, C. S.: Propos sur une nouvelle moutarde azotée. Experientia **16**, 351—352 (1960).
DUKE, P. S., DEMOPOULOS, H. B.: *In vivo* necrosis of large S-91 mouse melanomas by DL-β-phenyllactic acid plus L-cysteine. Life Sci. **6**, 951—957 (1967).
DUKE, P. S., YUEN, T. G. H., DEMOPOULOS, H. B.: *In vitro* growth inhibition of S-91 mouse melanomas by tyrosinase substrate analogs with and without L-cysteine. Cancer Res. **27**, 1783—1787 (1967).
DYM, H., BECKER, Y.: Effect of *p*-fluorophenylalanine on the replication of herpes simplex virus. Israel J. med. Sci. **5**, 1083—1086 (1969).
EDELSON, J., FISSEKIS, J. D., SKINNER, C. G., SHIVE, W.: 3-Cyclohexene-1-glycine, an isoleucine antagonist. J. Amer. chem. Soc. **80**, 2698—2700 (1958).
EDELSON, J., SKINNER, C. G., RAVEL, J. M., SHIVE, W.: 3-Cyclohexene-1-DL-alanine, an analog of leucine. Arch. Biochem. Biophys. **80**, 416—420 (1959).
EISENSTADT, J. M., GROSSMAN, L., KLEIN, H. P.: Inhibition of protein synthesis by D-aspartate and a possible site of its action. Biochim. biophys. Acta (Amst.) **36**, 292—294 (1959).
ELY, J. O., BATT, W. G.: The effect of ethionine on tumor growth, content and composition of fat of livers and tumor cells, and glycogen content of liver. J. Franklin Inst. **260**, 424—428 (1955).
FALKSON, G., FALKSON, H. C.: DL-Serine *bis*(2-chloropropyl)carbamate ester (CB-3210; NSC-37023) for treatment of cancer patients — preliminary results. Cancer Chemother. Rep. **49**, 31—46 (1965).
FARBER, E.: Carcinoma of the liver in rats fed ethionine. Arch. Pathol. **62**, 445—453 (1956).
FARBER, S., DIAMOND, L. K., MERCER, R. D., SYLVESTER, R. F., JR., WOLFF, J. A.: Temporary remissions in acute leukemia in children produced by folic acid antagonist, 4-aminopteroylglutamic acid (aminopterin). New Engl. J. Med. **238**, 787—793 (1948).
FEHER, I., DOKLEN, A., SELMECI, V.: Effect of amino acid esters on the growth of fibroblast cultures. Nature (Lond.) **191**, 494—495 (1961).
FEIGIN, R. D., KLAINER, A. S., BEISEL, W. R.: Circadian periodicity of blood amino-acids in adult men. Nature (Lond.) **215**, 512—514 (1967).
FISHBEIN, W. N., CARBONE, P. P., OWENS, A. H., JR., KELLY, M. G., RALL, D. P., TARR, N.: Preliminary studies with 5-*bis*(2-chloroethyl)amino-DL-tryptophan (NSC-62403) in animals and man. Cancer Chemother. Rep. **42**, 19—24 (1964).
FISHMAN, W. H., SIE, H.: L-Homoarginine; an inhibitor of serum "bone and liver" alkaline phosphatase. Clin. chim. Acta **29**, 339—341 (1970).
FOWDEN, L., LEWIS, D., TRISTRAM, H.: Toxic amino acids: their action as antimetabolites. Advanc. Enzymol. **29**, 89—163 (1967).
FRIEDMAN, O. M., RUTENBURG, A. M.: Possible usefulness of substituted amino acids for tumor growth inhibition. Proc. Soc. exp. Biol. (N. Y.) **74**, 764—766 (1950).
FRISCH, A. W.: Inhibition of antibody synthesis by cycloleucine. Biochem. Pharmacol. **18**, 256—260 (1969).
GALEGOV, G. A.: Metabolism of β-methylaspartic acid. Vopr. Med. Khim. **9**, 339—351 (1963). Chem. Abstr. **60**, 1955b (1964).
GALEGOV, G. A., BENYUMOVICH, M. S.: The inhibiting action of D,L-hexafluorvaline on the growth of HeLa cells. Dokl. Akad. Nauk SSSR **163**, 1484—1486 (1965).
GEIGY, J. R.: Substituted lysine esters for treating inflammatory and allergic diseases. Brit. Patent 1, 143, 186; Chem. Abstr. **70**, 106873 (1969).
GILLETTE, R. W., FINDLEY, A., CONWAY, H.: Prolonged survival of homografts in mice treated with EACA. Transplantation **1**, 116—117 (1963).
GOLD, J.: Proposed treatment of cancer by inhibition of gluconeogenesis. Oncology **22**, 185—207 (1968).

GOLD, J.: Inhibition of Walker 256 intramuscular carcinoma in rats by administration of L-tryptophan. Oncology **24**, 291—303 (1970).
GOSS, R. J.: Metabolic antagonists and prolonged survival of scale homografts in *Fundulus heteroclitus*. Biol. Bull. **121**, 162—172 (1961).
GRAHAME-SMITH, D. G.: Tryptophan hydroxylation in carcinoid tumors. Biochim. biophys. Acta **86**, 176—179 (1964).
GREER, M., ANTON, A. H., WILLIAMS, C. M.: Failure of enzyme inhibition therapy for malignant melanoma. Trans. Amer. Neurol. Ass. **94**, 273—275 (1969). Chem. Abstr. **73**, 2590 (1970).
GREGORY, F. J., FLINT, S. F., RUELIUS, H. W., WARREN, G. H.: Reversal of antileukemic action and toxicity of 1-aminocyclopentanecarboxylic acid in mice by L-valine. Cancer Res. **29**, 728—729 (1969).
GUALANDI, G., BERGAMINI, A.: Ethionine in the treatment of pancreatic carcinoma. Arch. maladies app. digest. et maladies nutrition **43**, 305—310 (1954). Excerpta Med. **9**, Sect. VI, 233 (1955).
GUROFF, G.: Irreversible *in vivo* inhibition of rat liver phenylalanine hydroxylase by *p*-chlorophenylalanine. Arch. Biochem. **134**, 610—611 (1969).
HALEY, E. E., FISCHER, G. A., WELCH, A. D.: The requirement for L-asparagine of mouse leukemia cells L5178Y in culture. Cancer Res. **21**, 532—536 (1961).
HALPERN, Y. S., GROSSOWICZ, N.: Hydrolysis of amides by extracts from mycobacteria. Biochem. J. **65**, 716—720 (1957).
HALVORSON, H. O., SPIEGELMAN, S.: The inhibition of enzyme formation by amino acid analogues. J. Bact. **64**, 207—221 (1952).
HANDSCHUMACHER, R. E., BATES, C. J., CHANG, P. K., ANDREWS, A. T., FISCHER, G. A.: 5-Diazo-4-oxo-L-norvaline: reactive asparagine analog with biological specificity. Science **161**, 62—63 (1968).
HASKELL, C. M., CANELLOS, G. P.: Asparagine biosynthesis in human KB tumor cells: inhibitor studies with asparagine and glutamine antagonists. Cancer Res. **30**, 1081—1083 (1970).
HEMPEL, K., LANGE, H. W., BIRKOFER, L.: ε-*N*-Trimethyllysin, eine neue Aminosäure in Histonen. Naturwissenschaften **55**, 37 (1968).
HERSH, E. M., BROWN, B. W.: Inhibition of immune responses by glutamine antagonism: effect of azotomycin on lymphocyte blastogenesis. Cancer Res. **31**, 834—840 (1971).
HEYMANN, H., GINSBERG, T., GULICK, Z. R., KONOPKA, E. A., MAYER, R. L.: The preparation and some biological properties of the asparagine analog L-2-amino-2-carboxyethanesulfonamide. J. Amer. chem. Soc. **81**, 5125—5128 (1959).
HIDVEGI, E. J., ARKY, J., ANTONI, F., KOTELESS, G. J., BALLWEG, H.: Effects of kinetin analogues on the nucleic acid metabolism of ascites tumour cells. Acta Unio Intern. Contra Cancrum **20**, 1037—1040 (1964).
HIREMATH, C. B., OLSON, G., ROSENBLUM, C.: Incorporation of L-*O*-ethylthreonine into chick muscle protein. Biochemistry **10**, 1096—1100 (1971).
HOURANI, B. T., DEMOPOULOS, H. B.: Inhibition of S-91 mouse melanoma metastases and growth by D-penicillamine. Lab. Invest. **21**, 434—438 (1969).
HRUBAN, Z., WISSLER, R. W.: Effect of β-3-thienylalanine and deoxypyridoxine on the growth of the Murphy-Sturm lymphosarcoma. Cancer Res. **20**, 1530—1537 (1960).
HRUBAN, Z., WISSLER, R. W., SLESERS, A.: Effects of β-3-thienylalanine and deoxypyridoxine on tumor growth. II. Effects on the tumor-bearing host. Lab. Invest. **11**, 382—394 (1962).
JACKSON, R. C., HANDSCHUMACHER, R. E.: *Escherichia coli* L-asparaginase. Catalytic activity and subunit nature. Biochemistry **9**, 3385—3590 (1970).
JACQUEZ, J. A., BARCLAY, R. K., STOCK, C. C.: Transamination in the metabolism of β-2-thienyl-DL-alanine in normal and neoplastic cells *in vitro*. J. exp. Med. **96**, 499—512 (1952).
JACQUEZ, J. A., MOTTRAM, F.: Tissue culture screening of amino acid analogs for selective damage to mouse sarcoma cells. Cancer Res. **13**, 605—609 (1953).
JACQUEZ, J. A., STOCK, C. C., BARCLAY, R. K.: Effect of β-2-thienyl-DL-alanine on the growth of sarcoma T241 in C57 black mice. Cancer **6**, 828—836 (1953).
JONES, N. F., WALKER, G., RUTHVEN, C. R. J., SANDLER, M.: α-Methyl-*p*-tyrosine in the management of phaeochromocytoma. Lancet **II**, 1105—1109 (1968).
JORGENSEN, E. C., WILEY, R. A.: Methyl-substituted tyrosines and related compounds as potential anticancer agents. J. pharm. Sci. **52**, 122—125 (1963).
KAKIMOTO, Y., AKAZAWA, S.: Isolation and identification of N^G, N^G- and N^G, N'^G-dimethylarginine, N^ε-mono, di-, and trimethyllysine, and glucosylgalactosyl- and galactosyl-δ hydroxylysine from human urine. J. biol. Chem. **245**, 5751—5758 (1970).
KARNOFSKY, D. A., CLIFFORD, G. O.: Selection of anticancer drugs for inclusion in Memorial Hospital formulary. Med. Clin. N. Amer. **50**, 857—868 (1966).
KEKOMÄKI, M., RAHIALA, E. L., RÄIHÄ, N. C. R.: Canaline: interfering with ornithine metabolism in the isolated perfused rat liver. Ann. med. exp. biol. Fenniae (HELSINKI) **47**, 33—38 (1969).

KEBLAS, S.: Comparative evaluation of the antitumor activity of derivatives of *p-bis*(2-chloroethyl)aminophenylacetic acid with certain α-amino acids. Vopr. Protivorak. Bor'by, Vilnyus, Sb. **1964**, 181—182. Chem. Abstr. **64**, 1231 (1966).

KLOPOTOWSKI, T., WIATER, A.: Synergism of aminotriazole and phosphate on the inhibition of yeast imidazole glycerol phosphate dehydratase. Arch. Biochem. Biophys. **112**, 562—566 (1965).

KOE, B.K., WEISSMAN, A.: *p*-Chlorophenylalanine: a specific depletion of brain serotonin. J. pharmacol. Exp. Ther. **154**, 499—516 (1966).

KOLC, J.: Amino acids and peptides. LXXXIX. Synthesis of L-4-azalysine, D-4-azalysine, and L-4-azalysine-6-^{14}C. Collect. Czech. Chem. Commun. **34**, 630—634 (1969). Chem. Abstr. **70**, 78350 (1969).

KRAKOFF, I.H.: The present status of cancer chemotherapy. Med. Clin. N. Amer. **55**, 683—701 (1971).

KRANT, M.J., ISZARD, D.M., ABADI, A., CAREY, R.W.: Treatment of multiple myeloma with 1-aminocyclopentanecarboxylic acid (NSC-1026). Cancer Chemother. Rep. **22**, 59—64 (1962).

KRUSE, P.F., JR., MCCOY, T.A.: The competitive effect of canavanine on utilization of arginine in growth of Walker carcinosarcoma 256 cells *in vitro*. Cancer Res. **18**, 279—282 (1958).

KRUSE, P.F., JR., MIEDEMA, E., CARTER, H.A.: Amino acid utilizations and protein synthesis at various proliferation rates, population densities, and protein contents of perfused animal cell and tissue cultures. Biochemistry **6**, 949—955 (1967).

KRUSE, P.F., JR., WHITE, P.B., CARTER, H.A., MCCOY, T.A.: Incorporation of canavanine into protein of Walker carcinosarcoma 256 cells cultured *in vitro*. Cancer Res. **19**, 122—125 (1959).

KUNG, F., NYHAN, W.L., ROSNER, F., CORTNER, J.A., CUTTNER, J., MOON, J.H., HOLLAND, J.F.: Tryptophan mustard (NSC-62403) in the treatment of acute leukemia and malignant solid tumors in children. Cancer Chemother. Rep. **52**, 445—450 (1968).

LALLIER, R.: Effects of L-asparaginase and of an analog of asparagine, L-2-amino-2-carboxyethanesulfonamide, on the development of the sea urchin egg. Life Sci. **7**, 801—804 (1968).

LAMPERT, F., NYHAN, W.L.: Effects of tryptophan mustard on incorporation of amino acids into proteins in tumor-bearing rats. J. Nat. Cancer Inst. **36**, 63—70 (1966).

LARIONOV, L.F., SPASSKAYA, I.G.: Anticancer activity of *N,N-bis*(β-chloroethyl) derivatives of lysine (lysepsin). Vopr. Onkol. **7**, 75—79 (1961). Chem. Abstr. **56**, 13512d (1962).

LA VIA, M.F., URIU, S.A., BARBER, N.D., WARREN, A.E.: Effect of β-3-thienylalanine on antibody synthesis. I. Preliminary *in vitro* and *in vivo* studies. Proc. Soc. exp. Biol. (N.Y.) **104**, 562—565 (1960).

LEVI, I., BLONDAL, H., LOZINSKI, E.: Serine derivative with antitumor activity. Science **131**, 666 (1960).

LEVIN, A.P., HARTMAN, P.E.: Action of a histidine analog, 1,2,4-triazole-3-alanine, in *Salmonella typhimurium*. J. Bacteriol. **86**, 820—828 (1963).

LEVIN, R.J.: Histamine synthesis in man: inhibition by 4-bromo-3-hydroxybenzyloxyamine. Science **154**, 1017—1019 (1966).

LEVINE, M., TARVER, H.: Studies on ethionine. III. Incorporation of ethionine into rat proteins. J. biol. Chem. **192**, 835—850 (1951).

LEVINTOW, L., THOREN, M.M., DARNELL, J.E., HOOPER, J.L.: Effect of *p*-fluorophenylalanine and puromycin on the replication of polio virus. Virology **16**, 220—229 (1962).

LEVY, H.M., MONTANEZ, G., MURPHEY, E.A., DUNN, M.S.: Effect of ethionine on tumor growth and liver amino acids in rats. Cancer Res. **13**, 507—512 (1953).

LEY, K.D., TOBEY, R.A.: Regulation of initiation of DNA synthesis in Chinese hamster cells. II. Induction of DNA synthesis and cell division by isoleucine and glutamine in G_1-arrested cells in suspension culture. J. Cell Biol. **47**, 453—459 (1970).

LINDENAUER, S.M., DOW, R.W., KOWALCZYK, R.S.: Distribution of 1-aminocyclopentanecarboxylic acid in the Rhesus monkey. J. surg. Res. **10**, 189—192 (1970).

LINN, B.S., GOLLAN, F.: Safer immunosuppression with epsilon-aminocaproic acid and prednisolone. Surg. Forum **17**, 254—255 (1966).

LITTMAN, M.L., TAGUCHI, T., SHIMIZU, Y.: Acceleration of growth of Sarcoma-180 with pyridoxamine and retardation with penicillamine. Proc. Soc. exp. Biol. (N.Y.) **113**, 667—674 (1963).

LITTMAN, M.L., TAGUCHI, T., SHIMIZU, Y.: Growth-retarding effect of oral L-penicillamine on Sarcoma-180. Nature (Lond.) **203**, 726—728 (1964).

LORINCZ, A.B., KUTTNER, R.E.: Suppression of advanced malignant disease by restricting phenylalanine intake. Fed. Proc. **25**, 360 (1966).

MAALØE, O., HANAWALT, P.C.: Thymine deficiency and the normal DNA replication cycle. I. J. molec. Biol. **3**, 144—155 (1961).

MACLEAN, S. J., HUBER, R. E.: The effects of DL-p-fluorophenylalanine and L-3-nitrotyrosine on the growth and biochemistry of the Taper liver tumor. Cancer Res. **31**, 1669—1672 (1971).
MAKINODAN, T., SANTOS, G. W., QUINN, R. P.: Immunosuppressive drugs. Pharmacol. Rev. **22**, 189—247 (1970).
MARTEL, F., BERLINGUET, L.: Impairment of tumor growth by unnatural amino acids. Can. J. biochem. Physiol. **37**, 433—439 (1959).
MATTHEWS R. E. F.: Biosynthetic incorporation of metabolite analogues. Pharmacol. Rev. **10**, 359—406 (1958).
MCCORD, T. J.: Some oxa and thia analogs of amino acids. Ph. D. Thesis, The University of Texas, Austin, Texas (1959).
MCCORD, T. J., BOOTH, L. D., DAVIS, A. L.: Some aza analogs of amino acids. J. med. Chem. **11**, 1077—1078 (1968).
MCCORD, T. J., COOK, D. E., SMITH, L. G.: The synthesis and biological activities of some aza analogs of amino acids. II. 4-Azalysine, an inhibitory analog of lysine. Arch. Biochem. Biophys. **105**, 349—351 (1964).
MCCORD, T. J., FOYT, D. C., KIRKPATRICK, J. L., DAVIS, A. L.: Diastereomers of 2-amino-3-methylaminobutyric acid, aza analogs of isoleucine. J. med. Chem. **10**, 353—355 (1967).
MCCORD, T. J., HOWELL, D. C., THARP, D. L., DAVIS, A. L.: 2-Amino-3-methylthiobutyric acid, an isoleucine antagonist. J. med. Chem. 8, 290—292 (1965).
MCCORD, T. J., RAVEL, J. M., SKINNER, C. G., SHIVE, W.: DL-4-Oxalysine, an inhibitory analog of lysine. J. Amer. chem. Soc. **79**, 5693—5696 (1957).
MCCOY, T. A., MAXWELL, M., KRUSE, P. F., JR.: The amino acid requirements of the Jensen sarcoma *in vitro*. Cancer Res. **19**, 591—595 (1959).
MCKAY, D. G., SHAPIRO, S. S.: Alterations in the blood coagulation system induced by bacterial endotoxin. J. Exp. Med. **107**, 353—367 (1958).
MCLAREN, A. D., KNIGHT, C. A.: Preparation and microbiological activity of a homolog of lysine. J. Amer. chem. Soc. **73**, 4478—4479 (1951).
MCLAREN, A. D., KNIGHT, C. A.: The response of *Leuconostoc mesenteroides* P-60 to some compounds related to lysine. J. biol. Chem. **204**, 417—422 (1953).
MICKELSON, M. N., FLIPPIN, R. S.: The use of an amino acid analogue in the therapy of mouse sarcoma 180. Arch. Biochem. Biophys. **64**, 246—248 (1956).
MIEDEMA, E., KRUSE, P. F., JR.: Effect of canavanine on proliferation and metabolism of human cells *in vitro*. Proc. Soc. exp. Biol. (N. Y.) **121**, 1220—1222 (1966).
MILNE, M. D.: Pharmacology of amino acids. Clin. Pharmacol. Ther. **9**, 484—516 (1968).
MIURA, M., HIRANO, M., KAKIZAWA, K., MORITA, A., UETANI, T., YAMADA, K.: Antitumor activity of L-β-aspartohydroxamic acid *in vivo*. Screening data of 21 L-asparagine related compounds. Prog. Antimicrobial Anticancer Chemother. **2**, 170—174 (1970a).
MIURA, M., HIRANO, M., KAKIZAWA, K., MORITA, A., UETANI, T., YAMADA, K.: Inhibitory effect of L-asparaginase in lymphocyte transformation induced by phytohemagglutinin. Cancer Res. **30**, 768—772 (1970b).
MOORE, T. C.: Histidine decarboxylase inhibitors and the survival of skin homografts. Nature (Lond.) **215**, 871—872 (1967).
MOR, G., LICHTENSTEIN, N.: Inhibitors of rat liver asparaginase. FEBS Let. **3**, 313—314 (1969).
MORGAN, J. F., MORTON, H. J., PASIEKA, A. E.: Arginine requirement of tissue cultures. I. Interrelationships between arginine and related compounds. J. biol. Chem. **233**, 664—667 (1958).
MORRISON, S. S., HIGGINS, G. M.: An attempt to block sources of methyl groups in the therapy of mouse leukemia. Cancer Res. **16**, 292—299 (1956).
MOYED, H. S.: Interference with the feed-back control of histidine biosynthesis. J. biol. Chem. **236**, 2261—2267 (1961).
MURRAY, K.: The occurrence of ε-*N*-methyl lysine in histones. Biochemistry **3**, 10—15 (1964).
NAGAI, K.: "GOBAB", an inflammatropic amino acid and its clinical implication. J. Nihon Univ. School Dent. **11**, 144—148 (1969).
NEUMAN, R. E., MCCOY, T. A.: The dual requirement of the Walker carcinosarcoma 256 *in vitro* for asparagine and glutamine. Science **124**, 124—125 (1956).
NORTON, S. J., CHEN, Y. T.: β-Aspartylhydroxamic acid: its action as a feedback inhibitor and a repressor of asparagine synthetase in *Lactobacillus arabinosus*. Arch. Biochem. Biophys. **129**, 560—566 (1969).
NOVIKOVA, M. A.: Amino acid derivatives of di-(2-chloroethyl)-amine: their effect on incorporation of heterologous amino acids in tumor and organ proteins. Vopr. Med. Khim. **9**, 250 (1963). Fed. Proc. **23**, T 1043—1046 (1964).
OHNUMA, T., BERGEL, F., BRAY, R. C.: Enzymes in cancer. Asparaginase from chicken liver. Biochem. J. **103**, 238—245 (1967).
OHNUMA, T., HOLLAND, J. F., FREEMAN, A., SINKS, L. F.: Biochemical and pharmacological studies with asparaginase in man. Cancer Res. **30**, 2297—2305 (1970).

OHNUMA, T., WALIGUNDA, J., HOLLAND, J.F.: Amino acid requirements *in vitro* of human leukemic cells. Cancer Res. **31**, 1640—1644 (1971).

PARDEE, A.B., PRESTIDGE, L.S.: The dependence of nucleic acid syntheses on the presence of amino acids in *Escherichia coli*. J. Bacteriol. **71**, 677—683 (1956a).

PARDEE, A.B., PRESTIDGE, L.S.: Incorporation of azatryptophan into proteins of bacteria and bacteriophage. Biochim. biophys. Acta **21**, 406—407 (1956b).

PATTERSON, M.K., JR., MAXWELL, M.D., CONWAY, E.: Studies on the asparagine requirement of the Jensen sarcoma and the derivation of its nutritional variant. Cancer Res. **29**, 296—300 (1969a).

PATTERSON, M.K., JR., ORR, G.R., CONWAY, E.: Studies on the aspartic acid "sparing effect" on the nutritional requirement of L-asparagine for tumors *in vitro*. Proc. Soc. exp. Biol. (N.Y.) **131**, 131—134 (1969b).

PILCHER, K.S., SOIKE, K.F., SMITH, V.H., TROSPER, F., FOLSTON, B.: Inhibition of multiplication of Lee influenza virus by canavanine. Proc. Soc. exp. Biol. (N.Y.) **88**, 79—86 (1955).

POPPER, H., DE LA HUERGA, J., YESINICK, C.: Hepatic tumors due to prolonged ethionine feeding. Science **118**, 80—82 (1953).

POTTER, V.R.: Sequential blocking of metabolic pathways *in vivo*. Proc. Soc. exp. Biol. (N.Y.) **76**, 41—46 (1951).

RABINOVITZ, M., FISHER, J.M.: Formation of a ribosomal lesion in rabbit reticulocytes by the lysine antagonist, *S*-(β-aminoethyl) cysteine. Biochem. biophys. Res. Commun. **6**, 449—451 (1962).

RABINOVITZ, M., MCGRATH, H.: Protein synthesis by rabbit reticulocytes. II. Interruption of the pathway of hemoglobin synthesis by a valine analogue. J. biol. Chem. **234**, 2091—2095 (1959).

RABINOVITZ, M., OLSON, M.E., GREENBERG, D.M.: Steric relationship between threonine and isoleucine as indicated by an antimetabolite study. J. Amer. chem. Soc. **77**, 3109—3111 (1955).

RABINOVITZ, M., TUVE, R.K.: Antimetabolite activity of lysine analogues on lysine incorporation into rat bone marrow protein *in vitro*. Proc. Soc. exp. Biol. (N.Y.) **100**, 222—224 (1959).

RANKI, M., KÄÄRIÄINEN, L.: Canavanine as an inhibitor of Semliki Forest virus growth. Ann. med. exp. Biol. Fenniae (Helsinki) **47**, 65—72 (1969).

RAY, P.D., FOSTER, D.O., LARDY, H.A.: Paths of carbon in gluconeogenesis and lipogenesis. IV. Inhibition by L-tryptophan of hepatic gluconeogenesis at the level of phosphoenolpyruvate formation. J. biol. Chem. **241**, 3904—3908 (1966).

RAY, P.D., HANSON, R.L.: Inhibition of gluconeogenesis by hydrazine. Fed. Proc. **28**., 411 (1969).

REGAN, J.D., VODOPICK, H., TAKEDA, S., LEE, W.H., FAULCON, F.M.: Serine requirement in leukemic and normal blood cells. Science **163**, 1452—1453 (1969).

REIS, H.E.: The role of immunosuppression in the genesis and growth of malignant tumors. Ger. Med. Monograph **1**, 16—21 (1971).

RENNERT, O.M., ANKER, H.S.: Effect of 5′,5′,5′-trifluoroleucine on a number of mouse leukaemias. Nature (Lond.) **203**, 1256—1257 (1964).

RICHMOND, M.H.: The effect of amino acid analogues on growth and protein synthesis in microorganisms. Bacteriol. Rev. **26**, 398—420 (1962).

RIZZOLI, C., CESTARI, A., DESSI, P., CONCILIO, A.: Richerche sugli omologhi superiori della metionina. Nota XX — Azione degli isomeri isopropilomocisteine sullo stipite HeLa. Ric. Sci. Sez. Biol. **2**, 52 (1962).

RIZZOLI, C., DESSI, P., CESTARI, A.: Metossinina e etossinina nel'accrescimento *in vitro* di stipiti di cellule umane in coltura continua. Arch. Ital. Sci. Farmacol. (Series III) **11**, (1961).

ROSENKRANZ, H.S., CARR, H.S., ZYROFF, J.: Synergism between cysteine and alkylating agents. J. Bacteriol. **102**, 672—676 (1970).

ROSENTHALE, M.E., GLUCKMAN, M.I.: Immunopharmacologic activity of 1-aminocyclopentane-1-carboxylic acid. Experientia **24**, 1229—1230 (1968).

ROSS, R.B., NOLL, C.I., ROSS, W.C.J., NADKARNI, M.V., MORRISON, B.H., JR., BOND, H.W.: Cycloaliphatic amino acids in cancer chemotherapy. J. med. pharm. Chem. **3**, 1—24 (1961).

ROWINSKI, W.A., HAGER, E.B.: Immunosuppressive effect of epsilon amino caproic acid (EACA). J. surg. Res. **6**, 58—63 (1966).

RYAN, W.L., ELLIOTT, J.A.: Fluorophenylalanine inhibition of tumors in mice on a phenylalanine-deficient diet. Arch. Biochem. Biophys. **125**, 797—801 (1968).

SAMAL, B.A., FRAZIER, L.E., MONTO, G., SLESERS, A., HRUBAN, Z., WISSLER, R.W.: Distribution of tritium labeled β-3-thienyl-L-alanine in tissues of adult male rats bearing Murphy-Sturm lymphosarcoma. Proc. Soc. exp. Biol. (N.Y.) **112**, 442—445 (1963).

Sartorelli, A.C., Kruse, P.F., Jr., Booth, B.A., Schoolar, E.J., Jr.: Combination chemotherapy: treatment of ascitic neoplasms by purine, amino acid, and vitamin analogs. Cancer Res. **20**, 495—503 (1960).

Schindler, R.: An analysis of cell function in serially propagated cell cultures as compared to studies of function in organ cultures. In: Dawe, C.J. (Ed.): Symposium on organ culture, Natl. Cancer Inst. Mon. No. 11. Washington, D.C.: U.S. Govt. Printing Office 1963.

Schlesinger, M., Grossowicz, N., Lichtenstein, N.: Anti-tumour activity of carbobenzoxy-L-asparagine. Experientia **25**, 14—15 (1969).

Schlesinger, M., Grossowicz, N., Lichtenstein, N.: Inhibition of murine tumors by carbobenzoxy derivatives of amino acids. Israel J. med. Sci. **7**, 547—552 (1971).

Schlesinger, S., Schlesinger, M.J.: The effect of amino acid analogues on alkaline phosphatase formation in *Escherichia coli* K-12. I. Substitution of triazolealanine for histidine. J. biol. Chem. **242**, 3369—3372 (1967).

Schmid, F.A., Fetzer, V.A., Smol, B.A., Tarnowski, G.S.: Effect of tryptophan and phenylalanine mustards on blood cells of tumor-free mice and mice with Ehrlich ascites carcinoma. Cancer Chemother. Rep. **49**, 9—13 (1965).

Schmid, F.A., Stern, B.R., Schmid, M.M., Tarnowski, G.S.: Effect of alanine, glycine, phenylalanine, and tryptophan mustards on Ehrlich ascites carcinoma and Ridgway osteogenic sarcoma. Cancer Chemother. Rep. **49**, 1—7 (1965).

Schmidt, C.G.: Stimulierung des Tumorwachstums durch Zufuhr von Asparaginsäure? Münch. med. Wschr. **112**, 1061—1062 (1970).

Schwartz, J.H., Cedar, H., Ehrman, M.: Synthesis and hydrolysis of β-aspartylhydroxamic acid catalyzed by L-asparaginase II of *E. coli*. Fed. Proc. **29**, 407 (1970).

Schwartz, R.S.: Are immunosuppressive anticancer drugs self-defeating? Cancer Res. **28**, 1452—1454 (1968).

Shani, M., Sheba, Ch.: Parachlorophenylalanine treatment in carcinoid syndrome. Brit. med. J. **4**, 784—785 (1970).

Shapiro, D.M., Fugmann, R.A.: Combination chemotherapy: synergism between a possible folic acid antagonist and ethionine on a "solid" tumor. J. nat. Cancer Inst. **18**, 201—207 (1957).

Sharon, N., Lipmann, F.: Reactivity of analogs with pancreatic tryptophan-activating enzyme. Arch. Biochem. Biophys. **69**, 219—227 (1957).

Shifrin, S., Ames, B.N., Gerroluzzi-Ames, G.: Effect of the α-hydrazino analogue of histidine on histidine transport and arginine biosynthesis. J. biol. Chem. **241**, 3424—3429 (1966).

Shiguera, H.T., Hen, A.C., Hiremath, C.B., Maag, T.A.: L-*O*-Ethylthreonine — an antagonist of L-isoleucine. Arch. biochem. Biophys. **135**, 90—96 (1969).

Shive, W.: The utilization of antimetabolites in the study of biochemical processes in living organisms. Ann. N.Y. Acad. Sci. **52**, 1212—1234 (1950).

Shive, W., Skinner, C.G.: Amino acid analogues. In: Hochster, R.M., Quastel, J.H. (Eds.): Metabolic Inhibitors, pp. 2—73. New York: Academic Press 1963.

Sjoerdsma, A.J.: Clinical implications of unnatural amino acids and amines. Fed. Proc. **30**, 908—911 (1971).

Skipper, H.E., Thomson, J.R.: A preliminary study of the influence of amino acid deficiencies on experimental cancer chemotherapy. In: Wolstenholme, G.E.W., O'Connor, C.M. (Eds.): Amino acids and peptides with antimetabolic activity, pp. 38—61, Ciba Foundation Symp. Boston: Little, Brown and Co. 1958.

Skipper, H.W., Thomson, J.R., Bell, M.: Attempts at dual blocking of biochemical events in cancer chemotherapy. Cancer Res. **14**, 503—507 (1954).

Smith, S.S., Bayliss, N.L., McCord, T.J.: The synthesis and biological activities of some aza analogs of amino acids. I. 4-Azaleucine, an inhibitory analog of leucine. Arch. Biochem. Biophys. **102**, 313—315 (1963).

Smolin, G., Keates, R.H.: Suppression of the corneal hypersensitivity reaction. Amer. J. Ophthalmol. **63**, 339—345 (1967).

Smulson, M.E., Rabinovitz, M., Breitman, T.R.: *O*-Methyl-threonine inhibition of growth and of threonine deaminase in *Escherichia coli*. J. Bacteriol. **94**, 1890—1895 (1967).

Spasskaya, I.G., Larionov, L.F.: Antitumor activity of ε,*N*,*N*-*bis*(β-chlorethyl)-L-lysine (lysepsin). Vopr. Onkol. **12**, 66—70 (1966). Chem. Abstr. **66**, 9849 (1967).

Spencer, R.P., Brody, K.R., Lutters, B.M.: Nontransport of certain substituted amino acid. Biochem. Pharmacol. **13**, 791—792 (1964).

Spencer, R.P., Brody, K.R., Mautner, H.G.: Intestinal transport of cystine analogs. Nature (Lond.) **207**, 418—419 (1965).

Spolter, P.D., Baldridge, R.C.: Effect of ethionine on histidine metabolism. Proc. Soc. exp. Biol. (N.Y.) **113**, 436—439 (1963).

Stapley, E.W., Miller, T.W., Mata, J.M., Hendlin, D.: L-4-Oxalysine, an antimetabolic antibiotic of microbial origin. Antimicrob. Agents Chemother. 401—406 (1967).

STOCK, J. A.: Amino acid and peptide derivatives with potential antitumor properties. In: WOLSTENHOLME, G. E. W., O'CONNOR, C.M. (Eds.): Amino acids and peptides with antimetabolic activity. pp. 89, Ciba Foundation Symp. Boston: Little, Brown and Co. 1958.
SUGIMURA, T., BIRNBAUM, S.M., WINITZ, M., GREENSTEIN, J.P.: Quantitative nutritional studies with water-soluble, chemically defined diets. VIII. The forced feeding of diets each lacking in one essential amino acid. Arch. Biochem. Biophys. **81**, 448—455 (1959).
SUMMERS, W.P., HANDSCHUMACHER, R.E.: L5178Y Asparagine-dependent cells and independent clonal sublines. Toxicity of 5-diazo-4-oxo-L-norvaline. Biochem. Pharmacol. **20**, 2213—2220 (1971).
SZENDE, B., TYIHAK, E.: Aspartic acid and cancer. Lancet **1**, 824 (1968).
SZENDE, B., TYIHAK, E., KOPPER, L., LAPIS, K.: The tumour growth promoting effect of 6-*N*-trimethyl lysine. Neoplasma **17**, 433—434 (1970).
TAGLIAMONTE, A., TAGLIAMONTE, P., GESSA, G. L., BRODIE, B. B.: Compulsive sexual activity induced by *p*-chlorophenylalanine in normal and pinealectomized male rats. Science **166**, 1433 (1969).
TANNENBAUM, A.: The role of nutrition in the origin and growth of tumors. Approaches to chemotherapy, pp. 96—127. Lancaster, Pa.: Am. Assoc. Advan. Sci., Science Press (1947).
TARNOWSKI, G. S., MOUNTAIN, I. M., STOCK, C. C.: Combination therapy of animal tumors with L-asparaginase and glutamine antagonists. Proc. Am. Assoc. Cancer Res. **10**, 92 (1969).
TARNOWSKI, G.S., MOUNTAIN, I.M., STOCK, C.C.: Combination therapy of animal tumors with L-asparaginase and antagonists of glutamine or glutamic acid. Cancer Res. **30**, 1118—1121 (1970).
TAYLOR, F. B., JR., FUDENBERG, H.: Inhibition of the C_1' component of complement by amino acids. Immunology **7**, 319—331 (1964).
THEUER, R. C.: Effect of essential amino acid restriction on the growth of female C57BL mice and their implanted BW10232 adenocarcinomas. J. Nutr. **101**, 223—232 (1971).
TOBEY, R. A., LEY, K. D.: Regulation of initiation of DNA synthesis in Chinese hamster cells. I. Production of stable, reversible G_1-arrested populations in suspension culture. J. cell Biol. **46**, 151—157 (1970).
TOBEY, R. A., LEY, K. D.: Isoleucine-mediated regulation of genome replication in various mammalian cell lines. Cancer Res. **31**, 46—51 (1971).
TOSA, T., PIZER, L. I.: Effect of serine hydroxamate on the growth of *Escherichia coli*. J. Bacteriol. **106**, 966—971 (1971a).
TOSA, T., PIZER, L. I.: Biochemical bases for the antimetabolite action of L-serine hydroxamate. J. Bacteriol. **106**, 972—982 (1971b).
TYRER, D. D., KLINE, I., GANG, M., GOLDIN, A., VENDITTI, J. M.: Effectiveness of antileukemic agents in mice inoculated with a leukemia L1210 variant resistant to 5-[3,3-*bis*(2-chloroethyl)-1-triazeno] imidazole-4-carboxamide (NSC 82196). Cancer Chemother. Rep. **53**, 229—241 (1969).
TYTELL, A. A., NEUMAN, R. E.: Growth response of stable and primary cell cultures to L-ornithine, L-citrulline, and L-arginine. Exp. cell Res. **20**, 84—91 (1960).
UDENFRIEND, S., ZALTZMAN-NIRENBERG, P., NAGATSU, T.: Inhibitors of purified beef adrenal tyrosine hydroxylase. Biochem. Pharmacol. **14**, 837—845 (1965).
UNGAR, G., YAMURA, T., ISOLA, J. B., KOBRIN, S.: Further studies on the role of proteases in the allergic reaction. J. exp. Med. **113**, 359—380 (1961).
WATSON, D. W., JOHNSON, A. G.: The clinical use of immunosuppression. Med. Clin. N. Amer. **53**, 1225—1241 (1969).
WEINBERG, A., BECKER, Y.: Effect of arginine deprivation on macromolecular processes in Burkitt's lymphoblasts. Exp. cell Res. **60**, 470—474 (1970).
WEINHOLD, P. A., RETHY, V. B.: Comparison of halogenated phenylalanine analogues as inhibitors as particle-bound and soluble tyrosine hydroxylase. Biochem. Pharmacol. **18**, 677—680 (1969).
WEISBERGER, A. S., LEVINE, B.: Incorporation of radioactive L-cystine by normal and leukemic leukocytes *in vivo*. Blood **9**, 1082—1094 (1954).
WEISBERGER, A. S., SUHRLAND, L. G.: The effect of a blocking analogue of cystine on leukemia. J. clin. Invest. **34**, 912—913 (1955).
WEISBERGER, A. S., SUHRLAND, L. G.: Studies on analogues of L-cysteine and L-cystine. II. The effect of selenium cystine on Murphy lymphosarcoma tumor cells in the rat. Blood **11**, 11—18 (1956a).
WEISBERGER, A.S., SUHRLAND, L.G.: Studies on analogues of L-cysteine and L-cystine. III. The effect of selenium cystine on leukemia. Blood **11**, 19—30 (1956b).
WEISBERGER, A.S., SUHRLAND, L.G., SEIFTER, J.: Studies on analogues of L-cysteine and L-cystine. I. Some structural requirements for inhibiting the incorporation of radioactive L-cystine by leukemic leukocytes. Blood **11**, 1—10 (1956).

WHITE, L. P., SHIMKIN, M. B.: Effects of DL-ethionine in six patients with neoplastic disease. Cancer **7**, 867—872 (1954).
WHITE, P. B., SMITH, C. W., KRUSE, P. F., JR.: Response of Jensen sarcoma cell cultures to some analogs, homologs, and peptides of arginine, ornithine, and citrulline. Cancer Res. **23**, 1051—1058 (1963).
WIELAND, T., DETERMANN, H.: The chemistry of peptides and proteins. Ann. Rev. Biochem. **35**, 651—690 (1966).
WILDE, C. E., JR.: The urodele neuroepithelium. II. The relation between phenylalanine metabolism and the differentiation of neural crest cells. J. Morphol. **97**, 313—344 (1955).
WILLIAMS, A. K., COX, S. T., EAGON, R. G.: Conversion of 3-amino-1,2,4-triazole into 3-amino-1,2,4-triazoyl alanine and its incorporation into protein by *Escherichia coli*. Biochem. biophys. Res. Commun. **18**, 250—258 (1965).
WILSON, J. E., IRVIN, J. L., SUGGS, J. E., LIU, K.: Inhibition of growth and protein biosynthesis in Ehrlich ascites carcinoma by α-hydroxylamino acids and α-oximino acids. Cancer Res. **19**, 272—276 (1959).
WISEMAN, G., GHADIALLY, F. N.: The inability of sarcoma RD3 to utilize D-histidine for protein synthesis. Cancer Res. **17**, 1108—1111 (1957).
WISEMAN, G., GHADIALLY, F. N.: A biochemical concept of tumour growth, infiltration, and cachexia. Brit. med. J. **2**, 18—21 (1958).
WISSLER, R. W., FRAZIER, L. F., SOULES, K. H., BARKER, P., BRISTOW, E. C.: The acute effects of beta-3-thienylalanine in the adult male albino rat. Arch. Pathol. **62**, 62—73 (1956).
WOODS, D. D.: The relation of *p*-aminobenzoic acid to the mechanism of the action of sulfanilamide. Brit. J. exp. Pathol. **21**, 74—90 (1940).
WOOLLEY, D. W.: 3-Methylaspartic acid as a potent antimetabolite of aspartic acid in pyrimidine biosynthesis. J. biol. Chem. **235**, 3238—3241 (1960).
ZEE-CHENG, K. Y., CHENG, C. C.: Experimental antileukemic agents. Preparation and structure-activity study of *S*-tritylcysteine and related compounds. J. Med. Chem. **13**, 414—418 (1970). Chem. Abstr. **72**, 133161 (1970).
ZWEIFACH, B. W., NAGLER, A. L., TROLL, W.: Some effects of proteolytic inhibitors on tissue injury and systemic anaphylaxis. J. Exp. Med. **113**, 437—450 (1962).

Chapter 55

Cytotoxic Analogs of Pyridine Nucleotide Coenzymes

L. S. DIETRICH

With 2 Figures

Introduction

NAD^+ and $NADP^+$ are among the most important coenzymes in biological systems. Aberrations in the regulation of their synthesis and metabolism could have profound effects on living systems because of the central role played by these coenzymes in intermediary metabolism.

NAD is synthesized in the nucleus of eukaryotic cells (HOGEBOOM and SCHNEIDER, 1952; BRANSTER and MORTON, 1956). NMN adenylyltransferase (EC 2.7.7.1) (reaction 3 in Fig. 1), the final step in pyridine dinucleotide synthesis, is located exclusively in the nucleus.

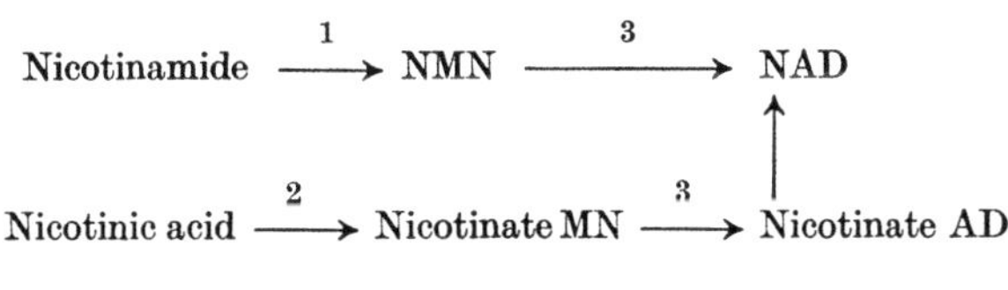

Fig. 1

This observation led to the proposal that NAD is involved in regulating growth (MORTON, 1958). This author reasoned that since the cell nucleus carries the genetic determination of cell behavior, it must "exercise control of cell division, growth, and differentiation, probably by means of a compound, or compounds, synthesized exclusively in the nucleus, but essential for cytoplasmic reactions". The coenzyme NAD meets this definition. MORTON and his collaborators postulated that cellular growth could be controlled by regulating the level of cellular pyridine nucleotides.

The concentration of pyridine dinucleotide in neoplastic tissue has been shown to be low as compared with normal tissue (JEDEIKIN and WEINHOUSE, 1955; GLOCK and MCLEAN, 1957). The work of MORTON (1958), together with the rationale that low levels of pyridine nucleotide in a tissue make it susceptible to chemotherapy employing compounds which would interfere with pyridine nucleotide metabolism, led to a search for compounds which would produce analogs of pyridine nucleotides with cytotoxic properties.

Exogenous NAD and NADP as such are not available for cellular metabolism, each cell having to synthesize the coenzyme *de novo* from smaller precursors.

Thus, to obtain fraudulent pyridine nucleotides intracellularly, one must administer analogs of pyridine nucleotide precursors. The structure of NAD is given in Fig. 2.

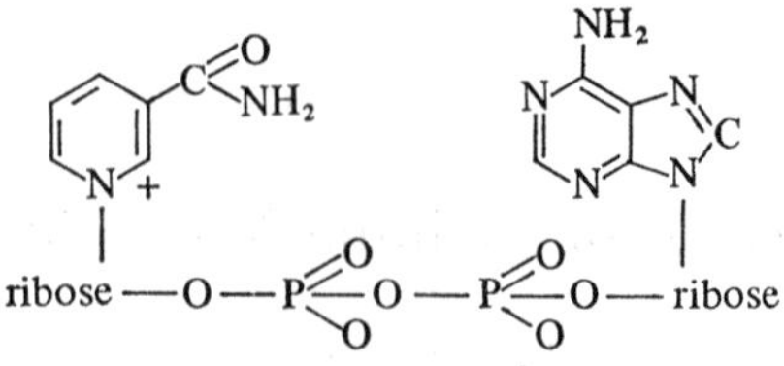

$$\text{ribose}-O-P(=O)(O)-O-P(=O)(O)-O-\text{ribose}$$

NH_2 C=O NH_2 N+ N N N C N

Fig. 2

Analogs of NAD

Theoretically, a cytotoxic analog of NAD should be one which binds the coenzyme at the appropriate catalytic site, but is incapable of carrying out the coenzyme function. The AMP moiety of pyridine nucleotide serves primarily in binding of the coenzyme to the appropriate enzyme while the nicotinamide portion of the molecule functions in coenzyme action.

Coenzyme analogs containing variations in the nicotinamide portion of the molecule would be candidates of choice in a search for cytotoxic pyridine nucleotide analogs. Studies in this direction were greatly facilitated by the observation that living cells contain an enzyme, NAD glycohydrolase (EC 3.2.2.5) (NADase), that converts NAD into nicotinamide and adenine diphosphoribose. ZATMAN et al. (1953) found that an NADase preparation from beef spleen was inhibited by nicotinamide in a reversible manner with respect to NAD. Using ^{14}C-labeled nicotinamide, these investigators were able to demonstrate an exchange reaction. They suggested that the following reaction was possible:

$$\underset{(\text{NAD}^+)}{\text{ARPPN}^+} + \text{X} \rightleftharpoons \text{ARPPX}^+ + \text{N},$$

where X is a molecule structurally similar to nicotinamide, and the product ($ARPPX^+$), an analog of NAD. The first analogs synthesized *in vitro* involved the use of isonicotinate hydrazide (ZATMAN et al., 1954). Good conversion of NAD into the isonicotinate hydrazide analog was observed. This analog, however, was neither reduced by NAD-requiring systems, nor did it interfere with the reduction of NAD by these systems. The first formation, *in vivo*, of a pyridine dinucleotide analog was demonstrated after the administration of the nicotinamide analog 3-acetylpyridine to tumor-bearing mice (KAPLAN et al., 1954). 3-Acetylpyridine adenine dinucleotide was isolated from the neoplastic tissue. These studies led to the synthesis of many pyridine nucleotide analogs in which substitutions of the carbonamide group of the nicotinamide moiety were made. All of these compounds can be reduced chemically and enzymatically, although the relative rate of enzymatic NAD analog reduction varies markedly depending on the enzyme being studied. These results are summarized in a review by SUND (1968). The fact that these NAD analogs can in part replace NAD *in vivo* probably accounts for the relatively low toxicity of the nicotinamide analogs employed.

The inhibition of folic acid reductase by the analog of NADP containing 3-acetylpyridine was described by HERKEN and TIMMLER (1965). A sensitive spectrofluorometric method for the determination of nucleotides containing 3-acetylpyridine in the cells of organs was indicated by HERKEN and NEUHOFF (1963). A summarizing description of reaction kinetics of different dehydrogenases with coenzymes containing 3-acetylpyridine as well as indications on the metabolism of 3-acetylpyridine (HARRIS and NEUHOFF, 1966; NEUHOFF and KÖHLER, 1966) was given by HERKEN (1968 a, b).

The most toxic nicotinamide analog known is 6-aminonicotinamide (6-AN). JOHNSON and McCOLL (1955) observed that nicotinamide or nicotinate protected mice from the lethal effect of 6-aminonicotinamide and that 6-aminonicotinamide adenine dinucleotide (6-ANAD) could be synthesized by pig brain NADase from NAD and 6-AN (JOHNSON and McCOLL, 1956). Subsequent work by DIETRICH et al. (1958a) demonstrated the synthesis of 6-AN analogs of NAD and NADP *in vivo* and *in vitro*. These 6-AN pyridine nucleotide analogs cannot be reduced chemically or enzymatically. Furthermore, the administration of 6-AN markedly affects the activity of NAD dependent dehydrogenases associated with mitochondrial function (DIETRICH et al., 1958a, b). That the inhibition of those systems dealing with high energy bond synthesis is operative *in vivo* was suggested by the observation that the administration of 6-AN resulted in a marked lowering of the levels of ADP and ATP and greatly increased the AMP level in adenocarcinoma 755. Adenocarcinoma 755 is very sensitive to 6-AN therapy (DIETRICH et al., 1958b; SHAPIRO et al., 1957). In addition, WOODS and BURK (1963) observed that 6-AN is an inhibitor of glycolysis in ascites cells, both *in vivo* and *in vitro*. The hypothesis advanced by DIETRICH et al. (1958a, b) concerning the inability of 6-AN analogs of NAD and NADP to function as normal electron carriers received confirmation and explanation from theoretical studies on the relationship between the electronic structure and the function of the respiratory enzymes (PULLMAN and PULLMAN, 1959). The quantum mechanical calculations of these authors indicate that 6-AN analogs of NAD and NADP do not possess the pronounced electron-acceptor properties of the true coenzyme and, thus, cannot function as electron carriers. In addition, 6-ANAD has been reported to interfere directly in oxidative phosphorylation (COPER and NEUBERT, 1964). Marked morphological changes in heart and liver mitochondria have been observed after 6-AN treatment (BACCINO, 1962). This suppression of mitochondrial function may account for the reported effect of 6-AN on cation transport (HERKEN et al., 1964, 1966).

The route of synthesis of 6-ANAD *in vivo* is via the NADase reaction and not via the biosynthetic pathway. 6-AN does not serve as a substrate for nicotinamide phosphoribosyltransferase (EC 2.4.2.12) (DIETRICH et al., 1968) (reaction 1, Fig. 1) and, although 6-aminonicotinate is an excellent substrate for nicotinate phosphoribosyltransferase (EC 2.4.2.11) (reaction 2, Fig. 1), the product of the reaction (6-aminonicotinate mononucleotide) is not a substrate for NMN adenylyltransferase (DIETRICH and FRIEDLAND, 1960).

Clinical trials with 6-AN have been disappointing. The compound is very toxic and has no significant tumoricidal properties at tolerated dosages (HERTER et al., 1961).

The mechanism of toxicity of 6-AN appears to differ significantly depending on whether the drug is given acutely or chronically. To produce the effect on mitochondrial respiration requires chronic treatment (2 to 4 mg/kg for 6 to 16 days) and even then only 3-phosphoglyceraldehyde dehydrogenase and the mitochondrial dehydrogenases are affected, while systems such as lactate dehydrogenase and glucose-6-phosphate dehydrogenase are not affected.

We have observed that acute toxicity produced by the administration of a single injection of 6-AN at 100 to 200 mg/kg (a lethal dose) produces no effect on the mitochondrial NAD-dependent dehydrogenases or 3-phosphoglyceraldehyde dehydrogenase despite the fact that large amounts of 6-ANAD and 6-ANADP are produced (DIETRICH, unpublished data). Similar results have been obtained by BRUNNEMANN et al. (1964). The time needed to produce the enzymatic effects observed after chronic administration of 6-AN is interpreted as a crude measure of the turnover of the tightly bound mitochondrial NAD and the rate of 6-ANAD penetration into mitochondria. These effects cannot be seen in chronically treated animals because they die before the lag phase is complete. REDETZKI and ALVAREZ-O'BOURKE (1962) are of the opinion that acute toxicity of 6-AN is due to direct central nervous system depression and not related to pyridine nucleotide metabolism. The cytotoxic effect of 6-AN given at chronic levels (cytotoxic pyridine dinucleotide analog effect) is markedly affected by hormone therapy (MARTIN et al., 1960; DIETRICH and MARTIN, 1961; DIETRICH, 1964; GREENGARD et al., 1966). 6-AN, presumably via pyridine dinucleotide analogs, has teratogenic activity (CHAMBERLAIN, 1966).

Pyridine dinucleotide analogs have been synthesized in which substitutions were made at the adenine portion of the molecule, e.g., hypoxanthine, 6-mercaptopurine, uracil, etc. These are reviewed by SUND (1968). In general, there is no clear evidence that substitutions at this part of the pyridine dinucleotide produce cytotoxic pyridine dinucleotides.

References

BACCINO, F. M.: Heart and liver cloudy swelling by 6-aminonicotinamide (6-AN) in rats. Sperimentale **112**, 61—73 (1962).

BRANSTER, M. V., MORTON, R. K.: Comparative rates of synthesis of diphosphopyridine nucleotide by normal and tumor tissue from mouse mammary gland: Studies with isolated nuclei. Biochem. J. **63**, 640—646 (1956).

BRUNNEMANN, A., COPER, H., NEUBERT, D.: Biosynthese und Wirkung des 6-Aminonicotinamid-adenindinucleotids (6-ANAD). Naunyn-Schmiedeberg's Arch. exp. Path. Pharmak. **246**, 437—451 (1964).

CHAMBERLAIN, J. G.: Effects of acute vitamin replacement therapy on 6-aminonicotinamide induced cleft palate late in rat pregnancy. Proc. Soc. exp. Biol. (N. Y.) **124**, 888—890 (1966).

COPER, H., NEUBERT, D.: Effect of 6-amino NAD and other NAD analogues on the formation of NADH ~ P and its transphosphorylation to ATP. Biochim. biophys. Acta (Amst.) **82**, 167—170 (1964).

DIETRICH, L. S.: Augmentation of 6-aminonicotinamide antagonism of tumor growth by compounds with estrogenic activity. Cancer Res. **24**, 61—63 (1964).

DIETRICH, L. S., FRIEDLAND, I. M.: 6-Aminonicotinamide and 6-aminonicotinic acid metabolism in nucleated and non-nucleated erythrocytes. Arch. Biochem. Biophys. **88**, 313—317 (1960).

DIETRICH, L. S., FRIEDLAND, I. M., KAPLAN, L. A.: Pyridine nucleotide metabolism: Mechanism of action of the niacin antagonist 6-aminonicotinamide. J. biol. Chem. **233**, 964—968 (1958a).

DIETRICH, L. S., KAPLAN, L. A., FRIEDLAND, I. M., MARTIN, D. S.: Quantitative biochemical differences between tumor and host tissue. VI. 6-Aminonicotinamide antagonism of DPN-dependent enzymatic systems. Cancer Res. **18**, 1272—1280 (1958b).

DIETRICH, L. S., MARTIN, D. S.: Augmentation of 6-aminonicotinamide antagonism of DPN-dependent enzymatic systems by diethylstilbesterol. Cancer Res. **21**, 361—364 (1961).

DIETRICH, L. S., MUNIZ, O., FARINAS, B., FRANKLIN, L.: 6-Aminonicotinamide-^{14}C utilization by the 755 tumor and host liver tissue. Cancer Res. **28**, 1652—1654 (1968).

GLOCK, G. E., McLEAN, P.: Levels of oxidized and reduced diphosphopyridine nucleotide and triphosphopyridine nucleotide in tumours. Biochem. J. **65**, 413—416 (1957).

GREENGARD, P., SIGG, E. B., FRATTA, I., ZAK, S. B.: Prevention and remission by adrenocortical steroids of nicotinamide deficiency disorders and of 6-aminonicotinamide toxicity in rats and dogs. J. Pharmacol. exp. Ther. **154**, 624—631 (1966).

HERKEN, H., SENFT, G., ZEMISCH, B.: Die Einschränkung des tubulären Natrium- und Kaliumtransportes durch Biosynthese 6-Aminonicotinsäureamid enthaltender Nucleotide. Naunyn-Schmiedeberg's Arch. exp. Path. Pharmak. **249**, 54—70 (1964).

HERKEN, H., SENFT, G., ZEMISCH, B.: Der Einfluß von 6-Aminonicotinsäureamid auf die Verteilung der Natrium- und Kaliumionen zwischen dem extra- und intracellulären Raum in der Leber und der Skelettmuskulatur. Naunyn-Schmiedeberg's Arch. exp. Path. Pharmak. **253**, 364—371 (1966).

HERTER, F. P., WEISSMAN, S. G., THOMPSON, H. G., JR., HYMAN, G., MARTIN, D. S.: Clinical experience with 6-aminonicotinamide. Cancer Res. **21**, 31—37 (1961).

HOGEBOOM, G. H., SCHNEIDER, W. C.: Cytochemical studies. VI. The synthesis of diphosphopyridine nucleotide by liver cell nuclei. J. biol. Chem. **197**, 611—620 (1952).

JEDEIKIN, L. A., WEINHOUSE, S.: Metabolism of neoplastic tissue. VI. Assay of oxidized and reduced diphosphopyridine nucleotide in normal and neoplastic tissues. J. biol. Chem. **213**, 271—280 (1955).

JOHNSON, W. J., MCCOLL, J. D.: 6-Aminonicotinamide — A potent nicotinamide antagonist. Science **122**, 834 (1955).

JOHNSON, W. J., MCCOLL, J. D.: Antimetabolite activity of 6-aminonicotinamide. Fed. Proc. **15**, 284 (1956).

KAPLAN, N. O., GOLDIN, A., HUMPHREYS, S. R., CIOTTI, M. R., VENDITTI, J. M.: Significance of enzymatically catalyzed exchange reactions in chemotherapy. Science **120**, 437—440 (1954).

MARTIN, D. S., DIETRICH, L. S., FUGMANN, R. A.: Hormonal augmentation of antimetabolite chemotherapy. Proc. Soc. exp. Biol. (N. Y.) **103**, 58—60 (1960).

MORTON, R. K.: Enzymic synthesis of coenzyme I in relation to chemical control of cell growth. Nature (Lond.) **181**, 540—542 (1958).

PULLMAN, B., PULLMAN, A.: Comment on the 6-aminonicotinamide antagonism of DPN-dependent enzymatic systems. Cancer Res. **19**, 337—338 (1959).

REDETZKI, H. M., ALVAREZ-O'BOURKE, F.: 6-Aminonicotinamide, a central nervous system depressant. J. Pharmacol. exp. Ther. **137**, 173—178 (1962).

SHAPIRO, D. M., DIETRICH, L. S., SHILS, M. E.: Quantitative biochemical differences between tumor and host as a basis for cancer chemotherapy. V. Niacin and 6-aminonicotinamide. Cancer Res. **17**, 600—604 (1957).

SUND, H.: The pyridine nucleotide coenzymes. In: SINGER, T. P. (Ed.): Biological oxidations, pp. 603—639. New York: Interscience 1968.

WOODS, M., BURK, D.: Formation of glycolytic inhibitor from 6-aminonicotinamide by ascites tumor cells *in vivo* and *in vitro*, and metabolic requirements for formation of this inhibitor. Biochem. Z. **338**, 381—392 (1963).

ZATMAN, L. J., KAPLAN, N. O., COLOWICK, S. P.: Inhibition of spleen diphosphopyridine nucleotidase by nicotinamide, an exchange reaction. J. biol. Chem. **200**, 197—212 (1953).

ZATMAN, L. J., KAPLAN, N. O., COLOWICK, S. P., CIOTTI, M. M.: The isolation and properties of the isonicotinic acid hydrazide analogue of diphosphopyridine nucleotide. J. biol. Chem. **209**, 467—484 (1954).

Further References

HARRIS, T., NEUHOFF, V.: Biosynthese, Verteilung und Ausscheidung von 3-Acetyl-6-pyridin, einem Metaboliten des 3-Acetylpyridins. Naunyn-Schmiedebergs Arch. exp. Path. Pharmak. **253**, 221-234 (1966).

HERKEN, H.: Drug-Induced Pathobiotic Effects. In: Proc. 3rd Intern. Pharmacol. Meeting, Vol. 4: Mechanism of Drug Toxicity, pp. 3-21. Oxford-New York: Pergamon Press 1968 a.

HERKEN, H.: Functional Discorders of the Brain Induced by Synthesis of Nucleotides Containing 3-Acetylpyridine. Z. klin. Chem. klin. Biochem. **6**, 357-367 (1968 b).

HERKEN, H., NEUHOFF, V.: Mikroanalytischer Nachweis von Acetylpyridin-adenin-dinucleotid und Acetylpyridin-adenin-dinucleotid-phosphat im Gehirn. Hoppe-Seyler's Z. physiol. Chem. **331**, 85-94 (1963).

HERKEN, H., TIMMLER, R.: Kinetik der Dihydrofolsäurereduktase aus Rattenleber und -gehirn mit 3-APADPH und H^+ als Wasserstoffdonator. Naunyn-Schmiedebergs Arch. exp. Path. Pharmak. **250**, 293-301 (1965).

NEUHOFF, V., KÖHLER, F.: Biochemische Analyse des Stoffwechsels von 3-Acetylpyridin. Naunyn-Schmiedebergs Arch. Pharmak. exp. Path. **254**, 301-326 (1966).

See also Addendum on page 891

Chapter 56

Triazenoimidazole Derivatives

Ti Li Loo

With 3 Figures

Introduction

To this day, the design and synthesis of cancer chemotherapeutic agents remain at best an art based more or less on enlightened empiricism. Triazenoimidazoles have been synthesized as latent forms of 5-diazoimidazole-4-carboxamide (DZC) (Shealy et al., 1962a), an unstable compound with antineoplastic activity in experimental tumors (Shealy et al., 1961). Also, since simpler phenyltriazenes are active (Clarke et al., 1955; Burchenal et al., 1956), the inclusion of an imidazolecarboxamide moiety may even potentiate this activity. Like that of most, if not all, anticancer agents, the mechanism of action of the triazeno-compounds remains to be elucidated. Nevertheless, at least one of them, 5-(3,3-dimethyl-1-triazeno) imid-azole-4-carboxamide (DIC, Fig. 1), has proven to be clinically useful in inducing temporary remissions in malignant melanoma (Luce et al., 1970).

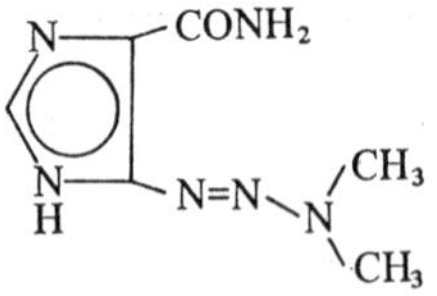

Fig. 1. 5-(3,3-Dimethyl-1-triazeno)imidazole-4-carboxamide or DIC

Chemistry

The triazenes are unsaturated derivatives of organic compounds with a chain of three nitrogen atoms, the triazanes. Completely aromatic triazenes, commonly named diazoamino compounds, are well-known. Organic compounds with a chain of nitrogen atoms usually become increasingly unstable as the chain is lengthened; however, some stability is conferred on them by the introduction of a double bond into the chain. Evidently, the stability of the triazenes is also highly dependent on the nature of the groups to which the nitrogen chain is attached. The completely alkyl triazenes, for example, are so unstable that relatively little is known about them. Depending on the location of the double bond, the mixed aryl alkyl triazenes readily decompose photochemically or in acid solution to give either an aryldiazonium salt and an alkylamine or an arylamine and the decomposition products of an alkyldiazonium salt (Sidgwick, 1966). Disubstituted triazenoimidazoles including DIC are essentially stable in the dark at pH 7 or in dilute acids for at least 24 h. On exposure to light, however, these solutions undergo decomposition to afford a secondary amine and DZC which cyclizes to 2-azahypoxanthine [imidazo-[4,5-*d*]-*v*-triazin-4(3*H*)-one] (SHEALY et al., 1962b). In fact, the photodecomposition of dialkyltriazenoimidazoles to DZC constitutes the basis of a method for the colorimetric determination of these triazenes (LOO, 1967). Simple monoalkyltriazenoimidazoles such as 5-(3-methyltriazeno)imidazole-4-carboxamide (MIC) decompose in aqueous and alcoholic solutions even in the dark with the formation of 5-aminoimidazole-4-carboxamide (AIC) and an unstable alkyldiazonium ion (SHEALY, 1966a). In addition to photodissociation, 5-[3,3-*bis*(2-chloroethyl)-1-triazeno]imidazole-4-carboxamide (BIC, Fig. 2), an agent capable of "curing" mouse leukemia L1210 (see below), undergoes an internal alkylation not only in solution

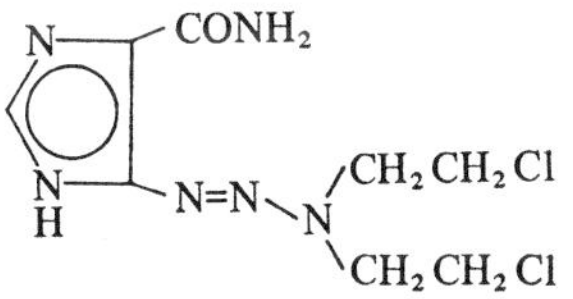

$CONH_2$

$N{=}N{-}N(CH_2CH_2Cl)_2$

Fig. 2. 5-[3,3-*bis*(2-chloroethyl)-1-triazeno]imidazole-4-carboxamide or BIC

but also slowly in solid state to 1-(5-carbomoylimidazol-4-yl)-3-(2-chloroethyl)-Δ^2-1,2,3-triazolinium chloride (SHEALY, 1966b, 1968; ABRAHAM, 1969). Monosubstituted triazenes are tautomeric; in solution as well as in solid state, the two tautomers are in dynamic equilibrium. In the monoalkyltriazenoimidazoles, however, the position of the equilibrium has not been established (SHEALY, 1966a). Geometric isomerism is expected in the unsymmetrically substituted triazenes which most likely exist normally in the *trans* form (LE FÈVRE, 1951). For experimental and clinical purposes, the best solvent for the triazenes is dilute acid; for instance, the solubility of both DIC and BIC in 0.1 *N* HCl is about 20 mg/ml.

5-(3,3-Dimethyl-1-Triazene)Imidazole-4-Carboxamide (DIC, NSC-45388)

In clinical cancer chemotherapy, DIC is by far the most important of the triazenoimidazoles. Consequently, most is known about its pharmacology and possible mode of action.

DIC is active against several experimental mouse tumors, including Sarcoma 180, adenocarcinoma 755, and leukemia L1210 (SHEALY, 1962a). In solid EHRLICH carcinoma, it shows an activity comparable to that of mitomycin C, cyclophosphamide, and 6-mercaptopurine at equimolar dose levels (HANO, 1965). Against the L1210 leukemia, treatment with DIC exhibits no schedule dependency (SCHABEL, F. M., JR., private communication). Recently it has been found that DIC is also active against mouse plasma cell tumor PC6 and lymphoma R1 (CONNORS, T. A., private communication). In combination with 5-fluorouracil, DIC has produced enhanced inhibition of leukemia L1210 (KLINE, 1971a).

Clinically, DIC has shown significant activity against malignant melanoma. Treatment with this drug has produced objective, but temporary, responses in 21 (19%) of 110 patients with melanoma (LUCE, 1970). This has since been confirmed by a number of investigators (SKIBBA, 1969; GOTTLIEB, 1971; BURKE, 1971; VOGEL, 1971a; COWAN, 1971). In other types of solid tumor, DIC is either devoid of activity or only slightly active (LUCE, 1970; SKIBBA, 1969; MOERTEL, 1970; MIZGERD, 1971; KINGRA, 1971). It has not received adequate trials in leukemia. The drug is usually administered intravenously at 250 mg/m^2 daily for 5 days, to be repeated at 3-week intervals. A major toxic effect of DIC is nausea and vomiting beginning 1 to 3 h after injection and lasting from 1 to 12 h. The nausea, most severe after the first dose, can sometimes be prevented or alleviated with phenothiazines and barbiturates. Another serious toxic effect is myelosuppression, leukopenia and thromobocytopenia. Other side effects include local pain at the site of injection, "flu-like" generalized aches and pains, and hepatoxicity (LUCE, 1970). DIC has also been successfully administered intra-arterially to eradicate localized melanoma (SAVLOV, 1971a, b).

In man, the gastrointestinal absorption of DIC is slow, incomplete, and variable. After intravenous injection, the plasma half-time of the drug is about 35 min in both man and dog; the apparent volume of distribution of DIC exceeds the total body water content in both species. The cumulative urinary excretion in 6 h is 43 % of the injected dose in man and 20 % in dogs. DIC is not appreciably bound to human plasma protein at concentrations above 5 μg/ml in plasma. In dilute solutions of 0.5 to 5 μg/ml in human plasma, it is about 20 % bound. In canine plasma, with solutions of 5 to 10 μg/ml, it is about 28 % bound. When DIC is given to the dog by constant intravenous infusion, the average cerebrospinal fluid to plasma concentration ratio is 1:7 at steady state (LOO, 1968a). The renal clearance of the drug exceeds the glomerular filtration rate (LOO, 1968b; SKIBBA, 1969). In the mouse, after an intraperitoneal injection of DIC labeled with ^{14}C in position-2 of the imidazole ring (DIC-2-^{14}C), 50 mg/kg, 55.8 % of the injected radioactivity is in the carcass at 15 min, diminishing to 4.7 % at 24 h. The small intestine with contents and the liver are the next greatest in radioactivity. Other organs contribute little to the distribution. Similar studies with DIC labeled with ^{14}C in the side chain methyl groups (DIC-DM-^{14}C) give comparable results with two important exceptions. First, 13.8 % of the dose was in the urine at 15 min and 43.5 % at 24 h; in contrast, the corresponding percentages with DIC-2-^{14}C were 5.9 % and 91.7 %, respectively. Second, about 10 % of the injected dose appeared in the expired air as $^{14}CO_2$ (HOUSHOLDER and LOO, 1971). Radioactive $^{14}CO_2$ as an *in vivo* metabolite of DIC-DM^{14}C has also been reported in man and the rat treated with the labeled drug. In these two species, pretreatment with phenobarbital, and probably with prochlorperazine also, increase the amount of $^{14}CO_2$ expired (SKIBBA, 1970a). Distribution of radioactivity in tumor-bearing mice was not greatly different from normal animals save that less $^{14}CO_2$ was produced (HOUSHOLDER and LOO, 1971). AIC is the only major metabolite of DIC that has been positively identified in man, dogs, and mice (HOUSHOLDER and LOO, 1969; SKIBBA, 1970b; HOUSHOLDER and LOO, 1971). Part of the AIC is excreted in the urine, and the rest enters normal metabolic pathways, eventually giving rise to hypoxanthine, xanthine, and uric acid (HOUSHOLDER and LOO, 1971). Methylation of nucleic acids and urinary excretion of radioactive 7-methyl-guanine by man and rats after administration of DIC-DM-^{14}C has been reported (SKIBBA, 1971). In the rat, DIC is concentratively excreted in the bile, probably by an active process (LOO, T. L., unpublished).

DIC prolongs the G_2 period of the mitotic cycle of mouse L1210 leukemia cells *in vivo*; the prolongation correlates with the dose and the magnitude of cell destruction (SHIRAKAWA, 1970). After oral administration to 24 female Sprague-Dawley weanling rats at 740 mg per rat for 14 weeks, DIC has induced mammary adenocarcinomas and thymic lymphosarcomas in all of the animals. Moreover, lymphosarcomas of the spleen, lymph nodes, and bone marrow, ependymomas of the brain, and pulmonary alveolar carcinomas have been induced in some of the rats (SKIBBA, 1970c). DIC inhibits cream xanthine oxidase (EC 1.2.3.2); however, in comparison with DZC, it is a much weaker inhibitor (IWATA, 1969). Using hypoxanthine as a substrate, the inhibition is competitive (LOO, T. L., unpublished data). Like DZC, but unlike other triazenoimidazoles, DIC is devoid of any effects on arterial blood pressure, peripheral blood vessels and isolated intestine of the rabbit (HANO, 1967). In man, DIC is only weakly immunosuppressive (HERSH, E. M., private communication). But in patients with malignant melanoma, DIC may inhibit the synthesis of tumor-associated antigens (NATHANSON, 1971).

Although many questions remain unanswered at present, a general consensus regarding the possible mechanism of action of DIC has gradually begun to emerge through the various different approaches of several laboratories. As mentioned previously, DIC is *N*-demethylated *in vitro* by rat liver microsomes (SKIBBA, 1970a). Also, in certain species, part of the dimethyl side chain is oxidized *in vivo* to CO_2 with the simultaneous formation of AIC (HOUSHOLDER, 1969, 1971; SKIBBA, 1970a, b). The *in vivo* methylation of the guanine moiety of nucleic acids in man and the rat after DIC administration has been described (SKIBBA, 1971). Moreover, in *Bacillus subtilis* (SAUNDERS, 1970) and also in mammalian cells in culture (LOO, 1971; GERULATH, 1971), DIC is more lethal in light than in darkness. A most interesting finding is that incubation of mammalian cells such as Chinese hamster ovary or human malignant melanoma cells with DIC-DM-^{14}C results in the labeling of cellular DNA only if light is excluded. On the other hand, with DIC-2-^{14}C, regardless of the presence or absence of light, both DNA and RNA become labeled (LOO, 1971; GERULATH and LOO, 1972). Furthermore, incubation of mammalian cells with DIC-DM-^{14}C in light causes the liberation of labeled dimethylamine but little or no $^{14}CO_2$. However, in darkness, three times as much $^{14}CO_2$ is formed as dimethylamine-^{14}C. Finally, with DIC-2-^{14}C, neither radioactive dimethylamine, nor radioactive CO_2 is evolved. Taken together, these observations tend to support the current generally accepted concept of the decomposition of triazenes (SHEALY, 1966a; PREUSSMANN, 1969, Fig. 3). Some of the reactions upon which this concept is based have been alluded to previously. In light, DIC rapidly undergoes photodecomposition to afford dimethylamine and DZC. The latter compound is a highly reactive species, and although it readily cyclizes to the relatively inactive 2-azahypoxanthine, it remains free long enough to interact with nucleic acids. In darkness, the decomposition is not entirely abolished, but is sufficiently retarded to allow the alternative mode of decomposition to display prominence. By the alternative pathway DIC loses a side chain methyl group, eventually as CO_2, through enzymic oxidative *N*-demethylation. The resultant monomethyl derivative of DIC, namely MIC or its tautomer, facilely cleaves to AIC and the precursor of the methyl carbonium ion. Like all alkylating agents, the methyl carbonium ion attacks DNA, ultimately leading to the formation of 7-methylguanine. Thus, biologically reactive intermediates are produced by either pathway. The methyl carbonium ion or its precursor has been recognized as being responsible not only for the antineoplastic activity of DIC, but also for the carcinogenicity of triazenes in general (PREUSSMANN, 1969, 1970; KRÜGER, 1970) and DIC in particular (SKIBBA, 1970c).

Biochemically and pharmacologically, DZC is yet another very reactive entity; many of its biological activities have recently been reported (IWATA, 1969, 1971; YAMAMOTO, 1970a, b). Similarly to DIC, it inhibits the growth of *Bacillus subtilis*. A DIC-resistant strain of *B. subtilis* is also resistant to DZC (SAUNDERS, 1970), thus suggesting a common underlying mechanism of action. Furthermore, both DIC and DZC are highly lethal to *Escherichia coli*; DZC probably exerts its antibacterial effect by inhibition of DNA synthesis (YAMAMOTO, 1969). In addition to these effects, DZC inhibits the growth of human epidermoid carcinoma cells in culture, the EHRLICH ascites carcinoma in mice, and the Walker 256 carcinosarcoma in rats (SHEALY, 1961). A potent electrophile, DZC is capable of interaction with nucleic acids, though the exact mechanism remains to be elucidated. Of the many possibilities, coupling with guanine at position-8, similar to benzene diazonium salts (ROBINS, 1967), is of particular interest because of the inherent biochemical repercussions at the molecular level. In summary, DIC may be a latent form of DZC in certain aspects.

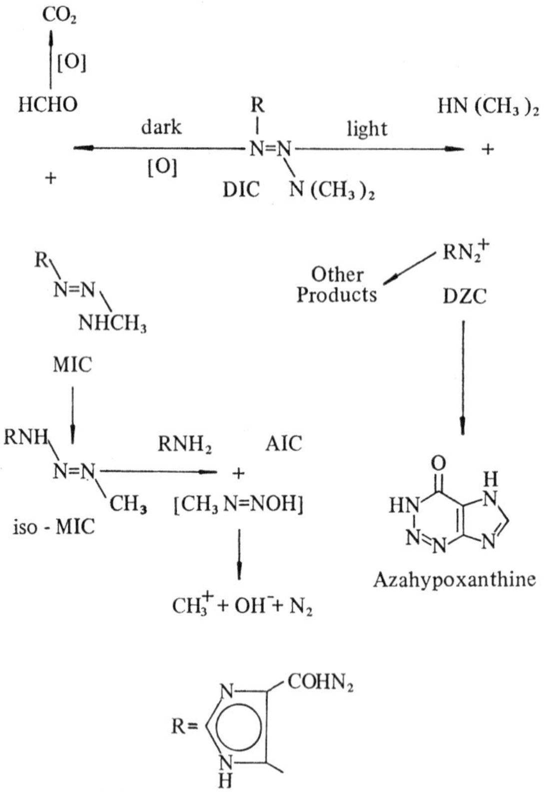

Fig. 3. The decomposition of DIC

5-[3,3-bis(2-Chloroethyl)-1-Triazeno] Imidazole-4-Carboxamide (BIC, NSC-82196)

Its status as an investigational agent notwithstanding, BIC deserves special attention for, thus far, it is the only triazenoimidazole derivative that has produced indefinite survivors in mouse leukemia L1210 (SHEALY, 1966b). In the L1210 system, whether administered orally or intraperitoneally, it is superior to DIC (HOFFMAN, 1968). A subline of the L1210 leukemia resistant to BIC is cross-resistant to DIC (TYRER, 1969), but another subline resistant to DIC is sensitive to BIC (KLINE, 1971b). Though extremely unstable and susceptible to internal alkylation with the formation of an isomeric triazolinium salt, even in solid state at room temperature, BIC is nevertheless stable for at least 22 months at $-15°$

to $-20°$ (SHEALY, 1968a). It is usually administered intravenously as a solution in 0.01 *N* HCl.

In human cancer, BIC has been disappointing thus far. In early studies, the drug was given orally; the ensuing erratic gastrointestinal absorption renders it difficult to interpret the observed clinical response and toxic effects (VOGEL, 1971b). In a recent study when BIC was injected intravenously, only 2 partial remissions were seen in 20 patients with metastatic melanoma. In these patients the development of myelosuppression as a result of BIC treatment is just as variable as in the early studies. Nausea and vomiting have been noted frequently, especially at doses above 900 mg/m^2 (GOTTLIEB, J.A., private communication).

As an anticancer drug, BIC is far more effective in mice than in man. This, though puzzling, is not unique. Attempts have been made to seek a solution to the paradox through comparative studies of the disposition of BIC in man and the mouse. By colorimetric assay, the average *in vitro* half-time of BIC in the plasma of both man and the mouse is about the same, 3.4 min and 3.7 min, respectively. In comparison, the average *in vivo* plasma half-time of BIC is 2.6 min in man (4 patients) and 2.9 min in mice (2 groups consisting of 40 BDF_1 mice each) (LOO, T. L., unpublished). However, this slight apparent difference between the *in vitro* and *in vivo* plasma half-time of BIC in the two species is probably statistically insignificant. Using BIC-2-^{14}C, the average plasma half-time of total radioactivity in 2 dogs is about 2 h (VOGEL, 1970). However, by the more specific colorimetric assay, the average plasma half-time of BIC in 6 dogs is only 3 min (LOO, T. L., unpublished). In both mice and dogs, no unchanged drug has been recovered in the urine after BIC-2-^{14}C administration. Most of the administered radioactivity is excreted in the urine as the isomeric triazolinium salt, with a small percentage as 2-azahypoxanthine. The remaining radioactivity resides in some unidentified metabolite(s) (VOGEL, 1970). There is no evidence at the present that the marked antitumor activity of BIC in mice, as compared with its relatively unimpressive activity in man, is attributable to species difference in the disposition of this drug. Part of the ineffectiveness of BIC is unquestionably a reflection of its instability.

BIC is more effective in suppressing experimental allergic encephalomyelitis than most immunosuppressive antitumor agents including DIC (VOGEL, 1969).

Structure-Activity Relationships

The antitumor activity of the triazenoimidazoles was first reported nearly 10 years ago (SHEALY, 1962). Since then a large number of triazenes with diverse structures have been synthesized and tested in experimental systems; this has recently been authoritatively reviewed (SHEALY, 1970a). In rodent tumors, some of the triazenes are, in fact, as active as, if not more so than, DIC. On the basis of these studies, certain conclusions regarding the structure-activity relationships among the triazenes can be drawn, with particular reference to the mechanism of action of the triazenoimidazoles. It must be emphasized that results obtained in experimental systems cannot always be successfully extrapolated to the clinical situation.

Antitumor activity is not uniquely associated with the attachment of the imidazole ring to the triazene side chain. Actually in DIC the imidazole ring may be exchanged with a phenyl (SHEALY, 1971b, c; LIN, 1972), pyrazole (NOELL, 1969; SHEALY, 1970b, 1971a), or a *v*-triazole ring (SHEALY, 1966c). Likewise, in many cases, the carboxamide moiety has been replaced with an ester (SHEALY, 1971a, c; LIN, 1972) or a hydrazide moiety (SHEALY, 1971c) without loss of activity. Also, in the phenyltriazenes, the relative position of the triazene chain with respect to the carboxamide or the carboxylic ester group is immaterial; *o*-, *m*-, or *p*-positions of the benzene ring are apparently equivalent (Lin, 1972). Moreover, though inactive against leukemia L1210, certain simple phenyltriazenes devoid of either the carboxamide or the ester group remain active in other experimental tumors (Burchenal, 1956). It therefore seems unlikely that the antineoplastic activity of DIC can be ascribed entirely to the close structural relationship between DIC and AIC.

Those dialkyltriazenoimidazole carboxamides and carboxylic esters having at least one methyl group in the dialkyl part are the most effective against leukemia L1210 (Shealy, 1968b, 1970a); MIC itself is active (Shealy, 1966a). However, against other experimental tumors, the methyl group does not appear to be indispensable (Shealy, 1968b). Certain monoaryltriazeno derivatives of imidazole carboxylic esters are modestly active against intramuscular Walker 256 carcinosarcoma, although inactive against leukemia L1210 (Shealy, 1970a). We may thus conclude that being the precursor of a methyl carbonium ion is not a prerequisite for antitumor activity in the triazene series.

In the L1210 system, BIC is far more effective than DIC. However, the fluoro analogs of BIC and its corresponding carboxylic methyl ester are merely comparable to DIC and its related carboxylic methyl ester as antileukemic agents. At the same time, these fluoro analogs are more toxic to the mouse than their parent chloro compounds. Nevertheless, the so-called mustard (2-haloethyl) groups are required for antitumor activity, since in 5[3,3-*bis*(2-acetoxyl)-1-triazeno]imidazole-4-carboxamide, an analog of BIC in which the chlorine atoms are replaced with acetoxyl groups, the activity is lost (Farquhar, D., unpublished work).

References

Abraham, D. J., Rutherford, J. S., Rosenstein, R. D.: Single crystal studies of chemotherapeutic agents. I. The structure of 1-(2-chloroethyl)-3-(5-carbamoylimidazol-4-yl)-Δ^2-1,2,3-triazolinium chloride. J. med. Chem. **12**, 189—190 (1969).

Burchenal, J. H., Dagg, M. K., Beyer, M., Stock, C. C.: Chemotherapy of leukemia. VII. Effect of substituted triazenes on transplanted mouse leukemia. Proc. Soc. exp. Biol. (N.Y.) **91**, 398—401 (1956).

Burke, P. J., McCarthy, W. H., Milton, G. W.: Imidazole carboxamide therapy in advanced malignant melanoma. Cancer **27**, 744—750 (1971).

Clarke, D. A., Barclay, R. K., Stock, C. C., Rondestvedt, C. S., Jr.: Triazenes as inhibitors of mouse sarcoma 180. Proc. Soc. exp. Biol. (N.Y.) **90**, 484—489 (1955).

Cowan, D. H., Bergsagel, D. E.: Intermittent treatment of metastatic malignant melanoma with high-dose 5-(3,3-dimethyl-1-triazeno)imidazole-4-carboxamide (NSC-45388). Cancer Chemother. Rep. **55**, 175—181 (1971).

Dagg, C. P., Karnofsky, D. A., Stock, C. C., Lacon, C. R., Roddy, J.: Effects of certain triazenes on chick embryos and on tumors explanted to the chorioallantois. Proc. Soc. exp. Biol. (N.Y.) **90**, 489—494 (1955).

Gerulath, A. H., Loo, T. L.: Mechanism of action of 5-(3,3-dimethyl-l-triazeno)imidazole-4-carboxamide in mammalian cells in culture. Biochem. Pharmacol. **21**, 2335—2343 (1972).

Gottlieb, J. A., Serpick, A. A.: Clinical evaluation of 5(3,3-dimethyl-1-triazeno)imidazole-4-carboxamide in malignant melanoma and other neoplasms: Comparison of twice-weekly and daily administration schedules. Oncology **25**, 225—233 (1971).

Hano, K., Akashi, A., Suzuki, Y., Yamamoto, I., Narumi, S., Iwata, H.: Pharmacological studies on 4(or 5)-aminoimidazole-5(or 4)-carboxamide (AICA) derivatives. Jap. J. Pharmacol. **17**, 668—677 (1967).

Hano, K., Akashi, A., Yamamoto, I., Narumi, S., Horri, Z., Ninomiya, I.: Antitumor activity of 4(or 5)-aminoimidazole-5(or 4)-carboxamide derivatives. Gann **56**, 417—420 (1965).

Hoffman, G. S., Kline, I., Gang, M., Tyrer, D. D., Venditti, J. M., Goldin, A.: Influence of treatment schedules and route of administration on the chemotherapy of murine leukemia L1210 with 5(or 4)-[3,3-*bis*(2-chloroethyl)-1-triazeno] imidazole-4(or 5)-carboxamide (NSC-82196). Cancer Chemother. Rep. **52**, 715—724 (1968).

Housholder, G.E., Loo, T.L.: Elevated urinary excretion of 4-aminoimidazole-5-carboxamide in patients after intravenous injection of 4-(3,3-dimethyl-1-triazeno)imidazole-5-carboxamide. Life Sci. 8, 533—536 (1969).

Housholder, G.E., Loo, T.L.: Disposition of 5-(3,3-dimethyl-1-triazeno) imidazole-4-carboxamide, a new antitumor agent. J. Pharmacol. exp. Ther. **179**, 386—395 (1971).

Iwata, H., Yamamoto, I., Muraki, K.: Potent xanthine oxidase inhibitors-4(or 5)-diazoimidazole-5(or 4)-carboxamide and two related compounds. Biochem. Pharmacol. **18**, 955—957 (1969).

Iwata, H., Yamamoto, I., Muraki, K.: Biological activity of diazonium compounds. Studies on the mechanism of action of 4(or 5)-diazoimidazole-5(or 4)-carboxamide on 5-hydroxytryptamine release from rabbit platelets — II. Comparative studies with *N*-ethylmaleimide *in vitro*. Biochem. Pharmacol. **20**, 297—304 (1971).

Kingra, G.S., Comis, R., Olson, K.B., Horton, J.: 5-(3,3-Dimethyl-1-triazeno)imidazole-4-carboxamide in the treatment of malignant tumors other than melanoma. Cancer Chemother. Rep. **55**, 281—283 (1971).

Kline, I., Woodman, R.J., Gang, M., Venditti, J.M.: Effectiveness of antileukemic agents in mice inoculated with leukemia L1210 variants resistant to 5-(3,3-dimethyl-1-triazeno)imidazole-4-carboxamide (NSC-45388) or 5-[3,3-*bis*(2-chloroethyl)-1-triazeno]imidazole-4-carboxamide (NSC-82196). Cancer Chemother. Rep. **55**, 9—28 (1971b).

Kline, I., Woodman, R.J., Gang, M., Waravdekar, V.S., Goldin, A., Venditti, J.M.: Enhanced response of leukemic (L1210) mice to combination chemotherapy with 5-(3,3-dimethyl-1-triazeno)imidazole-4-carboxamide (NSC-45388) and 5-fluorouracil (NSC-19893). Cancer **27**, 1363—1368 (1971a).

Krüger, F.W., Preussmann, R., Niepelt, N.: Mechanism of carcinogenesis with 1-aryl-3,3-dialkyltriazenes — III. *In vivo* methylation of RNA and DNA with 1-phenyl-3,3-[^{14}C]-dimethyltriazene. Biochem. Pharmacol. **20**, 529—533 (1971).

Le Fèvre, R.J.W., Liddicoet, T.H.: The possibility of geometrical isomerism among the 1-aryl-3:3-dimethyl-triazens. J. chem. Soc. 2743 (1951).

Lin, Y.T., Loo, T.L., Vadlamudi, S., Goldin, A.: Preparation and antitumor activity of derivatives of 1-phenyl-3,3-dimethyltriazene. J. med. Chem., **15**, 201—203 (1972).

Loo, T.L., Gerulath, A.H.: Studies of the mechanism of action of 5-(3,3-dimethyl-1-triazeno) imidazole-4-carboxamide. Proceedings of the VIIth International Chemotherapy Congress, Prague, 1971.

Loo, T.L., Luce, J.K., Jardine, J.H., Frei, E., III: Pharmacologic studies of the antitumor agent 5-(dimethyltriazeno)imidazole-4-carboxamide. Cancer Res. **28**, 2448—2453 (1968a).

Loo, T.L., Strasswender, E.A.: Colorimetric determination of dialkyltriazenoimidazoles. J. pharm. Sci. **56**, 1016—1018 (1967).

Loo, T.L., Tanner, B.B., Housholder, G.E., Shepard, B.J.: Some pharmacokinetic aspects of 5-(dimethyltriazeno)imidazole-4-carboxamide in the dog. J. pharm. Sci. **57**, 2126—2131 (1968b).

Luce, J.K., Thurman, W.G., Isaacs, B.L., Talley, R.W.: Clinical trials with the antitumor agent 5-(3,3-dimethyl-1-triazeno)imidazole-4-carboxamide. Cancer Chemother. Rep. **54**, 119—124 (1970).

Mizgerd, J.B., Amick, R.M., Hilal, H.M., Patno, M.E.: Clinical study of 5 (3,3-dimethyl-1-triazeno)imidazole-4-carboxamide (NSC-45388) in carcinoma of the lung. Cancer Chemother. Rep. **55**, 83—86 (1971).

Moertel, C.G., Reitmeier, R.J., Hahn, R.G., Schutt, A.J.: Study of 5-(3,3-dimethyl-1-triazeno)imidazole-4-carboxamide (NSC-45388) in patients with gastrointestinal carcinoma. Cancer Chemother. Rep. **54**, 471—473 (1970).

Nathanson, L., Jehn, U., Schwartz, R.S.: Disappearance of a tumor-associated antigen in malignant melanoma after imidazole carboxamide therapy. Cancer **27**, 411—415 (1971).

Noell, C.W., Cheng, C.C.: Pyrazoles. III. Antileukemic activity of 3-(3,3-dimethyl-1-triazeno)pyrazole-4-carboxamide. J. med. Chem. **12**, 545—546 (1969).

Preussmann, R., Von Hodenberg, A.: Mechanism of carcinogenesis with 1-aryl-3,3-dialkyltriazenes — II. *In vitro* alkylation of guanosine, RNA and DNA with aryl-monoalkyltriazenes to form 7-alkyl-guanine. Biochem. Pharmacol. **19**, 1505—1508 (1970).

Preussmann, R., Von Hodenberg, A., Hengy, H.: Mechanism of carcinogenesis with 1-aryl-3,3-dialkyltriazenes. Enzymatic dealkylation by rat liver microsomal fraction *in vitro*. Biochem. Pharmacol. **18**, 1—13 (1969).

Robins, R.K.: The purine and related ring systems. In: Elderfield, R.C. (Ed.): Heterocyclic compounds, Vol. 8, pp. 277—279. New York: Wiley 1967.

Saunders, P.P., Schultz, G.A.: Studies of the mechanism of action of the antitumor agent 5(4)-(3,3-dimethyl-1-triazeno)imidazole-4(5)-carboxamide in *Bacillus subtilis*. Biochem. Pharmacol. **19**, 911—919 (1970).

Savlov, E. D., Hall, T. C.: Response of localized melanoma to intra-arterial dimethyl triazeno imidazole carboxamide: a case report. J. surg. Oncol. **2**, 341—347 (1970).

Savlov, E. D., Hall, T. C., Oberfield, R. A.: Intra-arterial therapy of melanoma with dimethyl triazeno imidazole carboxamide. Cancer **28**, 1161—1164 (1971).

Shealy, Y. F.: Syntheses and biological activity of 5-aminoimidazoles and 5-triazenoimidazoles. J. pharm. Sci. **59**, 1533—1558 (1970a).

Shealy, Y. F., Krauth, C. A.: Imidazoles. II. 5(or 4)-(monosubstituted triazeno)imidazole-4(or 5)-carboxamides. J. med. Chem. **9**, 34—38 (1966a).

Shealy, Y. F., Krauth, C. A.: Complete inhibition of mouse leukemia L1210 by 5(or 4)-[3,3-*bis*(2-chloroethyl)-1-triazeno]imidazole-4(or 5)-carboxamide. (NSC-82196). Nature (Lond.) **210**, 208—209 (1966b).

Shealy, Y. F., Krauth, C. A., Clayton, S. J., Shortnacy, A. T., Laster, W. R., Jr.: Imidazoles. V. 5(or 4)-(3-Alkyl-3-methyl-1-triazeno)imidazole-4(or 5)-carboxamides. J. pharm. Sci. **57**, 1562—1568 (1968b).

Shealy, Y. F., Krauth, C. A., Holum, L. B., Fitzgibbon, W. E.: Synthesis and properties of the antileukemic agent 5(or 4)-[3,3-*bis*(2-chloroethyl)-1-triazeno]imidazole-4(or 5)-carboxamide. J. pharm. Sci. **57**, 83—86 (1968a).

Shealy, Y. F., Krauth, C. A., Montgomery, J. A.: Imidazoles. I. Coupling reactions of 5-diazoimidazole-4-carboxamide. J. org. Chem. **27**, 2150—2154 (1962b).

Shealy, Y. F., Krauth, C. A., Opliger, C. E., Guin, H. W., Laster, W. R., Jr.: Triazenes of phenylbutyric, hydrocinnamic, phenoxyacetic, and benzoylglutamic acid derivatives. J. pharm. Sci. **60**, 1192—1198 (1971b).

Shealy, Y. F., Montgomery, J. A., Laster, W. R., Jr.: Antitumor activity of triazenoimidazoles. Biochem. Pharmacol. **11**, 674—676 (1962a).

Shealy, Y. F., O'Dell, C. A.: Triazeno-*v*-triazole-4-carboxamides. Synthesis and antitumor evaluation. J. med. Chem. **9**, 733—737 (1966c).

Shealy, Y. F., O'Dell, C. A.: Imidazole and pyrazole *bis* (2-fluoroethyl)-triazenes. J. pharm. Sci. **59**, 1358—1360 (1970b).

Shealy, Y. F., O'Dell, C. A.: Synthesis, antileukemic activity, and stability of 3-(substituted-triazeno)pyrazole-4-carboxylic acid esters and 3-(substituted-triazeno)pyrazole-4-carboxamides. J. pharm. Sci. **60**, 554—560 (1971a).

Shealy, Y. F., O'Dell, C. A., Clayton, J. D., Krauth, C. A.: Benzene analogs of triazenoimidazoles. J. pharm. Sci. **60**, 1426—1428 (1971c).

Shealy, Y. F., Struck, R. F., Holum, L. B., Montgomery, J. A.: Synthesis of potential anticancer agent. XXIX. 5-Diazoimidazole-4-carboxamide and 5-diazo-*v*-triazole-4-carboxamide. J. org. Chem. **26**, 2396—2401 (1961).

Shirakawa, S., Frei, E., III: Comparative effects of the antitumor agents 5-(dimethyltriazeno) imidazole-4-carboxamide and 1,3-*bis*(2-chloroethyl)-1-nitrosourea on cell cycle of L1210 leukemia cell *in vivo*. Cancer Res. **30**, 2173—2179 (1970).

Sidgwick, N. V.: The Organic Chemistry of Nitrogen, 3rd ed., pp. 602—607 (Revised by Millar, I. T and Springall, H. D.). Oxford: Oxford University Press 1966.

Skibba, J. L., Beal, D. D., Ramirez, G., Bryan, G. T.: *N*-Demethylation of the antineoplastic agent 4(5)-(3,3-dimethyl-1-triazeno)imidazole-5(4)-carboxamide by rats and man. Cancer Res. **30**, 147—150 (1970a).

Skibba, J. L., Bryan, G. T.: Methylation of nucleic acids and urinary excretion of ^{14}C-labeled 7-methylguanine by rats and man after administration of 4(5)-(3,3-dimethyl-1-triazeno) imidazole-5(4)-carboxamide. Toxicol. appl. Pharmacol. **18**, 707—719 (1971).

Skibba, J. L., Ertürk, E., Bryan, G. T.: Induction of thymic lymphosarcoma and mammary adenocarcinomas in rats by oral administration of the antitumor agent 4(5)-(3,3-dimethyl-1-triazeno)imidazole-5(4)-carboxamide. Cancer **26**, 1000—1005 (1970c).

Skibba, J. L., Ramirez, G., Beal, D. D., Bryan, G. T.: Preliminary clinical trial and the physi. ologic disposition of 4(5)-(3,3-dimethyl-1-triazeno)imidazole-5(4)-carboxamide in man- Cancer Res. **29**, 1944—1951 (1969).

Skibba, J. L., Ramirez, G., Beal, D. D., Bryan, G. T.: Metabolism of 4(5)-(3,3-dimethyl-1-triazeno)imidazole-5(4)-carboxamide to 4(5)-aminoimidazole-5(4)-carboxamide in man. Biochem. Pharmacol. **19**, 2043—2051 (1970b).

Tyrer, D. D., Kline, I., Gang, M., Goldin, A., Venditti, J. M.: Effectiveness of antileukemic agents in mice inoculated with a leukemia L1210 variant resistant to 5-[3,3-*bis*(2-chloroethyl)-1-triazeno]imidazole-4-carboxamide (NSC-82196). Cancer Chemother. Rep. **53**, 229—241 (1969).

Vogel, C. L., Comis, R., Ziegler, J. L., Kiryabwire, J. W. M.: Clinical trials of 5-(3,3-dimethyl-1-triazeno)imidazole-4-carboxamide (NSC-45388) given intravenously in the treatment of malignant melanoma in Uganda. Cancer Chemother. Rep. **55**, 143—149 (1971a).

VOGEL, C. L., DENHAM, C., WAALKES, T. P., DE VITA, V. T.: The physiological disposition of the carcinostatic imidazole-4(or 5)-carboxamide, 5(or 4)-[3,3-*bis*(2-chloroethyl)-1-triazeno] (NSC 82196) (imidazole mustard) in mice and dogs. Cancer Res. **30**, 1651—1657 (1970).

VOGEL, C. L., DEVITA, V. T., DENHAM, C., FOLEY, H. T., FIELD, R. B., CARBONE, P. P.: Preliminary clinical trials and clinical pharmacologic studies with 5-[3,3-*bis*(2-chloroethyl)-1-triazeno]imidazole-4-carboxamide (NSC-82196) given orally. Cancer Chemother. Rep. **55**, 159—165 (1971b).

VOGEL, C. L., DEVITA, V. T., LISAK, R. P., KIES, M. W.: Suppression of experimental allergic encephalomyelitis by NSC 82196, a new imidazole carboxamide derivative. Cancer Res. **29**, 2249—2253 (1969).

YAMAMOTO, I.: 4(or 5)-Diazoimidazole-5(or 4)-carboxamide and related triazenoimidazoles as antibacterial agents: Their effects on nucleic acid metabolism of *Escherichia coli* B. Biochem. Pharmacol. **18**, 1463—1472 (1969).

YAMAMOTO, I., IWATA, H.: Biological activity of diazonium compounds: Studies on the mechanism of action of 4(or 5)-diazoimidazole-5(or 4)-carboxamide on 5-hydroxytryptamine release from rabbit platelets — I. Requirement for calcium ion. Biochem. Pharmacol. **19**, 1541—1550 (1970a).

YAMAMOTO, I., OKA, M., IWATA, H.: *In vitro* activation of monoamine oxidase in rat tissue homogenates by 4(or 5)-diazoimidazole-5(or 4)-carboxamide. Biochem. Pharmacol. **19**, 1831—1833 (1970b).

Chapter 57

Cytotoxic Inhibitors of Protein Synthesis

ARTHUR P. GROLLMAN

With 10 Figures

Introduction

Many antineoplastic agents exert profound inhibitory effects on protein synthesis. With few exceptions, such drugs are too toxic to be used for therapeutic purposes, but many have been employed as experimental tools in cell biology. Several reviews and symposia have been devoted to this topic (GOLDBERG, 1965; GOTTLIEB and SHAW, 1967; BUCHER and SIES, 1969; PESTKA, 1971; MUNOZ et al., 1972; GROLLMAN and HUANG, 1973), and this chapter will attempt to summarize current knowledge of the biochemical pharmacology of these drugs.

Classification of Inhibitors

Cytotoxic inhibitors of protein synthesis are conveniently grouped as inhibitors of initiation, peptide chain elongation, or chain termination, according to the functional events that they perturb. Initiation of protein synthesis includes those events that occur prior to formation of the complex between ribosome, mRNA, and methionyl-tRNA (Fig. 1, Stage III). Chain elongation involves binding of tRNA to the ribosome, peptide bond formation and translocation, a series of reactions (Fig. 1, Stages IV—VI) that repeats, sequentially, until the peptide chain is complete. Chain termination occurs when peptides are released from the ribosome and the ribosome-mRNA complex dissociates into its component parts. Several proteins and cofactors are involved in this series of reactions, as shown in Fig. 1.

Establishing the mechanism of action of any given inhibitor requires precise demarcation of the affected ribosomal function. This has been reported for a few drugs, such as puromycin; for others, only a functional description can be given (PESTKA, 1972; GROLLMAN and HUANG, 1973). Some inhibitors affect more than one step in protein synthesis, usually at different concentrations of drug.

Inhibitors of protein synthesis have also been classified according to their pattern of binding to ribosomes and ribosomal subunits (c.f. VAZQUEZ et al., 1969). Mammalian cells and other eukaryotes possess 80 S ribosomes composed of 60 S and 40 S subunits; prokaryotes have 70 S ribosomes composed of 50 S and 30 S subunits. Some inhibitors of eukaryotes bind only to ribosomes of the 80 S type; others bind to both 70 S and 80 S particles. Binding sites on either the larger or smaller ribosomal subunit can frequently be distinguished.

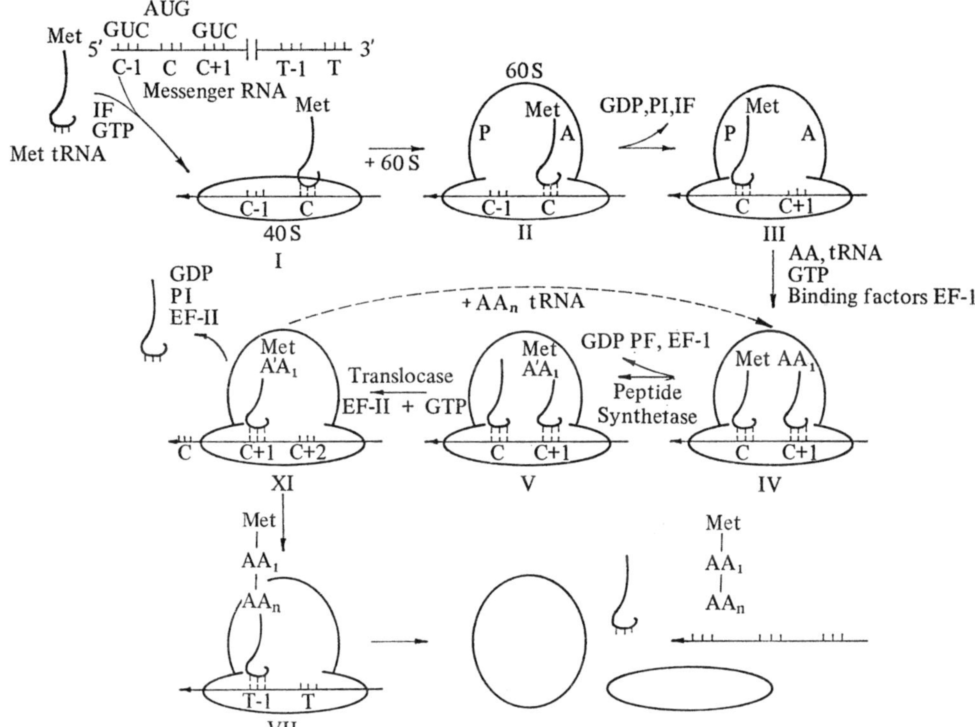

Fig. 1. Schematic repesentation of the reactions involved in protein synthesis. Abbreviations used: IF, initiation factors; EF, elongation factors; Met, methionyl; tRNA, transfer RNA; C, initiation codon; T, termination codon; PI, inorganic phosphate; AA, amino acid residue; P, peptidyl (or donor) site; A, aminoacyl (or acceptor) site

Effects on Protein Synthesis and Polyribosome Structure

Certain readily observed effects result from selective interruption of protein synthesis. For example, amino acid incorporation continues for several minutes in the presence of an inhibitor of initiation before the effect of the drug becomes apparent (Fig. 2). During this period of time, elongation and termination of peptide chains is unaffected. Inhibition of initiation is also characterized by sequential dissociation of polyribosomes into single ribosomes and subunits. Release of completed peptides serves to distinguish inhibitors of chain initiation from drugs, such as puromycin, that dissociate polyribosomes by inducing premature termination of peptide chains.

Kinetic experiments and changes in polyribosome structure can also be used to detect inhibitors of chain elongation. Such compounds inhibit amino acid incorporation almost immediately (Fig. 2); furthermore, these agents directly or indirectly prevent movement of mRNA along the ribosome. As a result, polyribosome structure is preserved for extended periods of time, and nascent peptide chains remain "frozen" to the polyribosome.

Protein synthesis is required for concurrent synthesis of DNA in animal cells; as a result, all inhibitors of protein synthesis simultaneously inhibit synthesis of DNA. Synthesis of RNA is not generally affected by these agents.

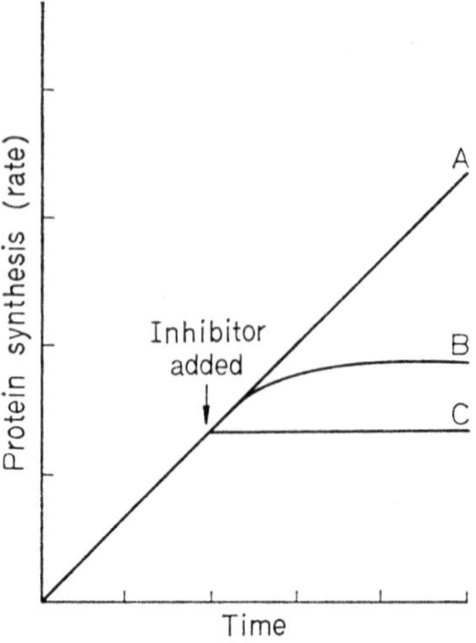

Fig. 2. Schematic representation of kinetics of amino acid incorporation. A, No inhibitor; B, inhibitor of initiation; C, inhibitor of elongation

Inhibitors

A. Harringtonine

I. General

Harringtonine (Fig. 3) is a cytotoxic alkaloid isolated from the seeds of *Cephalotoxus harringtonia* (POWELL et al., 1969). Several isomers of this alkaloid, including isoharringtonine and homoharringtonine, are obtained from the same source. The structure of the parent alkaloid, cephalotaxine, has been established by x-ray diffraction (ABRAHAM et al., 1969).

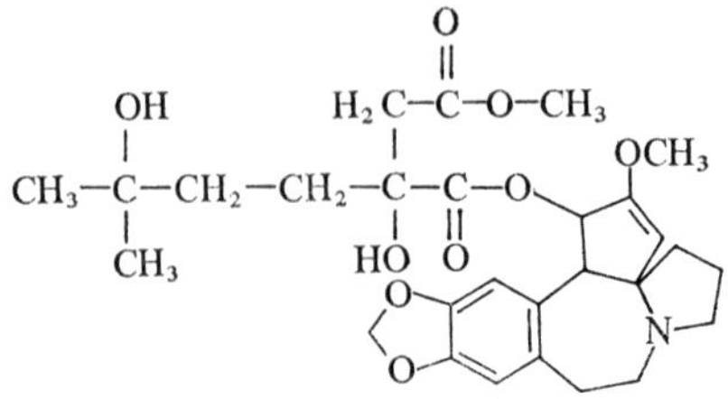

Fig. 3. Structure of harringtonine

II. Mechanism of Action

Harringtonine displays general characteristics of an inhibitor of chain initiation. After the drug is added, there is a short delay before effects on amino acid incorporation are observed; breakdown of polyribosomes occurs during this period of time (HUANG and GROLLMAN, 1972a). Harringtonine does not inhibit binding of mRNA or tRNA to ribosomes; thus, this agent appears primarily to affect the function and stability of the initiation complex. The effects of harringtonine on protein synthesis in HeLa cells are irreversible.

III. Other Cephalotaxus Alkaloids

Hydrolysis of harringtonine yields cephalotaxine and an unsaturated fatty acid. Neither of the hydrolysis products inhibit protein synthesis; however, the isomers, isoharringtonine and homoharringtonine, have activity equal to the parent compound. Small modifications in the side chain abolish biological activity

B. Pactamycin

I. General

Pactamycin is a cytotoxic antibiotic isolated from *Streptomyces pactum* (Bhuyan et al., 1961). The structure (Fig. 4) has recently been elucidated (Wiley et al., 1970). Pactamycin is cytotoxic to animal cells in tissue culture and inhibits the growth of gram-positive and gram-negative organisms (Bhuyan, 1967).

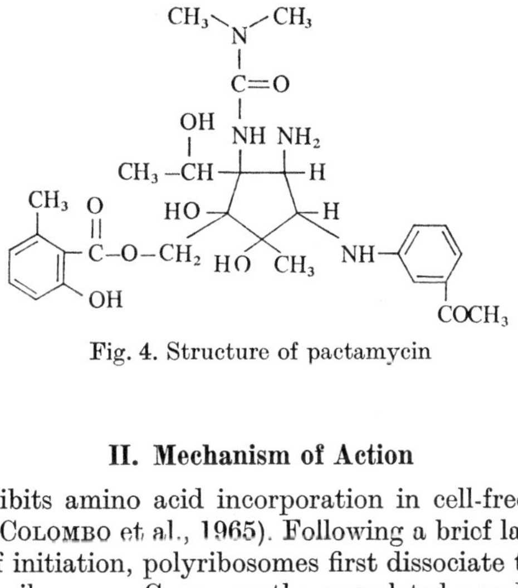

Fig. 4. Structure of pactamycin

II. Mechanism of Action

Pactamycin inhibits amino acid incorporation in cell-free extracts prepared from reticulocytes (Colombo et al., 1965). Following a brief lag period, characteristic of inhibitors of initiation, polyribosomes first dissociate to smaller units and eventually to single ribosomes. Concurrently, completed α and β globin chains are released from the ribosome. These observations indicate that pactamycin prevents formation of new polyribosomes while allowing translation of mRNA (cf. Goldberg et al., 1973).

Pactamycin binds to the smaller ribosomal subunit and to the 80 S ribosome, but not to the larger subunit or to polyribosomes (Goldberg et al., 1973). Single ribosomes derived from polyribosomes by treatment with ribonuclease do not bind pactamycin. 80 S ribosomes, produced by treatment with sodium fluoride, readily bind the antibiotic. Pactamycin does not prevent binding of initiation factors to 40 S subunits or attachment of synthetic mRNA to the ribosome. The ability of a "dissociation factor" to convert 80 S ribosomes into subunits is not affected by the antibiotic. These data suggest that pactamycin binds preferentially to free smaller ribosomal subunits, possibly before the initiation complex is formed.

In eukaryotes, pactamycin does not prevent formation of the initiation complex, but conversion of initiator methionyl-$tRNA_f$ into a puromycin-reactive form is blocked by the drug (GOLDBERG et al., 1973). In rabbit reticulocytes, puromycin induced release of peptides is inhibited if pactamycin is present during the binding-reaction. If the antibiotic is added after the binding reaction is complete, the reaction with puromycin is not significantly affected.

In the presence of pactamycin, the smaller ribosomal subunit is either unable to join with the 60 S subunit to form an active 80 S ribosome or forms an inactive and unstable monosome structure. Methionyl-$tRNA_f$ is bound to free 40 S particles that accumulate at the expense of the 80 S monosome. Polyribosome decay and release of nascent globin peptides are completed within two minutes after addition of pactamycin to reticulocyte lysates. These processes are not coordinated, suggesting premature release of incomplete polypeptide chains.

Pactamycin has been used by several groups to determine the gene order for the viral genome (SUMMERS and MAIZEL, 1971; TABER et al., 1971). By comparing the labeling pattern of virus-specific peptides that form at different times after the addition of the antibiotic, the order of synthesis for polio virus and encephalomyocarditis viral proteins was determined.

C. Emetine

I. General

The ipecac alkaloids (c.f. OPENSHAW, 1970) include some of the few cytotoxic inhibitors of protein synthesis to be used clinically. Ipecac, a mixture of these alkaloids, is principally used in the treatment of certain dysenteries and as an emetic; these therapeutic properties were recognized as early as the 17th century (c.f. LLOYD, 1921). Emetine (Fig. 5), an active principle of ipecac, was reported

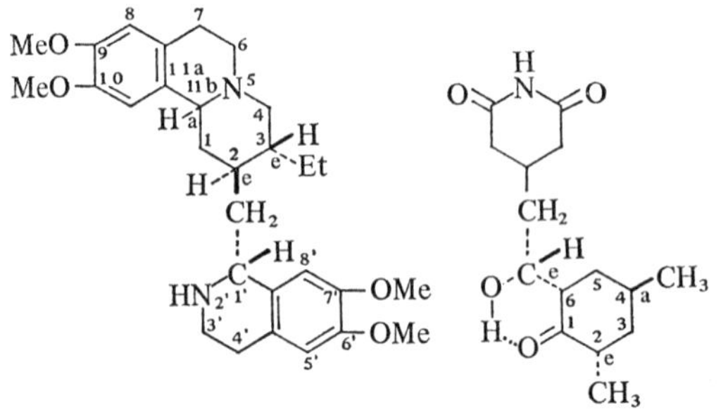

Fig. 5. Structure of emetine (left); structure of cycloheximide (right)

to be an amebicidal agent by VEDDER (1912) and was used in the treatment of neoplastic disease by VAN HOOSEN (1919). Much later, the drug proved beneficial in the therapy of nonspecific granulomas (GROLLMAN, 1965). The latter observation stimulated experiments on the mode of action of the ipecac alkaloids, which were found to inhibit protein synthesis irreversibly (GROLLMAN, 1966, 1968). These studies, in turn, led to an evaluation of the ipecac alkaloids as potential antineoplastic agents. Emetine or its analogs were reported to have significant antitumor (ABD-RABBO, 1969; JONDORF et al., 1971) and antiviral (GRUNBERG and PRINCE, 1966) activities. The well-established toxicities of emetine (KLATSKIN and FRIEDMAN, 1948) facilitated clinical studies, and Phase I experience with the drug as an antineoplastic agent has been reported (PANETTIERE and COLTMAN, 1971). Emetine may prove useful when used in combination with other chemotherapeutic agents, particularly since it seems not to be myelosuppressive. The general pharmacology and toxicology of emetine is described in various textbooks (GROLLMAN and GROLLMAN, 1970; ROLLO, 1970).

II. Mechanism of Action

Addition of emetine to HeLa cells or to crude reticulocyte lysates results in a decrease in the number of single ribosomes and a parallel increase in the number of polyribosomes (GROLLMAN, 1968). Nascent peptide remains attached to the polyribosome in the presence of the drug. If puromycin is added after prior incubation with emetine, nascent chains are released from the ribosome, but dissociation of polyribosomes is prevented.

When reticulocytes are incubated in the presence of 0.1 M sodium fluoride, polyribosomes dissociate to single ribosomes. If fluoride-treated cells are washed and resuspended in a buffer that contains components required for hemoglobin synthesis, polyribosomes reform. If this experiment is conducted in the presence of emetine, dimeric, trimeric, and tetrameric ribosomes form, but complete reassembly of polyribosomes does not occur (GROLLMAN and HUANG, 1973).

Specific protein factors (EF-I, EF-II and peptidyl transferase) are required for binding of aminoacyl-tRNA, translocation of peptidyl-tRNA and formation of peptide bonds, respectively. Puromycin reacts directly with peptidyl-tRNA located in the peptidyl (donor) site on the ribosome, causing premature termination and release of peptide chains from the polyribosome. This reaction, which does not require supernatant factors or GTP, has been used to examine the action of inhibitors of chain elongation. Established inhibitors of peptide bond formation, such as anisomycin (GROLLMAN, 1968; GROLLMAN and HUANG, 1973) and sparsomycin (GOLDBERG et al., 1973), inhibit puromycin-induced release of peptidyl-tRNA from polysomes. Emetine does not prevent this reaction nor does it affect the "fragment reaction," suggesting that the drug does not affect peptide bond formation. The activity of the binding enzyme, EF-I, is unaffected by emetine (GROLLMAN and HUANG, 1973).

The effect of emetine on translocation of peptidyl-tRNA has been determined by a two step assay, originally described by MCKEEHAN and HARDESTY (1969). This assay is based on the assumption that peptidyl-tRNA will be located at the donor (peptidyl) site following incubation of ribosomes in the presence of EF-II and GTP. Labeled aminoacyl-tRNA can then be bound to the aminoacyl site on the ribosome in the presence of sodium fluoride, an agent that prevents initiation of new globin peptides. Under these experimental conditions, further incorporation of amino acids into peptides is blocked by inhibitors of peptide bond formation, but not by inhibitors of translocation. Emetine has no effect at this stage of the reaction; however, if the drug is present prior to addition of EF-II and GTP, incorporation of amino acids is inhibited by approximately 50 % (GROLLMAN and HUANG, 1973). Assuming that nascent peptide is equally distributed between the aminoacyl and peptidyl sites on the ribosome, such partial inhibition would be anticipated by an agent that blocks translocation.

Puromycin releases 90 % of nascent peptide chains from the polyribosome, even in the presence of emetine. If translocation is inhibited by the drug, peptidyl-tRNA should accumulate in the aminoacyl site and, thus, be unable to react with puromycin. It would appear, therefore, that emetine chiefly affects that aspect of translocation that involves movement of mRNA along the ribosome.

Emetine inhibits protein synthesis in experimental animals; however, microsomes isolated from emetine-treated rats show enhanced rates of amino acid incorporation when tested *in vitro* (JONDORF and SZAPARY, 1968; JONDORF et al., 1969). Similar effects have been noted using cycloheximide and other glutarimide antibiotics (JONDORF et al., 1966; JONDORF and FILLER, 1968).

III. Structure-Activity Relationships

The availability of stereoisomers and derivatives of emetine allows demarcation of the structural requirements for inhibition of protein synthesis by members of this series (GROLLMAN, 1966, 1971). The (*R*) configuration at $C1'$ and the secondary nitrogen atom at the $2'$ position appear to be essential for inhibitory activity. This conclusion is based, in part, on the inactivity of the epimer with the (*S*) configuration at $C1'$ (isoemetine) and the loss of activity by creating an unsaturated $1'-2'$ position (*o*-methylpsychotrine) or by substitution of the secondary nitrogen (*N*-methylemetine). Unsaturation at the 2—3 position (dehydroemetine) destroys the asymmetry at carbons 2 and 3 without loss of biological activity, but further oxidation to 1,2,3,4,5,11*b*-trisdehydroemetine creates a positive charge at the tertiary nitrogen atom and results in inactivation of the compound. A *cis*-ethyl side chain is required for optimal activity, but the presence of this group is not essential since noremetine, *N*-propylemetine and even *des*-ethyl emetine retain some biological activity. If the ethyl side chain is present as the 2—3 transisomer, activity is markedly reduced. Inactivity of the 11*b* epimer of dehydroemetine may result from steric influences.

IV. Effects on Synthesis of RNA

The complex effects of emetine on RNA synthesis in HeLa cells include transient stimulation of RNA synthesis at very low (0.1 μM) concentrations of the drug (GROLLMAN, 1968). At concentrations sufficient to inhibit protein synthesis (1 μM), there is progressive decrease in the rate of RNA synthesis over a period of hours. At much larger concentrations (1 mM), synthesis of ribosomal RNA is inhibited (GILEAD and BECKER, 1971). This effect is reversible and may be related to a direct action of emetine on the DNA template.

The effects of emetine on RNA synthesis in viruses have also been reported. Synthesis of viral RNA in HeLa cells infected with polio virus, an RNA virus, is sensitive to the effects of low concentrations of the drug (GROLLMAN, 1968). Emetine has been reported to have selective antiviral action in experimental animals (GRUNBERG and PRINCE, 1966) and man (MELCHIOR, 1959; DEL PUERTO et al., 1968). RNA synthesis in the trachoma agent, an obligate prokaryotic parasite of eukaryotes, is resistant to concentrations of emetine that suppress RNA synthesis in the host cell. GILEAD and BECKER (1971) have used the drug to differentiate the two processes.

V. Mechanism of Cytotoxicity

The most important toxic effects of emetine relate to the cardiovascular system; these include hypotension, tachycardia, and various pathological and electrocardiographic abnormalities. The cardiotoxic effects have been attributed to inhibition of mitochondrial respiration evidenced by depletion of ATP and decreased oxygen consumption in emetine-treated cells (APPELT and HEIM, 1964, 1965). Emetine toxicity in cultures of embryonic chick heart cells was reversed by addition of NADH (WATKINS and GUESS, 1968). Selective damage of myocardial mitochondria has been observed (PEARCE et al., 1971).

GROLLMAN (1966) and others (BELLER, 1968) have suggested that inhibition of protein synthesis might be responsible for the cardiotoxicity of emetine. Emetine has been shown to inhibit the biosynthesis of actomyosin in rat heart (BELLER, 1968). In this regard, diphtheria toxin, a well known cardiotoxin, is also an established inhibitor of protein biosynthesis (STRAUSS and HENDEE, 1959; COLLIER and PAPPENHEIMER, 1964; HONJO et al., 1968; BASEMAN et al., 1970).

In addition to toxic effects on the myocardium, emetine therapy is associated with alterations in neuromuscular function. Emetine myopathy has been described (KLATSKIN and FRIEDMAN, 1948; DUANE and ENGEL, 1970), and the drug blocks both inhibitory and motor responses to sympathetic nerve stimulation (NG, 1966). The relationship of these observations to the biochemical effects of the alkaloid is unclear.

D. Cycloheximide

I. General

The cytotoxic activity and biological properties of cycloheximide (Fig. 5) are shared by a number of glutarimide antibiotics, including acetoxycycloheximide, streptimidone, and streptovitacin. The chemistry of this family of compounds is discussed in a comprehensive article by JOHNSON (1971), and the biochemical pharmacology has been reviewed by SISLER and SIEGEL (1967).

Cycloheximide is toxic to a wide variety of eukaryotes, including fungi, higher plants, and mammals, but is inactive against prokaryotes. The antibiotic has antitumor activity (WHITE, 1959), but proved too toxic for clinical use (FORD and KLOMPARENS, 1960). Cycloheximide was the most active of several hundred chemicals tested as inhibitors of tobacco mosaic virus multiplication (LINDER et al., 1959) and is one of the most effective rodent repellents known (WELCH, 1954).

Yeast grown in the presence of cycloheximide usually develop resistance to the antibiotic. A variety of genes confer resistance; in addition, recessive modifier genes have been found (WILKIE and LEE, 1965; CASKEY and BEAUDET, 1972). Resistance associated with the 60 S ribosomal subunit (RAO and GROLLMAN, 1967) may result from alterations in ribosomal proteins, as in the case of streptomycin-resistant strains of *E. coli*, or from changes in ribosomal conformation that alter the binding affinity of the ribosome for cycloheximide.

II. Mechanism of Action

Early studies on the mechanism of cycloheximide action have been reviewed by SISLER and SIEGEL (1967). LIN et al. (1966) showed that cycloheximide inhibited both peptide chain initiation and elongation by an effect on the donor site of the ribosome. Later studies (OBRIG et al., 1971) indicate that the drug blocks at or beyond the step in initiation (Fig. 1, Stage II) that is sensitive to sodium fluoride.

The action of cycloheximide on chain elongation bears many similarities to that described for emetine in the Section on Inhibitors (C, II). Inhibition of translocation was originally described by MCKEEHAN and HARDESTY (1969). BALIGA et al. (1969) suggested that the effect of cycloheximide was directed against EF-II; based, in part, on the protective effect of sulfhydryl compounds. Inhibition of chain elongation was observed at larger concentrations of drug than effects on chain initiation (OBRIG et al., 1971).

III. Structure-Activity Relationships

SIEGEL et al. (1966) have tested various glutarimide antibiotics for their capacity to inhibit protein synthesis. Replacement of the imide hydrogen of cycloheximide by a methyl group, esterification of the hydroxyl with acetate, or conversion of the ketone to an oxime, diminish or abolish biological activity, suggesting that the keto, hydroxyl, and imide groups are involved in a three-point attachment of the glutarimide antibiotics to their receptor. Since epicycloheximide was not available, the probable importance of the correct configuration of the carbon bearing the hydroxyl could not be demonstrated directly. Any modification of the spatial position of this hydroxyl group in relation to the cyclohexanone ring, however, as in neocycloheximide (which has an axially oriented side chain) or inactone (in which C_{5-6} is unsaturated), results in loss of biological activity. Available data support the suggestion of a hydrogen-bonded conformation in the biologically active forms; β-dihydrocycloheximide (in which intramolecular hydrogen-bonding is sterically prevented) is inactive, while α-dihydrocycloheximide (in which stronger hydrogen-bonding is demonstrable) has some activity. The active compound, streptimidone, which has an open chain in place of the cyclohexanone ring, would assume the conformation of cycloheximide if stabilized by intramolecular hydrogen-bonding.

IV. Topological Similarity to the Ipecac Alkaloids

The most significant conclusion to be drawn from the results of SIEGEL et al. (1966) and the structure-activity data described in the Section on Inhibition (C, III) is that groups required for biological activity in the glutarimide antibiotics correspond to essential positions for the ipecac alkaloids (GROLLMAN, 1966). In addition, there are topochemical similarities between cycloheximide and part of the emetine molecule (Fig. 5).

Interpretations of a necessarily tentative character may be useful in defining the possible interactions of these inhibitors with their biological receptor. One postulated receptor site would, presumably, bind the hydroxyl of cycloheximide or the secondary nitrogen of emetine. The loss of activity that accompanies the replacement of the hydrogens at these positions with methyl or acetyl groups is consistent with the view that these positions are involved in hydrogen-bonding to the receptor. Although an intramolecularly hydrogen-bonded conformation appears to be favored in cycloheximide, preferential bonding of the hydroxyl hydrogen to a receptor site is not precluded.

Additional testing of analogous compounds will be required to define fully the receptor site corresponding to the tertiary nitrogen of emetine or the imide nitrogen of cycloheximide. The imide grouping of cycloheximide is rendered inactive by *N*-methylation. This observation implies that the hydrogen atom on the imide nitrogen is involved in bonding, since the two adjacent carboxyl groups effectively prevent bonding through the π-electrons. If the tertiary nitrogen of emetine is hydrogen-bonded in a similar manner, the hydrogen atom must be supplied via the receptor. A bifunctional site in the receptor that could protonate, as well as accommodate a hydrogen atom, such as a hydroxyl or an imidazole group, would satisfy these requirements. Inactivity of trisdehydroemetine may result from repulsion by the positively charged nitrogen atom or from the effective removal of free electrons at this position. Steric effects also seem to be involved in the area of this nitrogen atom, since reversal of configuration at the adjacent 11*b* position [(+)-dehydroisoemetine] creates steric hindrance at the lower face of the molecule and is associated with a corresponding decrease in biological activity (BROSSI et al., 1962).

Although *C*1′ of emetine and the asymmetric carbon of the side chain of cycloheximide may be involved in binding to the receptor, it is more likely that they serve to fix the spatial position of the secondary nitrogen atom of emetine and the hydroxyl group of cycloheximide. The asymmetric carbon at *C*6 of cycloheximide would fulfill a similar function since, in order for the quasi ring of cycloheximide to correspond to the ring of emetine, the configuration at *C*6 must be such that the side chain is equatorial to the cyclohexanone ring.

Cycloheximide acts reversibly in the above biochemical reactions while the effects of emetine are irreversible. The action of streptovitacin A and acetoxycycloheximide, which differ from cycloheximide only in having an equatorial hydroxyl or acetoxy substitution at the *C*4 position, closely resembles emetine in being partially or totally irreversible (GROLLMAN, 1971). The property of irreversibility may be conferred by a secondary binding site that is not essential for inhibition of protein synthesis. Such secondary binding sites may also account for other reported functional differences between cycloheximide and emetine (JIMINEZ et al., 1972).

The usefulness of structure-function relationships in drug design is illustrated by a prediction of biological activity on the basis of the foregoing analysis. The postulated structure (I) common to the glutarimide antibiotics and ipecac alkaloids (Fig. 6) is found in the indole alkaloid, tubulosine (Fig. 6). Biological activity had not been reported for tubulosine. Subsequent biochemical studies (GROLLMAN, 1967b) established that the inhibitory action of tubulosine is: (1) species specific, being active against certain mammalian cells, protozoa, and yeast, but inactive against preparations of bacteria, (2) structurally specific, requiring a secondary nitrogen atom at the 2′-position and the (*R*) configuration at the 1′-carbon for activity, (3) selective, as RNA synthesis is unaffected at concentrations of tubulosine that totally inhibit protein synthesis, and (4) exerted during elongation of the peptide chain. Tubulosine proved to be equal to emetine in amebicidal activity when tested against several strains of *Entamoeba histolytica* (OPENSHAW, 1970).

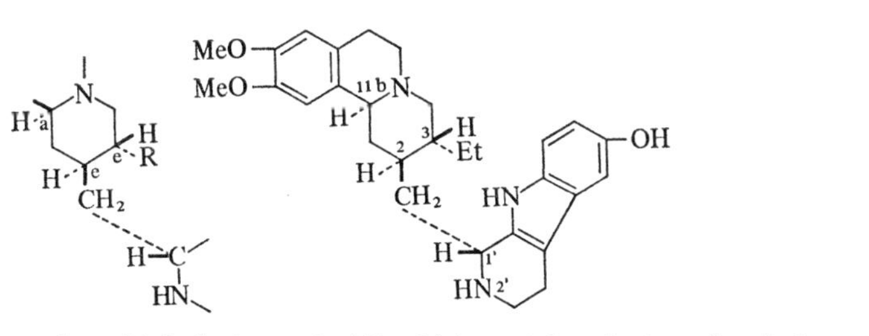

Fig. 6. Structural formulas of tubulosine and of I, which contains the topochemical requirements for inhibition of protein synthesis based on an analogy between the ipecac alkaloids and the glutarimide antibiotics (GROLLMAN, 1967b)

V. Effects on Synthesis of RNA

Within 15 min after administration of cycloheximide, synthesis of nucleolar 45 S RNA in rat liver is suppressed. The suppression increases for one hour, but does not exceed 80%. Synthesis of extranucleolar nuclear RNA is not inhibited prior to 60 min, at which time gradual inhibition occurs. These studies were interpreted as suggesting the presence of some short-lived proteins required for normal transcription of multinuclear genes (MURAMATSU et al., 1970).

E. Tylocrebrine

I. General

The phenanthroidolizidine alkaloids, tylophorine and tylocrebrine, and the phenanthroquinolizidine alkaloid, cryptopleurine, are vesicants isolated from *Tylophora crebriflora* and *Cryptocarya pleurosperma*. The structure of tylocrebrine (Fig. 7) has been established by GELLERT et al. (1962).

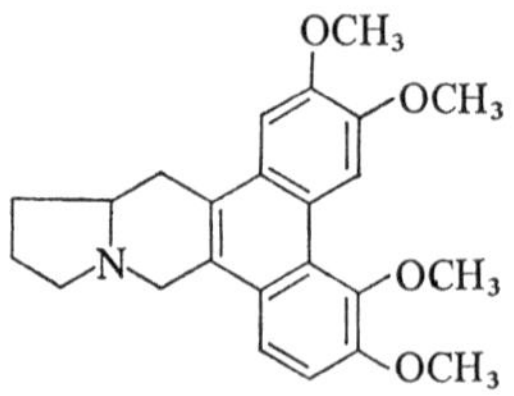

OCH_3 OCH_3 N OCH_3 OCH_3

Fig. 7. Structure of tylocrebrine

The phenanthrene alkaloids inhibit growth of L1210 leukemic cells and various experimental tumors in animals (GOLDIN et al., 1966). DONALDSON et al. (1968) reported that these compounds affected protein synthesis in animal cells, and detailed studies of the mode of action of tylocrebrine were subsequently reported by HUANG and GROLLMAN (1972b).

II. Mechanism of Action

The effect of tylocrebrine on protein synthesis generally resembles that of cycloheximide; however, certain differences have been observed (HUANG and GROLLMAN, 1972b). Cycloheximide reversibly inhibits protein synthesis while the action of tylocrebrine is irreversible. Under certain conditions, cycloheximide affects chain initiation; tylocrebrine does not appear to have this effect. Cycloheximide inhibits binding of deacylated tRNA to ribosomes while tylocrebrine markedly stimulates this reaction. Cycloheximide inhibits polyphenylalanine synthesis on reticulocyte ribosomes while tylocrebrine does not affect this process.

Ribosomes and EF-II require sulfhydryl compounds for maximal activity. The presence of mercaptoethanol and other sulfhydryl compounds diminishes the inhibitory effects of tylocrebrine (HUANG and GROLLMAN, 1972b). Sulfhydryl compounds have also been reported to protect against inhibitory effects of cycloheximide in cell-free systems prepared from rat liver (BALIGA et al., 1969). The exact mechanism of this effect remains obscure.

F. Anisomycin

I. General

Anisomycin, a pyrrolidine antibiotic isolated from cultures of various *Streptomyces* species, is toxic to plants, certain protozoa, yeast, and animal cells, but does not inhibit growth of bacteria (LYNCH et al., 1954). Like cycloheximide, anisomycin has limited clinical application as an antifungal agent; but proved too toxic for general use. The chemistry of anisomycin (Fig. 8) and related compounds has been reported (BEEREBOOM et al., 1965).

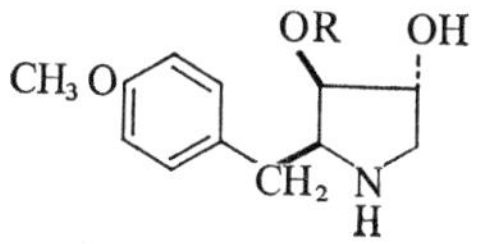

Fig. 8. Structure of anisomycin

II. Mechanism of Action

Anisomycin effectively inhibits protein synthesis in HeLa cells and intact rabbit reticulocytes at concentrations of 10^{-7} M (GROLLMAN, 1967a). The antibiotic is totally inactive against *E. coli* at concentrations of 10^{-3} M. In cell-free preparations of rabbit reticulocytes, larger concentrations of anisomycin were required to achieve the same degree of inhibition of protein synthesis as observed in intact cells.

Inhibition of protein synthesis by anisomycin is reversible (GROLLMAN, 1967a). HeLa cells were exposed to 10^{-5} M concentrations of the antibiotic for 2, 30, 60, and 120 min, then washed and resuspended in fresh medium. Following the reversal procedure, the rate of protein synthesis was 95 %, 83 %, 78 %, and 69 %, respectively, of that observed in control cultures subjected to similar manipulations.

Reversible inhibition of DNA synthesis was observed at low concentrations of the antibiotic; the maximum inhibition achieved was 60 to 70 % of control values. During the initial 10 min, inhibition of protein synthesis was greater than 90 % while inhibition of DNA synthesis was less than 40 %. Inhibition of protein synthesis was observed less than 30 sec after addition of anisomycin to the medium and preceded slightly the inhibition of DNA synthesis.

Using the assay of MCKEEHAN and HARDESTY (1969) and the puromycin reaction (MUNRO and MARCKER, 1967), a primary effect of anisomycin has been demonstrated on peptide bond formation (GROLLMAN and HUANG, 1973). VAZQUEZ et al. (1969) have reported that anisomycin inhibits the "fragment reaction," another measure of this effect.

III. Structure-Activity Relationships

The activity of certain analogs and isomers of anisomycin, as tested in intact rabbit reticulocytes and in reticulocyte lysates, has been reported (GROLLMAN, 1967a). Removal of the acetoxy group, acetylation or quaternization of the nitrogen atom, or bromination of the *p*-methoxyphenyl substituent, significantly reduced activity. None of the derivatives tested showed more than 1 % of the inhibitory activity of anisomycin.

G. Sparsomycin

I. General

Sparsomycin, a sulfur-containing antibiotic (Fig. 9) obtained from *Streptomyces sparsogenes*, is toxic to prokaryotic and eukaryotic cells (OWEN et al., 1962). COLOMBO et al. (1965) showed that sparsomycin inhibited protein synthesis and prevented breakdown of polyribosomes in animal cells while RNA synthesis was inhibited only slightly. Later, sparsomycin was shown to inhibit peptide bond formation in bacteria and, subsequently, in animal cells (Goldberg and Mitsugi, 1967a, b; Goldberg et al., 1973).

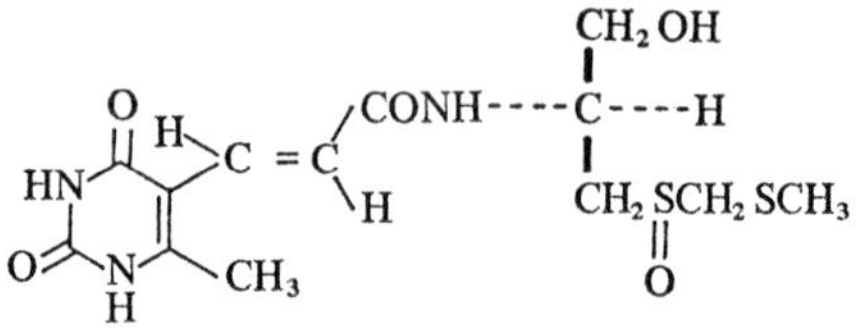

Fig. 9. Structure of sparsomycin

II. Mechanism of Action

Several model systems have been used to study the effects of sparsomycin on peptide bond formation independent of the other steps involved in polypeptide synthesis. Sparsomycin is a competitive inhibitor of the puromycin-induced release of polylysine bound to *E. coli* ribosomes. However, sparsomycin inhibition could not be overcome by increasing the concentration of tRNA (for which puromycin is considered to be an analog).

The so-called "fragment reaction", in which *N*-substitution of the aminoacyl group attached to a short fragment of tRNA is transferred to puromycin or another acceptor, requires the presence of the larger ribosomal subunit. This reaction, which involves peptidyl transferase, is sensitive to the effects of sparsomycin.

Sparsomycin also inhibits release of initiator-tRNA and peptidyl-tRNA from the P site on the ribosome. Taken together, these results suggest that sparsomycin interferes with the "acceptor" recognition site in peptidyl transferase (located on the larger ribosomal subunit), thereby blocking interaction with the aminoacyl end of an incoming aminoacyl-tRNA (or with the amino group of puromycin) and fixing peptidyl-tRNA in the donor site.

The structural basis for the action of sparsomycin is not known, but Goldberg et al. (1973) have speculated that the pseudouridine-like moiety of sparsomycin, which is attached to a peptide-like grouping, may play a role in its biological activity. It is of interest that the loop of tRNA that contains pseudouridine has a complementary sequence on the 5 S RNA which has been implicated in the function of peptidyl transferase (Erdmann et al., 1971).

H. Paederin

I. General

Paederin is a poisonous substance extracted from the insect *Paederus fuscipes* (Pavan and Bo, 1953). Its chemical structure (Fig. 10) was determined by Cardani et al. (1965). The LD_{50} for rodents is less than 2 μg per 100 g of body weight, and HeLa cells are sensitive to concentrations as low as 10 μM (Soldati et al., 1966).

II. Mechanism of Action

Brega et al. (1968) and Perani et al. (1968) have described the inhibitory action of paederin on protein synthesis in various mammalian cells and in cell-free extracts. BAGLIONI et al. (1972) and CARRASCO and VAZQUEZ (1972) have compared the effects of paederin to other inhibitors of protein synthesis. Paederin binds to the ribosome, inhibits initiation of protein synthesis at low concentrations (JACOBS-LORENA et al., 1971) and chain elongation (CARRASCO and VAZQUEZ, 1972) at high concentrations of drug. Paederin inhibits the reaction of *N*-formylmethionyl-tRNA with puromycin, but does not affect binding of mRNA or tRNA to the ribosome.

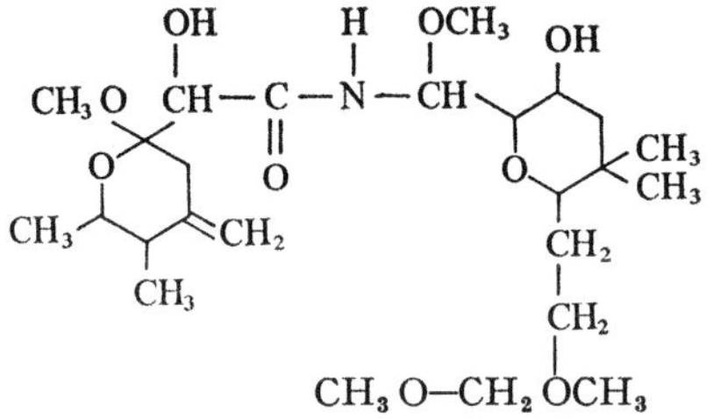

Fig. 10. Structure of paederin

References

ABD-RABBO, H.: Chemotherapy of neoplasia (cancer) with dehydroemetine. J. trop. Med. **72**, 287—290 (1969).

ABRAHAM, D. J., ROSENSTEIN, R. D., MCGANDY, E. L.: Single crystal x-ray structures of chemotherapeutic agents. II. The structure of cephalotaxine methiodide. Tetrahedron Let. **46**, 4085—4086 (1969).

APPELT, G. D., HEIM, H. C.: Effect of chronic poisoning by emetine on oxidative process in rat heart. I. Effects on lipid metabolism and oxidative phosphorylation. J. pharmacol. Sci. **53**, 1080—1083 (1964).

APPELT, G. D., HEIM, H. C.: Effect of chronic poisoning by emetine on oxidative process in rat heart. II. Effects on oxidation of citric acid cycle intermediates and nicotinamide adenine dinucleotide metabolism. J. pharmacol. Sci. **54**, 1621—1625 (1965).

BAGLIONI, C., JACOBS-LORENA, M., MEADE, H.: The site of action of inhibitors of initiation of protein synthesis in reticulocytes. Biochim. biophys. Acta (Amst.) **277**, 188—197 (1972).

BALIGA, B. S., PRONCZUK, A. W., MUNRO, H. N.: Mechanism of cycloheximide inhibition of protein synthesis in a cell-free system prepared from rat liver. J. biol. Chem. **244**, 4480—4489 (1969).

BASEMAN, J. B., PAPPENHEIMER, A. M., JR., GILL, D. M., HARPER, A. A.: Action of diphtheria toxin in the guinea pig. J. exp. Med. **132**, 1138 1152 (1070).

BEEREBOOM, J. J., BUTLER, K., PENNINGTON, F. C., SOLOMONS, I. A.: Anisomycin. I. Determination of the structure and stereochemistry of anisomycin. J. org. Chem. **30**, 2334—2342 (1965).

BELLER, B. M.: Observations of the mechanism of emetine poisoning of myocardial tissue. Circulat. Res. **22**, 501—505 (1968).

BHUYAN, B. K.: Edeine and pactamycin. In: GOTTLIEB, D., SHAW, P. D. (Eds.): Antibiotics I: Mechanism of action, p. 169. New York: Springer-Verlag 1967.

BHUYAN, B. K., DIETZ, A., SMITH, C. G.: Pactamycin, a new antitumor antibiotic. I. Discovery and biological properties. Antimicrob. Ag. Chemother. 184—197 (1961).

BREGA, A., FALASCHI, A., DECARLI, L., PAVAN, M.: Studies on the mechanism of action of pederine. J. cell Biol. **36**, 485—496 (1968).

BROSSI, A., BAUMANN, M., BURKHARDT, F., RICHIE, R., FREY, J. R.: Synthese Versuche in der Emetinreihe 9. Die absolute Konfiguration von (—)-2-Dehydro-Emetin. Helv. chim. Acta **45**, 2219—2226 (1962).

BUCHER, T., SIES, H.: Inhibitors, tools in cell research. New York: Springer-Verlag 1969.

CARDANI, C., GHIRINGHELLI, D., MONDELLI, R., QUILICO, A.: The structure of pederin. Tetrahedron Let. **29**, 2537—2545 (1965).

CARRASCO, L., VAZQUEZ, D.: Survey of inhibitors in different steps of protein synthesis by mammalian ribosomes. J. Antibiot. **25**, 732—737 (1972).

CASKEY, C. T., BEAUDET, A. L.: Antibiotic inhibitors of peptide chain termination. In: MUNOZ, E., GARCIA-FERRENDIZ, F., VAZQUEZ, D. (Eds.): Molecular mechanisms of antibiotic action on protein biosynthesis, p. 326. New York: American Elsevier 1972.

COLLIER, R. J., PAPPENHEIMER, A. M., JR.: Studies on the mode of action of diphtheria toxin. II. Effect of toxin on amino acid incorporation in cell-free systems. J. exp. Med. **120**, 1019—1039 (1964).

COLOMBO, B., FELICETTI, L., BAGLIONI, C.: Inhibition of protein synthesis by antibiotics in reticulocytes. I. Effect on polysomes. Biochim. biophys. Acta (Amst.) **119**, 109—119 (1965).

DEL PUERTO, B. M., TATO, J. C., KOLTAN, A., BURES, O. M., DE CHIERI, P. R., GARCIA, A., ESCARY, T. I., LORENZO, B.: Hepatitis viral en el nino con especial referencia a su tratamiento con emetina. Apart. Prensa Med. Argentina **55**, 818—834 (1968).

DONALDSON, G. R., ATKINSON, M. R., MURRAY, A. W.: Inhibition of protein synthesis in Ehrlich ascites tumour cells by the phenanthrene alkaloids tylophorine, tylocrebrine and crytopleurine. Biochem. biophys. Res. Commun. **31**, 104—109 (1968).

DUANE, D. D., ENGEL, A. G.: Emetine myopathy. Neurology **20**, 733—739 (1970).

ERDMANN, V. A., FAHNESTOCK, S., HIJO, K., NOMURA, M.: Role of 5 S RNA in the functions of 50 S ribosomal subunits. Proc. nat. Acad. Sci. (Wash.) **68**, 2932—2936 (1971).

FORD, J. H., KLOMPARENS, W.: Cycloheximide (acti-dione) and its nonagricultural uses. Antibiot. Chemother. **10**, 682—687 (1960).

GELLERT, E., GOVINDACHARI, T. R., LAKSHMIKANTHAM, M. V., RAGADE, I. S., RUDZUTS, R., VISWANATHAN, N.: The alkaloids of *Tylophora crebriflora*. J. chem. Soc. 10084—10140 (1962).

GILEAD, Z., BECKER, Y.: Effect of emetine on ribonucleic acid biosynthesis in HeLa cells. Europ. J. Biochem. **23**, 143—149 (1971).

GOLDBERG, I. H.: Mode of action of antibiotics. II. Drugs affecting nucleic acid and protein synthesis. Amer. J. Med. **39**, 722—752 (1965).

GOLDBERG, I. H., MITSUGI, K.: Sparsomycin inhibition of polypeptide synthesis promoted by synthetic and natural polynucleotides. Biochemistry **6**, 372—383 (1967a).

GOLDBERG, I. H., MITSUGI, K.: Inhibition by sparsomycin and other antibiotics of the puromycin-induced release of polypeptide from ribosomes. Biochemistry **6**, 383—391 (1967b).

GOLDBERG, I. H., STEWART, M. L., AYUSO, M., KAPPEN, L.: On the mechanism of polypeptide synthesis by the antibiotics sparsomycin and pactamycin. Fed. Proc. **32**, 1688—1697 (1973).

GOLDIN, A., SERPICK, A. A., MANTEL, N.: Experimental screening procedures and clinical predictability value. Cancer Chemother. Rep. **50**, 173—218 (1966).

GOTTLIEB, D., SHAW, P. D.: Antibiotics. I. Mechanism of action. New York: Springer-Verlag 1967.

GROLLMAN, A. P.: Emetine in the treatment of intra-abdominal and retroperitoneal nonspecific granulomas. Surg. Gynec. Obstet. **120**, 792—796 (1965).

GROLLMAN, A. P.: Structural basis for inhibition of protein synthesis by emetine and cycloheximide based on an analogy between ipecac alkaloids and glutarimide antibiotics. Proc. nat. Acad. Sci. (Wash.) **56**, 1867—1874 (1966).

GROLLMAN, A. P.: Inhibitors of protein biosynthesis. II. Mode of action of anisomycin. J. biol. Chem. **242**, 3226—3233 (1967a).

GROLLMAN, A. P.: Structural basis for the inhibition of protein biosynthesis: mode of action of tubulosine. Science **157**, 84—85 (1967b).

GROLLMAN, A. P.: Inhibitors of protein biosynthesis. V. Effects of emetine on protein and nucleic acid biosynthesis in HeLa cells. J. biol. Chem. **243**, 4089—4094 (1968).

GROLLMAN, A. P.: Inhibition of protein biosynthesis: its significance in drug design. In: ARIENS, E. J. (Ed.): Medicinal chemistry II. Drug design. New York: Academic Press 1971.

GROLLMAN, A. P., GROLLMAN, E. F.: Pharmacology and therapeutics, 7th ed. Philadelphia: Lea & Febiger 1970.

GROLLMAN, A. P., HUANG, M. T.: Inhibitors of protein synthesis in eukaryotes: tools in cell research. Fed. Proc. **32**, 1673—1678 (1973).

GRUNBERG, E., PRINCE, H. N.: Antiviral activity of emetine, 2-dehydroemetine and 2-dehydro-3-noremetine. Antimicrob. Ag. Chemother. 527—530 (1966).

HANISCH, J., VAJDA, G., BERTHA, I.: The mode of action of emetine. Acta chirurgica Acad. Sci. Hung. Tom. **7**, 51—54 (1966).

HONJO, T., NISHIZUKA, Y., HAYAISHI, O., KATO, I.: Diphtheria toxin-dependent adenosine diphosphate ribosylation of aminoacyl transferase II and inhibition of protein synthesis. J. biol. Chem. **243**, 3553—3555 (1968).

HUANG, M. T., GROLLMAN, A. P.: Harringtonine, a novel inhibitor of initiation of protein synthesis. Proceedings of the Fifth International Congress on Pharmacology, p. 109. 1972a,

HUANG, M. T., GROLLMAN, A. P.: Mode of action of tylocrebrine: effects on protein and nucleic acid synthesis. Molec. Pharm. **8**, 538—550 (1972b).

JACOBS-LORENA, M., BREGA, A., BAGLIONI, C.: Inhibition of protein synthesis in reticulocytes by antibiotics. V. Mechanism of action of pederine, an inhibitor of initiation and elongation. Biochim. biophys. Acta (Amst.) **240**, 263—272 (1971).

JIMINIZ, A., LITTLEWOOD, B., DAVIES, J.: Inhibition of protein synthesis in yeast. In: MUNOZ, E., GARCIA-FERRANDIZ, F., VAZQUEZ, D. (Eds.): Molecular mechanisms of antibiotic action on protein biosynthesis and membranes, p. 292. New York: American Elsevier 1972.

JOHNSON, F.: The chemistry of glutarimide antibiotics. In: HERZ, W., GRISEBACH, H., KIRBY, G.W. (Eds.): Progress in the chemistry of organic natural products. XXIX, p. 140. New York: Springer-Verlag 1971.

JONDORF, W.R., ABBOTT, B.J., GREENBERG, N.H., MEAD, J.A.R.: Increased lifespan of leukemic mice treated with drugs related to (—)-emetine. Chemotherapy **16**, 109—129 (1971).

JONDORF, W.R., DRASSNER, J.D., JOHNSON, R.K., MILLER, H.H.: Effect of various compounds related to emetine on hepatic protein synthesis in the rat. Arch. Biochem. Biophys. **131**, 163—169 (1969).

JONDORF, W.R., FILLER, R.S.: Further studies with glutarimide antibiotics. III. Changes in protein synthesis at the liver microsomal level in rats pretreated with streptimidone. Arch. Biochem. Biophys. **128**, 673—684 (1968).

JONDORF, W.R., SIMON, D.C., AVNIMELECH, M.: Further studies on the stimulation of L-(^{14}C)-amino acid incorporation with cycloheximide. Molec. Pharm. **2**, 506—517 (1966).

JONDORF, W.R., SZAPARY, D.: Enhanced protein synthesis at the liver microsomal level in emetine-pretreated rats. Arch. Biochem. Biophys. **126**, 892—904 (1968).

JORDA, V.V., LENFELD, J., ROTHSCHILD, L.: Zur Frage der Wirkung des Emetins bei Herpes Zoster. Z. Ges. Inn. Med. **13**, 71—76 (1958).

KLATSKIN, G., FRIEDMAN, H.: Emetine toxicity in man: studies on the nature of early toxic manifestations, their relation to dose level, and their significance in determining safe dosage. Ann. intern. Med. **28**, 892—915 (1948).

LINDER, R.C., KIRKPATRICK, H.C., WEEKS, T.E.: Comparative inhibition of virus multiplication by certain types of chemicals. Phytopathology **49**, 802—807 (1959).

LLOYD, J.R.: Ipecacuanha. In: Origin and history of all the pharmacopeial vegetable drugs, chemicals and preparations, p. 168, vol. 1. Cincinnati: Caxton Press 1921.

LYNCH, J.E., ENGLISH, A.R., BAUCK, H., DELIGIANIS, H.: Studies on the *in vitro* activity of anisomycin. Antibiot. Chemother. **4**, 844—848 (1954).

MCKEEHAN, W., HARDESTY, B.: The mechanism of cycloheximide inhibition of protein synthesis in rabbit reticulocytes. Biochem. biophys. Res. Commun. **36**, 625—630 (1969).

MELCHIOR, E.: Emetine: Seine Wirksamkeit auf schwere chirurgische Infekte. Stuttgart: Ferdinand Enke 1954.

MONRO, R.E., MARCKER, K.A.: Ribosome-catalysed reaction of puromycin with a formylmethionine-containing oligonucleotide. J. molec. Biol. **25**, 347—350 (1967).

MUNOZ, E.F., GARCIA-FERRANDIZ, F., VAZQUEZ, D.: Molecular mechanisms of antibiotic action on protein biosynthesis and membranes. New York: American Elsevier 1972.

MURAMATSU, M., SHIMADA, N., HIGASHINAKAGAWA, T.: Effect of cycloheximide on the nucleolar RNA synthesis in rat liver. J. molec. Biol. **53**, 91—106 (1970).

NG, K.K.F.: A new pharmacological action of emetine. Brit. med. J. 1278—1279 (1966).

OBRIG, T.C., CULP, W.J., MCKEEHAN, W.L., HARDESTY, B.: The mechanism by which cycloheximide and related glutarimide antibiotics inhibit peptide synthesis on reticulocyte ribosomes. J. biol. Chem. **246**, 174—181 (1971).

OPENSHAW, H.T.: The ipecacuanha alkaloids. In: PELLETIER, S.W. (Ed.): Chemistry of the alkaloids, p. 85. New York: Van Nostrand Reinhold 1970.

OWEN, S.P., DIETZ, A., CAMIENER, G.W.: Sparsomycin, a new antitumor antibiotic. I. Discovery and biological properties. Antimicrob. Ag. Chemother. 772—786 (1962).

PANETTIERE, F., COLTMAN, C.A.: Phase I experience with emetine hydrochloride (NSC 33669) as an antitumor agent. Cancer **27**, 835—841 (1971).

PAVAN, M., BO, G.: Pederin, toxic principle obtained in the crystalline state from the beetle *Paederus fuscipes curt.* Physiol. Comp. Oecol. **3**, 307 (1953).

PEARCE, M.B., BULLOCH, R.T., MURPHY, M.L.: Selective damage of myocardial mitochondria due to emetine hydrochloride. Arch. Pathol. **91**, 8—18 (1971).

PERANI, A., PARISI, B., DE CARLI, L., CIFERRI, O.: Incorporation of amino acids by a cell-free system prepared from human cells cultured *in vitro*. Biochim. biophys. Acta (Amst.) **161**, 223—231 (1968).

PESTKA, S.: Inhibitors of ribosome functions. Ann. Rev. Microbiol. **25**, 487—562 (1971).

PESTKA, S.: Inhibitors of ribosome functions. In: MUNOZ, E., GARCIA-FERRENDIZ, F., VAZQUEZ, D. (Eds.): Molecular mechanisms of antibiotic action on protein biosynthesis and membranes, p. 160. New York: American Elsevier 1972.

POWELL, R.G., WEISLEDER, D., SMITH, C.R., JR., WOLFF, I.A.: Structure of cephalotaxine and related alkaloids. Tetrahedron Let. **46**, 4081—4084 (1969).

RAO, S. S., GROLLMAN, A. P.: Cycloheximide resistance in yeast: a property of the 60 S ribosomal subunit. Biochem. biophys. Res. Commun. **29**, 696—704 (1967).
ROLLO, I. M.: Drugs used in the chemotherapy of amebiasis. In: GOODMAN, L. S., GILMAN, A. (Eds.): The pharmacological basis of therapeutics, 4th ed., p. 1125. New York: Macmillan 1970.
SIEGEL, M. R., SISLER, H. D., JOHNSON, F.: Relationship of structure to fungitoxicity of cycloheximide and related glutarimide derivatives. Biochem. Pharmacol **15**, 1213—1223 (1966).
SISLER, H. D., SIEGEL, M. R.: Cycloheximide and other glutarimide antibiotics. In: GOTTLIEB, D., SHAW, P. D. (Eds.): Antibiotics I. Mechanism of action, p. 283. New York: Springer-Verlag 1967.
SOLDATI, M., FIORETTI, A., GHIONE, M.: Cytotoxicity of pederin and some of its derivatives on cultured mammalian cells. Experientia (Basel) **22**, 176—178 (1966).
STRAUSS, N., HENDEE, E. D.: The effect of diphtheria toxin on the metabolism of HeLa cells. J. exp. Med. **109**, 145—163 (1959).
SUMMERS, D. F., MAIZEL, J. V., JR.: Determination of the gene sequence of poliovirus with pactamycin. Proc. nat. Acad. Sci. (Wash.) **68**, 2852—2856 (1971).
TABER, R., REKOSH, D., BALTIMORE, D.: Effect of pactamycin on synthesis of poliovirus proteins: a method for genetic mapping. J. Virology **8**, 395—401 (1971).
VAN HOOSEN, B.: Emetine hydrochloride in malignancy. Women's med. J. **29**, 101—116 (1919).
VAZQUEZ, D., BATTANER, E., NETH, R., HELLER, G., MONRO, R. E.: The function of 80 S ribosomal subunits and effects of some antibiotics. Cold Spr. Harb. Symp. Quant. Biol. **34**, 369—375 (1969).
VEDDER, E. B.: An experimental study of the action of ipecacuanha on amoebae. J. trop. Med. **15**, 313 (1912).
WATKINS, W. D., GUESS, W. L.: Toxicity of emetine to isolated embryonic chick-heart cells. J. pharm. Sci. **57**, 1968—1974 (1968).
WELCH, J. F.: Rodent control. A review of chemical repellents for rodents. J. Agr. food Chem. **2**, 142—149 (1954).
WHITE, F. R.: Actidione. Cancer Chemother. Rep. **5**, 48—52 (1959).
WILEY, P. F., JAHNKE, H. K., MAC KELLER, F., KELLEY, R. B., ARGOUDELIS, A. D.: The structure of pactamycin. J. org. Chem. **35**, 1420—1425 (1970).
WILKIE, D., LEE, B. K.: Genetic analysis of actidione resistance in *Saccharomyces cerevisiae*. Genet. Res. Camb. **6**, 130—138 (1965).

Chapter 58

Selective Interruption of RNA Metabolism by Chemotherapeutic Agents

HERBERT T. ABELSON and SHELDON PENMAN

With 2 Figures

Introduction

Chemotherapeutic agents have generally been considered to exert their cytotoxic effects by directly interacting with DNA metabolism or by inhibiting enzymatic steps within the multiple pathways of purine and pyrimidine nucleotide metabolism (for review, see ROY-BURMAN, 1970). It has now become increasingly clear that most agents have multiple effective sites or targets within the cell, and that their effect on macromolecular metabolism may be of prime importance. This chapter will deal only with ribonucleic acid (RNA) metabolism and how various RNA species can be selectively inhibited by drugs. In addition, where possible, suggestions will be given on how this selectivity may be strategically utilized in designing a rational basis for chemotherapy.

The past few years have seen rapid advances in the understanding of macromolecular metabolism in mammalian cells. Many of the important aspects of RNA synthesis and processing are now understood, and in many respects these differ significantly from the biochemistry of prokaryotes (for reviews see DARNELL, 1968; PENMAN et al., 1969, 1970; PERRY et al., 1970; WEINBERG, 1973). Fundamental to many of these advances has been the development of selective inhibitors of various macromolecular processes. These inhibitors serve in mammalian cell biology in a manner similar to that of genetic variants in prokaryotic biochemical investigation. The genetic information of the cell is encoded within DNA molecules. Before this information can be utilized, it must be transcribed into RNA. Several different types of RNA are known to be metabolically active in cellular processes. RNA species are described by a special nomenclature relating to the migration of RNA species in a centrifugal field; both the RNA size and secondary structure are involved in determining its unique sedimentation characteristics. RNA molecules are therefore characterized as having a certain number of SVEDBERGS (S), a measure of the RNA sedimentation coefficient. Molecular weights of various RNA species are related to their S values, but the relation is not linear. In mammalian cells, the major RNA component is ribosomal RNA, which comprises more than 80% of the total cellular RNA. Ribosomal RNA, in intimate association with structural proteins, comprises the ribosome, a cellular organelle which is the site at which protein synthesis occurs. The greater part of stable RNA in the mammalian cell is therefore destined to become a structural component of the ribosome. At least two other species of RNA are associated with protein synthesis, messenger RNA, and transfer RNA.

Since ribosomal RNA plays such a central role in normal cellular processes, agents that interfere with its metabolism produce serious defects in the integrity of the cell. A great deal is now known about the biogenesis of ribosomes in mammalian cells (PERRY, 1969); this process has been localized to the nucleolus.

Nucleolus

The nucleolus is the site of precursor ribosomal RNA (rRNA) synthesis and processing (PERRY, 1964; PENMAN et al., 1966; WEINBERG and PENMAN, 1970). The most precise description of nucleolar metabolism has been obtained using HeLa cells in tissue culture. The first event is transcription with simultaneous methylation of giant RNA molecules (45 S RNA) which are the precursor to rRNA. Transcription occurs from nucleolar DNA cistrons. The subsequent processing of this 45 S RNA precursor is nonconservative, with progressive loss of nonmethylated portions. Each 45 S RNA molecule gives rise to one 32 S RNA molecule and one 18 S RNA molecule. The 32 S RNA molecule undergoes further nonconservative processing with loss of nonmethylated regions to form a 28 S RNA molecule which is retained in the nucleus for a short period of time and then enters the cytoplasm as a portion of the large ribosomal subunit. The 18 S molecule is rapidly transported from the nucleolus to the cytoplasm, where it becomes incorporated into the small ribosomal subunit. A schematic representation of ribosomal precursor RNA synthesis and processing to mature cytoplasmic rRNA species is shown in Fig. 1.

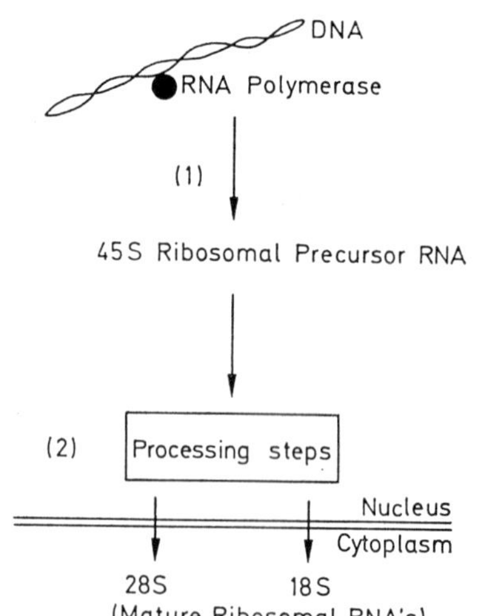

Fig. 1. Schematic synthesis and processing of ribosomal RNA (rRNA)

Agents which interfere with:

(1) formation of ribosomal precursor RNA (45 S)

Actinomycin D	Nitrogen Mustard
Daunomycin	Cordycepin
Mithramycin	3′-Deoxycytidine
CCNU	Ellipticine
Camptothecin	

(2) processing of 45 S RNA to cytoplasmic rRNA

Toyocamycin	Ellipticine
Sangivamycin	Proflavin
Formycin	Ethidium Bromide
BCNU	5-Fluorouridine
CCNU	5-Azacytidine

Drugs that inhibit the formation of rRNA can act either at the DNA template, thereby affecting the synthesis of the ribosomal precursor RNA (i.e., 45 S RNA), or by interfering with the processing of rRNA. In eukaryotic cells, the rRNA genes represent a small percentage of the total DNA, but this comprises a sensitive "target" for a number of agents. This may be possibly a reflection of the high G+C content of the rRNA genes, but more likely is related to a physical property, such as protein shielding, polymerase specificity, or, most likely, clustering of the rRNA genes (PERRY and KELLEY, 1968; PENMAN et al., 1968).

One of the first nucleolar-specific agents studied in detail was actinomycin D. Actinomycin D forms complexes with cellular DNA (KIRK, 1960) by specifically interacting with guanine moieties in the minor groove of helical DNA (for reviews see REICH et al., 1967; SOBELL et al., 1971). This interaction has the effect of inhibiting DNA-dependent RNA polymerases. The dose-dependent differential inhibition of actinomycin D on rRNA was first shown by PERRY (1962, 1963). This effect was later quantitated for various RNA species (PERRY and KELLY, 1970). The explanation for the extreme sensitivity of rRNA to inhibition by actinomycin D in comparison with other RNA species is not certain, but may involve a combination of factors: (1) high G+C content of rRNA genes and preferential binding of actinomycin D to guanine residues; (2) clustering of rRNA genes as evidenced from electron micrographs (MILLER and BEATTY, 1969). If a limited number of initiation sites for the RNA polymerase are present within a cluster of 45 S rRNA genes, then the binding of an actinomycin D molecule will inhibit transcription of all 45 S rRNA genes between that initiation site and the next, assuming that the polymerase reads sequentially and does not detach from the DNA template (PENMAN et al., 1968; PERRY and KELLY, 1970).

Selective inhibition of ribosomal precursor RNA or 45 S RNA has been reported for daunomycin (CROOK et al., 1972; DANØ et al., 1972; KANN and KOHN, 1972a), cordycepin (3′-deoxyadenosine) (SIEV et al., 1969; KANN and KOHN, 1972a), nogalamycin (BHUYAN and SMITH, 1965; ELLEM and RHODE, 1970), 3′-deoxycytidine (ABELSON and PENMAN, 1972b), mithramycin (ABELSON and PENMAN, 1972c), CCNU [1-(2-chloroethyl)-3-cyclohexyl-1-nitrosourea] (ABELSON et al., 1974), as well as actinomycin D (PERRY, 1962, 1963). Although somewhat less selective, preferential inhibition of 45 S RNA occurs with nitrogen mustard (ABELSON et al., 1974), camptothecin (ABELSON and PENMAN, 1972a), and ellipticine (ABELSON and PENMAN, 1972c; KANN and KOHN, 1972a). Inhibition of nucleolar RNA metabolism by nitrogen mustard and camptothecin has also been noted by KANN and KOHN (1972a), but they considered the effect to be primarily one of producing shortened RNA chains without selective inhibition of 45 S RNA synthesis. Other agents, such as anthramycin (KANN and KOHN, 1972b) and thalicarpine (ABELSON and PENMAN, 1972c), show no selective inhibition of RNA synthesis.

The mechanisms by which inhibition occurs are quite different and allow a partial classification of these agents. It is known that actinomycin D exerts its action at the level of transcription by inhibiting DNA-dependent RNA polymerase. The mode of action of CCNU is unknown, but it may selectively alkylate initiation sites for 45 S RNA synthesis (ABELSON et al., 1974).

Chain termination is a common mode of inhibiting nucleolar RNA, as demonstrated by cordycepin (3′-deoxyadenosine), 3′-deoxycytidine, and nitrogen mustard. In the latter class of compounds, a broad distribution of shortened RNA chains is found in the nucleolus rather than complete 45 S RNA molecules. This presumably occurs because the polymerase is prevented from transcribing the entire gene segment. In the case of the nucleoside analogs, the premature termination is probably due to the insertion into a growing RNA chain of the altered base, which will not allow further nucleotide addition (i.e., a blocked 3′ position occurs after the insertion 5′ → 3′ of the nucleotides of cordycepin or 3′-deoxycytidine). Nitrogen mustard may exert its effect by alkylating sites within the nucleolar DNA cistrons, thereby allowing only partial transcription. The effect of camptothecin on the nucleolus is specific in that a unique 24 S RNA species is synthesized and methylated rather than a broad distribution of shortened chains (ABELSON and PENMAN, 1972a). This appears to be a prematurely shortened 45 S precursor terminated at a specific site. With continuous labeling over long periods, little or no 45 S rRNA precursor is formed (ABELSON and PENMAN, 1972c).

Processing of 45 S RNA subsequent to synthesis can also be interrupted by several agents in different ways. The nucleoside analog, toyocamycin, and the related compounds, sangivamycin and formycin, are known to be incorporated into the growing 45 S rRNA precursor molecule and may exert their effects by physical alteration of the molecule. After treatment with these analogs, conversion of 45 S RNA to 32 S RNA is significantly inhibited and mature rRNA species are not found in the cytoplasm (TAVITIAN et al., 1969; SVERAK et al., 1970; ABELSON and PENMAN, 1973a). 5-Azacytidine may also be incorporated into the 45 S rRNA precursor molecule and inhibit processing, but its mode of action is quite different (JUROVČIK, 1965). After treatment with 5-azacytidine, the 45 S rRNA precursor molecule disappears in an actinomycin D "chase", the normal nucleolar products are not formed, and essentially no 32 S RNA is recoverable (REICHMAN et al., 1973). The processing is therefore nonconservative or destructive. 5-Fluorouridine has also been reported to inhibit processing (WILKINSON and PITOT, 1973). Compounds such as ellipticine, ethidium bromide, and proflavin also block processing. Since these are primarily intercalating agents, their modes of action may be by direct physical interference with processing (SNYDER et al., 1971b; ABELSON and PENMAN, 1972c). Other drugs which may also physically interfere with processing are the alkylating agents BCNU (1,3-*bis*(2-chloroethyl)-1-nitrosourea) (KANN et al., 1971; ABELSON et al., 1974) and CCNU (ABELSON et al., 1974).

Nuclear Heterogeneous RNA (HnRNA) and Messenger RNA (mRNA)

The HnRNA is now widely accepted as the precursor to cytoplasmic mRNA (KATES, 1970; DARNELL et al., 1971; EDMONDS et al., 1971; LEE et al., 1971; WALL and DARNELL, 1972). The HnRNA, found in the nucleoplasm, is transcribed as heterogeneously sedimenting RNA with S values from 20 S to greater than 100 S. *In vitro* experiments have identified several DNA-dependent RNA polymerases which have been distinguished by their location within the nucleus and by cation specificities (ROEDER and RUTTER, 1969, 1970; ZYLBER and PENMAN, 1971). Polymerase II is the major nucleoplasmic polymerase and can be inhibited by α-amanitin, while the nucleolar polymerase (Polymerase I) is not affected by the drug. There are no agents currently available which will selectively inhibit the synthesis of HnRNA in intact cells. However, some drugs will dramatically alter the size of the HnRNA formed, primarily by interrupting the formation of high molecular weight RNA. Camptothecin and nitrogen mustard both interfere with the synthesis of high molecular weight RNA and produce instead a distribution of HnRNA with an average sedimentation of about 26 S (WU et al., 1971; ABELSON and PENMAN, 1972a; KANN and KOHN, 1972a). Both drugs appear to interact with DNA and cause a premature termination of the transcription of HnRNA. In both cases, the size of the RNA produced is independent of the concentration of the drug once a threshold level has been reached. This suggests specific sites of interaction which become saturated with the larger drug concentrations. It is also interesting that the size of the RNA produced by the two agents is approximately the same, suggesting that, if indeed specific sites on the DNA are involved, they are similar for both compounds.

After longer labeling periods in the presence of camptothecin, the radioactive HnRNA increases in size and approaches a normal distribution in sedimentation values. This possibly reflects occasional breakthroughs of the inhibited sites by the polymerase. However, the effect is clearly a complex one and at present is not fully understood. It cannot be ascribed solely to a reduced rate of chain elongation. The ability of camptothecin to produce single-strand DNA fragments in alkaline sucrose gradients is also complex and may not be related to the shortened RNA segments (ABELSON and PENMAN, 1973b). In contrast, the size of the HnRNA labeled in the presence of nitrogen mustard is constant and apparently the alkylation of the DNA by this compound is irreversible and no readthrough occurs.

Both drugs completely suppress the appearance of labeled mRNA in the cytoplasm, presumably by preventing the completion of HnRNA and its subsequent processing to form mRNA for export from the nucleus. Even though some RNA of apparently normal size is produced in the nucleoplasm in the case of camptothecin, little or no mRNA results, implying that either very small amounts of this RNA are formed or the process is never normal.

Another class of agents interferes with the formation of mRNA at a step subsequent to the transcription of HnRNA. With cordycepin (PENMAN et al., 1970), formycin (ABELSON and PENMAN, 1973a), and BCNU (ABELSON et al., 1974), the synthesis of HnRNA appears to be normal. With each of these agents, however, mRNA appearance in the cytoplasm is inhibited to varying degrees. Since all of these agents allow the HnRNA to be synthesized in apparently normal size and amounts, and the HnRNA is precursor to cytoplasmic mRNA, then inhibition must occur at some post-transcriptional step.

It has now been firmly established that the HnRNA and cytoplasmic mRNA both contain a segment of polyadenylic acid [poly(A)] at their 3′ terminus (KATES, 1970; DARNELL et al., 1971; EDMONDS et al., 1971; LEE et al., 1971). A unique poly(A) segment has also been found to be associated with mitochondrial RNA (PERLMAN et al., 1973). An exception to the above is histone mRNA, which has been shown not to contain a poly(A) segment at its 3′ terminus (ADESNIK and DARNELL, 1972). No other RNA species within the cell has been found to have a poly(A) segment included in its structure. These poly(A) segments are approximately 150 to 200 nucleotides long, and are probably added to the HnRNA as a post-transcriptional modification (DARNELL et al., 1971; PHILIPSON et al., 1971). The function of the poly(A) is unknown, although it may have some importance as a signal for the subsequent cleavage and transport of the mRNA molecule to the cytoplasm. Cordycepin severely inhibits the formation of the poly(A) at concentrations which minimally affect the synthesis of HnRNA (PENMAN et al., 1970; ABELSON and PENMAN, 1972c; MENDECKI et al., 1972). The appearance of rapidly synthesized polysomal-associated RNA (i.e., mRNA) is less than 10% of the expected amount.

In the presence of BCNU, HnRNA is synthesized normally and there seems to be a normal component of poly(A) synthesized. The poly(A) is also found attached to the HnRNA. Since mRNA appearance in the cytoplasm is severely inhibited, BCNU seems to affect HnRNA molecules after poly(A) has been added (i.e., cleavage of the 5′ end of the molecule or transport of the mRNA to the cytoplasm) (ABELSON et al., 1974). At present, these possibilities cannot be distinguished.

The HnRNA, like nucleolar RNA, therefore seems to have a number of distinct processing steps which must proceed in an orderly fashion for mature mRNA to appear in the cytoplasm. The processing scheme for the HnRNA is only beginning to be elucidated. A schematic, and probably idealized, representation is found in Fig. 2. As is the case with nucleolar RNA, there are a number of steps in processing at which drugs may exert their inhibitory effects.

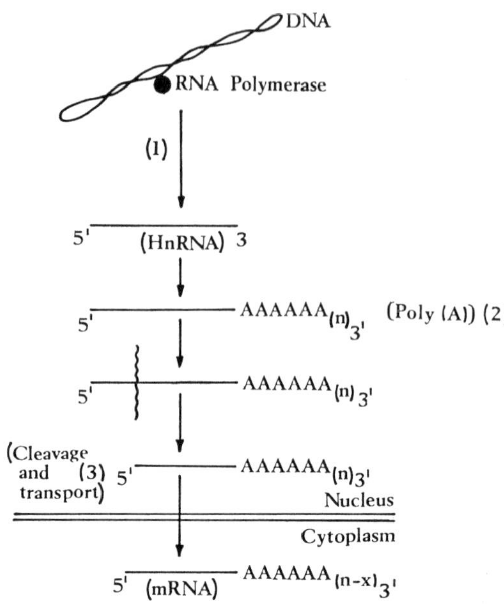

Fig. 2. Schematic synthesis and processing of nuclear heterogeneous RNA (HnRNA)

Agents which interfere with:
(1) transcription of giant HnRNA molecules
Actinomycin D — Nitrogen Mustard
Camptothecin — Anthramycin
(2) proper poly (A) formation
Cordycepin — Toyocamycin
Formycin — Sangivamycin
Camptothecin
(3) cleavage and/or transport of mRNA to the cytoplasm
BCNU — Cordycepin (?)

4S and 5S RNA

Most agents that have an effect on RNA synthesis will inhibit the formation of 4 S and 5 S RNA to some degree. One agent has been found that seems to exert a relatively selective inhibition of the synthesis of 4 S and 5 S RNA. Formycin, an adenosine analog, at concentrations that do not affect the synthesis of nucleolar RNA or HnRNA, significantly depresses the synthesis of 4 S and 5 S RNA (Abelson and Penman, 1973a). There is evidence from other systems that low molecular weight RNA may be synthesized by a separate polymerase activity (Price and Penman, 1972). The selective inhibition of 4 S and 5 S RNA by the drug formycin suggests that a possibly separate polymerase activity from those which transcribe HnRNA and nucleolar RNA is responsible for the transcription of 4 S and 5 S RNA.

Mitochondrial RNA

Mitochondrial RNA metabolism can be selectively inhibited with ethidium bromide (ZYLBER et al., 1969). Concentrations of ethidium bromide which will produce this selective inhibition are very low (1 μg/ml) and have no measurable effect on other cellular processes. At much larger concentrations, the drug has been reported to interfere with nucleolar processing (KANN and KOHN, 1972a).

Many of the compounds that interfere with nuclear RNA metabolism have no effect on mitochondria, either because of a failure to penetrate the mitochondrial membrane or a lack of sensitivity of the mitochondrial enzymatic components. An excellent example is the drug camptothecin, which completely suppresses the appearance of any nuclear RNA into the cytoplasm, but has no apparent effect on mitochondrial metabolism (BOSMAN, 1970; ABELSON and PENMAN, 1972a). Thus, detailed studies of mitochondrial RNA are possible by using this inhibitor.

An interesting example of the distinctiveness of mitochondrial RNA metabolism is afforded by the selective effects of cordycepin on mitochondrial RNA. It will be recalled that this drug has little effect on the transcription of HnRNA, but blocks the formation of poly(A). In contrast, mitochondrial transcription is blocked, presumably because the mitochondrial polymerase is sensitive to the altered nucleoside. However, poly(A) formation is unaffected and poly(A) continues to be added to preformed RNA long after transcription of DNA is completely suppressed (HIRSH and PENMAN, 1973).

This brief summary of agents which inhibit RNA metabolism is intended to point out that there exist specific macromolecular targets for some chemotherapeutic agents. Table 1 summarizes these effects. The selectivity with which these

Table 1. Species of RNA Inhibited

Drug	Ribosomal Precursor RNA (45 S)	Interference with Nucleolar Processing	Heterogeneous Nuclear RNA (HnRNA)	Messenger RNA (mRNA)	Poly(A)	Selective Inhibition of 4 S and 5 S RNA	Mitochondrial RNA
Actinomycin D	+++	—	+	—			+
Mithramycin	+++		+				
Daunorubricin	+++	—	+				
Cordycepin	+++	—	-	+++	+++		+++
3′-Deoxycytidine	+++	—	—	—	—		—
Nogalamycin	+++		+				
Camptothecin	+++	—	++	+++	+++		—
Anthramycin	++	—	++				
Formycin	—	++	—	++	+	++	
Toyocamycin	—	++	+		+++		
Sangivamycin	—	++	+		+++		
5-Azacytidine	—	++	—	—			
CCNU[a]	++	++	—	+			
BCNU[a]	+	++	—	++	—		
Nitrogen Mustard	+++	—	++	+++	+++		
Proflavin	+	++					
Ethidium Bromide	+	+					+++
Ellipticine	+++	+++	++				
5-Fluorouridine	+	++					

Key: Degree of Inhibition + mild, ++ moderate, +++ severe, — none

[a] Abbreviations used: CCNU,1-(2-chloroethyl)-3-cyclohexyl-1-nitrosourea; BCNU,1,3-*bis* (2-chloroethyl)-1-nitrosourea.

agents inhibit macromolecular processes has been exploited in the study of cell biology in order to focus upon distinct species of RNA.

Some Examples of the Use of Selective Inhibitors

Actinomycin D has been an invaluable agent for the study of mRNA. Its ability at low concentrations to inhibit the formation of rRNA, while leaving mRNA unaffected, has enabled the synthesis, kinetics, and decay of mRNA to be examined in detail (ROBERTS and NEWMAN, 1966; PENMAN et al., 1968). At concentrations which inhibit all DNA-dependent RNA polymerase activity, the use of actinomycin D has contributed greatly to our understanding of the processing of nucleolar RNA and transfer RNA (BERNHARDT and DARNELL, 1969; WEINBERG and PENMAN, 1970). After incorporation of a radioactive precursor, a "chase" experiment with actinomycin D allows the fate of ribosomal precursor RNA and pre-tRNA to be studied.

A separate series of metabolic pathways for DNA, RNA, and protein synthesis exists in mitochondria. The toxicity of some agents depends on whether they affect the mitochondria. The measurement of macromolecular metabolism in mitochondria is facilitated by potent selective inhibitors (i.e., ethidium bromide and chloramphenicol) which permit an unambiguous measurement of the effect of an unknown agent on mitochondrial DNA, RNA, and protein synthesis. On the other hand, camptothecin allows a critical study of mitochondrial RNA metabolism. The effect of camptothecin on RNA synthesis is dramatic and results in the selective interruption of synthesis of high molecular weight nuclear RNA. Therefore, no new messenger RNA or ribosomal RNA is synthesized in the presence of the drug, while mitochondrial macromolecular metabolism is not affected. This not only allows the isolation of mitochondrial macromolecules, but the latter are obtained free of contaminating cellular mRNA. This degree of selectivity was not previously attainable using actinomycin D or cell fractionation techniques. With nuclear contamination eliminated, it has become feasible to look within mitochondria for messenger-like RNA. A class of heterogeneous RNA containing a segment of poly(A) unique in size for eukaryotic cells has been identified, and this was associated with the mitochondrial protein-synthesizing structure. Association with a protein-synthesizing structure, the poly(A) segment (in eukaryotic cells, poly(A) is found only in the heterogeneous nuclear RNA or pre-messenger RNA and in cytoplasmic mRNA), and the fact that the messenger-like RNA can be released from the protein-synthesizing structure by puromycin, all lend support to the contention that this class of RNA is truly a mitochondrial mRNA (PERLMAN et al., 1973). Camptothecin has additional utility in that its effect on RNA metabolism is rapidly reversible (HORWITZ et al., 1971; KESSEL, 1971).

An agent like 3′-deoxycytidine may be of particular importance. Since this agent affects only nucleolar RNA synthesis, without affecting other macromolecular processes, it may have specificity for proliferating cells and therefore be useful as an immunosuppressive agent.

The major aim of any systematic characterization of chemotherapeutic agents by their effects on cellular macromolecular metabolism is to obtain knowledge of mechanisms which would make possible the beginnings of a theoretical basis for combination drug therapy. A rationale for synergism between agents should become possible when drug targets and their relative importance to cell survival are known. An example of drug synergism, which is not readily predictable by current means, is that found between BCNU and actinomycin D. BCNU has an inhibitory effect on protein synthesis and acts specifically at the initiation of translation

(ABELSON and PENMAN, 1972c). Polyribosomes rapidly disaggregate in the presence of this agent. This effect is partially reversible if the agent is removed, with the return of a normal polyribosome profile and incorporation of radioactive leucine into newly formed proteins. The reaggregation of polyribosomes can be blocked with low levels of actinomycin D.

Therapeutic regimes currently in use have evolved primarily through empirical observation. It is essential that means be established to examine systematically the effects of chemotherapeutic agents on cellular processes. Ultimately, it should prove possible to make use of biochemical and clinical findings to maximize the effect of agents on selected cellular targets while minimizing undesired toxicity. Once our understanding of drug and cellular metabolism has provided a rational basis for designing individual therapy, not only will morbidity and mortality be reduced, but strides will have been made toward the control of fundamental biological processes.

References

ABELSON, H. T., KARLAN, D., PENMAN, S.: A comparison of the effects of alkylating agents on HeLa cell macromolecular metabolism. Biochim. biophys. Acta (Amst.), in press (1974).

ABELSON, H. T., PENMAN, S.: Selective interruption of high molecular weight RNA synthesis in HeLa cells by camptothecin. Nature New Biol. **237**, 144—146 (1972a).

ABELSON, H. T., PENMAN, S.: Messenger RNA formation: resistance to inhibition by 3'-deoxycytidine. Biochim. biophys. Acta (Amst.) **277**, 129—133 (1972b).

ABELSON, H. T., PENMAN, S.: unpublished observations.

ABELSON, H. T., PENMAN, S.: Selective inhibition of 4 S and 5 S RNA synthesis and nucleolar processing by the adenosine analogue formycin. Biochim. biophys. Acta (Amst.) **312**, 292—296 (1973a).

ABELSON, H. T., PENMAN, S.: Induction of alkali labile links in cellular DNA by camptothecin. Biochem. biophys. Res. Commun. **50**, 1048—1054 (1973b).

ADESNIK, M., DARNELL, J. E.: Biogenesis and characterization of histone messenger RNA in HeLa cells. J. molec. Biol. **67**, 397—406 (1972).

BERNHARDT, D., DARNELL, J. E.: tRNA Synthesis in HeLa cells: a precursor to tRNA and the effects of methionine starvation on tRNA synthesis. J. molec. Biol. **42**, 43—56 (1969).

BHUYAN, B. K., SMITH, C. G.: Differential interaction of nogalamycin with DNA of varying base composition. Proc. nat. Acad. Sci. (Wash.) **54**, 566—572 (1965).

BOSMAN, H. B.: Camptothecin inhibits macromolecular synthesis in mammalian cells but not in isolated mitochondria or *E. coli*. Biochem. biophys. Res. Commun. **41**, 1412—1420 (1970).

CROOK, L. E., REES, K. R., COHEN, A.: Effect of daunomycin on HeLa cell nucleic acid synthesis. Biochem. Pharmacol. **21**, 281—286 (1972).

DANØ, K., FREDERIKSEN, S., HELLUNG-LARSEN, P.: Inhibition of DNA and RNA synthesis by daunorubicin in sensitive and resistant Ehrlich ascites tumor cells *in vitro*. Cancer Res. **32**, 1307—1314 (1972).

DARNELL, J. E., JR.: Ribonucleic acids from animal cells. Bact. Rev. **32**, 262—290 (1968).

DARNELL, J. E., PHILIPSON, L., WALL, R., ADESNIK, M.: Polyadenylic acid sequences: role in conversion of nuclear RNA into messenger RNA. Science **174**, 507—510 (1971).

DARNELL, J. E., WALL, R., TUSHINSKI, R.: An adenylic acid-rich sequence in messenger RNA of HeLa cells and its possible relationship to reiterated sites in DNA. Proc. nat. Acad. Sci. (Wash.) **68**, 1321—1325 (1971).

EDMONDS, M., VAUGHAN, M. H., NAKAZOTO, N.: Polyadenylic acid sequences in the heterogeneous nuclear RNA and rapidly-labeled polyribosomal RNA of HeLa cells: possible evidence for a precursor relationship. Proc. nat. Acad. Sci. (Wash.) **68**, 1336—1340 (1971).

ELLEM, K. A. O., RHODE, S. L., III: Selective inhibition of ribosomal RNA synthesis in HeLa cells by nogalamycin, a dA:dT binding antibiotic. Biochim. biophys. Acta (Amst.) **209**, 415—425 (1970).

HIRSH, M., PENMAN, S.: unpublished observations.

HORWITZ, S. B., CHANG, C., GROLLMAN, A. P.: Abstract in Pharmacologist **12**, 283 (1970).

JUROVČIK, M., RÁSKA, K., JR., ŠORMOVÁ, Z., ŠORM, F.: Anabolic transformation of a novel antimetabolite 5-azacytidine, and evidence for its incorporation into RNA. Coll. Czech. Chem. Commun. **30**, 3370—3376 (1965).

Kann, H. E., Jr., Kohn, K. W.: Effects of deoxyribonucleic acid-reactive drugs on ribonucleic acid synthesis in leukemia L1210 cells. Molec. Pharmacol. **8**, 551—560 (1972a).
Kann, H. E., Jr., Kohn, K. W.: Effects of anthramycin and actinomycin on RNA synthesis patterns in L1210 cells. J. cell Physiol. **79**, 331—342 (1972b).
Kann, H. E., Jr., Snyder, A. L., Kohn, K. W.: Effects of chemotherapeutic agents on RNA synthesis in L1210 cells. Proc. Amer. Assoc. Cancer Res. **12**, 59 (1971).
Kates, J.: Transcription of the vaccinia virus genome and the occurrence of polyriboadenylic acid sequences in messenger RNA. Cold Spr. Harb. Symp. Quant. Biol. **35**, 743—752 (1970).
Kessel, D.: Effects of camptothecin on RNA synthesis in leukemia L1210 cells. Biochim. biophys. Acta (Amst.) **246**, 225—232 (1971).
Kirk, J. M.: The mode of action of actinomycin D. Biochim. biophys. Acta (Amst.) **42**, 167—169 (1960).
Lee, S. Y., Mendecki, J., Brawerman, G.: A polynucleotide segment rich in adenylic acid in the rapidly-labeled polyribosomal RNA component of mouse sarcoma 180 ascites cells. Proc. nat. Acad. Sci. (Wash.) **68**, 1331—1335 (1971).
Mendecki, J., Lee, S. Y., Brawerman, G.: Characteristics of the polyadenylic acid segment associated with messenger ribonucleic acid in mouse sarcoma 180 ascites cells. Biochemistry **11**, 792—798 (1972).
Miller, O. L., Jr., Beatty, B. R.: Nucleolar structure and function, Chapter 24. In: Lima-de-Faira, A. (Ed.): Handbook of molecular cytology. Amsterdam: North-Holland 1969.
Penman, S., Fan, H., Perlman, S., Rosbash, M., Weinberg, R., Zylber, E.: Distinct RNA synthesis systems of the HeLa cell. Cold Spr. Harb. Symp. Quant. Biol. **35**, 561—575 (1970).
Penman, S., Rosbash, M., Penman, M.: Messenger and heterogeneous nuclear RNA in HeLa cells: differential inhibition by cordycepin. Proc. nat. Acad. Sci. (Wash.) **67**, 1878—1885 (1970).
Penman, S., Smith, I., Holtzman, E.: Ribosomal RNA synthesis and processing in a particulate site in the HeLa cell nucleus. Science **154**, 786—789 (1966).
Penman, S., Vesco, C., Penman, M.: Localization and kinetics of formation of nuclear heterodisperse RNA, cytoplasmic heterodisperse RNA and polyribosome-associated messenger RNA in HeLa cells. J. molec. Biol. **34**, 49—69 (1968).
Penman, S., Vesco, C., Weinberg, R., Zylber, E.: The RNA metabolism of nucleoli and mitochondria in mammalian cells. Cold Spr. Harb. Symp. Quant. Biol. **34**, 535—546 (1969).
Perlman, S., Abelson, H. T., Penman, S.: Mitochondrial protein synthesis: RNA with the properties of eukaryotic messenger RNA. Proc. nat. Acad. Sci. (Wash.) **70**, 350—353 (1973).
Perry, R. P.: The cellular sites of synthesis of ribosomal and 4 S RNA. Proc. nat. Acad. Sci. (Wash.) **48**, 2179—2186 (1962).
Perry, R. P.: Selective effects of actinomycin D on the intra-cellular distribution of RNA synthesis in tissue culture cells. Exp. Cell Res. **29**, 400—406 (1963).
Perry, R. P.: Role of the nucleolus in ribonucleic acid metabolism and other cellular processes. Nat. Cancer Inst. Monograph **14**, 73—89 (1964).
Perry, R. P.: Nucleoli: the cellular sites of ribosome production, Chapter 25. In: Lima-de-Faira, A. (Ed.): Handbook of molecular cytology. Amsterdam: North-Holland 1969.
Perry, R. P., Greenberg, J. R., Tartof, K. D.: Transcription of ribosomal, heterogeneous nuclear and messenger RNA in eukaryotes. Cold Spr. Harb. Symp. Quant. Biol. **35**, 577—587 (1970).
Perry, R. P., Kelley, D. E.: Inhibition of RNA synthesis by actinomycin D: characteristic dose-response of different RNA species. J. Cell Physiol. **76**, 127—140 (1970).
Philipson, L., Wall, R., Glickman, G., Darnell, J. E.: Addition of polyadenylate sequences to virus-specific RNA during adenovirus replication. Proc. nat. Acad. Sci. (Wash.) **68**, 2806—2809 (1971).
Price, R., Penman, S.: A distinct RNA polymerase activity synthesizing 5.5 S, 5 S and 4 S RNA in nuclei from adenovirus 2-infected HeLa cells. J. molec. Biol. **70**, 435—450 (1972).
Reich, E., Cerami, A., Ward, D. C.: Actinomycin. In: Gottlieb, D., Shaw, P. D. (Eds.): Antibiotics I: Mechanism of action. New York: Springer-Verlag 1967.
Reichman, M., Karlan, D., Penman, S.: Destructive processing of the 45 S ribosomal precursor in the presence of 5-azacytidine. Biochim. biophys. Acta (Amst.) **299**, 173—175 (1973).
Roberts, W. K., Newman, J. F. E.: Use of low concentrations of actinomycin D in the study of RNA synthesis in Ehrlich ascites cells. J. molec. Biol. **20**, 63—73 (1966).
Roeder, R. G., Rutter, W. J.: Multiple forms of DNA-dependent RNA polymerase in eukaryotic organisms. Nature (Lond.) **224**, 234—236 (1969).
Roeder, R. G., Rutter, W. J.: Specific Nucleolar and Nucleoplasmic RNA Polymerases. Proc. nat. Acad. Sci. (Wash.) **65**, 675—682 (1970).
Roy-Burman, P.: Analogues of nucleic acid components, Vol. 25 of Recent results in cancer research. New York: Springer-Verlag 1970.

SIEV, M., WEINBERG, R., PENMAN, S.: The selective interruption of nucleolar RNA synthesis in HeLa cells by cordycepin. J. Cell Biol. **41**, 510—520 (1969).
SNYDER, A.L., KANN, H.E., Jr., KOHN, K.W.: Inhibition of processing of ribosomal precursor RNA by intercalating agents. J. molec. Biol. **58**, 555—565 (1971).
SOBELL, H.M., JAIN, S.C., SAKORE, T.D.: Stereochemistry of actinomycin-DNA binding. Nature New Biol. **231**, 200—205 (1971).
SVERAK, L., BONAR, R.A., LANGLOIS, A.J., BEARD, J.W.: Inhibition by toyocamycin of RNA synthesis in mammalian cells and normal and avian tumor virus-infected chick embryo cells. Biochim. biophys. Acta (Amst.) **224**, 441—450 (1970).
TAVITIAN, A., URETSKY, S.C., ACS, G.: The effect of toyocamycin on cellular RNA synthesis. Biochim. biophys. Acta (Amst.) **179**, 50—57 (1969).
WALL, R., DARNELL, J.E.: Presence of cell and virus specific sequences in the same molecules of nuclear RNA from virus transformed cells. Nature New Biol. **232**, 73—76 (1971).
WEINBERG, R.A.: Nuclear RNA metabolism. Ann. rev. Biochem. **42**, 329—354 (1973).
WEINBERG, R.A., PENMAN, S.: Processing of 45 S nucleolar RNA. J. molec. Biol. **47**, 169—178 (1970).
WILKINSON, D.S., PITOT, H.C.: Inhibition of ribosomal ribonucleic acid maturation in Novikoff hepotoma cells by 5-fluorouracil and 5-fluorouridine. J. biol. Chem. **248**, 63—68 (1973).
WU, R.S., KUMAR, A., WARNER, J.R.: Ribosome formation is blocked by camptothecin, a reversible inhibitor of RNA synthesis. Proc. nat. Acad. Sci. (Wash.) **68**, 3009—3014 (1971).
ZYLBER, E.A., PENMAN, S.: Products of RNA polymerases in HeLa cell nuclei. Proc. nat. Acad. Sci. (Wash.) **68**, 2861—2865 (1971).
ZYLBER, E., VESCO, C., PENMAN, S.: Selective inhibition of the synthesis of mitochondrial associated RNA by ethidium bromide. J. molec. Biol. **44**, 195—204 (1969).

Chapter 59

Actinomycin D

IRVING H. GOLDBERG

With 2 Figures

Introduction

The actinomycins are a group of bright red, highly toxic, peptide-containing antibiotics that were discovered in 1940; they were the first antibiotics to be isolated from actinomycetes (WAKSMAN and WOODRUFF, 1940). The isolation, production, and chemistry, as well as the biological and clinical uses of actinomycin have recently been reviewed (WAKSMAN, 1968). Since the findings of KIRK (1960) that actinomycin C_1(D) (Fig. 1), one of the most potent agents in the group, complexes with DNA and selectively inhibits RNA synthesis in microorganisms, there has been considerable interest in the use of this antibiotic in the study of nucleic acid synthesis and function, and in the elucidation, in molecular terms, of the antibiotic binding site on DNA (REICH and GOLDBERG, 1964; GOLDBERG and FRIEDMAN, 1971). Complex formation between actinomycin and DNA appears to account for the primary toxicity of the antibiotic in both prokaryotic and eukaryotic cells.

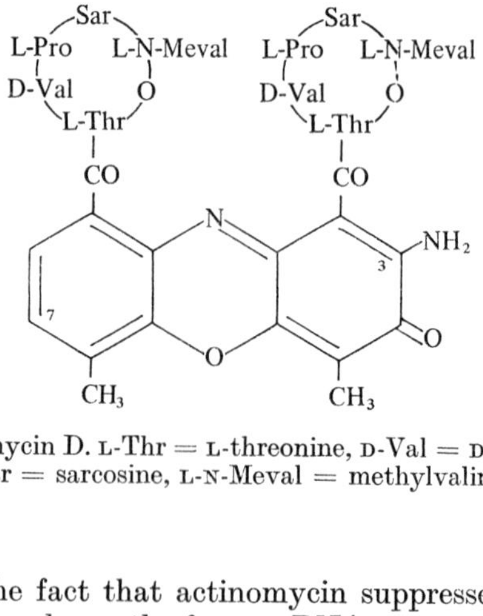

Sar Sar
L-Pro L-N-Meval L-Pro L-N-Meval
D-Val O D-Val O
L-Thr L-Thr
CO CO
N
NH_2
3
7
O
O
CH_3 CH_3

Fig. 1. Structure of actinomycin D. L-Thr = L-threonine, D-Val = D-valine, L-Pro = L-proline, Sar = sarcosine, L-N-Meval = methylvaline

This is suggested by the fact that actinomycin suppresses the growth of DNA viruses, but permits normal growth of many RNA viruses (REICH and GOLDBERG, 1964; REICH et al., 1961). Since synthesis of the DNA virus requires formation of new RNA using the entering DNA as template, whereas synthesis of many RNA viruses does not make use of cellular or other DNA for new RNA synthesis, it appears that the antibiotic affects only those cellular activities which require the direct participation of DNA itself. By complexing with DNA, actinomycin inhibits the DNA-dependent synthesis of RNA by intact cells (KIRK, 1960; REICH et al., 1961; HARBERS and MÜLLER, 1962) and by the isolated eukaryotic and prokaryotic RNA polymerase (GOLDBERG and RABINOWITZ, 1962; HURWITZ et al., 1962; REICH et al., 1962; HARTMANN et al., 1962), with RNA chain elongation, not initiation, being blocked (RICHARDSON, 1966; MAITRA et al., 1967; SENTENAC et al., 1968; HYMAN and DAVIDSON, 1970). DNA synthesis by intact cells or by the isolated DNA polymerase is inhibited by actinomycin, but considerably higher levels of the antibiotic are needed than for comparable inhibition of RNA synthesis, indicating that different mechanisms are involved. In fact, inhibition of the DNA polymerase is found only at concentrations of actinomycin which are large enough to stabilize the helical DNA structure against strand separation, normally required for DNA replication (REICH, 1964). Other cellular processes (see REICH and GOLDBERG, 1964) that require the direct participation of DNA, such as cell division, bacteriophage maturation, the growth of certain RNA viruses (influenza, tumor viruses), DNA modification (i.e., methylation) (GOLD and HURWITZ, 1964), repair, or degradation (SARKAR, 1967; SULKOWSKI and LASKOWSKI, 1968; KAGEYAMA et al., 1970), and maintenance of chromosome morphology, are all sensitive to the antibiotic. Thus, the DNA-dependent, but not the RNA-dependent DNA polymerases of RNA tumor viruses, such as Rous sarcoma virus, avian myeloblastosis virus, and Rauscher murine leukemia virus, are sensitive to actinomycin (McDONNELL et al., 1970; MÜLLER et al., 1971). This selectivity of action has resulted in the widespread use of actinomycin in the study of gene action, cellular differentiation, virus life-cycles, and the role of RNA synthesis in many biological systems, including enzyme induction and degradation, neoplastic transformation, and hormone and vitamin action (see REICH and GOLDBERG, 1964). As would be expected of an agent which acts by forming a complex with cellular DNA, resistance of both bacterial and mammalian cells to actinomycin has been found to be due to reduced permeability into the cells (SLOTNICK and SELLS, 1964; BIEDLER and RIEHM, 1970; BOSMANN, 1971). While actinomycin has been used widely to measure the half-life of cellular RNA by blocking the formation of new RNA, this use has been subject to criticism since the drug has been found both to accelerate mammalian nuclear RNA degradation (WIESNER et al., 1965; STEWART and FARBER, 1968; ROVERA et al., 1970), and to prolong the half-life of liver messenger RNA (ENDO et al., 1971).

Site of Action in Mammalian Cells

Actinomycin is selectively concentrated in the nucleus of the normal mammalian cell where it is found in association with the DNA (DINGMAN and SPORN, 1965). Actinomycin-treated cells show profound nuclear and nucleolar morphological changes (JOURNEY and GOLDSTEIN, 1961; HEINE et al., 1966; RECHER et al., 1971; GOLDSTEIN et al., 1960; REYNOLDS et al., 1964; STENRAM, 1964, 1965, 1966; PERRY, 1963; SCHOEFL, 1964; GOLDBLATT et al., 1969; HAZLETT, 1971; PHILLIPS and PHILLIPS, 1971; DE MAN and NOORDUYN, 1967) which include nuclear condensation, nucleolar segregation, and finally a disaggregation of nucleolar components. DNA isolated from animals treated with actinomycin functions poorly as template for *in vitro* transcription (BECKER, 1966). Tritiated actinomycin has been shown to bind to the chromosomes of several species of eukaryotes (EBSTEIN, 1967; CAMARGO and PLANT, 1967; SIMARD, 1967). Euchromatin binds more actinomycin than heterochromatin (HARBERS and VOGT, 1966; DESAI and TENCER, 1968; BERLOWITZ et al., 1969). The pattern of binding of labeled actinomycin to human chromosomes is nonrandom with some tendency for radioactivity to be concentrated at the ends of the chromosomes and near the centromere (MILES, 1970). It is of note, however, that while actinomycin induces breaks in human chromosomes (OSTERTAG and KERSTEN, 1965), the sites of the breaks do not correspond with the sites of the actinomycin label (MILES, 1970). Although the binding sites for actinomycin in purified DNA are qualitatively similar to those in deoxyribonucleoprotein preparations, there are more than twice as many sites available in DNA, suggesting that histone and other proteins in chromatin block these sites (DINGMAN and SPORN, 1964; JURKOWITZ, 1965; DESAI and TENCER, 1968; BERLOWITZ et al., 1969; RINGERTZ and BOLUND, 1969; KLEIMAN and HUANG, 1971). Of interest is the finding that the increase in actinomycin binding shows a more linear relationship with the removal of protein by salt than by acid (KLEIMAN and HUANG, 1971). The binding of actinomycin to DNA in intact cells suggests a correlation between the extent of binding and the growth activity (RNA synthetic activity) of the cells (see BOLUND, 1970 for a review), which may also be due to the transcriptional control by chromatin protein. It is possible, however, that permeability factors play a more important role in this phenomenon.

It is of interest that while the inhibitory action of actinomycin on RNA synthesis in mammalian cells correlates with tissue levels of the drug, cytotoxicity does not (SCHWARTZ et al., 1968). Instead, cytotoxicity appears to depend more on the prolonged retention of the antibiotic in the cell (SCHWARTZ et al., 1968; KESSEL and WODINSKY, 1968).

Actinomycin suppresses the formation of all cellular RNA fractions (REICH et al., 1961), although at concentrations of antibiotic that do not completely suppress RNA formation there is a differential inhibition of the various RNA classes, with ribosomal RNA being most susceptible (PERRY, 1962; GEORGIEV et al., 1963; FRANKLIN, 1963; REVEL and HIATT, 1964; YAMADA, 1965), and inhibition may be partially reversible in certain animal cells (SCHLUEDERBERG et al., 1971; BENEDETTO and DJACZENKO, 1972). Further, the greater sensitivity of the synthesis of ribosomal RNA appears to reside in the transcription process for this species of RNA and is not linked to the specific mechanism of action of the antibiotic, since several other unrelated inhibitors also cause a preferential block in ribosomal RNA synthesis (MACKEDONSKI and HADJIOLOV, 1970). This action of actinomycin has been related to the target size of the gene or operon being transcribed, since the sensitivity of *in vitro* RNA synthesis has been shown to be a function of the size of the RNA being made (BLEYMAN and WOESE, 1969). On the other hand, an adenylate-uridylate rich 45 S RNA made in nucleoli of Novikoff hepatoma ascites cells has been found to be relatively resistant to actinomycin compared with a similar RNA possessing a high guanylate-cytidylate content (CHOI and BUSCH, 1969). Of additional interest is the finding that a double-stranded RNA continues to be synthesized in animal cells exposed to high doses of actinomycin (STERN and FRIEDMAN, 1971).

Structural Features Required for Biological Activity

The actinomycins offer unique opportunities for correlating biological activity with molecular structure. Many different actinomycins have been isolated and characterized and a large number of chemically altered actinomycins, with various degrees of change in the phenoxazone chromophore or the cyclic pentapeptides have been prepared (see WAKSMAN, 1968; MÜLLER and CROTHERS, 1968, for the work of H. BROCKMANN). A strong correlation has been found between the ability of the antibiotics to complex with DNA and their inhibition of bacterial and mammalian cell growth and of the RNA polymerase reaction (REICH et al., 1962). Changes in different portions of the actinomycin molecule may affect its inhibitory properties to a greater or lesser extent but the integrity of several functional groups is essential for biological activity and ability to form stable complexes with DNA. These functional groups are: (1) the free amino group at position 3 of the chromophore, (2) the unreduced quinoidal oxygen, and (3) the intact, cyclic pentapeptide lactones. Although certain substitutions or modifications in the amino acid sequence of the cyclic peptides may cause only minor changes in actinomycin activity, other changes which produce major alterations in the conformational properties of the pentapeptides markedly affect antibiotic activity (see REICH and GOLDBERG, 1964; MÜLLER and CROTHERS, 1968; ASCOLI and SAVINO, 1968; ASCOLI et al., 1968).

Complex formation between DNA and actinomycin can be measured by changes in the visible spectrum of the antibiotic, by equilibrium dialysis with radioactive antibiotic, by the decrease in the buoyant density and increase in the melting temperature of the DNA, and by the inhibition of the template activity of the DNA in enzymic RNA synthesis. Actinomycin interacts with DNA, but not with single stranded DNA, RNA, or RNA-DNA hybrids (HASELKORN, 1964), to form stable but reversible complexes. A considerable body of evidence has been accumulated to show that complex formation requires that the DNA be helical and possess the 2-amino function of guanine residues (GOLDBERG et al., 1962; REICH and GOLDBERG, 1964; GOLDBERG, 1965; CERAMI et al., 1967). Although there are two classes of binding sites in DNA, the one involving the G-C (guanine-cytosine) base pair is the strongly binding one and is responsible for the biological activity of actinomycin. Thus, actinomycin does not form stable complexes with DNA's such as synthetic $d(\text{A-T})_n$ or $d(\text{I-C})_n$ (the strictly alternating deoxyadenylate-deoxythymidylate and deoxyinosinate-deoxycytidylate copolymers, respectively) which lack the 2-amino function of guanine, and these DNA's function as templates for the RNA polymerase with complete immunity to actinomycin. Naturally occurring and most synthetic DNA's containing even small amounts of guanine react with the antibiotic. On the other hand, the binding of actinomycin is less than expected if it were to be strictly proportional to the amount of guanine, especially in the middle and higher ranges of guanine contents in DNA (GELLERT et al., 1965). These data suggest that other factors may also determine actinomycin binding, such as steric hindrance by the bound antibiotic or local distortions in the DNA at the site of antibiotic binding which prevent the complexing of an adjacent actinomycin molecule. It is also possible that the binding site on the DNA may involve more than one base pair, one of which is G-C; however, the possibility that adjacent guanines (or adjacent guanine and other purine) on the *same* strand are required to create the strong binding site has been excluded (HYMAN and DAVIDSON, 1967; WELLS and LARSON, 1970; HYMAN and DAVIDSON, 1971).

The most direct demonstration that the presence of the 2-amino function of a purine in DNA is necessary for actinomycin binding comes from experiments with synthetic DNA's with identical primary structures except for the presence or absence of the purine 2-amino group (CERAMI et al., 1967). Synthetic DNA's possessing 2,6-diaminopurine instead of 6-aminopurine (adenine) as the only purine in the DNA were shown to form stable complexes with actinomycin, and their template activity with the RNA polymerase was sensitive to the antibiotic. On the other hand, the analogous DNA possessing adenine, which lacks the 2-amino group, did not interact with actinomycin at all. Recently, however, there have been reports on two synthetic DNA's, one lacking a purine with a 2-amino group and the other possessing guanine, which appear to bind and not bind, respectively, to actinomycin (WELLS and LARSON, 1970). The results have been interpreted to indicate that while guanine in DNA usually is responsible for creating a structure in the DNA for actinomycin binding, this need not always be so. Since the three dimensional structure of the polydeoxyribonucleotide is crucial as a determinant for actinomycin binding, the significance of these isolated findings for complex formation between actinomycin and natural DNA must await elucidation of their structures. Furthermore, a recent detailed analysis of the transcription process supports the role of G-C base pairs in actinomycin binding and action (HYMAN and DAVIDSON, 1970). A study of the rates of incorporation of the precursor nucleotides in the RNA polymerase reaction showed a selective effect of actinomycin on the utilization of CTP and GTP (not ATP and UTP). In fact, since the rate of utilization of CTP (coded by guanine in DNA) was inhibited twice as effectively as that of GTP (coded by cytosine in DNA), it appeared that the antibiotic interacts with DNA in an unsymmetrical way with respect to guanine and cytosine in the DNA.

Models of Actinomycin Binding Site on DNA

Two basically different types of models have been proposed to describe the molecular nature of the actinomycin binding site on DNA: (1) the outside binding model (HAMILTON et al., 1963) and (2) the intercalation model (MÜLLER and CROTHERS, 1968). In the outside binding model, actinomycin is considered to be located in the smaller (minor) of the two grooves of helical DNA with which it can form up to seven hydrogen bonds (HAMILTON et al., 1963). According to the model, one hydrogen bond is formed between the quinoidal oxygen of actinomycin and the 2-amino group (which projects into the minor groove of DNA) of guanine, and the 3-amino group of the actinomycin chromophore forms one hydrogen bond each with the ring nitrogen 3 and the ribose-ring oxygen of the deoxyguanosine. The cyclic peptides of actinomycin are packed into the minor groove of the DNA helix. The lactones presumably stabilize the peptide chains in a conformation permitting the formation of four additional hydrogen bonds between the four peptide-NH groups of actinomycin and the phosphodiester oxygens of the DNA strand opposite to that containing the guanine which interacts with the actinomycin chromophore. Recently, a variant of this type of model has been proposed in which the cyclic peptides lie *trans* to one another in the minor groove of DNA (GURSKY, 1969). In this model, the cyclic peptides occupy a region in the DNA minor groove equivalent to about 6 base pairs, thus excluding, by steric hindrance, the binding of another actinomycin molecule within this distance. Such a proposal is consistent with binding data that show that a maximum of about one actinomycin molecule is bound per 6 G-C base pairs in DNA's rich in G-C.

The outside binding model accounts for the structures in DNA on which complex formation depends. Thus, only guanine can furnish the 2-amino hydrogen in the DNA minor groove for which the actinomycin quinoidal oxygen can serve as acceptor. Furthermore, the model depends critically on the relative positions of the DNA constituents as they are disposed in helical DNA in its native conformation and thus is in accord with the fact that actinomycin binds poorly, if at all, to single-stranded DNA, and does not bind to DNA-RNA hybrids or double-stranded RNA, which are thought to exist in other conformations.

In the second type of model the actinomycin phenoxazone chromophore is postulated to be intercalated between adjacent base pairs in the DNA (MÜLLER and CROTHERS, 1968). MÜLLER and CROTHERS (1968) found that actinomycin increased the viscosity and decreased the sedimentation coefficient of low molecular weight DNA, but had opposite effects on DNA of high molecular weight. They interpreted these results to indicate that the length of the DNA is increased by complex formation as would be found with intercalation. Presumably actinomycin induces a sort of crosslinking of high molecular weight DNA (which is flexible enough to coil back on itself) by increasing the tendency of parts of the DNA to interact with each other. Furthermore, substitution of bulky groups on the 7 position of the actinomycin chromophore markedly slowed down the combination of actinomycin with DNA. This would not have been predicted by the outside binding model in which actinomycin lies on the outside of the DNA molecule, since the 7 position on the actinomycin chromophore would project away from the helix. These workers proposed that the actinomycin chromophore intercalates between the base pairs of DNA adjacent to any G-C pair. The chromophore is inserted from the minor groove, into which the peptide rings project. The specificity for guanine is attributed to electronic interactions in the π-complex formed in the intercalated structure; the actinomycin chromophore ring nitrogen would fall directly under the 2-amino group of the purine. In the most stable form of the actinomycin-DNA complex, the peptide rings undergo conformational changes that adapt their structure to interact specifically with the DNA backbone, one ring interacting with each strand of the double helix in the minor groove. The slow reversal of the peptide ring conformation is viewed as accounting for the slow dissociation of actinomycin from DNA and as being the basis for the high order of effectiveness of actinomycin on the RNA polymerase reaction as compared with simpler analogs of the antibiotic. It should be noted that in both of the proposed model types, the peptide rings of actinomycin lie in the minor groove of the DNA where the path of the advancing RNA polymerase might be blocked. MÜLLER and CROTHERS (1968) suggest that the selective resistance of the DNA polymerase reaction to actinomycin is due to the local denaturation immediately ahead of the enzyme that causes the antibiotic to dissociate much faster. Consistent with the intercalation model are experiments (WARING, 1970) in which actinomycin has been found to lead to the uncoiling of the replicative form (closed circular duplex DNA) of bacteriophage $\varphi \times 174$ in a manner similar to that of ethidium bromide, an intercalating dye.

Recently, a new model (Fig. 2), combining features of the two previous models, has been proposed for the actinomycin-DNA complex based on x-ray data obtained from a crystalline complex containing actinomycin and deoxyguanosine (SOBELL et al., 1971; SOBELL, 1972). In this model the phenoxazone ring system of actinomycin intercalates between adjacent G-C base pairs of DNA, where the guanine moieties are on opposite DNA strands, and the 2-amino groups of the guanines interact with both cyclic peptides through specific hydrogen bonds. As in the other models, the cyclic peptides lie in the minor groove of helical DNA. There is much to suggest that this model may be the correct one.

The actinomycin-deoxyguanosine complex contains one actinomycin, two deoxyguanosines, and ten water molecules. Both the actinomycin molecule and the complex formed with the two deoxyguanosine molecules have two-fold symmetry. The actinomycin chromophore extends outside and perpendicular to the peptide rings. In the complex, the two deoxyguanosine molecules interact with the two cyclic peptide residues by a strong hydrogen bond between the 2-amino group of guanine and the carbonyl oxygen of the L-threonine residue and stack on alternate sides of the phenoxazone ring system. A weaker hydrogen bond connects the guanine N3 ring nitrogen with the NH group on this same L-threonine residue. The sugar residues of both deoxyguanosine molecules are in close steric juxtaposition with the isopropyl groups of the L-methyl valine residues, and such hydro-

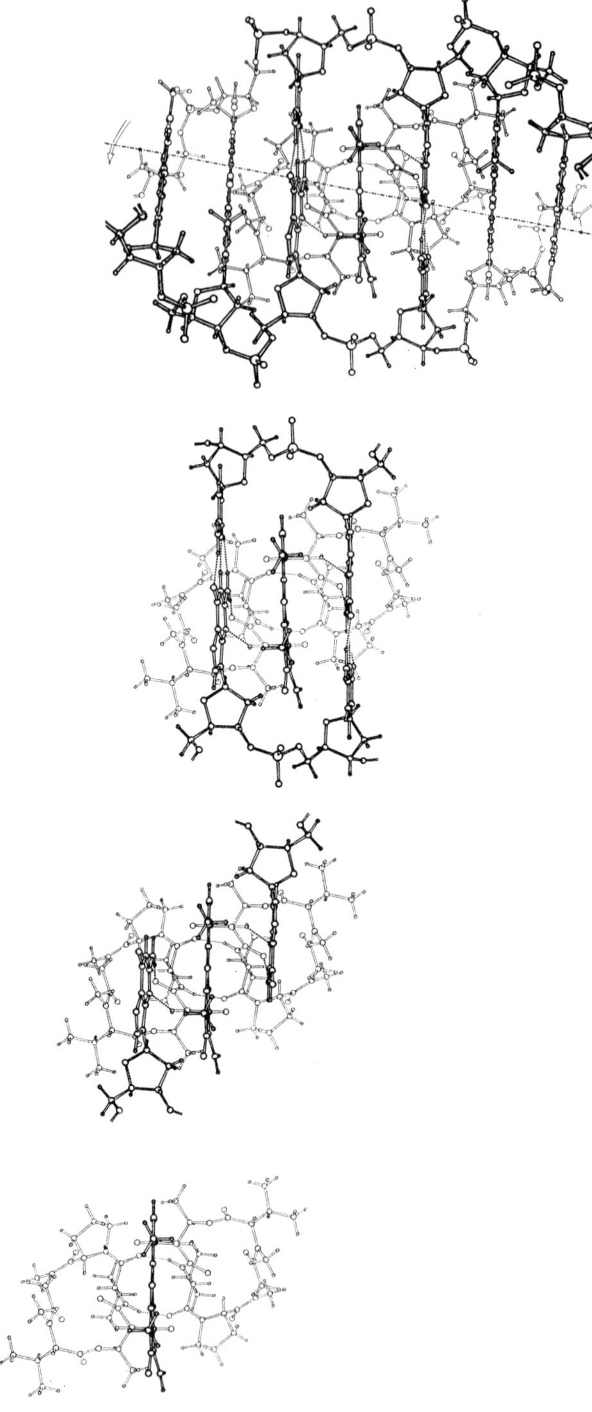

Fig. 2. Steps in the assembly of the actinomycin-DNA stereochemical model (after SOBELL, 1972). From left to right: actinomycin, viewed down its dyad axis; the actinomycin-deoxyguanosine complex, viewed down its dyad axis; the actinomycin-d-G_pC complex; and the actinomycin-d-$A_pT_pG_pC_pA_pT$ complex. A = adenosine, G = guanosine, C = cytosine, and T = thymidine. Dotted lines indicate hydrogen bonds. Arrows indicate 5′—3′ direction of DNA chains. Oligodeoxyribonucleotides are represented as double-stranded structures

phobic interactions, as well as the stacking of guanine and phenoxazone rings, provides stability to the complex, but it is the hydrogen-bonding which plays a key role in the association and explains the requirement for guanine in the binding of actinomycin with DNA.

In the proposed actinomycin-DNA model, both sugar residues on deoxyguanosine and deoxycytidine of the same strand are rotated so as to reduce the helix twist from 36° in the B form of DNA to about 15°, and this provides adequate space for intercalation of the actinomycin chromophore between the base pairs. This results in close steric juxtaposition of the 2-amino group on the chromophore residue to phosphate and the deoxycytidine furanose ring oxygen with hydrogen bonds being likely between them. This model predicts that poly $(G\text{-}C)_n$ (strictly alternating deoxyguanylate-deoxycytidylate) which contains the sequence $G_3'P_5'C$ should bind actinomycin best, although other sequences containing guanine can bind actinomycin, but with lower affinity and efficiency. This is supported by the binding data of WELLS and LARSON (1970) (although possibly not by those of GELLERT et al., 1965).

Clinical Uses of Actinomycin D

In addition to its widespread use in the study of various biological phenomena, actinomycin D has been of value clinically for immunosuppression and in the treatment of certain solid tumors. Actinomycin has been especially effective as an antitumor agent when administered in sequential combination with radiotherapy. It is possible, in fact, that the clinically observed synergism between actinomycin and ionizing radiation (D'ANGIO et al., 1959; BASES, 1959) is due to interference by actinomycin with the cellular repair of damage to DNA induced by x-rays. In the treatment of disseminated malignancies, actinomycin D has proven of particular value against Wilms' tumor, testicular tumors, and choriocarcinoma (see WAKSMAN, 1968; LIVINGSTON and CARTER, 1970, for review of clinical usage and toxicology). Actinomycin D has also been effective in the treatment of hypercalcemia associated with tumors producing parathormone-like substances (MUGGIA et al., 1968).

Carcinogenicity of Actinomycin D

Actinomycin D has been found to be a carcinogen. Thus, multiple intraperitoneal injections of the antibiotic in rats have been found to produce invasive, transplantable tumors which resemble mesotheliomas (SVOBODA et al., 1970). The biologically inactive analog, actinocylgramicidin S, which contains the same chromophore as actinomycin D but different peptides and which does not bind to DNA, is not oncogenic.

References

ASCOLI, F., SAVINO, M.: Interaction between model compounds of actinomycin D and DNA.: DNA dependent RNA synthesis. Nature (Lond.) **217**, 162 (1968).

ASCOLI, F., SAVINO, M., LIQUORI, A. M.: Interaction between model compounds of actinomycin and DNA: Physicochemical studies. Nature (Lond.) **217**, 162—164 (1968).

BASES, R. E.: Modification of the radiation response determined by single-cell technics: actinomycin D. Cancer Res. **19**, 1223—1229 (1959).

BECKER, F. F., MARGOLIS, A. A., TROLL, W.: *In vivo* complex formation of actinomycin D and deoxyribonucleic acid. Nature (Lond.) **211**, 84—85 (1966).

BENEDETTO, A., DJACZENKO, W.: 37 RC cells rapidly recover their RNA synthesis after inhibition with high doses of actinomycin D. J. Cell Biol. **52**, 171—174 (1972).

BERLOWITZ, L., PALLOTTA, D., SIBLEY, C. H.: Chromatin and histones: binding of tritiated actinomycin D to heterochromatin in mealy bugs. Science **164**, 1527—1529 (1969).

Biedler, J. L., Riehm, H.: Cellular resistance to actinomycin D in Chinese hamster cells *in vitro:* cross-resistance, radioautographic, and cytogenetic studies. Cancer Res. **30**, 1174—1184 (1970).
Bleyman, M., Woese, C.: Transcriptional mapping. I. Introduction to the method and the use of actinomycin D as a transcriptional mapping agent. Proc. nat. Acad. Sci. (Wash.) **63**, 532—539 (1969).
Bolund, L.: Actinomycin D binding to isolated deoxyribonucleoprotein and intact cells. Exp. Cell Res. **63**, 171—188 (1970).
Bosmann, H. B.: Mechanism of cellular drug resistance. Nature (Lond.) **233**, 566—569 (1971).
Camargo, E. P., Plaut, W. J.: The radioautographic detection of DNA with tritiated actinomycin D. J. Cell Biol. **35**, 713—716 (1967).
Cerami, A., Reich, E., Ward, D. C., Goldberg, I. H.: The interaction of actinomycin with DNA. Requirement for the 2-amino group of purines. Proc. nat. Acad. Sci. (Wash.) **57**, 1036—1042 (1967).
Choi, Y. C., Busch, H.: Effects of actinomycin D on the oligonucleotide composition of nucleolar 45 S RNA of Novikoff hepatoma ascites cells. Biochim. biophys. Acta (Amst.) **174**, 766—769 (1969).
D'Angio, G. J., Farber, S., Maddock, C. L.: Potentiation of x-ray effects by actinomycin D. Radiology **73**, 175—177 (1959).
De Man, J. C. H., Noorduyn, N. J. A.: Light and electron microscopic radioautography of hepatic cell nucleoli in mice treated with actinomycin D. J. Cell Biol. **33**, 489—496 (1967).
Desai, L., Tencer, R.: Effects of histones and polylysine on the synthetic activity of the giant chromosomes of salivary glands of dipteran larvae. Exp. Cell Res. **52**, 185—197 (1968).
Dingman, C. W., Sporn, M. B.: Studies on chromatin. Isolation and characterization of nuclear complexes of deoxyribonucleic acid, ribonucleic acid and protein from embryonic and adult tissues of the chicken. J. biol. Chem. **239**, 3483—3492 (1964).
Dingman, C. W., Sporn, M. B.: Actinomycin D and hydrocortisone: intracellular binding in rat liver. Science **149**, 1251—1254 (1965).
Ebstein, B. S.: Tritiated actinomycin D as a cytochemical label for small amounts of DNA. J. Cell Biol. **35**, 709—713 (1967).
Endo, Y., Tominaga, H., Natori, Y.: Effect of actinomycin D on turnover rate of messenger ribonucleic acid in rat liver. Biochim. biophys. Acta (Amst.) **240**, 215—217 (1971).
Franklin, R. M.: The inhibition of ribonucleic acid synthesis in mammalian cells by actinomycin D. Biochim. biophys. Acta (Amst.) **72**, 555—565 (1963).
Gellert, M., Smith, C. E., Neville, D., Felsenfeld, G.: Actinomycin binding to DNA. Mechanism and specificity. J. molec. Biol. **11**, 445—457 (1965).
Georgiev, G. P., Samarina, O. P., Lerman, M. I., Smirnov, M. N., Severtzov, A. N.: Biosynthesis of messenger and ribosomal ribonucleic acids in the nucleolochromosomal apparatus of animal cells. Nature (Lond.) **200**, 1291—1294 (1963).
Gold, M., Hurwitz, J.: The enzymatic methylation of ribonucleic acid and deoxyribonucleic acid. VI. Further studies on the properties of the deoxyribonucleic acid methylation reaction. J. biol. Chem. **239**, 3866—3874 (1964).
Goldberg, I. H.: Mode of action of antibiotics. II. Drugs affecting nucleic acid and protein synthesis. Amer. J. Med. **39**, 722—752 (1965).
Goldberg, I. H., Friedman, P. A.: Antibiotics and nucleic acids. Ann. Rev. Biochem. **40**, 775—810 (1971).
Goldberg, I. H., Rabinowitz, M.: Actinomycin D inhibition of nucleic acid dependent synthesis of ribonucleic acid. Science **136**, 315—316 (1962).
Goldberg, I. H., Rabinowitz, M., Reich, E.: Basis of actinomycin action. I. DNA binding and inhibition of RNA-polymerase synthetic reactions by actinomycin. Proc. nat. Acad. Sci. (Wash.) **48**, 2094 (1962).
Goldblatt, P. J., Sullivan, R. J., Farber, E.: Induction of partial nucleolar segregation in hepatic parenchymal cells by actinomycin D following inhibition of ribonucleic acid synthesis by ethionine. Lab. Invest. **20**, 283—291 (1969).
Goldstein, M. N., Slotnick, I. J., Journey, L. J.: *In vitro* studies with HeLa cell lines sensitive and resistant to actinomycin D. Ann. N. Y. Acad. Sci. **89**, 474—483 (1960).
Gursky, G. V.: Structure of DNA-actinomycin complex. Molek. Biol. (USSR) **3**, 749—757 (1969).
Hamilton, L., Fuller, W., Reich, E.: X-ray diffraction and molecular model binding studies of the interaction of actinomycin with nucleic acids. Nature (Lond.) **198**, 538—540 (1963).
Harbers, E., Müller, W.: On the inhibition of RNA synthesis by actinomycin. Biochem. biophys. Res. Commun. **7**, 107—110 (1962).
Harbers, E., Vogt, M.: Studies on the properties of nucleohistones. Proceedings of the International Symposium on Cell Nuclear Metabolism and Radiosensitivity, Rijswijk, The Netherlands, p. 165, 1966.

HARTMANN, G., COY, U., KNIESE, G.: Zum biologischen Wirkungsmechanismus der Actinomycine. Z. Physiol. Chem. **330**, 227—233 (1962).
HASELKORN, R.: Actinomycin D as a probe for nucleic acid secondary structure. Science **143**, 682—684 (1964).
HEINE, U., LANGLOIS, A. J., BEARD, J. W.: Ultrastructural alterations in avian leukemia myeloblasts exposed to actinomycin D *in vitro*. Cancer Res. **26**, 1847—1858 (1966).
HURWITZ, J., FURTH, J. J., MALAMY, M., ALEXANDER, M.: The role of deoxyribonucleic acid in ribonucleic acid synthesis. III. The inhibition of the enzymatic synthesis of ribonucleic acid and deoxyribonucleic acid by actinomycin D and proflavin. Proc. nat. Acad. Sci. (Wash.) **48**, 1222—1230 (1962).
HYMAN, R. W., DAVIDSON, N.: The binding of actinomycin to crab *d*AT. The nature of the DNA binding site. Biochem. biophys. Res. Commun. **26**, 116—120 (1967).
HYMAN, R. W., DAVIDSON, N.: Kinetics of the *in vitro* inhibition of transcription by actinomycin. J. molec. Biol. **50**, 421—438 (1970).
HYMAN, R. W., DAVIDSON, N.: The binding of actinomycin D to crab poly *d*AT poly *d*(T—A). II. On the nature of the DNA binding site. Biochim. biophys. Acta (Amst.) **228**, 38—48 (1971).
JOURNEY, L. J., GOLDSTEIN, M. N.: Electron microscope studies on HeLa cell lines sensitive and resistant to actinomycin D. Cancer Res. **21**, 929—932 (1961).
JURKOWITZ, L.: Actinomycin D binding by calf thymus deoxyribonucleic acid and nucleoprotein. Arch. biochem. Biophys. **111**, 88—95 (1965).
KAGEYAMA, M., HASEGAWA, M., INAGAKI, A., EGAMI, F.: Interaction of antibiotics with deoxyribonucleic acid. I. Sensitivity of the complexes to nucleolytic enzymes. J. Biochem. (Tokyo) **67**, 549—557 (1970).
KESSEL, D., WODINSKY, I.: Uptake *in vivo* and *in vitro* of actinomycin D by mouse leukemias as factors in survival. Biochem. Pharmacol. **17**, 161—164 (1968).
KIRK, J.: The mode of action of actinomycin D. Biochim. biophys. Acta (Amst.) **42**, 167—169 (1960).
KLEIMAN, L., HUANG, R. C. C.: Binding of actinomycin D to calf thymus chromatin. J. molec. Biol. **55**, 503—521 (1971).
LIVINGSTON, R. B., CARTER, S. K.: Single agents in cancer chemotherapy. New York-Washington-London: IFI/Plenum 1970.
MACKEDONSKI, V. V., HADJIOLOV, A. A.: Selective inhibition of ribosomal RNA synthesis in Ehrlich ascites tumor cells by a non-specific inhibitor, 2,4-dinitrophenol. Biochim. biophys. Acta (Amst.) **204**, 462—469 (1970).
MAITRA, U., NAKATA, Y., HURWITZ, J.: The role of deoxyribonucleic acid in ribonucleic acid synthesis. XIV. A study of the initiation of ribonucleic acid synthesis. J. biol. Chem. **242**, 4908—4918 (1967).
McDONNELL, J. P., GARAPIN, A. C., LEVINSON, W. E., QUINTRELL, N., FANSHIER, L., BISHOP, J. M.: DNA polymerases of Rous sarcoma virus: delineation of two reactions with actinomycin. Nature (Lond.) **228**, 433—435 (1970).
MILES, C. P.: Labeling and other effects of actinomycin D on human chromosomes. Proc. nat. Acad. Sci. (Wash.) **65**, 585—592 (1970).
MÜLLER, W., CROTHERS, D. M.: Studies on the binding of actinomycin and related compounds to DNA. J. molec. Biol. **35**, 251—290 (1968).
MÜLLER, W. E. G., ZAHN, R. K., SEIDEL, H. J.: Inhibitors acting on nucleic acid synthesis in an oncogenic RNA virus. Nature New Biol. **232**, 143—145 (1971).
MUGGIA, F. M., HEINEMANN, H. O., BELANGER, R., WEINSTEIN, I. B.: Hyperparathyroid-like hypercalcemia in neoplastic disease — treatment with dactinomycin. Clin. Res. **16**, 558a (1968).
OSTERTAG, W., KERSTEN, W.: The action of proflavin and actinomycin D in causing chromatid breakage in human cells. Exp. Cell Res. **39**, 296—301 (1965).
PERRY, R. P.: The cellular sites of synthesis of ribosomal and 4 S RNA. Proc. nat. Acad. Sci. (Wash.) **48**, 2179—2186 (1962).
PERRY, R. P.: Selective effects of actinomycin D on the intracellular distribution of RNA synthesis in tissue culture cells. Exp. Cell Res. **29**, 400—406 (1963).
PHILLIPS, S. G., PHILLIPS, D. M.: Nucleoli of diploid cell strains: their normal ultrastructure and the effects of toyocamycin and actinomycin D. J. Cell Biol. **49**, 785—802 (1971).
RECHER, L., BRIGGS, I. G., PARRY, N. T.: A re-evaluation of nuclear and nucleolar changes induced *in vitro* by actinomycin D. Cancer Res. **31**, 140—151 (1971).
REICH, E.: Actinomycin: correlation of structure and function of its complexes with purines and DNA. Science **143**, 684—689 (1964).
REICH, E., FRANKLIN, R. M., SHATKIN, A. J., TATUM, E. L.: Effect of actinomycin D on cellular nucleic acid synthesis and virus production. Science **134**, 556—557 (1961).

REICH, E., GOLDBERG, I. H.: Actinomycin and nucleic acid function. In: Progress in nucleic acid research and molecular biology, Vol. 3. New York: Academic Press 1964.
REICH, E., GOLDBERG, I. H., RABINOWITZ, M.: Structure activity correlations of actinomycins and their derivatives. Nature (Lond.) **196**, 743—748 (1962).
REVEL, M., HIATT, H. H.: Synthesis of transfer RNA in rat liver relatively resistant to actinomycin. Biochem. biophys. Res. Commun. **17**, 730—736 (1964).
REYNOLDS, R. C., MONTGOMERY, P. O., HUGHES, B.: Nucleolar "caps" produced by actinomycin D. Cancer Res. **24**, 1269—1277 (1964).
RICHARDSON, J. P.: The binding of RNA polymerase to DNA. J. molec. Biol. **21**, 83—114 (1966).
RINGERTZ, N. R., BOLUND, L.: Actinomycin binding capacity of deoxyribonucleoprotein. Biochim. biophys. Acta (Amst.) **174**, 147—154 (1969).
ROVERA, G., BERMAN, S., BASERGA, R.: Pulse labeling of RNA of mammalian cells. Proc. nat. Acad. Sci. (Wash.) **65**, 876—833 (1970).
SAKAR, N. K.: Effects of actinomycin D and mitomycin C on the degradation of deoxyribonucleic acid and polydeoxyribonucleotide by deoxyribonucleases and venom phosphodiesterase. Biochim. biophys. Acta (Amst.) **145**, 174 (1967).
SCHLUEDERBERG, A., HENDEL, R. C., CHAVANICH, S.: Actinomycin D: renewed RNA synthesis after removal from mammalian cells. Science **172**, 577—579 (1971).
SCHOEFL, G. I.: The effect of actinomycin D on the fine structure of the nucleolus. J. Ultrastruct. Res. **10**, 224—243 (1964).
SCHWARTZ, H. S., SODERGREN, J. E., AMBOYE, R. Y.: Actinomycin D — drug concentrations and actions in mouse tissues and tumors. Cancer Res. **28**, 192—197 (1968).
SENTENAC, A., SIMON, E. J., FROMAGEOT, P.: Initiation of chains by RNA polymerase and the effects of inhibitors studied by a direct filtration technique. Biochim. biophys. Acta (Amst.) **161**, 299—308 (1968).
SIMARD, R.: The binding of actinomycin D^3H to heterochromatin as studied by quantitative high resolution radioautography. J. Cell Biol. **35**, 716—722 (1967).
SLOTNICK, I. J., SELLS, B. H.: Actinomycin resistance in *Bacillus subtilis*. Science **146**, 407—408 (1964).
SOBELL, H. M.: The stereochemistry of actinomycin binding to DNA. In: Progress in nucleic acid research and molecular biology, Vol. 13A. New York: Academic Press 1972.
SOBELL, H. M., JAIN, S. C., SAKORE, T. D., NORDMAN, C. E.: Stereochemistry of actinomycin-DNA binding. Nature New Biol. **231**, 200—205 (1971).
STENRAM, U.: Radioautographic RNA and protein labeling and the nucleolar volume in rats following administration of moderate doses of actinomycin D. Exp. Cell Res. **36**, 242—255 (1964).
STENRAM, U.: Electron-microscopic study on liver cells of rats treated with actinomycin D. Z. Zellforsch. **65**, 211—219 (1965).
STENRAM, U.: Autoradiographic, biochemical and ultrastructural studies into the effect of actinomycin, 5-fluorouracil, and adenosine on nucleolar and cellular structure and function. Nat. Cancer Inst. Monogr. **23**, 379—390 (1966).
STERN, R., FRIEDMAN, R. M.: Ribonucleic acid synthesis in animal cells in the presence of actinomycin. Biochemistry **10**, 3635—3645 (1971).
STEWART, G. A., FARBER, E.: The rapid acceleration of hepatic nuclear ribonucleic acid breakdown by actinomycin but not by ethionine. J. biol. Chem. **243**, 4479—4485 (1968).
SULKOWSKI, E., LASKOWSKI, M.: Degradation of thymus DNA and crab poly *d*(A—T) by micrococcal nuclease in the presence of actinomycin D. Biochim. biophys. Acta (Amst.) **157**, 207—209 (1968).
SVOBODA, D., REDDY, J., HARRIS, C.: Invasive tumors induced in rats with actinomycin D. Cancer Res. **30**, 2271—2279 (1970).
WAKSMAN, S. A.: Actinomycin. New York: Interscience 1968.
WAKSMAN, S. A., WOODRUFF, H. B.: Bacteriostatic and bactericidal substances produced by a soil actinomyces. Proc. Soc. exp. Biol. (N.Y.) **45**, 609—614 (1940).
WARING, M.: Variation of the supercoils in closed circular DNA by binding of antibiotics and drugs: evidence for molecular models involving intercalation. J. molec. Biol. **54**, 247—279 (1970).
WELLS, R. D., LARSON, J. E.: Studies on the binding of actinomycin D to DNA and DNA model polymers. J. molec. Biol. **49**, 319—342 (1970).
WIESNER, R., ACS, G., REICH, E., SHAFIQ, A.: Degradation of ribonucleic acid in mouse fibroblasts treated with actinomycin. J. Cell Biol. **27**, 47—52 (1965).
YAMADA, T. A.: A demonstration of preferential inhibition of net synthesis of 23 S RNA in growing bacteria by actinomycin S. Biochim. biophys. Acta (Amst.) **108**, 158—159 (1965).

Chapter 60

Daunomycin (Daunorubicin) and Adriamycin

A. DiMarco

With 17 Figures

Introduction

Daunomycin (NSC-82151) is an antibiotic isolated from cultures of *Streptomyces peucetius* (DiMarco et al., 1963, 1964a, b). While weakly active against some gram positive microorganisms, the drug inhibits the multiplication of coliphages more than that of the host bacteria (Sanfilippo et al., 1964) and exhibits marked cytotoxic activity against normal and neoplastic cells (DiMarco et al., 1964).

The active product was isolated as the crystalline hydrochloride and was shown to be a glycosidic antibiotic of the anthracycline group such as rhodomycin, cinerubin, pyrromycin, and rutilantine (Arcamone et al., 1964).

A product with the same chemical composition was independently isolated from *Streptomyces coeruleorubidus* (Dubost et al., 1963) and named rubidomycin. The chromophore portion of daunomycin is present also in the rubomycin complex (Gause, 1966; Brachnikova, 1966). Other antibiotics related to daunomycin have been subsequently discovered, namely 14-hydroxydaunomycin (Adriamycin) (Arcamone et al., 1969a), 13-dihydrodaunomycin, and daunosaminyl-daunomycin (Arcamone et al., 1969b). Adriamycin (NSC-123127) is of particular importance because of its activity against a variety of tumors (Di Marco et al., 1969).

Chemistry

Daunomycin (Fig. 1) is hydrolyzed by dilute acids to give a lipid-soluble, red crystalline substance (daunomycinone), for which a partial structure was presented (Arcamone et al., 1964a), and a water-soluble basic compound (daunosamine), shown to be a new aminosugar, i.e., 2,3,6-trideoxy-3-amino-L-lyxohexose (Arcamone et al., 1964b). The structure and stereochemistry of daunosamine were later confirmed by the stereospecific synthesis of derivatives of the D-enantiomer (Richardson, 1967; Baer et al., 1969), and of daunosamine itself (Marsh et al., 1967). The structure and absolute configuration of daunomycin are now known in detail (Arcamone et al., 1968a, b), and are represented in Fig. 1.

Adriamycin (Fig. 1) is a metabolite of *S. peucetius* var. *caesius* (Arcamone et al., 1969a). This compound gives, on acid hydrolysis, the aglycone, adriamycinone, and the aminosugar, daunosamine; it differs from daunomycin only by substituting a hydrogen atom by a hydroxyl group in the acetyl radical (Fig. 1, Arcamone et al., 1969a).

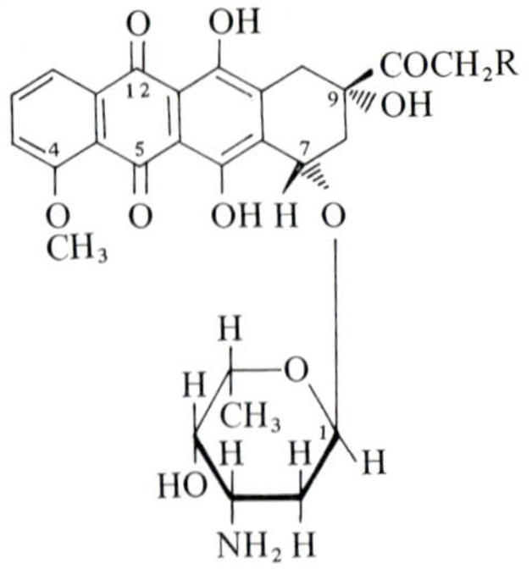

Fig. 1. Structure of daunomycin (R = H) and adriamycin (R = OH)

Activity on Normal and Neoplastic Cells *in Vitro*

Daunomycin has a strong inhibiting effect on the growth of mammalian cells *in vitro*; a 0.1 µg/ml concentration reduces considerably the mitotic activity of rat fibroblasts, HeLa, KB, and Helius-Lettré cells (DiMarco et al., 1963a) (Fig. 2). Cell damage induced by daunomycin is mainly nuclear, producing a finely granular appearance of the chromatin of resting cells and marked alterations in the shape and size of the nucleoli, while cytoplasmic changes, such as vacuolization, are

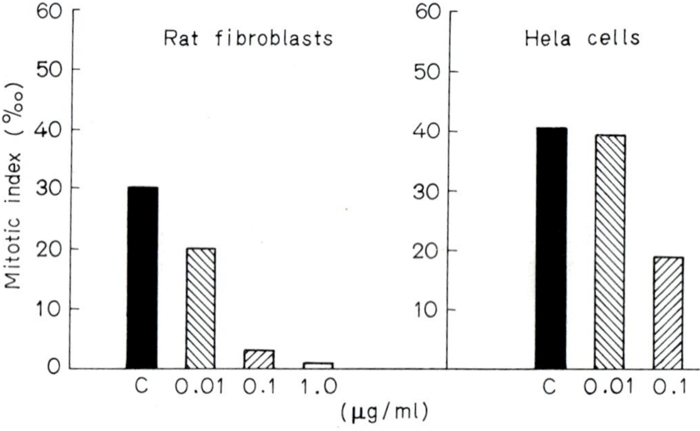

Fig. 2. Action of daunomycin on the mitotic index of *in vitro* cultures of rat fibroblasts and HeLa cells. Values of mitotic index found 24 h after treatment with daunomycin at a dose of 1, 0.1, and 0.01 µg/ml; C = control (DiMarco et al., 1963a)

moderate and appear only after prolonged treatment with large doses. The damage to the nucleolar structure appears rapidly after addition of daunomycin to the medium and can be followed by electron microscopy. Thus, HeLa cells after 2 h of incubation in the presence of 1 µg/ml of daunomycin in the medium show disorganization and fragmentation of the nucleolar filamentous structure with detachment of RNA granules (Fig. 3a, b) (Dorigotti et al., 1964). After 24 h of exposure to daunomycin the nucleolus is a very compact structure with the appearance of vacuoles (Fig. 4a, b). The injuries to the nucleolar structure

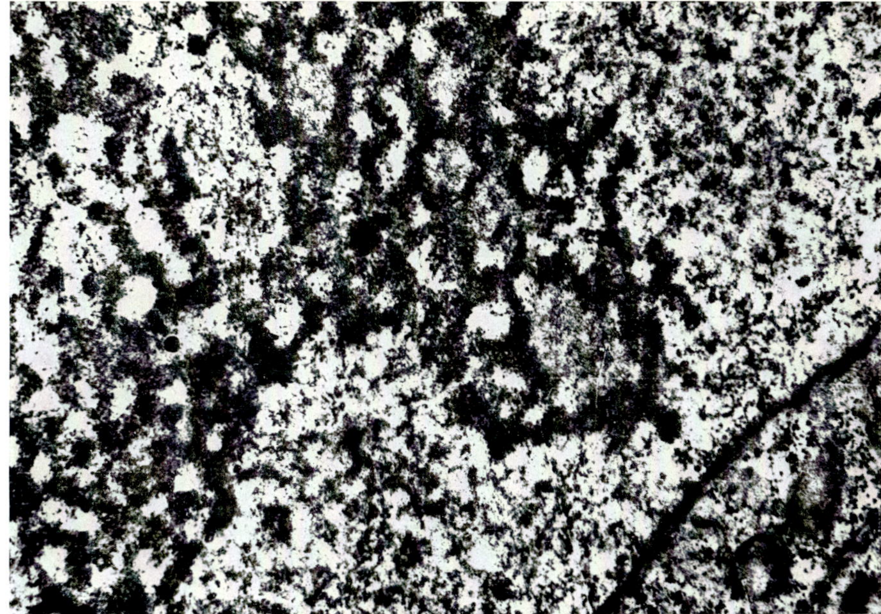

Fig. 3a. Control HeLa cell nucleolus showing filamentous appearance

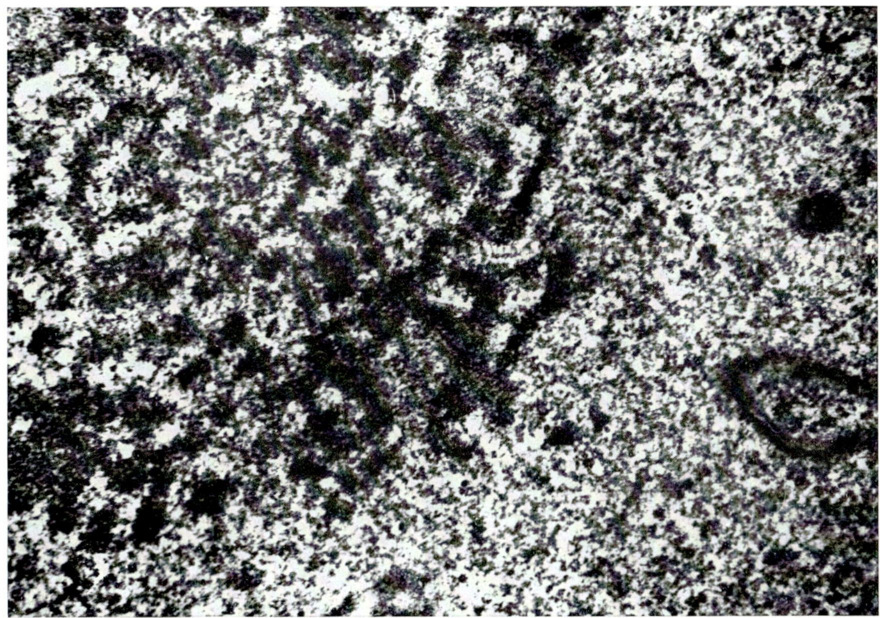

Fig. 3b. HeLa cell nucleolus after 2 h of exposure to 1 μg of daunomycin/ml. Nucleoloneme is fragmented and shows a progressive loss of RNA granules

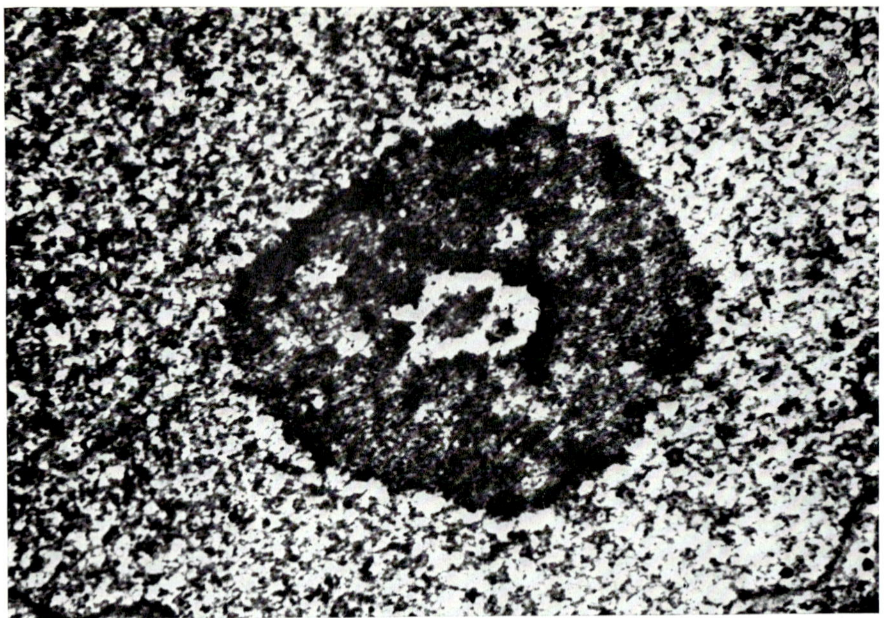

Fig. 4a. HeLa cell nucleolus after 18 h of exposure to 1 μg of daunomycin/ml. The nucleolus is changed into a dense and compact body showing large areas in which RNA granules have completely disappeared

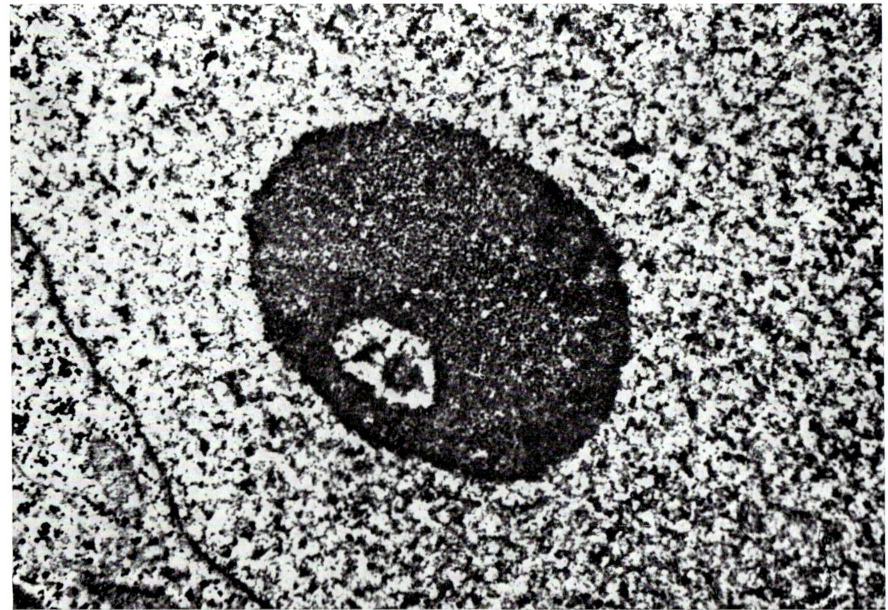

Fig. 4b. HeLa cell nucleolus after 48 h of exposure to 1 μg of Daunomycin/ml

should be considered a consequence of the inhibition of RNA synthesis produced by daunomycin. During mitosis chromosomal damage such as fragmentations and mitotic aberrations, mainly anaphasic bridges, have been described (DIMARCO et al., 1963).

If a sufficient amount of daunomycin is added to rat fibroblast cultures it is possible to observe, by phase contrast microscopy, an immediate block of the mitotic process and an anomalous scattering of the chromosomes within the cell.

With HeLa cells cultivated *in vitro*, adriamycin has a lesser effect on the mitotic index than daunomycin (ID_{50} after 8 h of treatment with daunomycin = 0.029 µg/ml and adriamycin = 0.14 µg/ml) and a lesser effect on proliferative activity (ID_{50} after 8 h of treatment and 40 h of recovery, for daunomycin = 0.3 µg/ml and for adriamycin = 0.64 µg/ml). The lack of parallelism between the dose-effect curves of the two antibiotics does not permit, however, the establishment of a precise ratio between the two antibiotics. Also, on different cell lines adriamycin shows a slightly lesser effect than daunomycin (NECCO and DASDIA, unpublished data).

Activity on Experimental Tumors

Daunomycin has a strong inhibitory effect on the Ehrlich ascites tumor (DI MARCO et al., 1964a, b). A single dose of 2 mg/kg produced a rapid drop in the mitotic index. After 48 h most of the mitoses showed aberrations such as anaphasic bridges, anomalous dispersion of chromosomes in the cytoplasm, and chromosomal fragmentation. Solid tumors show a lesser degree of susceptibility to daunomycin, as compared to the ascitic forms of these neoplasms. Daunomycin induces a significant increase of survival time in mice bearing L1210 leukemia (VENDITTI et al., 1966).

Adriamycin produces an increase in survival time which is greater than that of daunomycin in animals bearing either the Ehrlich ascites tumor (DIMARCO et al., 1969) or the L1210 leukemia (SANDBERG et al., 1970) and exerts a great inhibitory effect on the growth of many other experimental tumors (DIMARCO et al., 1969). The effectiveness of adriamycin against Sarcoma 180 is about twice that of daunomycin, the therapeutic index being 1.21 in the case of adriamycin and 0.67 in the case of daunomycin.

A significant antitumor effect is observed with different treatment schedules in transplantable and spontaneous mammary carcinoma of C3H mice (DIMARCO et al., 1972). In MSV-induced tumors in 16 day-old mice, large doses of daunomycin cause a transient inhibition of tumor growth, followed by strong recurrence of tumors, which progress up to death of the animals, while in untreated controls complete and permanent tumor regression is observed (CASAZZA et al., 1970, 1971). Tumor recurrence is rare after daunomycin treatment in 20 day-old mice and is absent after daunomycin or adriamycin treatment in mice 28 days-old at the time of implantation.

Tumor recurrence can be attributed to the action of daunomycin on the induction and multiplication of immunocompetent cells able to react with the virus or virus-induced antigens of tumor cells. When compared to daunomycin, adriamycin was more effective in inhibiting tumor growth, while tumor recurrence occurred later and to a lesser extent. When administered before tumor implantation only adriamycin did not inhibit tumor regression, thus, under these experimental conditions the difference between the two antibiotics is particularly evident.

Biochemical Effects and Mechanisms of Action

The most important metabolic effects of daunomycin are related to the processes of DNA transcription and replication and can be considered as consequences of its ability to bind to DNA. A brief summary of the experimental evidence seems to be appropriate (see also DiMarco, 1967).

The ability of daunomycin to react with DNA to form a physical complex can be demonstrated by:

(a) Changes in the spectral properties of daunomycin. In the presence of DNA, the absorption maximum around 480 nm shifts to a longer wavelength by about 25 nm, with a decrease in extinction (Fig. 5). The reaction between daunomycin and DNA is also revealed by the reduction of daunomycin's fluorescence (emission at 580 nm when excited at 485 nm (Fig. 6) and by disappearance of the polarographic reduction wave characteristic of anthraquinones (Calendi et al., 1965).

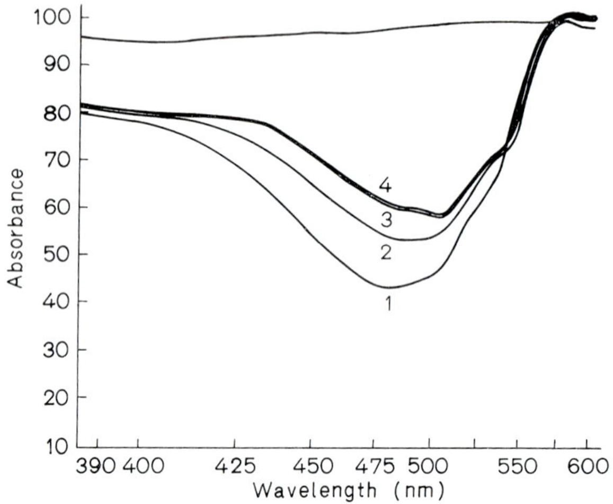

Fig. 5. Changes in the visible spectrum of daunomycin (35.6×10^{-6} M) at increasing DNA levels: (1) daunomycin, (2) daunomycin + DNA (155×10^{-6} M), (3) daunomycin + DNA (310×10^{-6} M), (4) daunomycin + DNA (620×10^{-6} M)

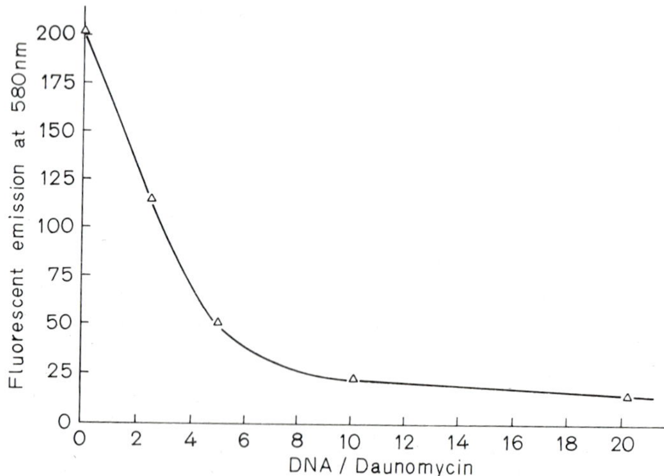

Fig. 6. Fluorescent emission of daunomycin (3.6×10^{-6} M) plotted against increasing DNA/daunomycin molar ratios

(b) Changes in physico-chemical properties of DNA such as increased relative viscosity of DNA and decreased sedimentation rate (CALENDI et al., 1965; KERSTEN et al., 1965a). The effect on DNA viscosity (ZUNINO, 1971) indicates a stiffening and an elongation of the DNA molecules (similar to that seen with amino-acridines) which could be caused by an intercalation of the ring system between base pairs of double helical DNA (LERMAN, 1961). This was in fact demonstrated by x-ray diffraction studies (WARING et al., 1968) and by drug-induced local uncoiling of the double helix (WARING, 1970).

The protecting effect of daunomycin against thermal denaturation of DNA is demonstrable by changes in optical rotation (CALENDI et al., 1965) or by a shift of the thermal transition point (KERSTEN and KERSTEN, 1965b) and indicates the formation of extra bonds between the two DNA strands and a consequent increase in the probability of rebuilding of the original native structure on cooling.

In this connection it should be noted that daunomycin does not appreciably modify the sedimentation behavior of single-stranded DNA of EC 9 bacteriophage. In addition, the absence of a specific increase in the viscosity of denatured DNA on interaction with daunomycin suggests that the increase in contour length on strong binding of daunomycin is a specific feature of the interaction with the intact double helical structure (ZUNINO et al., 1971). To establish a firm bond with DNA both the intercalation process and binding of the aminosugar residue to the backbone of the DNA helix are essential. A masking or a shift of the 3′-amino group appears to be critical for bond formation and for biological activity (DI MARCO et al., 1971).

From different types of physical measurement (i.e., optical titrations, low-shear viscosimetry, and thermal denaturation of DNA) it appears that the binding ability of adriamycin to double helical DNA is very similar to that of daunomycin (ZUNINO et al., 1971).

The fluorescence of daunomycin permits the demonstration of the penetration of this substance into the cell and its fixation to the nucleus (Fig. 7) and in particular to the nucleolar and the perinucleolar region. This binding pattern is con-

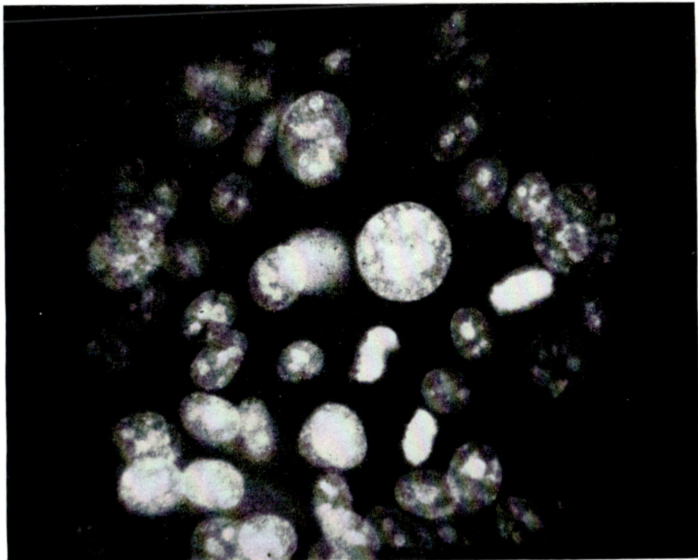

Fig. 7. Daunomycin fluorescence in HeLa cells treated for 5 min with 5 μg/ml

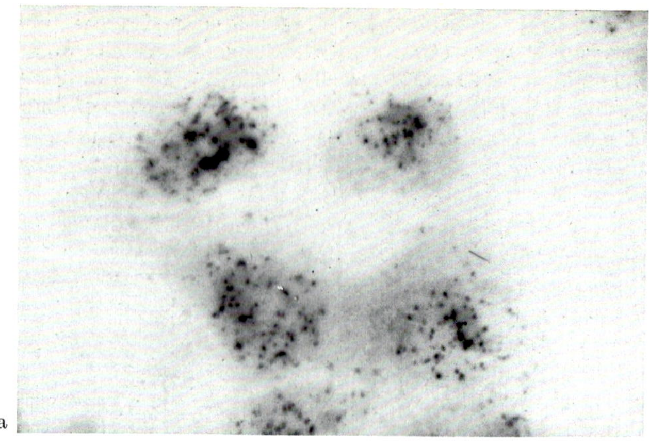

a

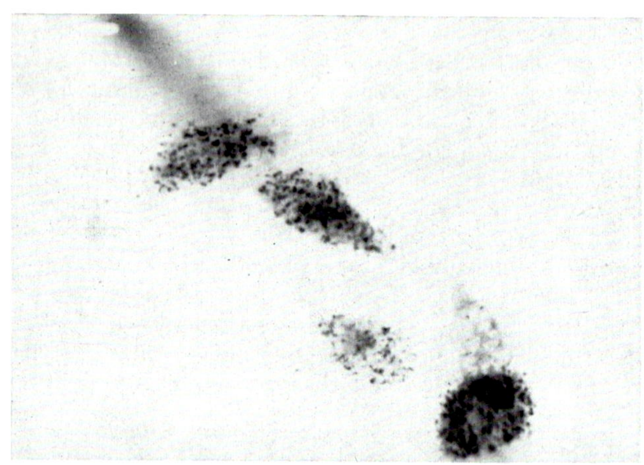

b

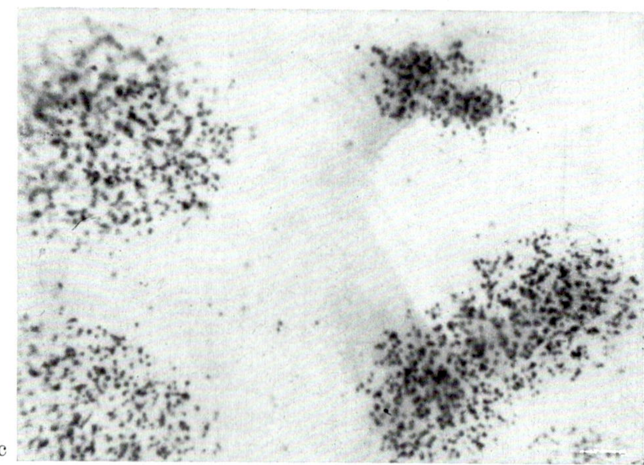

c

Fig. 8a—c. Autoradiography of ^{3}H-daunomycin uptake into (a) normal rat fibroblast cultures, (b) normal lymphoid cell cultures (C3H mouse strain), and (c) HeLa cells

firmed by autoradiography with tritiated daunomycin (Fig. 8). The uptake of daunomycin by HeLa cells is directly proportional to the concentration of the drug in the culture medium (RUSCONI and DIMARCO, 1969). The effect of different concentrations of daunomycin on adenine-8-C^{14} incorporation into DNA and RNA of HeLa cells is shown in Fig. 9 (RUSCONI and CALENDI, 1966). An attempt to

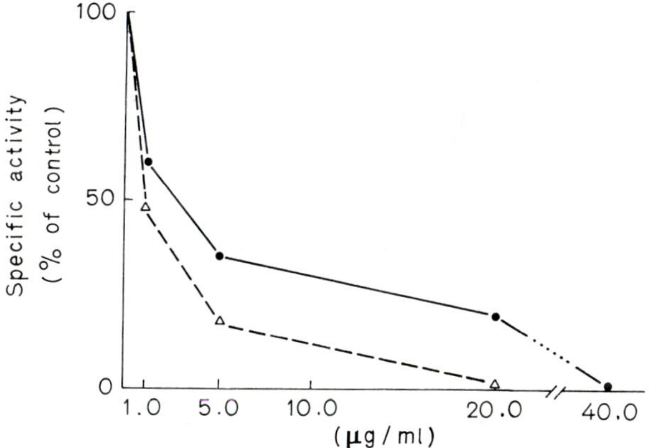

Fig. 9. Effect of increasing concentration of daunomycin on the incorporation of 8—C^{14}-adenine into DNA (△- - - -△) and RNA (●——●) extracted by NaCl method (RUSCONI and CALENDI, 1966)

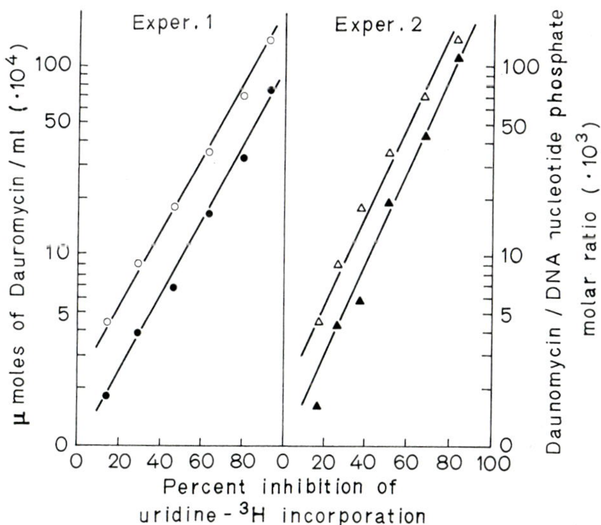

Fig. 10. Dose-response curves for HeLa cells incubated in the presence of ^{3}H-uridine and increasing concentrations of daunomycin (open symbols, ordinate, left scale). Values of daunomycin are expressed as μmol/ml. Under the same experimental conditions HeLa cells were incubated without ^{3}H-uridine in the presence of labeled daunomycin. The amount of the antibiotic taken up by cells is shown on the ordinate, right scale (closed symbols), expressed as moles of ^{3}H-daunomycin per mole of DNA nucleotide phosphate. Data on the ordinate are plotted against the percent inhibition of ^{3}H-uridine incorporation (abscissa). Cells incubated with ^{3}H-daunomycin were collected without any washing by centrifugation or by filtration through glass fiber discs (RUSCONI and DIMARCO, 1969)

calculate the quantitative relationship between the amount of daunomycin fixed to DNA and the degree of inhibition of uridine incorporation into RNA led to the conclusion that 50% inhibition was reached when one mole of daunomycin was fixed per 62.5 to 100 mol of DNA nucleotide phosphate (Fig. 10).

The interference with the incorporation of labeled precursor into RNA should be related to the inhibition exerted by daunomycin on the activity of DNA-dependent RNA polymerase (Hartmann et al., 1964; Ward et al., 1965) (Fig. 11).

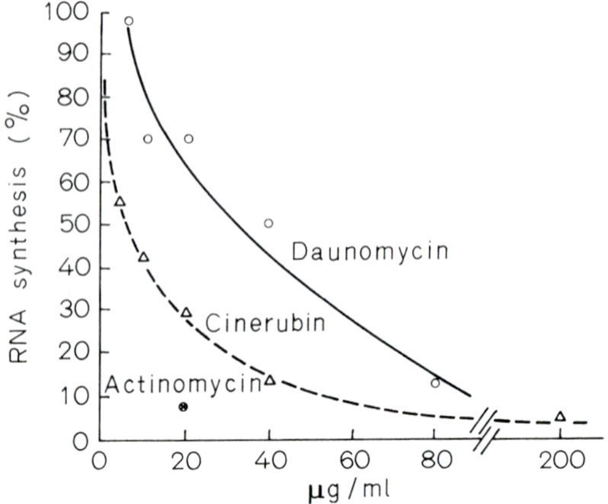

Fig. 11. Inhibition of DNA-dependent RNA synthesis by daunomycin, cinerubin, and actinomycin. The incubation system contained in a final volume of 0.5 ml: 100 μmol Tris-HCl, pH 7.8; 10 μmol $MgCl_2$, 1 μmol $MnCl_2$, 0.33 μmol each GTP, CTP, UTP; 0.06 μmol $AT^{32}P$ (15,000 cpm/mμmol); and 0.14 mg of enzyme (from *E. coli*). DNA nucleotide concentration: 0.82 μmol/ml. Incubation time: 10 min at 30°. The radioactivity incorporated into acid-insoluble material was measured. Results were expressed as radioactivity as a percent of that found in control sample (from Hartmann et al., 1964)

As observed for actinomycin, the inhibition of enzyme activity increases with the concentration of daunomycin, and the action of daunomycin can be antagonized by DNA. According to Ward et al. (1965), the effect of daunomycin occurs when the enzymatic polymerization reaction is primed by crab *d*AT, *d*G*d*C, or *d*I*d*C. It seems, therefore, that the linkage of daunomycin to DNA involves some groups which are present in all these pairs of bases. Recently, template specific inhibition of DNA polymerase from RNA tumor viruses by daunomycin and its derivatives has been reported (Chandra et al., 1972). The inhibition exerted by these antibiotics on the enzymatic activity is much more pronounced when poly (dA-dT) or poly rA oligo dT are used as primer-template, as compared to poly (dI.dC). These observations lead to conclusions similar to those obtained with nogalamycin (Bhuyan and Smith, 1965), suggesting a specific interaction of daunomycin with A-T base pairs of DNA.

Interference with DNA synthesis was also observed following the incorporation of adenine-8-C^{14} into nucleic acids of cell suspensions of Yoshida ascites hepatoma (Rusconi and Calendi, 1964) and with *in vitro* cultured HeLa cells (Rusconi et al., 1965). The inhibiting effect of daunomycin on the incorporation of nucleic acid precursors into DNA should be related to the observed interference exerted by this substance on the activity of DNA-dependent DNA polymerase (Hartman et al., 1964) (Fig. 12). The activities of some enzymes related to DNA synthesis such as thymidine kinase and deoxycytidine monophosphate deaminase increase and DNA polymerase is not reduced after treatment of HeLa cells with daunomycin; this indicates that the drug does not act on the formation of the latter

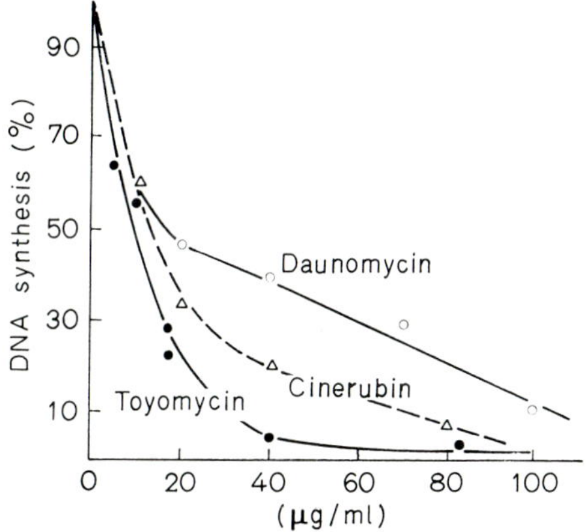

Fig. 12. Inhibition of DNA-dependent synthesis of DNA by daunomycin, cinerubin, and toyomycin. The incubation system contained 0.15 μmol of activated thymus DNA/ml and 50 μg of enzymatic protein (purified up to stage IV). The concentrations of the antibiotics are reported in the abscissa. Results are expressed as a percent of control value (from HARTMANN et al., 1964)

enzyme but, as pointed out by KIM et al. (1969), results in the unavailability of the template to the enzyme as a consequence of the interaction of the antibiotic with DNA.

Assuming that DNA polymerase starts its action on the 3′-hydroxy end of double stranded segments of DNA, partially opened by the activity of some endonuclease, and moves along the single stranded segment, the presence of the intercalating drug and its tendency to tie together the two strands of DNA could interrupt the process from the initial step.

Alternatively, it is possible that the binding of the antibiotic to DNA, and the consequent alteration in the stereochemical configuration of DNA, similar to that described for proflavine by WARING (1968), causes steric hindrance to the formation of the hypothetical DNA:DNA polymerase complex. The same mechanism should be operative for both DNA polymerase and DNA-dependent RNA polymerase since daunomycin, like proflavine and ethidium bromide, inhibits the two processes nearly equally. This differs from actinomycin, which is more active on DNA-dependent RNA polymerase. As RNA polymerase does not seem to require the preliminary opening of the helix, the latter hypothesis seems to be more satisfying.

Conflicting results were reported concerning the relative activity of the drug on the incorporation of labeled precursors into RNA and DNA *in vivo* or in cultured cells (RUSCONI et al., 1964, 1966; SILVESTRINI et al., 1963a, b; THEOLOGIDES et al., 1968).

In experiments on HeLa cells (RUSCONI and DIMARCO, 1969) it was demonstrated that experimental conditions, such as the time of addition of daunomycin to the medium and the cell population density, can affect the relative sensitivity of RNA and DNA syntheses to daunomycin (Fig. 13). A recent paper (Silvestrini et al., 1970) describes the effects of daunomycin on nucleic acid synthesis during the different phases of the cell cycle in cultures of rat fibroblasts synchronized by thymidine excess (Xeros, 1962; Bootsman et al., 1964; Firket, 1964). DNA and RNA syntheses were determined by autoradiographic methods using ^{3}H-thymidine, ^{3}H-deoxycytidine, and ^{3}H-uridine as labeled precursors. The effects of daunomycin

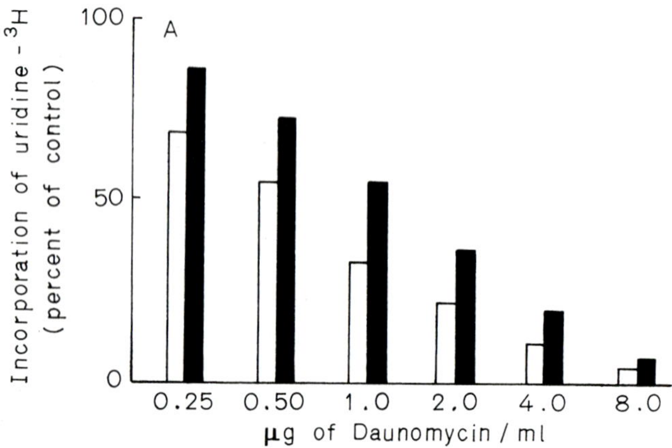

Fig. 13a. Action of increasing concentrations of daunomycin on the incorporation of ^{3}H-uridine into RNA. Shaded bars indicate that, in the same incubation volume, the number of cells (1.2×10^{5}) present was three times as great as in the experiment indicated by clear bars. The drug and the precursors were added at the beginning of the incubation time (60 min)

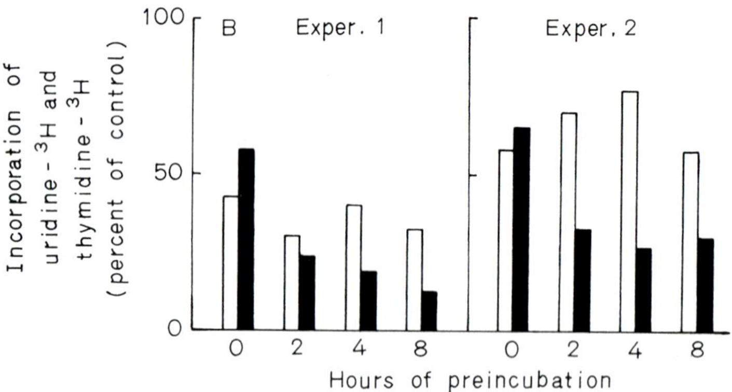

Fig. 13b. Action of daunomycin (1 µg/ml) on the incorporation of ^{3}H-uridine (clear bars) or ^{3}H-thymidine (shaded bars) into RNA and DNA, respectively. The precursors were added at the same time as the drug or after 2, 4, or 8 h of preincubation with the drug. The incubation time with the label was 60 min. Results obtained in replicate experiments are reported

were most evident on the DNA synthesis which occurs in late *S* phase, which is tentatively identified with heterochromatin duplication (Simard, 1967), and on RNA synthesis which occurs in the middle of G_1, and in the G_2 phase just before mitosis. Clearly, the inhibition of these metabolic events can explain the arrest of cell reproduction; there has been described, however, an immediate premitotic block which seems to be quite unrelated to the inhibition of DNA and RNA synthesis (SILVESTRINI et al., 1970; DI FRONZO et al., in press). In fact it has been observed by phase contrast microscopy that daunomycin can stop the mitotic activity of rat fibroblasts when added 20 min prior to the prophase stage, when DNA and premitotic RNA syntheses are completed. Furthermore, with HeLa cells and rat methylcholanthrene-induced sarcoma cells, a marked inhibition of mitotic index takes place with daunomycin doses inactive on ^{3}H-thymidine incorporation into DNA. The same is true for the *N*-acetyl-derivative of daunomycin; in this case the reduction of mitotic activity, dissociated from any effect on DNA synthesis, leads to cells with mean ^{3}H-thymidine incorporation greater than that of controls (DIMARCO et al., 1965). As the ability of this compound to bind to DNA is considerably reduced, the possibility of an antimitotic effect of daunomycin, unrelated to its effect on DNA synthesis, should be considered. KIM et al. (1968) observed that the lethal effect of daunomycin on a synchronously dividing population of HeLa cells is greater in *S* phase than in either G_1 or G_2 and, by analogy between the action of daunomycin and that of actinomycin D on HeLa cells, it was suggested that "accessibility of DNA in chromosomal structures and repair processes may vary during the division cycle and cell death may be the outcome of at least two reactions that would be differently affected by different DNA-binding drugs". As a strong binding of daunomycin to DNA occurs, under ordinary conditions with double stranded DNA, it could be tentatively presumed that only during the process of replication could the drug find access to the DNA (Fig. 14). In this case, a few molecules of drug could irreversibly damage all chromosomal structure.

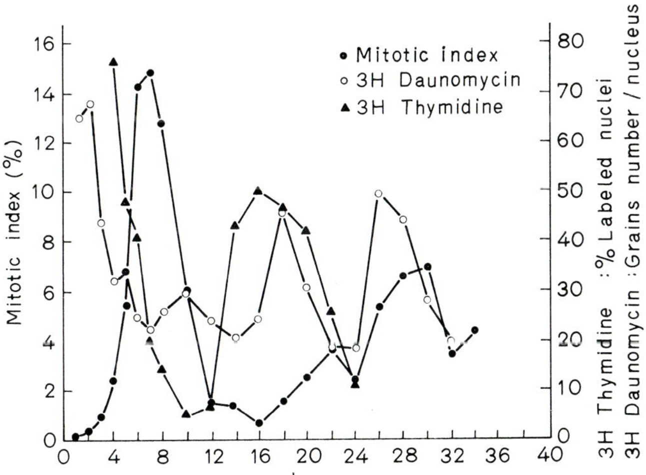

Fig. 14. Mitotic activity, ^{3}H-daunomycin uptake, and DNA synthesis in different phases of the proliferative cycle of synchronized cultures of rat fibroblasts (SILVESTRINI et al., 1970)

Until the present time very little was known about the precise mechanism of action of adriamycin; from studies on the binding ability to DNA and from the effect on DNA synthesis, as shown by the incorporation of ^{3}H-thymidine into the nucleus by autoradiographic methods (DIMARCO et al., 1971) it appears, however, very similar to that of daunomycin.

Resistance to Daunomycin

In chinese hamster cells cross-resistance was observed between actinomycin D and daunomycin (Biedler and Riehm, 1970), which seems noteworthy in view of the many similarities in the mechanism of action of the two antibiotics. However, cell lines resistant to actinomycin D are resistant also to other drugs such as mithramycin, vinblastine, vincristine, and pirromycin. The degree of resistance to actinomycin D was inversely related to the degree of nuclear labeling by ^{3}H-actinomycin D and to inhibition of uridine-^{3}H incorporation into RNA by the antibiotic. According to these authors, these results support the hypothesis that the development of resistance to actinomycin D in hamster cells is due to qualitative differences in the cell membrane resulting in decreased permeability to actinomycin D and other compounds. Cross-resistance between daunomycin and vinca alkaloids was observed *in vivo* in lines of the Ehrlich ascites tumor in which permanent resistance to daunomycin was developed as a result of long term treatment with subinhibitory doses (Danø, 1970).

The subline of leukemia P815 selected for resistance to vinblastine was also shown to be resistant to daunomycin (Kessel et al., 1968). These authors demonstrated also that there is a good correlation between daunomycin sensitivity *in vivo* of a transplantable murine leukemia (P388) and the ability of the cells to retain the drug. Neither cross-resistance nor collateral sensitivity to methotrexate or 6-mercaptopurine was observed by Danø et al. (1971) in Ehrlich ascites cells resistant to daunomycin; a collateral sensitivity to cytosine arabinoside and 1,3-*bis*(2-chloroethyl)nitrosourea was explained on the basis of the slower growth of the resistant line with respect to the sensitive one. The cross-resistance between daunomycin, actinomycin, and vinca alkaloids seems to be understandable as a result of limited permeability of the cells to these drugs. Other unknown factors may contribute, however, to the altered sensitivity of cells to the drug; in fact, in a resistant subline of the Ehrlich ascites tumor the difference in uptake of labeled daunomycin is not great enough to explain the difference in inhibition of nucleic acid synthesis (Danø et al., personal communication).

Complete cross-resistance to adriamycin was observed in resistant sublines of the L1210 leukemia (Hoshino et al., 1971), and this appears to confirm that the modes of action of the two antibiotics are very similar.

Antiviral Activity

Interference by daunomycin with the multiplication of bacteriophage was reported by Sanfilippo et al. (1964) and by Parisi and Soller (1964). These observations were confirmed by Calendi et al. (1966) who did not observe any inhibitory effect of daunomycin on the multiplication of two single stranded DNA bacteriophages (EC9 and S13) and on RNA bacteriophages at a concentration of daunomycin that gives a 99.9 % inhibition of the plaque formation caused by T6 double stranded DNA phage.

No explanation is available on the mechanism of inhibition of phage multiplication induced by daunomycin; it seems, however, that the interference is not related to either direct inactivation of phage particles or inhibition of their absorption to the bacterial cell (Sanfilippo et al., 1964; Parisi and Soller, 1964).

From the previously discussed data it appears that inhibition of the function or replication of the bacterial genome requires the formation of a stable bond between the antibiotic and the nucleic acids, and this is established only with double-helical DNA. The lack of activity against single-stranded DNA or RNA bacterial viruses appears to be a simple consequence of an inability to form this stable bond. The inhibiting effect of daunomycin is seen also with other double-stranded DNA viruses; thus, it was shown that daunomycin protects cells from herpes simplex virus (HSV) when given before or a few hours after infection, during the intracellular phase of virus replication (Fig. 15) (DIMARCO et al., 1968). Daunomycin was not effective when added 4 h after the infection, when mature virions are thought to appear.

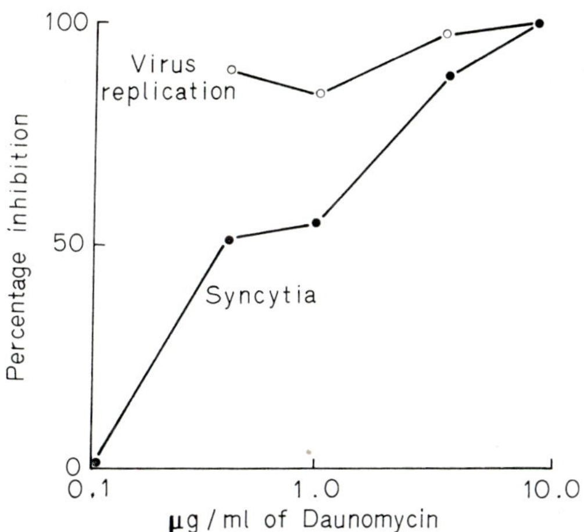

Fig. 15. Effect of daunomycin on syncytiogenesis and virus replication in KB cell cultures infected with herpes simplex virus. Treatment with different doses of daunomycin was carried out for 20 min, immediately after the infection

Autoradiographic studies of the interference by daunomycin of the rate of DNA and RNA synthesis in noninfected cells show that HSV replication is inhibited at doses active on nucleolar RNA, but not on extranucleolar RNA or on DNA synthesis.

The inhibiting effect of daunomycin on the replication of DNA viruses has been confirmed with herpes simplex and vaccinia virus by COHEN et al. (1969), who also noted absence of antiviral activity against influenza virus and a reduced virus production in HeLa cells infected with poliovirus. Daunomycin added to the incubation medium at different times before and after infection inhibits the multiplication of Moloney sarcoma virus (MSV) and the focus formation typical of this virus in mouse embryonal cells. The concentrations active on these processes have little effect on cellular proliferation (CASAZZA et al., 1972). A similar effect was reported for actinomycin D on the replication of Rous sarcoma virus (BARON et al., 1967; PAUKER et al., 1963; HALLUM et al., 1968; CHANY et al., 1967) and on murine leukemia virus (MINER et al., 1966; SONNABEND et al., 1967); these results indicate the presence of a DNA dependent step in virus multiplication. Daunomycin inhibits DNA and DNA-dependent RNA synthesis to essentially the same extent; therefore, the effect on viral multiplication and cellular transformation could be the result of interference with both of these processes. The inhibitory effect of daunomycin on virus replication is also compatible with the hypothesis originally proposed by TEMIN (1964) that single-stranded viral RNA serves as primer for the formation of the replicative form of the virus containing a complementary strand of DNA. The further conversion of the DNA-RNA hybrid into the DNA-DNA duplex demands a DNA-directed DNA polymerase. The recent finding that daunomycin and adriamycin inhibit the reverse transcriptase activity of RNA tumor viruses (Chandra et al., 1972) is, therefore, of major importance.

Exposure to white light of mixtures of daunomycin and some viruses such as vaccinia virus (VR) and HF strains of herpes simplex virus increases noticeably the virucidal activity of daunomycin (Verini et al., 1968). The increase is proportional to drug concentration and intensity of light; the virucidal activity is a linear function of the exposure to light. Similar results were observed by other authors studying photoinactivation of dye-sensitized DNA and RNA viruses (Baron et al., 1963; Baltimore, 1969; Ho et al., 1967; Friedman et al., 1967; Wheelock, 1965). While daunomycin has no activity when light is excluded, on RNA viruses such as Newcastle disease virus, the exposure to light induces the appearance of antiviral activity against this virus (Verini et al., 1968). If one recalls the preferential binding of daunomycin to double-stranded DNA and the different physicochemical behavior of the RNA-daunomycin complex, in comparison to the DNA-daunomycin complex (Calendi, 1964; Rusconi and Calendi, 1966) the observed effects could be explained by two possible mechanisms: (a) the photodynamic inactivation of viruses by daunomycin could be attributed to possible direct damage to nucleic acids (Simon et al., 1962); or (b) by the action of light, the molecule of daunomycin could undergo an alteration in its energy state such as to confer on it the ability to establish a different type of bond not only with DNA, but also with RNA. The formation of one covalent link per viral genome could be sufficient to produce virus inactivation and this could explain the increase in activity in comparison with that induced by the relatively reversible physical binding of the antibiotic to DNA which occurs under normal conditions.

Pharmacological and Toxicological Studies

The distribution and excretion of daunomycin and adriamycin have been studied using tritium-labeled drugs, as well as by taking advantage of the fluorescence characteristics of these antibiotics (Rusconi et al., 1968; Bachur et al., 1970; Di Fronzo et al., 1971; Di Fronzo and Gambetta, 1971; Picone et al., 1970; Dusonchet et al., in press; Yesair et al., 1971). Both drugs are rapidly cleared from the blood and fixed by the different tissues and organs. In rodents, high drug levels are maintained over a long period of time, especially in bone marrow, spleen, and lymphoid tissues. The two antibiotics do not appear to cross the blood-brain barrier. Both drugs are slowly excreted into the urine and the bile (Fig. 16). In rats, the excretion of adriamycin equivalents was about one-third that of daunomycin equivalents (Yesair et al., 1971). In mice, 50 % excretion of the drug occurs in about 24 h in the case of daunomycin, and in about 32 h in the case of adriamycin; moreover, drug accumulation in tissues after subacute treatment is more pronounced after adriamycin than after daunomycin (Di Fronzo et al., 1971). The calculated $C \times t$ (concentration $\times$ time) for adriamycin equivalents in all tissues has been demonstrated to be several times greater than that found for daunomycin or its metabolites (Yesair et al., 1971). Preliminary work (DiMarco et al., 1967; DiMarco, 1967a, b; DiMarco and Rusconi, 1967) provided evidence of extensive metabolism of daunomycin by liver homogenates. The main transformation product showed chromatographic and spectral properties very similar to those of the substance obtained from daunomycin by the action of sodium dithionite; it therefore was concluded that the metabolic transformation consisted of a reductive modification of the chromophore group associated with breakage of the glycosidic linkage. Besides the described transformation product, a small amount of another substance with a different Rf was observed, by thin-layer chromatography. More recent studies (BACHUR et al., 1971; BACHUR, 1971;

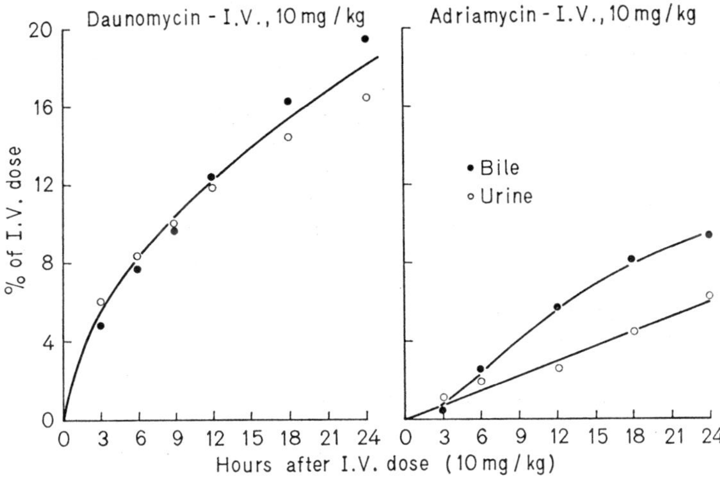

Fig. 16. Excretion of daunomycin or adriamycin equivalents by bile-duct cannulated rats (from YESAIR et al., 1971)

YESAIR et al., 1971) have elucidated the major pathway for daunorubicin metabolism in tissue homogenates (Fig. 17). Daunorubicinol is the only daunomycin metabolite present in the urine and bile of mice, rats and man (BACHUR, 1971). The presence of the hydroxyl group in the 14-position of the chromophore protects against metabolic transformation; in fact, no metabolic transformation product analogous to daunorubicinol was observed after incubation of adriamycin with tissue homogenates or in excreted materials (YESAIR 1971; DI FRONZO et al., 1971). These findings are consistent with the higher toxicity and activity of adriamycin *in vivo*. Daunorubicinol has significant cytotoxic activity *in vitro* and was also shown to be active *in vivo* against P388 lymphocytic leukemia (YESAIR, 1971); daunorubicinol could, therefore, contribute to the antitumor and pharmacological activity of daunomycin.

A number of studies on the toxicity of daunomycin (DIMARCO et al., 1964a,b, 1967) and adriamycin (BERTAZZOLI et al., 1970; DIMARCO et al., 1969) have been published. As could be expected for drugs which interfere with the synthesis of nucleic acids, the tissues most susceptible to the two antibiotics are rapidly proliferating tissues such as intestinal mucosa, lymphoid organs, and bone marrow. Few signs of cardiac toxicity have been observed in experimental animals; some EKG alterations have been noted in the hamster (HERMAN et al., 1969, 1970a,b) and in the monkey (BURKA et al., 1970), possibly mediated by a central mechanism involving the sympathetic nervous system (BURKA et al., 1970; HERMAN et al., 1970a,b). No impairment of oxidative phosphorylation by heart mitochondria has been observed. A lesion characteristic of daunomycin is the development of a nephrotic syndrome in rats given a large single dose of the drug (STERNBERG et al., 1967; Sternberg, 1970). Like most antitumor agents, daunomycin and adriamycin have been shown to be immunosuppressive (Natale et al., 1969; Casazza et al., 1970, 1971). When administered subcutaneously to infant mice and rats, both daunomycin and adriamycin induce fibrosarcomas at the injection site (Casazza et al., unpublished observations). When administered intravenously to young rats, daunomycin induces mammary and other carcinomas,

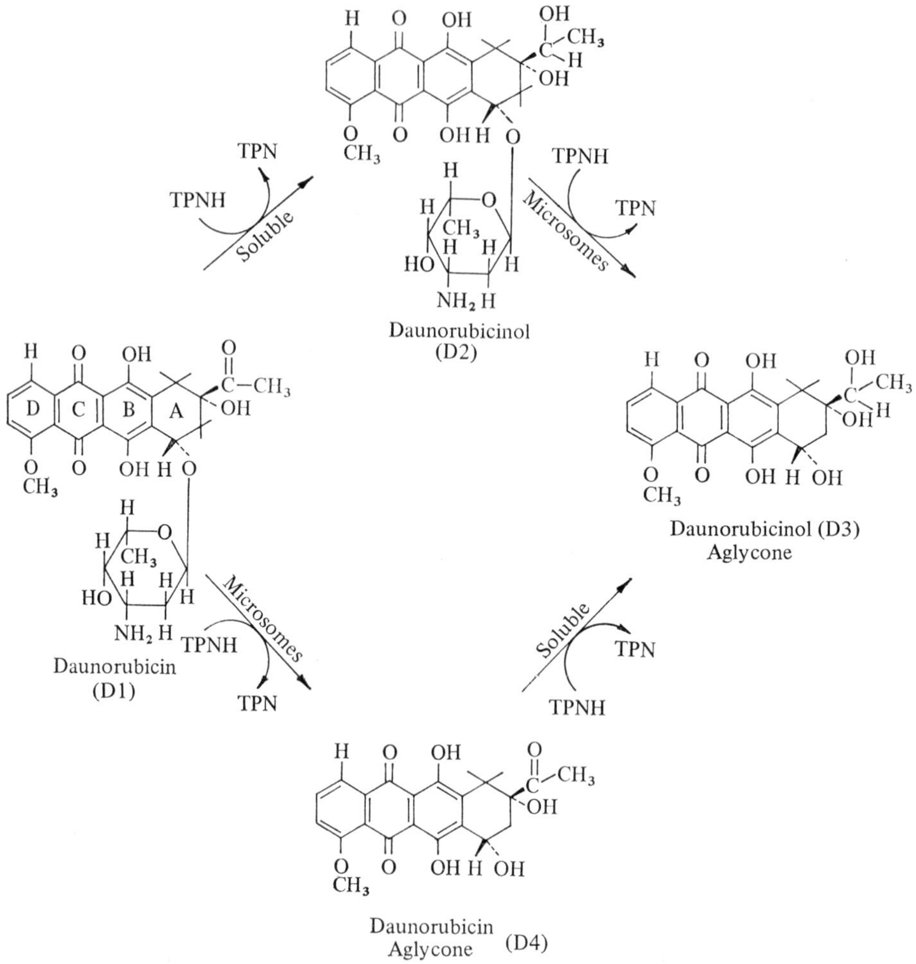

Fig. 17. Pathway for daunorubicin metabolism in mammalian liver fractions (from Bachur and Gee, 1971)

while in rats given adriamycin benign neoplasms are prevalent (Bertazzoli et al., personal communication). Both drugs have shown little or no teratogenic effects on chick, mouse, and rabbit embryos (Bertazzoli et al., personal communication).

References

ARCAMONE, F., CASSINELLI, G., FANTINI, G., GREIN, A., OREZZI, P., POL, C., SPALLA, C.: Adriamycin, 14-hydroxydaunomycin, a new antitumor antibiotic from *S. peucetius* var. *caesius*. Biotechnol. Bioeng. **11**, 1101 (1969a).

ARCAMONE, F., CASSINELLI, G., FRANCESCHI, F., OREZZI, P., MONDELLI, R.: The absolute stereochemistry of daunomycin. Tetrahedron Let. 3353 (1968b).

ARCAMONE, F., CASSINELLI, G., OREZZI, P., FRANCESCHI, F., MONDELLI, R.: Daunomycin. II. The structure and stereochemistry of daunosamine. J. Amer. chem. Soc. **86**, 5335 (1964b).

ARCAMONE, F., FRANCESCHI, G., OREZZI, P., CASSINELLI, G., BARBIERI, W., MONDELLI, R.: Daunomycin. I. The structure of daunomycinone. J. Amer. chem. Soc. **86**, 5335 (1964a).

ARCAMONE, F., FRANCESCHI, G., OREZZI, P., PENCO, S., MONDELLI, R.: The structure of daunomycin. Tetrahedron Let. 3349 (1968a).

ARCAMONE, F., FRANCESCHI, G., PENCO, S.: Substances antibiotiques et procédé pour leur préparation. Belg. 732.968 (November 13, 1969b).

BACHUR, N. R.: Daunorubicinol, a major metabolite of daunorubicin: isolation from human urine and enzymatic reactions. J. Pharmacol. exp. Therap. **177**, 573 (1971).

BACHUR, N. R., GEE, M.: Daunorubicinol metabolism by rat tissue preparations. J. Pharmacol. exp. Therap. **177**, 567 (1971).

BACHUR, N. R., MOORE, A. L., BERNSTEIN, J. B., LIU, A.: Tissue distribution and disposition of daunomycin (NSC-82151) in mice: fluorometric and isotopic methods. Cancer Chemother. Rep. **54**, 89 (1970).

BAER, H. H., CAPEK, K., COOK, M. C.: Synthesis of 3-acetamide 2,3,6-trideoxy-D-lyxo-hexose (*N*-acetyl-daunosamine) and its D-arabino isomer. Canad. J. Chem. **47**, 89 (1969).

BALTIMORE, D.: Virus growth and cell metabolism, Chap. 3. (H.B. LEVY, Ed.). New York: Dekker 1969.

BARON, S., BUCKLER, C. E.: Circulating interferon in mice after intravenous injection of virus. Science **141**, 1061 (1963).

BARON, S., BUCHLER, C. E., LEVY, H. B., FRIEDMAN, R. M.: Some factors affecting the interferon-induced antiviral state. Proc. Soc. exp. biol. (N.Y.) **125**, 1320 (1967).

BERTAZZOLI, C., CHIELI, T., GRANDI, M., RICEVUTI, G.: Adriamycin toxicity data. Experientia (Basel) **26**, 389 (1970).

BHUYAN, B. K., SMITH, C. G.: Differential inhibition of nogalamycin with DNA of varying base composition. Proc. nat. Acad. Sci. (Wash.) **54**, 566—572 (1965).

BIEDLER, J. L., RIEHM, H.: Cellular resistance to actinomycin D chinese hamster cells *in vitro:* cross-resistance, radioautographic and cytogenetic studies. Cancer Res. **30**, 1174 (1970).

BOOTSMA, D., BUDKE, L., VOS, O.: Studies on synchronous division of tissue culture cells initiated by excess thymidine. Exp. Cell Res. **33**, 301 (1964).

BRACHNIKOVA, M. G., KOSTANTINOVA, N. V., POMASKOVA, F. A., ZACHAROV, B. M.: Physicochemical properties of antitumor antibiotic rubidomycin, produced by *Act. coeruleorubidus*. Antibiotiki **11**, 763 (1966).

BURKA, B., HERMAN, E. H., VICK, J.: Role of the sympathetic nervous system in daunomycin-induced arrhythmia in the monkey. Brit. J. Pharmacol. **39**, 501 (1970).

CALENDI, E., DETTORI, R., NERI, M. G.: Filamentous sex-specific bacteriophages of *E. coli* K12. IV-Studies on physico-chemical characteristics of bacteriophage Ec 9. Giorn. Microbiol. **14**, 227 (1966).

CALENDI, E., DIMARCO, A., REGGIANI, M., SCARPINATO, B., VALENTINI, L.: On physico-chemical interactions between daunomycin and nucleic acids. Biochim. biophys. Acta (Amst.) **103**, 25 (1965).

CASAZZA, A. M., DIMARCO, A., DI CUONZO, G.: Interference of daunomycin and adriamycin on the growth and regression of murine sarcoma virus (Moloney)-induced tumors in mice. Cancer Res. **31**, 1971—1976 (1971).

CASAZZA, A. M., SCARPINATO, B., DI CUONZO, G.: Activity of adriamycin and daunomycin on primary and transplantable Moloney sarcoma virus-induced tumors. (Abstr.) 10th International Cancer Congress Houston, 391 (1970).

CASAZZA, A. M., SILVESTRINI, R., GAMBARUCCI, C.: Activity of daunomycin, adriamycin and some other daunomycin derivatives on the murine sarcoma virus (Moloney) MSV (M). Europ. J. clin. biol. Res. **17**, 622 (1972).

CHANDRA, P., ZUNIO, F., GÖTZ, A., GERICKE, D., THORBECK, R., DIMARCO, A.: Specific inhibition of DNA polymerases from RNA tumor viruses by some new daunomycin derivatives. FEBS Let. **21**, 264—268 (1972).

CHANY, C., BRAILOVSKY, C.: Stimulating interaction between viruses (stimulations). Proc. nat. Acad. Sci. (Wash.) **57**, 87 (1967).

COHEN, A., HARLEY, E. M., RESS, K. E.: Antiviral effect of daunomycin. Nature (Lond.) **222**, 36 (1969).

Danø, K.: Development of resistance to daunorubicin in experimental tumors. 10th International Cancer Congress, Houston, Texas (1970).
Di Fronzo, G., Gambetta, R. A.: *In vivo* studies on the distribution of ³H-daunomycin in tumors and in different tissues of the mouse. Europ. J. clin. Biol. Res. **16**, 50 (1971).
Di Fronzo, G., Gambetta, R. A., Lenaz, L.: Distribution and disposition of adriamycin: comparison with daunomycin. Europ. J. Clin. Biol. Res. **16**, 572 (1971).
Di Fronzo, G., Silvestrini, R., Scarpinato, B. M.: Correlations between ³H-daunomycin uptake and its antimitotic and antimetabolic activities in ascites sarcoma 180. Tumori **57**, 67 (1971).
DiMarco, A.: Daunomycin and related antibiotics. Antibiotics, Vol. I, p. 190. (Gottlieb, D., Shaw, P. D., Ed.) Berlin-Heidelberg-New York: Springer 1967a.
DiMarco, A.: Daunomycin pharmacological activity at the cellular level. Path. Biol. **15**, 897 (1967b).
DiMarco, A., Boretti, G., Rusconi, A.: Trasformazione metabolica della daunomicina da parte di estratti di tessuti. Il farmaco **7**, 535 (1967).
DiMarco, A., Gaetani, M., Dorigotti, L., Soldati, M., Bellini, O.: Daunomycin: a new antibiotic with antitumor activity. Cancer Chemother. Rep. **38**, 31 (1964a).
DiMarco, A., Gaetani, M., Orezzi, P., Scarpinato, B., Silvestrini, R., Soldati, M., Dasdia, T., Valentini, L.: Daunomycin, a new antibiotic of the rhodomycin group. Nature (Lond.) **201**, 706 (1964b).
DiMarco, A., Gaetani, M., Orezzi, P., Soldati, M.: Antitumor activity of a new antibiotic, daunomycin. Comm. IIIrd Congress International of Chemistry, Stuttgart, July 22—27, 1963.
DiMarco, A., Gaetani, M., Scarpinato, B.: Adriamycin (NSC-123, 127): a new antibiotic with antitumor activity. Cancer Chemother. Rep. **53**, 33—37 (1969).
DiMarco, A., Lenaz, L., Casazza, A. M., Scarpinato, B. M.: Activity of adriamycin (NSC-123127) and daunomycin (NSC-82151) on mouse mammary carcinoma. Cancer Chemother. Rep. **56**, 153 (1972).
DiMarco, A., Rusconi, A.: Action mechanism and metabolic transformation of daunomycin. Gann Monograph, 23, 1967.
DiMarco, A., Silvestrini, R., DiMarco, S., Dasdia, T.: Inhibiting effect of the cytotoxic antibiotic daunomycin on nucleic acids and mitotic activity of HeLa cells. J. cell. Biol. **27**, 545 (1965).
DiMarco, A., Soldati, M., Fioretti, A., Dasdia, T.: Ricerche sulla attività della daunomicina su cellule normali e neoplastiche coltivate *in vitro*. Tumori **49**, 4 (1963a).
DiMarco, A., Terni, M., Silvestrini, R., Scarpinato, B., Biagioli, E., Antonelli, A.: Effect of daunomycin on Herpes virus hominis in human cell. Giorn. Microbiol. **16**, 25 (1968).
DiMarco, A., Zunino, F., Silvestrini, R., Gambarucci, C., Gambetta, R. A.: Interaction of some daunomycin derivatives with DNA and their biological activity. Bioch. Pharmacol. **20**, 1323 (1971).
Dorigotti, L.: Studio al microscopio elettronico delle modificazioni indotte dalla daunomicina sulle cellule HeLa. Tumori **50**, 117 (1964).
Dubost, M., Ganter, P., Maral, R., Ninet, L., Pinnet, S., Preud Homme, J., Werner, G. H.: Un nouvel antibiotique à propriétés antitumorales. C. R. Acad. Sci. (Paris) **257**, 1813 (1963).
Dusonchet, L., Perbasi, F., Gebbia, N.: Spectrofluorophotometric characterization of adriamycin: a new antitumor drug. Experientia (Basel) (in press).
Firket, H.: Synchronization de cultures des cellules HeLa par un excess de thymidine. C. R. Soc. Biol. (Paris) **158**, 1408 (1964).
Friedman, R. M., Cooper, H. L.: Stimulation of interferon production in human lymphocytes by mitogens. Proc. Soc. exp. Biol. (N. Y.) **125**, 901 (1967).
Gause, G. F.: Aspects of antibiotics research. Chem. Ind. **36**, 1506 (1966).
Hallum, J. V., Youngner, J. S., Arnold, N. J.: Effect of pH on the protective action of interferon in L cells. J. Virol. **2**, 772 (1968).
Hartmann, G., Goller, H., Koschel, K., Kersten, W., Kersten, H.: Hemmung der DNA-abhängigen RNA- und DNA-synthese durch Antibiotica. Biochem. Z. **341**, 126 (1964).
Herman, E. H., Schein, P., Farmar, R. M.: Comparative cardiac toxicity of daunomycin in three rodent species. Proc. Soc. exp. Biol. (N. Y.) **130**, 1093 (1969).
Herman, E. H., Schein, P., Farmar, R. M.: Influence of pharmacologic or physiologic pretreatment on acute daunomycin cardiac toxicity in the hamster. Toxicol. appl. Pharmacol. **16**, 335 (1970a).
Herman, E. H., Schein, P., Taylor, C., Waravdekar, U. S.: Effect of various antiarrhythmic drugs on the daunomycin induced arrhythmia in the hamster. Proc. Soc. exp. Biol. (N. Y.) **133**, 69 (1970b).
Ho, M., Hohler, H.: Studies on human adenoviruses as inducers of interferon in chick cells. Arch. Ges. Virusforsch. **22**, 69 (1967).

HOSHINO, A., TAKETOSHI, K., HIROYUKI, A., KAZUO, O.: Antitumor effects of adriamycin on Yoshida rat sarcoma and L1210 mouse leukemia — cross resistance and combination chemotherapy. International Symposium on Adriamycin, Milano, Sept. 9—10, 1971.
KERSTEN, W., KERSTEN, H.: Die Bindung von Daunomycin, Cinerubin und Chromomycin A_3 and Nucleinsäuren. Biochem. Z. **341**, 174 (1965).
KESSEL, D., BOTTERIL, V., WODINSKY, L.: Uptake and retention of daunomycin by mouse leukemic cells as factors in drug response. Cancer Res. **28**, 938 (1968).
KIM, K. H., GELBARD, A. S., DJORDJEVIC, B., KIM, S. H., PEREZ, A. G.: Action of daunomycin on the nucleic acid metabolism and viability of HeLa cells. Cancer Res. **28**, 2437 (1968).
MARSH, J. P., JR., MOSHER, L. W., ACTON, E. M., GOODMAN, L.: The synthesis of daunosamine. Chem. Comm. 973 (1967).
MCDONNELL, J. P., GARAPIN, A. C., LEVINSON, W. E., QUINTRELL, N., FANSHIER, L., BISHOP, J. M.: DNA polymerases of Rous sarcoma virus: delineation of two reactions with actinomycin. Nature (Lond.) **228**, 433 (1970).
MINER, N., RAY, W. J., JR., SIMON, E. H.: Effect of interferon on the production and action of viral RNA polymerase. Biochem. biophys. Res. Comm. **24**, 264 (1966).
NATALE, N., MOCARELLI, P.: Depressione immunitaria di daunomicina. Tumori **55**, 409 (1969).
PARISI, B., SOLLER, A.: Studies on the antiphage activity of daunomycin. Giorn. Microbiol. **12**, 183 (1964).
PAUCKER, K., CANTELL, K.: Quantitative studies on viral interference in suspended L cells. Persistance of protection in growing cultures. Virology **31**, 22 (1963).
PICONE, M. A., TRAINE, A.: Pharmacokinetic characteristics of daunomycin, an antibiotic with antitumor action. Arzneim. Forsch. **20**, 88 (1970).
RICHARDSON, A. C.: The synthesis of *N*-benzoyl-D-daunosamine. Carbohyd. Res. **4**, 422 (1967).
RUSCONI, A., CALENDI, E.: Azione della daunomicina sulla sintesi nucleica in cellule di epatoma. Tumori **50**, 261 (1964).
RUSCONI, A., CALENDI, E.: Action of daunomycin on nucleic acid metabolism. Biochim. biophys. Acta (Amst.) **119**, 413 (1966).
RUSCONI, A., DI FRONZO, G., DIMARCO, A.: Distribution of tritiated daunomycin (NSC-82151) in normal rats. Cancer Chemother. Rep. **52**, 331 (1968).
RUSCONI, A., DIMARCO, A.: Inhibition of nucleic acid synthesis by daunomycin and its relationship to the uptake of the drug in HeLa cells. Cancer Res. **29**, 1508 (1969).
SANDBERG, J. S., HOWSDEN, F. L., DIMARCO, A., GOLDIN, A.: Comparison of the antileukemic effect in mice of Adriamycin (NSC 123127) with Daunomycin (82151). Cancer Chemoth. Rep. **54**, 1 (1970).
SANFILIPPO, A., MAZZOLENI, E.: Attività antifagica dello antibiotico daunomicina. Giorn. Microbiol. **12**, 83 (1964).
SILVESTRINI, R., DIMARCO, A., DASDIA, T.: Interference of daunomycin with metabolic events of the cell in synchronized cultures of rat fibroblasts. Cancer Res. **30**, 966 (1970).
SILVESTRINI, R., DIMARCO, A., DASDIA, T., DIMARCO, S.: The action of daunomycin on the metabolism of nucleic acids of normal and neoplastic cells growing *in vitro*. Tumori **49**, 399 (1963a).
SILVESTRINI, R., GAETANI, M.: The action of daunomycin on the metabolism of nucleic acids of Ehrlich ascites tumor cells. Tumori **49**, 389 (1963b).
SIMARD, R.: The binding of actinomycin D-^{3}H to heterochromatin as studied by quantitative high resolution radioautography. J. Cell Biol. **35**, 716 (1967).
SIMON, M. I., VAN VUNAKIS, H.: The photodynamic reaction of methylene blue with deoxyribonucleic acid. J. molec. Biol. **4**, 488 (1962).
SONNABEND, J. A., MARTIN, E. M., MESS, E., FANTES, K. H.: The effect of interferon on the synthesis and activity of an RNA polymerase isolated from chick cells infected with semliki forest virus. J. gen. Virol. **1**, 41 (1967).
STERNBERG, S. S.: Cross-striated fibrils and other ultrastructural alterations in glomeruli of rats with daunomycin nephrosis. Lab. Invest. **23**, 39 (1970).
STERNBERG, S. S., PHILIPS, F. S.: Biphasic intoxication and nephrotic syndrome in rats given daunomycin. Proc. Amer. Ass. Cancer Res. **8**, 64 (1967).
TEMIN, H. M.: Nature of the provirus of Rous sarcoma. Nat. Cancer Inst. Monograph **17**, 557 (1964).
THEOLOGIDES, A., YARBRO, J. M., KENNEDY, B. J.: Daunomycin inhibition of DNA and RNA synthesis. Cancer **21**, 16 (1968).
VENDITTI, J. M., ABBOTT, J. B., DIMARCO, A., GOLDIN, A.: Effectiveness of daunomycin (NSC-82151) against experimental tumors. Cancer Chemother. Rep. **50**, 659 (1966).
VERINI, M. A., CASAZZA, A. M., FIORETTI, A., RODENGHI, F., GHIONE, M.: Photodynamic action of daunomycin. II. Effect on normal viruses. Giorn. Microbiol. **16**, 55 (1968).

Ward, D. C., Reich, E., Goldberg, I. H.: Base specificity in the interaction of polynucleotides with antibiotic drugs. Science **149**, 1259 (1965).

Waring, M. J.: Drugs which affect the structure and function of DNA. Nature (Lond.) **219**, 1320 (1968).

Waring, M. J.: Variation of the supercoils in closed circular DNA by binding of antibiotics and drugs: evidence for molecular models involving intercalation. J. molec. Biol. **54**, 247 (1970).

Wheelock, E. F.: Interferon-like virus-inhibitors induced in human leukocytes by phytohemoagglutinin. Science **149**, 310 (1965).

Xeros, N.: Deoxyriboside control and synchronization of mitosis. Nature (Lond.) **194**, 692 (1962).

Yesair, D. W., Asbell, M. A., Bruni, R., Bullock, F. J., Schwartzbach, E.: Pharmacokinetics and metabolism of adriamycin and daunomycin. International Symposium on Adriamycin, Milano Sept. 9—10, 1971.

Zunino, F., Gambetta, R. A., Zaccara, A., DiMarco, A.: Interaction of daunomycin and its derivatives with DNA. FEBS Let. (in press).

Chapter 61

Chromomycin, Olivomycin, Mithramycin

G. F. Gause

With 2 Figures

Chemistry and Mechanism of Action

Olivomycin, chromomycin, and mithramycin are closely related chemically, as can be seen from the structures of these antibiotics (Fig. 1). Olivomycin is produced by *Streptomyces olivoreticuli*, mithramycin by *Streptomyces atroolivaceus*, and chromomycin by *Streptomyces griseus*. Olivomycin differs from the other two antibiotics in its aglycone, which is not methylated in position 7, and is named

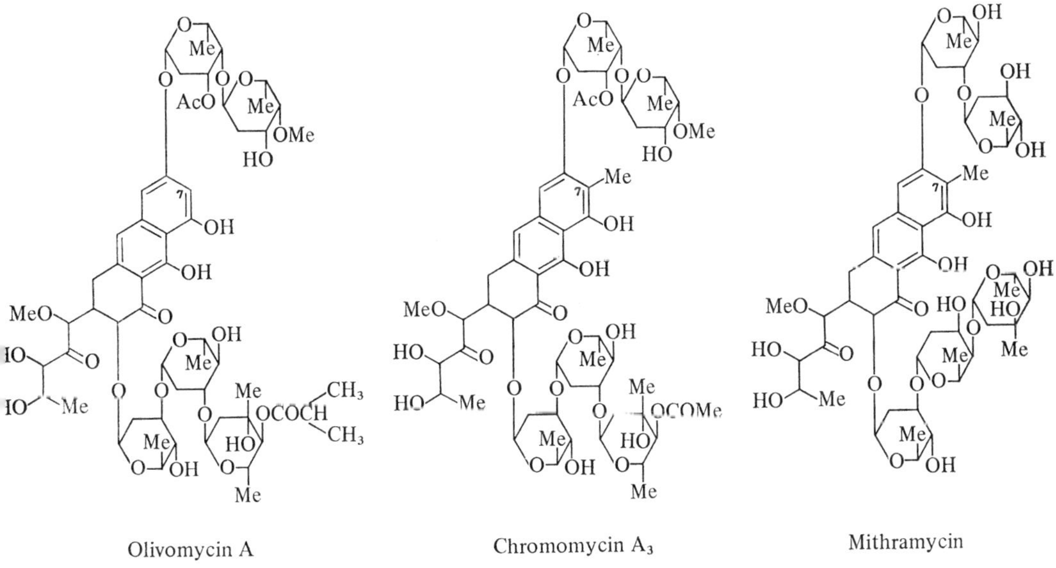

Olivomycin A | Chromomycin A_3 | Mithramycin

Fig. 1. Structures of olivomycin A, chromomycin A_3, and mithramycin. From Sedov et al. (1969)

olivine. The aglycones of chromomycin and mithramycin are identical. They are named chromomycinone and are methylated in position 7. The carbohydrate moieties of these antibiotics are listed in Table 1. Olivomycin and chromomycin have identical sugar contents. Mithramycin is different, and contains olivose and oliose, but not olivomose or olivomycose, the latter being replaced by its diastereomer, *d*-mycarose (Berlin et al., 1968).

Table 1. *Structural comparison of olivomycin, mithramycin, and chromomycin*

Antibiotic	Aglycone	Sugars				
		Olivo-mycose	D-Myca-rose	Olivo-mose	Oli-vose	Oli-ose
Olivomycin	Olivine	+	—	+	+	+
Chromomycin	Chromomycinone	+	—	+	+	+
Mithramycin	Chromomycinone	—	+	—	+	+

Similarities in the mechanisms of action of these antibiotics are suggested by the appearance of partial cross-resistance in both *Staphylococci* and tumor cells to olivomycin, mithramycin, and chromomycin (CHORIN and SHAPOVALOVA, 1966). *Staphylococcus aureus*, grown on media containing increasing concentrations of olivomycin, achieved a 125 fold increase in resistance after 10 passages. Tumor cells of Sarcoma 37 became 267 times more resistant to olivomycin after 16 passages in mice treated with increasing concentrations of the antibiotic. These olivomycin resistant strains of *Staphylococcus aureus* and Sarcoma 37 showed partial cross-resistance to chromomycin and mithramycin, as shown in Table 2.

Table 2. *Partial cross resistance in Staphylococcus aureus and Sarcoma 37 to olivomycin, mithramycin, and chromomycin*

Antibiotic	Fold Increase in resistance	
	Staphylococci	Sarcoma 37 cells
Olivomycin	125	267
Chromomycin	63	—
Mithramycin	17	25

The mechanism of action of these antibiotics has been studied in a number of systems. Of particular interest is an investigation of the *in vivo* effects of mithramycin on the 6C3HED lymphoma (YARBRO et al., 1966). In this system the drug appears to exert its cytotoxic action by inhibition of RNA synthesis. RNA synthesis has been studied at varying times following treatment with mithramycin in both the 6C3HED lymphoma and mouse liver. There was a marked difference between these two tissues in the rate of recovery from the inhibitory effects of mithramycin on RNA synthesis. Whereas liver rapidly recovered its capacity for RNA synthesis, the recovery by the tumor cells was considerably slower, suggesting some selectivity to the vulnerability of nucleic acid synthesis in tumor cells. Such a finding is of considerable interest in a consideration of the use of these antibiotics in cancer chemotherapy.

It has been observed that all three antibiotics preferentially inhibit the synthesis of RNA, and that this effect is due to complex formation between the antibiotic and DNA (GAUSE, 1967). Olivomycin, chromomycin, and mithramycin interact with DNA only in the presence of Mg^{++} ions, and it is the antibiotic-Mg^{++} complex which binds to DNA. The behavior of olivomycin and mithramycin is qualitatively indistinguishable from that of chromomycin in all spectral tests. BEHR et al. (1969) studied in some detail the interaction of chromomycin with DNA. Formation of a complex between chromomycin and DNA has been shown to depend on the guanine content and on base pairing with the polydeoxynucleotides. A limit of association is reached when one chromomycin molecule is bound per four nucleotide base pairs.

Chromomycin is much less inhibitory to RNA polymerase when heat-denatured DNA is used as a template. This observation suggests that a substantially reduced number of binding sites is present in denatured DNA, if complex formation is responsible for the inhibition. In support of this supposition, denatured DNA proved to be much less effective in producing shifts in the absorption spectrum of the antibiotic. BEHR et al. (1969) have found by spectrophotometric titration that heat-denatured calf thymus DNA contains only 0.07 apparent binding sites per base pair compared to 0.19 for native DNA. Similar findings have been obtained using equilibrium dialysis. Heat-denatured DNA contains considerable portions of base paired regions; consequently, such measurements do not allow a decision as to whether base pairing is absolutely required for complex formation. To resolve this question BEHR et al. (1969) studied the binding of chromomycin to poly(*d*G) · poly(*d*C) and its single-stranded components, poly *d*C and poly *d*G. As expected from the base specificity for complex formation (GAUSE, 1967), poly *d*C is completely inactive in producing changes in the absorption spectrum. On the other hand, poly *d*G, which fulfills the base requirement for binding, also does not cause a spectral shift on addition of this polynucleotide to a solution of chromomycin. In contrast to single-stranded polynucleotides, poly(*d*G) · poly(*d*C) interacts with one molecule of chromomycin per four base pairs. These results suggest that base pairing in DNA is necessary for complex formation with chromomycin, and are consistent with the hypothesis that the binding of the chromophore of the antibiotic involves intercalation between base pairs of the DNA helix, as has been proposed for the binding of actinomycin to DNA. However, WARING (1971) noted that interaction of chromomycin and mithramycin with DNA differed significantly from the pattern typically seen with intercalating drugs; such findings agree with the expectation that the very bulky sugar substituents on their chromophores make an intercalative mode of binding seem unlikely.

Antitumor Activity

CHORIN et al. (1962) studied in detail the antitumor action of olivomycin in various systems. This antibiotic strongly inhibits the growth of implanted mouse lymphosarcoma LYO 1, as is shown in Table 3. In optimal well-tolerated doses (a single intravenous injection of 5 mg/kg of the drug on the third day after the intramuscular transplantation of the tumor), olivomycin inhibited the growth of the tumor by 80 % on the 20th day. When given in toxic though sublethal doses (10 mg/kg), olivomycin completely prevented the development of the tumor.

Table 3. *Antitumor action of olivomycin on mouse lymphosarcoma LYO 1*

Olivomycin (mg/kg)	Inhibition of tumor weight (%)	Implantation as compared with controls (%)
2.7	43	74
3.5	52	56
4.0	75	60
5.0	80	23
7.5	90	18
10.0	100	0

Olivomycin also strongly inhibited the growth of subcutaneously implanted myeloleukosis of mice, as can be seen from the data presented in Table 4. In maximum tolerated doses the drug inhibited the development of this tumor by 73.7 % and increased the life span of mice with implanted myeloleukosis by 86 %. It should be pointed out that approximately 10 % of the animals treated with olivomycin did not die. This was never observed in untreated animals.

Table 4. *Antitumor action of olivomycin on myeloleukosis in mice*

Olivomycin (mg/kg)	Life span (days) Controls	Treated
3.0	15.7	15.9
5.0	16.9	24.1
7.5	15.1	28.2[a]

[a] Ten percent of animals are permanently cured; these are not included in the calculation of the life span.

Olivomycin is very active in inhibiting the growth of the Harding-Passey melanoma in mice (ROSSOLIMO, 1964) (Table 5). The complete disappearance of tumors was observed in some animals when treatment was started at an early stage of growth of the transplant, i.e., on the ninth day after the inoculation of tumor cells. Olivomycin also inhibited the growth of sarcomas in mice and rats induced by 9,10-dimethyl-1,2-benzanthracene.

Table 5. *Antitumor action of olivomycin on the Harding-Passey melanoma in mice*

Olivomycin (mg/kg)	Tumor weight[a] (gm)	Percent of permanently cured animals
0	1.44 ± 0.20	0
4	0.60 ± 0.16	0
6	0.30 ± 0.04	53

[a] Treatment was started on the 9th day after transplantation of the tumor, and the weight was estimated on the 24th day after transplantation.

The inhibitory action of chromomycin A_3 on transplantable tumors has been studied in detail by Japanese investigators. Chromomycin A_3 strongly inhibited the growth of several transplantable ascites tumors in rats, i.e., the Yoshida sarcoma (including Nitromin-resistant sublines) and hepatoma AH 130. In mice it inhibited the Ehrlich ascites carcinoma, Sarcoma 180 (ascites and solid forms), and the lymphatic leukemia SN-36 (KAZIWARA et al., 1961).

CHORIN and ROSSOLIMO (1965) carried out an interesting comparative study of the antitumor action of olivomycin and chromomycin A_3 on mouse lymphosarcoma LYO1 under identical experimental conditions. They observed that the chemotherapeutic index (LD_{50}/DIT_{50}) of olivomycin (2.35) is much more favorable than that of chromomycin A_3 (0.99). More information concerning the comparative antitumor activity of these two substances is presented in Fig. 2. The dose of each antibiotic is expressed in fractions of its corresponding LD_{50}. As can be seen from Fig. 2, an LD_{50} dose of olivomycin inhibits tumor growth by 88 %, while an equivalent dose of chromomycin A_3 inhibits the same tumor by only 49 %. On the other hand, inhibition of tumor growth by 50 % can be obtained with only a fraction (0.46) of the LD_{50} of olivomycin; in the case of chromomycin A_3 the same effect can be obtained by injecting more toxic doses of the drug, i.e., approaching one LD_{50} dose. These comparative data are of considerable interest, and SEDOV

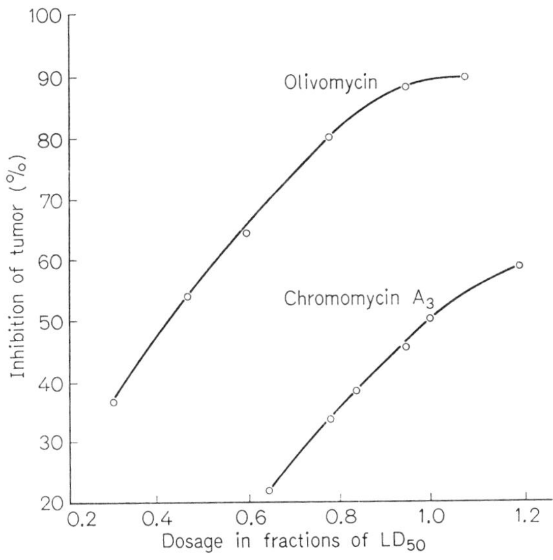

Fig. 2. Antitumor action of olivomycin and chromomycin A_3 on the growth of mouse lymphosarcoma LYO 1 in doses of equivalent toxicity. From CHORIN and ROSSOLIMO (1965)

et al. (1969) made a similar study of the effect of olivomycin A, chromomycin A_3, and mithramycin upon transplantable leukosis La in mice. It was observed that the same effect (the increase of the life span of mice by 25 %) can be attained with olivomycin A at $^1/_{103}$ of LD_{50}, with chromomycin A_3 at $^1/_{32}$ of LD_{50}, and with mithramycin at $^1/_4$ of LD_{50}. One can conclude that olivomycin appears to be therapeutically the most active member of this group of natural products.

Pharmacology

The pharmacology of olivomycin has been investigated in great detail and is described in a number of papers. The study of acute toxicity has shown that the LD_{50} in mice is 13.7 mg/kg (intravenous), 12.7 (intraperitoneal), and 15.6 (subcutaneous), as observed by GOLDBERG and KREMER (1962). Chromomycin is much more toxic and its LD_{50} intraperitoneally in mice is 2.1 mg/kg (KAZIWARA et al., 1961). MORRISON et al. (1967) reported that the acute intravenous toxicity of mithramycin in mice and rats was 2.14 and 1.74 mg/kg, respectively. Mithramycin was not toxic orally in mice or rats at the doses studied, and was essentially nontoxic when administered to dogs at 0.025 and 0.050 mg/kg/day and to monkeys at 0.025 mg/kg/day for a total of 24 doses over a 28 day period. Mithramycin was lethal to dogs and monkeys when administered intravenously at 0.1 mg/kg/day.

Dogs demonstrated marked thrombocytopenia. Necropsy findings were characterized by necrosis of lymphoid tissue and multiple hemorrhages throughout the body.

Shorin and Rossolimo (1965) compared the acute and chronic toxicity of olivomycin and chromomycin A_3 for mice under identical conditions. Their data are given in Table 6. The cumulation index shows the relation of the dose killing 50 % of the animals by a single intravenous injection to the total dose killing the same percentage of animals by four repeated intravenous injections at intervals of 72 h. Table 6 clearly shows that chromomycin A_3 is approximately 10 times more toxic than olivomycin, and also possesses greater cumulative toxicity, as revealed by the larger cumulation index.

Table 6. *Toxicity for mice (LD_{50} in mg/kg) of olivomycin and chromomycin A_3 by single intravenous injection and by four repeated intravenous injections at intervals of 72 h*

Antibiotic	Single injection	Four injections	Cumulation index
Olivomycin	10.00 (8.10—12.30)	8.00 (7.08—9.04)	1.25
Chromomycin A_3	1.21 (1.07—1.37)	0.75 (0.63—0.88)	1.61

The only practical route of administration of olivomycin and related antibiotics is by intravenous injection, since subcutaneous administration produces considerable tissue damage. Goldberg and Kremer (1962) observed that multiple intravenous injections of olivomycin into rabbits in toxic doses led to an abrupt increase in residual nitrogen in the blood shortly before death. No changes were observed in blood pressure within the first few hours following the administration of the antibiotic to rabbits and cats. Baumstein and Goldberg (1964) later studied in greater detail the effect of olivomycin on the functions of kidney and liver. Olivomycin changes neither the amount of residual nitrogen in the blood, nor the amount of glycogen and fat in the liver, when administered intraperitoneally to rats for a prolonged period of time in well tolerated doses (0.4 and 0.6 mg/kg). However, if the antibiotic is administered in a dose causing the death of some animals, the level of residual nitrogen in the blood increases 6 fold, and the amount of glycogen in the liver decreases 2 fold, as compared to control values.

The maintenance of blood levels of olivomycin was studied by Kunrat (1962). The disappearance of the antibiotic from the circulating blood of rabbits was rapid, and only traces were present in the blood 3 h after injection. Similar observations were reported by Kaziwara et al. (1961) for chromomycin A_3. The latter authors also mentioned accumulation of the antibiotic in lymph glands. Kunrat (1962) reported that olivomycin is excreted by rabbits in the urine in the amount of 31 to 34 % of the administered dose. This occurs within 3 to 4 h following the administration of the drug. Very small amounts (0.12 % of the administered dose) of olivomycin are also excreted by rabbits in the bile. Olivomycin is not bound by the proteins of the blood serum.

Vertogradova (1962) studied in detail the action of olivomycin on the blood of laboratory animals. Dogs and rabbits received olivomycin intravenously 25 to 30 times, at intervals of 48 h. At a well-tolerated dose (0.1 mg/kg per injection) no changes were found in the red or white blood cells of the animals, nor were alterations observed in the capillary permeability of the skin of rabbits and rats.

However, multiple administration of toxic doses of olivomycin caused a drop in thrombocytes and erythrocytes of rabbits and produced leucocytosis with relative lymphopenia. As a rule, thrombocytopenia was noted after the first few administrations of the drug, while the drop in erythrocyte count occurred not long before the death of the animal.

Clinical Investigations

SMIRNOVA (1969) summarized some results of treatment of tonsillar tumors with olivomycin, and ASTRAKHAN and GARIN (1970) reviewed their observations on olivomycin therapy of patients with malignant tumors of the testicle. It has been concluded that olivomycin gives favorable results in the treatment of testicular tumors (i.e., seminomas, embryonal carcinomas, and teratoblastomas) in the stage of generalized spread (with metastases), as well as in tonsillar tumors and in reticulocarcinomas affecting the peripheral nodes.

BROWN and KENNEDY (1965) and KENNEDY (1970) report that mithramycin is effective in the treatment of disseminated testicular neoplasms, which are refractory to the action of all other drugs available at present. ANSFIELD (1969) described a case of complete remission of metastasis of seminoma into the lung which continued for 9 years after 12 courses of treatment. REAM et al. (1968) used mithramycin therapy in disseminated germinal testicular cancer, and observed complete disappearance of metastases in lungs and lymphatic nodes. KOONS et al. (1966) reported that mithramycin induced complete remission of clinical evidence of embryonal cancer. They also reported that the major clinically limiting toxicity was a hemorrhagic diathesis associated with a precipitous thrombocytopenia. Further observations on the mechanism of hemorrhagic toxicity with mithramycin therapy were published by MONTO et al. (1969). These observations support the concept that the hemorrhagic diathesis associated with mithramycin therapy is produced by: (a) direct injury to the terminal vascular bed; (b) quantitative and qualitative alteration of platelets; (c) reduction of many (if not all) coagulation factors; and (d) enhancement of fibrinolytic activity. It is of considerable interest that hemorrhagic diathesis was not observed during the administration of the closely related derivative olivomycin in the treatment of testicular and tonsillar tumors.

References

ANSFIELD, F. J.: Clinical studies with mithramycin. Oncology **23**, 283—288 (1969).

ASTRAKHAN, V. I., GARIN, A. M.: Olivomycin in therapy of patients with malignant tumors of testicle. Antibiotiki **15**, 837—840 (1970).

BAUMSTEIN, V. E., GOLDBERG, L. E.: An experimental study of the effect of olivomycin on kidney and liver functions. Antibiotiki **9**, 252—258 (1964).

BEHR, W., HONIKEL, K., HARTMANN, G.: Interaction of the RNA polymerase inhibitor chromomycin with DNA. Europ. J. Biochem. **9**, 82—92 (1969).

BERLIN, Y. A., KISELEVA, O. A., KOLOSOV, M. N., SHEMYAKIN, M. M., SOIFER, V. S., VASINA, I. V., YARTSEVA, I. V.: Aureolic acid group of antitumor antibiotics. Nature (Lond.) **218**, 193—194 (1968).

BROWN, J. H., KENNEDY, B. J.: Mithramycin in the treatment of disseminated testicular neoplasms. New Engl. J. Med. **272**, 111—118 (1965).

CHORIN, V. A., ROSSOLIMO, O. K.: An experimental study of the antitumor effect of six antibiotics belonging to olivomycin group. Antibiotiki **10**, 48—53 (1965).

CHORIN, V. A., ROSSOLIMO, O. K., STANISLAVSKAYA, M. S., BLUMBERG, N. A., FILIPOSYAN, S. T., LEPESHKINA, G. N.: The antitumor activity of the antibiotic olivomycin. Antibiotiki **7**, 60—64 (1962).

CHORIN, V. A., SHAPOVALOVA, S. P.: Cross resistance in a group of antitumor antibiotics belonging to olivomycin-mithramycin type. Antibiotiki **11**, 239—242 (1966).

GAUSE, G. F.: Chromomycin, olivomycin and mithramycin. In: GOTTLIEB, D., SHAW, P. D. (Eds.): Antibiotics, Vol. I., pp. 246—258. New York: Springer 1967.

GOLDBERG, L. E., KREMER, V. E.: Pharmacological studies on the antibiotic olivomycin. Antibiotiki 7, 53—57 (1962).
KAZIWARA, K., WATANABE, J., KOMEDA, T., USUI, T.: Further observations on the inhibiting effects of chromomycin A_3 on transplantable tumors. Cancer Chemother. Rep. 13, 99—106 (1961).
KENNEDY, B. J.: Mithramycin therapy in advanced testicular neoplasms. Cancer 26, 755—766 (1970).
KENNEDY, B. J., YARBRO, J. W., KICKERTZ, V., SANDBERG-WOLLHEIM, M.: Effect of mithramycin on a mouse glioma. Cancer Res. 28, 91—97 (1968).
KOONS, C. R., SENSENBRENNER, L. L., OWENS, A. H., JR.: Clinical studies of mithramycin in patients with embryonal cancer. Bull. Johns Hopkins Hosp. 118, 462—475 (1966).
KUNRAT, I. A.: Absorption, circulation and excretion of olivomycin from the organism. Antibiotiki 7, 44—48 (1962).
MONTO, R. W., TALLEY, R. W., CALDWELL, M. J., LEVIN, W. C., GUEST, M. M.: Observations on the mechanism of hemorrhagic toxicity in mithramycin (NSC 24559) therapy. Cancer Res. 29, 697—704 (1969).
MORRISON, R. K., BROWN, D. E., OLESON, J. J.: A toxicologic study of mithramycin. Toxicol. appl. Pharmacol. 11, 468—481 (1967).
REAM, N. W., PERLIA, C. P., WOLTER, J., TAYLOR, S. G., III: Mithramycin therapy in disseminated germinal testicular cancer. J. Amer. med. Ass. 204, 1030—1036 (1968).
ROSSOLIMO, O. K.: The effect of olivomycin on the development of melanoma (Harding-Passey line) in mice. Antibiotiki 9, 249—252 (1964).
SEDOV, K. A., SOROKINA, I. B., BERLIN, Y. A., KOLOSOV, M. N.: Olivomycin and related antibiotics. XXIII. Effect of olivomycins, chromomycins and mithramycin on leucosis La of mice. Antibiotiki 14, 721—725 (1969).
SMIRNOVA, I. N.: Results of olivomycin treatment of tonsillar tumors. Antibiotiki 14, 271—274 (1969).
YARBRO, J. W., KENNEDY, B. J., BARNUM, C. P.: Mithramycin inhibition of ribonucleic acid synthesis. Cancer Res. 26, 36—39 (1966).
VERTOGRADOVA, T. P.: Effect of the antibiotic olivomycin on the blood of laboratory animals. Antibiotiki 7, 48—53 (1962).
WARING, M.: Binding of drugs to supercoiled circular DNA: evidence for and against intercalation. Progr. molec. subcell. Biol. 2, 216—231 (1971).

Chapter 62

Nogalamycin

B. K. BHUYAN and C. G. SMITH

With 1 Figure

Introduction

As part of a cooperative program carried out by the American pharmaceutical industry and the United States National Cancer Institute, a concerted effort was made to find unique cytotoxic antibiotics which inhibited macromolecule synthesis in, and growth of, cancer cells, to explore their potential as chemotherapeutic agents in the treatment of human malignant disease. During the course of this screening effort, the antibiotic, nogalamycin, an anthracyclinone produced by *Streptomyces nogalater var. nogalater*, was discovered because of its marked cytotoxicity against KB human epidermoid carcinoma cells growing in culture. Nogalamycin selectively inhibited the synthesis of ribonucleic acid (RNA) after binding to the deoxyribonucleic acid (DNA) template. Mammalian cells and bacteria *in vitro* and enzyme induction in rat liver all appeared to be inhibited by the same mechanism. When the antibiotic was found to inhibit the growth of several experimental animal tumors, it was considered for clinical trial as an anticancer agent, but unacceptable toxicity in animals precluded such investigations. The compound still provides an interesting tool to the biochemist for studying various aspects of the molecular mechanism of nucleic acid synthesis.

Chemistry of Nogalamycin

Discovery of nogalamycin was reported in 1965 by BHUYAN and DIETZ (1965) and BHUYAN et al. (1965). Detailed studies on its isolation, characterization, and degradation appeared in 1968 when the structural formula shown in Fig. 1 was reported (WILEY, 1969; WILEY and CARON, 1970; WILEY et al., 1968). These studies on the degradation of the molecule led to the preparation of several degradation products or derivatives of the parent substance also shown in Fig. 1. These investigators thus demonstrated that nogalamycin belongs to the broad family of anthracyclinone antibiotics which includes daunomycin, olivomycin, chromomycin, echinomycin, mithramycin, and cinnerubin, all of which have been differentiated from nogalamycin in one or more structural features and/or biological activities.

In Vitro Studies

A. Antibacterial Activity

Nogalamycin was markedly active against a variety of gram positive organisms. Thus, the minimum inhibitory concentration for *Bacillus subtilis* was 50 μg/ml, compared to 0.4 to 0.8 μg/ml needed to inhibit *Staphylococcus aureus*, *Streptococcus*

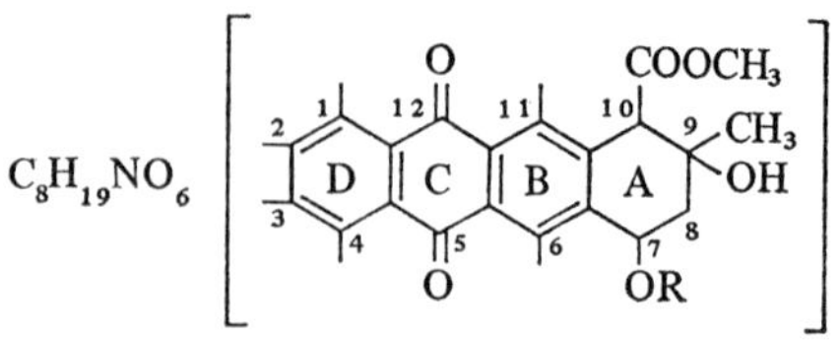

$C_8H_{19}NO_6$ [structure: rings D, C, B, A; positions 1–12; C=O at 12 and 5; COOCH$_3$ at 10; CH$_3$ and OH at 9; OR at 7]

Nogalamycin : R = nogalosyl = [structure with H, CH$_3$, O, CH$_3$, H, CH$_3$O, OCH$_3$, OCH$_3$, H]

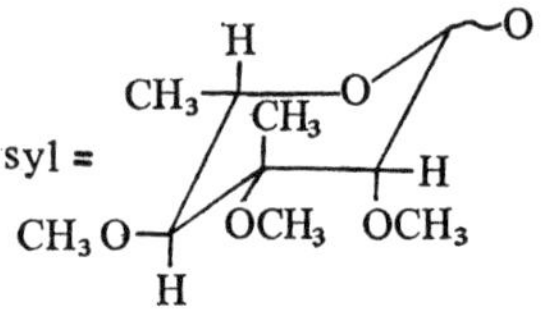

Nogalarol:	R = H
O-Methylnogalarol:	R = CH_3
7-Deoxynogalarol:	no OR on carbon 7 of Ring A
Nogalamycin *N*-oxide:	The N in nogalamycin has two CH_3 groups attached. In nogalamycin *N*-oxide the N also has an O attached.
Nogalarene:	Ring A becomes aromatic and the OH on carbon 9 and the OR on carbon 7 are absent.

This is a schematic representation in which the amino sugar moiety ($C_8H_{19}NO_6$) is attached to 2 adjacent positions of the 1, 2, 3, 4 group carbons and 2 hydroxyls are present in 2 positions of the 1, 4, 6, 11 group carbons.

Fig. 1. Structure of nogalamycin and analogs

faecalis, and *S. hemolyticus*. It was inactive against gram-negative organisms such as *Escherichia coli*, *Proteus vulgaris*, *Salmonella typhosa*, and *Klebsiella pneumoniae* at 100 µg/ml (BHUYAN and DIETZ, 1965).

The time course of inhibition of macromolecule synthesis in *S. aureus* indicated that nogalamycin inhibited both RNA and DNA synthesis equally well with significantly less effect on protein synthesis. In mammalian cells (discussed below) nogalamycin inhibited RNA synthesis significantly more than DNA synthesis with little or no inhibition of protein synthesis (BHUYAN and DIETZ, 1965). The toxicity of nogalamycin precluded serious consideration of this antibiotic as an antibacterial agent.

B. Cytotoxicity to Mammalian Cells

KB cell growth, measured as increase in cell protein, was inhibited 50 % for 3 days at 0.005 µg/ml of nogalamycin (BHUYAN and SMITH, 1965). RNA synthesis in KB cell monolayers was more sensitive to the antibiotic than DNA synthesis, while very little inhibition of the formation of protein was found (Table 1). The overall pattern of inhibition in both mammalian cells and bacteria was similar to that seen with actinomycin D, which is known to interact with the DNA template, thereby inhibiting RNA synthesis.

C. Characteristics of Nogalamycin - DNA Interaction

When nogalamycin and DNA were mixed *in vitro* the following effects indicated that nogalamycin was bound to DNA: (1) a change in the nogalamycin absorption spectrum, (2) a marked increase in the melting temperature (T_m) of DNA, and (3) the formation of an orange colored precipitate of the nogalamycin-DNA com-

Table 1. *Inhibition of growth and macromolecule synthesis by nogalamycin and its derivatives*

Drug	mμMole/ml for 50% inhibition		% Inhibition[a]		
	Growth[b]	RNA[a]	RNA	DNA	Protein
Nogalamycin	0.006	0.41	80	40	5
O-Methyl nogalarol	0.13	0.85	71	30	5
7-Deoxynogalarol	0.68	2.04	69	30	27
Nogalarol	0.17	3.18	72	39	15
Nogalarene	1.77	25	71	74	80
Nogalamycin-*N*-oxide	0.35	55.7	69	0	13

[a] The incorporation of thymidine-methyl-^{3}H into DNA, uridine-^{3}H into RNA, and valine-^{14}C into protein was determined after 2 h of incubation of KB cells, drug, and radioactive precursor. Drugs were added at a concentration suitable to inhibit RNA synthesis by 70 to 80%.

[b] The inhibition of growth was measured after 3 days of contact between cells and drug. From Bhuyan and Reusser (1970).

plex upon addition of streptomycin to the DNA-nogalamycin mixture. The nogalamycin-DNA complex precipitated by streptomycin was stable to several extractions with ethyl acetate and contained 175 μg of nogalamycin firmly bound per mg of DNA (Bhuyan and Smith, 1965).

It was further shown that: (1) the ΔT_m (i.e., the increase in T_m on mixing DNA with nogalamycin) increased with increasing AT content of DNA, in contrast to actinomycin D for which the ΔT_m decreased with increasing AT content; and (2) nogalamycin bound strongly to poly *d*AT with little binding to poly *d*G*d*C or poly *d*A*d*T (Table 2).

Table 2. *Effect of binding of actinomycin (Act.D) and nogalamycin (Nogal.) to synthetic DNA-like polymers on ΔT_m and inhibition of RNA polymerase*

Polymer	Effect on T_m[a]			Inhibition of RNA Polymerase[b]	
	T_m (°C)	ΔT_m (°C) Nogal.	ΔT_m (°C) Act. D	Substrate	% Inhibition
Poly *d*AT	38	27	0	ATP—H^3	99
Poly *d*G*d*C	84	1.8	0.2	CTP—H^3	3
Poly *d*G*d*C	—			GTP—H^3	3.5
Poly *d*A*d*T	43	3	—	UTP—H^3	0
Poly *d*A*d*T				ATP—H^3	1

[a] T_m experiments were conducted in 3×10^{-2} M NaCl and 3×10^{-4} M sodium citrate, pH 7. Polymer concentration was equivalent to 0.15 A_{260} units. Nogalamycin and actinomycin D were present at 2.5 and 4 μg/ml, respectively.

[b] *E. coli* RNA polymerase was isolated and the assay carried out by the method of Chamberlin and Berg in the laboratory of E. Reich. Nogalamycin was present at 10 μg/ml. From Bhuyan and Smith (1965).

These studies, indicating the preference of nogalamycin for adenine or thymine or both moieties in DNA, were confirmed and extended by Ward et al. (1965). These authors showed a marked difference in the binding of various anthracyclinones to different DNA primers (Table 3).

Table 3. *Inhibition of DNA-primed RNA synthesis by various drugs. RNA synthesis was measured for thirty minutes at 37°; eight units of enzyme protein were used. The concentrations of DNA-phosphorus used were: calf thymus, 120*µM; *crab d*AT *(0.018* A/ml *at 260* nm*), 3.0* µM; *synthetic d*AT, *6.0* µM; *d*A*d*T, *7.2* µM; *d*G*d*C, *53* µM; *and d*I*d*C, *16* µM. *The specific activity of the tritiated nucleoside triphosphates used was* 5.5×10^6 *counts* min^{-1} μmol^{-1}. *The labeled nucleoside triphosphate incorporated in the control reactions with each DNA preparation was in* µµmol: *calf thymus* (H^3-CTP), *1740; crab d*AT (H^3-ATP), *580; synthetic d*AT (H^3-ATP), *6830; d*A*d*T (H^3-ATP), [?]; *d*G*d*C (H^3-GTP), *410; d*G*d*C (H^3-CTP), *57; d*I*d*C (H^3-GTP), *3460; d*I*d*C (H^3-CTP), *1180*

Drug	Inhibition of various DNA primers (%)									
	Calf-thymus DNA						*d*G*d*C		*d*I*d*C	
	Amount (mµmol/ml)	Drug/DNA	% Inhib.	Crab *d*AT	*d*AT	*d*A*d*T	GTP[a]	CTP[b]	GTP[a]	CTP[b]
Ethidium	100	0.78	100	100	100		75.8	26.2	36.2	25.6
Daunomycin	71	0.55	95	100	97.3		17.9	17.9	18.2	30.9
Echinomycin	27.5	0.21	100	98.0	97.2		41.8	29.8	13.7	25.4
Nogalamycin	26.3	0.20	100	100	100	0	3.0	3.5	0	0
Chromomycin	100	0.78	96.5	1.5	4.0		53.4	70.2	5.0	0

[a] GTP refers to percentage inhibition of incorporation of labeled GTP as primed by *d*C strand of both *d*G*d*C and *d*I*d*C polymers.

[b] CTP refers to percentage inhibition of incorporation of labeled CTP as primed by the *d*G strand of the *d*G*d*C primer and the *d*I strand of the *d*I*d*C primer.

From WARD et al. (1965).

It was elegantly shown by WELLS and LARSON (1970) that actinomycin D also prefers certain nucleotide sequences in DNA. They found that the DNA isomer which contains both purines and pyrimidines in both strands binds more actinomycin than the isomer which contains all purines in one strand and all pyrimidines in the complementary strand. This is similar to the binding of nogalamycin to poly *d*AT, compared to the negligible binding with poly *d*A*d*T. Whether this specificity is a function of primary nucleotide sequence or a matter of DNA configuration cannot be determined at present.

The preference of nogalamycin for adenine or thymine or both moieties in DNA was questioned by KERSTEN et al. (1966). They reported that the shift in the buoyant density of DNA in the presence of nogalamycin or actinomycin D increased with greater G+C content of the DNA. However, equilibrium density centrifugation studies are of necessity performed in concentrated salt solutions. Such concentrated salt solutions may not only cause structural changes in DNA but also affect the affinity of nogalamycin and actinomycin D for DNA. Thus, the buoyant density studies of KERSTEN et al. (1966) indicate that denatured DNA binds more actinomycin than native DNA, which contradicts the observations of REICH and GOLDBERG (1964). Also, WELLS and LARSON (1970) observed that poly *d*I binds to actinomycin, as shown by spectral change and equilibrium dialysis experiments; however, cesium sulfate density gradient studies indicated that poly *d*I did not bind to actinomycin.

It has been suggested that planar polycyclic drugs can bind to DNA by 2 means. One is strong binding (i.e., "intercalation"), which involves the insertion of the drug molecule between adjacent base pairs in the DNA helix. A second weak binding is an ionic reaction between the drug molecule and the phosphate group of DNA (SAUNDERS et al., 1969). The following evidence suggested that nogalamycin intercalates with DNA: (1) Nogalamycin binding resulted in a marked increase in the viscosity of DNA (Table 4; KERSTEN et al., 1966) and decreased the sedimentation coefficient of DNA (KERSTEN et al., 1966). (2) Difference spectra measurements indicated that, like proflavin, nogalamycin-DNA binding was inhibited by high salt concentration (Table 5).

Table 4. *Effect of DNA-drug complex on the viscosity of DNA*[a]

Drug	[NaCl]	Intrinsic viscosity (dl/gm)
None	0.01 M	457
Nogalamycin	0.01 M	679
Actinomycin	0.01 M	386
None	0.1 M	301
Nogalamycin	0.1 M	396

[a] The drugs were added to T_4B phage DNA at a molar ratio of DNA—P:drug of 10:1. The measurements were done by P. Ross (NIH) with a ZIMM zero shear viscometer.

Table 5. *Effect of* NaCl *concentration on the spectral change caused by nogalamycin-DNA or actinomycin-DNA interaction*

[NaCl]	Nogalamycin ΔA	%[a]	Actinomycin ΔA	%
0.005 M	0.225	100	0.565	100
0.125 M	0.170	75.5	0.515	91
0.25 M	0.110	49	0.500	88.5
1.0 M	0.020	9	0.415	73.5

All substances were dissolved in 0.1 M *tris*-HCl, pH 7. One ml of 500 μg/ml of nogalamycin or actinomycin containing 0.01 to 2 M NaCl was mixed with 1 ml of calf thymus DNA (0.5 mg/ml) in 5 mM NaCl.

[a] The spectral change in 0.005 M NaCl is taken as 100%.

Further rigorous evidence for nogalamycin intercalation with DNA has come from the studies of WARING (1970). Intercalation results in the local uncoiling of tho DNA double helix which leads to the removal and reversal of the supercoils of circular ΦX174 DNA (replicative form). WARING (1970) found that proflavin, daunomycin, nogalamycin, and actinomycin affected the supercoils in the same qualitative manner as ethidium bromide, indicating that all these drugs intercalate with DNA. In contrast, nonintercalating compounds such as spermine, streptomycin, and mithramycin did not affect the supercoiling. A certain fraction of the bound intercalating drug molecules may be present in a nonintercalated state. This was zero for ethidium bromide, 0.05 for actinomycin, and 0.32 for nogalamycin.

The complexities of the macromolecular binding system are illustrated by the studies of SAUNDERS and coworkers (1969) in which the thermal stability enhancement (ΔT_m) of nogalamycin (and daunomycin, and ethidium bromide as well) was greater with calf-thymus DNA than it was with bacteriophage TP-84 DNA, although both nucleic acids contained 42 % G+C. Whether such discrepancies are due to differences in specific nucleotide sequences within the DNA or to more subtle differences in conformation of the macromolecule cannot be decided from the available data.

Nogalamycin, like actinomycin, binds to a greater extent to native DNA than to denatured DNA. Thus, heat denatured calf thymus DNA bound 80 μg nogalamycin/mg of DNA compared to 175 μg/mg of native DNA. SAUNDERS et al. (1969) reported on the renaturation of DNA after heating in the presence and absence of nogalamycin. They found that nogalamycin interacts with denatured TP-84 phage DNA and initiates an ordering of structure. However, the molecular conformation so obtained did not have the melting characteristics of native DNA.

D. Effects of Nogalamycin on RNA Synthesis

Nogalamycin inhibited RNA synthesis more than the formation of DNA or protein in mammalian cells (Table 1). In a similar manner the antibiotic inhibited RNA polymerase of KB cells to a greater extent than DNA polymerase (Table 6). However, the DNA and RNA polymerase enzymes of *E. coli* were about equally inhibited.

Table 6. *Effects of nogalamycin on DNA and RNA synthesis in Escherichia coli and in KB cell-free systems and KB cell cultures*[a]

Antibiotic	*E. coli* polymerases				KB Cell polymerases		Whole KB cells[b]	
	DNA polymerase		RNA polymerase		DNA Poly-merase	RNA Poly-merase	^{3}H-thym-idine incorp. into DNA	^{3}H-uridine incorp. into RNA
	Native DNA primer	Denat. DNA primer	Native DNA primer	Denat. DNA primer				
Nogalamycin	0.006	0.032	0.008	0.026	0.026	0.005[c]	0.0013	0.0004

[a] All results are expressed in micromoles of nogalamycin per milliliter necessary to cause 50% inhibition of the reaction.

[b] Labeled precursors were added simultaneously with nogalamycin, and the cells were harvested and processed after 1 h.

[c] The KB cell RNA polymerase assay was done by the method of GOLDBERG; the *E. coli* polymerase by the method of SUMMERS et al.
From REUSSER and BHUYAN (1967).

Cytochemical studies in intact mammalian cells in culture led ARRIGHI (1967) to conclude that nogalamycin, like actinomycin D, inhibited nucleolar RNA synthesis more than RNA synthesis in the chromatin (DUPRAT et al., 1967; JONES, 1967). The inhibition of nucleolar RNA synthesis led to nucleolar lesions consisting of a decrease in size and of a segregation and redistribution of the nucleolar components (SIMARD and BERNHARD, 1966).

The difference in the DNA-binding site between nogalamycin (i.e., *d*A or *d*T) and actinomycin D (i.e., *d*G) suggested that these antibiotics might show differences in the inhibition of synthesis of different species of RNA. However, ELLEM and RHODE (1970) found that both nogalamycin and actinomycin D inhibited the synthesis of nucleic acids in the following order: rRNA > tRNA, 5 S RNA > DNA-like RNA > DNA. Also, the rate of degradation of any nucleic acid species or the maturation of rRNA precursors was not affected. ELLEM and RHODE (1970) suggested that the preferential inhibition of rRNA synthesis by both antibiotics could be due to the much larger size of the rRNA precursor molecule (i.e., 4.5×10^{6} daltons) as compared to tRNA (i.e., 2×10^{4} daltons). Thus, the synthesis of a larger molecule would be more susceptible to a small number of randomly distributed interruptions to the progress of RNA polymerase than an equivalent weight of smaller molecules.

SENTENAC et al. (1968) found that both nogalamycin and actinomycin D inhibited RNA chain elongation rather than chain initiation. Since no selectivity was observed with respect to chains that were initiated by either ATP or GTP, these authors conclude that both initiation sites must be complex, both containing A-T as well as G-C pairs

Nogalamycin did not inhibit RNA synthesis directed by synthetic RNA polymers (WARD et al., 1965; REUSSER and BHUYAN, 1967).

E. Other Activities Inhibited by Nogalamycin

As is the case with actinomycin D, large nogalamycin levels inhibited DNA-directed DNA synthesis (BHUYAN and SMITH, 1965). At sufficiently large concentrations nogalamycin inhibited deoxyribonuclease action and displaced methyl green from its complex with DNA, presumably due to interaction with the macromolecule (ZELEZNICK and SWEENEY, 1967). Nogalamycin (0.05 μmole/ml) did not markedly inhibit respiration (<20%) or oxidative phosphorylation (0 to 40%) with glutamate or succinate as substrates (REUSSER and BHUYAN, 1967).

F. Phase Specificity of Nogalamycin

Using synchronized DON cells it was found that both nogalamycin and actinomycin D were most cytotoxic to cells in both M phase and at the G_1/S border (BHUYAN et al., 1970; MAURO and MADOC-JONES, 1970). The related inhibitor, daunomycin, however, was most cytotoxic to cells in S phase (MAURO and MADOC-JONES, 1970).

G. Comparative Biological Activity of Nogalamycin and Its Derivatives

When a series of derivatives of nogalamycin (structures shown in Fig. 1) was evaluated for effects on the growth of mammalian cells in culture and on the inhibition of macromolecular synthesis therein, the results shown in Table 1 were obtained (BHUYAN and REUSSER, 1970). These results indicate the following:

1. Nogalamycin is the most active compound of the series.
2. The order of activities of the compounds was the same in inhibiting RNA synthesis both in intact cells and in RNA polymerase systems and in increasing the T_m of DNA. This finding supports the concept that the inhibition of RNA synthesis is due to the binding of the drugs to DNA.
3. If inhibition of RNA synthesis causes inhibition of growth then the relative order of activity of the compounds should be the same regardless of whether growth inhibition or RNA synthesis is measured. However, the order of growth inhibition, namely nogalamycin > O-methyl nogalarol > nogalarol > nogalamycin-N-oxide > 7-deoxy nogalarol > nogalarene, is very different from the order of inhibition of RNA synthesis (see Table 1). It is probable, therefore, that while RNA synthesis may be the prime site of inhibition, in long term exposure of cells to drug, as when measuring growth inhibition, other inhibitory effects of the drug leading to inhibition of growth may be superimposed on the inhibition of RNA synthesis.
4. With nogalamycin, and most of the derivatives, RNA synthesis was inhibited more than DNA or protein synthesis. However, with nogalamycin-N-oxide DNA synthesis was not inhibited at all, while RNA synthesis was inhibited 69%. Nogalarene inhibited the biosynthesis of DNA, RNA, and protein equally; how-

ever, the ring structure of nogalarene is completely different from the other derivatives and so it is doubtful if nogalarene should be compared with these other agents.

Studies on the nature of the binding of the various compounds to DNA showed the following: (1) Although similar amounts of nogalamycin, nogalarol, and *O*-methyl nogalarol are bound per mg of DNA, nogalamycin stabilized DNA, as measured by an increase in T_m, to a much greater extent than the other two compounds. Nogalamycin, in contrast to nogalarol and *O*-methyl nogalarol, contains the sugar (nogalose) side chain. This indicates that, in addition to the OH groups on the chromophore, nogalose is also involved in binding of nogalamycin to DNA. (2) Unlike nogalamycin, nogalarol, or *O*-methyl nogalarol, 7-deoxynogalarol binds markedly to apurinic DNA and equally strongly to poly *d*I:*d*C and poly *d*AT (Table 7). The first three compounds preferentially bind to poly *d*AT. This change in the specificity of binding to polynucleotides could be due to the absence in 7-deoxynogalarol of the nonbinding electrons on the oxygen attached to carbon 7, or change in the conformation of the fourth ring due to removal of the OH or OR groups attached to carbon 7.

Table 7. *Inhibition of E. coli RNA polymerase activity primed by poly d*I:*d*C *and poly d*AT

Drug	Concentration (nmol/ml)	Inhibition (%)		
		Poly *d*AT	Poly *d*I:*d*C	Poly *d*G:*d*C
Nogalamycin	2.3	81	22	
Nogalarol	100	74	26	
O-Methylnogalarol	85	75	21	
7-Deoxynogalarol	110	73	82	
Nogalarene	55	75	69	
Actinomycin D	10	0	0	38

The assay mixtures (0.25 ml) contained: *Tris*-HCl (pH 7.9), 5 μmoles; $MgCl_2$, 1 μmole; mercaptoethanol, 3 μmole; $MnCl_2$, 0.25 μmole; GTP, UTP, CTP for poly *d*AT-primed reaction or ATP, CTP, UTP for poly *d*I:*d*C-primed reaction, 0.1 μmole each; the respective labeled nucleotide (ATP—^{14}C for poly *d*AT and GTP—^{14}C for poly *d*I:*d*C) contained 0.5 μCi ^{14}C/μmole; poly *d*AT, or poly *d*I:*d*C, 0.04 A_{260} unit; *E. coli* RNA polymerase, 35 μg. Reactions were run at room temperature for 15 min, tubes were then chilled in ice, and 3 ml cold 3.5% perchloric acid containing 60 mg Celite/100 ml were added. The acid-insoluble product was collected on 0.45 μ Millipore filters (type HA, Millipore Corp., Bedford, Mass.) and the filters were washed extensively with cold 0.1 N HCl. The filter discs were then dried and counted in 15 ml Diotol. In the *d*I:*d*C-primed reaction, the control (i.e., no drug) tube gave 1060 cpm compared to 200 cpm for the tube containing no primer. In the *d*AT-primed reaction, the control tube (i.e., no drug) gave 2600 cpm compared to 174 cpm for the tube containing no primer.
From Bhuyan and Reusser (1970).

In Vivo Studies

A. Enzyme Synthesis in Regenerating Liver

Gray et al. (1966) demonstrated in partially hepatectomized and sham-operated rats that nogalamycin exhibited the same pattern of inhibitory activity as that seen with mammalian cells in culture; namely, marked inhibition of RNA synthesis, inhibition of DNA synthesis only at larger drug levels and little or no inhibition of protein synthesis.

The antibiotic completely inhibited the hydrocortisone-induced increase in tryptophan pyrrolase, but had no effect on the substrate-induced increase in enzyme activity. These findings are consistent with the hypothesis that the primary action of the compound is on the inhibition of RNA synthesis, since the induction by hydrocortisone, but not substrate, is postulated to proceed via DNA transcription (GRAY et al., 1966).

B. Whole Animal Toxicity

Nogalamycin proved to be quite toxic when administered parenterally. Although the acute LD_{50} for mice was 18 mg/kg, dogs receiving 40 µg/kg/day for 16 days died from the toxic effects of the drug. Monkeys, however, tolerated up to 113 µg/kg/day for 20 days.

The following toxic effects were obtained by the Mason Research Institute (Worcester, Mass.): (1) venous occlusion, even when the drug (100 µg/ml) was infused into dogs over a period of 1 h to give a total daily dose of 40 µg/kg for 16 days; (2) renal toxicity with fluid retention and development of cystic tubular nephritis at a daily dose of 20 µg/kg/day given for 5 days to dogs (this was one of the primary toxic effects of the compound); (3) pulmonary thrombosis with inflammation and thrombus formation in the arterioles of the lung and inflammation of the surrounding lung tissue in dogs receiving 20 µg/kg/day for 5 days; and (4) liver damage and increased intraocular pressure.

Since the extent of binding of nogalamycin to DNA can be lessened by large concentrations of NaCl, two approaches were taken to prevent venous occlusion: (1) by mixing the nogalamycin with DNA before injection in the hope of carrying it past the venous wall at the injection site and (2) by infusing the antibiotic in hypertonic saline in an attempt to decrease cellular penetration and binding. Neither of these approaches showed any diminution of the phlebitic action.

C. Antitumor Activity

The antitumor activity of nogalamycin was determined under the auspices of the Cancer Chemotherapy National Service Center. Nogalamycin was active against both an adenocarcinoma of the duodenum producing 73 % inhibition and the Novikoff hepatoma causing 66 % inhibition (BHUYAN and DIETZ, 1965). It was inactive against several other tumors (BHUYAN and DIETZ, 1965).

Nogalamycin increased the life span (ILS) of L1210 leukemic mice by 32 % (marginally active), compared to a 32 % ILS for nogalarol and a 48 % ILS (active) for *O*-methyl nogalarol. Nogalarene, nogalamycin-*N*-oxide, and 7-deoxynogalarol were inactive (BHUYAN and REUSSER, 1970).

References

ARRIGHI, F.E.: Nucleolar RNA synthetic activity in Chinese hamster cells *in vitro* and the effects of actinomycin D and nogalamycin. J. cell. Physiol. **69**, 45—52 (1967).

BHUYAN, B.K., DIETZ, A.: Fermentation, taxonomic, and biological studies of nogalamycin. Antimicrob. Ag. Chemother. **1965**, 836—844 (1965).

BHUYAN, B.K., KELLY, R.B., SMITH, R.M.: Nogalamycin and its production. U.S. Patent **3**, 183, 157 (May 11, 1965).

BHUYAN, B.K., REUSSER, F.: Comparative biological activity of nogalamycin and its analogs. Cancer Res. **30**, 984—989 (1970).

BHUYAN, B.K., SCHEIDT, L.G., FRASER, T.J.: Cell cycle phase specificity of antitumor agents. Cancer Res. **32**, 398—407 (1972).

BHUYAN, B.K., SMITH, C.G.: Differential interaction of nogalamycin with DNA of varying base composition. Proc. nat. Acad. Sci. (Wash.) **54**, 566—572 (1965).

DUPRAT, A.M., MIQUEL, M.T., BEETSCHEN, J.C., ZALTA, J.P.: Effect of chromomycin A_3 and nogalamycin on urodelous amphibian embryo cells cultured *in vitro*; analogy with the effects of actinomycin D. C.R. Acad. Sci (Paris) D **265**, 2080—2083 (1967).

Ellem, K. A. O., Rhode, S. L., III: Selective inhibition of ribosomal RNA synthesis in HeLa cells by nogalamycin, a *d*A:*d*T binding antibiotic. Biochim. biophys. Acta (Amst.) **209**, 415—424 (1970).

Gray, G. D., Camiener, G. W., Bhuyan, B. K.: Nogalamycin effects in rat liver; inhibition of trytophan pyrrolase induction and nucleic acid biosynthesis. Cancer Res. **26**, 2419—2424 (1966).

Jones, K. W.: The induction of paracrystalline thread-complexes in the nuclei of amphibian cells by actinomycin D and other DNA-binding antibiotics. J. Ultrastruc. Res. **18**, 71—84 (1967).

Kersten, W., Kersten, H., Szybalski, W.: Physicochemical properties of complexes between deoxyribonucleic acid and antibiotics which affect ribonucleic acid synthesis (actinomycin, daunomycin, cinerubin, nogalamycin, chromomycin, mithramycin, and olivomycin). Biochemistry **5**, 236—244 (1966).

Mauro, F., Madoc-Jones, H.: Age responses of cultured mammalian cells to cytotoxic drugs. Cancer Res. **30**, 1397—1408 (1970).

Reich, E., Goldberg, I. H.: Actinomycin and nucleic acid function. Prog. nucleic Acid Res. molec. Biol. **3**, 184—234 (1964).

Reusser, F., Bhuyan, B. K.: Comparative studies with three antibiotics binding to deoxyribonucleic acid. J. Bact. **94**, 576—579 (1967).

Saunders, G. F., Reese, W. N., Saunders, P. P.: Differential reactivity of intercalative dyes with bacteriophage TP-84 DNA. Biochim. biophys. Acta (Amst.) **190**, 406—417 (1969).

Sentenac, A., Simon, E. J., Fromageot, P.: Initiation of chains by RNA polymerase and the effects of inhibitors studied by a direct filtration technique. Biochim. biophys. Acta (Amst.) **161**, 299—308 (1968).

Simard, R., Bernhard, W.: Nucleolar segregation. Specific action of certain antimetabolites. Int. J. Cancer **1**, 463—479 (1966).

Ward, D. C., Reich, E., Goldberg, I. H.: Base specificity in the interaction of polynucleotides with antibiotic drugs. Science **149**, 1259—1263 (1965).

Waring, M.: Variation of the supercoils in closed circular DNA by binding of antibiotics and drugs: evidence for intercalation. J. molec. Biol. **54**, 247—279 (1970).

Wells, R. D., Larson, J. E.: Studies on the binding of actinomycin to DNA and DNA model polymers. J. molec. Biol. **49**, 319—342 (1970).

Wiley, P. F.: Antibiotic nogalamycin *N*-oxide. U.S. Patent 3, 449, 490 (June 10, 1969).

Wiley, P. F., Caron, E. L., Jr.: Antibiotic nogalarol, *O*-methylnogalarol, and nogalarene. U.S. Patent **3**, 501, 569 (March 17, 1970).

Wiley, P. F., MacKellar, F. A., Caron, E. L., Kelly, R. B.: Isolation, characterization and degradation of nogalamycin. Tetrahedron Let. 663—668 (1968).

Zeleznick, L. D., Sweeney, C. M.: Inhibition of deoxyribonuclease action by nogalamycin and U-12,241 by their interaction with DNA. Arch. Biochem. Biophys. **120**, 292—295 (1967).

Chapter 63

Streptonigrin

William B. Kremer and John Laszlo

With 4 Figures

Introduction

Streptonigrin (SN) is an antibiotic which was isolated and prepared from broth filtrates of *Streptomyces flocculus* (Rao and Cullen, 1960). By the use of animal tumor screening tests it was determined that SN inhibited the growth of several transplantable rodent and human tumors grown in conditioned rats (Merker et al., 1961; Oleson et al., 1961). Its chemical structure was subsequently defined and it was found to resemble another antibiotic with antitumor activity, mitomycin C, in that it contained an amino quinone ring with a heterocyclic system (Fig. 1) (Rao et al., 1963).

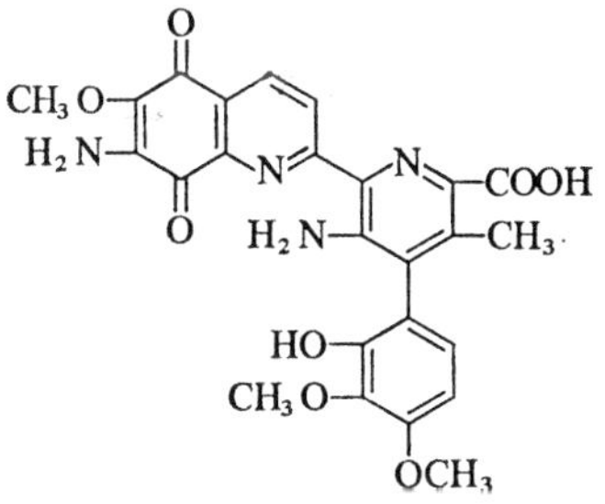

Streptonigrin (SN)

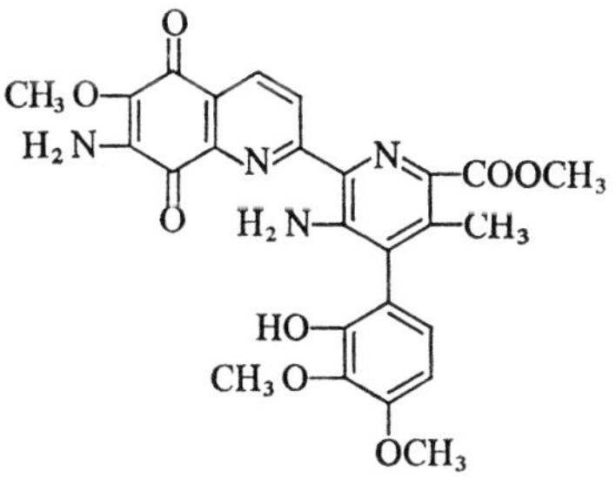

Methyl Streptonigrin (MeSN)

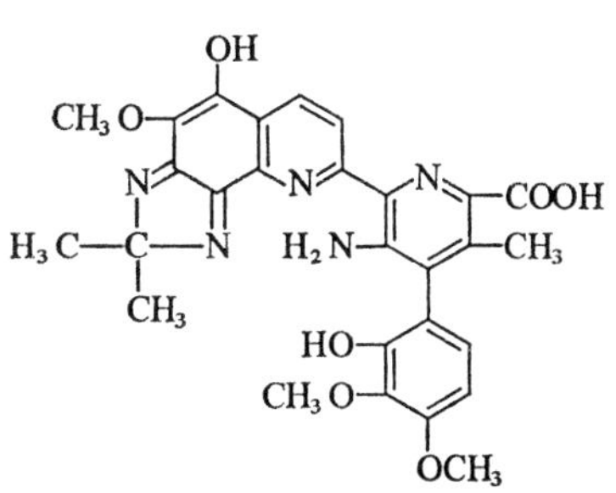

Isopropylidine Azastreptonigrin (IPAS)

Fig. 1. Structures of streptonigrin, methyl streptonigrin, and isopropylidine azastreptonigrin

Biological Properties

Early studies on the mechanism of action of SN centered around its effects on nucleic acid metabolism and bacterial death. Streptonigrin was found to stimulate induction of phage production in lysogenic bacteria while inhibiting the net synthesis of bacterial DNA; it had little effect on RNA and protein synthesis (LEVINE and BORTHWICK, 1963). Exposure of bacteria to SN resulted in marked degradation of DNA to acid soluble components, as well as in DNA single strand breaks (RADDING, 1963; SZYBALSKI, 1964).

When mammalian tissue culture cells are incubated with low levels of SN, their mitoses and replication are inhibited (YOUNG and HODAS, 1965; MIZUNO, 1965). In one report of mouse mammary tumor cells grown in suspension culture, SN exposure did not result in degradation of cellular DNA to acid-soluble components as in bacteria, but there was inhibition of DNA synthesis with subsequent inhibition of RNA and protein synthesis (MIZUNO, 1965). However, human leukemic leukocytes incubated with SN *in vitro* did yield less high molecular weight DNA than did untreated controls, indicating DNA degradation (MILLER et al., 1967). Although overall DNA synthesis, as measured by tritiated thymidine incorporation, was inhibited in this system, the DNA that was isolated had an increased specific activity, suggesting that the process of DNA repair accompanied DNA degradation (Table 1). Human leukocytes incubated with SN were found to have extensive chromosomal breakage and rearrangement (COHEN et al., 1963). SN also caused striking inhibition of mitosis and the types of chromosome abnormalies thus produced included chromatin breaks, isochromatin breaks, severe fragmentation, and degeneration of the entire chromatin material. Along with the high frequency of chromosome abnormalities in cultured leukocytes, SN treatment also resulted in polyploid and endoreduplicated mitoses (NASJLETI and SPENCER, 1967).

Table 1. *Recovery of leukocyte high molecular weight DNA*[a]

SN (μg/ml)	DNA Amount Isolated (mg)	DNA Specific Activity (cpm/μg)
none	12.3	380
10	7.4	490
50	5.7	750
200	2.1	1050

[a] Leukemic leukocytes were incubated with varying concentrations of streptonigrin (SN) plus ^{3}H-thymidine. After 4 h of incubation, high molecular weight DNA was isolated, quantitated, and its radioactivity determined. MILLER et al. (1967).

Biochemical Effects

The mechanism of the bactericidal effect of SN was further explored by WHITE and his colleagues (WHITE and WHITE, 1964, 1965a, 1966, 1968; WHITE and DEARMAN, 1965b). They determined that bacterial lethality was not dependent upon inhibition of DNA synthesis, since bacterial death occurred at drug concentrations which permitted the synthesis of DNA, RNA, and protein. However, with increasing concentrations of SN, DNA synthesis was preferentially inhibited. Bacterial death was accompanied by DNA degradation, and this required the intracellular reduction of SN in the presence of both an electron source and oxygen.

The addition of substances such as cyanide, which increased the reduction of the quinone ring of SN, increased the lethality of this agent, whereas phenazine methosulfate, an electron scavenger, inhibited this action by competing for electrons intracellularly. Lethality, although dependent on the presence of oxygen, was not accompanied by an increase in oxygen consumption, nor was hydrogen peroxide produced. It was concluded that a reaction product of oxygen and intracellularly reduced SN was the lethal agent, and that this may be in the form of a peroxy free radical or a peroxide modification of the antibiotic structure.

Utilizing a cell-free system, HOCHSTEIN et al. (1965) were able to demonstrate that SN caused the catalytic oxidation of intra- and extra-mitochondrial NADH and of extra-mitochondrial NADPH. Oxidation was found to be mediated by the enzyme NADH-NADPH diaphorase and was not coupled to phosphorylation, but led instead to the generation of hydrogen peroxide. As outlined in Fig. 2, it was proposed that SN, after reduction by NADH or NADPH by the diaphorase enzyme, underwent a rapid, metal catalyzed autoxidation which bypassed the electron transport system and resulted in the formation of hydrogen peroxide and in

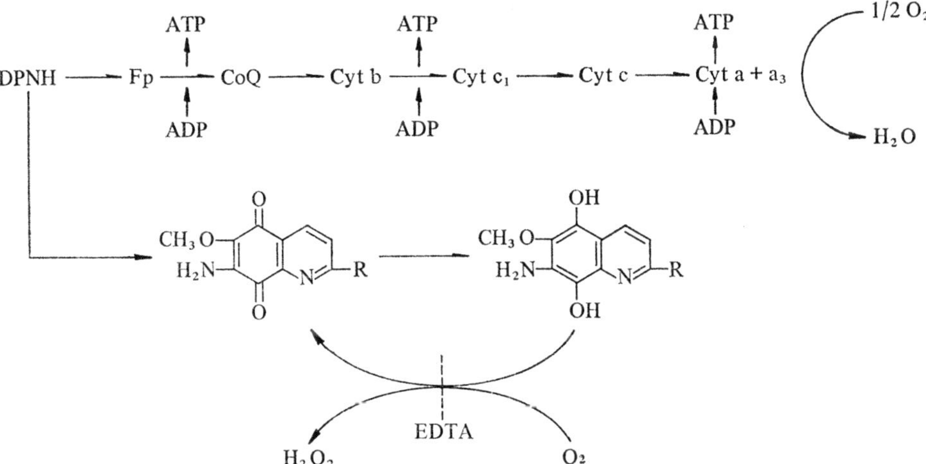

Fig. 2. A scheme for the oxidation of intramitochondrial NADH (DPNH) by catalytic amounts of streptonigrin. The upper portion of the scheme represents the normal pathway of NADH oxidation in mitochondria. The lower portion represents the reduction of SN to a phenolic form by NADH and its EDTA-sensitive autoxidation back to the quinoid form with the generation of hydrogen peroxide. DPNH (NADH), reduced diphosphopyridine nucleotide; SN, streptonigrin; EDTA, ethylenediamine tetraacetate; ATP, adenosine triphosphate; Fp, flavoprotein; CoQ, coenzyme Q; Cyt, cytochrome; ADP, adenosine diphosphate. From MILLER et al. (1967). (Reproduced with the kind permission of Cancer Research Inc.)

the regeneration of the quinoid form of SN, which was again available for enzymatic reduction. Further *in vivo* studies confirmed the marked interference with oxidative phosphorylation (MILLER et al., 1967). When leukemic leukocytes were incubated with SN there occurred a profound drop in cellular ATP levels, although oxygen uptake was unaffected (Fig. 3). The high-speed supernatant from disrupted leukemic cells was able to mediate the oxidation of NADH and generate the production of hydrogen peroxide. When SN was incubated with mature erythrocytes (cells lacking mitochondria), oxygen consumption and hydrogen peroxide production were conclusively demonstrated (KREMER and LASZLO, 1966).

From these experiments it was postulated that cellular toxicity could be due to (1) the depletion of cellular NADH and NADPH, (2) uncoupling of oxidative phosphorylation and depletion of cellular ATP, and (3) the formation of hydrogen peroxide. It was further suggested that the effects of SN on nucleic acid metabolism

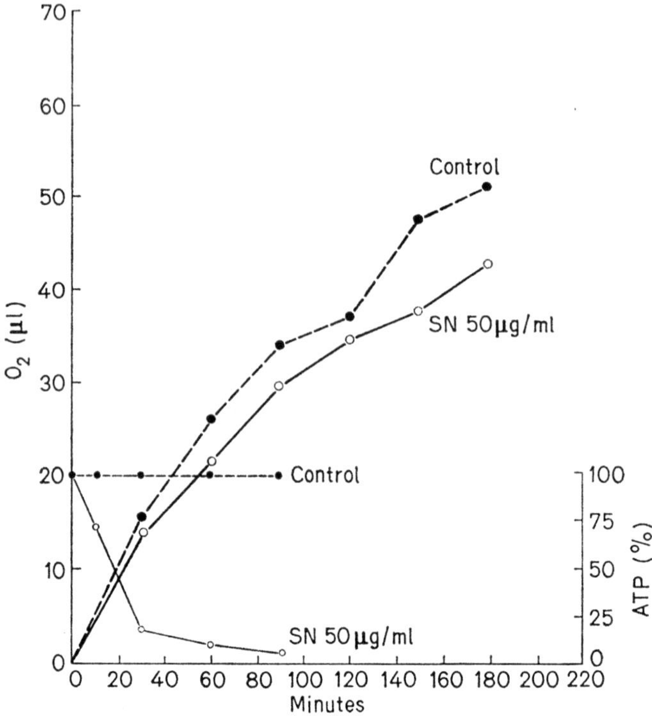

Fig. 3. Effect of streptonigrin (SN) on the oxygen consumption and adenosine triphosphate (ATP) content of human leukemic lymphocytes. Aliquots of cell suspension (2.5 ml each, 5.7×10^7 cells/ml) were incubated in manometer flasks and oxygen consumption was measured and expressed as cumulative µl of O_2 uptake. The control ATP (14.4 nmoles/ml cell suspension) is referred to as the 100% value. From MILLER et al. (1967). (Reproduced with the kind permission of Cancer Research Inc.)

and protein synthesis noted *in vivo* may be secondary to its effects on energy metabolism. For example, SN did not inhibit cell-free protein synthesis to which an ATP-generating system was added, but did markedly inhibit protein synthesis in intact leukemic cells (MILLER et al., 1967). The marked depletion of cellular ATP caused by SN is the likely cause of this inhibition. DNA degradation may also be a secondary effect resulting from the formation of hydrogen peroxide.

Streptonigrin interacts with DNA *in vitro* as evidenced by an increase in the T_m of the DNA thermal denaturation curve (WHITE and WHITE, 1966). Unlike mitomycin C, SN does not cross-link with DNA (Fig. 4) (MILLER et al., 1967). Radioactive SN binds tightly to calf thymus DNA *in vitro* and the binding is preferentially to the dCMP moiety (MIZUNO and GILBOE, 1970). There was no increase in binding with reduced SN, nor did the binding require oxidation, since it also occurred under anaerobic conditions. When intact mammalian cells were incubated with radioactive SN, the majority of bound radioactivity was found in the DNA fraction (MIZUNO, 1965). Although SN or reduced SN did not inactivate extracellular T1-phage or transforming DNA when incubated *in vitro* (IYER and SZYBALSKI, 1964), DNA treated with SN was defective as a template for both DNA and RNA polymerase (MIZUNO and GILBOE, 1970).

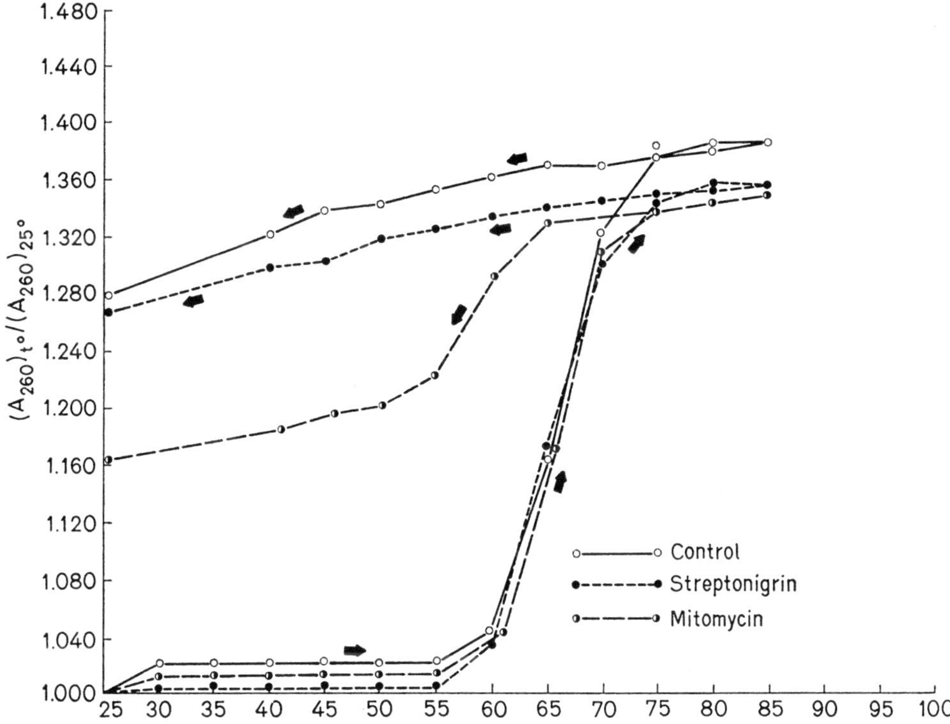

Fig. 4. The temperature melting curves of human leukemic DNA. Determinations were made on DNA extracted from cells incubated *in vitro* with streptonigrin, 200 μg/ml, or mitomycin C, 200 μg/ml. Values were determined on DNA dissolved in 0.015 M sodium chloride with 0.0015M sodium citrate. Note the cooling phase of control and streptonigrin treated DNA. There was no sharp descent in the area of the melting point ascent, indicating no cross-linking of the DNA. This contrasted with mitomycin C treated DNA. From MILLER et al. (1967). (Reproduced with the kind permission of Cancer Research Inc.)

WHITE and WHITE (1966) were able to demonstrate that when SN was reduced *in vitro* and incubated with isolated DNA over a prolonged period there occurred a decrease in the viscosity of the DNA solution, as well as the appearance of single strand breaks, similar to the DNA degradation noted in bacteria. MIZUNO and GILBOE (1970) were unable to confirm the degradation seen when DNA was incubated with SN or reduced SN *in vitro* but did confirm the occurrence of single strand breaks. Therefore SN does interact with DNA both *in vitro* and *in vivo*. The binding to DNA is stable, with the dCMP moiety preferred. SN need not be reduced, nor is oxygen required for binding to take place. It is not clear from the literature whether DNA degradation and single strand breaks resulting from incubation with SN *in vitro* require reduced SN and the presence of oxygen.

In conclusion, SN has unique biochemical effects among antitumor agents. This compound would be expected to be very toxic to all cells, since even minute concentrations have profound effects on energy metabolism. The drug catalyzes the oxidation of NADH and NADPH and undergoes rapid autoxidation resulting in the bypass of oxidative phosphorylation with depletion of cellular ATP, and this is accompanied by the production of hydrogen peroxide. The DNA degradation and chromosomal breakage which have been observed may be secondary to hydrogen peroxide formation and/or the interaction of SN (or a peroxide modification of the antibiotic) with DNA resulting in its damage. Interestingly, the *E. coli* mutant, B/r, which is resistant to x-irradiation, was also resistant to SN (WHITE and WHITE, 1968). In many ways the type of DNA breakdown observed with SN is similar to that produced by x-irradiation, which is felt to be mediated in part by the formation of free radicals.

Clinical Studies

After the initial observations that SN inhibited the growth of several transplantable mouse tumors, this agent was evaluated for its effect in human malignancy. Early exploratory studies revealed SN to be toxic at very low dosages (HACKETHAL et al., 1961; HUMPHREY and BLANK, 1961; WILSON et al., 1961). Nausea and vomiting occurred acutely with dosages as low as 0.2 to 0.5 mg given intravenously; more serious was the delayed bone marrow toxicity. Pancytopenia was recorded from 1 to 3 weeks after the discontinuation of therapy and in some cases persisted for as long as 2 months. Also noted at low doses was injury to the digestive tract with moderate diarrhea, anorexia, and weight loss occurring even after the discontinuation of therapy and lasting for several weeks. Initially there seemed to be little effect demonstrated against a spectrum of malignancies, except for HODGKIN's disease where a small number of patients with advanced disease had an objective response. Further investigation of this agent revealed that the oral form of this drug was as effective as the intravenous form, but was associated with more nausea and vomiting (HARRIS et al., 1965). Oral doses of 0.2 to 0.4 mg per day seemed to be tolerated for periods of up to 6 weeks. Bone marrow depression occurred as with the intravenous form, but appeared to be less pronounced and of shorter duration. Toxicity with the oral form also included mucous membrane ulcerations and rare instances of alopecia. In a wide spectrum of cancers in man SN appeared to produce objective responses (2 to 4 months) only in patients with lymphoid malignancy, including mycosis fungoides, lymphocytic lymphoma, and HODGKIN's disease. A phase II study of SN was performed by the Southeast Cancer Study Group and the results are illustrated in Table 2 (unpublished observations). In this study most patients with advanced neoplastic disease failed to respond to SN, but there was some indication that the drug is active in lymphoid malignancies.

Clinical trials of SN then advanced to the phase III level where it was compared with chlorambucil, a drug known to be active against lymphoproliferative diseases. Streptonigrin appeared to have the same effectiveness as a maximum dose of chlorambucil in patients with chronic lymphocytic leukemia (KUANG et al., 1969a). Objective responses were seen in the majority of patients and the quality of response was similar with the two compounds (Table 3). In several patients with Hodgkin's disease and other lymphomas, SN again appeared to have equal activity in inducing objective responses (Table 3) (KUANG et al., 1966b). It was concluded that although SN does have activity in lymphoid malignancies, it was not superior to chlorambucil, but was associated with a greater degree of toxicity. In view of the lack of therapeutic superiority and the increased risk from toxicity, SN has not been recommended for use in these diseases and at present is not used clinically.

Table 2. *Results of oral streptonigrin therapy*[a]

Disease	Response						Total Evaluable Patients
	Ex-cellent	Good	Fair	Ques-tionable	No Change	Worse	
HODGKIN's disease		2			4	1	7
Reticulum cell sarcoma			1	1	1	1	4
Lymphosarcoma		1			1	1	3
Chronic myelogenous leukemia		2	1	1	1		5
Chronic lymphocytic leukemia		1	3	1	2		7
Acute myelogenous leukemia				3	2		5
Multiple myeloma				1		1	2
Mycosis fungoides		2	1	1	2		6
Malignant melanoma					2	2	4
Miscellaneous malignancies				1		4	5

[a] Response of patients with various malignancies to maximally tolerated doses of streptonigrin. Southeast Cancer Study Group phase II study of streptonigrin (1965).

Table 3. *Comparison of streptonigrin with chlorambucil in lymphoid malignancies*[a]

		Objective Response	No Response	% Response
Chronic lymphocytic leukemia	CB	18	6	75
	SN	21	4	81
Malignant lymphoma	CB	12	23	34
	SN	11	22	34
HODGKIN's disease	CB	12	11	52
	SN	6	14	32

[a] Phase III study of streptonigrin (SN) versus chlorambucil (CB) in patients with chronic lymphocytic leukemia, malignant lymphoma, and HODGKIN's disease. KUANG et al. (1969a, b).

Derivatives of Streptonigrin

The clinical effectiveness of SN is often limited by its toxic effect on the gastrointestinal tract and by bone marrow depression, as has been described. Derivatives of SN, methyl streptonigrin (MeSN), and isopropylidine azastreptonigrin (IPAS), were developed in an effort to prepare a compound retaining effective antitumor properties but with fewer side effects. MeSN is identical to SN with the exception of the substitution of a methyl group for the hydrogen in the acid radical of the third ring, whereas IPAS differs from SN by modification of the quinone structure of the first ring (Fig. 1). Preclinical studies involving experimental animal tumor systems revealed that the maximum tolerable and the minimum lethal concentrations of MeSN were much greater than with SN, although at very high doses the toxicity was qualitatively similar to that of low doses of SN. The biochemical properties of MeSN resembled SN in that this agent was also able to oxidize NADH via NADH-NADPH diaphorase, accompanied by oxygen consumption and hydrogen peroxide formation (KREMER and LASZLO, 1966). In addition, MeSN-treated leukemic leukocytes exhibited depletion of cellular ATP, inhibition of protein synthesis, and DNA degradation, all of which were observed with SN. However, although the biochemical effects of the two drugs were similar, MeSN was considerably less potent in all systems studied. The differences were not solely due to cellular transport, since MeSN was also less active in cell-free systems. The biochemical findings correlated with studies in tissue culture and in animals, which demonstrated that MeSN was less toxic than an equimolar amount of SN (MIZUNO, 1967). Reduction of the biochemical effectiveness of MeSN thus appeared to explain the decreased toxicity of the drug. If the antitumor effects and the toxicity result from a common mechanism, then it would be expected that MeSN would not provide a more advantageous therapeutic ratio than its parent compound. In a large series of patients treated with MeSN the frequency and types of responses, as well as toxicity, were indeed similar to the experience with SN (RIVERS et al., 1966). Objective responses were observed in lymphoid malignancies, but these required a larger dose than SN and, at that larger dose, nausea, vomiting, and bone marrow depression were encountered.

IPAS, in contrast to MeSN, did not resemble SN, in that no cytotoxicity was observed in tissue culture cells (MIZUNO, 1967). Furthermore, IPAS did not resemble SN in its effects on NADH oxidation, oxygen consumption, or hydrogen peroxide formation; it also had no effect on leukemic cell ATP levels, protein synthesis, or recovery of high molecular weight DNA (KREMER and LASZLO, 1967). IPAS in concentrations 100 times that of SN did not interfere with nucleic acid synthesis of tissue culture cells (MIZUNO, 1967). It would appear that masking of the quinone group rendered the IPAS dissimilar to SN. These studies indicate that the biochemical properties and cytotoxic activity of SN are dependent on its quinone moiety, since modifying the quinone ring, as in IPAS, renders the derivative inactive. Clinical studies with IPAS have not been reported, nor would they appear indicated on the basis of preclinical studies and on the biochemical rationale described above.

References

COHEN, M. M., SHAW, M. W., CRAIG, A. P.: The effects of streptonigrin on cultured human leukocytes. Proc. nat. Acad. Sci. (Wash.) **50**, 16—24 (1963).

HACKETHAL, C. A., GOLBEY, R. B., TAN, G. T. C., KARNOFSKY, D. A., BURCHENAL, J. H.: Clinical observations on the effects of streptonigrin in patients with neoplastic disease. Antibiot. Chemother. **11**, 178—183 (1961).

HARRIS, M. N., MEDREK, T. J., GOLUMB, F. M., GUMPORT, S. L., POSTEL, A. H., WRIGHT, J. C.: Chemotherapy with streptonigrin in advanced cancer. Cancer **18**, 49—57 (1965).

HOCHSTEIN, P., LASZLO, J., MILLER, D.S.: A unique, dicoumarol-sensitive non-phosphorylating oxidation to DPNH and TPNH catalyzed by streptonigrin. Biochem. biophys. Res. Comm. **19**, 289—295 (1965).

HUMPHREY, E. W., BLANK, N.: Clinical experience with streptonigrin. Cancer Chemother. Rep. **12**, 99—103 (1961).

IYER, V. N., SZYBALSKI, W.: Mitomycin and porfiromycin: chemical mechanisms of activation and cross-linking of DNA. Science **145**, 55—58 (1964).

KREMER, W. B., LASZLO, J.: Biochemical effects of the methyl ester of streptonigrin. Biochem. Pharmacol. **15**, 1111—1118 (1966).

KREMER, W. B., LASZLO, J.: Comparison of biochemical effects of isopropylidine azastreptonigrin (NSC-62709) with streptonigrin (NSC-45383). Cancer Chemother. Rep. **51**, 19—24 (1967).

KUANG, D. T., WHITTINGTON, R. M., SPENCER, H. H., PATNO, M. E.: Comparison of chlorambucil and streptonigrin (NSC-45383) in the treatment of chronic lymphocytic leukemia. Cancer **23**, 597—600 (1969a).

KUANG, D. T., WHITTINGTON, R. M., SPENCER, H. H., PATNO, M. E.: Comparison of chlorambucil and streptonigrin (NSC-45383) in the treatment of malignant lymphomas. Cancer **23**, 1280—1283 (1969b).

LEVINE, M., BORTHWICK, M.: The action of streptonigrin on bacterial DNA metabolism and on induction of phage production in lysogenic bacteria. Virology **21**, 568—574 (1963).

MERKER, P. C., PEARCE, R. K., SARINO, J. S., WOOLEY, G. W.: The effect of streptonigrin and other antibiotics on a human epidermoid carcinoma, HEP No. 3, growing in conditioned Swiss mice. Antibiot. Chemother. **11**, 184—189 (1961).
MILLER, D. S., LASZLO, J., MCCARTY, K. S., GUILD, W. R., HOCHSTEIN, P.: Mechanism of action of streptonigrin in leukemia cells. Cancer Res. **27**, 632—638 (1967).
MIZUNO, N. S.: Effects of streptonigrin on nucleic acid metabolism of tissue culture cells. Biochim. biophys. Acta (Amst.) **108**, 394—403 (1965).
MIZUNO, N. S.: Comparative effects of streptonigrin derivatives on tissue culture cells. Biochem. Pharmacol. **16**, 933—940 (1967).
MIZUNO, N. S., GILBOE, D. P.: Binding of streptonigrin to DNA. Biochim. biophys. Acta (Amst.) **224**, 319—327 (1970).
NASJLETI, C. E., SPENCER, H. H.: Chromosome polyploidization in human leukocyte cultures treated with streptonigrin and cyclophosphamide. Cancer **20**, 31—35 (1967).
OLESON, J. J., CALDERELLA, L. A., MJOS, K. J., REITH, A. R., THIE, R. S., TOPLIN, I.: The effects of streptonigrin on experimental tumors. Antibiot. Chemother. **11**, 158—164 (1961).
RADDING, C. M.: Incorporation of H^3-thymidine by K12 (λ) induced by streptonigrin. Proc. XI int. Congr. Genetics **1**, 22 (1963).
RAO, K. V., BIEMANN, D., WOODWARD, R. B.: The structure of streptonigrin. J. Amer. chem. Soc. **85**, 2532—2533 (1963).
RAO, K. V., CULLEN, W. P.: Streptonigrin, an antitumor substance. Antibiot. Ann. 1959—1960, 950—953 (1960).
RIVERS, S. L., WHITTINGTON, R. M., MEDREK, T. J.: Treatment of malignant lymphomas with methyl ester of streptonigrin (NSC-45384). Cancer **19**, 1377—1385 (1966).
SZYBALSKI, W.: Structural modifications of DNA: cross-linking, circularization and single strand interruption. Abhandl. Deut. Wiss. Berlin **4**, 1—19 (1964).
WHITE, H. L., WHITE, J. R.: Interaction of streptonigrin with DNA *in vitro*. Biochim. biophys. Acta (Amst.) **123**, 648—651 (1966).
WHITE, H. L., WHITE, J. R.: Lethal action and metabolic effects of streptonigrin on *Escherichia coli*. Molec. Pharmacol. **4**, 549—565 (1968).
WHITE, J. R., WHITE, H. L.: Phenethylalcohol synergism with Mitomycin C, porfirmycin and streptonigrin. Science **145**, 1312—1313 (1964).
WHITE, J. R., WHITE, H. L.: Effect of intracellular redox environment on bactericidal action of mitomycin C and streptonigrin. Antimicrob. Agents Chemother. **1964**, 495—499 (1965a).
WHITE, J. R., DEARMAN, H. H.: Generation of free radicals from phenazine methosulfate, streptonigrin and rubiflavin in bacterial suspensions. Proc. nat. Acad. Sci. (Wash.) **54**, 887—891 (1965b).
WILSON, W. L., LABRA, C., BARRIST, E.: Preliminary observations on the use of streptonigrin as an antitumor agent in human beings. Antibiot. Chemother. **11**, 147—150 (1961).
YOUNG, C. W., HODAS, S.: Acute effects of cytotoxic compounds on incorporation of precursors into DNA, RNA and protein of HeLa monolayers. Biochem. Pharmacol. **14**, 205—214 (1965).

Chapter 64

Anthramycin

SUSAN B. HORWITZ

With 2 Figures

Introduction

Fermentation products of *Streptomyces refuineus* var. *thermotolerans* include a component with antitumor activity. This material was originally described by TENDLER and KORMAN (1963) as "refuin". The active principle responsible for the antitumor properties of "refuin" was eventually isolated by LEIMGRUBER et al. (1965b) and renamed anthramycin. The structure and stereochemistry of anthramycin (Fig. 1) and its analogs have been established (LEIMGRUBER et al., 1965a) and the total synthesis has been reported (LEIMGRUBER et al., 1968).

Anthramycin-11-methyl ether, a relatively stable and well characterized derivative, is isolated from hot methanol-water. In aqueous medium, this derivative is rapidly hydrolyzed to form an equilibrium mixture of anthramycin (I)[1], epianthramycin (II), and anhydroanthramycin (III) (LEIMGRUBER, W., personal communication).

The present chapter reviews the properties of anthramycin with particular reference to its interaction with deoxyribonucleic acid (DNA). The interaction of anthramycin with DNA presents fewer complexities than that of actinomycin since the former contains no large side chains. This interaction is of further interest because of the relatively unusual structure of anthramycin.

Cytotoxic, Antimicrobial, and Chemosterilant Properties

The antitumor properties of anthramycin in rodents and in man have been reported (ZBINDEN, 1964; KORMAN and TENDLER, 1965; COLE et al., 1966; GRUNBERG et al., 1966; ADAMSON et al., 1968). Anthramycin is active against the following tumors that have been transplanted into rodents: Ehrlich carcinoma, Sarcoma 180, Walker carcinosarcoma 256, human epidermoid carcinoma No. 3, and human adenoma No. 1 (GRUNBERG et al., 1966). The antibiotic increases the survival time of mice bearing the experimental leukemia P388 and the plasma cell tumor YPC-1 (ADAMSON et al., 1968). In animal experiments and in clinical trials, anthramycin exhibits marked irritating and necrotizing properties on direct contact with tissues (ZBINDEN 1964; SIGDESTAD et al., 1970a).

In vitro, anthramycin has a wide antibacterial spectrum (KORMAN and TENDLER, 1965) and exerts chemotherapeutic effects in experimental infections with *Trichomonas vaginalis*, *Endamoeba histolytica*, and *Syphacia obvelata* (GRUNBERG et al., 1966). At low concentrations, anthramycin penetrates the cell wall of certain bacteria and inhibits the growth of *Sarcina lutea*, *Bacillus subtilis*, and *E. coli B*.

[1] Roman numerals refer to the structural formulas in Fig. 1.

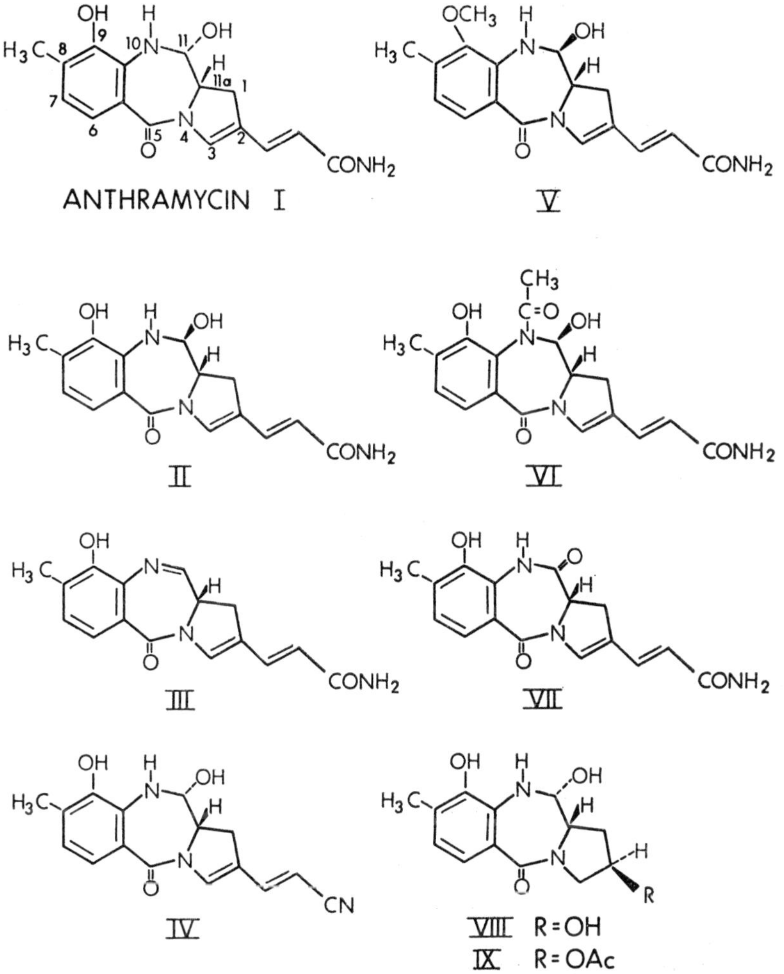

Fig. 1. Structural formulae of anthramycin and related derivatives

(Horwitz and Grollman, 1968). Anthramycin is also toxic to the growth of the alga, *E. gracilis* (Guttman and Tendler, 1966) and to the developing chick embryo (Lee, 1972).

Anthramycin inhibits the activity of purified DNA and RNA polymerases prepared from *E. coli* (Horwitz and Grollman, 1968). The antibiotic is a potent inhibitor of the DNA-dependent RNA polymerase of *E. coli*, inhibiting the enzyme more than 50 % at a concentration of 2 μM.

The chemosterilant properties of anthramycin have been demonstrated in *Drosophilia melanogaster* (Meigen) and in the housefly *Musca domestica L.* Anthramycin methyl ether induces complete and permanent sterilization of the female *D. melanogaster* (Barnes et al., 1969). The antibiotic is an active chemosterilant in both mature and newly emerged adults and sterilizes only the female. Other antitumor antibiotics such as actinomycin D, novobiocin, and echinomycin show no chemosterilant activity when tested under similar conditions (Barnes et al., 1969).

Anthramycin is a highly effective male chemosterilant when administered by intrathoracic injection to the male housefly (BOŘKOVEC et al., 1971). The estimated SD_{50} (the amount of drug that reduces hatching by 50 %) for anthramycin methyl ether in the male housefly is 0.03 μg per fly. The high activity of anthramycin methyl ether in sterilizing male houseflies was unexpected because of the antibiotic's inactivity in the male *D. melanogaster*. Variation in sex specificity in different species has not been previously observed with other chemosterilants.

Effects on Macromolecular Synthesis in Cultured Cells

Anthramycin inhibits the biosynthesis of nucleic acids in HeLa cells (HORWITZ and GROLLMAN, 1968), in L1210 leukemia cells (KOHN et al., 1968), in Ehrlich ascites carcinoma cells (BATES et al., 1969), in Sarcoma 180 ascites tumor cells, and in the proliferative cells of the intestinal epithelium of the mouse (SIGDESTAD et al., 1970b). In HeLa cells, anthramycin rapidly inhibits RNA and DNA synthesis at concentrations that do not affect protein synthesis. The rate of DNA synthesis is inhibited by 50 % at a concentration of 3 μM and the rate of RNA synthesis is inhibited by 50 % at a concentration of 1 μM. The rate of protein synthesis is unaffected by the antibiotic at concentrations of 80 μM. The effect of anthramycin on the synthesis of RNA in HeLa cells cannot be reversed by washing the cells and resuspending them in anthramycin-free medium (HORWITZ et al., 1971a).

KANN and KOHN (1972) have examined the effects of anthramycin on the synthesis of different classes of RNA in suspension cultures of mouse leukemia L1210 cells. These studies, using sucrose gradient sedimentation, demonstrated that anthramycin inhibits uridine incorporation into the nucleolar and nucleoplasmic fractions. RNA molecules synthesized in the presence of the drug are smaller. Reduction in length of the RNA synthesized could be explained by assuming premature termination of RNA chains.

Interaction of Anthramycin with DNA

Anthramycin appears to act by virtue of its ability to bind to DNA and to interfere with its function. The biological activities of the drug can be attributed to the resultant effects on nucleic acid synthesis. The direct interaction of anthramycin and DNA has been studied by several groups of investigators (KOHN, et al., 1968; STEFANOVIĆ, 1968; BATES et al., 1969; KOHN and SPEARS, 1970; HORWITZ, 1971).

Binding of anthramycin to DNA displays two unusual features that distinguish it from other small molecules. The rate of complex formation is slow, requiring approximately one hour for completion. Furthermore, the resulting complex is stable and can be isolated by alcohol precipitation or by gel filtration. The anthramycin-DNA complex is not appreciably dissociated by sodium lauryl sulfate, dialysis, or silver ion. Denaturation of the complex by alkali results in separated strands of DNA to which anthramycin remains bound (KOHN and SPEARS, 1970). The unusually tight binding of anthramycin to DNA and the slowness of the interaction have led to the suggestion that the formation of the complex may involve a covalent bond (KOHN et al., 1968).

When calf thymus DNA is added to a solution of anthramycin, there is a shift in the antibiotic's absorption maximum from 333 mμ to 343 mμ, and the absorption decreases by approximately 15 % (Fig. 2). The rate of the reaction is proportional to hydrogen ion concentration (KOHN and SPEARS, 1970). The spectrum of the antibiotic does not change when free bases or mononucleotides are mixed with anthramycin.

Anthramycin reacts with heat-denatured DNA, but much more slowly than with helical DNA. The alkaloid does not interact with RNA. The thermal denaturation temperature of calf thymus DNA is increased in the presence of anthramycin (KOHN et al., 1968; BATES et al., 1969). The change in the thermal denaturation temperature is also a time-dependent reaction that attains its maximum value only after one hour.

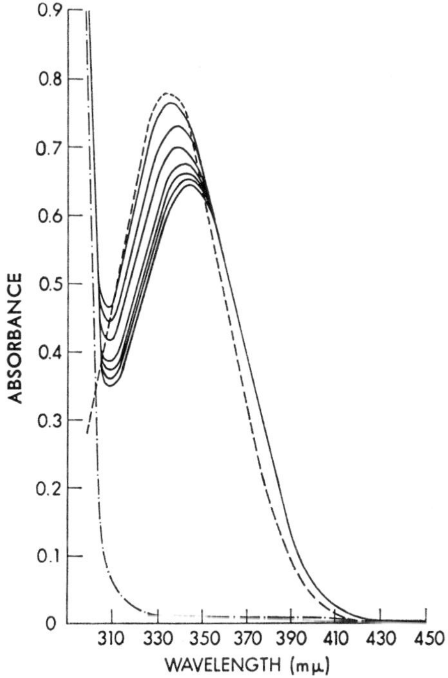

Fig. 2. Change in absorption spectrum of anthramycin at various times after the addition of DNA. (--------) 2.2×10^{-5} M anthramycin in 0.0015 M NaCl — 0.00015 M sodium citrate pH 7.0; (—·—·) 2×10^{-3} M calf thymus DNA in 0.0015 M NaCl — 0.00015 M sodium citrate pH 7.0; (———) a mixture of 2×10^{-3} M calf thymus DNA and 2.2×10^{-5} M anthramycin in 0.0015 M NaCl — 0.00015 M sodium citrate pH 7.0. Spectra shown were recorded at 1, 5, 10, 20, 30, 40, and 60 min. There was no further change in the spectrum after 60 min. (From HORWITZ, 1971. Reproduced by permission of Springer-Verlag)

The complex of *E. coli* DNA with anthramycin can also be characterized by a reduced buoyant density in cesium chloride (KOHN et al., 1968). Anthramycin binds to poly *d*G · poly *d*C, but not to poly *d*(A-T). This relationship is not simple since DNA with a high GC content does not interact more readily with anthramycin than a DNA with a low GC content. The conclusion from these studies is that there are at least two classes of binding sites, fast-reacting and slower-reacting (KOHN and SPEARS, 1970).

Inhibition of RNA polymerase activity by anthramycin was greatly diminished when heat-denatured DNA, poly *d*(A-T), or poly *d*G · poly *d*C were substituted for native calf thymus DNA as primer (HORWITZ, 1971). Since anthramycin affects the buoyant density of poly $dG \cdot$ poly dC, it is surprising that anthramycin does not inhibit the activity of RNA polymerase primed with this polymer.

Equilibrium dialysis studies, using a wide range of anthramycin concentrations and calf thymus DNA, have demonstrated that approximately one molecule of anthramycin is bound for every eight to nine base pairs of calf thymus DNA (Kohn and Spears, 1970; Horwitz, 1971). Binding of anthramycin to DNA alters the ability of DNA to act as a primer for DNA and RNA polymerases and decreases its rate of degradation by pancreatic deoxyribonuclease I and snake venom phosphodiesterase (Bates et al., 1969; Horwitz, 1971).

Structure-Activity Relationships

Derivatives and analogs of anthramycin have been tested for their abilities to inhibit the activity of *E. coli* RNA polymerase, to increase the thermal denaturation temperature of calf thymus DNA, and to alter the fertility of the male housefly (Table 1) (Horwitz, 1971; Horwitz et al., 1971b). Since inhibition of RNA polymerase activity and an increase in the thermal denaturation temperature of DNA by anthramycin reflects binding of this antibiotic to DNA, it has been proposed that the interaction of anthramycin with DNA may also account for its action as a chemosterilant. The results of these structure-activity studies are

Table 1. *Effect of anthramycin and its derivatives on E. coli RNA polymerase activity, thermal denaturation temperature (T_m) of calf thymus DNA, and fertility in the male housefly, Musca domestica, L.*

Derivative[a]	RNA polymerase Inhibition	ΔT_m	Egg Hatchability
	%	°C	%
Active			
Anthramycin I	>75	+7.0	0
II	>75	+7.0	1
III	>75	+7.0	0
IV	>50	+4.0	43
Inactive			
V	<10	<1.0	93
VI	<10	<1.0	91
VII	<10	+1.5	96
VIII	<10	<1.0	88
IX	<10	<1.0	88

[a] Roman numerals refer to the structural formulas in Fig. 1. The concentration of each inhibitor was 200 μM for the enzyme assay and 20 μM for the determination of T_m. Chemosterilant properties were determined by injecting ten newly emerged males with 0.5 μg/fly (1.0 μg/fly for compound VII) of the test compounds. The treated males were then caged with eight untreated virgin females of the same age. One or more batches of eggs were collected and their hatchability was scored. (Horwitz and Grollman, 1968; Horwitz, 1971; Horwitz et al., 1971b.)

closely correlated in the three assays. Only anthramycin (I) and the closely related derivatives II, III, and IV are active, although IV is definitely less active than I, II, and III. Analogs in which the phenolic function is methylated (V), the aniline nitrogen is acetylated (VI), the carbinolamine function is replaced by an amide group (VII), or the conjugated side chain is absent (VIII and IX) are devoid of biological activity in the three systems in which they have been tested. The activity observed with compounds II and III was not unexpected, since the two forms are in rapid equilibrium with anthramycin I in aqueous solution. The other active analog IV differs from anthramycin in that the primary amide group is replaced by a nitrile function.

A quantitative spectrophotometric method for the determination of anthramycin has been described (STEFANOVICH and CEPRINI, 1971). The interaction of anthramycin and some of its derivatives with DNA has been investigated by following the change in the spectrum of anthramycin that results from the formation of a complex between anthramycin and DNA. By this method it has been determined that substitutions on positions 9 and 10 of anthramycin interfere with the binding of the antibiotic to DNA (STEFANOVIĆ, 1968).

Conclusions

Anthramycin is an antibiotic with potent antitumor, antimicrobial, and chemosterilant activities. Its primary mode of action is inhibition of the synthesis of nucleic acids. The biological properties of anthramycin can be explained by its ability to bind to DNA and to interfere with the function of DNA. Structure-activity studies have established the involvement of at least three groups of the alkaloid in binding to DNA. The rate of reaction of anthramycin with DNA is relatively slow, but in the resulting complex, anthramycin is tightly bound to DNA. Although it has been suggested that covalent bonds are formed between anthramycin and DNA, the exact nature of this interaction is not clear.

References

ADAMSON, R. H., HART, L. G., DEVITA, V. T., OLIVERIO, V. T.: Antitumor activity and some pharmacologic properties of anthramycin methyl ether. Cancer Res. **28**, 343—347 (1968).

BARNES, J. R., FELLIG, J., MITROVIC, M.: The chemosterilant effect of anthramycin methyl ether in *Drosophila melanogaster*. J. Econ. Entomol. **62**, 902—904 (1969).

BATES, H. M., KUENZIG, W., WATSON, W. B.: Studies on the mechanism of action of anthramycin methyl ether, a new antitumor antibiotic. Cancer Res. **29**, 2195—2205 (1969).

BOŘKOVEC, A. B., CHANG, S. C., HORWITZ, S. B.: Chemosterilization of house flies with anthramycin methyl ether. J. Econ. Entomol. **64**, 983—984 (1971).

COLE, D. R., DREYER, B. B., ROUSSELOT, L. M., TENDLER, M. D.: The radioprotective and antitumor effect of mixed bacterial toxins and anthramycin. Am J. Roentgenol. Radium Ther. nuclear Med. **97**, 997—1002 (1966).

GRUNBERG, E., PRINCE, H. N., TITTSWORTH, E., BESKID, G., TENDLER, M. D.: Chemotherapeutic properties of anthramycin. Chemotherapia **11**, 249—260 (1966).

GUTTMAN, H. N., TENDLER, M. D.: Studies on anthramycin sensitivity in *Euglena*. Proc. Soc. exp. Biol. (N.Y.) **121**, 1140—1141 (1966).

HORWITZ, S. B.: Anthramycin. In: HAHN, F. (Ed.): Progress in molecular and subcellular biology, Vol. 2. Berlin-Heidelberg-New York: Springer 1971.

HORWITZ, S. B., CHANG, C., GROLLMAN, A. P.: Studies on camptothecin: I. Effects on nucleic acid and protein synthesis. Molec. Pharmacol. **7**, 632—644 (1971a).

HORWITZ, S. B., CHANG, S. C., GROLLMAN, A. P., BOŘKOVEC, A. B.: Chemosterilant action of anthramycin: a proposed mechanism. Science **174**, 159—161 (1971b).

HORWITZ, S. B., GROLLMAN, A. P.: Interactions of small molecules with nucleic acids. I. Mode of action of anthramycin. Antimicrob. Agents and Chemother. 21—24 (1968).

KANN, H. E., KOHN, K. W.: Effects of anthramycin and actinomycin on RNA synthesis patterns in L1210 cells. J. cell. Physiol. **79**, 331—342 (1972).

KOHN, K. W., BONO, V. H., JR., KANN, H. E., JR.: Anthramycin, a new type of DNA-inhibiting antibiotic: reaction with DNA and effect on nucleic acid synthesis in mouse leukemia cells. Biochim. biophys. Acta (Amst.) **155**, 121—129 (1968).

KOHN, K. W., SPEARS, C. L.: Reaction of anthramycin with deoxyribonucleic acid. J. molec. Biol. **51**, 551—572 (1970).

KORMAN, S., TENDLER, M. D.: Clinical investigation of cancer chemotherapeutic agents for neoplastic disease. J. New Drugs **5**, 275—285 (1965).

LEE, H.: Effects of anthramycin methyl ether on early chick embryos. Growth **36**, 1—16 (1972).

LEIMGRUBER, W., BATCHO, A. D., CZAJKOWSKI, R. C.: Total synthesis of anthramycin. J. Amer. chem. Soc. **90**, 5641—5643 (1968).
LEIMGRUBER, W., BATCHO, A. D., SCHENKER, F.: The structure of anthramycin. J. Amer. chem. Soc. **87**, 5793—5795 (1965a).
LEIMGRUBER, W., STEFANOVIĆ, V., SCHENKER, F., KARR, A., BERGER, J.: Isolation and characterization of anthramycin, a new antitumor antibiotic. J. Amer. chem. Soc. **87**, 5791—5793 (1965b).
SIGDESTAD, C. P., HAGEMANN, R. F., LESHER, S.: Biological effects of anthramycin methyl ether. I. Acute intestinal necrosis. Chemotherapy **15**, 286—296 (1970a).
SIGDESTAD, C. P., HAGEMANN, R. F., LESHER, S.: Biological effects of anthramycin methyl ether. II. Inhibition of DNA synthesis in the intestinal epithelium and Sarcoma 180 tumor cells. Chemotherapy **15**, 297—303 (1970b).
STEFANOVIĆ, V.: Spectrophotometric studies of the isolation of anthramycin with deoxyribonucleic acid. Biochem. Pharmacol. **17**, 315—323 (1968).
STEFANOVIĆ, V., CEPRINI, M. Q.: Spectrophotometric determination of anthramycin. J. pharm. Sci. **60**, 781—783 (1971).
TENDLER, M. D., KORMAN, S.: "Refuin": A non-cytotoxic carcinostatic compound proliferated by a thermophilic actinomycete. Nature (Lond.) **199**, 501 (1963).
ZBINDEN, G.: Fermentation products derived from a thermophilic streptomycete. In: PLATTNER, P. A. (Ed.): Chemotherapy of cancer, Proceedings of International Symposium. Amsterdam-London-New York: Elsevier 1964.

Chapter 65

Camptothecin

Susan B. Horwitz

With 5 Figures

Introduction

Camptothecin and its analogs are cytotoxic alkaloids, originally isolated from the bark and wood of *Camptotheca acuminata* (family Nyssaceae), a tree indigenous to China (Wall et al., 1966). Camptothecin was subsequently shown to have antitumor properties, and its structure (Fig. 1) has been established (Wall et al., 1966; McPhail and Sim, 1968).

The limited supply of the natural alkaloid and the prospects of using camptothecin for the treatment of human malignancies encouraged chemists to synthesize this compound. As a result, numerous efforts have been made to prepare camptothecin and its analogs (Wenkert et al., 1967; Kepler et al., 1969; Wani

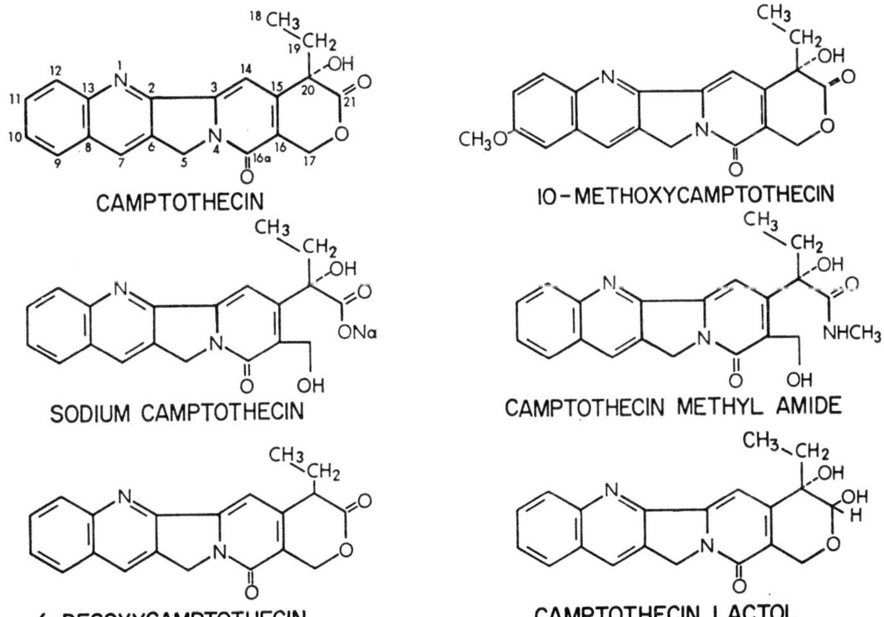

Fig. 1. Structural formulae of camptothecin and analogs. The numbering system is based on its biogenesis (Shamma, 1968). (From Horwitz et al., 1971. Reproduced by permission of Academic Press, Inc.)

et al., 1970; SHAMMA and NOVAK, 1969; KAMETANI et al., 1970; WINTERFELDT and RADUNZ, 1971; LIAO et al., 1971; BIESLER, 1971; DANISHEFSKY et al., 1971; WARNEKE et al., 1972; KENDE et al., 1970). Total synthesis of camptothecin has recently been accomplished in several laboratories (STORCK and SCHULTZ, 1971; VOLKMANN et al., 1971; WANI et al., 1972; BOCH et al., 1972).

Interest in camptothecin as an antitumor agent has stimulated investigations of its mode of action. The present chapter reviews these studies with particular emphasis on its effects on nucleic acid synthesis.

Pharmacokinetics

Some pharmacokinetic properties of camptothecin have been reported. A half-life of 35 min was established in mice bearing L1210 leukemia (KESSEL, 1971b) after injection of a single dose of camptothecin (25 mg/kg). In these studies the loss of camptothecin was followed from both ascitic fluid and ascitic cells. A sensitive fluorometric method for determining the alkaloid has been developed (HART et al., 1969) and used to determine the plasma and urine concentrations of the drug. The lower limit of detection by this technique is 0.005 μg/ml. Using this method, GOTTLIEB et al. (1970) demonstrated in patients that a high percentage of camptothecin is bound to plasma proteins after intravenous administration; this binding may account for the prolonged half-life of the drug in plasma. During the first 48 h after administration, the mean urinary recovery of the unmetabolized drug is 17%. Unmetabolized camptothecin was the only fluorescent compound identified in the urine.

Antitumor Properties

Camptothecin has potent antitumor properties in experimental animals. The drug is active against mouse leukemia L1210 and inhibits the growth of the solid Walker 256 carcinosarcoma in rats (VENDITTI and ABBOTT, 1967; DEWYS, 1968). Camptothecin is also active against various murine lymphocytic leukemias, including L5178Y, K1964, and P388, the plasma cell tumor YPC-1, the mast cell tumor P815, the Adamson reticulum cell sarcoma (A-RCS), and a number of murine leukemias resistant to other antitumor drugs (GALLO et al., 1971). In the early clinical trial of camptothecin, GOTTLIEB et al. (1970) reported encouraging results in patients with advanced gastrointestinal carcinoma and in one patient with melanoma. The study was designed to determine human tolerance to single doses of the agent, and the brief duration of response was attributed to the long interval required between doses. The considerable toxicity that accompanied therapy was not emphasized in this report.

Subsequent clinical trials with camptothecin in gastrointestinal cancer have been less encouraging and intolerable drug toxicity has been reported at doses used in the initial report. There were only two patients with objective responses among 61 patients with advanced gastrointestinal adenocarcinoma who received the drug for two months (MOERTEL et al., 1972). Camptothecin showed no clinical benefit in the treatment of fifteen patients with advanced disseminated melanoma (GOTTLIEB and LUCE, 1972).

Tolerance to weekly and daily schedules of camptothecin in patients with cancer has been evaluated. Clinical benefit was not observed in any of the patients receiving daily courses, while two of the fifteen patients receiving weekly courses showed transient objective responses (MUGGIA et al., 1972). In spite of the discouraging reports in gastrointestinal cancer and melanoma, camptothecin in weekly or biweekly doses should probably be further evaluated in a variety of other malignancies, including lymphomas and leukemias. However, the drug causes dose-dependent hematopoietic depression, diarrhea, alopecia, and cystitis, which restricts its potential usefulness when used alone or in combination with other cytotoxic agents.

Effects on Cultured Cells

Camptothecin is a potent inhibitor of nucleic acid synthesis in HeLa cells (HORWITZ et al., 1970). Synthesis of DNA and RNA is inhibited 50% by 5 μM camptothecin while the rate of protein synthesis is essentially unaffected by a 100 μM concentration of the alkaloid (Fig. 2). These effects on nucleic acid synthesis are observed immediately after the addition of the drug to the medium (HORWITZ et al., 1971). In one study, significant inhibition of nucleic acid synthesis was attained in HeLa cells only when using high concentrations (1 mg/ml) of camptothecin (BOSMANN, 1970).

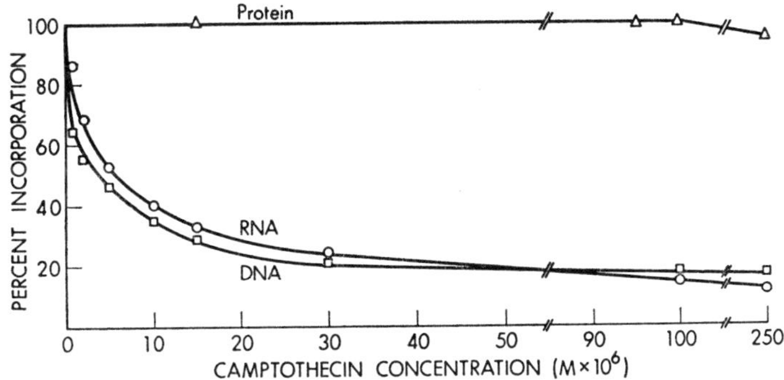

Fig. 2. Effect of various concentrations of camptothecin on synthesis of protein, RNA, and DNA in HeLa cells. Cells were incubated for 60 min at 37°, and the incorporation of radioactivity into TCA-insoluble material was used to calculate the rates of synthesis of protein (△——△), RNA (○——○), and DNA (□——□). (From HORWITZ et al., 1971. Reproduced by permission of Academic Press, Inc.)

An unusual characteristic of camptothecin is the rapid reversibility of its inhibitory effects on HeLa cells (HORWITZ et al., 1971). If cells are treated with camptothecin for as long as an hour, washed, and resuspended in drug-free medium, uridine incorporation into RNA resumes within min (Fig. 3). Inhibition of DNA synthesis is partially reversed by similar procedures, the extent of reversibility being dependent on the length of time the cells are exposed to the drug.

Analysis of the RNA of camptothecin-treated cells on sucrose density gradients showed that little 28 S and 18 S ribosomal RNA is formed while the synthesis of 4–5 S RNA is only partially inhibited (Fig. 4). Thus, camptothecin inhibits synthesis of ribosomal RNA to a far greater extent than of small RNA (HORWITZ et al., 1971). Other investigators (WU et al., 1971) have demonstrated differential effects on the synthesis and processing of the various classes of nuclear RNA and reported that synthesis of precursor ribosomal RNA in the nucleolus is more sensitive to camptothecin than that of heterogeneously sedimenting nuclear RNA. While the maturation of 45 S RNA to 32 S RNA occurs normally in the nucleolus, the appearance of 28 S RNA in the cytoplasm is inhibited. ABELSON and PENMAN (1972) confirmed that RNA synthesized in the presence of camptothecin consists partly

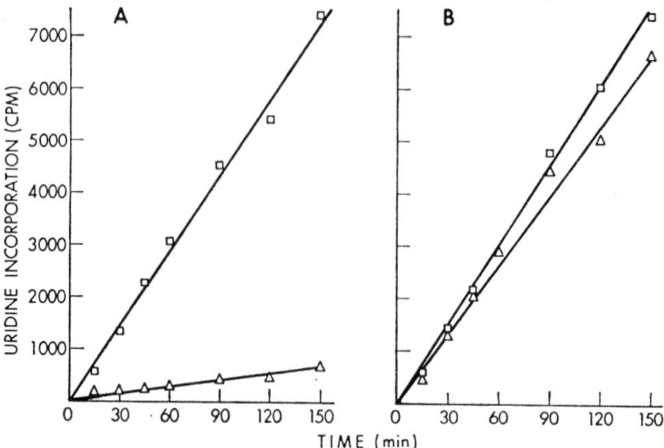

Fig. 3. Reversal of inhibition of RNA synthesis in HeLa cells. HeLa cells were incubated at 37° with 100 μM camptothecin (△——△) or in the absence of inhibitor (□——□). After 30 min, a 10 ml sample was removed from each culture, washed twice, and resuspended in medium with no additions. ^{14}C-Uridine (0.025 μCi) was added to 10 ml of the original culture (A) or the washed cells (B); 1 ml aliquots were removed at the indicated times, and the amount of uridine incorporation was measured. (From HORWITZ et al., 1971. Reproduced by permission of Academic Press, Inc.)

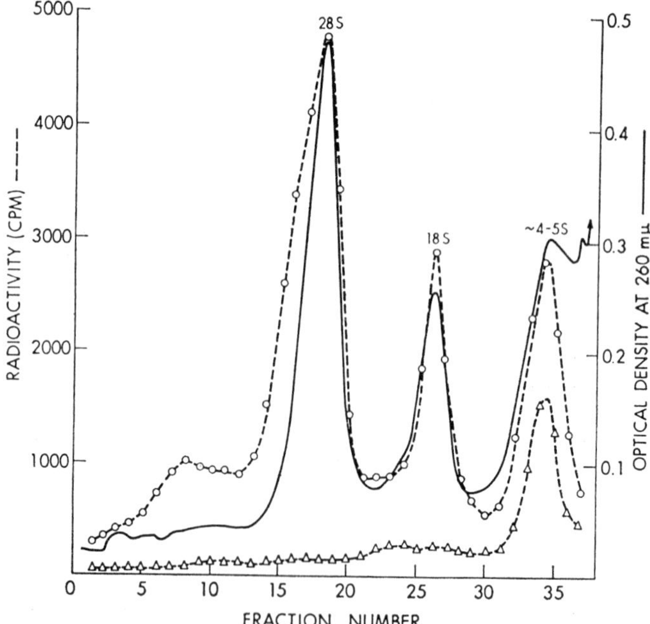

Fig. 4. Effect of camptothecin on ribosomal RNA synthesis. Cultures of HeLa cells were exposed to ^{14}C-uridine for 4 h in the presence (△——△) or absence (○——○) of 50 μM camptothecin. RNA was extracted from whole cells and analyzed by sucrose gradient sedimentation. The optical density is shown only for the control, as it was essentially the same in both cultures. (From HORWITZ et al., 1971. Reproduced by permission of Academic Press, Inc.)

of short RNA molecules of both heterogeneous nuclear RNA and nucleolar RNA. Camptothecin does not affect 5 S RNA synthesis in HeLa cells (ABELSON and PENMAN, 1972).

Camptothecin induces single strand breaks in cellular DNA when HeLa cells are incubated with the drug (HORWITZ and HORWITZ, 1971) (Fig. 5). Total DNA, measured as acid-insoluble material, remains unchanged in camptothecin-treated HeLa cells, but analysis on alkaline sucrose gradients demonstrates a conversion of cellular DNA to a lower molecular weight form. This degradation of cellular DNA can occur within 10 min after exposure of HeLa cells to camptothecin, even at 0° (HORWITZ et al., 1971). This process is reversible after removal of the drug. Camptothecin has essentially no effect on the uridine and thymidine nucleotide pools in HeLa cells, nor does it significantly affect the enzymatic activity of DNA and RNA polymerases prepared from HeLa cells, or of RNA polymerase prepared from *E. coli* (HORWITZ et al., 1971).

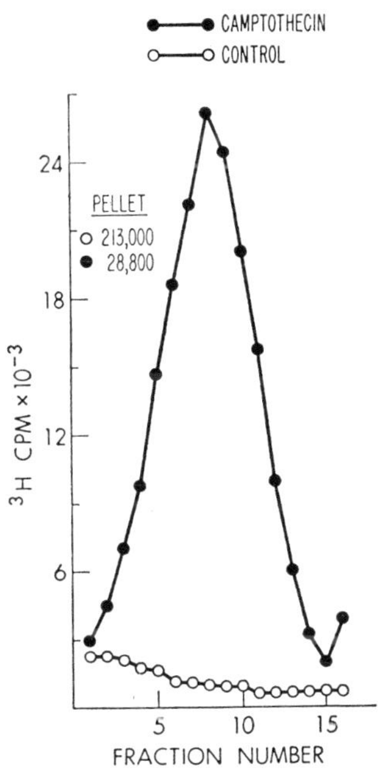

Fig. 5. Sedimentation of DNA from HeLa cells (○——○) and camptothecin-treated HeLa cells (●——●) in alkaline sucrose gradients. The "pellet" represents the acid-insoluble ^{3}H-thymidine in the 2.5 cm remaining at the bottom of the gradient. Sedimentation is from right to left. (From HORWITZ and HORWITZ, 1972. Reproduced by permission of Academic Press, Inc.)

The effects of camptothecin on macromolecular synthesis in leukemia L1210 cells have also been reported (KESSEL, 1971a,b). As in HeLa cells, the synthesis of RNA and DNA is inhibited by camptothecin and the effects on RNA synthesis are readily reversible. DNA in L1210 cells is degraded after treatment of these cells with camptothecin (SPATARO and KESSEL, 1972). There appear to be certain differences between the effects of camptothecin on HeLa cells and those on L1210 cells. Synthesis of ribosomal precursor RNA and of heterogeneous nuclear RNA was extensively inhibited in L1210 cells; however, maturation of 45 S RNA to cytoplasmic 18 S and 28 S RNA is unaffected by the drug (KESSEL, 1971b). This result differs from the reported effect of camptothecin on processing of 45 S RNA in HeLa cells (WU et al., 1971). It has also been stated that synthesis of 4 S and 5 S RNA in L1210 cells is unaffected by camptothecin (KESSEL, 1971b). Although there is no effect of camptothecin on 5 S RNA synthesis in HeLa cells, the synthesis of 4 S RNA is partially inhibited (ABELSON and PENMAN, 1972).

Camptothecin inhibits DNA synthesis in human lymphocytes stimulated by phytohemagglutin (GALLO et al., 1971). Cells are most sensitive to the lethal effects of camptothecin during the S phase of the cell cycle and even after removal of the drug the cells are incapable of subsequent division (KESSEL et al., 1972; LI et al., 1972; HORWITZ and HORWITZ, 1973). The induction of single strand breaks in cellular DNA by camptothecin and the repair of most of these breaks on removal of the drug occurs in both the S and G_1 phases of the cell cycle (HORWITZ and HORWITZ, 1973).

Camptothecin has no effect on nucleic acid synthesis in isolated rat liver mitochondria, rat brain mitochondria, or *E. coli* (BOSMANN, 1970).

Effects on Mammalian Viruses

Camptothecin is an effective inhibitor of replication of type 2 adenovirus (HORWITZ and BRAYTON, 1972) and vaccinia virus (HORWITZ et al., 1972). In both cases, the drug acts by inhibiting synthesis of viral DNA. In the presence of camptothecin, intracellular viral DNA is cleaved to smaller acid-insoluble pieces. After removal of the drug, fragmented viral DNA is rapidly repaired.

Synthesis of vaccinia messenger RNA is inhibited by camptothecin, but the activity of RNA polymerase, as tested in isolated vaccinia cores, is unaffected by the drug. Similar results were observed with polymerases isolated from HeLa cells.

Adenovirus and vaccinia virus are DNA viruses that replicate in the nucleus and cytoplasm, respectively. Camptothecin inhibits the replication of both viruses, but has essentially no effect on the replication of polio-virus, an RNA virus (HORWITZ et al., 1972). It seems likely that camptothecin exerts its effects principally on DNA viruses and is active only when DNA serves as a template for nucleic acid synthesis.

Structure-Activity Relationships

Derivatives and analogs of camptothecin (Fig. 1) were tested in HeLa cells to determine their inhibitory effects on RNA synthesis and ability to convert DNA to a lower molecular weight species (HORWITZ et al., 1971). Camptothecin, its sodium salt, the amide, and deoxy and methoxy analogs inhibited RNA synthesis in HeLa cells by 50 % or more at concentrations of 5 μM. At 20 μM these compounds also converted approximately 90 % of cellular DNA to lower molecular weight species. The lactol analog was the least active of the group but still inhibited the rate of RNA synthesis by 50 % at a concentration of 30 μM, and at 20 μM converted 20 % of cellular DNA to lower molecular weight species. These structure-activity relationships correspond closely to the ability of these compounds to suppress the growth of tumors in experimental animals (HARTWELL and ABBOTT, 1969; WALL, 1969). One discrepancy exists in the literature concerning the antitumor properties of deoxycamptothecin. The deoxy analog is stated to be totally inactive (WALL, 1969), although another report (HARTWELL and ABBOTT, 1970) has referred to it as an active agent. We find that deoxycamptothecin is active in HeLa cells and might be expected to be an active antitumor agent; however, intracellular metabolism to camptothecin has not been excluded.

Mechanism of Action

Although the precise mechanism of action of camptothecin is not fully understood, its properties differ from other established inhibitors of nucleic acid synthesis. The cytotoxic effects of the drug can be explained by the rapid inhibition of nucleic acid synthesis and the fragmentation of cellular DNA. The mechanism by which the postulated degradation of DNA occurs also remains unclear. The drug may directly induce cleavage of DNA or may bind to DNA, thus rendering it susceptible to the action of endonucleases. Fragmentation of DNA may create small pieces of template, inadequate for synthesis of DNA. Use of this altered template for RNA synthesis could be responsible for the abnormal RNA synthesized in the nucleus.

Conclusions

The plant alkaloid, camptothecin, displays potent antitumor properties and inhibits the synthesis of DNA and certain species of RNA in mammalian cells. RNA synthesized in the presence of camptothecin represents transfer RNA and short nucleoplasmic RNA. Inhibition of RNA synthesis is reversed by removing the drug from the medium. Cells treated with the drug during S do not undergo division even after removal of camptothecin. DNA, isolated from cells inhibited by camptothecin and analyzed on alkaline sucrose gradients, has a lower sedimentation constant than DNA isolated from untreated cells. Camptothecin inhibits replication of adenovirus and vaccinia virus. The properties of camptothecin make it a new and exciting tool for the study of macromolecular synthesis in animal cells and their DNA viruses.

References

Abelson, H. T., Penman, S.: Selective interruption of high molecular weight RNA synthesis in HeLa cells by camptothecin. Nature New Biol. **237**, 144—146 (1972).

Biesler, J. A.: Potential antitumor agents. I. Analogs of camptothecin. J. med. Chem. **14**, 1116—1118 (1971).

Boch, M., Korth, T., Nelke, J. M., Pike, D., Radunz, H., Winterfeldt, E.: Die biogenetisch orientierte Totalsynthese von DL-Camptothecin und 7-Chlor-camptothecin. Chem. Ber. **105**, 2126—2142 (1972).

Bosmann, H. B.: Camptothecin inhibits macromolecular synthesis in mammalian cells but not in isolated mitochondria or *E. coli*. Biochem. biophys. Res. Commun. **41**, 1412—1420 (1970).

Danishefsky, S., Etheredge, S. J., Volkmann, R., Eggler, J., Quick, J.: Nucleophilic additions to allenes. A new synthesis of α-pyridones. J. Amer. chem. Soc. **93**, 5575—5576 (1971).

DeWys, W. D., Humphreys, S. R., Goldin, A.: Studies on therapeutic effectiveness of drugs with tumor weight and survival time indices of Walker 256 carcinoma. Cancer Chemother. Rep. **52**, 229—242 (1968).

Gallo, R. C., Whang-Peng, J., Adamson, R. H.: Studies on the antitumor activity, mechanism of action, and cell cycle effects of camptothecin. J. nat. Cancer Inst. **46**, 789—795 (1971).

Gottlieb, J. A., Guarino, A. M., Call, J. B., Oliverio, V. T., Block, J. B.: Preliminary pharmacologic and clinical evaluation of camptothecin sodium (NSC-100880). Cancer Chemother. Rep. **54**, 461—470 (1970).

Gottlieb, J. A., Luce, J. K.: Treatment of malignant melanoma with camptothecin (NCS-100880). Cancer Chemother. Rep. **56**, 103—105 (1972).

Hart, L. G., Call, J. B., Oliverio, V. T.: A fluorometric method for determination of camptothecin in plasma and urine. Cancer Chemother. Rep. **53**, 211—214 (1969).

Hartwell, J. L., Abbott, B. J.: Antineoplastic principles in plants: recent developments in the field. Advanc. Pharmacol. Chemother. **7**, 137 (1969).

Horwitz, M. S., Brayton, C.: Effect of camptothecin on adenovirus DNA replication. Virology **48**, 690—698 (1972).

Horwitz, M. S., Horwitz, S. B.: Intracellular degradation of HeLa and adenovirus type 2 DNA induced by camptothecin. Biochem. biophys. Res. Commun. **45**, 723—727 (1971).

Horwitz, S. B., Chang, C., Grollman, A. P.: Mechanism of action of camptothecin. Pharmacologist **12**, 1283 (1970).

Horwitz, S. B., Chang, C., Grollman, A. P.: Studies on camptothecin: I. Effects on nucleic acid and protein synthesis. Molec. Pharmacol. **7**, 632—644 (1971).

Horwitz, S. B., Chang, C., Grollman, A. P.: Studies on camptothecin: II: Antiviral action. Antimicrob. Ag. Chemother. **2**, 395—401 (1972).

Horwitz, S. B., Horwitz, M. S.: Effects of camptothecin on the breakage and repair of DNA during the cell cycle. Cancer Res. **33**, 2834—2836 (1973).

Kametani, T., Nemoto, H., Takeda, H., Takano, S.: Studies on the synthesis of heterocyclic compounds — CCCXXI. Synthetic approach to camptothecin. Tetrahedron **26**, 5753—5755 (1970).

Kende, A. S., Draper, R. W., Kubo, I., Joyeux, M.: (Abstr.) 160th Amer. Chem. Soc. Meeting (Chicago) ORGN-10 (1970).

Kepler, J. A., Wani, M. C., McNaull, J. N., Wall, M. E., Levine, S. G.: Plant antitumor agents. IV. An approach toward the synthesis of camptothecin. J. Amer. chem. Soc. **34**, 3853—3858 (1969).

Kessel, D.: Effects of camptothecin on RNA synthesis in leukemia L1210 cells. Biochim. biophys. Acta (Amst.) **246**, 225—232 (1971a).
Kessel, D.: Some determinants of camptothecin responsiveness in leukemia L1210 cells. Cancer Res. **31**, 1883—1887 (1971b).
Kessel, D., Bosmann, H. B., Lohr, K.: Camptothecin effects on DNA synthesis in murine leukemia cells. Biochim. biophys. Acta (Amst.) **269**, 210—216 (1972).
Li, L. H., Fraser, T. J., Olin, E. J., Bhuyan, B. K.: Action of camptothecin on mammalian cells in culture. Cancer Res. **32**, 2643—2650 (1972).
Liao, T. K., Nyberg, W. H., Cheng, C. C.: Total synthesis of camptothecin. I. Synthesis of ethyl 8-(α-chlorobutyryloxymethyl)-7,9-dioxo-7,8,9,11-tetrahydroindolizino [1,2-a] quinoline-8-carboxylate and related tetracyclic compounds (1). J. heterocycl. Chem. **8**, 373—377 (1971).
McPhail, A. T., Sim, G. A.: The structure of camptothecin: x-ray analysis of camptothecin iodoacetate. J. chem. Soc. (B), 923—928 (1968).
Moertel, C. G., Schutt, A. J., Reitemeier, R. J., Hahn, R. G.: Phase II study of camptothecin (NSC-100880) in the treatment of advanced gastrointestinal cancer. Cancer Chemother. Rep. **56**, 95—101 (1972).
Muggia, F. M., Creaven, P. J., Hansen, H. H., Cohen, M. H., Selawry, O. S.: Phase I clinical trial of weekly and daily schedules of camptothecin sodium (NSC-100880): correlation with preclinical studies. Cancer Chemother. Rep. **56**, 515—521 (1972).
Shamma, M.: A numbering system for camptothecin based on its biogenesis. Experientia (Basel) **24**, 107 (1968).
Shamma, M., Novak, L.: Synthetic approaches to camptothecin. Tetrahedron **25**, 2275—2279 (1969).
Shamma, M., Novak, L.: The preparation of some tricyclic analogs of camptothecin. Collect. Czech. Chem. Commun. **35**, 3280—3286 (1970).
Spataro, A., Kessel, D.: Studies on camptothecin-induced degradation and apparent reaggregation of DNA from L1210 cells. Biochem. biophys. Res. Commun. **48**, 643—648 (1972).
Stork, G., Schultz, A. G.: The total synthesis of *dl*-camptothecin. J. Amer. chem. Soc. **93**, 4074—4075 (1971).
Venditti, J. M., Abbott, B. J.: Studies on oncolytic agents from natural sources. Correlations of activity against animal tumors and clinical effectiveness. Lloydia **30**, 332—348 (1967).
Volkmann, R., Danishefsky, S., Eggler, J., Solomon, D. M.: A total synthesis of *dl*-camptothecin. J. Amer. chem. Soc. **93**, 5576—5577 (1971).
Wall, M. E.: Alkaloids with anti-tumor activity. In: International symposium on the biochemistry and physiology of alkaloids, Halle. Berlin: Academic Press 1969.
Wall, M. E., Wani, M. C., Cook, C. E., Plamer, K. H., McPhail, A. T., Sim, G. A.: Plant antitumor agents. I. The isolation and structure of camptothecin, a novel alkaloidal leukemia and tumor inhibitor from *Camptotheca acuminata*. J. Amer. chem. Soc. **88**, 3888—3890 (1966).
Wani, M. C., Kepler, J. A., Thompson, J. B., Wall, M. E., Levine, S. G.: Plant antitumor agents: alkaloids: synthesis of a pentacylic camptothecin precursor. Chem. Comm. 404 (1970).
Wani, M. C., Campbell, H. F., Brine, G. A., Kepler, J. A., Wall, M. E., Levine, S. G.: Plant antitumor agents. IX. The total synthesis of *dl*-camptothecin. J. Amer. chem. Soc. **94**, 3631—3632 (1972).
Warneke, J., Winterfeldt, E.: Die autoxydative Indol-chinolon-Umwandlung eines Camptothecin-Modells. Chem. Ber. **105**, 2120—2125 (1972).
Wenkert, E., Dave, K. G., Lewis, R. G., Sprague, P. W.: General methods of synthesis of indole alkaloids. VI. Synthesis of *dl*-corynantheidine and a camptothecin model. J. Amer. chem. Soc. **89**, 6741—6745 (1967).
Winterfeldt, E., Radunz, H.: A convenient route to the camptothecin chromophore. Chem. Comm. 374—375 (1971).
Wu, R. S., Kumar, A., Warner, J. R.: Ribosome formation is blocked by camptothecin, a reversible inhibitor of RNA synthesis. Proc. nat. Acad. Sci. (Wash.) **68**, 3009—3014 (1971).

Chapter 66

3′-Deoxyadenosine and Other Polynucleotide Chain Terminators

Sune Frederiksen and Hans Klenow

Introduction

At present only one principle for enzyme reactions responsible for synthesis of polynucleotide chains is known. It consists of extension of chains in the 5′ → 3′ direction by a nucleophilic attack of the 3′-OH group of the 3′-terminal nucleotidyl group on the phosphorus atom of the α-phosphate group of a nucleoside di- or triphosphate, resulting in extension of the chain by a further nucleoside monophosphate. The incorporation into a polymer by this type of reaction of a nucleoside monophosphate lacking the free 3′-OH group in the ribose configuration would prevent further chain elongation since no further 3′,5′-phosphodiester linkage can be formed. This expectation has been experimentally confirmed. Any nucleoside or nucleotide containing this type of sugar moiety could, therefore, be regarded as a potential polynucleotide chain growth terminator, and will be the topic of the present chapter.

Although 3′-deoxyadenosine triphosphate and some related compounds employed in experiments with isolated RNA polymerases have been found to function as terminators of polynucleotide chain synthesis, the addition of these compounds to cell suspensions would be expected to have no effect on nucleic acid synthesis, since cell membranes usually are impermeable to nucleotides. In contrast, nucleosides usually permeate cell membranes readily. The potential of nucleoside analogs like 3′-deoxyadenosine to stop polynucleotide chain elongation depends, therefore, on their metabolic fate in the cells. If the anabolic enzymatic activities leading to the formation of the corresponding phosphates dominate over the catabolic enzyme activities like deaminase activity, phosphorylated derivatives will accumulato. This may result in termination of nucleotide chain growth, provided that the nucleoside phosphate analogs formed are substrates for one or more nucleic acid polymerases in the cell.

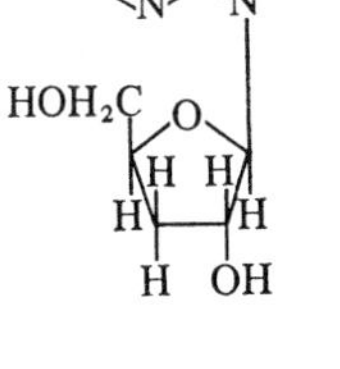

Structure of cordycepin (3′-deoxyadenosine).

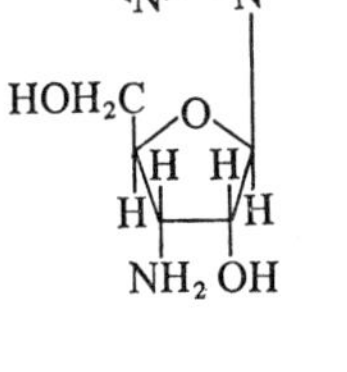

Structure of 3′-amino-3′-deoxyadenosine.

Two nucleosides lacking the 3'-OH group, 3'-deoxyadenosine (TODD and ULBRICHT, 1960) and 3'-amino-3'-deoxyadenosine (REIST and BAKER, 1958), were prepared by chemical synthesis before the existence in nature of compounds with identical or similar structure was recognized. 3'-Deoxyadenosine was isolated in 1951 as the first nucleoside antibiotic from a natural source (CUNNINGHAM et al., 1951). It was prepared from culture filtrates of *Cordyceps militaris* and given the name cordycepin. Several procedures for the isolation have been published (KREDICH and GUARINO, 1960; FREDERIKSEN et al., 1965; CHASSY and SUHADOLNIK, 1969). The yield of cordycepin may be increased considerably by addition of adenine to the growth medium, while the addition to the medium of a number of pyrazolopyrimidines and benzimidazoles does not result in the accumulation of the corresponding 3'-deoxyribosides (CURTIS and THOMAS, 1962). Cordycepin is also produced by *Aspergillus nidulans* (KACZKA et al., 1964a). The identification of cordycepin as 3'-deoxyadenosine by KACZKA et al. (1964b) was based on comparison of infrared and NMR spectra with those of the authentic compound (TODD and ULBRICHT, 1960; LEE et al., 1961; WALTON et al., 1964). The identification has been confirmed by infrared spectra (FREDERIKSEN et al., 1965) and mass spectra (HANESSIAN et al., 1966). 3'-Amino-3'-deoxyadenosine has been isolated from culture filtrates of *Helminthosporium* (AMMANN and SAFFERMAN, 1958; GERBER and LECHEVALIER, 1962), the mycelium of *Cordyceps militaris* (GUARINO and KREDICH, 1963) and from *Aspergillus nidulans* (SUHADOLNIK, unpublished results). The structure has been determined by chemical methods (GERBER and LECHEVALIER, 1962) and by mass spectra (SUHADOLNIK et al., 1969). A large number of other potential nucleoside chain terminators have been prepared, mainly by chemical synthesis. Those with biological effect will be mentioned below.

For other reviews on nucleoside antibiotics the readers are referred to FOX et al. (1966), GUARINO (1967), and SUHADOLNIK (1970).

Enzymatic Studies

A. Deamination

Partially purified adenosine deaminase from intestinal mucosa catalyzes the deamination of 3'-deoxyadenosine (CODDINGTON, 1965), xylosyladenine, arabinosyladenine, 3'-amino-2',3'-dideoxyadenosine, 2',3'-dideoxyadenosine, 3'-amino-3'-deoxyadenosine, 2'-amino-2',3'-dideoxyadenosine, and arabinosyladenine. The K_m values (FREDERIKSEN, 1966) vary from 0.6 to 12-fold that of adenosine in the order of the compounds mentioned (see also CORY and SUHADOLNIK, 1965; LEPAGE and JUNGA, 1965; KOSHIURA and LEPAGE, 1968). With extracts of *E. coli* the rate of deamination of 3'-deoxyadenosine and 2',3'-dideoxyadenosine was about 14 and 25 fold lower, respectively, than that of 2'-deoxyadenosine (TOJI and COHEN, 1970).

B. Phosphorylation

A large number of adenosine analogs are phosphorylated by adenosine kinase. Partially purified rabbit liver enzyme catalyzes the phosphorylation of the following potential chain terminator nucleosides, 3'-deoxyadenosine, 3'-amino-3'-deoxyadenosine, xylofuranosyladenine, 2'-amino-2',3'-dideoxyadenosine (LINDBERG et al., 1967), N^6-methyl-3'-amino-3'-deoxyadenosine, and 3'-deoxy-3-isoadenosine (LINDBERG, 1969). All of the compounds have a K_m value which is greater (300 to 2×10^4 fold) than that for adenosine. With adenosine kinase from H. Ep. 2 cells the phosphorylation of 3'-deoxyadenosine proceeds fairly slowly (SCHNEBLI et al., 1967). Enzymatic formation of triphosphates from the corresponding monophosphates in the presence of ATP and muscle myokinase was obtained for the following potential chain terminators: xylofuranosyladenine, 3'-deoxyadenosine, 3'-amino-3'-deoxyadenosine (LINDBERG et al., 1967), N^6-methyl-3'-amino-3'-deoxyadenosine, and 3'-deoxy-3-isoadenosine (LINDBERG, 1969).

Effects of Phosphorylated Derivatives

3'-Deoxy AMP, which is dephosphorylated in the presence of 5'-nucleotidase from snake venom (KLENOW, 1963a), inhibits the phosphoribosylpyrophosphate amidotransferase from *B. subtilis* and pigeon liver (ROTTMAN and GUARINO, 1964c). 3'-Deoxy ADP functions as a phosphate acceptor in the pyruvate kinase reaction (KLENOW, 1963a) and 3'-deoxy ATP as a phosphate donor in the fructokinase reaction (ADELMAN et al., 1967). 3'-Deoxy ATP is not a substrate for ribonucleoside triphosphate reductase from *L. leichmannii*, but it has a marked stimulatory effect on the reduction of CTP to 2'-deoxy CTP. The effect under optimal conditions is, however, smaller than that obtained with 2'-dATP. Similarly, the reduction of ATP is inhibited by 3'-deoxy ATP, but the effect is smaller than that obtained with 2'-deoxy ATP. 3'-Deoxy ATP also functions as an effector for the ribonucleoside diphosphate reductase from *E. coli*. It especially inhibits the reduction of ADP, but again to a smaller extent than 2'-deoxy ATP (CHASSY and SUHADOLNIK, 1968, SUHADOLNIK et al., 1968). Both 3'-deoxy ATP (OVERGAARD-HANSEN, 1964) and xylosyl ATP (ELLIS and LEPAGE, 1965a, b) are potent inhibitors of the enzymatic formation of 5-phosphoribosyl pyrophosphate from ATP and ribose-5-phosphate as catalyzed by extracts of Ehrlich ascites tumor cells.

Chain growth terminating effects as studied with isolated enzymes have been shown for a number of compounds. The triphosphates of 3'-deoxyadenosine and 3'-amino-3'-deoxyadenosine inhibit RNA synthesis as catalyzed by RNA polymerase from *Micrococcus lysodeicticus* (SHIGEURA et al., 1966). The formation of polyadenylic acid, but not that of polyuridylic acid, is inhibited by 3'-dATP (SHIGEURA and GORDON, 1965). Experiments with ^{14}C-3'-deoxy ATP have shown that the corresponding monophosphate is incorporated almost exclusively into the 3'-end group of RNA chains as expected for a true chain terminator (SHIGEURA and BOXER, 1964). Both 3'-dATP and 3'-amino-3'-deoxy ATP block RNA synthesis as catalyzed by the DNA-dependent RNA polymerase from Ehrlich ascites tumor cells. The type of kinetics obtained is as expected for inhibitors which function as chain growth terminators (KLENOW and FREDERIKSEN, 1964; SHIGEURA et al., 1966; TRUMAN and KLENOW, 1968). SENTENAC et al. (1968) have found that the RNA chains formed in the presence of 3'-dATP as catalyzed by RNA polymerase from *E. coli* are very short (i.e. 10 to 40 nucleotides), as compared to chains formed in the absence of 3'-deoxy ATP.

2',3'-Dideoxyadenosine triphosphate inhibits the exchange between pyrophosphate and 2'-deoxyribonucleoside triphosphates and it blocks DNA synthesis irreversibly as catalyzed by DNA polymerase from *E. coli* (polymerase I). In the latter reaction, the monophosphate was incorporated in the 3'-terminal position (TOJI and COHEN, 1969).

In a similar manner, 2',3'-dideoxy TTP is incorporated as the corresponding monophosphate into the 3'-end group of various types of DNA molecules in the presence of DNA polymerase I from *E. coli*. 2',3'-Didehydro-2',3'-dideoxy TTP was as effective as an inhibitor of chain growth in this system as 2',3'-dideoxy ATP, while 3'-iodo-2',3'-dideoxy TTP was much less effective. Oligo *d*(T) with a terminal 2′,3′-dideoxy TMP was degraded more slowly by the exonuclease moiety of the polymerase than was a normal oligo *d*(T) molecule (ATKINSON et al., 1969). 2′,3′-Dideoxy TTP also inhibits the reverse transcriptase from avian myeloblastosis virus (VERMA et al., 1971).

The structure of arabinosyl-nucleoside triphosphates does not necessarily suggest that they may function as chain terminators. Cytosine arabinoside 5′-triphosphate has, however, been shown to inhibit DNA synthesis and the corresponding monophosphate is incorporated almost exclusively into the 3′-end group of DNA as catalyzed by DNA polymerase from calf thymus (MOMPARLER, 1969). Both arabinosyl ATP and arabinosyl CTP inhibit DNA synthesis by isolated nuclei from rat liver or thymus (WAQAR et al., 1971). REDDY et al. (1971) have found that araCTP is a potent inhibitor for DNA polymerase II, but not for polymerase I from *E. coli*. Polymerase III is inhibited to some extent.

Effects on Whole Cells

A. Growth

I. 3′-Deoxyadenosine and 3′-Amino-3′-Deoxyadenosine

3′-Deoxyadenosine inhibits growth of an avian-tubercle bacillus and *B. subtilis* (CUNNINGHAM et al., 1951; ROTTMAN and GUARINO, 1964a), Ehrlich ascites cells *in vivo* (JAGGER et al., 1961; FREDERIKSEN and RASMUSSEN, 1967) and H. Ep. 1 cells grown in culture (RICH et al., 1965), but the compound does not inhibit the growth of *Staphylococcus aureus* Oxf. H, *Sarcina lutea*, *E. coli*, *B. proteus*, *Streptococcus hemolyticus*, *S. flexneri*, *S. faecalis*, or *Pasteurella septica* (CUNNINGHAM et al., 1951).

3′-Deoxyadenosine has been shown to inhibit the growth of several strains of *Saccharomyces cerevisiae*. The compound does not induce petite mutants, but effectively prevents the induction of petite mutants by 5-fluorouracil (D.H. WILLIAMSON, 1970).

The effect of 3′-deoxyadenosine on the protozoon giving rise to sleeping sickness in cattle and man has been investigated by WILLIAMSON (1966, 1969, 1970, 1972) and MACADAM and WILLIAMSON (1969). Infections in mice of *Trypanosoma congolense*, *Trypanosoma rhodesiense*, and *Trypanosoma cruzi* are inhibited to different extents by 3′-deoxyadenosine and infection may be prevented if the animal is treated with 3′-deoxyadenosine in multiple small doses early after infection (WILLIAMSON, 1972). The trypanosome differs from other cells that are affected by cordycepin in its inability to synthesize adenine (LITTLE and OLESON, 1951; WILLIAMSON and ROLLO, 1952).

The effect of 3′-deoxyadenosine on malaria parasites has been investigated by TRIGG et al. (1971) who found that the growth *in vitro* of *Plasmodium knowlesi* and *Plasmodium berghei berghei* was inhibited. *Plasmodium berghei berghei* was likewise inhibited *in vivo* in mice by 3′-deoxyadenosine, although no curative effect was obtained due to the toxic effect of larger doses.

3′-Amino-3′-deoxyadenosine has also been found to inhibit a variety of cell types: ascites tumors of mice (PUGH et al., 1962; PUGH and GERBER, 1963), J-tumor and ascites cell forms of adenocarcinoma, Ehrlich carcinoma, Gardner lymphosarcoma, and Sarcoma 180 (BLOCH and NICHOL, 1964), *Cryptococcus neoformans* 4806, *Candida albicans*, and protoplasts from *Saccharomyces cerevisiae* LK 2612, whereas the nucleoside was not inhibitory to bacteria (GERBER and LECHEVALIER, 1962).

II. 3′-Deoxyinosine and 3′-Deoxyadenosine N¹-Oxide

The inhibitory effect of 3′-deoxyadenosine may be reduced considerably in cells that have a high content of adenosine deaminase, since the compound is a good substrate for the deaminase (see above). The product of deamination (i.e. 3′-deoxyinosine) is without effect on nucleic acid synthesis in Ehrlich cells (KLENOW, 1963b) and must be present in much greater concentration than 3′-deoxyadenosine in order to inhibit growth of *B. subtilis* (ROTTMAN and GUARINO, 1964a). 3′-Deoxyadenosine N^1-oxide is not deaminated by adenosine deaminase from calf intestine (FREDERIKSEN, 1966) or by intact Ehrlich cells, but will give rise to an inhibition of RNA and DNA synthesis in the cells. 3′-Deoxyadenosine N^1-oxide is slowly deoxygenated within the cell to yield 3′-deoxyadenosine which following phosphorylation inhibits nucleic acid synthesis (FREDERIKSEN, 1963). 3′-Deoxyadenosine N^1-oxide also inhibits the replication of Ehrlich cells *in vivo* to a greater extent than molar equivalent amounts of 3′-deoxyadenosine (FREDERIKSEN and RASMUSSEN, 1967).

III. Other 3′-Deoxyribonucleosides

The 3′-deoxyribonucleosides of 2,6-diaminopurine, purine, purine-6-thiol, 6-methylaminopurine, 6-ethylaminopurine, 6-dimethylaminopurine (WALTON et al., 1965), and guanine (JENKINS et al., 1965) have been synthetically prepared. None of these nucleosides were phosphorylated to the triphosphate level (SHIGEURA et al., 1966). The effect of these nucleosides was tested on KB cells and chick fibroblasts; they were found to be less potent inhibitors than 3′-deoxyadenosine (GITTERMAN et al., 1965).

IV. 3′-Amino Substituted Compounds

3′-Acetamido-3′-deoxyadenosine was isolated from *Helminthosporium* sp. 215 by SUHADOLNIK et al. (1969), and homocitrullylaminoadenosine (KREDICH and GUARINO, 1961), and lysylamino adenosine (GUARINO and KREDICH, 1964) from *Cordyceps militaris*. 3′-Acetamido-3′-deoxyadenosine does not inhibit the growth of bacteria, yeast, or Ehrlich ascites cells (SUHADOLNIK et al., 1969). A possible reason for this inactivity could be a lack of phosphorylation, since the compound is not a substrate for a purified adenosine kinase from rabbit liver (LINDBERG et al., 1967). Lysylaminoadenosine and homocitrullylaminoadenosine have, to our knowledge, not been tested as inhibitors of cell growth, but homocitrullylaminoadenosine, which structurally resembles puromycin, inhibits the incorporation of amino acids into proteins in cell-free extracts of *E. coli* and rat liver, but not as strongly as puromycin (GUARINO et al., 1963).

3′-Amino-3′-deoxyadenosine has been converted to 3′-amino-3′-deoxyinosine enzymatically and has been oxidized to 3′-amino-3′-deoxyadenosine N^1-oxide. Neither of the two latter compounds inhibited the growth of several different strains of bacteria or fungi (GERBER, 1964).

V. 3′-Halogen Substituted Compounds

3′-Deoxy-3′-fluorothymidine and 3′-deoxy-3′-chlorothymidine inhibit the incorporation of $^{32}P_i$ into DNA of Ehrlich ascites cells *in vitro*, but 3′-deoxythymidine is completely inactive (LANGEN et al., 1969). This result is in agreement with the findings of TOJI and COHEN (1970). 3′-Deoxy-3′-chlorothymidine is only half as effective as 3′-deoxy-3′-fluorothymidine as an inhibitor of $^{32}P_i$ incorporation into DNA. The latter compound also strongly inhibits the growth of Ehrlich ascites cells. Indirect evidence is provided to support the conclusion that the inhibition of the synthesis of DNA is due to incorporation of 3'-deoxy-3'-fluorothymidine into a terminal position, but this remains to be proved.

VI. 2',3'-Dideoxyribonucleosides

2',3'-Dideoxythymidine, 2',3'-dideoxyuridine, 2',3'-dideoxycytidine, and 2',3'-dideoxyadenosine have been synthetically prepared (Horwitz et al., 1966; McCarthy et al., 1966; Robins et al., 1966; Russell and Moffatt, 1969). 2',3'-Dideoxyadenosine inhibits the growth of *E. coli*, but the bacteria are insensitive to the three other 2',3'-dideoxynucleosides (Doering et al., 1966; Toji and Cohen, 1970). No effects of the 2',3'-dideoxynucleosides have been obtained on mammalian cells (Toji and Cohen, 1970). The authors suggest that this inactivity is due to a lack of phosphorylation and for 2',3'-dideoxyadenosine this suggestion is in agreement with results obtained with adenosine kinase from rabbit liver, which does not use this compound as a substrate (Lindberg et al., 1967).

B. Mitosis and Chromosomes

Treatment of root tips from *Vicia faba* with 3'-deoxyadenosine or xylosyladenine results in inhibition of the function of the mitotic spindle and produces extreme chromosome contraction. A high frequency of breaks, but no exchanges, were produced in the nucleolar constriction (Kihlman and Odmark, 1966). Root tips of *Allium cepa* were treated with 3'-deoxyadenosine and the redistribution of nucleolar morphological components (i.e., the nucleolar segregation) was studied by electron microscopy. The rate of development of nucleolar segregation induced by 3'-deoxyadenosine was dependent on the time during interphase at which the cells were treated (Stockert et al., 1970). Cells treated with 3'-deoxyadenosine in late interphase reached prophase but were unable to initiate metaphase, and cells treated in prophase remained in prophase, whereas cells treated in metaphase were able to finish mitosis, as well as the subsequent mitosis, normally (Gonzalez-Fernandez et al., 1970). Further analysis of the effects of 3'-deoxyadenosine have shown that the compound blocks the rupture of the nuclear membrane giving rise to a process of endomitosis (Giménez-Martin et al., 1971).

3'-Amino-3'-deoxyadenosine produced a strong antimitotic effect in onion root tips (Ammann and Safferman, 1958).

C. Uptake and Metabolism

3'-Deoxyadenosine and 3'-amino-3'-deoxyadenosine are rapidly taken up by Ehrlich ascites cells, as seen from the accumulation of the corresponding mono-, di-, and triphosphates (Klenow, 1963a; Shigeura et al., 1966a; Shigeura and Sampson, 1967a; Truman and Klenow, 1968). The effect of 3'-deoxyadenosine on the uptake of uridine, cytidine, and adenosine into Novikoff hepatoma cells has been studied by Plagemann (1971). 3'-Deoxyadenosine inhibits the transport of uridine and adenosine competitively when present in a 20 to 40 fold excess. The inhibitory effect under these conditions on the incorporation of adenosine into the nucleic acids is, however, much greater, indicating that the primary effect of this agent is not on cellular uptake. Even with this high ratio of 3'-deoxyadenosine to adenosine, the conversion of adenosine to ATP was not inhibited. This is probably explained by the 300 fold greater K_m value for 3'-deoxyadenosine than for adenosine with adenosine kinase (Lindberg et al., 1967). When Ehrlich carcinoma cells are incubated with large amounts of 3'-deoxyadenosine (i.e., 15 to 25 μmol per gram of cells wet weight) the phosphorylation of 3'-deoxyadenosine to its phosphate esters is accompanied by a concomitant exhaustion of the adenine ribonucleotide pool (KLENOW, 1963b).

In *B. subtilis*, 3'-deoxyadenosine inhibits the incorporation of formate and glycine into nucleic acids, but does not affect the incorporation of 5-amino-4-imidazolecarboxamide into these macromolecules (ROTTMAN and GUARINO, 1964b). In Ehrlich cells, 3'-deoxyadenosine inhibits the incorporation into RNA and DNA of orthophosphate (KLENOW, 1963b), uridine (FREDERIKSEN and KLENOW, 1964), adenine (KLENOW and OVERGAARD-HANSEN, 1964), formate, glycine, hypoxanthine, adenine, and guanine (SHIGEURA and GORDON, 1965); 3'-amino-3'-deoxyadenosine inhibits the incorporation into the polynucleotides of hypoxanthine and orotic acid (SHIGEURA et al., 1966), and uridine and adenine (TRUMAN and KLENOW, 1968). 3'-Deoxyadenosine inhibits the utilization of adenosine for nucleic acid synthesis in H. Ep. 1 cells (RICH et al., 1965) and uridine and adenosine for nucleic acids in Novikoff hepatoma cells (PLAGEMANN, 1971).

The number of pathways inhibited and the difference in degree of inhibition suggest that several enzymatic processes are affected by the nucleoside analogs. In *B. subtilis* incubated with 3'-deoxyadenosine, the monophosphate was found to accumulate and this nucleotide inhibits the phosphoribosylpyrophosphate amidotransferase from *B. subtilis* and pigeon liver (ROTTMAN and GUARINO, 1964c). Using extracts of Ehrlich cells, OVERGAARD-HANSEN (1964) showed that 3'-deoxyadenosine triphosphate inhibits the formation of 5-phosphoribosyl-1-pyrophosphate and a similar inhibition was found in intact L5178Y lymphoma cells (TYRSTED and SARTORELLI, 1968). The finding that 3'-amino-3'-deoxyadenosine inhibits the formation of 5-phosphoribosylamine is in agreement with the results described above (SHIGEURA et al., 1966).

N^6-Methyl-3'-deoxyadenosine is phosphorylated to the monophosphate level in Ehrlich ascites cells, which inhibits the formation of 5-phosphoribosylamine (SHIGEURA et al., 1966), but in KB cells the nucleoside is demethylated to 3'-deoxyadenosine (SHIGEURA and SAMPSON, 1967b).

RNA Synthesis

A. Ehrlich Ascites Cells

3'-Deoxyadenosine gives rise to a differential inhibition of the synthesis of different RNA species. RNA from Ehrlich ascites cells may be separated into three fractions consisting of mainly cytoplasmic RNA, as well as nuclear RNA I and nuclear RNA II. Their labeling with ^{32}P was inhibited to different degrees by 3'-deoxyadenosine, nuclear RNA being inhibited little or not at all (FREDERIKSEN and KLENOW, 1964). By further fractionation of the cytoplasmic RNA on sucrose gradients, it was found that the incorporation of uridine into 28 S RNA was inhibited to a greater extent than was the incorporation into 18 S RNA, and the 4 to 5 S RNA peak was the least inhibited by this agent; furthermore, the nuclear heterodisperse RNA was only slightly inhibited under these conditions (TRUMAN and FREDERIKSEN, 1969). A differential inhibitory effect on the synthesis of different RNA fractions was also obtained with 3'-amino-3'-deoxyadenosine (TRUMAN and FREDERIKSEN, 1969). After separation of the cytoplasmic RNA on methylated albumin kieselguhr columns, tRNA was found to be less inhibited by this agent than was ribosomal RNA, and two low molecular weight RNA components were least inhibited (FREDERIKSEN et al., 1971). The inhibitory effects of 3'-deoxyadenosine on the synthesis of low molecular weight RNA components was further investigated after separation of these components on polyacrylamide gels; components designated D and C (migrating slower than 5 S RNA in 10% gels) were inhibited to a lesser degree than the small RNA component in the H region (migrating between tRNA and 5 S RNA) (HELLUNG-LARSEN and FREDERIKSEN, 1972).

B. HeLa Cells

The differential inhibitory effects of 3′-deoxyadenosine on RNA synthesis have been used in the study of RNA metabolism of HeLa cells. 3′-Deoxyadenosine inhibits the incorporation of uridine into RNA of HeLa cells under conditions in which the incorporation of thymidine and amino acids into acid-insoluble material was not affected (SIEV et al., 1969). The synthesis of nucleoplasmic heterogeneous RNA was unaffected by 3′-deoxyadenosine, but the synthesis of nucleolar 45 S RNA was strongly depressed; furthermore, the labeling of cytoplasmic 18 S RNA was inhibited less than was the 28 S RNA.

The synthesis of two low molecular weight nuclear RNA components in HeLa cells, components D and C, is inhibited by 3′-deoxyadenosine, with component C being more sensitive than component D (WEINBERG and PENMAN, 1969). The synthesis of mitochondrial 12 S and 21 S RNA is depressed by 3′-deoxyadenosine, but in this case shorter RNA chains are not formed (PERLMAN and PENMAN, 1970; ZYLBER et al., 1971). The synthesis of messenger RNA (mRNA) [i.e., rapidly labeled RNA released from the polysomes by ethylenediamine tetraacetic acid (EDTA)] is inhibited by 3′-deoxyadenosine, but the transport from the nucleus to the cytoplasm of mRNA synthesized before exposure to drug is not affected (PENMAN et al., 1970a). The effect of 3′-deoxyadenosine on RNA metabolism in HeLa cells is summarized by PENMAN et al. (1970b). Further information on the inhibitory effect of 3′-deoxyadenosine on the appearence of mRNA on the polyribosomes was provided by DARNELL et al. (1971) who showed that 3′-deoxyadenosine produced a tenfold reduction in adenosine incorporation into poly A linked to heterogeneous nuclear RNA and to mRNA. After infection of HeLa cells with adenovirus, the virus specific mRNA is attached to poly A before transport into the cytoplasm. 3′-Deoxyadenosine also inhibits the synthesis of poly A in this instance and, thereby, interferes with the appearance of labeled virus mRNA in the cytoplasm (PHILIPSON et al., 1971).

Since 45 S and 32 S ribosomal RNA precursors were found not to be influenced by 3′-deoxyadenosine or actinomycin in metaphase-arrested HeLa cells, it was concluded that these precursors were not synthesized during mitoses but that they were stabilized as ribonucleoprotein particles (FAN and PENMAN, 1971).

C. H.Ep. Cells

It should be emphasized that although the effect of 3′-deoxyadenosine in the experiments described above can best be explained by this agent functioning as a chain terminator, results obtained with H. Ep. 1 cells incubated with 3′-deoxyadenosine-^{3}H have shown that very small amounts of 3′-deoxyadenosine were incorporated into internal positions of RNA and DNA, which implies that abnormal 2′,5′-linkages are formed (CORY et al., 1965).

References

ADELMAN, R. C., BALLARD, F. J., WEINHOUSE, S.: Purification and properties of rat liver fructokinase. J. biol. Chem. **242**, 3360—3365 (1967).

AMMANN, C. A., SAFFERMAN, R. S.: The onion test as a possible screening method for antitumor agents. Antibiot. and Chemother. 8, 1—7 (1958).

ATKINSON, M.R., DEUTSCHER, M.P., KORNBERG, A., RUSSELL, A.F., MOFFATT, J.G.: Enzymatic synthesis of deoxyribonucleic acid. XXXIV. Termination of chain growth by a 2′,3′-dideoxyribonucleotide. Biochemistry 8, 4897—4904 (1969).

BLOCH, A., NICHOL, C.A.: Nucleoside antibiotics related to adenosine. Antimicrob. Agents Chemother. 530—539 (1964).

CHASSY, B.M., SUHADOLNIK, R.J.: Nucleoside antibiotics. II. Biochemical tools for studying the structural requirements for interaction at the catalytic and regulatory sites of ribonucleotide reductase from *Escherichia coli*. J. biol. Chem. **243**, 3538—3541 (1968).

CHASSY, B.M., SUHADOLNIK, R.J.: Nucleoside antibiotics. IV. Metabolic fate of adenosine and cordycepin by *Cordyceps militaris* during cordycepin biosynthesis. Biochim. biophys. Acta (Amst.) **182**, 307—315 (1969).

CODDINGTON, A.: Some substrates and inhibitors of adenosine deaminase. Biochim. biophys. Acta (Amst.) **99**, 442—451 (1965).

CORY, J.G., SUHADOLNIK, R.J.: Structural requirements of nucleosides for binding by adenosine deaminase. Biochemistry **4**, 1729—1732 (1965).

CORY, J.G., SUHADOLNIK, R.J., RESNICK, B., RICH, M.A.: Incorporation of cordycepin (3′-deoxyadenosine) into ribonucleic acid and deoxyribonucleic acid of human tumor cells. Biochim. biophys. Acta (Amst.) **103**, 646—653 (1965).

CUNNINGHAM, K.G., HUTCHINSON, S.A., MANSON, W., SPRING, F.S.: Cordycepin, a metabolic product from cultures of *Cordyceps militaris* (linn.) link. Part I. Isolation and characterization. J. chem. Soc. **3**, 2299—2300 (1951).

CURTIS, P.J., THOMAS, D.R.: The metabolism of exogenous adenine and purine analogues by fungi. Biochem. J. **82**, 381—384 (1962).

DARNELL, J.E., PHILIPSON, L., WALL, R., ADESNIK, M.: Polyadenylic acid sequences: role in conversion of nuclear RNA into messenger RNA. Science **174**, 507—510 (1971).

DOERING, A.M., JANSEN, M., COHEN, S.S.: Polymer synthesis in killed bacteria: lethality of 2′,3′-dideoxyadenosine. J. Bact. **92**, 565—574 (1966).

ELLIS, D.B., LE PAGE, G.A.: The effect of β-xylosyl adenine on the formation of 5-phosphoribosyl-1-pyrophosphate by cell-free extract of TA3 ascites cells. Canad. J. Biochem. **43**, 617—619 (1965a).

ELLIS, D.B., LE PAGE, G.A.: Some inhibitory effects of 9-β-D-xylofuranosyladenine, an adenosine analog, on nucleotide metabolism in ascites tumor cells. Molec. Pharmacol. **1**, 231—238 (1965b).

FAN, H., PENMAN, S.: Regulation of synthesis and processing of nucleolar components in metaphase-arrested cells. J. molec. Biol. **59**, 27—42 (1971).

FOX, J.J., WATANABE, K.A., BLOCH, A.: In: DAVIDSON, J.N., COHN, W.E. (Eds.): Progress in nucleic acid research and molecular biology, p. 251—313. New York: Academic Press 1966.

FREDERIKSEN, S.: Inhibition of ribonucleic acid and deoxyribonucleic acid synthesis in Ehrlich ascites cells by cordycepin-N^1-oxide. Biochim. biophys. Acta (Amst.) **76**, 366—371 (1963).

FREDERIKSEN, S.: Specificity of adenosine deaminase toward adenosine and 2′-deoxyadenosine analogues. Arch. Biochem. Biophys. **113**, 383—388 (1966).

FREDERIKSEN, S., KLENOW, H.: Differential inhibition by 3′-deATP of nuclear and cytoplasmic RNA fractions of Ehrlich ascites tumor cells *in vitro*. Biochem. biophys. Res. Commun. **17**, 165—170 (1964).

FREDERIKSEN, S., MALLING, H., KLENOW, H.: Isolation of 3′-deoxyadenosine (Cordycepin) from the liquid medium of *Cordyceps militaris* (L. EX FR.) link. Biochim. biophys. Acta (Amst.) **95**, 189—193 (1965).

FREDERIKSEN, S., RASMUSSEN, A.H.: Effect of the N^1-oxides of adenosine, 2′-deoxyadenosine, and 3′-deoxyadenosine on tumor growth *in vivo*. Cancer Res. **27**, 385—391 (1967).

FREDERIKSEN, S., TØNNESEN, T., HELLUNG-LARSEN, P.: Isolation of two small molecular weight RNA components by MAK column chromatography. Arch. Biochem. Biophys. **142**, 238—246 (1971).

GERBER, N.N.: Aminonucleosides II. 3′-Amino-3′-deoxyinosine and 3′-amino-3′-deoxyadenosine 1-N-oxide. J. Med. Chem. **7**, 204—207 (1964).

GERBER, N.N., LECHEVALIER, H.A.: 3′-Amino-3′-deoxyadenosine, an antitumor agent from Helminthosporium sp.[1]. J. org. Chem. **27**, 1731—1732 (1962).

GIMENEZ-MARTIN, G., GONZALEZ-FERNANDEZ, A., DE LA TORRE, C., FERNANDEZ-GOMEZ, M.E.: Partial initiation of endomitosis by 3′-deoxyadenosine. Chromosoma **33**, 361—371 (1971).

GITTERMAN, C.O., BURG, R.W., BOXER, G.E., MELTZ, D., HITT, J.: Relation of structure to activity of purine 3′-deoxynucleosides in KB cell and chick embryo fibroblast cell cultures. J. med. Chem. 8, 664—667 (1965).

GONZALEZ-FERNANDEZ, A., FERNANDEZ-GOMEZ, M.E., STOCKERT, J.C., LOPEZ-SAEZ, J.F.: Effect produced by inhibitors of RNA synthesis on mitosis. Exp. Cell Res. **60**, 320—326 (1970).

GUARINO, A. J.: In: GOTTLIEB, D., SHAW, P. D. (Eds.): Antibiotics, Vol. 1, p. 468—480. Berlin-Heidelberg-New York: Springer 1967.
GUARINO, A. J., IBERSHOF, M. L., SWAIN, R.: Inhibition of protein synthesis in cell-free systems by homocitrullylamino adenosine. Biochim. biophys. Acta (Amst.) **72**, 62—68 (1963).
GUARINO, A. J., KREDICH, N. M.: Isolation and identification of 3′-amino-3′-deoxyadenosine from *Cordyceps militaris*. Biochim. biophys. Acta (Amst.) **68**, 317—319 (1963).
GUARINO, A. J., KREDICH, N. M.: Isolation and identification of lysylamino adenosine from *Cordiceps militaris*. Fed. Proc. **23**, 371 (1964).
HANESSIAN, S., DE JONGH, D. C., MCCLOSKEY, J. A.: Further evidence on the structure of cordycepin. Biochim. biophys. Acta (Amst.) **117**, 480—482 (1966).
HELLUNG-LARSEN, P., FREDERIKSEN, S.: Small molecular weight RNA compounds in Ehrlich ascites tumor cells. Biochim. Biophys. Acta (Amst.) **262**, 290—307 (1972).
HORWITZ, J. P., CHUA, J., DA ROOGE, M. A., NOEL, M., KLUNDT, I. L.: Nucleosides. IX. The formation of 2′,3′-unsaturated pyrimidine nucleosides via a novel β-elimination reaction. J. org. Chem. **31**, 205—211 (1966).
JAGGER, D. V., KREDICH, N. M., GUARINO, A. J.: Inhibition of Ehrlich mouse ascites tumor growth by cordycepin. Cancer Res. **21**, 216—220 (1961).
JENKINS, S. R., HOLLY, F. W., WALTON, E.: 3′-Deoxynucleosides. III. 3′D-eoxyguanosine. J. org. Chem. **30**, 2851—2852 (1965).
KACZKA, E. A., DULANEY, E. L., GITTERMAN, C. O., WOODRUFF, H. B., FOLKERS, K.: Isolation and inhibitory effects on KB cell cultures of 3′-deoxyadenosine from *Aspergillus nidulans* (eidam) wint. Biochem. biophys. Res. Commun. **14**, 452—455 (1964a).
KACZKA, E. A., TRENNER, N. R., ARISON, B., WALKER, R. W., FOLKERS, K.: Identification of cordycepin, a metabolite of *Cordyceps militaris*, as 3′-deoxyadenosine. Biochem. biophys. Res. Commun. **14**, 456—457 (1964b).
KIHLMAN, B. A., ODMARK, G.: Effects of adenine nucleosides on chromosomes, cell division and nucleic acid synthesis in *Vicia faba*. Hereditas **56**, 71—82 (1966).
KLENOW, H.: Formation of the mono-, di-, and triphosphate of cordycepin in Ehrlich ascites-tumor cells *in vitro*. Biochim. biophys. Acta (Amst.) **76**, 347—353 (1963a).
KLENOW, H.: Inhibition by cordycepin and 2-deoxyglucose of the incorporation of ^{32}P orthophosphate into the nucleic acids of Ehrlich ascites-tumor cells *in vitro*. Biochim. biophys. Acta (Amst.) **76**, 354—365 (1963b).
KLENOW, H., FREDERIKSEN, S.: Effect of 3′-deoxyATP (cordycepin triphosphate) and 2′-deoxyATP on the DNA-dependent RNA nucleotidyltransferase from Ehrlich ascites tumor cells. Biochim. biophys. Acta (Amst.) **87**, 495—498 (1964).
KLENOW, H., OVERGAARD-HANSEN, K.: Effect of cordycepin triphosphate on the incorporation of [8-^{14}C] adenine and [^{32}P] orthophosphate into the acid-soluble ribotides of Ehrlich ascites tumor cells *in vitro*. Biochim. biophys. Acta (Amst.) **80**, 500—504 (1964).
KOSHIURA, R., LEPAGE, G. A.: Some inhibitors of deamination of 9-β-D-arabinofuranosyladenine and 9-β-D-xylofuranosyladenine by blood and neoplasms of experimental animals and humans. Cancer Res. **28**, 1014—1020 (1968).
KREDICH, N. M., GUARINO, A. J.: An improved method of isolation and determination of cordycepin. Biochim. biophys. Acta (Amst.) **41**, 363—365 (1960).
KREDICH, N. M., GUARINO, A. J.: Homocitrullylaminoadenosine, a nucleoside isolated from *Cordyceps militaris*. J. biol. Chem. **236**, 3300—3302 (1961).
LANGEN, P., ETZOLD, G., HINTSCHE, R., KOWOLLIK, G.: 3′-Deoxy-3′-fluorothymidine, a new selective inhibitor of DNA-synthesis. Acta biol. med. germ. **23**, 759—766 (1969).
LEE, W. W., BENITEZ, A., ANDERSON, C. D., GOODMAN, L., BAKER, B. R.: Potential anticancer agents. LV. Synthesis of 3′-amino-2′,3′-dideoxyadenosine and related analogs. J. Amer. chem. Soc. **83**, 1906—1911 (1961).
LEPAGE, G. A., JUNGA, I. G.: Metabolism of purine nucleoside analogs. Cancer Res. **25**, 46—52 (1965).
LINDBERG, B.: Some additional properties of partially purified mammalian adenosine kinase. Biochim. biophys. Acta (Amst.) **185**, 245—247 (1969).
LINDBERG, B., KLENOW, H., HANSEN, K.: Some properties of partially purified mammalian adenosine kinase. J. biol. Chem. **242**, 350—356 (1967).
LITTLE, P. A., OLESON, J. J.: The cultivation of *Trypanosoma cruzi*. J. Bact. **61**, 709—714 (1951).
MACADAM, R. F., WILLIAMSON, J.: Lesions in the fine structure of *Trypanosoma rhodesiense* specifically associated with drug treatment. Trans. Roy. Soc. trop. Med. Hyg. **63**, 421 (1969).
MCCARTHY, J. R. Jr., ROBINS, M. J., TOWNSEND, L. B., ROBINS, R. K.: Purine nucleosides. XIV. Unsaturated furanosyl adenine nucleosides prepared via base-catalyzed elimination reactions of 2′-deoxyadenosine derivatives. J. Amer. chem. Soc. **88**, 1549—1553 (1966).
MOMPARLER, R. L.: Effect of cytosine arabinoside 5′-triphosphate on mammalian DNA polymerase. Biochem. biophys. Res. Commun. **34**, 465—471 (1969).

Overgaard-Hansen, K.: The inhibition of 5-phosphoribosyl-1-pyrophosphate formation by cordycepin triphosphate in extracts of Ehrlich ascites tumor cells. Biochim. biophys. Acta (Amst.) **80**, 504—507 (1964).

Penman, S., Fan, H., Perlman, S., Rosbash, M., Weinberg, R., Zylber, E. A.: Distinct RNA synthesis systems of the HeLa cell. Cold Spr. Harb. Symp. quant. Biol. **35**, 561—575 (1970b).

Penman, S., Rosbash, M., Penman, M.: Messenger and heterogeneous nuclear RNA in HeLa cells: differential inhibition by cordycepin. Proc. nat. Acad. Sci. (Wash.) **67**, 1878—1885 (1970a).

Perlman, S., Penman, S.: Mitochondrial protein synthesis: resistance to emetine and response to RNA synthesis inhibitors. Biochim. biophys. Res. Commun. **40**, 941—948 (1970).

Philipson, L., Wall, R., Glickman, G., Darnell, J. E.: Addition of polyadenylate sequences to virus-specific RNA during adenovirus replication. Proc. nat. Acad. Sci. (Wash.) **68**, 2806—2809 (1971).

Plagemann, P. G.: Effects of 3′-deoxyadenosine (cordycepin) and 2′-deoxyadenosine on nucleoside transport, macromolecular synthesis, and replication of cultured Novikoff hepatoma cells. Arch. Biochem. Biophys. **144**, 401—412 (1971).

Pugh, L. H., Gerber, N. N.: The effect of 3′-amino-3′-deoxyadenosine against ascitic tumors of mice. Cancer Res. **23**, 640—647 (1963).

Pugh, L. H., Lechevalier, H. A., Solotorovsky, M.: Antitumor activity of a substance produced by a strain of Helminthosporium. Antibiot. and Chemother. **12**, 310—317 (1962).

Reddy, G. V. R., Goulian, M., Hendler, S. S.: Inhibition of *E. coli* DNA polymerase II by ara-CTP. Nature (Lond.) **234**, 286—288 (1971).

Reist, E. J., Baker, B. R.: Potential anticancer agents. III. 3′-Amino-3′-deoxyadenosine. J. org. Chem. **23**, 1083 (1958).

Rich, M. A., Meyers, P., Weinbaum, G., Cory, J. G., Suhadolnik, R. J.: Inhibition of human tumor cells by cordycepin. Biochim. biophys. Acta (Amst.) **95**, 194—204 (1965).

Robins, M. J., McCarthy, J. R., Jr., Robins, R. K.: Purine nucleosides. XII. The preparation of 2′,3′-dideoxyadenosine, 2′,5′-dideoxyadenosine, and 2′,3′,5′-trideoxyadenosine from 2′-deoxyadenosine. Biochemistry **5**, 224—231 (1966).

Rottman, F., Guarino, A. J.: Studies on the inhibition of *Bacillus subtilis* growth by cordycepin. Biochim. biophys. Acta (Amst.) **80**, 632—639 (1964a).

Rottman, F., Guarino, A. J.: The inhibition of purine biosynthesis de novo in *Bacillus subtilis* by cordycepin. Biochim. biophys. Acta (Amst.) **80**, 640—647 (1964b).

Rottman, F., Guarino, A. J.: The inhibition of phosphoribosyl-pyrophosphate amidotransferase activity by cordycepin monophosphate. Biochim. biophys. Acta (Amst.) **89**, 465—472 (1964c).

Russell, A. F., Moffatt, J. G.: Synthesis of some nucleotides derived from 3′-deoxythymidine. Biochemistry **8**, 4889—4896 (1969).

Schnebli, H. P., Hill, D. L., Bennett, L. L., Jr.: Purification and properties of adenosine kinase from human tumor cells of type H. Ep. No. 2. J. biol. Chem. **242**, 1997—2004 (1967).

Sentenac, A., Ruet, A., Fromageot, P.: Initiation de chaines de RNA par la RNA polymérase *in vitro*. European. J. Biochem. **5**, 385—394 (1968).

Shigeura, H. T., Boxer, G. E.: Incorporation of 3′-deoxyadenosine-5′-triphosphate into RNA by RNA polymerase from *Micrococcus lysodeicticus*. Biochem. biophys. Res. Commun. **17**, 758—763 (1964).

Shigeura, H. T., Boxer, G. E., Meloni, M. L., Sampson, S. D.: Structure-activity relationship of some purine 3′-deoxyribonucleosides. Biochemistry **5**, 994—1004 (1966).

Shigeura, H. T., Gordon, C. N.: The effects of 3′-deoxyadenosine on the synthesis of ribonucleic acid. J. biol. Chem. **240**, 806—810 (1965).

Shigeura, H. T., Sampson, S. D.: Structural basis for phosphorylation of adenosine congeners. Nature (Lond.) **215**, 419—420 (1967a).

Shigeura, H. T., Sampson, S. D.: Utilization of 6-methylamino-9-(3′-deoxy-β-D-ribofuranosyl) purine by KB cells. Biochim. biophys. Acta (Amst.) **138**, 26—34 (1967b).

Siev, M., Weinberg, R., Penman, S.: The selective interruption of nucleolar RNA synthesis in HeLa cells by cordycepin. J. cell. Biol. **41**, 510—520 (1969).

Stockert, J. C., Fernandez-Gomez, M. E., Sogo, J. M., Lopez-Saez, J. F.: Nucleolar segregation by adenosine 3′-deoxyriboside (Cordycepin) in root-tip cells of *Allium cepa*. Exp. Cell Res. **59**, 85—89 (1970).

Suhadolnik, R. J.: Nucleoside Antibiotics. New York-London-Sydney-Toronto: John Wiley & Sons 1970.

Suhadolnik, R. J., Chassy, B. M., Waller, G. R.: Nucleoside antibiotics. III. Isolation, structural elucidation and biological properties of 3′-acetamido-3′-deoxyadenosine from Helminthosporium sp. 215. Biochim. biophys. Acta (Amst.) **179**, 258—267 (1969).

Suhadolnik, R. J., Finkel, S. I., Chassy, B. M.: Nucleoside antibiotics. I. Biochemical tools for studying the structural requirements for interaction at the catalytic and regulatory sites of ribonucleotide reductase from *Lactobacillus leichmannii*. J. biol. Chem. **243**, 3532—3537 (1968).

Todd, A., Ulbricht, T. L. V.: Deoxynucleoside and related compounds. Part IX. A synthesis of 3′-deoxyadenosine. J. chem. Soc. **5**, 3275—3277 (1960).

Toji, L., Cohen, S. S.: The enzymatic termination of polydeoxynucleotides by 2′,3′-dideoxyadenosine triphosphate. Proc. nat. Acad. Sci. (Wash.) **63**, 871—877 (1969).

Toji, L., Cohen, S. S.: Termination of deoxyribonucleic acid in *Escherichia coli* by 2′,3′-dideoxyadenosine. J. Bact. **103**, 323—328 (1970).

Trigg, P. I., Gutteridge, W. E., Williamson, J.: The effects of cordycepin on malaria parasites. Trans. roy. Soc. trop. Med. Hyg. **65**, 514—520 (1971).

Truman, J. T., Frederiksen, S.: Effect of 3′-deoxyadenosine and 3′-amino-3′-deoxyadenosine on the labelling of RNA sub-species in Ehrlich ascites tumor cells. Biochim. biophys. Acta (Amst.) **182**, 36—45 (1969).

Truman, J. T., Klenow, H.: Effect of 3′-amino-3′-deoxyadenosine on nucleic acid synthesis in Ehrlich ascites tumor cells. Molec. Pharmacol. **4**, 77—86 (1968).

Tyrsted, G., Sartorelli, A. C.: Inhibition of the synthesis of 5-phosphoribosyl-1-pyrophosphate by 3′-deoxyadenosine and structurally related nucleoside analogs. Biochim. biophys. Acta (Amst.) **155**, 619—622 (1968).

Verma, I. M., Meuth, N. L., Bromfeld, E., Manly, K. F., Baltimore, D.: Covalently linked RNA—DNA molecule as initial product of RNA tumour virus DNA polymerase. Nature (Lond.) **233**, 131—134 (1971).

Walton, E., Holly, F. W., Boxer, G. E., Nutt, R. F., Jenkins, S. R.: 3′-Deoxynucleosides. II. Purine 3′-deoxynucleosides. J. med. Chem. **8**, 659—663 (1965).

Walton, E., Nutt, R. F., Jenkins, S. R., Holly, F. W.: 3′-Deoxynucleosides. I. A synthesis of 3′-deoxyadenosine. J. Amer. chem. Soc. **86**, 2952 (1964).

Waqar, M. A., Burgoyne, L. A., Atkinson, M. R.: Deoxyribonucleic acid synthesis in mammalian nuclei. Incorporation of deoxyribonucleotides and chain-terminating nucleotide analogues. Biochem. J. **121**, 803—809 (1971).

Weinberg, R., Penman, S.: Metabolism of small molecular weight monodisperse nuclear RNA. Biochim. biophys. Acta (Amst.) **190**, 10—29 (1969).

Williamson, D. H.: The effect of environmental and genetic factors on the replication of mitochondrial DNA in yeast. Symp. Soc. exp. Biol. **23**, 247—276 (1970).

Williamson, J.: Cordycepin, an antitumour antibiotic with trypanocidal properties. Trans. roy. Soc. trop. Med. Hyg. **60**, 8—9 (1966).

Williamson, J.: The activity of drugs on *Trypanosoma congolense in vitro* at 37 °C. Trans. roy. Soc. trop. Med. Hyg. **63**, 422 (1969).

Williamson, J.: Nucleoside trypanocides and *Trypanosoma congolense*. Trans. roy. Soc. trop. Med. Hyg. **64**, 179 (1970).

Williamson, J.: Further experiments with the nucleoside trypanocide cordycepin. Trans. roy. Soc. trop. Med. Hyg. **66**, 354—355 (1972).

Williamson, J., Rollo, I. M.: Stimulating effect of amino-acids on the survival at 37 °C of *Trypanosoma rhodesiense* in a serum-free synthetic medium. Nature (Lond.) **170**, 376—377 (1952).

Zylber, E. A., Perlman, S., Penman, S.: Mitochondrial RNA turnover in the presence of cordycepin. Biochim. biophys. Acta (Amst.) **240**, 588—593 (1971).

Addendum

The following papers which have appeared after completion of this manuscript are of relevance to the topic described:

Synthesis and Purification:

Jenkins, S. R., Walton, E.: Synthesis of 9-(3-deoxy-3-C-methyl-β-D-xylofuranosyl)adenine: A branched-chain sugar analog of cordycepin. Carbohydrate Res. **26**, 71—81 (1973).

Melling, J., Belton, F. C., Kitching, D., Stones, W. R.: Production of pure cordycepin (3′-deoxyadenosine) from *Cordyceps militaris*. J. Pharm. Pharmacol. **24**, suppl. 125 P (1972).

Nagpal, K. L., Horwitz, J. P.: Nucleosides XIV. Synthesis of 3′-deoxyadenosine and 9-(-3-deoxy-α-L-threopentofuranosyl)adenine. J. org. Chem. **36**, 3743—3745 (1971).

Biochemical Effects:

Abelson, H. T., Penman, S.: Messenger RNA formation: resistance to inhibition by 3′-deoxycytidine. Biochim. biophys. Acta (Amst.) **277**, 129—133 (1972).

BUTCHER, F. R., BUSHNELL, D. E., BECKER, J. E., POTTER, V. R.: Effect of cordycepin on introduction of tyrosine aminotransferase employing hepatoma cells in tissue culture. Exptl. Cell Res. **74**, 115—123 (1972).
CHU, L. L. H., EDELMAN, I. S.: Cordycepin and α-aminitin: Inhibitors of transcription as probes of aldosterone action. J. memb. Biol. **10**, 291—310 (1972).
CORNUDELLA, L., FAIFERMAN, I., POGO, A. O.: Polyadenylic acid sequences in ascites nuclear particles and membrane-bound messenger RNA. Biochim. biophys. Acta (Amst.) **294**, 541—546 (1973).
FIUME, L., NARDI, I., BUCCI, S., MANCINO, G.: Effects of cordycepin on morphology and RNA synthesis of amphibian lampbrush chromosomes. Exptl. Cell Res. **75**, 11—14 (1972).
FRASER, T. H., RICH, A.: Synthesis and aminoacylation of 3′-amino-3′-deoxy transfer RNA and its activity in ribosomal protein synthesis. Proc. nat. Acad. Sci. (Wash.) **70**, 2671—2675 (1973).
FREDERIKSEN, S., PEDERSEN, I. R., HELLUNG-LARSEN, P., ENGBERG, J.: Metabolic studies of small molecular weight nuclear RNA components in BHK-21 cells. Biochim. biophys. Acta (Amst.) **340**, 64—76 (1974).
GIMÉNEZ-MARTIN, G., DE LA TORRE, C., FERNÁNDEZ-GÓMEZ, M. E., GONZÁLES-FERNÁNDEZ, A.: Effect of cordycepin on the nucleolar cycle. Caryologia **25**, 43—58 (1972).
GOPALAN, H. N. B.: Cordycepin inhibits induction of puffs by ions in chironomus salivary gland chromosomes. Experienta **20**, 724—726 (1973).
GRAHN, B., LØVTRUP-REIN, H.: The effect of cordycepin on nuclear RNA synthesis in nerve and glial cells. Acta physiol. Scand. **82**, 28—34 (1971).
GRAYSON, S., BERRY, S. J.: Estimation of the half-life of a secretory protein message. Science **180**, 1071—1072 (1973).
JELINEK, W., ADESNIK, M., SALDITT, M., SHEINESS, D., WALL, R., MOLLOY, G., PHILIPSON, L., DARNELL, J. E.: Further evidence on the nuclear origin and transfer to the cytoplasm of polyadenylic acid sequences in mammalian cell RNA. J. mol. Biol. **75**, 515—532 (1973).
KANN, H. E., JR., KOHN, K. W.: Effect of deoxyribonucleic acid-reactive drugs on ribonucleic acid synthesis in leukemia L1210 cells. Mol. Pharmacol. 8, 551—560 (1972).
MAHY, B. W. J., COX, N. J., ARMSTRONG, S. J., BARRY, R. D.: Multiplication of influenza virus in the presence of cordycepin, an inhibitor of cellular RNA synthesis. Nature (Lond.) **243**, 172—174 (1973).
MENDECKI, J., LEE, S. Y., BRAWERMAN, G.: Characteristics of the polyadenylic acid segment associated with messenger ribonucleic acid in mouse sarcoma 180 ascites cells. Biochemistry **11**, 792—798 (1972).
MOMPARLER, R. L.: Inhibition of cytotoxic action of 1-β-D-arabinofuranosylcytosine on S-phase HeLa cells by 5-fluorodeoxyuridine. Cancer Res. **33**, 1754—1758 (1973).
ODMARK, G.: True or apparent inhibition of nucleic acid synthesis by the chromosome-breaking purine derivatives adenine and 8-ethoxycaffeine. Mutation Res. **14**, 123—126 (1972).
PODOBED, O. V., LEITIN, V. L., BRYKINA, E. V., MANT'EVA, V. L., LERMAN, M. I.: Effect of cordycepin on the synthesis of nuclear and cytoplasmic RNA in the liver and Ehrlich ascites cells of the mouse. Mol. Biol. (Moscow) **7**, 343—352 (1973).
RIZZO, A. J., KELLY, C., WEBB, T. E.: Effect of cordycepin on ribosome formation and enzyme induction in rat liver. Can. J. Biochem. **50**, 1010—1015 (1972).
SLATER, D. W., SLATER, I., GILLESPIE, D.: Post-fertilization synthesis of polyadenylic acid in sea urchin embryos. Nature (Lond.) **240**, 333—337 (1972).
SMUCKLER, E. A., HADJIOLOV, A. A.: Inhibition of hepatic deoxyribonucleic acid-dependent ribonucleic acid polymerases by the exotoxin of *Bacillus thuringiensis* in comparison with the effects of α-amanitin and cordycepin. Biochem. J. **129**, 153—166 (1972).
SPRINZL, M., CRAMER, F.: Accepting site for aminoacylation of $tRNA^{Phe}$ from yeast. Nature (Lond.) **245**, 3—5 (1973).
SPRINZL, M., SCHEIT, K.-H., STERNBACH, H., VON DER HAAR, F., CRAMER, F.: In vitro incorporation of 2′-deoxyadenosine and 3′-deoxyadenosine into yeast $tRNA^{Phe}$ using tRNA nucleotidyl transferase and properties of $tRNA^{Phe}$-C-C-2′-dA and $tRNA^{Phe}$-C-C-3′-dA. Biochem. biophys. Res. Commun. **51**, 881—887 (1973).
STERN, R., TWANMOH, A., COOPER, H. L.: Site of actinomycin-resistant RNA synthesis in animal cells. Exptl. Cell Res. **78**, 136—142 (1973).
WU, A. M., TING, R. C., PARAN, M., GALLO, R. C.: Cordycepin inhibits induction of murine leukovirus production by 5-iodo-2′-deoxyuridine. Proc. natl. Acad. Sci. (Wash.) **69**, 3820—3824 (1972).

Chapter 67

Vinca Alkaloids and Colchicine

WILLIAM A. CREASEY

With 2 Figures

Introduction

The vinca alkaloids and the colchicine derivatives, although of widely disparate chemical structure, may be considered to constitute a single class of agents in view of the many similarities in their biochemical and biological actions, most notably in their ability to produce metaphase arrest. This resemblance extends to certain other unrelated compounds, including griseofulvin and podophyllotoxin.

Colchicine was isolated in the late nineteenth century, although final confirmation of its structure was obtained only in 1950. In the form of various preparations from plants of the genus *Colchicum*, colchicine represents one of the few modalities from the ancient Egyptian materia medica to have survived to the present day. In the *Ebers papyrus*, written about 1500 B.C., the seeds of saffron plants belonging to this genus were recommended to be eaten on bread for relief of acute joint pain; such seeds of *Colchicum autumnale* may contain up to 4 g per kg of colchicine. The use of *Colchicum lingulatum* (Ephemeron) for the treatment of tumors that had not widely metastasized was first described by DIOSCORIDES in the first century A.D.; he considered this preparation safer than that from *Colchicum autumnale*.

The vinca alkaloids, on the other hand, have been available for clinical use for little more than a decade. It is true that the periwinkle plant, *Vinca rosea* Linn., or more correctly *Catharanthus roseus* G. Don, from which the alkaloids are derived, was widely used in herbal medicine for treating gingivitis and diabetes and for arresting bleeding, a use described by CULPEPER in *The Complete Herbal* (1653). There is, however, no sound evidence for the effectiveness of the plant in such applications. Nevertheless, it was during testing of the purported hypoglycemic activity that leukopenic and antineoplastic potential was first noted (BEER, 1955; JOHNSON et al., 1959). In contrast to the high levels of colchicine in its source plants, the vinca alkaloids occur in very low concentrations, one kg of dried periwinkle leaves yielding, for example, only 3 mg of vincristine.

The resin of the may-apple, *Podophyllum peltatum* Linn., was long used as a cathartic and as a remedy for treating warts; more recently it has been employed as a topical cytotoxic agent for condylomata acuminata. From this resin podophyllotoxin was isolated and many derivatives subsequently synthesized. Podophyllotoxin and other compounds of this group have antineoplastic action, but most have proven rather toxic. Griseofulvin, an antifungal agent effective in certain skin infections, is derived from the mold *Penicillium griseofulvum* Dierckx (OXFORD et al., 1939). These two latter compounds will receive mention in this chapter only insofar as studies with them have helped in understanding the actions of colchicine and the vinca alkaloids.

Various aspects of the isolation, chemistry, and early evaluation of the vinca alkaloids as antitumor agents have been rather completely covered in the reviews of JOHNSON et al. (1963) and NEUSS et al. (1964). Colchicine has been the subject of a monograph by EIGSTI and DUSTIN (1955) that provides a large amount of background material. KELLY and HARTWELL (1953) have published a review on podophyllum, while a substantial amount of information regarding griseofulvin may be found in the article by BENT and MOORE (1966). The pharmacology of antimitotic agents in general has been discussed by DUSTIN (1963), SAVEL (1966), SARTORELLI and CREASEY (1969), and CREASEY (in press). It will not be the concern of this chapter to cover the background areas in depth, but rather to concentrate on recent studies that have shed light on the mechanisms of action of this interesting group of drugs. Developments have occurred in two distinct areas, one primarily cytological, but presently reaching to the molecular level, and the other purely biochemical.

Basic Considerations

A. Chemical Nature and Structure-Activity Relationships

I. Vinca Alkaloids

The vinca alkaloids possess a basic structure comprising an indole and a dihydroindole nucleus linked together in complex relationship with other ring systems (Fig. 1). The term dimeric has been applied to this structure, although the two portions of the molecule are not identical. Of the large number of compounds occurring in the periwinkle plant that are based on this structure or its component parts, only four have been found to inhibit the growth of tumors. These are vinblastine, vincristine, vinleurosine, and vinrosidine; of these, only the first two have proven clinical value; the others are rather more toxic and unpredictable in effect. The sulfate salt is the commonest form in which these agents are available, but vinleurosine has been employed as the methiodide which was more active against experimental mouse tumors. In addition to these natural alkaloids, a number of semisynthetic compounds have been prepared, of which two, dihydrovinblastine and vinglycinate, appear to have potential. Certain features of the alkaloids with antitumor activity cannot be modified without loss of activity:

1. Change of the basic indole nitrogen in the catharanthine structure, as by amide formation, so as to reduce the compounds to only one pK value from the normal two, leads to total loss of activity. Many of the naturally occurring alkaloids such as catharine, neoleurocristine, and neorosidine exhibit this change.

2. All of the naturally occurring active alkaloids possess an acetyl group at *C*-4 of the vindoline moiety. Removal of this group from vinblastine yields 4-desacetyl vinblastine, which is inactive. However, the substituent group need not be acetyl; a wide variety of 4-acyl and 4-aminoacetyl functions can be substituted to give compounds of varying activity (JOHNSON et al., 1966). One of the most active of these derivatives is the 4-dimethylamino acetyl derivative of desacetylvinblastine, vinglycinate, which has reached clinical trial.

3. Acetylation of the free hydroxyl functions of vinblastine yields the corresponding acetates, which are inactive.

4. Reduction of vinblastine or vinleurosine with $LiAlH_4$ to the stage of the carbinols causes complete loss of activity. However, reduction of only the double bond between C-6 and C-7 does not completely destroy the activity, but instead

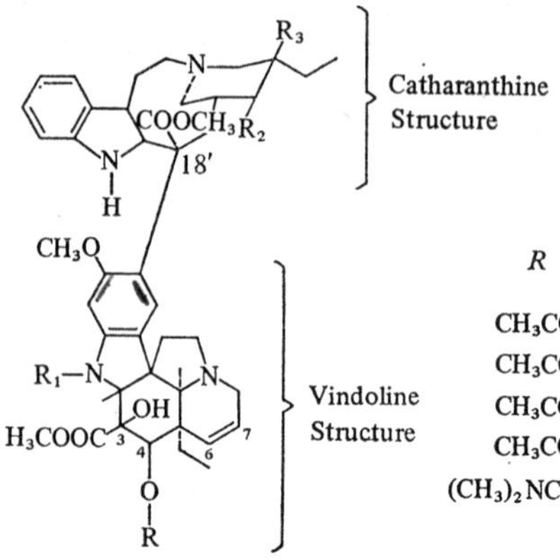

Catharanthine Structure / Vindoline Structure

R	R_1	R_2	R_3	Name
CH_3CO	CHO	H	OH	Vincristine
CH_3CO	CH_3	H	OH	Vinblastine
CH_3CO	CH_3	OH	H	Vinrosidine
CH_3CO	CH_3	H		Vinleurosine
$(CH_3)_2NCH_2CO$	CH_3	H	OH	Vinglycinate

R_1	R_2	Name
$COCH_3$	OCH_3	Colchicine
CH_3	OCH_3	Colcemid
H	OCH_3	Deacetylamino-Colchicine
$COCH_3$	$NHCH_2CH_2N<$	Colchicinamide Derivatives

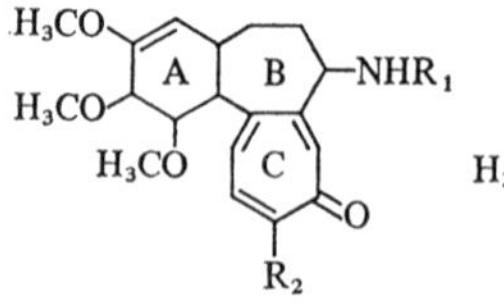

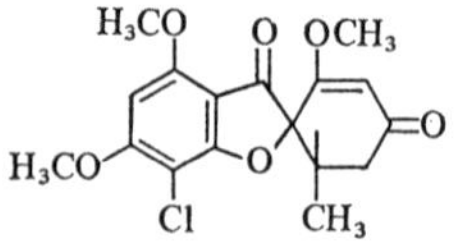

Griseofulvin

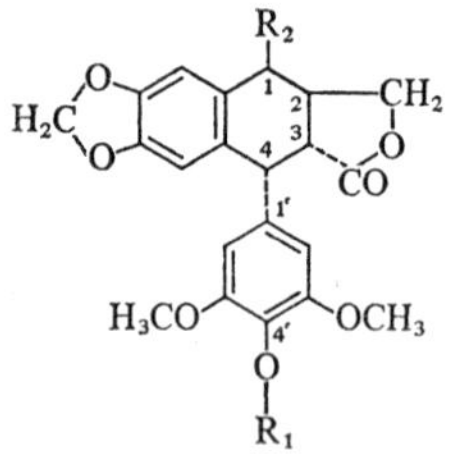

R_1	R_2	2, 3, 4 Positions	Name
CH_3	---OH	As shown	Podophyllotoxin
CH_3	---OH	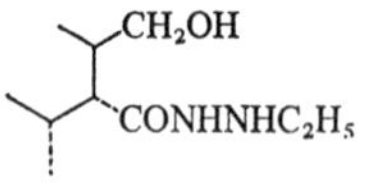 CH_2OH, $CONHNHC_2H_5$	Podophyllic Acid Ethyl Hydrazide
H	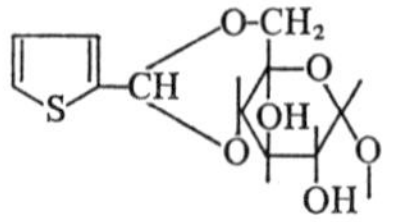	As shown	VM-26

Fig. 1. Structural formulas of antimitotic agents

gives a less potent derivative, dihydrovinblastine, with some differences from the parent alkaloid in both toxicity and dose-response relationships (NOBLE et al., 1967).

MONCRIEF and HELLER (1967) have suggested that the $-COOCH_3$ groups at positions 3 and 18′ enable the vinca alkaloids to function as biological acylating agents. While such activity can be demonstrated in chemical systems it has not yet been shown to occur *in vivo*.

II. Colchicine Derivatives

Colchicine is a tropolone derivative containing three rings (Fig. 1). Several derivatives of colchicine have been prepared, of which the most useful clinically is deacetyl-*N*-methylcolchicine or colcemid (demecolcine), which is now more extensively used than the parent compound. Structure-activity relations have been rather extensively studied; EIGSTI and DUSTIN (1955) and DUSTIN (1963) have summarized many of the findings, which are for the most part based on assay of the ability to produce mitotic arrest. Three main points may be noted:

1. Ring A should possess at least one methoxy group for the compound to retain activity.
2. It is necessary that ring C be 7-membered.
3. A substituent on ring C is necessary, but considerable latitude exists as to the substituting group, which may be methoxy, an esterified amino group, or sulfhydryl with or without substituents. DA RE et al. (1966) synthesized several basic colchicinamides, including the dimethylaminoethylamine and morpholinoethylamine derivatives that proved considerably more active than colchicine itself.

Substitution of the B ring does not appear to be critical, since removal of the *N*-acetyl group to yield the free amino function gives a more active compound, deacetylamino colchicine. The retention of activity on removal of this acetyl group contrasts with the situation for the vinca alkaloids in which such a group is essential for activity.

III. Podophyllotoxin and Griseofulvin

The structural features of these compounds and some derivatives appear in Fig. 1. Among the more recent podophyllin derivatives are podophyllic acid ethyl hydrazide, which has undergone clinical trial in the treatment of cancer (VAITKEVICIUS and REED, 1966), and 4'-demethylepipodophyllotoxin thenylidene glucoside (VM-26). Griseofulvin has not been employed for treating neoplastic disease.

B. Biological Activity

I. Mitotic Arrest

The most characteristic action of all these agents is the arrest of cell division in metaphase, first observed with colchicine by LITS (1934). VM-26, the podophyllin derivative, is exceptional in that a preprophase action predominates over mitotic arrest (STÄHELIN, 1970). The duration and extent of mitotic arrest produced by these antimitotic agents have been compared by many laboratories. Among these studies might be mentioned those of PALMER et al. (1963) and CARDINALI et al. (1961). Vinblastine has generally proved to be the most active compound, while vincristine appears to possess a degree of irreversibility that distinguishes it from the other agents (GEORGE et al., 1965; JOURNEY et al., 1968). Mitotic arrest is not, however, a simple fixation of the mitotic apparatus in the metaphase configuration. Rather, the action consists in an attack on the spindle structure itself leading to its dissolution; chromosome damage and breakage, in so far as it occurs, is a secondary effect (SENTEIN, 1964). In the absence of a complete spindle the chromosomes may be dispersed throughout the cytoplasm (exploded mitosis) or adopt various unusual groupings (ball, star mitoses).

Provided that exposure to the drug has not been too prolonged, a large proportion of the arrested cells are able to resume mitotic activity on removal of the agent. KRISHAN (1968) has described the reversal of mitotic arrest in Earle's L cells exposed to vinblastine. In this example, many metaphase-blocked and multimicronucleate cells resumed division within 4 h after removal of the alkaloid, although the subsequent incidence of abnormal configurations during mitosis was rather high. A particularly elegant demonstration of the reversibility of spindle dissolution has been provided by Malawista et al. (1968) using the oöcytes of the marine annelid *Pectinaria gouldi*. Vinblastine, colcemid, and griseofulvin produced rapid attrition and disappearance of the spindle within minutes, followed by rapid reappearance on washing away the drugs with sea water; this cycle could be repeated almost indefinitely. With vincristine and podophyllotoxin, recovery was incomplete however, a finding that recalls the data of Journey et al. (1968) obtained with cultures of HeLa cells and Chinese hamster fibroblasts exposed to vincristine. Reversible mitotic arrest by colchicine, colcemid, and vinblastine has come to be widely employed as a method for obtaining synchronous cell populations (Kim and Stambuk, 1966; Pfeiffer and Tolmach, 1967). In addition, the rate of accumulation of mitotic figures, especially ones that have incorporated radiolabeled thymidine into DNA, is a useful method for studying cell kinetics. Kinetic data obtained by this method should be interpreted with caution, however, as there have been conflicting reports as to effects of these agents on nonmitotic stages of the cell cycle. Bruchovsky et al. (1965), using vinblastine as an inhibitor of the proliferation of L cells in partial synchrony, could find no evidence of retardation other than during mitosis. On the other hand, in grasshopper neuroblast cultures exposed to colchicine (Mueller et al., 1971), and L1210 cells removed from mice treated with vinca alkaloids (Cardinali et al., 1968), there appeared to be a reduction in rate of entry into prophase. This could relate to the report of Madoc-Jones and Mauro (1968) that in HeLa and Chinese hamster cells, in the presence of somewhat higher concentrations of vinblastine than are normally required to arrest mitosis, both the later G_1 and S phases showed enhanced sensitivity to drug. Some of the conflicting data could arise from factors such as a marked dependence on the position in the cell cycle at which drug exposure occurs, as has been demonstrated in synchronized cultures of *Tetrahymena pyriformis* (Wunderlich and Peyk, 1969) treated with colchicine. On the other hand, this data could reflect a very low level of activity, by colchicine and the vinca alkaloids, of the same preprophase type as that which is predominant for VM-26 (Stähelin, 1970).

A final aspect of mitotic arrest concerns its modification by other agents. Marsland (1968), studying the first cleavage division of the fertile eggs of the echinoderm *Lytechinus variegatus*, noted that reducing the temperature from 25° to 15°, or applying high pressure, potentiated the antimitotic effect of colchicine; similar effects have been seen in other systems. In contrast, several authors have claimed an antagonism between colchicine or colcemid and cortisone, an example described by De Harven and Dustin (1956) being the mitotic activity of rat bone marrow eosinophils. Division of these cells did not seem to be greatly affected by colcemid in normal animals, but in adrenalectomized rats, mitotic arrest was pronounced unless cortisone was administered. A similar antagonism was discussed by Dustin (1963) for Ehrlich ascites carcinoma growing in mice that received injections of cortisone and vinblastine. Although these data are suggestive of a simple antagonism, De Harven (1956) has raised the possibility that in fact cortisone acts by facilitating the recovery of the damaged spindle. Another hormonal antagonism described by Cutts (1968) is the finding that diethylstilbestrol protected rats from vinblastine toxicity. Among other compounds that have been found to reduce the degree of mitotic arrest are ATP, which may actually act as a nonspecific inhibitor of cell division (see Dustin, 1963), tryptophan, and glutamic acid (Cutts, 1961). The two latter compounds brought about a reduction in the percentage of arrested mitoses in Ehrlich ascites tumor seen after treatment with vinblastine. This effect, which resulted from a less complete degree of mitotic arrest, since cells were proceeding into post-metaphase stages, was temporary in that after 24 h there was no difference between the cell populations exposed to vinblastine alone, and those treated with the alkaloid plus the antagonists. In the case of glutamic acid, recent data published by CREASEY et al. (1971) indicate that this amino acid acts as a competitive inhibitor of the uptake of tritiated vinblastine by human leukocyte preparations. If this applies to other cells, it affords an explanation for the ability of glutamic acid to antagonize the antimitotic effects of vinblastine.

II. Antitumor Effects

Colchicine, colcemid, the vinca alkaloids, and the podophyllotoxin derivatives all inhibit the growth of various experimental tumors. JOHNSON et al. (1963) have listed the tumors responsive to the vinca alkaloids; EIGSTI and DUSTIN (1955) and LUDFORD (1945) have described some findings of antitumor activity by colchicine, while STÄHELIN and CERLETTI (1964) found 5 tumors that were sensitive to podophyllotoxin derivatives.

III. Anti-Inflammatory Action

The traditional use of the colchicine derivatives is in the treatment of acute episodes of gouty arthritis. Although able to effect rapid relief of pain in this disease, these drugs are generally only weak anti-inflammatory agents without clinical value in most other inflammatory disorders. MALAWISTA (1968a) has discussed aspects of this activity and reviewed evidence that it results from an underlying mechanism of action common to mitotic arrest. This is compatible with the fact that other antimitotic agents such as vinblastine (KRAKOFF, 1965) and griseofulvin (SLONIM et al., 1962) are also effective in treating gout. We will return to this topic in connection with the microtubule interactions discussed below.

VI. Other Biological Effects

Neurological toxicity may be produced by any of the colchicine-vinca alkaloid family of agents and is especially characteristic of vincristine. Colchicine modifies the process of axon-sprouting in denervated muscles by a nonmitotic mechanism (HOFFMAN, 1952), and when locally infused into the sciatic nerve of the mouse produces axonal degeneration and demyelination (ANGEVINE, 1957). Inhibition of axonal transport of protein has also been reported (KARLSSON and SJÖSTRAND, 1969). Vinblastine causes a retraction of terminal expansion and of the undulating membrane of spinal ganglion neurons in culture (BARASA et al., 1970). In the case of vincristine, neurological toxicity is the dose-limiting factor. In mice, administration of vincristine leads to degeneration of dorsal root cells and the myelin sheath, and inhibition of Schwann cell proliferation (UY et al., 1967). Interference with deep tendon reflexes, noted during vincristine therapy, may be the result of depression of muscle spindle function (TOBIN and SANDLER, 1966). In rats this drug may produce degenerative changes in the motor end plates (ANDERSON et al., 1967).

Among the miscellaneous biological effects produced by these agents are changes in movement and cytological appearance of mast cells, including displacement of the cell nucleus and anisodiametry of the cytoplasm (PADAWER 1963, 1966). Possibly related to this is the ability of colchicine to inhibit motility (MALAWISTA, 1968b) and chemotactic response (CANER, 1965) of human polymorphonuclear leukocytes and also to interfere with lysosomal degranulation and formation of digestive vacuoles during phagocytosis by these cells (MALAWISTA, 1968a); these effects may be components of the anti-inflammatory action of this drug. As might be anticipated for compounds with the ability to interfere with cell division and growth, the vinca alkaloids have been shown to be teratogenic in rats (COHLAN and

Kitay, 1965) and hamsters (Ferm, 1963); in the latter animals colchicine produced similar effects. Among the deformities observed were exencephaly, microphthalmia, anophthalmia, spina bifida, rib fusions, and gastroschisis. Finally, in rats, vinblastine and vincristine suppressed both the formation of antibodies to serum albumin, as measured by the tanned sheep cell hemagglutination technique, and delayed hypersensitivity (Aisenberg, 1963).

C. Microtubule Interaction

With the introduction of glutaraldehyde as a fixative for electron microscopy, it became possible to visualize many more structural details of cells. Among one of the most ubiquitous elements found by the improved techniques are microtubules. These structures, with diameters of about 250 Å, and often many microns in length, appear to be derived from fibrillar subunits (Ledbetter and Porter, 1964). Microtubules are especially abundant in neuronal processes (Gonatas and Robbins, 1965), the cortical cytoplasm and cellular microspikes (Taylor, 1966), and flagella and cilia of both plants (Manton, 1959; Rice and Laetsch, 1967) and animals (Afzelius, 1959). In cilia these microtubules are arranged in a characteristic 9 + 2 pattern (Fig. 2). The mitotic spindle is itself at least partially composed of aggregated and organized microtubules (Harris, 1962); the remainder may constitute a contractile actomyosin system of which the actin portion has been identified (Gawadi, 1971; Behnke et al., 1971). Among the many cells in which these structures have been demonstrated are human leukocytes (Malawista and Bensch, 1967), *Coleus* cells (Newcomb and Hepler, 1964), crane fly spermatids (Behnke and Forer, 1967), and the cells around the bordered pits of angiosperms (Robards and Humpherson, 1967). Much recent work with cytoplasmic filaments and microtubules has been summarized by Adelmann et al. (1968) in an excellent review. These organelles seem to be associated with regions of the cell that are involved in motion or in stabilization of cellular structure (Porter, 1966; Adelmann, 1968), although they themselves cannot be regarded as motile elements. The relationship of the microtubules to the smaller microfilaments of diameter 30 to 40 Å is unclear. It has been considered that the latter are components of the microtubules, but more probably they are alternative structures composed of the same subunits. This is certainly suggested by the data from studies with *Ameba* (Morgan, 1971). Figure 2 presents in schematic form some of the concepts of microtubule interrelationships.

A well authenticated effect of the antimitotic agents is the disappearance of microtubules from treated cells. This has been observed in HeLa cells (Robbins and Gonatas, 1964), the heliozoan *Actinosphaerium nucleophilum* (Tilney, 1965), human leukocytes (Malawista and Bensch, 1967), and blood platelets (Sneddon, 1971). In *Tetrahymena*, adaptation to colchicine is accompanied by the reassembly in the macronuclei of microtubules initially disorganized by drug (Wunderlich and Speth, 1970). Dissolution of microtubules leads to secondary effects such as inhibition of regeneration of protozoan cilia (Rosenbaum and Carlson, 1969) and reduction of certain types of cell motility, such as saltatory movements, but not ameboid motion (Freed et al., 1968; Spooner et al., 1971), which seems to be a function of the microfilament system. These changes in intracellular and cellular motility could underlie the changes in activity of phagocytes in joints that lead to relief of the pain of gouty arthritis.

Another type of interaction between antimitotic drugs and the microtubule system involves only the vinca alkaloids and not colchicine; this is the formation of cytoplasmic inclusion bodies described as microtubule crystals. In L-strain fibroblasts and human leukocytes, vinca alkaloids cause the appearance of uniaxial birefringent crystals, with sides as long as 8 μ, which consist of regular aggregates of microtubular bodies sharing their walls in common in a hexagonal arrangement; these tubules are somewhat larger in diameter than normal microtubules (BENSCH

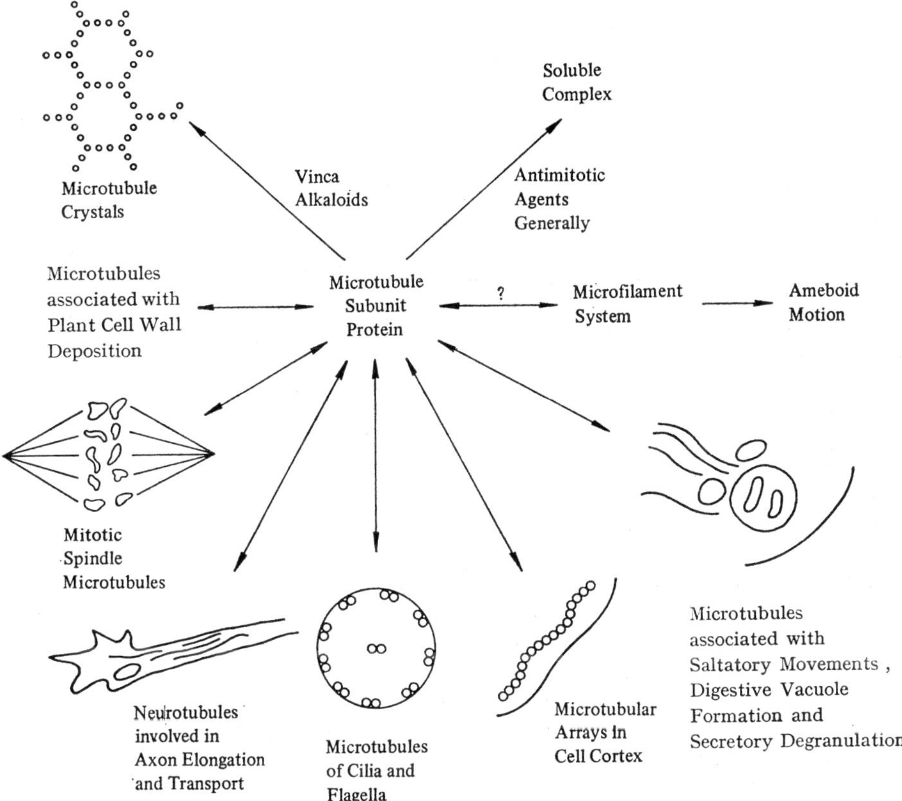

Fig. 2. The microtubule system: possible interrelationships and the displacements produced by antimitotic agents. It is probable that the system is in dynamic equilibrium between subunit protein and microtubule-containing structures. Antimitotic agents would tend to deplete the pool of subunits leading to dissolution of the organized tubules

and MALAWISTA, 1969; MARANTZ and SHELANSKI, 1970). Rather similar pseudo-crystalline aggregates have been reported in starfish oöcytes (MALAWISTA and SATO, 1969) exposed to vinblastine, and in human (SCHOCHET et al., 1968) and rabbit neurons (KOTORII et al., 1971) after intrathecal or intracisternal administration of vincristine. Inclusions of a noncrystalline nature have been described in platelets after treatment with colchicine or the vinca alkaloids (WHITE, 1968), but these may be of a different nature.

While these investigations were continuing, isotopically labeled colchicine and vinblastine became available for use in studying these interactions in more detail. The most extensive of these studies has been undertaken in the laboratory of TAYLOR in Chicago using tritiated colchicine (TAYLOR, 1965; BORISY and TAYLOR, 1967a, b; SHELANSKI and TAYLOR, 1967; WEISENBERG et al., 1968). A protein in the supernatant fraction obtained by high speed centrifugation of cell homogenates was able to bind colchicine noncovalently. This protein, which had a sedimentation coefficient of 6 S, was widely distributed among different cells, but was present in larger amounts in dividing cells, the mitotic apparatus, cilia, sperm tails, and brain tissue, precisely where concentration of microtubules occurs. Wilson and Friedkin (1967) identified a similar binding protein of molecular weight 105,000 in grasshopper embryos. Binding of tritiated colchicine was a time and temperature dependent process. The complex was destroyed by urea, and its formation was inhibited by podophyllotoxin and stimulated by vinblastine. Creasey and his coworkers (Creasey, 1967, in press; Creasey and Chou, 1968; Creasey et al., 1969, 1971) have studied the binding of tritiated colchicine, griseofulvin, and vinblastine by Sarcoma 180 cells and by human normal and leukemic leukocytes. A similar soluble binding protein occurs in these cells, and apparently interacts differently with labeled colchicine and vinblastine. The linkage with colchicine is sensitive to urea, but not to high salt concentrations, whereas the opposite relation holds for the complex with vinblastine. Vinca alkaloids increase the amount of labeled colchicine that is bound, and colchicine and griseofulvin affect vinblastine binding similarly. As further evidence for a generalized binding of antimitotic agents, Georgatsos et al. (1968) have found that soluble proteins in mouse mammary tumors bind tritiated podophyllic acid ethyl hydrazide in a similar fashion.

Colchicine binding protein has been isolated from several sources, including the sperm tails of the sea urchin *Strongylocentrotus purpuratus* (Shelanski and Taylor, 1967), porcine brain (Weisenberg et al., 1968), human blood platelets (Puszkin et al., 1971), and chick embryo brain (Wilson, 1970). Many of the properties of these proteins have been described, but the actual sites at which interaction occurs have yet to be identified. It would appear that the stimulations and inhibitions of binding produced by various antimitotics result from the presence of sites of different specificity. Binding at two or more sites leads to stabilization of the protein, while agents that bind to the same site will presumably compete. Evidence suggests that two sites per molecule of protein are normally occupied by guanosine triphosphate (Weisenberg and Taylor, 1968; Weisenberg et al., 1968; Bryan, 1972). The type of interaction involved in the case of the vinca alkaloids is presumably ionic or at least sensitive to high ionic strength. The heterodimer contains one such site. On the other hand, colchicine, griseofulvin, and podophyllotoxin may interact at the other site (one per molecule) at which binding is urea sensitive. It is of interest that the association to form a complex occurs *in vitro* with both purified protein and crude cell supernatant, and in the case of the vinca alkaloids may lead to the formation of aggregates somewhat resembling the crystals formed *in vivo* (Marantz et al., 1969; Bensch et al., 1969; Weisenberg and Timasheff, 1969; Marantz and Shelanski, 1970; Olmsted et al., 1970). However, it should be noted that vinblastine is able to cause other types of aggregation, as for example of ribosomes (Krishan, 1970) and erythrocyte membrane proteins (Wilson et al., 1970), so that the aggregates of colchicine binding protein are likely to contain other components. Under appropriate conditions of ionic strength, microtubule subunit protein from the sperm tails of *Arbacia punctulata* will aggregate spontaneously to reform microtubules (Stephens, 1968); this presumably reflects a normal process of association occurring *in vivo*.

Experiments with the intracellular microtubule crystals, in which labeled alkaloids are employed, suggest not only that vinblastine forms an integral part of the crystals it induces, but also that colchicine binding sites remain free. Thus in radioautographs of starfish oöcytes exposed to tritiated vinblastine there is an apparent concentration of grains over the crystals (Malawista et al., 1969), while autoradiographic studies of mammalian cells in culture show that crystals induced by vincristine may contain bound tritiated colchicine (KRISHAN and HSU, 1971).

Thus, it is reasonable to suggest that microtubule interactions can go far toward explaining most of the biological actions of the antimitotic agents. Dissolution of the spindle, interference with some phases of phagocytosis, changes in morphology and motility, and neurologic effects might all be reasonably expected to result from displacements in the equilibria governing the microtubule system. Such displacements would naturally follow binding of microtubules or their subunit proteins by drugs, or their aggregation into abnormal crystalline structures.

D. Biochemical Effects

The antimitotic agents were in clinical use before significant knowledge of their biochemical actions was available; their cytotoxic action was thus ascribed to mitotic arrest. A reversible phenomenon, as is mitotic arrest, may not be adequate, however, as a sole basis for potent cytotoxic action, especially as one study by FREI et al. (1964) with the vinca alkaloids failed to disclose any correlation between cytotoxicity and metaphase arrest in human and rat bone marrow. Among the earliest biochemical findings concerning these agents was the partial protection afforded by certain amino acids, including glutamic acid, against the mitotic and cytotoxic effects of the vinca alkaloids (CUTTS, 1961, 1964). This effect has been mentioned previously, and is most probably a reflection of competition for transport into cells rather than an indication of possible sites of action. The development of various biochemical studies may best be described under the headings of the major metabolic areas.

I. Nucleic Acid Biosynthesis

Perhaps the earliest observation in this area was made by McGEER and McGEER (1963), who found that after administration of vinblastine to rats there was a reduction in the urinary excretion of 4(5)-amino-5(4)-imidazolecarboxamide, possibly indicative of interference with purine nucleotide biosynthesis *de novo*. Although later experiments have suggested that vinblastine produces a greater inhibition of the synthesis of DNA purines than of pyrimidine bases in rat thymus cells (JONES et al., 1966), no definitive studies on purine nucleotide biosynthesis after treatment with the alkaloid have been made.

The earliest attempts to screen for inhibitory action of the vinca alkaloids on the biosynthesis of nucleic acids generally resulted in negative results (JOHNSON et al., 1963), in agreement with the earlier findings of BEER (1961) who reported only DNA synthesis in marrow to be affected. Subsequent studies, however, have implicated inhibition of the synthesis of these macromolecules as major effects of all the antimitotic drugs. The cytological study of SUGÁR (1963) established, with the help of polarizing and flourescence microscopy, that treatment of tumor cells with vinblastine reduced the amount of nucleic acid. At about the same time it was found that colchicine, and to a much lesser extent colcemid, inhibit the incorporation of thymidine into DNA by isolated pieces of skin from guinea pig ears (HELL and COX, 1963). Colchicine also affected DNA synthesis by several normal mammalian tissues *in vivo* and by the pupas of *Tenebrio molitor* (ILAN and QUASTEL, 1966). RICHARDS et al. (1966) compared the activity of the four naturally occurring vinca alkaloids on the incorporation of labeled formate into nucleic acids by suspensions of isolated rat thymus cells. Vinblastine was the most active and vinrosidine the least active inhibitor in this system, in contrast to findings with Ehrlich ascites cells in which very high levels of vinblastine were required to inhibit thymidine incorporation *in vitro*, and no effect was seen *in vivo* (CREASEY and MARKIW, 1964a). However, at least *in vivo*, DNA synthesis in the Ehrlich tumor was sensitive to vincristine and colchicine (CREASEY, 1968a). When rats were treated with vinblastine and the incorporation of tritiated thymidine into DNA studied in the spleen and bone marrow (VAN LANCKER et al., 1966) and regenerating liver (LUYCKX and VAN LANCKER, 1966), marked depression of DNA synthesis was evident. The period of minimum synthesis extended from 12 to 48 h in the spleen and marrow; effects on RNA synthesis were minimal. A similar finding of marked inhibition of DNA biosynthesis with only small changes in the incorporation of uridine into RNA was reported by SLOTNICK et al. (1966) for the protozoan *Tetrahymena pyriformis* treated with vincristine. These workers found that the inhibitory effect was prevented by riboflavin, flavin mononucleotide, and flavin adenine dinucleotide. It would appear, however, that these antagonists act by catalyzing the photochemical inactivation of vincristine (HAKALA, 1969). DESJARDINS et al. (1967), examining the effects of uracil mustard, actinomycin D, and vinblastine on the incorporation of thymidine into tumor DNA of rats bearing the Walker tumor, found that in contrast to the other agents, the vinca alkaloid showed a specificity for nucleolar DNA whose synthesis was suppressed to a greater extent than that of extranucleolar material.

In contrast to these reports, other workers have described changes in RNA biosynthesis as being more prominent. Thus, LOVE (1964) found a reduction of cytoplasmic RNA, with an apparent accumulation of nucleolar ribonucleoprotein, in Ehrlich ascites cells treated with colchicine *in situ*. In rats treated with vinblastine, there was a reduction in RNA and ribonuclease of both the thymus and lymphosarcoma P1798 at 4 and 22 h after treatment; levels of DNA either remained unchanged or rose somewhat (WIERNIK and MCLEOD, 1965). Our own studies with mice bearing Ehrlich ascites carcinoma showed that vinblastine produced a time-dependent reduction of the incorporation of tritiated uridine into total phenol-extractable RNA. Synthetic rates reached a minimum at 6 h and did not recover for 18 to 24 h; the soluble or transfer component of the RNA appeared to be most sensitive to the alkaloid (CREASEY and MARKIW, 1964a). This apparent sensitivity of transfer RNA may be an artifact, however, since WAGNER and ROIZMAN (1968) have found that in HEp-2 cells, there is an additional component, separable from transfer RNA only by acrylamide gel electrophoresis, whose synthesis was extremely sensitive to vinblastine. Such a component would not have been separated from RNA in our studies. Although we did not find the synthesis of DNA by Ehrlich ascites cells to be sensitive to vinblastine, in Sarcoma 180, a tumor which in many respects resembles the Ehrlich carcinoma, both RNA and DNA synthesis were inhibited (CREASEY, in press). Colchicine and vincristine seemed much less selective than vinblastine in that their inhibitory action on RNA synthesis by Ehrlich ascites carcinoma extended to all RNA subfractions (CREASEY and MARKIW, 1964b). In this latter study, pretreatment with large doses of glutamic acid reduced the inhibition of RNA synthesis produced by the alkaloids. Inhibition of incorporation of uridine into RNA by suspensions of ascites cells required rather prolonged preincubation, at least one hour in our experiments. Vinblastine was more active in this system than vincristine or colchicine (CREASEY and MARKIW, 1965). In contrast to normal human leukocytes, in which incorporation of uridine into RNA is not affected by antimitotic agents until levels of about 2×10^{-4} M are attained (CREASEY et al., 1971), incorporation of precursors into both RNA and DNA by leukemic leukocytes is inhibited at concentrations at least fivefold lower (CREASEY, 1968a). CLINE (1968) has found that human acute lymphoblastic leukemic leukocytes, clinically very sensitive to vincristine, when incubated for periods of up to 24 h with this drug, may show inhibition of RNA synthesis at levels as low as 7×10^{-9} M. In one clinical study, with acute granulocytic leukemia, attempts were made to correlate enzyme activities with incorporation of precursors into nucleic acids during treatment with vincristine. Levels of thymidylate synthetase and dihydrofolic reductase, and incorporation of thymidine into DNA, were well correlated, showing an initial rise and then a depression at 24 and 48 h; thymidine and uridine kinases correlated with each other, but not with the other parameters (ROBERTS et al., 1969). The pronounced neurological toxicity of vincristine has been found to be associated with marked reduction of the incorporation of intracranially administered uridine into mouse brain (AGUSTIN and CREASEY, 1967). It cannot be said, however, that this is the definitive mechanism of such toxicity, especially in view of the microtubular and other forms of damage induced in the nervous system by vincristine (SHELANSKI and WISNIEWSKI, 1968).

Of the podophyllin derivatives, VM-26 has been found to be most active as an inhibitor of DNA synthesis in P-815 cells in culture (STÄHELIN, 1970), but podophyllic acid ethyl hydrazide also has activity in this respect, since, when administered to mice it inhibited the incorporation of precursors into the nucleic acids of mammary tumors (GEORGATSOS and KAREMFYLLIS, 1968). Griseofulvin caused substantial inhibition of the incorporation of ^{14}C-labeled uridine and thymidine into the nucleic acids of *Microsporum gypseum* (EL-NAKEEB et al., 1965).

Solid evidence regarding the mechanisms involved in these inhibitory actions is, unfortunately rather scanty, so that there is need for further work in this area. It has been found that indirect mediation of these effects through release of adrenal steroids as a result of treatment with vinblastine is unlikely (CHUNG and GABOUREL, 1968). Another change induced by vinca alkaloids, which could relate to inhibition of nucleic acid biosynthesis, is a reduction in transport of uridine into cells. This cannot be a general phenomenon for all nucleosides, however, since the uptake of deoxycytidine is not affected (CREASEY, 1968a, 1969). Thus, direct inhibition of the polymerase system, or effects on the template, remain as viable possibilities. Although direct inhibition of RNA nucleotidyl transferase by vincristine has been reported (CLINE, 1968; CREASEY, 1968b), the drug levels required were rather high and the effects not highly reproducible. In regard to drug interaction with templates, GEORGATSOS et al. (1968) produced data consistent with a weak binding of podophyllic acid ethyl hydrazide by nucleic acids. Interestingly enough, ILAN and QUASTEL (1966) reported changes in the optical rotation of solutions of colchicine and DNA on being mixed, suggestive of an interaction between them, while EL NAKEEB and LAMPEN (1964), using various techniques including gel filtration, found that labeled griseofulvin was bound by the RNA of sensitive, but not resistant fungi. Thus, association of these drugs with nucleic acids presents itself, by analogy with the antitumor antibiotics, as a possible mechanism for inhibition of nucleic acid biosynthesis.

An interesting footnote to this discussion of the inhibition of nucleic acid biosynthesis by antimitotic agents, is the report that in dense cultures of mouse embryo fibroblasts, in which proliferation and DNA synthesis had been inhibited by cell surface changes, low levels (0.05 to 0.4 μg/ml) of colcemid, colchicine, or vinblastine initiate the incorporation of thymidine into DNA (VASILIEV et al., 1971). The mechanism of this effect is at present unclear.

II. Protein Biosynthesis

Effects of this type on the synthesis of nucleic acids would be expected to lead to interference with the fabrication of protein. Such inhibitory effects have been reported to occur in Ehrlich ascites carcinoma cells (Creasey and Markiw, 1964b, 1965) and in human leukemic leukocytes (Cline, 1968) at concentrations that produce a similar degree of suppression of RNA synthesis. However, the situation may not be as simple as it first appears. Warnecke and Seeber (1968) described protein biosynthesis as being the parameter in leukemic lymphocytes most sensitive to vinblastine and vincristine. Similarly, in our own laboratory, inhibition of the incorporation of valine into protein by normal human leukocytes occurs at concentrations of vinca alkaloids that do not affect RNA biosynthesis, indicating that the effect is not mediated through the latter action (Creasey et al., 1971). One factor possibly involved in such an effect is the change in uptake of glutamic acid, but not of glycine, by Ehrlich ascites cells inhibited by vinblastine, and we have subsequently extended such studies to normal human leukocytes in which vinblastine and glutamic acid exhibit competition for uptake by the cells (Creasey et al., 1971). In recent unpublished data we have found three patterns for the effect of vinblastine on transport of amino acids by leukocytes. The uptake of amino acids such as glutamic acid is more sensitive to drug than is the subsequent incorporation into protein. Valine presents a pattern of equivalent effects on the two processes, while with lysine, protein synthesis is more sensitive to the drug than is the transport of this amino acid. Thus, neither inhibition of uptake of amino acids, nor suppression of protein synthesis, can each by itself explain these results. It is evident that more work needs to be done in order to arrive at a satisfactory explanation for these findings.

III. Lipid Metabolism

Evidence for effects of vinca alkaloids and colchicine on lipid metabolism, although not abundant, is sufficiently convincing. Neurological toxicity from both colchicine (Angevine, 1957) and vincristine (Adamson et al., 1965; Uy et al., 1967; Gottschalk et al., 1968) is characteristically accompanied by degeneration of the myelin sheath which is rich in phospholipids. Again, an indirect indication of lipid involvement might be the cross-resistance between vincristine and the phthalanilides (Kensler, 1963), which are known to form complexes with lipids (Yesair et al., 1966); it should be realized, however, that this is not indicative of an identical interaction with lipids; other processes such as a common transport mechanism could be responsible. In studies of the turnover of labeled phosphate in rat gastrocnemius muscle, vincristine depressed the synthesis of phospholipids without affecting the metabolism of organic acid-soluble phosphates (Graff et al., 1967). Vinleurosine, both *in vivo* and *in vitro*, specifically inhibited the synthesis of phospholipids in Sarcoma 180 ascites cells (Creasey, 1969). A similar specific effect on phospholipids was seen with vincristine; these effects were obtained at lower drug levels than those that inhibited nucleic acid synthesis (Creasey, in press).

IV. Miscellaneous Biochemical Effects

Changes in the areas of respiration and carbohydrate metabolism were among the earliest effects ascribed to vinblastine and vincristine. Such effects included modifications in lactic acid production and suppression of the Pasteur effect (Johnson et al., 1963; Hunter, 1963). Obrecht and Fusenig (1966) found that vinblastine inhibited anaerobic glycolysis in the Jensen sarcoma, Yoshida ascites cells, hepatoma AH 130, and jejunal mucosa cells; nicotinamide was able to abolish this effect temporarily. Both colchicine and vinblastine suppress the burst of elevated respiration and glucose oxidation that accompanies phagocytosis by human polymorphonuclear leukocytes (GOLDFINGER et al., 1965; MALAWISTA, 1968). It should be borne in mind, however, that all of these changes could be secondary in nature, and not indicative of basic mechanisms of action, especially since similar effects have been attributed to a number of unrelated chemotherapeutic agents (KATCHMAN et al., 1963).

In an early report it was claimed that administration of a relatively crude preparation containing the vinca alkaloids was able to reduce the level of coenzyme A in rat liver; the decrease was prevented by pantothine, but not pantothenate or pantothenylcysteine (MASCITELLI-CORIANDOLI and LANZANI, 1963). If confirmed, such a lesion could be important in producing secondary effects on lipid and carbohydrate metabolism.

Changes in serum levels of various ions have been reported. BARIETY and GADJOS (1965) found that after treatment of rabbits with vinblastine there was an elevation in serum copper and iron content. Since the latter occurred in the absence of changes in incorporation of iron into protoporphyrin, it presumably reflects a hemolytic process. SLATER et al. (1969) have described hyponatremia in a child with acute lymphoblastic leukemia treated with vincristine; the authors suggested that the fall in serum sodium, which was accompanied by urinary hypertonicity, might result from an effect of the alkaloid on the sites of antidiuretic hormone formation or storage in the central nervous system.

The vinca alkaloids are indole derivatives and, like reserpine, might be expected to release catecholamines, and in some instances histamine, from their storage sites. However, vinblastine inhibited rather than stimulated the release of histamine by mast cells (GILLESPIE et al., 1968), while vincristine did not alter blood pressure and blood pressure response to histamine, epinephrine, norepinephrine, or acetylcholine (ADAMSON et al., 1965). On the other hand, UEDA et al. (1969) have described an elevation of blood pressure in cats, dogs, rabbits, and guinea pigs treated with vincristine. This effect, which was abolished by α-adrenergic blockade or pretreatment with reserpine, appeared to involve central vasomotor excitation leading to release of norepinephrine. Interestingly, colchicine, which does not possess an indole structure, is able to delay the degenerative release of transmitter in sectioned sympathetic nerves of the rat (LUNDBERG, 1970). The same drug in high concentrations *in vitro* was able to cause accumulation of norepinephrine in lumbar sympathetic ganglia (DAHLSTRÖM, 1968).

E. Metabolism and Distribution

The metabolism and distribution of the antimitotic agents, especially in man, are not very well understood. Of the vinca alkaloids, most is known about vinblastine, which has been available as tritium-labeled material. Bioassay methods that involve inhibition of the growth of KB or L cells have also been devised and applied to the determination of plasma levels of vinblastine and vincristine. NOBLE (1961) found that in rats given vinblastine at a dosage of 5 mg/kg, the alkaloid was undetectable by bioassay in serum samples collected more than 5 min after injection. Less than one percent of the administered dose was recovered as urinary vinblastine (BEER, 1961). In humans, serum levels of less than 0.05 μg/ml were found after 0.2 mg/kg of the same alkaloid (SMITH et al., 1965). Data obtained with tritiated vinblastine are compatible with the bioassay findings. In rats less than 1.5 % of the intravenously administered radioactivity was in the blood after 30 min. This rapid disappearance was not due to fast urinary clearance since only 6.6 % was excreted by this route in 24 h. It appeared that biliary excretion was the major pathway for clearance of drug and that only about 2 % of this passed out as unchanged vinblastine (BEER et al., 1964). After intraperitoneal injection, maximum plasma concentrations of tritiated vinblastine in rats were attained in 1 to 2 h. Approximately 75 % of the blood radioactivity was associated with the buffy coat and still present as unchanged vinblastine (GREENIUS et al., 1968). The concentration in the buffy coat was possibly a reflection of the high affinity of platelets for vinblastine (HEBDEN et al., 1970).

In dogs and monkeys, serum vincristine levels (by bioassay) after intravenous injection of drug at a dosage of 1 mg/kg fell from an initial range of 0.3 to 1.0 μg/ml to 0.02 to 0.05 μg/ml by 6 h. Rats evidently disposed of the drug more rapidly, since it was undetectable within 3 h (DIXON et al., 1969). About 50 % of a group of children treated with vincristine (0.1 mg/kg) showed measurable blood levels (0.005 to 0.05 μg/ml) some 4 h after injection (MORASCA et al., 1969).

As with the vinca alkaloids, biliary excretion is the major route of elimination of colchicine. Thus BRUES (1942), using colorimetric and biological assays, found a rapid initial drop in blood levels in rats to a relatively constant value which was achieved in a few min. About 50 % was still present in the body after 16 h, while in the first few h 10 to 25% had been eliminated into the intestine. BACK and WALASZEK (1953) found that after injection of biosynthetically ^{14}C-labeled colchicine into mice, 18 to 46 % was present in the intestine, 22 to 31 % in the kidney, and 7 to 26 % in the liver. High levels in the spleen (39 to 47 %) were found in normal mice, but not those bearing ascitic tumors. In human subjects receiving therapeutic doses of colchicine-^{14}C, the plasma half life was 19.3 min. Intracellular concentrations within the leukocytes were between 3 and 17 times greater than the maximum plasma levels of drug (ERTEL et al., 1969).

Podophyllotoxin labeled with ^{14}C has been isolated from *Podophyllum* plants grown in the presence of $^{14}CO_2$. This material was given to mice by subcutaneous injection; 4 h later 26 % was in the liver, gall bladder, and intestine as unchanged drug, and 22 % in the urine. Conversion to the very insoluble picropodophyllin probably accounted for low overall recoveries (KOCSIS et al., 1957). Such conversion to an insoluble, inactive derivative probably accounts for the very low recoveries of podophyllotoxin in the bioassays of rat and canine urine and feces reported by KELLY et al. (1951). STÄHELIN and CERLETTI (1964) have found that in dogs, rats, mice, and man, the highest concentrations of radioactivity from labeled podophyllic acid ethyl hydrazide are in the liver and kidney; significant concentrations were found in human brain and bronchogenic tumors.

It is evident that much work needs to be done on the metabolism and distribution of these agents, particularly in man. The fact that radiolabeled representatives of all the classes of antimitotic drugs are now available should facilitate such studies. The knowledge gained would provide guidance for optimum dosage scheduling and might help to indicate desirable features that might be incorporated into the design of derivatives with reduced susceptibility to metabolic degradation.

Clinical Considerations

In the field of cancer chemotherapy the vinca alkaloids are the only antimitotic agents to have earned themselves a place among the truly valuable drugs. Although the new podophyllum derivatives, VM-26 and podophyllic acid ethyl hydrazide, are currently of interest and have been receiving clinical trials, agents of this class have not in the past proved to be especially useful in the treatment of cancer. Colchicine, trimethylcolchicinic acid, and colcemid have also undergone sporadic use in the clinic as antineoplastic agents. However, in the management of advanced lymphomas and Hodgkin's disease they are clearly inferior to the vinca alkaloids, and find their more valuable application as anti-inflammatory agents. Thus, we shall restrict this discussion to the vinca alkaloids. The elements of human pharmacology to be considered are human toxicity, therapeutic indications, and the pharmacological basis for use in combination therapy. Knowledge of the metabolism and distribution of these agents, normally a major portion of clinical pharmacology, is in a very rudimentary state, and for this reason the available data have been considered in the section on metabolism and distribution.

A. Drugs, Dosage, and Administration

Of the naturally occurring vinca alkaloids only vinblastine and vincristine are of established clinical value. Vinleurosine has been subject to rather intensive clinical trial (HODES et al., 1963; MATHÉ et al., 1965; GAILANI et al., 1966), with the finding that it is generally inferior to the other alkaloids, and produces a shock-like syndrome when injected rapidly by the intravenous route. Vinrosidine, despite the promise shown when used against experimental tumors, has evinced toxicity without therapeutic benefit in the clinic (GAILANI et al., 1966). Vinglycinate, a synthetic derivative of vinblastine, has been used by ARMSTRONG et al. (1967) with some success in the treatment of Hodgkin's disease, lymphosarcoma and bronchogenic carcinoma. It resembles vinblastine, except that tenfold higher dosages are required, and it apparently lacks cross-resistance to vincristine and vinblastine. There have, however, been problems in the stability of preparations (JOHNSON, 1968).

All the alkaloids are normally in the form of the sulfates, which are chemically more stable than the free bases, but vinleurosine has also been used as the methiodide (HODES et al., 1963), which in preclinical trials appeared more active (JOHNSON et al., 1963). Vincristine sulfate (Oncovin) is normally supplied as 1 or 5 mg ampoules for intravenous injection, containing in addition 10 or 50 mg of lactose, respectively. Vinblastine sulfate (Velban) for intravenous use is supplied in 10 mg ampoules without excipient. It has also been available as oral preparations to obviate the necessity for injection. Initially, uncoated tablets of vinblastine were used, but absorption from the gastrointestinal tract was erratic (JOHNSON et al., 1963). Subsequently, enteric-coated 5 mg tablets have given more satisfactory absorption, as determined by therapeutic results, but the large doses of this expensive drug that must be used render the oral route impractical.

An incremental approach to dosage levels has been employed with these drugs. For vinblastine, an initial dose of 0.1 mg/kg has been recommended, followed by weekly doses in 0.05 mg/kg increments up to 0.3 mg/kg. However, this range is strictly circumscribed by regular observation of toxicity based on peripheral leucocyte count and by tumor response; most patients require weekly doses in the range of 0.15 to 0.2 mg/kg. JOHNSON et al. (1963) described an interesting case of a woman who, while receiving testosterone, was unable to tolerate more than 0.05 mg/kg of vinblastine. After cessation of androgen therapy, her tolerance to the alkaloid rose to normal values. Because of the biliary excretion of this drug, impaired liver function may also give rise to reduced tolerance. On the other hand, at the Yale-New Haven Medical Center, one subject did not develop signs of toxicity until a dose of 1.2 mg/kg was administered. A similar pattern is used with vincristine, a common starting dose for adults being 0.02 mg/kg, and for children, who have greater tolerance, 0.05 mg/kg. There follows a carefully titrated increase in dosage to 0.05 mg/kg for adults and 0.075 mg/kg (approximately 2 mg/M^2) or more in children. A tingling of the extremities followed by numbness is the normal signal for reducing the dose.

Although the use of weekly injections is standard with these agents, experiments carried out with transplantable mouse tumors show that daily injections produce antitumor effects clearly superior to those of single large doses (Johnson et al., 1963; Creasey, 1966). Furthermore, the theoretical considerations of Valeriote et al. (1966) also suggest that optimal effects of vinblastine require significant lengths of exposure to critical drug concentrations. However, in the clinic, toxicity has soared with more frequent injection, and this has discouraged exploration of other dose regimens.

B. Toxicity

The major toxic manifestations of therapy with the vinca alkaloids are indicated in Table 1. Perhaps the most striking feature is that leukopenia, the most prominent side-effect of vinblastine, is relatively uncommon with vincristine,

Table 1. *Human Toxicity of the Vinca Alkaloids*

Percentage incidence	Vinblastine	Vincristine
Above 50		Paresthesias
30—50	Leukopenia	Loss of deep tendon reflex
10—30	Nausea Vomiting Anorexia	Constipation Hoarseness
5—10	Neurotoxicity Hair loss	Weakness Hair loss Slapping gait
Below 5	Stomatitis Diarrhea Constipation Lethargy and depression Phlebitis Ileus	Abdominal pain Muscle cramps Depression Phlebitis Cranial nerve palsy

From De Conti and Creasey (in press).

which produces a range of neurologic and neuromuscular symptoms. Features of this neurotoxicity have already been mentioned in this chapter with regard to preclinical studies. Tobin and Sandler (1966, 1968), Sandler et al. (1969), and Gottschalk et al. (1968) have described the clinical changes encountered. The most consistent finding is depression and finally loss of the Achilles deep tendon reflex. Most studies have not indicated changes in conduction velocity, but there is one report that this is slowed (McLeod and Penny, 1969). In general, it would appear that there is a selective effect on the muscle spindle (Sandler et al., 1969), together with axonal degeneration and demyelination comparable to that seen experimentally (Gottschalk et al., 1968; McLeod and Penny, 1969; Bradley et al., 1970). Many of these neurologic symptoms could result from the biochemical and microtubular interactions discussed earlier.

Although vinblastine is considered to be a marrow depressant, it is evidently selective in its action since thrombocytopenia is relatively rare. Indeed, there are reports of thrombocytosis accompanying therapy with both vinblastine and vincristine (Hwang et al., 1969; Robertson and McCarthy, 1969). Vinblastine (Hertz et al., 1960) and vincristine have been shown to be capable of suppressing erythropoiesis (MORSE and STOHLMAN, 1966). Phlebitis, another of the less frequent complications, is primarily the result of extravasation and irritation at the injection site. Among the more interesting of the rare toxic side effects of vincristine is hyponatremia, apparently resulting from inappropriate antidiuretic hormone secretion (FINE et al., 1966). Alopecia is rather more frequent during treatment with vincristine than with vinblastine. Constipation and even paralytic ileus are common side effects of vincristine; adequate precautions can minimize this serious problem.

The Place of the Vinca Alkaloids in the Chemotherapy of Cancer

The vinca alkaloids are established agents in the treatment of lymphomas, especially Hodgkin's disease, childhood acute leukemias, choriocarcinoma, and embryonal or mesenchymal carcinomas such as Wilms' tumor, neuroblastoma, rhabdomyosarcoma, and carcinoma of the testis. Responses have been obtained with some frequency in such other diseases as mycosis fungoides, Letterer-Siwe disease, oat cell carcinoma of the lung, breast carcinoma, the blastic crisis stage of chronic myelocytic leukemia, and some central nervous system neoplasms. This of course does not represent an exhaustive list, but rather an indication of the areas of most useful application. It should also be stressed that there are significant differences in the spectra of activity of vinblastine and vincristine. Vinblastine is somewhat more effective than vincristine in the treatment of advanced Hodgkin's disease, whereas the latter drug is the more active against lymphosarcoma and reticulum cell sarcoma. More striking, however, is that vincristine is of value in the therapy of acute lymphoblastic leukemia, a disease for which vinblastine is ineffective. Considerably more clinical information regarding the uses of these drugs may be found in the reviews of JOHNSON et al. (1963) and NEUSS et al. (1964), in the proceedings of the Symposium on Vincristine (1968), and in the chapter by DE CONTI and CREASEY (in press).

In the last few years it has become evident that the future of the vinca alkaloids, and possibly of most other types of anticancer drugs, lies in their integration into intensive schedules of combination therapy. At the present time considerable progress is being made in devising and applying drug combinations to clinical disease; many of the most successful of these protocols involve the vinca alkaloids. The major principles behind the selection of components, apart from activity against the disease, are avoidance of cumulative toxicity by use of agents with differing limiting side-effects, and employment of drugs of different mechanisms of action in the hope of inflicting a variety of metabolic lesions on the target cells. Further improvements are to be expected when increased knowledge of the human pharmacology of these agents is obtained and applied to determining logical combinations. The reader is referred for detailed consideration of various aspects of combination chemotherapy to the reviews of FREI and FREIREICH (1965), HENDERSON and SAMAHA (1969), HOLLAND (1968), SARTORELLI (1965), SARTORELLI and CREASEY (1973), and VENDITTI and GOLDIN (1964). However, it is only when such multiagent schedules have evolved to encompass other modalities such as surgery, radiation, and immunotherapy in a concerted approach to cancer, that therapeutic benefits such as are now obtained in only a few diseases will be achieved in all neoplasia.

References

ADAMSON, R. H., DIXON, R. L., BEN, M., CREWS, L., SHOHET, S. B., RALL, D. P.: Some pharmacologic properties of vincristine. Arch. int. Pharmacodyn. **157**, 299—311 (1965).

ADELMANN, M. R., BORISY, G. G., SHELANSKI, M. L., WEISENBERG, R. C., TAYLOR, E. W.: Cytoplasmic filaments and tubules. Fed. Proc. **27**, 1186—1193 (1968).
AFZELIUS, B.: Electron microscopy of the sperm tail. Results obtained with a new fixative. J. biophys. biochem. Cytol. **5**, 269—278 (1959).
AGUSTIN, B. M., CREASEY, W. A.: Effects of vinca alkaloids on the synthesis of RNA in mouse brain. Nature (Lond.) **215**, 965—966 (1967).
AISENBERG, A. C.: Suppression of immune response by vincristine and vinblastine. Nature (Lond.) **200**, 484 (1963).
ANDERSON, P. J., SONG, S. K., SLOTWINER, P.: The fine structure of spheromembranous degeneration of skeletal muscle induced by vincristine. J. Neuropathol. exp. Neurol. **26**, 15—24 (1967).
ANGEVINE, J. B., JR.: Nerve destruction by colchicine in mice and golden hamsters. J. exp. Zool. **136**, 363—391 (1957).
ARMSTRONG, J. G., DYKE, R. W., FOUTS, P. J., HAWTHORNE, J. J., JANSEN, C. J, JR., PEABODY, A. M.: Initial clinical experience with vinglycinate sulfate, a molecular modification of vinblastine. Cancer Res. **27**, 221—227 (1967).
BACK, A., WALASZEK, E. J.: Studies with radioactive colchicine. I. The influence of tumors on the tissue distribution of radioactive colchicine in mice. Cancer Res. **13**, 552—555 (1953).
BARASA, A., MACCOTTA, V., FILOGAMO, G., CANAVESE, B.: Azione della vincaleucoblastina (VLB) sui prolungamenti, centrale e periferico, dei neuroni dei gangli spinali coltivati *in vitro*. Boll. Soc. Ital. Biol. Sper. **46**, 860—864 (1970).
BARIÉTY, M., GADJOS, A.: Action de 3 substances antimitotiques sur la sidérémie et la cuprémie du lapin. Press Med. **73**, 921 (1965).
BEER, C. T.: The leukopenic action of extracts of *Vinca rosea*. A.R. Brit. Emp. Cancer Campaign **33**, 487—488 (1955).
BEER, C. T.: Biochemical studies with vincaleukoblastine. Canad. Cancer Conf. **4**, 355—361 (1961).
BEER, C. T., WILSON, M. L., BELL, J.: A preliminary investigation of the fate of tritiated vinblastine in rats. Canad. J. Physiol. Pharmacol. **42**, 368—373 (1964).
BEHNKE, O., FORER, A.: Evidence for four classes of microtubules in individual cells. J. cell Sci. **2**, 169—192 (1967).
BEHNKE, O., FORER, A., EMMERSEN, J.: Actin in sperm tails and meiotic spindles. Nature (Lond.) **234**, 408—410 (1971).
BENSCH, K. G., MALAWISTA, S. E.: Microtubule crystals in mammalian cells. J. Cell Biol. **40**, 95—107 (1969).
BENSCH, K. G., MARANTZ, R., WISNIEWSKI, H., SHELANSKI, M.: Induction *in vitro* of microtubular crystals by vinca alkaloids. Science **165**, 495—496 (1969).
BENT, K. J., MOORE, R. H.: The mode of action of griseofulvin. In: NEWTON, B. A., REYNOLDS, P. E. (Eds.): Biochemical studies of antimicrobial drugs. London: Cambridge University Press 1966.
BORISY, G. G., TAYLOR, E. W.: The mechanism of action of colchicine. Binding of colchicine-^{3}H to cellular protein. J. Cell Biol. **34**, 525—533 (1967a).
BORISY, G. G., TAYLOR, E. W.: Colchicine binding to sea urchin eggs and the mitotic apparatus. J. Cell Biol. **34**, 535—548 (1967b).
BRADLEY, W. G., LASSMAN, L. P., PEARCE, G. W., WALTON, J. N.: The neuromyopathy of vincristine in man. Clinical, electrophysiological and pathological studies. J. neurol. Sci. **10**, 107—131 (1970).
BRUCHOVSKY, N., OWEN, A. A., BECKER, A. J., TILL, J. E.: Effects of vinblastine on the proliferative capacity of L cells and their progress through the division cycle. Cancer Res. **25**, 1232—1237 (1965).
BRUES, A. M.: The fate of colchicine in the body. J. clin. Invest. **21**, 646—647 (1942).
BRYAN, J.: Definition of three classes of binding sites in isolated microtubule crystals. Biochemistry **11**, 2611—2616 (1972).
CANER, J. E. Z.: Colchicine inhibition of chemotaxis. Arthritis Rheum. **8**, 757—760 (1965).
CARDINALI, G., CARDINALI, G., CENTURELLI, G.: The *Catharanthus roseus (Vinca rosea)* alkaloids: a new class of stathmokinetic agents. Acta Genet. med. Gemellolog. (Roma) **17**, 197—208 (1968).
CARDINALI, G., CARDINALI, G., HANDLER, A. H., AGRIFOGLIO, M. F.: Comparative effects of colchicine and vincaleukoblastine on bone marrow mitotic activity in Syrian hamster. Proc. Soc. exp. Biol. (N.Y.) **107**, 891—892 (1961).
CHUNG, L., GABOUREL, J. D.: Adrenal steroid release by vinblastine and its contribution to vinblastine effect on rat thymus. Fed. Proc. **27**, 760 (1968).
CLINE, M. J.: Effect of vincristine on synthesis of ribonucleic acid and protein in leukaemic leucocytes. Brit. J. Haematol. **14**, 21—29 (1968).

COHLAN, S. Q., KITAY, D.: The teratogenic effect of vincaleukoblastine in the pregnant rat. J. Pediat. **66**, 541—544 (1965).
CREASEY, W. A.: Tumor-inhibitory effects of combinations of the vinca alkaloids with actinomycin D. Biochem. Pharmacol. **15**, 367—375 (1966).
CREASEY, W. A.: The binding of antimitotic agents by cell-free extracts of tumor cells. Pharmacologist **9**, 192 (1967).
CREASEY, W. A.: Modifications in biochemical pathways produced by the vinca alkaloids. Cancer Chemother. Rep. **52**, 501—507 (1968a).
CREASEY, W. A.: Effect of the vinca alkaloids on RNA synthesis in relation to mitotic arrest. Fed. Proc. **27**, 760 (1968b).
CREASEY, W. A.: Biochemical effects of the vinca alkaloids — IV. Studies with vinleurosine. Biochem. Pharmacol. **18**, 227—232 (1969).
CREASEY, W. A.: Biochemistry of dimeric *Catharanthus* alkaloids. In: TAYLOR, W. I., FARNSWORTH, N. R. (Eds.): The *Catharanthus* Species: botany, chemistry and biological activity. New York: Marcel Dekker, in press.
CREASEY, W. A., BENSCH, K. G., MALAWISTA, S. E.: Binding of antimitotic agents as the basis for mitotic inhibition and anti-inflammatory action. Fed. Proc. **28**, 362 (1969).
CREASEY, W. A., BENSCH, K. G., MALAWISTA, S. E.: Colchicine, vinblastine and griseofulvin. Pharmacological studies with human leukocytes. Biochem. Pharmacol. **20**, 1579—1588 (1971).
CREASEY, W. A., CHOU, T. C.: The binding of colchicine by Sarcoma 180 cells. Biochem. Pharmacol. **17**, 477—480 (1968).
CREASEY, W. A., MARKIW, M. E.: Biochemical effects of the vinca alkaloids — I. Effects of vinblastine on nucleic acid synthesis in mouse tumor cells. Biochem. Pharmacol. **13**, 135—142 (1964a).
CREASEY, W. A., MARKIW, M. E.: Biochemical effects of the vinca alkaloids — II. A comparison of the effects of colchicine, vinblastine and vincristine on the synthesis of ribonucleic acids in Ehrlich ascites carcinoma cells. Biochim. biophys. Acta (Amst.) **87**, 601—609 (1964b).
CREASEY, W. A., MARKIW, M. E.: Biochemical effects of the vinca alkaloids — III. The synthesis of ribonucleic acid and the incorporation of amino acids in Ehrlich ascites cells *in vitro*. Biochim. biophys. Acta (Amst.) **103**, 635—645 (1965).
CUTTS, J. H.: Changes in mitosis in ascites tumors and normal bone marrow induced by vincaleukoblastine *in vivo*. Canad. Cancer Conf. **4**, 363—372 (1961).
CUTTS, J. H.: Effects of other agents on the biologic responses to vinca-leukoblastine. Biochem. Pharmacol. **13**, 421—431 (1964).
CUTTS, J. H.: Protective action of diethylstilbestrol on toxicity of vinblastine in rats. J. nat. Cancer Inst. **41**, 919—922 (1968).
DAHLSTRÖM, A.: Effect of colchicine on transport of amine storage granules in sympathetic nerves of rat. European J. Pharmacol. **5**, 111—113 (1968).
DA RE, P., MANCINI, V., COLOMBO, G., MICCIARELLI, A.: Antimitotic effects of some basic colchicinamides on mammalian cells *in vitro*. Life Sci. **5**, 211—213 (1966).
DE CONTI, R. C., CREASEY, W. A.: Clinical aspects of the dimeric *Catharanthus* alkaloids. In: TAYLOR, W. I., FARNSWORTH, N. R. (Eds.): The *Catharanthus* species: botany, chemistry and biological activity. New York: Marcel Dekker, in press.
DE HARVEN, E.: Action de la colchicine et de certaines hormones corticosurrénaliennes sur les mitoses des follicules pileux du rat. Rev. Belge Pathol. **25**, 277—285 (1956).
DE HARVEN, E., DUSTIN, P., JR.: La régulation hormonale de l'éosinophilie. II. Antagonisme entre certains poisons stathmocinétiques et la cortisone au niveau des myélocytes éosinophiles du rat. Rev. Hématol. **11**, 131—139 (1956).
DESJARDINS, R., GROGAN, D. E., ARENDELL, J. P., BUSCH, H.: Effects of antitumor agents on the synthesis of nucleolar DNA. Cancer Res. **27**, 159—164 (1967).
DIXON, G. J., DULMADGE, E. A., MULLIGAN, L. T., MELLETT, L. B.: Cell culture bioassay for vincristine sulfate in sera from mice, rats, dogs and monkeys. Cancer Res. **29**, 1810—1813 (1969).
DUSTIN, P., JR.: New aspects of the pharmacology of antimitotic agents. Pharmacol. Rev. **15**, 449—480 (1963).
EIGSTI, O. J., DUSTIN, P., JR.: Colchicine, in agriculture, medicine, biology and chemistry. Ames: Iowa College Press 1955.
EL-NAKEEB, M. A., LAMPEN, J. O.: Formation of complexes of griseofulvin and nucleic acids of fungi and its relation to griseofulvin sensitivity. Biochem. J. **92**, 59P—60P (1964).
EL-NAKEEB, M. A., MCLELLAN, W. L., JR., LAMPEN, J. O.: Antibiotic action of griseofulvin on dermatophytes. J. Bact. **89**, 557—563 (1965).
ERTEL, N., OMOKOKU, B., WALLACE, S. L.: Colchicine concentrations in leukocytes. Arthritis Rheum. **12**, 293 (1969).

FERM, V. H.: Congenital malformations in hamster embryos after treatment with vinblastine and vincristine. Science **141**, 426 (1963).

FINE, R. N., CLARKE, R. R., SHORE, N. A.: Hyponatremia and vincristine therapy. Syndrome possibly resulting from inappropriate antidiuretic hormone secretion. Amer. J. Dis. Child. **112**, 256—259 (1966).

FREED, J. J., BHISEY, A. N., LEBOWITZ, M. M.: The relation of microtubules and microfilaments to the motility of cultured cells. J. Cell Biol. **39**, 46A—47A (1968).

FREI, E., III, FREIREICH, E. J.: Progress and perspectives in the chemotherapy of acute leukemia. In: GOLDIN, A., HAWKING, F., SCHNITZER, R. J. (Eds.): Advances in Chemotherapy, Vol. 2. New York: Academic Press 1965.

FREI, E., III, WHANG, J., SCOGGINS, R. B., VAN SCOTT, E. J., RALL, D. P., BEN, M.: The stathmokinetic effect of vincristine. Cancer Res. **24**, 1918—1925 (1964).

GAILANI, S. D., ARMSTRONG, J. G., CARBONE, P. P., TAN, C., HOLLAND, J. F.: Clinical trial of vinleurosine sulfate (NSC-90636): a new drug derived from *Vinca rosea* Linn. Cancer Chemother. Rep. **50**, 95—103 (1966).

GAWADI, N.: Actin in the mitotic spindle. Nature (Lond.) **234**, 410 (1971).

GEORGATSOS, J. G., KAREMFYLLIS, T.: Action of podophyllic acid on malignant tumors — II. Effects of podophyllic acid ethyl hydrazide on the incorporation of precursors into the nucleic acids of mouse mammary tumors and liver *in vivo*. Biochem. Pharmacol. **17**, 1489—1492 (1968).

GEORGATSOS, J. G., KAREMFYLLIS, T., SYMEONIDIS, A.: Action of podophyllic acid on malignant tumors — I. Distribution of tritiated podophyllic acid ethyl hydrazide in subcellular fractions of mouse mammary tumors. Biochem. Pharmacol. **17**, 1485—1488 (1968).

GEORGE, P., JOURNEY, L. J., GOLDSTEIN, M. N.: Effect of vincristine on the fine structure of HeLa cells during mitosis. J. nat. Cancer Inst. **35**, 355—375 (1965).

GILLESPIE, E., LEVINE, R. J., MALAWISTA, S. E.: Histamine release from rat peritoneal mast cells: inhibition by colchicine and potentiation by deuterium oxide. J. Pharmacol. exp. Therap. **164**, 158—165 (1968).

GOLDFINGER, S. E., HOWELL, R. R., SEEGMILLER, J. E.: Suppression of metabolic accompaniment of phagocytosis by colchicine. Arthritis Rheum. **8**, 1112—1122 (1965).

GONATAS, N. K., ROBBINS, E.: The homology of spindle tubules and neurotubules in the chick embryo retina. Protoplasma **59**, 377—391 (1965).

GOTTSCHALK, P. G., DYCK, P. J., KIELY, J. M.: Vinca alkaloid neuropathy: nerve biopsy studies in rats and in man. Neurology **18**, 875—882 (1968).

GRAFF, G. L. A., GUEUNING, C., HILDEBRAND, J.: Action du sulfate de vincristine sur le gastrocnémien de rat — I. Mis en évidence de deux compartiments, metaboliquement distincts, pour le phosphate inorganique; effets sur les phosphates organiques acidosolubles et les phospholipides. C. R. Soc. Biol. (Paris) **161**, 2645—2651 (1967).

GREENIUS, H. F., MCINTYRE, R. W., BEER, C. T.: The preparation of vinblastine-4-acetyl-*t* and its distribution in the blood of rats. J. med. Chem. **11**, 254—257 (1968).

HAKALA, M. T.: Photochemical inactivation of *Vinca rosea* alkaloids catalyzed by riboflavin. Fed. Proc. **28**, 856 (1969).

HARRIS, P.: Some structural and functional aspects of the mitotic apparatus in sea urchin embryos. J. Cell Biol. **14**, 475—487 (1962).

HEBDEN, H. F., HADFIELD, J. R., BEER, C. T.: The binding of vinblastine by platelets in the rat. Cancer Res. **30**, 1417—1424 (1970).

HELL, E., COX, D. G.: Effects of colchicine and colcemid on synthesis of deoxyribonucleic acid in the skin of the guinea pig's ear *in vitro*. Nature (Lond.) **197**, 287—288 (1963).

HENDERSON, E. S., SAMAHA, R. J.: Evidence that drugs in multiple combinations have materially advanced the treatment of human malignancies. Cancer Res. **29**, 2272—2280 (1969).

HERTZ, R., LIPSETT, M. B., MOY, R. H.: Effect of vincaleukoblastine on metastatic choriocarcinoma and related trophoblastic tumors in women. Cancer Res. **20**, 1050—1053 (1960).

HODES, M. E., ROHN, R. J., BOND, W. H., YARDLEY, J.: Clinical trials with leurosine methiodide, an alkaloid from *Vinca rosea* Linn. Cancer Chemother. Rep. **28**, 53—55 (1963).

HOFFMAN, H.: Acceleration and retardation of the processes of axon-sprouting in partially denervated muscles. Austral. J. exp. Biol. med. Sci. **30**, 541—566 (1952).

HOLLAND, J. F.: Progress in the treatment of acute leukemia, 1966. In: DAMESHEK, W., DUTCHER, R. M. (Eds.): Perspectives in leukemia. New York: Grune and Stratton 1968.

HUNTER, J. C.: Effects of vincaleukoblastine sulfate on metabolism of thioguanine-resistant L1210 leukemia cells. Biochem. Pharmacol. **12**, 283—291 (1963).

HWANG, Y. F., HAMILTON, H. E., SHEETS, R. F.: Vinblastine-induced thrombocytosis. Lancet **2**, 1075—1076 (1969).

ILAN, J., QUASTEL, J. H.: Effect of colchicine on nucleic acid metabolism during metamorphosis of *Tenebrio molitor* L. and in some mammalian tissues. Biochem. J. **100**, 448—457 (1966).

JOHNSON, I. S.: Historical background of vinca alkaloid research and areas of future interest. Cancer Chemother. Rep. **52**, 455—461 (1968).
JOHNSON, I. S., ARMSTRONG, J. G., GORMAN, M., BURNETT, J. P., JR.: The vinca alkaloids: a new class of oncolytic agents. Cancer Res. **23**, 1390—1427 (1963).
JOHNSON, I. S., HARGROVE, W. W., HARRIS, P. N., WRIGHT, H. F., BODER, G. B.: Preclinical studies with vinglycinate, one of a series of chemically derived analogs of vinblastine. Cancer Res. **26**, 2431—2436 (1966).
JOHNSON, I. S., WRIGHT, H. F., SVOBODA, G. H.: Experimental basis for clinical evaluation of antitumor principles derived from *Vinca rosea* Linn. J. Lab. clin. Med. **54**, 830 (1959).
JONES, R. G. W., RICHARDS, J. F., BEER, C. T.: Biochemical studies with the vinca alkaloids II. Effect of vinblastine on the biosynthesis of nucleic acids and their precursors in rat thymus cells. Cancer Res. **26**, 882—887 (1966).
JOURNEY, L. J., BURDMAN, J., GEORGE, P.: Ultrastructural studies on tissue culture cells treated with vincristine (NSC-67574). Cancer Chemother. Rep. **52**, 509—516 (1968).
KARLSSON, J. O., SJÖSTRAND, J.: The effect of colchicine on the axonal transport of protein in the optic nerve and tract of the rabbit. Brain Res. **13**, 617—619 (1969).
KATCHMAN, B. J., ZIPF, R. E., MURPHY, J. P. F.: The effect of chemotherapeutic agents upon the metabolism of intact human cancer cells. An *in vitro* technic for cell sensitivity. Clin. Chem. **9**, 511—529 (1963).
KELLY, M. G., HARTWELL, J. L.: The biological effects and the chemical composition of podophyllin. A review. J. nat. Cancer Inst. **14**, 967—1010 (1953).
KELLY, M. G., LEITER, J., BOURKE, A. R., SMITH, P. K.: Fate and distribution of podophyllotoxin in animals. Cancer Res. **11**, 263 (1951).
KENSLER, C. J.: Chemotherapeutic activity of phthalanilide derivatives. An approach to anticodic therapy? Cancer Res. **23**, 1353—1363 (1963).
KIM, J. H., STAMBUK, B. K.: Synchronization of HeLa cells by vinblastine sulfate. Exp. cell Res. **44**, 631—634 (1966).
KOCSIS, J. J., WALASZEK, E. J., GEILING, E. M.: Disposition of biosynthetically labeled ^{14}C podophyllotoxin in normal and tumor-bearing mice. Arch. int. Pharmacodyn. **111**, 134—144 (1957).
KOTORII, K., MORI, H., YOSHIDA, M.: A peculiar crystalline structure in neurons of rabbits treated with vincristine. Kurume med. J. **18**, 57—63 (1971).
KRAKOFF, I. H.: Discussion of conference on gout and purine metabolism. Arthritis Rheum. 8, 760 (1965).
KRISHAN, A.: Time lapse and ultrastructure studies on the reversal of mitotic arrest induced by vinblastine sulfate in Earle's L. cells. J. nat. Cancer Inst. **41**, 581—595 (1968).
KRISHAN, A.: Ribosome-granular material complexes in human leukemic lymphoblasts exposed to vinblastine sulfate. J. Ultrastructure Res. **31**, 272—281 (1970).
KRISHAN, A., HSU, D.: Binding of colchicine-^{3}H to vinblastine- and vincristine-induced crystals in mammalian tissue culture cells. J. Cell Biol. **48**, 407—410 (1971).
LEDBETTER, M. C., PORTER, K. R.: Morphology of microtubules of plant cells. Science **144**, 872—874 (1964).
LITS, F.: Contribution a l'études des réactions cellulaires provoquées par la colchicine. C. R. Soc. Biol. (Paris) **115**, 1421—1423 (1934).
LOVE, R.: Studies on the cytochemistry of nucleoproteins. I. Effect of colchicine on the ribonucleoproteins of the cell. Exp. Cell Res. **33**, 216—231 (1964).
LUDFORD, R. J.: Colchicine in the experimental chemotherapy of cancer. J. Nat. Cancer Inst. **6**, 89—101 (1945).
LUNDBERG, D.: Colchicine-induced delay of the degenerative release of sympathetic transmitter in the conscious rat. Acta physiol. scand. **80**, 430—432 (1970).
LUYCKX, A., VAN LANCKER, J. L.: Metabolic effects of vinblastine. II. The effect of vinblastine on deoxyribonucleic acid and ribonucleic acid synthesis of regenerating liver. Lab. Invest. **15**, 1301—1303 (1966).
MADOC-JONES, H., MAURO, F.: Interphase action of vinblastine and vincristine: differences in their lethal action through the mitotic cycle of cultured mammalian cells. J. Cell Physiol. **72**, 185—196 (1968).
MALAWISTA, S. E.: Colchicine: a common mechanism for its anti-inflammatory and antimitotic effects. Arthritis Rheum. **11**, 191—197 (1968a).
MALAWISTA, S. E.: Vinblastine: colchicine-like effects on human blood leukocytes. Arthritis Rheum. **11**, 108—109 (1968b).
MALAWISTA, S. E., BENSCH, K. G.: Human polymorphonuclear leukocytes: demonstration of microtubules and effect of colchicine. Science **156**, 521—522 (1967).
MALAWISTA, S. E., SATO, H.: Vinblastine produces uniaxial, birefringent crystals in starfish oocytes. J. Cell Biol. **42**, 596—599 (1969).

MALAWISTA, S. E., SATO, H., BENSCH, K. G.: Vinblastine and griseofulvin reversibly disrupt the living mitotic spindle. Science **160**, 770—772 (1968).
MALAWISTA, S. E., SATO, H., CREASEY, W. A., BENSCH, K. G.: Vinblastine produces uniaxial birefringent crystals in starfish oocytes. Fed Proc. **28**, 875 (1969).
MANTON, I.: Observations on the microanatomy of the spermatozoid of the bracken fern *(Pteridium aquilinum)*. J. biophys. biochem. Cytol. **6**, 413—418 (1959).
MARANTZ, R., SHELANSKI, M.: Structure of microtubule crystals induced by vinblastine *in vitro*. J. Cell Biol. **44**, 234—238 (1970).
MARANTZ, R., VENTILIA, M., SHELANSKI, M.: Vinblastine-induced precipitation of microtubule protein. Science **165**, 498—499 (1969).
MARSLAND, D.: Cell division-enhancement of the anti-mitotic effects of colchicine by low temperature and high pressure in the cleaving eggs of *Lytechinus variegatus*. Exp. Cell Res. **50**, 369—376 (1968).
MASCITELLI-CORIANDOLI, E., LANZANI, P.: Effects of *Vinca rosea* Linn. alkaloids on the liver coenzyme A and pantothenic acid. Arzneimittel-Forsch. **13**, 1011—1012 (1963).
MATHÉ, G., SCHNEIDER, M., BAND, P., AMIEL, J. L., SCHWARZENBERG, L., CATTAN, A., SCHLUMBERGER, J. R.: Leurosine sulfate (NSC-90636) in treatment of Hodgkin's disease, acute lymphoblastic leukemia, and lymphoblastic lymphosarcoma. Cancer Chemother. Rep. **49**, 47—49 (1965).
MCGEER, P. L., MCGEER, E. G.: Effect of amethopterin and vincaleukoblastine on urinary 4-amino-5-imidazolecarboxamide. Biochem. Pharmacol. **12**, 297—298 (1963).
MCLEOD, J. G., PENNY, R.: Vincristine neuropathy: an electrophysiological and histological study. J. Neurol. Neurosurg. Psychiat. **32**, 297—304 (1969).
MONCRIEF, J. W., HELLER, K. S.: Acylation: a proposed mechanism of action for various oncolytic agents based on model chemical systems. Cancer Res. **27**, 1500—1502 (1967).
MORASCA, L., RAINISIO, C., MASERA, G.: Duration of cytotoxic activity of vincristine in the blood of leukemic children. European J. Cancer **5**, 79—80 (1969).
MORGAN, J.: Microfilaments from ameba proteins. Exp. Cell Res. **65**, 7—16 (1971).
MORSE, B. S., STOHLMAN, F., JR.: Regulation of erythropoiesis. XVIII. The effect of vincristine and erythropoietin on bone marrow. J. clin. Invest. **45**, 1241—1250 (1966).
MUELLER, G. A., GAULDEN, M. E., DRANE, W.: The effects of varying concentrations of colchicine on the progression of grasshopper neuroblasts into metaphase. J. Cell Biol. **48**, 253—265 (1971).
NEUSS, N., JOHNSON, I. S., ARMSTRONG, J. G., JANSEN, C. J., JR.: The vinca alkaloids. In: GOLDIN, A., HAWKING, F., SCHNITZER, R. J. (Eds.): Advances in Chemotherapy, Vol. 1. New York: Academic Press 1964.
NEWCOMB, E. H., HEPLER, P. K.: Microtubules and fibrils in the protoplasm of *Coleus* cells undergoing secondary wall deposition. J. Cell Biol. **20**, 529—533 (1964).
NOBLE, R. L.: Symposium on vincaleukoblastine (VLB). Canad. Cancer Conf. **4**, 333—338 (1961).
NOBLE, R. L., BEER, C. T., MCINTYRE, R. W.: Biological effects of dihydrovinblastine. Cancer **20**, 885—890 (1967).
OBRECHT, P., FUSENIG, N. E.: Die Wirkung von Vincaleukoblastin (Velbe) auf die Glykolyse von Tumorzellen. Europ. J. Cancer, **2**, 109—115 (1966).
OLMSTED, J. B., CARLSON, K., KLEBE, R., RUDDLE, F., ROSENBAUM, J. L.: Isolation of microtubule protein from cultured mouse neuroblastoma cells. Proc. nat. Acad. Sci. (Wash.) **65**, 129—136 (1970).
OXFORD, A. E., RAISTRICK, H., SIMONET, P.: Studies in the biochemistry of microorganisms: LX. Griseofulvin: $C_{17}H_{17}O_6Cl$, a metabolic product of *Penicillium griseofulvum* Dierckx. Biochem. J. **33**, 240—248 (1939).
PADAWER, J.: Quantitative studies with mast cells. Ann. N.Y. Acad. Sci. **103**, 87—138 (1963).
PADAWER, J.: Induction of cellular movements in mast cells by colchicine treatment. J. Cell Biol. **29**, 176—180 (1966).
PALMER, C. G., WARREN, A. K., SIMPSON, P. J.: A comparison of the cytologic effects of leurosine methiodide and vinblastine in tissue culture. Cancer Chemother. Rep. **31**, 1—2 (1963).
PFEIFFER, S. E., TOLMACH, L. J.: Selecting synchronous populations of mammalian cells. Nature (Lond.) **213**, 139—142 (1967).
PORTER, K. R.: Cytoplasmic microtubules and their functions. In: CIBA Foundation Symposium, Principles of biomolecular organization. Boston: Little, Brown 1966.
PUSZKIN, E., PUSZKIN, S., ALEDORT, L. M.: Colchicine-binding protein from human platelets and its effect on muscle myosin and platelet myosin-like thrombosthenin-M. J. biol. Chem. **246**, 271—276 (1971).
RICE, H. V., LAETSCH, W. M.: Observations on the morphology and physiology of MARSILEA sperm. Amer. J. Bot. **54**, 856—866 (1967).

RICHARDS, J.F., JONES, R.G.W., BEER, C.T.: Biochemical studies with the vinca alkaloids. I. Effect on nucleic acid formation by isolated cell suspensions. Cancer Res. **26**, 876—881 (1966).
ROBARDS, A.W., HUMPHERSON, P.G.: Microtubules and angiosperm bordered pit formation. Planta (Berlin) **77**, 233—238 (1967).
ROBBINS, E., GONATAS, N.K.: Histochemical and ultrastructural studies on HeLa cell cultures exposed to spindle inhibitors with special reference to the interphase cell. J. Histochem. Cytochem. **12**, 704—711 (1964).
ROBERTS, D.W., HALL, T.C., ROSENTHAL, D.: Coordinated changes in thymidine-5′-monophosphate metabolism of leukocytes following vincristine administration to patients with acute granulocytic leukemia. Cancer Res. **29**, 789—794 (1969).
ROBERTSON, J.H., MCCARTHY, G.M.: Periwinkle alkaloids and the platelet-count. Lancet II, 353—355 (1969).
ROSENBAUM, J.L., CARLSON, K.: Cilia regeneration in *Tetrahymena* and its inhibition by colchicine. J. Cell Biol. **40**, 415—425 (1969).
SANDLER, S.G., TOBIN, W., HENDERSON, E.S.: Vincristine-induced neuropathy. A clinical study of fifty leukemic patients. Neurology **19**, 367—374 (1969).
SARTORELLI, A.C.: Approaches to the combination chemotherapy of transplantable neoplasms. Proc. exp. Tumor Res. **6**, 228—288 (1965).
SARTORELLI, A.C., CREASEY, W.A.: Cancer chemotherapy. Ann. Rev. Pharmacol. **9**, 51—72 (1969).
SARTORELLI, A.C., CREASEY, W.A.: Combination chemotherapy. In: HOLLAND, J.F., FREI, E. III. (Eds.): Cancer Medicine. Philadelphia: Lea and Febiger 1973.
SAVEL, H.: The metaphase-arresting plant alkaloids and cancer chemotherapy. Progr. exp. Tumor Res. **8**, 189—224 (1966).
SCHOCHET, S.S., LAMPERT, P.W., EARLE, K.M.: Neuronal changes induced by intrathecal vincristine sulfate. J. Neuropathol. exp. Neurol. **27**, 645—658 (1968).
SENTEIN, P.: Action de la vincaleukoblastine sur l'oeuf en segmentation et analyse du mécanisme mitotique. C.R. Acad. Sci. (Paris) **258**, 4854—4857 (1964).
SHELANSKI, M.L., TAYLOR, E.W.: Isolation of a protein subunit from microtubules. J. cell Biol. **34**, 549—555 (1967).
SHELANSKI, M.L., WISNIEWSKI, H.: Neurofibrillary degeneration induced by vinca alkaloids: clinical and experimental. Trans. Amer. Neurol. Ass. **93**, 137—140 (1968).
SLATER, L.M., WAINER, R.A., SERPICK, A.A.: Vincristine neurotoxicity with hyponatremia. Cancer **23**, 122—125 (1969).
SLONIM, R.R., HOWELL, D.S., BROWN, H.E., JR.: Influence of griseofulvin upon acute gouty arthritis. Arthritis Rheum. **5**, 397—404 (1962).
SLOTNICK, I.J., DOUGHERTY, M., JAMES, D.H., JR.: Vincristine inhibition of DNA synthesis in *Tetrahymena pyriformis*. Cancer Res. **26**, 673—675 (1966).
SMITH, C.G., GRADY, J.E., KUPIECKI, F.P.: Blood and urine levels of antitumor agents determined with cell culture methods. Cancer Res. **25**, 241—245 (1965).
SNEDDON, J.M.: Effect of mitosis inhibitors on blood platelet microtubules and aggregation. J. Physiol. **214**, 145—158 (1971).
SPOONER, B.S., YAMADA, K.M., WESSELLS, N.K.: Microfilaments and cell locomotion. J. Cell Biol. **49**, 595—613 (1971).
STÄHELIN, H.: 4′-Demethyl-epipodophyllotoxin thenylidene glucoside (VM-26), a podophyllin compound with a new mechanism of action. European J. Cancer. **6**, 303—311 (1970).
STÄHELIN, H., CERLETTI, A.: Experimentelle Ergebnisse mit den Podophyllumcytostatica SP-1 und SP-G. Schweiz. Med. Wschr. **94**, 1490—1502 (1964).
STEPHENS, R.E.: Reassociation of microtubule protein. J. molec. Biol. **33**, 517—519 (1968).
SUGÁR, J.: Nucleic acid changes in tumour cells following chemotherapeutics studied under the polarization and fluorescence microscope. Acta histochem. (Jena) **16**, 382—392 (1963).
SYMPOSIUM ON VINCRISTINE. Pediatric Division, Southwest Cancer Chemotherapy Study Group. Cancer Chemother. Rep. **52**, 453—535 (1968).
TAYLOR, A.C.: Microtubules in the microspikes and cortical cytoplasm of isolated cells. J. Cell Biol. **28**, 155—168 (1966).
TAYLOR, E.W.: The mechanism of colchicine inhibition of mitosis. I. Kinetics of inhibition and the binding of ^{3}H-colchicine. J. Cell Biol. **25**, 145—160 (1965).
TILNEY, L.G.: Microtubules in the heliozoan *Actinosphaerium nucleophilum* and their relation to axopod formation and motion. J. Cell Biol. **27**, 107A (1965).
TOBIN, W.E., SANDLER, S.G.: Depression of muscle spindle function with vincristine. Nature (Lond.) **212**, 90—91 (1966).
TOBIN, W.E., SANDLER, S.G.: Neurophysiologic alterations induced by vincristine (NSC-67574). Cancer Chemother. Rep. **52**, 519—526 (1968).

UEDA, M., SAWAI, M., KAWAKAMI, M., MINESITA, T., TAKEDA, H.: Pressure mechanism of vincristine sulfate. Jap. J. Pharmacol. **19**, 324—325 (1969).

UY, Q. L., MOEN, T. H., JOHNS, R. J., OWENS, A. H., JR.: Vincristine neurotoxicity in rodents. Johns Hopkins med. J. **121**, 349—360 (1967).

VAITKEVICIUS, V. K., REED, M. L.: Clinical studies with podophyllum compounds SPI-77 (NSC-72274) and SPG-827 (NSC-42076). Cancer Chemother. Rep. **50**, 565—571 (1966).

VALERIOTE, F. A., BRUCE, W. R., MEEKER, B. E.: A model for the action of vinblastine *in vivo*. Biophys. J. **6**, 145—152 (1966).

VAN LANCKER, J. L., FLANGAS, A. L., ALLEN, J.: Metabolic effects of vinblastine. I. The effect of vinblastine on nucleic acid synthesis in spleen and bone marrow. Lab. Invest. **15**, 1291—1300 (1966).

VASILIEV, J. M., GELFAND, I. M., GUELSTEIN, V. I.: Initiation of DNA synthesis in cell cultures by colcemid. Proc. nat. Acad. Sci. (Wash.) **68**, 977—979 (1971).

VENDITTI, J. M., GOLDIN, A.: Drug synergism in antineoplastic chemotherapy. In: GOLDIN, A., HAWKING, F., SCHNITZER, R. J. (Eds.): Advances in chemotherapy, Vol. 1. New York: Academic Press 1964.

WAGNER, E. K., ROIZMAN, B.: Effect of the vinca alkaloids on RNA synthesis in human cells *in vitro*. Science **162**, 569—570 (1968).

WARNECKE, P., SEEBER, S.: Angriffspunkte von Vinca-alkaloiden im Protein- und Nucleinsäurestoffwechsel. Z. Krebsforsch. **71**, 361—367 (1968).

WEISENBERG, R. C., BORISY, G. G., TAYLOR, E. W.: The colchicine-binding protein of mammalian brain and its relation to microtubules. Biochemistry **7**, 4466—4478 (1968).

WEISENBERG, R. C., TAYLOR, E. W.: The binding of guanosine nucleotide to microtubule subunit protein purified from porcine brain. Fed. Proc. **27**, 299 (1968).

WEISENBERG, R. C., TIMASHEFF, S.: Aggregation of microtubule protein induced by vinblastine. Biophys. J. **9**, 174A (1969).

WHITE, J. G.: Effects of colchicine and vinca alkaloids on human platelets. II. Changes in the dense tubular system and formation of an unusual inclusion in incubated cells. Amer. J. Pathol. **53**, 447—461 (1968).

WIERNIK, P. H., MCLEOD, R. M.: Vinblastine effect on nucleic acids and ribonuclease of lymphoid tissue. Proc. Soc. exp. Biol. (N.Y.) **119**, 118—120 (1965).

WILSON, L.: Properties of colchicine binding protein from chick embryo brain. Interaction with vinca alkaloids and podophyllotoxin. Biochemistry **9**, 4999—5007 (1970).

WILSON, L., BRYAN, J., RUBY, A., MAZIA, D.: Precipitation of proteins by vinblastine and calcium ions. Proc. nat. Acad. Sci. (Wash.) **66**, 807—814 (1970).

WILSON, L., FRIEDKIN, M.: The biochemical events of mitosis. II. The *in vivo* and *in vitro* binding of colchicine in grasshopper embryos and its possible relation to inhibition of mitosis. Biochemistry **6**, 3126—3135 (1967).

WUNDERLICH, F., PEYK, D.: Antimitotic agents and macronuclear division of ciliates. III. The effect of colchicine on synchronized *Tetrahymena pyriformis* GL. Experientia (Basel) **25**, 1278—1280 (1969).

WUNDERLICH, F., SPETH, V.: Antimitotic agents and macronuclear division of ciliates. IV. Reassembly of microtubules in macronuclei of *Tetrahymena* adapting to colchicine. Protoplasma (Wien) **70**, 139—152 (1970).

YESAIR, D. W., KOHNER, F. A., ROGERS, W. I., BARONOWSKY, P., KENSLER, C. J.: Relationship of phthalanilide-lipid complexes to uptake and retention of 2-chloro-4′,4″-di(2-imidazolin-2-yl) terephthalanilide (NSC-60339) by sensitive and resistant P388 leukemia cells. Cancer Res. **26**, 202—207 (1966).

Chapter 68

L-Asparaginase: Basic Aspects

M. K. PATTERSON, JR.

Introduction

L-Asparaginase (L-asparagine amidohydrolase, E.C. 3.5.1.1) catalyzes the hydrolysis of L-asparagine to yield L-aspartic acid and ammonia. The enzyme was first reported by LANG (1904), who demonstrated its activity in various beef tissues. Confirmatory observations with tissues from horse and pig were reported a few years later by VON FURTH and FRIEDMANN (1910). The observation most pertinent to the current discussion, however, was that of CLEMENTI (1921, 1922), who found that of numerous blood sera tested only that of the guinea pig showed L-asparaginase activity.

In 1953, KIDD (1953a, b) reported that injections of guinea pig serum caused regression of certain transplanted mouse and rat tumors (i.e., the 6C3HED lymphoma of C3H mice, the Lorenz lymphoma II of strain A mice, and the Murphy-Sturm lymphosarcoma of the rat). The guinea pig serum was being used as a source of complement to enhance the activity of heterologous antiserum made against the tumors. The tumor inhibitory action of the serum, however, could not be explained on an immunological basis. Moreover, sera other than guinea pig failed to cause tumor regressions. Subsequent studies using transplanted ACMCA2 fibrosarcoma (JAMESON et al., 1956), Murphy-Sturm lymphosarcoma (JAMESON et al., 1958), and Walker 256 carcinoma (KWAK et al., 1961) in rats confirmed these observations. Studies by NEUMAN and McCOY (1956) showed that certain tumor cells had a nutritional requirement for L-asparagine. In attempts to cultivate Walker 256 carcinoma cells in tissue culture, they found that the amino acids described by EAGLE (1955) as essential for cells in culture failed to support cell proliferation and that a yeast extract was an essential supplement. Fractionation of the extract revealed L-asparagine to be the active constituent. A similar requirement for L-asparagine by the Jensen sarcoma (McCOY et al., 1959a) and the L5178Y mouse leukemia (HALEY and FISCHER, 1961) was subsequently demonstrated. These early observations and basic considerations have been reviewed by BROOME (1968a), MARQUARDT (1968), ADAMSON and FABRO (1968a), BAUER (1969), LABOUREUR (1969), KIDD (1970), COONEY and HANDSCHUMACHER (1970), and WEINBERGER (1971).

On the basis of CLEMENTI's earlier findings that guinea pig serum contained L-asparaginase activity while other sera did not, BROOME (1961, 1963a) compared the properties of the tumor inhibitory agent of the serum with those of its L-asparaginase. In all properties tested, the two were identical. Thus, BROOME concluded that L-asparaginase of guinea pig serum was responsible for its antilymphoma effect. Confirmatory studies were provided by HOLMQUIST (1962) using Agouti serum, by MASHBURN and WRISTON (1963) using partially purified guinea pig serum L-asparaginase, and by OLD et al. (1963) using sera from three distinct genera other than the guinea pig. Furthermore, BOYSE et al. (1963) reported that a number of mouse leukemias, including some spontaneous ones, were sensitive to suppression by guinea pig serum.

Studies on the Jensen sarcoma (McCOY et al., 1959b) and the 6C3HED mouse lymphosarcoma (BROOME, 1963b) in cell culture showed that continued cultivation of these cells in the absence of L-asparagine resulted in a cell population that no longer showed a requirement for the amino acid. Moreover, the "variant" 6C3HED cells, when transplanted *in vivo*, were resistant to the regressive effects of guinea pig serum. PATTERSON et al. (1965) also showed that the "variant" Jensen sarcoma cells were resistant to the serum in a culture system and that addition of the guinea pig serum to Jensen sarcoma cells ultimately resulted in a "variant" population. On the basis of these studies it was concluded that L-asparaginase catalyzed the hydrolysis of exogenous L-asparagine, thus creating a nutritional deficiency of the amino acid. Similar "variants" of the 6C3HED lymphosarcoma had previously been reported by KIDD (1958) in mice bearing the tumor and injected with "subcurative" doses of guinea pig serum. DOLOWY et al. (1968) have also reported development of a resistant "variant" of the Walker 256 carcinoma in rats treated with guinea pig serum.

Impetus for further research on L-asparaginase as a practical therapeutic measure was provided by the observation of MASHBURN and WRISTON (1964) that L-asparaginase from *Escherichia coli* (TSUJI, 1957) also inhibited tumor growth. Efficacy of the enzyme at the clinical level was supplied by the studies of a group of physicians at the University of Recife in Brazil who first treated a patient with Agouti serum (DEBARROS et al., 1965; cf. OLD et al., 1968), by DOLOWY et al. (1966) using partially purified guinea pig serum L-asparaginase, by OETTGEN et al. (1967) and by HILL et al. (1967) using *E. coli* L-asparaginase preparations. The results were encouraging and provided a foundation for subsequent research in "amino acid depletion" therapy.

In addition to its antitumor effect, the enzyme has recently been shown to have beneficial properties in autoimmune disease therapy (see Section on Immunological effects) and to inhibit the multiplication of certain viruses (e.g., Rous sarcoma virus) (LI et al., 1970) and vaccinia and myxoma poxviruses (MARAL and WERNER, 1971).

Assay of Enzyme Activity

The most commonly used assay for L-asparaginase is that published by MEISTER (1955) in which enzyme, L-asparagine, and sodium borate buffer (pH 8.5) are incubated at 37° for 5 to 60 min. The reaction is stopped by addition of trichloroacetic acid (TCA); released ammonia is determined by microdiffusion and nesslerization or by a direct method using alkaline-hypochlorite reagent (CHANEY and MARBACH, 1962). A more direct and sensitive (0.01 I.U./ml) method involving the spectrophotometric measurement at 274 mμ of the decomposition of 5-diazo-4-oxo-4-norvaline by the enzyme has been reported by JACKSON and HANDSCHUMACHER (1970). Adaptations of methods designed for the assay of L-asparagine, in which rate-limiting amounts of the enzyme are used, followed by measurements of the loss of substrate or appearance of product, have also been used for measuring L-asparaginase activity. The most sensitive (0.001 I.U./ml) of the methods appears to be a coupled reaction that measures aspartic acid in the presence of excess glutamic-oxaloacetate transaminase, α-ketoglutarate, and malic dehydrogenase (KOJIMA and WACKER, 1969; COONEY et al., 1970) or the reductive amination of α-ketoglutaric acid by ammonia in the presence of L-glutamic dehydrogenase (COONEY et al., 1971) and recording at 340 mμ the rate of oxidation of NADH.

A similar procedure where the decrease of NADH is measured fluorometrically has also been reported (NAHORSKI, 1971). Other methods used to measure substrate disappearance of product formation are: automated ion exchange columns (BENSON et al., 1967), formate ion exchange columns (PATTERSON et al., 1963; PATTERSON and ORR, 1967; PRUSINER and MILNER, 1970), and alumina gels (RAVEL et al., 1962; HOLCENBERG, 1969), as well as ion exchange paper (SCHWARTZ, J.H. et al., 1966) and electrophoresis, either directly (BROOME, 1968b) or of the trinitrophenyl derivatives of L-asparagine and L-aspartic acid (BROOME, 1966). EHRMAN et al. (1971) and FROHWEIN et al. (1971) have measured the disappearance of L-aspartyl-β-hydroxamic acid, a substrate for asparaginase, using acidic ferric chloride as an assay system.

Distribution and Antitumor Activity

L-Asparaginase has been found widely distributed in nature. Extracts of plant rootlets (GROVER and CHIBNALL, 1927; LEES and BLAKENEY, 1970) and seedlings (KRETOVICH, 1958), tissues of fish (STEENSHOLT, 1944), birds (CLEMENTI, 1922), pigs and horses (VON FURTH and FRIEDMAN, 1910), and rodents (GREENSTEIN and CARTER, 1946; BONETTI et al., 1969) show activity. In blood sera, enzyme activity has been found only in certain rodents of the superfamily Cavioidea (OLD et al., 1963) and in new world monkeys, but not in old world monkeys (BROOME, 1968a; PETERS et al., 1970). Those asparaginases which have been tested for antitumor activity are included in Table 1.

Table 1. *Antitumor activity of various L-asparaginases*

L-Asparaginase source	Antitumor activity	Tumor tested	Reference
Aspergillus terreus	+	Walker 256	DE-ANGELI et al. (1970)
Bacillus coagulans	—	6C3HED	MASHBURN and WRISTON (1964)
Erwinia aroidea	+	Not specified	PETERSON et al. (1969b)
Erwinia cartovora	+	6C3HED	WADE et al. (1968)
Escherichia coli	±	(see text)	(see text)
Fusarium tricinctum	—	6C3HED	SCHEETZ et al. (1971)
Mycobacterium:			
tuberculosis, $H_{37}R_a$	+	Yoshida	JAYARAM et al. (1968)
tuberculosis, $H_{37}R_v$	+	Yoshida	REDDY et al. (1969)
Serratia marcescens	+	6C3HED—RG-1	BOYD and PHILLIPS (1971)
			HEINEMANN and HOWARD (1969)
			ROWLEY and WRISTON (1967)
Yeast	—	6C3HED	BROOME (1965)
Chicken liver	+	6C3HED	OHNUMA et al. (1967)
Guinea pig — sera	+	6C3HED	SULD and HERBUT (1965)
Guinea pig — liver	+	6C3HED	SULD and HERBUT (1965)

Bacteria possessing activity are: *Mycobacteria phlei* (HALPERN, 1957), *Pseudomonas fluorescens* (DEGROOT and LICHTENSTEIN, 1960), *Brucella abortus* (ALTENBERN and HOUSEWRIGHT, 1954), *Pseudomonas species* (EVSEEV and NIKOLAEV, 1968), *Streptococcus mitis* (KRZEMINSKI, 1969), *Staphylococcus aureus* (MIKUCKI et al., 1968), *Bacterium cadaveris* (EREMENKO et al., 1968), and *Alcaligenes eutrophus* (ALLISON et al., 1971), as well as certain fungi, *Penicillium camemberti* (DOX, 1909) and *Aspergillus niger* (BOCH, 1928). Those tested for antitumor activity are included in Table 1. Mass screening by BILIMORIA (1969) of 28 coliforms and by

PETERSON and CIEGLER (1969a) of 123 strains representing 44 bacterial species have demonstrated the wide distribution of asparaginase, with varying levels of enzyme activity in bacteria.

The most extensively studied of the bacterial groups have been the various strains of *E. coli* (GALAEV and KHARATS, 1969). Following the initial studies of MASHBURN and WRISTON (1964) on *E. coli* B, it was shown that two L-asparaginases (ROBERTS et al., 1966) designated EC-1 and EC-2 by CAMPBELL et al. (1967) were present in the extracts, with only one (EC-2) showing antitumor activity. Similarly, two asparaginases have been found in *E. coli* K-12 (SCHWARTZ, J.H. et al., 1966; CEDAR and SCHWARTZ, 1967), though various strains exhibited wide quantitative differences in the two (ROBINSON and BERK, 1969). Moreover, wide differences in the ratios of EC-1 and EC-2 activities have been shown to result from varying the culture media and conditions (BILIMORIA, 1969). *Aerobacter aerogenes* and *Pseudomonas* species, however, had EC-1 activity, but no detectable EC-2 activity. Avirulent *Mycobacterium tuberculosis* $H_{37}R_a$ also possessed two asparaginases with only one showing antitumor activity, while the virulent strain, $H_{37}R_v$, possessed only one asparaginase which was inactive against tumor and was identical to the inactive enzyme in the $H_{37}R_a$ strain (JAYARAM et al., 1968; REDDY et al., 1969). Two asparaginases, one isolated from *E. coli* strain ATCC 9637 and another from strain ATCC 11303 and designated asparaginase A and B, respectively, were of the EC-2 type only (ARENS et al., 1970). There was no sign of the EC-1 type, though it might have been lost in the extraction procedure. Two asparaginases were found in rat liver (GREENSTEIN and PRICE, 1949), one of which was activated by phosphate ion, but not by α-keto acids, while the other required the presence of an α-keto acid for activity. Neither of the asparaginases in *E. coli* B (CAMPBELL et al., 1967) nor the asparaginase of *M. tuberculosis* $H_{37}R_v$ (JAYARAM et al., 1968) required α-keto acids or were affected by phosphate ion.

Isolation and Purification

Isolation of L-asparaginase from microorganisms has been achieved by harvesting mass cultures and subjecting them to cell rupture and fractionation with ammonium sulfate, chromatography, and organic solvents. Though highly purified preparations were obtained through use of gel filtration and ion exchange techniques (ROBERTS et al., 1968; WHELAN and WRISTON, 1969; WRISTON, 1970), the stability of the enzyme in organic solvents (RAUENBUSCH et al., 1970) has resulted in procedures yielding crystalline materials. Suitable crystallizing solvents, such as ethanol (HO, P.P.K. et al., 1969, 1970; TANAKA et al., 1970), 2-methylpentane-2,4-diol (ARENS et al., 1970), and polyethyleneglycol (WAGNER et al., 1969a) have been reported. A possibly faster and simpler purification method using affinity chromatography based on specific adsorption and desorption on a matrix (Sepharose 6 B) covalently linked to a spacer (putrescine or hexamethylenediamine) and enzyme inhibitor (D-asparagine) has recently been described (KRISTIANSEN et al., 1970).

Though limited in utility as a source of L-asparaginase for therapeutic purposes, guinea pig serum enzyme has certain properties that differ from the enzyme derived from microorganisms that may be desirable. A 7-fold purification of guinea pig serum was reported by MEISTER (1955), a 138-fold purification by MARDASHEV and SHAO-HUA (1962), a 220-fold purification by TOWER et al. (1963), a 400-fold purification by MASHBURN and WRISTON (1970), a 1419-fold purification by SULD and HERBUT (1965), and recently a 3000-fold purification by SULD and HERBUT (1970a). Both the 900-fold and the 3000-fold, but not the 1419-fold preparation, appeared to be similar when judged by the same physical criteria, but differed in their amino acid composition (see Section on Properties and Structure). Attempts to fractionate a 50-fold purified guinea pig liver asparaginase by methods similar to that used in obtaining the 3000-fold purified serum asparaginase were unsuccessful (SULD and HERBUT, 1970a). Digestion of the liver preparation with papain, however, yielded enzyme similar in all parameters tested, including antitumor effects, to that of the purified serum asparaginase. Attempts to purify guinea pig liver and serum asparaginase by immunological techniques have also been described by SULD and HERBUT (1970b). Essentially quantitative recovery of the enzyme with retention of enzyme activity in the antigen-antibody complex was obtained, but concomitant losses of activity occurred when attempts were made to dissociate the immune complex and separate the enzyme and antibody moieties. The L-asparaginase-antibody complexes, solubilized by digestion with papain and purified by DEAE-cellulose chromatography, were effective against "Gardner lymphosarcoma".

Properties and Structure

Some properties of L-asparaginase derived from various sources are shown in Table 2. It now appears that the *E. coli* enzyme has an approximate molecular weight of 133,000 (cf. WRISTON, 1971a). Recent studies by WRISTON (1971b) and ARENS et al. (1970) using end group analysis indicate that the enzyme has four subunits (molecular weight 33,000) rather than six (molecular weight 22,000), as had previously been reported (WHELAN and WRISTON, 1969). Moreover, the

Table 2. *Properties of L-asparaginases derived from various sources*

Property	*E. coli*[a]	*M. tuberculosis*, $H_{37}R_a$[c]	*E. carotovora*[d]	*F. tricinctum*[e]	G. pig[f]
Molecular wt.	120—141,000		130,000	160—171,000	138,000
K_m(M)	$1.15—1.25 \times 10^{-5}$	2.0×10^{-3}		5.2×10^{-4}	7.2×10^{-5}
Isoelectric point	4.9—5.2		8.79	5.18	3.6—4.5
pH optimum	7.2—8.4	9.6		7.5—8.7	7.5—8.5
Sed. coeff.	7.5—7.9		7.43		6.55
D-Asparaginase	6—9%[b]	none	5%	none	yes
L-Glutaminase	1—4%	none	yes	none	none
Carbohydrate	none				yes (?)[g]

[a] Range of values. WHELAN and WRISTON, 1969; WRISTON, 1970, 1971; HO, P.P.K. et al., 1970; FRANK et al., 1970; ARENS et al., 1970; TANAKA et al., 1970; RAUENBUSCH et al., 1971; LABOURER et al., 1971.
[b] MASHBURN and LANDIN, 1970.
[c] JAYARAM et al., 1968; REDDY et al., 1969.
[d] NORTH et al., 1969; MILLER, D.S. et al., 1971.
[e] SCHEETZ et al., 1971.
[f] YELLIN and WRISTON, 1966; WRISTON, 1970.
[g] SULD and HERBUT, 1970a.

stoichiometry of binding of 5-C^{14}-diazo-4-oxo-L-norvaline (DONV), which acts as a substrate and binds irreversibly to inactivate the catalytic sites of the enzyme, indicates that there are four active sites per molecule (JACKSON and HANDSCHUMACHER, 1970). Studies by ARENS et al. (1970) on asparaginases A and B isolated from *E. coli* strains ATCC 9637 and 11303, respectively, have suggested that both enzymes consist of isoenzymes with different isoelectric points, with asparaginase B containing the more acidic isoenzymes. Whether this is characteristic of all asparaginases must await further study, since GREENQUIST and WRISTON (1970) have reported that the subunits of the *E. coli* B enzyme are identical. The difference may reside in the amide content of the subunits.

An interesting property of L-asparaginase is the ease with which it will reconstitute after being dissociated and denatured. KIRSCHBAUM et al. (1969) showed the enzyme dissociated either by dilution (1 mg/ml or less), by lowering the pH to 4, by raising it above pH 11, by increasing the ionic strength, or by adding sodium dodecyl sulfate or cysteine. WHELAN and WRISTON (1969) also observed dissociation of the enzyme by dilution and by urea. Reconstitution occurred following dialysis or by simple dilution of the urea-protein solution (FRANK et al., 1970). In contrast, however, these last investigators were unable to dissociate their crystalline enzyme by dilution to concentrations as low as 15 μg/ml. Reversible dissociation also occurs in the presence of guanidinium chloride, lithium chloride, or sodium perchlorate (RAUENBUSCH et al., 1971). Studies on the effects of these denaturing agents on the enzyme to determine the number of polypeptide chains which constitute the native enzyme and to define its dissociate behavior have confirmed the presence of four disulfide bonds (HO, P. P. K. et al., 1970), and have indicated that dissociation occurs prior to reduction of disulfide linkages (FRANK et al., 1970; LABOUREUR et al., 1971). The disulfide linkages appear, therefore, to be intramolecular and not intermolecular. Recent attempts have been made to maintain subunits (HANDSCHUMACHER, 1971) as an adjunct to therapy through permeation of the enzyme into extravascular spaces. Dissociation of the enzyme followed by ultrafiltration through a semipermeable membrane and treatment with tetranitromethane, however, have been unsuccessful (LIU and HANDSCHUMACHER, 1971).

While the relatively wide range of isoelectric points of L-asparaginase may reflect differences in techniques of measurement, the studies of MASHBURN and LANDIN (1970) suggest that they may be attributed to variations in *E. coli* strains and purification procedures. Moreover, these studies suggest that a therapeutic advantage of longer *in vivo* half life are obtained from low isoelectric point preparations. An exception is found, however, with preparations from *Erwinia carotovora*.

The sedimentation coefficient, intrinsic viscosity, and low ultraviolet circular dichroic spectrum of L-asparaginase are in the range of values expected for a globular protein (FRANK et al., 1970). The spectrum is also suggestive of an α-helix-like form. Similar characteristics of *E. carotovora* asparaginase have been reported (MILLER, D. S. et al., 1971).

An apparent intrinsic property of L-asparaginase is its hydrolysis of carbon-nitrogen bonds of the *N*-carboxyl, hydrazide, diazoketone, and nitrile type, as well as ω-ester bonds. The various substrates tested and found to be reactive are:

A. D-Asparagine

Both bacterial (cf. MASHBURN and LANDIN, 1970) and guinea pig serum enzyme (TOWER et al., 1963) hydrolyze D-asparagine at rates that are 5 to 9 % and 5 %, respectively, of that seen for L-asparagine hydrolysis. With crystalline *E. coli* preparations, competitive inhibition by D-asparagine of the hydrolysis of the L-isomer indicates a common enzyme site.

B. Glutamine

E. coli, but not guinea pig serum enzyme, hydrolyzes L-glutamine at a level of 1 to 4 % of the rate of that of L-asparagine (cf. MASHBURN and LANDIN, 1970). These amidase activities have not been separated by several different methods of enzyme purification, by electrofocusing, or by partial heat inactivation (CAMPBELL et al., 1967; CAMPBELL and MASHBURN, 1969); furthermore, titration of the active center with DONV eliminates both enzyme activities (cf. COONEY and HANDSCHUMACHER, 1970). The two activities, however, have different pH optima, the glutaminase activity being 6-fold greater at pH 8.7 than at pH 5.0, while asparaginase activity is almost constant over this pH range. As a result of these studies, MILLER, H. K. and BALIS (1969) concluded that pH dependency is due to differences in the ionic environment of the enzyme such that L-glutamine hydrolysis requires the removal of a proton from a grouping near the catalytic site. Minimal D-glutamine hydrolysis (0.1 %) has also been reported (NAKAMURA et al., 1971).

C. 5-Diazo-4-Oxo-L-Norvaline (DONV)

This analog of asparagine appears to react with *E. coli* asparaginase in three distinct ways (JACKSON and HANDSCHUMACHER, 1970): it binds covalently at or near the catalytic site, causing irreversible inactivation of the enzyme, it binds to sites other than the catalytic site, and it is decomposed to form 5-hydroxyl-4-oxo-L-norvaline and nitrogen. L-β-Cyanoalanine competitively inhibits the latter reaction and suggests that the two substrates are hydrolyzed at the same active site.

D. L-β-Cyanoalanine

L-Asparaginase from guinea pig serum or *E. coli* catalyzes the hydrolysis of L-β-cyanoalanine to aspartic acid and ammonia (LAUINGER and RESSLER, 1970). D-Asparagine, carbobenzoxy-L-asparagine, and L-aspartic acid effectively inhibit this nitrilase activity. Moreover, the L-β-cyanoalanine inhibits L-asparaginase activity.

E. β-Aspartylhydroxamate

The hydrolysis of β-aspartylhydroxamate proceeds at a maximal rate that is 1.6-fold greater than the rate for hydrolysis of L-asparagine (EHRMAN et al., 1971). The enzyme also catalyzes the synthesis of the hydroxamate from hydroxylamine and asparagine or aspartic acid. These reactions suggest a mechanism involving a β-aspartyl-enzyme intermediate and are consistent with product formation proceeding by a "ping-pong" mechanism.

F. β-Methyl-L-Aspartate

Crystalline L-asparaginase from *E. coli* A-1-3 hydrolyzes β-methyl-L-aspartate to release aspartate at about 0.3 % of the rate of L-asparagine (NAKAMURA et al., 1971).

G. Macromolecules

L-Asparaginase reportedly releases carbohydrate from fetuim, a glycoprotein with an *N*-glycoside bond between asparagine and a carbohydrate moiety, but not from porcine submaxillary gland glycoprotein, which has an *O*-glycoside bond between serine or threonine and a carbohydrate moiety (BOSMANN and KESSEL, 1970). Such intramolecular hydrolytic activity of the enzyme deserves further study because of implications relating to serum and membrane glycoproteins.

KESSEL (1971) has also reported conversion of asparaginyl-tRNA^{asn} to aspartyl-tRNA^{asn} in the presence of L-asparaginase.

These findings are consistent with the possibility that the amidase activity (L- and D-asparagine and L-glutamine), diazo-4-oxo-L-norvaline decomposition, and nitrilase activity are all catalyzed at the same site. Both guinea pig serum and *M. tuberculosis* $H_{37}R_a$ asparaginases are effective antitumor preparations, but the *Fusarium tricinctum* preparation is not effective; none of the three has shown either L-glutaminase or D-asparaginase activity (Table 2). *A. eutrophus* enzyme, on the other hand, has broad substrate specificity with relative activities of 100, 53, 90, and 103% for L-asparagine, D-asparagine, L-glutamine, and L-alanyl-L-asparagine, respectively (ALLISON et al., 1971).

E. coli L-asparaginase is stable in aqueous solutions at neutral pH, but loses its activity at 60° within 1 h (RAUENBUSCH et al., 1970). Polyethyleneglycol and glycine, however, stabilize the enzyme at this temperature. L-Asparagine appears to accelerate thermal denaturation, while tryptone broth protects the enzyme (COONEY and DAVIS, 1970). Partial resistance to inactivation is also observed following treatment with picric acid, trichloroacetic acid, and perchloric acid.

The amino acid composition for L-asparaginase derived from various sources is shown in Table 3. The values reported for *E. coli* (columns 1—5) agree reasonably well, with the exception of tryptophan and cystine. Since both are present in such low amounts and are difficult to determine with accuracy, this exception is not surprising. The data would seem most consistent with the presence of one tryptophan and one cystine residue per subunit enzyme. The absence of sulfhydryl groups is consistent with the lack of effect of *p*-chloromercuribenzoate, *N*-ethyl-

Table 3. *Amino acid composition of L-asparaginase*[a]

Amino acid	(1)	(2)	(3)[b]	(4)[b]	(5)[b]	(6)	(7)	(8)[b]
Alanine	120	132	114	125	112	184	72	111
Arginine	36	28	29	30	27	46	45	57
Aspartic acid	180	204	177	202	172	166	90	106
Cystine/2	6	8	6	0	5	—	18	62
Glutamic acid	84	76	74	74	63	166	108	129
Glycine	108	116	97	107	108	157	90	126
Histidine	12	12	11	11	10	37	27	29
Isoleucine	48	48	46	46	39	111	45	56
Leucine	84	88	80	88	79	111	116	239
Lysine	84	84	74	84	79	64	54	52
Methionine	24	16	17	22	19	18	9	34
Phenylalanine	36	32	29	30	29	55	36	38
Proline	48	44	46	50	42	64	90	70
Serine	60	60	57	62	51	101	108	116
Threonine	120	132	114	133	109	111	81	78
Tryptophane	12	4	6	4	tr.	—	9	32
Tyrosine	48	44	40	44	40	46	18	—
Valine	120	140	114	124	100	120	90	104

[a] References in parentheses.
[b] Calculated to nearest integer and data normalized for molecular wt. reported by author.
References: (1) WHELAN and WRISTON, 1969, mol/133,000 g, *E. coli* B, E.C.2.; (2) Ho, P.P.K. et al., 1970, mol/133,200 g, *E. coli* B (ATCC 13706); (3) ARENS et al., 1970; IRION and ARENS, 1970, calculated mol/120,000 g, *E. coli* (ATCC 9637 and 11303); (4) TANAKA et al., 1970, calculated mol/141,000 g, *E. coli*, HAP; (5) HILL et al., 1970, calculated mol/139,500 g, *E. coli*, HAP; (6) SCHEETZ et al., 1971, mol/165,000 g, *F. tricinctum*; (7) YELLIN and WRISTON, 1966, mol/140,000 g, 900 × guinea pig; (8) SULD and HERBUT, 1970a, calculated mol/140,000 g, 3000 × guinea pig.

maleimide, and iodoacetamide, as well as other specific sulfhydryl inhibitors (cf. ARENS et al., 1970). A recent report that 50 μmoles acrolein/ml, but not 5 μmoles/ml, causes 30 to 40 % inhibition of *E. coli* enzyme activity is an apparent exception and must await further explanation (BILIMORIA and NISBET, 1971). In contrast, guinea pig serum enzyme is inhibited by β-chloromercurisulfonate and $HgCl_2$, but not by *N*-ethylmaleimide (TOWER et al., 1963).

The amino acid composition of *F. tricinctum* L-asparaginase, a preparation without antitumor effect, is shown in Table 3 for comparative purposes. Notably greater levels of glutamic acid, histidine, and isoleucine are present compared to the *E. coli* enzyme (SCHEETZ et al., 1971). Moreover, both galactosamine and glucosamine are present, while no carbohydrate is detectable in the latter enzyme (ARENS et al., 1970). Guinea pig serum asparaginase also appears to be a glycoprotein (SULD and HERBUT, 1970a).

Amino acid sequence studies of *E. coli* asparaginase have shown leucine to be *N*-terminal and the following sequence (ARENS et al., 1970): Leu-Pro-Asn-Ile-Thr-Ile-Leu-Ala-Thr-Gly-(Gly ?, Val, Ile, Ala)... Tyrosine appears to be *C*-terminal and on the basis of carboxypeptidase A digestion, is sequentially followed by glycine, isoleucine, phenylalanine, and asparaginase (WRISTON, 1971b). *Erwinia aroidea* L-asparaginase, which has antitumor activity and no immunological cross reactivity with *E. coli* L-asparaginase, has L-alanine as the *N*-terminal amino acid (STAERK et al., 1971).

Attempts to identify the amino acid residues associated with the active site by modification of the residues with chemicals such as glyoxal for the arginine residue, tetranitromethane for the tyrosine residue, peroxide-dioxane for the tryptophane residue, and monochlorotrifluoro-*p*-quinone for the amino group have been reported (NISHIMURA et al., 1971). Their results suggest that the modification of four amino groups in the enzyme molecule results in inactivation without dissociation into subunits. This is consistent with the previously related findings of JACKSON and HANDSCHUMACHER (1970) that the enzyme has four active sites. It is of interest, however, that treatment of asparaginase with nitrous acid, which results in removal of the α-NH_2 groups of lysine, does not affect enzyme activity (WAGNER et al., 1969b).

Pharmacological Effects

Most evidence supports a concept that the basis for the effect of L-asparaginase as a therapeutic agent is the hydrolysis of L-asparagine in extracellular spaces, mainly in plasma. Cells dependent upon extracellular L-asparagine, when deprived of the amino acid, cease metabolic functions and die. Studies using sensitive and resistant tumors in rats and mice have shown below-normal asparagine levels in the sera of animals bearing the sensitive tumors and a more rapid clearance of large intravenous doses of the amino acid (MILLER, H.K. et al., 1970). Following a single parenteral administration of enzyme, circulating L-asparagine is rapidly cleared from the plasma (BROOME, 1968b, c; MILLER, H.K. et al., 1969; COONEY et al., 1970; OHNUMA, 1970). Glutamine levels also drop, reaching zero levels after asparagine levels have done so, but in contrast to asparagine begin to reappear even though relatively high serum asparaginase levels are present (MILLER, H.K. et al., 1969). Additionally, in leukemic patients, the concentration of virtually every other amino acid in the sera reportedly increases 20 to 400 % by 2 to 6 h after asparaginase injection (100 I.U./kg) (RUDMAN et al., 1971).

An important factor in the efficacy of asparaginase as an antitumor agent against sensitive tumors is the clearance rate of the enzyme from the plasma. The rate of clearance appears to be dependent upon the recipient species (Table 4). In the same species, however, other factors effect changes in the clearance rate. For instance, *E. coli* preparations having low isoelectric points also have slower clearance rates (Mashburn and Landin, 1970), while *Serratia marcescens* enzyme is cleared 2 to 3 times more slowly than *E. coli* enzyme (Boyd and Phillips, 1971).

Table 4. *Plasma half-life of* L-*asparaginase*[a]

Animal	Condition	Enzyme source	Plasma half-life (h)
Dog	Normal	*E. coli*	18—23 (10, 13)
Guinea pig	Normal	*E. coli*	4.5 (13)
Human	Tumor	*E. coli*	12—24 (6, 7, 8, 9, 10, 13)
Monkey	Normal	*E. coli*	8.0 (12)
Mouse	Normal	*E. coli*	2.5—6.0 (2, 4, 11, 13)
		S. marcescens	6—8 (1)
		G. pig	19—26 (2, 3, 9)
		Yeast	0.5 (3)
	LDH virus	*E. coli*	25 (10)
	Tumor	*E. coli*	18.7—29.7 (4)
Rabbit	Normal	*E. coli*	4 (10)
Rat	Normal	*E. coli*	1.5—3.0 (5, 10, 13)
	Normal	*E. carotovora*	1.5 (5)
Sheep	Normal	*E. coli*	5.0 (5)
	Normal	*E. carotovora*	2.0 (5)

[a] References in parentheses.

References: (1) Boyd and Phillips, 1971. (2) Boyse et al., 1967. (3) Broome, 1965. (4) Broome, 1968. (5) Hall, 1970. (6) Haskell et al., 1970. (7) Hill et al., 1969. (8) Mashburn and Landin, 1970. (9) Ohnuma et al., 1967. (10) Pütter, 1970. (11) Riley et al., 1970. (12) Schein, 1969. (13) Schwartz, M.K., 1970; Schwartz, M.K. et al., 1970.

Asparaginase preparations not showing antitumor effects, such as *F. tricinctum* (Scheetz et al., 1971) and yeast (Broome, 1965) both have half-lives of approximately 30 min. Riley (1970) has shown that a benign LDH-elevating virus, which is limited to mice as hosts, markedly impairs the clearance of the enzyme. Moreover, mice implanted with EARAD 1 tumors and intentionally infected with LDH virus show 100 % survival after a single dose of asparaginase at 30 days (Riley et al., 1970); a 5 % survival is seen in asparaginase-injected animals bearing the tumor without virus. This effect does not appear to be entirely due to clearance rate, since simulation of virus-impaired clearance by injecting enzyme at 4 h intervals failed to give the expected therapeutic effect. Analysis of the disappearance of amino acids from the plasma suggests that LDH virus potentiates the glutaminase activity of the enzyme, since in virus-infected animals both asparagine and glutamine completely disappear, whereas in the absence of the virus only asparagine completely disappears. The studies of Miller, H. K. et al. (1969), however, showed complete hydrolysis of both amides in plasma of humans following asparaginase therapy. The possibility that potentiating viruses were present in the latter studies, or that a virus interferes with adaptive glutamine synthesis in the former, was not eliminated.

The mechanism of plasma clearance of asparaginase appears to be immunological, though some clearance probably reflects migration into the extravascular fluids and ultimately sequestration in organs. Studies by Pütter (1970) show that following injection of *E. coli* asparaginase into dogs, all tissues except the brain show increased levels of the enzyme. Also, 24 h after treating mice with asparaginase, BROOME (1968b) reported only small amounts remained in blood or spleen, but five times more asparaginase activity was found in the liver than in untreated controls. The studies by PÜTTER (1970) strongly suggest that "immune-elimination" is largely responsible for the plasma clearance of the enzyme. Clearance rate of the enzyme accelerated following a second injection given after a 1-week interval. Antibodies were detected after a third or fourth injection. They also note, however, that dogs given larger doses of asparaginase did not show an immune response, nor was their clearance rate affected.

A recent report suggests a method of administering L-asparaginase which avoids the clearance and immune response problems. Growth of 6C3HED lymphosarcoma cells was effectively suppressed when the host was given intra-abdominal injections of microencapsulated enzyme (CHANG, 1971).

Immunological Studies

L-Asparaginase has diverse effects on the immunological processes. It is a protein and therefore immunogenic, but because of its enzymic activity it is also potentially immunosuppressive. It is not surprising, therefore, that both phenomena have been observed and appear to be dose dependent.

Immunogenicity relates adversely to the use of asparaginase as a therapeutic agent by development of hypersensitivity reactions, ranging from mild allergic reactions to anaphylactic shock (cf. CAPIZZI et al., 1970; COONEY and HANDSCHUMACHER, 1970; PETERSON, R.G. et al., 1971). Formation of titrating antibodies to the enzyme was first reported by ROBERTS et al. (1966). Treatment with enzyme before tumor implantation renders continued therapy with the enzyme ineffective; when accompanied by cyclophosphamide, an immunosuppressant, activity was retained (VADLAMUDI et al., 1971). In small single doses (e.g., 9 to 15 I.U./mouse) humoral precipitating antibodies to the enzyme form (VADLAMUDI et al., 1970).

Immunosuppression by the enzyme adversely affects its therapeutic efficacy by affecting the natural barrier to metastasis (FIDLER, 1970, 1971; DEODHAR, 1971) or to malignant cell proliferation (NICOLIN and NAPOLI, 1969).

Suppression of humoral antibody formation by asparaginase during the primary immune response has been demonstrated by a number of investigations (SCHWARTZ, R.S., 1969; OHNO and HERSH, 1970a; PRAGER and DERR, 1970; LAUENSTEIN et al., 1970; MARAL et al., 1970). Maximum suppressive effect is seen when asparaginase is given before or immediately after exposure to an antigen (BERENBAUM, 1970; CHAKRABARTY and FRIEDMAN, 1970) and at levels above 200 to 500 I.U./kg (MIURA et al., 1971; KHAN and HILL, 1970). Moreover, while suppression of primary responses by the enzyme is routinely observed, secondary immune responses are not suppressed (MIURA et al., 1971; NELSON et al., 1970).

Suppression of cell-bound immune response was first reported by BERTELLI et al. (1968), who observed an increase in the survival time of skin allografts and xenografts in mice treated with asparaginase. Facilitated grafts of transplanted tumors (SCHULTEN et al., 1969; SCHULTEN and GIRALDO, 1970; BRAMBILLA et al., 1970; MIURA et al., 1971) and skin allografts (HOBIK, 1969; BRAMBILLA et al., 1970; LAUENSTEIN et al., 1970; SHONS et al., 1970; NELSON et al., 1970) into incompatible hosts have been observed. Treatment of the recipients is normally for 1 or 2 weeks before grafting and thereafter until the grafts are rejected. The enzyme is more effective than azathioprine (BRAMBILLA et al., 1970), but less so than antilymphocyte serum (SCHULTEN and GIRALDO, 1970), in inhibiting graft rejections. In contrast to these investigators, St. Pierre et al. (1970) failed to observe prolongation of growth of skin allografts in mice or heart grafts in dogs, even though the recipients were treated with 1000 I.U./kg/day for 7 and 5 days, respectively, before transplantation.

Supporting evidence for suppression of cell-bound immunity by asparaginase is provided by studies of effects, both *in vivo* and *in vitro*, of the enzyme on the immunological reaction of human peripheral blood lymphocytes. Astaldi et al. (1969a) first reported that *E. coli* L-asparaginase inhibited the blast transformation of lymphocyte cultures stimulated by phytohaemagglutinin (PHA). A similar inhibition is observed if the enzyme is given intravenously and the subject's lymphocytes added to PHA and serum from the same subject (McElwain and Hayward, 1969) or if lymphocytes from uninjected subjects are added to PHA and serum from the injected subjects (Astaldi et al., 1969b; Ohno and Hersh, 1970b). Blastogenic response of lymphocytes is not totally lost, since the cells from injected subjects in the presence of serum from uninjected subjects and PHA undergo a normal amount of blastogenesis (Astaldi et al., 1969b). This finding would confirm the observation of Schrek et al. (1967) that L-asparaginase is relatively nontoxic to normal lymphocytes. Similar inhibition of blastogenesis by the enzyme is observed using stimulating antigenic systems such as mixed lymphocyte cultures (Astaldi et al., 1969c), poke weed mitogen (Astaldi et al., 1970), lymphocyte-irradiated fibroblast cultures (Berenbaum et al., 1970), or several specific antigens (Ohno and Hersh, 1970b; Benezra et al., 1970). The timing of the addition of the enzyme to the cultures as well as the concentration are important factors. Maximal inhibition of blastogenesis is obtained when L-asparaginase is added to the cultures at the same time or within several hours after the addition of the antigen (Berenbaum et al., 1970; Burgio et al., 1970) and at concentrations greater than 10 I.U./ml of culture medium (Ohno and Hersh, 1970b; Burgio et al., 1970). A correlation between serum levels of asparaginase and the extent of blastogenesis of lymphocyte cultures has also been established (De Barbieri et al., 1970). After a single injection of 500 I.U./kg, a subject's serum inhibits the lymphocyte transformation within 5 to 10 min after the injection; blastogenesis in the presence of the serum then progressively increases, reaching the original value only after about 2 weeks.

Histological studies have shown that 4 to 8 h following the injection of 1000 I.U. of asparaginase into mice, transient necrosis of lymphoid cells in thymic cortex and the germinal centers of lymph nodes and spleen occurs (Berenbaum, 1970), normal appearance being restored by 24 h. In spite of the widespread cell death, however, the germinal centers of the latter do not lose their hemolytic activity, suggesting that asparaginase is toxic to cells other than those producing antibody (Berenbaum and Bondurant, 1971). Smaller doses of the enzyme (1000 to 2000 I.U./kg total over 1 to 2 weeks) injected into rabbits result in a decrease in the lymphocyte collars and finally a disappearance in the lymphatic follicles of spleen, with a progressive enlargement of the germinal centers (Astaldi et al., 1970, 1971). Similar dosages also produce an increase in the number of plasma cells and a decrease in the number of lymphocytes in the bone marrow (Micou et al., 1970). These observations support the contention that cellular and humoral immunities originate from two separate lymphoid systems. That the two systems react differently to asparaginase injections is further suggested by the observation of Miura et al. (1971) that the ratio of tumor-effective dose to immunosuppressive dose is approximately 1:6 for the suppression of humoral antibody production and 1:50 for successful tumor allograft.

The mechanism of action by which L-asparaginase is immunosuppressive is not clear and several divergent views have been expressed. Moreover, the role of the

L-glutaminase activity of L-asparaginase is uncertain. L-Asparagine has been shown to enhance *in vitro* antibody production (Osoba, 1969) and to be required for PHA-stimulated lymphocyte blastogenesis (Weiner et al., 1969). Addition of the amino acid or of L-glutamine to PHA-lymphocyte cultures reportedly partially reverses the inhibitory effects of L-asparaginase (Ohno and Hersh, 1970b; Miura et al., 1970a; Burgio et al., 1970), suggesting that both amidase activities are involved. In one study, the addition of glutaminase to lymphocyte cultures produced no difference in the proportion of transformed cells or mitosis compared with controls (Dartnall, 1969). Recent studies by Hersh (1971), however, show that *E. coli* L-glutaminase inhibits the response of lymphocytes to PHA, streptolysin O, and allogeneic leukocytes. The inhibition was reversed by L-glutamine but not by L-asparagine. Azotomycin, a glutamine antagonist, also inhibits the blastogenic response to mitogens (Hersh and Brown, 1971). Moreover, certain dosage combinations of the drug and L-asparaginase are synergistic. Thus, with the observation that arginine deaminase resulting from mycoplasma contamination (Simberkoff et al., 1969) also causes inhibition of blastogenesis, it would appear that deletion of an essential amino acid results in immunosuppression. In contrast, the studies of Prager and Derr (1971) have shown that lymphoid tissue incorporates glutamate, glutamine, aspartate, and asparagine into cell protein, but asparagine incorporated 1.3 to 6.3 times as readily as aspartate, whereas glutamate and glutamine were incorporated to the same degree. Asparagine synthetase was barely detectable while glutamine synthetase was 2200 times as high and glutamic-oxalacetic transaminase was 7000 times as great.

Guinea pig serum and the L-asparagine analog β-aspartylhydroxamate inhibit PHA-stimulated lymphocyte blastogenesis (Miura et al., 1970a) and Agouti serum enhances the growth of an allografted tumor in histoincompatible recipient mice (Schulten et al., 1969). In conflict with these results are those of Simberkoff et al. (1969) who have shown that in contrast to the *E. coli* enzyme, Agouti serum did not inhibit blastogenesis and antibody production *in vitro*, and those of Simberkoff and Thomas (1970) who have shown that addition of glutamine to culture media preincubated with *E. coli* L-asparaginase and then heat-inactivated prevented the inhibition of lymphocyte mitotic activity. Inhibition was not reversed by additions of L-asparagine under these conditions. In neither study, however, was it possible to obtain reversal by direct addition of the amino acids to the *E. coli* system.

It is not yet clear which of two types of lymphocytes (thymus-derived or bone marrow-derived) that appear to cooperate in the sequence of events leading to antibody synthesis (cf. Abdou and Richter, 1970) is primarily affected by asparaginase. Evidence cited by Weksler and Weksler (1971) supporting a primary effect on thymus-derived lymphocytes are (1) their studies that the enzyme produced lymphocytopenia and a reduction in thymus mass (Weksler and Weksler, 1971); (2) the thymus has large concentrations of asparagine, compared to other tissues (Broome, 1968c); (3) the enzyme is more cytotoxic to thymocytes than to lymphocytes (Dolowy et al., 1967); (4) the response of lymphocytes to phytohaemagglutinin is dependent upon thymus-derived lymphocytes (Weksler and Weksler, 1971); (5) the enzyme affects the primary but not the secondary response to sheep red blood cells (Nelson et al., 1970) as does thymectomy (Sinclair and Elliott, 1968); and finally (6) the immune mechanisms suppressed by enzyme (e.g., graft versus host reaction and skin graft rejection) are highly thymic dependent (Miller, J. F. A. P. and Mitchell, 1969). However, studies by Friedman (1971) have suggested the major target for the immunosuppressive activity of the enzyme to be the marrow cell population. Thymus or bone marrow cells alone, from either normal or enzyme-treated donors (20 I.U./day for 4 days),

constant (SEEBER et al., 1969). Similarly, injections of the enzyme do not affect DNA or RNA polymerase of rat liver though labeling of nuclear DNA is significantly inhibited (SEEBER and WESER, 1970). Injection of L-asparaginase into rats at the time of hepatectomy inhibits the early mitotic wave (ca. 30 h), but not the secondary wave (ca. 50 h) (BECKER and BROOME, 1967). While DNA synthesis of dividing tissues such as intestinal mucosa and lymphoid cells is delayed by 10 h following enzyme injection, renal tubular cells stimulated to divide by nephrectomy or administration of folic acid, and salivary acinar cells stimulated by isoproterenol are not affected (BECKER et al., 1970). The intranuclear increase in RNA polymerase activity usually seen in normal regenerating liver is delayed following injection of L-asparaginase. The period of delay was similar to the delay in mitosis and DNA synthesis that occurred after enzyme injection (BECKER and BROOME, 1969). This suggests a functional relationship between the two events.

In 6C3HED tumors, derived from mice injected with asparaginase, an 80% increase in alkaline ribonuclease (RNase) occurs within 2 h, and within 18 h a 43% increase in acid RNase occurs (MASHBURN and WRISTON, 1966). No change in levels of either enzyme is seen in asparaginase-resistant strains of the tumor. In the P1798 lymphosarcoma, neither enzyme is elevated 2 or 4 h after injection of of asparaginase, but by 18 h significant increases are observed (MASHBURN and LANDIN, 1968). On the basis of the long delay in the increase of both RNases observed in the latter studies, it is proposed that the effect could be on the aggregation of polysomes or on the destruction of cytoplasmic RNA. It was earlier proposed that asparaginase might, by removal of inhibitors of RNase, result in an increase in activities of the enzymes (MASHBURN and WRISTON, 1966).

Toxicological Effects

In acute toxicity studies of L-asparaginase in experimental animals, the LD_{50} was found to exceed 200,000 I.U./kg in the mouse and rat and to be about 50,000 I.U./kg in cats and dogs; but, in rabbits, some animals died after receiving 500 or 1000 I.U./kg while others survived 10,000 I.U./kg (LORKE and TETTENBORN, 1970). In all five species, decreased motility, anorexia, weakness, and weight loss were observed; in cats and dogs, vomiting was also observed. In subchronic studies, where animals were given 200, 800, and 3000 I.U./kg five times a week for 3 months, no biochemical or hematological effects were found in rats, but clear signs of toxicity were observed in dogs. In addition to the symptoms seen in the acute toxicity studies, thymic atrophy and slight fatty infiltration of liver cells were found. SCHEIN et al. (1969) reported the dog resistant to all toxic effects other than reversible anemia, whereas the monkey demonstrated varying degrees of toxicity. It is of interest that a number of the toxic effects disappear with continued therapy (cf. COONEY and HANDSCHUMACHER, 1970).

Embryotoxicity of the enzyme in rabbits (ADAMSON and FABRO, 1968b) resulted in 100% resorption of fetuses following injections (50 to 100 I.U./kg) of *E. carotovora* enzyme and 70% resorption using *E. coli* preparations (ADAMSON et al., 1970). Although numerous malformations of the fetuses occurred, normal karyotypes were found. In contrast, pregnant Sprague-Dawley rats given larger doses (1000 I.U./kg) than those used in the rabbit study did not reveal any embryopathic properties. In dams given 300 to 10,000 I.U./kg, however, LORKE and TETTENBORN (1970) reported a diminished number of fetuses and increased malformations, which were dose-related, and a marked influence on fetus resorption.

In general, it would appear that extrapolation of toxic effects of the enzyme in higher experimental animals to man is valid, although certain manifestations such as coagulopathy seen in man have not been observed in lower animals.

Asparagine Synthetase

Any consideration of the therapeutic aspects of L-asparaginase should include a discussion of asparagine biosynthesis, since the two now appear related. This became apparent when it was demonstrated that those cells having a nutritional requirement for L-asparagine were sensitive to the effects of L-asparaginase and possessed an inherently low and nonadaptive level of asparagine synthetase activity.

Despite the wide occurrence of L-asparagine in mammalian tissue proteins, little was known of its biosynthesis until recently. Several mechanisms had, however, been proposed (MEISTER, 1965). LEVINTOW (1957) showed that the glutamine amide nitrogen (N^{15}), but not ammonia (N^{15}), was incorporated as asparagine amide nitrogen in growing HeLa cell cultures. ARFIN (1967) reported an asparagine synthesizing system in embryonic chick livers that required both mitochondrial and supernatant fractions and decreased during maturation of the chick. PATTERSON and ORR (1967) described an assay system which included the pH 5 enzyme from tissue, Mg^{++}, ATP, and glutamine. They demonstrated that Jensen sarcoma variant cells, which show no nutritional requirement for L-asparagine (McCOY et al., 1959b), had a 2- to 3-fold increase in L-asparagine synthetase activity over parent Jensen sarcoma cells that require the amino acid for proliferation. Novikoff hepatoma, however, showed a 68-fold higher activity than did the variant tumor, whereas normal liver had activities below that found in parent Jensen sarcoma cells. Studies by BROOME and SCHWARTZ, J.H. (1967), BROOME (1968a), and HOROWITZ et al. (1968) showed that a spectrum of mouse lymphomas and leukemias that were L-asparaginase-sensitive were either devoid of or had low asparagine synthetase activities, while resistant tumors had high synthetase activities. Normal tissues elicited low and intermediate activities. In their studies, BROOME and SCHWARTZ (1967) observed that resistant cells responded to deprivation of exogenous asparagine by increasing their rate of asparagine synthesis. Similarly, resistant 6C3HED lymphomas responded to asparaginase by increased asparagine synthetase activities of 5- to 19-fold; sensitive tumors elicited a transient response, and a moderate increase was observed in normal mouse tissues (PRAGER and BACHYNSKY, 1968a, b). These studies, those of ARFIN (1967) where the synthetase decreased with maturation, as well as the observations of BREUER et al. (1964) that weanling rats adapted to an asparagine-deficient diet following a short lag in growth rate, suggested that asparagine synthetase was an adaptive enzyme. Additionally, the previously cited studies of BECKER and BROOME (1967) on delayed mitosis of regenerating liver following asparaginase injections suggested that normal liver responded to asparagine deprivation by increased synthesis of the amino acid. Subsequently, it was shown that synthetase activity of rat liver was enhanced during liver regeneration, tumor growth, injections of asparaginase, and by nutritional deprivation of asparagine (PATTERSON and ORR, 1969). In human leukemic cells, pretreatment levels of synthetase were similar, but in those patients not responding to asparaginase therapy, synthetase levels increased 5- to 7-fold following treatment (HASKELL and CANELLOS, 1969; CANELLOS and HASKELL, 1970). The mechanism of adaptation appears to involve new enzyme synthesis (PATTERSON, 1970, 1971). Normal rat liver and asparaginase-resistant Jensen sarcoma cells in culture showed a 2- to 3-fold increase in synthetase activity following treatment with asparaginase. Inhibitors of protein and RNA synthesis blocked the increase and immunochemical evidence supported increased enzyme amounts. Studies of GALLO et al. (1970) would support such a mechanism through a process of "derepression" of enzyme synthesis. Asparaginase-sensitive mouse leukemias showed the presence of an additional asparagine-tRNA ("peak 4") over that seen in resistant leukemic cells. They suggest that such a tRNA may act as a unique repressor of asparagine synthetase biosynthesis.

The adaptive nature of asparagine synthetase has suggested a mechanism of developed resistance of tumor cells ultimately seen during asparaginase therapy. While resistant cells and normal tissues appear to respond by such a mechanism, evidence that sensitive cells respond in a similar manner is lacking. Studies by PATTERSON et al. (1969) on the derivation of an asparaginase-resistant variant of the Jensen sarcoma suggest that the resistant population is derived by a cell selection process. The resistant cells, however, originate via mutations which were apparently unrelated to the deprivation of L-asparagine. A similar conclusion has also been reached for the derivation of a Walker 256 carcinoma "variant" by MORROW (1971). Other mechanisms, however, have been proposed. CONNORS and JONES (1970) suggest that "it could be a result of an extension of cell generation time, or perhaps, a retardation of growth when the enzyme (i.e., asparaginase) is present in high concentrations, until the cells can induce sufficient amounts of asparagine synthetase". Recently, SERRA (1970) proposed that "graded differences (in asparagine synthetase levels in tissues) are not typical of mutation, but of genetic changes which develop during differentiation, biochemical and otherwise, and have been termed treptions".

Asparagine synthetase has been isolated and partially purified from a variety of tissues [e.g., Novikoff hepatoma (PATTERSON and ORR, 1968), guinea pig liver (HOLCENBERG and PEASE, 1968; HOLCENBERG, 1969), RADA1 mouse leukemia cells (HOROWITZ et al., 1970), and 6C3HED (RG1) mouse lymphoma (CHOU and HANDSCHUMACHER, 1970)]. Its reaction requires aspartic acid, ATP, Mg^{++}, and either glutamine or ammonia. The K_m for the latter is, however, about 10 to 100 times greater than that observed when glutamine is the amide donor (Table 5).

Table 5. *Kinetic properties of asparagine synthetase*

Property	Enzyme source Rat tumor[a]	 Mouse tumor[b]	 G. pig liver[c]
pH optimum	6.6—8.0	7.6	8.0
K_m (M)			
Aspartate	5.8×10^{-4}	8.0×10^{-4}	9×10^{-3}
Glutamine	1.1×10^{-3}	1.2×10^{-3}	
Ammonia	0.12	1.0	
ATP	1.1×10^{-4}	1×10^{-4}	3×10^{-3}
Mg^{++}	2.3×10^{-2}		
K_i			
Asparagine		2×10^{-3}	1.5×10^{-4}
PP_i		2.0	

[a] Novikoff hepatoma; PATTERSON and ORR, 1968.
[b] RADA1 mouse leukemic cells; HOROWITZ et al., 1970.
[c] HOLCENBERG, 1969.

The studies by PATTERSON and ORR (1968) and HOLCENBERG (1969) suggest a single enzyme site for the two substrates. Using L-2-amino-4-oxo-5-chloropentanoic acid, an irreversible inhibitor which reportedly binds to the glutamine site, HOROWITZ and MEISTER (1971) have shown, however, that the enzyme was no longer active with glutamine, while the K_m value for NH_4^+ was unaffected.

CHOU and HANDSCHUMACHER (1970), using a combinatorial equation for pattern analysis of multisubstrate reactions, have proposed a reaction sequence for substrate and asparagine synthetase. They propose that enzyme and glutamine interact, releasing glutamic acid; the aminated enzyme interacts with ATP, releasing PP, yielding an aminated and adenylated enzyme. The modified enzyme then appears to react with aspartic acid and to release asparagine and AMP.

On the basis of the substrate requirement for the synthesis of asparagine and the requirement for the amino acid in cellular metabolism, a number of analogs have been tested as potential inhibitors (cf. MIURA et al., 1970b). These are discussed elsewhere in this book (Chapter on Cytotoxic Amino Acid Analogs).

References

ABDOU, N. I., RICHTER, M.: The role of bone marrow in the immune response. Advanc. Immunol. **12**, 201—270 (1970).

ADAMSON, R. H., FABRO, S.: Antitumor activity and other biologic properties of L-asparaginase (NSC-109229) — A review. Cancer Chemother. Rep. **52**, 617—626 (1968a).

ADAMSON, R. H., FABRO, S.: Embryotoxic effect of L-asparaginase. Nature (Lond.) **218**, 1164—1165 (1968b).

ADAMSON, R. H., FABRO, S., HAHN, M. A., CREECH, C. E., WHANG-PENG, J.: Evaluation of the embryotoxic activity of L-asparaginase. Arch. int. Pharmacodyn. **186**, 310—320 (1970).

ALLISON, J. P., MANDY, W. J., KITTO, G. B.: The substrate specificity of L-asparaginase from *Alcaligenes eutrophus*. FEBS Let. **14**, 107—108 (1971).

ALTENBERN, R. A., HOUSEWRIGHT, R. D.: Stereospecific asparaginases in smooth *Brucella abortus* strain 19. Arch. Biochem. Biophys. **49**, 130—137 (1954).

ARENS, A., RAUENBUSCH, E., IRION, E., WAGNER, O., BAUER, K., KAUFMANN, W.: Isolation and properties of L-asparaginase from *Escherichia coli*. Hoppe-Seylers Z. Physiol. Chem. **351**, 197—212 (1970).

ARFIN, S. M.: Asparagine synthesis in the chick embryo liver. Biochim. biophys. Acta (Amst.) **136**, 233—244 (1967).

ASTALDI, G., BURGIO, G. R., BISCATTI, G., ASTALDI, A., JR., FERFOGLIA, L.: L-Asparaginase and blastogenesis. Lancet **II**, 643—644 (1969b).

ASTALDI, G., BURGIO, G. R., KRC, J., GENOVA, R., ASTALDI, A., JR.: L-Asparaginase and blastogenesis. Lancet **I**, 423 (1969a).

ASTALDI, G., MICU, D., ASTALDI, A., JR., BURGIO, G. R., KRČ, I.: Further investigations on L-asparaginase and immune reactions. Colloq. Intern. Centre Natl. Rech. Scien. (Paris) **197**, 205—219 (1971).

ASTALDI, G., MICU, D., ASTALDI, A., JR., BURGIO, G. R.: Immunosuppressive action of L-asparaginase. Lancet **II**, 1357 (1969c).

ASTALDI, G., MICU, D., ASTALDI, A., JR., BURGIO, G. R.: Immunological effect of *E. coli* L-asparaginase. Blut **21**, 273—282 (1970).

BAUER, K.: Zur Biochemie der Asparaginase. Med. Klin. **64**, 9—12 (1969).

BECKER, F. F., BASERGA, R., BROOME, J. D.: Effect of L-asparaginase on DNA synthesis in regenerating liver and in other dividing tissues. Cancer Res. **30**, 133—137 (1970).

BECKER, F. F., BROOME, J. D.: L-Asparaginase: inhibition of early mitosis in regenerating rat liver. Science **156**, 1602—1603 (1967).

BECKER, F. F., BROOME, J. D.: L-Asparaginase: inhibition of endogenous RNA polymerase activity in regenerating liver. Arch. Biochem. Biophys. **130**, 332—336 (1969).

BEGEMANN, H., KABOTH, W., FINK, U., THEML, H.: Clinical studies on treatment of autoimmunological disorders with L-asparaginase. Colloq. Intern. Centre Natl. Rech. Scien. (Paris) **197**, 195—198 (1971).

BENEZRA, D., HOCHMAN, A., PITARO, R.: L-Asparaginase and blastogenesis. Lancet **I**, 1235—1236 (1970).

BENSON, J. V., JR., GORDON, M. J., PATTERSON, J. A.: Accelerated chromatographic analysis of amino acids in physiological fluids containing glutamine and asparagine. Anal. Biochem. **18**, 228—240 (1967).

BERENBAUM, M. C.: Immunosuppression by L-asparaginase. Nature (Lond.) **225**, 550—552 (1970).

BERENBAUM, M. C., BONDURANT, S.: Effect of L-asparaginase on germinal centre haemolysin. Nature (Lond.) **231**, 318—319 (1971).

BERENBAUM, M. C., GINSBURG, H., GILBERT, D. M.: Effects of L-asparaginase on lymphocyte-target cell reactions *in vitro*. Nature (Lond.) **227**, 1147—1148 (1970).

Bertelli, A., Donati, L., Trabucchi, E., Jr.: Prolonged survival of allo- and xeno-grafts of skin by means of an antitumoral compound: the L-asparaginase. Arch. ital. pat. **11**, 475—479 (1968).

Bilimoria, M. H.: Conditions for the production of L-asparaginase 2 by coliform bacteria. Appl. Microbiol. **18**, 1025—1030 (1969).

Bilimoria, M. H., Nisbet, M. A.: The effect of acrolein on L-asparaginase 2 from *Escherichia coli*. Proc. Soc. exp. Biol. (N.Y.) **136**, 698—700 (1971).

Boch, D.: Les conditions d'action de l'asparaginase de *l'Aspergillus niger*. C.R. Soc. Biol. (Paris) **187**, 955—956 (1928).

Bonetti, E., Abbondanza, A., Corte, E. D., Stirpe, F.: The regulation of L-asparaginase activity in rats and mice. Biochem. J. **115**, 597—601 (1969).

Bosmann, H. B.: Asparaginase action: Inhibition of protein synthesis in rat liver mitochondria and microsomes and brain mitochondria and inhibition of glycoprotein synthesis in liver and brain mitochondria by asparaginase. Life Sci. **9**, 851—859 (1970).

Bosmann, H. B., Kessel, D.: inhibition of glycoprotein synthesis in L5178Y mouse leukaemic cells by L-asparaginase *in vitro*. Nature (Lond.) **226**, 850—851 (1970).

Boyd, J. W., Phillips, A. W.: Purification and properties of L-asparaginase from *Serratia marcescens*. J. Bact. **106**, 578—587 (1971).

Boyse, E. A., Old, L. J., Campbell, H. A., Mashburn, L. T.: Suppression of murine leukemias by L-asparaginase. J. exp. Med. **125**, 17—31 (1967).

Boyse, E. A., Old, L. J., Stockert, E.: Inhibitory effect of guinea pig serum on a number of new leukaemias in mice. Nature (Lond.) **198**, 800 (1963).

Brambilla, G., Parodi, S., Cavanna, M., Caraceni, C. E., Baldini, L.: The immunodepressive activity of *Escherichia coli* L-asparaginase in some transplantation systems. Cancer Res. **30**, 2665—2670 (1970).

Breuer, L. H., Warner, R. G., Benton, D. A., Loosli, J. K.: Dietary requirement for asparagine and its metabolism in rats. J. Nutr. **88**, 143—150 (1966).

Broome, J. D.: Evidence that the L-asparaginase activity of guinea pig serum is responsible for its antilymphoma effects. Nature (Lond.) **191**, 1114—1115 (1961).

Broome, J. D.: Evidence that the L-asparaginase of guinea pig serum is responsible for its antilymphoma effects. I. Properties of the L-asparaginase of guinea pig serum in relation to those of the antilymphoma substance. J. exp. Med. **118**, 99—120 (1963a).

Broome, J. D.: Evidence that the L-asparaginase of guinea pig serum is responsible for its antilymphoma effects. II. Lymphoma 6C3HED cells cultured in a medium devoid of L-asparagine lose their susceptibility to the effects of guinea pig serum *in vivo*. J. exp. Med. **118**, 121—148 (1963b).

Broome, J. D.: Antilymphoma activity of L-asparaginase *in vivo:* clearance rates of enzyme preparations from guinea pig serum and yeast in relation to their effect on tumor growth. J. nat. Cancer Inst. **35**, 967—974 (1965).

Broome, J. D.: A method for estimating free asparagine and glutamine in biological fluids as trinitrophenyl derivatives. Nature (Lond.) **211**, 602—604 (1966).

Broome, J. D.: L-Asparaginase: the evolution of a new tumor inhibitory agent. Trans. N.Y. Acad. Sci. **30**, 690—704 (1968a).

Broome, J. D.: Factors which may influence the effectiveness of L-asparaginases as tumor inhibitors. Brit. J. Cancer **22**, 595—602 (1968b).

Broome, J. D.: Studies on the mechanism of tumor inhibition by L-asparaginase. J. exp. Med. **127**, 1055—1072 (1968c).

Broome, J. D., Schwartz, J. H.: Differences in the production of L-asparagine in asparaginase-sensitive and resistant lymphoma cells. Biochim. biophys. Acta (Amst.) **138**, 637—639 (1967).

Brown, C. H., III, Canellos, G. P., Carbone, P. P.: Effect of L-asparaginase on mouse bone marrow, assayed by *in vitro* culture. Blood **36**, 385—389 (1970).

Burgio, G. R., Astaldi, A., Jr., Krc, I., Micu, D., Astaldi, G.: With reference to blastogenesis inhibition by L-asparaginase. Recent Res. Cancer Res. **33**, 288—295 (1970).

Campbell, H. A., Mashburn, L. T.: L-Asparaginase EC-2 from *Escherichia coli*. Some substrate specificity characteristics. Biochemistry 8, 3768—3775 (1969).

Campbell, H. A., Mashburn, L. T., Boyse, E. A., Old, L. J.: Two L-asparaginases from *Escherichia coli* B. Their separation, purification, and antitumor activity. Biochemistry **6**, 721—730 (1967).

Canellos, G. P., Haskell, C. M.: Studies of resistance to L-asparaginase in human leukemia. Recent Res. Cancer Res. **33**, 188—193 (1970).

Canellos, G. P., Haskell, C. M., Arseneau, J., Carbone, P. P.: Hypoalbuminemic and hypocholesterolemic effect of L-asparaginase (NSC-109, 229) treatment in man — a preliminary report. Cancer Chemother. Rep. **53**, 67—69 (1969).

CAPIZZI, R. L., BERTINO, J. R., HANDSCHUMACHER, R. E.: L-Asparaginase. Ann. Rev. Med. **21**, 433—444 (1970).
CEDAR, H., SCHWARTZ, J. H.: Localization of the two L-asparaginases in anaerobically grown *Escherichia coli*. J. biol. Chem. **242**, 3753—3755 (1967).
CHAKRABARTY, A. K., FRIEDMAN, H.: L-Asparaginase-induced immunosuppression: effects on antibody-forming cells and serum titers. Science **167**, 869—870 (1970).
CHANEY, P. L., MARBACH, E. P.: Modified reagents for determination of urea and ammonia. Clin. Chem. **8**, 130—132 (1962).
CHANG, T. M. S.: The *in vivo* effects of semipermeable microcapsules containing L-asparaginase on 6C3HED lymphosarcoma. Nature (Lond.) **229**, 117—118 (1971).
CHOU, T. C., HANDSCHUMACHER, R. E.: Kinetic mechanism of L-asparagine synthetase of 6C3HED—RG1 tumor. Fed. Proc. **29**, 407 (1970).
CLEMENTI, A.: La désamidation enzymatique de l'asparagine chez les différentes espèce-animales et la signification physiologique de sa présence dans l'organisme. Arch. int. Physiol. **19**, 369—398 (1922).
CONNORS, T. A., JONES, M.: The effect of asparaginase on some animal tumors. Recent Res. Cancer Res. **33**, 181—187 (1970).
COONEY, D. A., CAPIZZI, R. L., HANDSCHUMACHER, R. E.: Evaluation of L-asparagine metabolism in animals and man. Cancer Res. **30**, 929—935 (1970).
COONEY, D. A., DAVIS, R. D.: The stability of L-asparaginase with respect to protein denaturants. Biochim. biophys. Acta (Amst.) **212**, 134—138 (1970).
COONEY, D. A., DAVIS, R. D., VAN ATTA, G.: A spectrophotometric method for the simultaneous measurement of L-glutamine and L-asparagine in biological materials. Anal. Biochem. **40**, 312—326 (1971).
COONEY, D. A., HANDSCHUMACHER, R. E.: L-Asparaginase and L-asparagine metabolism. Ann. Rev. Pharmacol. **10**, 421—440 (1970).
DARTNALL, J. A.: L-Asparaginase and blastogenesis. Lancet **II**, 1357—1358 (1969).
DE-ANGELI, L. C., POCCHIARI, F., RUSSI, S., TONOLO, A., ZURITA, V. E., CIARANFI, E., PERIN, A.: Effect of L-asparaginase from *Aspergillus terreus* on ascites sarcoma in the rat. Nature (Lond.) **225**, 549—550 (1970).
DE BARBIERI, A., ASTALDI, A., JR., MICU, D., MISTRETTA, A. P., ASTALDI, G., BURGIO, G. R.: Relationship between L-asparaginase blood level and inhibition of lymphocyte blastogenesis. Boll. Ist. sieroter. Milan. **49**, 382—389 (1970).
DE BARROS, T., FILHO, M. C., FERREIRA DE SANTANA, C., VALENCA, M., PEREIRA DA SILVA, M., GUEDES, J., DE CARVALHO, A. R. L.: Utilizacao de L'asparaginase em paciente humano portador de neoplasia malignana. An. Fac. Med. Recife **25**, 21—28 (1965).
DE GROOT, N., LICHTENSTEIN, N.: The action of *Pseudomonas fluorescens* extracts on asparagine and asparagine derivatives. Biochim. biophys. Acta (Amst.) **40**, 99—110 (1960).
DEODHAR, S. D.: Enhancement of metastases by L-asparaginase in a mouse tumour system. Nature (Lond.) **231**, 319—321 (1971).
DEUTSCH, E., FISCHER, M., FRISCHAUF, H., HONETZ, N., LECHNER, K., PESENDORFER, F., STYCH, H., WEISSMANN, A.: Blood coagulation changes under L-asparaginase therapy. Recent Res. Cancer Res. **33**, 331—341 (1970).
DOLOWY, W. C., ELROD, L. M., AMMERAAL, R. N., SCHREK, R.: Toxicity of L-asparaginase to resistant and susceptible lymphoma cells *in vitro*. Proc. Soc. exp. Biol. (N. Y.) **125**, 598—601 (1967).
DOLOWY, W. C., HENSON, D., CORNET, J., SELLIN, H.: Toxic and antineoplastic effects of L-asparaginase. Cancer **19**, 1813—1819 (1966).
DOLOWY, W. C., SCHREK, R., HENSON, D., CORNET, J., BROWN, E.: Effects of guinea-pig serum on the Walker 256 carcinosarcoma. Nature (Lond.) **218**, 1028—1031 (1968).
DOX, A. W.: The intracellular enzymes of lower fungi, especially those of *Penicillium camemberti*. J. biol. Chem. **6**, 461—467 (1909).
EAGLE, H.: The specific amino acid requirements of a mammalian cell (strain L) in tissue culture. J. biol. Chem. **214**, 839—852 (1955).
EHRMAN, M., CEDAR, H., SCHWARTZ, J. H.: L-Asparaginase II of *Escherichia coli*. Studies on the enzymatic mechanism of action. J. biol. Chem. **246**, 88—94 (1971).
ELLEM, K. A. O., FABRIZIO, A. M., JACKSON, L.: The dependence of DNA and RNA synthesis on protein synthesis in asparaginase-treated lymphoma cells. Cancer Res. **30**, 515—527 (1970).
EREMENKO, V. V., EVSEEV, L. P., NIKOLAEV, A. Y.: Asparaginaza *Bacterium cadaveris*. Mikrobiologiya **37**, 207—212 (1968).
EVSEEV, L. P., NIKOLAEV, A. Y.: Indutsirovannoe obrazovanie sintetaz asparagina i gliutamina u *Pseudomonas sp.* Biokhimiya **33**, 1106—1110 (1968).
FIDLER, I. J.: L-Asparaginase and metastasis. Lancet **I**, 777—778 (1970).
FIDLER, I. J.: Duration of *in vivo* effects of L-asparaginase on experimental metastasis. Nature (Lond.) **229**, 564 (1971).

FINK, U., BEGEMANN, H.: Clinical studies with L-asparaginase in dermatomyositis. Recent Res. Cancer Res. **33**, 329—330 (1970).

FRANK, B. H., PEKAR, A. H., VEROS, A. J., HO, P. P. K.: Crystalline L-asparaginase from *Escherichia coli* B. II. Physical properties, subunits, and reconstitution behavior. J. biol. Chem. **245**, 3716—3724 (1970).

FRIEDMAN, H.: L-Asparaginase induced immunosuppression: inhibition of bone marrow derived antibody precursor cells. Science **174**, 139—141 (1971).

FROHWEIN, Y. Z., FRIEDMAN, M., REIZER, J., GROSSOWICZ, N.: Sensitive and rapid assay for L-asparaginase. Nature New Biol. **230**, 158—159 (1971).

GALAEV, Y. V., KHARATS, K. S.: Izuchenie aktinvnosfi L-asparaginazy u kishechnol palochki razlichnykh tipov. Zh. Mikrobiol. (mosk.) **46**, 127—131 (1969).

GALLO, R. C., LONGMORE, J. L., ADAMSON, R. H.: Asparaginyl-tRNA and resistance of murine leukaemias to L-asparaginase. Nature (Lond.) **227**, 1134—1136 (1970).

GREENQUIST, A. C., WRISTON, J. C., JR.: On the structure of L-asparaginase from *Escherichia coli* B. Fed. Proc. **29**, 882 (1970).

GREENSTEIN, J. P., CARTER, C. E.: Influence of α-keto acids on the desamidation of amino acid amides. J. nat. Cancer Inst. **7**, 57—60 (1946).

GREENSTEIN, J. P., PRICE, V. E.: α-Keto acid-activated glutaminase and asparaginase. J. biol. Chem. **178**, 695—705 (1949).

GROVER, C. E., CHIBNALL, A. C.: The enzymic deamidation of asparagine in the higher plants. Biochem. J. **21**, 857—868 (1927).

GUARINO, A. M., SCHROEDER, D. H., ADAMSON, R. H., CALL, J. B., GRAM, T. E.: Studies of hepatic microsomal enzymes, serum proteins, and serum cholesterol after treatment of rats with L-asparaginase alone or in combination with phenobarbital. J. nat. Cancer Inst. **45**, 783—787 (1970).

HALEY, E. E., FISCHER, G. A., WELCH, A. D.: The requirement for L-asparagine of mouse leukemia cells L5178Y in culture. Cancer Res. **21**, 532—536 (1961).

HALL, J. G.: The partitioning of L-asparaginase between blood and lymph. Rec. Res. Cancer Res. **33**, 75—80 (1970).

HALPERN, Y. S., GROSSOWICZ, N.: Hydrolysis of amides by extracts from mycobacteria. Biochem. J. **65**, 716—720 (1957).

HANDSCHUMACHER, R. E.: Asparaginase: chemical structure and its relation to disposition and therapeutic efficacy. Colloq. Intern. Centre Nat. Rech. Scien. (Paris) **197**, 377—386 (1971).

HARRIS, J. E.: Effect of L-asparaginase on the ability of normal mouse bone marrow to form soft agar colonies. Nature (Lond.) **223**, 850—851 (1969).

HASKELL, C. M., CANELLOS, G. P.: L-Asparaginase resistance in human leukemia-asparagine synthetase. Biochem. Pharmacol. **18**, 2578—2580 (1969).

HASKELL, C. M., CANELLOS, G. P., COONEY, D. A., HANSEN, H. H.: Biochemical and pharmacologic effects of L-asparaginase in man. J. Lab. clin. Med. **75**, 763—770 (1970).

HEENE, D. L., LÖFFLER, H.: The hemostatic defect induced by treatment with asparaginase in leukemia. Recent Res. Cancer Res. **33**, 342—343 (1970).

HEINEMANN, B., HOWARD, A. J.: Production of tumor-inhibitory L-asparaginase by submerged growth of *Serratia marcescens*. Appl. Microbiol. **18**, 550—554 (1969).

HERSH, E. M.: L-Glutaminase: suppression of lymphocyte blastogenic responses *in vitro*. Science **172**, 736—738 (1971).

HERSH, E. M., BROWN, B. W.: Inhibition of immune responses by glutamine antogonism: effect of azotomycin on lymphocyte blastogenesis. Cancer Res. **31**, 834—840 (1971).

HILL, J. M., LOEB, E., HILL, N. O., MACLELLAN, A., KHAN, A., ALEXANDER, T. R., ADACHI, M.: Treatment of acute leukemia with L-asparaginase. Progr. Antimicrob. Anticancer Chemother. **2**, 667—678 (1970).

HILL, J. M., LOEB, E., MACLELLAN, A., KHAN, A., ROBERTS, J., SHIELDS, W. F., HILL, N. O.: Response to highly purified L-asparaginase during therapy of acute leukemia. Cancer Res. **29**, 1574—1580 (1969).

HILL, J. M., ROBERTS, J., LOEB, E., KHAN, A., MACLELLAN, A., HILL, R. W.: L-Asparaginase therapy for leukemia and other malignant neoplasms. J. Amer. med. Assoc. **202**, 882—888 (1967).

HO, D. H. W., WHITECAR, J. P., JR., LUCE, J. K., FREI, E., III: L-Asparagine requirement and the effect of L-asparaginase on the normal and leukemic human bone marrow. Cancer Res. **30**, 466—472 (1970).

HO, P. P. K., FRANK, B. H., BURCK, P. J.: Crystalline L-asparaginase from *Escherichia coli* B. Science **165**, 510—512 (1969).

HO, P. P. K., MILIKIN, E. B., BOBBITT, J. L., GRINNAN, E. L., BURCK, P. J., FRANK, B. H., BOECK, L. D., SQUIRES, R. W.: Crystalline L-asparaginase from *Escherichia coli* B. I. Purification and chemical characterization. J. biol. Chem. **245**, 3708—3715 (1970).

HOBIK, H. P.: Immunosuppressive Wirkung von L-asparaginase in der Graft-Versus-Host Reaktion. Naturwissenschaften **56**, 217 (1969).
HOLCENBERG, J. S.: Guinea pig asparagine synthetase. Biochim. biophys. Acta (Amst.) **185**, 228—238 (1969).
HOLCENBERG, J. S., PEASE, J.: Asparagine synthesis in guinea-pig liver. Biochim. biophys. Acta (Amst.) **158**, 500—502 (1968).
HOLMQUIST, N. D.: Effect of normal agouti serum on 6C3HED lymphoma *in vivo*. Fed. Proc. **21**, 166 (1962).
HOROWITZ, B., MADRAS, B. K., MEISTER, A., OLD, L. J., BOYSE, E. A., STOCKERT, E.: Asparagine synthetase activity of mouse leukemias. Science **160**, 533—535 (1968).
HOROWITZ, B., MEISTER, A.: Asparagine synthetase from RADA1 leukemia cells. Colloq. Intern. Centre nat. Rech. Scien. (Paris) **197**, 87—91 (1971).
HOROWITZ, B., NELSON, J. A., MEISTER, A.: Asparagine synthetase (tumor cells). Meth. Enzymol. **17**, 726—732 (1970).
IRION, E., ARENS, A.: Biochemical characterization of L-asparaginases from *E. coli*. Recent Res. Cancer Res. **33**, 39—47 (1970).
JACKSON, R. C., HANDSCHUMACHER, R. E.: *Escherichia coli* L-asparaginase. Catalytic activity and subunit nature. Biochemistry **9**, 3585—3590 (1970).
JAHNES, W. G., LI, C. P., TAURASO, N. M.: Studies on inhibition of viral oncogenesis. II. Inhibitory effect of L-asparaginase, clam liver extract and methotrexate on Rous virus focus formation. Arch. ges. Virusforsch. **32**, 236—243 (1970).
JAMESON, E., AINIS, H., RYAN, R. M.: Action of guinea pig serum and human gamma globulin on growth of a rat tumor. Science **124**, 980—981 (1956).
JAMESON, E., AINIS, H., RYAN, R. M.: The inhibition by guinea pig serum of the growth of the Murphy-Sturm lymphosarcoma. Cancer Res. **18**, 866—868 (1958).
JAYARAM, H. N., RAMAKRISHNAN, T., VAIDYANATHAN, C. S.: L-Asparaginases from *Mycobacterium tuberculosis* strains $H_{37}R_v$ and $H_{37}R_a$. Arch. Biochem. Biophys. **126**, 165—174 (1968).
KESSEL, D.: Asparaginyl-transfer RNA: a substrate for L-asparaginase. Biochim. biophys. Acta (Amst.) **240**, 554—557 (1971).
KESSEL, D., BOSMANN, H. B.: Effects of L-asparaginase on protein and glycoprotein synthesis. FEBS Let. **10**, 85—88 (1970).
KHAN, A., HILL, J. M.: Suppression of skin hypersensitivity and antibody formation by L-asparaginase. J. Immunol. **104**, 679—684 (1970).
KHAN, A., HILL, J. M., ADACHI, M.: L-Asparaginase in experimental auto-immune disease: inhibition of allergic encephalomyelitis. J. Immunol. **105**, 256—258 (1970).
KIDD, J. G.: Regression of transplanted lymphomas induced *in vivo* by means of normal guinea pig serum. I. Course of transplanted cancers of various kinds in mice and rats given guinea pig serum, horse serum, or rabbit serum. J. exp. Med. **98**, 565—582 (1953a).
KIDD, J. G.: Regression of transplanted lymphomas induced *in vivo* by means of normal guinea pig serum. II. Studies on the nature of the active serum constituent: histological mechanism of the regression: tests for effects of guinea pig serum on lymphoma cells *in vitro:* discussion. J. exp. Med. **98**, 583—606 (1953b).
KIDD, J. G.: Effects of arsenic-azoproteins on mouse lymphoma cells *in vivo* with observations on the effects of other "anti-lymphoma" agents, and on the susceptibility to these effects of lymphoma cells of various types. J. exp. Med. **108**, 665—684 (1958).
KIDD, J. G.: Asparaginase and cancer - yesterday and today. Rec. Res. Cancer Res. **33**, 3—14 (1970).
KIRSCHBAUM, J., WRISTON, J. C., JR., RATYCH, O. T.: Subunit structure of L-asparaginase from *Escherichia coli* B. Biochim. biophys. Acta (Amst.) **194**, 161—169 (1969).
KOJIMA, Y., WACKER, W. E. C.: An enzymatic method for the measurement of asparagine and a new assay of asparaginase activity. J. Lab. clin. Med. **74**, 521—526 (1969).
KRETOVICH, W. L.: The biosynthesis of dicarboxylic amino acids and enzymic transformations of amides in plants. Advanc. Enzymol. **20**, 319—340 (1958).
KRISTIANSEN, T., EINARSSON, M., SUNDBERG, L., PORATH, J.: Purification of L-asparaginase from *E. coli* by specific adsorption and desorption. FEBS Let. **7**, 294—296 (1970).
KRZEMINSKI, Z.: Dalsze badania nad dezaminacja aminokwasów drzez Streptococcus mitis. 2. Dezeminacja asparaginy. Cz. Stomat. **22**, 249—254 (1969).
KWAK, K. S., JAMESON, E., RYAN, R. M., KURTZ, H. M.: The effect of varying implant cell numbers on the inhibitory activity of guinea pig serum on Walker carcinosarcoma 256 in the rat. Cancer Res. **21**, 44—47 (1961).
LABOUREUR, P.: Biochimie de L'asparaginase. Propriétés du système asparaginase et activité biologique. Pathol. Biol. **17**, 885—908 (1969).
LABOUREUR, P., LANGLOIS, C., LABROUSSE, M., BOUDON, M., EMERAUD, J., SAMAIN, J. F.: Differentes formes d'asparaginases de *E. coli*. Colloq. int. Centre nat. Rech. Scien. (Paris) **197**, 43—53 (1971).

LAJOLO, D., ASTALDI, A., JR., PECCO, P., BERT, G., ASTALDI, G.: Electrophoretical mobility of human lymphocytes in the presence of *E. coli* L-asparaginase. Exp. cell Res. **60**, 458—459 (1970).

LANG, S.: Über Desamidierung im Tierkörper. Beitr. chem. Physiol. Path. **5**, 321—345 (1904).

LAUENSTEIN, K., GRUNDMANN, E., HOBIK, H. P., MADAUS, W. P.: Experimental immunosuppression with L-asparaginase. Recent Res. Cancer Res. **33**, 170—173 (1970).

LAUINGER, C., RESSLER, C.: β-Cyanoalanine as a substrate for asparaginase. Stoichiometry, kinetics, and inhibition. Biochim. biophys. Acta (Amst.) **198**, 316—323 (1970).

LEES, E. M., BLAKENEY, A. B.: The distribution of asparaginase activity in legumes. Biochim. biophys. Acta (Amst.) **215**, 145—151 (1970).

LEVINTOW, L.: Evidence that glutamine is a precursor of asparagine in a human cell in tissue culture. Science **126**, 611—612 (1957).

LIU, Y. P., HANDSCHUMACHER, R. E.: Chemical modification of L-asparaginase. Proc. Amer. Ass. Cancer Res. **12**, 99 (1971).

LORKE, D., TETTENBORN, D.: Experimental studies on the toxicity of crasnitin in animals. Recent Res. Cancer Res. **33**, 174—180 (1970).

MARAL, R., GUYONNET, J. C., JULOU, L., DE RATULD, Y., WERNER, G. H.: Studies on the immunosuppressive activity of L-asparaginase. Rec. Res. Cancer Res. **33**, 160—169 (1970).

MARAL, R., WERNER, G. H.: Antiviral activity of L-asparaginase. Nature New Biol. **232**, 187—188 (1971).

MARDASHEV, S. R., SHAO, H. W.: Purification of guinea pig serum asparaginase by chromatography on a diethylaminoethyl cellulose column. Dokl. Akad. Nauk. S.S.S.R. **142**, 21—24 (1967).

MARQUARDT, H.: L-Asparaginase — das erste spezifische Cytostaticum. Arzneimittel-Forsch. **18**, 1380—1386 (1968).

MASHBURN, L. T., GORDON, C. S.: The effects of L-asparaginase on the amino acid incorporation of mouse lymphoid tumors. Cancer Res. **28**, 961—967 (1968).

MASHBURN, L. T., LANDIN, L. M.: Changes in ribonuclease activities in P1798 lymphosarcoma after asparaginase treatment. Arch. Biochem. Biophys. **125**, 721—726 (1968).

MASHBURN, L. T., LANDIN, L. M.: Some physicochemical aspects of L-asparaginase therapy. Recent Res. Cancer Res. **33**, 48—57 (1970).

MASHBURN, L. T., WRISTON, J. C., JR.: Tumor inhibitory effect of L-asparaginase. Biochem. biophys. Res. Commun. **12**, 50—55 (1963).

MASHBURN, L. T., WRISTON, J. C., JR.: Tumor inhibitory effect of L-asparaginase from *Escherichia coli*. Arch. Biochem. Biophys. **105**, 450—452 (1964).

MASHBURN, L. T., WRISTON, J. C., JR.: Change in ribonuclease concentrations in L-asparaginase-treated lymphosarcomata. Nature (Lond.) **211**, 1403—1404 (1966).

McCOY, T. A., MAXWELL, M., IRVINE, E., SARTORELLI, A. C.: Two nutritional variants of cultured Jensen sarcoma cells. Proc. Soc. exp. Biol. (N.Y.) **100**, 862—865 (1959b).

McCOY, T. A., MAXWELL, M., KRUSE, P. F., JR.: The amino acid requirements of the Jensen sarcoma *in vitro*. Cancer Res. **19**, 591—595 (1959a).

McELWAIN, T. J., HAYWARD, S. K.: L-Asparaginase and blastogenesis. Lancet **I**, 527 (1969).

MEISTER, A.: Glutaminase, asparaginase, and α-keto acid-ω-amidase. B. L-Asparaginase from guinea pig serum. Meth. Enzymol. **2**, 383—385 (1955).

MEISTER, A.: Intermediary metabolism of the amino acids. In: MEISTER, A. (Ed.): Biochemistry of the Amino Acids, Vol. II, 2nd. Edition, pp. 606—617. New York: Academic Press 1965.

MEISTER, A., SOBER, H. A., TICE, S. V., FRASER, P. E.: Transamination and associated deamidation of asparagine and glutamine. J. biol. Chem. **197**, 319—330 (1952).

MICOU, D., ASTALDI, G., ASTALDI, A., JR., MIHAILESCO, E., LISIEWICZ, J.: L'effet de la L-asparaginase sur les cellules de la série plasmocytaire. Schweiz. med. Wschr. **100**, 1997—1999 (1970).

MIKUCKI, J., SZARAPIŃSKA-KWASZEWSKA, J., KRZEMIŃSKI, Z.: Aktywność asparaginazy u antybiotykoopornych *gronkowców ziocistych*. Med. Doswiadczalna Mikrobiol. **20**, 227—231 (1968).

MILLER, D. S., MARLBOROUGH, D. I., CAMMACK, K. A.: Physical properties and subunit structure of L-asparaginase isolated from *Erwinia carotovora*. Colloq. int. Centre nat. Rech. Scien. (Paris) **197**, 55—71 (1971).

MILLER, H. K., BALIS, M. E.: Glutaminase activity of L-asparagine amidohydrolase. Biochem. Pharmacol. **18**, 2225—2232 (1969).

MILLER, H. K., KRAKOFF, I. H., SALSER, J. S., BALIS, M. E.: Sensitivity to L-asparaginase and amino acid metabolism. J. nat. Cancer Inst. **44**, 1129—1139 (1970).

MILLER, H. K., SALSER, J. S., BALIS, M. E.: Amino acid levels following L-asparagine amidohydrolase (EC. 3.5.1.1) therapy. Cancer Res. **29**, 183—187 (1969).

MILLER, J. F. A. P., MITCHELL, G. F.: Thymus and antigen reactive cells. Transplant. Rev. **1**, 3—42 (1969).

MIURA, M., HIRANO, M., KAKIZAWA, K., MORITA, A., UETANI, T., YAMADA, K.: Inhibitory effect of L-asparaginase in lymphocyte transformation induced by phytohemagglutinin. Cancer Res. **30**, 768—772 (1970a).

MIURA, M., HIRANO, M., KAKIZAWA, K., MORITA, A., UETANI, T., YAMADA, K.: Antitumor activity of L-β-aspartohydroxamic acid *in vivo*. Screening data of 21 L-asparagine related compounds. Progr. antimicrob. anticancer Chemotherapy **2**, 170—174 (1970b).

MIURA, M., KAWASHIMA, K., UETANI, T., HIRANO, M., KAKIZAWA, H., OHNO, R., MORITA, A., NISHIWAKI, H., YAMADA, K.: Influence of L-asparaginase on antibody production and growth of tumors in allogeneic mice. Cancer Res. **31**, 114—121 (1971).

MORROW, J.: Mutation rate from asparagine requirement to asparagine non-requirement. J. cell. Physiol. **77**, 423—425 (1971).

NAHORSKI, S. R.: Fluorometric measurement of glutamine and asparagine using enzyme methods. Anal. Biochem. **42**, 136—142 (1971).

NAKAMURA, N., MORIKAWA, Y., TANAKA, M.: L-Asparaginase from *Escherichia coli*. II. Substrate specificity studies. Agr. biol. Chem. **35**, 743—751 (1971).

NELSON, S. D., LEE, M. B., BRIDGES, J. M.: Immunosuppressive activity of L-asparaginase in mice. Transplantation **9**, 566—570 (1970).

NEUMAN, R. E., MCCOY, T. A., The dual requirement of the Walker carcinosarcoma 256 *in vitro* for asparagine and glutamine. Science **124**, 124—125 (1956).

NICOLIN, A., NAPOLI, P. A.: Azione favorente delia levo-asparaginasi sulla crescita del carcinoma ascite di Ehrlich (in animali normali o in animali previamente "vaccinati" verso lo stesso tumore ascitico). Arch. ital. Pat. **12**, 177—187 (1969).

NISHIMURA, Y., MAKINO, H., TAKENAKA, O., INADA, Y.: Amino acid residues in asparaginase (*Escherichia coli* HAP) associated with its enzymic activity. Biochim. biophys. Acta (Amst.) **227**, 171—179 (1971).

NORTH, A. C. T., WADE, H. E., CAMMACK, K. A.: Physiochemical studies of L-asparaginase from *Erwinia carotovora*. Nature (Lond.) **224**, 594—595 (1967).

OETTGEN, H. F., OLD, L. J., BOYSE, E. A., CAMPBELL, H. A., PHILIPS, F. S., CLARKSON, B. D., TALLAL, L., LEEPER, R. D., SCHWARTZ, M. K., KIM, J. H.: Inhibition of leukemias in man by L-asparaginase. Cancer Res. **27**, 2619—2631 (1967).

OHNO, R., HARRIS, J. E., HERSH, E. M.: L-Asparaginase: suppression of the immune response of mice to sheep red blood cells. Clin. exp. Immunol. **7**, 221—227 (1970).

OHNO, R., HERSH, E. M.: Immunosuppressive effects of L-asparaginase. Cancer Res. **30**, 1605—1611 (1970a).

OHNO, R., HERSH, E. M.: The inhibition of lymphocyte blastogenesis by L-asparaginase (LA). Blood **35**, 250—262 (1970b).

OHNUMA, T., BERGEL, F., BRAY, R. C.: Enzymes in cancer. Asparaginase from chicken liver. Biochem. J. **103**, 238—245 (1967).

OHNUMA, T., HOLLAND, J. F., FREEMAN, A., SINKS, L. F.: Biochemical and pharmacological studies with asparaginase in man. Cancer Res. **30**, 2297—2305 (1970).

OLD, L. J., BOYSE, E. A., CAMPBELL, H. A.: L-Asparagine and leukemia. Sci. Amer. **219**, 34—40 (1968).

OLD, L. J., BOYSE, E. A., CAMPBELL, H. A., DARIA, G. M.: Leukaemia-inhibiting properties and L-asparaginase activity of sera from certain South American rodents. Nature (Lond.) **198**, 801 (1963).

OSOBA, D.: Restriction of the capacity to respond to two antigens by single precursors of antibody-producing cells in culture. J. exp. Med. **129**, 141—152 (1969).

PATTERSON, M. K., JR.: Studies on the control of asparagine biosynthesis in mammalian tissues. Rec. Res. Cancer Res. **33**, 22—30 (1970).

PATTERSON, M. K., JR.: Effects of L-asparaginase on asparagine synthetase levels of normal and malignant tissues. Colloq. int. Centre nat. Rech. Scien. (Paris) **197**, 107—113 (1971).

PATTERSON, M. K., JR., CONWAY, E., WHITTLE, W., MCCOY, T. A.: *In vitro* effects of guinea pig serum on the Jensen, JA-1 and JA-2 sarcomas. Proc. Soc. exp. Biol. (N.Y.) **119**, 5—9 (1965).

PATTERSON, M. K., JR., MAXWELL, M. D.: Effects of L-asparagine deprivation on the cell cycle of the Jensen sarcoma. Cancer Res. **30**, 1064—1067 (1970).

PATTERSON, M. K., JR., MAXWELL, M. D., CONWAY, E.: Studies on the asparagine requirement of the Jensen sarcoma and the derivation of its nutritional variant. Cancer Res. **29**, 296—300 (1969).

PATTERSON, M. K., JR., ORR, G.: L-Asparagine biosynthesis by nutritional variants of the Jensen sarcoma. Biochem. biophys. Res. Commun. **26**, 228—233 (1967).

PATTERSON, M. K., JR., ORR, G. R.: Asparagine biosynthesis by the Novikoff hepatoma. Isolation, purification, property, and mechanism studies of the enzyme system. J. biol. Chem. **243**, 376—380 (1968).

PATTERSON, M. K., JR., ORR, G. R.: Regeneration, tumor, dietary, and L-asparaginase effects on asparagine biosynthesis in rat liver. Cancer Res. **29**, 1179—1183 (1969).
PATTERSON, M. K., JR., ORR, G. R., MCCOY, T. A.: Asparagine-C^{14} and glutamine-C^{14} from animal cell protein and their chemical degradation. Anal. Biochem. **6**, 543—548 (1963).
PETERS, J. H., LIN, S. C., BERRIDGE, B. J., JR., CHAO, W. R., CUMMINGS, J. G.: Circulatory L-asparaginase activity in primates. Life Sci. **9**, 431—436 (1970).
PETERSON, R. E., CIEGLER, A.: L-Asparaginase production by various bacteria. Appl. Microbiol. **17**, 929—930 (1969a).
PETERSON, R. E., CIEGLER, A.: L-Asparaginase production by *Erwinia aroideae*. Appl. Microbiol. **18**, 64—67 (1969b).
PETERSON, R. G., HANDSCHUMACHER, R. E., MITCHELL, M. S.: Immunological responses to L-asparaginase. J. clin. Invest. **50**, 1080—1090 (1971).
PRAGER, M. D., BACHYNSKY, N.: Asparagine synthetase in asparaginase resistant and susceptible mouse lymphomas. Biochem. biophys. Res. Commun. **31**, 43—47 (1968a).
PRAGER, M. D., BACHYNSKY, N.: Asparagine synthetase in normal and malignant tissues; correlation with tumor sensitivity to asparaginase. Arch. Biochem. Biophys. **127**, 645—654 (1968b).
PRAGER, M. D., DERR, I.: Inhibition of primary antibody response by *E. coli* asparaginase. Nature (Lond.) **225**, 952 (1970).
PRAGER, M. D., DERR, I.: Metabolism of asparagine, aspartate, glutamine, and glutamate in lymphoid tissue: basis for immunosuppression by L-asparaginase. J. Immunol. **106**, 975—979 (1971).
PRUSINER, S., MILNER, L.: A rapid radioactive assay for glutamine synthetase, glutaminase, asparagine synthetase and asparaginase. Anal. Biochem. **37**, 429—438 (1970).
PÜTTER, J.: Pharmacokinetic behavior of L-asparaginase in men and in animals. Recent Res. Cancer Res. **33**, 64—74 (1970).
RAUENBUSCH, E., BAUER, K., KAUFMANN, W., WAGNER, O.: Isolation and crystallization of L-asparaginase from *E. coli*. Recent Res. Cancer Res. **33**, 31—38 (1970).
RAUENBUSCH, E., IRION, E., ARENS, A.: The subunits of L-asparaginase from *Escherichia coli*. Colloq. int. Centre nat. Rech. Scien. (Paris) **197**, 31—42 (1971).
RAVEL, J. M., NORTON, S. J., HUMPHREYS, J. S., SHIVE, W.: Asparagine biosynthesis in *Lactobacillus arabinosus* and its control by asparagine through enzyme inhibition and repression. J. biol. Chem. **237**, 2845—2849 (1962).
REDDY, V. V. S., JAYARAM, H. N., SIRSI, M., RAMAKRISHNAN, T.: Inhibitory activity of L-asparaginase from *Mycobacterium tuberculosis* on Yoshida ascites sarcoma in rats. Arch. Biochem. Biophys. **132**, 262—267 (1969).
RILEY, V.: Influence of a benign virus upon mouse leukemia during asparaginase therapy. Path. et Biol. **18**, 757—764 (1970).
RILEY, V., SPACKMAN, D. H., FITZMAURICE, M. A.: Critical influence of an enzyme-elevating virus upon long-term remissions of mouse leukemia following asparaginase therapy. Recent Res. Cancer Res. **33**, 81—101 (1970).
ROBERTS, J., BURSON, G., HILL, J. M.: New procedures for purification of L-asparaginase with high yield from *Escherichia coli*. J. Bact. **95**, 2117—2123 (1968).
ROBERTS, J., PRAGER, M. D., BACHYNSKY, N.: The antitumor activity of *Escherichia coli* L-asparaginase. Cancer Res. **26**, 2213—2217 (1966).
ROBISON, R. S., BERK, B.: L-Asparaginase synthesis by *Escherichia coli* B. Biotechnol. Bioeng. **11**, 1211—1225 (1969).
ROWLEY, B., WRISTON, J. C., JR.: Partial purification and antilymphoma activity of *Serratia marcescens* L-asparaginase. Biochem. biophys. Res. Commun. **28**, 160—165 (1967).
RUDMAN, D., VOGLER, W. R., HOWARD, C. H., GERRON, G. G.: Observations on the plasma amino acids of patients with acute leukemia. Cancer Res. **31**, 1159—1165 (1971).
RYAN, W. L., DWORAK, J. E.: Amino acids of the 6C3HED lymphosarcoma following treatment with asparaginase. Cancer Res. **30**, 1206—1209 (1970).
RYAN, W. L., SORNSON, H. C.: Glycine inhibition of asparaginase. Science **167**, 1512—1513 (1970).
ST. PIERRE, R. L., TENNENBAUM, J. I., FOLK, R. M.: L-Asparaginase and allograft immunity. Lancet **II**, 1365—1366 (1970).
SCHEETZ, R. W., WHELAN, H. A., WRISTON, J. C., JR.: Purification and properties of an L-asparaginase from *Fusarium tricinctum*. Arch. Biochem. Biophys. **142**, 184—189 (1971).
SCHEIN, P. S., RAKIETEN, N., GORDON, B. M., DAVIS, R. D., RALL, D. P.: The toxicity of *Escherichia coli* L-asparaginase. Cancer Res. **29**, 426—434 (1969).
SCHREK, R., DOLOWY, W. C., AMMERAAL, R. N.: L-Asparaginase: toxicity to normal and leukemic human lymphocytes. Science **155**, 329—330 (1967).
SCHULTEN, H. K., GIRALDO, G.: Influence of L-asparaginase preparations of *E. coli* and Agouti serum on the homograft reactivity in the mouse. Recent Res. Cancer Res. **33**, 155—159 (1970).

SCHULTEN, H.K., GIRALDO, G., BOYSE, E.A., OETTGEN, H.F.: Immunosuppressive action of L-asparaginase. Lancet **II**, 644—645 (1969).
SCHWARTZ, J.H., REEVES, J.Y., BROOME, J.D.: Two L-asparaginases from *E. coli* and their action against tumors. Proc. nat. Acad. Sci. (Wash.) **56**, 1516—1519 (1966).
SCHWARTZ, M.K.: The distribution and clearance of L-asparaginase. Recent Res. Cancer Res. **33**, 58—63 (1970).
SCHWARTZ, M.K., LASH, E.D., OETTGEN, H.F., TOMAO, F.A.: L-Asparaginase activity in plasma and other biological fluids. Cancer **25**, 244—252 (1970).
SCHWARTZ, R.S.: Immunosuppression by L-asparaginase. Nature (Lond.) **224**, 275—276 (1969).
SEEBER, S., WARNECKE, P., STRAUB, O.C.: Zum Einfluß von *E. coli*-L-asparaginase auf den Nucleinsäurestoffwechsel lymphatischer Rinderleukämiezellen. Arzneimittel-Forsch. **19**, 1745—1748 (1969).
SEEBER, S., WESER, U.: Inhibition of ^{3}H-thymidine incorporation into rat liver nuclei by *E. coli* L-asparaginase. Nature (Lond.) **225**, 652—653 (1970).
SERRA, J.A.: Regulatory genetic changes in the origin of asparaginase-sensitive leukemias. Tenth International Cancer Congress, Abstr. 359—360 (1970).
SHAW, M.T., BARNES, C.C., MADDEN, F.J.F., BAGSHAWE, K.D.: L-Asparaginase and pancreatitis. Lancet **II**, 721 (1970).
SHONS, A., JETZER, T., NAJARIAN, J.S.: Prolongation of skin homograft survival by L-asparaginase. Transplantation **10**, 280—281 (1970).
SIMBERKOFF, M.S., THOMAS, L.: Reversal by L-glutamine of the inhibition of lymphocyte mitosis caused by *E. coli* asparaginase. Proc. Soc. exp. Biol. (N.Y.) **133**, 642—644 (1970).
SIMBERKOFF, M.S., THORBECKE, G.J., THOMAS, L.: Studies of PPLO infection. V. Inhibition of lymphocyte mitosis and antibody formation by mycoplasmal extracts. J. exp. Med. **129**, 1163—1181 (1969).
SINCLAIR, N.R.ST.C., ELLIOTT, E.V.: Neonatal thymectomy and hemolysin responses in inbred mice. J. Immunol. **101**, 251—255 (1968).
SOBIN, L.H., KIDD, J.G.: A metabolic difference between two lines of lymphoma 6C3HED cells in relation to asparagine. Proc. Soc. exp. Biol. (N.Y.) **119**, 325—327 (1965).
SOBIN, L.H., KIDD, J.G.: Alterations in protein and nucleic acid metabolism of lymphoma 6C3HED—OG cells in mice given guinea pig serum. J. exp. Med. **123**, 55—74 (1966).
STAERK, J., ZWISLER, O., RONNEBERGER, H.: A comparison of L-asparaginase from *Erwinia aroideae* and from *Escherichia coli:* biochemical and biological properties. Experientia (Basel) **27**, 250—252 (1971).
STEENSHOLT, G.: On the distribution of asparaginase. Acta physiol. scand. **8**, 342—347 (1944).
SULD, H.M., HERBUT, P.A.: Guinea pig serum and liver asparaginases. Purification and antitumor activity. J. biol. Chem. **240**, 2234—2241 (1965).
SULD, H.M., HERBUT, P.A.: Guinea pig serum and liver L-asparaginases. Comparison of serum and papain-digested liver L-asparaginases. J. biol. Chem. **245**, 2797—2801 (1970a).
SULD, H.M., HERBUT, P.A.: Immunological studies on guinea pig serum and liver L-asparaginases. Purification of L-asparaginases by antibody precipitation. J. biol. Chem. **245**, 2802—2808 (1970b).
TANAKA, M., KAGAWA, T., TATANO, T., MOCHIZUKI, K., NAKAMURA, N., KOHAGURA, M., HILL, J.M.: Antineoplastic crystalline L-asparaginase from *E. coli.* Progr. antimicrob. anticancer Chemother. **2**, 260—200 (1970).
TOWER, D.B., PETERS, E.L., CURTIS, W.C.: Guinea pig serum L-asparaginase. Properties, purification, and application to determination of asparagine in biological samples. J. biol. Chem. **238**, 983—993 (1963).
TSUJI, Y.: Amidase action of bacteria. Naika Hokan. **4**, 222—223 (1957).
UBUKA, T., MEISTER, A.: Studies on the utilization of asparagine by mouse leukemia cells. J. nat. Cancer Inst. **46**, 291—298 (1971).
VADLAMUDI, S., PADARATHSINGH, M., BONMASSAR, E., WARAVDEKAR, V., GOLDIN, A.: Studies on neutralization of L-asparaginase activity *in vitro* and *in vivo.* Cancer **27**, 1321—1327 (1971).
VADLAMUDI, S., PADARATHSINGH, M., WARAVDEKAR, V.S., GOLDIN, A.: Factors influencing the therapeutic activity of L-asparaginase (NSC 109229) in leukemic (L5178Y) mice. Cancer Res. **30**, 1467—1472 (1970).
VON FURTH, O., FRIEDMANN, M.: Über die Verbreitung asparaginspaltender Organfermente. Biochem. Z. **26**, 435—440 (1910).
WADE, H.E., ELSWORTH, R., HERBERT, D., KEPPIE, J., SARGEANT, K.: A new L-asparaginase with antitumour activity. Lancet **II**, 776—777 (1968).
WAGNER, O., BAUER, K., IRION, E., RAUENBUSCH, E., KAUFMANN, W., ARENS, A.: Polyäthylenglykol zur Anreicherung und Kristallisation von L-Asparaginase. Angew. Chem. **81**, 904—905 (1969a).

WAGNER, O., IRION, E., BAUER, K.: Partially deaminated L-asparaginase. Biochem. biophys, Res. Commun. **37**, 383—392 (1969b).

WEINBERGER, S.: L-Asparaginase as an antitumor agent. Enzyme **12**, 143—159 (1971).

WEINER, M. S., WAITHE, W. I., HIRSCHHORN, K.: L-Asparaginase and blastogenesis. Lancet II, 748 (1969).

WEKSLER, M. E., WEKSLER, B. B.: Studies on the immunosuppressive properties of asparaginase. Immunology **21**, 137—150 (1971).

WHELAN, H. A., WRISTON, J. C., JR.: Purification and properties of asparaginase from *Escherichia coli* B. Biochemistry **8**, 2386—2393 (1969).

WHITECAR, J. P., JR., BODEY, G. P., HILL, C. S., JR., SAMAAN, N. A.: Effect of L-asparaginase on carbohydrate metabolism. Metabolism **19**, 581—586 (1970).

WOODS, J. S., LEE, I. P., DIXON, R. L.: Asparagine incorporation into the DNA of hepatic and 6C3HED murine lymphosarcoma cells. Cancer Res. **30**, 1210—1211 (1970).

WRISTON, J. C., JR.: Asparaginase. Meth. Enzymol. **17**, 732—742 (1970).

WRISTON, J. C., JR.: L-Asparaginase. Enzymes **4**, 101—121 (1971a).

WRISTON, J. C., JR.: On the structure of *E. coli* B asparaginase. Colloq. int. Centre nat. Rech. Scien. (Paris) **197**, 25—29 (1971b).

YELLIN, T. O., WRISTON, J. C., JR.: Purification and properties of guinea pig serum asparaginase. Biochemistry **5**, 1605—1612 (1966).

Chapter 69

L-Asparaginase: Current Status of Clinical Evaluation

HERBERT F. OETTGEN

Introduction

The advances that led to the use of L-asparaginase in cancer therapy were (1) the discovery that guinea pig serum inhibits certain transplanted leukemias of the mouse (KIDD, 1953), (2) the finding that the cells of some tumors die *in vitro* unless supplied with L-asparagine (NEUMANN and McCOY, 1956; HALEY et al., 1961), (3) the demonstration that the enzyme L-asparaginase is the antileukemic factor in guinea pig serum (BROOME, 1961, 1963a, b), (4) the demonstration that the inhibitory effect of asparaginase is not restricted to mouse leukemias with a long history of transplantation (i.e., does not depend on histoincompatibility) (BOYSE et al., 1963, 1967), (5) the finding that asparaginase with antileukemic activity can be isolated from *E. coli*, a potentially inexhaustible source (MASHBURN and WRISTON, 1964), and (6) the successful use of *E. coli* L-asparaginase in the treatment of primary lymphosarcoma of the dog (OLD et al., 1967). In 1967, it was first reported that treatment with *E. coli* L-asparaginase induces complete remissions in patients with acute lymphoblastic leukemia (HILL et al., 1967; OETTGEN et al., 1967). Since then, therapeutic trials have been conducted in many centers in more than 1000 patients. It is the purpose of this report to review the results.

Properties of the Enzyme Preparation

E. coli L-asparaginase EC-2 (L-asparagine amidohydrolase, EC. 3.5.1.1) is quite stable in aqueous solution in the pH range from 5 to 9. At room temperature the enzyme activity is preserved for weeks; at 60° the enzyme loses its activity within 1 h. The preparations that are now available for clinical use have 90% or more of the maximal specific activity. This does not mean that they contain 10% of contaminating proteins, but rather that asparaginase tends to aggregate. Aggregates are found in all lyophilized and even in crystalline preparations. As shown by precipitation in gel, the purest preparations contain traces of impurities. Contamination with endotoxin, a problem with earlier, less purified preparations, has been largely eliminated. The molecular weight, according to analysis in the ultracentrifuge, is 127000. In 8 M urea, however, smaller subunits have been found, and a lower molecular weight has also been calculated on the basis of amino acid analysis. One can therefore assume that aggregation and dissociation takes place. Asparaginase EC-2 has its maximal activity at pH 6 to 8. It has some glutaminase activity that, being constant (3 to 4%) in preparations of different purity, is thought to be due to a less than perfect "fit" rather than to the presence of another enzyme (MASHBURN and WRISTON, 1964; CAMPBELL et al., 1967; WHELEN and WRISTON, 1969; BAUER, 1969; IRION and ARENS, 1970; RAUENBUSCH et al., 1970; CAPIZZI et al., 1970). Insoluble, matrix-supported EC-2 has been prepared for possible use in extracorporeal filters (HASSELBERGER et al., 1970). L-Asparaginase from *Erwinia carotovora* has also been used in clinical trials; its molecular weight has been estimated to be 130000 (NORTH et al., 1969).

Distribution and Elimination

After intravenous injection, *E. coli* L-asparaginase is distributed in the total plasma volume. Generally, the disappearance curve is monophasic, although in some cases, a biphasic curve has been observed. The mean half-life time in the plasma was 22.6 h for the Merck preparation and 11.2 h for the Bayer preparation (Table 1) (SCHWARTZ, 1970; SCHWARTZ et al., 1970a; OHNUMA et al., 1970). *E. coli* enzymes with a shorter half-life (Bayer, Lilly) have 3 to 4 different iso-

Table 1. *Half-life of E. coli* L-*asparaginase in human blood after intravenous injection* (SCHWARTZ et al., 1970a)

Diagnosis	Source	Dose IU/kg	*t* 1/2 (h) fast segment	slow segment
Acute lymphoblastic leukemia	Bayer	200	—	8.2
Acute myeloblastic leukemia		200	—	11.7
Acute myeloblastic leukemia		200	—	12.5
Melanoma		200	—	6.2
Carcinoma breast		200	—	10.5
Acute lymphoblastic leukemia		1000	—	11.3
Acute myeloblastic leukemia		1000	3.2	7.8
Chronic lymphocytic leukemia		1000	8.6	14.3
Choriocarcinoma		1000	—	13.3
Melanoma		1000	—	10.1
Melanoma		1000	6.3	14.8
Carcinoma tonsil		1000	7.9	13.2
Acute lymphoblastic leukemia	Merck	200	11.8	28.5
Melanoma		200	4.0	16.8
Carcinoma maxilla		200	11.2	21.1
Carcinoma rectum		200	—	17.4
Acute lymphoblastic leukemia		1000	—	21.3
Acute myeloblastic leukemia		1000	—	26.8
Lymphosarcoma		1000	—	26.3

electric points near pH 5.5, while preparations with a longer half-life (Squibb, Merck) are focused as a more homogeneous species with one isoelectric point near pH 4.95 (MASHBURN and LANDIN, 1970). Interestingly, the removal of the α-amino group of the *N*-terminal leucine and of one equivalent of the ε-amino groups of the lysine residues from the short-lived material (Bayer) leads to both increased acidity (isoelectric point 4.65) and increased half-life in the blood plasma (24 h) without any loss of enzymatic activity (PUTTER, 1969, 1970). The maximum plasma levels obtained during therapy with different preparations reflect the differences in half-life (Table 2) (SCHWARTZ, 1970; SCHWARTZ et al., 1970a). After intramuscular injection, plasma levels were lower, but persisted longer.

Asparaginase was not found in the urine even when blood levels were high. Only rarely, at higher blood levels, were small amounts of enzyme demonstrable in the cerebrospinal fluid. After intrathecal administration, the enzyme disappeared rapidly from the cerebrospinal fluid and entered the blood (SCHWARTZ, 1970; SCHWARTZ et al., 1970a). Assays of bile or lymph have not yet been performed in

Table 2. *Plasma levels of E. coli L-asparaginase* (SCHWARTZ, 1970)

Patients	Dose IU/kg/day	Plasma levels[a] (IU/ml, Mean ± S.D.) Squibb	Bayer	Merck
Children	10	(9)[b] 0.4 ± 0.1	—	—
	200	(21) 5.8 ± 2.6	(11) 2.7 ± 2.1	—
	1000	(5) 22.7 ± 3.4	(21) 6.5 ± 4.0	(5) 14.5 ± 2.2
	5000	—	(14) 21.6 ± 13.3	(12) 57.0 ± 18.1
Adults	10	(13) 0.4 ± 0.2	—	—
	200	(9) 5.8 ± 2.5	(19) 2.6 ± 1.6	—
	1000	(1) 21.8	(30) 8.8 ± 5.4	(12) 26.7 ± 9.8
	5000	—	(8) 25.5 ± 8.8	(6) 70.1 ± 38.9

[a] Maximum plasma levels measured during each course of therapy. The blood samples were drawn 18 to 22 h after the preceding injection of asparaginase.
[b] The numbers in parentheses are the number of patients in each group.

man (in rats and sheep, only small amounts of enzyme appear in the lymph). Asparaginase was not found in erythrocytes of patients under therapy or in tissues obtained at autopsy (after correction for their blood content) (SCHWARTZ, 1970a; SCHWARTZ et al., 1970b). It seems likely that much of the enzyme is removed from the circulation by the reticuloendothelial system (this view is supported by the fact that clearance from the plasma is delayed in mice infected with the LDH virus).

Dose and Route of Administration

In most cases the enzyme preparation was administered by daily intravenous injection. Occasionally, the injections were given three times, twice, or once a week, or twice daily. A small number of patients received intramuscular or intrathecal injections. The duration of treatment was generally on the order of 4 weeks. In some patients treatment was discontinued earlier because of progressing disease or toxicity. Others received maintenance therapy for periods up to 8 months. The daily dose ranged from 10 to 5000 IU per kg; higher single doses were given on rare occasions.

Effects of Asparaginase Therapy on Plasma Amino Acid Levels

In patients treated at a dose of 200 IU/kg/day both asparagine and glutamine levels rapidly fell to zero, while glutamate levels increased temporarily. Complete amino acid analysis revealed no remarkable changes in the concentration of other amino acids. On maintenance therapy with 10 or 50 IU/kg/day glutamine levels returned to normal, but asparagine could not be detected (CAPIZZI et al., 1969; MILLER et al., 1969). A dose as small as 0.2 IU/kg injected intradermally produced a substantial fall of plasma asparagine (OHNUMA et al., 1970). By contrast, extensive removal of asparagine from the blood by hemodialysis did not lower plasma asparagine levels (COONEY et al., 1970).

Therapeutic Effects

A. Spectrum of Response (Tables 3—5)

The patients who responded best to asparaginase therapy were children and adults with acute lymphoblastic leukemia. Seventeen groups of investigators reported 214 complete or partial remissions (54 %) in 395 patients (HILL et al., 1969;

Table 3. *Results of asparaginase therapy reported in the literature*

Ref.	Diagnosis	Number of patients	Number of responses
	Acute lymphoblastic leukemia		
Beard et al. (1970) Carbone et al. (1970) Fairley et al. (1970) Gerhartz and Begemann (1970) Goudemand and Bauters (1970) Hill et al. (1969) Jacquillat et al. (1970) Jaffe et al. (1971) Loeb et al. (1970) Marmont and Damasid (1970) Mathé et al. (1970) Mayer and Holton (1971) Ohnuma et al. (1971) Pratt and Holton (1970) Storti and Quaglino (1970) Sutow et al. (1971) Whitecar et al. (1969)	Asparaginase alone	289	162
Aur et al. (1971) Capizzi et al. (1969) Goudemand and Bauters (1970) Haghbin et al. (1970) Jacquillat et al. (1970) Loeb et al. (1970) Leventhal and Henderson (1971) Leventhal et al. (1970) Rausen and Glidewell (1970) Sutow et al. (1971)	Combination	96	70
	Acute myeloblastic leukemia		
Beard et al. (1970) Carbone et al. (1970) Fairley et al. (1970) Hill et al. (1969) Jacquillat et al. (1970) Loeb et al. (1970) Marmont and Damasid (1970) Mathé et al. (1970) Ohnuma et al. (1969) Ohnuma et al. (1971) Schmidt and Gallmeier (1968) Storti and Quaglino (1970) Whitecar et al. (1969)	Asparaginase alone	100	34
Crowther et al. (1970) Fairley et al. (1970) Goudemand and Bauters (1970) Leventhal and Henderson (1971) Mathé et al. (1970)	Combination	29	14
	Acute leukemia, other types		
Marmont and Damasid (1970) Schmidt and Gallmeier (1968) Storti and Quaglino (1970) Whitecar et al. (1969)		69	6
	Chronic myelogenous leukemia, blastic		
Carbone et al. (1970) Marmont and Damasid (1970) Whitecar et al. (1969)	Asparaginase alone	8	1

Table 3 (cont.)

Ref.	Diagnosis	Number of patients	Number of responses
MATHÉ et al. (1970)	Combination	5	1
CARBONE et al. (1970) SCHMIDT and GALLMEIER (1968)	Chronic myelogenous leukemia	4	3
CARBONE et al. (1970)	Chronic lymphocytic leukemia	3	2
	Leukosarcoma		
STORTI and QUAGLINO (1970)	Asparaginase alone	3	1
MATHÉ et al. (1970)	Combination	4	3
BEARD et al. (1970) CARBONE et al. (1970) MARMONT and DAMASID (1970)	Lymphosarcoma	10	6
SCHMIDT and GALLMEIER (1968)	Brill-Symmers' Disease	1	0
CARBONE et al. (1970) JAFFE et al. (1971)	Burkitt's lymphoma	9	0
CARBONE et al. (1970) SCHMIDT and GALLMEIER (1968)	Multiple myeloma	3	0
CARBONE et al. (1970) JAFFE et al. (1971)	Hodgkin's Disease	5	0
	Melanoma		
BEARD et al. (1970) CARBONE et al. (1970) FAIRLEY et al. (1970) JAFFE et al. (1971) MARMONT and DAMASID (1970)	Asparaginase alone	17	1
MATHÉ et al. (1970)	Combination	12	0
CARBONE et al. (1970) JAFFE et al. (1971)	Osteogenic sarcoma	3	0
CARBONE et al. (1970)	Teratocarcinoma	1	0
CARBONE et al. (1970)	Hypernephroma	1	0
CARBONE et al. (1970)	Undifferentiated carcinoma	2	0
CARBONE et al. (1970)	Carcinoma of the lung	1	0
CARBONE et al. (1970)	Carcinoma of the breast	1	0
JAFFE et al. (1971)	Neuroblastoma	2	0
JAFFE et al. (1971)	Rhabdomyosarcoma	1	0
JAFFE et al. (1971)	Ewing's sarcoma	1	0
JAFFE et al. (1971)	Wilm's tumor	1	0
WHITECAR et al. (1969)	Various solid tumors	15	0

BEARD et al., 1970; CARBONE et al., 1970; FAIRLEY et al., 1970; GERHARTZ and BEGEMANN, 1970; GOUDEMAND and BAUTERS, 1970; JACQUILLAT et al., 1970; LOEB et al., 1970; MARMONT and DAMASID, 1970; MATHÉ et al., 1970; PRATT and HOLTON, 1970; STORTI and QUAGLINO, 1970; WHITECAR et al., 1970; JAFFE et al., 1971; MAYER and HOLTON, 1971; OHNUMA et al., 1971; SUTOW et al., 1971). This is in good agreement with our own experience of 37 complete remissions (41 %) and 11 good partial remissions (12 %) in 89 patients (OETTGEN et al., 1967, 1970; OETTGEN and SCHULTEN, 1969; CLARKSON et al., 1970; TALLAL et al., 1970).

In 200 patients with acute leukemia of non-lymphoblastic types, 42 complete or partial remissions (21 %) have been reported by others (SCHMIDT and GALL-

Table 4. *Results of asparaginase therapy in children treated at Memorial Hospital, New York*

Diagnosis	Number of patients		Number of responses [a]
	total	treated for 2 weeks or longer	
Acute lymphoblastic leukemia			
Asp. alone, first course	91	78	42
Asp. alone, second course	17	17	3
In remission	9	9	—
Combination	38	33	25
Acute myelo(mono)blastic leukemia			
Asp. alone, first course	12	8	0
Combination, first course	7	7	4
Combination, second course	1	1	0
Chronic granulocytic leukemia	1	1	0
Hodgkin's disease	7	6	0
Lymphosarcoma	5	2	0
Embryonal rhabdomyosarcoma	4	3	0
Neuroblastoma	5	5	0
Ewing's sarcoma	1	1	0
Osteogenic sarcoma	1	1	0
Wilm's tumor	3	2	0
Hepatoma	1	1	0
Melanoma	1	1	0
Embryonal adenocarcinoma	1	1	0

[a] For acute leukemia: complete remission or good partial remission with M1-bone marrow. For lymphomas and solid tumors: Category I (see Appendix).

MEIER, 1968; HILL et al., 1969; OHNUMA et al., 1969; BEARD et al., 1970; CARBONE et al., 1970; FAIRLEY et al., 1970; GERHARTZ and BEGEMANN, 1970; GOUDEMAND and BAUTERS, 1970; JACQUILLAT et al., 1970; LOEB et al., 1970; MARMONT and DAMASID, 1970; MATHÉ et al., 1970; STORTI and QUAGLINO, 1970; WHITECAR et al., 1970; OHNUMA et al., 1971). We have seen only 4 remissions in 32 patients (12 %) (OETTGEN and SCHULTEN, 1969; CLARKSON et al., 1970; OETTGEN et al., 1970b; TALLAL et al., 1970). A strikingly high remission rate of 50 %, reported by one group (HILL et al., 1967, 1969), accounts for the difference and underlines the difficulties that beset the morphological classification of acute leukemias. In one dramatic case, a complete remission was induced with a single dose of 1000 IU/kg (OHNUMA et al., 1969). In several instances a high leukocyte count fell sharply at the beginning of therapy, only to rise again a week or so later; no effect on the bone marrow was seen (CLARKSON et al., 1970).

While the criteria for a remission in acute leukemia are well defined, albeit not rigorously applied by all investigators, the term "response" in the case of chronic leukemias, lymphomas, and solid tumors is rather vague and does not necessarily imply the destruction of most neoplastic cells. Nine responses were seen in 29 patients with lymphosarcoma or leukosarcoma. Seven patients with Burkitt's tumor (6 of them from Uganda) did not respond. The only responses in the group of patients with other solid tumors were observed in two of the 41 patients with melanoma. One of these patients responded to at least three and perhaps four separate courses of therapy over a total period of two years. The finding that 30 to 50 % of melanomas are sensitive to asparaginase *in vitro* (OLD et al., 1968; OETTGEN and SCHULTEN, 1969; ALEXANDER et al., 1970) has given rise to the speculation that the need of melanoma cells for asparagine may be met *in vivo*

Table 5. *Results of asparaginase therapy in adults treated at Memorial Hospital, New York*

Diagnosis	Number of patients total	Number of patients treated for 2 weeks or longer	Number of responses [a]
Acute lymphoblastic leukemia			
Asp. alone, first course	15	11	6
Asp. alone, second course	4	4	1
In remission	9	9	—
Combination	10	9	7
Combination, in remission	4	4	—
Acute myelo(mono)blastic leukemia			
Asp. alone, first course	35	22	4
Asp. alone, seond course	6	5	0
In remission	1	1	—
Combination	10	8	0
Combination in remission	1	1	—
Acute undifferentiated leukemia			
Asp. alone, first course	4	2	0
Leukosarcoma			
Asp. alone, first course	19	8	2
Combination	5	5	4
Chronic granulocytic leukemia, blastic			
Asp. alone, first course	9	4	0
Combination	2	2	2
Chronic granulocytic leukemia	1	1	0
Chronic lymphocytic leukemia	3	3	0
Chronic monocytic leukemia	1	1	0
Lymphosarcoma or reticulum cell sarcoma	12	6	0
Mycosis fungoides	1	1	0
Hodgkin's disease	8	7	0
Malignant melanoma	33	24	1
Neuroblastoma	2	2	0
Embryonal rhabdomyosarcoma	2	2	0
Spindle cell sarcoma	2	0	—
Leiomyosarcoma	2	2	0
Osteogenic sarcoma	2	1	0
Ewing's sarcoma	2	2	0
Testicular tumor	4	0	—
Trophoblastic tumor	3	3	0
Hepatoma	3	3	0
Carcinoma head and neck	8	4	0
Carcinoma thyroid	2	1	0
Carcinoma lung	4	0	—
Carcinoma prostate	1	0	—
Carcinoma colon	4	2	0
Carcinoma anus	1	0	—
Carcinoma breast	6	2	0
Carcinoma cervix	1	0	—
Carcinoma ovary	1	1	0
Carcinoma kidney	2	2	0

[a] For acute leukemia: Complete remission or good partial remission with M1-bone marrow. For lymphomas and solid tumors: Category I (see Appendix).

by asparagine-producing stroma cells growing in close association in the tumor nodule. No response was observed in patients with any other type of solid tumor. However, the numbers in each group are small. Thus, considering that only 2 of 40 patients with melanoma responded, one cannot say that other solid tumors are never sensitive to asparaginase (OETTGEN et al., 1967; SCHMIDT and GALLMEIER, 1968; OETTGEN and SCHULTEN, 1969; BEARD et al., 1970; CARBONE et al., 1970; CLARKSON et al., 1970; FAIRLEY et al., 1970; MASHBURN and LANDIN, 1970; OETTGEN et al., 1970; STORTI and QUAGLINO, 1970; TALLAL et al., 1970; WHITECAR et al., 1970; JAFFE et al., 1971).

B. Relation of Incidence and Duration of Remissions to Dose and Schedule of Administration of Asparaginase

Since different investigators have employed somewhat different criteria to define complete and partial remissions and to determine the duration of remissions, and since it is not always evident at what stage of the disease the patients were treated, the following analysis is largely restricted to children with acute lymphoblastic leukemia who were treated at Memorial Hospital, New York.

Of the total number of 91 children, 78 were treated for 2 weeks or longer. In only 15 of these had the diagnosis of leukemia been made one month or less before asparaginase therapy. Twenty-nine patients were treated during the first year and 32 patients during the second year of their illness. The remaining 17 patients had been ill for more than 2 years. Only 11 of the 78 patients had no chemotherapy before they were treated with asparaginase. All others had received prednisone previously, many had been treated with methotrexate, vincristine, and 6-mercaptopurine and about one-third had also received daunomycin or arabinosyl cytosine. Thirty-two of the 78 patients achieved complete remissions (M1, H1, P1, S1: see appendix). In 10 additional patients the bone marrow rating was M1, but they did not qualify for a complete remission because their hemoglobin levels were not in the normal range. The total number of patients whose bone marrow was rated M1 (i.e., normal with respect to both cellularity and differential count) was 42 of 78 patients or 54%. As far as these small numbers go, there was little difference in remission rates between the groups treated at a dose of 10, 200, 1000, or 5000 IU per kg per day (Table 6). In a randomized study of children with advanced acute lymphoblastic leukemia the incidence of remissions was reported to be higher for the group that was treated with 5000 IU/kg once weekly for three weeks (i.e., 10 of 15) than for the group that received 1000 IU/kg/day on 5 days per week for three weeks (i.e., 6 of 15) (RAUSEN and GLIDEWELL, 1970). Considering the small number of cases and their probable differences with respect to duration of disease and previous therapy it is not yet certain whether the first schedule is in fact more effective. Its disadvantages with respect to hypersensitivity reactions are discussed below.

Table 6. *Incidence of remissions obtained with asparaginase therapy in children with acute lymphoblastic leukemia*

Dose IU/kg/day	Number of patients	Number of CR[a]	Number of GPR-M1[b]	Percent remissions
10	12	4	1	42
200	28	13	5	64
1000	22	12	0	55
5000	16	3	4	44
Total	78	32	10	54

[a] CR: complete remission.
[b] GPR-M1: good partial remission with M1-bone marrow rating (see Appendix).

Table 7. *Duration of remissions obtained with asparaginase therapy in children with acute lymphoblastic leukemia*

Therapy		Remissions[a]			
Dose IU/kg/day	Duration	Number	Duration (days)		
			Range	Mean	Median
10	Maintained	5	38—145	79	61
200→50	Maintained	5	28—247	98	50
200	28 days	6	19—104	67	64
200	Maintained	4	40—104	67	63
1000	28 days	12	58—424	158	122
5000	28 days	7	20—158	98	129

[a] Complete or good partial remissions with M1-bone marrow.

All remissions were temporary. The duration ranged from less than three weeks to more than one year. The median was 60 days for patients who received 10 or 200 IU per kg per day and 120 days for patients who were treated with 1000 or 5000 IU per kg per day (Table 7). Although suggestive, these figures do not necessarily indicate that the larger dose produces longer lasting remissions. This becomes evident when we examine the correlation between the duration of asparaginase-induced remissions and factors other than asparaginase therapy. The duration of the disease prior to therapy is one of these factors. The median duration of remissions was 142 days for patients who had been ill for one month or less, 60 days for patients whose disease had existed from one month to 2 years (calculated from the time of diagnosis), and 114 days for patients who had leukemia for more than 2 years (Table 8). Seven of the 10 remissions in the first group were obtained by treatment with 1000 IU/kg/day. A related, though not identical, factor that can be considered is the number of chemotherapeutic agents used prior to asparaginase therapy. The median duration was 146 days for untreated patients, 99 days for patients who had been treated previously with 1 to 4 other agents, and 63 days for those who had received 5 to 10 other agents (Table 8). Again, the majority of the patients who achieved remissions in the first group were treated at the dose of

Table 8. *Correlation of duration of disease and of previous therapy with duration of asparaginase-induced remissions*

Ref.	Number of patients	Number of remissions					Median duration (days)
		Total	10	200 (IU/kg/day)	1000	5000	
Duration of Disease							
< 1 month	15	10	1		7	2	142
1—12 months	14	7		4	3		58
1— 2 years	32	13	3	8	1	1	63
> 2 years	17	12	1	6	1	4	114
Previous Therapy							
None	11	9	1		6	2	146
1— 4 agents[a]	25	12		6	5	1	99
5—10 agents[a]	42	21	4	12	1	4	63

[a] Agents used prior to asparaginase were prednisone, vincristine, methotrexate, 6-mercaptopurine, daunomycin, arabinosyl cytosine, cytoxan, BCNU, nitrogen mustard, and actinomycin D.

1000 IU/kg/day. Clearly, the question of what is the optimal dose and schedule of asparaginase administration for patients with acute lymphoblastic leukemia can only be answered by comparing the results obtained in groups of closely matched patients. Results of this type are not yet available.

C. Central Nervous System Leukemia

Meningeal leukemic infiltrates in 7 of 14 children with asparaginase-sensitive acute lymphoblastic leukemia responded to intravenous administration of asparaginase (Tan and Oettgen, 1969; Clarkson et al., 1970). This has also been observed by others (Hill et al., 1969; Jacquillat et al., 1970), and the response clearly occurs in the absence of measurable enzyme levels. It has been shown, however, that asparagine levels decrease sharply in the spinal fluid after intravenous asparaginase administration, although the enzyme cannot be detected (Schulten, H. K., unpublished observations). In 9 cases asparaginase was given intrathecally (Clarkson et al., 1970; Tallal et al., 1970; Tan and Oettgen, 1970). While intrathecal administration was tolerated and effective, it cannot yet be considered as a superior method of treating meningeal leukemia with asparaginase.

D. Combination Therapy

Since drug combinations have produced better results than their single components in the treatment of acute leukemia, it is not surprising that asparaginase has also been used in combination with other drugs. Agents that have been used in various combinations are prednisone, vincristine, daunomycin, arabinosyl cytosine, thioguanine, 6-mercaptopurine, methotrexate, and cytoxan (Carbone et al., 1970; Crowther et al., 1970; Fairley et al., 1970; Goudemand and Bauters, 1970; Haghbin et al., 1970; Hardisty and McElwain, 1970; Jacquillat et al., 1970; Leventhal et al., 1970; Mathé et al., 1970; Oettgen et al., 1970; Rausen and Glidewell, 1970; Aur et al., 1971; Leventhal and Henderson, 1971; Sutow et al., 1971). Whether a synergistic effect is obtained cannot yet be said with assurance. The combination of asparaginase with the glutamine antagonists, azaserine or azotomycin (glutamine donates the amino group that converts aspartic acid to asparagine in the presence of asparagine synthetase), did not give better results than asparaginase alone in patients with acute lymphoblastic leukemia (Leventhal et al., 1970; Leventhal and Henderson, 1971). Asparaginase has also been given at the beginning of a remission induced by other drugs. Some of the results obtained at Memorial Hospital, New York, with combination therapy are summarized in Table 9. Asparaginase was given at the dose of 1000 IU/kg/day

Table 9. *Combination therapy of acute lymphoblastic leukemia*

Therapy	Number of cases	Median duration of disease (months)	Number of remissions	Duration of remissions (days)	
				Range	Median
Asparaginase 1000 IU/kg/day × 28					
(1) *With* prednisone, vincristine, methotrexate, and daunomycin.					
First asparaginase treatment	15	1	10	33—264+	110
Second asparaginase treatment	8	10	7	60—286+	125
(2) *After* remission inductions with other agents.	9	13		61—555+	152
(3) *Alone*	22	7	12	58—424	112

I.V. for 28 days. Three groups are compared, namely (1) patients who received asparaginase simultaneously with prednisone, vincristine, methotrexate, and daunomycin, (2) patients who were treated with asparaginase after a remission had been induced with other agents, and (3) patients who received asparaginase only. The first group was subdivided into patients who had been treated with asparaginase before and thus were less likely to respond again to the enzyme (see below) and patients who received asparaginase for the first time. The patients in groups 2 and 3 had not been given asparaginase previously. All but 4 patients in group 1 had received one or more of the other agents of the combination prior to this trial. While the incidence of remissions was, of course, greater in group 1 than in group 3, there was no striking difference in the duration of the remissions between the groups. At present, the merits of using asparaginase in combination therapy are explored in clinical trials with previously untreated patients. In designing these studies, advantage can be taken of the fact that asparaginase has little myelo-suppressive activity, and therefore can, and perhaps should, be given during a period of bone marrow depression induced by other drugs. Such a regimen would not only make good use of an interval during which most other agents cannot be given, but also deprive the remaining leukemia cells in the bone marrow of asparagine at a time when "feeding" by normal bone marrow cells should be minimal. Promising attempts of this sort have been reported (CANELLOS and HASKELL, 1970).

E. Resistance

Sooner or later, all patients with primarily responsive disease develop resistance to asparaginase. Without exception, the patients who relapsed during maintenance therapy did not respond to an increased dose of the enzyme preparation. When relapse occurred after an unmaintained remission or after a remission induced and maintained with other drugs, however, a second remission was obtained occasionally by treatment with asparaginase. At Memorial Hospital, New York, 14 patients with acute lymphoblastic leukemia and 3 patients with acute myeloblastic leukemia received a second course of asparaginase, preceded by desensitization (Table 10). Second remissions were induced in one child and in one adult with acute lymphoblastic leukemia. The adult patient had relapsed, 10.5 months earlier, after a remission induced and maintained for 6 months with asparaginase. During the interval he was treated with other drugs. The child received no other treatment during the 4 month-remission that followed the first course of asparaginase. The second remission also lasted 4 months. A third course of asparaginase did not produce a remission.

It is known that sensitive tumor cells have a lower capacity to synthesize asparagine than resistant variants (BROOME and SCHWARTZ, 1967; PRAGER et al., 1969). *In vitro* studies have shown that the cells of responsive human leukemias often require asparagine and that an increased ability to synthesize asparagine may also be the basis of clinical resistance (OETTGEN et al., 1967; OLD et al., 1968; OETTGEN and SCHULTEN, 1969; CANELLOS and HASKELL, 1970; HASKELL and CANELLOS, 1970; HO et al., 1970; OHNUMA et al., 1970; CAPIZZI et al., 1969; SHREK and DOLOWY, 1971). It has not been possible, however, to predict on the basis of *in vitro* tests whether a patient will respond to asparaginase therapy. During treatment a rise of asparagine synthetase levels was found in leukemia cells from patients with refractory disease, but not in cells from patients with responsive disease (CANELLOS and HASKELL, 1970). The ability of asparaginase-resistant cells to utilize endogenous asparagine for protein synthesis with higher efficiency is demonstrated by the finding that intracellular asparagine levels decrease to the

Table 10. *Results of a second course of asparaginase in patients who had responded to asparaginase therapy before*

Diagnosis	Number of cases	Duration of interval without asparaginase (days)		Number of remissions
		Range	Median	
Acute lymphoblastic leukemia				
Children	11	48—365	99	1
Adults	3	15—319	172	1
Acute myeloblastic leukemia				
Adults	3	55—124	99	0

same extent in sensitive and resistant cells during asparaginase therapy. This indicates that, in resistant cells, protein synthesis continues at intracellular levels of free asparagine which are inadequate for sensitive cells, and that there is a close linkage between asparagine synthesizing and utilizing systems (BROOME, 1968). Attempts to find an explanation for the greater ability of the resistant cell to utilize endogenous asparagine have led to experiments examining cellular transfer RNA (BROOME, 1970). It has been speculated that asparagine-tRNA may serve as a corepressor for asparagine synthetase in sensitive cells.

Toxic Effects

Asparaginase therapy produced a large variety of toxic effects (Table 11). Their incidence in the patients treated at Memorial Hospital, New York, is shown in Table 12.

Table 11. *Toxic effects of E. coli L-asparaginase*

Toxic Effect
General (fever, anorexia, nausea, vomiting, weight loss): AUR et al. (1971), BEARD et al. (1970), CAPIZZI et al. (1969), CARBONE et al. (1970), DEUTSCH et al. (1970), FAIRLEY et al. (1970), GERHARTZ and BEGEMANN (1970), GOUDEMAND and BAUTERS (1970), HASKELL et al. (1969), JACQUILLAT et al. (1970), JAFFE et al. (1971), LOEB et al. (1970), LEVENTHAL and HENDERSON (1971), LEVENTHAL et al. (1970), MARMONT and DAMASID (1970), MATHÉ et al. (1970), MAYER and HOLTON (1971), OETTGEN et al. (1967, 1970a, b), OETTGEN and SCHULTEN (1969), OHNUMA et al. (1969, 1970, 1971), PRATT and HOLTON (1970), SCHMIDT and GALLMEIER (1968), WHITECAR et al. (1969, 1970)
Liver (SGOT, SGPT increased, alkaline phosphatase increased, 5′-nucleotidase increased, bilirubin increased, BSP retention increased, fatty infiltration): BEARD et al. (1970), CAPIZZI et al. (1969), CARBONE et al. (1970), DEUTSCH et al. (1970), FAIRLEY et al. (1970), GERHARTZ and BEGEMANN (1970), GOUDEMAND and BAUTERS (1970), HASKELL et al. (1969), JACQUILLAT et al. (1970), JAFFE et al. (1971), LOEB et al. (1970), LEVENTHAL and HENDERSON (1971), LEVENTHAL et al. (1970), MARMONT and DAMASID (1970), MAYER and HOLTON (1971), OETTGEN and SCHULTEN (1969), OETTGEN et al. (1970a,b), OHNUMA et al. (1969, 1970, 1971), PRATT and HOLTON (1970), PRATT and JOHNSON (1971), STORTI and QUAGLINO (1970), WHITECAR et al. (1969, 1970)
Proteins (Albumin decreased, other serum proteins decreased, edema, immunoglobulins increased, chorionic gonadotropin decreased, insulin decreased): AUR et al. (1971), BEARD et al. (1970), CARBONE et al. (1970), DEUTSCH et al. (1970), FAIRLEY et al. (1970), FATEH-MOGHADAM et al. (1970), FINK and BEGEMANN (1970), GERHARTZ and BEGEMANN (1970), HASKELL et al. (1969), JACQUILLAT et al. (1970), LOEB et al. (1970), LEVENTHAL et al. (1970), MARMONT and DAMASID (1970), MATHÉ et al. (1970), OERKERMANN et al. (1970), OETTGEN et al. (1970a,b), OHNUMA et al. (1969), PRATT and HOLTON (1970), SCHMIDT and GALLMEIER (1968), WHITECAR et al. (1969, 1970)

Table 11 (cont.)

Toxic Effect
Coagulation (fibrinogen decreased, consumption coagulopathy): Aur et al. (1971), Beard et al. (1970), Bettigole et al. (1970), Burgio et al. (1970), Deutsch et al. (1970), Fink and Begemann (1970), Gerhartz and Begemann (1970), Goudemand and Bauters (1970), Gralnick and Henry (1969), Hasselberger et al. (1970), Jacquillat et al. (1970), Loeb et al. (1970), Leventhal and Henderson (1971), Leventhal et al. (1970), Marmont and Damasid (1970), Mathé et al. (1970), Mayer and Holton (1971), Oettgen and Schulten (1969), Oettgen et al. (1970a, b), Ohnuma et al. (1969), Pratt and Holton (1970), Storti and Quaglino (1970), Whitecar et al. (1969, 1970)
Lipids (serum lipids decreased, serum lipids increased): Aur et al. (1971), Canellos et al. (1969), Carbone et al. (1970), Deutsch et al. (1970), Fateh-Moghadam et al. (1970), Gerhartz and Begemann (1970), Goudemand and Bauters (1970), Haskell et al. (1969), Jacquillat et al. (1970), Lash et al. (1968), Mathé et al. (1970), Oettgen and Schulten (1969), Oettgen et al. (1970b), Ohnuma et al. (1969), Pratt and Holton (1970), Storti and Quaglino (1970), Whitecar et al. (1969, 1970)
Carbohydrates (glucose increased): Aur et al. (1971), Deutsch et al. (1970), Jaffe et al. (1971), Oettgen et al. (1970a, b), Ohnuma et al. (1969), Whitecar et al. (1970)
Pancreatitis (or elevated amylase): Aur et al. (1971), Capizzi et al. (1970), Carbone et al. (1970), Loeb et al. (1970), Leventhal and Henderson (1971), Leventhal et al. (1970), Oettgen et al. (1970a, b), Ohnuma et al. (1969, 1970, 1971), Whitecar et al. (1970)
Prerenal or renal (ammonia increased, blood urea nitrogen increased, renal failure): Aur et al. (1971), Carbone et al. (1970), Gerhartz and Begemann (1970), Haskell et al. (1969), Jaffe et al. (1971), Mayer and Holton (1971), Oettgen et al. (1970a, b), Ohnuma et al. (1969, 1970, 1971), Pratt and Holton (1970), Rausen and Glidewell (1970), Whitecar et al. (1970)
Central nervous system (somnolence, lethargy, confusion, delirium, Parkinson syndrome): Carbone et al. (1970), Gerhartz and Begemann (1970), Haskell et al. (1969), Jacquillat et al. (1970), Loeb et al. (1970), Marmont and Damasid (1970), Oettgen et al. (1970a, b), Ohnuma et al. (1969, 1970, 1971), Pratt and Holton (1970), Storti and Quaglino (1970), Whitecar et al. (1970)
Bone marrow (hemoglobin decreased, leukocytes decreased, platelets decreased): Carbone et al. (1970), Fink and Begemann (1970), Jaffe et al. (1971), Lash et al. (1968), Marmont and Damasid (1970), Mathé et al. (1970), Mayer and Holton (1971), Oettgen et al. (1970a, b)
Immunosuppression (delayed hypersensitivity, lymphocyte stimulation, antibody production, complement activity): Astaldi et al. (1969a, b), Benezra et al. (1970), Burgio et al. (1970), Delage et al. (1971), Fink and Begemann (1970), Jackson et al. (1970), McElwain and Hayward (1969), Miura et al. (1970), Ohno and Hersh (1970a, b), Schwartz et al. (1970)
Sensitization (anaphylaxis (mild-severe), serum sickness, circulating antibodies): Beard et al. (1970), Capizzi et al. (1969), Carbone et al. (1970), Dahlwitz et al. (1970), Eigner et al. (1970), Fairley et al. (1970), Gerhartz and Begemann (1970), Haskell et al. (1969), Jaffe et al. (1971), Khan and Hill (1969), Loeb et al. (1970), Leventhal and Henderson (1971), Mathé et al. (1970), Ohnuma et al. (1970, 1971), Peterson et al. (1971), Pinsky et al. (1970), Rausen and Glidewell (1970), Schmidt and Gallmeier (1968), Whitecar et al. (1970)

With the highly purified products that are now available, fever due to contamination with endotoxin is no longer as serious a problem as it was in the early trials. Anorexia, nausea, and vomiting have also become less prominent. Liver toxicity was indicated by increased levels of transaminases, alkaline phosphatase, 5'-nucleotidase and bilirubin and by an increased retention of bromsulfophthalein (BSP). In biopsy and autopsy specimens, fatty infiltration of the liver was noted. Hypoalbuminemia was noted frequently, was occasionally severe enough to cause

Table 12. *Incidence of toxic effects in patients treated at Memorial Hospital, New York*

Toxic effect	Number of cases evaluated	Percent abnormal
Fever	197	54
Anorexia, nausea, vomiting	303	54
Weight loss	221	69
Increased serum GOT	244	55
Increased serum alkaline phosphatase	240	39
Increased serum 5′-nucleotidase	163	22
Increased serum bilirubin	190	40
Increased BSP-retention	124	62
Decreased serum albumin	144	76
Edema	267	6
Decreased plasma fibrinogen	33	97
Decreased serum cholesterol	221	83
Increased blood glucose	68	19
Glucosuria	303	10
Increased blood urea nitrogen	283	60
Proteinuria	303	10
Lethargy, somnolence, confusion	303	39
Decreased leukocyte count [a]	116	25
Decreased platelet count [a]	116	12
Hypersensitivity	247	30
Precipitating antibodies	105	71

[a] Only hematologically normal patients with solid tumors were evaluated.

generalized edema, and probably explains the low serum calcium levels. The serum levels of at least 15 other individual serum proteins were found to decrease during treatment. The concentrations of IgM, IgA, and IgG, on the contrary (Table 13), increased. Levels of hormones such as insulin and chorionic gonadotropin (in patients with choriocarcinoma) also decreased. A decrease in plasma fibrinogen was observed in almost every patient. In patients with solid tumors who did not respond to asparaginase therapy, this was clearly due to decreased synthesis rather than accelerated consumption, as shown in studies measuring the survival of

Table 13. *Changes in serum protein levels during asparaginase therapy*

Protein	Percent of pretreatment level (Median) [a]	Protein	Percent of pretreatment level (Median) [a]
IgM	196	Hemopexin	51
IgA	189	Transferrin	50
IgG	150	β_{1A}-globulin	48
α-Acid glycoprotein	120	β_2-glycoprotein I	47
α-Antichymotrypsin	89	Anti GcGlobulin	45
α_2-Macroglobulin	81	α_2-Antithrombin	37
β_2-Glycoprotein II	79	β_2-Glycoprotein III	29
α-Antitrypsin	74	Haptoglobin	25
α_1-Lipoprotein	74	Ceruloplasmin	20
β-Lipoprotein	69		

[a] Sera from 8 children and 8 adults were examined before therapy and after 2 to 4 weeks of therapy by means of quantitative radial immunodiffusion.

autologous ^{131}I-fibrinogen. In these patients, factor V, VIII, euglobulin lysis time, thrombin time, prothrombin time, and partial thromboplastin time did not change. This has been confirmed, but others have also reported findings indicative of an intravascular coagulation syndrome in patients with acute leukemia, not surprising if one considers that this type of clotting defect has been observed in leukemia patients who did not receive asparaginase therapy. Hypolipidemia with

Table 14. *Biochemical and hematological changes during asparaginase therapy*

Test	Results (mean) Days of Therapy						
	0	1	3	7	14	21	28
SGOT (Karmen Units) [a]	40			67	99	112	145
Alkaline phosphatase (Bodansky Units) [a]							
Children	6.2			9.2	14.0	16.0	17.8
Adults	3.5			4.5	11.0	15.0	9.7
5′-Nucleotidase (Campbell Units) [a]	8			9	24	20	23
Bilirubin (mg/100 ml) [a]	0.5			1.7	1.9	2.0	2.3
Albumin (% of pre-treatment levels)	100			85	78	76	76
α_1-Globulin (% of pre-treatment levels)	100			96	94	93	97
α_2-Globulin (% of pre-treatment levels)	100			78	68	67	68
β- Globulin (% of pre-treatment levels)	100			78	72	76	76
γ- Globulin (% of pre-treatment levels)	100			131	146	163	173
Cholesterol (mg/100 ml)	169			102	88	100	107
BUN (mg/100 ml)							
Children	11	18	16	13	12		11
Adults	14	27	23	22	20		18
Leukocytes (per μl × 1000) [a]	5.9			4.1	3.2	4.6	7.6
Thrombocytes (per μl × 1000) [a]	293			266	156	223	280

[a] Only patients who developed abnormal levels during asparaginase therapy are included.

decreased serum levels of cholesterol, phospholipids, and total lipids was found in the majority of patients. On rare occasions patients developed hyperlipidemia of the mixed exogenous and endogenous type, with chylomicrons, an increase of pre-β-lipoprotein, a decrease of β-lipoprotein, and low lipoprotein lipase levels. Rarely was the blood glucose found elevated, and clinical diabetes without ketonuria developed in isolated instances only. Although we have not yet observed a case of fulminant clinical pancreatitis, as have some other groups, we have seen microscopic foci of inflammation in the pancreas at autopsy. Transient and apparently prerenal azotemia during the first days of therapy was found in many patients, irrespective of whether or not they responded to therapy. On rare occasions, however, patients developed acute renal failure with tubular necrosis in a setting that can only be described as a general metabolic catastrophe. Asparaginase produced leukopenia or thrombocytopenia in a small proportion of patients. The biochemical and hematological changes were usually not progressive throughout the period of therapy, but tended to maintain a plateau after the second week or even become less marked. The magnitude of some of the changes and their time course are shown in Table 14. It made little or no difference whether asparaginase was given at a dose of 10, 200, 1000, or 5000 IU per kg per day. By contrast, the effects on the central nervous system (i.e., lethargy, somnolence, and confusion) were more severe when larger doses were given. Another effect on normal tissues was immunosuppression, documented *in vivo* as a reduced capacity to develop a cellular or humoral immune response to new antigens, and *in vitro* as a decreased lymphocyte response to phytohemagglutinin (BENEZRA et al., 1970; JACKSON et al., 1970; MIURA et al., 1970; OHNO and HERSH, 1970a, b; SCHWARTZ et al., 1970b). Reduction of complement activity *in vitro* was also noted (DELAGE et al., 1971). Improvement of skin lesions was seen in a patient with dermatomyositis, an "autoimmune" disease, under asparaginase therapy (FINK, 1970).

When considering these effects of *E. coli* L-asparaginase on normal tissues, one has to keep in mind that the enzyme preparation possesses a low but definite glutaminase activity. Although glutamine levels in the blood decreased below measurable values during the first days of asparaginase therapy and increased subsequently while treatment was continued (in contrast to asparagine levels), this has been studied only in patients treated with low doses of the enzyme preparation. It is conceivable that, at larger dose levels, the compensatory mechanisms are no longer adequate to cope with the increased rate of glutamine destruction. That the inhibition of human cells in tissue culture by *E. coli* L-asparaginase can be due to its glutaminase activity has been clearly shown (KIM et al., 1968; OERKERMANN et al., 1970).

Another group of side effects was the consequence of sensitization to the enzyme preparations. Most patients produced antibodies. Precipitating antibodies of two types were found: one type was directed against the enzyme itself and was not found in the presence of measurable plasma enzyme levels, while the other type was directed against other *E. coli* components. Antibodies of this type were found in the serum both during (with measurable plasma enzyme levels) and after therapy and, in some instances, even before therapy. While there was cross-reactivity between *E. coli* asparaginases from different sources, the enzyme prepared from *Erwinia carotovora* was of different antigenic structure. Antibodies were responsible for an accelerated elimination of asparaginase in some patients, and they produced hypersensitivity reactions in approximately one third of the patients. These reactions were usually of the anaphylactic type, namely, urticaria, abdominal cramps, respiratory distress, hypotension, or facial edema. The clinical syndrome of serum sickness was seen only rarely. We have not observed a fatal anaphylactic reaction (PINSKY et al., 1970). With respect to anaphylaxis, intermittent therapy is expected to carry a greater risk than daily administration of the enzyme preparation. The longer the interval, the more likely it is to include a period when there is no asparaginase (which can be measured) or contaminants (which cannot be measured) left in the circulation. During this period, anaphylactic antibodies continue to be produced and to be fixed to tissues, giving rise to a magnified response when antigen is introduced again with the next injection. A case of fatal anaphylaxis was reported to have occurred in a group of patients treated at weekly intervals (RAUSEN and GLIDEWELL, 1970). In one study, antibodies to L-asparaginase, as measured by passive hemagglutination, were found in the serum of all patients at least one day before an allergic reaction occurred, but not in the serum of patients who did not develop allergy. It was suggested that titration of antibodies by passive hemagglutination may provide a means of predicting impending anaphylaxis, particularly when coupled with a sudden decrease in circulating L-asparaginase levels (PETERSON et al., 1971).

To summarize, asparaginase therapy is certainly not without side effects. However, the toxicity differs from that observed with many other agents in several respects. First, the bone marrow is not the most severely affected organ; toxic effects on other tissues are more pronounced. Second, the tendency of the abnormalities to maintain a plateau or even to become somewhat less marked as treatment progresses indicates that adaptive mechanisms may come into play, such as, for instance, a compensatory increase of asparagine synthetase levels in normal cells. The sum of the side effects seen at a dose of 5000 units per kg per day represents a clear hazard for many adults. That children fare somewhat better at this dose may again indicate the importance of adaptation. If one considers that much smaller doses are effective in the treatment of responsive neoplasms, it should be possible to treat the majority of patients without serious side effects.

When asparaginase was given in combination with other agents it was noted that the patients were more susceptible to the toxic effects of vincristine, and perhaps also to those of arabinosyl cytosine, thioguanine, and daunomycin. Two possible explanations come to mind. First, the catabolism of cytotoxic agents may be depressed in a liver that is affected by asparaginase. If this were so, effective blood and tissue levels could be maintained with lower doses of these agents. Second, the metabolic demands made on normal tissues by an asparagine deficiency may make them more susceptible to the toxic effects of cytotoxic agents. In this case, the therapeutic index of these agents would be reduced and the patients might actually be deprived of some of their therapeutic activity. At present, a course of asparaginase after therapy with other agents appears more attractive than simultaneous combination therapy.

Conclusions

What, then, are our conclusions as to the present and possible future value of asparaginase in the treatment of human cancer? At present, the enzyme is often useful as a temporarily effective agent in patients with acute lymphoblastic leukemia, less commonly in patients with acute myeloblastic leukemia, and more rarely still in patients with other types of cancer.

No doubt, this is less than had been hoped for. However, a wider spectrum of activity could not really be expected if one considers the specificity of the characteristic that makes cells sensitive to the action of the enzyme. On the contrary, it surprises one that the cells of acute lymphoblastic leukemia have this characteristic so often. The fact that the lack of one amino acid can kill certain cancer cells is still exciting, and we hope that asparagine-dependence will not remain the only example. What can we do to improve the therapeutic results within the spectrum of sensitive neoplasms?

The initial hope that larger doses might be more effective has to be abandoned because the largest doses that have been used did not give better results and produced a degree of toxicity which clearly prohibits the administration of yet larger doses. This indicates that the difference in the requirement for asparagine between sensitive neoplastic cells and some normal tissues is quantitative rather than qualitative (i.e., that normal cells can adapt faster and better than sensitive neoplastic cells to asparagine deficiency). It remains to be seen, and clearly deserves further exploration, whether asparaginase potentiates the therapeutic effects of other agents and thus adds to the ever increasing life span of patients with acute leukemia. In the small number of responsive patients with severe hypersensitivity reactions to the *E. coli* enzyme the usefulness of asparaginase therapy might be extended if preparations with different antigenic properties were available. The enzyme prepared from *Erwinia carotovora* appears to satisfy this requirement. We may hope, in terms of increasing the spectrum of responsive tumors and of obtaining more prolonged remissions, for successful attempts to modify the enzyme molecule so that its distribution throughout all intercellular compartments becomes more favorable. This could be of importance if one considers that sanctuaries may exist where asparagine-dependent cells are provided with asparagine. It is doubtful that the theoretically crucial condition, namely isolation of each and every neoplastic cell in the body from an extracellular source of asparagine within a period short enough to preclude adaptation, has ever been achieved. In view of our ignorance as to whether acquired resistance is selective or adaptive, we must recognize that the potential value of asparagine deprivation may not really have been tested and possibly cannot be tested adequately with present asparaginase therapy.

Appendix

Criteria of Response Used in the Evaluation of Patients Treated at Memorial Hospital, New York

HEWLETT, J. S., BETTLE, J. D., JR., BISHOP, R. C., FOWLER, W. M., SCHWARTZ, S. O., HAGEN, P. S., LOUIS, J.: Cancer Chemother. Rep. 42, 27 (1964).

1. Criteria for Rating Categories

Qualitative or quantitative changes which appear to be the operation of normal homeostatic mechanisms, or physiologic responses of the patients to nonleukemic stimuli rather than a part of the disease, should not be considered abnormalities (e.g., secondary to medication or the normoblastic hyperplasia seen in early phases of remission, etc.).

1.1. Bone Marrow (Category M)

1.1.1. Ratings for Parameters

Type leukemia	ALL	Lymphocytic[a]	Granulocytic + other types
Parameter	Blast cells[b]	Lymphocytes + blast cells[b]	Leukemic + blast cells[b]
Parameter rating			
1	0— 5	0—40	0— 5
2	6—25	41—69	6—39
3	25	69	39

[a] Include childhood undifferentiated leukemia with the lymphocytic group. Percentage values given for Parameter Rating represent percentage of all marrow elements.

[b] This term includes blast cells, as well as all cells which cannot be classified as either blast cells or more mature *normal* elements, and includes "leukemic cells", "pathologic lymphocytes", and "stem cells".

1.1.2. Ratings for Category M

Rating of this category will be determined by the most abnormal parameter found. Bone marrows qualifying for M 1 ratings must contain qualitatively and quantitatively normal erythropoiesis, granulopoiesis, and megakaryopoiesis.

1.2. Hemogram (Category H)

1.2.1. Ratings for Parameters

Rating	Hemoglobin Child <2	Hemoglobin Child >2	Hemoglobin adults M	Hemoglobin adults F	Neutrophilic Granulocytes	Blasts[a]	Platelets
1	10	11	12	10	1500	0	100,000 (phase) or normal
2					500 to 1499	<5%	<100,000 or decreased
3	<7				<500	>5%	<25,000 or 25% of normal

[a] This term includes blast cells, as well as all cells which cannot be classified as either blast cells or more mature normal elements, and includes "leukemic cells", "pathologic lymphocytes", and "stem cells".

1.2.2. Ratings for Category H

The rating for category H is determined by the sum of the ratings for all of the parameters (hemoglobin, neutrophilic granulocytes, blast[a] cells and platelets). Ratings indicating improvement in this category must not be ascribable to transfusion of any blood elements. Mononuclear cells must not exceed 7000 cells/mm^3 (10000 for <2 years) for an H1 rating. The appearance of 1 to 2% blast cells on an isolated count will not preclude an H1 rating.

Rating	Sum of parameter ratings
1	4
2	8
3	>8

1.3. Category P — Physical Findings

1.3.1. Ratings for Each Parameter

Each physical finding constitutes a measurable parameter. The degree of abnormality for each parameter will be rated as follows:

a) *Liver*
1 = within normal limits for age
2 = definite enlargement (to umbilicus)
3 = enlargement below umbilicus

b) *Spleen*
1 = within normal limits for age
2 = definite enlargement (to umbilicus)
3 = enlargement below umbilicus

c) *Lymph Nodes*
1 = within normal limits
2 = definite enlargement
3 = massive enlargement (grossly visible)

d) *Other Leukemic Organ Involvement*
(If present, note and score separately: skin, CNS, kidney, lungs etc.)
1 = none
2 = definite
3 = marked

1.3.2. Ratings for Category P

The final rating for Category P is based on the sum of the numerical values given to each Parameter.

Category P rating	Sum of parameter rating
1	4
2	5—8
3	>8

1.4. Category S — Symptoms

Rating for Category S is determined by the performance activity of the patient ratings listed below.

1 = Asymptomatic and normal activity
2 = Symptomatic with normal or limited activity but less than 50% of normal waking hours in bed.
3 = Symptomatic with more than 50% of time in bed.

2. Criteria for Rating Disease Status

A. *No Evident Disease:*	A rating of 1 in all categories (M1, H1, P1, S1)
B. *Moderate Disease:*	A rating of 2 in one or more categories, but no rating of 3 in any category.
C. *Extensive Disease:*	A rating of 3 in one or two categories.
D. *Extreme Disease:*	A rating of 3 in more than two categories.

3. Terms for Describing the Response to Therapy

A. *Complete Remission* (CR):	Improvement to disease status A.
B. *Good Partial Remission* (GR):	Improvement to disease status B.
C. *Poor Partial Remission* (PR):	Improvement to disease status C.
D. *No Remission* (NR):	No change in any status.
E. *Progressive Disease* (PD):	Deterioration from initial disease status, or if initially in status D, documented deterioration in any category.

Lymphomas and solid tumors

Category I = Clinical benefit with favorable objective changes in all measurable criteria of disease for more than one month.

References

ALEXANDER, P., FAIRLEY, G. H., HUNTER-CRAIG, I. D., ILONOPISOV, R. L., LEWIS, M. G.: Inhibition by L-asparaginase from *E. coli* of human malignant melanoma cells growing *in vitro*. In: GRUNDMANN, E., OETTGEN, H. F. (Eds.): Experimental and clinical effects of L-asparaginase. New York-Heidelberg-Berlin: Springer 1970.

ASTALDI, G., BURGIO, G. R., BISCATTI, G., ASTALDI, A. JR., FERFOGLIA, L.: L-Asparaginase and blastogenesis. Lancet 643—644 (1969a).

ASTALDI, G., BURGIO, G. R., KRČ, J., GENOVA, R., ASTALDI, A., JR.: L-Asparaginase and blastogenesis. Lancet, 423 (1969b).

AUR, R. J. A., SIMONE, J. V., PRATT, C. B.: Successful remission induction in children with acute lymphocytic leukemia at high risk for treatment failure. Cancer **27**, 1332—1336 (1971).

BAUER, K.: Zur Biochemie der Asparaginase. Med. Klin. **64**, 2—11 (1969).

BEARD, M. E. J., CROWTHER, D., GALTON, D. A. G., GUYERS, R. G., FAIRLEY, G. H., KAY, H. E. M., KNAPTON, P. J., MALPAS, J. S., SCOTT, R. B.: L-Asparaginase in treatment of acute leukemia and lymphosarcoma. Brit. med. J., 191—195 (1970).

BENEZRA, D., HOCHMAN, A., PITARO, R.: L-Asparaginase and blastogenesis. Lancet, 1235—1236 (1970).

BETTIGOLE, R. E., HIMELSTEIN, E. S., OETTGEN, H. F., CLIFFORD, G. O.: Hypofibrinogenemia due to L-asparaginase: studies of fibrinogen survival using autologous ^{131}I-fibrinogen. Blood **35**, 195—200 (1970).

BOYSE, E. A., OLD, L. J., CAMPBELL, H. A., MASHBURN, L. T.: Suppression of murine leukemia by L-asparaginase. J. exp. Med. **125**, 17—31 (1967).

BOYSE, E. A., OLD, L. J., STOCKERT, E.: Inhibitory effect of guinea pig serum on a number of new leukemias in mice. Nature (Lond.) **198**, 800—801 (1963).

BROOME, J. D.: Evidence that the L-asparaginase activity of guinea pig serum is responsible for its antilymphoma effects. Nature (Lond.) **191**, 1114—1115 (1961).

BROOME, J. D.: Evidence that the L-asparaginase of guinea pig serum is responsible for its antilymphoma effects. I. Properties of the L-asparaginase of guinea pig serum in relation to those of the antilymphoma substance. J. exp. Med. **118**, 99—120 (1963a).

BROOME, J. D.: Evidence that the L-asparaginase of guinea pig serum is responsible for its antilymphoma effect. II. Lymphoma 6C3HED cells cultured in a medium devoid of L-asparagine lose their susceptibility to the effects of guinea pig serum *in vivo*. J. exp. Med. **118**, 121—148 (1963b).

BROOME, J. D.: Studies on the mechanism of tumor inhibition by L-asparaginase. Effects of the enzyme on asparagine levels in the blood, normal tissues, and 6C3HED lymphomas in mice: Differences in asparagine formation and utilization of asparaginase-sensitive and resistant lymphoma cells. J. exp. Med. **127**, 1055—1072 (1968).

BROOME, J. D.: L-Asparaginase: early findings and current studies on the metabolism of L-asparaginase in lymphoma cells. In: GRUNDMANN, E., OETTGEN, H. F. (Eds.): Experimental and clinical effects of L-asparaginase. New York-Heidelberg-Berlin: Springer 1970.

BROOME, J. D., SCHWARTZ, J. H.: Differences in the production of L-asparagine in asparaginase-sensitive and resistant lymphoma cells. Biochim. biophys. Acta (Amst.) **138**, 637—639 (1967).

BURGIO, G. R., ASTALDI, A., JR., KRČ, J., ASTALDI, G.: With reference to blastogenesis inhibition by L-asparaginase. In: GRUNDMANN, E., OETTGEN, H. F. (Eds.): Experimental and clinical effects of L-asparaginase. New York-Heidelberg-Berlin: Springer 1970.

CAMPBELL, H. A., MASHBURN, L. T., BOYSE, E. A., OLD, L. J.: Two L-asparaginases from *Escherichia coli* B: their separation, purification and antitumor activity. Biochemistry **6**, 721—730 (1967).

CANELLOS, G. P., HASKELL, C. M.: Studies of resistance to L-asparaginase in human leukemia. In: GRUNDMANN, E., OETTGEN, H. F. (Eds.): Experimental and clinical effects of L-asparaginase. New York-Heidelberg-Berlin: Springer 1970.

CANELLOS, G. P., HASKELL, C. M., ARSENEAU, J., CARBONE, P. P.: Hypoalbuminemic and hypocholesterolemic effect of L-asparaginase (NSC-109, 229) treatment in man — a preliminary report. Cancer Chemotherapy Rep. **53**, 67—69 (1969).

CAPIZZI, R. L., BERTINO, J. R., HANDSCHUMACHER, R. E.: L-Asparaginase. Ann. Rev. Med. **21**, 433—444 (1970).

CAPIZZI, R. L., PETERSON, R., COONEY, D. A., CREASEY, W. A., HANDSCHUMACHER, R. E.: L-Asparaginase therapy of acute leukemia: biochemical and clinical observations. Proc. Amer. Ass. Cancer Res. **10**, 12 (1969).

CARBONE, P. P., HASKELL, C. M., LEVENTHAL, B. G., BLOCK, J. B., SELAWRY, O. S.: Clinical experience with L-asparaginase. In: GRUNDMANN, E., OETTGEN, H. F. (Eds.): Experimental and clinical effects of L-asparaginase. New York-Heidelberg-Berlin: Springer 1970.

CLARKSON, B. D., KRAKOFF, I. H., BURCHENAL, J. H., KARNOFSKY, D. A., GOLBEY, R. B., DOWLING, M. D., OETTGEN, H. F., LIPTON, A.: Clinical results of treatment with *E. coli* L-asparaginase in adults with leukemia, lymphosarcoma and solid tumors. Cancer **25**, 279—305 (1970).

COONEY, D. A., CAPIZZI, R. L., HANDSCHUMACHER, R. E.: Evaluation of L-asparagine metabolism in animals and man. Cancer Res. **30**, 929—935 (1970).

CROWTHER, D., BATEMAN, C. J. T., VARTAN, C. P., WHITEHOUSE, J. M. A., SCOTT, R. B.: Combination chemotherapy using L-asparaginase, daunorubicin and cytosine arabinoside in adults with acute myelogenous leukemia. Brit. med. J. **28**, 513—517 (1970).

DAHLWITZ, A., FRANZEN, S., HOLMGREN, A., KILLANDER, A., KILLANDER, D., WIDE, L., AHSTROM, L.: Studies of antibody formation in patients treated with L-asparaginase. In: GRUNDMANN, E., OETTGEN, H. F. (Eds.): Experimental and clinical effects of L-Asparaginase. New York-Heidelberg-Berlin: Springer 1970.

DELAGE, J. M., SIMARD, J., LEHNER-NETSCH, G., BARRY, A.: L-Asparaginase and complement. Nature (Lond.) **233**, 485—486 (1971).

DEUTSCH, E., FISCHER, M., FRISCHAUG, H., HONETZ, N., LECHNER, K., PESENDORFER, F., STYCH, H., WEISSMANN, A.: Blood coagulation changes under L-asparaginase therapy. In: GRUNDMANN, E., OETTGEN, H. F. (Eds.): Experimental and clinical effects of L-asparaginase. New York-Heidelberg-Berlin: Springer 1970.

DUNNICLIFF, M. A., EIGNER, E. A., JAFFE, N., TRAGGIS, D., ROSENOER, V. M.: Plasma asparaginase concentrations and the prediction of anaphylactic reactions. Proc. Amer. Ass. Cancer Res. **11**, 22 (1970).

FAIRLEY, G. H., MALPAS, J. S., GALTON, D. A. G.: Clinical experience with L-asparaginase. In: GRUNDMANN, E., OETTGEN, H. F. (Eds.): Experimental and clinical effects of L-asparaginase. New York-Heidelberg-Berlin: Springer 1970.

FATEH-MOGHADAM, A., LAMERZ, R., SCHWANDT, P., HORNUNG, B., EHRHARDT, J.: Quantitative Veränderungen der Serumproteine und -lipide im Verlauf der Asparaginase-Therapie maligner Tumoren und Haemoblastosen. Klin. Wschr. **48**, 116—125 (1970).

FINK, U., BEGEMANN, H.: Clinical studies with L-asparaginase in dermatomyositis. In: GRUNDMANN, E., OETTGEN, H. F. (Eds.): Experimental and clinical effects of L-asparaginase. New York-Heidelberg-Berlin: Springer 1970.

GERHARTZ, H., BEGEMANN, H.: Results of a collective study with L-asparaginase in human leukemias. Report of the section "oncology" of the Paul Ehrlich Society of Chemotherapy. In: GRUNDMANN, E., OETTGEN, H. F. (Eds.): Experimental and clinical effects of L-asparaginase. New York-Heidelberg-Berlin: Springer 1970.

GOUDEMAND, M., BAUTERS, F.: Clinical trials of asparaginase therapy in chemoresistant acute leukemias. In: GRUNDMANN, E., OETTGEN, H. F. (Eds.): Experimental and clinical effects of L-asparaginase. New York-Heidelberg-Berlin: Springer 1970.

GRALNICK, H. R., HENRY, P. H.: L-Asparaginase induced coagulopathy. Proc. Amer. Ass. Cancer Res. **10**, 32 (1969).

HAGHBIN, M., TAN, C., TALLAL, L., WOLLNER, N., ROSENSTOCK, J., BURCHENAL, J. H.: L-Asparaginase combination therapy of childhood acute leukemia. Proc. Amer. Ass. Cancer Res. **11**, 33 (1970).

HALEY, E. E., FISCHER, G. A., WELCH, A. D.: The requirements for L-asparagine of mouse leukemia cells L5178Y in culture. Cancer Res. **21**, 532—536 (1961).

HARDISTY, R. M., MCELWAIN, T. J.: Use of L-asparaginase in conjunction with cytosine arabinoside in acute leukemia in children. In: GRUNDMANN, E., OETTGEN, H. F. (Eds.): Experimental and clinical effects of L-asparaginase. New York-Heidelberg-Berlin: Springer 1970.

HASKELL, C. M., CANELLOS, G. P.: Asparagine biosynthesis in human KB tumor cells: inhibitor studies with asparagine and glutamine antagonists. Cancer Res. **30**, 1081—1083 (1970).

HASKELL, C. M., CANELLOS, G. P., LEVENTHAL, B. G., CARBONE, P. P., SERPICK, A. A., HANSEN, H. H.: L-Asparaginase toxicity. Cancer Res. **29**, 974—975 (1969).

HASSELBERGER, F. X., BROWN, H. D., CHATTOPADHYAY, S. K., MATHER, A. N., STASIW, R. O., PATEL, A. B., PENNINGTON, S. N.: The preparation of insoluble, matrix-supported derivatives of asparaginase for use in cancer therapy. Cancer Res. **30**, 2736—2738 (1970).

HEENE, D. L., LOEFFLER, H.: The hemostatic defect induced by treatment with asparaginase in leukemia. In: GRUNDMANN, E., OETTGEN, H. F. (Eds.): Experimental and clinical effects of L-asparaginase. New York-Heidelberg-Berlin: Springer 1970.

HILL, J. M., LOEB, E., MACLELLAN, A., KHAN, A., ROBERTS, J., SCHIELDS, W. F., HILL, N. O.: Response to highly purified L-asparaginase during therapy of acute leukemia. Cancer Res. **29**, 1574—1580 (1969).

HILL, J. M., ROBERTS, J., KHAN, A., MACLELLAN, A., HILL, R. W., LOEB, E.: L-Asparaginase therapy for leukemia and other malignant neoplasms. J. Amer. med. Ass. **202**, 882—888 (1967).

HO, D. H. W., WHITECAR, J. P., JR., LUCE, J. K., FREI, E., III.: L-Asparagine requirement and the effect of L-asparaginase on the normal and leukemic human bone marrow. Cancer Res. **30**, 466—472 (1970).

IRION, E., ARENS, A.: Biochemical characterization of L-asparaginase from *E. coli*. In: GRUNDMANN, E., OETTGEN, H. F. (Eds.): Experimental and clinical effects of L-asparaginase. New York-Heidelberg-Berlin: Springer 1970.

JACKSON, L., BARR, M., WEISS, A.: Lymphocyte mitotic and chromosomal changes in patients treated with L-asparaginase. Proc. Amer. Ass. Cancer Res. **11**, 40 (1970).

JACQUILLAT, C., WEIL, M., BUSSEL, A., LOISEL, J. P., ROUSSE, J., LARRIEU, M. J., BOIRON, M., DREYFUS, B., BERNARD, J.: Treatment of acute leukemia with L-asparaginase-preliminary results of 84 cases. In: GRUNDMANN, E., OETTGEN, H. F. (Eds.): Experimental and clinical effects of L-asparaginase. New York-Heidelberg-Berlin: Springer 1970.

JAFFE, N., TRAGGIS, D., DAS, L., MOLONEY, W. C., HANN, H. W., KIM, B. S., NAIR, R.: L-Asparaginase in the treatment of neoplastic diseases in children. Cancer Res. **31**, 942—949 (1971).

KHAN, A., HILL, J.M.: Neutralizing precipitin in the serum of a patient treated with L-asparaginase. J. Lab. clin. Med. 73, 846—852 (1969).
KIDD, J.G.: Regression of transplanted lymphomas induced *in vivo* by means of normal guinea pig serum. I. Course of transplanted cancers of various kinds in mice and rats given guinea pig serum, horse serum, or rabbit serum. J. exp. Med. 98, 565—581 (1953).
KIM, J.H., BOYSE, E.A., OLD, L.J., CAMPBELL, H.A.: Inhibition of HeLa cell cultures by preparations of *Escherichia coli* L-asparaginase. Biochim. biophys. Acta (Amst.) 158, 476—479 (1968).
LASH, E., SCHWARTZ, M.K., TALLAL, L., OETTGEN, H.F.: Serum lipids in patients receiving L-asparaginase. XII. Congress International Society of Hematology, New York (1968).
LEVENTHAL, B.G., HENDERSON, E.S.: Therapy of acute leukemia with drug combination which includes asparaginase. Cancer 28, 825—829 (1971).
LEVENTHAL, B.G., SKEEL, R.T., YANKEE, R.A., HENDERSON, E.S.: L-Asparaginase (NSC-109229) plus azaserine (NSC-742) in acute lymphatic leukemia. Cancer Chemother. Rep. 54, 4751 (1970).
LOEB, E., HILL, J.M., MACLELLAN, A., KHAN, A., ALEXANDER, T.R., ADACHI, M.: Treatment of acute leukemia with L-asparaginase. In: GRUNDMANN, E., OETTGEN, H.F. (Eds.): Experimental and clinical effects of L-asparaginase. New York-Heidelberg-Berlin: Springer 1970.
MARMONT, A.M., DAMASID, E.E.: Some clinical observations on the treatment with L-asparaginase of the acute leukemias. In: GRUNDMANN, E., OETTGEN, H.F. (Eds.): Experimental and clinical effects of L-asparaginase. New York-Heidelberg-Berlin: Springer 1970.
MASHBURN, L.T., LANDIN, L.M.: Some physiochemical aspects of L-asparaginase therapy. In: GRUNDMANN, E., OETTGEN, H.F. (Eds.): Experimental and clinical effects of L-asparaginase. New York-Heidelberg-Berlin: Springer 1970.
MASHBURN, L.T., WRISTON, J.C., JR.: Tumor inhibitory effect of L-asparaginase from *Escherichia coli*. Arch. Biochem. Biophys. 105, 450—452 (1964).
MATHÉ, G., AMIEL, J.L., CLARYSSE, A., HAYAT, M., SCHWARTZENBERG, L.: The place of L-asparaginase in the treatment of acute leukemia. In: GRUNDMANN, E., OETTGEN, H.F. (Eds.): Experimental and clinical effects of L-asparaginase. New York-Heidelberg-Berlin: Springer 1970.
MAYER, C.M., HOLTON, C.P.: Multiple course therapy with L-asparaginase in acute childhood leukemia. Clin. Res. 19, 227 (1971).
MCELWAIN, T.J., HAYWARD, S.K.: L-Asparaginase and blastogenesis. Lancet I, 527 (1969).
MILLER, H.K., SALSER, J.S., BALIS, M.E.: Amino acid levels following L-asparagine amidohydrolase (EC.3.5.1.1) therapy. Cancer Res. 29, 183—187 (1969).
MIURA, M., HIRANO, M., KAKIZAWA, K., MORITA, A., UETANI, T., YAMADA, K.: Inhibitory effect of L-asparaginase in lymphocyte transformation induced by phytohemagglutinin. Cancer Res. 30, 768—772 (1970).
NEUMAN, R.E., MCCOY, R.A.: Requirements of Walker carcinosarcoma 256 *in vitro* for asparagine and glutamine. Science 124, 124—125 (1956).
NORTH, A.C.T., WADE, H.E., CAMMACK, K.A.: Physicochemical studies of L-asparaginase from *Erwinia carotovora*. Nature (Lond.) 224, 594—595 (1969).
OERKERMANN, H., HIRSCHMANN, W.D., CROSS, R.: Studies on the glutaminase activity of *E. coli* asparaginase in tissue culture. In: GRUNDMANN, E., OETTGEN, H.F. (Eds.): Experimental and clinical effects of L-asparaginase. New York-Heidelberg-Berlin: Springer 1970.
OETTGEN, H.F., OLD, L.J., BOYSE, E.A., CAMPBELL, H.A., PHILIPS, F.S., CLARKSON, B.D., TALLAL, L., LEEPER, R.D., SCHWARTZ, M.K., KIM, J.H.: Inhibition of leukemia in man by L-asparaginase. Cancer Res. 27, 2619—2631 (1967).
OETTGEN, H.F., SCHULTEN, H.K.: Hemmung maligner Neoplasien des Menschen durch L-asparaginase. Klin. Wschr. 4, 65—71 (1969).
OETTGEN, H.F., STEPHENSON, P., SCHWARTZ, M.K., LEEPER, R.D., TALLAL, L., TAN, C.C., CLARKSON, B.D., GOLBEY, R.B., KRAKOFF, I.H., KARNOFSKY, D.A., MURPHY, M.L., BURCHENAL, J.H.: The toxicity of *E. coli* L-asparaginase in man. Cancer 25, 253—278 (1970a).
OETTGEN, H.F., TALLAL, L., TAN, C.C., MURPHY, M.L., CLARKSON, B.D., GOLBEY, R.B., KRAKOFF, I.H., KARNOFSKY, D.A., BURCHENAL, J.H.: Clinical experience with L-asparaginase. In: GRUNDMANN, E., OETTGEN, H.F. (Eds.): Experimental and clinical effects of L-asparaginase. New York-Heidelberg-Berlin: Springer 1970b.
OHNO, R., HERSH, E.M.: The inhibition of lymphocyte blastogenesis by L-asparaginase. Blood 35, 250—262 (1970a).
OHNO, R., HERSH, E.M.: Immunosuppressive effects of L-asparaginase. Cancer Res. 30, 1605—1611 (1970b).
OHNUMA, T., HOLLAND, J.F., FREEMAN, A., SINKS, L.F.: Biochemical and pharmacological studies with asparaginase in man. Cancer Res. 30, 2297—2305 (1970).
OHNUMA, T., HOLLAND, J.F., NAGEL, J., ST. ARNEAULT, G.: Effects of L-asparaginase in acute myelocytic leukemia. J. Amer. med. Ass. 210, 1919—1921 (1969).

OHNUMA, T., BOSNER, F., LEVY, R. N., CUTTNER, J., MOON, J. H., SILVER, R. T., BLOM, J., FALKSON, G., BURNINGHAM, R., GLIDEWELL, O., HOLLAND, J. F.: Treatment of adult leukemia with L-asparaginase (NSC-109229). Cancer Chemother. Rep. **55**, 269—275 (1971).
OLD, L. J., BOYSE, E. A., CAMPBELL, H. A., BRODEY, R. S., FIDLER, J., TELLER, J.: Treatment of lymphosarcoma in the dog with L-asparaginase. Cancer **20**, 1066—1070 (1967).
OLD, L. J., KIM, J. H., BETH, E., BOYSE, E. A., OETTGEN, H. F., CAMPBELL, H. A., BURCHENAL, J. H.: Identification of asparagine-sensitive human neoplasms by tests *in vitro*. XII. Congress of International Society of Hematology, New York 1968.
PETERSON, R. G., HANDSCHUMACHER, R. E., MITCHELL, M. S.: Immunological responses to L-asparaginase. J. clin. Invest. **50**, 1080—1090 (1971).
PINSKY, C. M., MITCHELL, S., OETTGEN, H. F., SCHWARTZ, M. K.: Immune reactions to L-asparaginase in man. Proc. Amer. Ass. Cancer Res. **11**, 63 (1970).
PRAGER, M. D., PETERS, P. C., JANES, J. O., DERR, I.: Asparagine synthetase activity in malignant and non-malignant human kidney and prostate specimens. Nature (Lond.) **221**, 1064—1065 (1969).
PRATT, C. B., HOLTON, C. P.: Comparison of weekly and twice weekly L-asparaginase in the treatment of childhood lymphocytic leukemia. Proc. Amer. Ass. Cancer Res. **11**, 64 (1970).
PRATT, C. B., JOHNSON, W. W.: Duration and severity of fatty metamorphosis of the liver following L-asparaginase therapy. Cancer **28**, 361—364 (1971).
PUTTER, J.: Pharmacokinetic behavior of L-asparaginase in men and animals. In: GRUNDMANN, E., OETTGEN, H. F. (Eds.): Experimental and clinical effects of L-asparaginase. New York-Heidelberg-Berlin: Springer 1970.
PUTTER, J., GEHRMAN, G.: Blutspiegelverlauf beim Menschen nach Gabe von zwei verschiedenen L-asparaginasen. Klin. Wschr. **47**, 1324—1326 (1969).
RAUENBUSCH, E., BAUER, K., KAUFMANN, W., WAGNER, O.: Isolation and crystallization of L-asparaginase from *E. coli*. In: GRUNDMANN, E., OETTGEN, H. F. (Eds.): Experimental and clinical effects of L-asparaginase. New York-Heidelberg-Berlin: Springer 1970.
RAUSEN, A. R., GLIDEWELL, O. J.: L-Asparaginase (L-Asp) in advanced childhood leukemia: comparative trial of drug schedules singly and in combination. Proc. Amer. Ass. Cancer Res. **11**, 66 (1970).
REIS, H. E., SCHMIDT, C. G.: The antigenicity of *E. coli*-asparaginase. In: GRUNDMANN, E., OETTGEN, H. F. (Eds.): Experimental and clinical effects of L-asparaginase. New York-Heidelberg-Berlin: Springer 1970.
SCHMIDT, C. G., GALLMEIER, W.: Zur Enzymtherapie der Leukemien. Dtsch. med. Wschr. **93**, 2299—2309 (1968).
SCHREK, R., DOLOWY, W. C.: *In vitro* test for sensitivity of leukemic cells to L-asparaginase. Cancer Res. **31**, 523—526 (1971).
SCHWARTZ, G. H., STENZEL, K. H., RUBIN, A. L.: Asparaginase effects on human lymphocytes. Clin. Res. **18**, 433 (1970b).
SCHWARTZ, M. K.: The distribution and clearance of L-asparaginase. In: GRUNDMANN, E., OETTGEN, H. F. (Eds.): Experimental and clinical effects of L-asparaginase. New York-Heidelberg-Berlin: Springer 1970.
SCHWARTZ, M. K., LASH, E. D., OETTGEN, H. F., TOMAO, F. A.: L-Asparaginase activity in plasma and other biological fluids. Cancer **25**, 244—252 (1970a).
STIER, H. W., GALLMEIER, W. M., SCHMIDT, C. G.: Über Störungen des Blutgerinnungssystems im Verlauf der Enzymtherapie maligner Tumoren und Haemoglastosen. Dtsch. med. Wschr. **94**, 253—260 (1969).
STORTI, E., QUAGLINO, D.: Dysmetabolic and neurological complications in leukemia patients treated with L-asparaginase. In: GRUNDMANN, E., OETTGEN, H. F. (Eds.): Experimental and clinical effects of L-asparaginase. New York-Heidelberg-Berlin: Springer 1970.
SUTOW, W. W., GARCIA, F., STARLING, K. A., WILLIAMS, T. E., LANE, D. M., GEHAN, E. A.: L-Asparaginase therapy in children with advanced leukemia. Cancer **28**, 819—824 (1971).
TALLAL, L., TAN, C. C., OETTGEN, H. F., WOLLNER, N., MCCARTHY, M., HELSON, L., BURCHENAL, J. H., KARNOFSKY, D. A., MURPHY, M. L.: *E. coli* L-asparaginase in the treatment of leukemia and solid tumors in 131 children. Cancer **25**, 306—320 (1970).
TAN, C. C., OETTGEN, H. F.: Clinical experience with L-asparaginase administered intrathecally. Proc. Amer. Ass. Cancer Res. **10**, 92 (1969).
WHELAN, H. A., WRISTON, J. C., JR.: Purification and properties of asparaginase from *E. coli*. B. Biochemistry **8**, 2386 (1969).
WHITECAR, J. P., BODEY, G. P., HARRIS, J. E., FREIREICH, E. J.: L-Asparaginase. New Engl. J. Med. **282**, 732—734 (1970).
WHITECAR, J. P., JR., HARRIS, J. E., BODEY, G. P., FREIREICH, E. J.: Host effects of L-asparaginase treatment. Clin. Res. **17**, 408 (1969).

Chapter 70

Procarbazine

DONALD J. REED

With 2 Figures

Introduction

Certain methylhydrazine derivatives constitute a class of antitumor substances whose mechanism of action appears to be different from that of other cytotoxic agents. These compounds were originally tested as monoamine oxidase inhibitors (ZELLER et al., 1963; BOLLAG and GRUNBERG, 1963) and subsequently were included in a survey for antitumor activity (BOLLAG, 1963a; 1964). Systematic variation of substituents on 1-methyl-2-benzylhydrazine revealed that antitumor activity was found among those compounds possessing the general formula $CH_3-NH-NH-CH_2R$. However, the biological properties of agents within this group showed a marked variation depending on the chemical nature of the R group and an absolute dependency upon the methyl group. Procarbazine (Matulane, natulan, ibenzmethyzin, Ro4-6467, NSC-77213), which is *N*-isopropyl-α-(2-methylhydrazino)-*p*-toluamide monohydrochloride,

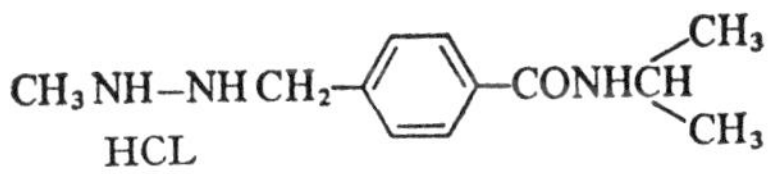

$$CH_3NH-NHCH_2-C_6H_4-CONHCH(CH_3)_2 \cdot HCL$$

is the most promising derivative and is now clinically available for the palliative treatment of Hodgkin's disease. In distinct contrast to other antineoplastic drugs, procarbazine has a rather specific effect upon this type of cancer.

Reviews on procarbazine include PLATTNER (1964), JELLIFFE and MARKS (1965), STOCK (1967), SARTORELLI and CREASEY (1969), CARTER (1970), and OLIVERIO (1973). A review on the metabolic fate of hydrazines, including procarbazine and hydrazides has been written by COLVIN (1969).

Tumor Inhibition

Procarbazine has tumor inhibitory activity against a wide variety of transplanted tumors in animals (Table 1). In addition to the tumors listed in Table 1, investigators have reported the antitumor activity of procarbazine with the solid form of advanced mast cell P815 in CD_2F_1 mice and Dunning leukemia in Fischer rats (OLIVERIO et al., 1964), the advanced LPC-1 plasma cell tumor in Balb/c mice (ABRAHAM et al., 1967), and a spontaneous mammary tumor in C3H mice (GELZER and LOUSTALOT, 1967).

Chemical Properties

Procarbazine is a white to pale yellow crystalline substance, which is soluble, but unstable in water or aqueous solutions. In aqueous solutions containing dissolved oxygen it slowly undergoes autoxidation to azo procarbazine and hydrogen

Table 1. *Activity of methylhydrazine derivatives against susceptible tumors*

Tumor and species[a]	Compound†	Dose[b]	Period of treatment (doses/days)	T/C[c]	% Inhibition	Body wt. change (g) T/C	Ref.
Hamster							
*HAd No. 1	III	60 (sc)	14	0.37	20% surviving	—20	Grunberg and Prince (1966)
		30 (sc)	14	0.43	80% surviving	—6	Grunberg and Prince (1966)
Mice							
EC (s.c.)	III	200	5/7	50/529 (mg)	91[d]	—2.2/+1.2	Bollag (1963b, 1964)
	III	200 (p.o.)	5/7	103/374 (mg)	72.5[e]	—2.2/+2.2	Bollag (1963b, 1964)
	IV	200 (p.o.)	5/7	141/735 (mg)	81[f]	—	Bollag and Grunberg (1963)
	V	200	5/7	350/791 (mg)	56[g]	—0.8/+3.8	Bollag (1964)
ECA	III	400	7/9	S[h]40.8/10.2	PS[i]300[j]	—	Bollag (1963b, 1964)
	III	400 (p.o.)	7/9	S40.6/10	PS310[k]	—	Bollag (1963b)
	IV	300 (p.o.)	7/9	S52.6/14.5	PS263[l]	—	Bollag and Grunberg (1963)
	V	400	7/9	S27.8/11.0	PS150	—	Bollag (1964)
S180	III	200	5/7	413/950 (mg)	57[m]	—2.0/+1.8	Bollag (1963b, 1964)
	III	400	5/7	281/1554 (mg)	82[n]	—4.0/+0.8	Bollag (1963b, 1964)
	III	200 (p.o.)	5/7	356/571 (mg)	38[o]	—2.0/+1.8	Bollag (1963b)
	III	400 (p.o.)	5/7	191/733 (mg)	74[p]	—3.2/+1.3	Bollag (1963b)
	IV	400 (p.o.)	5/7	921/2314 (mg)	60[q]	—	Bollag and Grunberg (1963)
	V	100	5/7	1221/1756 (mg)	30.5[r]	+1.6/+5.6	Bollag (1964)
	V	400	5/7	1022/1432 (mg)	29[s]	—1.0/+5.0	Bollag (1964)
L5178Y	III	300 (i.p.)	1	—	("inhibition")	—	Sartorelli and Tsunamura (1965)
	III	7.5—120 (i.p.)	6	—	("inhibition")	—	
P815 (7-day)	III	450	3/7	2.3 (S)	PS130	—7.3 (T)	
	III	450 (p.o.)	3/7	2.0 (S)	PS100	—8.0 (T)	
YPC (plasma cell; 7-day)							
L1210 (s.c.; 5-day)	III	320	5/8	1.5 (S)	PS50	—5.1 (T)	Oliverio and Kelly (1964)
	III	320 (s.c.)	5/8	1.5 (S)	PS50	—5.5 (T)	
L1210 (intracranial; 4-day)	III	200	3/7	1.4 (S)	PS40	—5.2 (T)	
	III	300	2/7	1.4 (S)	PS40	—5.1 (T)	
	III	450	1/7	1.4 (S)	PS40	—3.8 (T)	
*C57BL/6	III	50 (i.p.)	12	0.12	9/16 surviving	—2.9	Grunberg and Prince (1969)
*ED771		25	12	0.22	13/16 surviving	—3.8	

Rats							
W256	III	10	6/8	0/4905 (mg)	100[t]	+20.7/+22.6	BOLLAG (1963b)
	III	10 (p.o.)	6/8	0/8135 (mg)	100[u]	+16.4/+18.9	BOLLAG (1963b)
	IV	10 (p.o.)	6/8	0/6920 (mg)	100[v]	—	BOLLAG and GRUNBERG (1963)
	V	10	6/8	0/16314 (mg)	100[w]	+16.2/+15.0	BOLLAG (1964)
W256 (estab.)	III	50[x]	5/wk.	0.10[y]; 0.02[z] (vol.)	—	—	BOLLAG (1963b)
UE-T8	III (expt. 1)	50	9/11	6817/15,083 (mg)	57[a1]	—2.2/+27.3	BOLLAG (1963b)
	III (expt. 2)	10	6/8	0/22,496 (mg)	100[b1]	+6.2/+10.6	BOLLAG (1964)
	IV	100 (p.o.)	9/11	1097/15,647 (mg)	93[c1]	—	BOLLAG and GRUNBERG (1963)
	V	5	6/8	0/8478 (mg)	100[d1]	+19.2/+33.3	BOLLAG (1964)
JS (estab.)	III	200[e1]	1 dose	—	CR[f1]	—	OBRECHT et al. (1964)
	III	300[g1]	1 dose	10.8/55 (g)[h1]	—	—	OBRECHT et al. (1964)
DL (3-day)	III	40	3/7	1.5 (S)	PS50	—42.0 (T)	OLIVERIO and KELLY (1964)
*HEr No. 3	III	100 (s.c.)	8	0.23	50% surviving	—32%	GRUNBERG and PRINCE (1966)
*Murphy-Sturm	III	50 (i.p.)	14	0.42	3/8 surviving	—7	GRUNBERG and PRINCE (1969)
*Flexner-Jobling	III	50 (i.p.)	14	0.48	17/24 surviving	+3.4	GRUNBERG and PRINCE (1969)

[a] For meaning of abbreviations, see Introduction (STOCK, 1967); [S], survival; (T), treated.
[b] mg/kg/day, beginning day after implantation except with established tumors; given intraperitoneally unless indicated otherwise (p.o., orally; s.c., subcutaneously).
[c] Average tumor size in treated animals/average tumor size in controls.
[d] 100, 300, 400 mg/kg gave 70, 92.5, 93% inhibition, respectively.
[e] 100, 300, 400 mg/kg gave 61, 77, and 80% inhibition.
[f] 100, 300 mg/kg gave 83, 90% inhibition.
[g] 100, 300, 400 mg/kg gave 52, 81.5, 80% inhibition.
[h] Average survival time, days.
[i] Percent prolongation of S (survival).
[j] 100, 200, 300 mg/kg gave 80, 130, 310% PS.
[k] 100, 200, 300 mg/kg gave 100, 220, 290 PS.
[l] 100, 200 mg/kg gave 70, 187% PS.
[m] 100 mg/kg gave 16% inhibition.
[n] 300 mg/kg gave 62% inhibition.
[o] 100 mg/kg gave 13.5% inhibition.
[p] 300 mg/kg gave 49% inhibition.
[q] 500 mg/kg gave 70% inhibition.
[r] 200 mg/kg gave 5% inhibition.
[s] 300 mg/kg gave 23% inhibition.
[t] 5, 20, 30 mg/kg gave 81, 100, 100% inhibition.
[u] 5, 20, 30 mg/kg gave 85, 100, 100% inhibition.
[v] 5 mg/kg gave 93% inhibition.
[w] 5, 20 mg/kg gave 80, 100% inhibition.
[x] Treatment began 5th day after implantation.
[y] At 5th day of treatment (9th day after implantation); 10, 20, 30 mg/kg doses gave values of 0.22, 0.19, 0.17 at this time.
[z] At 9th day of treatment; 10, 20, 30 mg/kg gave values of 0.16, 0.09, 0.05 at this time.

[a1] 25 mg/kg gave 11% inhibition in this experiment.
[b1] 2.5, 5 mg/kg gave 69, 81% inhibition.
[c1] 50, 75 mg/kg gave 31.5, 77% inhibition.
[d1] 2.5 mg/kg gave 63% inhibition.
[e1] Tumors weighed 3 to 4 g at time of treatment.
[f1] Complete regression.
[g1] Tumors 5.4 g wet wt. at time of treatment.
[h1] 10th day after treatment.

* Data added to a table reproduced by permission STOCK, J.A. (1967) Table II pp. 350—351.

† $CH_3NHNHCH_2$—⟨benzene ring⟩—CONHR.
(III) R = $(CH_3)_2CH$— (as hydrochloride); Ro4-6467/1 (procarbazine).
(IV) R = H_2NCO— (as hydrobromide); Ro4-6824.
(V) R = $HOCH_2CH_2$— (as hydrochloride); Ro4-6658.

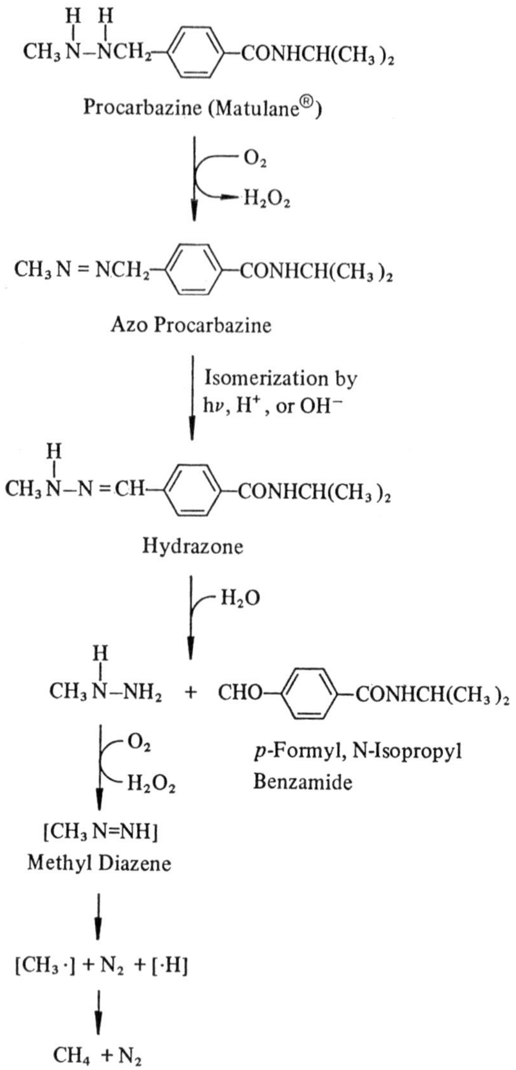

$CH_3NH{-}NHCH_2{-}C_6H_4{-}CONHCH(CH_3)_2$

Procarbazine (Matulane®)

O_2 → H_2O_2

$CH_3N=NCH_2{-}C_6H_4{-}CONHCH(CH_3)_2$

Azo Procarbazine

Isomerization by $h\nu$, H^+, or OH^-

$CH_3NH{-}N=CH{-}C_6H_4{-}CONHCH(CH_3)_2$

Hydrazone

H_2O

$CH_3NH{-}NH_2$ + $CHO{-}C_6H_4{-}CONHCH(CH_3)_2$

p-Formyl, N-Isopropyl Benzamide

O_2 → H_2O_2

$[CH_3N{=}NH]$

Methyl Diazene

$[CH_3\cdot] + N_2 + [\cdot H]$

$CH_4 + N_2$

Fig. 1. Chemical reactions of the degradation of procarbazine and possible metabolic intermediates in procarbazine metabolism. Brackets denote postulated but unidentified intermediates

peroxide (Fig. 1). Azo procarbazine, which can be readily synthesized by mercuric oxide oxidation of procarbazine, has a very limited solubility in water, but it is readily soluble in most organic solvents. In the presence of light, azo procarbazine in solution slowly isomerizes to the hydrazone of monomethylhydrazine (MMH) and *p*-formyl *N*-isopropylbenzamide. A rapid isomerization occurs at pH 1 to 2 which is followed by a rapid hydrolysis of the hydrazone to monomethylhydrazine (MMH) and *p*-formyl *N*-isopropyl benzamide. Acid treatment of azo procarbazine gives essentially a quantitative yield of these products and less than 1 % yield of the formaldehyde hydrazone which hydrolyzes to formaldehyde and *N*-isopropyl-*p*-carbamoyl benzylhydrazine. The quantitative analysis of procarbazine and several of its degradation products is based on solvent extraction techniques and ultraviolet absorption spectrometry (OLIVERIO et al., 1964; BAGGIOLINI et al., 1969; PROUGH et al., 1970).

AEBI et al. (1965a, b) studied in detail the autoxidation of procarbazine and other methylhydrazine derivatives. In 0.05 M phosphate buffer, pH 7.0, procarbazine is relatively stable, but in the presence of various metal ions, especially Cu(II) ion, oxidation occurs which can be measured by oxygen uptake and hydrogen peroxide formation (BERNEIS et al., 1964; AEBI et al., 1965a, b). Metalloproteins, such as siderophilin, myoglobin, and to a lesser extent hemoglobin, also catalyze procarbazine oxidation (AEBI et al., 1965a, b).

Monomethylhydrazine (MMH) is formed *in vivo* from procarbazine (CHABNER et al., 1969) and possesses the methyl group which is required for biological activity of procarbazine (BOLLAG, 1964, 1965). All monoalkylhydrazines are easily oxidized, especially at alkaline pH, in the presence of molecular oxygen. Such oxidation results in the formation of the corresponding monoalkyldiazenes which have very limited stability. TSUJI and KOSOWER (1971) have prepared methyl-, ethyl-, isopropyl-, and tert-butyl diazene among other diazenes and found them all to react rapidly and disappear in a bimolecular process. Methyldiazene was the least reactive, having a rate constant of 0.03 M^{-1} sec^{-1} at 25° in ethanol, with the major product being methane; ethyldiazene was 13 times more reactive and isopropyl diazene about 19 times. All monoalkyldiazenes rapidly decompose after exposure to oxygen and unless molecules such as reduced glutathione are present to compete for free radicals, the product of the chain reaction is the hydrocarbon (TSUJI and KOSOWER, 1971).

$$\begin{aligned} RN = NH + O_2 &\rightarrow RN = N\cdot + HO_2\cdot, \\ RN = N\cdot &\rightarrow R\cdot + N_2, \\ RN = NH + R\cdot &\rightarrow RH + RN = N\cdot, \\ RN = N\cdot &\rightarrow R\cdot + N_2. \end{aligned}$$

Azo procarbazine, being a disubstituted diazene, does not appear to react with molecular oxygen when in aqueous solution at room temperature.

Pharmacology

Procarbazine, like many other cytotoxic agents, has a variety of biological effects including leukopenia, thrombopenia, immunosuppression, carcinogenesis, teratogenesis, and depression of spermatogenesis. The drug is absorbed well by both parenteral and oral routes of administration, resulting in a rapid distribution throughout the body including the cerebrospinal fluid in dogs and man.

The oral LD_{50} of procarbazine in mice, rats, and rabbits is given as 1,320 ± 66 mg/kg body wt, 785 ± 34 mg/kg, and 145 ± 11.5 mg/kg, respectively (Roche Laboratories, 1969).

Procarbazine has numerous toxic side effects which occur in 50 to 70% of all patients treated with the drug. These effects include nausea, vomiting, leukopenia, and thrombocytopenia. If daily doses of procarbazine do not exceed about 300 mg in adults, central nervous system side effects are largely avoided. Recommended dosage to adults is single or divided doses of 100 to 200 mg daily for the first week. Daily dosage should then be maintained at 300 mg or less until the white blood count falls below 4000 per cmm or the platelets fall below 100000 per cmm or until maximum response is obtained (Roche Laboratories, 1969). When maximum response is obtained, the dose may be maintained at 50 to 100 mg daily. Hematologic toxicity must be monitored very closely since maximum response is generally dependent upon the success of controlling this parameter with individual patients.

Certain of the central nervous system effects may arise from decreased pyridoxal phosphate levels (CHABNER et al., 1969) or monoamine oxidase inhibition (DEVITA et al., 1965).

Suppression of immunological reactions by procarbazine was first noted by BOLLAG (1963) who reported that with heterologous tumors in rats the heterograft rejection is retarded. FLOERSHEIM (1963) also found extended survival of skin homografts in mice treated with procarbazine and he concluded that the drug was more effective than most drugs known to suppress transplantation immunity. AMIEL et al. (1964) found that procarbazine depressed immune reactions in mice most markedly if the drug is given after the antigenic stimulus, and was particularly effective in the rejection of allogenic skin grafts.

In more recent work, CERILLI and GIDEON (1969) reported prolongation of the survival of skin xenografts from hamsters to mice from 4.5 days in untreated controls to 12.5 days in procarbazine-treated animals (25 to 50 mg/kg). STEWART and COHEN (1969) using procarbazine, FLOERSHEIM and BRUNE (1970) using procarbazine and antilymphocyte serum, and FLOERSHEIM et al. (1970) using 1-methyl-2-*p*-allophanoylbenzylhydrazine hydrochloride and antilymphocyte serum, have achieved marked prolongation of mouse skin allograft survival.

MACDONALD et al. (1971) performed renal allografts in 46 unrelated adult mongrel dogs of both sexes. The dogs were divided into 5 treatment groups: no therapy either pre- or post-kidney transplant, 5 mg/kg of azathioprine and prednisone beginning 2 days prior to transplantation and continuing thereafter, five pairs of dogs given 5 mg/kg of procarbazine for 5, 4, 3, 2, or 1 day pretransplantation and continuously thereafter, 3 pairs pretreated for 13, 7, or 6 days with procarbazine 2.5 to 5 mg/kg/day pretransplant and continuously with both procarbazine and azathioprine following kidney exchange. Procarbazine alone or with azathioprine, in the dosages used, did not prolong renal homograft survival and larger doses could not be tolerated because of bone marrow toxicity.

STEWART and BELL (1970) compared the immunosuppressive activity of procarbazine using the survival of skin grafts in strains of mice. Incompatible (H_2 locus) grafts survived 20.8 days compared to 10.3 days in controls, while compatible (H_2 locus) grafts survived 51.3 days compared to 12.4 days for controls. Prolongation of second set skin allografts was for a mean of 32 days compared to 7.0 days with the controls. MAKINODAN et al. (1970) have reviewed immunosuppressive drugs and have tentatively classified procarbazine as a Class III agent, a type of drug which may be immunosuppressive if given either before or after the antigenic stimulus and thus shares properties with both Class I and Class II agents. Certainly, much more knowledge is needed about the immunosuppressive properties of procarbazine.

Procarbazine shows multipotential carcinogenic activity by its ability to produce lung adenomas, leukemia, and mammary adenocarcinomas in rodents (KELLY et al., 1964, 1968, 1969). Chronic administration of procarbazine has caused the induction of acute myelogenous leukemia in two Rhesus monkeys (*Macaca mulatta*) (O'GARA et al., 1971).

CHAUBE and MURPHY (1964, 1969) have described teratogenic effects in pregnant rats when single intraperitoneal injections of procarbazine were administered on the 5th to 12th, 14th, and 17th days of gestation. Doses ranged from 5 to 550 mg/kg with malformations occurring even in 21 day fetuses exposed to doses of 250 mg/kg on the 17th day or 12 mg/kg once on the 12th day. Doses of 25, 50, and 75 mg/kg were lethal and teratogenic to some offspring after a single treatment on the 5th, 6th, 9th, and 12th days, but essentially of no effect on the 14th

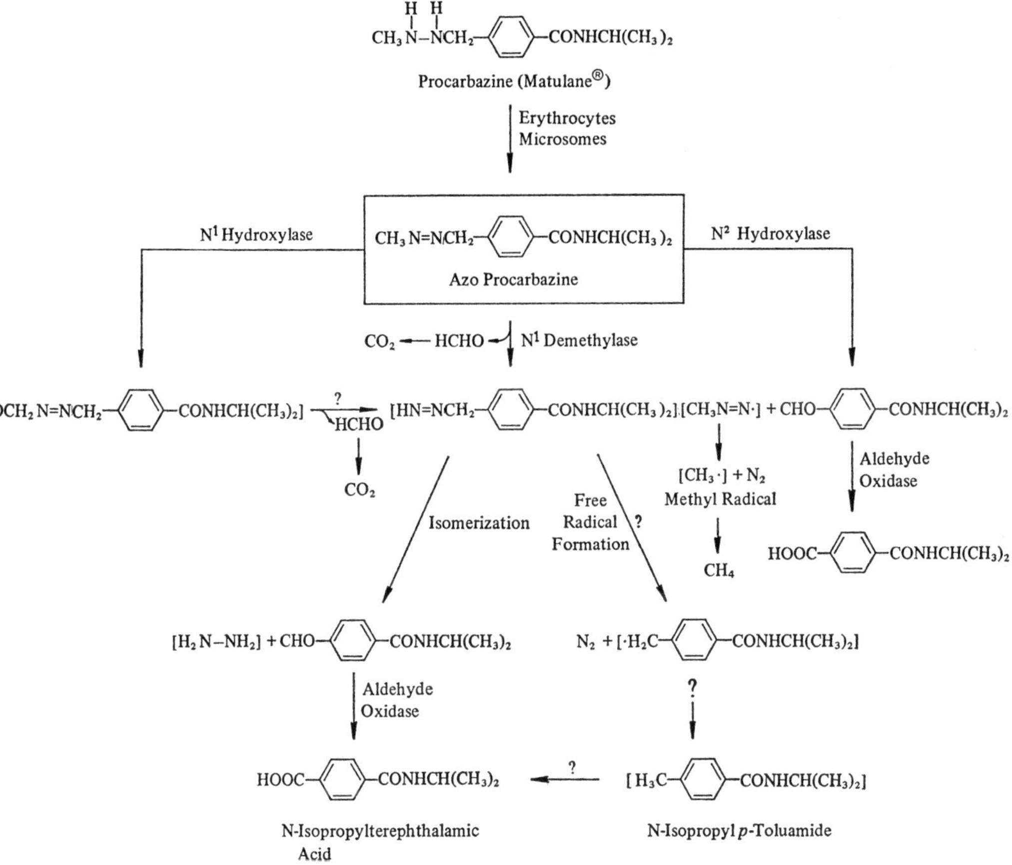

Fig. 2. Other possible metabolic pathways of procarbazine metabolism. Brackets denote postulated but unidentified intermediates

or 17th day of gestation. Types of malformations included malpositioned and shortened appendages and tail, and defects of digits, jaw, palate, and face.

Procarbazine treatment of rats caused a marked depression of spermatogenesis and atrophy of the testis (BOLLAG and THEISS, 1964; HILSCHER and REICHELT, 1968). Male rats mated after procarbazine treatment were sterile from the second week and fertility did not recover (FOX and FOX, 1967). DIXON and LEE (1971) have reported that with mouse spermatogenic cells, procarbazine caused an immediate cessation of DNA, RNA, and protein synthesis, with subsequent recovery of thymidine incorporation, but not uridine or leucine incorporation. Fertility was decreased dramatically.

Metabolism

The metabolic fate of procarbazine is still somewhat in question. The initial metabolic step, conversion of procarbazine to azo procarbazine [*N*-isopropyl-α-(2-methyldiazeno)-*p*-toluamide] occurs very rapidly *in vivo*, as measured by the loss of procarbazine from the blood. In man, the half life of procarbazine is about 7 to 10 min (OLIVERIO, 1972). Azo procarbazine, a biologically active intermediate (BOLLAG, 1964, 1965) has several possible metabolic fates as shown in Figs. 1 and 2.

However, the major urinary metabolite, *N*-isopropylterephthalamic acid, which represents nearly 70 % of the administered radioactivity, is excreted within 24 h after administering carbonyl-^{14}C procarbazine (BOLLAG, 1965). KLEIBEL (1965) used ^{3}H-labeled procarbazine to study the fate of procarbazine in rats with the Walker 256 tumor and found high levels of radioactivity in the ovaries three hours after injection.

Using ^{14}C-carbonyl labeled, *N*-methyl-^{14}C labeled and *N*-methyl-^{3}H labeled procarbazines, SCHWARTZ et al. (1967c) studied the distribution of radioactivity in rat and man and excretion in rat, dog, and man. The largest concentration of radioactivity was found in the liver and kidneys 30 and 60 min after administration of each of the labeled forms of procarbazine. Respiratory and excretion patterns verified the release of the *N*-methyl group as CO_2 (30 %) and excretion of terephthalamic acid (67 to 70 %). Erythrocytes and liver endoplasmic reticulum are thought to be primarily responsible for the conversion of procarbazine to azo procarbazine *in vivo*. OLIVERIO et al. (1964) and RAAFLAUB and SCHWARTZ (1965) have proposed that procarbazine metabolism proceeds in a similar pattern in man, dog, rat, and mice to form *N*-isopropyl terephthalamic acid essentially according to the scheme shown in Fig. 1.

The *in vitro* conversion of procarbazine to azo procarbazine by liver microsomes requires NADPH (PROUGH et al., 1970; BAGGIOLINI and DEWALD, 1969). Indirect evidence for azo procarbazine formation by erythrocytes has been reported by MORTENSEN (1965) and AEBI and SUTER (1965). DEWALD et al. (1969) have studied procarbazine metabolism and have found in perfused rat liver an accumulation of azo procarbazine due to a greater rate of procarbazine oxidation than of *N*-isopropyl terephthalamic acid formation. SKF 525-A (diethylaminoethyl 2,2-diphenylvalerate HCl) slightly decreased and 3-methylcholanthrene slightly increased the rate of procarbazine disappearance from the perfusion medium (BAGGIOLINI and DEWALD, 1966; DEWALD et al., 1969). Formation of $^{14}CO_2$ from *N*-methyl-^{14}C-procarbazine indicates microsomal dependent *N*-demethylation (BAGGIOLINI et al., 1965; BAGGIOLINI and BICKEL, 1966; AEBI et al., 1966; DEWALD et al., 1969). Formaldehyde formation by rat liver microsomes, first observed by WEITZEL et al. (1967), occurs at a more rapid rate with azo procarbazine than with procarbazine (WITTKOP et al., 1969; PROUGH et al., 1970). PROUGH et al. (1970) also found that while 1-methyl-2-benzylhydrazine was not a substrate, azo 1-methyl-2-benzylhydrazine was nearly as good a substrate as azo procarbazine. In addition, these workers noted from microsomal induction and CO inhibition experiments that two types of *N*-demethylases exist in rat liver which can catalyze *N*-demethylation of various *N*-methylhydrazines.

The *N*-methyl group of procarbazine is rapidly converted *in vivo* to methane in addition to formaldehyde (REED and DOST, 1966; DOST and REED, 1967). When ^{14}C- or ^{3}H-*N*-methyl-labeled procarbazine was administered intraperitoneally to rats at 20 and 200 mg/kg within an 8 hour period, 7 to 10 % of the methyl group was converted to respired methane and 11 to 22 % to respiratory CO_2.

SCHWARTZ et al. (1967a, b) confirmed the metabolic formation of methane from ^{14}C-labeled MMH and methyl-^{14}C-labeled procarbazine in rats. Peak methane production from MMH occurred in 10 min, but with procarbazine the peak was much less intense. Methane formation within 60 min after drug administration was 20 % and 5 % of the dose for MMH and procarbazine, respectively.

A comparison was made of *in vivo* released methane and CO_2 from azo procarbazine, the methylhydrazine hydrazone of procarbazine, MMH, and 1,1-dimethylhydrazine (Table 2) (REED, 1971, unpublished results). From this and

Table 2. *In vivo formation of methane-^{14}C and $^{14}CO_2$ from N-methyl-^{14}C-procarbazine and related compounds by rats*

N—$^{14}CH_3$ compound	Dose (μmoles/kg)	Percent recovery (8 h) $^{14}CO_2$	$^{14}CH_4$	Percent total recovery
Procarbazine[a]	78	21.2	8.3	29.5
Azo procarbazine	78	15.5	9.9	25.4
Procarbazine hydrazone	78	24.3	20.4	44.7
MMH[b]	120	6.3	25.0	31.3
1,1-Dimethylhydrazine[b]	13	26.5	0	26.5
1,1-Dimethylhydrazine[b]	330	15.2	0	15.2

REED (1971), [a] DOST and REED (1967), [b] DOST et al. (1966).

other evidence, procarbazine appears to be almost entirely converted to azo procarbazine and the latter compound has at least three pathways of metabolism.

One pathway, possibly a minor one, is via the hydrazone to MMH and *p*-formyl-*N*-isopropyl benzamide. This pathway must exist because CHABNER et al. (1969) have isolated the methylhydrazone of pyridoxal from mice that had been pretreated intraperitoneally with pyridoxal 30 min prior to a single subcutaneous injection of procarbazine. In other experiments, these workers gave mice procarbazine by intraperitoneal injection and observed a rapid and prolonged fall in plasma levels of pyridoxal phosphate. Similar observations were noted when mice were administered MMH. *p*-Formyl-*N*-isopropyl benzamide is rapidly converted to *N*-isopropyl terephthalamic acid by aldehyde oxidase present in perfused liver and liver microsomes (BAGGIOLINI et al., 1969).

A second pathway, which may be the major route of procarbazine metabolism, is an inducible pathway involving the N^1-demethylation or N^1-methyl hydroxylation of azo procarbazine to yield formaldehyde and an unstable intermediate which would form *N*-isopropyl terephthalamic acid directly or via the aldehyde *p*-formyl-*N*-isopropyl benzamide (Fig. 2). This pathway would explain the high yield of $^{14}CO_2$ from both *N*-methyl-^{14}C procarbazine and *N*-methyl-^{14}C-azo procarbazine which is about two-fold greater than methane formation (Table 2). *N*-methyl-^{14}C hydrazone, in contrast, gives a high yield of both $^{14}CO_2$ and ^{14}C-methane, which indicates that it is a good substrate for *N*-demethylation and that it is also undergoing isomerization to yield MMH which gives a much higher yield of methane than CO_2.

A third pathway has been proposed by BAGGIOLINI et al. (1969) which involves a microsomal hydroxylase attacking the N^2-C bond of azo procarbazine to yield methyldiazene free radical and *p*-formyl-*N*-isopropyl benzamide. Such a pathway was proposed by these workers because of greater *N*-isopropyl terephthalamic acid formation than of CO_2 release from the *N*-methyl group, as well as the lack of azo procarbazine isomerization by liver microsomes. The data in Table 2 preclude this route being the major pathway because of the greater yield of CO_2 than of methane from the *N*-methyl group of either procarbazine or azo procarbazine. This pathway could be the major pathway if a great portion of the methyldiazene radicals from azo procarbazine, and not from MMH, methylated cellular constituents rather than undergoing hydrogen abstraction to form methane. Large yields of methane have been reported by TSUJI and KOSOWER (1971) for chemical decomposition of methyldiazene in the presence of oxygen.

The fate of the postulated methyldiazene may be the most important aspect of procarbazine metabolism, since methyldiazene may in fact represent the active intermediate in the pharmacology of the parent drug. Specificity of the methyl group for biological activity may be related to the greater stability of the methyl group against isomerization compared to the ethyl or other alkyl groups, preventing rapid formation of the corresponding hydrazone. Certainly the ethyl azo derivative would very rapidly form the biologically inactive hydrazone. Evidence for a certain degree of hydrazone formation by azo procarbazine is provided by the data of CHABNER et al. (1969) which demonstrate the formation of MMH from procarbazine *in vivo*. An unconfirmed report of methylamine being a metabolite of procarbazine and methylhydrazine in rats indicates a reductive cleavage of the *N-N* bond (SCHWARTZ, 1966). However, BAGGIOLINI and BICKEL (1966) have presented evidence that methylamine is not an intermediate in $^{14}CO_2$ production from methyl-^{14}C procarbazine and that the cleavage of the *N-N* bond does not occur to a measurable extent in the isolated perfused rat liver.

WEITZEL et al. (1967) observed that a mild oxidizing agent such as potassium hexacyanoferrate caused procarbazine and other methylhydrazine derivatives to be cleaved with concomitant formaldehyde formation. They have suggested that intermediates such as azo methines and *N*-hydroxymethyl derivatives are formed which can function as alkylating agents (WEITZEL et al., 1964a, b, 1968).

Mode of Action of Procarbazine

While the metabolism of procarbazine has been extensively investigated, the question remains as to whether the biological activities of this agent are due to the parent drug or its metabolites; it seems probable that metabolites are involved.

Cytological studies have revealed that procarbazine exerts a marked influence on the mitotic cycle of cell division. In Ehrlich ascites carcinoma cells, a suppression of mitosis brought about by a prolongation of interphase has been demonstrated (RUTISCHAUSER and BOLLAG, 1963). An important characteristic of the cytological effects of procarbazine is the appearance of numerous chromatid breaks (RUTISCHAUSER and BOLLAG, 1963). The treatment of cells with the drug over many transplant generations resulted in the formation of resistant cell lines (BOLLAG and GRUNBERG, 1963).

The mechanism of action has been compared with the indirect effects of ionizing radiation (BERNEIS et al., 1963a). These workers (BERNEIS et al., 1963b, 1965, 1966) reported synergism between the effects of ionizing radiation and procarbazine upon the *in vitro* degradation of DNA. RAO (1967) examined the effects of x-rays and procarbazine on the Ehrlich ascites tumor in mice and concluded that the *in vivo* cytostatic effects were additive but not synergistic.

SARTORELLI and TSUNAMURA (1965, 1966) grew L5178Y ascites cells in the peritoneal cavity of adult male C57BL X DBA F_1 mice for 5 days and then gave a single intraperitoneal dose (300 mg/kg) of procarbazine. At selected intervals after exposure to the drug, cells were removed quantitatively and counted. The volume was measured and the cellular content of DNA, RNA, and protein determined. Total numbers of cells decreased markedly while cellular volume increased slightly. Average cellular DNA content remained essentially constant (intervals to 120 h) while RNA accumulated significantly. The rate of incorporation of labeled specific precursors indicated a pronounced inhibition of thymidine incorporation into DNA thymine, which reached a maximum of about 70% when the thymidine-^3H was administered from one to three hours after procarbazine. By 24 h after the drug, inhibition of DNA synthesis appeared to be relieved completely. Treatment of cells with procarbazine did not influence the rate of loss of thymine-^3H from prelabeled

DNA. RNA synthesis was also markedly depressed by procarbazine; however, the cells appeared to recover from the inhibition within 12 h after administration of the drug. The onset of inhibition of protein synthesis was delayed and the maximum decrease in synthesis occurred 12 h after procarbazine.

GALE et al. (1967) found that freshly prepared solutions of procarbazine are virtually without effect on DNA, RNA, or protein synthesis in Ehrlich ascites tumor cells *in vitro*. Upon exposure of 10^{-2} M solutions of procarbazine to air in a dark moisture chamber at 37° for three days, degradation of the drug occurred with the formation of one or more products that were inhibitory. The formation of H_2O_2 was measured and the concentration attained at three days (10^{-5} M) was almost ten-fold lower than that needed for 50% inhibition of DNA synthesis. Measurement of the time course of DNA inhibition indicated that the active compound is a labile intermediate in the degradation of procarbazine, rather than a compound which accumulates during storage as was noted for H_2O_2. The inhibitory action was approximately equally manifest against DNA and RNA synthesis. The inhibition of protein synthesis was delayed in onset and may reflect a diminished rate of nucleic acid synthesis. Neither DNA, RNA, nor nucleosides antagonized the inhibition of DNA synthesis. The washing of drug treated cells with Eagle's minimum essential medium containing Hank's balanced salt solution freed them of the drug and reversed the inhibition. One can speculate that washing of the cells not only removed the drug, but also any oxidized glutathione, as well as possibly replenishing reduced glutathione. This would be in agreement with the suggestion of GALE et al. (1967) that the inhibition of DNA synthesis is an antianabolic effect rather than a manifestation of depolymerization of preexisting DNA as would be caused by H_2O_2. However, there is little evidence that procarbazine has a limiting effect upon cellular respiration and glycolysis of neoplastic cells (FUSENIG et al., 1966; OBRECHT et al., 1967).

GUTTERMAN et al. (1969), have confirmed the findings of GALE et al. (1967), that freshly prepared solutions of procarbazine do not affect the incorporation of thymidine-^{3}H, uridine-^{3}H, and arginine-^{3}H into acid-insoluble material of Ehrlich cells treated *in vitro*. Treatment of tumor-bearing mice with a single subcutaneous dose of the drug (200 mg/kg) resulted in a noticeable prolongation of the survival time of the mice. Inhibition of DNA synthesis reached a maximum of 35 to 40% when the cells were pulse-labeled *in vitro* with thymidine-^{3}H at 4 to 8 h after *in vivo* exposure to procarbazine. After 4 to 8 h, thymidine utilization gradually returned to its normal level, as was observed by SARTORELLI and TSUNAMURA (1966). Onset of inhibition of protein synthesis was observed at 8 h after administration of procarbazine with maximum depression at 16 h and noticeable recovery at 24 h. In contrast to the findings of SARTORELLI and TSUNAMURA (1966), GUTTERMAN et al. (1969) observed that procarbazine consistently produced a marked but transitory enhancement of the incorporation of uridine-^{3}H into RNA. The stimulation became maximal between 8 and 16 h after procarbazine treatment. These workers developed a line of cells resistant to procarbazine and observed that resistance was induced much more rapidly when procarbazine was administered in coincidence with periods of normal DNA synthesis. Resistance developed more slowly when the drug was given over a period in which DNA synthesis was depressed. The resistant line was characterized by the appearance of two new metacentric chromosomes in each cell in mitosis. HUANG and KREMER (1969) purified an active derivative of procarbazine, possibly azo procarbazine, and at a concentration of 3×10^{-4} M prevented lymphocyte transformation and suppressed the synthesis of DNA, RNA, and protein. When the drug was added within the first 24 h of culture, blastogenesis was completely suppressed. Once DNA synthesis had begun, the drug was without effect. The authors concluded that azo procarbazine is an inhibitor which is active in the early phase of cell division.

KOBLET and DIGGELMAN (1966, 1968) treated rats with procarbazine (1 to 4×200 mg/kg i.p. every second day), isolated the livers, and examined protein synthesis in perfused liver preparations. They concluded that protein synthesis comes nearly to a complete stop, but could not decide if procarbazine acts *in vivo* on DNA or on the biosynthesis of mRNA, rRNA, or tRNA. The ability of amino-acyl-tRNA synthetases to load tRNA and the capacity of tRNA to accept labeled amino acids were both normal; loaded tRNA's of pretreated animals were able to enter polysomes isolated from control animals. Incorporation of L-leucine-1-^{14}C into protein was significantly decreased when polysomes of livers of pretreated animals were used, as compared to those of untreated rats.

KREIS and YEN (1965), KREIS (1966, 1970), and KREIS et al. (1966, 1968) have observed the transfer *in vivo* with P815 mouse ascites cells of the intact *N*-methyl group of procarbazine into cytoplasmic RNA. The degree of methylation of cytoplasmic RNA was compared between specifically labeled procarbazine, methionine, and formate. Trace amounts of radioactive methylated bases, identified as 7-methylguanine (the major methylated base), thymine, 5-methylcytosine, 1-methylguanine, and 1-methyladenine (tentatively) were found in cytoplasmic RNA, with likely predominance in transfer RNA, of ascites cells 2 and 4 h after intraperitoneal injection of the labeled procarbazine into mice bearing the P815 ascites tumor. Experiments with a mixture of L-methionine-C^3H_3 and methyl-^{14}C procarbazine indicated transfer of the intact *N*-methyl group, as well as a slight selective "over methylation" when compared to the normal pattern of methylation of RNA. KREIS (1970) suggested that this disturbance may be a part of the biological effect of procarbazine.

The role of methylation of the nucleic acids by procarbazine in the antitumor activity of this drug remains to be clarified. BROOKES (1965) examined the degree of methylation of DNA, RNA, and protein of mice after administration of *N*-methyl-^{3}H-procarbazine. He concluded that, although methylation did occur, the level was such that it would not be expected to produce significant cell toxicity unless a high specificity of reaction exists with a vital site(s) within the cell.

Incubation of washed human erythrocytes in isotonic saline, pH 7.4, and procarbazine (25 µmoles/ml of suspension) at 37° caused no decrease in reduced glutathione levels in the erythrocytes during the first 60 min, whereupon a linear decrease ensued, which continued until essentially complete disappearance of reduced glutathione was observed at 180 min. Reduced glutathione levels remained unchanged in untreated erythrocytes (MORTENSEN, 1965).

Formation of methemoglobin occurred at linear rates which were dependent upon procarbazine concentration at 25 µmoles/ml; 20 % methemoglobin was formed in 3 h. Procarbazine caused a large increase in erythocyte osmotic fragility which occurred during the first hour of incubation in 0.46 % sodium chloride solution. Less than 3 % hemolysis occurred in control erythrocytes, while procarbazine caused 40 to 50 % hemolysis.

The role of free radicals possibly derived from procarbazine in the biological activity of this drug remains uncertain. Methane formation most logically would involve a free radical intermediate(s), with reduced glutathione being a major donor of hydrogen radicals and concomitant glutathione free radicals, forming oxidized glutathione. Oxidation of intracellular reduced glutathione by free radicals can cause severe hemolysis of red cells (KOSOWER and KOSOWER, 1969).

Inhibition of protein synthesis occurs with levels of oxidized glutathione as low as 5×10^{-5} M even in the presence of reduced glutathione (KOSOWER et al., 1971). Much remains to be understood about the effects of procarbazine, as well as those of the nitrosoureas, and their effects upon thiol compounds in cells.

Clinical Aspects

MARTZ et al. (1963) reported the first clinical trial of procarbazine chemotherapy. Significant responses were observed with 16 of 17 patients with malignant lymphoma, while 14 patients with solid tumors were therapeutic failures. From 1963 until 1969 over 1000 patients were treated with procarbazine (MILLER, 1970). Of these, 480 were evaluable patients with Hodgkin's disease and 273 (i.e., 57 %) obtained objective and subjective response for at least one month (IA under the Karnofsky classification) (MILLER, 1970). Approximately 95 % of the patients had become refractory to other forms of therapy. These results give further indication that procarbazine is not cross-resistant with other therapeutic agents.

BONADONNA et al. (1969) have evaluated the responses of patients with generalized Hodgkin's disease to sequential therapy ending with procarbazine chemotherapy. A 46.4 % objective improvement for more than one month was obtained after procarbazine in 28 patients. These authors compiled similar information from the published literature (Table 3).

Combination chemotherapy with nitrogen mustard, vincristine, procarbazine, and prednisone is highly effective in the treatment of Hodgkin's disease (Table 4) (DEVITA et al., 1969, 1970). A complete response was obtained in 35 of 43 patients

Table 3. *Patient improvement of greater than 1 month duration (Category 1) after procarbazine therapy in Hodgkin's disease as estimated from published literature by* BONADONNA et al. (1969)

No. patients treated	Previous therapy (No. cases)		Responsive cases		Duration of response in months		Ref.
	Yes	No	Category 1	(%)	Mean	Median	
33	RT,[a] 13 alkyl. VLB[b]		23	69	3		KENIS et al. (1965)
33	20 RT, chemotherapy	13	23	69	not specified		FIORENTINO and FINOTTO (1968)
24	RT, chemotherapy		15	62.5	3.3		TODD (1965)
22	Some with RT, alkyl. agents, VLB	7	15	68	not specified		MATHÉ (1963)
20	18 chemotherapy	2	12	60	4.5		BRUNNER and YOUNG (1965)
18	14 RT, chemotherapy	4	10	55	not specified		OBRECHT et al. (1966)
17	RT, alkyl. agents, VLB		10	59	not specified		FAIRLEY et al. (1966)
14	11 RT, chemotherapy	3	14	100	2		MARTZ et al. (1963)
11	RT, alkyl. agents, VLB		8	72		4	SAMUELS et al. (1967)
28	RT, chemotherapy		13	46	5.7	4	BONADONNA et al. (1969)

[a] Radiotherapy. [b] Vinblastine.

Table 4. *Schedule of drug administration (one cycle)*

Day 1	2 3 4 5 6 7	8	9 10 11 12 13 14	15 to 28
Nitrogen Mustard 6 mg/m² i.v.		Nitrogen Mustard 6 mg/m² i.v.		No therapy
Vincristine 1.4 mg/m² i.v.		Vincristine 1.4 mg/m² i.v.		No therapy
Procarbazine 100 mg/m² p.o.	———	———	———→	No therapy
Prednisone 40 mg/m² p.o.	———	———	———→	No therapy

Therapy consisted of 6,2-week cycles of nitrogen mustard, 6 mg/m² i.v., and vincristine, 1.4 mg/m² i.v., on days 1 and 8 of each cycle; procarbazine, 100 mg/m² p.o., daily for each cycle and prednisone, 40 mg/m² p.o., daily for cycles 1 and 4. One cycle of therapy is shown in Table 4. A 2-week interval is employed between each cycle. Therapy took about 6 months to complete and patients received no maintenance therapy after the course of treatment was completed. The drugs were given at full dosages unless toxicity was prohibitive (DEVITA et al., 1970).

Table 5. *Response of Hodgkin's disease to combination chemotherapy (43 patients)*

Mean duration of treatment	5.8 months
Deaths during treatment	2
Responded but failed to achieve a complete remission	6
Achieved a complete remission	35 (81%)
Mean time to complete remission	3 months
Median duration of complete remission (from the cessation of all therapy)	29—42 months
Number who have relapsed	18 of 31 (51%)
Median time to relapse	11 months
(DEVITA et al., 1970)	

treated, with a mean response duration of 24 + months (Table 5). This combination chemotherapy treatment has given 7 complete remissions and 5 partial remissions in 15 patients with generalized lymphosarcoma. Among 8 reticulum cell sarcoma patients, 3 achieved complete remission and 2 achieved partial remission (LOWENBRAUN et al., 1970).

References

ABRAHAM, D., CARBONE, P. P., VENDITTI, J. M.: Evaluation of chemical agents against the plasma cell tumor LPC-1 in mice. Biochem. Pharmacol. **16**, 665—673 (1967).

AEBI, H., BAGGIOLINI, M., BICKEL, M. H., MESSIHA, F. S.: Untersuchungen über die *N*-Demethylierung des Cytostaticums Ibenzmethyzin (Natulan). Helv. physiol. pharmacol. Acta **24**, 1—14 (1966).

AEBI, H., DEWALD, B., SUTER, H.: Autoxydation *N*²-substituierter Methylhydrazine; Beeinflussung der Cu- und Fe-Katalyse durch Proteine, Desoxyribonucleinsäure (DNS) und EDTA. Helv. chim. Acta **48**, 656—674 (1965a).

AEBI, H., DEWALD, B., SUTER, H.: Peroxidbildung bei der Autoxydation *N*²-substituierter Methylhydrazine. Helv. chim. Acta **48**, 1380—1394 (1965b).

AEBI, H., SUTER, H.: Wirkung peroxybildender Cytostatica auf Methaemoglobin- und Glutathiongehalt normaler und akatalatischer Erythrocyten. Verh. Schweiz. Ver. Physiol., physiol. Chem., Pharmakol., 65th Meeting, Lausanne, May 1—2, 1965; Helv. physiol. pharmacol. Acta **23**, C9—C11 (1965).

AMIEL, J.-L., BREZIN, C., SEKIGUCHI, M., MERY, A.-M., HOERNI, B., GARATTINI, S., DAGUET, G., MATHÉ, G.: Depression des reactions immunitaires par une methyl hydrazine. Rev. franc. Etud. clin. biol. **9**, 636—638 (1964).

BAGGIOLINI, M., BICKEL, M. H.: Demethylation of ibenzmethyzin (natulan), monomethylhydrazine and methylamine by the rat *in vivo* and by the isolated perfused rat liver. Life Sci. **5**, 795—802 (1966).

BAGGIOLINI, M., BICKEL, M. H., MESSIHA, F. S.: Demethylation *in vivo* of natulan, a tumour-inhibiting methylhydrazine derivative. Experientia (Basel) **21**, 334—336 (1965).

BAGGIOLINI, M., DEWALD, B.: Induktion und Hemmung der Demethylierung von Ibenzmethyzin (Natulan) und Monomethylhydrazin in der isoliert perfundierten Rattenleber. 68th Meet. Verhandl. Schweiz. Vereins Physiol., physiol. Chemie Pharmakol., Zürich, Nov. 5, 1966; Helv. physiol. pharmacol. Acta **24**, C72—C74 (1966).

BAGGIOLINI, M., DEWALD, B.: NADPH-dependent oxidation of an alkyl, aralkyl hydrazine to the azo derivative by rat liver microsomes. International Congress on Pharmacology, 4th, Basel, July 14—18, 1969, pp. 229—230.

BAGGIOLINI, M., DEWALD, B., AEBI, H.: Oxidation of *p*-(N^1-methylhydrazino methyl)-*N*-isopropyl benzamide (procarbazine) to the methylazo derivative and oxidative cleavage of the N^2-C bond in the isolated perfused rat liver. Biochem. Pharmacol. **18**, 2187—2196 (1969).

BERNEIS, K., BOLLAG, W., KOFLER, M., LEUTHY, H.: Synergism between ionizing radiation and a cytotoxic methylhydrazine derivative: effect on DNA-degradation. Experientia (Basel) **21**, 318—320 (1965).

BERNEIS, K., BOLLAG, W., KOFLER, M., LEUTHY, H.: The enhancement of the after effect of ionizing radiation by a cytotoxic methylhydrazine derivative. Europ. J. Cancer **2**, 43—49 (1966).

BERNEIS, K., KOFLER, M., BOLLAG, W.: Die Auslösung von Fenton-Reaktionen durch cytotoxische Methylhydrazin-Verbindungen. Helv. chim. Acta **47**, 1903—1911 (1964).

BERNEIS, K., KOFLER, M., BOLLAG, W., KAISER, A., LANGEMANN, A.: The degradation of deoxyribonucleic acid by new tumor inhibiting compounds: the intermediate formation of hydrogen peroxide. Experientia (Basel) **19**, 132—133 (1963a).

BERNEIS, K., KOFLER, M., BOLLAG, W., ZELLER, P., KAISER, A., LANGEMANN, A.: Der prooxydative Effect tumorhemmender Methylhydrazin-Verbindungen. Helv. chim. Acta **46**, 2157—2167 (1963b).

BOLLAG, W.: Suppression of the immunological reaction by methylhydrazines, a new class of antitumour agents. Experientia (Basel) **19**, 304—305 (1963a).

BOLLAG, W.: The tumor-inhibitory effects of the methylhydrazine derivative Ro 4-6467/1 (NSC-77213). Cancer Chemother. Rep. **33**, 1—4 (1963b).

BOLLAG, W.: Investigations with methylhydrazine derivatives. In: PLATTNER, P. A. (Ed.): Proceedings of the international symposium on the chemotherapy of cancer, Lugano, April 28—May 1, 1964, pp. 191—197. Amsterdam-London-New York: Elsevier 1964.

BOLLAG, W.: Experimental studies with a methylhydrazine derivative — ibenzmethyzin. In: JELLIFFE, A. M., MARKS, J. (Eds.): Report of the proceedings of the symposium, Downing College, Cambridge, June 22, 1965, sponsored by Roche Products Limited; Natulan (Ibenzmethyzin), pp. 1—8. Bristol: John Wright & Sons, Ltd. 1965.

BOLLAG, W., GRUNBERG, E.: Tumour inhibitory effects of a new class of cytotoxic agents: methylhydrazine derivatives. Experientia (Basel) **19**, 130—131 (1963).

BOLLAG, W., THEISS, E.: Methylhydrazine derivatives. In: PLATTNER, P. A. (Ed.): Proceedings of the international symposium on the chemotherapy of cancer, Lugano, April 28—May 1, 1964, pp. 311—313. Amsterdam-London-New York: Elsevier 1964.

BONADONNA, G., MONFARDINI, S., OLDINI, C.: Comparative effects of vinblastine and procarbazine in advanced Hodgkin's disease. Europ. J. Cancer **5**, 393—402 (1969).

BROOKES, P.: Studies on the mode of action of ibenzmethyzin. In: JELLIFFE, A. M., MARKS, J. (Eds.): Report of the proceedings of the symposium, Downing College, Cambridge, June 22, 1965, sponsored by Roche Products Limited; Natulan (Ibenzmethyzin), pp. 9—12. Bristol: John Wright & Sons, Ltd. 1965.

BRUNNER, K. W., YOUNG, C. W.: A methylhydrazine derivative in Hodgkin's disease and other malignant neoplasms. Therapeutic and toxic effects studied in 51 patients. Ann. intern. Med. **63**, 69—86 (1965).

CARTER, S. K. (Ed.): Procarbazine (matulane: NSC-77213): Development and application, Bethesda: Cancer Therapy Evaluation Branch, National Cancer Institute 1970, p. 109. (U.S. Government Printing Office: 1971 0 - 440 - 316.)

CERILLI, G. J., GIDEON, L.: Successful long term inhibition of xenograft rejection. Surg. Forum **20**, 284—285 (1969).

CHABNER, B. A., DEVITA, V. T., CONSIDINE, N., OLIVERIO, V. T.: Plasma pyridoxal phosphate depletion by the carcinostatic procarbazine. Proc. Soc. exp. Biol. (N. Y.) **132**, 1119—1122 (1969).

CHAUBE, S., MURPHY, M. L.: The teratogenic effects of 1-methyl-2-para (isopropylcarbamoyl) benzylhydrazine. HCl MHl. Proc. Amer. Ass. Cancer Res. **5**, 11 (1964).

Chaube, S., Murphy, M. L.: Fetal malformations produced in rats by *N*-isopropyl-α-(2-methylhydrazino)-*p*-toluamide hydrochloride (procarbazine). Teratology **2**, 23—32 (1969).

Colvin, L. B.: Metabolic fate of hydrazines and hydrazides. J. pharm. Sci. **58**, 1433—1443 (1969).

DeVita, V. T., Hahn, M. A., Oliverio, V. T.: Monoamine oxidase inhibition by a new carcinostatic agent, *N*-isopropyl-α-(2-methylhydrazino)-*p*-toluamide (MIH). Proc. Soc. exp. Biol. (N. Y.) **120**, 561—565 (1965).

DeVita, V. T., Serpick, A., Carbone, P. P.: Combination chemotherapy of advanced Hodgkin's disease (HD): the NCI program, a progress report. Proc. Amer. Ass. Cancer Res. **10**, 19 (1969).

DeVita, J. R., Serpick, A. A., Carbone, P. P.: Combination chemotherapy in the treatment of advanced Hodgkin's disease. Ann. intern. Med. **73**, 881—895 (1970).

Dewald, B., Baggiolini, M., Aebi, H.: *N*-Demethylation of *p*-(N^1-methylhydrazino methyl)-*N*-isopropyl benzamide (procarbazine), a cytostatically active methylhydrazine derivative, in the intact rat and in the isolated perfused rat liver. Biochem. Pharmacol. **18**, 2179—2186 (1969).

Dixon, R. L., Lee, I. P.: Antineoplastic drug effects on spermatogenesis studied by velocity sedimentation cell separation and serial mating. Pharmacologist **13**, 294 (1971).

Dost, F. N., Reed, D. J.: Methane formation *in vivo* from *N*-isopropyl *alpha*(2-methylhydrazino)-*p*-toluamide hydrochloride, a tumor-inhibiting methylhydrazine derivative. Biochem. Pharmacol. **16**, 1741—1746 (1967).

Dost, F. N., Reed, D. J., Wang, C. H.: The metabolic fate of monomethylhydrazine and unsymmetrical dimethylhydrazine. Biochem. Pharmacol. **15**, 1325—1332 (1966).

Fairley, G. H., Patterson, M. J. L., Scott, R. B.: Chemotherapy of Hodgkin's disease with cyclophosphamide, vinblastine, and procarbazine. Brit. med. J. **2**, 75—78 (1966).

Fiorentino, M., Finotto, E.: Action de la procarbazine dans les lymphomes malins. Presse med. **76**, 992 (1968).

Floersheim, G. L.: Verlängerte Überlebenszeit von Hauthomotransplantaten bei Mäusen durch ein Methylhydrazinderivat. Experientia (Basel) **19**, 546—547 (1963).

Floersheim, G. L., Brune, K.: Abstracts of the third international congress of the transplantation society. The Hague 1970.

Floersheim, G. L., Taub, R. N., Phillips-Quagliata, J. M., Levey, R. H.: Induction of tolerance to skin homografts with a methylhydrazine derivative. Synergism with antilymphocytic serum and morphologic responses of the lymphoid system. Agents and Actions **1**, 115—123 (1970).

Fox, B. W., Fox, M.: Biochemical aspects of the actions of drugs on spermatogenesis. Pharmacol. Rev. **19**, 21—57 (1967).

Fusenig, N. E., Obrecht, P., Strickstrock, K. H.: Zur Biochemie der sogenannten cytostatischen Nebenwirkungen. Vergleichende Untersuchungen. I. Mitteilung: NAD, TP und FDP in Duenndarmschleimhaut, Hoden und Leber nach Trenimon, Velbe und Natulan. Klin. Wschr. **44**, 1335—1339 (1966).

Gale, G. R., Simpson, J. G., Smith, A. B.: Studies of the mode of action of *N*-isopropyl-α-(2-methylhydrazino)-*p*-toluamide. Cancer Res. **27**, 1186—1191 (1967).

Gelzer, J., Loustalot, P.: Biological and chemotherapeutic studies on primary mammary tumors in C3H and C3HO mice. Int. J. Cancer **2**, 179—187 (1967).

Grunberg, E., Prince, H. N.: The activity of ibenzmethyzin hydrochloride against the human transplantable tumors human epithelioma No. 3 and human adenoma No. 1. Experientia (Basel) **22**, 324—325 (1966).

Grunberg, E., Prince, H. N.: Further studies on the tumor-inhibitory and tumor-inducing properties of *N*-isopropyl-α-(2-methylhydrazino)-*p*-toluamide hydrochloride(procarbazine hydrochloride). Chemotherapy **14**, 65—76 (1969).

Gutterman, J. A., Huang, A. T., Hochstein, P.: Studies on the mode of action of *N*-isopropyl-α-(2-methylhydrazino)-*p*-toluamide (MIH). Proc. Soc. exp. Biol. (N. Y.) **130**, 797—802 (1969).

Hilscher, W., Reichelt, P.: Untersuchungen am Samenepithel der Ratte nach Gaben von "Endoxan" und "Natulan". Beitr. path. Anat. **137**, 452—478 (1968).

Huang, A. T., Kremer, W. B.: Inhibition of lymphocyte transformation by an active derivative of MIH. Proc. Amer. Ass. Cancer Res. **10**, 41 (1969).

Jelliffe, A. M., Marks, J. (Eds.): Natulan (ibenzmethyzin). Bristol: John Wright & Sons, Ltd. 1965.

Kelly, M. G., O'Gara, R. W., Gadekar, K., Yancey, S. T., Oliverio, V. T.: Carcinogenic activity of a new antitumor agent, *N*-isopropyl-α-(2-methyl-hydrazino)-*p*-toluamide, hydrochloride (NSC-77213). Cancer Chemother. Rep. **39**, 77—80 (1964).

KELLY, M. G., O'GARA, R. W., YANCEY, S. T., BOTKIN, C.: Induction of tumors in rats with procarbazine hydrochloride. J. nat. Cancer Inst. **40**, 1027—1051 (1968).

KELLY, M. G., O'GARA, R. W., YANCEY, S. T., GADEKAR, K., BOTKIN, C., OLIVERIO, V. T.: Comparative carcinogenicity of *N*-isopropyl-α-(2-methylhydrazino)-*p*-toluamide HCl (procarbazine hydrochloride), its degradation products, other hydrazines, and isonicotinic acid hydrazide. J. nat. Cancer Inst. **42**, 337—344 (1969).

KENIS, Y., WERLI, J., HILDEBRAND, J., TAGNON, H. J.: Action d'un dérivé de la methylhydrazine, le Ro 4-6467, dans la maladie de Hodgkin, dans d'autres lymphomes malins et dans des leucémies. Europ. J. Cancer **1**, 33—40 (1965).

KLEIBEL, F.: Untersuchungen mit ^{3}H-markierten Methylhydrazinderivaten. In: HOFFMANN, G., SCHEER, K. E. (Eds.): Radionuklide in Klin. und Exp. Onkologic; Nuclear-Med. Vol. 2, pp. 63—67 (Suppl. 3). Stuttgart: Schattauer 1965.

KOBLET, H., DIGGELMANN, H.: On the action of ibenzmethyzin (*N*-isopropyl-alpha-(2-methylhydrazino)-*p*-toluamide hydrochloride, natulan, IMTH) on protein biosynthesis, p. 344. 9th International Cancer Congress, Tokyo, Oct. 23—29, 1966.

KOBLET, H., DIGGELMANN, H.: Action of ibenzmethyzin (*N*-isopropyl-α-(2-methyl-hydrazino)-*p*-toluamid-hydrochlorid, natulan®, IMTH) on protein synthesis in the rat liver. Europ. J. Cancer **4**, 45—58 (1968).

KOSOWER, E. M., KOSOWER, N. S.: Lest I forget thee, glutathione. Nature (Lond.) **224**, 117—120 (1969).

KOSOWER, N. S., VANDERHOFF, G. A., BENEROFE, B., HUNT, T., KOSOWER, E. M.: Inhibition of protein synthesis by glutathione disulfide in the presence of glutathione. Biochem. biophys. Res. Comm. **45**, 816—821 (1971).

KREIS, W.: Studies on the metabolism and reaction mechanism of a methylhydrazine derivative in BDF P815-leukemic mice. Proc. Amer. Ass. Cancer Res. **7**, 39 (1966).

KREIS, W.: Metabolism of an antineoplastic methylhydrazine derivative in a P815 mouse neoplasm. Cancer Res. **30**, 82—89 (1970).

KREIS, W., BURCHENAL, J. H., HUTCHISON, D. J.: Influence of a methylhydrazine derivative on the *in vivo* transmethylation of the *S*-methyl group of methionine onto purine and pyrimidine bases of RNA. Proc. Amer. Ass. Cancer Res. **9**, 38 (1968).

KREIS, W., PIEPHO, S. B., BERNHARD, H. V.: Studies of the metabolic fate of the ^{14}C-labeled methyl group of a methylhydrazine derivative in P815 mouse leukemia. Experientia (Basel) **22**, 431—433 (1966).

KREIS, W., YEN, W.: An antineoplastic C^{14}-labeled methylhydrazine derivative in P815 mouse leukemia. A metabolic study. Experientia (Basel) **21**, 284—286 (1965).

LOWENBRAUN, S., DEVITA, V. T., SERPICK, A. A.: Combination chemotherapy with nitrogen mustard, vincristine, procarbazine and prednisone in lymphosarcoma and reticulum cell sarcoma. Cancer **25**, 1018—1025 (1970).

MACDONALD, A. S., CHAN, C. C., FALVEY, C. F.: Use of procarbazine hydrochloride (natulan) and procarbazine hydrochloride and azathioprine in canine renal allografts. Transplanation **11**, 103—104 (1971).

MAKINODAN, T., SANTOS, G. W., QUINN, R. P.: Immunosuppressive drugs. Pharmacol. Rev. **22**, 189—247 (1970).

MARTZ, G.: Clinical results with a methylhydrazine derivative. In: PLATTNER, P. A. (Ed.): Proceedings of the international symposium on the chemotherapy of cancer, Lugano, April 28—May 1, 1964, pp. 198—203. Amsterdam-London-New York: Elsevier 1964.

MARTZ, G., D'ALLESSANDRI, A., KEEL, H. J.: Preliminary clinical results with a new antitumor agent Ro 4-6467. Cancer Chemother Rep. **33**, 5—14 (1963).

MATHÉ, G., BERUMEN, L., SCHWEISGUTH, O., BRULE, G., SCHNEIDER, M., CATTAN, A., AMIEL, J. L., SCHWARZENBERG, L.: Methyl-hydrazine in treatment of Hodgkin's disease. Lancet **II**, 1077—1080 (1963).

MILLER, E.: Development of procarbazine. In: CARTER, S. K. (Ed.): Procarbazine (matulane: NSC-77213): development and application, pp. 3—8. Bethesda: Cancer Therapy Evaluation Branch, National Cancer Institute 1970.

MORTENSEN, E.: Some effects of 1-methyl-2-*p*-(isopropylcarbamoyl)-benzyl-hydrazine and Mannomustine on the metabolism of human erythrocytes *in vitro*. Scand. J. Haematol. **2**, 288—304 (1965).

OBRECHT, P., STRICKSTROCK, K.-H., FUSENIG, N.: Die Wirkung von Natulan auf den Energiestoffwechsel. Z. Krebsforsch. **69**, 25—36 (1967).

OBRECHT, P., STRICKSTROCK, K. H., WEISSLEDER, H.: Klinische und lymphographische Verlaufskontrollen bei Lymphogranulomatose und Retothelsarkom unter Behandlung mit Natulan. Europ. J. Cancer **2**, 59—68 (1966).

Obrecht, P., Strickstrock, K. H., Woenckhaus, J. W.: Zur Frage der biochemischen Wirkung eines neuen Zytostatikum, Ro 4-6467, aus der Klasse der Methylhydrazinderivate. Chemotherapia 8, 106—113 (1964).

O'Gara, R. W., Adamson, R. H., Kelly, M. G., Dalgard, D. W.: Neoplasma of the hematopoietic system in nonhuman primates: report of one spontaneous tumor and two leukemias induced by procarbazine. J. nat. Cancer Inst. 46, 1121—1130 (1971).

Oliverio, V. T.: Derivatives of triazenes and hydrazines. In: Holland, J. F., Frei, E., III (Eds.): Cancer medicine. Philadelphia: Lea and Febiger 1973.

Oliverio, V. T., Denham, C., DeVita, V. T., Kelly, M. G.: Some pharmacologic properties of a new antitumor agent, *N*-isopropyl-α-(2-methylhydrazino)-*p*-toluamide, hydrochloride (NSC-77213). Cancer Chemother. Rep. 42, 1—7 (1964).

Oliverio, V. T., Kelly, M. G.: Contributions to the biological and clinical effect of a methylhydrazine derivative. II. Some preliminary observations on its physiological disposition, antitumor activity and carcinogenicity. In: Plattner, P. A. (Ed.): Proceedings of the international symposium on the chemotherapy of cancer, Lugano, April 28—May 1, 1964, pp. 221—227. Amsterdam-London-New York: Elsevier Publishing Co. 1964.

Plattner, P. A. (Ed.): Proceedings of the international symposium on the chemotherapy of cancer, Lugano, April 28—May 1, 1964, p. 324. Amsterdam-London-New York: Elsevier 1964.

Prough, R., Wittkop, J., Reed, D. J.: Evidence for the hepatic metabolism of some monoalkylhydrazines. Arch. Biochem. Biophys. 131, 369—373 (1969).

Prough, R., Wittkop, J., Reed, D. J.: Further evidence on the nature of microsomal metabolism of procarbazine and related hydrazines. Arch. Biochem. Biophys. 140, 450—458 (1970).

Raaflaub, J., Schwartz, D. E.: Über den Metabolism eines cytostatisch wirksamen Methylhydrazin-Derivates (Natulan). Experientia (Basel) 21, 44—45 (1965).

Rao, K. R.: Interaction between the carcinostatic effects of x-rays and ibenzmethyzin on Ehrlich ascites carcinoma in mice. Strahlentherapie 134, 574—584 (1967).

Reed, D. J.: Unpublished observations (1971).

Reed, D. J., Dost, F. N.: Methane and CO_2 formation by rats during metabolism of a methylhydrazine (natulan). Proc. Amer. Ass. Cancer Res. 7, 57 (1966).

Roche Laboratories: Package insert for Matulane capsules by Roche Laboratories Division of Hoffmann-La Roche Inc. Nutley, N. J. August 1969.

Rutishauser, A., Bollag, W.: Cytological investigations with a new class of cytotoxic agents: methylhydrazine derivatives. Experientia (Basel) 19, 131—132 (1963).

Samuels, M. L., Leary, W. V., Alexanian, R., Howe, C. D., Frei, E., III: Clinical trials with *N*-isopropyl-alpha-(2-methylhydrazino)-*p*-toluamide hydrochloride in malignant lymphoma and other disseminated neoplasia. Cancer 20, 1187—1194 (1967).

Sartorelli, A. C., Creasey, W. A.: Cancer chemotherapy. Ann. Rev. Pharmacol. 9, 51—72 (1969).

Sartorelli, A. C., Tsunamura, S.: Metabolic alterations in L5178Y lymphoma cells induced by *N*-isopropyl-α-(2-methylhydrazino)-*p*-toluamide. Proc. Amer. Ass. Cancer Res. 6, 55 (1965).

Sartorelli, A. C., Tsunamura, S.: Studies on the biochemical mode of action of a cytotoxic methylhydrazine derivative, *N*-isopropyl-α-(2-methylhydrazino)-*p*-toluamide. Molec. Pharmacol. 2, 275—283 (1966).

Schwartz, D. E.: Comparative metabolic studies with natulan, methylhydrazine and methylamine in rats. Experientia (Basel) 22, 212—213 (1966).

Schwartz, D. E., Bollag, W., Obrecht, P.: Distribution and excretion studies of procarbazine in animals and man. Arzneimittel-Forsch. 17, 1389—1393 (1967c).

Schwartz, D. E., Brubacher, G. B., Vecchi, M.: Metabolic formation of methane from *N*-methyl-substituted hydrazine compounds and carcinostatic activity. J. labelled Compounds 111, 487—488 (1967a).

Schwartz, D. E., Brubacher, G. B., Vecchi, M.: Metabolic formation of methane from *N*-methyl-substituted hydrazine compounds and carcinostatic activity, pp. 65—66. International conference on the use of radioactive isotopes in pharmacology, Geneva, Sept. 20—23 (1967b).

Stewart, P. B., Bell, R.: Procarbazine as an immunosuppressant in animals. J. Immunology 105, 1271—1277 (1970).

Stewart, P. B., Cohen, V.: Antiserum to lymphocytes and procarbazine compared as immunosuppressants in mice. Science 164, 1082—1083 (1969).

Stock, J. A.: Other antitumor agents. Exp. chemotherapy 5, 333—416 (1967).

Todd, I. D. H.: Natulan in management of late Hodgkin's disease, other lymphoreticular neoplasms, and malignant melanoma. Brit. med. J. 1, 628—631 (1965).

TSUJI, T., KOSOWER, E. M.: Diazenes, VI. Alkyldiazenes. J. Amer. chem. Soc. **93**, 1992—1999 (1971).
WEITZEL, G. L., SCHNEIDER, F., FRETZDORFF, A. M.: Cytostatischer Wirkungsmechanismus der Methylhydrazine. Experientia (Basel) **20**, 38—39 (1964a).
WEITZEL, G. L., SCHNEIDER, F., FRETZDORFF, A. M., DURST, J., HIRSCHMANN, W.: Untersuchungen zum cytostatischen Wirkungsmechanismus der Methylhydrazine, II. Z. Physiol. Chem. **348**, 433—442 (1967).
WEITZEL, G. L., SCHNEIDER, F., FRETZDORFF, A. M., SEYNSCHE, K., FINGER, H.: Untersuchungen zum cytostatischen Wirkungsmechanismus der Methylhydrazine. Z. Physiol. Chem. **336**, 271—282 (1964b).
WEITZEL, G. L., SCHNEIDER, F., KUMMER, D., OCHS, H.: Cytostatischer Wirkungsmechanismus von Natulan. Z. Krebsforsch. **70**, 354—365 (1968).
WITTKOP, J. A., PROUGH, R. A., REED, D. J.: Oxidative demethylation of *N*-methylhydrazines by rat liver microsomes. Arch. Biochem. Biophys. **134**, 308—315 (1969).
ZELLER, P., GUTMANN, H., HEGEDUS, B., KAISER, A., LANGEMANN, A., MUELLER, M.: Methylhydrazine derivatives, a new class of cytotoxic agents. Experientia (Basel) **19**, 129 (1963).

Chapter 71

Bis-Guanylhydrazones

E. Mihich

With 2 Figures

Introduction

Although the synthesis of certain aliphatic *bis*(guanylhydrazones) was described long ago (Thiele and Dralle, 1898), the biological activities of *bis*(guanylhydrazones) were studied only during the last 15 years, following the report that methylglyoxal-*bis*(guanylhydrazone) had significant antitumor action (Freedlander and French, 1958). These compounds form a relatively heterogeneous group comprising distinct classes of chemicals with different pharmacological characteristics. Common to most of them, however, is their marked basicity and the fact that their chemical structure consists of two polar aminoguanidine groups separated by an aliphatic or aromatic skeleton. The basicity and the polarity of *bis*(guanylhydrazones) is due to the stabilization of the protonated terminal guanidino groups by resonance. In this sense, *bis*(guanylhydrazones) are similar to diamidines and *bis*(guanidines) (Fastier, 1962). Also, from a general pharmacological point of view, aliphatic and aromatic *bis*(guanylhydrazones) and diamidines, aliphatic *bis*(guanidines), and terephthalanilides have some features in common. In fact, within each of these groups, compounds were found that exert trypanocidal, antibacterial, antitumor, immunosuppressive, hepatotoxic, hypoglycemic, or cardiovascular action.

Two *bis*(guanylhydrazones) are discussed herein as examples of aliphatic and aromatic derivatives, respectively: methylglyoxal-*bis*(guanylhydrazone) (CH_3—G)[1], which has antitumor activity in man, and 4,4′-diacetyldiphenylurea-*bis*(guanylhydrazone) (DDUG), which is the most potent *bis*(guanylhydrazone) tested against mouse leukemia L1210. (For chemical structures, see Charts 1 and 2). Congeners of the two prototypes are compared when relevant. The early studies with CH_3—G have been reviewed (Mihich, 1965) and only selected aspects of this material are discussed in detail. The reader is also referred to other sources for information on diamidines (Fastier, 1962), stilbamidines (Schoenbach and Greenspan, 1948), *bis*(guanidines) (Hollunger, 1955; Duncan and Baird, 1960), terephthalanilides (Bennett, 1965; and Chapt. 75 of this volume) and physiological polyamines (Herbst and Bachrach, 1970; Cohen, 1971).

Methylglyoxal-*bis* (Guanylhydrazone) and Aliphatic Derivatives

Of the aliphatic analogs tested to date, CH_3—G is the most effective against mouse leukemia L1210. The drug has activity in patients with acute myelocytic

1 Methylglyoxal-*bis*(guanylhydrazone) has been also indicated by different authors as methyl—GAG, CH_3GAG, Me—GAG, MGBG, MGGH, and NSC 32946. The "Chemical Abstract" name for this compound is 1,1′[(methylethane diylidene)-dinitrilo] diguanidine.

leukemia and lymphomas. Although its mode of action is still unknown, it seems in part related to the function of the physiological polyamines.

A. Effects on Experimental Tumors

I. Tumor Sensitivity

The activity of CH_3—G against the L1210 leukemia was first reported by Freedlander and French (1958) and was soon repeatedly confirmed (see Mihich, 1965). After oral, subcutaneous, or intraperitoneal administration, the drug was active against the L1210 tumor inoculated intraperitoneally, subcutaneously, or intracerebrally, as well as against advanced leukemia. Also inhibited by CH_3—G, were lymphocytic leukemias P388, B82T, and B8174, mast cell leukemia P815, reticular cell sarcoma P329, lymphomas 4, P288, P1798, and Sarcoma 180 ascites in mice, and Dunning-Schmidt leukemia in rats. Several tumor sublines resistant to a variety of drugs were also sensitive to CH_3—G. In particular, CH_3—G was active against L1210 cells resistant to DDUG or to 2-chloro-4′,4″-*bis*(2-imidazolin-2-yl)-terephthalanilide (Mihich et al., 1970a). The drug was not active against the solid sarcomas and carcinomas tested, against mouse lymphocytic leukemias AK_4, L4946, and L5178 Y_F (see Mihich, 1965) or against mouse melanoma B_{16} (Schepartz, 1971). Thus, with the exception of Sarcoma 180 ascites, all sensitive tumors were leukemias.

Against the L1210 leukemia, CH_3—G appeared to be less active than methotrexate, but more active than 6-mercaptopurine, 5-fluorouracil, or 5-fluorodeoxyuridine when each of these compounds was given intraperitoneally at the LD_{10} dose. In BDF_1 mice, the ratio between LD_{90} and LD_{10} was 1.3 for CH_3—G and between 1.8 and 2.3 for methotrexate, 6-mercaptopurine, 5-fluorouracil, thio-TEPA, and chlorambucil (Griswold et al., 1963). In mice with advanced L1210 leukemia, CH_3—G was more toxic, without change in optimal dose and with decreased therapeutic effect, when given subcutaneously in 50% DMSO, in contrast with the observed improvement in therapeutic effectiveness of methotrexate in 20 to 50% DMSO (Kline et al., 1971). The relatively narrow therapeutic index of CH_3—G found in mice (Mihich, 1963a) was confirmed in man (see below).

Resistance of L1210 cells to CH_3—G developed rapidly, in 1 to 3 transfer generations (Freedlander and French, 1958; Mihich, 1967a). No consistent

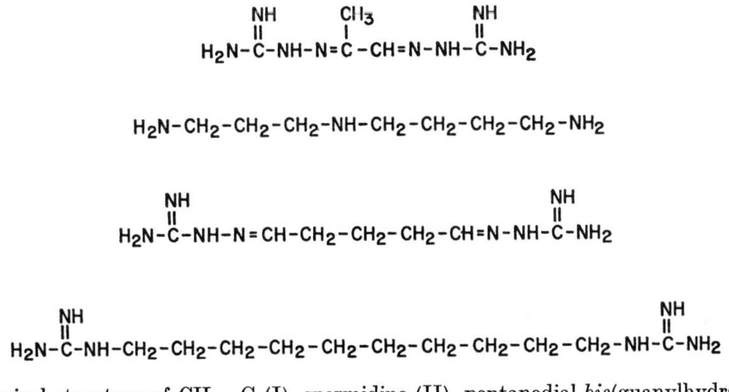

I $H_2N-C(=NH)-NH-N=C(CH_3)-CH=N-NH-C(=NH)-NH_2$

II $H_2N-CH_2-CH_2-CH_2-NH-CH_2-CH_2-CH_2-CH_2-NH_2$

III $H_2N-C(=NH)-NH-N=CH-CH_2-CH_2-CH_2-CH=N-NH-C(=NH)-NH_2$

IV $H_2N-C(=NH)-NH-CH_2-CH_2-CH_2-CH_2-CH_2-CH_2-CH_2-CH_2-CH_2-CH_2-NH-C(=NH)-NH_2$

Fig. 1. Chemical structure of CH_3—G (I), spermidine (II), pentanedial-*bis*(guanylhydrazone) (III), and decamethylene-*bis*(guanidine) (Synthalin) (IV)

pattern of cross-resistance could be identified (see MIHICH, 1965). For instance, P815/MTX was sensitive to CH_3—G, whereas L1210/MTX was resistant to it, and P815/VCR was sensitive to CH_3—G, whereas P388/VCR was not. It is of interest that L1210 cells resistant to CH_3—G were sensitive to DDUG (MIHICH and MULHERN, 1968), decamethylene-*bis*(guanidine) (Synthalin) and hydroxystilbamidine alone or in combination with other *bis*(guanylhydrazones) (MIHICH, 1967a).

In DBA/2 mice, arabinosylcytosine, carzinostatin, and 2-chloro-4',4''-*bis*(2-imidazolin-2-yl)-terephthalanilide, but not methotrexate, had greater therapeutic effects against an L1210 variant resistant to CH_3—G than against parent L1210 tumor, this effect being a reflection of the greater immunogenicity of the resistant leukemia (MIHICH, 1969b; MIHICH and KITANO, 1971) due to the presence of more and different antigens on the resistant cells (KITANO et al., 1972; CAREY et al., 1972). These differences may be an expression of biochemical changes related to the development of resistance to CH_3—G or may result from the selection of pre-existing clones of more antigenic cells.

II. Structure-Activity Relationships

Glyoxal-*bis*(guanylhydrazone) also had activity against the L1210 leukemia, but was not superior to CH_3—G (FREEDLANDER and FRENCH, 1958). The effects of the so-called hydroxymethylglyoxal-*bis*(guanylhydrazone) were actually due to CH_3—G (DAVIDSON et al., 1963). Of more than 200 other *bis*(guanylhydrazones) none had significant antileukemic activity (MONTGOMERY, 1965). These included homologs of the methylglyoxal moiety, where an alkyl group replaces the methyl group as in ethylglyoxal-*bis*(guanylhydrazone), and of the guanylhydrazone moiety, where a methyl group replaces one or more hydrogens in one or both of the guanylhydrazone moieties (PODREBARAC et al., 1963; FRENCH and BLANZ, 1971). Dimethylglyoxal-*bis*(guanylhydrazone), and compounds where the two guanylhydrazonyl groups are separated by a three carbon or longer aliphatic chain, also had no activity (BAIOCCHI et al., 1963). Thus, steric factors seem important in determining the antileukemic action of CH_3—G. Even trifluoromethylglyoxal-*bis*(guanylhydrazone) (PODREBARAC and CHENG, 1964) was inactive against the L1210 leukemia (MIHICH, unpublished data). Diacetylated CH_3—G (LIAO et al., 1965) was active (MIHICH, 1963a), probably subsequent to cleavage of the acetyl groups in the animal. No aliphatic monoguanylhydrazone has been reported to have antileukemic action.

The structural requirements for the hypoglycemic and trypanocidal activity of CH_3—G do not seem to be as strict as outlined above (MIHICH, 1965; JAFFE, 1965). For instance, whereas CH_3—G caused antileukemic, hypoglycemic, and trypanocidal effects, dimethylglyoxal-*bis*(guanylhydrazone) caused hypoglycemic and trypanocidal effects, and ethylglyoxal-*bis*(guanylhydrazone) caused only hypoglycemic effects (MIHICH, 1965).

III. Combination Treatments

The effects of CH_3—G in combination with other compounds have been studied mainly in mouse leukemias P815 and L1210. Synergistic effects were noted with 2-chloro-4',4''-*bis*(2-imidazolin-2-yl)-terephthalanilide, 6-mercaptopurine, methotrexate, Synthalin, stilbamidine, or hydroxystilbamidine (see MIHICH, 1965). The most pronounced synergism was in combination with hydroxystilbamidine. The synergism with the terephthalanilide was not confirmed on Sarcoma 180 cells in culture, where the two drugs only had additive effects (HAKALA, 1971). The effects of CH_3—G and vincristine on the L1210 leukemia were additive (BURCHENAL et al., 1963).

Synergism between CH_3—G and DDUG was evident both with L1210 cells in mice (MIHICH and HAKALA, 1968) and with Sarcoma 180 cells in culture (HAKALA, 1971). Except for this synergism, which was confirmed in preirradiated mice, all of the other combinations mentioned were studied only in nonirradiated mice, under conditions in which the complicating participation of host defenses directed against the leukemia cannot be excluded (GRINDEY et al., 1972).

The effects of CH_3—G on the L1210 leukemia were prevented by spermidine, and, in part, by thymidine (MIHICH, 1963a, b, 1965).

B. Effects on Microorganisms

I. Bacteria and Protozoa

CH_3—G was found to inhibit the growth of *L. leichmannii* ATCC 7830, but not that of *E. coli* B (see MIHICH, 1965). The drug was effective against *T. equiperdum* in Swiss mice, and its action was not prevented by spermidine (JAFFE, 1965). Effective in this system also were analogs that had no activity on the L1210 leukemia. The growth of *Crithidia fasciculata* in a defined medium was moderately inhibited by CH_3—G (see MIHICH, 1965).

II. Viruses

In vivo, CH_3—G was more potent than guanidine in inhibiting polio virus, both in terms of replication and cytopathic effects (FERRARI et al., 1964). No damage to human amnion cells was detected at concentrations effective on virus. The drug was active on guanidine-resistant strains and could not replace guanidine in a guanidine-dependent strain. Preincubation of sensitive virus with excess CH_3—G did not modify infectivity. The unsubstituted *bis*(guanylhydrazone) moiety seems to be essential for antipolio activity, since *N*-methylated derivatives were inactive. Both CH_3—G and guanidine also inhibited Coxsackie B_3 and Echo 6 viruses.

C. Pharmacological Studies

I. Toxicological Effects

The toxic effects of CH_3—G have been studied in mice, rats, rabbits, dogs, and monkeys (MIHICH, 1963a, 1965). The LD_{50}, after repeated (5 to 15) intraperitoneal or intravenous injections, ranged from less than 10 mg/kg/day in the monkey to 123 mg/kg/day in the mouse. In man, 5 mg/kg/day for 5 to 67 (median 10) days, possibly contributed to death in 15 cases (LEVIN et al., 1965; REGELSON and HOLLAND, 1961). When these doses were expressed as a function of body surface area, they varied from 115 mg/m^2 in the monkey to 458 mg/m^2 in the rat. In man the toxic dose became 150 mg/m^2. Thus, the maximum difference between lethal doses across species was reduced from a 24-fold to a 4-fold difference.

In animals, sharp increases in toxicity occurred as a result of small increments of dosage. Parallel observations were made in humans (see below). The slight reduction of CH_3—G lethality seen in rats bearing the Walker carcinosarcoma 256 (MIHICH, 1963a) or in AKD_2F_1 mice bearing the L1210 leukemia, which were also treated with folinic acid (HOLLAND et al., 1962), are difficult to interpret.

The toxicological effects of CH_3—G were of three general types, namely, acute pharmacodynamic effects, hepatic, cardiac, and renal toxicity, and antiproliferative effects (MIHICH et al., 1962; MIHICH, 1965). The acute effects were seen primarily with large doses and were either lethal or readily reversible. The hepatic, cardiac, and renal toxicity were not prevented by spermidine. The antiproliferative effects were all prevented by nontoxic doses of spermidine.

The acute effects were noted in all animal species studied, and consisted of ataxia, loss of postural tone, salivation, and diarrhea. Death followed parenteral doses three times the LD_{50} or greater within minutes, and was related to respiratory failure.

Hepatic necrosis, hypoglycemia, and renal tubular necrosis were less marked in the dog than in the rat, rabbit, or monkey. Cardiotoxicity was pronounced in the dog; sinus tachycardia with premature supraventricular contractions and ectopic premature ventricular beats appeared only after 2 to 4 days of treatment and was initially reversible, but ultimately led to frank ventricular fibrillation and death. Since no histological signs of myocardial damage were found, the cumulative effects noted seem functional in nature. The guanylhydrazonyl moiety may be responsible for cardiac effects when linked to appropriate structures. Several mono- and *bis*(guanylhydrazones) were found to exert digitalis-like action in experimental systems (WOLLERT, 1969).

The antiproliferative effects consisted of marked gastrointestinal, bone marrow, and lymphoid toxicity which occurred in all species. Lymphoid depression also occurred in adrenalectomized rats and thus was not related to non-specific stress (MIHICH, 1963a). In mice, the drug inhibited hemagglutinin production, and both skin allograft (MIHICH, 1964) and tumor allograft rejection (MIHICH et al., 1970b). In man, primary antibody response was also inhibited (HERSH et al., 1965).

Both cardiac and antiproliferative effects appeared to contribute to the lethal toxicity of CH_3—G. Dogs in which bone marrow and gastrointestinal toxicity were prevented by spermidine still developed cardiac toxicity and died of demonstrable ventricular fibrillation. Conversely, while most dogs showed both cardiotoxicity and antiproliferative effects, some had no EKG evidence of terminal ventricular fibrillation.

II. Disposition and Cellular Uptake

The tissue distribution and disposition of CH_3—G have been studied in mice, rats, dogs, and monkeys (OLIVERIO et al., 1963) using compound labeled with ^{14}C in both guanyl groups (OLIVERIO and DENHAM, 1963). In mice and rats radioactivity was present in all tissues within two hours after parenteral injection, but was mostly in the liver, salivary glands, gonads, and seminal vesicles. In the liver, radioactivity was greater and lasted longer in rats than in mice, consistent with the greater hepatotoxicity seen in rats. The drug was excreted primarily in urine after parenteral injection, and in feces after oral administration. No significant biliary excretion was noted. Urinary excretion was most rapid in mice, where 70% of the label was recovered in 48 h, and, in decreasing order, it was less rapid in rats, monkeys, and dogs. In all species studied urinary radioactivity represented unchanged CH_3—G. In mice the CO_2 expired within 24 h contained less than 0.01% of the radioactivity injected, consistent with a lack of demonstrable drug biotransformation. In man, within 3 weeks from a single intravenous infusion, about 60% of the label was recovered in urine as the intact compound, whereas only 20% was in feces. After oral administration most of the radioactivity was found in feces, further demonstrating limited drug absorption by this route. Also, in man no radioactivity was found in expired CO_2 (OLIVERIO and ZUBROD, 1965). The rate of CH_3—G elimination in man was closer to that occurring in dogs than to that in rodents.

The cellular uptake of ^{14}C-labeled CH_3—G has been studied *in vitro* using various types of mammalian and amphibian cells (BLOCK et al., 1964; FIELD et al., 1964; DAVE et al., 1971c) and in rodents bearing sensitive or resistant L1210 leukemic cells (ADAMSON et al., 1966; DAVE et al., 1971c). The studies by DAVE and his coworkers have been carried out with CH_3—G labeled in two of the three carbons of the methylglyoxal moiety (ZAKRZEWSKI, personal communication).

In vitro, the drug accumulated in cells against a concentration gradient in normal and leukemic human leukocytes, rabbit reticulocytes, frog and skate erythrocytes, and mouse leukemia L1210. The accumulation was greatest in HeLa cells. The drug was not concentrated in human and rabbit erythrocytes. The differences between mammalian erythrocytes and reticulocytes, and those between mammalian erythrocytes and nucleated amphibian erythrocytes, may reflect metabolic differences related to the presence and/or functions of nucleic acids. As mentioned below, CH_3—G was found to bind to DNA of Sarcoma 180 ascites cells (SARTORELLI et al., 1965).

The accumulation of CH_3—G in nucleated cells seemed to be energy-dependent, since it was reduced at 4° and it was impaired at 37° by iodoacetate and *p*-aminomercurichlorobenzoate, as measured after 1 to 5 h of incubation (FIELD et al., 1964). Other metabolic inhibitors, however, such as sodium fluoride, dinitrophenol, and potassium cyanide, had variable and inconsistent effects. More recently the kinetics of initial uptake of CH_3—G by L1210 cells were shown to satisfy the criteria for a saturable facilitated diffusion process with a K_m of 40 nmoles/ml and V_{max} of 4 *p*moles/mg cell/min (DAVE et al., 1971c) and with a Q_{10} of 2.4; the rate of uptake at 37° was not significantly affected by *p*-aminomercurichlorobenzoate during the first 60 min of incubation, but was markedly reduced afterwards (DAVE and CABALLES, 1973). Spermidine competitively prevented CH_3—G uptake by human CML cells (FIELD et al., 1964) and mouse L1210 cells (DAVE and CABALLES, 1973). In the human cells, closely related CH_3—G analogs, such as ethylglyoxal-*bis*(guanylhydrazone) and dimethylglyoxal-*bis*(guanylhydrazone), were as effective as unlabeled CH_3—G in reducing the uptake of the labeled compound. Ethylglyoxal-*bis*(guanylhydrazone) itself was taken up by L1210 cells at a rate one-third that of CH_3—G (ADAMSON et al., 1966). The most effective inhibitors of CH_3—G uptake were 1,4-dialdehydobenzene-*bis*(guanylhydrazone) and two related analogs (FIELD et al., 1964). Derivatives, such as dimethylglyoxal-*bis*(guanylhydrazone), which are chemotherapeutically inactive and prevent the antileukemic effects of CH_3—G (MIHICH, 1955), may inhibit primarily the uptake of CH_3—G; others, such as 1,4-dialdehydobenzene-*bis*(guanylhydrazone), which have some activity against the L1210 leukemia (MIHICH, 1967b), may also compete for intracellular sites of action.

The uptake of CH_3—G by human leukemic cells increased when the pH of the incubation medium decreased from 8.0 to 6.5 (BLOCK et al., 1964). Since the pKa of the guanylhydrazonyl groups of CH_3—G is about 7.9, the drug seems to be taken up or bound in ionized form.

Loss of CH_3—G from human leukemic cells occurred after 2 to 3 h of incubation without any evidence of cellular damage. A concurrent loss of other gradients may be related to this effect. In fact, increases in extracellular potassium from 0 to 150 mmoles per liter greatly decreased the ratio of intracellular to extracellular drug concentration after 90 min incubation at 37° (BLOCK et al., 1964).

In mice both increased loss of drug and reduced uptake have been implicated as possible bases for resistance to CH_3—G in different lines of L1210 leukemia grown subcutaneously (Adamson et al., 1966). Intracellular drug distribution was similar in sensitive and resistant leukemia, however. Drug levels were greatest in the nuclear fraction (600 × g), followed, in decreasing order, by those in the supernatant fraction (72000 × g), mitochondria (9000 × g), and microsomes (72000 × g, sediment).

The relative importance of cellular transport versus intracellular binding to receptors in determining antileukemic action among aliphatic *bis*(guanylhydrazones) is not known. The structural alterations which modify the effects of CH_3—G may do so by affecting the influx of the drug into cells, its intracellular binding, or its efflux. The lack of antileukemic action of some close analogs of CH_3—G cannot be readily explained by a lack of drug entry into cells because they exert synergism in combination with hydroxystilbamidine (see below).

III. Therapeutic Effects in Man

The early clinical studies of CH_3—G have been carried out primarily at Roswell Park Memorial Institute (Regelson and Holland, 1961) and at the United States National Cancer Institute (Freireich et al., 1962). The overall results obtained by these two groups in more than 150 patients (Regelson and Holland, 1963; Levin et al., 1965) have shown that CH_3—G has definite activity in acute myelocytic leukemia and malignant lymphomas, albeit at the cost of severe toxicity. These findings were confirmed repeatedly (Mathé et al., 1964; Boiron et al., 1965; Weil et al., 1969; see also Mihich, 1965).

Among 83 patients with acute myelocytic leukemia (Levin et al., 1965), complete bone marrow remission was obtained in 1 of 12 subjects given daily intravenous doses of less than 100 mg/m² for a median duration of 30 days, in 4 of 23 patients given 100 to 125 mg/m² for 38 days, in 14 of 36 patients given 126 to 160 mg/m² for 28 days, and in only 1 of 12 patients given 160 to 300 mg/m² for 18 days. Of the 20 patients who underwent complete bone marrow remission, 18 also developed clinical remission; all of these had received an average daily dose of 150 mg/m² of CH_3—G. Marrow remission occurred within 13 to 70 days, with a median of 29 days. It became apparent that the doses causing the greatest incidence of remissions were more toxic than the minimum active ones, and that moderate increases beyond optimal daily doses led to greater toxicity and lower incidence of remissions.

In various reports (see Mihich, 1965) the incidence of bone marrow remission varied, ranging from 69 to 7%. This variation was attributed to differences in patient selection and supportive care. Thus, a three to five fold greater incidence of remission occurred in patients with acute myelocytic leukemia having Auer rods or granulation in their marrow leukemic cells than in the rest of the cases. Because of the narrow range of safety of CH_3—G, supportive care may permit the establishment of more effective regimens.

Abnormal cells in the bone marrow disappeared more rapidly with CH_3—G than with 6-mercaptopurine (Levin et al., 1963). With CH_3—G, but not with 6-mercaptopurine, prednisone, or antifolates, there was a dichotomy between early myeloid maturation and slow erythroid recovery.

The dramatic side effects of CH_3—G in man included gastrointestinal toxicity, marrow depression, hypoglycemia, intractable generalized infection, as well as laryngitis, cytomegalic disease, balanitis, bronchopneumonia, mucocutaneous lesions, vasculitis, and cardiac disturbances. Efforts were made to improve the range of safety of CH_3—G by varying doses and schedules, and by using the drug in combination with other agents. Initially, CH_3—G was studied in combination with 6-mercaptopurine, mostly in patients with acute myelocytic leukemia (LEVIN et al., 1965; BOIRON et al., 1965). BOIRON et al. (1965) gave CH_3—G intramuscularly or by intravenous infusion three times a week at doses of 250 or 350 mg/m^2, in combination with 6-mercaptopurine at 250 mg/m^2 intravenously twice a week, or 100 mg/m^2 orally every day. Complete remission was obtained in 33 % of the cases, with much less toxicity than previously noted. More recently (WEIL et al., 1969), the same doses and schedule of CH_3—G were given to 30 adults and 7 children, in quadruple combination with 6-mercaptopurine, 90 mg/m^2, and prednisone, 40 mg/m^2, both given daily orally, and with arabinosylcytosine, 30 mg/m^2, given intravenously either daily or 2 to 3 times a week. Eight adults and 5 children underwent complete remission, 11 for a median time of 5 months, and 2 (1 adult and 1 child) for more than 24 months. Gastrointestinal and mucocutaneous toxicity were moderate. These results indicate that the drug can be usefully employed in combination with other agents in the treatment of acute myelocytic leukemia.

Recently, CH_3—G was found to cause objective responses in 10 of 21 patients with advanced carcinoma of the esophagus, with clinical remissions in 8 of them (FALKSON, 1971). It seems possible that solid tumors originating from other tissues, such as the colon, may also be sensitive to appropriate treatments with the drug.

D. Mechanism of Action

Based on the data available, it would seem that CH_3—G interferes with nuclear and mitochondrial metabolism, and that many of its actions are related to the functions and/or metabolism of the physiological polyamines, particularly spermidine. The antiproliferative effects of the drug may have a different mechanism than cardiotoxicity, hepatotoxicity, and nephrotoxicity. In fact, in mammalian tissues, all, and only, the antiproliferative effects can be prevented by spermidine. Moreover, as mentioned earlier, the strict structural specificity of the CH_3—G molecule relates to antileukemic effects, and not to hepatotoxicity and hypoglycemia. Such specificity is not as strict for the trypanocidal action, which is the only "antiproliferative" effect that could not be prevented by spermidine and related polyamines.

I. Relationships to Spermidine

The effects of CH_3—G on L1210 leukemic cells were prevented by the concurrent administration of spermidine (MIHICH, 1963a, b), spermine, or putrescine (MIHICH, 1963b). Spermidine did not affect the antileukemic action of methotrexate, 6-mercaptopurine, decamethylene-*bis*(guanidine) (MIHICH, 1963b), pentanedial-*bis*(guanylhydrazone), 1,4-dialdehydobenzene-*bis*(guanylhydrazone), hydroxystilbamidine, or DDUG (MIHICH, 1967a). The immunosuppressive effects of CH_3—G in mice were also prevented by spermidine (MIHICH, 1964), as were gastrointestinal toxicity and bone marrow depression in dogs (MIHICH, 1963b, 1965).

The results of x-ray and neutron diffraction studies (HAMILTON and LAPLACA, 1968) are compatible with a structural similarity between CH_3—G and spermidine. At least two types of interaction between these two compounds are indicated by the data available, namely competition for a common transport carrier and intracellular site of binding (FIELD et al., 1964; BLOCK et al., 1964; DAVE and CABALLES, 1973) and inhibition of spermidine synthesis by the drug (WILLIAMS-ASHMAN and SCHENONE, 1972; CORTI et al., 1973, 1974).

It is unlikely that competition between CH_3—G and spermidine for uptake is the only basis for the prevention of drug action by the polyamine, because this would imply either that drug transport is different in proliferating and nonproliferating cells, or that the concentration of drug sufficient to cause an effect is much smaller in resting than in dividing cells. A competition at an intracellular site might imply that CH_3—G interferes with the role of polyamines in dividing cells. Both putrescine and spermidine levels increase in liver after partial hepatectomy (RAINA et al., 1966; RUSSELL et al., 1970), in developing embryos (CALDARERA et al., 1965; RUSSELL et al., 1969), and in leukemia L1210 (RUSSELL and LEVY, 1971). By binding to polynucleotides and nucleic acids (NEWTON, 1970), polyamines may exert diversified effects in various cell types and under different conditions (TABOR and TABOR, 1964). Thus, while spermine stimulated DNA polymerase in isolated nuclei of *Physarum polycephalum* (BREWER and RUSCH, 1946), it inhibited partially purified DNA polymerase in the presence of a primer of native DNA (O'BRIEN et al., 1960). Glyoxal-*bis*(guanylhydrazone) stimulated nucleohistone-primed DNA polymerase activity in pea embryo (SCHWIMMER, 1968). It is obvious that a possible interference by CH_3—G with polyamine function deserves investigation.

The inhibition of spermidine synthesis by CH_3—G in a cellfree system was reported recently (WILLIAMS-ASHMAN and SCHENONE, 1972). The putrescine-activated *S*-adenosylmethionine decarboxylase of rat ventral prostate, liver, and baker's yeast was markedly inhibited by CH_3—G, 50% inhibitory concentrations being as low as 0.0015 mM. This enzyme catalyzes a key reaction in the biosynthesis of spermidine and spermine (COHEN, 1971). The magnesium ion-activated *S*-adenosylmethionine decarboxylase of *E. coli*, which is insensitive to putrescine, was affected by CH_3—G only at very high concentrations (0.1 to 1.0 mM). The activities of ornithine decarboxylase, spermidine synthase, and spermine synthase were not inhibited, thus indicating specificity of drug effect (WILLIAMS-ASHMAN et al., 1973). Aminoguanidine had no inhibitory effect at 1 mM. Inactive also were the CH_3—G derivatives methylated on the terminal nitrogen of the two guanylhydrazonyl moieties, as well as propanedial- and pentanedial-*bis*(guanylhydrazone). In contrast, ethylglyoxal-*bis*(guanylhydrazone) and dimethylglyoxal-*bis*(guanylhydrazone) were inhibitory (CORTI et al., 1974). These compounds are not active against leukemia L1210, and inhibit CH_3—G uptake (see above).

Following the initial observations by WILLIAMS-ASHMAN and SCHENONE (1972), the inhibition of S-adenosylmethionine decarboxylase activity by CH_3—G has been confirmed with enzyme preparations from rat liver and kidney (PEGG, 1973), plant lectin-stimulated lymphocytes (FILLINGAME and MORRIS, 1973a; KAY and PEGG, 1973), and mouse leukemia L1210 cells (CORTI et al., 1973; HEBY and RUSSELL, 1973). The S-adenosylmethionine decarboxylase from *Physarum polycephalum*, which does not require amine or metal cofactor, was also inhibited by the drug (MITCHELL and RUSCH, 1973).

In lymphocytes from bovine lymph nodes stimulated with concanavalin A *in vitro*, CH_3—G inhibited the synthesis of spermidine and spermine with concurrent accumulation of putrescine (FILLINGAME and MORRIS, 1973a, b). It is of interest that no change was noted in the synthesis, processing, and accumulation of RNA in these cultures, nor in the specific activity of the ATP pool (FILLINGAME and MORRIS, 1973b). Essentially similar results were concurrently obtained using human lymphocytes stimulated with phytohemagglutinin in culture (KAY and PEGG, 1973). In rat liver and kidney, the incorporation of putrescine into spermidine was markedly inhibited 8 h after the i.p. injection of 80 mg/kg of CH_3-G (PEGG, 1973). This inhibition was no longer evident 20 h after drug administration; however, putrescine continued to accumulate during this period. Since, in stimulated lymphocytes (FILLINGAME and MORRIS, 1973a), in rat thymus and regenerating liver (HOLTTA et al., 1973), and in leukemia L1210 cells (HEBY et al., 1973), the activity of ornithine decarboxylase is also increased after exposure to CH_3-G, the increase in putrescine levels noted in most cell types (FILLINGAME and MORRIS, 1973a, b; HEBY and RUSSELL, 1973; HOLTTA et al., 1973; KAY and PEGG, 1973; PEGG, 1973) after treatment with the drug may be due to both an inhibition of putrescine utilization for spermidine synthesis and an increase in putrescine formation. It is of interest that in rat liver and thymus no significant decreases in spermidine and spermine levels could be seen after injection of single CH_3-G doses in the LD_{50} range (HOLTTA et al., 1973).

The early inhibition of putrescine stimulated S-adenosylmethionine decarboxylase in kidney, ventral prostate, and testis of rats treated with CH_3-G is followed in a few hours by a marked increase in the activity of this enzyme (PEGG et al., 1973). Similar results were obtained in concanavalin A stimulated bovine lymphocytes (FILLINGAME and MORRIS, 1973c), leukemia L1210 cells (HEBY et al., 1973), and rat regenerating liver and thymus (HOLTTA et al., 1973). In the rat and bovine cells this increase was found to be related to a prolongation of the half-life of the enzyme, from 40–120 min to about 20 h (FILLINGAME and MORRIS, 1973c; HOLTTA et al., 1973; PEGG et al., 1973). It was postulated that this prolongation in half-life of the enzyme is related to a stabilization of the protein molecule occurring as a result of the binding of the drug (FILLINGAME and MORRIS, 1973c; HOLTTA et al., 1973; PEGG et al., 1973) in analogy with the methotrexate stabilization of dihydrofolate reductase against proteolytic inactivation observed by others (HAKALA and SUOLINNA, 1966; BERTINO et al., 1970; JACKSON and HUENNEKENS, 1973).

In studies of the nature of the inhibition of putrescine-activated S-adenosylmethionine decarboxylase by CH_3-G, it was found that the drug seems to act as a competitive inhibitor for S-adenosylmethionine (HOLTTA et al., 1973; CORTI et al., 1974) and as an uncompetitive inhibitor of putrescine (HOLTTA et al., 1973). Inhibition by the drug also depends on the nature of the aliphatic amine used as a stimulator of the rat prostate enzyme (CORTI et al., 1974). In rat thymus the drug also inhibited diamine oxidase (EC 1.4.3.6) and in this system CH_3-G was a noncompetitive inhibitor with respect to putrescine (HOLTTA et al., 1973).

The effects of CH_3-G were further studied in mice, in attempts to clarify the possible role of the drug-induced inhibition of polyamine metabolism in the antileukemic effects of the drug (MIHICH et al., 1973, 1974; CORTI et al., 1974). A marked inhibition of the activity of putrescine activated S-adenosylmethionine decarboxylase was caused by CH_3-G in crude extracts from heart, kidney, spleen, salivary glands, thymus, brain, and from L1210, as well as L1210/CH_3-G cells (CORTI et al., 1974). In intact leukemic cells, and in mouse liver, salivary gland, and spleen (MIHICH et al., 1974), the drug did not cause any change in spermidine levels after a single administration of a therapeutic dose (50 mg/kg), in analogy with the results obtained in rat liver and thymus (HOLTTA et al., 1973). After five repeated doses, however, a 70% decrease in the spermidine level occurred in L1210 cells but not in L1210/CH_3-G cells (MIHICH et al., 1974). These findings, and those of DAVE and CABALLES (1973), indicating a reduced uptake and retention of

CH_3-G in L1210/CH_3-G cells, suggest that resistance to the drug is related to reduced drug uptake rather than to a difference in target enzyme sensitivity. In view of the fact that the levels of spermidine are reduced in L1210 cells after treatment with therapeutic drug regimes, the question still needs to be answered as to whether the antiproliferative effects of CH_3-G are related to an interference with polyamine metabolism.

II. Relationships to Nucleic Acids

The possibility that CH_3-G interferes with nucleic acid metabolism was initially considered on the basis of the observation that thymidine reduces the antineoplastic effects of the drug on the L1210 leukemia (MIHICH, 1963a, 1965). In trypanosomes, the incorporation of labeled thymidine into DNA was selectively impaired by CH_3-G, and a marked inhibition of orotic decarboxylase by the drug was also observed (JAFFE, 1965). In mice, CH_3-G inhibited the incorporation of thymidine into DNA of Sarcoma 180 ascites cells by a maximum of 43 %, and that of orotic acid into RNA uracil by a maximum of 30 % (SARTORELLI et al., 1965). These effects occurred at 5 and 2 h, respectively. *In vitro*, the incorporation of thymidine into DNA of L1210 cells was inhibited by CH_3-G at 1 h, at drug concentrations about ten times greater than those required to obtain a comparable inhibition with DDUG within 10 min (DAVE et al., 1971c). Thus, in tumor cells CH_3-G was a relatively weak inhibitor of thymidine incorporation into DNA.

CH_3-G binds to DNA *in vitro* (SARTORELLI et al., 1965). Binding was reduced in the presence of magnesium ions, suggesting the existence of ionic bonds between drug and DNA. One molecule of CH_3-G was bound per 6 to 9 nucleotide residues. The drug also bound to heat denaturated DNA and deoxyribonucleosides. Interference by spermidine was not reported.

The DNA-dependent DNA polymerase reaction in a cellfree system was only moderately inhibited by CH_3-G (DAVE et al., 1971a). Glyoxal-*bis*(guanylhydrazone) did not interfere with pea embryo DNA-dependent DNA polymerase (SCHWIMMER, 1968). Although binding to DNA and inhibition of DNA polymerase may contribute to the mode of action of CH_3-G, these effects are relatively weak, especially if compared to those of DDUG (see below).

III. Relationships to Mitochondrial Functions

The hypoglycemic effects of CH_3-G and Synthalin are similar in many respects. Both compounds cause an initial hyperglycemic response, liver glycogen depletion, increase in blood lactic acid concurrently with delayed hypoglycemia, decreased glucose utilization for glycogen synthesis and prevention of the hyperglycemic responses to glucagon and epinephrine (MIHICH, 1963a). In view of these similarities, it was suggested that a site of action of CH_3-G might be related to oxidative phosphorylation.

In coupled mitochondria from rat liver, guanidine and alkyl guanidines inhibited energy transfer in oxidative phosphorylation (PRESSMAN, 1963), and this effect was also exhibited by CH_3-G (PRESSMAN, personal communication). In medium containing glucose, respiration of L1210 cells was inhibited by CH_3-G at concentrations much lower than those required to inhibit glycolysis and endogenous respiration (BURK et al., 1962). Respiration of L1210 cells was also inhibited in mice (PINE and DIPAOLO, 1966), while the Crabtree effect and anaerobic glycolysis were not affected. In bone marrow and peripheral blood leukocytes from normal and leukemic subjects, however, anaerobic glycolysis was moderately inhibited in the presence of 1 mg/ml of CH_3—G (KOLMEIER et al., 1966). In L1210 cells, acetate incorporation into lipids was inhibited selectively, and ATP levels were decreased by 42 % after 3 daily treatments with CH_3—G (PINE and DIPAOLO, 1966). It seems unlikely that these effects are the basis of the antileukemic action of the drug. Their relevance to toxicity in nonproliferating tissues requires exploration.

4,4'-Diacetyl-Diphenyl-Urea-*bis* (Guanylhydrazone) (DDUG) and Other Aromatic *bis* (Guanylhydrazones)

Against the L1210 leukemia, DDUG is the most potent *bis*(guanylhydrazone) found to date. No therapeutic effect was seen in the initial clinical study which was carried out in 21 patients with terminal neoplastic disease, including 5 with acute leukemia (HOLLAND, personal communication). While the drug still awaits conclusive evaluation in man, its therapeutic potential does not seem as promising as expected on the basis of the outstanding activity seen in animals. Antileukemic aromatic *bis*(guanylhydrazones) have pharmacological characteristics different from those of CH_3—G and related aliphatic analogs (see Table 1).

A. Effects on Experimental Tumors

I. Spectrum of Tumor Sensitivity

In mice, DDUG had marked activity against leukemias L1210, P288, P388, P1534JS and L5178Y, lymphoma AK_4, mastocytoma P815, Ehrlich ascites carcinoma and primary mammary tumors of the C3H and DBA/2Ha strain (MIHICH, 1966, 1967b; MARXER, 1967; GELZER et al., 1967; MIHICH and MULHERN, 1968; MIHICH and GELZER, 1968). In addition, DDUG was active against L1210 cells resistant to CH_3—G, arabinosylcytosine, or methotrexate, but not against an L1210 variant resistant to 2-chloro-4',4''-*bis*(2-imidazolin-2-yl)-terephthalanilide (MIHICH and MULHERN, 1968; MIHICH et al., 1970a). The compound had no effects against mouse Sarcoma 180, Adenocarcinoma 755, Adenocarcinoma EO771, solid Ehrlich carcinoma, and against rat uterus epithelioma T-8 Guerin, Flexner-Jobling carcinoma, Dunning leukemia R3323, and Walker carcinosarcoma 256 (MIHICH and GELZER, 1968).

Intraperitoneal six day treatments of DBA/2Ha-DD female mice bearing early L1210 leukemia caused 50 day cures in up to 40 % of the animals. The incidence of cures was lower in male mice. Similar treatments caused only prolongation of survival without cures in DBA/2J mice, or in DBA/2Ha DD mice with advanced leukemia. The effectiveness of delayed treatment could be increased by changes in drug schedules (MIHICH, 1967c). DDUG was effective by parenteral or oral routes against L1210 cells inoculated intraperitoneally or subcutaneously, but not against L1210 leukemia inoculated intracerebrally (MIHICH and MULHERN, 1968). The curative effects of DDUG in DBA/2 mice bearing leukemia L1210 were mediated by host defenses directed against the leukemia (MIHICH, 1969a). In fact, no cures occurred in preirradiated mice; the cured mice were resistant to reinoculation of 10^3 L1210 cells in the absence of drug treatment, and this state of resistance could be transferred from cured mice to mice previously not exposed to L1210 cells by the transfer of spleen cells or serum. In the absence of drug treatment, the immunological responses to leukemia L1210 are very inefficient, since 100 % of DBA/2 mice die after the inoculation of as few as 10 leukemic cells.

L 1210 leukemic cells resistant to DDUG developed in three transfer generations (MIHICH, 1967b). The resistant subline was sensitive to CH_3—G, Synthalin (MIHICH, 1967a), methotrexate and carcinostatin (MIHICH, unpublished data), but was resistant to 2-chloro-4′,4″-*bis*(2-imidazolin-2yl)-terephthalanilide (MIHICH and HAKALA, 1968) and to hydroxystilbamidine alone or in combination with pentanedial-*bis*(guanylhydrazone) (MIHICH and MULHERN, 1968), or with 1,4-dialdehydobenzene-*bis*(guanylhydrazone) (MIHICH, 1967b). In tissue culture, a subline of Sarcoma 180 resistant to DDUG was sensitive to CH_3—G, but resistant to a terephthalanilide (HAKALA, 1971). In this system, DDUG and vincristine were not cross-resistant.

The DDUG-resistant subline of the L1210 leukemia was more sensitive to arabinosylcytosine than the parent L1210 tumor in nonirradiated, but not in preirradiated DBA/2Ha-DD mice (MIHICH and KITANO, 1971). Thus, in a manner similar to the subline resistant to CH_3—G, this subline is also more immunogenic than leukemia L1210 in the DBA/2 mouse.

II. Structure-Activity Relationships

Among analogs closely related to DDUG, four (MARXER and GELZER, 1967) have been tested against leukemia L1210 in mice (MIHICH and HAKALA, 1968) and six on TA3 mammary carcinoma cells in tissue culture (KORYTNYK, et al., 1973).

V $H_2N-C(=NH)-NH-N=C(CH_3)-C_6H_4-NH-C(=O)-NH-C_6H_4-C(CH_3)=N-NH-C(=NH)-NH_2$

VI $H_2N-C(=NH)-NH-N=CH-C_6H_4-C_6H_4-CH=N-NH-C(=NH)-NH_2$

VII $H_2N-C(=NH)-NH-N=CH-C_6H_4-CH=N-NH-C(=NH)-NH_2$

VIII $H_2N-C(=NH)-NH-N=C_6H_4=N-NH-C(=NH)-NH_2$

IX $H_2N-C(=NH)-C_6H_4-CH=CH-C_6H_3(OH)-C(=NH)-NH_2$

X $(H_2C-N)(H_2C-NH)C-C_6H_4-NH-C(=O)-C_6H_3(Cl)-C(=O)-NH-C_6H_4-C(N-CH_2)(NH-CH_2)$

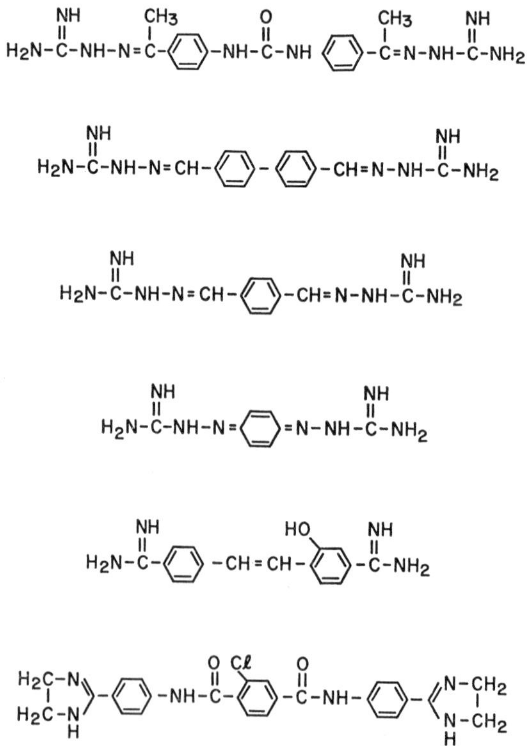

Fig. 2. Chemical structure of DDUG (V), 4,4′-diphenyl-*bis*(guanylhydrazone) (VI), 1,4-dialdehydobenzene-*bis*(guanylhydrazone) (VII), *p*-benzoquinone-*bis*(guanylhydrazone) (VIII), hydroxystilbamidine (IX), and 2-chloro-4′,4″-*bis*(2-imidazolin-2yl)-terephthalanilide (X)

Six compounds modified in the urea moiety were less effective than DDUG; the thiourea and the guanidine derivatives were more toxic than DDUG, but less effective on the L1210 tumor; whereas, compounds with one or both urea nitrogens methylated, or with a methylene group separating one or both urea nitrogens from the corresponding phenyl ring, were 10 to 100-times less active than DDUG in tissue culture. Diphenyl-urea-*bis*(guanylhydrazone) and 3,3'-diacetyldiphenyl-urea-*bis*(guanylhydrazone) were both about one-half as effective and more toxic than DDUG in mice with leukemia L1210. Two pyridine derivatives, where in one or both rings a nitrogen substitutes for a carbon atom in the ortho-position with respect to the urea moiety, were both as active as DDUG in tissue culture. The structural requirements for antiproliferative action seem relatively less strict for DDUG than for the CH_3—G molecule.

Several diphenyl-*bis*(guanylhydrazone) derivatives had antibacterial activity (CAVALLINI et al., 1961). Of the three analogs tested against leukemia L1210, the 4,4'-diphenylether and the 4,4'-diphenylsulfone derivatives were inactive (MIHICH, unpublished data), whereas the 4,4'-diphenyl analog had some activity (MIHICH, 1967a). This latter compound also caused hepatotoxicity and hypoglycemia in rats.

p-Benzoquinone-*bis*(guanylhydrazone), 2-methyl-*p*-benzoquinone-*bis*(guanylhydrazone), 1,4-dialdehydobenzene-*bis*(guanylhydrazone), and 1,4-diacetylbenzene-*bis*(guanylhydrazone) showed some activity against leukemia L1210, the 1,4-dialdehydobenzene derivative being the most active (MIHICH, 1967a). The benzene, but not the benzoquinone, derivatives had synergistic antileukemic effects in combination with hydroxystilbamidine (MIHICH, 1967a, b).

Of 14 aromatic monoguanylhydrazone analogs of the diphenyl and benzyl series tested in this laboratory, none had antileukemic effects. Several monoguanylhydrazone derivatives of polyhalo-substituted benzophenones were effective against *Plasmodium berghei* in mice (DOAMAREL et al., 1971).

III. Combination Treatments

Treatments with DDUG and arabinosylcytosine in combination were therapeutically synergistic against leukemia L1210 in DBA/2 mice and also caused 50 day cures of DBA/2J mice and of DBA/2Ha-DD mice with advanced leukemia (MIHICH and MULHERN, 1968). The two drugs had only additive effects, however, in preirradiated mice (MIHICH, unpublished data) and in cultures of L1210 cells (GRINDEY, personal communication). In contrast, the therapeutic synergism between DDUG and CH_3—G against leukemia L1210 (MIHICH and HAKALA, 1968) was confirmed in preirradiated mice (MIHICH, unpublished data) and in Sarcoma 180 cultures (HAKALA, 1971). In this system DDUG had additive effects in combination with 2-chloro-4',4''-*bis*(2-imidazolin-2-yl)-terephthalanilide. Against the L1210 leukemia, DDUG was not synergistic in combination with pentanedial-*bis*(guanylhydrazone), 6-mercaptopurine, or methotrexate. In non-irradiated mice, more than additive effects were seen in combination with Synthalin (MIHICH, unpublished data).

Hydroxystilbamidine had synergistic effects in combination with CH_3—G against leukemias P815 (BURCHENAL et al., 1963) and L1210 (MIHICH, 1965). Combinations of hydroxystilbamidine with other *bis*(guanylhydrazones) are of particular interest because they provide examples of marked therapeutic synergism between compounds which are only moderately or very slightly active when given alone (MIHICH, 1967a, b). Therapeutic synergism was seen with DDUG in admixture with pentanedial-*bis*(guanylhydrazone), 1,4-dialdehydrobenzene-*bis*(guanylhydrazone) or 1,4-diacetylbenzene-*bis*(guanylhydrazone). These synergisms were not evaluated in preirradiated mice or in tissue culture. Hydroxystilbamidine in combination with pentanedial-*bis*(guanylhydrazone) was also active against L1210 cells resistant to CH_3—G, but not against an L1210 variant resistant to DDUG (MIHICH and MULHERN, 1968) or to 2-chloro-4′,4″-*bis*(2-imidazolin-2-yl)-terephthalanilide (MIHICH et al., 1970a).

No prevention of antileukemic effects by spermidine was seen with DDUG, hydroxystilbamidine in combination with the *bis*(guanylhydrazones) tested other than CH_3—G, or Synthalin (MIHICH, 1967a).

B. Pharmacological Studies

I. Toxicological Effects

The toxicological effects of DDUG were studied in mice, rats, rabbits, dogs, and monkeys (MIHICH et al., 1969a). In each species acute lethal doses caused rapid paralysis and apnea. Toxicity occurred at the site of injection. The drug was inactive by the oral route, and was not readily absorbed by the intraperitoneal route. Hepatotoxicity, pulmonary edema, and lymphoid depression occurred in rats, dogs and monkeys. In rats, hypoglycemia was demonstrated only terminally, after repeated treatments. Bone marrow depression was minor and infrequent.

Because of the acute effects seen in animals, the drug was given to man by 1 h intravenous infusions (SENN and HOLLAND, personal communication). Nausea and vomiting occurred in 10 patients given 60 to 200 mg/m² of DDUG and in 3 of 6 patients given 20 to 40 mg/m². The diarrhea observed in 3 of the 10 patients treated with the larger doses was much milder than that caused by CH_3—G. Changes in serum glutamate oxalacetate transaminase (SGOT), serum alkaline phosphatase, or bromsulfophthalein (BSP) indicative of hepatotoxicity were seen in 16 cases, being marked and concurrent in 6 of the 10 patients treated with the larger doses. Neurological symptoms were observed in 3 patients at doses of 120 to 150 mg/m². Myelosuppression was minor.

II. Disposition and Cellular Uptake

In mice, rats, and dogs, DDUG, uniformly labeled with ^{14}C in the phenyl rings, accumulated primarily in liver and kidney after intravenous injection; in rodents radioactivity was also great in the intestines, salivary glands, and lungs (MIHICH et al., 1969b). Retention of radioactivity in these organs was long, more than 50% being present 11 to 21 days after treatment. In all three species no radioactivity could be detected in the blood 4 to 5 h after administration and more was found in the bile than in the urine within 15 to 60 min; in rats, 70% of radioactivity from DDUG was recovered in the feces and only 9% in the urine within 50 days. No detectable $^{14}CO_2$ was expired within 30 h. Liver extracts from treated rats contained ^{14}C—DDUG as the only radioactive compound detectable by thin-layer chromatography. No evidence for DDUG biotransformation was found in either sensitive or resistant L1210 cells (DAVE et al., 1970; DAVE and MIHICH, 1972). In 5 patients, patterns of DDUG disposition were similar to those found in animals (MIHICH et al., 1969b).

The cellular uptake and intracellular distribution of DDUG were studied using Sarcoma 180 cells in culture (HAKALA, 1970, 1971) and P815 (GELZER et al., 1967) or L1210 cells (DAVE et al., 1970; DAVE and MIHICH, 1972) *in vitro* and in mice. DDUG was taken up by first order passive diffusion and was accumulated against an apparent concentration gradient as a consequence of firm binding, primarily to nuclei and mitochondrial fractions. In the L1210 cells, the rate of uptake was similar to the rate of binding to intracellular organelles. Uptake was reduced by about 30 to 50% in drug resistant cells. In Sarcoma 180 cells, the uptake of DDUG was inhibited by 2-chloro-4,4''-*bis*(2-imidazolin-2-yl)-terephthalanilide and by Janus Green, both of which bind to lipoproteins. The partition of DDUG between methanol-water and chloroform-water phases in the presence of various phospholipids was consistent with the concept that the drug may be attracted by negatively charged phosphate residues in phospholipids, unless these are shielded or neutralized by positively charged choline (HAKALA, 1971). The competition between DDUG and the terephthalanilide conceivably could occur at sites of binding to lipid moieties. Alterations in such binding sites might be responsible for resistance (HAKALA, 1971).

Treatment of DDUG-sensitive Sarcoma 180 cells with neuraminidase or ribonuclease decreased sensitivity to growth inhibition by DDUG (WEISS and HAKALA, 1971). This change might reflect a decrease in initial drug binding to the cell surface, possibly due to reduced ionic attraction, and consequent reduced cellular uptake. Indeed in L1210 cells, the actual uptake of drug was preceded by a rapid phase of adsorption to the cell surface (DAVE and MIHICH, 1972).

C. Mechanism of Action

The incorporation of both thymidine and formate into the DNA of L1210 cells was inhibited by DDUG to a comparable extent (SOUČEK et al., 1970; DAVE et al., 1971a), as was the incorporation of phenylalanine into protein (SOUČEK et al., 1970). These effects occurred within one hour after exposure of neoplastic cells to DDUG and were followed by inhibition of uridine incorporation into RNA (SOUČEK et al., 1970). DDUG decreased the incorporation of thymidine into nucleotides in leukemia L1210 cells, but had no effect on thymidine kinase or thymidine triphosphate phosphorylase from these cells (DAVE et al., 1973). The drug also had no significant effect on precursor incorporation in DDUG-resistant L1210 cells (SOUČEK et al., 1970).

The DNA-dependent DNA polymerase reaction in a cell-free system with enzyme from drug-sensitive or -resistant L1210 cells was equally inhibited by DDUG (SOUČEK et al., 1970). This inhibition was strictly dependent on the DDUG-DNA ratio and was not reversed by the addition of enzyme or excess Mg^{++} (DAVE et al., 1971a). A 50% inhibition was seen at a molar ratio of DDUG to DNA phosphorus of 1 to 10 (DAVE et al., 1971b, 1972). Spectral studies indicated that two types of interactions occur between drug and DNA. One caused a hypochromic shift and occurred when the ratio of DDUG to DNA phosphorus was varied from 40:1 to 1:1. This shift also occurred with excess citrate in the absence of DNA and thus may correspond to an ionic interaction. A hyperchromic shift occurred when the drug to DNA phosphorus ratio varied from 1:1 to 1:2. Since this shift was ion-insensitive and urea-sensitive, it may correspond to a "nonionic" interaction. With RNA, only the "ionic" interaction occurred. It should be noted that 3,3'-dimethyl-4,4'-diacetyldiphenyl-*bis*(guanylhydrazone), a compound with digitalis-like action (WOLLERT, 1969), also binds through "ionic" interactions to yeast RNA (REICHERT and WOLLERT, 1971). 4,4'-Diacetyldiphenylurea did not interact with DNA, whereas its monoguanylhydrazone derivative showed evidence only for "ionic" interactions (DAVE et al., 1971b, 1972). Aromatic diamidines also bind to nucleic acids (NEWTON, 1970).

Binding of DDUG to DNA may be responsible for the antiproliferative actions of the drug. It explains the observed inhibition of DNA polymerase. This inhibition occurs at drug concentrations comparable to those interfering with precursor incorporation into DNA in whole cells and to those required for antileukemic action in mice. Since incorporation of precursors into DNA is not inhibited in resistant L1210 cells, this inhibition seems relevant to drug action. Furthermore, since the rate of DDUG uptake and binding to nuclei is less in DDUG-resistant cells than in susceptible cells, and DNA polymerase reactions with enzyme from either sensitive or resistant cells are equally susceptible to inhibition by the drug, the reduced inhibition of precursor incorporation into DNA of resistant cells seems related to reduced drug concentration at the site of action rather than to reduced sensitivity of target metabolic sites.

Table 1. *Some differences between* CH_3—G *and* DDUG

Parameter	CH_3—G	DDUG
L1210 i.p. or s.c.	Prolongation of survival	50-Day cures
Therapeutic index	Low	High
L1210 intracerebrally	Prolongation of survival	No effect
Advanced L1210 leukemia	Prolongation of survival	Prolongation of survival
Tumor spectrum in rodents	Leukemias and Sarcoma 180	Leukemias, Sarcoma 180, mammary carcinomas
CH_3-G or DDUG	Synergism, cross-sensitivity	Synergism, cross-sensitivity
Hydroxystilbamidine	Synergism, cross-sensitivity	Additive effect, cross-resistance
Spermidine	Antagonism	No effect
Terephthalanilide	Synergism, cross-sensitivity	Additive effect, cross-resistance
Gastrointestinal toxicity	Severe, prevented by spermidine	Minor, not affected by spermidine
Immunosuppression	Marked, prevented by spermidine	Minor, not affected by spermidine
Hypoglycemia and cardiotoxicity	Severe	Slight and inconsistent
Cellular uptake	Carrier mediated, prevented by spermidine	Passive diffusion, not affected by spermidine
Excretion	Urinary	Biliary
Inhibition of thymidine incorporation into DNA	Slight	Marked
Inhibition of DNA polymerase	Slight	Marked
Binding to DNA	Ion sensitive	Ion and urea sensitive
Structural specificity for inhibition of leukemia L1210	Extremely strict	Moderately strict
Clinical activity	Acute myelocytic leukemia, lymphoma, carcinoma of esophagus	Not seen

Conclusions

CH_3—G and DDUG are both quantitatively and qualitatively different from each other. Some of these differences are listed in Table 1. In DBA/2 mice bearing leukemia L1210 and treated shortly after tumor inoculation, the therapeutic index of DDUG is about 20 times greater than that of CH_3—G. This apparent advantage of DDUG over CH_3—G is not as clear in the treatment of advanced leukemia; moreover, against intracerebral leukemia L1210, CH_3—G is effective, whereas DDUG is not. Clinically, the antitumor action of CH_3—G is well established, whereas that of DDUG does not seem promising.

On the basis of studies of sensitivity, cross-resistance, synergisms, and antagonisms by spermidine, it would appear that DDUG, CH_3—G, and Synthalin are each chemotherapeutically different. Although it is not possible to propose unifying concepts on structural requirements for antileukemic action among aromatic *bis*-(guanylhydrazones), it is likely that DDUG, biphenyl-, and benzyl-derivatives, as well as hydroxystilbamidine, belong to the same general pharmacological group. Similarities with the terephthalanilides are apparent, especially in terms of cross-resistance, and have also been pointed out on the basis of physicochemical characteristics (CAIN et al., 1969).

While the clinical activity of DDUG needs to be conclusively evaluated and its limitations explained, the possibility seems real that new aromatic *bis*(guanylhydrazone) derivatives can be found with improved antileukemic activity. This possibility is more remote in the case of aliphatic analogs because in this case the structural specificity for antileukemic action seems exceptionally strict. The clinical activity of CH_3—G deserves further exploration, towards developing more effective combination treatments and schedules and identifying additional potentially sensitive tumor types. Studies on the mode of action of CH_3—G should be pursued further; the observed interactions with spermidine may be relevant to the antitumor action of the drug and may also provide an insight into the role of physiological polyamines in cell proliferation.

References

ADAMSON, R. H., DENHAM, C., OLIVERIO, V. T.: Studies of resistance to methylglyoxal-*bis*(guanylhydrazone) and its metabolic fate in tumor-bearing rodents. Arch. int. Pharmacodyn. **161**, 364—374 (1966).

BAIOCCHI, F., CHENG, C. C., HAGGERTY, W. J., JR., LEWIS, L. R., LIAO, T. K., NYBERG, W. H., O'BRIEN, D. E., PODREBARAC, E. G.: Studies on methylglyoxal-*bis*-(guanylhydrazone) analogs. II. Structural variations on methylglyoxal-*bis*(guanylhydrazone). J. med. Chem. **6**, 431—435 (1963).

BENNETT, L. L., JR.: Phthalanilides and some related dibasic and polybasic compounds: a review of biological activities and mode of action. Progr. exp. Tumor Res. (Basel) **7**, 259—325 (1965).

BERTINO, J. R., CASHMORE, A. R., HILLCOAT, B. L.: "Induction" of dihydrofolate reductase: purification and properties of the "induced" human erythrocyte and leukocyte enzymes and normal bone marrow enzyme. Cancer Res. **30**, 2372—2378 (1970).

BLOCK, J. B., FIELD, M., OLIVERIO, V. T.: Cellular accumulation of methylglyoxal-*bis*(guanylhydrazone) *in vitro*. II. Studies on the mechanism of accumulation in leukemic leukocytes. Cancer Res. **24**, 1947—1951 (1964).

BOIRON, M., JACQUILLAT, C., WEIL, M., BERNARD, J.: Combination of methylglyoxal-*bis*(guanylhydrazone) (NSC 32946) and 6-mercaptopurine (NSC 755) in acute granulocytic leukemia. Cancer Chemother. Rep. **45**, 69—73 (1965).

BREWER, E. N., RUSCH, H. P.: Control of DNA replication: effect of spermine on DNA polymerase activity in nuclei isolated from *Physarum polycephalum*. Biochem. biophys. Res. Commun. **25**, 579—584 (1966).

BURCHENAL, J. H., PURPLE, J. R., BUCHOLZ, E., STRAUB, P. W.: Potentiation of methylglyoxal-*bis*(guanylhydrazone) by stilbamidine in transplanted mouse leukemias. Cancer Chemother. Rep. **29**, 85—89 (1963).

BURK, D., EVANS, W., HUNTER, J., WOODS, M.: Primary inhibition of respiration by methylglyoxal-*bis*(guanylhydrazone) in L1210 leukemia and other cells with implications for multiple chemotherapy. Proc. Amer. Ass. Cancer Res. **3**, 308 (1962).

CAIN, B. F., ATWELL, G. J., SEELYE, R. N.: Potential Antitumor Agents. X. *Bis*-quaternary salts. J. med. Chem. **12**, 199—206 (1969).

CALDARERA, C. M., BARBIROLI, B., MORUZZI, G.: Polyamines and nucleic acids during development of the chick embryo. Biochem. J. **97**, 84—88 (1965).

CAREY, T., MAWAS, C., KITANO, M., MIHICH, E.: Cytotoxic antibody against leukemia L1210 in DBA/2Ha-DD mice. Proc. Amer. Ass. Cancer Res. **13**, 91 (1972).

CAVALLINI, G., MASSARANI, E., NARDI, D., MAURI, L., MANTEGAZZA, P.: Antibacterial agents. Some new guanylhydrazone derivatives. J. med. pharm. Chem. **4**, 177—182 (1961).

Cohen, S.S.: Introduction to the polyamines. Englewood Cliffs, N.J.: Prentice Hall 1971.

Corti, A., Dave, C., Williams-Ashman, H.G., Mihich, E., Schenone, A.: Specific inhibition of the enzymic decarboxylation of S-adenosylmethionine by methylglyoxal-*bis*(guanylhydrazone) and related substances. Biochem. J. **139**, 351—357 (1974).

Corti, A., Schenone, A., Williams-Ashman, H.G., Dave, C., Mihich, E.: Inhibition of adenosylmethionine decarboxylases (AMEDC) by methylglyoxal-*bis*-(guanylhydrazone) (CH_3G) and its congeners. Fed. Proc. **32**, 512 (1973).

Dave, C., Caballes, L.: Studies on the uptake of methylglyoxal-*bis*-(guanylhydrazone) (CH_3G) and spermidine (Spd) in mouse leukemia L1210 sensitive and resistant to CH_3G (L1210/CH_3G). Fed. Proc. **32**, 736 (1973).

Dave, C., Ehrke, M.J., Mihich, E.: Mechanism of resistance to 4,4′-diacetyl-diphenyl-urea-*bis*-guanylhydrazone (DDUG) in leukemia L1210. Pharmacologist **12**, 302 (1970).

Dave, C., Ehrke, M.J., Mihich, E.: Inhibition of DNA replication in leukemia L1210 by 4,4′-diacetyldiphenylurea-*bis*(guanylhydrazone) (DDUG). Proc. Amer. Ass. Cancer Res. **12**, 40 (1971a).

Dave, C., Ehrke, J., Mihich, E.: Mechanism of inhibition of DNA biosynthesis in leukemia L1210 cells by 4,4′-diacetyl-diphenylurea-*bis*(guanylhydrazone). Cancer Res. **33**, 2129—2134 (1973).

Dave, C., Ehrke, J., Soucek, J., Mihich, E.: Molecular basis for the inhibition of DNA synthesis by 4,4′-diacetyl-diphenyl-urea-*bis*(guanylhydrazone) (DDUG), an agent with activity against experimental leukemia. Abstract B-1.4/12 Vol. II, VIIth Int. Congr. Chemother., Prague (1971b).

Dave, C., Ehrke, J., Soucek, J., Mihich, E.: Differences in the action of methylglyoxal-*bis*-(guanylhydrazone) (CH_3—G), 4,4′-diacetyl-diphenyl-urea-*bis*(guanylhydrazone) (DDUG) and related analogs. Fed. Proc. **30**, 628 (1971c).

Dave, C., Ehrke, J., Soucek, J., Mihich, E.: Molecular basis for the inhibition of DNA synthesis by 4,4′-diacetyl-diphenyl-urea-*bis*-guanylhydrazone, an agent with activity against experimental leukemia. In: Proc. 7th Intl. Congress of Chemotherapy, pp. 127—129. München: Urban and Schwarzenberg 1972.

Dave, C., Mihich, E.: Uptake and intracellular distribution of 4,4′-diacetyl-diphenyl-urea-*bis*(guanylhydrazone) in sensitive and resistant leukemia L1210 cells. Biochem. Pharmacol. **21**, 2681—2696 (1972).

Davidson, J.D., Engle, R.R., Mancuso, R.W.: Hydroxymethylglyoxal-*bis*(guanylhydrazone). Cancer Chemother. Rep. **31**, 3—6 (1963).

DoAmaral, J.R., French, F.A., Blanz, E.J., Jr., French, D.A.: Antimalarial activity of guanylhydrazone salt of aromatic ketones. 2. Development of active polyhalo derivatives. J. med. Chem. **14**, 862—866 (1971).

Duncan, L.J.P., Baird, J.D.: Compounds administered orally in the treatment of diabetes mellitus. Pharmacol. Rev. **12**, 91—158 (1960).

Falkson, G.: Methyl—GAG (NSC-32946) in the treatment of esophagus cancer. Cancer Chemother. Rep. **55**, 209—212 (1971).

Fastier, F.N.: Structure-activity relationships of amidine derivatives. Pharmacol. Rev. **14**, 37—90 (1962).

Ferrari, W., Loddo, B., Gessa, G.L., Spanedda, A., Brotzu, G.: *In vitro* antipolio activity of methylglyoxal-*bis*-(guanylhydrazone). Life Sci. **3**, 755—758 (1964).

Field, M., Block, J.B., Oliverio, V.T., Rall, D.P.: Cellular accumulation of methylglyoxal-*bis*(guanylhydrazone) *in vitro*. I. General characteristics of cellular uptake. Cancer Res. **24**, 1939—1946 (1964).

Fillingame, R.H., Morris, D.R.: Accumulation of polyamines and its inhibition by methyl glyoxal *bis*(guanylhydrazone) during lymphocyte transformation. In: Polyamines in normal and neoplastic growth, pp. 249—260 (Russell, D.H., Ed.). New York: Raven Press 1973a.

Fillingame, R.H., Morris, D.R.: Polyamine accumulation during lymphocyte transformation and its relation to the synthesis, processing, and accumulation of ribonucleic acid. Biochemistry **12**, 4479—4487 (1973b).

Fillingame, R.H., Morris, D.R.: S-Adenosyl-L-methionine decarboxylase during lymphocyte transformation: decreased degradation in the presence of a specific inhibitor. Biochem. biophys. Res. Commun. **52**, 1020—1025 (1973c).

Freedlander, B.L., French, F.A.: Carcinostatic action of polycarbonyl compounds and their derivatives. II. Glyoxal *bis* (guanylhydrazone) and derivatives. Cancer Res. **18**, 360—363 (1958).

FREIREICH, E. J., FREI, E., III, KARON, M.: Methylglyoxal-*bis*(guanylhydrazone) (Methyl—GAG), a new active agent against adult human leukemia. Cancer Chemother. Rep. **16**, 183—186 (1962).

FRENCH, F. A., BLANZ, E. J., JR.: Chemotherapy studies on experimental mouse tumors. IX. Cancer Chemother. Rep. **2**, 177—197 (1971).

GELZER, J., MARXER, A., SCHMID, K.: Studies on the cytostatic action of 4,4'-diacetyl-diphenyl-urea-*bis*-guanyl-hydrazone (DDUG or CIBA 32, 248 B-Ba). In: Proceedings 5th international congress of chemotherapy, Vol. 2, pp. 197—202 (SPITZY, K. H., HASCHEK, H., Eds.). Vienna: Wiener Medizinischen Akademie 1967.

GRINDEY, G. B., MIHICH, E., NICHOL, C. A.: Evaluation of combination chemotherapy *in vivo* and in culture using 1-β-D-arabinofuranosylcytosine and 1-formylisoquinoline thiosemicarbazone. Cancer Res. **32**, 522—526 (1972).

GRISWOLD, D. P., JR., LASTER, W. R., SNOW, M. Y., SCHABEL, F. M., JR., SKIPPER, H. E.: Experimental evaluation of potential anticancer agents. XII. Quantitative drug response of the SA180. CA755, and leukemia L1210 system to a "standard list" of "active" and "inactive" agents. Cancer Res. **23**, 271—521 (1963).

HAKALA, M. T.: Uptake and binding of 4,4'-diacetyl-diphenyl-urea-*bis*(guanylhydrazone) (DDUG) in sarcoma 180 cells *in vitro*. Proc. 6th int. congress chemotherapy, Tokyo, Vol. 2, pp. 185—189 (1970).

HAKALA, M. T.: Uptake and distribution of 4,4'-diacetyl-diphenyl-urea-*bis*-guanylhydrazone in sensitive and resistant sarcoma 180 cells *in vitro*. Biochem. Pharmacol. **20**, 81—95 (1971).

HAKALA, M. T., SUOLINNA, E-M. R.: Specific protection of folate reductase against chemical and proteolytic inactivation. Molecular Pharmacol. **2**, 465—480 (1966).

HAMILTON, W. C., LAPLACA, S. J.: The crystal and molecular structure of anti-leukemic drug: methylglyoxal bisguanylhydrazone dihydrochloride monohydrate, $C_5N_8H_{12} \cdot 2HCl \cdot H_2O$. Neutron and x-ray diffraction studies. Acta Cryst. **B24**, 1147—1156 (1968).

HEBY, O., RUSSELL, D. H.: Changes in polyamine metabolism in tumor cells and host tissues during tumor growth and after treatment with various anticancer agents. In: Polyamines in normal and neoplastic growth, pp. 221—237 (RUSSELL, D. H., Ed.). New York: Raven Press 1973.

HEBY, O., SAUTER, S., RUSSELL, D. H.: Stimulation of L-ornithine decarboxylase activity and inhibition of S-adenosyl-L-methionine decarboxylase activity in leukemic mice by methylglyoxal-*bis*(guanylhydrazone). Biochem. J. **136**, 1121—1124 (1973).

HERBST, E. J., BACHRACH, V. (Eds.): Metabolism and biological functions of polyamines. Ann. N.Y. Acad. Sci. **171**, 691—1009 (1970).

HERSH, E. M., CARBONE, P. P., WONG, V. G., FREIREICH, E. J.: Inhibition of the primary immune response in man by anti-metabolites. Cancer Res. **25**, 997—1001 (1965).

HOLLAND, J. F., BARDOS, T. J., BRYANT, B., MIHICH, E.: Relation of methylglyoxal-*bis*-guanylhydrazone to folic acid metabolism. Proc. Amer. Ass. Cancer Res. **3**, 330 (1962).

HOLLUNGER, G.: Guanidines and oxidative phosphorylations. Acta pharmacol. (Kbh.) **11**, 1—82 (1955).

HOLTTA, E., HANNONEN, P., PISPA, J., JANNE, J.: Effect of methylglyoxal *bis*(guanylhydrazone) on polyamine metabolism in normal and regenerating rat liver and rat thymus. Biochem. J. **136**, 669—676 (1973).

JACKSON, R. C., HUENNEKENS, F. M.: Turnover of dihydrofolate reductase in rapidly dividing cells. Arch. biochem. Biophys. **154**, 192—198 (1973).

JAFFE, J. J.: Trypanocidal activity of methylglyoxal-*bis*(guanylhydrazone) (CH_3—G) and congeners. Fed. Proc. **24**, 455 (1965).

KAY, J. E., PEGG, A. E.: Effect of inhibition of spermidine formation on protein and nucleic acid synthesis during lymphocyte activation. FEBS Letters **29**, 301—304 (1973).

KITANO, M., MIHICH, E., PRESSMAN, D.: Antigenic differences between leukemia L1210 and a subline resistant to methylglyoxal-*bis*-guanylhydrazone. Cancer Res. **32**, 181—186 (1972).

KLINE, I., GANG, M., TYRER, D. D., VENDITTI, J. M., ARTIS, E. W., GOLDIN, A.: Evaluation of antileukemic agents in advanced leukemia L1210 in mice. IX. Cancer Chemother. Rep. **2**, 65—133 (1971).

KOLMEIER, K. H., SILVERSTEIN, M. N., FLEISHER, G. A.: Anaerobic glycolysis in normal and leukemic bone marrow leukocytes: effect of methyl-glyoxal-*bis*-guanylhydrazone dihydrochloride. Cancer **19**, 1195—1199 (1966).

KORYTNYK, W., GHOSH, A. C., ANGELINO, N., DAVE, D.: Guanylhydrazones with potential antileukemic activity. 1. Aza analogs of 4,4'-diacetyl-diphenylurea-*bis*(guanylhydrazone). J. Med. Chem. **16**, 959—961 (1973).

LEVIN, R. H., BRITTIN, G. M., FREIREICH, E. J.: Different patterns of remissions in acute myelocytic leukemia. A comparison of the effects of methylglyoxal-*bis*-(guanylhydrazone) and 6-mercaptopurine. Blood **21**, 689—698 (1963).

LEVIN, R. H., HENDERSON, E., KARON, M., FREIREICH, E. J.: Treatment of acute leukemia with methylglyoxal-*bis*(guanylhydrazone) (Methyl—GAG). Clin. Pharmacol. Ther. **6**, 31—42 (1965).

LIAO, T. K., BAIOCCHI, F., CHENG, C. C.: Studies on methylglyoxal-*bis*(guanylhydrazone) analogs. IV. Acetylation studies. J. org. Chem. **30**, 560—562 (1965).

MARXER, A.: A new *bis*(guanylhydrazone) with antileukemic properties. Experientia (Basel) **23**, 173—174 (1967).

MARXER, A., GELZER, J.: Über ein neues *bis*-guanylhydrazon mit antileukämischer Wirkung. In: SPITZY, K. H., HARSCHEK, H. (Eds.): Proceedings of the 5th international congress of chemotherapy, Vol. 2, pp. 277—280. Vienna: Wiener Medizinischen Akademie 1967.

MATHÉ, G., SCHNEIDER, M., CATTAN, A., AMIEL, J. L., SCHWARTZENBERG, L.: Clinical trials with methylglyoxal-*bis*(guanylhydrazone) and with *N*-isopropyl-α-(2-methylhydrazino)*p*-toluamide in various leukemias and hematosarcomas. In: PLATTNER, P. A. (Ed.): Chemotherapy of cancer, pp. 204—214. Amsterdam: Elsevier 1964.

MIHICH, E.: Current studies with methylglyoxal-*bis*(guanylhydrazone). Cancer Res. **23**, 1375—1389 (1963a).

MIHICH, E.: Prevention of the antitumor activity of methylglyoxal-*bis*(guanylhydrazone) (CH_3—G) by spermidine. Pharmacologist **5**, 270 (1963b).

MIHICH, E.: Impairment of host defenses by methylglyoxal-*bis*(guanylhydrazone) (CH_3—G). Fed. Proc. **23**, 388 (1964).

MIHICH, E.: Methylglyoxal-*bis*(guanylhydrazone), an agent with activity in acute myelocytic leukemia and lymphomas. Arch. Ital. Patol. Clin. Tumori **8**, 153—206 (1965).

MIHICH, E.: Antileukemic action of *bis*(guanylhydrazone) derivatives. Proc. 9th int. cancer congress, Tokyo, p. 317 (1966).

MIHICH, E.: Recent studies with new antileukemic bis guanylhydrazones. Gann Monograph 2, 167—176 (1967a).

MIHICH, E.: Antileukemic action of new aromatic bisguanylhydrazone derivatives. Cancer **20**, 880—884 (1967b).

MIHICH, E.: Studies of the antileukemic action of 4,4′-diacetyl-diphenyl-urea-*bis*(guanylhydrazone) (DDUG). Pharmacologist **9**, 192 (1967c).

MIHICH, E.: Combined effects of chemotherapy and immunity against leukemia L1210 in DBA/2 mice. Cancer Res. **29**, 848—854 (1969a).

MIHICH, E.: Modification of tumor regression by immunologic means. Cancer Res. **29**, 2345—2350 (1969b).

MIHICH, E., BROSS, I., MIHICH, R. M., NICHOL, C. A.: A model system for detecting drug impairment of antitumor host defenses. Cancer Res. **30**, 1376—1383 (1970b).

MIHICH, E., DAVE, C., SOUČEK, J., MULHERN, A. I., EHRKE, M. J.: Comparative studies on the antileukemic action of 4,4′-diacetyl-diphenyl-urea-*bis*(guanylhydrazone and methylglyoxal-*bis*(guanylhydrazone). Proc. 6th intl. congress of chemotherapy, Tokyo, Vol. 2, pp. 190—192 (1970a).

MIHICH, E., DAVE, C., WILLIAMS-ASHMAN, H. G.: Antiproliferative actions of antileukemic agent, methylglyoxal-*bis*(guanylhydrazone) (CH_3—G): relationship to spermidine (Spd). Abstracts, 8th intl. congr. chemotherapy, Athens, B-184 (1973).

MIHICH, E., DAVE, C., WILLIAMS-ASHMAN, H. G.: Antiproliferative actions of the antileukemic agent, methylglyoxal-*bis*-guanylhydrazone (CH_3—G): relationships to spermidine (Spd.). Proc. 8th intl. congr. chemotherapy, Athens, in press.

MIHICH, E., GELZER, J.: Effects of 4,4′-diacetyl-diphenyl-urea-*bis*(guanylhydrazone) on a spectrum of mouse and rat tumors. Cancer Res. **28**, 553—558 (1968).

MIHICH, E., HAKALA, M. T.: Differences between the antitumor action of 4,4′-diacetyl-diphenyl-urea-*bis*-(guanylhydrazone) (DDUG) and methylglyoxal-*bis*(guanylhydrazone) (CH_3—G). Proc. Amer. Ass. Cancer Res. **9**, 48 (1968).

MIHICH, E., KITANO, M.: Differences in the immunogenicity of leukemia L1210 sublines in DBA/2 mice. Cancer Res. **31**, 1999—2003 (1971).

MIHICH, E., MULHERN, A. I.: Antileukemic effects of 4,4′-diacetyl-diphenyl-urea-*bis*(guanylhydrazone). Cancer Res. **28**, 354—362 (1968).

MIHICH, E., MULHERN, A. I., SENN, H., DAVE, C., AHRENS, H.: Studies on the disposition of 4,4′-diacetyl-diphenyl-urea-*bis*(guanylhydrazone) (DDUG) in animals and man. Proc. Amer. Ass. Cancer Res. **10**, 58 (1969b).

MIHICH, E., SIMPSON, C. L., LOTH, L., MULHERN, A. I.: Toxic and pathologic effects of 4,4'-diacetyl-diphenyl-urea-*bis*(guanylhydrazone), a new antileukemic agent. Cancer Res. **29**, 1056—1061 (1969a).

MIHICH, E., SIMPSON, C. L., MULHERN, A. I.: Pharmacology of methylglyoxal-*bis*(guanylhydrazone) (CH_3—G). 1. Toxic and pathologic effects. Cancer Res. **22**, 962—972 (1962).

MITCHELL, J. L. A., RUSCH, H. P.: Regulation of polyamine synthesis in *Physarum polycephalum* during growth and differentiation. Biochim. biophys. Acta **297**, 503—516 (1973).

MONTGOMERY, J. A.: On the chemotherapy of cancer. Progr. Drug Res. **8**, 431—507 (1965).

NEWTON, B. A.: Chemotherapeutic compounds affecting DNA structure and function. Adv. Pharmacol. Chemoth. **8**, 149—184 (1970).

O'BRIEN, R. L., OLENICK, J. G., HAHN, F. E.: Reactions of quinine, chloroquine and quinacrine with DNA and their effects on the DNA and RNA polymerase reactions. Proc. nat. Acad. Sci. (Wash.) **55**, 1511—1517 (1960).

OLIVERIO, V. T., ADAMSON, R. H., HENDERSON, E. S., DAVIDSON, J. D.: The distribution, excretion, and metabolism of methylglyoxal-*bis*(guanylhydrazone)-C^{14}. J. pharm. exp. Therap. **141**, 149—156 (1963).

OLIVERIO, V. T., DENHAM, C.: Synthesis of methylglyoxal-*bis*(guanylhydrazone)-C^{14}. J. pharm. Sci. **52**, 202—203 (1963).

OLIVERIO, V. T., ZUBROD, C. G.: Clinical pharmacology of the effective antitumor drugs. Ann. Rev. Pharmacol. **5**, 335—356 (1965).

PEGG, A. E.: Inhibition of spermidine formation in rat liver and kidney by methylglyoxal-*bis*-(guanylhydrazone). Biochem. J. **132**, 537—540 (1973).

PEGG, A. E., CORTI, A., WILLIAMS-ASHMAN, H. G.: Paradoxical enhancement of S-adenosylmethionine decarboxylase in rat tissues following administration of the specific inhibitor methyl glyoxal-*bis* (guanylhydrazone). Biochem. biophys. Res. Commun. **52**, 696—701 (1973).

PINE, M. J., DIPAOLO, J. A.: The antimitochondrial action of 2-chloro-4,4'-*bis*(2-imidazolin-2-yl) terephthalanilide and methylglyoxal *bis*(guanylhydrazone). Cancer Res. **26**, 18—25 (1966).

PODREBARAC, E. G., CHENG, C. C.: Studies on methylglyoxal-*bis*(guanylhydrazone) analogs. III. Trifluoromethylglyoxal-*bis*(guanylhydrazone) and 1,2-*bis*(guanidinoamino)-propane. J. med. Chem. **7**, 806—808 (1964).

PODREBARAC, E. G., NYBERG, W. H., FRENCH, F. A., CHENG, C. C.: Studies on methylglyoxal-*bis*(guanylhydrazone) analogs. I. Homologs of methylglyoxal-*bis*(guanylhydrazone). J. med. Chem. **6**, 283—288 (1963).

PRESSMAN, B. C.: The effects of guanidine and alkylguanidines on the energy transfer reactions of mitochondria. J. biol. Chem. **238**, 401—409 (1963).

RAINA, A., JANNE, J., SIIMES, M.: Stimulation of polyamine synthesis in relation to nucleic acids in regenerating rat liver. Biochim. biophys. Acta (Amst.) **123**, 197—201 (1966).

REGELSON, W., HOLLAND, J. F.: Initial clinical study of parenteral methylglyoxal-*bis*(guanylhydrazone) diacetate. Cancer Chemother. Rep. **11**, 81—86 (1961).

REGELSON, W., HOLLAND, J. F.: Clinical experience with methylglyoxal-*bis*(guanylhydrazone) HCL (methyl—GAG), a new agent with clinical activity in acute myelocytic leukemia and the lymphomas. Cancer Chemother. Rep. **27**, 15—26 (1963).

REICHERT, M., WOLLERT, U.: Über die Wechselwirkung herzwirksamer Substanzen mit Ribonucleinsäure. Naunyn-Schmiedebergs Arch. exp. Path. Pharmak. **268**, 148—160 (1971).

RUSSELL, D. H., LEVY, C. C.: Polyamine accumulation and biosynthesis in a mouse L1210 leukemia. Cancer Res. **31**, 248—251 (1971).

RUSSELL, D. H., MEDINA, V. J., SNYDER, S. H.: Presence and biosynthesis of putrescine and polyamines in amphibian embryos. Life Sci. **8**, 1247—1254 (1969).

RUSSELL, D. H., MEDINA, V. J., SNYDER, S. H.: Polyamine turnover in normal and regenerating rat liver and brain. J. biol. Chem. **245**, 6732—6738 (1970).

SARTORELLI, A. C., IANNOTTI, A. T., BOOTH, B. A., SCHNEIDER, F. H., BERTINO, J. R., JOHNS D. G.: Complex formation with DNA and inhibition of nucleic acid synthesis by methylglyoxal-*bis*(guanylhydrazone). Biochem. biophys. Acta (Amst.) **103**, 174—176 (1965).

SCHEPARTZ, S. A.: Screening. Cancer Chemother. Rep. **2**, 3—8 (1971).

SCHOENBACH, E. B., GREENSPAN, E. M.: The pharmacology, mode of action and therapeutic potentialities of stilbamidine, pentamidine, propamidine and other aromatic diamidines. A review. Medicine **27**, 327—377 (1948).

SCHWIMMER, S.: Differential effects of putrescine, cadaverine, and glyoxal-*bis*(guanylhydrazone) on DNA- and nucleohistone-supported DNA synthesis. Biochem. biophys. Acta (Amst.) **166**, 251—254 (1968).

SOUČEK, J., EHRKE, M. J., MIHICH, E.: Effects of 4,4'-diacetyldiphenylurea-*bis*(guanylhydrazone) on the incorporation of precursors into nucleic acid and protein of leukemia L1210. Cancer Res. **30**, 2187—2194 (1970).

Tabor, H., Tabor, C. W.: Spermidine, spermine and related amines. Pharmacol. Rev. **16**, 245—300 (1964).

Thiele, J., Dralle, E.: Zur Kenntnis des Amidoguanidins. I. Condensationsprodukte des Amidoguanidins mit Aldehyden und Ketonen der Fettreihe. Annalen der Chemie (Liebig) **302**, 275—299 (1898).

Weil, M., Jacquillat, C., Boiron, M., Bernard, J.: Combination of arabinosyl cytosine, methylglyoxal *bis*(guanylhydrazone), 6-mercaptopurine and prednisone in the treatment of acute myelocytic leukemia. Europ. J. Cancer **5**, 271—275 (1969).

Weiss, L., Hakala, M. T.: The anionic nature of sarcoma 180 cell surfaces and sensitivity to 4,4′-diacetyldiphenylurea-*bis*(guanylhydrazone). Cancer Res. **31**, 1369—1372 (1971).

Williams-Ashman, H. G., Coppoc, G. L., Schenone, A., Weber, G.: Aspects of polyamine biosynthesis in normal and malignant eukaryotic cells. In: Polyamines in normal and neoplastic growth, p. 188, (Russell, D. H., Ed.). New York: Raven Press 1973.

Williams-Ashman, H. G., Schenone, A.: Methyl-glyoxal-*bis*(guanylhydrazone) as a potent inhibitor of mammalian and yeast S-adenosylmethionine decarboxylases. Biochem. biophys. Res. Commun. **46**, 288—295 (1972).

Wollert, V. U.: Pharmakologische Eigenschaften von Mono- und *Bis*guanylhydrazonen. Arzneimittel-Forschung (Drug Res.) **19**, 680—683 (1969).

Chapter 72

Clinical and Pharmacologic Effects of Hydroxyurea

IRWIN H. KRAKOFF

Introduction

Hydroxyurea was synthesized more than 100 years ago. It is a simple compound structurally related to urea. In 1963 it was found to have activity against leukemia L1210 in mice (STEARNS et al., 1963) and clinical trials began that same year. It was found to produce responses in patients with chronic granulocytic leukemia (KRAKOFF et al., 1964), metastatic malignant melanoma (BLOEDOW, 1964) and, occasionally, other tumors. It has not gained a prominent place in cancer chemotherapy, since its activity is not unique and it does not appear to have a specific advantage over other agents used in the treatment of chronic granulocytic leukemia. Its effectiveness in other neoplastic diseases in man is inconsistent. By the use of hydroxyurea, it is possible to cause a very rapid fall in the peripheral leukocyte count of patients with chronic granulocytic leukemia; this is a distinct advantage in some patients in whom marked elevation of leukocyte count makes a rapid decrease desirable. In addition, when hydroxyurea administration is discontinued, the depressed leukocyte count rises very rapidly. This provides a measure of safety in relation to the possibility of serious myelosuppression. This property has also been exploited to provide a reservoir for granulocytes in programs in which granulocyte donors are needed. The withdrawal of hydroxyurea therapy from patients with chronic granulocytic leukemia results within a few days in the availability of large numbers of apparently functional granulocytes. The usual dose is 40 mg/kg daily by mouth.

Another clinical role for hydroxyurea is in the treatment of the nonneoplastic disease, psoriasis, a condition in which there is marked proliferation of the epidermis (YARBRO, 1969). Hydroxyurea has been effective at relatively low doses, causing no serious toxicity and apparently producing prolonged useful control of this disabling skin disease.

Fate and Distribution

Hydroxyurea is absorbed well from the gastrointestinal tract. After a single oral or intravenous dose, there is a prompt peak in the level of hydroxyurea in the blood which then falls rapidly (DAVIDSON and WINTER, 1963; KRAKOFF et al., 1964). When given intravenously, the maximum blood level occurs in ten minutes and the principal excretion within the first hour after drug administration. When given orally, the maximum blood level is achieved at 2.5 h, the greatest excretion occurs in the second hour, and one-half of the total administered dose is found in the urine within 3.5 h. In various studies, from 35 to 75 % of administered doses have been recovered in the urine; the remainder is presumably degraded in the liver.

Teratogenic Effects

Hydroxyurea is markedly teratogenic to the rat fetus when given from the ninth to the twelfth day of gestation (CHAUBE and MURPHY, 1966). It is also inconsistently teratogenic in the four-day chick embryo and the echinoderm embryo (CHAUBE et al., 1963; MURPHY and CHAUBE, 1964).

Mechanism of Action

Hydroxyurea and several related compounds have been found to inhibit the synthesis of DNA, but not that of RNA or protein in cultures of mammalian cells (YOUNG and HODAS, 1964), bacteria (GALE et al., 1964), and regenerating rat liver (SCHWARTZ et al., 1967). In all of these systems this biologic effect of hydroxyurea is rapidly reversible. The possibility that hydroxyurea inhibits the formation of deoxyribonucleotides from ribonucleotides was studied using the highly purified ribonucleoside diphosphate reductase of *E. coli* (KRAKOFF et al., 1968). Hydroxyurea produces 70 percent inhibition of the *E. coli* reductase at a concentration of 3×10^{-3} M. Hydroxyurea was found to produce an irreversible inactivation of one of the two protein subunits (B_2) of the reductase complex. There was, however, negligible irreversible binding of hydroxyurea to protein B_2. Considerable evidence is available to suggest that the effect of hydroxyurea or hydroxylamine is due to an interaction with the nonheme iron portion of this specific protein (BROWN et al., 1968, 1969). It has also been shown (BROCKMAN et al., 1972) that the iron chelating agent, deferoxamine, augments the inhibition of DNA synthesis and of growth produced by hydroxyurea in Adenocarcinoma 755 cells. This augmentation is prevented by an excess of iron. In similar studies using a mammalian (i.e., Novikoff hepatoma) enzyme MOORE (1969) demonstrated 50-percent inhibition at a hydroxyurea concentration of 3×10^{-4} M. With this mammalian enzyme, inhibition could be partially reversed by the addition of ferrous iron, also suggesting that an interaction between hydroxyurea and iron might be responsible for inhibition of ribonucleoside diphosphate reductase.

Other mechanisms of action have been proposed for the cytotoxic effect of hydroxyurea. BORENFREUND et al. (1964) have suggested a direct effect on chromosomes of hyponitrite derived from hydroxyurea degradation. ROSENCRANZ (1966) has suggested that hydroxyurea may have a direct effect on cellular DNA, or that it may interact with other DNA synthesizing enzymes. YARBRO (1967) found that the addition of mixed deoxyribonucleosides failed to correct the inhibition by hydroxyurea of DNA synthesis and concluded that ribonucleoside diphosphate reductase was not the principal target for hydroxyurea. All of these effects, however, required concentrations considerably in excess of the 10^{-3} M concentration of hydroxyurea which inhibits the *E. coli* reductase enzyme and the even smaller concentration which inhibits the mammalian ribonucleoside diphosphate reductase. The weight of evidence, therefore, appears to favor inhibition of ribonucleoside diphosphate reductase as the primary site of action responsible for the cytotoxic effect of hydroxyurea, although other effects can clearly be demonstrated.

Hydroxyurea has also been shown to inhibit the growth of DNA viruses [i.e., polyoma (NORDENSKJOLD and KRAKOFF, 1968); vaccinia (NII et al., 1966); and herpes simplex (ROSENCRANZ et al., 1966)] suggesting that a ribonucleoside diphosphate reductase system is necessary for DNA synthesis in the viruses. However, DNA synthesis and cell replication of uninfected cells are more sensitive to inhibition by hydroxyurea than are DNA synthesis and viral replication in polyoma-infected cells.

Cell Cycle Specificity

Hydroxyurea is one of several compounds whose effects on cell proliferation appear to be restricted to the *S* (i.e., DNA synthesis) phase of cell growth (SKIPPER, 1970). Such compounds produce little effect on resting cells, but cells that are actively synthesizing DNA may be highly sensitive. This suggests that the design of dose schedules may be very important in producing optimum therapeutic responses; this conclusion is confirmed in studies with L1210 leukemia in mice in which hydroxyurea given at maximally tolerated doses once daily is less effective than fractionated administration.

Conclusions

Hydroxyurea is an active chemotherapeutic agent in man, although it does not appear to be uniquely active against any tumor. It does not appear to have a specific role in cancer chemotherapy, but is of continuing interest because of its ability to inhibit DNA synthesis markedly, promptly, and in the intact animal, reversibly. It is highly teratogenic in various animal systems. It has also been shown to be immunosuppressive in experimental systems although this property has not been exploited clinically.

References

BLOEDOW, C. E.: Phase II studies of hydroxyurea (NSC-32065) in adults: miscellaneous tumors. Cancer Chemother. Rep. **40**, 39—41 (1964).

BORENFREUND, E., KRIM, M., BENDICH, A.: Chromosomal aberrations induced by hyponitrite and hydroxylamine derivatives. J. Nat. Cancer Inst. **32**, 667—669 (1964).

BROCKMAN, R. W., SHADDIX, S., STRINGER, V., ADAMSON, D.: Enhancement by deferoxamine of inhibition of DNA synthesis by ribonucleotide reductase inhibitors. Proc. Amer. Ass. Cancer Res. **13**, 88 (1972).

BROWN, N. C., ELIASSON, R., REICHARD, P., THELANDER, L.: Non-heme iron as a cofactor in ribonucleotide reductase from *E. coli*. Biochem. biophys. Res. Commun. **30**, 522—527 (1968).

BROWN, N. C., ELIASSON, R., REICHARD, P., THELANDER, L.: Protein spectrum and iron content of protein B_2 from ribonucleoside diphosphate reductase. Europ. J. Biochem. **9**, 512 (1969).

CHAUBE, S., LACON, C., SIMMEL, E.: Hydroxyurea, a chemical teratogen. Proc. Amer. Ass. Cancer Res. **4**, 37 (1963).

CHAUBE, S., MURPHY, M. L.: The effects of hydroxyurea and related compounds on the rat fetus. Cancer Res. **26**, 1448—1457 (1966).

DAVIDSON, J. D., WINTER, T. S.: A method of analyzing for hydroxyurea in biological fluids. Cancer Chemother. Rep. **27**, 97—110 (1963).

GALE, G. R., KENDALL, S. M., MCCLAIN, H. H., DUBOIS, S.: Effect of hydroxyurea on *Pseudomonas aeruginosa*. Cancer Res. **24**, 1012—1019 (1964).

KRAKOFF, I. H., BROWN, N. C., REICHARD, P.: Inhibition of ribonucleoside diphosphate reductase by hydroxyurea. Cancer Res. **28**, 1559—1565 (1968).

KRAKOFF, I. H., SAVEL, H., MURPHY, M. L.: Phase II studies of hydroxyurea (NSC-32065) in adults: clinical evaluation. Cancer Chemother. Rep. **40**, 53—55 (1964).

MOORE, E. C.: The effect of ferrous iron and dithioerythritol on inhibition by hydroxyurea of ribonucleotide reductase. Cancer Res. **29**, 291—295 (1969).

MURPHY, M. L., CHAUBE, S.: Hydroxyurea (NSC-32065) as a teratogen. Cancer Chemother. Rep. **40**, 1—7 (1964).

NII, S., MORGAN, C., ROSE, H. M., ROSENCRANZ, H. S.: Effect of hydroxyurea on the development of herpes simplex virus. Fed. Proc. **25**, 311 (1966).

NORDENSKJOLD, B. A., KRAKOFF, I. H.: Effects of hydroxyurea on polyoma virus replication. Cancer Res. **28**, 1686—1691 (1968).

ROSENCRANZ, H. S., ROSE, H. M., MORGAN, C., HSU, K. C.: The effect of hydroxyurea on virus development. II. Vaccinia virus. Virology **28**, 510—519 (1966).

SCHWARTZ, H. S., GAROFALO, M., STERNBERG, S. S., PHILIPS, F. S.: Hydroxyurea: inhibition of deoxyribonucleic acid synthesis in regenerating liver in rats. Cancer Res. **25**, 1867—1870 (1967).

SKIPPER, H. E.: Leukocyte kinetics in leukemia and lymphoma. In: Leukemia and lymphoma. Chicago: Year Book Medical Publishers 1962.

STEARNS, B., LOSEE, K. A., BERNSTEIN, J.: Hydroxyurea. A new type of potential anti-tumor agent. J. med. Chem. (Abstr.) **6**, 201 (1963).

YARBRO, J. W.: The effect of deoxyribonucleoside and ribonucleoside addition on the inhibiting effect of hydroxyurea on deoxyribonucleic acid synthesis. Biochem. J. **104**, 52C—54C (1967).

YARBRO, J. W.: Hydroxyurea in the treatment of refractory psoriasis. Lancet **2**, 846—847 (1969).

YOUNG, C. W., HODAS, S.: Hydroxyurea: inhibiting effect on DNA metabolism. Science **146**, 1172—1174 (1964).

Handbook Expt. Pharm. 38/2, Springer-Verlag, Berlin 1975.
Antineoplastic and Immunosuppressive Agents II
ed. A.C. Sartorelli + D.G. Johns.

Chapter 73

α-(*N*)-Heterocyclic Carboxaldehyde Thiosemicarbazones

KRISHNA C. AGRAWAL and ALAN C. SARTORELLI

With 2 Figures

Introduction

To combat neoplastic disease forms effectively, it is essential to have available a variety of medicaments with different biochemical mechanisms of action. Since deoxyribonucleotides are present in relatively low levels in mammalian cells, a particularly critical step in the biosynthesis of DNA is the reductive conversion of ribonucleotides to deoxyribonucleotides by the enzyme ribonucleoside diphosphate reductase. The importance of this enzyme to cell reproduction was demonstrated by ELFORD et al. (1970) in a series of rat hepatomas with different rates of cellular proliferation; these tumors exhibited an absolute correlation between tumor growth rate and the activity of ribonucleoside diphosphate reductase, while two other enzymes involved in DNA synthesis, thymidylate synthetase and thymidine kinase, did not demonstrate such a close degree of correlation with tumor growth rate. Thus, it seems reasonable that a potent inhibitor of ribonucleoside diphosphate reductase would be an important addition to the chemotherapeutic arsenal for the treatment of rapidly growing cancers. In support of this, three different types of drugs with relatively weak inhibitory potency for ribonucleoside diphosphate reductase [i.e., hydroxyurea (KRAKOFF, 1973), guanazole (BROCKMAN, 1970), and 5-hydroxy-2-formylpyridine thiosemicarbazone (5-HP) (SARTORELLI et al., 1969; BROCKMAN et al., 1970a; MOORE et al., 1971)] have all demonstrated some, although clearly minimal, activity in man; see, for example, the references for hydroxyurea (BLOEDOW, 1964; MOERTEL et al., 1965; KENNEDY and YARBRO, 1966) and 5-HP (DE CONTI et al., 1971, 1972; ETCUBANAS et al., 1971).

Antineoplastic Activity

The initial observation of the antileukemic activity in mice of an α-(*N*)-heterocyclic carboxaldehyde thiosemicarbazone was made by BROCKMAN et al. (1956). They demonstrated that administration of 2-formylpyridine thiosemicarbazone (PT) significantly increased the life span of mice with L1210 leukemia. These results were confirmed and extended to a number of derivatives of glyoxal *bis*(thiosemicarbazone) that were inhibitory to Sarcoma 180 in mice (FRENCH and FREEDLANDER, 1958). Among these are the thiosemicarbazones of methylglyoxal and of 3-ethoxy-2-oxobutyraldehyde (Kethoxal) which are discussed elsewhere in these volumes. A number of related *bis*(N^4-methylthiosemicarbazones) of diketones, dialdehydes, and ketoaldehydes, in which the carbonyl functions are separated by varied methylene groups, are active agents against Sarcoma 180 (BARRY et al., 1967). A series of thiosemicarbazones of oxypolysaccharides has also been reported (BARRY et al., 1966).

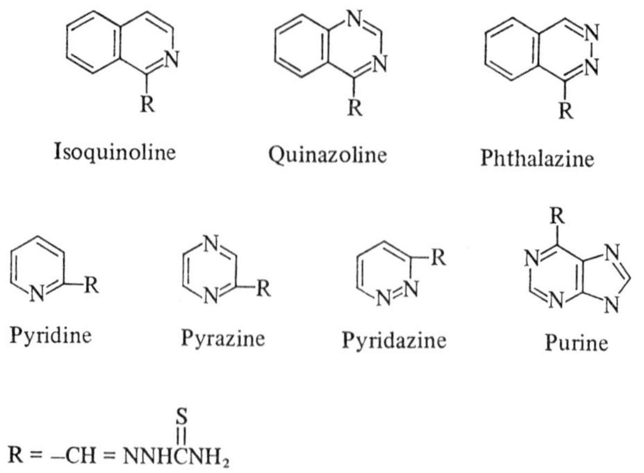

Isoquinoline Quinazoline Phthalazine

Pyridine Pyrazine Pyridazine Purine

$R = -CH = NNHC(=S)NH_2$

Fig. 1. α-(*N*)-Heterocyclic carboxaldehyde thiosemicarbazones with antineoplastic activity

The antineoplastic activity of a variety of α-(*N*)-heterocyclic carboxaldehyde thiosemicarbazones was described by FRENCH and BLANZ (1966) who reported a series of derivatives from 16 different heterocyclic ring systems. A conjugate $N^*-N^*-S^*$ tridentate ligand system was found to be a common feature of compounds with carcinostatic potency. Employing structure-activity relationships, it was postulated that (a) the π electron density at the point of attachment of the formyl thiosemicarbazone side chain should be low, and (b) the ring nitrogen should be a reasonably good donor to the transition metals for formation of coordination compounds (chelates). It was also deemed necessary that the carbonyl attachment be in a position α to the heteroaromatic nitrogen atom; compounds where the side chain was attached at the β or γ positions to the heterocyclic *N* atom were found to be inactive as antitumor agents. Thus, a variety of heterocyclic ring systems (Fig. 1) carrying the thiosemicarbazone side chain α to the heteroaromatic nitrogen are active antineoplastic agents, each having the following general features:

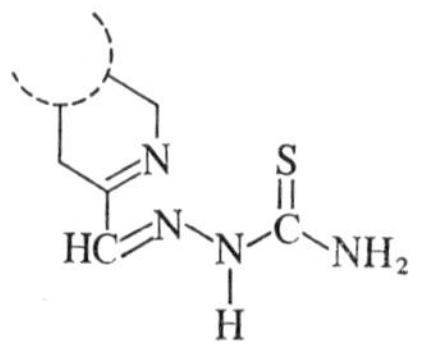

AGRAWAL and SARTORELLI (1969) have made a number of modifications in the formyl thiosemicarbazone side chain of 1-formylisoquinoline thiosemicarbazone (IQ-1) to ascertain the importance of this part of the molecule for antineoplastic activity; tumor-inhibitory potency and host toxicity of these compounds were assessed in mice bearing Sarcoma 180 ascites cells. Substitutions made on the different positions of the side chain resulted in either a diminution or a total loss of tumor-inhibitory activity, indicating that the intactness of this portion of the molecule was essential for IQ-1 to function as an inhibitor of the growth of malignant cells.

A. Correlation of Ring Substitution with Tumor-Inhibitory Potency

The first systematic approach to evaluate the effects of various substituents in the heterocyclic ring on biological activity of these agents was undertaken by AGRAWAL et al. (1968). The most likely candidate for such a study was IQ-1, since it was the most biochemically active agent of the series and has been shown to cause pronounced inhibition of the growth of a relatively wide spectrum of transplanted rodent tumors (FRENCH and BLANZ, 1965); in addition, IQ-1 has also been shown to cause tumor regression in spontaneous lymphomas of dogs (CREASEY et al., 1970, 1972). This study of substituent effects was followed by a series of papers on both the isoquinoline (AGRAWAL et al., 1970, 1972; FRENCH et al., 1970) and pyridine series (BLANZ et al., 1970); a detailed compilation has been published (FRENCH and BLANZ, 1971). The effect of various substituents on the antitumor activity is shown in Tables 1 and 2. The data indicate that no simple parametric

Table 1. *The effect of substituents on the pyridine ring on the antineoplastic activity of 2-formylpyridine thiosemicarbazone*

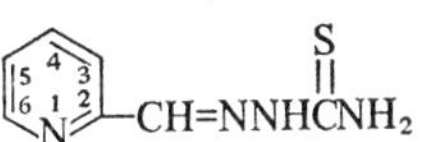

Substitution	Antitumor Activity Sarcoma 180 (ascites)	L1210	Lewis Lung Carcinoma
None	—	+	—
3-OH	+++	+++	+++
3-OC_2H_5	+	+	—
3-CH_3	—	+	—
3-F	—	+	+
3-COOH	—	—	—
4-OH	—		
4-CH_3	—	+	—
5-OH	++++	++++	+
5-OAc	—	+	+++
5-OCF_3	—	—	—
5-OC_2H_5	—	+	—
5-NH_2	+	+	—
5-$N(CH_3)_2$	++	++	+
5-CH_3	—	+	—
5-C_2H_5	—	++	+
5-F	+	+	++
5-Cl	—	+	++
5-Br	+	—	—
5-I	—	—	—
5-SO_2CH_3	—	—	—
6-CH_3	—	±	+
3-OC_2H_5, 5-OC_2H_5	—	—	—
3-OH, 6-CH_3	—	—	—
3-OH, 1-CH_3, Iodide	—	—	—

Antitumor activity of derivatives is indicated in % as follows: the L1210 leukemia and Sarcoma 180 are given as increases in survival time of tumor-bearing mice and the Lewis Lung Carcinoma as decreases in tumor size.

	+	++	+++	++++
Lewis Lung Carcinoma	$\leqq$ 30	$\leqq$ 15	$\leqq$ 5	$<$ 1
L1210 leukemia	$\geqq$ 125	$\geqq$ 160	$\geqq$ 180	$\geqq$ 200
Sarcoma 180	$\geqq$ 150	$\geqq$ 200	$\geqq$ 250	$\geqq$ 300

— Indicates no activity.
A blank space indicates that the compound has not been tested in that system.

Table 2. *The effect of substituents on the isoquinoline ring on the antineoplastic activity of 1-formylisoquinoline thiosemicarbazone*

(Structure: isoquinoline ring, positions 1–8, N at 2; at position 1: CH=NNHC(=S)NH$_2$)

Substitution	Antitumor Activity Sarcoma 180 (ascites)	L1210	Lewis Lung Carcinoma
None	++++	++	+++
2-oxide	+	—	—
3-CH_3	+	—	
4-CH_3		+	
4-OH	+++	+	—
4-ONa	+++	+++	
4-$OCOCH_3$	+++	+	—
5-CH_3		—	
5-OH	++++	+	
5-ONa	++++	+++	
5-$OCOCH_3$	++++	+	—
5-NH_2	++++		
5-NO_2	+++	+	—
5-SO_3H	—	—	—
5-SO_3NH_4	—	—	—
5-COOH	—	—	—
5-CN	—	—	—
5-Cl	++	+	—
5-F	++	++	++
5-CF_3	+	+	+
5-C_3F_7	—	—	—
6-OCH_3	—	—	—
7-OH	—	—	—
7-$OCOCH_3$	++	—	—
7-OCH_3	+++	+	—
7-F	++++	+	—
7-Cl	—	—	—
8-F	+++	+	—

Antitumor activity of derivatives is indicated in % as follows: the L1210 leukemia and Sarcoma 180 are given as increases in survival time of tumor-bearing mice and the Lewis Lung Carcinoma as decreases in tumor size.

	+	++	+++	++++
Lewis Lung Carcinoma	$\leqq$ 30	$\leqq$ 15	$\leqq$ 5	< 1
L1210 leukemia	$\geqq$ 125	$\geqq$ 160	$\geqq$ 180	$\geqq$ 200
Sarcoma 180	$\geqq$ 150	$\geqq$ 200	$\geqq$ 250	$\geqq$ 300

— Indicates no activity.
A blank space indicates that the compound has not been tested in that system.

rationale (electronic, steric, hydrophilic, or hydrophobic) explains the effect of various substituents on activity of these agents against neoplastic cells in different test systems. Also, the sensitivity of different cell lines varies to a great extent with these agents e.g., Sarcoma 180 ascites cells were most sensitive to isoquinoline derivatives, while the Lewis lung carcinoma was the least responsive of the three test systems listed (Table 2). Alternatively, pyridine derivatives were better agents against the L1210 leukemia and the Lewis lung carcinoma (Table 1). Some generalizations can still be made within one test system, although they may not hold true in all cell lines. AGRAWAL et al. (1968) have reported that the introduction of electron donating groups such as NH_2 or OH at the 5-position of IQ-1 resulted in compounds retaining high activity against Sarcoma 180 ascites cells and that 5-OH and 5-$OCOCH_3$ substituted derivatives possessed higher therapeutic indices than IQ-1. Introduction of OH and $OCOCH_3$ groups at the 4-position of the isoquinoline ring in IQ-1 resulted in less effective antineoplastic agents against Sarcoma 180 ascites cells in mice; however, the sodium salt of the 4-OH derivative was considerably more efficacious than IQ-1 on the L1210 leukemia (AGRAWAL et al., 1970a). Introduction of electron withdrawing groups such as NO_2, SO_3H, and CO_2H has generally resulted in a lowering of antineoplastic activity. Possibly hydrophilic groups such as NH_2 or OH, aside from their electron donating effect, might assist in better distribution of the resultant derivatives in tumor-bearing animals because of increased water solubility. This conclusion, however, could not be made for the pyridine series, where the 5-NH_2 derivative is much less active than either the 3- or 5-OH derivative, which were found to be potent antineoplastic agents (FRENCH and BLANZ, 1966a, 1967, 1968).

Several monomethylated derivatives of both the isoquinoline and pyridine series have been prepared to define the molecular dimensions compatible with antineoplastic activity (AGRAWAL et al., 1972c). These were the thiosemicarbazones of 3-, 4-, and 5-methylisoquinoline-1-carboxaldehyde and of 3-, 4-, 5-, and 6-methylpyridine-2-carboxaldehyde. Tests for tumor-inhibitory potency against the L1210 leukemia demonstrated that introduction of a 6-methyl group in the pyridine ring and of an analogous 3-methyl substituent in the isoquinoline structure resulted in compounds with no antineoplastic activity, indicating an apparent intolerance to substitution at the α' position to the heterocyclic N atom for inhibitory action (SARTORELLI et al., 1971). Whether this reduction in activity is due to steric hindrance resulting in possible lower chelation affinity or due to the low bulk tolerance of the enzyme ribonucleoside diphosphate reductase at this locus is yet to be distinctly defined.

Based on these findings, AGRAWAL et al. (1972a) have introduced several groups, potentially capable of alkylating the enzyme ribonucleoside diphosphate reductase at a polar region of the inhibitor-binding site of the enzyme, at the 5-position of the isoquinoline ring. Two series of compounds were made using either 5-NH_2 or 5-OH derivatives of IQ-1 to yield corresponding amides [$-NHSO_2CH_3$, $-NHCOC_6H_4$ (m- or p-SO_2F)] or esters [$-OSO_2CH_3$, $-OCO_2C_2H_5$, $-OCO_2C_6H_5$, $-OCOC_6H_4$ (m- or p-SO_2F), $-OSO_2C_6H_4$ (o-, m-, or p-SO_2F)]. Only two derivatives, those containing an $-OCO_2C_2H_5$ or an $-OCO_2C_6H_5$ moiety, were shown to have potent tumor-inhibitory activity in mice bearing Sarcoma 180 ascites cells. However, there is no evidence yet that these groups (carboethoxy or carbophenoxy, respectively) are involved in irreversible inhibition of the enzyme, though it has been shown that duration of inhibition of DNA synthesis lasted longer with these agents (AGRAWAL et al., 1972). Introduction of a group with high chemical reactivity [i.e., *bis*(β-chloroethyl)amino] at the 5-position of the isoquinoline ring did not result in any appreciable tumor-inhibitory effect, although the compound inhibited the enzyme ribonucleoside diphosphate reductase effectively *in vitro* (AGRAWAL et al., 1972). This suggests a high probability of nonselective reaction of the nitrogen mustard group with diverse nucleophilic centers available *in vivo*, thus limiting the availability of this drug for the target enzyme.

Studies of the interaction of α-(N)-heterocyclic carboxaldehyde thiosemicarbazones with the enzyme ribonucleoside diphosphate reductase have suggested a region of hydrophobic bonding at the inhibitor binding site (SARTORELLI et al.,

1971). The possible existence of this hypothetical hydrophobic bonding zone has been explored by AGRAWAL et al. (1972b) in an effort to synthesize agents with greater affinity for the target enzyme. Hydrophobic groups such as phenyl or benzyl were introduced at various positions of the pyridine nucleus. Though these derivatives were found to be potent inhibitors of the enzyme *in vitro*, only one isomer, 4-*m*-aminophenyl-2-formylpyridine thiosemicarbazone, was found to possess potent antitumor activity against Sarcoma 180 ascites cells in mice. A similar approach has also been attempted by MOONEY et al. (1972), by introducing an alkyl chain in the 5-amino group of the isoquinoline ring system. Syntheses of meta- and para-substituted 3- and 5-benzyloxy derivatives of 2-formylpyridine thiosemicarbazone have been reported (LIN et al., 1972). These were synthesized in order to increase (a) the relatively short-lived activity and (b) low potency for the target enzyme of 5-HP. 3-(*m*-Aminobenzyloxy)-2-formylpyridine thiosemicarbazone was found to be a potent antitumor agent, increasing the life span of Sarcoma 180 ascites tumor-bearing mice over untreated animals by a factor of 2.4.

It must be emphasized that these correlations of heterocyclic ring substitution with tumor inhibitory potency are based on data that were obtained in most cases with a single daily dose mode of administration. AGRAWAL and SARTORELLI (1968) have reported that multiple daily dosage regimens caused a greater prolongation of the survival time of mice bearing the L1210 leukemia, and also, that monosodium salts of compounds bearing a phenolic OH, especially of isoquinoline derivatives, were much more active than the free phenolic compounds. SKIPPER et al. (1970) have also reported that about 50% of mice inoculated with 10^5 L1210 leukemia cells can be cured with the 5-hydroxypyridine derivative (5-HP) if therapy is given every 3 h for 8 doses on days 2, 6, 10, and 14 after tumor transplantation.

B. Correlative Studies of Chelating Potential with Antitumor Activity

α-(*N*)-Heterocyclic carboxaldehyde thiosemicarbazones are excellent coordinating agents for a number of transition metals including divalent iron, cobalt, nickel, copper, zinc, and manganese (FRENCH and BLANZ, 1966). The exceptionally strong affinity of 2-formylpyrazine thiosemicarbazone for ferrous ions *in vivo* was demonstrated by the finding that administration of a 100 mg/kg dose of this compound to mice removed about 11 μg of iron in 24 h (FRENCH et al., 1965).

It has been hypothesized that the biological activity of these compounds is associated with the chelation of iron. As will be described in more detail later in this chapter, MOORE et al. (1970, 1971) have postulated that IQ-1 and PT interact with ribonucleoside diphosphate reductase either by coordination of iron in the metal-bound enzyme or that the iron chelate of these agents is the active inhibitory form. Direct correlation between antitumor activity and the chelating ability of these compounds was shown by MICHAUD and SARTORELLI (1968). They demonstrated that the capacity of IQ-1 to prolong the survival time of mice bearing Sarcoma 180 ascites cells and to inhibit the formation of DNA in these cells was decreased considerably by the substitution of an imino group for the sulfur atom in the thiosemicarbazone side chain, and was eliminated completely by replacing the sulfur with an oxygen atom. These findings were correlated with the abilities of these derivatives to coordinate ferrous ions; IQ-1 had the highest chelation affinity, followed by the guanylhydrazone; the semicarbazone did not appear to bind ferrous ions. Similar results have been shown by AGRAWAL et al. (1970) in the pyridine series where the 5-hydroxy analog (5-HP) was found to be a more active antineoplastic agent than its selenosemicarbazone analog, and the guanylhydrazone and semicarbazone derivatives were ineffective. The chelating potential of these agents correlated with biological activity: 5-HP was shown to be the most effective ligand in this series, the selenosemicarbazone was about 1/8th as effective, while the other two analogs, the guanylhydrazone and semicarbazone, were found to have very low chelation potential. These results also correlated with the degree of inhibition of DNA synthesis by these compounds in transplanted neoplastic cells. Administration of 5-HP to man has been reported to result in significant amounts of iron (2 to 11 mg/24 h) excretion in urine, probably in chelate form with 5-HP (DeConti et al., 1972). Serum iron and total iron-binding capacity of the serum was also increased. However, urinary and serum calcium, copper, and zinc values remained within normal limits during treatment.

C. Combination Chemotherapy

Various studies have indicated the superiority of combination chemotherapy for the treatment of cancer (Venditti and Goldin, 1964; Sartorelli, 1965, 1969; Henderson and Samaha, 1969). For this reason, α-(*N*)-heterocyclic carboxaldehyde thiosemicarbazones have been tested in combination with other antineoplastic agents. Grindey and Nichol (1972) have employed the combination of several inhibitors of DNA synthesis with IQ-1, which could be expected to act at sequential or concurrent steps, to determine whether increased effectiveness occurred in suspension cultures of leukemia L1210. They reported that combination of IQ-1 with methotrexate yielded slight antagonism, while its combination with 5-fluorodeoxyuridine was either additive or slightly synergistic. Also, the combination of 9-β-D-arabinofuranosyladenine with IQ-1 was found to be additive. Mihich (1969) and Grindey et al. (1972) have also reported that combination of IQ-1 with 1-β-D-arabinofuranosylcytosine (ara-C) resulted in synergistic effects against the L1210 leukemia in DBA/2Ha-DD mice. However, they obtained only additive effects with this combination against irradiated mice and in cell cultures, indicating that the therapeutic synergism *in vivo* resulted in part from host defenses directed against the tumor.

Another derivative of the α-(*N*)-heterocyclic carboxaldehyde thiosemicarbazone series which has been tried in combination chemotherapy is 5-HP. Burchenal et al. (1970) have reported that 5-HP acts synergistically with L-asparaginase. They obtained about 70 to 80% 50-day "cures" of leukemia L5178Y in mice with a combination of asparaginase and 5-HP.

Thus, these studies indicate that combination of one of the active α-(*N*)-heterocyclic carboxaldehyde thiosemicarbazones with other antineoplastic agents results in either additive or synergistic antitumor effects.

D. Clinical Studies

5-HP was the derivative of this series of α-(*N*)-heterocyclic carboxaldehyde thiosemicarbazones to be studied in man. The selection of 5-HP for clinical trials was due to (a) its considerable activity against transplanted tumors (French and Blanz, 1967; Blanz and French, 1968) and a spontaneous dog lymphoma (Creasey et al., 1972) and (b) its ease of parenteral administration as its sodium salt (Agrawal and Sartorelli, 1968). Etcubanas et al. (1971) administered 5-HP to 14 children and 8 adults (15 with leukemia, 7 with solid tumors) in doses ranging from 0.5 to 76 mg/kg/day by single injection, or by 1 to 2 h of continuous infusions. They reported that 3 out of 12 patients with leukemia had partial remissions of 7 to 41 days. Relapses were found to occur either while continuing or shortly after treatment. DECONTI et al. (1972) have reported the administration of 5-HP to 13 patients (5 with leukemia, 8 with solid tumors) in doses ranging from 1 to 16 mg/kg, either by a Volutrole in approximately 6 min, or by slow continuous i.v. infusion. No antitumor effects were noted in 8 patients with solid tumors. Transient decreases in blast counts were observed in 3 of 5 patients with acute leukemia, although no remissions were obtained. In both studies the administration of drug was limited by gastrointestinal toxicity; severe nausea and vomiting and fever occurred in all patients.

Antiviral Activity

The initial observation of HAMRE et al. (1950) of the activity of *p*-aminobenzaldehyde thiosemicarbazone on vaccinia virus replication prompted the synthesis of a wide variety of thiosemicarbazones. Of particular significance are the studies of THOMPSON et al. (1953, 1953a), which led to the synthesis of isatin β-thiosemicarbazone. BAUER and SADLER (1960) examined structure-activity correlations in the isatin series and concluded that 1-alkyl derivatives of isatin β-thiosemicarbazone were the most active compounds against vaccinia. These investigations have been reviewed by PRUSOFF (1967). Recently, 5-cyanothiophene-2-carboxaldehyde thiosemicarbazone, a compound with the thiosemicarbazone side chain in the α-position to the heterocyclic sulfur atom, has been reported to be more active than methisazone, the *N*-methyl isatin derivative (ROLLY and WINKELMANN, 1971). Isatin thiosemicarbazones have not been reported active against cytomegalovirus, a member of the herpes group; however, SIDWELL et al. (1969) demonstrated that 6-formylpurine thiosemicarbazone (a member of the class of α-(*N*)-heterocyclic carboxaldehyde thiosemicarbazones), which possesses structural features essential for antitumor activity, was an effective inhibitor of cytomegalovirus in cell culture. This prompted BROCKMAN et al. (1970) to compare selected α-(*N*)-heterocyclic carboxaldehyde thiosemicarbazones for activity against herpes simplex virus in H.EP.2 cells and human cytomegalovirus in WI-38 cells. They found that all the derivatives of this class, which were tested, had moderate to marked activity against both viruses. A correlation was also observed between antiviral activity and inhibition of ribonucleoside diphosphate reductase activity in H.Ep.2 cells, suggesting that the activity of ribonucleoside diphosphate reductase may be a limiting factor in the replication of certain members of the herpes virus group.

Distribution and Metabolism

Various aspects of the distribution and metabolism of α-(*N*)-heterocyclic carboxaldehyde thiosemicarbazones have been studied in mice, dogs, and man. The tissue distribution of IQ-1 was studied in mice (CREASEY et al. 1970, 1972) after intraperitoneal injection of IQ-1 labeled with either 1-^{14}C, 3'-^{14}C, or ^{35}S. The greatest amount of radioactivity occurred in the intestine (24 to 40 %), liver (4 to 12 %) and stomach (2 to 6 %). Lesser amounts were present in other tissues and about 40 % was found in the residual carcass at the end of an 8 h period. The relatively large amounts of radioactivity from IQ-1 present in the tissues of the gastrointestinal tract of the mouse have also been reported for 5-HP in the dog (COFFEY et al., 1972); these findings suggest that localization of these agents in the gastrointestinal tract may be in part associated with the nausea, vomiting, and diarrhea that characterize the toxicity of 5-HP in man (DECONTI et al. 1971, 1972; ETCUBANAS, 1971). It is also tempting to speculate that the affinity of this class of agents for intestinal tissue is due to the extensive stores of iron contained therein.

CREASEY et al. (1972) demonstrated that 20 % of the radioactivity from 3'-^{14}C—IQ-1 was excreted in the urine of mice and 2.8 % in the feces in 16 h. During an 8 h period about 2 % of the radioactivity was present in the respiratory CO_2 when side-chain labeled (3'-^{14}C), but not ring labeled (1-^{14}C) IQ-1, was administered. Furthermore, these workers found that in dogs, the half-life of radioactivity in the blood from labeled IQ-1 was about 4 h, and between 28 and 46 % of the label was excreted in the urine during a 48 h period. Investigation of urinary metabolites indicated great complexity in the degradative pattern of IQ-1. The proposed metabolic pathways of IQ-1 are shown in Fig. 2. Little unchanged drug was pres-

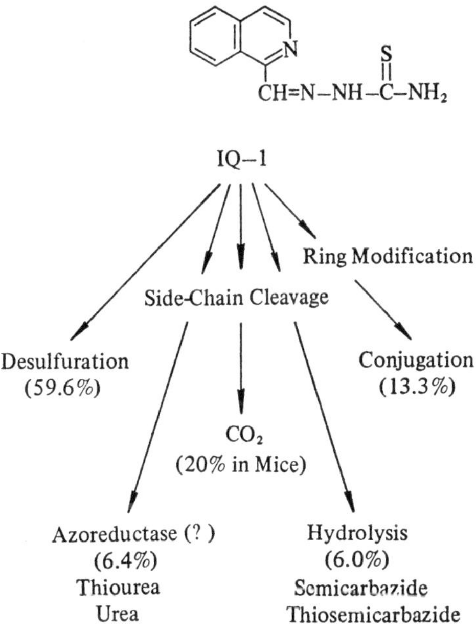

Fig. 2. Outline of metabolic pathways for IQ-1 tentatively identified in the present studies (From CREASEY et al., 1972)

ent in urine, indicating the completeness of breakdown. A major contributor to the process is desulfuration and about 60 % of the excreted derivatives of IQ-1 undergo such alteration. This change should lead to loss of antitumor potency since 1-formylisoquinoline semicarbazone was reported to be inactive against sensitive transplanted tumors (AGRAWAL and SARTORELLI, 1969). Metabolic cleavage of the side chain of IQ-1 was shown by CREASEY et al. (1972) to be of lesser importance, accounting for 11 to 16 % of the total urinary metabolites in the dog and about 15 % in the mouse. Two types of cleavage occur, one on the =N—N-linkage, presumably the result of the action of azoreductase, and the other on the —CH=N-bond. About 4 % of urinary radioactivity was in the form of urea, and somewhat less as thiourea, indicating that desulfuration need not precede side-chain cleavage. Significant amounts of semicarbazide and thiosemicarbazide were also found, providing evidence that hydrolytic attack proceeds at a rate similar to that of azoreductase action. The finding in the mouse that greater than 2 % of side chain-^{14}C was excreted as CO_2 indicates that complete catabolism of a portion of the side chain can take place.

The water solubility of urinary metabolites of IQ-1, which contrasts with that of the parent compound, suggests that modification of the ring occurred. This was supported by the finding of (a) a hydroxyl infrared band in an acidic metabolite and (b) 13.3 % of urinary radioactivity in glucuronide forms.

COFFEY et al. (1972) reported that following intravenous administration of 5-HP to the dog, drug-derived radioactivity appeared in both bile and urine, where two unidentified metabolites were separated.

In man, plasma levels of 5-HP decayed in a biphasic mode with an initial half-life of 2.5 to 10 min (DECONTI et al., 1972). This is shorter than the $t^1/_2$ of 15 min for this drug in mice (TOMCHICK and MEAD, 1970). Of the dose of 5-HP administered to patients with cancer, 47 to 75 % was excreted within 24 h (DECONTI et al., 1972). In contrast to the metabolic fate of IQ-1, 50 to 74 % of the urinary radioactivity was in the form of glucuronide conjugates. The major glucuronide form was that of 5-HP itself and the other was of an unknown compound. No degradation of the thiosemicarbazide portion of 5-HP appears to occur in man, as was demonstrated with IQ-1 in the dog (CREASEY et al., 1972). This does not appear to be a species difference, but a reflection of contrasting metabolic susceptibilities of various α-(N)-heterocyclic carboxaldehyde thiosemicarbazones, since the release of $^{14}CO_2$ in expired air from 3'-^{14}C—5-HP was 10 to 20 times lower in the mouse than that released from 3'-^{14}C—IQ-1 (DECONTI et al., 1972).

Biochemical Mechanism of Action

An understanding of the biochemical basis for the carcinostatic activity of α-(N)-heterocyclic carboxaldehyde thiosemicarbazones is necessary for (a) the rational design of a clinically more effective agent and (b) the effective utility of this class of compounds in admixture with other clinically useful carcinostatic agents. α-(N)-Heterocyclic carboxaldehyde thiosemicarbazones are primarily inhibitors of the synthesis of DNA in neoplastic cells (SARTORELLI, 1967; SARTORELLI et al., 1972; DECONTI et al., 1972) and therefore are active in the S phase of the cell cycle (BHUYAN et al., 1972; KARON and BENEDICT, 1972). For example, in non-replicating Sarcoma 180 ascites cells *in vitro*, the incorporation of ^{3}H-thymidine into DNA was inhibited approximately 50 % by a concentration of IQ-1 of 2×10^{-7} M. Under these conditions, the incorporation of ^{3}H-uridine and ^{14}C-leucine into RNA and protein, respectively, was unaffected by 4×10^{-5} M IQ-1, and respiration was resistant to concentrations of this agent as great as 5×10^{-4} M (SARTORELLI et al., 1972). In growing Sarcoma 180 cells *in vivo*, inhibition of the synthesis of RNA and protein by α-(N)-heterocyclic carboxaldehyde thiosemicarbazones can be demonstrated; however, these processes are considerably less sensitive than is the biosynthesis of DNA (SARTORELLI, 1967; MOORE et al., 1970, 1971; BOOTH et al., 1971; SARTORELLI et al., 1972). Interference with the biosynthesis of DNA by these agents was shown to be due to inhibition of the enzyme ribonucleoside diphosphate reductase (SARTORELLI et al., 1969; MOORE et al., 1970, 1971; BROCKMAN et al., 1970). α-(N)-Heterocyclic carboxaldehyde thiosemicarbazones constitute, as a class, the most potent known inhibitors of ribonucleoside diphosphate reductase, being 80 to 5,000 times more potent than hydroxyurea as inhibitors of the activity of the mammalian enzyme (for appropriate references see SARTORELLI, 1969).

The kinetic mechanism of inhibition of ribonucleoside diphosphate reductase by α-(N)-heterocyclic carboxaldehyde thiosemicarbazones is not clear. The concentrations of the nucleoside diphosphate substrate, the allosteric activator ATP, or magnesium ion do not influence the inhibition of the enzyme produced by all of the thiosemicarbazones tested to date. Interesting differences exist, however, between the ring hydroxylated and nonhydroxylated α-(*N*)-heterocyclic carboxaldehyde thiosemicarbazones with respect to the dithiols, used as model substrates in place of the natural substrate thioredoxin, and to iron. IQ-1 and PT are similar in action; both are partially competitive with the dithiol substrate and both prevent any stimulation of reductase activity by iron. It has been hypothesized (Moore et al., 1970, 1971) that inhibition by these derivatives is the result of either coordination of iron in the metal-charged enzyme by the inhibitor, or formation of an iron chelate of IQ-1, which acts as the true inhibitor at the site functionally occupied by thioredoxin.

The hydroxylated derivatives, 5-HP and 3-hydroxy-2-formylpyridine thiosemicarbazone, show a different pattern of inhibition (Moore et al., 1971). They appear "competitive" with iron and either noncompetitive or uncompetitive with the dithiol substrate; the imprecise nature of the assay did not allow a choice between these alternatives. The failure of the dithiol to reverse inhibition of ribonucleoside diphosphate reductase by the hydroxylated derivatives implies that the interaction of these inhibitors with the enzyme occurs at a site different from that involved in the action of PT and IQ-1. The impure nature of this complex enzyme system, however, makes it impossible to explain fully these differences and further advances will require the availability of a highly purified enzyme.

Some of the structural features required for inhibition of ribonucleoside diphosphate reductase have been determined (Sartorelli et al., 1971). Comparisons of the inhibitory activity of PT and its derivatives have indicated that the introduction of a methyl group at either the 3, 4, or 5 positions of PT enhanced inhibitory activity. In addition, IQ-1, which can be visualized as PT with a benzene ring fused across the 3 and 4 positions of the pyridine ring, was approximately 2.5-fold more inhibitory to ribonucleoside diphosphate reductase than was PT. These findings suggested the possible existence of a hydrophobic bonding zone adjacent to the inhibitor binding site of the enzyme. The introduction of a methyl group at the 6-position of the pyridine ring of PT reduces both inhibitory potency toward ribonucleoside diphosphate reductase and antitumor activity, as does fusion of a benzene ring across the 5 and 6 positions of the pyridine ring (2-formylquinoline thiosemicarbazone); the decreased activity results presumably from low bulk tolerance by the enzyme for substituents in this position or from interference by the substituent with the coordination of iron in the ribonucleoside diphosphate reductase molecule or from both.

Karon and Benedict (1972) showed that 5-HP caused chromatid breaks principally during *S* phase in hamster fibroblasts and that the addition of iron did not prevent the induction of chromatid breakage.

The ribonucleoside diphosphate reductase enzyme of *Escherichia coli*, although similar in mechanism of action to the catalyst derived from mammalian sources, is resistant to the inhibitory action of α-(*N*)-heterocyclic carboxaldehyde thiosemicarbazones (Moore et al., 1970, 1971), even though the growth of *E. coli* is retarded by these agents. Thus, the biochemical mechanism responsible for the cytotoxicity of α-(*N*)-heterocyclic carboxaldehyde thiosemicarbazones differs in mammalian and bacterial systems. The primary site of cytostatic action in *E. coli* appears to be on the RNA biosynthetic pathways; RNA polymerase and pyrimidine nucleoside monophosphate kinase are the sites of the lesions on RNA synthesis, with blockade of the latter enzyme apparently being more critical (Hochman et al., 1972, 1972a). The locus of the inhibitory action of α-(*N*)-heterocyclic carboxaldehyde thiosemicarbazones on the RNA synthetic pathways in mammalian cells is unknown, as is the relative contribution of the action of these compounds on the biosynthesis of RNA to cytotoxicity.

Conclusions

The impressive antineoplastic potency of 5-HP in animal systems has not been achieved in man. The reasons for inactivity in man appear to be two-fold. First, 5-HP has relatively low inhibitory potency for the target enzyme ribonucleoside diphosphate reductase, being approximately 100-fold less active at the enzymatic level than the most active member of this series, IQ-1, a derivative with apparently little clinical potential due to extreme insolubility (MOORE et al., 1970, 1971); second, 5-HP has a relatively short-lived activity in man (DECONTI et al., 1971, 1972). This latter factor results from a difference in the rate of excretion of 5-HP between mice and man, and may well be the significant feature which explains the striking antitumor potency of this agent in rodents, but not in the clinic. Thus, 20 % of a therapeutic dose of 5-HP is excreted in the urine of mice within 24 h (TOMCHICK and MEAD, 1970), whereas man excretes this agent at 2 to 3.5 times the rate occurring in the mouse (DECONTI et al., 1972). This was reflected by (a) a more rapid disappearance of labeled 5-HP from the blood of patients receiving this agent than from mice and (b) an inability to achieve and maintain the degree of blockade of DNA synthesis in leukemic cells that was attained with murine neoplasms (BOOTH et al., 1971; DECONTI et al., 1972). Forty-one to 62 % of the 5-HP excreted in the urine of man was in the form of glucuronide of the unchanged drug, and 3 to 15 % appeared to be a glucuronide of an unknown metabolite (DECONTI et al., 1972). These findings suggest that an α-(*N*)-heterocyclic carboxaldehyde thiosemicarbazone with clinical utility might result by preventing or minimizing *o*-glucuronide formation.

References

AGRAWAL, K. C., BOOTH, B. A., MICHAUD, R. L., SARTORELLI, A. C., MOORE, E. C.: Comparative studies on the action of 5-hydroxy-2-formylpyridine thiosemicarbazone and its selenosemicarbazone, guanylhydrazone and semicarbazone analogs. Proc. Amer. Ass. Cancer Res. **11**, 3 (1970).

AGRAWAL, K. C., BOOTH, B. A., MOORE, E. C., SARTORELLI, A. C.: Studies on the action of possible irreversible inhibitors of ribonucleotide reductase. Proc. Amer. Ass. Cancer Res. **13**, 492 (1972).

AGRAWAL, K. C., BOOTH, B. A., MOORE, E. C., SARTORELLI, A. C.: Potential antitumor agents. 6. Possible irreversible inhibitors of ribonucleoside diphosphate reductase. J. med. Chem. **15**, 1154—1158 (1972a).

AGRAWAL, K. C., BOOTH, B. A., SARTORELLI, A. C.: Potential antitumor agents. I. A series of 5-substituted 1-formylisoquinoline thiosemicarbazones. J. med. Chem. **11**, 700—703 (1968).

AGRAWAL, K. C., BOOTH, B. A., WHEATON, J. R., MOORE, E. C., SARTORELLI, A. C.: Potential antitumor agents. 9. Design of inhibitors of ribonucleotide reductase. Abstracts of Papers, MEDI 45, 164th Am. Chem. Soc. National Meeting, New York City, New York, August (1972b).

AGRAWAL, K. C., CUSHLEY, R. J., LIPSKY, S. R., WHEATON, J. R., SARTORELLI, A. C.: Potential antitumor agents. 5. Methylated α-(*N*)-heterocyclic carboxaldehyde thiosemicarbazones. J. med. Chem. **15**, 192—195 (1972c).

AGRAWAL, K. C., CUSHLEY, R. J., MCMURRAY, W. J., SARTORELLI, A. C.: Potential antitumor agents. IV. 4-Substituted 1-formylisoquinoline thiosemicarbazones. J. med. Chem. **13**, 431—434 (1970a).

AGRAWAL, K. C., SARTORELLI, A. C.: Potential antitumor agents. III. Sodium salts of α-(*N*)-heterocyclic carboxaldehyde thiosemicarbazones. J. pharm. Sci. **57**, 1948—1951 (1968).

AGRAWAL, K.C., SARTORELLI, A.C.: Potential antitumor agents. II. Effects of modifications in the side chain of 1-formylisoquinoline thiosemicarbazone. J. med. Chem. **12**, 771—774 (1969).

BARRY, V.C., CONALTY, M.L., MCCORMICK, J.E., MCELHINNEY, R.S., O'SULLIVAN, J.F.: Anticancer agents. I. Structure-activity relationships in a series of oxypolysaccharide thiosemicarbazide derivatives. Proc. roy. Irish Acad. **64**, 335—354 (1966).

BARRY, V.C., CONALTY, M.L., O'CALLAGHAN, C.N., TWOMEY, D.: Anticancer agents. 3. Synthesis and anticancer activity of some *bis*-thiosemicarbazones and thiosemicarbazides. Proc. roy. Irish Acad. **65**, 309—324 (1967).

BAUER, D.J., SADLER, P.W.: The structure-activity relationships of the antiviral chemotherapeutic activity of isatin β-thiosemicarbazone. Brit. J. Pharmacol. Chemother. **15**, 101—110 (1960).

BHUYAN, B.K., SCHEIDT, L.G., FRASER, T.J.: Cell-cycle phase specificity of antitumor agents. Cancer Res. **32**, 398—407 (1972).

BLANZ, E.J., JR., FRENCH, F.A.: The carcinostatic activity of 5-hydroxy-2-formylpyridine thiosemicarbazone. Cancer Res. **28**, 2419—2422 (1968).

BLANZ, E.J., JR., FRENCH, F.A., DOAMARAL, J.R., FRENCH, D.A.: Carcinostatic activity of thiosemicarbazones of formyl heteroaromatic compounds. VII. 2-Formylpyridine derivatives bearing additional ring substituents. J. med. Chem. **13**, 1124—1130 (1970).

BLOEDOW, C.E.: Phase II. Studies of hydroxyurea (NSC-32065) in adults: miscellaneous tumors. Cancer Chemother. Rep. **40**, 39—41 (1964).

BOOTH, B.A., MOORE, E.C., SARTORELLI, A.C.: Metabolic effects of some tumor-inhibitory pyridine carboxaldehyde thiosemicarbazones. Cancer Res. **31**, 228—234 (1971).

BROCKMAN, R.W., SHADDIX, S., LASTER, W.R., JR., SCHABEL, F.M., JR.: Inhibition of ribonucleotide reductase, DNA synthesis, and L1210 leukemia by guanazole. Cancer Res. **30**, 2358—2368 (1970).

BROCKMAN, R.W., SIDWELL, R.W., ARNETT, G., SHADDIX, S.: Heteroxyclic thiosemicarbazones: correlation between structure, inhibition of ribonucleotide reductase, and inhibition. Proc. Soc. exp. Biol. (N.Y.) **133**, 609—614 (1970a).

BROCKMAN, R.W., THOMSON, J.R., BELL, M.J., SKIPPER, H.E.: Observations on the antileukemic activity of pyridine-2-carboxaldehyde thiosemicarbazone and thiocarbohydrazone. Cancer Res. **16**, 167—170 (1956).

BURCHENAL, J.H., BENVENISTI, D., STEFFA, M., TALLAL, L., TAN, C.: Potentiation of the antileukemic activity of asparaginase. Abtr. 10th International Cancer Congress No. 715, Houston (1970).

COFFEY, J.J., KELLEY, S.A., PALM, P.E., MEAD, J.A.R., KENSLER, C.J.: Pharmacokinetics and metabolism of 5-hydroxypicolinaldehyde thiosemicarbazone (NSC 107392) in the dog. Proc. Amer. Ass. Cancer Res. **13**, 44 (1972).

CREASEY, W.A., AGRAWAL, K.C., CAPIZZI, R.L., STINSON, K.K., SARTORELLI, A.C.: Studies of the antineoplastic activity and metabolism of α-(N)-heterocyclic carboxaldehyde thiosemicarbazones in dogs and mice. Cancer Res. **32**, 565—572 (1972).

CREASEY, W.A., AGRAWAL, K.C., STINSON, K.K., SARTORELLI, A.C.: Antineoplastic effects and metabolism of α-(N)-heterocyclic carboxaldehyde thiosemicarbazones in dogs and mice. Fed. Proc. **29**, 681 (1970).

DECONTI, R.C., CREASEY, W.A., AGRAWAL, K.C., BERTINO, J.R., JATLOW, P.I., MEAD, J.A.R., SARTORELLI, A.C.: Clinical pharmacologic studies with 5-hydroxy-2-formylpyridine thiosemicarbazone (5-HP). Proc. Amer. Ass. Cancer Res. **12**, 58 (1971).

DECONTI, R.C., TOFTNESS, B.R., AGRAWAL, K.C., TOMCHICK, R., MEAD, J.A.R., BERTINO, J.R., SARTORELLI, A.C., CREASEY, W.A.: Clinical and pharmacologic studies with 5-hydroxy-2-formylpyridine thiosemicarbazone. Cancer Res. **32**, 1455—1462 (1972).

ELFORD, H.L., FREESE, M., PASSAMANI, E., MORRIS, H.P.: Ribonucleotide reductase and cell proliferation. J. biol. Chem. **245**, 5228—5233 (1970).

ETCUBANAS, E., TAN, C., WOLLNER, N., BETHUNE, V., KRAKOFF, I.H., BURCHENAL, J.H.: Preliminary clinical trials of 5-hydroxy-2-formylpyridine thiosemicarbazone (5-HP). Proc. Amer. Ass. Cancer Res. **12**, 38 (1971).

FRENCH, F.A., BLANZ, E.J., JR.: The carcinostatic activity of α-(N)-heterocyclic carboxaldehyde thiosemicarbazones. I. Isoquinoline-1-carboxaldehyde thiosemicarbazone. Cancer Res. **25**, 1454—1458 (1965).

FRENCH, F.A., BLANZ, E.J., JR.: The carcinostatic activity of thiosemicarbazones of formyl heteroaromatic compounds. III. Primary correlation. J. med. Chem. **9**, 585—589 (1966).

FRENCH, F.A., BLANZ, E.J., JR.: The carcinostatic activity of α-(N)-heterocyclic carboxaldehyde thiosemicarbazones. II. 3-Hydroxypyridine-2-carboxaldehyde thiosemicarbazone. Cancer Res. **26**, 1638—1640 (1966a).

FRENCH, F. A., BLANZ, E. J., JR.: Carcinostatic hydrazones: some design principles, data, and correlations. Gann 2, 51—57 (1967).
FRENCH, F. A., BLANZ, E. J., JR.: Chemotherapy studies on experimental mouse tumors. X. Cancer Chemother. Rep. 2, 199—235 (1971).
FRENCH, F. A., FREEDLANDER, B. L.: Carcinostatic action of polycarbonyl compounds and their derivatives. IV. Glyoxal *bis*(thiosemicarbazone) and derivatives. Cancer Res. 18, 1290—1300 (1958).
FRENCH, F. A., LEWIS, A. E., SHEENA, A. H., BLANZ, E. J., JR.: Pyrazine-2-carboxaldehyde thiosemicarbazone (PCT), an iron eliminating agent with antitumor activity. Fed. Proc. 24, 402 (1965).
GRINDEY, G. B., MIHICH, E., NICHOL, C. A.: Evaluation of combination chemotherapy *in vivo* and in culture with 1-β-D-arabinofuranosylcytosine and 1-formylisoquinoline thiosemicarbazone. Cancer Res. 32, 522—526 (1972).
GRINDEY, G. B., NICHOL, C. A.: Interactions of drugs inhibiting different steps in the synthesis of DNA. Cancer Res. 32, 527—531 (1972).
HAMRE, D., BERNSTEIN, J., DONOVICK, R.: Activity of *p*-aminobenzaldehyde 3-thiosemicarbazone on vaccinia virus in the chick embryo and in the mouse. Proc. Soc. exp. Biol. (N.Y.) 73, 275—278 (1950).
HENDERSON, E. S., SAMAHA, R. J.: Evidence that drugs in multiple combinations have materially advanced the treatment of human malignancies. Cancer Res. 29, 2272—2280 (1969).
HOCHMAN, H. I., AGRAWAL, K. C., SARTORELLI, A. C.: Biochemical studies of the effects of 1-formylisoquinoline thiosemicarbazone in *Escherichia coli* B. Biochem. Pharmacol. 21, 3213—3221 (1972).
HOCHMAN, H. I., AGRAWAL, K. C., SARTORELLI, A. C.: The localization in *Escherichia coli* B of two enzymatic sites of action by 1-formylisoquinoline thiosemicarbazone (IQ-1) on RNA biosynthetic pathways. Biochem. Pharmacol. 21, 3223—3233 (1972a).
KARON, M., BENEDICT, W. F.: Chromatid breakage: differential effect of inhibitors of DNA synthesis during G_2 phase. Science 178, 62 (1972).
KENNEDY, B. J., YARBRO, J. W.: Metabolic and therapeutic effects of hydroxyurea in chronic myeloid leukemia. J. Amer. med. Assoc. 195, 1038—1043 (1966).
KRAKOFF, I. H.: Clinical and pharmacological effects of hydroxyurea. In: SARTORELLI, A. C., JOHNS, D. G. (Eds.): Handbook of experimental pharmacology. New York: Springer 1974.
LIN, A. J., AGRAWAL, K. C., SARTORELLI, A. C.: Potential antitumor agents. 8. Derivatives of 3- and 5-benzyloxy-2-formylpyridine thiosemicarbazone. J. med. Chem. 15, 615—618 (1972).
MICHAUD, R. L., SARTORELLI, A. C.: Antitumor and metal-coordinating activities of the thiosemicarbazone, semicarbazone and guanylhydrazone of 1-formylisoquinoline. Abstracts of Papers, 155th Amer. Chem. Soc. National Meeting, No. NO54, San Francisco, April (1968).
MIHICH, E.: Modification of tumor regression by immunologic means. Cancer Res. 29, 2345—2350 (1969).
MOERTEL, C. G., REITEMEIER, R. J., HAHN, R. G.: Evaluation of hydroxyurea (NSC-32065) by parenteral infusion. Cancer Chemother. Rep. 49, 27—29 (1965).
MOONEY, P. D., BOOTH, B. A., MOORE, E. C., AGRAWAL, K. C., SARTORELLI, A. C.: Potential antitumor agents. 10. Synthesis of 5-substituted monoalkylamino, dialkylamino and *N*-alkylacetamido 1-formylisoquinoline thiosemicarbazones. Abstracts of Papers, MEDI 46, 164th Am. Chem. Soc. National Meeting, New York City, New York, August (1972).
MOORE, E. C., BOOTH, B. A., SARTORELLI, A. C.: Inhibition of deoxyribonucleotide synthesis by pyridine carboxaldehyde thiosemicarbazones. Cancer Res. 31, 235—238 (1971).
MOORE, E. C., ZEDECK, M. S., AGRAWAL, K. C., SARTORELLI, A. C.: The inhibition of ribonucleoside diphosphate reductase by 1-formylisoquinoline thiosemicarbazone and related compounds. Biochemistry 9, 4492—4498 (1970).
PRUSOFF, W. H.: Recent advances in chemotherapy of viral diseases. Pharmacol. Rev. 19, 209—250 (1967).
ROLLY, H., WINKELMANN, E.: A new thiosemicarbazone active *in vivo* against vaccinia virus. Seventh International Congress on Chemotherapy, Prague, Czechoslovakia, Abstract A-5/13, August (1971).
SARTORELLI, A. C.: Approaches to the combination chemotherapy of transplantable neoplasms. Progr. exp. Tumor Res. (Basel) 6, 228—288 (1965).
SARTORELLI, A. C.: Effect of chelating agents upon the synthesis of nucleic acids and protein: inhibition of DNA synthesis by 1-formylisoquinoline thiosemicarbazone. Biochem. biophys. Res. Communs. 27, 26—32 (1967).
SARTORELLI, A. C.: Some approaches to the therapeutic exploitation of metabolic sites of vulnerability of neoplastic cells. Cancer Res. 29, 2292—2299 (1969).

SARTORELLI, A. C., AGRAWAL, K. C., BOOTH, B. A., MOORE, E. C.: Inhibition of ribonucleotide diphosphate reductase by substituted α-(N)-heterocyclic aldehyde thiosemicarbazones, p. 195. Abstract, Fourth International Congress Pharmacology, Basel, Switzerland (1969).

SARTORELLI, A. C., AGRAWAL, K. C., MOORE, E. C.: Mechanism of inhibition of ribonucleoside diphosphate reductase by α-(N)-heterocyclic aldehyde thiosemicarbazones. Biochem. Pharmacol. **20**, 3119—3123 (1971).

SARTORELLI, A. C., BOOTH, B. A., MOORE, E. C.: Studies on the site of action of pyridine aldehyde thiosemicarbazones. Proc. Amer. Ass. Cancer Res. **10**, 76 (1969).

SARTORELLI, A. C., HILTON, J., BOOTH, B. A., AGRAWAL, K. C., DONNELLY, T. E., JR., MOORE, E. C.: Studies on the mechanism of action of α-(N)-heterocyclic carboxaldehyde thiosemicarbazones. Advanc. Biol. Skin **12**, 271—285 (1972).

SIDWELL, R. W., ARNETT, G., DIXON, G. J., SCHABEL, F. M., JR.: Purine analogs as potential anticytomegalovirus agents. Proc. Soc. exp. Biol. (N. Y.) **131**, 1223—1230 (1969).

SKIPPER, H. E., SCHABEL, F. M., JR., MELLETT, L. B., MONTGOMERY, J. A., WILCO, L. J., LLOYD, H. H., BROCKMAN, R. W.: Implications of biochemical, cytokinetic, pharmacologic, and toxicologic relationships in the design of optimal therapeutic schedules. Cancer Chemother. Rep. **54**, 431—450 (1970).

THOMPSON, R. L., DAVIS, J., RUSSELL, P. B., HITCHINGS, G. H.: Effect of aliphatic oxime and isatin thiosemicarbazones on vaccinia infection in the mouse and in the rabbit. Proc. Soc. exp. Biol. (N. Y.) **84**, 496—499 (1953).

THOMPSON, R. L., MINTON, S. A., JR., OFFICER, J. E., HITCHINGS, G. H.: Effects of heterocyclic and other thiosemicarbazones on vaccinia infection in the mouse. J. Immunol. **70**, 229—234 (1953a).

TOMCHICK, R., MEAD, J. A. R.: A method for the determination of 5-hydroxypyridine-2-carboxaldehyde thiosemicarbazone (NSC-107,392) in biological material. Biochem. Med. **4**, 13—23 (1970).

VENDITTI, J. M., GOLDIN, A.: Drug synergism in antineoplastic chemotherapy. In: GOLDIN, A., HAWKING, F., SCHNITZER, R. J. (Eds.): Advances in chemotherapy, Vol. 1, pp. 387—498. New York: Academic Press 1964.

Chapter 74

1-(*o*-Chlorophenyl)-1-(*p*-Chlorophenyl)-2,2-Dichloroethane (*o,p'*-DDD), an Adrenocorticolytic Agent

JAMES A. STRAW and MICHAEL M. HART

With 1 Figure

Introduction

The compound 1-(*o*-chlorophenyl)-1-(*p*-chlorophenyl)-2,2-dichloroethane, best known by its trivial name *o,p'*-DDD, has been assigned the generic name Mitotane and is available in the United States under the trade name Lysodren.

o,p'-DDD is unique among the anticancer agents in that it demonstrates a high degree of selective toxicity. The fact that it is selectively toxic to the adrenal cortex limits its use as an anticancer agent to the treatment of tumors of adrenal origin. The effects of *o,p'*-DDD on responsive adrenal tumors and on normal adrenocort-

o, p' – DDD

m, p' – DDD

p, p' – DDD

p, p' – DDT

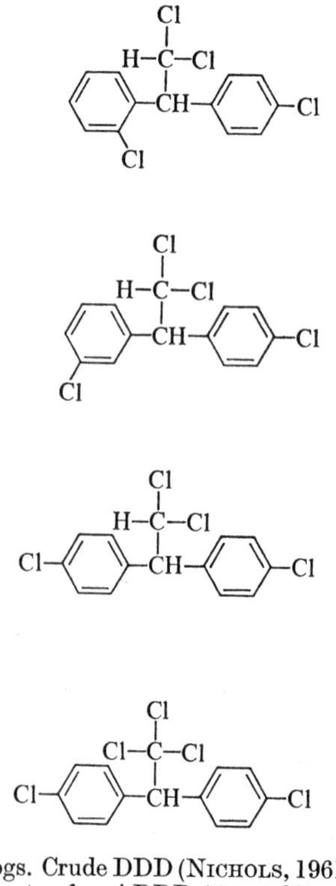

Fig. 1. Structures of *o,p'*-DDD and analogs. Crude DDD (NICHOLS, 1961) consists of primarily *p,p'*-DDD (90 to 92%) and varying amounts of *o,p'*-DDD (5 to 7%) and *m,p'*-DDD (<2%).

ical tissue appear to be qualitatively similar. In brief, these effects consist of inhibition of steroid synthesis followed by cellular death and atrophy of the gland.

As shown in Fig. 1, *o,p'*-DDD is a structural analog of the insecticide DDT [1,1-*bis*-(*p*-chlorophenyl)-2,2,2-trichloroethane] and is one of the constituents of another insecticide "Rothane" or crude DDD. Our knowledge of the adrenocorticolytic action of crude DDD dates to the toxicological studies of NELSON and WOODWARD (1949). Resolution of the constituents of crude DDD was achieved by NICHOLS and HENNIGAR (1956) and by CUETO and BROWN (1958). The question of relative potency of the 3 structural isomers is not resolved; however, comparison of the results of an early clinical trial (ZIMMERMAN et al., 1956) using crude DDD, with subsequent studies using *o,p'*-DDD, strongly suggest that the latter compound has a greater therapeutic index. There is insufficient data on *m,p'*-DDD to make a definitive statement, but both animal and human studies suggest that it is at least as effective as *o,p'*-DDD (NICHOLS et al., 1961).

Pharmacology

A. Absorption

Absorption of DDD from the gastrointestinal tract of the rat, dog (FINNEGAN et al., 1949), and man (MOY, 1961) is poor, thus accounting for the necessity of administering large doses of *o,p'*-DDD orally in order to affect the adrenal cortex. The absorption of *o,p'*-DDD by patients being treated for adrenal cortical carcinoma was estimated by means of stool analysis. At doses of 5 to 15 grams/day, only 30 to 40 % of the drug was absorbed. Blood levels of *o,p'*-DDD and an alkaline-soluble metabolite, probably *o,p'*-DDA [1-(*o*-chlorophenyl)-1-(*p*-chlorophenyl)acetic acid], were determined during and following drug administration. The number of days on therapy ranged from 14 to 210. Serum levels of both substances rose continuously during the treatment period; however, there appeared to be no correlation between blood levels and therapeutic or toxic effects. The highest serum level obtained on oral dosage was 140 µg/ml after 1900 grams of *o,p'*-DDD was given to a ten year old girl who did not respond to therapy. When the drug was discontinued, blood levels fell to an undetectable level within 6 to 9 weeks.

B. Distribution

Following long term oral administration of *o,p'*-DDD to rats and dogs (FINNEGAN et al., 1949) the drug was concentrated in body fat, with high concentrations also being found in the adrenals. A similar distribution of *o,p'*-DDD has been found in humans (MOY, 1961). A large number of tissues was examined in one patient and *o,p'*-DDD was found in all. In biopsy and autopsy material from 8 patients under long term therapy with *o,p'*-DDD, drug concentration was greatest in fat (1270 to 8750 µg/gram wet weight), with moderate amounts in adrenals (20 to 30 % of fat value), and minimal amounts in liver (3 to 5 % of fat value) and brain (1 % of fat value).

DIGIULIO and BEIERWALTES (1968) showed that a radioiodinated derivative of *p,p'*-DDD was concentrated in the adrenal glands of rabbits and dogs 1 to 4 h after intravenous (i.v.) administration. At early time periods the adrenal to fat ratio was 3.8, but by 48 h the drug was redistributed to body fat. This observation, as well as those of MOY (1961), indicate that the adrenocorticolytic action of *o,p'*-DDD cannot be attributed to selective concentration of the drug in adrenocortical tissue.

C. Metabolism

The metabolism of *o,p'*-DDD has not been adequately studied in humans. The elucidation of the biochemical pathway of *o,p'*-DDD metabolism in animals has been a by-product of investigation of the metabolism of DDT (DATTA, 1970). In rats, available evidence suggests that the dichloro-containing carbon of the aliphatic segment of the DDD molecule is oxidized to the organic acid, DDA, through a series of complex steps involving hepatic and renal enzymes (DATTA and NELSON, 1970) and bacteria in the gastrointestinal tract, or both (WEDEMEYER, 1967).

Two groups of investigators were unable to demonstrate *in vitro* *o,p'*-DDD inhibition of adrenal systems, which were dramatically inhibited after *in vivo* administration of the drug (CAZORLA and MONCLOA, 1962; GRADY et al., 1965). These observations suggested that *o,p'*-DDD was metabolized peripherally to an active metabolite which in turn acted on the adrenal. However, a series of experiments by HART and STRAW (1971a) showed that extra-adrenal metabolism was not required for the blocking action of *o,p'*-DDD on ACTH-induced steroidogenesis.

D. Excretion

MOY (1961) found that *o,p'*-DDD itself was not excreted in either urine or bile; a metabolite, probably DDA, was excreted in these fluids. Only about 25 % and 2 % per day of the absorbed dose of *o,p'*-DDD was excreted in the urine and feces, respectively. Thus, considerable amounts of the drug are retained in the body, at least during the initial stages of treatment. Excretion of metabolite(s) continued after discontinuation of the drug. One month after the end of an intensive, intermittent course of *o,p'*-DDD treatment (50 days, 95 grams of drug), urinary excretion of metabolite(s) was half of the peak urinary excretion found during treatment.

Effects on Adrenocortical Tissue

The adrenocorticolytic effects of *o,p'*-DDD are species specific. Dogs are the most responsive, man is apparently less responsive, and other species which have been tested, such as rats, rabbits, and the Rhesus monkey are essentially nonresponsive (NELSON and WOODWARD, 1949).

It is convenient to separate the adrenocorticolytic effects of *o,p'*-DDD into effects on steroid synthesis and effects resulting in cellular death and adrenal necrosis. However, it is possible that the former effect is an early manifestation of a direct cytotoxic effect that eventually results in cellular death. In addition to inhibiting steroid production, *o,p'*-DDD also modifies the peripheral metabolism of corticosteroids, which complicates the interpretation of changes in measured levels of urinary corticosteroids. The effects on peripheral metabolism are discussed in a subsequent section.

A. Histologic and Ultrastructural Changes

NELSON and WOODWARD (1949) reported that the oral administration of crude DDD produced gross atrophy of the adrenals and histologic evidence of degenerative necrosis of the innermost zones of the dog adrenal cortex. Subsequent studies in dogs have shown that these effects of DDD are not due to ACTH deficiency (NICHOLS and GREEN, 1954), and probably result from both (a) a direct cytotoxic action of the drug on the adrenal cortical cell, and (b) the ability of the drug to block the trophic actions of ACTH on the adrenal cell (NICHOLS, 1961). A number of studies in humans have revealed that *o,p'*-DDD is effective in causing atrophy of normal (LUBITZ et al., 1973), hyperactive (SOUTHREN et al., 1961; WALLACE et al., 1961), and tumorous (BERGENSTAL et al., 1960; MOLNAR et al., 1963; FISHER et al., 1963; SOUTHREN et al., 1966; HUTTER and KAYHOE, 1966; LUBITZ et al., 1973) adrenals. Presumably, the cause(s) of the DDD-induced atrophy is the same in man as in the dog.

Marked ultrastructural changes in the dog adrenal cortex appear before histologic changes become evident. As early as 2 h after the i.v. injection of 60 mg/kg of *o,p'*-DDD (HART et al., 1973) and 12 h after the oral administration of 200 mg/kg of crude DDD (KAMINSKY et al., 1962), mitochondria of the cells in the zonas fasciculata-reticularis become swollen, undergo internal dissolution, and eventually rupture. Other cytoplasmic and nuclear membranes are unaltered at these times. Eventually (18 h — i.v. *o,p'*-DDD, and 12 days — oral crude DDD), cells of the inner two zones become shrunken with altered nuclei, altered lipid, and sparse intracellular organelles.

Both histologic and ultramicroscopic evidence suggest that *o,p'*-DDD does not damage the aldosterone-secreting cells of the zona glomerulosa with the same uniformity, severity, and onset of action with which it destroys the glucocorticoid secreting cells of the zonas fasciculata-reticularis. However, long-term treatment of dogs (KAMINSKY et al., 1962) and humans (BERGENSTAL et al., 1960) with *o,p'*-DDD has shown that the zona glomerulosa can be severely damaged, resulting in a poor response to sodium restriction and the necessity of appropriate replacement therapy.

Each of the three structural isomers of DDD has been found to cause similar histologic and ultrastructural changes in the dog adrenal cortex following i.v. administration (HART et al. 1973). However, the rate of onset differs markedly, being most rapid with *m,p'*-DDD, slightly less rapid with *o,p'*-DDD, and much less rapid with *p,p'*-DDD.

B. Effects on Steroid Production

Characterization of the biochemical effects of *o,p'*-DDD on steroid production by the human adrenal is obviously difficult. However, the available information indicates that responses in the dog qualitatively mimic the responses in humans and consist initially of blockade of the response to ACTH followed by a depression in base-line secretion rates.

When cortisol production was measured in dogs using the adrenal vein cannulation technique, i.v. administration of *o,p'*-DDD was shown to depress cortisol secretion rates to 10% of control values within 2 h (HART and STRAW, 1971a). Adrenal slices prepared from glands removed 2 h after i.v. administration of *o,p'*-DDD and incubated *in vitro* did not respond to ACTH, but demonstrated normal baseline levels of steroid production (HART and STRAW, 1971b). In patients with Cushing's disease, TEMPLE et al. (1969) observed that several weeks of treatment with *o,p'*-DDD had little effect on basal rates of cortisol secretion, but that the ability to respond to ACTH was lost. With continued administration of *o,p'*-DDD, baseline rates of secretion are depressed.

The histological evidence that *o,p'*-DDD tends to spare the zona glomerulosa is substantiated by *in vivo* studies of steroid secretion rates. TEMPLE et al. (1969) measured the secretion rates of cortisol and aldosterone in patients with Cushing's disease. Treatment with *o,p'*-DDD reduced initially high cortisol secretion rates to subnormal levels, but had essentially no effect on aldosterone secretion rates. In addition, the treated patients responded to a low sodium diet by increasing aldosterone secretion rates and decreasing urinary excretion of sodium. It should be noted that in these studies the doses of *o,p'*-DDD were regulated to achieve suppression of excess production of cortisol. On the other hand, when *o,p'*-DDD is used in large doses, as in the treatment of adrenocortical cancer, adrenocortical insufficiency has been observed (BERGENSTAL et al., 1960). In addition, prolonged treatment of dogs with *o,p'*-DDD produces death as the result of complete destruction of the adrenal cortex.

From the available evidence it would appear that *o,p'*-DDD produces the following time and dose dependent effects on steroid production by the adrenal cortex.

(1) Blockade of the response to ACTH.
(2) Depression of basal levels of cortisol secretion.
(3) Depression of aldosterone secretion.

If one assumes that successful treatment of adrenocortical cancer requires the destruction of all adrenocortical tissue, it follows that a depression in aldosterone secretion should prove to be the more reliable indicator of a favorable clinical response.

C. Mechanism of Action of *o,p'*-DDD

The exact mechanism by which *o,p'*-DDD exerts its adrenocorticolytic action is not yet fully understood. However, the following studies have led to the definition of the site of inhibition of ACTH-induced steroidogenesis. *o,p'*-DDD does not interfere with ACTH production (NICHOLS, 1961), nor does it act by preventing the formation of cyclic-AMP in response to ACTH (HART and STRAW, 1971c). Furthermore, the step in ACTH-mediated steroidogenesis which is postulated to involve protein synthesis is not affected, as evidenced by the failure of *o,p'*-DDD to inhibit the incorporation of radioactive amino acids into adrenal protein (HART and STRAW, 1971d).

HART and STRAW (1971c) showed that the action of *o,p'*-DDD to block ACTH-induced steroidogenesis was due to inhibition of the intramitochondrial conversion of cholesterol to pregnenolone. Another intramitochondrial step in steroid synthesis, 11-β-hydroxylation, was also inhibited, but consideration of relative reaction rates excluded this as a primary site of action (HART et al., 1971). These workers also showed that the addition of an NADPH-generating system partially reversed the effects of *o,p'*-DDD on these two steps in steroid synthesis. Furthermore, CAZORLA and MONCLOA (1962) showed that the generation of NADPH by glucose-6-phosphate dehydrogenase was depressed in adrenals from *o,p'*-DDD-treated dogs. Therefore, it is possible that the action of *o,p'*-DDD in blocking intramitochondrial hydroxylations is due to a lack of availability of NADPH to the mitochondria. However, the ultrastructural evidence of damage to mitochondria suggests a mitochondrial action of *o,p'*-DDD which is difficult to relate to an effect on cytoplasmic generation of NADPH. Thus, it seems reasonable that *o,p'*-DDD might exert a direct toxic effect on mitochondria, in addition to its action on glucose-6-phosphate dehydrogenase.

MARTZ and STRAW (1973) reported that *o,p'*-DDD caused extensive damage to several components of the adrenal electron transport system. This damage consisted of a loss of microsomal and mitochondrial cytochrome P 450 in adrenals removed from dogs 3 h following treatment with *o,p'*-DDD (60 mg/kg, i.v.). These changes in P 450 were accompanied by an even greater loss of heme, in addition to a reduction of microsomal protein concentration. GREENE et al. (1969) have reported that CCl_4 produced similar effects in rat liver. This similarity suggests that the adrenotoxicity of DDD may be related to its metabolism in the adrenal to a reactive intermediate, in a manner similar to the hepatic activation of CCl_4 into a hepatotoxic substance.

Extra-Adrenal Effects

A. Effects on Steroid Metabolism

The reductive pathway for steroid metabolism is accomplished by enzymes present in the soluble fraction of a liver homogenate. In man, the products of the reductive pathway are tetrahydrocortisol (THF), allotetrahydrocortisol (ATHF), and tetrahydrocortisone (THE). These three products are conjugated with glucuronic acid and normally constitute about 90% of the urinary 17-hydroxycorticoids (17-OH—CS). Routine clinical laboratory determination of urinary 17-OH—CS is performed by hydrolysis with beta-glucuronidase followed by extraction into dichloromethane and measurement as Porter-Silber chromogens. An alternate pathway for steroid metabolism is the oxidative pathway which is accomplished by hepatic microsomal enzymes. This enzyme system may be part of the microsomal enzyme system which is involved in drug metabolism (CONNEY et al., 1967). The major product of the oxidative pathway is the 17-OH—CS,6-β-hydroxycortisol (6-β-F). This polar metabolite is not extracted by dichloromethane and consequently is not measured in routine determinations of urinary 17-OH—CS (BLEDSOE et al., 1964).

Therapy with *o,p'*-DDD alters the relative amounts of cortisol metabolized by the two pathways. BLEDSOE et al. (1964) and, later, SOUTHREN et al. (1966) showed that the apparent decrease in urinary 17-OH—CS seen during the first weeks of *o,p'*-DDD therapy could be accounted for by an almost quantitative increase in urinary 6-β-F. These changes occurred at a time when cortisol secretion rates and plasma cortisol levels were unchanged from pretreatment values. In addition, the half-life of cortisol was not altered. FUKUSHIMA et al. (1971) showed that this action of *o,p'*-DDD to increase urinary excretion of 6-β-F is not due to its secretion by the adrenal, but is secondary to enhanced peripheral production from cortisol. *o,p'*-DDD has been shown to induce hepatic drug metabolizing enzymes in several species; and phenobarbital, a typical inducer of hepatic drug metabolism, increases the production of 6-β-F in man (BURSTEIN and KLAIBER, 1965). Thus, it would appear that the effects of *o,p'*-DDD on the metabolism of cortisol may be explained by the induction of hepatic microsomal enzymes involved in the oxidative pathway.

Because of the effects of *o,p'*-DDD on cortisol metabolism it is obvious that determination of urinary 17-OH—CS by the usual method does not give an accurate indication of the adrenal effects of the drug. BLEDSOE et al. (1964) have described a modification of the extraction procedure which permits the measurement of total urinary 17-OH—CS, including 6-β-F. A decrease in urinary 17-OH—CS measured by the modified technique should prove to be a better indicator of a favorable disease response to *o,p'*-DDD.

B. Effects on Drug Metabolism

The effects of *o,p'*-DDD on drug metabolism have not been studied in man. In animals the effects are species specific, and in part are secondary to adrenal effects. Chronic administration to rats or guinea pigs, at doses which have no effects on adrenal function, induces hepatic microsomal enzymes which metabolize a variety of drugs (STRAW et al., 1965; KUPFER and PEETS, 1966). Treatment of dogs with adrenocorticolytic doses of *o,p'*-DDD results in a decreased rate of metabolism of pentobarbital, secobarbital, and phenylbutazone (AZARNOFF et al., 1966). This effect is secondary to the adrenocorticolytic effects, since it can be prevented by the concomitant administration of glucocorticoids. In contrast to chronic administration of *o,p'*-DDD, acute administration to either rats or dogs results in generalized inhibition of drug metabolism. *In vitro* studies indicate that this is the result of competitive inhibition of drug metabolizing enzymes and occurs only at relatively high concentrations of *o,p'*-DDD (MARTZ and STRAW, 1972).

In summary, human studies which indicate that *o,p'*-DDD induces the oxidative pathway for steroid metabolism suggest that a similar increase would occur in drug metabolizing enzymes. However, studies in dogs show that both large concentrations of *o,p'*-DDD in the liver, as well as adrenal suppression, result in a decreased ability to metabolize barbiturates. Caution in the use of barbiturates in patients being treated with *o,p'*-DDD is recommended. Clinical studies of drug metabolism in such patients are required before more positive guidelines can be provided.

C. Effects on Thyroxine Binding Globulin

DANOWSKI et al. (1964) observed that administration of *o,p'*-DDD resulted in a decrease in serum protein bound iodine (PBI). MARSHALL and TOMPKINS (1968) showed that this effect could be explained by competition of *o,p'*-DDD with thyroxine for binding sites on thyroxine binding globulin. Although patients treated with *o,p'*-DDD had PBI levels normally associated with hypothyroidism, there was no clinical evidence of hypothyroidism, and thyroidal uptake and binding of ^{131}I was normal. Thus, it would appear that thyroid function is normal in patients treated with *o,p'*-DDD and that plasma levels of "free" thyroxine are not depressed.

Clinical Studies

Clinical trial of *o,p'*-DDD has been attempted in five conditions: adrenocortical carcinoma, Cushing's disease (TEMPLE et al., 1969), interstitial cell carcinoma of the testis (ABELSON et al., 1966; TAMONEY and NARIEGA, 1969), malignant lipid cell tumor of the ovary (LIPSETT et al., 1970), and steroid-dependent carcinomas of the breast (WEISENFELD et al., 1964). However, extensive trials have been completed only against the adrenocortical carcinoma and to a lesser extent in Cushing's disease. Only those involving the former will be discussed here.

BERGENSTAL et al. (1960) reported that the administration of *o,p'*-DDD to patients with functioning adrenocortical carcinoma resulted in significant regression of measurable metastatic lesions and a reduction of the abnormally high levels of urinary steroids. Based on these data, the United States National Cancer Institute initiated studies by supplying *o,p'*-DDD to selected investigators for use in patients with this disease. The results of these studies have established the clinical usefulness of this drug.

HUTTER and KAYHOE (1966a, b) described the clinical features and the results of the treatment of 138 patients with adrenocortical carcinoma with *o,p'*-DDD. At the time of their report, which included the period up to June, 1965, the results of treatment of 48 patients with *o,p'*-DDD had already been cited in the literature, and were compared to those from the 138 patients in their study. The second and most recent report of this study covers the period from June, 1965 through January, 1969, during which time 115 additional patients were treated (LUBITZ et al., 1973). Isolated case reports have also appeared in the literature since 1965 (SAKAUCHI et al., 1969; COPE, 1969).

A general description of the patient population, drug treatment, clinical results, and side effects described in these studies follows.

A. Patient Population

The disease incidence-population ratio of adrenocortical carcinoma is approximately 2:1 million. It seems to occur at all ages and to reflect the racial composition of the population. It is not clear if there is a sex-related difference in incidence; however, in the two United States National Cancer Institute-sponsored studies, females predominated 2:1. Tumors occurred almost exclusively in one adrenal. Metastases were most frequent in adjacent structures, but were also commonly found in the lungs and liver. The largest proportion of patients had a functional adrenal malignancy as indicated by excessive urinary steroid excretion and/or physical symptoms resulting from adrenal steroid synthesis. The exact nature of the symptoms depends on the type of hormone produced in excess. Cushing's syndrome (52 %), virilization (35 %), and feminization (11 %) were observed. A few patients (6 %) had nonfunctional adrenal neoplasms. The median time from diagnosis to initiation of *o,p'*-DDD treatment was 7 months in the most recent large study, with a range from less than one week to 18 years. In all cases inoperable metastatic malignancy was considered the indication for *o,p'*-DDD therapy.

B. Drug Treatment

The dosage form of *o,p'*-DDD most commonly used was a 0.5 gram scored tablet administered orally. Two other techniques of administration have been attempted, but sufficient data are not available to evaluate their effectiveness. Brown et al. (1959) dissolved crude DDD in oil and administered it orally, and Moy (1961) dissolved *o,p'*-DDD in a phospholipid emulsion for injection, i.v. Generally, the least toxicity following oral administration was encountered when the patients were started on divided daily doses of from 1 to 6 grams. The dosage was increased until significant adverse reaction occurred. In the United States National Cancer Institute study 72 % of the 250 patients received 5 to 10 grams/day as maximum dosage with doses ranging from 0.5 to 20 grams/day. The duration of treatment with *o,p'*-DDD was quite variable, ranging from 21 days to 36 months. Lubitz et al. (1971) reported that 16 and 4 % of the 115 patients received *o,p'*-DDD for more than 1 and 2 years, respectively, as of the data cutoff date of January, 1969. Drug treatment was terminated when the tumor regressed, when no clinical benefit could be determined over a period of months, or when severe adverse drug reactions were encountered.

C. Clinical Results

The effectiveness of *o,p'*-DDD in treating adrenocortical carcinoma was evaluated with respect to measurable disease response (MDR), measurable steroid response (MSR), clinical response, and mean survival time. MDR refers to a quantitative estimate of a reduction in tumor size by the investigator, involving either palpation of a metastatic mass, or an x-ray for estimate of tumor size. MSR means a decrease during treatment of more than 30 % in the urinary steroid excretion from pretreatment values. Clinical response refers to an overall improvement related to *o,p'*-DDD therapy regardless of other parameters. A compilation of available information concerning the effect of *o,p'*-DDD on these parameters is

Table 1. *Responsiveness and toxicity of o,p'-DDD in adrenocortical carcinoma*

Category	Literature 1962—1963 48 patients	Hutter and Kayhoe 1960—1965 138 patients	Lubitz et al. 1965—1969 115 patients
Measurable disease response			
% responders	37	34	61
onset — mean		9 weeks	8 weeks
— median		6 weeks	4 weeks
— range		2—28 weeks	2—76 weeks
duration — mean		10.2 months	10.3 months
— median		7 months	6 months
— range		1.5—46[a] months	1—36[a] months
% responders with steroid drop		100	94
Measurable steroid response			
% responders	70	72	89
onset		within 30 days	17 days
duration		4.8 months	
% responders with measurable disease response		42	
Clinical response — %		35	54
Mean survival time			
non-responders			2.4 months
responders			10.3[a] months
Side effects			
All types — %	93	88	83
type — %			
gastrointestinal	93	78	74
neuromuscular	49	37	60
dermal	17	16	13
miscellaneous	2	15	21

[a] This figure indicates the duration disease response as of the date of paper preparation. A number of patients have lived for longer periods (years) in apparent tumor-free states.

shown in Table 1. For a number of reasons, measurable disease response appears to be a more accurate indicator of clinical benefit to the patient than a measurable steroid response. First, the data concerning MDR is not similar to that of the MSR. Fewer patients showed a disease response than showed a steroid decrease. Also, a disease response occurred later and lasted longer than a steroid response. Furthermore, a good steroid response occurred in all patients who were measurable disease responders; however, the converse was not true. MDR was approximately the same in steroid responders as in the entire drug tested group. Investigation of individual patient records revealed that the same patients who had a measurable disease response had a high clinical response. On the other hand, a steroid response could not be correlated with increased survival, did not indicate a measurable disease response and was associated with a lower clinical response rate than was measurable disease response. It is likely that a steroid response primarily reflects the extra-adrenal action of *o,p'*-DDD to alter hepatic steroid catabolism. The direct actions of *o,p'*-DDD on the adrenal undoubtedly cause regression of tumor mass and decreased steroid synthesis. This accounts for the observation that disease response is always accompanied by a steroid response.

It is particularly encouraging that 61 % of all patients treated with *o,p'*-DDD in the recent United States National Cancer Institute-sponsored study had a measurable disease response. Fifty-six percent of all patients in this study were still living at the data cutoff date. Age, site of tumor, and location of metastases did not appear to be factors which influence the chances of a beneficial effect.

D. Side Effects and Toxicity

Under the conditions of use which involved increasing the dose until toxicity appeared, a very high percentage of patients showed at least one side effect or toxicity. Only 7 to 17 % of all patients had no toxicity attributable to *o,p'*-DDD. Toxicity was of three general forms: gastrointestinal (74 to 93 %), usually anorexia, nausea, and vomiting; neuromuscular (37 to 60 %), usually central nervous system depression manifested as lethargy and somnolence; and dermal (13 to 17 %), generally a skin rash. This drug demonstrates a remarkable lack of hepatic and bone marrow toxicity.

In some cases, the toxicity disappeared while the patients were maintained on the drug, but usually the dose of drug was decreased or stopped temporarily. Although about 90 % of the patients had the first onset of toxicity at a dose level of 10 grams/day or less, a full 50 % did not develop toxicity until they did achieve 10 grams/day. Thus, a significant proportion of patients probably could receive greater amounts and, indeed, a number of patients have received considerably higher dosages.

References

ABELSON, D., BULASCHENKO, H., TROMMER, P. R., VALDES-DAPENA, A.: Malignant interstitial-cell tumor of the testis treated with *o,p'*-DDD. Metabolism **15**, 242—256 (1966).

AZARNOFF, D. L., GRADY, H. J., SVOBODA, D. J.: The effect of DDD on barbiturate and steroid-induced hypnosis in the dog and rat. Biochem. Pharmacol. **15**, 1985—1993 (1966).

BERGENSTAL, D. M., HERTZ, R., LIPSETT, M. B., MOY, R. H.: Chemotherapy of adrenocortical cancer with *o,p'*-DDD. Ann. int. Med. **53**, 672—682 (1960).

BLEDSOE, T., ISLAND, D. P., KEY, R. L., LIDDLE, G. W.: An effect of *o,p'*-DDD on the extra-adrenal metabolism of cortisol in man. J. clin. Endocrinol. **24**, 1303—1311 (1964).

BROWN, J. H. U., PREEDY, J. R. K., BROWN, C. H., HALLMAN, B. L.: Action of an adrenocorticolytic drug in man. Lancet **I**, 1208—1209 (1959).

BURSTEIN, S., KLAIBER, E. L.: Phenobarbital-induced increase in 6β-hydroxycortisol excretion: clue to its significance in human urine. J. clin. Endocrinol. **25**, 293—296 (1965).

CAZORLA, A., MONCLOA, F.: Action of 1,1,dichloro-2-*p*-chlorophenyl-ethane on dog adrenal cortex. Science **136**, 47 (1962).

CONNEY, A. H., WELCH, R. W., KUNTZMAN, R.: Effects of pesticide on drug and steroid metabolism. Clin. Pharmacol. Ther. **8**, 2—10 (1967).

COPE, C. L.: The case of the persistent pituitary. Brit. med. J. **2**, 557—560 (1969).

CUETO, C., BROWN, J. H. A.: Biological studies on an adrenocorticolytic agent and the isolation of the active components. Endocrinology **62**, 334—339 (1958).

DANOWSKI, T. S., SARVER, M. E., MOSES, C., BONESSI, J. V.: *o,p'*-DDD therapy in Cushing's syndrome and in obesity with cushingoid changes. Amer. J. Med. **37**, 235—250 (1964).

DATTA, P. R.: *In vivo* detoxification of *p,p'*-DDT via *p,p'*-DDE to *p,p'*-DDA in rats. Indust. Med. **39**, 190—194 (1970).

DATTA, P. R., NELSON, M. J.: *p,p'*-DDT detoxication by isolated perfused rat liver and kidney. Indust. Med. **39**, 195—198 (1970).

DIGIULIO, W., BEIERWALTES, W. H.: Tissue localization studies of a DDD analog. J. nucl. Med. **9**, 634—637 (1968).

FINNEGAN, J. K., HAAG, H. B., LARSON, P. S.: Tissue distribution and elimination of DDD and DDT following oral administration to dogs and rats. Proc. Soc. exp. Biol. (N. Y.) **72**, 357—360 (1949).

FISHER, D. A., PANOS, T. C., MELBY, J. C.: Therapy of adrenocortical cancer with *o,p'*-DDD in two children. J. clin. Endocrinol. **23**, 218—221 (1963).

FUKUSHIMA, D. K., BRADLOW, H. L., HELLMAN, L.: Effects of *o,p'*-DDD on cortisol and 6-beta-hydroxycortisol secretion and metabolism in man. J. clin. Endocrinol. **32**, 192—200 (1971).

GRADY, H. J., AZARNOFF, D. L., CREAGER, R., HUFFMAN, D. H., NICHOLS, J.: Specificity of enzyme inhibition by DDD. Proc. Soc. exp. Biol. (N.Y.) **119**, 238—241 (1965).

GREENE, F. E., STRIPP, B., GILLETTE, J. R.: The effect of carbon tetrachloride on heme components and ethylmorphine metabolism in rat liver microsomes. Biochem. Pharmacol. **18**, 1531—1533 (1969).

HART, M. M., REAGAN, R. L., ADAMSON, R. H.: The effect of isomers of DDD on the ACTH-induced steroid output, histology and ultrastructure of the dog adrenal cortex. Toxicol. Appl. Pharmacol. **24**, 101—113 (1973).

HART, M. M., STRAW, J. A.: Effect of 1-(*o*-chlorophenyl)-1-(*p*-chlorophenyl)-2,2-dichloroethane on adrenocorticotropic hormone-induced steroidogenesis in various preparations *in vitro* of dog adrenal cortex. Biochem. Pharmacol. **20**, 1679—1688 (1971a).

HART, M. M., STRAW, J. A.: Effect of 1-(*o*-chlorophenyl)-1-(*p*-chlorophenyl)-2,2-dichloroethane *in vivo* on baseline and adrenocorticotropic hormone-induced steroid production in dog adrenal slices. Biochem. Pharmacol. **20**, 1689—1691 (1971b).

HART, M. M., STRAW, J. A.: Studies on the site of action of *o,p'*-DDD in the dog adrenal cortex. I. Inhibition of ACTH-mediated pregnenolone synthesis. Steroids **17**, 559—574 (1971c).

HART, M. M., STRAW, J. A.: Effects of 1-(*o*-chlorophenyl)-1-(*p*-chlorophenyl)-2,2-dichloroethane and puromycin on adrenocorticotropic hormone-induced steroidogenesis and on amino acid incorporation in slices of dog adrenal cortex. Biochem. Pharmacol. **20**, 257—263 (1971d).

HART, M. M., SWACKHAMER, E. S., STRAW, J. A.: Studies on the site of action of *o,p'*-DDD in the dog adrenal cortex. II. TPNH- and corticosteroid precursor-stimulation of *o,p'*-DDD inhibited steroidogenesis. Steroids **17**, 575—586 (1971).

HUTTER, A. M., KAYHOE, D. E.: Adrenal cortical carcinoma — Clinical features of 138 patients. Amer. J. Med. **41**, 572—580 (1966a).

HUTTER, A. M., KAYHOE, D. E.: Adrenal cortical carcinoma — Results of treatment with *o,p'*-DDD in 138 patients. Amer. J. Med. **41**, 581—592 (1966b).

KAMINSKY, N., LUSE, S., HARTROFT, P.: Ultrastructure of adrenal cortex of the dog during treatment with DDD. J. nat. Cancer Inst. **29**, 127—159 (1962).

KUPFER, D., PEETS, L.: The effects of *o,p'*-DDD on cortisol and hexobarbital metabolism. Biochem. Pharmacol. **15**, 573—581 (1966).

LIPSETT, M. B., KIRSCHNER, M. A., WILSON, H., BARDIN, C. W.: Malignant lipid cell tumor of the ovary. Clinical, biochemical and etiologic considerations. J. clin. Endocrinol. **30**, 336—344 (1970).

LUBITZ, J. A., FREEMAN, L., OKUN, R.: Mitotane use in inoperable adrenal cortical carcinoma. J. Amer. med. Ass. **233**, 1109—1112 (1973).

MARSHALL, J. A., TOMPKINS, L. S.: Effect of *o,p'*-DDD and similar compounds on thyroxine binding globulin. J. clin. Endocrinol. **24**, 386—392 (1968).

MARTZ, F., STRAW, J. A.: Effects of Mitotane (*o,p'*-DDD) on hepatic drug metabolism in dogs. Fed. Proc. **31**, 581 (1972).

MARTZ, F., STRAW, J. A.: Mitotane decreases adrenal cortical heme and P_{450}. Fed. Proc. **32**(3), 734 (1973).

MOLNAR, G. D., MATTOX, V. R., BAHN, R. C.: Clinical and therapeutic observations in adrenal cancer. A report on 7 patients treated with *o,p'*-DDD. Cancer **16**, 259—268 (1963).

MOY, R. H.: Studies of the pharmacology of *o,p'*-DDD in man. J. Lab. clin. Med. **58**, 296—304 (1961).

NELSON, A. A., WOODWARD, G.: Severe adrenal cortical atrophy (cytotoxic) and hepatic damage produced in dogs by feeding 2,2-*bis*(para-chlorophenyl)-1,1-dichloroethane (DDD or TDE). Arch. Path. **48**, 387—394 (1949).

NICHOLS, J.: Studies on an adrenal cortical inhibitor. In: MOON, H. D. (Ed.): The adrenal cortex. Int. Acad. of Path. Monograph. New York: Harper and Brothers 1961.

NICHOLS, J., GREEN, H. D.: Effect of DDD treatment on metabolic response of dogs to ACTH injection. Amer. J. Physiol. **176**, 374—376 (1954).

NICHOLS, J., HENNIGAR, G.: Studies on DDD, 2,2-*bis*-(parachlorophenyl)-1,1-dichloroethane. Exp. Med. Surg. **15**, 310—316 (1957).

NICHOLS, J., PRESTLEY, W. F., NICHOLS, F.: Effects of *m,p'*-DDD in a case of adrenal corticol carcinoma. Curr. Ther. Res. **3**, 266—271 (1961).

SAKAUCHI, N., KUMAOKA, S., NARUKE, T., ABE, O., KUSAMA, M., TAKATANI, O.: A case of adrenocortical cancer treated with *o,p'*-DDD. Endocrinology **16**, 287—290 (1969).

SOUTHREN, A. L., TOCHIMOTO, S., STROM, L., RATUSCHNI, A., ROSS, R., GORDON, G.: Remission in Cushing's syndrome with *o,p'*-DDD. J. clin. Endocrinol. **26**, 268—278 (1966).

Southren, A. L., Weisenfeld, S., Laufer, A., Goldner, M. G.: Effect of *o,p'*-DDD in a patient with Cushing's syndrome. J. clin. Endocrinol. **21**, 201—208 (1961).

Straw, J. A., Waters, I. W., Fregly, M. J.: Effect of *o,p'*-DDD on hepatic metabolism of pentobarbital in rats. Proc. Soc. exp. Biol. **118**, 391—394 (1965).

Tamoney, H. J., Jr., Noriega, A.: Malignant interstitial cell tumor of the testis. Cancer **24**, 547—551 (1969).

Temple, T. E., Jones, D. J., Liddle, G. W., Dexter, R. N.: Treatment of Cushing's disease. Correction of hypercortisolism by *o,p'*-DDD without induction of aldosterone deficiency. N. Engl. J. Med. **281**, 801—805 (1969).

Wallace, E. Z., Silverstein, J. N., Villadolid, L. S., Weisenfeld, S.: Cushing's syndrome due to adrenocortical hyperplasia. N. Engl. J. Med. **265**, 1088—1093 (1961).

Wedemeyer, G.: Dechlorination of 1,1,1-trichloro-2,2-*bis*(*p*-chlorophenyl)ethane by *Aerobacter aerogenes*. Appl. Microbiol. **15**, 569—574 (1967).

Weisenfeld, S., Hecht, A., Leichter, D., Goldner, M.: *o,p'*-DDD in the treatment of advanced mammary carcinoma. Cancer **17**, 1258—1266 (1964).

Zimmerman, B., Bloch, H. L., Williams, W. L., Hitchcock, C. R., Hoelscher, B.: The effects of DDD [1,1-dichloro-2,2-*bis*(*p*-chlorophenyl)ethane] on the human adrenal. Cancer **9**, 940—948 (1956).

Chapter 75

The Phthalanilides

DAVID W. YESAIR and CHARLES J. KENSLER

With 2 Figures

Introduction

A decade ago, HIRT and BERCHTOLD (1962) described a new class of compounds, the phthalanilides, which they regarded as "phosphatide blockers". These investigators employed a simple biophysical model: lecithin dissolved in carbon tetrachloride promotes the transport of cationic dyes from an aqueous solution into the lipid phase. They showed that the phthalanilides maximally inhibited dye transfer when at least two strongly basic groups are connected by several coplanar rings and by carbonamide groups. When several derivatives of this series were shown to have activity against an experimental neoplasm, a large number of these structurally related compounds was synthesized (HIRT and BERCHTOLD, 1962; ATWELL and CAIN, 1967, 1968; RAUEN et al., 1965, 1966). See Fig. 1 for structures.

Tumor-Inhibitory Activity and Toxicity

Many phthalanilide congeners were shown to have potent activity against a broad spectrum of murine leukemias and lymphomas (BENNETT, 1965; BURCHENAL et al., 1962; PITTILLO et al., 1962; SCHEPARTZ et al., 1962; VENDITTI et al., 1962; KENSLER, 1963; LAW, 1962; ATWELL and CAIN 1967, 1968). The chemotherapeutic activity of the phthalanilides relative to classical agents is noteworthy (WODINSKY, personal communication): for example, the phthalanilides, NSC 60339 and NSC 57153, were active against 19 of 20 experimental tumors, a result superior to that found for methotrexate (17 of 19), for 6-mercaptopurine (6 of 19), and for cytoxan (15 of 19). In addition, many phthalanilides were active against several microorganisms (THAYER and GORDON, 1962; PINE et al., 1963; RAUEN et al., 1965, 1966), but like most chemotherapeutic agents, resistance to them developed. Interestingly, experimental vinca alkaloid-resistant tumors were cross-resistant to the phthalanilides (KENSLER, 1963; BURCHENAL et al., 1963; BURCHENAL and LYMAN, 1963; HUTCHISON, 1965).

In clinical trials, several phthalanilides were evaluated in man after other therapeutic efforts with vinca alkaloids and other drugs had failed. These new agents were inactive, perhaps owing to the prior development of resistant cells, but one of the terephthalanilides did produce objective response against Burkitt's lymphoma (OETTGEN et al., 1963). Early clinical toxicity such as oculomotor paralysis and thrombophlebitis with 2-chloro-4′,4″-di(2-imidazolin-2-yl)terephthalanide dihydrochloride (NSC 38280) limited the clinical evaluation of this group of compounds against human neoplasms (LOUIS, 1962; LYMAN et al., 1962; OETTGEN et al., 1963; LOUIS et al., 1963). It is noteworthy that the three clinically evaluated

NSC No.	Molecular weight of base	Name and structure of base
35843	452	4′,4″-Di(2-Imidazolin-2-yl)Terephthalanilide Dihydrochloride 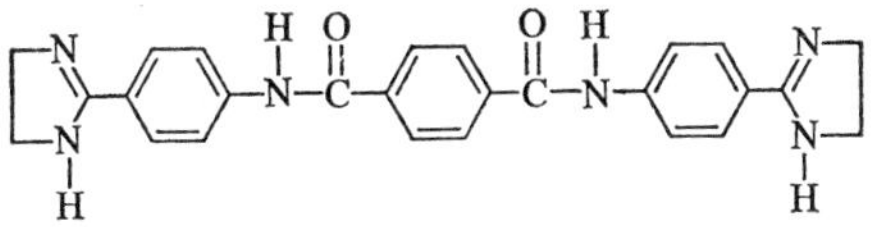
60339	487	2-Chloro-4′, 4″-Di(2-Imidazolin-2-yl)Terephthalanilide 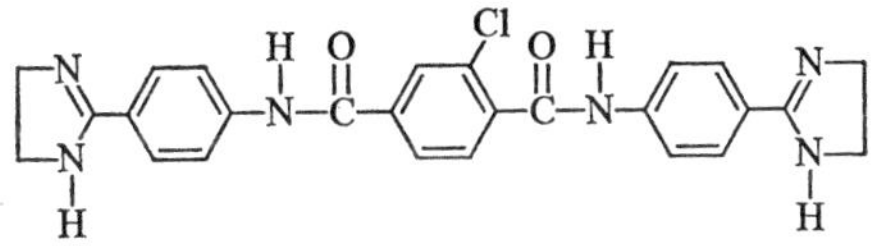
38280	487	Dihydrochloride of NSC 60339
50469	467	2-Amino-4′, 4″-Di(2-Imidazolin-2-yl)Terephthalanilide Dihydrochloride 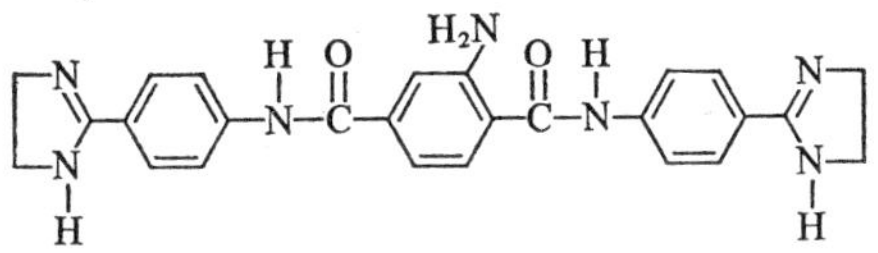
57153	480	4′,4″-*Bis*(1,4,5,6-Tetrahydro-2-pyrimidinyl)Terephthalanilide Dihydrochloride 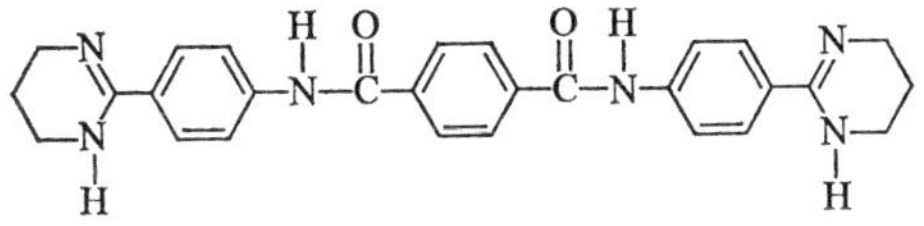
57155	426	*N′*, *N″*-*Bis*[*p*(*N′*-Methylamidino)Phenyl]Therephthalamidine Tetrahydrochloride 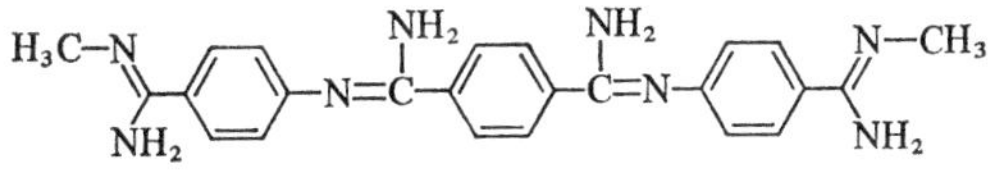
57143	182	1,1′-*p*-Phenylene *Bis*[3-(*m*-2-Imidazolin-2-yl phenyl)]Urea Dihydrochloride 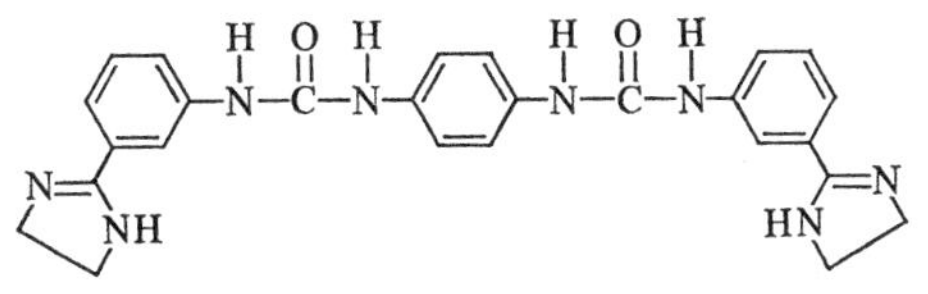
57142	482	1,1′-*m*-Phenylene *Bis*[3-(*p*-2-Imidazolin-2-yl phenyl)]Urea Dihydrochloride 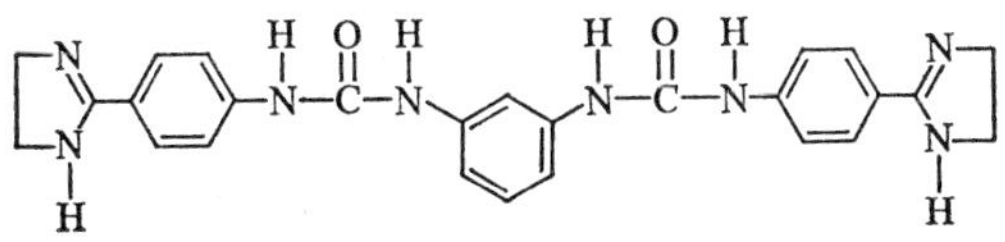

Fig. 1. Structures of terephthalanilides and related compounds

drugs were ones that produced extensive thrombi and emboli in the hamster cheek pouch assay (York et al., 1963). Other phthalanilides which produced negligible thromboembolism in this experimental system have not been evaluated clinically.

Other side effects encountered with the phthalanilides were impairment of renal and hepatic functions. It has been found that low doses of several of these agents produced renal damage which was not apparent until several weeks after the last dose (Kensler et al., 1965). The delayed and/or chronic renal toxicity seen with several phthalanilides in animals was also apparent in man (see personal communications in Kensler et al., 1965). However, several other phthalanilides looked promising, notably NSC 60339 [2-chloro-4′,4″-di(2-imidazolin-2-yl)terephthalanilide] and *N*′,*N*″-*bis*[*p*(*N*′-methylamidino)phenyl]-terephthalamidine tetrahydrochloride (NSC 57155), which have not shown this effect in the clinic or in animals. In general, it was found that those organs which accumulated the highest concentrations of phthalanilide are affected adversely and that the principal target organs have been liver, kidney, and oculomotor muscles.

Some effort was made to minimize the toxic effects of the phthalanilides without sacrificing chemotherapeutic activity. Burchenal and coworkers showed that the acute and chronic toxicity of several phthalanilides can be prevented by complexing the phthalanilides with sulfonic and phosphoric compounds, but all these agents, except suramin, also blocked the antileukemic activity of the phthalanilides in mice (Burchenal et al., 1965a, b, c). Suramin, a polysulfonate compound, reduced acute, chronic, and delayed toxicity without preventing the chemotherapeutic efficacy of three terephthalanilides (Burchenal et al., 1965a, b, c). It was subsequently shown (Yesair et al., 1968) that the administration of suramin does not affect the uptake of 4′,4″-*bis*(1,4,5,6-tetrahydro-2-pyrimidinyl)terephthalanilide dihydrochloride (NSC 57153), a tetrahydropyrimidinyl terephthalanilide, in P815 cells, but does result in lower drug concentrations in the kidney and liver of tumor-bearing mice. The drug in these tissues is complexed primarily with lipids as in P815 cells. Since suramin itself is not deposited in any particular tissue, it probably enhances the excretion of drug, as a suramin-complex before deposition of NSC 57153 as a lipid complex in tissues. Therefore, better scheduling of drug and suramin administration may enhance their complex formation *in vivo* and, thus, may increase excretion of the drug prior to its deposition in tissues. Such enhancement of drug excretion may be of value in improving the therapeutic value of the phthalanilides.

Metabolism

Gellhorn et al. (1964) first suggested that 2-amino-4′,4″-di(2-imidazolin-2-yl)terephthalanilide dihydrochloride (NSC 50469) may be converted *in vivo* into an active form. Booth et al. (1964) searched for metabolites hoping that they would be less toxic than the unchanged drug, but were largely unsuccessful. They did note, however, that the phthalanilide complexed with lipid. Investigation of the metabolism of another imidazole terephthalanilide (NSC 60339) in animals and the amidine congener (NSC 57155) in man indicate that these drugs are not biologically modified (Booth et al., 1964; Kreis et al., 1965; Rogers et al., 1962, 1966). There is some evidence that the deschloroimidazole analog (NSC 35943) is metabolized (Sivak et al., 1964) and that the ureido congeners (NSC 57142, NSC 57143) undergo nonbiological degradation (Rogers et al., 1963). A report has been presented (Yesair et al., 1969) showing that the imidazole terephthalanilide (NSC 60339) is extensively metabolized in man. High-resolution mass spectrometry data indicate that the metabolites contain 2-chloroterephthalic acid, *p*-aminobenzoic

Infused drug

IMA-CP*-IMA

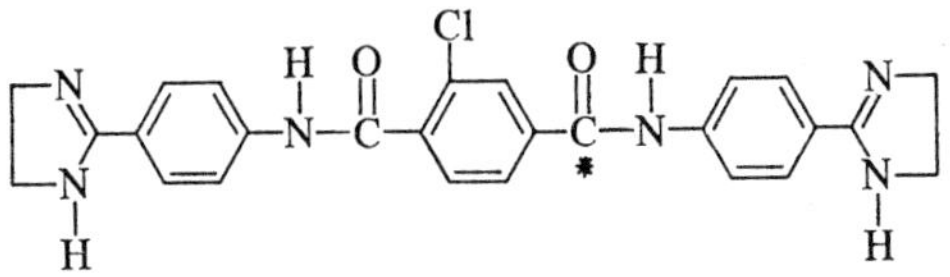

Probable Anionic Metabolites

IMA-CP*

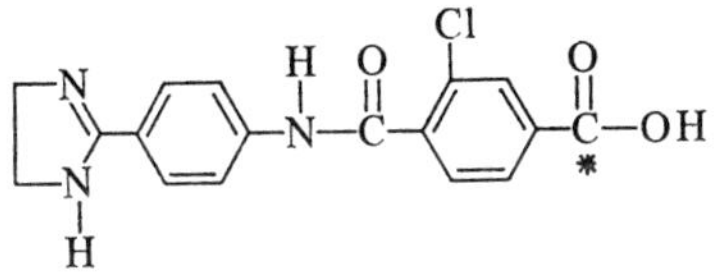

IMA-CP*-ABA

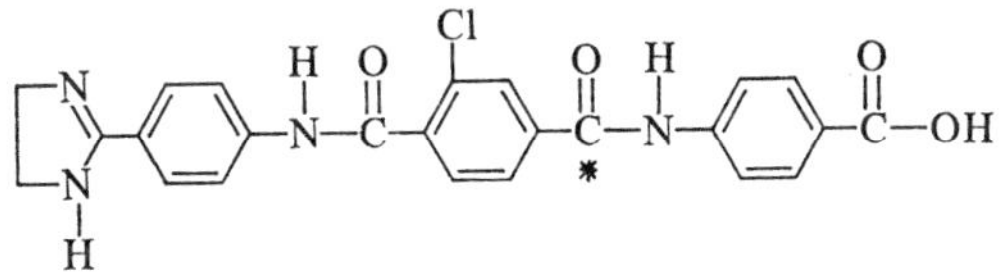

ABA-CP*-ABA

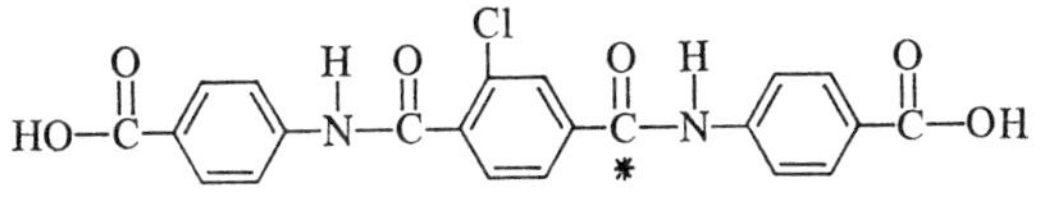

ABA-CP*

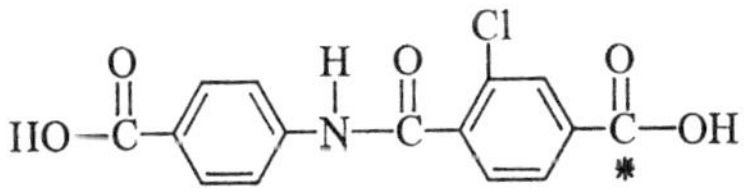

Fig. 2. Probable anionic metabolites of ^{14}C-NSC 60339 in urine of cancer patients (Yesair et al., 1969): IMA, imidazolinyl aniline; CP, 2-chloroterephthalic acid; ABA, *p*-aminobenzoic acid. The asterisk designates the radioactive carbon

acid and/or imidazolinylaniline (Fig. 2). The extent of this metabolism in man may contribute to the ineffectiveness of chemotherapy and/or to the toxicity of the terephthalanilides in man.

Biochemical Mechanism of Action

After the introduction of these drugs in 1962, investigations into the mechanism of action of the phthalanilides were numerous, principally in the areas of nucleic acids (Sivak et al., 1963, 1965; Rauen et al., 1966), protein (Pine et al., 1963; Ochoa et al., 1964), and lipids (Gellhorn et al., 1964; Yesair et al., 1967). The phthalanilides, which are cationic at neutral pH, form ionic complexes with many biological components *in vitro*, e.g., nucleic acids (Sivak et al., 1963, 1965; Rauen et al., 1965, 1966), protein (Rogers et al., 1962), and lipids (Booth et al., 1964; Yesair et al., 1966). However, evidence for these ionic complexes *in situ* has not been obtained. The imidazole and tetrahydropyrimidinyl terephthalanilides are extracted from tissues, tumor cells, nuclei, and mitochondria of tumor cells and *E. coli* B, primarily as ionic drug-lipid complexes (YESAIR et al., 1966a, b, 1967, 1971; YESAIR and HOFOOK, 1968), whereas the amidino terephthalanilides were extracted primarily as "free" drug (YESAIR et al., 1971). Interestingly, "active" imidazole and amidino compounds, which produce an increase in lifespan of 125 % or more in tumor-bearing mice, and "inactive" compounds which produce lesser increases in lifespan, complex equally well with nucleic acids and lipids *in vitro* (SIVAK et al., 1963, 1965), inhibit growth and biosynthetic capabilities of tumor cells growing in suspension culture, and show the same pattern of inhibition of several biosynthetic pathways (YESAIR et al., 1971).

Biochemical studies have indicated that DNA, RNA, protein, and lipid synthesis were inhibited after phthalanilide treatment of leukemia cells, either in culture or in mice (KENSLER, 1963; PINE et al., 1963; BOOTH et al., 1964; OCHOA et al., 1964; KREIS et al., 1965; JONDORF et al., 1965; YESAIR et al., 1967). Since many biochemical functions are inhibited by both "active" and "inactive" phthalanilides, it is unlikely that there is only one locus for phthalanilide action at the molecular level. Indeed, several proposed mechanisms have been reviewed by BENNETT (1965) and by KENSLER et al. (1965). The unique intracellular distribution of drug [it is extracted primarily as lipid complexes from the nuclear and mitochondrial fraction, but not from the microsomal or supernatant fractions of tumors (SIVAK et al., 1964; YESAIR et al., 1966)] suggests that the physiologic site of drug activity is probably in the nucleus and mitochondria.

The drug-binding lipids from sensitive or resistant tumors are chemically similar to a new class of phospholipids that was isolated from dog brain (YESAIR et al., 1966). The new phospholipids are characterized by their unusual glycerol:fatty acid:phosphorus:nitrogen ratio, by their unidentified ninhydrin-positive components and by their presumed large molecular weight. The concentration of extractable imidazole and tetrahydropyrimidinyl terephthalanilide-lipid complexes is generally highest in tissues and tumors that are adversely affected by phthalanilide treatment (PALM et al., 1965; YESAIR et al., 1966a, b, 1967; YESAIR and HOFOOK, 1968). Therefore, it is likely that phospholipids represent important loci for phthalanilide activity in mitochondrial and nuclear fractions.

The importance of lipids for mitochondrial function and especially for oxidative phosphorylation is well documented. Phthalanilides as lipid complexes in the mitochondria probably account for the observed inhibition of oxidative phosphorylation (SIVAK et al., 1967). These same investigators suggested that the extent of this inhibition, which is like that produced by oligomycin, may be related to the observed inhibition of the adenosine triphosphate-dependent biosyntheses (note above).

The lipid content and composition of cell nuclei and intranuclear fractions have been described for a variety of tissues (STONEBURG, 1939; LEVINE and CHARGAFF, 1952; CHAYEN et al., 1959a, b; BIEZINSKI and SPAET, 1961; GETZ and BARTLEY, 1961; GURR et al., 1963; REES et al., 1963; ALTMANN et al., 1964; ROSE and FRENSTER, 1965; FRENSTER, 1965). FRENSTER (1965) and ROSE and FRENSTER (1965) have shown that the chromatin fraction, active in RNA synthesis, is rich in phospholipids and have suggested that phospholipids, along with nonhistone protein, may function as derepressors by affecting the histone-DNA interaction. It is known that DNA is rendered less effective as a template for RNA synthesis *in vitro* when histones are added (HUANG and BONNER, 1962; ALLFREY et al., 1964) and that removal of histones from chromatin preparations stimulates template activity (FRENSTER, 1965; DAHMAS and BONNER, 1965). Gangliosides, which are anionic glycolipids, form complexes with basic proteins and histones (BOOTH, 1962; MCILWAIN, 1963) and can compete with DNA for its associated histones (MERSLER and MCCLUEN, 1966). A protein moiety, extracted as a proteolipid from *Staphylococcus epidermidis* has been shown to form a complex with DNA or RNA (BERGH et al., 1965). Also, a DNA-lipid-protein-containing material was isolated from calf thymus nuclear chromatin (JACKSON et al., 1968).

We have suggested that the new phospholipids, extracted primarily from the nucleus and mitochondria and presumed to have a large molecular size, may be an integral component of a phospholipid (possibly as lipoprotein)-histone-DNA interaction (YESAIR et al., 1967). The chemotherapeutic and biochemical response to the phthalanilides may be interpreted with reference to the phthalanilides affecting a phospholipid-histone-DNA equilibrium. Substantial inhibition of DNA and protein synthesis occurs at drug concentrations which do not depress lipid and RNA synthesis or result in cell death. Therefore, these inhibitions must have been reversible, possibly because new lipid is synthesized to replenish the lipid-complex with the phthalanilides, and/or because newly synthesized lipids complex with the phthalanilides which may be associated with nucleic acids. Thus, the phospholipid (possibly as lipoprotein)-histone-DNA equilibrium is affected reversibly, and biochemical processes, e.g., DNA, messenger RNA, and protein synthesis associated with this equilibrium are also not affected irreversibly. However, when lipid synthesis is extensively inhibited, the equilibrium of the phospholipid (protein)-histone-DNA system may be shifted to favor the histone-DNA complex and/or a phthalanilide-DNA complex. In either case, DNA synthesis may then be irreversibly inhibited and the cells cannot divide.

It has been shown that the "active" and "inactive" imidazole terephthalanilides are taken up more readily by cells than the amidino terephthalanilides (YESAIR et al., 1971). Once taken up, the former show a greater tendency to form lipid complexes, whereas the amidino terephthalanilides were extracted primarily as "free" drug. Yet cell kill was possible with both "active" and "inactive" imidazole or amidino congeners. In terms of the proposed mechanism of action of the phthalanilides, the pair of imidazole analogs extracted as a lipid complex, may shift the lipid (protein)-histone-DNA equilibrium towards a histone-DNA complex, whereas the amidino analogs extracted primarily as "free" drugs, may affect chemotherapy or toxicity by forming a terephthalanilide-DNA complex.

This difference in extractability and proposed mechanism of action between imidazole and amidino congeners suggests that combination chemotherapy with the two types of drugs, or with drugs with both types of functional groups, might have been fruitful. Although none of the phthalanilides contained mixed basic groups, a new series of compounds the basic structure of which resembles the phthalanilides, two strongly basic groups connected with several coplanar rings and by carbonamide groups, contains mixed, basic functional groups. These compounds are active against murine tumors and we recently found (YESAIR and CALLAHAN, unpublished data) that they, as the phthalanilides, partition to the aqueous phase of a chloroform:methanol:water biphasic solvent system, partition to the same aqueous phase in the presence of lipids from egg yolk, but partition to the non-aqueous phase in the presence of lipids from brain. Further, cations can displace these compounds from the lipids. The characteristics of these complexes suggest that the lipid may be the new class of phospholipids already observed to complex with the phthalanilides. If so, the extraction of these compounds from tumor cells may show roughly equivalent complexing with lipid and with nucleic acids.

Conclusions

The phthalanilides represent a unique class of cancer chemotherapeutic agents which still have great promise. Unfortunately, the representatives which were first chosen for clinical evaluation had adverse side effects. Such side effects, however, were not universal for all members of this series. These compounds also showed variations in their metabolism and may have specific differences in their mechanisms of action. It has been proposed that the chemotherapeutic and biochemical responses to the phthalanilides may be associated with their effect on a phospholipid-histone-DNA equilibrium.

References

ALLFREY, V. G., FAULKNER, R., MIRSKY, A. E.: Acetylation and methylation of histones and their possible role in the regulation of RNA synthesis. Proc. nat. Acad. Sci. (Wash.) **51**, 786—794 (1964).

ALTMANN, F. P., HAMPSON, S. E., CHAYEN, R.: Phospholipids in formalin extracts of nuclei isolated from sheep lungs. Nature (Lond.) **202**, 1215—1216 (1964).

ATWELL, G. J., CAIN, B. F.: Potential antitumor agents. V. Bisquaternary salts. J. med. Chem. **10**, 706—713 (1967).

ATWELL, G. J., CAIN, B. F.: Potential antitumor agents. VI. Bisquaternary salts. J. med. Chem. **11**, 295—305 (1968).

BENNETT, L. L., JR.: Phthalanilides and some related dibasic and polybasic compounds: a review of biological activities and modes of action. In: HOMBURGER, F. (Ed.): Progress in experimental tumor research. New York: Hafner Publishing Company, Inc. 1965.

BERGH, A. K., WEBB, S. J., MCARTHUR, C. S.: A histone-like fraction bound to lipid in *Staphylococcus epidermidis*. Can. J. Biochem. **43**, 625—633 (1965).

BIEZINSKI, J. J., SPAET, T. H.: Phospholipid content of subcellular fractions in adult rat organs. Biochim. biophys. Acta (Amst.) **51**, 221—226 (1961).

BOOTH, D. A.: The isolation and assay of gangliosides and their interactions with basic proteins. J. Neurochem. **9**, 265—276 (1962).

BOOTH, J., BOYLAND, E., GELLHORN, A.: Search for metabolites of anti-leukemic phthalanilides, 2-chloro-4′,4″-di(2-imidazolin-2-yl) terephthalanilide (NSC 60339) and 2-amino-4′,4″-di(2-imidazolin-2-yl) terephthalanilide dihydrochloride (NSC 50469). Cancer Chemother. Rep. **43**, 11—18 (1964).

BURCHENAL, J. H., ADAMS, H. H., LANCASTER, S., HIRT, R.: Selective antagonism of toxicity but not antileukemic effect of terephthalanilides by suramin. Fed. Proc. **24**, 443 (Abstract 1745) (1965a).

BURCHENAL, J. H., COLEY, V., PURPLE, J. R., BUCHOLZ, E., LYMAN, M. S., KREIS, W.: Studies on the mechanisms of action of various phthalanilide derivatives by cross-resistance and tissue culture. Cancer Res. **23**, 1364—1374 (1963).

BURCHENAL, J. H., GREGGS, V. C., LANCASTER, S. P., HIRT, R., BERCHTOLD, R., FISCHER, R., BALSIGER, R.: Prevention by sulfonic and phosphoric analogs of the terephthalanilide inhibition of leukemia P815Y *in vitro*. Cancer Res. **25**, 469—471 (1965b).

BURCHENAL, J. H., SPOONER, E., LANCASTER, S.: Blocking of chronic toxicity and antileukemic activity of terephthalanilides in mice. Proc. Amer. Assoc. Cancer Res. **6**, 9 (Abstract 33) (1965c).

BURCHENAL, J. H., LYMAN, M. S.: Lack of cross resistance to the amidino and the ureido derivatives in mouse leukemia made resistant to 4′,4″-*bis*(2-imidazolin-2-yl)-2-chloro-terephthalanilide dihydrochloride (NSC 38280). Canad. Cancer Conf. **5**, 439—448 (1963).

BURCHENAL, J. H., LYMAN, M. S., PURPLE, J. R., COLEY, V., SMITH, S., BUCHOLZ, E.: Therapeutic, combination and resistant studies on certain imidazolin phthalanilide derivatives in mouse leukemia. Cancer Chemother. Rep. **19**, 19—29 (1962).

CHAYEN, J., GAHAN, P. B., LACOUR, L. F.: The nature of a chromosomal phospholipid. Quart. J. microscop. Sci. **100**, 279—284 (1959a).

CHAYEN, J., GAHAN, P. B., LACOUR, L. F.: The masked lipids of nuclei. Quart. J. microscop. Sci. **100**, 325—327 (1959b).

DAHMAS, M. E., BONNER, J.: Increased template activity of liver chromatin, a result of hydrocortisone administration. Proc. nat. Acad. Sci. (Wash.) **54**, 1370—1375 (1965).

FRENSTER, J. H.: Nuclear polyanions as de-repressors of synthesis of ribonucleic acid. Nature (Lond.) **206**, 680—683 (1965).
GELLHORN, A., WAGNER, M., RICHLER, M., KOREN, A., BENJAMIN, W.: The effect of a phthalanilide derivative on lipid metabolism in L1210 leukemia cells. Cancer Res. **24**, 400—408 (1964).
GETZ, G. S., BARTLEY, W.: The intracellular distribution of fatty acids of intracellular compartments. Biochem. J. **78**, 307—312 (1961).
GURR, M. I., FINEAN, J. B., HAWTHORNE, J. N.: The phospholipids of liver-cell fractions. I. The phospholipid composition of the liver-cell nucleus. Biochim. biophys. Acta (Amst.) **70**, 406—416 (1963).
HIRT, R., BERCHTOLD, R.: Biophysical studies with synthetic lecithin as a road to new chemotherapeutic agents. Cancer Chemother. Rep. **18**, 5—7 (1962).
HUANG, R. C., BONNER, J.: Histone, a suppressor of chromosomal RNA synthesis. Proc. nat. Acad. Sci. (Wash.) **48**, 1216—1222 (1962).
HUTCHISON, D. J.: Studies on cross-resistant and collateral sensitivity (1962—1964). Cancer Res. **25**, 1581—1595 (1965).
JACKSON, V., EARNHARDT, J., CHALKLEY, R.: A DNA-lipid protein containing material isolated from calf thymus nuclear chromatin. Biochem. biophys. Res. Commun. **33**, 253—259 (1968).
JONDORF, W. R., SPECTOR, A., CHAIKEN, S. J.: The effect of two carcinostatic agents on the chemically induced stimulation of amino acid incorporation in a mammalian system. Biochem. biophys. Res. Commun. **20**, 787—792 (1965).
KENSLER, C. J.: Chemotherapeutic activity of phthalanilide derivatives: an approach to anticodic therapy? Cancer Res. **23**, 1353—1363 (1963).
KENSLER, C. J., PALM, P. E., DAY, H. M., BATTISTA, S. P., ROGERS, W. I., YESAIR, D. W., WODINSKY, I.: Toxicology of antileukemic agents with special reference to phthalanilide derivatives. Cancer Res. **25**, 1622—1667 (1965).
KREIS, W., ELLISON, R. R., LYMAN, M. S., BURCHENAL, J. H., BLOCK, R., WARKENTIN, D. L.: Clinical investigation of the physiologic disposition of a phthalanilide (NSC 38280) and a phthalanilide derivative (NSC 57155) in 7 patients. Cancer Res. **25**, 402—407 (1965).
LAW, L. W.: Studies of inhibitory effects of terephthalanilide derivatives against several variants of leukemia L1210. Cancer Chemother. Rep. **19**, 13—18 (1962).
LEVINE, C., CHARGAFF, E.: Phosphatide composition in different liver cell fractions. Exp. Cell Res. **3**, 154—162 (1952).
LOUIS, J.: Coordinated phase I studies for cooperative chemotherapy groups. Cancer Chemother. Rep. **16**, 99—105 (1962).
LOUIS, J., TAYLOR, H., SUTOW, W., LYMAN, M. S., BURCHENAL, J. H.: Phase I evaluation of terephthalamidine [*N′,N″-bis,p-(N′*-methylamidino)phenyl, tetrahydrochloride, trihydrate] NSC 57155. Proc. Amer. Ass. Cancer Res. **4**, 40 (Abstract 155) (1963).
LYMAN, M., WOLLNER, N., ELLISON, R. R., KRAKOFF, I., FREI, E. III., CLOSE, H., BURCHENAL, J. H.: Effects of NSC 38280 in man. Proc. Amer. Ass. Cancer Res. **3**, 340 (Abstract 165) (1962).
MCILWAIN, H.: Chemical Exploration of the Brain. New York: Elsevier, 1963.
MERSLER, M. H., MCCLUEN, R. H.: Nucleohistone dissociation by ganglioside micelles. Science **154**, 896—897 (1966).
OCHOA, M., JR., GELLHORN, A., BENJAMIN, W. B.: Phthalanilide inhibition of protein synthesis in a cell-free L1210 mouse ascites leukemia system. Cancer Res. **24**, 480—484 (1964).
OETTGEN, H. F., CLIFFORD, P., BURCHENAL, J. H.: Malignant lymphoma involving the jaw in African children: treatment with 2-chloro-4′,4″-di-2-imidazolin-2-yl terephthalanilide dihydrochloride. Cancer Chemother. Rep. **27**, 45—54 (1963).
PALM, P. E., ROGERS, W. I., YESAIR, D. W., KENSLER, C. J.: Studies on the delayed toxicity of phthalanilides and other compounds. Toxicol. appl. Pharmacol. **7**, 494 (Abstract 50) (1965).
PINE, M. J., HARZEWSKI, E., WISSLER, F. C.: Action of the phthalanilide drugs on *Escherichia coli*. Cancer Res. **23**, 932—937 (1963).
PITTILLO, A. F., BENNETT, L. L., JR., SHORT, W. A., TOMISEK, A. J., DIXON, G. J., THOMSON, J. R., LASTER, W. R., JR., TRADER, M., METTIL, L., ALLAN, P., BOWDON, B., SCHABEL, F., JR., SKIPPER, H. E.: Preliminary studies on some terephthalanilides — a new class of antitumor drugs. Cancer Chemother. Rep. **19**, 41—53 (1962).
RAUEN, H. M., HAAR, H., UNTERBERG, W.: Coplanare Heterooligobasen (pthalanilide) und ihr cytostatischer Wirkungsmechanismus. Arzneimittel-Forschg. **16**, 533—541 (1966).
RAUEN, H. M., NOROTH, K., UNTERBERG, W.: Coplanare Heterooligobasen (phthalanilide) hochaktive Cytostatica. Experientia (Basel) **21**, 300—304 (1965).
REES, K. R., ROWLAND, G. F., VARCOE, J. S.: The metabolism of isolated rat-liver nucleoli and other subnuclear fractions. The active site of amino acid incorporation in the nucleus. Biochem. J. **86**, 130—136 (1963).

ROGERS, W. I., SIVAK, A., YORK, I. M.: Stability of 1,1′-*m*-phenylene *bis* [3-(*p*-2-imidazolin-2-yl phenyl)urea] and 1,1′-*p*-phenylene *bis* [3-(*m*-2-imidazolin-2-yl phenyl)urea] and effect of degradation products on the circulation of the hamster cheek pouch. Cancer Chemother. Rep. **29**, 77—83 (1963).
ROGERS, W. I., YESAIR, D. W., KENSLER, C. J.: Physiological disposition of 4′,4″-*bis*(1,4,5,6-tetrahydro-2-pyrimidinyl)-terephthalanilide and 4-(1,4,5,6-tetrahydro-2-pyrimidinyl)-4′-[*p*-(1,4,5,6-tetrahydro-2-pyrimidinyl)phenyl]carbamoylbensanilide in dogs, monkeys, rats, and mice. J. Pharmacol. exp. Therap. **152**, 139—150 (1966).
ROGERS, W. I., YORK, I. M., KENSLER, C. J.: Physiological disposition studies of 4′,4″-*bis*(2-imidazolin-2-yl)terephthalanilide. Cancer Chemother. Rep. **19**, 67—74 (1962).
ROSE, H. G., FRENSTER, J. H.: Composition and metabolism of lipids within repressed and active chromatin of interphase lymphocytes. Biochim. biophys. Acta (Amst.) **106**, 577—591 (1965).
SCHEPARTZ, S. A., WODINSKY, I., LEITER, J.: Phthalanilides — a new group of potential anti-tumor agents. Cancer Chemother. Rep. **19**, 1—3 (1962).
SIVAK, A., MAHONEY, A. J., ROGERS, W. I.: Studies on the intracellular localization and effects of 2-chloro-4′,4″-di(2-imidazolin-2-yl)terephthalanilide on mitochondria from P388 lymphocytic leukemia and rat liver. Biochem. Pharmacol. **16**, 1919—1931 (1967).
SIVAK, A., ROGERS, W. I., KENSLER, C. J.: Phthalanilide interaction with nucleic acids. Biochem. Pharmacol. **12**, 1056—1058 (1963).
SIVAK, A., ROGERS, W. I., WODINSKY, I., KENSLER, C. J.: Distribution and effects of 4′,4″-di(2-imidazolin-2-yl)terephthalanilide dihydrochloride hemihydrate and its 2-chloro analogue in lymphocytic leukemias L1210 and P388. J. nat. Cancer Inst. **33**, 457—465 (1964).
SIVAK, A., ROGERS, W. I., WODINSKY, I., KENSLER, C. J.: Studies on the formation of phthalanilide-deoxyribonucleic acid complexes and their relationship to chemotherapeutic activity. Cancer Res. **25**, 902—909 (1965).
STONEBURG, C. A.: Lipids of the cell nuclei. J. biol. Chem. **129**, 189—196 (1939).
THAYER, P. S., GORDON, H. C.: Protection of *Escherichia coli* against the growth-inhibiting effects of terephthalanilides by purines, pyrimidines and amino acids. Cancer Chemother. Rep. **19**, 55—57 (1962).
VENDITTI, J. M., GOLDIN, A., KLINE, I.: Studies on the effectiveness of 4′,4″-di(2-imidazolin-2-yl)terephthalanilides against mouse leukemia L1210 and resistant variants. Cancer Chemother. Rep. **19**, 5—11 (1962).
YESAIR, D. W., HOFOOK, C.: The retention or efflux of phthalanilide (NSC 60339)-lipid complexes by sensitive or resistant murine tumor cells and *Escherichia coli* B. Cancer Res. **28**, 314—319 (1968).
YESAIR, D. W., KOHNER, F. A., ROGERS, W. I., BARONOWSKY, P. E., KENSLER, C. J.: Relationship of phthalanilide-lipid complexes to uptake and retention of 2-chloro-4′,4″-di(2-imidazolin-2-yl)terephthalanilide (NSC 60339) by sensitive and resistant P388 leukemia cells. Cancer Res. **26**, 202—207 (1966a).
YESAIR, D. W., LEVINS, P., CARAGAY, A., SHUCK, D., FUNKHOUSER, J. T.: Identification of metabolites of 2-chloro-4′,4″-di(2-imidazolin-2-yl)terephthalanilide (NSC 60339) from cancer patients with high resolution mass spectroscopy. Proc. Amer. Ass. Cancer Res. **10**, 101 (Abstract 402) (1969).
YESAIR, D. W., ROGERS, W. I., BARONOWSKY, P. E., WODINSKY, I., THAYER, P. S., KENSLER, C. J.: Relationship of uptake and binding of an antileukemic phthalanilide to its biochemical and chemotherapeutic effects on P388 lymphocytic leukemia cells. Cancer Res. **27**, 314—321 (1967).
YESAIR, D. W., ROGERS, W. I., FUNKHOUSER, J. T., KENSLER, C. J.: Purification and characterization of phthalanilide-lipid complexes from tissues. J. Lipid Res. **7**, 492—500 (1966b).
YESAIR, D. W., THAYER, P. S., KENSLER, C. J.: Comparative studies of drug uptake, viability, and biosynthetic capabilities of P388 cells treated with "active" or "inactive" terephthalanilides. Ann. N.Y. Acad. Sci. **172**, 653—666 (1971).
YESAIR, D. W., WODINSKY, I., ROGERS, W. I., KENSLER, C. J.: The effect of suramin-phthalanilide complexes on the chemotherapeutic activity and toxicity of 4′,4″-*bis*(1,4,5,6-tetrahydro-2-pyrimidinyl)terephthalanilides (NSC 57153). Biochem. Pharmacol. **17**, 305—313 (1968).
YORK, I. M., ROGERS, W. I., KENSLER, C. J.: The production of thrombi and emboli in the hamster cheek pouch by phthalanilides and related compounds. J. Pharmacol. exp. Therap. **141**, 36—49 (1963).

Chapter 76

Platinum Compounds

GLEN R. GALE

With 1 Figure

Introduction

In an investigation of the possible effects of an electric field on growth processes in bacteria, ROSENBERG et al. (1965) noted that the amplified output from an audio oscillator, delivered at 1000 cycles/sec at 2 amperes between platinum electrodes immersed in a liquid culture, induced cells of *Escherichia coli* to form long filaments up to 300 times the normal length. Subsequent investigations revealed that this pattern of unbalanced growth was not due to the electrical current *per se*, but to one or more long-lived chemical species of platinum released from the presumably inert electrodes in the presence of ammonium and chloride ions. In a continuous culture system, about 8 parts per million of platinum went into solution in the steady state, and the principal complex was tentatively identified as $[PtCl_6]^{2-}$. Attempts to induce filamentous growth in synthetic medium using authentic $(NH_4)_2[PtCl_6]$ were initially unsuccessful and yielded only bacteriostasis without filament formation. However, it was soon observed (ROSENBERG et al., 1967a) that these solutions of $(NH_4)_2[PtCl_6]$, when left standing for several days exposed to light, conferred cytological changes in bacteria identical with those seen in the initial experiments using an electric current. Studies showed subsequently that the $[PtCl_6]^{2-}$ ion in solution in the nutrient medium was bactericidal. When the solution was irradiated with light, one or more of the ligand chloride ions of the complex was replaced by NH_3. The negative charge on the complex decreased by one for each replacement. The neutral species attained did not inhibit growth, but completely inhibited cell division. The identity of the neutral species was confirmed by synthesis, and found to be the *cis* form of the doubly substituted complex, $[PtCl_4(NH_3)_2]^\circ$. The photochemical reaction is described by the equation

$$[PtCl_6]^{2-} + nNH_4^+ \xrightarrow{h\nu} [PtCl_{(6-n)}(NH_3)_n]^{(2-n)^-} + nH^+ + nCl^-. \tag{1}$$

The corresponding *trans* isomer of the complex was virtually devoid of activity, and substitution of NO_2 for NH_3 yielded an inactive product (ROSENBERG et al., 1967a). Of all organisms tested, gram-negative bacilli were the most sensitive to the effects of the complex, and resumption of cell division was observed following removal of the compound from the medium (ROSENBERG et al., 1967b). HOWLE and GALE (1970a) examined with an electron microscope the filamentous forms of *E. coli* grown in the presence of the dichlorodiammine complex and found ribosomal aggregation, loss of the discrete nucleoid-ribosomal border, and concentration of electron density in the aggregated nucleoprotein.

Tumor-Inhibitory Activity

In the initial assays of platinum compounds against experimental tumors, ROSENBERG et al. (1969) tested the neutral complexes *cis*-tetrachlorodiammine-platinum(IV), *cis*-dichlorodiammineplatinum(II) (NSC-119875), tetrachloro(ethylenediamine)platinum(IV), and dichloro(ethylenediamine)platinum(II) (Fig. 1) against Sarcoma 180. The most active compound was NSC-119875, which restricted the extent of tumor development to only 2 % of that of untreated controls when given at 2 mg/kg/day for 10 days. This same compound, when administered

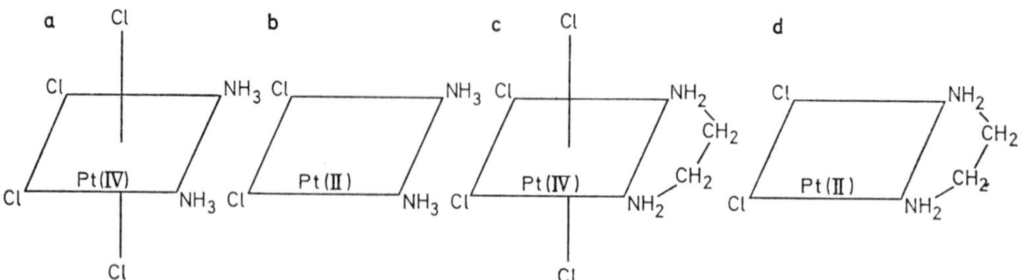

Fig. 1a—d. (a) *cis*-Tetrachlorodiammineplatinum(IV). (b) *cis*-Dichlorodiammineplatinum(II) (NSC-119875). (c) Tetrachloro(ethylenediamine)platinum(IV). (d) Dichloro(ethylenediamine) platinum(II)

to mice bearing the L1210 leukemia, increased the survival times of the animals over 80 % when given either at 1.25 mg/kg/day for 9 days or at 10 mg/kg on day 1 only. Three of 10 mice in the group receiving only a single injection were alive and free of tumor when discarded on day 30. NSC-119875 also caused regression of large (i.e., day 8 after implantation) solid Sarcoma 180 tumors in 63 to 100 % of treated animals with no apparent irreversible damage to the hosts (ROSENBERG and VAN CAMP, 1970). The optimum dosage regimen appeared to be 8 mg/kg on day 8, or 4 mg/kg on days 8 and 17. Other transplantable rodent tumors which are quite sensitive to NSC-119875 include the Dunning ascitic leukemia and the Walker 256 carcinosarcoma (KOCIBA et al., 1970), a virus-induced reticulum cell sarcoma (TALLEY, 1970), a 7,12-dimethylbenzanthracene-induced mammary tumor (WELSCH, 1971), and the Ehrlich ascites carcinoma (HOWLE and GALE, 1970b). Currently unpublished data from several laboratories[1] indicate that the following animal tumors are also sensitive to NSC-119875: B-16 melanosarcoma, leukemia P388, ADJ/PC6, SV40, and certain autochthonous dog tumors.

In a system designed to detect combination therapies of potential clinical usefulness, SIRICA et al. (1971) gave NSC-119875 and cyclophosphamide (NSC-26271) intraperitoneally, alone or in combination, on days 1, 3, or 5 only after intraperitoneal implantation with various numbers of L1210 cells. In two experiments, day 3 combination therapy of mice implanted with 10^5 cells produced 50 % and 75 % 63-day survivors, as compared with 0 % and 37 % for cyclophosphamide alone and 0 % and 0 % for NSC-119875 alone. Against day 5 L1210 leu-

1 Presented at the International Symposium on the Bacterial, Viral, and Anti-Tumor Activities of Platinum Compounds, Kellogg Center for Continuing Education, Michigan State University, East Lansing, Michigan, September 23—25, 1970.

kemia, the combination elicited an increased life span 47 % greater than cyclophosphamide alone and 142 % greater than NSC-119875 alone. Day 1 combination therapy of mice implanted with 4×10^4 to 3×10^6 L1210 cells was also superior to treatment with either drug alone. For example, combination therapy after an inoculum of 3.3×10^5 cells produced 100 % 36-day survivors, compared with 38 % and 12 % obtained with cyclophosphamide and NSC-119875 alone, respectively.

As regards possible similarities in the mode of action between NSC-119875 and certain alkylating agents, workers at the Chester Beatty Institute found that a strain of Walker 256 tumor with an acquired resistance to melphalan was totally cross-resistant, not only to other alkylating agents, but to NSC-119875 as well. This resistant strain retained its original sensitivity to antineoplastic agents which are active by mechanisms other than alkylation, such as 6-mercaptopurine and methotrexate (CONNORS, personal communication).

Toxicity of Platinum Compounds

Acute toxicological investigations of NSC-119875 in the rat have been reported by THOMPSON and GALE (1970, 1971) and by KOCIBA and SLEIGHT (1971). The former authors observed impressive reticulocytopenia and lymphocytopenia in animals that received 1, 2, or 3 mg/kg/day for 3 days and were sacrificed on the fifth day. Neutrophiles and erythrocytes were unaffected during this period of observation. Similar changes were seen in animals given a single injection of 15 mg/kg and sacrificed on the third day. With this latter treatment, peripheral reticulocytes and lymphocytes were reduced to 4 % and 13 % of the respective control values. Thymic atrophy was a striking finding upon necropsy; a reduction of over 50 % of the thymus weight to body weight ratio was recorded following treatment at 3 mg/kg/day for 3 days. Histologic aberrations included a reduction of the number of thymocytes and the appearance of numerous pycnotic nuclei in the thymic cortices, a diminution of red cell precursors in the marrow, a diminished size of lymphoid follicles, and a virtual absence of megakaryocytes in the spleen. All animals incurred a dose-dependent reduction of weight gain. The vivid thymic changes were not merely secondary to a nonspecific stress reaction, since these changes were also observed in adrenalectomized rats.

KOCIBA and SLEIGHT (1971) determined the LD_{50} of NSC-119875 to be 12.0 mg/kg in male rats of the Spartan variety, Sprague-Dawley strain; the 95 % confidence limits extended from 7.5 to 19.1 mg/kg. They consequently studied the histologic, hematologic, and serum chemistry alterations after intraperitoneal injections of 12.2 mg/kg. Histologic changes were most evident in those tissues containing cellular constituents with rapid turnover times and consisted of generalized lymphoid depletion, intestinal epithelial damage, and bone marrow depression 2 to 4 days after injection. Sloughing of the renal tubular epithelium also occurred, possibly as a concomitant of the urinary excretion of the drug and its metabolites. Regeneration of the cellular constituents of affected tissues occurred in those animals which survived the intoxication. Panleukocytopenia, reticulocytopenia, and thrombocytopenia were severe at 3 days and were followed by regenerative increases in survivors. Total serum proteins were depressed coincident with maximal lymphoid depression, and blood urea nitrogen levels were elevated due to renal tubular damage. Other alterations of serum components were attributed to dehydration as a result of enteritis.

Extensive studies at the Mason Research Institute (HEYMAN et al., 1971; SCHAEPPI, U., personal communication) initiated as a preclinical pharmacological evaluation of NSC-119875 have established the minimum lethal dose for the dog as a single intravenous injection of 2.5 mg/kg or 5 daily injections of 0.75 mg/kg. The minimum lethal dose for the monkey was 5 daily doses of 2.5 mg/kg. Treatment elicited severe morbidity in both species within 5 to 17 days and its rapidity of onset was dose related. Toxicity included severe hemorrhagic enterocolitis, hypocellularity of the bone marrow and lymphoid tissues, and prominent renal lesions. These latter occurred as renal tubular necrosis in the dog and as nephrosis in the monkey, and were accompanied by azotemia, hypochloremia, proteinuria, cylindruria, and the appearance of urinary erythrocytes and leukocytes. Occasional findings were pancreatitis in the dog, myocarditis in the monkey, and testicular degeneration in both species. Apparently total recovery occurred in 60 to 120 days in those animals which survived.

Distribution of Tumor-Inhibitory Platinum Compounds

The first study of the distribution of an antitumor platinum compound in a living system was reported by RENSHAW and THOMSON (1967). They bombarded iridium metal with protons and obtained ^{191}Pt, which has a half-life of 3 days and decays by electron capture. This was extracted from the iridium and immediately converted to a solution of $(NH_4)_2[PtCl_6]$. The latter was added to a synthetic broth culture medium and irradiated with a mercury lamp to obtain the neutral tetrachlorodiammineplatinum(IV) complex [structure (a) in Fig. 1]. Growth of filamentous forms of *E. coli* occurred in this irradiated medium; fractionation of the cells showed that the platinum metal was associated with metabolic intermediates, nucleic acids, and cytoplasmic proteins. Nonirradiated $(NH_4)_2[^{191}PtCl_6]$, which did not force filamentous growth, was associated only with cytoplasmic proteins. The neutral complex *cis*-$[^{191}Pt(NH_3)_2Cl_4]^0$ did not penetrate the cell wall of *Bacillus cereus* or *Staphylococcus aureus*.

In a study of the distribution of NSC-119875 in mice, TOOTH-ALLEN, J. and ROSENBERG, B.[1] used the method of neutron activation analysis to detect levels of platinum in various tissues at intervals after a single injection. Greatest concentrations were found in the organs of excretion and filtration (i.e., kidney, intestine, liver, and spleen), but the amounts found did not indicate a selective uptake by any organ; in no case was the accumulation greater than that computed on the basis of homogenous distribution, and no appreciable accumulation occurred in tumor tissue. No material was found in the brain. The total recovered at 6 days from the organs examined was a small fraction of that which was administered, implying virtually total excretion.

ROSENBERG and VAN CAMP (1970) reported that mice that were treated with NSC-119875 8 days after implantation with Sarcoma 180 extruded the tumor rather than resorbing it; the skin at the site formed a flap which healed with subsequent overgrowth of hair. Animals thus cured consistently rejected a reimplantation of the tumor. The authors considered as one possible mode of action of the drug a stimulation of the immune mechanism of the host. Workers in other laboratories, however, have found NSC-119875 to be an immunosuppressive agent. Dr. MARVIS RICHARDSON at Michigan State University (personal communication) immunized rabbits with killed cells of *Brucella abortus*, and 10 to 24 months later prepared spleen cell suspensions to assess the effects of NSC-119875 on secondary stimulation *in vitro*. Anti-Brucella agglutinin levels of the medium were measured

1 Personal communication

8 to 11 days after the secondary stimulus. With graded concentrations of NSC-119875, the reciprocals of the agglutinin titers were: 0 μg/ml, 160; 0.75 μg/ml, 20; and 1.5 μg/ml, <10. On a weight basis, NSC-119875 was more active than cyclophosphamide, methotrexate, 6-mercaptopurine, or puromycin, but less active than actinomycin D or cycloheximide. BERENBAUM (1971) gave formalinized sheep red cells intravenously to mice and 2 days later administered various doses of NSC-119875, its tetrachloro analog, or one of the bidentate ethylenediamine congeners. Five days after injection of antigen he counted the direct hemolytic plaque-forming cells in the spleens. The two inorganic compounds were active inhibitors of antibody-forming cells, and NSC-119875 was the more active of the two; a single injection of 10 mg/kg yielded almost 90 % inhibition. The exponential nature of the dose-response curve obtained with NSC-119875 suggested a random hit mode of action similar to the response obtained with ionizing radiation or alkylating agents, as opposed to the hyperbolic response customarily obtained with agents that act competitively, such as antimetabolites. The ethylenediamine derivatives were relatively much less active. A similar study by KHAN and HILL (1971) yielded virtually identical results with NSC-119875. Inferential evidence of an immunosuppressive action of NSC-119875, as manifest by its inhibition of DNA synthesis in cultured human lymphocytes stimulated with phytohemagglutinin, was reported by HOWLE et al. (1971).

Biochemical Mechanism of Action

In a study designed to detect the biochemical mode of action of NSC-119875, HOWLE and GALE (1970b) incubated a suspension of Ehrlich ascites tumor cells in Eagle's medium *in vitro* with the drug at 10^{-4} M. At intervals after the addition of platinum to the cells, thymidine-methyl-^{3}H, uridine-5-^{3}H, or L-leucine-^{14}C were added and the incorporation of each into the acid-insoluble fraction of the cells after a 20 min pulse labeling period was monitored. A time-dependent onset of inhibitory action against the incorporation of each precursor was observed, with maximal inhibition occurring at 4 to 6 h after addition of NSC-119875. Only a moderately greater action against thymidine incorporation into acid-insoluble material was noted in these *in vitro* experiments, as compared with the action of the drug on uridine or L-leucine incorporation into macromolecules. The same authors administered the drug as a single injection of 10 mg/kg to mice bearing well-developed Ehrlich ascites tumors. At intervals up to 4 days, 3 to 4 animals were sacrificed, the tumor cells were pooled, and the cell count was adjusted to 10^{6} cells/ml. Tumor cells from mice which received only vehicle, adjusted to the same cell concentration, served as controls. An incidental observation was that when equal volumes of standardized [10^{6} cells/ml] cell suspension from control and treated animals were sedimented in microhematocrit tubes, the packed volume of cells from the treated animals was about 40 % greater than that from control animals. Radioactively labeled thymidine, uridine, and L-leucine were then added to aliquots of each suspension, and the extent of incorporation of each was measured after a 20 min pulse period. The rates of incorporation of uridine and L-leucine into cells from treated animals were impaired about 40 to 50 % at 12 to 24 h after injection, but these rates returned to control values when measured 48 to 72 h after treatment. The rate of incorporation of thymidine was more severely impeded (i.e., 75 to 80 %), and remained depressed during the entire 96 h post-treatment observation period. It was concluded that the persistent and ultimately selective inhibition of DNA synthesis may be the biochemical mode of action of the drug, and the time-dependent onset of action *in vitro* and *in vivo* was considered possibly to be a reflection of a requirement for transformation of an initially inactive compound to an inhibitory product.

HOWLE et al. (1971) found that NSC-119875 was a potent inhibitor of the phytohemagglutinin-induced blastogenic response of cultured human peripheral lymphocytes. Fifty percent inhibition, as assessed by the rate of incorporation of thymidine-methyl-^3H into the acid-insoluble fraction of the cells, was attained at a platinum concentration of 10^{-7} M. As was found with Ehrlich ascites tumor cells, onset of maximal inhibition at any concentration required several hours, and at low concentration considerable selectivity against DNA synthesis was noted. For example, with the drug at 3×10^{-6} M added 24 h prior to a 2 h pulse period, the respective rates of incorporation of thymidine, L-leucine, and uridine were inhibited 88 %, 40 %, and 22 %. Inhibition of thymidine incorporation was not reversed upon washing and resuspending the cells in fresh medium devoid of platinum. No resolvable cytologic lesion coincident with drug action was observed by electron microscopy. The authors suggested that NSC-119875 may undergo two sequential transformations, with the loss of one Cl^- ion at each step, and that the resultant platinum species may act bifunctionally to cross-link adjacent nucleophilic centers through covalent binding.

In an *in vitro* study using human amnion AV_3 cells in culture, HARDER and ROSENBERG (1970) compared the effects of the three antitumor platinum-containing compounds, NSC-119875, *cis*-$[Pt(NH_3)_2Cl_4]^0$, and $[Pt(NH_3)_2(CH_2)_2Cl_2]^0$ (b, a, and d, respectively, in Fig. 1) with two platinum compounds devoid of antitumor action, $[Pt(NH_3)_4]Cl_2$ and *trans*-$[Pt(NH_3)_2Cl_4]^0$. A correlation was established between the relative antitumor effectiveness of the first three compounds and the extent of their inhibitory effects on the syntheses of DNA, RNA, and protein. The two compounds without antitumor effectiveness had no remarkable action on macromolecular synthesis when added at pharmacologically realistic concentrations. As noted by HOWLE and GALE (1970b) in the case of Ehrlich ascites tumor cells treated *in vivo*, and by HOWLE et al. (1971) in the case of human lymphocytes *in vitro*, DNA synthesis was the most sensitive of the parameters measured; NSC-119875 inhibited DNA synthesis at concentrations below 5×10^{-6} M. In AV_3 cells the onset of inhibition was also time-dependent, and once established could not be reversed appreciably by washing and resuspending the cells in fresh medium free of inhibitor. The authors also considered that the slow onset of inhibition may have been related to a requisite conversion of an inactive to an active agent. One postulate which they offered differed subtly from one proposed by HOWLE and GALE (1970b), but they also suggested alternate possibilities. HARDER (1971) hypothesized that NSC-119875 substitutes at the $C6$ or at both the $C6$ and $N7$ positions of two adjacent purines, thereby creating an intrastrand DNA crosslink.

Other actions of NSC-119875 on AV_3 cells described by HARDER (1970) include the induction of giant cell formation, a moderate inhibition of formate-^{14}C incorporation into purines of DNA and RNA, and a concentration dependent enhancement of DNA polymerase activity from cells treated with the drug. However, when the platinum compound was added to assay systems containing extracts prepared from untreated cells, inhibition of DNA polymerase as well as deoxyribonuclease activity was observed. There was no effect on DNA-dependent RNA polymerase from *Pseudomonas putida*. The author noted a close parallel between the actions of NSC-119875 and those of bifunctional alkylating agents, especially mechlorethamine. HARDER (1970) also cited as personal communications the unpublished results of other investigators relating to the following actions of NSC-

119875: inactivation of bacteriophages (DROBNIK, J., KREKULOVA, A., and KUBELKOV, A), induction of lysogenic strains of *E. coli* (RESLOVA, S.), and a lowering of the melting temperature of DNA (HORACEK, P. and DROBNIK, J.).

More recently, GALE et al. (1970), realizing the potential usefulness of an organic platinum antitumor derivative with an abundant content of carbon and hydrogen amenable to radioisotopic labeling, synthesized *cis*-dichloro(dipyridine)-platinum(II) (*cis*-$[PtPy_2Cl_2]^0$) by the method of KAUFFMAN (1963). Using pyridine-^1H in the initial synthesis, the authors compared the actions of this organic analog with those of NSC-119875. The parameters assessed were its effects on bacterial cell division, on the development of the Ehrlich ascites carcinoma *in vivo*, on nucleic acid and protein synthesis in ascites tumor cells *in vitro*, and on phytohemagglutinin-induced blastogenesis of human lymphocytes in culture. The aryl derivative was shown to force filamentous growth of *E. coli* and to retard markedly the rate of tumor development *in vivo*. Of the regimens examined, one injection at 25 mg/kg on day 1 yielded the optimal response; this dose increased the mean survival time 147 %, and permitted 2 of 10 mice to survive over 50 days. Only 3 mice of one group of 10 died as an obvious result of toxicity; these were in a group given 100 mg/kg on day 1. DNA, RNA, and protein synthesis in ascites tumor cells *in vitro* were sensitive to the action of this derivative, but only after a period of about 3 h of preincubation with the inhibitor. DNA synthesis was again the most sensitive of the three processes, with 50 % inhibition occurring at a *cis*-$[PtPy_2Cl_2]^0$ concentration of about 2×10^{-5} M. The rate of uptake of thymidine-methyl-^3H into human lymphocytes undergoing blastogenic transformation was reduced 50 % at a concentration of about 5×10^{-6} M. The authors concluded that the actions of the aryl derivative were similar to the actions of NSC-119875, but that the compound was somewhat less potent than the totally inorganic compound. However, the toxicity in mice of the organic derivative was less by almost an order of magnitude than that of NSC-119875.

Following this study, pyridine-^3H was substituted for pyridine-^1H (HOWLE and GALE, 1971, unpublished data). The tritiated derivative bound tenaciously with intact Ehrlich ascites tumor cells *in vitro* at 2° and 37° and resisted dissociation by vigorous washing or by repetitive precipitation with trichloroacetic acid followed by solubilization in alkali. The maximal accumulation of radioactivity at the end of 4 h incubation corresponded to 4.3×10^{-4} μμmoles of platinum per cell. Dialysis experiments showed that in unbuffered aqueous solution the compound also bound firmly to calf thymus DNA, yeast high molecular weight RNA, and bacterial and yeast transfer RNA, but not to dextran, bovine serum albumin, or purified erythrocyte membranes. One gram of DNA was found to bind 30 μmoles of platinum during a 2 h dialysis period, which corresponded to approximately 1 atom of platinum per 2 nucleotides. In these experiments, using a nonliving system, the presence of Cl^- ion suppressed markedly the extent of binding with the otherwise susceptible molecules, indicating that dissociation of chloride from the neutral complex is a prerequisite for chemical interaction. The homopolymers polyadenylate and polycytidylate bound to *cis*-$[PtPy_2Cl_2]^0$ to the same extent as did RNA on a weight basis; polyguanylate and polyuridylate were bound to a greater extent. Whereas prior exposure of DNA to NSC-119875 reduced the subsequent accumulation of the labeled pyridine analog, prior alkylation of the DNA with mechlorethamine did not influence the subsequent rate or extent of binding of *cis*-$[PtPy_2Cl_2]^0$.

THOMPSON and GALE (unpublished data) studied the distribution and excretion of the tritiated analog in rats. Largest amounts were recovered from kidney and liver, but no accumulation was observed in excess of the amount predicted on the basis of homogenous distribution. None was found in brain. The amount excreted in urine in the first 24 h after injection was 30 % of the total administered dose. The total amount recovered in three experiments at the end of 5 days was 70 ± 14 %, and 25 % of the total given was recovered from feces.

Compounds of the type $PtCl_2A_2$, where A_2 is two ammine ligands, two amine ligands, or the bidentate ethylenediamine ligand, are known to lose both chloride atoms in aqueous solution in successive aquation reactions (see Coley and Frigerio, 1969), i.e.,

$$[PtCl_2A_2]^0 + H_2O = [PtCl(H_2O)A_2]^+ + Cl^-, \quad (2)$$

$$[PtCl(H_2O)A_2]^+ + H_2O = [Pt(H_2O)_2A_2]^{2+} + Cl^-. \quad (3)$$

The concentration equilibrium quotients for these reactions, K_1 and K_2, are related to the total complex concentration, A, and to the equilibrium chloride concentration, T, by the expression (Sanders and Martin, 1961)

$$T^3 + K_1T^2 + (K_1K_2 - AK_1)T - 2AK_1K_2 = 0. \quad (4)$$

The analogy of (2) and (3) above to the cyclic immonium ion formation by the nitrogen mustards evokes speculation that the two classes of compounds may have qualitatively similar modes of action, but the molecular sites of attachment to the DNA molecule may differ.

NSC-119875 is now available for clinical trials; at this writing at least seven institutions are participating in phase I investigations.

In the only published report of antitumor actions of a platinum compound which did not stem directly from the original observations of Rosenberg et al. (1965), Kirschner et al. (1965) described the preparation of a number of organic complexes with metals, including platinum. The platinum (IV) complex with 6-mercaptopurine, $Na_2[Pt(6\text{-mercaptopurine})_2Cl_4] \cdot 2H_2O$, was active against adenocarcinoma 755 and Sarcoma 180, but the relative contribution of 6-mercaptopurine to the observed activity was not clear.

Addendum

Since submission of the above manuscript, a number of reports have appeared concerned with the pharmacologic properties of antitumor platinum compounds and with the clinical antitumor activity of NSC-119875 (*cis*-diamminedichloroplatinum(II)).

Zak et al. (1972a, b) monitored changes in the bone marrow of rats for up to 28 days after a single intraperitoneal injection of NSC-119875 at 8.0 mg/kg. Beginning at one hour after injection, mitotic index and total cell count decreased and reached nadirs at 24 h and 72 h, respectively. Normal values were reestablished following oscillatory fluctuations. Erythroblasts were only slightly affected, but more mature normoblasts decreased on day 3 and later returned to normal values. Oscillatory changes were noted in the number of lymphocytes, monocytes, and megakaryocytes, and were characterized by a rise immediately after injection of NSC-119875, a subsequent decline below control values, and finally a return to normal. The authors likened the observed changes to those following low doses of x-irradiation.

Khan and Hill (1971) studied the blastogenic response of cultured lymphocytes in the presence of NSC-119875. Control cultures yielded 43 % blast forms, while cultures containing NSC-119875 at 0.625, 1.25, and 2.5 μg/ml of the drug contained 38, 24, and 5 % blasts, respectively. The graft-versus-host reaction was also found to be suppressed (KHAN and HILL, 1972), and there was prolonged survival of skin grafts against H_2 histocompatibility (KHAN et al., 1972).

VARKARAKIS and MURPHY (1972) administered NSC-119875 to mature dogs bearing fistulas which permitted prostatic fluid collections. Even at doses of 1.5 mg/kg/day for 5 days, which resulted in the death of all animals, histologic examination of the prostates revealed no abnormalities. Selected parameters (e.g., composition, enzymatic activity) of prostatic fluid were virtually unchanged following treatment with these clearly toxic doses.

HORACEK and DROBNIK (1971) reported that NSC-119875 changes the absorption spectrum of calf thymus DNA, with a shift of the absorption maximum from 259 to 264 nm, and found that hyperchromicity was readily observed at room temperature. They also found that the interaction of the drug with DNA facilitated renaturation of the latter. ROBERTS and PASCOE (1972) reported a concentration-dependent cross-linking of HeLa cell DNA by NSC-119875. The authors cultured cells for one generation in the presence of 5-bromo-2'-deoxyuridine and produced a hybrid DNA consisting of one "light" strand and one "heavy" strand. Cesium chloride gradient centrifugation of DNA from cells exposed to NSC-119875 yielded three peaks, representing a light, a heavy, and an intermediate or cross-linked species. At 2×10^{-3} M platinum, over 60 % of the DNA was cross-linked, but only about 20 % at 2.5×10^{-4} M platinum. Since even this latter concentration (75 mg/l) is greater by over an order of magnitude than anticipated levels in body fluids after nonlethal doses of NSC-119875, the contribution of cross-linking to the antineoplastic action of this drug remains equivocal. SHOOTER and MERRIFIELD (1972) also studied the binding of NSC-119875 to DNA. They found an increased sedimentation coefficient following binding of the compound to denatured DNA which was accounted for in terms of the increased molecular weight and decreased partial specific volume. The expansion of the denatured DNA molecule usually observed in alkali was inhibited by the binding, a fact which the authors attributed to cross-linking of the chain in hydrogen-bonded regions. Binding of dichloro(ethylenediamine)platinum(II) to native DNA induced a marked change in conformation of the molecule, and this change was reversed to a large extent upon denaturation in alkali. The *trans* isomer of NSC-119875 induced no detectable conformational change in native DNA.

SHOOTER et al. (1972) also reported characteristics of the interaction of platinum compounds with bacteriophages T7 and R17. Quantitative comparisons showed that at the mean lethal dose, 1.5 molecules of platinum compound were bound to each R17 phage and 5 molecules to each T7 particle. Over 95 % of the compound bound to R17 was bound to RNA and 76 % of that bound to T7 was bound to DNA. Cross-linking of complementary strands of DNA occurred with each of the three platinum compounds studied; however, in each case it was a relatively rare reaction and accounted for only about 3 % of the bound molecules. The authors considered intrastrand linking of nucleic acid bases to be the most important inactivating reaction.

ROBINS (1973) used the ^{14}C-labeled ethylenediamine derivative to study its reaction in 0.1 M $NaClO_4$ with purine and pyrimidine bases, nucleosides, and nucleotides. Adenine, guanine, and cytosine and their nucleosides and nucleotides reacted with the platinum compound under these conditions, but thymine and its derivatives did not. Guanine derivatives reacted at the most rapid rate. In double-labeling experiments using tritiated bases, a platinum:base ratio of about unity was generally found. The exception was ATP, with which an additional product was detected with a platinum: base ratio of 2. A comparison of guanine and its derivatives in which the *N*7, *N*9, or both positions were blocked indicated that probably more than one site is available for reaction with this platinum congener.

GALE et al. (1973) extended the earlier studies of HOWLE et al. (1972) of the interaction of the tritiated dipyridine derivative with cells, to determine if an enzymatic mechanism is involved in transport across cell membranes or in the aquation of the molecule. Binding of the compound to Ehrlich ascites tumor cells occurred at the same rate at 0° as at 37°, but was enhanced several-fold at 60°. The maximum number of binding sites per cell at this latter temperature was found to be approximately 7 billion. The extent of binding was also increased upon increasing the hydrogen ion concentration of the suspending medium. Double-reciprocal plots of pg of platinum bound per cell as a function of extracellular *cis*-($PtPy_2Cl_2$) concentration extrapolated to infinity on the ordinate, indicating no rate-limiting factor in binding other than the concentration of the platinum compound. Almost 50 chemicals and drugs were tested for their effects on binding. None reduced the rate or extent of binding, but certain heavy metals and compounds that increase membrane permeability enhanced markedly the amount of platinum bound per cell. The binding characteristics of the dipyridine compound were virtually the same with human and bovine lymphocytes as with Ehrlich ascites tumor cells; however, both types of lymphocytes bound much more platinum per unit cell volume. Entry of the compound into all three cell types appeared to proceed by passive diffusion.

VONKA et al. (1972) treated EB3 cells with NSC-119875 at a concentration of 1.0 to 10 μM and observed an increased number of cells reactive in the indirect immunofluorescence test with human sera containing Epstein-Barr virus antibody. Increases of 2- to 3-fold were noted after 3 to 7 days. Concurrent addition of cytosine arabinoside or 5-bromo-2′-deoxyuridine prevented the increase, indicating that DNA synthesis is necessary for the effect. A similar enhancement was not observed in P3J cells.

CLEARE and HOESCHELE (1973) have reviewed the structure-activity relationships of a number of organoplatinum congeners in which both ammines and chlorides of the original NSC-119875 have been substituted with various organic groups. Substitution of a malonyl group for the two chlorides has yielded several compounds with notable activity against Sarcoma 180, and a number of cyclic aliphatic amine substitutions for the ammines have produced compounds with quite impressive action against the ADJ PC6 plasma cell tumor. For example, dichlorobis(cyclohexylamine)platinum has been shown to cause 90% remission of this tumor when given at 12 mg/kg, while its LD_{50} dose is more than 3200 mg/kg. The resulting therapeutic index of more than 267 contrasts with a value of 8.1 obtained with NSC-119875. So far as this writer is aware, this activity has not yet been demonstrated against the L1210 leukemia. Unexpectedly, a number of derivatives, notably aquo complexes, possess neuromuscular toxicity properties, resulting in violent convulsions.

HILL et al. (1972) have administered NSC-119875 to 63 patients. Tumor regression of more than 50% was seen in 9 patients, including carcinomas of the endometrium, ovary, breast, larynx, and esophagus, one case of acute granulocytic leukemia, and 4 of lymphosarcoma. Lesser regressions were observed in lung carcinoma, late Hodgkins disease, multiple myeloma, and carcinoma of the colon. Notable side effects were nausea, vomiting, and marrow depression, and the authors emphasized that severe renal tubular damage and deafness may occur following a single dose greater than 3.0 mg/kg. ROSSOF et al. (1972) reported evidence of antitumor activity in 5 of 31 patients treated with NSC-119875 at dosages ranging from 7.5 to 200 mg/m^2 of body surface area. The tumors responding were a mucin-producing adenocarcinoma, a sarcoma with metastases, a breast carcinoma, a poorly differentiated carcinoma of probable renal origin, and a case of stage IV-B Hodgkins disease. This latter case was the most impressive of the 5; there was complete remission 4 days after treatment, and the patient was free of disease 4 months after the last dose. Drug-related toxicity was severe in patients with abnormal excretory function. In addition to nausea and vomiting, the authors observed hyperuricemia, nephrotoxicity, leukopenia, and thrombocytopenia, as well as a slowly progressive normocytic anemia with marrow erythroid hypoplasia. Audiologic impairment above the frequency range of normal speech was detected by audiometry.

References

BERENBAUM, M. C.: Immunosuppression by platinum diammines. Brit. J. Cancer **25**, 208—211 (1971).

CLEARE, M. J., HOESCHELE, J. D.: Anti-tumor platinum compounds: relationship between structure and activity. Platinum Metals Rev. **17**, 2—13 (1973).

COLEY, R. F., FRIGERIO, N. A.: Least squares adjustment of hydrolysis data for antitumor compounds of platinum (II). ANL-7635, U.S. A.E.C. Argonne Nat. Lab. 150-1, Dec. 1969.

GALE, G. R., HOWLE, J. A., WALKER, E. M., JR.: Antitumor and antimitogenic properties of *cis*-dichloro(dipyridine)platinum(II). Cancer Res. **31**, 950—952 (1971).

GALE, G. R., MORRIS, C. R., ATKINS, L. M., SMITH, A. B.: Binding of an antitumor platinum compound to cells as influenced by physical factors and pharmacologically active agents. Cancer Res. **33**, 813—818 (1973).

HARDER, H. C.: Molecular effects of tumor-inhibiting platinum compounds in mammalian cells *in vitro:* investigations into their possible mechanisms of action. Thesis, Department of Biophysics, Michigan State University (1970).

HARDER, H. C.: Platinum coordinated purine dimers: a hypothesis of the mechanism of action of tumor-inhibitory platinum compounds. Biophys. Soc. Abstr. **11**, 299a (1971).

HARDER, H. C., ROSENBERG, B.: Inhibitory effects of anti-tumor platinum compounds on DNA, RNA and protein syntheses in mammalian cells *in vitro*. Int. J. Cancer **6**, 207—216 (1970).

HEYMAN, I. A., THOMPSON, G. R., SCHAEPPI, U. H., ROSENKRANTZ, H., FLEISCHMAN, R. W., ILIEVSKI, V., COONEY, D. A., DAVIS, R. D.: Report no. MRI-CCO 2-71-19, Mason Research Institute, Worcester, Mass. (1971).

HILL, J. M., LOEB, E., SPEER, R. J., MACLELLAN, A., HILL, N. O.: *cis*-Platinous diammino dichloride (P.D.D.) therapy of various malignant diseases. Proc. Amer. Ass. Cancer Res. **13**, 20 (1972).

HORACEK, P., DROBNIK, J.: Interaction of *cis*-dichlorodiammineplatinum(II) with DNA. Biochim. biophys. Acta (Amst.) **254**, 341—347 (1971).

HOWLE, J. A., GALE, G. R.: *cis*-Dichlorodiammineplatinum(II): cytological changes induced in *Escherichia coli*. J. Bact. **103**, 258—259 (1970a).

HOWLE, J. A., GALE, G. R.: *cis*-Dichlorodiammineplatinum(II): persistent and selective inhibition of deoxyribonucleic acid synthesis *in vivo*. Biochem. Pharmacol. **19**, 2757—2762 (1970b).

HOWLE, J. A., GALE, G. R.: Bonding of *cis*-dichloro(dipyridine)-platinum(II) to polynucleotides. Pharmacologist **13**, 210 (1971).

HOWLE, J. A., GALE, G. R., SMITH, A. B.: A proposed mode of action of antitumor platinum compounds based upon studies with *cis*-dichloro([G—^{3}H]dipyridine)-platinum(II). Biochem. Pharmacol. **21**, 1465—1475 (1972).

HOWLE. J. A., THOMPSON, H. S., STONE, A. E., GALE, G. R.: *cis*-Dichlorodiammineplatinum(II): inhibition of nucleic acid synthesis in lymphocytes stimulated with phytohemagglutinin. Proc. Soc. exp. Biol. (N.Y.) **137**, 820—825 (1971).

KAUFFMAN, G. B.: *cis*- and *trans*-Dichloro(dipyridine)platinum(II). In: KLEINBERG, J. (Ed.): Inorganic syntheses, Vol. 7, pp. 249—253. New York: McGraw-Hill 1963.

KHAN, A., ALBAYRAK, A., HILL, J. M.: Effect of *cis*-platinous diamminodichloride on graft rejection: prolonged survival of skin grafts against H_2 histocompatibility. Proc. Soc. exp. Biol. Med. (N.Y.) **141**, 7—9 (1972).

KHAN, A., HILL, J. M.: Immunosuppression with *cis*-platinum(II)-diamminodichloride: effect on antibody plaque-forming spleen cells. Infect. Immun. **4**, 320—321 (1971a).

KHAN, A., HILL, J. M.: Inhibition of lymphocyte blastogenesis by platinum compounds. J. Surg. Oncol. 3, 565—567 (1971b).

KHAN, A., HILL, J. M.: Suppression of graft-versus-host reaction by *cis*-platinum(II)diamminodichloride. Transplantation 13, 55—57 (1972).

KIRSCHNER, S., WEI, Y.-K., FRANCIS, D., BERGMAN, J. G.: Anticancer and potential antiviral activity of complex inorganic compounds. J. med. Chem. 9, 369—372 (1966).

KOCIBA, R. J., SLEIGHT, S. D.: Acute toxicologic and pathologic effects of *cis*-dichlorodiammineplatinum (NSC-119875) in the male rat. Cancer Chemother. Rep. 55, 1—8 (1971).

KOCIBA, R. J., SLEIGHT, S. D., ROSENBERG, B.: Inhibition of Dunning ascitic leukemia and Walker 256 carcinosarcoma with *cis*-diamminedichloroplatinum (NSC-119875). Cancer Chemother. Rep. 54, 325—328 (1970).

RENSHAW, E., THOMSON, A. J.: Tracer studies to locate the site of platinum ions within filamentous and inhibited cells of *Escherichia coli*. J. Bact. 94, 1915—1918 (1967).

ROBERTS, J. J., PASCOE, J. M.: Cross-linking of complementary strands of DNA in mammalian cells by antitumour platinum compounds. Nature (Lond.) 235, 282—284 (1972).

ROBINS, A. B.: The reaction of ^{14}C-labelled platinum ethylenediamine dichloride with nucleic acid constituents. Chem. Biol. Interact. 6, 35—45 (1973).

ROSENBERG, B., RENSHAW, E., VAN CAMP, L., HARTWICK, J., DROBNIK, J.: Platinum-induced filamentous growth in *Escherichia coli*. J. Bacteriol. 93, 716—721 (1967b).

ROSENBERG, B., VAN CAMP, L.: The successful regression of large solid Sarcoma 180 tumors by platinum compounds. Cancer Res. 30, 1799—1802 (1970).

ROSENBERG, B., VAN CAMP, L., GRIMLEY, E. B., THOMSON, A. J.: The inhibition of growth or cell division in *Escherichia coli* by different ionic species of platinum(IV) complexes. J. biol. Chem. 242, 1347—1352 (1967a).

ROSENBERG, B., VAN CAMP, L., KRIGAS, T.: Inhibition of cell division in *Escherichia coli* by electrolysis products from a platinum electrode. Nature (Lond.) 205, 698—699 (1965).

ROSENBERG, B., VAN CAMP, L., TROSKO, J. E., MANSOUR, V. H.: Platinum compounds: a new class of potent antitumour agents. Nature (Lond.) 222, 385—386 (1969).

ROSSOF, A. H., SLAYTON, R. E., PERLIA, C. P.: Preliminary clinical experience with *cis*-diamminedichloroplatinum(II) (NSC 119875, CACP). Cancer 30, 1451—1456 (1972).

SANDERS, C. I., MARTIN, D. S., JR.: Acid hydrolysis of $[PtCl_4]^{=}$ and $[PtCl_3(H_2O)]^{-}$. J. Amer. chem. Soc. 83, 807—810 (1961).

SHOOTER, K. V., HOWSE, R., MERRIFIELD, R. K., ROBINS, A. B.: The interaction of platinum II compounds with bacteriophages T7 and R17. Chem. Biol. Interact. 5, 289—307 (1972).

SHOOTER, K. V., MERRIFIELD, R. K.: Changes in the hydrodynamic properties of DNA induced by interaction with platinum(II) compounds. Biochim. biophys. Acta (Amst.) 287, 16—27 (1972).

SIRICA, A., VENDITTI, J. M., KLINE, I.: Enhanced survival response of L1210 leukemic mice to single combination treatment with *cis*-platinum(II) diamminodichloride (*cis*-PtII; NSC-119875) plus cyclophosphamide (CY; NSC-26271). Proc. Amer. Ass. Cancer Res. 12, 4 (1971).

TALLEY, R. W.: Chemotherapy of a mouse reticulum cell sarcoma with platinum salts. Proc. Amer. Ass. Cancer Res. 11, 78 (1970).

THOMPSON, H. S., GALE, G. R.: *cis*-Dichlorodiammineplatinum(II): hematopoietic toxicity in rats. Pharmacologist 12, 281 (1970).

THOMPSON, H. S., GALE, G. R.: *cis*-Dichlorodiammineplatinum(II): hematopoietic effects in rats. Toxicol. appl. Pharmacol. 19, 602—609 (1971).

VARKARAKIS, M. J., MURPHY, G. P.: Prostatic effects of *cis*-diamine-chloroplatinum in the dog. Res. Common. chem. Path. Pharmacol. 4, 433—438 (1972).

VONKA, V., KUTINOVA, L., DROBNIK, J., BRÄUEROVA, J.: Increase of Epstein-Barr-virus-positive cells in EB3 cultures after treatment with *cis*-dichloro-diammine-platinum(II). J. nat. Cancer Inst. 48, 1277—1281 (1972).

WELSCH, C. W.: Effects of *cis*-platinum diamminodichloride(II) on growth of 7,12-dimethylbenzanthracene (DMBA)-induced mammary tumors in female rats. Proc. Amer. Ass. Cancer Res. 12, 25 (1971).

ZAK, M., DROBNIK, J., REZNY, Z.: The effect of *cis*-platinum(II)diamminodichloride on bone marrow. Cancer Res. 32, 595—599 (1972a).

ZAK, M., DROBNIK, J., REZNY, Z.: The effect of *cis*-dichlorodiammineplatinum(II) on cytological and morphological changes in bone marrow of mice (long-term observations). Neoplasma 19, 305—310 (1972b).

Chapter 77

Metal Chelates of 3-Ethoxy-2-Oxobutyraldehyde *Bis* (Thiosemicarbazone), H_2KTS

DAVID H. PETERING and HAROLD G. PETERING

With 1 Figure

Introduction

Interest in the chemotherapeutic activity of thiosemicarbazones stems from the discovery of DOMAGK et al. (1946) that certain monothiosemicarbazones have antitubercular action. Since then, a great many mono- and dithiosemicarbazones have been synthesized and assayed for possible chemotherapeutic activity in a number of systems. Among these compounds are a number of *bis*(thiosemicarbazones) of α-ketoaldehydes or diketones which have been found to show antimicrobial, antiparasitic, and antitumor activities (BARRETT et al., 1965; MICHAELS et al., 1962; FRENCH and FREEDLANDER, 1958; BARRY et al., 1970).

The antineoplastic activity of dithiosemicarbazones was first reported by FRENCH and FREEDLANDER (1958) in a study of glyoxal *bis*(thiosemicarbazones) and of several substituted analogs. In a subsequent paper in which screening data of fifty *bis*(thiosemicarbazones) were reported, FRENCH and FREEDLANDER (1960) found only four with significant activity against Sarcoma 180 in mice, among which was 3-ethoxy-2-oxo-butyraldehyde *bis*(thiosemicarbazone) (H_2KTS). PETERING and BUSKIRK (1962) confirmed the antineoplastic activity of H_2KTS in a study of its analogs and methylglyoxal derivatives, and in a later paper PETERING et al. (1964) presented evidence of the superiority of H_2KTS as a chemotherapeutic agent against several rat tumors.

The pronounced transition metal-binding properties of both mono- and dithiosemicarbazones have been recognized since the turn of the century, when NEUBERG and NEIMANN (1902) found this property in a number of thiosemicarbazones of simple aldehydes and ketones. Since then the coordination chemistry of thiosemicarbazones has been studied by a number of investigators, among them BÄHR (1952, 1953), GINGRAS et al. (1960, 1961, 1962), and PETERING (1972a). Scientists investigating the chemotherapeutic action of both mono- and dithiosemicarbazones have been cognizant of the possible importance of complex formation and chelation of transition metals to an understanding of the mechanism of action of these compounds. FRENCH and FREEDLANDER (1958), for example, suggested that the antineoplastic activity of glyoxal *bis*(thiosemicarbazone) might be due to the binding of key metal ions which may be specifically important in tumor growth. However, in none of the early work was there evidence indicating which metal(s) may be involved in the mechanism of action of mono- or dithiosemicarbazones.

The extensive studies of PETERING et al. (1963, 1964, 1966a, 1967) led these authors to conclude that the action of the *bis*(thiosemicarbazones) was due not to the sequestering of essential or heavy metal ions, but rather to *in vivo* formation of the copper chelates, which in themselves were responsible for the antitumor activity. They concluded that Cu(II)KTS[3-ethoxy-2-oxobutyraldehyde *bis*(thiosemicarbazonato) copper(II)] was the active agent formed *in vivo*.

Antineoplastic Activity of H_2KTS

In their screening tests of hundreds of compounds from seventeen categories of chemical structures, FRENCH and FREEDLANDER (1960) found that significant activity against Sarcoma 180 in mice (more than 70 % inhibition of growth of the tumor when treatment was begun on the day of implantation) resided in only four thiosemicarbazones. These compounds were 3-ethoxy-2-oxobutyraldehyde *bis*(thiosemicarbazone) (H_2KTS), 3-ethoxy-2-oxobutyraldehyde *bis*(N^4-methylthiosemicarbazone) (H_2KTSM), glyoxal *bis*(N^4-allylthiosemicarbazone), and methoxymethylglyoxal *bis*(N^4-methylthiosemicarbazone).

PETERING and BUSKIRK (1962) reported that H_2KTS had pronounced activity when it was given orally to rats bearing the Walker 256 carcinosarcoma (W-256), Jensen sarcoma, or Murphy Sturm lymphosarcoma, and showed that this drug caused the complete regression of established tumors. Subsequently, PETERING et al. (1964) compared the activity of H_2KTS with four active analogs, including pyruvaldehyde *bis*(thiosemicarbazone), which exhibited *in vitro* cytotoxic activity against KB cells in culture equal to that of H_2KTS. Their data clearly showed the superiority of H_2KTS to the other analogs in causing inhibition and regression of the above mentioned tumors in rats when it was administered either orally or intraperitoneally. Later, PETERING et al. (1966c) reported the preparation of three new thiosemicarbazones with *in vivo* activity against a nitrogen mustard (HN_2) resistant variant of W-256 (W-256/HN_2), and more recently, MIHICH and SIMPSON (1968) found that 3-butyryloxy-2-oxobutyraldehyde *bis*(thiosemicarbazone) (H_2BGTS) had activity similar to that of H_2KTS against Sarcoma 180 in mice. The chemical structures of the *bis*(thiosemicarbazones) which have significant *in vivo* activity in the various studies are shown in Fig. 1.

$$\begin{array}{l} R - C = N{-}NH{-}CS{-}NX_2 \\ \quad\;\; | \\ \quad HC = N{-}NH{-}CS{-}NX_2 \end{array}$$

I.	$R = CH_3 \cdot CH(OC_2H_5);\ X_2 = H_2$	(H_2KTS)
II.	$R = CH_3 \cdot CH(OC_2H_5);\ X_2 = H,CH_3$	(H_2KTSM)
III.	$R = CH_3 \cdot CH(OCH_3);\ X_2 = H_2$	(H_2KMTS)
IV.	$R = CH_3 \cdot CH(OCOCH_3);\ X_2 = H_2$	(H_2KATS)
V.	$R = CH_3 \cdot CH(CH_3OC_2H_4O);\ X_2 = H_2$	(H_2MKTS)
VI.	$R = H;\ X_2 = H,(H_2C = CH - CH_2)$	(- - - - - -)
VII.	$R = CH_3OCH_2;\ X_2 = H,CH_3$	(- - - - - -)
VIII.	$R = CH_3;\ X_2 = H, CH_3$	(H_2PTSM)
IX.	$R = CH_3 \cdot CH(OCOC_3H_7);\ X_2 = H_2$	(H_2BGTS)

Fig. 1. Structures of *bis*(thiosemicarbazones) with significant *in vivo* antineoplastic activity

The detailed study of PETERING et al. (1964) showed that H_2KTS exhibited dose-response relationships upon oral administration to rats bearing five-day transplants of W-256/HN_2 tumors with respect to *percent* inhibition, complete regressions, and weight gain. These authors also reported that H_2KTS had significant activity against a C3H spontaneous mammary tumor in mice, and against cells from a human adenocarcinoma and two canine adenocarcinomas, as well as against W-256 cells in an *in vitro* cytotoxicity test. MIHICH and NICHOL (1965) reported that the drug was highly active against a spontaneous mammary tumor in DBA_2 mice, and against transplants of adenocarcinoma 755, the Ridgeway osteosarcoma, the Mecca lymphosarcoma, and carcinoma 1025 in mice. They also found that a significant number of complete regressions occurred with Sarcoma 180 and W-256 tumors.

MIHICH and NICHOL (1965) reported that feeding mice bearing Sarcoma 180 tumors a vitamin B_6-deficient diet enhanced the activity of H_2KTS, a finding similar to that previously reported for enhancement of activity of pyruvaldehyde *bis*(4-methylthiosemicarbazone) against Sarcoma 180 by MIHICH and NICHOL (1961). It was found that H_2KTS was equally active against HN_2 sensitive and resistant variants of W-256 (PETERING et al., 1964), and that enhancement of antitumor activity against a number of tumors in mice and rats was found when H_2KTS and uracil mustard combinations were given (MIHICH and NICHOL, 1965; PETERING et al., 1966a). MARTIN (1963) reported that administration of H_2KTS to CD_8F_1 mice bearing spontaneous mammary tumors enhanced the cure rate usually obtained with surgery, and JOHNSTON and PETERING (1962, unpublished) found that powdering H_2KTS into the surgical wounds following enucleation of W-256 tumors of rats led to greatly enhanced cure rates.

These reports clearly established the potent antitumor activity of H_2KTS and suggested the importance of initiating clinical investigations of the drug. Up to the present time, preclinical pharmacology studies have been reported by MIHICH et al. (1965) and only one Phase I clinical study has been initiated by REGELSON et al. (1967). The latter investigators did not find the delayed hepatic, pancreatic, myocardial, and adrenal toxicity reported by MIHICH et al. (1965) in animals given very large and lethal doses of the drug. Many of the toxic symptoms reported by REGELSON et al. (1967) can readily be attributed to interference with copper metabolism. These studies and the information obtained on the antitumor activity of metal chelates of H_2KTS suggest that further clinical studies of the *bis*(thiosemicarbazones) and their metal chelates are warranted.

Metal Chelation and Antitumor Activity of H_2KTS (Activity of Cu(II) KTS and ZnKTS)

Early in their search to define the optimal conditions for the therapeutic action of H_2KTS, PETERING et al. (1963) found that the mineral content of the diets fed tumor-bearing animals was a most important factor in influencing the antitumor activity of the drug. They found that of a number of metal ions tested *in vitro*, only copper and zinc enhanced the low cytotoxicity of H_2KTS. The findings shown in Table 1 are from unpublished data of VAN GIESSEN et al. (1973); they show the effect of a number of metal ions on the cytotoxic action of H_2KTS against W-256 tumor cells in suspension, and confirm the pronounced effect of the Cu(II) ion in enhancing the activity of the drug. These data also show that in the case of those metals with little or no potentiating effects, the further addition of a small concentration of cupric ion to the medium raised the cytotoxicity of H_2KTS to its maximum. Similar results were obtained when W-256/HN_2, Harding-Passey melanoma, and L5178Y tumor cells were used. By itself, H_2KTS had insignificant cytotoxic activity *in vitro*.

Subsequently, PETERING et al. (1965) reported that of a number of chelates of transition metals, which were made and tested on W-256 cells in the same cytotoxicity test system, only the cupric chelate, Cu(II)KTS, had the activity necessary to explain the potentiating activity of Cu(II) ion. Among the other chelates tested and found to have little activity were those of Co(II), Fe(III), Ni(II), and Zn(II). MIHICH and MULHERN (1965) at the same time confirmed the pronounced *in vivo* antitumor activity of Cu(II)KTS.

Following these reports, detailed information was adduced to establish the unique role of Cu(II) *in vivo* in the antitumor action of H_2KTS and the probable formation of Cu(II)KTS as the active intermediate metabolite. PETERING and VAN GIESSEN (1966b) and PETERING et al. (1967) showed that the drug was devoid of antitumor activity when given orally at 25 mg per kg to rats bearing the W-256 tumor and fed a semipurified diet low in copper. When, however, copper was given in the drinking water to other rats receiving the drug, inhibition of tumor growth and regression occurred readily. Control rats, on the other hand, which received only copper in the water, exhibited no inhibition of tumor growth. A typical dose-response was shown for antitumor activity with respect to copper concentration in the drinking water of rats bearing W-256 tumors when 25 mg per kg of H_2KTS was given orally. When zinc was given to rats bearing the same tumor, but fed a diet deficient in zinc and adequate in copper, there was no reduction in the activity of the drug. CRIM and PETERING (1967) further demonstrated that Cu(II)KTS had potent antitumor activity regardless of the copper content of the diets and that the zinc chelate (ZnKTS) had minimal activity on a stock diet containing copper and none when copper was eliminated. These data established *in vivo* that H_2KTS required copper for activity and did not require zinc. In fact, PETERING et al. (1967) showed that zinc is essential to tumor growth, a finding confirmed by McQUITTY et al. (1970).

BOOTH and SARTORELLI (1966) also examined the effect of H_2KTS in the presence and absence of cupric ions on Sarcoma 180 (ascites) in mice and found that i.p. administration of a combination of the drug and $CuCl_2$ prolonged the life of the mice, whereas neither agent alone had any significant effect on life span. This is in contrast to the reported activity of H_2KTS alone at much higher doses against the solid form of Sarcoma 180 (FRENCH and FREEDLANDER, 1960; MIHICH and NICHOL, 1965) and may indicate that under the conditions of solid tumor growth copper was available, while it was not when ascites tumors were used.

The lack of ascites tumor response to the low levels of the drug and the marked potentiation of activity when Cu(II) was present are similar to the *in vitro* cytotoxicity findings of PETERING and VAN GIESSEN (1966b) and VAN GIESSEN et al. (1973; cf. Table 1). A reasonable explanation for the observation that ascites tumors treated by direct injection of the drug into the peritoneum are not responsive is that there is an inadequate supply of available copper for reaction with H_2KTS prior to its encounter with the target tumor cells, even though the diet may contain adequate copper for normal function of the mice. In fact, BOOTH and SARTORELLI (1967) substantiated this point of view when they noted that the drug alone did not stimulate the uptake of copper by the ascites cells *in vivo*, but that when Cu(II)KTS was given there was a pronounced uptake of copper. In the solid tumor systems, in which the drug alone is active when the diet contains copper, the drug must make its way to the tumor site from a distant point of entry into the organism, whether it is given orally or parenterally. This provides many opportunities for interaction with available copper before the target tumor mass is reached. This line of reasoning would explain the fact that MIHICH and NICHOL (1965) found the drug inactive against the L1210 leukemia in ascites form, although these cells in culture systems containing copper are sensitive to the drug.

Even though there is some disagreement about the efficacy of ZnKTS *in vivo*, it would appear that its activity, as well as that of H_2KTS can be explained by

Table 1. *Effect of transition metal ions on cytotoxicity*[a] *of* H_2KTS *on* W-256/HN_2 *cells*

Metal Ion Added	Cytotoxicity of Metal Ion Alone μg/ml	Level Used for H_2KTS Cytotoxicity μg/ml	Cytotoxicity of H_2KTS with Metal μg/ml	Cytotoxicity of H_2KTS with Metal $+0.4$ μg/ml Cu^{2+} μg/ml
None (H_2KTS alone)	—	—	800	0.8
Cu^{2+}	1.6 to 3.2	0.4	0.8	—
Zn^{2+}	100	40	25	1.6
Ni^{2+}	100	20	200	25
Co^{2+}	200	40	400	1.6
Fe^{3+}	200	40	400	0.8
Mn^{2+}	200	40	400	0.2

[a] The ARAI and SUZUKI (1956) method was used. Cytotoxicity was determined as amount of drug $\pm$ metal ion which would reduce respiratory activity (using methylene blue) of cells equivalent to rate of 80% of control. ($\leq$ 1.6 μg/ml of drug is highly active; 3.2 to 12.5 μg/ml of drug is moderately active; 25 to 50 μg/ml of drug is slightly active; and $\geqq$ 100 μg/ml of drug is inactive.)

Data of VAN GIESSEN et al., 1973.

the probable interaction of these agents with available copper in the organism bearing the tumor to form Cu(II)KTS as the necessary intermediate. This conclusion is in harmony with the chemical properties of H_2KTS, which have been described by PETERING and VAN GIESSEN (1966b) and VAN GIESSEN and PETERING (1968). These authors and PETERING (1972a) have pointed out that H_2KTS, as well as other related *bis*(thiosemicarbazones), react with first transition series divalent metal ions readily to form 1:1 chelates as described in Eq. (1):

$$\begin{array}{l} R-C=N-NH-CS-NH_2 \\ \quad | \\ HC=N-NH-CS-NH_2 \end{array} + M^{2+} \longrightarrow \begin{array}{l} R-C=N-N=C-NH_2 \\ \quad | \qquad \searrow \quad\; | \\ \quad | \qquad\quad M \!\!<\!\! \begin{array}{l} S \\ S \end{array} \\ \quad | \qquad \nearrow \quad\; | \\ HC=N-N=C-NH_2 \end{array} \tag{1}$$

H_2KTS is an excellent chelating agent for a variety of heavy metals. In particular, it forms a thermodynamically strong complex with copper(II). At pH 7.4, the association constant of Cu(II)KTS is $10^{18.8}$, much larger than those of putative cellular ligands such as amino acid mixtures (PETERING, 1972a). In the presence of reactive copper, such as is found in plasma, therefore, H_2KTS is expected to exist entirely as its copper chelate. The association constant of ZnKTS has also been determined at pH 7.0 (PETERING, 1974). Its value of $10^{5.1}$ indicates that at low concentration measurable portions of the complex are dissociated and that in the presence of cupric ion or bound copper available to H_2KTS, the zinc chelate will be converted quantitatively to Cu(II)KTS.

These results strengthen the view that the mechanism of action of H_2KTS or ZnKTS depends upon the initial formation of the very stable complex, Cu(II)KTS (PETERING and VAN GIESSEN, 1966b).

Studies on the Mechanisms of Action of Cu (II) KTS

Several reports have appeared which present data bearing on the possible mechanism of antitumor action of Cu(II)KTS (or Cu^{2+} + H_2KTS). These will be summarized here and related briefly to the experimental facts presented previously.

The cytotoxicity of Cu(II)KTS must depend upon the net chemical reaction of this chelate with some cellular component. Generally, copper complexes participate in three types of reactions; namely, ligand exchange, adduct formation, and oxido-reductions. These are illustrated in the following equations.

$$\mathrm{Cu(II)KTS} + 2\mathrm{HL} \longrightarrow \mathrm{Cu(II)L_2} + \mathrm{H_2KTS} \qquad (2)$$

$$\mathrm{Cu(II)KTS} + \mathrm{L} \longrightarrow \underset{\displaystyle \mathrm{L}}{\overset{}{\mathrm{Cu(II)KTS}}} \qquad (3)$$

$$\mathrm{Cu(II)KTS} + \mathrm{L(Reduced)} \longrightarrow \mathrm{Cu(I)KTS} + \mathrm{L(Oxidized)} \qquad (4)$$

The extremely great thermodynamic stability of Cu(II)KTS and its negligible ability to form stable adducts militate against hypotheses based on Eqs. (2) and (3) (PETERING, 1972a). However, PETERING (1972b) has shown that Cu(II)KTS is a selective agent for the controlled oxidation of thiols according to the following reaction:

$$\mathrm{Cu(II)KTS} + 2\mathrm{RSH} \longrightarrow \mathrm{Cu(I)SR} + 1/2\,\mathrm{RSSR} + \mathrm{H_2KTS} \qquad (5)$$

A variety of cellular sulfhydryl compounds, such as lipoic acid, glutathione, coenzyme A, and cysteine, undergo this reaction, which occurs sluggishly in comparison with the reaction between a number of other common copper complexes and sulfhydryl compounds. This anomalous behavior may be important in that it allows Cu(II)KTS to be transported to target cells before being dissociated by reaction with thiols *en route*, as would be expected with more rapidly reacting copper chelates. This reaction also is the only one known that could account for the dissociation of Cu(II)KTS within tumor cells, a process that has been demonstrated by BOOTH and SARTORELLI (1967). The utility of chemical studies alongside investigations of biological mechanisms resides in the fact that they provide a basis for and a check on the hypotheses being formulated concerning the biochemical mechanisms of action.

BOOTH et al. (1966, 1967, 1968, 1971) have examined the effects of H_2KTS, Cu(II)KTS, H_2KTS plus Cu^{2+}, $CuCl_2$, ZnKTS, and $ZnCl_2$ on some of the metabolic functions of Sarcoma 180 ascites cells. In studying the influence of these agents upon the incorporation of precursors into DNA, RNA, and protein, these authors suggested that the primary action of Cu(II)KTS and H_2KTS is the inhibition of DNA synthesis; these agents also depress RNA and protein synthesis but to a lesser extent. However, the inhibition pattern for DNA is quite nonspecific, both in terms of the wide spectrum of processes inhibited by each agent and in the similar degrees of inhibition caused by Cu(II)KTS, H_2KTS, and $CuCl_2$ in a variety of cases (BOOTH and SARTORELLI, 1966, 1967). In particular, considering the percent inhibition of incorporation of various precursors into DNA, with only one precursor out of five is the difference in inhibition between equal amounts of cellular copper, delivered either by $CuCl_2$ or Cu(II)KTS, greater than 25%. The broad similarity of activity of Cu(II)KTS, $CuCl_2$, and $Cu(stearate)_2$ holds also for RNA precursors and for the incorporation of amino acids into protein (cf., Table 3 and Fig. 6 of BOOTH and SARTORELLI, 1967). This similarity of action extends to the effects of H_2KTS, ZnKTS, and $ZnCl_2$ (BOOTH and SARTORELLI, 1968; BOOTH et al., 1971). Furthermore, the effects of ZnKTS and $ZnCl_2$ on DNA and RNA synthesis by ascites cells are similar and do not provide a basis for localizing the metabolic site associated with antitumor activity.

On the other hand, in a variety of animal experiments already delineated above, including those of BOOTH and SARTORELLI (1966), the results are all consistent with the conclusion that Cu(II)KTS is the sole active cytotoxic entity. Hence, the finding of broad and similar activity with respect to DNA synthesis by Cu(II)KTS, ZnKTS, Cu(II) salts, and $ZnCl_2$ suggests strongly that the effect of Cu(II)KTS on DNA synthesis may be a secondary effect and not the primary antitumor action.

The results of these investigators do not support the view that H_2KTS simply serves as a delivery system for copper (BOOTH and SARTORELLI, 1967). Although copper uptake by ascites cells occurs when $CuCl_2$ or copper stearate is given, there is no evidence that copper alone in these forms produces genuine antineoplastic action *in vivo*, as evidenced by prolongation of survival or tumor inhibition and regression. Therefore, one must conclude from these interesting studies that the form in which copper enters the cell, not just the quantity, is of critical importance to the development of antitumor activity.

An alternative hypothesis which needs exploration is that the primary activity of Cu(II)KTS is on the energy transport mechanism of tumor cells. This is implicit in the cytotoxicity results of VAN GIESSEN et al. (1973) and PETERING and VAN GIESSEN (1966b). Its possibility has been further enhanced by the findings of COATS et al. (unpublished) that Cu(II)KTS uncouples oxidative phosphorylation of liver mitochondria, and inhibits the Crabtree effect and the respiration of Ehrlich ascites cells at levels which could be realized in *in vivo* experiments. Inhibition of the energy transport system could be related to the reaction of Cu(II)KTS with thiols and could inhibit the biosynthetic capacity of the tumor cells.

Editor's Comments (ACS). In the opinion of the Editors there is no unequivocal proof that ZnKTS does not have inherent cytotoxic activity against susceptible transplanted neoplastic cells. Furthermore, the findings of BOOTH and SARTORELLI (1967) and BOOTH et al. (1968, 1971) clearly indicate that the patterns of inhibition of DNA, RNA, and protein by H_2KTS, ZnKTS, and Cu(II)KTS are different, suggesting the production by these agents of different metabolic lesions. With both metal chelates, the synthesis of DNA was found to be more sensitive to inhibition than was the formation of RNA or protein; however, no evidence is available to directly implicate alterations of these metabolic pathways with antitumor activity. Evidence to support the concept that the cellular toxicity of Cu(II)KTS is probably due to copper was presented by BOOTH and SARTORELLI (1967). Cu(II)KTS, a relatively lipid-soluble form of copper, was demonstrated to serve effectively to transport copper to sensitive cellular sites. Apparently greater affinity of intracellular components for copper leads to the dissociation of the chelate and deposition of the metal within tumor cells. The ligand portion of the molecule, H_2KTS, is then rapidly eliminated from cells, while the copper is retained for much longer periods. The use of several radioactive precursors of DNA led to findings that suggested that the intracellular localization of copper from Cu(II)KTS differed to some extent from that of $CuCl_2$.

References

BÄHR, G.: Über Emprotide Schwermetall-Inner-Complexe der α-Diketon-dithiosemicarbazone (thiazone). I. Z. f. Anorg. Allg. Chemie **268**, 351—363 (1952).

BÄHR, G.: Über Emprotide Schwermetall-Inner-Complexe der α-Diketon-dithiosemicarbazone (thiazone). II. Z. f. Anorg. Allg. Chemie **273**, 325—332 (1953).

BARRETT, P.A., BEVERIDGE, E., BRADLEY, P.L., BROWN, C.G.D., BUSHBY, S.R.M., CLARKE, M.L., NEAL, R.A., SMITH, R., WILDE, J.K.H.: Biological activities of some α-dithiosemicarbazones. Nature (Lond.) **206**, 1340—1341 (1965).

BARRY, V. C., CONALTY, M. L., MCCORMICK, J. E., MCELHENNEY, R. S., MCINERNEY, M. R., O'SULLIVAN, J. F.: Anticancer agents. IV. The antitumor activity of some 1,4- and 1,5-(*bis*thiosemicarbazones) and of related heterocycles. J. med. Chem. **13**, 421—427 (1970).

BOOTH, B. A., DONNELLY, T. E., JR., ZETTNER, A., SARTORELLI, A. C.: Metabolic effects of zinc in intact cells — comparative studies of zinc chloride and the zinc chelate of kethoxal *bis*-(thiosemicarbazone). Biochem. Pharmacol. **20**, 3109—3118 (1971).

BOOTH, B. A., JOHNS, D. G., BERTINO, J. R., SARTORELLI, A. C.: Sites of inhibition of DNA synthesis by kethoxal *bis*(thiosemicarbazone). Nature (Lond.) **217**, 250—251 (1968).

BOOTH, B. A., SARTORELLI, A. C.: Synergistic interaction of kethoxal *bis*(thiosemicarbazone) and cupric ions in Sarcoma 180. Nature (Lond.) **210**, 104—105 (1966).

BOOTH, B. A., SARTORELLI, A. C.: Metabolic effects of copper in intact cells: comparative activity of cupric chloride and the cupric chelate of kethoxal *bis*(thiosemicarbazone). Molec. Pharmacol. **3**, 290—302 (1967).

CRIM, J. A., PETERING, H. G.: The antitumor activity of Cu(II)KTS, the copper (II) chelate of 3-ethoxy-2-oxobutyraldehyde *bis*(thiosemicarbazone). Cancer Research **27**, 1278—1285 (1967).

DOMAGK, G., BEHNISCH, R., MIETZSCH, F., SCHMIDT, H.: Über eine neue, gegen Tuberkelbazillen *in vitro* wirksame Verbindungsklasse. Naturwissenschaften **33**, 315 (1946).

FRENCH, F. A., FREEDLANDER, B. L.: Carcinostatic action of polycarbonyl compounds and their derivatives. IV. Glyoxal *bis*(thiosemicarbazone) and derivatives. Cancer Res. **18**, 1298—1300 (1958).

FRENCH, F. A., FREEDLANDER, B. L.: Chemotherapy studies on transplanted tumors. Cancer Res. **21**, 505—538 (1960).

GINGRAS, B. A., HORNAL, R. W., BAYLEY, C. H.: The preparation of some thiosemicarbazones and their copper complexes. I. Canad. J. Chem. **38**, 712—719 (1960).

GINGRAS, B. A., SOMARJAI, R. L., BAYLEY, C. H.: The preparation of some thiosemicarbazones and their copper complexes. II. Canad. J. Chem. **39**, 973—985 (1961).

GINGRAS, B. A., SUPRUNCHUK, T., BAYLEY, C. H.: The preparation of some thiosemicarbazones and their copper complexes. III. Canad. J. Chem. **40**, 1053—1059 (1962).

MARTIN, D. S.: Combination adjuvant therapy after surgery for spontaneous breast tumors. Proc. Amer. Ass. Cancer. Res. **4**, 42 (1963).

MCQUITTY, J. T., DEWYS, W. D., MONACO, L., STRAIN, W. H., ROB, C. G., APGAR, J., PORIES, W. J.: Inhibition of tumor growth by dietary zinc deficiency. Cancer Res. **30**, 1387—1390 (1970).

MICHAELS, R. M., PETERSON, L. J., STAHL, G. L.: The activity of substituted thiosemicarbazones against *T. vaginalis* and *T. foetus in vitro* and in experimental animals. J. Parasitol. **48**, 891—897 (1962).

MIHICH, E., MULHERN, A. I.: Comparative potency of kethoxal *bis*(thiosemicarbazone) (KTS) and its copper II chelate (KTS—Cu) in rodents. Fed. Proc. **24**, 454 (1965).

MIHICH, E., NICHOL, C. A.: Enhanced inhibition of Sarcoma 180 (S180) caused by methylglyoxal-*bis*(N^4-methylthiosemicarbazone) (CH_3—GMS) and dietary pyridoxine deficiency. Proc. Amer. Ass. Cancer Res. **3**, 250 (1961).

MIHICH, E., NICHOL, C. A.: Kethoxal *bis*(thiosemicarbazone). I. Effects against experimental tumors. Cancer Res. **25**, 1410—1416 (1965).

MIHICH, E., SIMPSON, C. L.: Comparative study of α-n-butyryloxyethylglyoxal *bis*(thiosemicarbazone) (BGTS) and kethoxal-*bis*(thiosemicarbazone) (KTS). Pharmacologist **10**, 171 (1968).

MIHICH, E., SIMPSON, C. L., MULHERN, A. I.: Kethoxal *bis*(thiosemicarbazone). II. Toxic and pathologic effects. Cancer Res. **25**, 1417—1431 (1965).

NEUBERG, C., NEIMANN, W.: Eine Methode zur Isolierung von Aldehyden und Ketonen. Ber. **35**, 2049—2056 (1902).

PETERING, D. H.: CuKTS. I. Physico-chemical properties of the antitumor agent. Bioinorg. Chem. I, 255—271 (1972a).

PETERING, D. H.: CuKTS. II. Reactions with thiols. Bioinorg. Chem., I, 273—288 (1972b).

PETERING, D. H.: The role of zinc in the antitumor activity of 3-ethoxy-2-oxobutyraldehyde *bis*(thiosemicarbazonato)zinc (II) and related compounds. Biochem. Pharmacol. **23**, 567—576 (1974).

PETERING, H. G., BUSKIRK, H. H.: The antitumor activity of 2-keto-3-ethoxybutyraldehyde *bis*(thiosemicarbazone) and related compounds. Fed. Proc. **21**, 163 (1962).

PETERING, H. G., BUSKIRK, H. H., CRIM, J. A.: Activity of combinations of uracil mustard (NSC-34462) and 3-ethoxy-2-oxobutyraldehyde *bis*(thiosemicarbazone) (KTS, NSC-82116) against murine tumors. Cancer Chemother. Rep. **50**, 557—563 (1966a).

PETERING, H. G., BUSKIRK, H. H., CRIM, J. A.: The effect of dietary mineral supplements of the rat on the antitumor activity of 3-ethoxy-2-oxobutyraldehyde *bis*(thiosemicarbazone). Cancer Res. **27**, 1115—1121 (1967).

PETERING, H. G., BUSKIRK, H. H., CRIM, J. A., VAN GIESSEN, G. J.: The effect of essential metal ions on the antitumor activity of kethoxal *bis*(thiosemicarbazone) (KTS). Pharmacologist **5**, 271 (1963).

PETERING, H. G., BUSKIRK, H. H., KUPIECKI, F.: Chelate formation and antitumor activity of KTS. Fed. Proc. **24**, 454 (1965).

PETERING, H. G., BUSKIRK, H. H., UNDERWOOD, G. E.: The antitumor activity of 2-keto-3-ethoxybutyraldehyde *bis*(thiosemicarbazone) and related compounds. Cancer Res. **24**, 367—372 (1964).

PETERING, H. G., VAN GIESSEN, G. J.: The essential role of cupric ion in the biological activity of 3-ethoxy-2-oxobutyraldehyde *bis*(thiosemicarbazone), a new antitumor agent. In: PIESACH, AISEN, BLUMBERG (Eds.): The biochemistry of copper, pp. 197—210. New York: Academic Press 1966b.

PETERING, H. G., VAN GIESSEN, G. J., CRIM, J. A., BUSKIRK, H. H.: The synthesis and antitumor activity of several thiosemicarbazones related to kethoxal *bis*(thiosemicarbazone). J. med. Chem. **9**, 420—421 (1966c).

REGELSON, W., HOLLAND, J. F., TALLEY, R. W.: Clinical pharmacologic study of kethoxal *bis*-(thiosemicarbazone) (NSC-82116) in advanced cancer. Cancer Chemother. Rep. **51**, 171—177 (1967).

SARTORELLI, A. C., WELCH, A. D., BOOTH, B. A.: Biochemical effects of kethoxal *bis*(thiosemicarbazone) and its cupric chelate. Fed. Proc. **24**, 454 (1965).

VAN GIESSEN, G. J., CRIM, J. A., PETERING, D. H., PETERING, H. G.: Effect of heavy metals on the *in vitro* cytotoxicity of 3-ethoxy-2-oxobutyraldehyde *bis*(thiosemicarbazone) and related compounds. J. nat. Cancer Inst. **51**, 139—146 (1973).

VAN GIESSEN, G. J., PETERING, H. G.: Metal complexes of 3-ethoxy-2-oxobutyraldehyde *bis*-(thiosemicarbazone) and related ligands as antitumor agents. J. med. Chem. **11**, 695—699 (1968).

Chapter 78

Phleomycin and Bleomycin

PAUL PIETSCH

With 7 Figures

Introduction

Strains of *Streptomyces verticillus* native to the soil of the coal mining country of Fukuoka Prefecture, Japan can elaborate heterogeneous antibiotic substances (i.e., phleomycin and bleomycin) with a capacity to block DNA synthesis, inhibit proliferation of replicative RNA's, and prevent higher cells from entering meiotic or mitotic division. These actions can occur separately, possibly because they depend on different specific compounds present in phleomycin and bleomycin. These actions were discovered at different times and in different laboratories during independent investigations. Reported separately, they created a confusing and conflicting literature on the action of phleomycin-bleomycin.

In part, this circumstance can be attributed to variations among the components of different batches of material. *S. verticillus*, after all, would be confronted with many different kinds of competitors, including bacteria, DNA and RNA viruses, and roots of plants. To survive in nature, presumably it had to be flexible, to have the capacity to adjust its toxic mixtures in accord with the realities of the milieu. In the laboratory, these inherent traits would and did produce differently constituted batches, depending on the medium.

In addition, *S. verticillus* had to escape the effects of its own strategy. For the actions of the elaborated antibiotics against replication would be expected to be directed against fundamental ubiquitous mechanisms shared by the organism itself. Receptors, at least for DNA replication, had to be general enough to persist through the broad diverse course of evolution. Yet those sites could scarcely present a ready passive target for the active moieties of phleomycin and bleomycin or *S. verticillus* would rapidly have become an extinct species. *S. verticillus* seems to have solved the problem by manufacturing compounds that match up with receptors only under circumscribed conditions and only at critical moments. Presumably, among wild *S. verticillus*, those moments would seem to arrive after phleomycin and bleomycin have filtered off into the soil. In addition, had receptive moments been set to a rigid schedule, bacteria soon would have evolved an harmonic escape; but, *S. verticillus* seems to have solved this problem with compounds aimed at receptors that turn on and off in response to internal conditions of the cell under attack. Thus, observations in the laboratory vary, not merely because different workers have studied different antibiotic mixtures, but because the underlying dynamics defy any single-minded, simplistic, linear view of the subject.

UMEZAWA and MAEDA (1955) initiated patent applications on phleomycin in 1955, but the cobalt blue material received very modest attention until the early 1960's when its antitumor properties became evident. Then research intensified, and in 1963 TANAKA et al. (1963a, b, c) published an account of the mechanism by which phleomycin arrested DNA synthesis without any manifest effect on transcription or protein manufacture. For a brief period, this seemed like the only action; however, that view soon required major modification. A number of other independent investigations have reproduced the essential findings of TANAKA et al., and it appears as though these workers, fortuitously, observed this most interesting action taking place by itself. Once the antitumor properties of phleomycin became evident, UMEZAWA et al. devoted major effort to its study. Initially they were encouraged by its lack of delayed lethality in mice; however, they soon discovered that phleomycin induces kidney malfunctions. Similar experiences with the kanamycins prompted them to search among substrains of *S. verticillus* for a batch of material without the kidney effects. This was obtained in the form of bleomycin (UMEZAWA, 1966).

General Properties

Specific compounds responsible for the main actions of phleomycin and bleomycin have not yet been characterized as to structure. But from all the evidence in the literature and from my laboratory during the past several years, it is abundantly clear that phleomycin and bleomycin represent a single general class of antibiotics. In fact, were it not for nephrotoxicity and the warning implied by phleomycin, I would urge that one term be used.

A. Composition

Phleomycin and bleomycin precipitate from the aqueous phase of strain 843 *S. verticillus* cultures upon the addition of most organic solvents, methanol being an important exception (MAEDA et al., 1956; UMEZAWA et al., 1966a). Molecular formulae have varied with virtually every new report. Carbon, hydrogen, nitrogen, and oxygen are always present. Copper, a native constituent, varies in amount, depending on the culture medium. Usually cupric, it can occur in cuprous form without loss of activity. Its removal generally increases potency and reduces toxicity (TAKITA, 1959; ISHIZUKA et al., 1967). Sulfur has been regularly identified in bleomycin samples, but its significance is equivocal, and, herein, may lie important clues.

Patent applications and early reports describe phleomycin as highly unstable in acid (UMEZAWA, 1955; MAEDA et al., 1956). PIETSCH and ENG (1969) could not support this claim after subjecting phleomycin-909[1] to hydrolysis in HCl. The acid-treated product showed 6 to 7 times the braking effect on growth of the parent material and about a four-fold drop in acute toxicity. Phleomycin-909 contains sulfur, as have other lots since the early days of this research (cf. IKEKAWA et al., 1964; PIETSCH, 1969a). Hydrolysis reduced the sulfur content of phleomycin-909 by a factor of five, suspiciously comparable to the drop in toxicity and rise in potency. Bleomycin has been characterized as being stable in acid (UMEZAWA et al., 1966a). Taking this into account, PIETSCH and ENG (1969) proposed that the apparent discrepancy must have involved sulfur present in phleomycin-909, but either absent or minute among earlier Japanese batches. They suggested that sulfurous constituents in phleomycin-909, antagonistic to growth-arresting effects and responsible for lethality, reacted in the presence of HCl, utilized free energy, and protected active sites that, otherwise, would have been stripped away.

1 These numbers come from suffixes of Bristol Laboratories' phleomycin lot numbers. Prefixes are A9331. Numbers used in connection with bleomycin represent chromatographic fractions.

The importance of sulfur sharpens in connection with monomers found in a chromatographic fraction of bleomycin, identified as A2. Nine such have been identified (TAKITA et al., 1968, 1969; KOYAMA et al., 1968; MURAOKA et al., 1970; cf. Table 1), three containing sulfur.

Table 1. *Monomers identified in bleomycin A2 (see references in text); Roman numerals used in literature*

CH–CH–CH–COOH (OH, NH) L-threonine I	CH_2–CH–COOH (N, N, NH_2, HOOC, NH_2, CH_3) β-(4-amino-6-carboxy-5-methyl pyrimidine-2-yl)alanine II	CH_3–CH–CH–CH–COOH (NH_2, OH, CH_3) 4-amino-3-hydroxy-2-methyl-*n*-valeric acid III
N, N, H –CH—C–COOH (COOH, NH_2) β-carboxyhistidine IV	H_2N–CH_2–CH–COOH (NH_2) L-β-aminoalanine V	H_2N–H_2C–H_2C– (N, S, N, S) –COOH 2-(2-aminoethyl)-2,4′-bithiazole -4-carboxylic acid VI
H_2N–CH_2–CH_2–S + $(CH_3)_2$ X unnamed VII	HOH_2C, OH, O, ~ OH, OH, O, H L-gulose VIII	CH_2OH, HO, O, HO, H_2NCO, O, ~ OH 3-0-carbamoyl-D-mannose IX

B. Physical Properties

Phleomycin and bleomycin separate into a dozen or more fractions on Sephadex columns (IKEKAWA et al., 1964; UMEZAWA et al., 1966b). Fractions can vary from each other and the parent sample in biological activity and spectral characteristics. Main constituents average 1300 to 1800 in molecular weight, as judged by column chromatography. Mass spectroscopy (GOHLKE, personal communication) indicates essentially the same molecular weight; i.e., a crude working estimate of 1500. GORMAN (personal communication) has retrieved relatively low molecular weight components (200 to 300 daltons) with biological activity and spectral features quite unlike fractions in the 1500 range.

C. Spectral Features

Phleomycin and bleomycin have broad ultraviolet absorption bands around 245 and 290 nm (Fig. 1; cf. also UMEZAWA, 1967). Phleomycins 909 and 616 may exhibit peaks at 197 nm (PIETSCH, 1969a).

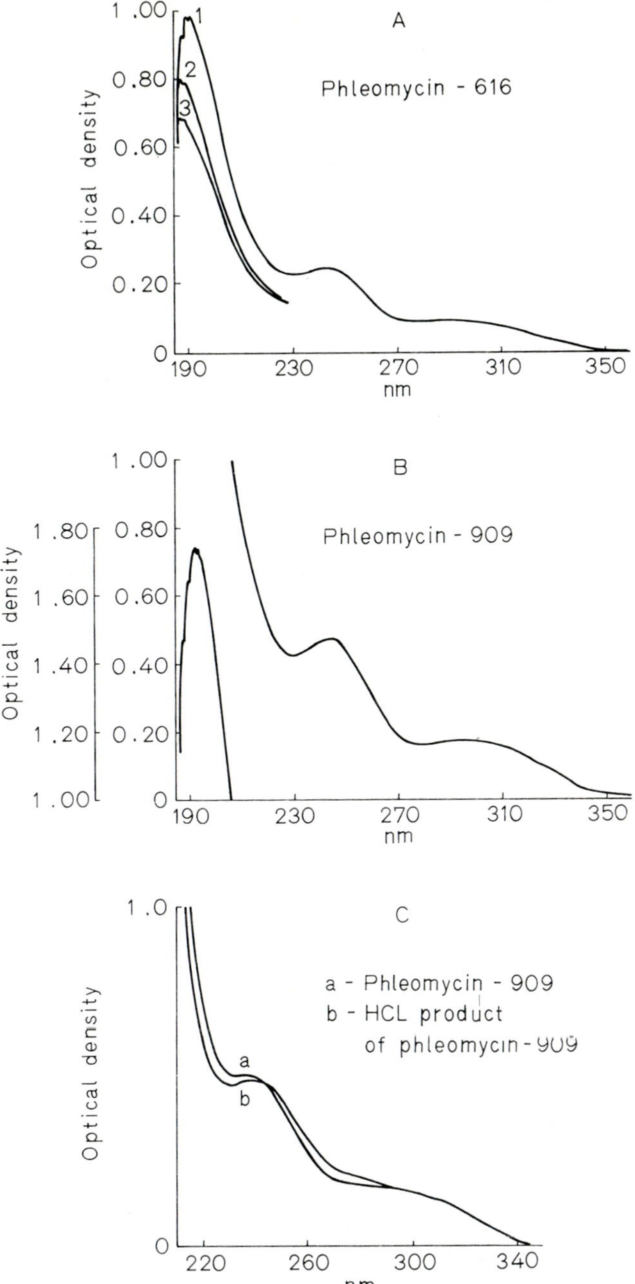

Fig. 1. Ultraviolet absorption of various phleomycin samples. A and B were recorded on a spectrophotometer equipped to scan low wave lengths. Numerals in A represent dilutions to test Beer's law, also performed with phleomycin-909, but not shown in B. C represents equal weights of phleomycin-909 before and after dissolution in concentrated HCl, carried out slowly in the cold to quench heat. Data of PIETSCH (1969a) and PIETSCH and ENG (1969)

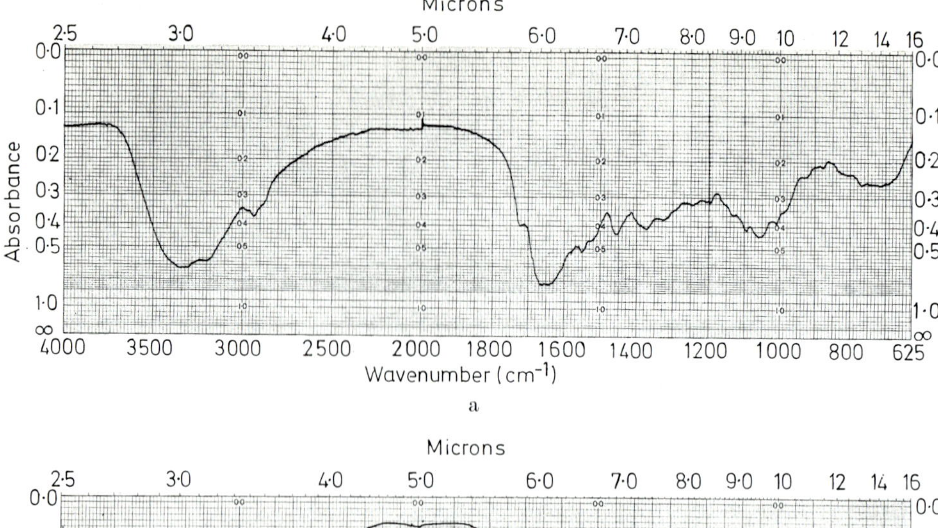

a

b

Fig. 2a and b. The upper record (a) is phleomycin-909 as available. The general features are more like samples designated bleomycin than phleomycin-616, shown in Fig. 3. The lower record (b) is the acid product of phleomycin-909. Data of Pietsch (1969a) and Pietsch and Eng (1969).

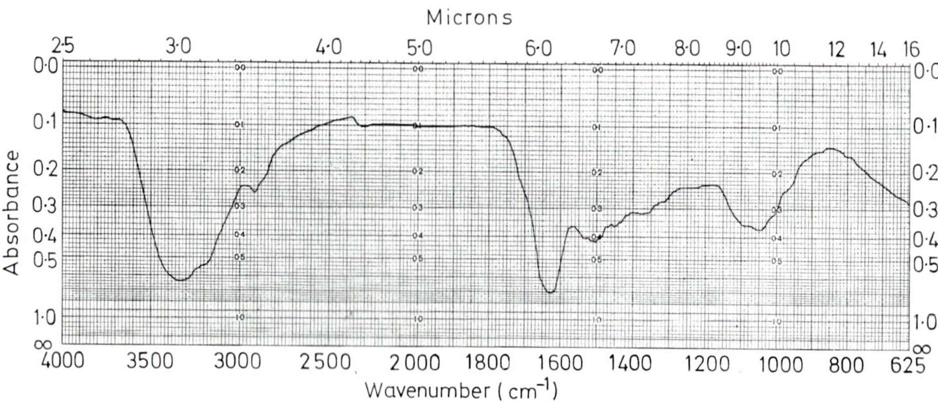

Fig. 3. Infrared spectrum of phleomycin-616. Data of Pietsch (1969a)

Infrared spectroscopy reveals many contaminants. Phleomycin-909, for example, produces records more like those of bleomycin than it does of phleomycin-616, although both clearly contain the same major components (compare Figs. 2 and 3 with UMEZAWA, 1967).

Likenesses between phleomycin and bleomycin are observed by infrared spectroscopy. Fingerprints of the most active fractions of both form near-perfect overlays (compare data of IKEKAWA et al., 1964 and UMEZAWA et al., 1966b). Not surprisingly, therefore, phleomycin preempts specific binding sites and blocks reactions of bleomycin with DNA (SUZUKI, H. et al., 1969).

D. Permeability

UMEZAWA et al. (1967, 1968) learned that phleomycin and bleomycin pass quickly into the tissues of animals after intravenous injections. Material tends to persist longer in skin than in other organs. PIETSCH et al. (1969) found that phleomycin filters readily through dialysis membranes *in vitro*, and diffuses with ease *in vivo*. Clearance via the kidney in mice, judged both by neutron activation analysis and bioassay, follows simple diffusion laws. Phleomycin had a 22 min body half-life in mice. The amount excreted bore a direct, linear relationship to dose above 2.5 mg/kg of body weight. Below that level, the relationship became nonlinear, possibly because of binding and pooling in target organs, such as the skin.

The microorganisms studied in my laboratory have been extremely permeable to phleomycin. Still, no thorough studies of this issue have been carried out, and the question of permease systems remains to be explored.

E. Range of Biological Activity

Phleomycin and bleomycin have inhibited growth among virtually all forms and subforms of life. These include bacteriophages (PITTS and SINSHEIMER, 1965; WATANABE and AUGUST, 1968; PIETSCH, 1969a), viruses cultivated in animal cells including DNA types (TEVETHIA and RAPP, 1969; IWATI and CONSIGLI, 1971), as well as replicative RNA's (HECHT and SUMMERS, 1970; KOCH, 1971).

Bacteria and fungi exhibit a broad variable range of sensitivities to phleomycin (MAEDA et al., 1956; TAKEUCHI et al., 1963; ISHIZUKA et al., 1966; cf., Table 2). Absolute values vary considerably among reports, reflecting batch variations. Published relative values, however, have been reliable. Data on bleomycin follow the same trend as those on phleomycin (UMEZAWA et al., 1966a, 1967, 1968a; ICHIKAWA et al., 1967; ISHIZUKA et al., 1967).

Phleomycin has inhibited bean rust (SMALE et al., 1961), safflower rust (ZIMMER, 1965), trypanosomes (JAFFE, 1967), free-living nematodes (PASTERNAK and SAMOILOFF, 1970), and some but not all experimental tumors cells (BRADNER and PINDELL, 1962, 1965, 1966; UMEZAWA et al., 1962; PRICE et al., 1964, 1965a, b; ISHIZUKA et al., 1966). Bleomycins exhibit a similar picture, but appear to be more efficient (ICHIKAWA et al., 1966; UMEZAWA et al., 1967, 1968a; TAKEUCHI and YAMAMOTO, 1968; ISHIZUKA et al., 1967; TERASIMA and UMEZAWA, 1970; KANNO et al., 1970). Fraction A2 of bleomycin seems to have the best therapeutic index, and such fractions are often employed in combinations (ICHIKAWA et al., 1967; ISHIZUKA et al., 1967).

Hasegawa et al. (1970) have found that bleomycin is a potent inhibitor of metastasis, more so by several fold than mitomycin C, snake venom, or some dozen other such agents.

Bleomycin has been studied as a chemotherapy agent; this activity will be discussed below.

Table 2. *Sensitivity of Representative Microorganisms to Phleomycin*

Organism	A+T/G+C[a]	Maeda et al. (1956)	Takita (1959)	Pietsch and Chambers (Unpublished)
B. subtilis	0.57—1.38	5.4	0.26	< 0.1
E. coli	0.86—1.07	10.7—21.3	0.26	0.1—8
S. lutea	0.35—0.56	> 42.5	0.52	—
S. aureus	1.88—2.09	21.3—42.5	0.52	0.5
Ps. aeruginosa	0.59—0.51	> 42.5	—	> 750
S. typhosa	0.93	21.3	1.0	> 10
A. aerogenes		—	—	< 40
M. phlei	0.49—0.50	0.3	0.05	—
C. albicans		> 42.5	> 500	—
R. nigricans		—	—	1000

[a] cf. Sober (1968).

Actions

Phleomycin and bleomycin inhibit DNA synthesis, cancel infectivity of replicative RNA viruses, block mitosis and meiosis, cause mutations in certain bacteria, induce chromosome damage, prevent transcription, and provoke certain toxicological side effects. Despite this range, their principal actions appear to be directed against facets of cell replication. But even these actions can occur specifically, to the exclusion of any other detectable effect, as though each depended upon different active sites and different receptors. Moreover, when one action becomes conspicuous, others tend to be decreased and often eliminated. Some effects can be attributed to the specific test sample. Others, particularly the arrest of DNA synthesis, depend upon "off-on" rhythms of receptors, and this in turn can undergo considerable change in response to intracellular conditions.

A. Selective Inhibition of DNA Synthesis

Tanaka et al. (1963a, b, c) initially showed that phleomycin blocked DNA synthesis in *E. coli* and HeLa cells. In the bacteria, at least, it arrested neither RNA nor protein synthesis. In addition, *E. coli* DNA did not undergo disintegration, an effect induced by mitomycin C, thus leading Tanaka et al. (1963a, b, c) to postulate nondestructive processes underlying inhibition.

The following year Falaschi and Kornberg (1964) showed that phleomycin inhibited DNA polymerase activity in cell-free enzyme systems (see also Tanaka, 1965, 1970). RNA polymerase activity remained at control levels up to phleomycin concentrations that exerted a 70% effect on DNA polymerase. Even at concentrations of inhibitor approaching the extreme range, RNA polymerase sustained only modest effects. Thus, the selectivity observed *in vivo* seemed fully substantiated by enzymatic studies. Falaschi and Kornberg (1964) also showed that phleomycin interacted with DNA, and that the amount bound bore a relationship to the ultimate effect.

Using phleomycin, ADAMS et al. (1965) virtually expunged DNA synthesis in cultured rabbit cells. They also tested for DNA polymerase activity in extracts of these cells and found that treated cells assayed at control levels. Thus, phleomycin prevented neither the production of polymerase enzymes nor their capacity to function, given an operative template. ADAMS et al. (1966) also demonstrated that cytosine is converted to dCMP despite arrest of DNA replication by phleomycin. Thus, phleomycin inhibited the synthesis of polymeric DNA, but proved harmless to the enzymes operating the precursor pool and to the transcription and translation underlying them.

There was other evidence of the escape of transcription. Yoshida rat sarcoma cells, for example, inhibited by phleomycin, nevertheless carried out glycolysis (HORI et al., 1963).

HIGUCHI et al. (1965) showed that phleomycin did not interfere with enzyme induction in *R. spheroides*. TEPPER et al. (1967) found that phleomycin-inhibited *Fraxinus* seeds still manufactured α-amylase, something they could not do in the presence of actinomycin D. GIESE (1970) matched the effects of phleomycin against puromycin and actinomycin D in experiments involving regeneration of the protozoan, *Blepharisma*. Protein synthesis appears to dominate this response. While puromycin and actinomycin D inhibited regeneration, phleomycin's effects were marginal. Along the same general line, YAMAI et al. (1969) have found little if any immunosuppressive activity in response to bleomycin.

TEVETHIA and RAPP (1969) performed an illuminating study on papovavirus SV40 in green monkey kidney cells. After demonstrating the arrest of viral DNA replication at low concentrations of antibiotic, they assayed for two proteins. One, a structural capsid, develops only if replication proceeds. The other, a so-called T antigen, develops independently of DNA synthesis. Phleomycin arrested capsid formation, but failed to affect the production of T. PIETSCH and MCCOLLISTER (1965) also learned that phleomycin inhibited actomyosin synthesis during regeneration of mouse muscle. However, injections of phleomycin had to be accurately timed to catch a particular wave of DNA synthesis that seems to trigger and entrain differentiation. Injections at other times, even during periods vulnerable to actinomycin D, did not affect manufacture of the contractile protein complex.

FALASCHI and KORNBERG (1964) detected a relationship between A—T content of the template and efficiency of phleomycin. TEVETHIA and RAPP (1969) also explored this relationship with viral DNA's of varying base compositions and found, likewise, a correlation between A—T content and the degree of inhibition of ^{3}H thymidine incorporation into DNA by phleomycin.

IWATA and CONSIGLI (1971), too, have recently observed 96% inhibition of mouse embryo DNA replication without any evidence of curtailed protein or RNA synthesis.

Of reports that vindicated TANAKA et al. (1963a, b, c), a short, provocative one by PITTS and SINSHEIMER (1965) ranks among the most important. They investigated ΦX174 bacteriophage. A single-stranded killer of *E. coli*, this DNA phage reproduces in three distinct steps: (1) early in the infection, it adds a complementary strand, phages assuming the double-helix or replicative form; (2) semiconservative replication; (3) conservative replication, towards the end of infection, to produce new, single-stranded progeny, a step roughly analogous to transcription in cells. This third step also requires a fresh round of protein synthesis and can be expunged by chloramphenicol. In contrast, a phleomycin inhibited phage production when it was introduced during steps 1 and 2. But late in the infective cycle, when the system demands the interplay of transcription and translation, phleomycin proved harmless.

A number of equivocal reports have appeared in the literature since 1963; these will be discussed following consideration of the rhythm attending specific inhibition of DNA synthesis and reactions with receptor sites.

B. Receptivity of Target Sites

Phleomycin and bleomycin bind to DNA, as already mentioned, and as will be discussed below. Thus, receptors must be occupied before drug action can occur. With respect to inhibition of DNA synthesis, such occupation does not occur on an ad hoc basis and, concerning this action in particular, the receptor provides anything but a static target. Indeed, this may ultimately prove to be the single most important property of those compounds that mediate a selective block on DNA replication, for the underlying rhythms can vary among cells of the very same animal, independently of any simple conventional explanation or cause.

After first encountering variations in receptivity, Pietsch and McCollister (1965) initially tried to dismiss their observations on methodological grounds, but did not succeed. In mice, transplanted rhabdomyosarcomas, melanomas, myeloid leukemia, breast adenocarcinomas, spleens, and presumptive regenerating myoblasts at different stages of development all had shown different levels of acute response to phleomycin in terms of DNA synthesis. But population turnover rate, DNA content per cell, permeability, or concentration of material in the tissue did not explain the results; however, variations in replication did. Pietsch and Clapper (1969) showed that receptivity is determined as a logical subset of replication. They explain variations in receptivity by showing vectorlike differences (differences that can be stated in vector rather than scalar terms) among cells while replication is actually in progress. Those workers estimate that a mouse nucleus has over a million random choices of specific receptivities.

Neubert (1966) has shown, too, that phleomycin can inhibit nuclear DNA replication without affecting that of mitochondria. Iwata and Consigli (1971) demonstrated a profound change in susceptibility of replication after viral infections. Receptivity clearly changes with changing internal conditions. Pietsch (1967a) drew correlations between the duration of receptivity and complexity of proteins later synthesized in developing cells: the number of ribosomes per polysome correlates with the degree of acute inhibition of DNA synthesis. His data are limited, however, to only a few cell types.

Receptivity is also periodic in microorganisms (Pietsch and Clapper, 1969). Receptivity can lap half a generation cycle, as in *Pseudomonas aeruginosa*, or it can be exceedingly brief; but, pulses of phleomycin exert no effect when the receptive moments are missed. *Bacillus subtilis* or *E. coli*, for example, pass through a short receptive interval toward the very end of replication. Accordingly, when challenged with phleomycin 909 at concentrations a thousand fold above the dose that inhibits organisms on agar, cultures continue to grow as though no antibiotic were in the medium. They complete the cycle, and as the time arrives for another round of growth, the challenged cultures brake smoothly and decelerate asymptotically over several generations. The trend is obvious in tabular data of Tanaka et al. (1963a, b, c; see also Pietsch and Corbett, 1968).

Theoretical implications aside, it behooves anyone designing experiments with phleomycin and bleomycin to take into account the near impossibility of predicting, *a priori*, just how a cell population or bacterial culture will respond, i.e., whether it will have long periods with patent receptors or be refractory most of the time. One inescapable feature of reports in which phleomycin attacked DNA synthesis selectively has been that experimental design guaranteed a period of receptivity with antibiotic in the environment.

C. Selective Inhibition of Cell Division

KAJIWARA et al. (1966), studying the effects of phleomycin on HeLa cells, discovered the second important and selective action of this class of antibiotics, namely the arrest of mitosis, in the absence of inhibition not only of RNA and protein synthesis, but of DNA synthesis as well. DJORDJEVIC and KIM (1967) have confirmed this finding, as have KUNIMOTO et al. (1967). HOTTA and STERN (1969) extended the observation to include meiosis. Recently, NAGATSU et al. (1971) have shown that bleomycin A2 also can block entry of transplanted rabbit tumor cells into mitosis without preventing increases in nuclear DNA content. HOTTA and STERN (1969) correlated their findings with progressive structural changes in chromosomes. MATTINGLY (1967) had previously drawn attention to chromosomal aberrations following phleomycin treatment (see also KIHLMAN et al., 1967a, b; JAGIELLO, 1968; JACOBS et al., 1969). This effect may relate to the fact that phleomycin and bleomycin break and incise bacterial chromosomes (GRIGG, 1969, 1970; PIETSCH and GARRETT, 1969a, b; SUZUKI, H. et al., 1969).

Specific arrest of mitosis seems to occur at the expense of other effects (see data of HOTTA and STERN, 1969) and has been observed in studies using sulfur-containing samples. As already mentioned, acid hydrolysis removes sulfur and increases specific replication inhibiting potency in bacteria. Sulfur may provide a handy label to follow and assess the action of the drug against mitosis and meiosis.

D. Inhibition of Replicative RNA

WATANABE and AUGUST (1968) discovered phleomycin's ability to inhibit replication of the RNA phage, R23, both during infection of *E. coli* and in cell-free systems. They also showed that the antibiotic binds to this replicative RNA. PIETSCH (1969a) observed that the phleomycin-616 used by those workers inhibited Ms 2 phage at concentrations far below the sensitivity of the host. This was not true of phleomycin-909.

HECHT and SUMMERS (1971), using rather massive concentrations of phleomycin-909 (200 μg/ml), inhibited poliovirus infections (also RNA) in HeLa cells. Although the concentration of phleomycin was relatively large, the challenge had to come during the first 90 min of infection, i.e., during a phase roughly comparable to steps 1 and 2 in bacteriophage ΦX 174. In other words, despite the fact that one virus was of an RNA and the other of a DNA type, both showed phase-dependent responses. This periodic feature fits the same overall pattern as receptivity on the part of cells. Selective inhibition of replicative RNA, thus, may be very similar mechanistically to that of DNA. The picture, however, is complicated by equivocal results from different laboratories.

TEVETHIA and RAPP (1969) found no inhibition of poliovirus at 50 μg/ml of phleomycin-648, many times the effective dose with papovavirus. KOCH (1971), working with phleomycin-616, showed that as little as 2 μg/ml inactivated poliovirus 99 % when he exposed single RNA strands prior to infection; however, intact viruses continued to be fully infective after 200 μg/ml.

Pietsch (1969a) found the C:N:H:S ratios of phleomycin-909 and 616 to be quite different. But of greater importance, both samples contained conjugated nitriles, 909 in barely detectable traces, but 616 in appreciable amounts. Rakieten et al. (1969) report that immediate death in mammals following large doses of phleomycin-616 occurs from respiratory failure. In my own experience, lethal doses of phleomycin-909 kill mice in a manner resembling cyanide poisoning. Acid treatment of phleomycin-909, in addition to removing sulfur, eradicates nitriles, leaving nitrates in their stead, and dramatically reduces toxicity (Pietsch and Eng, 1969). There is a nitrile analog of anthramycin, and it is a potent inhibitor of messenger RNA synthesis (Horwitz et al. 1971). *S. verticillus* may be capable of producing, if not anthramycins, certainly, compounds with similar active sites. The production of such compounds may vary; therefore, batches of phleomycin would then require different doses to reveal these compounds. In this same connection, phleomycin-616, like the anthramycins, inhibits transcription *per se* (Watanabe and August, 1968). These workers also found that phleomycin-616 inhibited ΦX174 phage during the protein-dependent phase, which Pitts and Sinsheimer (1966) had previously found to be unaffected by phleomycin.

If replicative RNA's are vulnerable to this class of antibiotics, the question that must arise is whether these materials influence RNA-dependent DNA synthesis. As of this writing, the question awaits study.

E. Arrest of Transcription

Inhibition of RNA or protein synthesis has been reported following phleomycin and bleomycin treatment of bacteria or animal cells (Pietsch and McCollister, 1965; Kunimoto et al., 1967; Palmer and Fridhandler, 1968; Watanabe and August, 1968; Terasima and Umezawa, 1970). Many of the observations reflect dependence on replication to trigger and entrain the round of peptide formation. Barring this and general cell poisoning, there still remains precedence for an effect on transcription. Phleomycin and bleomycin can inhibit RNA polymerase, albeit at high concentrations (Falaschi and Kornberg, 1964; Tanaka, 1965; Watanabe and August, 1968). Tanaka (1970) has studied the effects of bleomycin on transcription from phage DNA. While he could demonstrate inhibition in cell-free systems, he found that bleomycin did not block transcription with phage infecting their hosts.

The simplest view is that effects on transcription do not represent primary actions of this class of antibiotics. Yet such a hasty conclusion might be costly in terms of insight. A loose connection between effects on transcription and concentrations of phleomycin required to bring about inhibition of replicative RNA's has been shown to exist. Fortuitously, nitriles were a concomitant of these correlations. They could serve as a guide that in turn might reveal transcription required for replication.

F. Toxicity

Lethal doses of phleomycin and bleomycin are much greater than those required to inhibit replication of cell division. But, once again, sample variations reveal their significance. Consider LD_{50} values in mice, for example. Intravenous and intraperitoneal injections beget identical results (Ishizuka et al., 1966, 1967), no doubt because of rapid transit across membranes. But similarities stop there. In early patent applications phleomycin's LD_{50} was put at 15 mg/kg (Umezawa and MAEDA, 1955). Later TAKITA (1959) stated that copper phleomycin had an LD_{50} of 40 to 50 mg/kg. Removing the metal yielded an LD_{50} of 150 mg/kg. RAKIETEN et al. (1969) placed the LD_{50} of phleomycin-616 at 20.4 mg/kg. ISHIZUKA et al. (1966) set the LD_{50} range for phleomycin-648 at 12.5 to 25 mg/kg. Native phleomycin-909 tested out at 67.1 mg/kg, whereas acid products showed an LD_{50} of 240 to 270 mg/kg (PIETSCH and ENG, 1969). Heterogeneous bleomycin's LD_{50} lies between 125 to 150 mg/kg (ISHIZUKA et al., 1967). Clearly, the batch of drug is a significant variable even in toxicology. In fact, no chromatographic fraction of phleomycin and bleomycin has the toxicity of the parent material, emphasizing that the total effect is made up of several individual components.

Acute toxicity and potency do not necessarily correlate in native samples. With mice and chick embryos *in vivo*, phleomycin-909 was at least 30% more efficient in arresting DNA synthesis than was phleomycin-616 (PIETSCH, unpublished). After acid hydrolysis of phleomycin-909, PIETSCH and ENG (1969) found six-fold increases in growth inhibiting effect. But the action was quantitative, not qualitative, the organisms responding merely as though dose had been increased. Thus, at least some secondary toxic effects can be dissociated from primary actions. If it is true of some toxicities, the possibility exists for others, and this is of practical importance.

One of the early promising things about phleomycin was that it either killed mice outright or the animals survived without any obvious untoward effects or delayed deaths. Unfortunately, repetitive administration induced kidney lesions in dogs that, once manifest, turned out to be irreversible (cf. ISHIZUKA et al., 1967). RAKIETEN et al. (1969) found essentially the same thing in dogs, as well as monkeys. Azotemia was a reliable index, and histopathology suggested that the distal portions of the nephron bore the lesion. Dogs and monkeys tolerated 0.08 mg/kg/day × 28 (phleomycin-616) without symptoms. Low-grade but irreversible damage appeared at 0.16 mg/kg/day × 28 and became progressively worse with larger doses. Results of ISHIZUKA et al. (1966) follow this general trend for phleomycin-648, although the two protocols do not permit precise comparison of batches. The latter investigator estimated that eight 0.3 mg/kg doses of phleomycin given semiweekly can be tolerated by dogs. (They evidently cured canine lymphosarcoma on the regimen.)

Bleomycin does induce liver damage, but it appears to be reversible (ISHIZUKA et al., 1967).

RAKIETEN et al. (1969) have also studied cardiovascular effects and cholinergic signs following phleomycin. Doses of 5 mg/kg of phleomycin quickly induce a fall in systolic pressure and produce marked hypotension. Smaller doses, even repetitive, did not bring on the change. Cholinergic symptoms appeared at 2.5 mg/kg of drug, but could be blocked with atropine given 15 min in advance of phleomycin. "Pharmacological" effects may relate to phleomycin's chelating capacity. BITTAR (1966, 1967) influenced sodium efflux in crab muscle directly injected with phleomycin or immersed in 5 mg/ml, a massive dose. With more modest doses he did not observe such an effect (BITTAR et al., 1966), nor did FANESTIL (1969) using 77 µg/ml of phleomycin on toad bladder.

Much remains to be done on the toxicology of phleomycin and bleomycin. The agents responsible for renal malfunction should be carefully identified and studied. Just as batches of phleomycins have varied, manufacturing procedures may one day induce renal toxins in company with bleomycin. As unknowns, they could occur without warning in the clinic.

G. Effects on Genes

Phleomycin can promote lysogeny (LEIN et al., 1962; PRICE et al., 1962, 1965) and enhance pyocin production in some strains of *Ps. aeruginosa* (IKEDA and EGAMI, 1966). Bleomycin induces pectolytic enzymes in *Erwinia aroides* (TOMIZAWA et al., 1971). Whether inductive effects depend, secondarily, on other actions or the direct binding of antibiotic to DNA or replicative RNA has not been studied, to my knowledge.

The same seems true of mutagenesis, where research has started. MITSUHASHI and TAKAHASHI (1964) observed that phleomycin cancelled the transmissible resistance to tetracycline, chloramphenicol, and streptomycin in *E. coli*, *S. newington*, and *Sh. flexneri*. At the same time, it did not affect all organisms, nor did it excise *E. coli's* F-episome (i.e., the sex factor) (IKEDA et al., 1967), indicating that the antibiotic, whether working directly or indirectly, did not sweep the genome generally.

Recently, IIJIMA and IKEDA (1970) have found certain strains of *E. coli* and *B. subtilis* that acquire resistance to phleomycin. Mutations turned out to be highly unstable, resistance declining in the next generation. The latter workers found evidence that resistance depends on regions of the genome near those that depress sensitivity to streptomycin. These results would seem to be at odds with those of MITSUHASHI and TAKAHASHI (1964). Some differences may relate to strain. In fact, one would anticipate strain-dependent mutations from what PIETSCH and GARRETT (1969a) deduced about DNA binding. Phleomycin, they believe, polymerizes on contiguous runs of thymine, as discussed subsequently. For DNA to serve as a template for phleomycin, there would have to be some minimum number of thymines. A strategically placed point mutation, resulting in a G—C in the progeny, could excise one entire receptor unit from the organism, reducing efficiency of phleomycin binding when the next generation entered an actively receptive period. Conversely, visualize a string of A—T's, one base pair short of the minimum. Again, a point mutation could alter efficiency in the next generation, now in an upward direction. How readily such changes might take place would depend on the precise genetic make-up of the organism, i.e., how many receptor units exist and how many sequences of thymine need just one more of their number to become a receptor.

Reactions with DNA and Considerations of Mechanisms

The literature contains hypotheses about the mechanism employed by phleomycin and bleomycin to halt DNA replication. If there is anything about these antibiotics to command attention, certainly it is their capacity to interact with DNA and directly interfere with replication while sparing transcriptive processes. That this might take place only sometimes makes this class of antibiotics a tool of inestimable value in discovering facts about the function of DNA, not only in replication, but in transcription as well.

A. Reactions

Phleomycin and bleomycin react with DNA *in vitro* (FALASCHI and KORNBERG, 1964; TANAKA, 1964, 1970; PIETSCH, 1966, 1969b; PIETSCH and GARRETT, 1968, 1969a, b; NAGAI et al., 1968, 1969; SUZUKI, H. et al., 1969a, 1970; IWATA and CONSIGLI, 1971). Under such conditions, two general classes (i.e., I and II) of interactions can be demonstrated (PIETSCH, 1969b). Class I appears to involve hydrogen bonding with the carbonyl oxygen at the 2 position of thymine (PIETSCH and GARRETT, 1968). This same site appears to serve as the receptor *in vivo* (PIETSCH and CORBETT, 1968). However, the *in vitro* class I binding utilizes a much greater surface of DNA than reactions that lead to complete arrest of replication *in vivo* (PIETSCH and GARRETT, 1969a, PIETSCH and CLAPPER, 1969). Thus, class I binding cannot be considered to be the reaction underlying biological effects.

The two *in vitro* types of binding can be differentiated on the basis of the spectral changes they exert on DNA. Class I quantitatively increases absorption without shifting the DNA peak. Class II only appears as class I binding approaches saturation, indicating that its receptor sites compete poorly with the 2 position of thymine. Class II interaction progressively shifts absorption to lower wave lengths and, above threshold amounts, reduces optical density as a linear function of the phleomycin concentration. This class manifests itself abruptly, with a jump discontinuity in the equation representing effect versus concentration. The jump, estimated by Fourier analysis, seems to occur at the phleomycin: DNA mass ratio of 0.27. In molar terms, this approximated the saturation level of all of the 2 positions of thymine in the system.

Class II binding can be inhibited by elevating salt concentration, introducing divalent copper, or by histones covering the major groove surface of DNA. Class I interaction occurs equally well in nucleoprotein and naked DNA preparations, indicating, again, that the minor groove is the seat of binding.

In vivo, phleomycin has been retrieved in company with the DNA of animal and bacterial cells (PIETSCH and GARRETT, 1969a; PIETSCH and CLAPPER, 1969). The amount of antibiotic extracted along with the DNA of a given cell population corresponded 1:1 with acute inhibition of replication. This conclusion was based on relative values between different DNA's of the same animal or bacterial cultures in different stages of growth (i.e., from coefficients representing inhibition of DNA synthesis versus assay values for phleomycin). Absolute values are less reliable because of imprecise standard solutions, but, in both the mouse and *E. coli*, phleomycin associated itself with approximately one percent of the base pairs in homologous DNA molecules.

SUZUKI, H. et al. (1969a, 1970), likewise, find two classes of reactions between bleomycin A2 and DNA. Under well-controlled *in vitro* conditions they observed bleomycin: nucleotide ratios of 1:350 for what they describe as the selective class of interaction. This is very close to the values of PIETSCH and GARRETT (1969a) and suggests the possibility of studying the physical chemistry of the reaction under *in vitro* conditions.

PIETSCH and GARRETT (1969a) reported nodules on *E. coli* chromosomes as a result of phleomycin treatment *in vivo* (Fig. 4). Their distribution and characteristics suggested that they were receptor units. The nodules were strung out at unequal distances along fragments of bacterial chromosomes, but they occurred at the same locations on different chromosomes and contributed to a total of one percent of the fragment length, a value consistent with bioassay. In chromosomal pairs still joined by a short common segment, one sister contained nodules, whereas the other did not. Unbranched, circular DNA (i.e., nonreplicating chromosomes) never contained nodules. In addition, as will be discussed subsequently, phleomycin and bleomycin break *E. coli* chromosomes. Breaks were always present as a concomitant of nodules, whereas the anodular sisters remained intact. In addition, replication does not terminate abruptly in *E. coli*. Rather it decelerates asymptotically as though exponential growth can no longer occur. This suggests that one-half of the cells dividing at any cycle will not execute replication in the next round. Phleo-

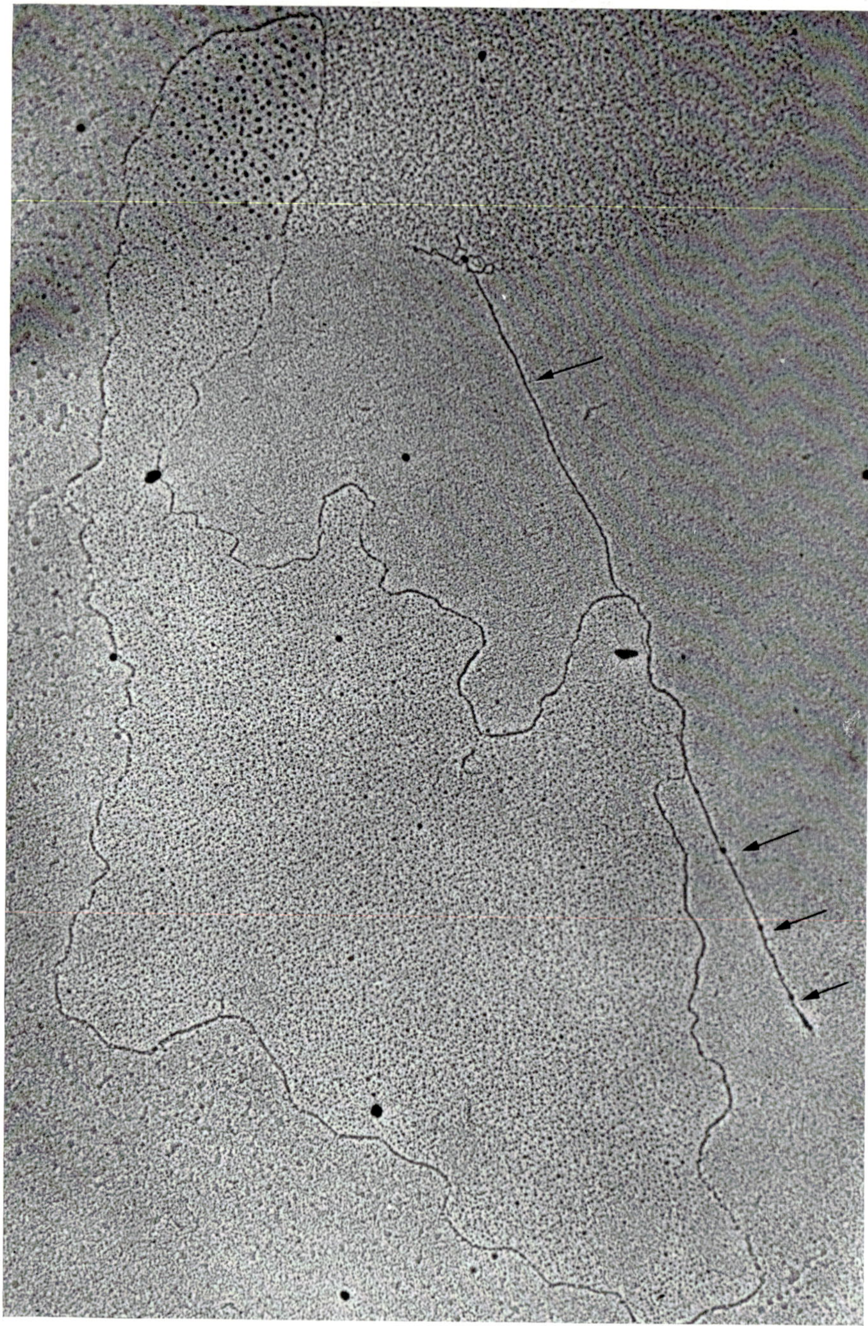

Fig. 4. Chromosome from phleomycin treated *E. coli*. Two replicates still joined by a short common piece. Intact sister on the left had no nodules. Fragmented sister on the right shows nodules at arrows. See Fig. 5 for magnified view of nodules (cf. Pietsch and Garrett, 1969a)

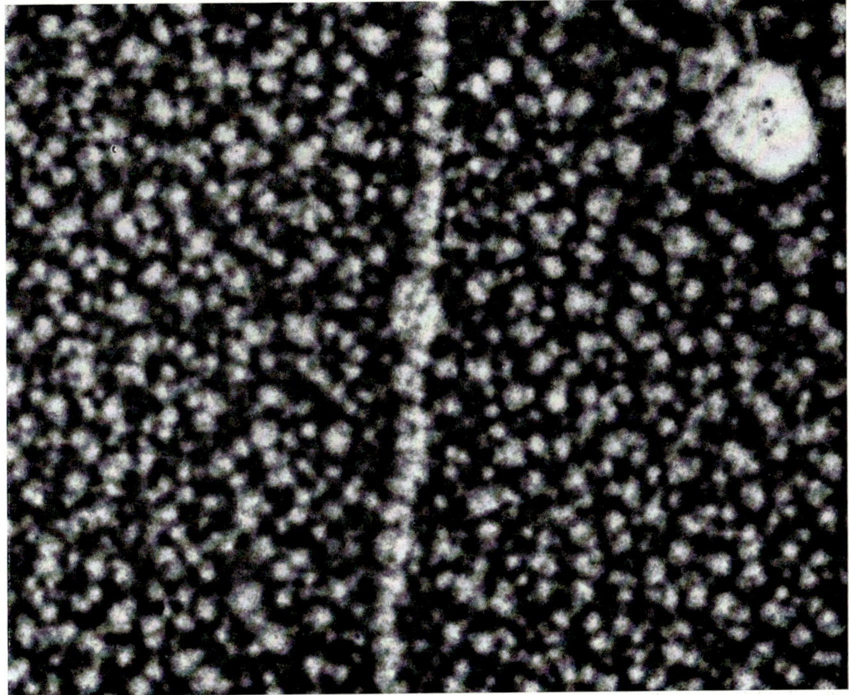

Fig. 5. Nodule on *E. coli* chromosome after challenge with phleomycin (cf. Fig. 4). Notice periodicity change over anodular region. This change is simulated optically in Fig. 6 (PIETSCH and GARRETT, 1969a)

mycin on one sister, but absent on the other, would beget just such a result. Finally, working *in vitro*, PIETSCH and GARRETT (1968, 1969b) stained phleomycin following reactions with DNA by means of mercury substitution and under the electron microscope observed heavy dark spots reminiscent in size and distribution of the nodules on *E. coli* chromosomes.

The internal pattern of nodules presented an interesting feature. At sharp resolution, periodicity ran longitudinally, at approximately right angles to that in anodular segments of the bacterial chromosome (Fig. 5). The pattern could be simulated optically by (a) creating a moiré pattern from two systems of coarse black and white stripes; (b) photographing the image in the hyperplane, to simulate loss of dimension (see Fig. 6). PIETSCH and GARRETT (1969a) found it impossible to reconstruct the molecular geometry of nodules from optical data; but, they were able to deduce one important thing: least divisible transverse subunits of the nodule must be identical. If thymine plus phleomycin lie at one level, the same would be true of the next, and so on. On the strength of this they inferred that a given receptor unit must consist of poly A—T or T—A, but not both in a contiguous array. This condition could account for one sister chromosome being anodular, for phleomycin would have to exist in the nodule in highly regular form. This in turn would mean polymerization and, perhaps, stereoregularity in the way each phleomycin approaches the 2 position of thymine.

Concerning receptors collectively, FALASHI and KORNBERG (1964) first pointed out the importance of A—T to the binding of phleomycin. TEVETHIA and RAPP

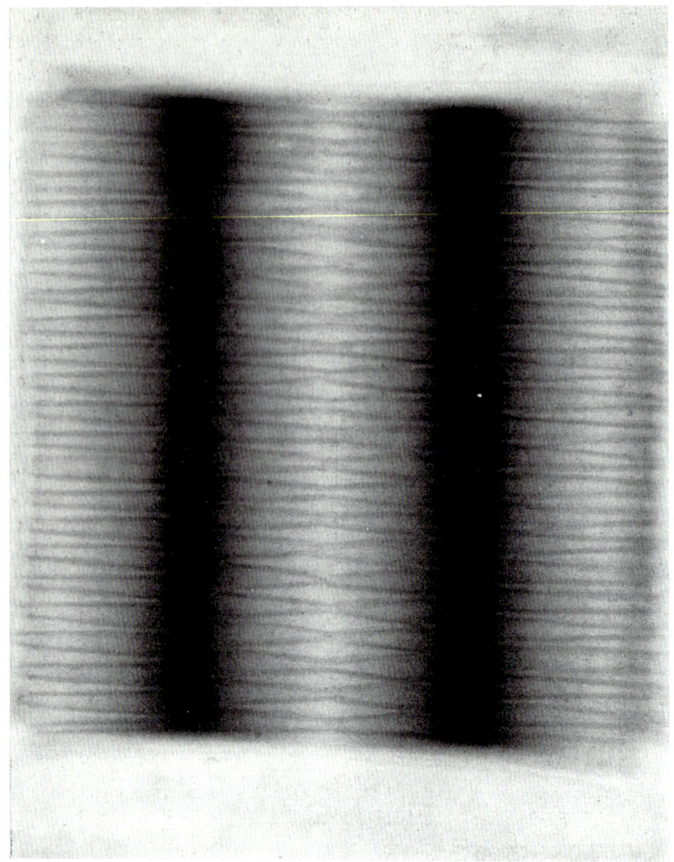

Fig. 6. Optical simulation of nodule anatomy. This is the pattern produced when two sets of coarse horizontal stripes are applied at a low angle and then viewed at reduced resolution. The interaction produces a new species of periodicity and, as in the nodule, creates five zones of alternating optical density that run vertically. The two interacting bars at any given level, representing vector sums or least whole units, produce the binary values for all levels. If thymine plus phleomycin occur at one level in the nodule, Pietsch and Garrett (1969a) reasoned, the structure must consist of polyphleomycin and poly T

(1969) extended this to cellular conditions. However, gross A—T content does not account for the reaction *in vivo*, as can be seen readily in comparing sensitivity of microorganisms with base ratios (cf. Table 2). The important consideration appears to be the number of A—T's in regular array. Of course, the more A—T the better the chance of having a receptor site. This may influence efficiency of the response.

B. Polyphleomycin Model

Pietsch (1967b) proposed the hypothetical model of polyphleomycin—poly A—T shown in Fig. 7. Built to satisfy the optical simulations discussed above, its dimensions were derived indirectly from the nodules (i.e., by normalizing the observed thickness of chromosomes with crystallographic data on diameter of DNA). The indirect approach minimized the impact of supercoiling on the problem.

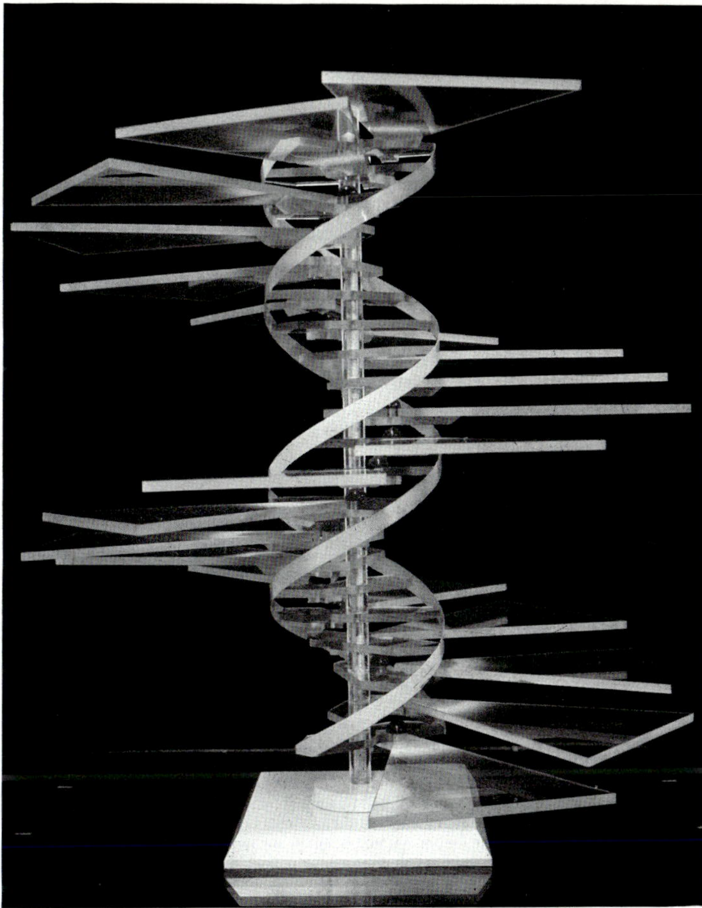

Fig. 7. Hypothetical model of a receptor unit with polyphleomycin attached (PIETSCH, 1969b; GORMAN and PIETSCH, 1969)

Each monomeric phleomycin is represented by an isosceles triangle postulated from these considerations: (a) to fit in the minor groove, phleomycins would have to be narrow on one end; (b) to achieve order peripherally, phleomycins would have to interact. This, in turn, meant that the other end had to be broadened; (c) a bisymmetrical wedge 30 Å in height and projecting laterally would account for the diameter at the nodule, and (d) phleomycin should have a very small amount of hydrophobic surface, just enough to mediate stacking in a sequential array. The postulated shape also allows for this.

Thomas Gorman has calculated Fourier transforms of the model's copper helices (cf. GORMAN and PIETSCH, 1969). The equations point to a rigorous test of the model. They also indicate how errors between the prediction and the data can be harmonized to build a correct model.

PIETSCH (1967b), using the model, suggested that position of poly A—T alone would permit most transcription without interference from phleomycins. Poly A—T would contain little by way of encoded information and seldom would be called upon to assemble messages. Segments bordering on receptor units might occasionally suffer the consequence of the drug. Indeed, some of the reported instances of inhibited transcription may reflect this.

Pietsch (1969b) later proposed another possible action, based on (a) location of phleomycin in the minor groove and (b) phleomycin's effects on replication apparently being the reciprocal of those exerted by certain 5-halogenated analogs of thymidine. After cells incorporate 5-iododeoxyuridine and 5-bromodeoxyuridine into their DNA, transcription ceases but replication continues for a period (see Pietsch, 1969b, for references). Cavaleri (cf. 1963) once suggested that transcription and replication might employ opposite grooves. Pietsch and Gorman (1969) found that bases can swing in and out of the helix without breaking bonds in the sugar phosphate skeleton.

Pietsch (1969b) examined the feasibility of this scheme with reference to possible actions of phleomycin by studying molecular models of DNA containing 5-halogenated pyrimidine nucleotides. He found that an iodine or a bromine overlapping the space-filling distances between neighboring bases would hinder rotation towards the minor groove. At the same time, the halogenated base has no difficulty exiting the core of the dyad via the major groove. With a bulky phleomycin in the minor groove, the exact opposite would occur. Phleomycin would lock thymine in the core and thus might prevent it from assuming a template configuration. If the receptor unit were the starting point in a replicon, replication would not begin. With a unit in the middle of a replicon, replication would be interrupted by the absence of one side of the template. Scission then would occur and the newly formed polynucleotide no doubt would separate and be rapidly broken up by deoxyribonuclease. Meanwhile, so long as DNA did not attempt to replicate, the bases would be free to come around into the minor groove for transcription.

C. Cleaving of DNA

Tanaka et al. (1963a, b, c) reported some liberation of nucleotides from *E. coli* after phleomycin treatment, but the amounts were small compared with the action of mitomycin C and certainly not enough to suggest disintegration of DNA. Grigg (1969), in contrast, did find extensive breakdown in the same organism. He also found that caffeine enhanced the breaking effect many fold (Grigg, 1970). More recently, he and his colleagues (personal communication) have found that other compounds, too, can amplify the effect, providing they have an affinity for single strands of DNA. Grigg (1969) attributes his observations to enhanced excision-endonuclease activity. Reminiscent of his findings are the observations of Tsuboi and Terasima (1970) on mouse L cells following combined treatment with x-irradiation and phleomycin. The latter workers studied the effects of various agents on repair of radiation-induced single strand breaks. Phleomycin partially interfered with repair when irradiated cells were incubated in its presence for 30 min. Tsuboi and Terasima (1970) also found that phleomycin had scission-producing effects of its own. However, these effects appeared only after a lag period of an hour or more (i.e., after the period of observation for the repair-blocking effect). Interference with the repair process may entail the same final mechanism as inhibition of replication *per se*. Recent research suggests that repair synthesis and replication involve different enzymes (see Werner, 1971). A corollary of these facts, observations, and inferences is that phleomycin and bleomycin must have an accidental rather than a causal relationship to polymerases. In other words, they are not likely to reap their net results by any primary effect on the enzyme. Obviously, if the formation of polynucleotide is the end-point in assaying polymerase activity, then blocking it will depress the assay index. But this should not be confused with the mechanism of action of these compounds, for it is a consequence, not an antecedent. Thus, it may be misleading to refer to bleomycin and phleomycin as polymerase inhibitors.

But what about the disparity between these observations and those of TANAKA et al. (1963a, b, c)? Again, ancillary sulfurous components may underlie the findings. GRIGG (1969, 1970) employed phleomycin-648 in his studies (personal communication). IKEKAWA et al. (1964) found sulfur in that sample. TSUBOI and TERASIMA (1970) employed both that lot and phleomycin-909, although they fail to stipulate which was being used in a given experiment. Phleomycin-909 contains sulfur (PIETSCH, 1969a). The earlier batches of phleomycin contained little if any sulfur (TAKITA, 1959).

Bleomycin A2, also highly sulfurous, can cause single strand scissions *in vitro* in the presence of hydrogen peroxide or 2-mercaptoethanol (NAGAI et al., 1969a, b, c; SUZUKI, H. et al., 1969). A potential clue seems to exist in this observation. SUZUKI, H. et al. (1970) found that bleomycin reacted with DNA in the presence or absence of 2-mercaptoethanol. With the latter present, bleomycin reacted in two ways. Mercaptoethanol appeared to attach first and set up a bridge with bleomycin. The second reaction did not involve mercaptoethanol. The latter workers observed that excess divalent cations inhibited scission, implicating phosphates in the breaks, for the following reasons. Large concentrations of phleomycin precipitate DNA fibers, and half-wave polarographic potentials show that copper reacts with phosphates (CLAPPER, personal communication). CLAPPER (unpublished) found that he could inhibit precipitation by introducing excess cupric ions. Together, these facts suggest that bleomycin establishes something on the order of a span, reinforced by sulfur linkages, across diester bonds in the sugar phosphate skeleton. Preventing free rotation around the 3′ or 5′ linkage would induce chain breakage. Bases "breathe" as they engage in hydrogen exchange (cf. in this connection discussions in PRINTZ and VON HIPPEL, 1965; PIETSCH and GORMAN, 1969; HANSON, 1971). "Strangled," the base no longer satisfies entropy by moving out of the dyad. This effect can be simulated with molecular models (cf. PIETSCH and GORMAN, 1969); i.e., entropy considerations would virtually insure scission. Phleomycin does not manifestly incise DNA *in vitro*. This may reflect a relative abundance among bleomycins of those compounds capable of establishing necessary bridges.

PIETSCH and GARRETT (1969a) saw broken *E. coli* chromosomes with the electron microscope after phleomycin treatment, with breaks having a random distribution. Strand dissociations and unwinding occurred for a short variable distance from the breaks. Of course, such DNA fragments would have been vulnerable to acid hydrolysis, the liberation of free nucleotides and, eventually, strand scission. In other words, breakdown of DNA might reflect increased fragility to handling procedures rather than destructive processes *per se*. Also, during the extraction of DNA in the presence of phleomycin and bleomycin, it is important to keep in mind that these agents form chelates. WELSH and VYSKA (1970) have shown that EDTA (ethylene diamine tetraacetic acid) cleaves certain high molecular weight DNA molecules. Such an effect, mediated by free phleomycin or bleomycin during extraction, could thereby alter the outcome of an experiment.

Bleomycin in Cancer Chemotherapy

LEIN et al. (1962) predicted antitumor activity for phleomycin from a screening technique involving lysogeny (cf. also HEINEMANN and HOWARD, 1965a, b). BRADNER and PINDELL (1962) tested and proved the hypothesis, and, shortly thereafter,

Umezawa et al. (1962) confirmed the result. By the time bleomycin had been isolated, those with an interest in these compounds knew that not all transplanted tumors would respond equally well (cf. Bradner and Pindell, 1965, 1966). But because phleomycin acted directly on neoplastic cells, bleomycin, too, would probably have its best chance of arresting tumors among tissues that tended to retain it. Therefore, Umezawa and his colleagues elected to track the fate of bleomycin, *in vivo*. They found that bleomycin accumulated in skin (Ichikawa et al., 1967; Ishizuka et al., 1967; Umezawa et al., 1967), and, therefore, predicted efficacy against epidermoid carcinoma in particular. Indeed, not long afterwards, Ichikawa and Umezawa (1967) reported on the successful treatment of squamous cell carcinoma (cf. Ichikawa, 1968, 1969a, b, c; Ichikawa et al., 1969).

Other similar accounts soon followed. Head, neck, and oral carcinomas responded to bleomycin treatment (Nakamura et al., 1969; Ueno, 1969; Nanjo and Suga, 1970; Suzuki, Y. and Miyake, 1969; Inuyama and Machukawa, 1969; Honda et al., 1969), as have those of male and female genitals (Suzuki, M. et al., 1969a, b, 1970; Mitsuya et al., 1969; Kato et al., 1969; Fukatsu and Yoshida, 1969; cf. also Ichikawa et al., 1969; Dold and Schmidt, 1971).

Oka et al. (1969) believed that squamous cell carcinoma of the lung, too, should be responsive. Accordingly, they treated six patients with 15 to 30 mg of bleomycin (Nippon Kayaku Company, Tokyo) twice a week for five weeks. Observation lasted one year. Therapy had no net effect in two cases. But the other four showed either slight or marked improvement. These findings approximate the general trend of all studies involving epidermoid carcinomas, remissions running about 50 to 70 %, with some showing no response at all. Clinical investigators rate most untoward side effects as slight. These include dermatitis, transitory hair loss, and nausea. Pulmonary fibrosis, however, is produced by bleomycin and is the toxicity which limits the utility of this agent.

Some investigators report bleomycin is particularly valuable in conjunction with other therapy; however, Takeda et al. (1970), in a study of 145 skin malignancies, indicate that their best results occur in new cases without radiation. During this study, tumors disappeared completely in 29 cases, while 76 showed modest to marked improvement.

Redon (1970) investigated 237 patients on bleomycin therapy. His original intention was merely to assess drug tolerance. But the findings were so remarkable that he continued long enough to make a preliminary assessment of efficacy. His report states that bleomycin was more effective than any previously employed chemotherapy agent in arresting melanoma and squamous cell carcinoma of the penis, vulva, esophagus, and uterine cervix (although data in Suzuki et al., 1970, show very marginal results with this important malignancy and breast cancer). Redon (1970) rated bleomycin at least as effective as other agents in treating testicular dysembryoma, choriocarcinoma, and oropharyngeal tumors. The latter responded especially well when bleomycin was administered via arteries supplying the region.

Redon (1970) found hemopoietic cancer refractory to bleomycin treatment, but Yamagata et al. (1968), in a parenthetical reference to bleomycin, said that lymphatic leukemias and reticulosarcoma were responsive. In addition, Kimura et al. (1969), motivated by the effectiveness of phleomycin and bleomycin against canine lymphosarcoma (cf. Umezawa et al., 1967; Ishisuka et al., 1966), tried the latter against malignant lymphoma. Of 21 cases, five showed partial and six showed complete remissions.

The clinical picture bears striking resemblance to what has emerged from the laboratory: in general a response, but in particular, seemingly unpredictable results. This seems to reguire attention in designing therapy.

PIETSCH and McCOLLISTER (1965) found transplanted myeloid leukemias to be quite refractory to acute inhibition of DNA synthesis by phleomycin. Believing this finding to be a result of a low incidence of receptiveness, CORBETT, ENG, and PIETSCH (unpublished) have treated mice (i.p.) bearing the transplanted myeloid leukemia for a period of four days. The mice were divided into sublots, and the dose was held constant, but the times of day of treatment were varied. Unpredictable variation in response was obtained. Although time-dependent effects are common in therapy, with bleomycin this is perhaps the most important single consideration, for, to miss a period of receptivity is to render essentially no therapy. Where the receptive period appears to be difficult to hit, as in blood neoplasias, raising the dose may have only marginal effects on the malignancy, for phleomycin and bleomycin clear the body rapidly (cf. PIETSCH et al., 1969). Moreover, receptivity seems to depend upon several superimposed rhythms, that must, in turn, relate to delicately balanced sets of initial conditions.

It appears from the clinical literature that the full theoretical potentialities of bleomycin have not been approached; furthermore, they probably will never be realized without due regard for receptivity. In practical terms, this would mean tailoring therapy to the individual patient rather than to a fixed regimen.

Finally, the laboratory has been a good indicator of clinical efficacy. Mouse rhabdomyosarcoma showed considerable acute response to random dosing (PIETSCH and McCOLLISTER, 1965; cf. PIETSCH and CLAPPER, 1969). Also, KANNO et al. (1970) have assayed bleomycin in mouse brain and brain tumors. They found at least four times as much antibiotic in neoplastic as in surrounding normal brain tissue. Thus, these workers predict efficacy in human disease.

References

ADAMS, R. L. P., ABRAMS, R., LIEBERMAN, I.: Rise in deoxyribonucleic acid polymerase activity in the absence of deoxyribonucleic acid synthesis in cultured kidney cells. Nature (Lond.) **206**, 512—513 (1965).

ADAMS, R. L. P., ABRAMS, R., LIEBERMAN, I.: Deoxycytidylate synthesis and entry into the period of deoxyribonucleic acid replication in rabbit kidney cells. J. biol. Chem. **241**, 903—905 (1966).

BITTAR, E. E.: Effect of aldosterone on Na efflux in single *Maia* fibers. Biochem. biophys. Res. Comm. **23**, 868—873 (1966).

BITTAR, E. E.: Insulin and the sodium pump of the *Maia* muscle fiber. Nature (Lond.) **214**, 726—727 (1967).

BITTAR, E. E., DICK, D. A. T., FRY, D. J.: Effects of aldosterone on Na efflux in single oocytes of *Bufo bufo*. J. Physiol. **184**, 23P (1966).

BRADNER, W. T., PINDELL, M. H.: Antitumor properties of phleomycin. Nature (Lond.) **196**, 683—684 (1962).

BRADNER, W. T., PINDELL, M. H.: Strain of stimulated regression of Sarcoma 180. Cancer Res. **25**, 859—864 (1965).

BRADNER, W. T., PINDELL, M. H.: Myeloid leukemia C149P as a screen for cancer chemotherapeutic agents. Cancer Res. **26**, 375—390 (1966).

CAVALIERI, L. F.: Nucleic acids and information transfer. J. cell. comp. Physiol. **62**, 111—122 (1963).

DJORDJEVIC, B., KIM, J. H.: Lethal effect of phleomycin in different stages of the division cycle of HeLa cells. Cancer Res. **27**, 2255—2260 (1967).

DOLD, U., SCHMIDT, C. G.: Cytostatically active antibiotics. Internist **12**, 136—142 (1971).

Falaschi, A., Kornberg, A.: Phleomycin, an inhibitor of DNA polymerase. Fed. Proc. **23**, 940—945 (1964).

Fanestil, D.: The mechanism of action of aldosterone on sodium transport; effect of inhibitors of DNA synthesis. Life Sci. **7**, 191—195 (1968).

Fukatsu, H., Yoshida, K.: Three cases of penile cancer — clinical use of a new antineoplastic antibiotic, bleomycin. Iryo. **23**, 694—697 (1969) (in Japanese).

Giese, A. C.: Macromolecular synthesis during regeneration in *Blepharisma* determined by specific inhibitors and incorporation of carbon-14 labeled tracers. Exp. cell. Res. **61**, 91—102 (1970).

Gorman, T., Pietsch, P.: Strategy for crystallographic analysis of phleomycin-DNA complexes: Fournier transforms. Physiol. Chem. Phys. **1**, 312—316 (1969).

Grigg, G. W.: Induction of DNA breakdown and death in *Escherichia coli* by phleomycin. Its association with dark-repair processes. Molec. gen. Genetics **104**, 1—11 (1969).

Grigg, G. W.: Amplification of phleomycin induced death and DNA breakdown by caffeine in *Escherichia coli*. Molec. gen. Genetics **107**, 162—172 (1970).

Hanson, C. V.: A study of rapid hydrogen exchange in nucleic acids. J. molec. Biol. **58**, 847—863 (1971).

Hasegawa, Y., Irikura, T., Mizuno, D.: Screening test for the prevention of metastasis produced by Ehrlich carcinoma cells. Chem. pharm. Bull. **18**, 810—814 (1970).

Hecht, T., Summers, D. F.: Effect of phleomycin on poliovirus RNA replication. Virology **40**, 441—447 (1970).

Heinemann, B., Howard, A. J.: Antiphage properties of compounds possessing both antitumor and inducing activities. Antimicrob. Ag. Chemother. **1964**, 126—130 (1965a).

Heinemann, B., Howard, A. J.: Effect of compounds with both antitumor and bacteriophage-inducing activities on *Escherichia coli* nucleic acid synthesis. Antimicrob. Ag. Chemother. **1964**, 488—492 (1965b).

Higuchi, M., Goto, K., Fujimoto, M., Namiki, O., Kikuchi, G.: Effect of inhibitors of nucleic acid and protein synthesis on the induced synthesis of bacteriochlorophyll and δ-aminlevulinic acid synthesis by *Rhodopseudomonas spheroides*. Biochim. biophys. Acta (Amst.) **95**, 94—110 (1965).

Honda, Y., Ohmori, K., Yoshida, K., Arai, K.: Experimental treatment of papilloma with bleomycin. Oto-Rhino-Laryngol. (Tokyo) **12**, 247—252 (1969) (in Japanese).

Hori, M., Ito, E., Umezawa, H.: Inhibitory effects of antitumor substances on growth and glycolysis of Yoshida rat sarcoma cells. J. Antibiot. **A 16**, 1—6 (1963).

Horwitz, S. B., Chang, S. C., Grollman, A. P., Bořkovec, A. B.: Chemosterilant action of anthramycin: a proposed mechanism. Science **174**, 159—161 (1971).

Hotta, Y., Stern, H.: Action of phleomycin on meiotic cells. Cancer Res. **29**, 1699—1706 (1969).

Ichikawa, T.: On an antineoplastic agent, bleomycin. Naika **22**, 630—633 (1968) (in Japanese).

Ichikawa, T., Nakano, I., Hirokawa, I.: Bleomycin treatment of the tumors of penis and scrotum. J. Urol. **102**, 699—707 (1969).

Ichikawa, T.: A new antineoplastic agent, bleomycin — its effect on squamous cell carcinoma. J. Jap. med. Assoc. **61**, 487—497, (1969a) (in Japanese).

Ichikawa, T.: New antineoplastic agent, bleomycin, with special reference to its notable effect on squamous cell carcinoma. Jap. J. clin. Med. **27**, 1618—1626 (1969b).

Ichikawa, T.: Discovery of the effect of bleomycin on squamous cell carcinoma and development of its research. J. Jap. med. Assoc. **62**, 153—158 (1969c) (in Japanese).

Ichikawa, T., Matsuda, A., Miyamoto, K., Tsubosaki, M., Kaihara, T., Sakamoto, K., Umezawa, H.: Biological studies on bleomycin A. J. Antibiot. **20**, 149—155 (1967).

Ichikawa, T., Umezawa, H.: Clinical study on a new antitumor antibiotic, bleomycin. Proc. 5th Int. Congr. Chemotherapy **507** (1967).

Iijima, T., Ikeda, Y.: Mutability of the phleomycin-resistant mutants of *Bacillus subtilis*. I. Isolation of genetically unstable mutants. J. gen. appl. Microbiol. **16**, 419—427 (1970).

Ikeda, K., Egami, F.: Effects of antibiotics and antimetabolites on the induced formation of pyocin R. Z. Allg. Mikrobiol. **6**, 219—225 (1966).

Ikeda, Y., Iijema, T., Tajima, K.: Elimination of F-episome from a male strain of *Escherichia coli* by treatment with sarkomycin and a related antibiotic. J. gen. appl. Microbiol. **13**, 247—254 (1967).

Ikekawa, T., Iwami, F., Hiranaka, H., Umezawa, H.: Separation of phleomycin components and their properties. J. Antibiot. **A 17**, 194—199, 1964.

Inuyama, Y., Machukawa, J.: Effect of 5-fluorouracil and bleomycin on malignant head and neck tumors. Otolaryngol. **41**, 901—909 (1969) (in Japanese).

Ishizuka, M., Takayama, H., Takeuchi, T., Umezawa, H.: Studies on antitumor activity, antimicrobial activity and toxicity of phleomycin. J. Antibiot. **A 19**, 260—271 (1966).

Ishizuka, M., Takayama, H., Takeuchi, T., Umezawa, H.: Activity and toxicity of bleomycin. J. Antibiot. **A 20**, 15—24 (1967).

Iwata, A., Consigli, R. H.: Effect of phleomycin on polyoma virus synthesis in mouse embryo cells. J. Virol. **7**, 29—40 (1971).

Jacobs, N. F., Neu, R. L., Gardner, L. T.: Phleomycin-induced mitotic inhibition and chromosomal abnormalities in cultured human leukocytes. Mutat. Res. **7**, 251—253 (1969).

Jaffe, J.: Sensitivity of *Trypanosoma equiperdum* to the action of tumor-inhibitory antibiotics *in vivo*. Nature (Lond.) **213**, 704—705 (1967).

Jagiello, G. M.: Action of phleomycin on the meiosis of the mouse ovum. Mutat. Res. **6**, 289—295 (1968).

Kajiwara, K., Kim, U. H., Mueller, G. C.: Phleomycin, an inhibitor of replication of HeLa cells. Cancer Res. **26**, 233—236 (1966).

Kanno, T., Kudo, T., Nakazawa, T., Takeuchi, T., Umezawa, H.: Bleomycin as an anti-brain tumor antibiotic. II. The distribution of ^3H bleomycin A 2 (—Cu) in the experimental brain tumor of the mouse. Clin. Neurol. (Tokyo) **10**, 501—506 (1970) (in Japanese).

Kato, S., Hara, I., Abe, H., Ikeda, T., Yamagami, K., Uchiya, M., Shimomura, G.: Treatment for cancer of the female genital organs with an antineoplastic agent, bleomycin. Sanfujinka no Jissai **19**, 204—215 (1970) (in Japanese).

Kihlman, B. A., Odmark, G., Hartley, B.: Studies on the effects of phleomycin on chromosome structure and nucleic acid synthesis in *Vicia faba*. Mutat. Res. **4**, 783—790 (1967).

Kimura, K., Sakai, Y., Konda, T., Kashiwada, N., Kitahara, T., Inagaki, J., Sakano, K., Fujita, H., Iizuka, N., Mikuni, M.: Chemotherapy of malignant lymphoma, with special reference to the effect of bleomycin. Jap. J. clin. Med. **27**, 1593—1601 (1968) (in Japanese).

Koch, G.: Differential effect of phleomycin on the infectivity of poliovirus and poliovirus-induced ribonucleic acids. J. Virol. **8**, 28—34 (1971).

Koyama, G., Nakamura, H., Muraoka, Y., Takita, T., Maeda, K., Umezawa, H.: The chemistry of bleomycin. II. The molecular and crystal structure of a sulfur-containing chromophoric amino acid. Tetrahedron Let. **44**, 4635—4638 (1968).

Kunimoto, T., Hori, M., Umezawa, H.: Modes of action of phleomycin, bleomycin, and formycin on HeLaS_3 cells in synchronized culture. J. Antibiot. **A 20**, 277—281 (1967).

Lein, J., Heinemann, B., Gourevitch, A.: Induction of lysogenic bacteria as a method of detecting potential antitumor agents. Nature (Lond.) **196**, 783—784 (1962).

Maeda, K., Kosaka, H., Yagishita, K., Umezawa, H.: A new antibiotic, phleomycin. J. Antibiot. **A 9**, 82—85 (1956).

Mattingly, E.: Induction of chromosome and chromatid type aberrations by phleomycin. Mutat. Res. **4**, 51—57 (1967).

Mitsuhashi, S., Takahashi, H.: Drug-resistance of enteric bacteria 19. Stability of the transmissible drug-resistance (R) factor in the host cell. Gunma J. med. Sci. **13**, 129—134 (1964).

Mitsuya, H., Kondo, A., Senda, H., Yamanchi, T.: (Clinical study with bleomycin on penile cancer: experience in 5 cases.) Nishinihon J. Urol. **31**, 270—272 (1969) (in Japanese).

Muraoka, Y., Takita, T., Maeda, K., Umezawa, H.: Chemistry of bleomycin. IV. Structure of amine component II of bleomycin A_2. J. Antibiot. **23**, 252—253 (1970).

Nagai, K., Suzuki, H., Tanaka, N., Umezawa, H.: Decrease of melting temperature and single strand scission of DNA by bleomycin in the presence of 2-mercaptoethanal. J. Antibiot. **A 22**, 569—573 (1969a).

Nagai, K., Suzuki, H., Tanaka, N., Umezawa, H.: Decrease of melting temperature and single strand scission of DNA by bleomycin in the presence of hydrogen peroxide. J. Antibiot. **A 22**, 624—628 (1969b).

Nagai, K., Yamaki, H., Suzuki, H., Tanaka, N., Umezawa, H.: The combined effects of bleomycin and sulfhydryl compounds on the thermal denaturation of DNA. Biochim. biophys. Acta (Amst.) **179**, 165—171 (1968).

Nagatsu, M., Okagaki, T., Richart, R. M., Lambert, A.: Effects of bleomycin on nuclear DNA in transplantable VX-2 carcinoma of rabbit. Cancer Res. **31**, 992—996 (1971).

Nakamura, S., Murakami, Y., Hashiguchi, T., Kuga, G., Yanagi, Y., Fujimoto, N., Masuda, Y.: (Clinical and pathological observations on malignant tumors of the head and neck region treated with bleomycin.) Otolaryngol. **41**, 465—477 (1969) (in Japanese).

Nanjo, S., Suga, A.: (Case report of lingual papilloma — electron microscopic observation of bleomycin.) J. Otolaryngol. Jap. **73**, 237—244 (1970) (in Japanese).

Neubert, D.: Vergleichende Untersuchungen über die Nucleinsäuresynthese in Zellkernen und Mitochondrien und ihre Beeinflußbarkeit durch Pharmaka. Arch. exp. Pathol. Pharmakol. **253**, 152—176 (1966).

Oka, S., Sato, K., Nakai, Y., Kurita, K., Hashimoto, K., Oshibe, M.: Treatment of lung cancer with bleomycin. Sci. Rep. Res. Inst. Tahoku Univ. **16**, 30—36 (1969).

Palmer, W. M., Fridhandler, L.: Effects of growth-inhibiting antibiotics on macromolecule biosynthesis in preimplantation rabbit conceptus. Fertil. Steril. **19**, 273—285 (1968).

Pasternak, J., Samoiloff, M. R.: The effect of growth inhibitors on post-embryonic development in the free-living nematode, *Pangrellus silusiae*. Comp. Biochem. Physiol. **33**, 27—38 (1970).

Pietsch, P.: Differences in DNA synthesis as reflected in variations in the acute inhibition of replication by the antibiotic, phleomycin. Anat. Rec. **157**, 301 (1967a).

Pietsch, P.: A structural hypothesis concerning the general mode of action of phleomycin, a specific inhibitor of DNA synthesis. Anat. Rec. **157**, 402 (1967b).

Pietsch, P.: Phleomycin: biological and chemical variations in different batches. Microbios. **1**, 387—392 (1969a).

Pietsch, P.: Structural events in DNA in transcription and replication: the influence of histones on *in vitro* reactions of actinomycin-D and phleomycin-909. Cytobios. **4**, 375—391 (1969b).

Pietsch, P., Clapper, G.: Receptivity of DNA to phleomycin. Cytobios. **1**, 145—152 (1969).

Pietsch, P., Corbett, C.: Competitive effects of phleomycin and mercuric chloride *in vivo*. Nature (Lond.) **219**, 933—934 (1968).

Pietsch, P., Corbett, C., Briden, D. W., Jewett, G.: Diffusability of phleomycin studied by means of neutron activation analysis. Physiol. chem. Phys. **1**, 232—236 (1969).

Pietsch, P., Eng, R.: Phleomycin: enhancement of properties by treatment with acid. Microbios. **1**, 213—231 (1969).

Pietsch, P., Garrett, H.: Primary site of reaction in the *in vitro* complex of phleomycin in DNA. Nature (Lond.) **219**, 488—489 (1968).

Pietsch, P., Garrett, H.: Phleomycin: evidence of *in vivo* binding to DNA. Cytobios. **1**, 7—15 (1969a).

Pietsch, P., Garrett, H.: Phleomycin induced changes in the ultrastructure of DNA. Biophys. J. **A9**, 126 (1969b).

Pietsch, P., McCollister, S. B.: Replication and the activation of muscle differentiation. Nature (Lond.) **208**, 1170—1173 (1965).

Pitts, J., Sinsheimer, R. L.: Effect of phleomycin on replication of bacteriophage ΦX174. J. molec. Biol. **15**, 676—680 (1966).

Price, K. E., Bradner, W. T., Buck, R. E., Lein, J.: Synergistic antimicrobial and antitumor effects of phleomycin and fluorinated pyrimidines. Antimicrob. Ag. Chemother. **1964**, 481—487 (1965).

Price, K. E., Buck, R. E., Lein, J.: System for detecting inducers of lysogenic *Escherichia coli* W1709 (λ) and its applicability as a screen for antineoplastic antibiotics. Appl. Microbiol. **12**, 428—435 (1964).

Price, K. E., Buck, R. E., Lein, J.: Incidence of antineoplastic activity among antibiotics found to be inducers of lysogenic bacteria. Antimicrob. Ag. Chemother. **1964**, 505—517 (1965).

Printz, M. P., von Hippel, P. H.: Hydrogen exchange studies of DNA structure. Proc. nat. Acad. Sci. (Wash.) **53**, 363—370 (1965).

Rakieten, N., Nadkarni, M. V., Rakieten, M. L., Gordon, B. S.: Toxicologic and pharmacologic evaluation of phleomycin, including special studies on its nephrotoxicity. Toxicol. appl. Pharmacol. **14**, 590—602 (1969).

Redon, H.: Study of the clinical efficiency of bleomycin in human cancer. Brit. med. J. **2**, 643—645 (1970).

Richmond, J. E., Glaeser, R. M., Todd, P.: Protein synthesis and aggregation of embryonic cells. Exp. Cell Res. **52**, 43—58 (1968).

Smale, B. C., Montgillion, M. D., Pridham, T. G.: Phleomycin, an antibiotic markedly effective for control of bean rust. Plant Dis. Rep. **45**, 244 (1961).

Sober, H. A.: Handbook of Biochemistry. Selected data for molecular biology. Cleveland: The Chemical Rubber Co. 1968.

Suzuki, H.: On the mechanism of action of bleomycin: scission of DNA strands *in vitro* and *in vivo*. J. Antibiot. **22**, 446—448 (1969b).

Suzuki, H., Nagai, K., Akutsu, E., Yamaki, H., Tanaka, N., Umezawa, H.: Mechanism of action of bleomycin. Strand scission of DNA caused by bleomycin and its binding to DNA *in vitro*. J. Antibiot. **23**, 473—480 (1970).

Suzuki, H., Nagai, K., Yamaki, H., Tanaka, N., Umezawa, H.: Mechanism of action of bleomycin. Studies with the growing culture of bacterial and tumor cells. J. Antibiot. **A21**, 379—386 (1968).

Suzuki, H., Nagai, K., Yamaki, H., Tanaka, N., Umezawa, H.: On the mechanism of action of bleomycin: scission of DNA strands *in vitro* and *in vivo*. J. Antibiot. **22**, 446—468 (1969a).

Suzuki, M., Murai, A., Watanabe, A., Nunokawa, O.: Treatment of cancer of the female genital organs with a new anti-cancer agent, bleomycin. Acta med. biol. **17**, 259—275 (1970).

Suzuki, M., Nomura, H., Ito, M., Kasamatu, T., Nakanishi, K., Yamaoka, S., Misoo, Y., Takamisawa, Y., Suzuki, T., Takeda, T., Iizima, H., Kuto, J., Kinoshita, S., Moriya, K., Murai, J., Hasegawa, K., Watanabe, K., Ootake, S., Fushekawa, O.: Therapy of cancer of the female genitalia with a new antineoplastic drug, bleomycin — basic study of bleomycin. Sanfujin Jissai **18**, 375—379 (1969a) (in Japanese).

Suzuki, M., Nomura, H., Ito, M., Kasamatu, T., Nakanishi, K., Yamaoka, S., Misoo, Y., Takamisawa, Y., Suzuki, T., Takeda, T., Iizima, H., Kuto, J., Kinoshita, S., Moriya, K., Murai, J., Hasegawa, K., Watanabe, K., Ootake, S., Fushekawa, O.: Therapy of gynecologic tumors with a new antineoplastic agent, bleomycin — clinical study. Sanfujin Jissai **18**, 574—581 (1969b) (in Japanese).

Suzuki, Y., Miyake, K.: Clinical use of bleomycin in malignant tumor of the head and neck. J. Jap. med. Assoc. **62**, 112—117 (1969) (in Japanese).

Takeda, K., Sawawa, Y., Arakawa, T.: Therapeutic effects of bleomycin for skin tumors. Gann **61**, 207—218 (1970) (in Japanese).

Takeuchi, M., Yamamoto, T.: Effects of bleomycin on mouse transplantable tumors. J. Antibiot. **A 21**, 631—637 (1968).

Takeuchi, T.: Inhibition of resistant dysentery bacilli by phleomycin. J. Antibiot. **A 16**, 172 (1963).

Takita, T.: Studies on purification and properties of phleomycin. J. Antibiot. **A 12**, 285—289 (1959).

Takita, T., Maeda, K., Umezawa, H.: Chemistry of bleomycin. III. The sugar moieties of bleomycin A_2. J. Antibiot. **A 22**, 237—239 (1969).

Takita, T., Muraoka, Y., Maeda, K., Umezawa, H.: Chemical studies on bleomycin. I. The acid hydrolysis products of bleomycin A_2. J. Antibiot. **A 21**, 79—80 (1968).

Tanaka, N.: Effect of phleomycin on DNA polymerase of tumor origin. J. Antibiot. **A 18**, 111 (1965).

Tanaka, N.: Inhibition of transcription by pluramycin and bleomycin. J. Antibiot. **A 23**, 523—530 (1970).

Tanaka, N., Yamaguchi, H., Umezawa, H.: Mechanism of action of phleomycin. J. Antibiot. **A 16**, 86—91 (1963a).

Tanaka, N., Yamaguchi, H., Umezawa, H.: Mechanism of action of angustmycins, mikamycins, and phleomycin. Jap. J. med. Sci. Biol. **16**, 240—246 (1963b).

Tanaka, N., Yamaguchi, H., Umezawa, H.: Mechanism of action of phleomycin, a tumor-inhibitory antibiotic. Biochem. biophys. Res. Commun. **10**, 171—174 (1963c).

Tepper, H. B., Hollis, C. A., Galson, E. C., Sondheimer, E.: Germination of *Fraxinus ornus* embryos with and without phleomycin. Plant Physiol. **42**, 1483—1486 (1967).

Terasima, T., Umezawa, H.: Lethal effect of bleomycin on cultured mammalian cells. J. Antibiot. **A 23**, 300—304 (1970).

Tevethia, F., Rapp, F.: Effect of phleomycin on the replication of papovavirus SV40 and other DNA viruses in simian cells. Cancer Res. **29**, 912—917 (1969).

Tomizawa, H., Takahashi, H.: Stimulation of pectolytic enzyme formation of *Erwinia aroides* by nalidixic acid, mitomycin C and bleomycin. Agr. Biol. Chem. **35**, 191—200 (1971).

Tsuboi, A., Terasima, T.: Rejoining of single breaks of DNA induced by x-rays in mammalian cells: effects of metabolic inhibitors. Molec. gen. Genetics **108**, 117—128 (1970).

Ueno, M.: Clinical use of bleomycin in cases of cancer of the oral cavity. J. Jap. med. Assoc. **62**, 117—126 (1969) (in Japanese).

Umezawa, H.: Bleomycin and other antitumor antibiotics of high molecular weight. Antimicrob. Ag. Chemother. **1965**, 1079—1085 (1966).

Umezawa, H.: Index of antibiotics from actinomycetes. Tokyo: University Park Press and University of Tokyo Press 1967.

Umezawa, H., Hori, M., Ishizuka, M., Takeuchi, T.: Studies on antitumor effect of phleomycin. J. Antibiot. **A 15**, 274—275 (1962).

Umezawa, H., Ishizuka, M., Hori, S., Chimura, H., Takeuchi, T., Komai, T.: The distribution of ^{3}H-bleomycin in mouse tissue. J. Antibiot. **A 21**, 638—642 (1968b).

Umezawa, H., Ishizuka, M., Kimura, K., Iwanaga, J., Takeuchi, T.: Biological studies on individual bleomycins. J. Antibiot. **A 21**, 592—602 (1968a).

Umezawa, H., Ishizuka, M., Maeda, K., Takeuchi, T.: Studies on bleomycin. Cancer **20**, 891—895 (1967).

Umezawa, H., Maeda, K.: Phleomycin, a new antibiotic substance. Japanese patent publication 2598/59, filed December 22, 1955 (translated by Kawase and Okada, Tokyo, 1959).
Umezawa, H., Maeda, K., Takeuchi, T., Okami, Y.: New antibiotics, bleomycin A and B. J. Antibiot. **A19**, 200—209 (1966a).
Umezawa, H., Suhara, Y., Ikekawa, T., Ishizuka, M., Hori, M., Maeda, K., Tanaka, N., Takeuchi, T.: Antitumor substances selected from streptomyces products. Int. Congr. Chemother. **1963**, 974—978 (1964).
Umezawa, H., Suhara, Y., Takita, T., Maeda, K.: Purification of bleomycins. J. Antibiot. **A19**, 210—215 (1966b).
Watanabe, M., August, J. T.: Replication of RNA bacteriophage R23. II. Inhibition of phage-specific RNA synthesis by phleomycin. J. molec. Biol. **33**, 21—33 (1968).
Welsh, R., Vyska, K.: Properties of a new form of DNA from whole calf thymus nuclei: evidence for reactive special sites in DNA. Arch. Biochem. Biophys. **142**, 132—143 (1971).
Werner, R.: Nature of DNA precursors. Nature New Biol. **233**, 99—103 (1971).
Yamagata, S., Uzuka, Y., Kurokawa, Y., Yonahara, M.: Cancer chemotherapy. Current status and prospects. J. Jap. Soc. Cancer Ther. **3**, 8—17 (1968) (in Japanese).
Yamaki, H., Tanaka, N., Umezawa, H.: Effects of several tumor-inhibitory antibiotics on immunological responses. J. Antibiot. **A22**, 315—321 (1969).
Zimmer, D. E.: Efficacy of some antifungal substances for control of seedling safflower rust. Plant Dis. Rep. **49**, 623—626 (1965).

Chapter 79

Pharmacology of Newer Antineoplastic Agents

RICHARD H. ADAMSON

With 9 Figures

Introduction

Within the last 2 to 3 years a number of drugs from different sources and with diverse structures have shown antitumor activity in experimental animal systems, and several of these are presently in clinical trial or ready to enter phase I clinical trial. Much of our knowledge of the pharmacology of these drugs is fragmentary, but with regard to several of the agents known information includes the mechanism of action, the metabolic fate, and structure-activity relationships. Some of the agents to be discussed are at the preclinical stage and therefore are of potential rather than proven value to cancer chemotherapy, but several of the agents have shown activity in limited clinical trials.

The agents discussed in this chapter include guanazole, gallium, hycanthone, ellipticine and 9-methoxyellipticine, alanosine, rifamycin SV, tilorone, ICRF 159, isophosphamide, and cyclocytidine.

Guanazole

Guanazole (3,5-diamino-1,2,4-triazole) (Fig. 1), a compound synthesized in 1894 (PELLIZZARI, 1894), is active against leukemia L1210, leukemia K1964, mast cell tumor P815, as well as other experimental tumors (BROCKMAN et al., 1970; HAHN and ADAMSON, 1970, 1972). Guanazole was found to be more effective in prolonging

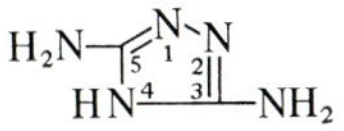

H_2N — N—N — HN — NH_2

Guanazole

Fig. 1

the life span of leukemic mice when it was administered as 2 or more divided doses daily rather than on a once per day schedule. In addition, guanazole was significantly more effective when given i.p. to mice 8 times at 3 h intervals on days 2, 6, and 10 after tumor cell inoculation, with 35 % of the mice on this schedule being long term survivors. Thus, dose scheduling is an important factor for maximal antitumor activity with this agent, at least in experimental animal systems.

The mechanism of action of guanazole has been investigated by studying the activity of various antitumor drugs against a variant of leukemia L1210 made resistant to guanazole and by studies on the effects of guanazole on the incorporation of precursors into macromolecules (BROCKMAN et al., 1970; SCHABEL et al., 1971; HAHN and ADAMSON, 1972). The folic acid antagonists, 1-β-D-arabinofuranosyl cytosine (ara-C), the nitrosoureas, and cyclophosphamide are active against leukemia L1210 made resistant to guanazole, whereas guanazole was active against variants made resistant to dichloromethotrexate, ara-C, and nitrosoureas. However, guanazole was cross-resistant to a tumor line made resistant to hydroxyurea. In studies on DNA, RNA, and protein synthesis, guanazole was found to inhibit DNA synthesis in L1210 tumor cells to a greater extent than RNA synthesis, while protein synthesis was not affected. Furthermore, guanazole inhibited the reduction of ribonucleotides to deoxyribonucleotides catalyzed by enzyme preparations from human epidermoid carcinoma cells. In general, the effects of guanazole on DNA synthesis and on ribonucleoside diphosphate reductase were similar to those found with hydroxyurea.

Structure activity studies *in vitro* against leukemia L1210 revealed that substitutions on the 1,2,4-triazole moiety other than amino groups in positions 3 and 5 resulted in a loss of cytotoxicity or in a compound with equal cytotoxic activity *in vitro*, but unacceptable toxicity *in vivo* (HAHN and ADAMSON, 1972). Thus, out of a series of substituted triazoles guanazole was the only compound of promise as an antitumor agent.

Studies on the disposition of guanazole utilizing a ^{14}C label in positions 3 and 5 have been reported (HAHN and ADAMSON, 1970; ADAMSON and HAHN, 1973). These studies revealed that one reason for the frequent dosing required for optimal activity is that guanazole is rapidly excreted by the mouse and rat, with greater than 90 % appearing in mouse urine three hours following an antitumor dose and 80 % excreted by the rat in the same time period. Tissue distribution studies in the mouse revealed that ^{14}C-guanazole was generally found in organs involved in urinary excretion. In addition, guanazole did not readily cross the blood-brain barrier of mice or dogs. This was not unexpected since guanazole is a highly polar compound having a heptane or chloroform/aqueous partition coefficient of < 0.0001. However, guanazole was absorbed after oral administration to mice, since 70 % of the radioactivity appeared in the urine four hours after administration while only 6 % was present in the feces.

Chromatographic studies on the urine from guanazole treated mice, rats, and dogs did not reveal any radioactivity other than in the parent compound. In addition, no radioactive CO_2 was found in the expired air after administration of ^{14}C-guanazole to mice. Preliminary studies in patients with malignant disease indicate that guanazole is rapidly excreted with little or no metabolism. These disposition studies along with the cytotoxic data obtained with guanazole *in vitro*, the structural specificity of the 3,5-diamino substitution for maximal activity, and the ability to extrapolate *in vivo* doses from tissue culture cytotoxicity data, strongly suggest that the active molecule for antitumor activity is guanazole per se.

Guanazole has received an evaluation in adult acute leukemia, being given by i.v. administration over a 5 day period at a dose of 7.5 to 25 grams/m^2/day. Three courses were given every 14 days and at least three courses were needed for an adequate trial. Complete remission rate was 16 % (5/31) for evaluable patients and 25 % (5/20) for patients with adequate trials (3 or more courses). These remissions occurred in AML or in the acute stage of CML and the major toxicity seen was myelosuppression. Thus, guanazole is an active agent for remission induction in adult acute leukemia (HEWLETT, 1972).

Gallium

Since gallium is a bone seeking element, radionuclides of this element have been of clinical interest as diagnostic screening agents for bone tumors (DUDLEY, 1949; HAYES et al., 1965). In addition, carrier-free gallium-67 citrate has been found to localize in nonosseous tumors in patients with Hodgkin's disease, lymphomas, and in "soft-tissue" slowly growing tumors such as reticulum cell sarcoma, carcinomas of the lung, breast, colon, and kidney (EDWARDS and HAYES, 1969, 1970). These observations prompted studies on the concentration of ^{67}Ga in various experimental animal tumors. Seven nonosseous rat and mouse carcinomas and sarcomas showed variable but distinct localization of ^{67}Ga (HAYES et al., 1970).

Recently, various gallium salts (gallium nitrate, gallium chloride and gallium sulfate) demonstrated antitumor activity in several experimental systems (HART and ADAMSON, 1971; HART et al., 1971). Gallium nitrate gave better than 90% inhibition of growth of several experimental solid tumors in animals, including an osteosarcoma, a reticulum cell sarcoma, and a lymphosarcoma. However, gallium nitrate showed little or no antitumor activity when evaluated against three murine leukemias (i.e., leukemias L1210, K1964 and P388).

The toxicity and antitumor activities of periodically related Group IIIa metal salts of aluminum (Al), indium (In) and thallium (Tl) were also investigated. The order of decreasing effectiveness of the Group IIIa salts against subcutaneously transplanted solid neoplasms was generally found to be $Ga(NO_3)_3 > Al(NO_3)_3 \geq In(NO_3)_3 > TlCl_3$. $Ga(NO_3)_3$ was by far the superior agent, being greater than 90% effective against 6 of 8 solid tumors. When tested against 8 i.p. transplanted tumors, these compounds were active in only one, the Walker carcinosarcoma 256. Substitution of other anions for the nitrate moiety did not alter the antitumor activity of the Group IIIa metal cations against the Walker carcinosarcoma 256.

These results suggest that gallium might be useful as an antitumor agent in the treatment of various solid tumors in humans, but would be ineffective in the treatment of leukemias.

Tracer doses of gallium (^{67}Ga) have been used for the study of its distribution and excretion in patients. These studies revealed a two component whole body retention curve with a shorter retention in the plasma (T 1/2 of 0.7 days) and a prolonged retention in tissue (T 1/2 of 13.8 days). Excretion of ^{67}Ga occurred by both urinary and fecal routes (ARSENEAU et al., 1972). Disposition studies using pharmacologic doses await clinical trial of gallium in human malignancy.

Hycanthone

Hycanthone is a drug with potent antischistosomal activity against *Schistosoma mansoni* and *S. haematobium* in both animals and man. Clinical trials in Africa and South America have shown that hycanthone is efficacious and relatively nontoxic (MARITZ, 1970; CLARKE et al., 1969; KATZ et al., 1968).

Hycanthone is the hydroxymethyl derivative (Fig. 2) of lucanthone (Miracil D), an antischistosomal agent in use for several decades. In addition to its antischistosomal activity, lucanthone has been reported to have antitumor activity in a number of experimental murine tumors including Sarcoma 180, leukemia L1210, and adenocarcinomas 755 and EO771 (HIRSCHBERG et al., 1959). There is evidence that one of the metabolites of lucanthone, rather than lucanthone per se, may be responsible for its antischistosomal activity and this active metabolite may be hycanthone (ROSI et al., 1965; BERBERIAN et al., 1967). Also, metabolic conversion of lucanthone to a more active metabolite appears necessary for antitumor activity

(HIRSCHBERG et al., 1964). The possibility that the antitumor activity of lucanthone, like its antischistosomal activity, was due to its metabolite hycanthone and certain structural features of hycanthone, prompted its evaluation for antitumor activity. Hycanthone was found to be cytotoxic *in vitro* against leukemia L1210, Walker 256 carcinosarcoma, and Novikoff hepatoma cells. In addition, hycanthone exhibited antitumor activity *in vivo* against leukemias L1210 and P388, mast cell tumor P815, and Walker 256 carcinosarcoma (ADAMSON, 1971a; SIEBER et al., 1973).

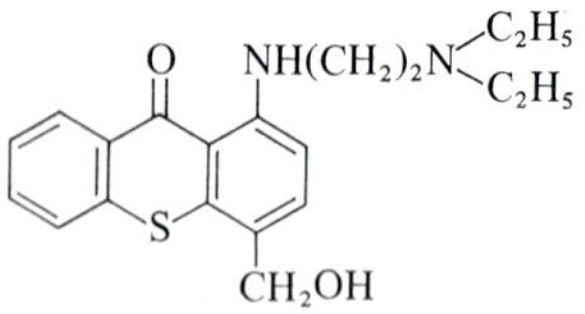

O NH(CH$_2$)$_2$N(C$_2$H$_5$)$_2$

S

CH$_2$OH

Hycanthone

Fig. 2

Studies on the effects of hycanthone on macromolecular synthesis showed that hycanthone inhibited the DNA and RNA synthesis of rapidly dividing, phytohemagglutinin (PHA)-stimulated lymphocytes, whereas inhibition of protein synthesis occurred only at larger concentrations (SIEBER et al., 1973). However, in HeLa cells, hycanthone inhibited RNA synthesis without affecting either DNA or protein synthesis (WITTNER et al., 1971). In L1210 cells *in vitro*, hycanthone inhibited DNA and RNA synthesis (HIRSCHBERG and WEINSTEIN, 1971). On the basis of its ability to increase the melting temperature and relative viscosity of native calf thymus DNA and to uncoil the helix of circular duplex DNA of bacteriophage ΦX174, it has been postulated that hycanthone may interact with DNA by intercalation (WARING, 1970; HIRSCHBERG and WEINSTEIN, 1971).

A large number of analogs of lucanthone and hycanthone have been synthesized and studies thus far indicate that for optimal antitumor activity, as well as for complexing with DNA, it is necessary for the molecule to have an intact 10-thiaxanthenone ring containing a compact substituent in the 4-position and a diamino side chain with a unsubstituted proximal nitrogen (BLANZ and FRENCH, 1963; WEINSTEIN and HIRSCHBERG, 1971).

The absorption, distribution, and excretion of hycanthone have been studied in rats and rhesus monkeys, using tritiated hycanthone at doses recommended for man for treatment of schistosomiasis (3 mg/kg). Peak blood and tissue concentration occurred 30 to 60 min after a single intramuscular dose. The largest concentrations were observed in the liver, spleen, kidneys and adrenals and decreased rapidly with greater than 80 % of the dose being excreted in 48 to 72 h. In monkeys, a large concentration of the compound was found in the bile, probably conjugated with glucuronic acid. Radiochromatography demonstrated only unchanged drug in the blood and tissues, except in the liver where rapid conversion occurred to the sulfoxide in the rat and to the deethyl analog in the monkey. In addition, the main metabolite formed *in vitro* with rat liver preparations was the sulfoxide, and deethyl hycanthone with monkey and human liver microsomes. The evidence, therefore, suggests that biotransformation of hycanthone in man would be similar to that observed in the monkey (HERNANDEZ et al., 1971).

Evidence for the antitumor activity of hycanthone (or one of its analogs) in man awaits clinical trial.

Ellipticine and 9-Methoxyellipticine

Various Australian plants have been evaluated for antitumor activity. Extracts of two botanically related species, *Ochrosia moorei* F. Muell and *Excavatia coccinea* were found to have activity against Sarcoma 180, adenocarcinoma 755, and leukemia L1210 *in vivo* and to be cytotoxic against human carcinoma of the nasopharynx in tissue culture (KB cells). This activity was found to be associated with the alkaloids of these plants, mainly by the two alkaloids, ellipticine and 9-methoxyellipticine (Fig. 3) (CULVENOR and LODER, 1966; DALTON et al., 1967; SVOBODA et al., 1968). A relatively broad spectrum of antitumor activity has been seen with 9-methoxyellipticine, 10 of 17 mouse neoplasms tested having responded. In addition, significant activity was seen against both the solid and the ascitic forms of Walker 256 carcinosarcoma in the rat (SVOBODA et al., 1968).

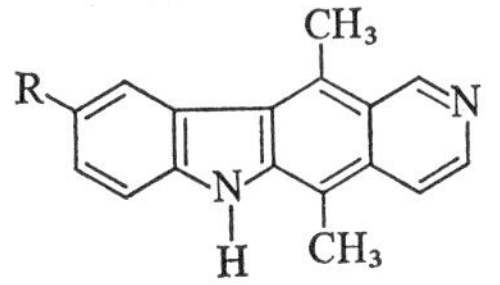

R = H Ellipticine
R = OCH_3 9-Methoxyellipticine

Fig. 3

In tissue culture, ellipticine inhibited DNA and RNA synthesis to a greater extent than protein synthesis in both Chinese hamster (DON) cells and L1210 cells (BHUYAN et al., 1972). The related compound, 9-methoxyellipticine, inhibited DNA synthesis in normal human fibroblast cultures, although a pronounced inhibitory effect on RNA and protein synthesis also occurred (GARCIA-GIRALT and MACIEIRA-COELHO, 1970). In a study on the ability of synchronized Chinese hamster cells to traverse the cell cycle, ellipticine inhibited initiation of DNA synthesis and completion of G_2, but was ineffective in preventing DNA synthesis in cells already in S at the time of drug addition (TOBEY, 1972). Ellipticine resembles proflavin in molecular size, shape, and charge and, like proflavin, increases the viscosity of DNA solutions. In addition, ellipticine inhibits the processing of 45 S nucleolar RNA to other RNA species in the ribosomal RNA maturation sequence in leukemia L1210 cells (SNYDER et al., 1971). The evidence, therefore, suggests that ellipticine binds to nucleic acid helices by intercalation.

In a search for active analogs of ellipticine, several compounds have been synthesized and evaluated for antitumor activity. The active analogs are 9-methoxyellipticine (described above), 11-desmethylellipticine, thiaellipticine (the 5-isostere), 6-methylellipticine, and 9-methoxy-6-methylellipticine. The following analogs were inactive against leukemia L1210 *in vivo*: 9-bromoellipticine, 9-methylellipticine, 1,2,3,4-tetrahydro-9-methoxy-2-methylellipticine, isoellipticine, 7,10-dimethylellipticine, 3-methylellipticine, 3,4-dihydroisoellipticine, oxaellipticine, and isothiaellipticine (HARTWELL and ABBOTT, 1969; FUJIWARA et al., 1969; DALTON et al., 1967).

Studies on the disposition of ellipticine have been reported in mice, rats, and dogs using both a sensitive photometric method and 1-^{14}C-labeled ellipticine (CHADWICK et al., 1971; HARDESTY et al., 1972). After administration to mice the drug was found to be widely distributed, concentrations in tissues being dependent on route of administration. The largest and smallest tissue levels were observed after administration to mice i.p., in solution and suspension, respectively. The major portion of excreted ellipticine was present in the feces; only trace amounts were found in the urine. After administration to rats, 11 and 13 % of the dose were found in the 24 h and 96 h urine, respectively, one-tenth as ellipticine and the remainder being metabolites. Rats secreted up to 70 % by the biliary route in 24 h, of which less than one-tenth was parent compound. Dogs excreted less than 5 % of the dose in the urine 24 h after administration and the presence of large concentrations of ellipticine equivalents in bile from gall bladder and intestinal contents also implicated a biliary route of secretion in dogs. Drug equivalents in dog tissues decreased between 1 and 24 h and by 24 h consisted primarily of metabolite(s).

A preliminary clinical trial of 9-methoxyellipticine has been carried out in 34 patients with Hodgkin's disease, acute lymphoblastic leukemia, or acute myeloblastic leukemia. Although the drug exhibited little or no effect in patients with Hodgkin's disease or acute lymphoblastic leukemia, 9 of 12 patients with acute myeloblastic leukemia showed some response with 3 patients achieving complete remission (MATHÉ et al., 1970). The activity of this compound in other neoplastic diseases and of other analogs must be decided after further clinical evaluation.

Alanosine

Alanosine [L(—)2-amino-3-nitrosohydroxylaminopropionic acid] is an antibiotic which was isolated from *Streptomyces alanosinicus* (ATCC No. 15710). This compound (Fig. 4) has inhibitory activity against several viruses *in vitro* and *in vivo* and induces regression of a transplanted fibrosarcoma (MURTHY et al., 1966). The DL-form also has antitumor activity against Walker 256 carcinosarcoma and, at doses approaching lethality, has activity against leukemia L1210.

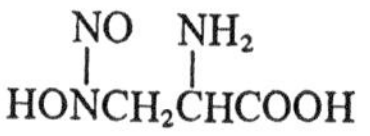

$$\begin{array}{c} \text{NO} \quad \text{NH}_2 \\ | \qquad | \\ \text{HONCH}_2\text{CHCOOH} \end{array}$$

DL-Alanosine

Fig. 4

Studies of the mechanism of action of the L-isomer have been carried out utilizing *Candida albicans*. The growth of this organism is inhibited by alanosine and this inhibition is antagonized by aspartate. The incorporation of ^{14}C-aspartate into RNA pyrimidines was inhibited by this drug, while the incorporation of ^{3}H-uridine was enhanced. Alanosine also depressed the rate of incorporation of ^{14}C-formate into RNA adenine, but increased the rate of its incorporation into RNA guanine. Incorporation of ^{14}C-formate into acid-soluble adenine nucleotides also was inhibited. These studies suggest that alanosine inhibited the activity of aspartate transcarbamylase and adenylosuccinate synthetase (GALE and SMITH, 1968; GALE et al., 1968).

Further studies with this interesting antibacterial, antiviral, and antitumor agent await preclinical toxicology as well as clinical trial.

Rifamycin SV and Derivatives

Rifamycin SV (Fig. 5) is one of a group of several semisynthetic rifamycins derived from an antibiotic isolated from the fermentation broth of *Streptomyces mediterranei*. Rifamycin SV and analogs have activity *in vitro* and *in vivo* against gram-positive microorganisms and mycobacteria, especially *Mycobacterium tuberculosis*. Although this agent is not active orally, the hydrazone or *N*-methylpiperazine derivative of rifamycin SV, called rifampin or rifampicin, was active on oral administration and is currently used primarily for the treatment of tuberculosis, especially in patients characterized as therapeutic failures and excreting tubercle bacilli resistant to standard drugs (BERGAMINI and FOWST, 1965; ARIOLI et al., 1967; RIVA and SILVESTRI, 1972; LESTER, 1972; WEHRLI and STAEHELIN, 1971).

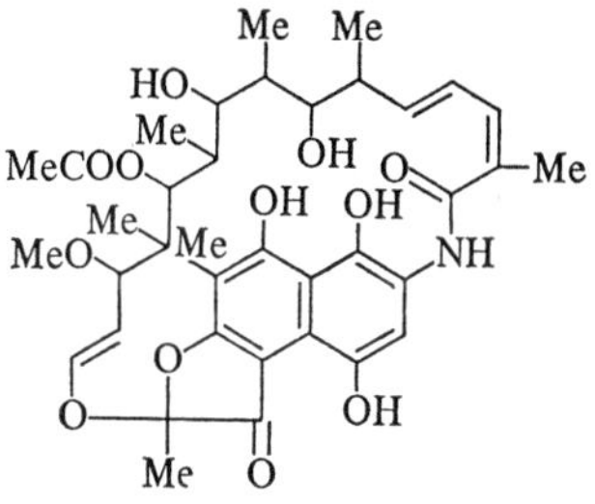

Rifamycin SV

Fig. 5

The rifamycins have been of interest to oncologists for three reasons: first, their antiviral, cytotoxic, and marginal antitumor activity; second, the high specificity of action of some of these compounds against the enzymes involved in the synthesis of polynucleotides; and third, the great number of possible chemical modifications of the molecule (over 1000 derivatives have been made). Rifamycin SV has cytotoxic activity in tissue culture against leukemias L1210 and L5178Y and the Novikoff hepatoma. In addition, Rifamycin SV has antitumor activity *in vivo* against Walker 256 carcinosarcoma, but not against leukemia L1210 or leukemia P388 (ADAMSON, 1971b). Rifamycin SV has cytotoxic activity against human leukemic cells *in vitro* (SMITH et al., 1972).

A number of rifamycin derivatives have been examined for their toxic effects against fresh human leukemia cells and normal cells. In general, those derivatives that were more toxic to fresh human leukemia cells than to normal proliferating blood cells were also better inhibitors of DNA polymerases of human and viral (RNA tumor virus) origin (SMITH et al., 1972). In a study of over 200 rifamycin derivatives tested for inhibitory activity against human lymphocyte and murine leukemia virus DNA polymerases, two had greater inhibitory effects against viral reverse transcriptase than against DNA polymerase I or II from normal human cells. In addition, these two derivatives, 3-(2,4-dinitrophenylhydrazonomethyl)-rifamycin SV and 3-piperazinoiminomethylrifamycin SV (*N*-demethyl rifampicin) preferentially inhibited leukemic DNA polymerase II over normal DNA polymerase, though inhibition was not as great as with reverse transcriptase (YANG et al., 1972). The activity of these two derivatives and other analogs against viral and nonviral experimental tumors remains to be demonstrated.

Rifamycin SV has received limited clinical trial in five patients with acute leukemia (2 ALL, 3 AML). This compound was evaluated even though other derivatives have greater inhibitory activity against reverse transcriptase because of its cytotoxic effect against murine and human leukemia cells at concentrations that could be achieved in human serum and because of the widespread previous use of this drug in tuberculosis, so that extensive preclinical toxicology studies were not necessary, as would have been the case with the other derivatives. These five patients had not responded or were refractory to other chemotherapeutic agents. One patient showed transient improvement with a reduction in circulating blasts. Reversible hepatotoxicity appeared in all patients following prolonged treatment at doses up to 1700 mg/m^2/every eight hours (HENDERSON, E.S., personal communication). Thus, the idea of further exploiting the inhibition of reverse transcriptase in man for either remission in acute lymphocytic leukemia or for maintenance of remission still awaits evaluation by the use of other derivatives of rifamycin.

Tilorone Hydrochloride

Various rodent tumors have been shown to be inhibited by exogenous interferon and inducers of interferon, including statolon, pyran copolymer, and poly I · poly C (see review by ADAMSON et al., 1972). Reports that tilorone hydrochloride (2,7-*bis*[2-(diethylamino)ethoxy]fluoren-9-one), a synthetic low molecular weight compound (Fig. 6), induced interferon and exhibited broad spectrum antiviral activity (MAYER and KRUEGER, 1970) prompted evaluation of tilorone for antitumor activity (ADAMSON, 1971c). Tilorone inhibited focus formation by Moloney sarcoma virus and exerted an effect against mice inoculated with Friend leukemia virus (ADAMSON and TING, 1971; BARKER et al., 1971). In addition, tilorone has cytotoxic effects *in vitro* and antitumor activity against a reticulum cell sarcoma in mice and the rat Walker 256 carcinosarcoma (ADAMSON, 1971c). Tilorone has little or no activity against mice bearing leukemias L1210 or P388. The mechanism of action of the antitumor effect of tilorone has not been fully elucidated, but is probably related to its interferon inducing ability, its stimulation of 19 S antibody production, and its stimulation of phagocytic response (ADAMSON, 1971c; HOFFMAN et al., 1971; MUNSON et al., 1972).

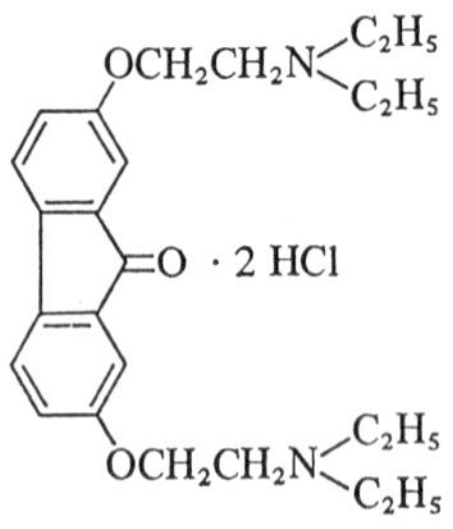

$OCH_2CH_2N(C_2H_5)_2$

$=O \cdot 2\,HCl$

$OCH_2CH_2N(C_2H_5)_2$

Tilorone Hydrochloride

Fig. 6

A number of analogs of tilorone have been synthesized and thus far 5 of these have been examined for antitumor activity and effects on the immune system (MUNSON et al., 1972). Although conclusive structure-activity relationships have not been elucidated at the present time, one analog [DEAA fluorene or 2,7-*bis*(2-diethylaminoacetyl)fluorene] was very effective against both the Friend virus and the Ehrlich carcinoma (MUNSON et al., 1972).

In a phase I study of tilorone in 10 patients treated with the drug for 2 weeks or longer, 8 had evaluable disease. Two patients with metastatic melanoma had partial responses and 6 patients exhibited no change. Tilorone did not depress the bone marrow, but to the contrary, appeared to stimulate platelet production. The primary toxic effect seen with tilorone was lethargy, but nausea and vomiting, weakness, dizziness, headache, and insomnia were also observed at larger doses (WAMPLER et al., 1973). The usefulness of tilorone and/or its analogs in the treatment of neoplasms awaits further investigation.

ICRF 159

ICRF 159, (±)-1,2-*bis*-(3,5-dioxopiperazin-1-yl)propane, was one of a series of ethylenediamine tetraacetic acid (EDTA) derivatives which were synthesized to examine the rationale that non-polar derivatives of EDTA might exert antitumor activity by virtue of their ability to cross cell membranes and chelate vulnerable metal-containing intracellular sites (CREIGHTON et al., 1969). ICRF 159 (Fig. 7) has antitumor activity against a variety of experimental tumors including Sarcoma 180 and leukemia L1210 (CREIGHTON et al., 1969). In addition, although ICRF 159 has little effect on the primary implant of Lewis lung carcinoma, it inhibited metastases to the lungs of mice bearing the primary implant. The authors suggested that this finding "adds a new and serious challenge to other considerations in accepting the predictive value of tests where inhibition of the primary tumor is the sole criterion to select compounds for the control of malignant growth" (HELLMANN and BURRAGE, 1969).

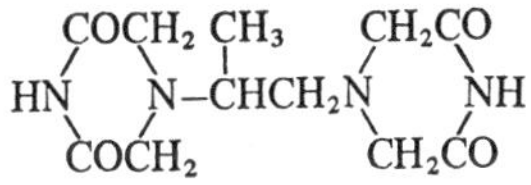

```
 COCH2 CH3    CH2CO
 /    \  |    /    \
HN     N-CHCH2N     NH
 \    /        \    /
 COCH2          CH2CO
```

ICRF 159

Fig. 7

ICRF 159 was found to block the entry of cultured human lymphocytes into mitosis and to arrest dividing cells in prophase and early metaphase (SHARP et al., 1970). In studies utilizing mouse embryo fibroblasts *in vitro*, ICRF 159 was shown to be a potent inhibitor of DNA synthesis while having relatively little effect on RNA or protein synthesis. The time course for the inhibition of ^{3}H-thymidine uptake into DNA by ICRF 159 was similar to that for ionizing radiation and radiomimetic drugs. All three showed a recovery taking place approximately four hours after the initial treatment, followed later by a more substantial and permanent inhibition. It is possible therefore that ICRF 159 exerts its effect by acting as a mono- or bifunctional acylating agent (CREIGHTON and BIRNIE, 1970).

Structure-activity studies have shown that the methyl and ethyl esters of EDTA had no antitumor activity and that antitumor activity was confined to a group of compounds having structures similar to ICRF 159. However, substitution on the central ethylene chain was not necessary for activity, and methyl substitution did not alter activity (ICRF 159), although ethyl substitution abolished activity. Optical isomers of ICRF 159 were active, but a series of acyclic analogs, including *N*,*N*'-dicarboxamidomethyl-*N*,*N*'-dicarboxymethyl-1,2-diaminoethane, the product of hydrolysis of ICRF 154 (i.e., no substitution on the central ethylene chain) was inactive (CREIGHTON et al., 1969).

The rate of clearance of ICRF-159 from the blood of rats after i.p. or i.v. administration was determined using the ^{14}C-labeled drug and a bioassay system of cultured Chinese hamster cells. The curve of clearance of radioactivity showed two components: a rapid exponential phase with a half-time of 25 min and a slow component probably representing the clearance of a degradation product. The bioassay method confirmed that the rapid exponential phase represented the clearance of active compound (FIELD et al., 1971).

Clinical trials of ICRF 159 have shown that the drug has activity in acute lymphocytic leukemia and lymphoma. The major toxicity seen thus far with this drug is leukopenia and, to a lesser extent, thrombocytopenia. Other toxicity observed has been pharyngitis and stomatitis, mild nausea and vomiting, and alopecia (HELLMANN et al., 1969; HELLMANN, 1970). Further clinical trials are necessary before the value of ICRF 159 in clinical chemotherapy can be ascertained.

Isophosphamide

Isophosphamide, 3-(2-chloroethyl)2-(2-chloroethylamine)tetrahydro-2*H*-1,3,2-oxaphosphorine-2-oxide (ifosfamide), is structurally related to cyclophosphamide (Fig. 8). Although alkyl substitution on the ring nitrogen of cyclophosphamide (cytoxan) generally reduces or abolishes activity, isophosphamide was found to be as active as cytoxan in several animal systems and demonstrated greater activity than cytoxan with the Yoshida ascites sarcoma, the DS carcinosarcoma, and the TA nephroblastoma (Chem. Abstracts, 1969; Asta-Werke Information, 1969). Isophosphamide was also active against leukemia L1210 and Lewis lung carcinoma, and was active when administered by either oral or parenteral administration.

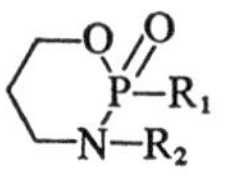

$R_1 = N(CH_2CH_2Cl)_2$, $R_2 = H$ } Cyclophosphamide

$R_1 = HNCH_2CH_2Cl$, $R_2 = CH_2CH_2Cl$ } Isophosphamide

Fig. 8

Isophosphamide, like cyclophosphamide, was inactive *in vitro* and for activity requires metabolism by hepatic microsomal enzymes. However, isophosphamide was metabolized (activated) less rapidly by liver microsomes than cyclophosphamide. The active metabolites seemed to be excreted in the urine with peak urinary activity occurring in 8 to 16 h, but continuing for 72 to 96 h.

Clinical trials in Germany and South Africa have demonstrated that isophosphamide is active in a variety of tumors including bronchogenic carcinoma (especially small cell carcinoma), ovarian carcinoma, Hodgkin's disease, and breast cancer (Astra-Werke Information, 1969; G. FALKSON, personal communication). Further trials of isophosphamide are underway in Europe, South Africa, and the United States.

Cyclocytidine

The cyclonucleosides were initially synthesized in 1956 (BROWN et al., 1956), but until 1971 2,2′-*O*-cyclocytidine (Fig. 9) remained untested for potential antitumor activity. HOSHI et al. (1971) evaluated 2,2′-*O*-cyclocytidine in an attempt to find analogs of 1-β-D-arabinofuranosylcytosine (ara-C) which were resistant to deamination by nucleoside deaminase. Cyclocytidine was found to be active against several experimental tumors including leukemia L1210, leukemia C-1498, adenocarcinoma 755, Sarcoma 180, and the Ehrlich ascites carcinoma. In a number of these experimental tumors cyclocytidine had a better therapeutic index than ara-C (HOSHI et al., 1972a; NAKAHARA and TOKUZEN, 1972).

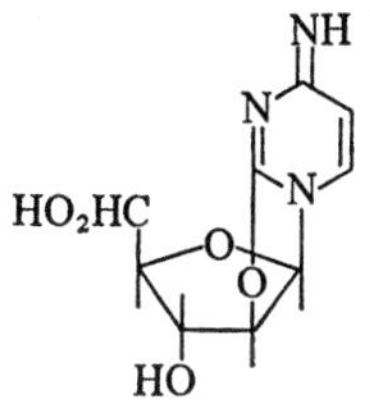

Cyclocytidine

Fig. 9

Studies on the mechanism of action of cyclocytidine have shown that it is active *in vitro* as well as *in vivo*, and *in vitro* depresses DNA synthesis in a manner similar to that for ara-C. Further experiments demonstrated that this depression was due to formation of ara-C, as ascertained by thin layer chromatography, and therefore cyclocytidine can be considered to be a transport form of ara-C with low toxicity (HOSHI et al., 1972b). Other studies have shown that cyclocytidine has no antitumor activity and no effect on DNA synthesis in mice bearing a variant of leukemia L1210 resistant to ara-C.

In preliminary clinical studies in thirteen patients, partial remissions were seen in three patients with acute myelogenous leukemia, in the only patient treated with acute lymphocytic leukemia, in two patients with lymphosarcoma, and in one patient with parotid carcinoma (SAKAI et al., 1972; Kohjin Co. data on cyclocytidine KJ-101). Further studies on this agent are in progress in Japan and the United States.

References

ADAMSON, R. H.: Antileukaemic activity of hycanthone. Lancet II, 1206 (1971a).

ADAMSON, R. H.: Evaluation of the antitumor activity of rifamycin SV. Arch. Int. Pharmacodyn. **192**, 61—65 (1971b).

ADAMSON, R. H.: Antitumor activity of tilorone hydrochloride against some rodent tumors: preliminary report. J. nat. Cancer Inst. **46**, 431—434 (1971c).

ADAMSON, R. H., HAHN, M. A.: The disposition of the antitumor agent 3,5-diamino-1,2,4-triazole (Guanazole) in mice, rats, and dogs. Xenobiotica **3**, 247—255 (1973).

ADAMSON, R. H., LEVY, H. B., BARON, S.: The interferon system. In: RUBIN, A. A. (Ed.): Search for new drugs, pp. 292—316. New York: Marcel Dekker 1972.

ADAMSON, R. H., TING, R. C.: The antitumor activity of the interferon inducer tilorone hydrochloride. Bact. Proc. 71st. Mtg., 196 (1971).

ARIOLI, V., PALLANZA, R., FURESZ, S., CARNITI, G.: Rifampicin: a new rifamycin. I. Bacteriological studies. Arzneim. Forsch. **17**, 523—529 (1967).

ARSENEAU, J., ADAMSON, R. H., HART, M. M., LARSON, S., AAMODT, R., JOHNSON, G., CANELLOS, G. P.: Experimental and clinical studies of gallium. Proc. Amer. Ass. Cancer Res. **13**, 40 (1972).

Asta-Werke, A. G., Chem. Fabrik: Summary of information for clinical investigators. Brackwede, Germany (1969).

BARKER, A. D., RHEINS, M. S., WILSON, H. E.: Tilorone hydrochloride: its effects on Friend virus leukemia in mice. Bact. Proc. 188 (1971).

BERBERIAN, D. A., FREELE, H., ROSI, D., DENNIS, E. W., ARCHER, S.: Schistosomicidal activity of lucanthone hydrochloride, hycanthone and their metabolites in mice and hamsters. J. Parasitol. **53**, 306—311 (1967).

BERGAMINI, N., FOWST, G.: Rifamycin SV — a review. Arzneim. Forsch. **15**, 951—1002 (1965).
BHUYAN, B. K., FRASER, T. J., LI, L. H.: Cytotoxic effects of ellipticine (NSC-71795) on DON (Chinese hamster) and L1210 cells in culture. Proc. Amer. Ass. Cancer Res. **13**, 60 (1972).
BLANZ, E. J., JR., FRENCH, F. A.: A systematic investigation of thiaxanthen-9-ones and analogs as potential antitumor agents. J. med. Chem. **6**, 185—191 (1963).
BROCKMAN, R. W., SHADDIX, S., LASTER, W. R., JR., SCHABEL, F. M., JR.: Inhibition of ribonucleotide reductase, DNA synthesis and L1210 leukemia by guanazole. Cancer Res. **30**, 2358—2368 (1970).
BROWN, D. M., TODD, A. R., VARADARAJAN, S.: Nucleotides. Part XXXVII. The structure of uridylic acids a and b, and a synthesis of spongouridine (3-β-D-arabofuranosyluracil). J. chem. Soc. Part **2**, 2388—2393 (1956).
CHADWICK, M., PLATZ, B. B., LISS, R. H.: Physiological disposition of ellipticine in dogs and rats. Proc. Amer. Ass. Cancer Res. **12**, 34 (1971).
Chemical Abstracts: Cyclic derivatives of phosphorodiamidic and phosphorodiamidothionic acids. Fr. Pat. 1530962. June 28, 1968; Chem. Abstr. **71**, 49998 M (1969).
CLARKE, V. D., BLAIR, D. M., WEBER, M. C.: Field trial of hycanthone (Etrenol Winthrop) in the treatment of urinary and intestinal bilharziasis. Cont. Afr. J. Med. **15**, 1—6 (1969).
CREIGHTON, A. M., BIRNIE, G. D.: Biochemical studies on growth-inhibitory *bis* dioxopiperazines. I. Effect on DNA, RNA and protein synthesis in mouse-embryo fibroblasts. Int. J. Cancer **5**, 47—54 (1970).
CREIGHTON, A. M., HELLMANN, K., WHITECROSS, S.: Antitumor activity in a series of *bis*-diketopiperazines. Nature (Lond.) **222**, 384—385 (1969).
CULVENOR, C. C. J., LODER, J. W.: Ellipticine alkaloids from Ochrosia and Excavatia species. Isolation and synthesis. Abstr. 152nd Meeting of the American Chemical. Society, New York, N. Y. (1966).
DALTON, L. K., DEMERAC, S., ELMES, B. C., LODER, J. W., SWAN, J. M., TEITEI, T.: Synthesis of the tumor inhibitory alkaloids, ellipticine, 9-methoxyellipticine, and related pyrido [4,3-*b*] carbazoles. Austr. J. Chem. **20**, 2715—2727 (1967).
DUDLEY, H. C.: Determination of gallium in biological materials. J. Pharmacol. exp. Therap. **95**, 482—486 (1949).
EDWARDS, C. L., HAYES, R. L.: Tumor scanning with ^{67}Ga citrate. J. nucl. Med. **10**, 103—105 (1969).
EDWARDS, C. L., HAYES, R. L.: Scanning malignant neoplasms with gallium^{67}. J. Amer. med. Ass. **212**, 1182—1190 (1970).
FIELD, E. O., MAURO, F., HELLMANN, K.: Blood clearance of ICRF 159 (NSC-129943). Cancer Chemother. Rep. **55**, 527—530 (1971).
FUJIWARA, A. N., ACTON, E. M., GOODMAN, L.: Ellipticine analogs: oxygen and sulfur isosteres. J. Heterocyclic Chem. **6**, 379—387 (1969).
GALE, G. R., OSTRANDER, W. E., ATKINS, L. M.: Effects of alanosine on purine and pyrimidine synthesis. Biochem. Pharmacol. **17**, 1823—1832 (1968).
GALE, G. R., SMITH, A. B.: Alanosine and hadacidin — comparison of effects on adenylosuccinate synthetase. Biochem. Pharmacol. **17**, 2495—2498 (1968).
GARCIA-GIRALT, E., MACIEIRA-COELHO, A.: Methoxy-9-ellipticine. II. Analysis *in vitro* of the mechanism of action. Europ. J. clin. Biol. Res. **15**, 539—541 (1970).
HAHN, M. A., ADAMSON, R. H.: Certain aspects of the pharmacology of guanazole — a new antitumor agent. Pharmacologist **12**, 282 (1970).
HAHN, M. A., ADAMSON, R. H.: Pharmacology of 3,5-diamino-1,2,4-triazole (guanazole). I. Antitumor activity of guanazole. J. nat. Cancer Inst. **48**, 783—790 (1972).
HARDESTY, C. T., CHANEY, N. A., MEAD, J. A. R.: The effect of route of administration on the distribution of ellipticine in mice. Cancer Res. **32**, 1884—1889 (1972).
HART, M. M., ADAMSON, R. H.: Antitumor activity and toxicity of salts of inorganic group IIIa metals: aluminum, gallium, indium, and thallium. Proc. nat. Acad. Sci. (Wash.) **68**, 1623—1626 (1971).
HART, M. M., SMITH, C. F., YANCEY, S. T., ADAMSON, R. H.: Toxicity and antitumor activity of gallium nitrate and periodically related metal salts. J. nat. Cancer Inst. **47**, 1121—1127 (1971).
HARTWELL, J. L., ABBOTT, B. J.: Antineoplastic principles in plants: recent developments in the field. In: GARATTINI, S., GOLDIN, A., HAWKING, F., KOPIN, I. J. (Eds.): Advances in Pharmacology and Chemotherapy, Vol. 7, pp. 117—209. New York-London: Academic Press 1969.
HAYES, R. L., CARLTON, J. E., BYRD, B. L.: Bone scanning with gallium-68: a carrier effect. J. nucl. Med. **6**, 605—610 (1965).
HAYES, R. L., NELSON, B., SWARTZENDRUBER, D. C., CARLTON, J. E., BYRD, B. L.: Gallium-67 localization in rat and mouse tumors. Science **167**, 289—290 (1970).

HELLMANN, K.: Further clinical experiences with ICRF 159. In: MATHÉ, G. (Ed.): Advances in the treatment of acute (blastic) leukemias, pp. 52—53. New York: Springer 1970.
HELLMANN, K., BURRAGE, K.: Control of malignant metastases by ICRF 159. Nature (Lond.) **224**, 273—275 (1969).
HELLMANN, K., NEWTON, K. A., WHITMORE, D. N., HANHAM, I. W. F., BOND, J. V.: Preliminary clinical assessment of ICRF 159 in acute leukemia and lymphosarcoma. Brit. med. J. **1**, 822—824 (1969).
HENDERSON, E. S.: Personal communication.
HERNANDEZ, P., DENNIS, E. W., FARAH, A.: Metabolism of the schistosomicidal agent hycanthone by rats and rhesus monkeys. Bull. World Health. Org. **45**, 27—34 (1971).
HEWLETT, J. S.: Intermittent guanazole (NSC-1895) in the treatment of adult acute leukemia. Proc. Amer. Ass. Cancer Res. **13**, 119 (1972).
HIRSCHBERG, E., BRINDLE, S. D., SEMENTE, G.: Development and properties of mouse leukemia L1210 resistant to miracil D. Cancer Res. **24**, 1733—1737 (1964).
HIRSCHBERG, E., GELLHORN, A., MURRAY, M. R., ELSLAGER, E. F.: Effects of miracil D, amodiaquin, and a series of other 10-thiaxanthenones and 4-aminoquinolines against a variety of experimental tumors *in vitro* and *in vivo*. J. nat. Cancer Inst. **20**, 567—579 (1959).
HIRSCHBERG, E., WEINSTEIN, I. B.: Comparative ability of hycanthone and miracil D to interact with DNA. Science **174**, 1147—1148 (1971).
HOFFMAN, P. F., RITTER, H. W., KRUEGER, R. F.: Tilorone hydrochloride stimulation of the primary immune response of mice. Presented at the VIIth International Congress of Chemotherapy, Prague, August 23—28, 1971.
HOSHI, A., KANZAWA, F., KURETANI, K.: Antitumor activity of cyclocytidine in a variety of tumors. Gann. **65**, 353—360 (1972a).
HOSHI, A., KANZAWA, F., KURETANI, K., SANEYOSHI, M., ARAI, Y.: 2,2'-*O*-Cyclocytidine, an antitumor cytidine analog resistant to cytidine deaminase. Gann. **62**, 145—146 (1971).
HOSHI, A., YOSHIDA, M., KANZAWA, F., KURETANI, K., KANAI, T., ICHINO, M.: Specific inhibition of DNA synthesis by cyclocytidine. Chem. pharm. Bull. **20**, 2286—2287 (1972b).
KATZ, N., PELLEGRINO, J., FERREIRA, M. T., OLIVEIRA, C. A., DIAS, C. B.: Preliminary clinical trials with hycanthone, a new antischistosomal agent. Amer. J. trop. Med. Hyg. **17**, 743—746 (1968).
KOHJIN CO., LTD.: Data on cyclocytidine KJ-101. Kohjin Co., Ltd. Tokyo, Japan.
LESTER, W.: Rifampin: a semisynthetic derivative of rifamycin — a prototype for the future. Ann. Rev. Microbiol. **26**, 85—102 (1972).
MARITZ, J. C.: Hycanthone therapy in bilharziasis. S. Afr. med. J. **44**, 126—128 (1970).
MATHÉ, G., HAYAT, M., DE VASSAL, F., SCHWARZENBERG, L., SCHNEIDER, M., SCHLUMBERGER, J. R., JASMIN, C., ROSENFELD, C.: Methoxy-9-ellipticine lactate. III. Clinical screening: its action in acute myeloblastic leukemia. Europ. J. clin. Biol. Res. **15**, 541—545 (1970).
MAYER, G. D., KRUEGER, R. F.: Tilorone hydrochloride: mode of action. Science **169**, 1213—1214 (1970).
MUNSON, A. E., MUNSON, J. A., REGELSON, W., WAMPLER, G. L.: Effect of tilorone hydrochloride and congeners on reticuloendothelial system, tumors, and the immune response. Cancer Res. **32**, 1397—1403 (1972).
MURTHY, Y. K. S., THIEMANN, J. E., CORONELLI, C., SENSI, P.: Alanosine, a new antiviral and antitumor agent isolated from a Streptomyces. Nature (Lond.) **211**, 1198—1199 (1966).
NAKAHARA, W., TOKUZEN, R.: Effect of 2,2'-*O*-cyclocytidine on transplanted lymphocytic sarcoma and reticulum cell sarcoma in mice. Gann **63**, 379—381 (1972).
PELLIZZARI, G.: Guanazole and its derivatives. L'Orosi **17**, 143—155, 185—192 (1894).
RIVA, S., SILVESTRI, L. G.: Rifamycins: a general view. Ann. Rev. Microbiol. **26**, 199—224 (1972).
ROSI, D., PERUZZOTTI, G., DENNIS, E. W., BERBERIAN, D. A., FREELE, H., ARCHER, S.: A new active metabolite of miracil D. Nature (Lond.) **208**, 1005—1006 (1965).
SAKAI, Y., KONDA, C., SHIMOYAMA, M., KITAHARA, T., SAKANO, T., KIMURA, K.: Cyclocytidine — A phase I study. Jap. J. clin. Oncol. **6**, 57—64 (1972).
SCHABEL, F. M., JR., LASTER, W. R., JR., TRADER, M. W.: Specific DNA inhibitors *vs* leukemia L1210. Development of resistance to ara-C and ribonucleotide reductase inhibitors. Proc. Amer. Ass. Cancer Res. **12**, 67 (1971).
SHARPE, H. B. A., FIELD, E. O., HELLMANN, K.: Mode of action of the cytostatic agent ICRF 159. Nature (Lond.) **226**, 524—526 (1970).
SIEBER, S. M., WHANG-PENG, J., JOHNS, D. G., ADAMSON, R. H.: Effects of hycanthone on rapidly proliferating cells. Biochem. Pharmacol. **22**, 1253—1262 (1973).
SMITH, R. G., WHANG-PENG, J., GALLO, R. C., LEVINE, P., TING, R. C.: Selective toxicity of rifamycin derivatives for leukaemic human leukocytes. Nature New Biol. **236**, 166—171 (1972).

SNYDER, A. L., KANN, H. E., JR., KOHN, K. W.: Inhibition of the processing of ribosomal precursor RNA by intercalating agents. J. molec. Biol. **58**, 555—565 (1971).

SVOBODA, G. H., POORE, G. A., MONTFORT, M. L.: Isolation of the alkaloids and study of the antitumor properties of 9-methoxyellipticine. J. pharm. Sci. **57**, 1720—1725 (1968).

TOBEY, R. A.: A simple rapid technique for determination of the effects of chemotherapeutic agents on mammalian cell-cycle traverse. Cancer Res. **32**, 309—316 (1972).

WAMPLER, G. L., KUPERMINC, M., REGELSON, W.: Phase I study of tilorone, a non-marrow depressing antitumor agent. Cancer Chemother. Rept. **57**, 209—217 (1973).

WARING, M. J.: Drugs and DNA: uncoiling of the DNA double helix as evidence of intercalation. Humangenetik **9**, 234—236 (1970).

WEHRLI, W., STAEHELIN, M.: Actions of the rifamycins. Bact. Rev. **35**, 290—309 (1971).

WEINSTEIN, I. B., HIRSCHBERG, E.: Mode of action of miracil D. In: HAHN, F. E. (Ed.): Progress in molecular and subcellular biology, Vol. 2, pp. 232—246. Berlin-Heidelberg-New York: Springer 1971.

WITTNER, M., TANOWITZ, H., ROSENBAUM, R. M.: Studies with the schistosomacide hycanthone: inhibition of macromolecular synthesis and its reversal. Exp. Molec. Pathol. **14**, 124—133 (1971).

YANG, S. S., HERRERA, F. M., SMITH, R. G., REITZ, M. S., LANCINI, G., TING, R. C., GALLO, R. C.: Rifamycin antibiotics: inhibitors of Rauscher murine leukemia virus reverse transcriptase and of purified DNA polymerases from human normal and leukemic lymphoblasts. J. nat. Cancer Inst. **49**, 7—25 (1972).

Addendum to

Cytotoxic Analogs of Pyridine Nucleotide Coenzymes

L. S. DIETRICH

(see pages 539—543)

New findings on the mechanism of the cytotoxic effects of 6-AN have been reported recently. Intracellularly synthesized 6-ANADP is an extremely effective inhibitor of the 6-phosphogluconate dehydrogenase [K_i 6-ANADP $= 1.3 \times 10^{-7}$M (brain)] (HERKEN, 1971; HERKEN et al., 1974). In the concentration attained, 6-phosphogluconate inhibits the 6-phosphoglucose isomerase which occupies a key position in the Embden-Meyerhoff pathway (HERKEN et al., 1969). The highest concentrations of 6-phosphogluconate were found in those regions of the central nervous system that also showed the most severe cell lesions. In the spinal cord they amounted to almost 400 times the normal value (HERKEN et al., 1973). In the animals treated with 6-AN, characteristic deviations were observed in the carbohydrate metabolism of the central nervous system (LANGE et al., 1972; KELLER et al., 1972; HERKEN et al., 1974) and above all, a decrease in lactate concentration. The accumulation of 6-phosphogluconate in the brain of mice with blockade of the pentose phosphate pathway after administration of 6-AN was confirmed by KAUFFMAN (1970). KAUFFMAN (1970) and KAUFFMAN and JOHNSON (1974) found a decrease in ribulose-5-phosphate to 50% of the normal values.

Electronmicroscopic studies on the spinal cord revealed a primary lesion of the oligodendroglial and astroglial cells, disrupting the functional relations between glial and nerve cells in the spinal grisea (SCHNEIDER, 1971; HERKEN et al., 1973; SCHNEIDER and CERVOS-NAVARRO, 1974). Morphologically recognizable cytotoxic effects were above all found in those cells, which are largely dependent for their nutrition on the glucose supply (brain and embryonic tissue).

Recent studies on the carbohydrate metabolism of ascites tumour cells also revealed a blockade of the pentose phosphate pathway after application of 6-AN (OFORI-NKANSAH and v. BRUCHHAUSEN, 1972).

References

HERKEN, H.: Antimetabolic action of 6-aminonicotinamide on the pentose phosphate pathway in the brain. In: ALDRIDGE, W.N. (Ed.): Mechanisms of toxicity, pp. 189—203. London: MacMillan 1971.

HERKEN, H., KELLER, K., KOLBE, H., LANGE, K., SCHNEIDER, H.: Experimentelle Myelopathie — Biochemische Grundlagen ihrer cellulären Pathogenese. Klin. Wschr. **51**, 644—657 (1973).

HERKEN, H., LANGE, K., KOLBE, H.: Brain disorders induced by pharmacological blockade of the pentose phosphate pathway. Biochem. biophys. Res. Commun. **36**, 93—100 (1969).

HERKEN, H., LANGE, K., KOLBE, H., KELLER, K.: Antimetabolic action on the pentose phosphate pathway in the central nervous system induced by 6-aminonicotinamide. In: GENAZZANI, E., HERKEN, H. (Eds.): Central nervous system—studies on metabolic regulations and function, pp. 41—54. Berlin-Heidelberg-New York: Springer 1974.

KAUFFMAN, F. C.: Effects of 6-aminonicotinamide on NADP+-dependent enzymes and metabolism in mouse brain. Pharmacologist **12**, 222 (1970).

KAUFFMAN, F. C., JOHNSON, E. C.: Cerebral energy reserves and glycolysis in neural tissue of 6-aminonicotinamide-treated mice. J. Neurobiol. **5**, 379—392 (1974).

KELLER, K., KOLBE, H., LANGE, K., HERKEN, H.: Behaviour of the glycolytic system of rat brain and kidney *in vivo* after inhibition of the glucose phosphate isomerase. II. Substrate concentration under the influence of ischemia, 6-aminonicotinamide, and 2-deoxyglucose. Hoppe-Seyler's Z. physiol. Chem. **353**, 1389—1400 (1972).

LANGE, K., KOLBE, H., KELLER, K., HERKEN, H.: Behaviour of the glycolytic system of rat brain and kidney *in vivo* after inhibition of the glucose phosphate isomerase. I. Kinetic studies on rat brain glucose phosphate isomerase. Hoppe-Seyler's Z. physiol. Chem. **353**, 1385—1388 (1972).

OFORI-NKANSAH, N., BRUCHHAUSEN, F. v.: Metabolic alterations in Yoshida ascites tumour cells caused by 6-aminonicotinamide and prevented by nicotinamide. Naunyn-Schmiedebergs Arch. Pharmacol. **272**, 156—168 (1972).

SCHNEIDER, H.: Elektronenmikroskopische Befunde bei selektiven Läsionen der spinalen grauen Substanz. Untersuchungen am Modell der 6-Aminonikotinamid-Intoxikation und der temporären Ischämie. Habilitationsschr. Fachber. Klin.-Theor. Med., Freie Univ. Berlin (1971).

SCHNEIDER, H., CERVOS-NAVARRO, J.: Acute gliopathy in spinal cord and brainstem induced by 6-aminonicotinamide. Acta neuropath. (Berl.) **27**, 11—23 (1974).

Author Index

Page numbers in *italics* refer to the bibliography

Aakvaag, A., see Tveter, K.J. 149, *157*
Aakvaag, A., see Unhjem, O. 150, *157*
Aamodt, L., Goz, B. 305, *327*
Aamodt, R., see Arseneau, J. 879, *887*
Aaron, H. 19, *30*
Aaronson, S. 495, *503*
Aaronson, S.A., Todaro, G. T., Scolnick, E.M. 308, *327*
Abadi, A., see Krant, M.J. 523, *533*
Abartiene, D. 517, *529*
Abbondanza, A., see Bonetti, E. 697, *714*
Abbott, B.J., see Hartwell, J.L. 654, *655*, 881, *888*
Abbott, B.J., see Jondorf, W.R. 558, *569*
Abbott, B.J., see Venditti, J.M. 597, *613*, 650, *656*
Abbott, J., Holtzer, H. 311, *327*
Abbott, J., see Anderson, H. C. 311, *327*
Abdou, N.I., Richter, M. 707, *713*
Abd-Rabbo, H. 558, *567*
Abe, H., see Kato, S. 870, *873*
Abe, M., Chibata, I., Hirokawa, H., Kameda, Y., Mizuno, D. 522, *529*
Abe, M., Tomizawa, J.I. 300, *327*
Abe, O., see Rooks, W.H. 145, *156*
Abe, O., see Sakauchi, N. 814, *818*
Abelson, D., Bulaschenko, H., Trommer, P.R., Valdes-Dapena, A. 814, *817*
Abelson, H.T., Karlan, D., Penman, S. 573, 574, 575, *579*
Abelson, H.T., Penman, S. 573, 574, 575, 576, 577, 579, *579*, 651, 653, *655*, *668*
Abelson, H.T., see Perlman, S. 575, 578, *580*
Ablondi, F.B., Hagen, J.J., Phillips, M., Derenzo, E. C. 527, *529*
Abraham, D., Carbone, P.P., Venditti, J.M., 747, *760*
Abraham, D.J., Rosenstein, R.D., McGandy, E.L. 556, *567*
Abraham, D.J., Rutherford, J.S., Rosenstein, R.D. 545, *550*
Abrams, R., Bentley, M. 489, 496, *503*
Abrams, R., see Adams, R. L.P. 857, *871*
Abshire, C.J. 523, *529*
Ackman, D., see Egger, G. 410, *420*
Acs, G., Reich, E., Mori, M. 436, 437, 438, 439, *452*
Acs, G., see Greengard, O. 120, 121, *129*
Acs, G., see Kapuler, A.M. 437, *454*
Acs, G., see Tavitian, A. 439, *456*, 574, *581*
Acs, G., see Uretsky, S.C. 437, 438, *456*
Acs, G., see Wiesner, R. 583, *592*
Acton, E.M., see Fujiwara, A.N. 881, *888*
Acton, E.M., see Iwamoto, R.H. 388, *400*
Acton, E.M., see Marsh, J. P., Jr. 593, *613*
Acton, E.M., see Ryan, K.J. 196, *230*
Adachi, M., see Hill, J.M. 702, *716*
Adachi, M., see Loeb, E. 726, 727, 728, 734, 735, *745*
Adair, F.E., Bagg, H.J. 18, *30*
Adams, H.H., see Burchenal, J.H. 198, *224*, 822, *826*
Adams, J.B., Wong, M.S.F. 178, 179, *188*
Adams, R.L.P., Abrams, R., Lieberman, I. 857, *871*
Adamson, D., see Brockman, R.W. 790, *791*
Adamson, D.J., see Wheeler, G.P. 76, 77, *84*
Adamson, R.H. 880, 883, 884, *887*
Adamson, R.H., Denham, C., Oliverio, V.T. 771, 772, *783*
Adamson, R.H., Dixon, R. L., Ben, M., Crews, L., Shohet, S.B., Rall, D.P. 682, 683, *687*
Adamson, R.H., Fabro, S. 695, 710, *713*
Adamson, R.H., Fabro, S., Hahn, M.A., Creech, C. E., Whang-Peng, J. 710, *713*
Adamson, R.H., Hahn, M. A. 878, *887*
Adamson, R.H., Hart, L.G., DeVita, V.T., Oliverio, V.T. 642, *647*
Adamson, R.H., Levy, H.B., Baron, S. 884, *887*
Adamson, R.H., Ting, R.C. 884, *887*
Adamson, R.H., see Arseneau, J. 879, *887*
Adamson, R.H., see Bray, D.A. 68, 77, *80*
Adamson, R.H., see Dixon, R.L. 235, 238, *251*, 261, *268*
Adamson, R.H., see Gallo, R.C. 650, 653, *655*, 711, *716*
Adamson, R.H., see Guarino, A.M. 709, *716*
Adamson, R.H., see Hahn, M.A. 877, 878, *888*
Adamson, R.H., see Hart, M.M. 811, *818*, 879, *888*
Adamson, R.H., see Henderson, E.S. 471, 472, 473, 474, *481*
Adamson, R.H., see O'Gara, R.W. 752, *764*

Adamson, R. H., see Oliverio, V. T. 69, 72, *82*, 770, *787*
Adamson, R. H., see Sieber, S. M. 880, *889*
Adamson, R. H., see Vogel, C. L. 478, *482*
Addison, I. E., Berenbaum, M. C. 38, *42*
Adelberg, E. A., see Driskell-Zamenhof, P. J. 58, *60*
Adelman, R. C., Ballard, F. J., Weinhouse, S. 659, *664*
Adelmann, M. R., Borisy, G. G., Shelanski, M. L., Weisenberg, R. C., Taylor, E. W. 676, *688*
Adesnik, M., Darnell, J. E. 575, *579*
Adesnik, M., see Darnell, J. E. 574, 575, *579*, 664, *665*
Adesnik, M., see Jelinek, W. *669*
Adye, J. C., Gots, J. S. 461, *464*
Aebi, H., Baggiolini, M., Bickel, M. H., Messiha, F. S. 754, *760*
Aebi, H., Dewald, B., Suter, H. 751, *760*
Aebi, H., Suter, H. 754, *760*
Aebi, H., see Baggiolini, M. 751, 755, *761*
Aebi, H., see Dewald, B. 754, *762*
Afkham, J., see Druckrey, H. 78, *80*
Afzelius, B. 676, *688*
Agarwal, K. C., Parks, R. E., Jr. 461, *464*
Agarwal, R. P., Scholar, E. M., Agarwal, K. C., Parks, R. E., Jr. *464*
Agarwal, K. C., see Agarwal, R. P. *464*
Agarwal, D. P., Eickhoff, K., Goedde, H. W. 283, *327*
Agrawal, K. C., Booth, B. A., Michaud, R. L., Sartorelli, A. C., Moore, E. C. 795, 798, *804*
Agrawal, K. C., Booth, B. A., Moore, E. C., Sartorelli, A. C. 795, 798, *804*
Agrawal, K. C., Booth, B. A., Moore, E. C., Sartorelli, A. C. 797, *804*
Agrawal, K. C., Booth, B. A., Sartorelli, A. C., 795, 797, *804*
Agrawal, K. C., Booth, B. A., Wheaton, J. R., Moore, E. C., Sartorelli, A. C. 798, *804*
Agrawal, K. C., Cushley, R. J., Lipsky, S. R., Wheaton, J. R., Sartorelli, A. C. 797, *804*
Agrawal, K. C., Cushley, R. J., McMurray, W. J., Sartorelli, A. C. 797, *804*
Agrawal, K. C., Sartorelli, A. C. 794, 798, 799, 801, *804*, *805*
Agrawal, K. C., see Creasey, W. A. 795, 799, 800, 801, 802, *805*
Agrawal, K. C., see DeConti, R. C. 793, 799, 800, 802, 804, *805*
Agrawal, K. C., see Hochman, H. I. 803, *806*
Agrawal, K. C., see Lin, A. J. 798, *806*
Agrawal, K. C., see Mooney, P. D. 798, *806*
Agrawal, K. C., see Moore, E. C. 798, 803, 804, *806*
Agrawal, K. C., see Sartorelli, A. C. 793, 797, 802, 803, *807*
Agrawal, K. C., see Wolpert, M. K. 393, *403*
Agrifoglio, M. F., see Cardinali, G. 673, *688*
Agustin, B. M., Creasey, W. A. 681, *688*
Ahearn, M. J., Lewis, C. W., Campbell, L. A., Luce, J. K. 236, *249*
Ahnström, G., Ehrenberg, L., Hussain, S., Natarajan, A. T. 314, *327*
Ahren, D., Hamberger, L. 176, *188*
Ahrens, H., see Mihich, E. 780, *786*
Ahstrom, L., see Dahlwitz, A. 735, *743*
Ainis, H., see Jameson, E. 695, *717*
Aisen, see Piesach *849*
Aisenberg, A. C. 676, *688*
Aizawa, S., Haidaka, T., Otake, N., Yonehara, H., Isono, K., Igarashi, N., Suzuki, S. 441, 444, *452*
Aizawa, S., see Otake, N. 441, *455*
Aizawa, Y., Mueller, G. C. 118, *125*
Aizawa, Y., see Mueller, G. C. 119, *133*
Akashi, A., see Hano, K. 545, 547, *550*
Akazawa, S., see Kakimoto, Y. 518, *532*
Akhtar, M., see Munday, K. A. 121, *134*
Akutsu, E., see Suzuki, H. 862, 863, 869, 870, *874*
Albach, H. R., Shaffer, J. G. 53, 54, *60*
Albala, M. M., see Leone, L. A. 477, *481*
Albayrak, A., see Khan, A. 837, *839*
Alberga, A., see Baulieu, E. E. 114, 115, *126*
Alberici, M., see DeRobertis, E. 499, *504*
Alberstadt, N., see Burchenal, J. H. 389, *398*
Albert, A., see Blackburn, C. M. 144, *153*, 173, *188*
Aledort, L. M., see Puszkin, E. *692*
Alexander, M., see Hurwitz, J. 583, *591*
Alexander, P., Fairly, G. H., Hunter-Craig, I. D., Ilonopisov, R. L., Lewis, M. G. 728, *742*
Alexander, P., see Goldenberg, G. J. 40, *44*
Alexander, T. R., see Hill, J. M. 702, *716*
Alexander, T. R., see Loeb, E. 726, 727, 728, 734, 735, *745*
Alexandre, G. P. J., Morelle, J., Haxhe, J. J., Michelsen, P., Ypersele, C. v., Michaux, M., Kestens, P. 502, *503*
Alexandre, G. P. J., Murray, J. E., Dammin, G. J., Nolan, B. 407, 409, *419*, 502, *503*
Alexandre, G. P. J., see Calne, R. Y. 409, *420*
Alexandre, G. P. J., see Haxhe, J. J. 410, *421*, 502, *505*
Alexanian, R., see Samuels, M. L. 759, *764*
Alford, C. A., see Ch'ien, L. T. 428, *432*
Allan, J. D., Ireland, J. T., Milner, J., Moss, A. D. 529, *529*
Allan, P., see Pittillo, A. F. 820, *827*

Allan, P. W., Bennett, L. L., Jr. 388, 395, *397*
Allan, P. W., Schnebli, H. P., Bennett, L. L., Jr. 386, *397*
Allan, P. W., see Bennett, L. L., Jr. 386, 391, *398*, 436, *452*
Allen, E. 108, *125*
Allen, E., Doisy, E. A. 104, 108, *125*
Allen, E., Francis, B. F., Robertson, L. L., Colgate, C. E., Johnston, C. G., Doisy, E. A., Kountz, W. B., Gibson, H. V. 108, *125*
Allen, J., see Van Lancker, J. L. 680, *694*
Allen, R. E., see Shelton, R. S. 105, *136*
Allen, W. M., see Noall, M. W. 113, *134*
Allfrey, V. G., Faulkner, R., Mirsky, A. E. 824, *826*
Allfrey, V. G., Pogo, B. G. T., Pogo, A. O., Kleinsmith, L. J., Mirsky, A. E. 89, *100*
Allinson, P. S., see Kimball, A. P. 429, 430, *432*
Allison, A. J., see Schroeder, D. D. 496, 498, *509*
Allison, J. P., Mandy, W. J., Kitto, G. B. 697, 702, *713*
Alpen, E. L., see Mandel, H. G. 459, 460, *466*
Altanerová, V. 363, *364*
Altanerová, V., see Rada, B. 355, *369*
Altenbern, R. A., Housewright, R. D. 697, *713*
Altman, R. L., see Mandel, H. G. 463, *466*
Altmann, F. P., Hampson, S. E., Chayen, R. 824, *826*
Altshtein, A. D., see Omelchenkov, T. N. 302, 304, 307, *341*
Altwerger, L., see Uretsky, S. C. 437, 438, *456*
Alvarez, B., see Perper, R. J. 408, *423*
Alvarez-O'Bourke, F., see Redetzki, H. M. 541, *543*
Amaleo, K., see Kimura, G. *337*
Ambellan, E., Hollander, V. P. 94, *100*
Amboye, R. Y. see Schwartz, H. S. 584, *592*
Ambrose, C. T. 89, *100*
Ames, B. N., see Shifrin, S. 517, 529, *536*
Amick, R. M., see Mizgerd, J. B. 546, *551*
Amiel, J.-L., Brezin, C., Sekiguchi, M., Mery, A.-M., Hoerni, B., Garattini, S., Daguet, G., Mathé, G. 752, *760*
Amiel, J.-L., see Mathé, G. 685, *692*, 726, 727, 728, 732, 734, 735, *745*, 759, *763*, 772, *786*
Amiel, J.-L., see Schwarzenberg, L. 474, *482*
Amirkhanian, J. D., see Jost, E. 37, *44*
Ammann, C. A., Safferman, R. S. 658, 662, *664*
Ammeraal, R. N., see Dolowy, W. C. 707, *715*
Ammeraal, R. N., see Schrek, R. 706, *720*
Amsterdam, E., see Gitlin, D. 314, 318, *334*
Anderson, B., see Kundig, W. 93, *101*
Anderson, B., see Simoni, R. D. 93, *103*
Anderson, C. D., see Lee, W. W. 658, *666*
Anderson, E. P., Brockman, R. W. 487, 488, 489, 490, 496, *503*
Anderson, E. P., Jacquez, J. A. 495, *503*
Anderson, E. P., Law, L. W. 458, *464*
Anderson, E. P., see Brockman, R. W. 292, 384, 387, 392, *398*, 458, *465*, 485, 495, *503*
Anderson, H. C., Chacko, S., Abbott, J., Holtzer, H. 311, *327*
Anderson, J. H., Jr., see Miech, R. P. 388, 394, 395, *401*
Anderson, K. M., Liao, S. 149, *153*, 177, *188*
Anderson, K. M., see Fang, S. 149, 150, *153*, 164, *167*
Anderson, L. L., Collins, G. J., Ojima, Y., Sullivan, R. D. 472, *479*
Anderson, M. M., see Diamond, I. 38, *43*
Anderson, P. J., Song, S. K., Slotwiner, P. 675, *688*
Anderson, S. W., see Heidelberger, C. 198, 219, *226*
Anderson, S. W., see Nizhizawa, Y. 197, *229*
Andervont, H. B., see Nathanson, J. T. 173, *191*
Andoh, T., Chargaff, E. 206, 210, *223*
André, J., see Schwartz, R. S. 384, *402*, 407, 410, *423*
Andrews, A. T., see Handschumacher, R. E. 515, *532*
Andrews, E. R., see Shelton, R. S. 105, *136*
Andrews, F. N., Beeson, W. M., Harper, C. 113, *125*
Andrews, F. N., see Dinusson, W. E. 113, *128*
Andrews, G. A., see Nelson, B. M. 39, *45*
Andrews, J. R., see Berry, R. J. 301, 307, 319, *328*
Andrews, R. E., see Clegg, R. E. 120, *127*
Angelino, N., see Korytnyk, W. 778, *785*
Angermann, J., see Munyon, W. 302, 304, 306, 307, *341*
Angevine, J. B., Jr. 675, 682, *688*
Anken, M., see Dubbs, D. R. 298, *331*
Anker, H. S., see Rennert, O. M. 524, *535*
Anonymous 387, *397*
Ansari, A. Q., see Munday, K. A. 121, *134*
Ansfield, F. J. 500, *503*, 561, *621*
Ansfield, F. J., Ramirez, G. 219, *223*
Ansfield, F. J., Ramirez, G., Davis, H. L., Jr., Korbitz, B. C., Vermund, H., Gollin, F. F. 221, *223*
Ansfield, F. J., Ramirez, G., Korbitz, B. C., Davis, H. L., Jr. 221, *223*
Ansfield, F. J., Ramirez, G., Mackman, S., Bryan, G. T., Curreri, A. R. 220, *223*
Ansfield, F. J., Ramirez, G., Skibba, J. L., Bryan, G. T., Davis, H. L., Wirtanen, G. W. 221, *223*
Ansfield, F. J., see Bisel, H. F. 440, *453*
Ansfield, F. J., see Clifton, K. H. 289, 291, *330*
Ansfield, F. J., see Curreri, A. R. 220, *224*
Ansfield, F. J., see Dexter, D. L. 222, 223, *224*
Ansfield, F. J., see Heidelberger, C. 193, 219, *226*

Ansfield, F. J., see Mukherjee, K. L. 221, *228*
Ansfield, F. J., see Olson, K. B. 183, *191*
Ansfield, F. J., see Schroeder, J. M. 394, 397, *402*, 500, *510*
Ansfield, F. J., see Wolberg, W. H. 217, *231*
Anton, A. H., see Greer, M. 520, *532*
Antonelli, A., see DiMarco, A. 607, *612*
Antoni, F., see Hidvegi, E. J. 518, *532*
Antonoglou, O., see Georgatos, J. G. 280, *333*
Aoki, K., see MacMahon, B. 178, *190*
Aoki, Y., Moore, G. E. 389, *397*
Aoyagi, T., see Takeuchi, T. 444, 445, *456*
Apgar, J., see McQuitty, J. T. 844, *848*
Aposhian, H. V., Blair, R. M., Morris, M., Smithson, C. H. 523, *529*
Apostoloff, E., see Heine, K. M. 416, *421*
Appelt, G. D., Heim, H. C. 560, *567*
Appleyard, G., Westwood, J. C. N. 303, *327*
Arai, Suzuki 845
Arai, K., see Honda, Y. 870, *872*
Arai, Y., see Hoshi, A. 234, *252*, 266, 267, *269*, 886, *889*
Arakawa, T., see Takeda, K. 870, *875*
Arcamone, F., Cassinelli, G., Fantini, G., Grein, A., Orezzi, P., Pol, C., Spalla, C. 593, *611*
Arcamone, F., Cassinelli, G., Franceschi, F., Orezzi, P., Mondelli, R. 593, *611*
Arcamone, F., Cassinelli, G., Orezzi, P., Franceschi, F., Mondelli, R. 593, *611*
Arcamone, F., Franceschi, G., Orezzi, P., Cassinelli, G., Barbieri, W., Mondelli, R. 593, *611*
Arcamone, F., Franceschi, G., Orezzi, P., Penco, S., Mondelli, R. 593, *611*
Arcamone, F., Franceschi, G., Penco, S. 593, *611*
Arcangeli, G., see Nervi, C. 478, *482*
Archer, S., see Berberian, D. A. 879, *887*
Archer, S., see Rosi, D. 879, *889*
Arden, G. M., Grant, D. J. W., Partridge, M. W. 517, *529*
Arendell, J. P., see Desjardins, R. 680, *689*
Arens, A., Rauenbusch, E., Irion, E., Wagner, O., Bauer, K., Kaufmann, W. 698, 699, 702, 703, *713*
Arens, A., see Irion, E. 702, *717*, 723, *744*
Arens, A., see Rauenbusch, E. 699, 700, *720*
Arens, A., see Wagner, O. 698, *721*
Arfin, S. M. 711, *713*
Argoudelis, A. D., see Herr, R. R. 65, *81*
Argoudelis, A. D., see Wiley, P. F. 557, *570*
Ariëns, E. J., Van Rossum, J. M., Simonis, A. M. 462, *464*
Arinoviche, R., Loewi, G. 408, *419*
Arioli, V., Pallanza, R., Furesz, S., Carniti, G. 883, *887*
Arison, B., see Kaczka, E. A. 658, *666*
Arky, J., see Hidvegi, E. J. 518, *532*
Armstrong, J. A., see Kjellen, L. 302, 307, *338*
Armstrong, J. A., see Plowright, W. 302, *342*
Armstrong, J. G., Dyke, R. W., Fouts, P. J., Hawthorne, J. J., Jansen, C. J., Jr., Peabody, A. M. 685, *688*
Armstrong, J. G., see Gailani, S. D. 685, *690*
Armstrong, J. G., see Johnson, I. S. 671, 675, 679, 682, 685, 686, 687, *691*
Armstrong, J. G., see Neuss, N. 671, 687, *692*
Armstrong, S. J., see Mahy, B. W. J. *669*
Arneson, V. G., see Szybalski, W. 48, *63*
Arnett, G., see Brockman, R. W. 793, *805*
Arnett, G., see Sidwell, R. W. 302, *344*, 428, *433*, 800, *807*
Arnold, H., Bourseaux, F. 29, *30*
Arnold, H., Bourseaux, F., Brock, N. 29, *30*
Arnold, N. J., see Hallum, J. V. 607, *612*
Arnstein, H. R. V., see Hipkiss, A. R. 209, *226*
Aronow, A., see Dingman, C. W. 121, *128*
Aronow, A., see O'Malley, B. W. 121, *134*
Aronow, L., see Brewer, H. B. 27, *31*
Aronow, L., see Gabourel, J. D. 86, 87, *100*
Aronow, L., see Gray, J. G. 91, *100*
Aronow, L., see Hackney, J. F. 97, 99, *100*
Aronow, L., see Pratt, W. B. 87, 88, 90, *102*
Aronow, L., see Tomizawa, S. 396, *403*
Aronsen, K. F., Husberg, B., Pihl, B. 410, *419*
Aronson, A. I. 206, 211, *223*
Arora, O. P., Shah, V. C., Rao, S. R. V. 57, *60*
Arrighi, F. E. 628, *631*
Arseneau, J., Adamson, R. H., Hart, M. M., Larson, S., Aamodt, R., Johnson, G., Canellos, G. P. 879, *887*
Arseneau, J., see Canellos, G. P. 709, *714*, 735, *743*
Artis, E. W., see Kline, I. 767, *785*
Asadullaev, T. A., see Bukrinskaya, A. G. 354, *364*
Asajima, T., see Kunimoto, T. 444, *454*
Asbell, M. A., see Yesair, D. W. 608, 609, *614*
Ascoli, F., Kahan, F. M. 274, *327*
Ascoli, F., Savino, M. 585, *589*
Ascoli, F., Savino, M., Liquori, A. M. 585, *589*
Ashenbrucker, H., see Mauer, A. M. 23, *33*
Ashida, T., see Mizuno, H. 279, *341*
Ashkenazi, A. 302, 308, *327*
Ashton, D. M., see Caskey, C. T. 390, *398*
Ashton, D. M., see McCollister, R. J. 390, 395, *401*
Ashton, H., Beveridge, G. W., Stevenson, C. J. 384, *397*
Astaldi, A., Jr., see Astaldi, G. 706, *713*, 735, *742*

Astaldi, A., Jr., see Burgio, G.R. 706, 707, *714*, 735, *743*
Astaldi, A., Jr., see DeBarbieri, A. 706, *715*
Astaldi, A., Jr., see Lajolo, D. *718*
Astaldi, A., Jr., see Micu, D. 706, *718*
Astaldi, A.A., see Astaldi, C. 526, *529*
Astaldi, G., Burgio, G.R., Krč, J., Genova, R., Astaldi, A., Jr. 526, *529*
Astaldi, G., Burgio, G.R., Biscatti, G., Astaldi, A., Jr., Ferfoglia, L. 706, *713*, 735, *742*
Astaldi, G., Burgio, G.R., Krč, J., Genova, R., Astaldi, A., Jr. 706, *713*, 735, *742*
Astaldi, G., Micu, D., Astaldi, A., Jr., Burgio, G.R. 706, *713*
Astaldi, G., Micu, D., Astaldi, A., Jr., Burgio, G.R., Krč, J. 706, *713*
Astaldi, G., see Burgio, G.R. 706, 707, *714*, 735, *743*
Astaldi, G., see DeBarbieri, A. 706, *715*
Astaldi, G., see Lajolo, D. *718*
Astaldi, G., see Micu, D. 706, *718*
Astrakhan, V.I., Garin, A. M. 621, *621*
Astwood, E.B. 108, *125*
Atger, M., see Milgrom, E. 162, *168*
Athens, J.W., see Mauer, A. M. 23, *33*
Atkins, L.M., see Gale, G.R. 838, *839*, 882, *888*
Atkinson, C., Stacey, K.A. 235, 241, *249*
Atkinson, M.R., Deutscher, M.P., Kornberg, A., Russell, A.F., Moffatt, J. G. 660, *665*
Atkinson, M.R., Eckermann, G., Stephenson, J. 386, *397*
Atkinson, M.R., Morton, R. K., Murray, A.W. 392, 395, *397*
Atkinson, M.R., Murray, A. W. 389, *398*
Atkinson, M.R., see Chalmers, A.H. 411, 412, *420*
Atkinson, M.R., see Donaldson, G.R. 564, *568*
Atkinson, M.R., see Tay, B. S. 390, 391, *403*
Atkinson, M.R., see Waqar, M.A. 660, *668*
Attardi, G., see Gros, F. 210, *225*
Attramadal, A. 114, *125*
Attramadal, A., see Sander, S. 117, *135*
Atwell, G.J., Cain, B.F. 820, *826*
Atwell, G.J., see Cain, B.F. 783, *783*
Auerbach, C., Robson, J.M., Carr, J.G. 21, *30*
Auerbach, R., see VanScott, E.S. 479, *482*
August, J.T., see Watanabe, M. 855, 859, 860, *876*
Aur, R.J.A., Simone, J.V., Pratt, C.B. 726, 732, 734, 735, *742*
Aurelian, L., see Roizman, B. 302, 303, *343*
Ausman, J.I., see Shapiro, W.R. 69, *83*
Avakyan, A.A., see Omelchenkov, T.N. 302, 304, 307, *341*
Avnimelech, M., see Jondorf, W.R. 560, *569*
Awapara, J., see Tapia, R. 497, *511*
Awdry, P.N., see Wellings, P.C. 195, 200, 219, *231*
Axelrad, A.A., Leblond, C. P. 171, *188*
Axelrod, J., see Eisenfeld, A. J. 114, 116, 117, *128*
Axelrod, L.R., Goldzieher, J.W. 106, 107, *125*
Axman, M.C., see Gorski, J. 119, *129*
Ayengar, P., Roberts, E. 496, *503*
Ayuso, M., see Goldberg, I. H. 557, 558, 559, 566, *568*
Azadova, N.B., see Demidova, S.A. 354, *365*
Azarnoff, D.L., Grady, H. J., Svobda, D.J. 814, *817*
Azarnoff, D.L., see Grady, H.J. 810, *818*
Azcurra, J.M., see Sellinger, O.Z. 499, *510*

Baba, T., see Yamada, T. 28, *34*
Babington, R.G., Wedeking, P.W. 408, *419*
Baccino, F.M. 541, *542*
Bach, J.F. 406, *419*
Bach, J.F., Dardenne, M. 406, 410, 413, 414, *419*
Bach, J.F., Dardenne, M., Crosnier, J. 414, *419*
Bach, J.F., Dardenne, M., Davies, A.J.S. 406, *419*
Bach, J.F., Dardenne, M., Fournier, C. 406, 414, *419*
Bach, J.F., Dardenne, M., Goldstein, A.L., Guha, A., White, A. 410, 413, 414, *419*
Bach, J.F., see Bach, M.A. 406, *419*
Bach, J.F., see Fournier, C. 405, *420*
Bach, J.F., see Hamburger, J. 407, 410, *421*
Bach, M.A., Bach, J.F. 406, *419*
Bach, M.A., see Fournier, C. 405, *420*
Bach, M.K. 247, *249*, 265, *267*
Bachrach, V., see Herbst, E. J. 766, *785*
Bachur, N.R. 609, *611*
Bachur, N.R., Gee, M. 609, 610, *611*
Bachur, N.R., Moore, A.L., Bernstein, J.B., Liu, A. 608, *611*
Bachynsky, N., see Prager, M.D. 711, *720*
Bachynsky, N., see Roberts, J. 698, 705, *720*
Bacigalupo, G., see Heise, E. 145, *154*
Bacila, M., Barron, E.S.G. 91, *100*
Bacila, M., see Kit, S. 86, *101*
Back, A., Walaszek, E.J. 684, *688*
Backus, E.J., see DeVoe, S. E. 486, 496, *504*
Bacon, R.L., see Kirkman, H. 175, *190*
Bacon, R.L., see Matthews, V.S. 175, *191*
Bacq, Z.M., see Koch, G. 40, *44*
Bader, J.P. 237, *249*, 306, 307, *327*
Bähr, G. 841, *847*
Baer, H.H., Capek, K., Cook, M.C. 593, *611*
Bagg, H.J., see Adair, F.E. 18, *30*
Baggett, B., Engel, L.L., Bolderas, L., Lanonan, G. 106, *125*

Baggett, B., see Marsh, J. M. 106, 107, *132*
Baggett, B., see Martin, L. 113, *133*
Baggett, B., see Savard, K. 140, *156*
Baggett, B., see Stone, G. M. 113, 117, *136*
Baggiolini, M., Bickel, M. H. 754, 756, *760*
Baggiolini, M., Bickel, M. H., Messiha, F. S. 754, *761*
Baggiolini, M., Dewald, B. 751, 754, 755, *761*
Baggiolini, M., Dewald, B., Aebi, H. 751, 755, *761*
Baggiolini, M., see Aebi, H. 754, *760*
Baggiolini, M., see Dewald, B. 754, *762*
Baglioni, C., Jacobs-Lorena, M., Meade, H. 567, *567*
Baglioni, C., see Colombo, B. 557, 565, *568*
Baglioni, C., see Jacobs-Lorena, M. 567, *569*
Bagshaw, M. A., Doggett, R. L. S. 319, 324, *327*
Bagshaw, M. A., Doggett, R. L. S., Smith, K. C., Kaplan, H. S., Nelson, T. S. 291, 319, 324, *327*
Bagshaw, M. A., see Doggett, R. L. S. 324, *331*
Bagshawe, K. D., see Currie, G. A. 24, *31*
Bagshawe, K. D., see Shaw, M. T. 709, *721*
Baguley, B. C., Falkenhaug, E. M. 234, 238, *249*, 262, *267*
Bahn, R. C., see Molnar, G. D. 811, *818*
Baiocchi, F., Cheng, C. C., Haggerty, W. J., Jr., Lewis, L. R., Liao, T. K., Nyberg, W. H., O'Brien, D. E., Podrebarac, E. G. 768, *783*
Baiocchi, F., see Liao, T. K. 768, *786*
Baird, J. D., see Duncan, L. J. P. 766, *784*
Bajkovič, N., see Crkvenjakov, R. 363, *365*
Baker, B. R. 289, *327*, 469, *479*, 488, 489, *503*
Baker, B. R., Bzeszotarski, W. 289, *327*
Baker, B. R., Ho, B. T., 469, *479*
Baker, B. R., see Lee, W. W. 427, *433*, 658, *666*
Baker, B. R., see Reist, E. J. 426, 427, 429, *433*, 658, *667*
Baker, C., see Werthessen, N. T. 106, *138*
Baker, H. T., Bennett, L. L., Jr. 392, *398*
Baker, R. G., see Rotenberg, A. D. 289, 314, *343*
Baker, W. H., see Kelley, R. M. 186, *190*
Bakhle, Y. S., Prusoff, W. H. 281, 285, 287, 301, 315, *327*
Bakhle, Y. S., Prusoff, W. H., McCrea, J. F. 273, 314, *327*
Bakhle, Y. S., see Prusoff, W. H. 289, 292, 293, 302, 303, 304, 305, *342*
Balazs, C., see Nagy, G. 36
Baldini, L., Brambilla, G. 524, 527, *529*, *530*
Baldini, L., Brambilla, G., Cavanna, M., Parodi, S. 237, *249*
Baldini, L., see Brambilla, G. 527, *530*, 705, *714*
Baldridge, R. C., see Spolter, P. D. *536*
Baldwin, R. L., Milligan, L. P. 123, *125*
Baldwin, R. L., Shooter, E. M. 294, *327*
Baldwin, R. L., see Davis, D. R. 293, *330*
Baldwin, R. L., see Inman, R. B. 293, 294, *336*
Baldwin, R. W., Partridge, M. W., Stevens, M. F. G. 517, *530*
Baliga, B. S., Hender, S., Srinivasan, P. R. 209, *223*
Baliga, B. S., Pronczuk, A. W., Munro, H. N. 561, 564, *567*
Balin, H., Glasser, S. 104, *125*
Balis, M. E. 384, 392, *398*
Balis, M. E., see Miller, H. K. 493, *507*, 701, 703, 704, *718*, 725, *745*
Balis, M. E., see Salser, J. S. 392, *402*
Ball, C. R. 28, *30*
Ball, C. R., Connors, T. A., Cooper, E. H., Topping, N. E. 23, *30*
Ball, C. R., Roberts, J. J. 13, *15*
Ballard, F. J., see Adelman, R. C. 659, *664*
Ballweg, H., see Hidvegi, E. J. 518, *532*
Ballweg, H., see Krüger, F. W. 70, *81*
Balo, J., see Vargha, L. 36, *46*
Balsiger, R., see Burchenal, J. H. 822, *826*
Baltimore, D. 608, *611*
Baltimore, D., see Taber, R. 558, *570*
Baltimore, D., see Verma, I. M. 660, *668*
Band, P., see Mathé, G. 685, *692*
Banfield, R. E. W., see Inman, D. R. 114, *131*
Barasa, A., Maccotta, V., Filogamo, G., Canavese, B. 675, *688*
Barber, N. D., see La Via, M. F. 513, 526, *533*
Barbieri, W., see Arcamone, F. 593, *611*
Barbiroli, B., see Billing, R. J. 120, *126*
Barbiroli, B., see Caldarera, C. M. 148, *153*, 774, *783*
Barclay, R. K., Garfinkel, E., Phillipps, M. A. 487, 489, *503*
Barclay, R. K., Phillipps, M. A. 487, 489, 491, 496, *503*
Barclay, R. K., see Clarke, D. A. 544, *550*
Barclay, R. K., see Jacquez, J. A. 519, *532*
Barclay, R. K., see Krenitsky, T. A. 289, *338*
Bardin, C. W., see Falk, R. J. 160, 162, *167*
Bardin, C. W., see Lipsett, M. B. 814, *818*
Bardos, T. J., Chmielewicz, Z. F., Hebborn, P. 20, 29, *30*
Bardos, T. J., see Holland, J. F. 769, *785*
Barg, W., Boggiano, E., Sloan, N., De Renzo, E. C. 488, *503*
Barham, F. W., see Kono, T. 95, *101*
Bariety, M., Gadjos, A. 683, *688*
Barker, A. D., Rheins, M. S., Wilson, H. E. 884, *887*
Barker, K. L. 124, *125*
Barker, K. L., Warren, J. C. 119, 124, *126*
Barker, K. L., see O'Dorisio, M. S. 124, *134*

Barker, P., see Wissler, R. W. 525, 526, *538*
Barker, S. A., Bassham, J. A., Calvin, M., Quarck, U. C. 493, *503*
Barker, T. L., see Bennett, L. L., Jr. 391, *398*
Barner, H. D., see Cohen, S. S. 21, *31*, 199, 203, 204, 218, *224*, 289, *330*
Barnes, C. C., see Shaw, M. T. 709, *721*
Barnes, J. R., Fellig, J., Mitrovic, M. 643, *647*
Barnett, E. V., see Levy, J. 407, *422*
Barnum, C. P., see Yarbro, J. W. 616, *622*
Baron, S., Buchler, C. E. 608 *611*
Baron, S., Buchler, C. E., Levy, H. B., Friedman, R. M. 607, *611*
Baron, S., see Adamson, R. H. 884, *887*
Baronowsky, P. E., see Coffey, J. J. 523, *530*
Baronowsky, P. E., see Yesair, D. W. 682, *694*, 823, 824, 825, *828*
Barr, M., see Jackson, L. 735, 738, *744*
Barranco, S. C., Humphrey, R. M. 76, 77, *79*, 396, *398*
Barrett, H. W., Munavalli, S. N., Newmark, P. 283, *327*
Barrett, H. W., West, R. A. 282, 283, *327*
Barrett, H. W., see Newmark, P. 283, *341*
Barrett, P. A., Beveridge, E., Bradley, P. L., Brown, C. G. D., Bushby, S. R. M., Clarke, M. L., Neal, R. A., Smith, R., Wilde, J. K. H. 841, *847*
Barrist, E., see Wilson, W. L. 638, *641*
Barron, E. S. G., Huggins, C. 151, *153*
Barron, E. S. G., see Bacila, M. 91, *100*
Barron, E. S. G., see Kit, S. 86, *101*
Barry, A., see Delage, J. M. 735, 738, *744*
Barry, J., Gorski, J. 119, *126*
Barry, R. D., Ives, D. R., Gruickshank, J. G. *328*
Barry, R. D., see Mahy, B. W. J. *669*
Barry, V. C., Conalty, M. L., McCormick, J. E., McElhinney, R. S., O'Sullivan, J. F. 793, *805*
Barry, V. C., Conalty, M. L., McCormick, J. E., McElhinney, R. S., McInerney, M. R., O'Sullivan, J. F. 841, *848*
Barry, V. C., Conalty, M. L., O'Callaghan, C. N., Twomey, D. 793, *805*
Bartlett, D., Morita, Y., Munck, A. 91, *100*
Bartley, W., see Getz, G. S. 824, *827*
Barton, B. W., Tobin, J. O. H. 323, *328*
Barton, B. W., see Conchie, A. F. 323, *330*
Barton, R. W., see Liao, S. 148, *155*
Bartuska, V. J., see Lee, W. W. 429, 430, 431, *433*
Bartuska, V. J., see Reist, E. J. 430, *433*
Bartz, Q. R., Elder, C. C., Frohardt, R. P., Fusari, S. A., Haskell, T. H., Johannessen, D. W., Ryder, A. 485, *503*
Bartz, Q. R., see Dion, H. W. 485, *504*
Bartz, Q. R., see Fusari, S. A. 485, *505*
Barwolf, D., see Preussel, B. 289, *342*
Barwolff, D., see Langen, P. 289, *339*
Basch, R. S., see Karnofsky, D. A. 310, *337*
Baseman, J. B., Pappenheimer, A. M., Jr., Gill, D. M., Harper, A. A. 561, *567*
Baserga, R., see Becker, F. F. 710, *713*
Baserga, R., see Rovera, G. 583, *592*
Bases, R. E. 396, *398*, 585, *589*
Basilio, C., see Wahba, A. J. 214, *231*
Bass, R., see Neubert, D. 280, *341*
Bassham, J. A., see Barker, S. A. 493, *503*
Bassham, J. A., see Van der Meulen, P. Y. F. 493, *511*
Basten, A., see Miller, J. F. A. P. 405, *422*
Basu, S. K., Chakrabarty, A. M., Roy, S. C. 56, *60*
Batcho, A. D., see Leimgruber, W. 642, *648*
Bateman, C. J. T., see Crowther, D. 726, 732, *743*
Bateman, J. R., Pugh, R. P., Cassidy, F. R., Marshall, G. J., Irwin, L. E. 221, *223*
Bateman, J. R., see Jacobs, E. M. 220, *226*
Bates, C. J., see Handschumacher, R. E. 515, *532*
Bates, H. M., Kuenzig, W., Watson, W. B. 644, 645, 646, *647*
Batt, W. G., see Ely, J. O. 521, *531*
Battaglini, J. W., see Hilf, R. 124, *130*
Battaner, E., see Vazquez, D. 554, 565, *570*
Battema, W., see Wittliff, J. L. 117, *138*
Battista, S. P., see Kensler, C. J. 822, 824, *827*
Bauck, H., see Lynch, J. E. 564, *569*
Bauer, D. J., Sadler, P. W. 800, *805*
Bauer, K. 695, *713*, 723, *742*
Bauer, K., see Arens, A. 698, 699, 702, 703, *713*
Bauer, K., see Rauenbusch, E. 698, 702, *720*, 723, *746*
Bauer, K., see Wagner, O. 698, 703, *721*, *722*
Bauer, V., Čapek, R. 359, *364*
Bauerova, J., Sebesta, K., Šorm, F., Šormova, Z. *328*
Bauerova, J., Šormova, Z. 283
Bauerova, J., see Sebesta, K. 283, *344*
Baugnet-Mahieu, L., Goutier, R. 280, 315, *328*
Baulieu, E. E., Alberga, A., Jung, I. 114, *126*
Baulieu, E. E., Alberga, A., Jung, I., LeBeau, M. C., Mercier-Bodard, C., Milgrom, E., Raynaud, J. P., Raynaud-Jammet, C., Rochefort, H., Truong, H., Robel, P. 115, *126*
Baulieu, E. E., Jung, I. 150, *153*, 164, *167*
Baulieu, E. E., Lasnitzki, I., Robel, P. 161, *167*

Baulieu, E.E., Raynaud, J. P. 114, 115, *126*
Baulieu, E.E., see Milgrom, E. 162, *168*
Baulieu, E.-E., see Raynaud-Jammet, M. 119, *134*
Baulieu, E.E., see Robel, P. 160, *168*
Baulieu, E.E., see Rochefort, H. 114, *135*
Baumann, M., see Brossi, A. 563, *567*
Baumstein, V.E., Goldberg, L.E. 620, *621*
Bauters, F., see Goudemand, M. 726, 727, 728, 732, 734, 735, *744*
Bautz, E., Freeze, E. 11, *15*
Baxter, D., see Cohen, J.L. 221, *224*
Baxter, J.D., Harris, A.W., Tomkins, G.M., Cohn, M. 97, 99, *100*
Baxter, J.D., Tomkins, G. M. 164, *167*
Bayley, C.H., see Gingras, B.A. 841, *848*
Bayliss, N.L., see Smith, S.S. 524, *536*
Beacham, L.M.III., see DeMiranda, P. 412, *420*
Beal, D.D., see Skibba, J.L. 545, 546, 547, *552*
Beard, J.W., see Heine, U. 583, *591*
Beard, J.W., see Riman, J. 440, *455*
Beard, J.W., see Sverak, L. 574, *581*
Beard, M.E.J., Crowther, D., Galton, D.A.G., Guyers, R.G., Fairley, G.H., Kay, H.E.M., Knapton, P.J., Malpas, J.S., Scott, R.B. 726, 727, 728, 730, 734, 735, *743*
Beato, M., Biesewig, D., Brandle, W., Sekeris, C. E. 164, *167*
Beatson, G.T. 111, *126*
Beatty, B.R., see Miller, O. L., Jr. 573, *580*
Beatty, E.C., Jr., see Sullivan, M.P. 397, *403*
Beaudet, A.L., see Caskey, C.T. 561, *568*
Beck, C., see Kit, S. 301, 302, *337*
Beck, G., Hentzen, D., Ebel, J.-P. 121, *126*
Becker, A.J., see Bruchovsky, N. 59, *60*, 674, *688*
Becker, F.F., Baserga, R., Broome, J.D. 710, *713*
Becker, F.F., Broome, J.D. 710, 711, *713*
Becker, F.F., Margolis, A. A., Troll, W. 583, *589*
Becker, J.E., see Butcher, F.R. *669*
Becker, Y., see Dym, H. 519, *531*
Becker, Y., see Gilead, Z. 560, *568*
Becker, Y., see Weinberg, A. 529, *537*
Beckett, V.L., Brennan, M. J. 173, *188*
Beer, C.T. 670, 679, 683, *688*
Beer, C.T., Gallagher, T.F. 108, *126*
Beer, C.T., Wilson, M.L., Bell, J. 684, *688*
Beer, C.T., see Greenius, H. F. 684, *690*
Beer, C.T., see Hebden, H. F. 684, *690*
Beer, C.T., see Jones, R.G. W. 679, *691*
Beer, C.T., see Noble, R.L. 672, *692*
Beer, C.T., see Richards, J. F. 679, *693*
Beereboom, J.J., Butler, K., Pennington, F.C., Solomons, I.A. 565, *567*
Beeson, W.M., see Andrews, F.N. 113, *125*
Beeson, W.M., see Dinusson, W.E. 113, *128*
Beetschen, J.C., see Duprat, A.M. 628, *631*
Begemann, H., Kaboth, W., Fink, U., Theml, H. 708, *713*
Begemann, H., see Fink, U. 708, *716*, 734, 735, 738, *744*
Begemann, H., see Gerhartz, H. 726, 727, 728, 734, 735, *744*
Behnisch, R., see Domagk, G. 841, *848*
Behnke, O., Forer, A. 676, *688*
Behnke, O., Forer, A., Emmersen, J. 676, *688*
Behr, W., Honikel, K., Hartmann, G. 616, 617, *621*
Beierwaltes, W.H., see Digiulio, W. 809, *817*
Beisel, W.R., see Feigin, R. D. 529, *531*
Bekleshova, A.Iu., see Terskikh, I.I. 354, *371*
Belanger, R., see Muggia, F. M. 589, *591*
Beldotti, L., see Schwartz, R.S. 408, *423*
Belham, J.E., Neal, G.E., Williams, D.C. 149, *153*
Beljanski, M., Beljanski, M. 375, *381*
Beljanski, M., Beljanski, M., Bourgarel, P., Chassagne, J. 376, *381*
Beljanski, M., Bourgarel, P., Beljanski, M. 376, *381*
Beljanski, M., Bourgarel, P., Beljanski, M. 376, *381*
Beljanski, M., see Beljanski, M. 375, 376, *381*
Belkhode, M.L., see Gotto, A.M. 216, *225*, 280, 290, 291, *334*
Bell, C., see Hilf, R. 117, 119, 123, *130*, 144, *154*
Bell, E. 242, *249*
Bell, J., see Beer, C.T. 684, *688*
Bell, J.P., see Gisler, R.H. 430, *432*
Bell, J.P., see LePage, G.A. 429, *433*
Bell, M., see Skipper, H.W. 522, *536*
Bell, M.J., see Brockman, R. W. 793, *805*
Bell, P.H., see Florini, J.R. 434, *453*
Bell, R., see Stewart, P.B. 752, *764*
Bell, W., see Block, J.B. 236, *249*, 261, *267*
Bell, W.R., Whang, J.J., Carbone, P.P., Brecher, G., Block, J.B. 236, *249*, 261, *267*
Bellamy, D., Phillips, J.G., Jones, I.C., Leonard, R. A. 96, *100*
Beller, B.M. 561, *567*
Bellini, O., see DiMarco, A. 593, 597, 609, *612*
Belsan, I., see Rašková, H. 361, *369*
Belton, F.C., see Melling, J. *668*
Beltz, R.E., Visser, D.W. 272, *328*, 376, 379, 380, *381*
Ben, M., see Adamson, R.H. 682, 683, *687*
Ben, M., see Frei, E., III. 679, *690*
Ben, T., see Stewart, S.E. 308, *345*

Bendich, A., see Borenfreund, E. 790, *791*
Bendich, A., see Fox, J.J. 232, *251*
Benditt, E.P., see Cannon, P.R. 526, *530*
Benedetto, A., Djaczenko, W. 584, *589*
Benedict, W.F., Harris, N., Karon, M. 236, *249*, 261, *267*
Benedict, W.F., Karon, M. 237, *249*, 261, *267*
Benedict, W.F., see Karon, M. 802, 803, *806*
Benerofe, B., see Kosower, N.S. 759, *763*
Benezra, D., Hochman, A., Pitaro, R. 706, *713*, 735, 738, *743*
Benezra, F.M., see Elion, G.B. 412, 413, *420*
Bengtsson, G., see Ullberg, S. 114, *137*
Ben-Ishai, R., Volcani, B.E. 377, *381*
Ben-Ishai, R., see Spiegelman, S. 377, *382*
Benitez, A., see Lee, W.W. 427, *433*, 658, *666*
Benitez, A., see Reist, E.J. 426, 427, 429, *433*
Benjamin, W., see Gellhorn, A. 822, 823, *827*
Benjamin, W.B., see Ochoa, M., Jr. 823, 824, *827*
Bennett, K.J., see Hansen, H.J. 500, 502, *505*
Bennett, L.L., Jr. 766, *783*, 820, 824, *826*
Bennett, L.L., Jr., Allan, P.W. 386, 391, *398*
Bennett, L.L., Jr., Brockman, R.W., Schnebli, H.P., Chumley, S., Dixon, G.J., Schabel, F.M., Jr., Dulmadge, E.A., Skipper, H.E., Montgomery, J.A., Thomas, H.J. 386, *398*
Bennett, L.L., Jr., Schabel, F.M., Jr., Skipper, H.E. 486, 495, *503*
Bennett, L.L., Jr. Schnebli, H.P., Vail, M.H., Allan, P.W., Montgomery, J.A. 436, *452*
Bennett, L.L., Jr., Simpson, L., Golden, J., Barker, T.L. 391, *398*
Bennett, L.L., Jr., Skipper, E., Mitchell, J.H., Sugiura, K. 463, *464*
Bennett, L.L., Jr., Smithers, D. 437, *452*, 487, *503*
Bennett, L.L., Jr., see Allan, P.W. 386, 388, 395, *397*
Bennett, L.L. Jr., see Baker, H.T. 392, *398*
Bennett, L.L., Jr., see Brockman, R.W. 385, *398*, 460, *465*
Bennett, L.L., Jr., see Hill, D.L. 390, 391, *400*, 437, *454*
Bennett, L.L., Jr., see Pittillo, A.F. 820, *827*
Bennett, L.L., Jr., see Schnebli, H.P. 436, 442, *455*, 659, *667*
Bennett, L.L., Jr., see Simpson, L. 392, *402*
Bennett, L.L., Jr., see Skipper, H.E. *402*, 458, *467*, 486, *510*
Bennett, S.J., see Hansen, H.J. 386, *399*
Ben-Porat, T., McBrown, K., Kaplan, A.S. 242, *249*
Ben-Porat, T., see Kamiya, T. 304, *336*
Ben-Porat, T., see Kaplan, A.S. 241, 242, *252*, 295, 302, 303, 304, 305, 306, *337*
Ben-Porat, T., see Kasamaki, A. 300, *337*
Bensch, K.G., Malawista, S.E. 677, *688*
Bensch, K.G., Marantz, R., Wisniewski, H., Shelanski, M. 678, *688*
Bensch, K.G., see Creasey, W.A. 678, 680, 682, *689*
Bensch, K.G., see Malawista, S.E. 674, 676, *691*
Benson, J.V., Jr., Gordon, M.J., Patterson, J.A. 697, *713*
Bent, K.J., Moore, R.H. 671, *688*
Bentinck, R.C., see Gordan, G.S. 91, *100*
Bentley, M., see Abrams, R. 489, 496, *503*
Benton, D.A., see Breuer, L.H. 711, *714*
Benua, S., see Eidinoff, M.L. 283, 295, 314, *332*
Benvenisti, D., see Burchenal, J.H. 799, *805*
Benyumovich, M.S., see Galegov, G.A. 524, *531*
Benyumovich, M.S., see Lerman, M.I. 56, *61*
Benzer, S., Freese, E. 295, *328*
Benzer, S., see Champe, S.P. 214, *224*
Beránek, J. 350, *364*
Beránek, J., Pitha, J. 349, *364*
Beránek, J., Šorm, F. 349, 350, *364*
Beránek, J., see Farkaš, J. 350, *366*
Beránek, J., see Grafnetterová, J., 357, 358, 359, *366*
Beránek, J., see Wieczorkowski, J. 350, *371*
Berard, C.W., see Krueger, G.R.F. 417, *422*
Berberian, D.A., Freele, H., Rosi, D., Dennis, E.W., Archer, S. 879, *887*
Berberian, D.A., see Rosi, D. 879, *889*
Berchtold, R., see Burchenal, J.H. 822, *826*
Berchtold, R., see Hirt, R. 820, *827*
Berecz, A., Goldin, C. 521, *530*
Bereczky, E., see Munyon, W. 302, 304, 306, 307, *341*
Berenbaum, M.C. 24, *30*, 384, 389, 396, *398*, 409, *419*, 525, *530*, 705, 706, *713*, 833, *839*
Berenbaum, M.C., Bondurant, S. 706, *713*
Berenbaum, M.C., Brown, I.N. 24, *30*
Berenbaum, M.C., Ginsburg H., Gilbert, D.M. 706, *713*
Berenbaum, M.C., Timmis, G.M., Brown, I.N. 38, *42*
Berenbaum, M.C., see Addison, I.E. 38, *42*
Berenblum, I. 18, *30*
Berends, A., see Beukers, R. 52, *60*
Berens, K., Shugar, D. 275, 296, *328*
Berg, P., see Jones, O.W. 326, *336*
Berg, P., see Slapikoff, S. 208, *231*
Bergamini, A., see Gualandi, G. 521, 522, *532*
Bergamini, N., Fowst, G. 883, *888*
Bergel, F., see Currie, R. 389, *398*
Bergel, F., see Ohnuma, T. *534*, 697, 704, *719*

Bergenstal, D. M., Hertz, R., Lipsett, M. B., Moy, R. H. 811, 812, 814, *817*
Bergenstal, D. M., see Huggins, C. 176, *189*
Berger, J., see Leimgruber, W. 642, *648*
Bergfeld, W. F., see Roenigk, H. H. 475, *482*
Bergh, A. K., Webb, S. J., McArthur, C. S. 825, *826*
Bergman, J. G., see Kirschner, S. 836, *840*
Bergman, W., Stempien, M. F., Jr. 435, *452*
Bergmann, M., see Golumbic, C. 19, *31*
Bergmann, W., Burke, D. C. 232, *249*, 426, *431*
Bergmann, W., Feeney, R. J. 232, *249*
Bergquist, P. L., see Lowrie, R. J. 209, 210, *228*
Bergsagel, D. E., see Cowan, D. H. 545, *550*
Bering, E. A., see Rubin, R. C. 472, *482*
Berk, B., see Robison, R. S. 698, *720*
Berlin, Y. A., Kiseleva, O. A., Kolosov, M. N., Shemyakin, M. M., Soifer, V. S., Vasina, I. V., Yartseva, I. V. 615, *621*
Berlin, Y. A., see Sedov, K. A. 615, 619, *622*
Berliner, D. L., see Sweat, M. L. 106, *136*
Berlinguet, L., see Martel, F. 523, *534*
Berlowitz, L., Pallotta, D., Sibley, C. H. 583, 584, *589*
Berman, L. D., Hayes, J., Sibay, T. 78, *79*
Berman, S., see Rovera, G. 583, *592*
Bermek, E., Kramer, W., Monkemeyer, H., Matthaei, H. 375, *381*
Bernard, J., Boiron, M., Jacquillat, C., Lortholary, P., Weiel, M. 260, *267*
Bernard, J., see Boiron, M. 773, *783*
Bernard, J., see Ellison, R. R. 260, *268*
Bernard, J., see Jacquillat, C. 726, 727, 728, 732, 734, 735, *744*
Bernard, J., see Weil, M. 772, 773, *788*
Berne, T., see Deshpande, N. 117, *127*
Berneis, K., Bollag, W., Kofler, M., Leuthy, H. 756, *761*
Berneis, K., Kofler, M., Bollag, W. 751, *761*
Berneis, K., Kofler, M., Bollag, W., Kaiser, A., Langemann, A. 756, *761*
Berneis, K., Kofler, M., Bollag, W., Zeller, P., Kaiser, A., Langemann, A. 756, *761*
Bernfeld, M. R., see Mäenpää, P. H. 121, *132*
Bernhard, H. V., see Kreis, W. 758, *763*
Bernhard, W., see Simard, R, 494, *510*, 628, *632*
Bernhardt, D., Darnell, J. E. 578, *579*
Bernstein, J., see Hamre, D. 800, *806*
Bernstein, J., see Stearns, B. 789, *792*
Bernstein, J. B., see Bachur, N. R. 608, *611*
Berridge, B. J., Jr., see Peters, J. H. 697, *720*
Berry, R. J., Andrews, J. R. 301, 307, 319, *328*
Berry, S. J., see Grayson, S. *669*
Berswordt-Wallrabe, R. von, see Neumann, F. 146, *155*
Bert, G., see Lajolo, D. *718*
Bertani, L. E. 199, *223*
Bertani, L. E., Haggmark, A., Reichard, P. 277, *328*
Bertazzoli, C., Chieli, T. Grandi, M., Ricevuti, G. 609, 610, *611*
Bertelli, A., Donati, L., Trabucchi, E., Jr. 705, *714*
Bertha, I., see Hanisch, J. *568*
Bertino, J. R. 468, *479*
Bertino, J. R., Booth, B. A., Cashmore, A., Bieber, A. L., Sartorelli, A. C. 468, 472, *479*
Bertino, J. R., Cashmore, A., Fink, M., Calabresi, P., Lefkowitz, E. 473, *479*
Bertino, J. R., Cashmore, A. R., Hillcoat, B. L. 775, *783*
Bertino, J. R., DeConti, R. C., Mosher, M. 477, 479, *479*
Bertino, J. R., Hillcoat, B. L., Johns, D. G. 528, *530*
Bertino, J. R., Johns, D. G. 474, *479*
Bertino, J. R., see Booth, B. A. 846, 847, *848*
Bertino, J. R., see Capizzi, R. L. 477, 479, *480*, 705, *715*, 723, 735, *743*
Bertino, J. R., see Chello, P. 469, *480*
Bertino, J. R., see Cleveland, J. C. 474, 478, *480*
Bertino, J. R., see DeConti, R. C. 793, 799, 800, 802, 804, *805*
Bertino, J. R., see Fischer, G. A. 471, *480*
Bertino, J. R., see Hellman, S. 477, *481*
Bertino, J. R., see Hryniuk, W. M. 469, 470, 473, 475, 476, *481*
Bertino, J. R., see Johns, D. G. 196, *226*, 472, 473, *481*
Bertino, J. R., see Levitt, M. 478, *481*
Bertino, J. R., see McDonald, C. J. 479, *482*
Bertino, J. R., see Mitchell, M. S. 237, *253*, 474
Bertino, J. R., see Nahas, A. 470, 471, *482*
Bertino, J. R., see Perkins, J. P. 469, *482*
Bertino, J. R., see Sartorelli, A. C. 771, 776, *787*
Bertino, J. R., see Skeel, R. T. 477, *482*
Berumen, L., see Mathé, G. 759, *763*
Beskid, G., see Grunberg, E. 642, *647*
Bessada, R., see Erdos, T. 114, 115, *128*
Bessman, J. J., Lehman, I. R., Simms, E. S., Kornberg, A. 281, *328*
Bessman, M. J., see Lehman, I. R. 274, *339*
Best-Belpomme, M., see Erdos, T. 115, *128*
Bestmann, H. J., see Weygand, F. 485, *511*
Beth, E., see Old, L. J. 728, 733, *746*
Bethune, V., see Etcubanas, E. 793, 799, 800, *805*
Bettigole, R. E., Himelstein, E. S., Oettgen, H. F., Clifford, G. O. 735, *743*
Bettle, J. D., Jr., see Hewlett, J. S. 740

Betz, B., see Groth, D.P. 74, *81*, 264, *269*
Beukers, R., Berends, A. 52, *60*
Beuving, G., Gruber, M. 120, *126*
Bevelander, G., see Karnofsky, D.A. 495, *506*
Bever, A.F., see Velardo, J. T. 110, *137*
Beveridge, E., see Barrett, P.A. 841, *847*
Beveridge, G.W., see Ashton, H. 384, *397*
Beyer, M., see Burchenal, J. H. 544, 550
Beyer, R., see Zahn, R.K. 244, *256*
Bhargava, P.M., see Heidelberger, C. *226*
Bhisey, A.N., see Freed, J. J. 676, *690*
Bhose, A., see Mukherjee, S. 109, *133*, *134*
Bhuyan, B.K. 73, 76, 77, *79*, 557, *567*
Bhuyan, B.K., Dietz, A. 623, 624, 631, *631*
Bhuyan, B.K., Dietz, A., Smith, C.G. 557, *567*
Bhuyan, B.K., Fraser, T.J., Li, L.H. 881, *888*
Bhuyan, B.K., Kelly, R.B., Smith, R.M. 623, *631*
Bhuyan, B.K., Reusser, F. 625, 629, 631, *631*
Bhuyan, B.K., Scheidt, L. G., Fraser, T.J. 75, 76, *80*, 218, *223*, 629, *631*, 802, *805*
Bhuyan, B.K., Smith, C.G. 573, *579*, 602, *611*, 624, 625, 629, *631*
Bhuyan, B.K., see Gray, G. D. 630, 631, *632*
Bhuyan, B.K., see Li, L.H. 362, *367*, 653, *656*
Bhuyan, B.K., see Reusser, F. 628, 629, *632*
Biagioli, E., see Di Marco, A. 607, *612*
Bianchi, A., see Lerner, L.J. 123, *132*, 146, *154*, 183, *190*
Bickel, M.H., see Aebi, H. 754, *760*
Bickel, M.H., see Baggiolini, M. 754, 756, *760*, *761*
Bickers, J.N., see Frei, E. III. 260, 262, *269*
Bieber, A.L., see Bertino, J. R. 468, 472, *479*
Bieber, A.L., see Sartorelli, A.C. 487, 500, *509*
Bieber, C.P., see Stinson, E. B. 416, *424*
Bieber, S., Dietrich, L.S., Elion, G.B., Hitchings, G.H., Martin, D.S. 386, 393, *398*
Bieber, S., Elion, G.B., Hitchings, G.H., Hooper, D.C., Nathan, H.C. 309, *328*
Bieber, S., see Elion, G.B. 404, 408, 409, 410, 411, *420*
Bieber, S., see Nathan, H.C. 407, 409, *422*
Biedler, J.L., Riehm, H. 583, *590*, 606, *611*
Biemann, D., see Rao, K.V. 633, *641*
Bierman, H.R., Kelly, K. H., Maekawa, T., Timmis, G.M. 36, *42*
Biesele, J.J., see Izutsu, K. 300, *336*
Biesewig, D., see Beato, M. 164, *167*
Biesler, J.A. 650, *655*
Biezinski, J.J., Spaet, T.H. 824, *826*
Bikbulatova, R.M., see Galegov, G.A. 354, *366*
Bikbulatova, R.M., see Galegov, G.A. *366*
Bilimoria, M.H. 697, 698, *714*
Bilimoria, M.H., Nisbet, M. A. 703, *714*
Billen, D., see Hsu, T.C. 300, *336*
Billeter, J.R., see Heer, J. 106, *130*
Billing, R.J., Barbiroli, B., Smellie, R.M.S. 120, *126*
Bills, C.E., see Hess, A.F. 120, *130*
Birch, A.J., Wright, J.J. 446, *453*
Bird, H.H., see Florini, J.R. 434, *453*
Bird, T.J., see Gots, J.-S. 494, *505*
Birkinshaw, J.H., Raistrick, H., Ross, D.J. 446, *453*
Birkofer, L., see Hempel, K. 518, *532*
Birnbaum, S.M., see Sugimura, T. 528, *537*
Birnie, G.D., Kroeger, H., Heidelberger, C. 203, 215, *223*, 315, 318, *328*
Birnie, G.D., see Creighton, A.M. 885, *888*
Birnie, G.D., see Heidelberger, C. 203, 215, *226*
Birtch, A.G., see Murray, J. E. 502, *508*
Biscatti, G., see Astaldi, G. 706, *713*, 735, *742*
Bischoff, K.B., Dedrick, R. L., Zaharko, D.S. 472, *479*
Bischoff, R., Holtzer, H. 311, 312, *328*
Bisel, H.F., Ansfield, F.J., Mason, J.H., Wilson, W. L. 440, *453*
Bishop, C.F., see Melnykovych, G. 96, *102*
Bishop, J.M., see Levinson, W.E. 307, *339*
Bishop, J.M., see McDonnell, J.P. 583, *591*, *613*
Bishop, R.C., see Hewlett, J.S. 740
Biskind, G.S., see Biskind, M.S. 171, *188*
Biskind, M.S., Biskind, G.S. 171, *188*
Biswas, D.K., see Talwar, G.P. 114, *137*
Bitman, J., Trezise, L.A., Cecil, H.C. 125, *126*
Bitman, J., see Cecil, H.C. 125, *127*
Bitoon, M., see Rosenkranz, H.S. 73, *83*
Bittar, E.E. 861, *871*
Bittar, E.E., Dick, D.A.T., Fry, D.J. 861, *871*
Black, F.L., see Fischer, D. S. 308, *333*
Black, P.H., see Hirsch, M. S. 418, *421*
Blackburn, C.M., Albert, A. 144, *153*, 173, *188*
Blackford, R.W., see Lee, W.W. 429, 430, 431, *433*
Bláha, V., see Šmahel, O. 361, *370*
Blair, D.M., see Clarke, V. D. 879, *888*
Blair, R.M., see Aposhian, H.V. 523, *529*
Blakeney, A.B., see Lees, E. M. 697, *718*
Blancuzzi, V., Elion, G.B. 409, *419*
Blank, N., see Humphrey, E.W. 638, *640*
Blanz, E.J., Jr., French, F. A. 799, *805*, 880, *888*
Blanz, E.J., Jr., French, F. A., DoAmaral, J.R., French, D.A. 795, *805*
Blanz, E.J., Jr., see DoAmaral, J.R. 779, *784*

Blanz, E. J., Jr., see French, F. A. 768, *785*, 794, 795, 797, 798, 799, *805*, *806*
Blaškovič, D., see Jasińska, S. 354, *367*
Blaškovič, D., see Rada, B. 302, 306, *342*, 354, *369*
Blattner, R. J., Williamson, A. P., Simonsen, L. 493, *503*
Bledsoe, T., Island, D. P., Key, R. L., Liddle, G. W. 813, *817*
Bleyman, M., Woese, C. 584, *590*
Bligh, E. G., see Heard, R. D. 106, *130*
Bloch, A. *453*
Bloch, A., Leonard, R. J., Nichol, C. A. 436, 437, 438, 439, 444, *453*
Bloch, A., Mihich, E., Leonard, R. J., Nichol, C. A. 444, 445, *453*
Bloch, A., Nichol, C. A. 436, 448, 449, *453*, 660, *665*
Bloch, A., see Fox, J. J. 434, 435, 436, *453*, 658, *665*
Bloch, A., see Nichol, C. A. 445, *455*
Bloch, H. L., see Zimmerman, B. 809, *819*
Block, G. E., see Jensen, E. V. 85, 95, *101*, 117, *131*
Block, J., see Fallon, H. J. 352, 359, *365*
Block, J. B., Bell, W., Whang, J., Carbone, P. P. 236, *249*, 261, *267*
Block, J. B., Field, M., Oliverio, V. T. 771, 774, *783*
Block, J. B., see Bell, W. R. 236, *249*, 261, *267*
Block, J. B., see Carbone, P. P. 726, 727, 728, 730, 732, 734, 735, *743*
Block, J. B., see Field, M. 771, 774, *784*
Block, J. B., see Gottlieb, J. A. 650, *655*
Block, R., see Kreis, W. 822, 824, *827*
Bloedow, C. E. 789, *791*, 793, *805*
Blohm, T. R., Kariya, T., Laughlin, M. W. 105, *126*
Blom, J., see Ellison, R. R. 260, *268*
Blom, J., see Ohnuma, T. 726, 727, 728, 734, 735, *746*
Blomgren, S. E., Wolberg, W. H., Kisken, W. A. 201, *223*
Blondal, H., Levi, I., Latour, J. P. A., Fraser, W. D. 524, *530*
Blondal, H., see Levin, I. 524, *533*
Bloom, B. R., Jimenez, L., Marcus, P. I. 417, *419*
Bloom, H. J. G. 186, *188*
Bloom, H. J. G., Dukes, C. E., Mitchley, B. C. V. 175, 186, *188*
Blossom, D. R., see Loo, T. L. 386, *401*
Blow, J. G., see Simpson-Herren, L. 78, *83*
Blum, G., see Druckrey, H. 78, *80*
Blumberg, see Piesach *849*
Blumberg, N. A., see Chorin, V. A. 617, *621*
Blumenthal, G., see Greenberg, D. M. 501, *505*
Blumenthal, H. J., see Ghosh, S. 493, *505*
Bo, G., see Pavan, M. 566, *569*
Bo, W., Smith, M. S. *126*
Board, J. A., Lee, H. M., Draper, D. A., Hume, D. M. 415, *419*
Bobbitt, J. L., see Ho, P. P. K. 698, 699, 700, 702, 708, *716*
Bobek, M., Farkaš, J., Šorm, F. 349, *364*
Boch, D. 697, *714*
Boch, M., Korth, T., Nelke, J. M., Pike, D., Radunz, H., Winterfeldt, E. 650, *655*
Bock, F. G., see Dao, T. L. 112, *127*
Boder, G. B., see Johnson, I. S. 671, *691*
Bodey, G. P., Coltman, C. A., Freireich, E. J., Bonnet, D., Gehan, E. A., Haut, A. B., Hewlett, J. S., McCredie, K. B., Saiki, J. H., Wilson, H. E. 264, *268*
Bodey, G. P., Freireich, E. J., Monto, R. W., Hewlett, J. S. 260, 261, 263, *268*
Bodey, G. P., Rodriguez, V., Hart, J. S., Freireich, E. J. 263, *268*
Bodey, G. P., see Freireich, E. J. 260, 262, 265, *269*, 397, *399*
Bodey, G. P., see Hersh, E. M. 264, *269*
Bodey, G. P., see Wang, J. J. 262, *271*
Bodey, G. P., see Whitecar, J. P., Jr. 263, *271*, 709, *722*, 723, 727, 728, 730, 734, 735, *746*
Bodmer, W. F., see Laird, C. D. 280, *338*
Boeck, L. D., see Ho, P. P. K. 698, 699, 700, 702, 708, *716*
Boeck, L. D., see Williams, R. H. 446, *457*
Boedtker, H., see Doty, P. 292, *331*
Boesen, E., Davis, W. 19, *30*
Böttger, M., see Wunderlich, V. 70, *84*
Bogart, R., Lesley, J. F., Mayer, D. T. 113, *126*
Boggiano, E., see Barg, W. 488, *503*
Bohonos, N., see DeVoe, S. E. 486, 496, *504*
Boileau, G., see Lahiri, S. R. 220, *228*
Boiron, A. M., see Ellison, R. R. 260, *268*
Boiron, M., Jacquillat, C., Weil, M., Bernard, J. 773, *783*
Boiron, M., see Bernard, J. 260, *267*
Boiron, M., see Jacquillat, C. 726, 727, 728, 732, 734, 735, *744*
Boiron, M., see Manteuil, S. 439, *454*
Boiron, M., see Weil, M. 772, 773, *788*
Boissier, J. R., Levine, P., DeRudder, J., Privat de Garilke, M. 430, *432*
Bolaffi, J. L., see Rich, M. A. 199, *229*
Bolderas, L., see Baggett, B. 106, *125*
Boldrey, E. B., see Wilson, C. B. 69, *84*
Boll, I., Klimas, J., Willigerodt, B. 405, *419*
Bollag, W. 39, *42*, 747, 748, 749, 751, 752, 753, 754, *761*
Bollag, W., Grunberg, E. 747, 748, 749, 756, *761*
Bollag, W., Theiss, E. 753, *761*

Bollag, W., see Berneis, K. 751, 756, *761*
Bollag, W., see Rutishauser, A. 756, *764*
Bollag, W., see Schwartz, D. E. 754, *764*
Bolte, E., Mancuso, S., Eriksson, G., Wiqvist, N., Diczfalusy, E. 107, *126*
Bolund, L. 584, *590*
Bolund, L., see Ringertz, N. R. 584, *592*
Bonadonna, G., Monfardini, S., Oldini, C. 759, *761*
Bonar, A., see Riman, J. 440, *455*
Bonar, R. A., see Sverak, L. 574, *581*
Bonasera, N., Mangione, G., Bonavita, V. 491, *503*
Bonavita, V., see Bonasera, N. 491, *503*
Bonavita, V., see Narrod, S. A. 491, *508*
Bond, H. W., see Ross, R. B. 523, *535*
Bond, J. V., see Hellmann, K. 886, *889*
Bond, S. B., see Kriss, J. P. 282, 283, 289, *338*
Bond, V. P., see Feinendegen, L. E. 283, 314, 315, 316, *332*
Bond, V. P., see Rubini, J. R. 280, 314, *343*
Bond, W. H., see Hodes, M. E. 685, *690*
Bondurant, S., see Berenbaum, M. C. 706, *713*
Bonessi, J. V., see Danowski, T. S. 814, *817*
Bonetti, E., Abbondanza, A., Corte, E. D., Stirpe, F. 697, *714*
Bonmassar, E., Castagnone, D., Celi, M. L., Melan, F. 528, *530*
Bonmassar, E., Celi, M. L., Melan, F., Testorelli, C. 527, *530*
Bonmassar, E., Melan, F., Testorelli, C. 528, *530*
Bonmassar, E., see Vadlamudi, S. 362, *371*, 705, *721*
Bonner, J., see Dahmas, M. E. 825, *826*
Bonner, J., see Huang, R. C. 824, *827*
Bonnet, J. D., see Bodey, G. P. 264, *268*
Bono, V. H., Weissman, S. M., Frei, E., III 352, *364*
Bono, V. H., Jr., see Kohn, K. W. 644, 645, *647*
Bono, V. H., Jr., see Handschumacher, R. E. 355, 358, 359, 360, 361, *366*
Bonomi, U., Tenconi, L. T. 520, 529, *530*
Boohar, J., see Heidelberger, C. 202, 203, 205, 215, 219, *226*
Boohar, J., see Mukherjee, K. L. 221, *228*
Booth, B. A., Donnelly, T. E., Jr., Zettner, A., Sartorelli, A. C. 846, 847, *848*
Booth, B. A., Johns, D. G., Bertino, J. R., Sartorelli, A. C. 846, 847, *848*
Booth, B. A., Moore, E. C., Sartorelli, A. C. 802, 804, *805*
Booth, B. A., Sartorelli, A. C. 301, *328*, 844, 846, 847, *848*
Booth, B. A., see Agrawal, K. C. 795, 797, 798, *804*
Booth, B. A., see Bertino, J. R. 468, 472, *479*
Booth, B. A., see Johns, D. G. 196, *226*, 473, *481*
Booth, B. A., see Mooney, P. D. 798, *806*
Booth, B. A., see Moore, E. C. 793, 798, 802, 803, 804, *806*
Booth, B. A., see Sartorelli, A. C. 487, 496, 500, 501, *509*, 516, 519, *530*, 771, 776, *787*, 793, 802, *807*, *849*
Booth, D. A. 825, *826*
Booth, J., Boyland, E., Gellhorn, A. 822, 823, 824, *826*
Booth, L. D., see McCord, T. J. 524, *534*
Bootsma, D., Budke, L., Vos, O. 604, *611*
Borberg, H., see Kreis, W. 247, 249, *253*
Borč, K., see Rašková, H. 361, *369*
Borek, E., Miller, H. K., Sheiness, P., Waelsch, H. 499, *503*
Borek, E., see Thomasz, A. 201, *230*
Borel, Y., Fauconnet, M., Miescher, P. A. 407, *419*
Borel, Y., Schwartz, R. *419*
Borenfreund, E., Krim, M., Bendich, A. 790, *791*
Boretti, G., see DiMarco, A. 608, *612*
Borges, P. R. F., see Roberts, E. 485, *509*
Boris, A., DeMartino, L., Trmal, T. 146, *153*
Borisy, G. G., Taylor, E. W. 677, *688*
Borisy, G. G., see Adelmann, M. R. 676, *688*
Borisy, G. G., see Weisenberg, R. C. 677, 678, *694*
Borkovec, A. B. 24, *30*
Bořkovec, A. B., Chang, C., Horwitz, S. B. 644, *647*
Bořkovec, A. B., see Horwitz, S. B. 646, *647*, 860, *872*
Borman, A., see Hilf, R. 110, 123, *130*
Borman, A., see Lerner, L. J. 146, *154*, 183, *190*
Bors, F. H., see Wellings, P. C. 195, 200, 219, *231*
Borsa, J., Whitmore, G. F. 469, 470, *479*
Borsa, J., Whitmore, G. F., Valeriote, F. A., Collins, D., Bruce, W. R. 234, 238, *250*
Borthwick, M., see Levine, M. 634, *640*
Borun, T. W., Scharff, M. D., Robbins, E. 245, *250*
Bosch, L., Harbers, E., Heidelberger, C. 203, 204, 206, *223*
Bosmann, H. B., 577, *579*, 583, *590*, 651, 654, *655*, 709, *714*
Bosmann, H. B., Kessel, D. 701, 708, 709, *714*
Bosmann, H. B., see Kessel, D. 653, *656*, 709, *717*
Bosner, F., see Ohnuma, T. 726, 727, 728, 734, 735, *746*
Bostwick, L., see Evans, J. S. 235, 236, *251*, 259, 263, 264, *268*
Botkin, C., see Kelly, M. G. 752, *763*
Botteril, V., see Kessel, D. *613*
Bottoms, G., Goetsch, D. D. 96, *100*
Boudon, M., see Laboureur, P. 699, 700, *717*
Bourgarel, P., see Beljanski, M. 376, *381*
Bourgarel, P., see Beljanski, M. 376, *381*

Bourke, A. R., see Kelly, M. G. 684, *691*
Bourseaux, F., see Arnold, H. 29, *30*
Bow, T. M., see Spencer, R. P. 495, *510*
Bowden, B., see Pittillo, A. F. 820, *827*
Bowdon, B. J., Wheeler, G. P. 73, *80*
Bowdon, B. J., see Wheeler, G. P. 66, 68, 69, 74, 75, 76, 77, *84*, 264, *271*
Bowen, J. M., Elliott, A. Y., Sykes, J. A., Dmochowski, L. L. 302, 307, *328*
Bowen, J. M., Hughes, R. G., Dmochowski, L. L. 302, *328*
Bowers, C. Y., see Segaloff, A. 173, 183, *191*
Bowman, B., see Kimball, A. P. 234, 241, *253*, 429, 430, *432*
Bowman, B., see LePage, G. A. 384, 396, *400*
Boxer, G. E., see Gitterman, C. O. 661, *665*
Boxer, G. E., see Shigeura, H. T. 659, 661, 663, *667*
Boxer, G. E., see Walton, E. 661, *668*
Boyce, R. P., Howard-Flanders, P. 12, *15*, 53, 54, *60*
Boyce, R. P., Setlow, R. B. 290, *328*
Boyd, G. S. 109, *126*
Boyd, G. S., McGuire, W. B. 109, *126*
Boyd, G. S., see Sulimovici, S. I. 139, 140, *156*
Boyd, J. W., Phillips, A. W. 697, 704, *714*
Boyd, T. C., see De Voe, S. E. 486, 496, *504*
Boyland, E., see Booth, J. 822, 823, 824, *826*
Boyse, E. A., Old, L. J., Campbell, H. A., Mashburn, L. T. 704, *714*, 723, *743*
Boyse, E. A., Old, L. J., Stockert, E. 696, *714*, 723, *743*
Boyse, E. A., see Campbell, H. A. 698, 701, *714*, 723, *743*
Boyse, E. A., see Horowitz, B. 711, *717*
Boyse, E. A., see Kim, J. H. 738, *745*
Boyse, E. A., see Oettgen, H. F. 696, *719*, 723, 727, 730, 733, 734, *745*
Boyse, E. A., see Old, L. J. 695, 696, 697, *719*, 723, 728, *746*
Boyse, E. A., see Schulten, H. K. 705, 707, *721*
Brachnikova, M. G., Kostantinova, N. V., Pomaskova, F. A., Zacharov, B. M. 593, *611*
Bradbury, J. T. 109, *126*
Bradley, P. L., see Barrett, P. A. 841, *847*
Bradley, W. G., Lassman, L. P., Pearce, G. W., Walton, J. N. 686, *688*
Bradlow, H. L., see Fukushima, D. K. 813, *817*
Bradner, W. T., Pindell, M. H. 855, 869, 870, *871*
Bradner, W. T., see Price, K. E. 862, *874*
Bradshaw, W. S., see Rutter, W. J. 311, *343*
Bräuerova, J., see Vonka, V. 838, *840*
Bragshaw, M. A., see Goffinet, D. R. 319, *334*
Brailovsky, C., see Chany, C. 607, *611*
Brakier, L., Verly, W. G. 10, *15*, 41, *42*
Brakier, L., see Verly, W. G. 10, *17*
Brambilla, G., Parodi, S., Cavanna, M., Baldini, L. 527, *530*
Brambilla, G., Parodi, S., Cavanna, M., Caraceni, C. E., Baldini, L. 705, *714*
Brambilla, G., see Baldini, L. 237, *249*, 524, 527, *529*, *530*
Brammer, K. W. 274, *328*
Brandle, W., see Beato, M. 164, *167*
Branster, M. V., Morton, R. K. 539, *542*
Bratzel, R. P., Ross, R. B., Goodridge, T. H., Huntress, W. T., Flather, M. T., Johnson, D. E. 18, *30*
Braunsberg, H., Irvine, W. T., James, V. H. T. 117, *126*
Braunwald, J., see Jacobs, E. M. 220, *226*
Brawerman, G., see Lee, S. Y. 574, 575, *580*
Brawerman, G., see Mendecki, J. *580*, *669*
Bray, D. A., DeVita, V. T., Adamson, R. H., Oliverio, V. T. 68, 77, *80*
Bray, R. C., see Currie, R. 389, *398*
Bray, R. C., see Ohnuma, T. *534*, 697, 704, *719*
Brayton, C., see Horwitz, M. S. 654, *655*
Brecher, G., see Bell, W. R. 236, *249*, 261, *267*
Brecher, P. I., see Jensen, E. V. 104, 110, 114, 115, *131*
Breeden, C. J., Hall, T. C., Tyler, H. R. 323, *328*
Brega, A., Falaschi, A., DeCarli, L., Pavan, M. 566, *567*
Brega, A., see Jacobs-Lorena, M. 567, *569*
Breitman, T. R., Perry, S., Cooper, R. A. 280, *328*
Breitman, T. R., see Smulson, M. E. 524, *536*
Bremerskov, V., Kaden, P., Mittermayer, C. 234, 241, *250*
Brendel, M., Khan, N. A., Haynes, R. H. 41, *42*
Brendler, H., see Edelman, J. C. 151, *153*
Brennan, M. J., see Beckett, V. L. 173, *188*
Brennan, M. J., see Loo, R. V. 261, *270*
Brent, T. P., see Roberts, J. J. 13, *16*, 21, 25, 27, *33*
Bresciani, F., see Puca, G. A. 114, 117, *134*
Bresnick, E. 404, 412, *419*
Bresnick, E., Thompson, U. B. 281, 285, *328*
Bresnick, E., Williams, S. S. 203, *223*
Breuer, L. H., Warner, R. G., Benton, D. A., Loosli, J K. 711, *714*
Brewen, J. G. 236, *250*, 261, *268*
Brewen, J. G., Christie, N. T. 236, *250*, 261, *268*
Brewer, E. N., Rusch, H. P. 774, *783*
Brewer, H. B., Aronow, L. 27, *31*
Brezin, C., see Amiel, J.-L. 752, *760*
Briden, D. W., see Pietsch, P. 855, 871, *874*
Bridges, B. A., Munson, R. J. 41, *42*
Bridges, J. M., see Nelson, S. D. 705, 707, *719*
Briggs, I. G., see Recher, L. 583, *591*
Briggs, M. H., Brotherton, J. 146, *153*

Brihaye, J., see Rappel, M. 324, *343*
Brillantes, F. P., see Huggins, C. 117, *131*
Brindle, S. D., see Hirschberg, E. 880, *889*
Brine, G. A., see Wani, M. C. 650, *656*
Brink, J. J., LePage, G. A. 427, 428, 429, *432*
Bristow, E. C., Wissler, R. W. 519, *530*
Bristow, E. C., see Wissler, R. W. 525, 526, *538*
Britten, R. J., Roberts, R. B., French, E. F. 513, *530*
Brittin, G. M., see Levin, R. H. 772, *786*
Brittle, N., see Vincent, P. C. 59, *63*
Briziarelli, G., see Huggins, C. 112, *131*, 181, *189*
Brock, M. L., see Brock, T. D. 495, *503*
Brock, N., Hohorst, H. J. 29, *31*
Brock, N., see Arnold, H. 29, *30*
Brock, N., see Hohorst, H. J. 29, *32*
Brock. T. D., Brock, M. L. 495, *503*
Brockman, R. W. 384, 385, 389, 390, 392, 393, 394, *398*
Brockman, R. W., Anderson, E. P. 292, *382*, 384, 387, 392, *398*, 458, *465*, 485, 495, *503*
Brockman, R. W., Bennett, L. L., Jr., Simpson, M. S., Wilson, A. R., Thomson, J. R., Skipper, H. E. 385, *398*, 460, *465*
Brockman, R. W., Chumley, S. 390, 391, *398*, 487, *503*
Brockman, R. W., Davis, J. M., Stutts, P. 217, *223*
Brockman, R. W., Pittillo, R. F., Shaddix, S., Hill, D. L. 496, *503*
Brockman, R. W., Shaddix, S., Laster, W. R., Jr., Schabel, F. M., Jr. 793, 800, *805*, 877, 878, *888*
Brockman, R. W., Shaddix, S., Stringer, V., Adamson, D. 790, *791*
Brockman, R. W., Sidwell, R. W., Arnett, G., Shaddix, S. 793, *805*
Brockman, R. W., Sparks, M. C., Hutchison, D. J., Skipper, H. E. 460, *465*
Brockman, R. W., Sparks, M. C., Simpson, M. S. 460, *465*
Brockman, R. W., Thomson, J. R., Bell, M. J., Skipper, H. E. 793, *805*
Brockman, R. W., see Anderson, E. P. 487, 488, 489, 490, 496, *503*
Brockman, R. W., see Bennett, L. L., Jr. 386, *398*
Brockman, R. W., see Sidwell, R. W. 302, *344*
Brockman, R. W., see Skipper, H. E. 235, *255*, 798, *807*
Brockman, R. W., see Stutts, P. 387, *403*
Brockmann, H. 584
Brodey, R. S., see Old, L. J. 723, *746*
Brodie, B. B., see Tagliamonte, A. 519, *537*
Broder, L., see Carter, S. K. 65, *80*
Brody, K. R., see Spencer, R. P. 521, 523, *536*
Bromfeld, E., see Verma, I. M. 660, *668*
Brooke, M. S. 407, *419*
Brookes, P. 758, *761*
Brookes, P., Lawley, P. D. 7, *15*, 22, 26, 27. *31*, 41, *42*
Brookes, P., see Lawley, P. D. 7, 8, 13, *16*, 25, 27, *32*, 49, 50, *61*, 71, *81*, 278, *339*
Brooks, S. C., see Rao, K. V. 486, 496, *509*
Brooks, V., see Dao, T. L. 184, *188*
Brooks, W. F., Jr., Wittliff, J. L. 115, *126*
Brooks, W. F., Jr., see Wittliff, J. L. 117, 118, *138*
Brooksby, J. B. 143, *153*
Broome, J. D. 695, 696, 697, 703, 704, 705, 707, 708, 711, *714*, 723, 734, *743*
Broome, J. D., Schwartz, J. H. 711, *714*, 733, *743*
Broome, J. D., see Becker, F. F. 710, 711, *713*
Broome, J. D., see Schwartz, J. H. 697, 698, *721*
Broschard, R. W., see Patrick, J. B. 48, *62*
Broschard, R. W., see Webb, J. S. 47, *64*
Bross, I., see Mihich, E. 770, *786*
Brossi, A., Baumann, M., Burkhardt, F., Richie, R., Frey, J. R. 563, *567*
Brotherton, J., see Briggs, M. H. 146, *153*
Brotzu, G., see Ferrari, W. 769, *784*
Brouček, J., see Čihák, A. 362, 363, *364*
Brown, B. W., see Hersh, E. M. 503, *506*, 527, *532*, 707, *716*
Brown, C. G. D., see Barrett, P. A. 841, *847*
Brown, C. H., see Brown, J. H. U. 815, *817*
Brown, C. H., III., Canellos, G. P., Carbone, P. P. 708, *714*
Brown, D. C., see Wellings, P. C. 195, 200, 219, *231*
Brown, D. E., see Morrison, R. K. 619, *622*
Brown, D. M., Todd, A. R., Varadarajan, S. 273, *328*, 886, *888*
Brown, D. W., see Palmer, D. L. 416, *423*
Brown, E., see Dolowy, W. C. 696, *715*
Brown, G. B., Roll, P. M., Plentl, A. A., Cavalieri, L. F. 458, *465*
Brown, G. B., Weinfeld, H., Roll, P. M. 318, *328*
Brown, G. F., see Sugiura, K. 36, *46*
Brown, G. M. 436, *453*
Brown, H. D., see Hasselberger, F. X. 724, 735, *744*
Brown, H. E., Jr., see Slonim, R. R. 675, *693*
Brown, I. N., see Berenbaum, M. C. 24, *30*, 38, *42*
Brown, J. B., see MacMahon, B. 178, *190*
Brown, J. B., see Strong, J. A. 178, *192*
Brown, J. E., see Wolpert, M. K. 393, *403*
Brown, J. H., Kennedy, B. J. 621, *621*
Brown, J. H. A., see Cueto, C. 809, *817*
Brown, J. H. U., Preedy, J. R. K., Brown, C. H., Hallman, B. L. 815, *817*
Brown, J. M., Goffinet, D. R., Cleaver, J. E., Kallman, R. F. 319, *329*

Brown, J.M., see Goffinet, D.R. 319, *334*
Brown, J.R., see Farnsworth, W.E. 149, *153*
Brown, McK., see Ben-Porat, T. 242, *249*
Brown, McK., see Kaplan, A.S. 241, 242, *252*
Brown, N.C., Eliasson, R., Reichard, P., Thelander, L. 790, *791*
Brown, N.C., see Krakoff, I.H. 790, *791*
Brown, N.C., see Nordenskjöld, B.A. 242, *254*
Brown, P.R., see Scholar, E.M. 391, *402*
Brown, R.R. 523, *530*
Brown, W.E., Wold, F. 73, *80*
Brownstone, A.D. 273, *329*
Brubacher, G.B., see Schwartz, D.E. 754, *764*
Brubaker, C.A., see Heyn, R.M. 397, *400*, 500, *506*
Bruce, J., see Strong, J.A. 178, *192*
Bruce, S.A., see Silagi, S. 311, *344*
Bruce, W.R. 469, *479*
Bruce, W.R., Meeker, B.E. 218, *223*
Bruce, W.R., Meeker, B.E., Valeriote, F.A. 21, *31*, 474, *479*, 494, *504*
Bruce, W.R., Valeriote, F.A. 76, *80*, 218, *223*
Bruce, W.R., see Borsa, J. 234, 238, *250*
Bruce, W.R., see Madoc-Jones, H. 217, 218, *228*
Bruce, W.R., see Rotenberg, A.D. 289, 314, *343*
Bruce, W.R., see Valeriote, F.A. 686, *694*
Bruchovsky, N., Owen, A.A., Becker, A.J., Till, J.E. 59, *60*, 674, *688*
Bruchovsky, N., Wilson, J.D. 85, *100*, 149, 150, *153*, 161, *167*, 177, *188*
Bruckner, H., see Zaharko, D.S. 473, *483*
Brues, A.M. 684, *688*
Brule, G., see Mathé, G. 759, *763*
Brune, K., see Floersheim, G.L. 752, *762*
Bruni, R., see Yesair, D.W. 608, 609, *614*
Brunnemann, A., Coper, H., Neubert, D. 541, *542*
Brunner, K.W., Young, C.W. 759, *761*
Bruns, R., see Kessel, D. 217, *227*
Brush, M.G., see Edwards, R. 160, *167*
Bryan, G.T., see Ansfield, F.J. 220, 221, *223*
Bryan, G.T., see Skibba, J.L. 71, *83*, 545, 546, 547, *552*
Bryan, J. 678, *688*
Bryan, J., see Wilson, L. 678, *694*
Bryant, B., see Holland, J.F. 769, *785*
Bryant, B.J. 314, *329*
Brykina, E.V., see Podobed, O.V. *669*
Bryson, M.J., see Sweat, M.L. 106, *136*
Bucci, S., see Fiume, L. *669*
Buchanan, J.M., see Dawid, I.B. 487, 488, *504*
Buchanan, J.M., see French, T.C. 487, 488, *505*
Buchanan, J.M., see Hartman, S.C. 486, 487, *505*
Buchanan, J.M., see Levenberg, B. 486, 487, 488, 490, 496, 497, *507*
Buchanan, J.M., see Schroeder, D.D. 496, 498, *509*
Buchanan, R.A., see Ch'ien, L.T. 428, *432*
Bucher, T., Sies, H. 554, *567*
Bucholz, E., see Burchenal, J.H. 779, *783*, 820, *826*
Buck, L.L., Pfau, C.J. 354, *364*
Buck, R.E., see Price, K.E. 496, *508*, 855, 862, *874*
Buckler, C.E., see Baron, S. 607, 608, *611*
Buckley, P., see Furusawa, E. 302, 307, *333*
Buděšínsky, Z., Jelínek, U., Přikryl, J. 196, *223*
Budke, L., see Bootsma, D. 604, *611*
Budman, D.R., Pardee, A.B. 290, *329*
Budy, A.M. 113, *126*
Bui, N.M., Gillett, R., Dumont, P. 273, *329*
Bujard, H., Heidelberger, C. 208, 214, *224*
Bukrinskaya, A.G., Asadullaev, T.A. 354, *364*
Bulaschenko, H., see Abelson, D. 814, *817*
Bulbrook, R.D., Greenwood, F.C. 178, *188*
Bulbrook, R.D., Greenwood, F.C., Hayward, J.L. 179, *188*
Bulbrook, R.D., see Deshpande, N. 117, *127*
Bulbrook, R.D., see Hayward, J.L. 179, *189*
Bull, F.E., see Coe, R.O. *480*
Bulloch, R.T., see Pearce, M.B. 560, *569*
Bullock, F.J., see Yesair, D.W. 608, 609, *614*
Bunting, S.L., see Dingman, C.W. 121, *128*
Burch, M.R., see Smith, C.G. 437, 440, 441, 445, *456*
Burchall, J.J. 469, *479*
Burchall, J.J., Hitchings, G.H. 469, *480*
Burchenal, J.H. 219
Burchenal, J.H., Adams, H., Lancaster, S., Hirt, R. 822, *826*
Burchenal, J.H., Adams, H.H., Newell, N.S., Fox, J.J. 198, *224*
Burchenal, J.H., Benvenisti, D., Steffa, M., Tallal, L., Tan, C. 799, *805*
Burchenal, J.H., Coley, V., Purple, J.R., Bucholz, E., Lyman, M.S., Kreis, W. 820, *826*
Burchenal, J.H., Dagg, M.K., Beyer, M., Stock, C.C. 544, 550, *550*
Burchenal, J.H., Dollinger, M.R. 264, *268*
Burchenal, J.H., Ellison, R.R., Murphy, M.L., Karnofsky, D.A., Sykes, M.P., Tan, T.C., Mermann, A.C., Yuceoglu, M., Myers, W.P.L., Krakoff, I., Alberstadt, N. 389, *398*
Burchenal, J.H., Greggs, V.C., Lancaster, S.P., Hirt, R., Berchtold, R., Fischer, R., Balsiger, R. 822, *826*
Burchenal, J.H., Holmberg, E.A.D., Fox, J.J., Hemphill, S.C., Reppert, J.A. 198, *224*
Burchenal, J.H., Lyman, M.S. 820, *826*

Burchenal, J.H., Lyman, M.S., Purple, J.R., Coley, V., Smith, S., Bucholz, E. 820, *826*
Burchenal, J.H., Murphy, M.L., Ellison, R.R., Sykes, M.P., Tan, T.C., Leone, L.A., Karnofsky, D.A., Craver, L.F., Dargeon, H.W., Rhoads, C.P. 384, 389, *398*
Burchenal, J.H., Oettgen, H.F., Reppert, J.A., Coley, V. *329*
Burchenal, J.H., Purple, J.R., Bucholz, E., Straub, P.W. 779, 783
Burchenal, J.H., Spooner, E., Lancaster, S. 822, *826*
Burchenal, J.H., Wiggins, R., Butterbaugh, J. 233, *250*
Burchenal, J.H., see Clarkson, B.D., 727, 728, 730, 732, *743*
Burchenal, J.H., see Dollinger, M.R. 233, 234, 239, *251*
Burchenal, J.H., see Duschinsky, R. 197, *225*
Burchenal, J.H., see Ellison, R.R. 394, *399*, 500, *504*
Burchenal, J.H., see Etcubanas, E. 793, 799, 800, *805*
Burchenal, J.H., see Hackethal, C.A. 638, *640*
Burchenal, J.H., see Haghbin, M. 726, 732, *744*
Burchenal, J.H., see Heyn, R.M. 397, *400*, 500, *506*
Burchenal, J.H., see Kreis, W. 758, *763*, 822, 824, *827*
Burchenal, J.H., see Louis, J. 820, *827*
Burchenal, J.H., see Lyman, M. 820, *827*
Burchenal, J.H., see Magill, G.B. 500, *507*
Burchenal, J.H., see Murphy, M.L. 394, *401*
Burchenal, J.H., see Oettgen, H.F. 727, 728, 730, 732, 734, 735, *745*, 820, *827*
Burchenal, J.H., see Old, L.J. 728, 733, *746*
Burchenal, J.H., see Tallal, L. 727, 728, 730, 732, *746*
Burchenal, J.H., see Yung, N.C. 196, *231*, 272, *347*
Burck, P.J., see Ho, P.P.K. 698, 699, 700, 702, 708, *716*
Burdeshaw, J.A., see Wilkoff, L.J. 235, *256*, 260, 263, *271*, 494, *511*
Burdman, J., see Journey, L.J. 673, 674, *691*
Bures, O.M., see Del Puerto, B.M. 560, *568*
Burford, B.O., see Sanders, F.K. 78, *83*
Burg, R.W., see Gitterman, C.O. 661, *665*
Burgen, M.W., see Cooper, A.D. 309, *330*
Burgi, E., see Elion, G.B. 389, *399*, 459, *465*
Burgio, G.R., Astaldi, A., Jr., Krč, J., Astaldi, G. 735, *743*
Burgio, G.R., Astaldi, A., Jr., Krč, I., Micu, D., Astaldi, G. 706, 707, *714*
Burgio, G.R., see Astaldi, G. 526, *529*
Burgio, G.R., see Astaldi, G. 706, *713*, 735, *742*
Burgio, G.R., see De Barbieri, A. 706, *715*
Burgoyne, L.A., see Waqar, M.A. 660, *668*
Burk, D., Evans, W., Hunter, J., Woods, M. 776, *783*
Burk, D., see Lineweaver, H. 115, *132*
Burk, D., see Woods, M. *543*
Burka, B., Herman, E.H., Vick, J. 609, *611*
Burke, D.C., see Bergmann, W. 232, *249*, 426, *431*
Burke, K., see Heiniger, H.J. 314, *335*
Burke, P.J., McCarthy, W.H., Milton, G.W. 545, *550*
Burke, P.J., Serpick, A.A., Carbone, P.P., Tarr, N.A. 260, 261, 262, *268*
Burke, P.J., see Henderson, E.S. 261, *269*
Burke, P.J., see Steuart, C.D. 247, *255*, 265, *271*
Burkhardt, F., see Brossi, A. 563, *567*
Burki, K., Shaer, J.C., Schindler, R. 318, *329*
Burkitt, D.P. 476, 478, *480*
Burman, P.R. 458, *465*
Burnett, J.P., Jr., see Johnson, I.S. 671, 675, 679, 682, 685, 686, 687, *691*
Burningham, R., see Ohnuma, T. 726, 727, 728, 734, 735, *746*
Burns, J., see Pittillo, R.F. 79, *82*, 494, *508*
Burrage, K., see Hellmann, K. 885, 886, *889*
Burris, R.H., see Delhumeau-Arrecillas, G. 493, *504*
Burrows, H. 175, *188*
Burrows, J.H., Talley, R.W., Drake, E.H., San Diego, F.J., Tucker, W.G. 478, *480*
Burson, G., see Roberts, J. 698, *720*
Burstein, S., Gut, M. 139, *153*
Burstein, S., Klaiber, E.L. 813, *817*
Busch, H., see Choi, Y.C. 584, *590*
Busch, H., see Desjardins, R. 680, *689*
Busch, H., see Smith, S.J. 25, *33*
Busch, K.A., see Katchman, B.J. 25, *32*
Buselmeier, T.J., see Simmons, R.L. 414, *424*
Bush, P.S., see Kimball, A.P. 234, 241, *253*, 429, *432*
Bushby, S.R.M., see Barrett, P.A. 841, *847*
Bushnell, D.E., see Butcher, F.R. *669*
Buskirk, H.H., Crim, J.A., Petering, H.G., Merritt, K., Johnson, A.G. 24, *31*, 237, *250*, 525, *530*
Buskirk, H.H., see Li, L.H. 362, *367*
Buskirk, H.H., see Petering, H.G. 841, 842, 843, 844, *848*, *849*
Buskirk, H.H., see Smith, C.G. 238, *255*
Bussard, A., Naono, S., Gros, F., Monod, J. 212, *224*
Busse, V., see Hampel, K.E. 415, *421*
Bussel, A., see Jacquillat, C. 726, 727, 728, 732, 734, 735, *744*
Butcher, F.R., Bushnell, D.E., Becker, J.E., Potter, V.R. *669*
Butel, J.S., see Rapp, F. 302, 303, 304, *343*

Butenandt, A. 104, *126*, 170, *188*
Buthala, D.A. 237, *250*
Butler, G.C., see Gimlin, D.M. 308, *334*
Butler, K., see Beereboom, J.J. 565, *567*
Butler, T.P., Pearson, O.H. 112, *127*
Butler, T.P., see Pearson, O.H. 112, *134*, 174, 183, *191*
Butler, W.W.S., Schade, A.L. 151, *153*
Butterbaugh, J., see Burchenal, J.H. 233, *250*
Buttoo, A.S., Israëls, M.C.G., Wilkinson, J.F. 352, 356, 359, *364*
Buttoo, A.S., see Elves, M.W. 361, *365*
Byrd, B.L., see Hayes, R.L. 879, *888*
Byrd, D.M. 326, *329*
Byvoet, P., see Clarkson, D.R. 283, 284, *330*
Bzeszotarski, W., see Baker, B.R. 289, *327*

Caballes, L., see Dave, C. 771, 774, 775, *784*
Cahn, R.D., see Lasher, R. 311, *339*
Cain, B.F., Atwell, G.J., Seelye, R.N. 783, *783*
Cain, B.F., see Atwell, G.J. 820, *826*
Cain, J.C., see Merits, I. 284, *340*
Calabresi, P. 313, 324, *329*
Calabresi, P., Cardoso, S.C., Finch, S.C., Kligerman, M.M., von Essen, C.F., Chu, M.Y., Welch, A.D. 283, 284, 314, 319, 323, 324, *329*
Calabresi, P., Creasey, W.A., Prusoff, W.H., Welch, A.D. 238, *250*, 302, 323, *329*
Calabresi, P., McCollum, R.W., Welch, A.D. 291, 324, *329*
Calabresi, P., Turner, R.W. 361, *364*
Calabresi, P., Welch, A.D. 324, *329*
Calabresi, P., see Bertino, J.R. 473, *479*
Calabresi, P., see Conn, H.O. 355, *365*
Calabresi, P., see Creasey, W.A. 234, 238, 240, 241, 242, 244, *251*, 258, 259, *268*, 359, *365*
Calabresi, P., see DeConti, R.C. 361, *365*
Calabresi, P., see Handschumacher, R.E. 355, 358, 359, 360, 361, *366*
Calabresi, P., see Heppner, G.H. 237, *252*
Calabresi, P., see Huebner, R.J. 308, *336*
Calabresi, P., see Kaplan, S.R. 264, *270*, 502, *506*
Calabresi, P., see Lefkowitz, E.R. 389, *400*, 500, *507*
Calabresi, P., see Mark, J.B.D. 313, *340*
Calabresi, P., see Mitchell, M.S. 237, *253*
Calabresi, P., see Papac, R.J. 236, 238, *254*
Calabresi, P., see Rosenberg, S. 502, *509*
Calabresi, P., see Turner, R.W. 361, *371*
Calabresi, P., see Vogel, C.L. 502, *511*
Caldarera, C.M., Barbiroli, B., Moruzzi, G. 148, *153*, 774, *783*
Caldarera, C.M., Moruzzi, M.S., Barbiroli, B., Moruzzi, G. 148, *153*
Calderella, L.A., see Oleson, J.J. 496, *508*, 633, *641*
Caldwell, I., see Lett, J.T. 319, *339*
Caldwell, I.C. 385, 386, *398*
Caldwell, I.C., Henderson, J.F., Paterson, A.R.P. 368, *398*, 442, 444, *453*
Caldwell, I.C., see Henderson, J.F. 368, *400*, 442, 445, *453*
Caldwell, M.J., see Monto, R.W. 621, *622*
Calendi, E. 608
Calendi, E., Dettori, R., Neri, M.G. 606, *611*
Calendi, E., DiMarco, A., Reggiani, M., Scarpinato, B., Valentini, L. 598, 599, *611*
Calendi, E., see Rusconi, A. 601, 602, 603, 608, *613*
Calhoun, D.W., see Edgren, R.A. 110, *128*
Calkins, D.F., see Reist, E.J. 431, *433*
Call, J.B., see Gottlieb, J.A. 650, *655*
Call, J.B., see Guarino, A.M. 709, *716*
Call, J.B., see Hart, L.G. 650, *655*
Callahan, see Yesair, D.W. 825
Callahan, S.W., see Elion, G.B. 384, 387, 389, *399* 404, 408, 409, 410, 411, *420*
Callantine, M.R., see Reel, J.R. 158, *168*
Callentine, M.R., Humphrey, R.R., Lee, S.L., Windsor, B.L., Schottin, N.H., O'Brien, O.P. 110, *127*
Callentine, M.R., Humphrey, R.R., Nesset, B.L. 109, *127*
Calne, R.Y. 407, 410, 414, *419*
Calne, R.Y., Alexandre, G.P.J., Murray, J.E. 409 *420*
Calvin, M., see Barker, S.A. 493, *503*
Camargo, E.P., Plant, W.J. 583, *590*
Came, P., see Lyons, M.J. 306, *340*
Camerman, N., Trotter, J. 279, 286, *329*
Camiener, G.W. 239, *250* 262, 268
Camiener, G.W., Smith, C.G. 238, 239, *250*, 259, 262, 266, *268*
Camiener, G.W., see Gray, G.D. 237, *252*, 630, 631, *632*
Camiener, G.W., see Owen, S.P. 565, *569*
Cammack, K.A., see Miller, D.S. 699, 700, *718*
Cammack, K.A., see North, A.C.T. 699, *719*, 724, *745*
Campbell, H.A., Mashburn, L.T. 701, *714*
Campbell, H.A., Mashburn, L.T., Boyse, E.A., Old, L.J. 698, 701, *714*, 723, *743*
Campbell, H.A., see Boyse, E.A. 704, *714*, 723, *743*
Campbell, H.A., see Kim, J.H. 738, *745*
Campbell, H.A., see Oettgen, H.F. 696, *719*, 723 727, 730, 733, 734, *745*
Campbell, H.A., see Old, L.J. 695, 696, 697, *719*, 723, 728, *746*
Campbell, H.F., see Wani, M.C. 650, *656*

Campbell, L. A., see Ahearn, M. J. 236, *249*
Campbell, L. D., Yu, J. Y.-L., Stothers, S. C., Marquardt, R. R. 125 *127*
Canavese, B., see Barasa, A. 675, *688*
Canellakis, E. S. 274, *329*
Canellakis, E. S., Gottesman, M. E., Kammen, H. O. 274, *329*
Canellakis, E. S., Mantsavinos, R. 274, *329*
Canellos, G. P., Haskell, C. M. 711, *714*, 733, *743*
Canellos, G. P., Haskell, C. M., Arseneau, J., Carbone, P.P. 709, *714*, 735, *743*
Canellos, G. P., see Arseneau, J. 879, *887*
Canellos, G. P., see Brown, C. H., III. 708, *714*
Canellos, G. P., see Haskell, C. M. 733, *744*
Canellos, G. P., see Haskell, C. M. 491, *505*, 514, *532*, 704, 711, *716*, 734, 735, *744*
Caner, J. E. Z. 675, *688*
Cann, M. C., see Heard, R. D. 106, *130*
Cannalakis, E. S., see Reichard, P. 243, *254*
Cannalakis, Z. N., see Reichard, P. 243, *254*
Cannon, P. R. 525, *530*
Cannon, P. R., Wissler, R. W., Woolridge, R. L., Benditt, E. P. 526, *530*
Cantarow, A., see Rutman, R. J. 193, *230*, 283, *343*
Cantell, K., see Paucker, K. 607, *613*
Cantelmo, F., see Heiniger, H. J. 314, *335*
Capek, K., see Baer, H. H. 593, *611*
Čapek R., see Bauer, V. 359, *364*
Čapek, R., see Janků, I. 349, 359, *367*
Capizzi, R. L. 471, 475, *480*
Capizzi, R. L., Bertino, J. R. 479, *480*
Capizzi, R. L., Bertino, J. R., Handschumacher, R. E. 705, *715*, 723, 735, *743*
Capizzi, R. L., DeConti, R. C., Marsh, J. C., Bertino, J. R. 477, *480*
Capizzi, R. L., Peterson, R., Cooney, D. A., Creasey, W. A., Handschumacher, R. E. 725, 726, 733, 734, *743*
Capizzi, R. L., Summers, W. P., Bertino, J. R. *480*
Capizzi, R. L., see Cooney, D. A. 514, *530*, 696, 703, *715*, 725, *743*
Capizzi, R. L., see Creasey, W. A. 795, 799, 800, 801, 802, *805*
Capizzi, R. L., see Nahas, A. 470, *482*
Caplan, R. M., Dossetor, J. B., Maughan, G. B. 415, *420*
Carabasi, R., see Segaloff, A. 184, *191*
Caraceni, C. E., see Brambilla, G. 705, *714*
Caragay, A., see Yesair, D. W. 822, 823, *828*
Carbone, P. P., Frei, E., III., Owens, A. H., Jr., Olson, K. B., Miller, S. P. 394, *398*
Carbone, P. P., Haskell, C. M., Leventhal, B. G., Block, J. B., Selawry, O. S. 726, 727, 728, 730, 732, 734, 735, *743*
Carbone, P. P., see Abraham, D. 747, *760*
Carbone, P. P., see Bell, W. R. 236, *249*, 261, *267*
Carbone, P. P., see Block, J. B. 236, *249*, 261, *267*
Carbone, P. P., see Brown, C. H., III. 708, *714*
Carbone, P. P., see Burke, P. J. 260, 261, 262, *268*
Carbone, P. P., see Canellos, G. P. 709, *714*, 735, *743*
Carbone, P. P., see DeVita, V. T. 759, 760, *762*
Carbone, P. P., see Fishbein, W. N. 521, *531*
Carbone, P. P., see Gailani, S. D. 685, *690*
Carbone, P. P., see Haskell, C. M. 734, 735, *744*
Carbone, P. P., see Hersh, E. M. 770, *785*
Carbone, P. P., see Vogel, C. L. 549, *553*
Cardani, C., Ghiringhelli, D., Mondelli, R., Quilico, A. 566, *567*
Cardeilhac, P. T., Cohen, S. S. 243, 244, *250*
Cardinali, G., Cardinali, G., Centurelli, G. 674, *688*
Cardinali, G., Cardinali, G., Handler, A. H., Agrifoglio, M. F. 673, *688*
Cardinali, G., see Cardinali, G. 674, *688*
Cardoso, S., see Haus, E. 249, *252*
Cardoso, S. C., see Calabresi, P. 283, 284, 314, 319, 323, 324, *329*
Cardoso, S. S., see Grisolia, S. 283, *334*
Carey, R. W., Ellison, R. R. 260, 261, *268*
Carey, R. W., see Krant, M. J. 523, *533*
Carey, T., Mawas, C., Kitano, M., Mihich, E. 768 *783*
Cargille, C. M., see Ross, G. T. 160, *168*
Carim, H., see Djerassi, I. 478, *480*
Carlo, P. E., Mandel, H. G. 459, *465*
Carlsen, E. N., Trelle, G. J., Schjeide, O. A. 121, *127*
Carlsen, E. N., see Schjeide, O. A. 120, *135*
Carlsen, R. A., see Morris, J. M. 357, *368*
Carlson, K., see Olmsted, J. B. 678, *692*
Carlson, K., see Rosenbaum, J. L. 676, *693*
Carlson, R. G., see Smith, C. G. 437, 445, *456*
Carlson, R. G., see Talley, R. W. 451, *456*
Carlton, J. E., see Hayes, R. L. 879, *888*
Carman, W. W., see Newell, G. W. 499, *508*
Carminatti, H., see DeAsua, L. J. 124, 125, *127*
Carniti, G., see Arioli, V. 883, *887*
Caron, E. L., see Wiley, P. F. 623, *632*
Caron, E. L., Jr., see Wiley, P. F. 623, *632*
Carpenter, A., see Constantopoulos, G. 139, *153*
Carpenter, C. B., see Hirsch, M. S. 418, *421*
Carpenter, C. B., see Murray, J. E. 502, *508*
Carpenter, D. G., see Nyhan, W. L. 414, *423*
Carr, H. S., see Rosenkranz, H. S. 73, *83*, 522, *535*
Carr, J. G., see Auerbach, C. 21, *30*
Carrasco, L., Vazquez, D. 567, *567*

Carrese, M., see Nervi, C. 478, *482*
Carrier, E., see Stein, K. F. 145, *156*
Carrier, W. L., see Setlow, R. B. 12, *17*, 52, *62*
Carrington, L. O., see Elion, G. B. 412, 413, *420*
Carrington, M. J., see Hilf, R. 123, *130*
Carter, C. E., see Greenstein, J. P. 238, *252*, 697, *716*
Carter, C. H., see Nyhan, W. L. 414, *423*
Carter, H. A., see Kruse, P. F., Jr. 515, 525, *533*
Carter, S. B., Franklin, T. J., Jones, D. F., Leonard, B. J., Mills, S. D., Turner, R. W., Turner, W. B. 446, 450, 451, *453*
Carter, S. K. 48, *60*, 193, 219, *224*, 496, *504*, 747, *761*
Carter, S. K., Livingston, R. B. 261, *268*
Carter, S. K., Schabel, F. M., Jr., Broder, L., Johnston, T. P. 65, *80*
Carter, S. K., see Livingston, R. B. 19, *32*, 232, *253*, 261, *270*, 477, *482*, 485, 500, *507*, 589, *591*
Cartwright, G. E., see Clarysse, A. M. *480*
Cartwright, G. E., see Mauer, A. M. 23, *33*
Carvalho, A. R. L. de, see De Barros, T. 696, *715*
Carvalho, R. P. S., see Dalldorf, G. 417, *420*
Casale, C., see Nervi, C. 478, *482*
Casazza, A. M., DiMarco, A., DiCuonzo, G. 597, 610, *611*
Casazza, A. M., Scarpinato, B., DiCuonzo, G. 597, 610, *611*
Casazza, A. M., Silvestrini, R., Gambarucci, C. 607 610, *611*
Casazza, A. M., see DiMarco, A. 597, *612*
Casazza, A. M., see Verini, M. A. 608, *613*
Casey, T. P. 417, *420*
Cashmore, A. R., see Bertino, J. R. 468, 472, 473, *479*, 775, *783*
Cashmore, A. R., see Chello, P. 469, *480*
Cashmore, A. R., see Johns, D. G. 472, 473, *481*
Casida, J. E., see Nizhizawa, Y. 197, *229*
Caskey, C. T., Ashton, D. M., Wyngaarden, J. B. 390, *398*
Caskey, C. T., Beaudet, A. L. 561, *568*
Caspersson, T., Farber, S., Foley, G. E., Killander, D. 21, *31*
Caspersson, T., Farber, S., Foley, G. E., Kudynowski, J., Modest, E. J., Simonsson, E., Wagh, U., Zech, L. 6, *15*
Cassell, E., see Meites, J. 174, *191*
Cassidy, E. P., see Fischer, D. S. 237, *251*, 309, 323, *333*, 356, 362, *366*
Cassidy, F. R., see Bateman, J. R. 221, *223*
Cassinelli, G., see Arcamone, F. 593, *611*
Cassouto, J., see Gallagher, T. F. 178, *189*
Cassouto, J., see Zumoff, B. 178, *192*
Castagnone, D., see Bonmassar, E. 528, *530*
Cate, T. R., see Knight, V. *338*
Cathey, W. J., see Clarysse, A. M. *480*
Cattan, A., see Mathé, G. 685, *692*, 759, *763*, 772, *786*
Cattan, A., see Schwarzenberg, L. 474, *482*
Caudi, R. B., see Knight, V. *338*
Cavalieri, L. F. 868, *871*
Cavalieri, L. F., see Brown, G. B. 458, *465*
Cavalieri, L. F., see Sugiura, K. 459, *467*
Cavallini, G., Massarani, E., Nardi, D., Mauri, L., Mantegazza, P. 779, *783*
Cavanna, M., see Baldini, L. 237, *249*
Cavanna, M., see Brambilla, G. 527, *530*, 705, *714*
Cavins, J. A., Hall, T. C., Olson, K. B., Khung, C. L., Horton, J., Colsky, J., Shadduck, R. K. 440 *453*
Cazorla, A., Moncloa, F. 810, 812, *817*
Cecil, H. C., Bitman, J. 125, *127*
Cecil, H. C., see Bitman, J. 125, *126*
Cedar, H., Schwartz, J. H. 698, *715*
Cedar, H., see Ehrman, M. 697, 701, *715*
Cedar, H., see Schwartz, J. H. 515, *536*
Celi, M. L., see Bonmassar, E. 527, 528, *530*
Centurelli, G., see Cardinali, G. 674, *688*
Ceprini, M. Q., see Stefanović, V. 647, *648*
Cerami, A., Reich, E., Ward, D. C., Goldberg, I. H. 585, *590*
Cerami, A., see Reich, E. 573, *580*
Cerami, A., see Ward, D. C. 442, 443, *456*
Cerdá-Olmeda, E., Hanawalt, P. C., Guerola, N. 8, *15*
Čerey, K., Elis, J., Raškorá, H. 350, *364*
Cerilli, G. J., Gideon, L. 752, *761*
Cerletti, A., see Stähelin, H. 675, 684, *693*
Černěckij, V., Chládek, S., Šorm, F., Smrt, J. 349, *364*
Černěckij, V., see Šorm, F. *370*
Černoch, A., see Šmahel, O. 361, *370*
Cestari, A., Concilio, C., Dessi, P., Rizzoli, C. 522, *530*
Cestari, A., see Rizzoli, C. 522, *535*
Cevik, W., see Howard, J. P. 261, *269*
Cha, S., Parks, R. E., Jr. 461, *465*
Chabner, B. A., DeVita, V. T., Considine, N., Oliverio, V. T. 751, 752, 754, 756, *761*
Chabaud, J. P., see DeSombre, E. R. 115, *127*
Chacko, S., Holtzer, S., Holtzer, H. 311, *329*
Chacko, S., see Anderson, H. C. 311, *327*
Chacko, S., see Holthausen, H. S. 311, *335*
Chadwick, M., Platz, B. B., Liss, R. H. 881, *888*
Chadwick, M., Rogers, W. L. 216, *224*
Chagoya, V., see Green, M. *334*
Chaiken, S. J., see Jondorf, W. R. 824, *827*
Chaikoff, I. L., see Goldberg, R. C. 171, *189*

Chakrabarty, A.K., Friedman, H. 705, *715*
Chakrabarty, A.M., see Basu, S.K. 56, *60*
Chakraborty, K.P., Hurlbert, R.B. 490, *504*
Chalkley, H.W., see Greenstein, J.P. 238, *252*
Chalkley, R., see Jackson, V. 825, *827*
Chalmers, A.H., Knight, P. R., Atkinson, M.R. 411, 412, *420*
Chamberlain, J.G. 542, *542*
Chamness, G.C., see McGuire, W.L. 99, *102*, 117, *133*
Champe, S.P., Benzer, S. 214, *224*
Chan, C.C., see MacDonald, A.S. 752, *763*
Chan, G.Y., Stone, R.L. 405, *420*
Chan, S.C., Leh, F. 68, *80*
Chandra, P., Zunio, F., Götz, A., Gericke, D., Thorbeck, R., Di Marco, A. 602, 608, *611*
Chandross, R., Rich, A. 197, *224*
Chanes, R.E., see Condit, P. T. 473, *480*
Chaney, N.A., see Hardesty, C.T. 881, *888*
Chaney, P.L., Marbach, E. P. 696, *715*
Chang, C., see Bořkovec, A.B. 644, *647*
Chang, C., see Horwitz, S.B. 578, *579*, 644, 646, *647*, 649, 651, 652, 653, 654, *655*, 860, *872*
Chang, E., Dao, T.L., Mittelman, A. 178, *188*
Chang, E., Mittelman, A., Rosen, F. 99, *100*
Chang, P., see Voytek, P. 281, 285, 286, 287, 320, 322, 325, *346*
Chang, P.K. 273, 274, *329*
Chang, P.K., Welch, A.D. 272, 273, 291, *329*
Chang, P.K., see Cramer, J. W. 291, *330*
Chang, P.K., see Handschumacher, R.E. 515, *532*
Chang, P.K., see Johns, D. G. 472, *481*
Chang, P.K., see Prusoff, W.H. 282, 287, *342*
Chang, T.M.S. 705, *715*
Chantrenne, H., Devreux, S. 463, *465*
Chany, C., Brailovsky, C. 607, *611*
Chao, W.R., see Peters, J. H. 697, *720*
Charache, S., Condit, P.T. Humphreys, S.R. 472 *480*
Chargaff, E., see Andoh, T. 206, 210, *223*
Chargaff, E., see Horowitz, J. 206, 208, 211, 212, *226*
Chargaff, E., see Levine, C. 824, *827*
Charipper, H.A., see Finkelstein, G. 145, *153*
Charipper, H.A., see Vollmer, E.P. 145, *157*
Chassagne, J., see Beljanski, M. 376, *381*
Chassy, B.M., Sugimori, T., Suhadolnik, R.J. 447, *453*
Chassy, B.M., Suhadolnik, R.J. 440, *453*, 658, 659, *665*
Chassy, B.M., see Suhadolnik, R.J. 437, 440, *456*, 658, 659, 661, *667*, *668*
Chatterton, R.T., Jr. *167*
Chattopadhyay, S.K., see Hasselberger, F.X. 724, 735, *744*
Chaube, S., see Murphy, M.L. 790, *791*
Chaube, S., Kreis, W., Uchida, K., Murphy, M. L. 237, 244, *250*, 261, *268*
Chaube, S., Lacon, C., Simmel, E. 790, *791*
Chaube, S., Murphy, M.L. 200, *224*, 310, *329*, 752, *761*, *762*, 790, *791*
Chaudhuri, N.K., Montag, B.J., Heidelberger, C. 202, 207, 208, 219, *224*
Chaudhuri, N.K., Mukherjee, K.L., Heidelberger, C. 202, 215, *224*, 283, *329*
Chaudhuri, N.K., see Harbers, E. 202, 203, 206, 208, 211, *225*
Chaudhuri, N.K., see Heidelberger, C. 193, 198, *226*
Chaudhury, R.R., see Saksena, S.K. 357, *369*
Chavanich, S., see Schluederberg, A. 584, *592*
Chayen, J., Gahan, P.B., Lacour, L.F. 824, *826*
Chayen, R., see Altmann, F. P. 824, *826*
Cheer, S., Tchen, T.T. 56, *60*
Cheers, C., see Miller, J.F. A.P. 405, *422*
Chello, P., Cashmore, A.R., Jacobs, S.A., Bertino, J. R. 469, *480*
Chen, F.P., see Mellett, L. B. 259, *270*
Chen, Y.T., see Norton, S. J. 515, *534*
Cheng, C.C., see Baiocchi, F. 768, *783*
Cheng, C.C., see Liao, T.K. 650, *656*, 768, *786*
Cheng, C.C., see Noell, C.W. 549, *551*
Cheng, C.C., see Podrebarac, E.G. 768, *787*
Cheng, C.C., see Zee-Cheng, K.Y. 523, *538*
Cheng, C.J., Fujimura, S., Grunberger, D., Weinstein, I.B. 68, 70, *80*
Cheong, L., Rich, M.A., Eidinoff, M.L. 272, 273, 298, *329*
Cheong, L., see Eidinoff, M. L. 283, 295, 314, *332*, 490, *504*
Cheong, L., see Rich, M.A. 199, *229*
Chermburkar, P.B., see Garrett, E.R. 275, 276, *333*
Chevremont, M. 40, *42*
Chibata, I., see Abe, M. 522, *529*
Chibnall, A.C., see Grover, C.E. 697, *716*
Chieli, T., see Bertazzoli, C. 609, 610, *611*
Ch'ien, L.T., Glazko, A.J., Buchanan, R.A., Alford, C.A. 428, *432*
Chiga, M., see Parkin, I.L. 59, *62*
Chimura, H., see Umezawa, H. *875*
Chin, M.L., see Notari, R.E. 232, *254*
Chiu, H., see Malamud, D. 410, *422*
Chiu, Y.W., see Hollander, N. 98, 99, *101*
Chládek, S., see Černěckij, V. 349, *364*
Chmielewicz, Z.F., see Bardos, T.J. 20, 29, *30*
Choi, Y.C., Busch, H. 584, *590*

Chorin, V. A., Rossolimo, O. K. 618, 619, 620, *621*
Chorin, V. A., Rossolimo, O. K., Stanislavskaya, M. S., Blumberg, N. A., Filiposyan, S. T., Lepeshkina, G. N. 617, *621*
Chorin, V. A., Shapovalova, S. P. 616, *621*
Chou, T. C., Handschumacher, R. E. 712, 713, *715*
Chou, T. C., see Creasey, W. A. 678, *689*
Christensen, A. K., see Palmiter, R. 121, *134*
Christensen, H. N., Jones, J. C. 523, *530*
Christie, N. T., see Brewen, J. G. 236, *250*, 261, *268*
Chu, E. H. Y. 261, *268*
Chu, E. H. Y., see Smith, D. B. 246, 247, *255*
Chu, L. C., see DeMiranda, P. 412, *420*
Chu, L. L. H., Edelman, I. S. *669*
Chu, L. L. H., see Swaneck, G. E. 164, *168*
Chu, M. Y. 245, *250*
Chu, M. Y., Fischer, G. A. 233, 235, 240, 241, 242, 244, 245, 246, *250*, 261, 264, *268*
Chu, M. Y., see Calabresi, P. 283, 284, 314, 319, 323, 324, *329*
Chu, M. Y., see Momparler, R. L. 247, *253*, 265, *270*
Chu, S. Y., see Henderson, J. F. 386, *400*
Chua, J., see Horwitz, J. P. 273, *336*, 662, *666*
Chumley, S., see Bennett, L. L., Jr. 386, *398*
Chumley, S., see Brockman, R. W. 390, 391, *398*, 487, *503*
Chumley, S., see Wheeler, G. P. 68, *84*
Chun, E. H. L., Gonzales, L., Lewis, F. S., Jones, J., Rutman, R. J. 14, *15*, 28, *31*
Chung, L., Gabourel, J. D. 681, *688*
Church, R. B., see Hahn, W. E. 121, *129*, 165, *167*
Church, R. H., McCarthy, B. J. 119, *127*
Chutkov, N. A., see Terskikh, I. I. 354, *371*
Chytil, F., see Spelsberg, T. C. *168*
Ciampor, F., see Omelchenkov, T. N. 302, 304, 307, *341*
Ciaranfi, E., see De-Angeli, L. C. 697, *715*
Ciegler, A., see Peterson, R. E. 697, 698, *720*
Ciferri, O., see Perani, A. 566, *569*
Čihák, A., Brouček, J. 362, 363, *364*
Čihák, A., Seifertová, M., Veselý, J. 363, *364*
Čihák, A., Škoda, J., Šorm, F. 350, *364*
Čihák, A., Šorm, F. 351, 361, *364*
Čihák, A., Veselý, J., Šorm, F. 362, 363, *364*, *365*
Čihák, A., Veselý, J., Inoue, H., Pitot, H. C. 363, *365*
Čihák, A., Wilkinson, D., Pitot, H. C., 213, *224*
Čihák, A., see Seifertová, M. *370*
Čihák, A., see Škoda, J. 350, *370*
Čihák, A., see Šorm, F. 351, 362, *370*
Čihák, A., see Veselý, J. 351, 362, 363, *371*
Čihák, A., see Wilkinson, D. S. 206, 207, 210, 211, 213, *231*
Ciotti, M. M., see Zatman, L. J. 540, *543*
Ciotti, M. R., see Kaplan, N. O. 540, *543*
Citri, N., see Zyk, N. 449, *457*
Clancy, T. P., see Levin, V. A. 69, *81*
Clapper, G. 869
Clapper, G., see Pietsch, P. 855, 858, 863, 871, *874*
Clark, D. A., see Stinson, E. B. 416, *424*
Clark, I., Stoerk, H. C. 86, *100*
Clark, J., see Meites, J. 174, *191*
Clark, J. H., Gorski, J. 115, 116, *127*
Clark, J. J., see Duncan, G. W. 110, *128*
Clark, N. B. 120, *127*
Clark, P. J., see Huggins, C. 170, 172, *189*
Clark, W. R., see Rutter, W. J. 311, *343*
Clarke, D. A., Barclay, R. K., Stock, C. C., Rondestvedt, C. S., Jr. 544, *550*
Clarke, D. A., Philips, F. S., Sternberg, S. S., Stock, C. C., Elion, G. B., Hitchings, G. H. 396, *398*
Clarke, D. A., Reilly, H. C., Stock, C. C. 391, *398*, 500, 501, *504*
Clarke, D. A., see Philips, F. S. 389, 394, *401*
Clarke, M. L., see Barrett, P. A. 841, *847*
Clarke, R. R., see Fine, R. N. 687, *690*
Clarke, V. D., Blair, D. M., Weber, M. C. 879, *888*
Clarkson, B., O'Connor, A., Winston, L., Hutchison, D. 222, *224*
Clarkson, B. D., Krakoff, I. H., Burchenal, J. H., Karnofsky, D. A., Golbey, R. B., Dowling, M. D., Oettgen, H. F., Lipton, A. 727, 728, 730, 732, *743*
Clarkson, B. D., see Gee, T. S. *269*, 394, 397, *399*
Clarkson, B. D., see Karnofsky, D. A. 458, *466*
Clarkson, B. D., see Oettgen, H. F. 696, *719*, 723, 727, 728, 730, 733, 734, 735, *745*
Clarkson, B. D., see Van Dyk, J. J. 197, *231*
Clarkson, D. R., Oppelt, W. W., Byvoet, P. 283, 284, *330*
Clarkson, D. R., see Oppelt, W. W. 282, *341*
Clarysse, A., see Mathé, G. 726, 727, 728, 732, 734, 735, *745*
Clarysse, A. M., Cathey, W. J., Cartwright, G. E., Wintrobe, M. N. *480*
Claybourn, B. E., see Hadler, H. I. 374, *381*
Clayton, J. D., see Shealy, Y. F. 434, *455*, 549, *552*
Clayton, S. J., see Shealy, Y. F. 550, *552*
Cleare, M. J., Hoeschele, J. D. 838, *839*
Cleaver, J. E. 242, *250*
Cleaver, J. E., see Brown, J. M. 319, *329*
Clegg, R. E., Sanford, R. E., Hein, P. E., Andrews, R. E., Hughes, A. C., Mueller, C. D. 120, *127*
Clement, D., see Kaplan, S. R. 264, *270*
Clementi, A. 695, 697, *715*
Clermont, Y., Harvey, S. C. 23, *31*

Clermont, Y., see Leblond, C.P. 37, *44*
Cleveland, J.C., Johns, D. G., Farnham, G., Bertino, J.R. 474, 478, *480*
Clifford, G.O., see Bettigole, R.E. 735, *743*
Clifford, G.O., see Karnofsky, D.A. 512, *532*
Clifford, P., see Oettgen, H. F. 820, *827*
Clifton, K.H., Szybalski, W., Heidelberger, C., Gollin, F.F., Ansfield, F. J., Vermund, H. 289, 291, *330*
Clifton, K.H., Yatvin, M.B. 314, 316, 318, *330*
Cline, J.C., see Williams, R. H. 446, *457*
Cline, M.J. 246, *250*, 680, 681, 682, *688*
Cline, M.J., Rosenbaum, E. 246, *250*
Cline, R.E., see Fink, K. 283, *333*
Close, H., see Lyman, M. 820, *827*
Coddington, A. 658, *665*
Coe, R.O., Bull, F.E. *480*
Coffey, D.S., Ichinose, R. R., Shimazaki, J. Williams-Ashman, H.G. 151, *153*
Coffey, J.J., Kelley, S.A., Palm, P.E., Mead, J.A. R., Kensler, C.J. 800 802, *805*
Coffey, J.J., Palm, P.E., Denine, E.P., Baronowsky, P.E., Kensler, C.J. 523, *530*
Coggin, J.H., Larson, V.M., Hilleman, M.R. 298, 308, *330*
Coggin, J.H., Jr., Martin, W. R. 491, 495, *504*
Coggin, L., see Moulton, J. 302, *341*
Cohen, A., Harley, E.M., Ress, K.E. 607, *611*
Cohen, A., see Crook, L.E. 573, *579*
Cohen, J.L., Krant, M.J., Shnider, B.I., Matias, P. I., Horton, J., Baxter, D. 221, *224*
Cohen, L.H., Parks, R.E., Jr. 461, *465*
Cohen, L.S., Studzinski, G. P. 21, *31*
Cohen, L.S., see Studzinski, G.P. 54, *63*
Cohen, M.H., see Muggia, F. M. 650, *656*
Cohen, M.M., Shaw, M.W. 56, *60*
Cohen, M.M., Shaw, M.W., Craig, A.P. 634, *640*
Cohen, M.M., see Shaw, M. W. 57, *62*
Cohen, N., see Hilf, R. 124, *130*
Cohen, R.A., see Rawls, W. F. 302, *343*
Cohen, S. 470, *480*
Cohen, S.S. 232, 234, 244, *250*, *330*, 426, *432*, 766, 774, *784*
Cohen, S.S., Barner, H.D. 21, *31*
Cohen, S.S., Flaks, J.G., Barner, H.D., Loeb, M. R., Lichtenstein, J. 199, 203, 204, 218, *224*, 289, *330*
Cohen, S.S., see Cardeilhac, P.T. 243, 244, *250*
Cohen, S.S., see Doering, A. M. 244, *251*, 662, *665*
Cohen, S.S., see Furth, J.J. 241, 243, 244, *251*, 261, *269*, 427, *432*
Cohen, S.S., see Hubert-Habart, M. 427, 429, *432*
Cohen, S.S., see Moore, E.C. 243, *254*
Cohen, S.S., see Pizer, L.I. 237, *254*
Cohen, S.S., see Toji, L. 658, 659, 661, 662, *668*
Cohen, S.S., see Tono, H. 237, 244, *255*
Cohen, V., see Stewart, P.B. 752, *764*
Cohlan, S.Q., Kitay, D. 675, 676, *689*
Cohn, M., see Baxter, J.D. 97, 99, *100*
Colby, C., Edlin, G. 242, *250*
Cole, D.R., Dreyer, B.B., Rousselot, L.M., Tendler, M.D. 642, *647*
Cole, D.R., see Rousselot, L.M. 221, *230*
Cole, L.J., see Davis, W.E. 318, *330*
Cole, L.J., see Miller, J.J. 408, *422*
Cole, P., see MacMahon, B. 178, *190*
Cole, Q.P., see Roblin, R.O., Jr. 458, *467*
Cole, W.H. 19, *31*
Coleman, A.W., Coleman, J. R., Kankel, D., Werner, I. 311, *330*
Coleman, A.W., see Coleman, J.R. 311, *330*
Coleman, J.R., Coleman, A. W., Hartline, E.J.H. 311, *330*
Coleman, J.R., see Coleman, A.W. 311, *330*
Coles, N.W., Gross, R. 56, *60*
Colessides, C., see Stevens, W. *103*
Coley, R.F., Frigerio, N.A. 836, *839*
Coley, V., see Burchenal, J. H. *329*, 820, *826*
Colgate, C.E., see Allen, E. 108, *125*
Collier, R.J., Pappenheimer, A.M., Jr. 561, *568*
Collins, D., see Borsa, J. 234, 238, *250*
Collins, G.J., see Anderson, L.L. 472, *479*
Colombo, B., Felicetti, L., Baglioni, C. 557, 565, *568*
Colombo, C., see Perper, R. J. 408, *423*
Colombo, G., see Da Re, P. 673, *689*
Colowick, S.P., see Zatman, L.J. 540, *543*
Colsky, J., Shnider, B.I., Franzino, A., Perez, J. 500, *504*
Colsky, J., see Cavins, J.A. 440, *453*
Coltman, C.A., see Bodey, G.P. 264, *268*
Coltman, C.A., see Panettiere, F. 558, *569*
Colucci, V., see Jensen, E.V. 114, *131*
Colvin, L.B. 747, *762*
Comis, R., see Kingra, G.S. 546, *551*
Comis, R., see Vogel, C.L. *553*
Commerford, S.L. 274, 314, 315, 316, *330*
Commerford, S.L., Gitlin, D., Hughes, W.L. 283, 318, *330*
Commerford, S.L., see Gitlin, D. 314, 318, *334*
Commerford, S.L., see Hughes, W.L. 280, 281, 283, 284, 314, 315, 316, *336*
Commerford, S.L., see Krueger, R.C. 283, 314, 315, *338*

Commerford, S. L., see Smith, H. H. 314, *344*
Common, R. H., Mok, C. C. 121, *127*
Common, R. H., see McCully, K. A. 121, *133*
Common, R. H., see Mok, C.-C. 121, *133*
Common, R. H., see Vanstone, W. E. 120, *137*
Comstock, J. P., see Gabourel, J. D. 89, *100*
Conalty, M. L., see Barry, V. C. 793, *805*, 841, *848*
Conchie, A. F., Barton, B. W., Tobin, J. O. H. 323, *330*
Concilio, A., see Rizzoli, C. 522, *535*
Concilio, C., see Cestari, A. 522, *530*
Condie, R. M., see Page, A. R. 384, *401*
Condit, P. T. 474, *480*
Condit, P. T., Chanes, R. E., Joel, W. 473, *480*
Condit, P. T., Eliel, L. 477, *480*
Condit, P. T., Shnider, B. J., Owens, A. H., Jr. 474, *480*
Condit, P. T., see Charache, S. 427, *480*
Conn, H. O., Creasey, W. A., Calabresi, P. 355, *365*
Connell, G. M., Eik-Nes, K. B. 140, *153*
Conney, A. H., Welch, R. W., Kuntzman, R. 813, *817*
Connon, A. F. 415, *420*
Connors 831
Connors, see Mandel 26
Connors, T. A. 545
Connors, T. A., Elson, L. A., Haddow, A., Ross, W. C. J. 523, *530*
Connors, T. A., Elson, L. A., Leese, C. L. 20, 28, *31*
Connors, T. A., Jeney, A., Jones, M. 20, 28, *31*
Connors, T. A., Jones, M. 712, *715*
Connors, T. A., Roe, F. J. C. 22, *31*
Connors, T. A., see Ball, C. R. 23, *30*
Considine, N., see Chabner, B. A. 751, 752, 754, 756, *761*
Consigli, R. H., see Iwata, A. 855, 857, 858, 862, *873*
Constantopoulos, G., Carpenter, A., Satoh, P. S., Tchen, T. T. 139 *153*
Constantopoulos, G., Tchen, T. T. 54, *60*, 139, *153*
Constantopoulos, G., see Satoh, P. G. 139, *156*
Conte, A. J., see Rousselot, L. M. 221, *230*
Conway, E., see Patterson, M. K., Jr. 514, *535*, 696, 712, *719*
Conway, H., see Gillette, R. W. 527, *531*
Cook, C. E., see Wall, M. E. 649, *656*
Cook, D. E., see McCord, T. J. 518, *534*
Cook, J. M., see Franklin, T. J. 450, 451, *453*
Cook, J. W., Dodds, E. C., Hewett, C. L. 105, *127*
Cook, M. C., see Baer, H. H. 593, *611*
Cooke, R. A., see Heard, B. E. 39, *44*
Coolsma, J. W., Gruber, M., Gruber, T. 121, *127*
Cooney, D. A., Capizzi, R. L., Handschumacher, R. E. 514, *530*, 696, 703, *715*, 725, *743*
Cooney, D. A., Davis, R. D. 696, 702, *715*
Cooney, D. A., Davis, R. D., Van Atta, G. 696, *715*
Cooney, D. A., Handschumacher, R. E. 501, *504*, 695, 696, 701, 705, 710, *715*
Cooney, D. A., see Capizzi, R. L. 725, 726, 733, 734, *743*
Cooney, D. A., see Haskell, C. M. 704, *716*
Cooney, D. A., see Heyman, I. A. 832, *839*
Cooney, D. A., see Livingston, R. B. 485, 500, *507*
Coons, A. H., see O'Brien, T. F. 310, *341*
Cooper, A. D., Burgen, M. W., White, C. W., Herrmann, R. L. 309, *330*
Cooper, D. Y., see Omura, T. 139, *155*
Cooper, D. Y., see Simpson, E. R. 140, *156*
Cooper, E. H., see Ball, C. R. 23, *30*
Cooper, E. R. A., Jackson, H. 37, *42*
Cooper, G. M., Dunning, W. F., Greer, S. 216, *224*
Cooper, G. M., Greer, S. 290, *330*
Cooper, G. M., Greer, S. *330*
Cooper, H. L., see Friedman, R. M. 608, *612*
Cooper, H. L., see Stern, R. *669*
Cooper, P. D. 200, *224*
Cooper, R. A., see Breitman, T. R. 280, *328*
Cooper, S., Zinder, N. D. 58, *60*
Cooper, W. C., see Murray, J. E. 502, *508*
Cope, C. L. *817*
Coper, H., Neubert, D. 541, *542*
Coper, H., see Brunnemann, A. 541, *542*
Coppoc, G. L., see Williams-Ashman, H. G. 774, *788*
Corbett, C., Eng, Pietsch 871
Corbett, C., see Pietsch, P. 855, 863, 871, *874*
Corner, G. W. 158, *167*
Cornet, J., see Dolowy, W. C. 696, *715*
Cornudella, L., Faiferman, I., Pogo, A. O. *669*
Coronelli, C., see Murthy, Y. K. S. 882, *889*
Corte, E. D., see Bonetti, E. 697, *714*
Corti, A., Dave, C., Williams-Ashman, H. G., Mihich, E., Schenone, A. 774, 775, *784*
Corti, A., Schenone, A., Williams-Ashman, H. G., Dave, C., Mihich, E. 774, *784*
Corti, A., see Pegg, A. E. 775, *787*
Cortner, J. A., see Iriarte, P. V. 69, *81*
Cortner, J. A., see Kung, F. 521, *533*
Corvol, P. L., see Sherman, M. R. 85, *103*, 163, 164, *168*, 187, *191*
Cory, J. G., Suhadolnik, R. J. 448, *453*, 658, 664, *665*
Cory, J. G., Suhadolnik, R. J., Resnick, B., Rich, M. A. 658, 664, *665*
Cory, J. G., see Rich, M. A. 660, 663, *667*
Costa, G., Holland, J. F., Pickren, J. W. 451, *453*
Costa, J., see Hayes, D. M. 394, 397, *399*, 500, *505*
Cosulich, D. B., see Patrick, J. B. 48, *62*

Cosulich, D. B., see Webb, J. S. 47, *64*
Cowan, D. H., Bergsagel, D. E. 545, *550*
Cox, D. G., see Hell, E. 679, *690*
Cox, N. J., see Mahy, B. W. J. *669*
Cox, R. I., see Emmens, C. W. 110, *128*
Cox, R. I., see Martin, L. 110, *133*
Cox, S. M., see Rosenkrantz, J. G. 415, *423*
Cox, S. T., see Williams, A. K. 517, *538*
Coy, U., see Hartmann, G. 583, *591*
Coyle, M., see Strauss, B. 13, *17*
Craddock, V. M. 71, 72, *80*
Craddock, V. M., see Lawley, P. D. 71, *81*
Craig, A. P., see Cohen, M. M. 634, *640*
Craig, A. W., Garrett, J. V., Jackson, I. M. 318, *330*
Craig, A. W., see Edwards, K. 35, 40, *43*
Craig, A. W., see Fox, B. W. 39, *43*
Craig, A. W., see Jackson, H. 37, 38, *44*
Craig, I. M., see Griffiths, C. T. 175, 179, *189*
Cramblett, H. G., see Heyn, R. M. 397, *400*, 500, *506*
Cramer, F., see Sprinzl, M. *669*
Cramer, F., see Sprinzl, M. *669*
Cramer, G. T., Sartorelli, A. C. 496, *504*
Cramer, J. W. 300
Cramer, J. W., Morris, N. R. 299, *330*
Cramer, J. W., Prusoff, W. H., Welch, A. D., Sartorelli, A. C., Delamore, I. W., von Essen, C. F., Chang, P. K. 291, *330*
Cramer, J. W., Wacker, A., Welch, A. D. 301, 302, 303, 306, *330*
Cramer, J. W., see Morris, N. R. 298, 299, *341*
Crathorn, A. R., see Roberts, J. J. 13, 14, *16*, *17*, 21, 25, 27, *33*, 70, 76, 78, *83*
Craver, L. F., see Burchenal, J. H. 384, 389, *398*
Creager, R., see Grady, H. J. 810, *818*
Creagh, T., see De Miranda, P. 412, *420*
Creaser, E. H. 463, *465*
Creasey, W. A. 238, 239, *250*, 671, 675, 678, 680, 681, 682, 686, *689*
Creasey, W. A., Agrawal, K. C., Capizzi, R. L., Stinson, K. K., Sartorelli, A. C. 795, 799, 800, 801, 802, *805*
Creasey, W. A., Agrawal, K. C., Stinson, K. K., Sartorelli, A. C. 795, 800, *805*
Creasey, W. A., Bensch, K. G., Malawista, S. E. 678, 680, 682, *689*
Creasey, W. A., Chou, T. C. 678, *689*
Creasey, W. A., DeConti, R. C., Kaplan, S. R. 233, 238, 240, 241, 242, 244, *251*
Creasey, W. A., Fink, M. E., Handschumacher, R. E., Calabresi, P. 359, *365*
Creasey, W. A., Flanigan, S., McCollum, R. W., Calabresi, P. 238, 240, 241, 242, 244, *251*
Creasey, W. A., Markiw, M. E. 680, 682, *689*
Creasey, W. A., Papac, R. J., Markiw, M. E., Calabresi, P., Welch, A. D., 234, 238, 242, 244, *251*, 258, 259, *268*
Creasey, W. A., see Agustin, B. M. 681, *688*
Creasey, W. A., see Calabresi, P. 238, *250*, 302, 323, *329*
Creasey, W. A., see Capizzi, R. L. 725, 726, 733, 734, *743*
Creasey, W. A., see Conn, H. O. 355, *365*
Creasey, W. A., see DeConti, R. C. 686, 687, *689*, 793, 799, 800, 802, 804, *805*
Creasey, W. A., see Lefkowitz, E. R. 389, *400*, 500, *507*
Creasey, W. A., see Malawista, S. E. *692*
Creasey, W. A., see Papac, R. J. 236, 238, *254*
Creasey, W. A., see Sartorelli, A. C. 196, *230*, 232, 236, *254*, 671, 687, *693*, 747, *764*
Creasey, W. H. 291, *330*
Creaven, P. J., see Muggia, F. M. 650, *656*
Creech, C. E., see Adamson, R. H. 710, *713*
Creech, H. J., see Sugiura, K. 377, *382*
Creighton, A. M., Birnie, G. D. 885, *888*
Creighton, A. M., Hellmann, K., Whitecross, S. 885, *888*
Crews, L., see Adamson, R. H. 682, 683, *687*
Crim, J. A., Petering, H. G. 844, *848*
Crim, J. A., see Buskirk, H. H. 24, *31*, 237, *250*, 525, *530*
Crim, J. A., see Petering, H. G. 841, 842, 843, 844, *848*, *849*
Crim, J. A., see Van Giessen, G. J. 843, 844, 845, 847, *849*
Crist, D. R., Leonard, N. J. 3, *5*
Cristescu, C. 349, *365*
Crkvenjakov, R., Bajkovič, N., Glišin, V. 363, *365*
Cronkite, E. P., see Feinendegen, L. E. 314, 315, *332*
Cronkite, E. P., see Rubini, J. R. 280, 314, *343*
Crook, L. E., Rees, K. R., Cohen, A. 573, *579*
Crooks, H. M., Jr., see Westland, R. D. 485, *511*
Crosnier, J., see Bach, J. F. 414, *419*
Crosnier, J., see Hamburger, J. 407, 410, *421*
Cross, R., see Oerkermann, H. 734, 738, *745*
Crothers, D. M., see Müller, W. 584, 585, 586, 587, *591*
Crowley, L. G., see Marmorston, J. 178, *191*
Crowther, D., Bateman, C. J. T., Vartan, C. P., Whitehouse, J. M. A., Scott, R. B. 726, 732, *743*
Crowther, D., see Beard, M. E. J. 726, 727, 728, 730, 734, 735, *743*
Cruz, O., see Heidelberger, C. 198, *226*
Crusberg, T. C., Leary, R., Kisliuk, R. L. *480*
Csapo, A. 158, *167*
Cseh, G., Marosvari, I., Harmath, A. 94, *100*
Cucchia, G., see Lauro, V. 415, *422*

Cudkowicz, G., Upton, A.C., Smith, L.H., Gosslee, D. G., Hughes, W.L. 314, *330*
Cueto, C., Brown, J.H.A. 809, *817*
Cullen, W.P., see Rao, K.V. 633, *641*
Culp, W.J., see Obrig, T.C. 561, *569*
Culvenor, C.C.J., Loder, J. W. 881, *888*
Cummings, D.J. 56, *60*, 235, 241, *251*
Cummings, J.G., see Peters, J.H. 697, *720*
Cunningham, J., see Dethlefsen, L.A. 314, 315, *331*
Cunningham, K.G., Hutchinson, S.A., Manson, W., Spring, F.S. 658, 660, *665*
Curreri, A.R., Ansfield, F.J., McIver, F.A., Waisman, H.A., Heidelberger, C. 220, *224*
Curreri, A.R., see Ansfield, F.J. 220, *223*
Curreri, A.R., see Mukherjee, K.L. 202, 215, 221, *228*
Curreri, A.R., see Schroeder, J.M. 394, 397, *402*, 500, *510*
Currie, G.A., Bagshawe, K. D. 24, *31*
Currie, R., Bergel, F., Bray, R.C. 389, *398*
Curry, J., Greenberg, J. 494, *504*
Curtis, J.E., see Gutterman, J.U. 265, *269*
Curtis, P.J., Thomas, D.R. 658, *665*
Curtis, W.C., see Tower, D. B. 698, 700, 703, *721*
Cushley, R., Wempen, I., Fox, J.J. 197, *224*
Cushley, R.J., see Agrawal, K.C. 797, *804*
Cutting, W., see Furusawa, E. 302, 307, *333*
Cuttner, J., see Ellison, R. R. 260, *268*
Cuttner, J., see Kung, F. 521, *533*
Cuttner, J., see Ohnuma, T. 726, 727, 728, 734, 735, *746*
Cutts, J.H. 521, *530*, 674, 679, *689*
Cysyk, R., Prusoff, W.H. 281, 320, 322, 325, *330*
Czajkowski, R.C., see Leimgruber, W. 642, *648*
Czochralska, B., see Wrona, M. 321, *347*

Dagg, C.P., Karnofsky, D. A. *504*
Dagg, C.P., Karnofsky, D. A., Stock, C.C., Lacon, C.R., Roddy, J. *550*
Dagg, M.K., see Burchenal, J.H. 544, 550, *550*
Daguet, G., see Amiel, J.-L. 752, *760*
Dahl, J.L., see Goldberg, N. D. 201, *225*
Dahl, J.L., see Roy, J.K. 463, *467*
Dahl, J.L., see Way, J.L. 461, *467*
Dahlström, A. 683, *689*
Dahlwitz, A., Franzen, S., Holmgren, A., Killander, A., Killander, D., Wide, L., Ahstrom, L. 735, *743*
Dahmas, M.E., Bonner, J. 825, *826*
Dale, D.G., see Vanstone, W.E. 120, *137*
Dalgard, D.W., see O'Gara, R.W. 752, *764*
Dalldorf, G., Carvalho, R.P. S., Jamara, M., Frost, P., Ehrlich, D., Marigo, C. 417, *420*
D'Alessandri, A., see Martz, G. 759, *763*
Dalton, A., see Morris, H.P. 171, *191*
Dalton, L.K., Demerac, S., Elmes, B.C., Loder, J. W., Swan, J.M., Teitei, T. 881, *888*
Damarackis, B. 522, *530*
Damasid, E.E., see Marmont, A.M. 726, 727, 728, 734, 735, *745*
Dameshek, W., see Kyle, R. A. 39, *44*
Dameshek, W., see Schwartz, R.S. 407, *423*
Damle, S.P., see Wolpert, M.K. 393, *403*
Dammin, G.J., see Alexandre, G.P.J. 407, 409, *419*, 502, *503*
Dammin, G.J., see Murray, J.E. 407, *422*, 502, *508*
Dammin, G.J., see Sheil, A. G.R. 502, *510*
D'Angelo, J.M., see Groth, D.P. 74, *81*, 264, *269*
D'Angio, G.J., Farber, S., Maddock, C.L. 589, *590*
Daniel, J.C., Jr., see O'Farrell, P.H. 117, *134*
Daniel, P.M., Gale, M.M., Pratt, O.E. 314, *330*
Danielli, G.A., see Levis, A. G. 22, *32*
Danielli, J.F., see Hawkins, R. 28, *32*
Danielli, J.F., see Hebborn, P. 29, *32*
Danishefsky, S., Etheredge, S.J., Volkmann, R., Eggler, J., Quick, J. 650, *655*
Danishefsky, S., see Volkmann, R. 650, *656*
Danneberg, P.B., Montag, B.J., Heidelberger, C. 204, 205, *224*
Danneberg, P., see Heidelberger, C. 193, 198, 204, 217, *226*
Danø, K. 606, *612*
Danø, K., Frederiksen, S., Hellung-Larsen, P. 573, *579*
Danowski, T.S., Sarver, M. E., Moses, C., Bonessi, J.V. 814, *817*
Danziger, R.M., Hayon, E., Langmuir, M.E. 319, *330*
Dao, T.L. 112, *127*, 171, 173, 178, 180, 184, *188*
Dao, T.L., Bock, F.G., Greiner, M. 112, *127*
Dao, T.L., Huggins, C. 176, *188*
Dao, T.L., Sunderland, H. 112, *127*
Dao, T.L., Tan, E., Brooks, V. 184, *188*
Dao, T.L., Varela, R., Morreal, C. 178, 179, *188*
Dao, T.L., see Chang, E. 178, *188*
Dardenne, M., see Bach, J. F. 406, 410, 413, 414, *419*
Dardenne, M., see Fournier, C. 405, *420*
Da Re, P., Mancini, V., Colombo, G., Micciarelli, A. 673, *689*
Dareer, S., see Struck, R.F. 29, *33*
Dargeon, H.W., see Burchenal, J.H. 384, 389, *398*
Daria, G.M., see Old, L.J. 695, 697, *719*
Darlix, J.L., Fromageot, P., Reich, E. 462, *465*

Darnall, K. R., Townsend, L. B., Robins, R. K. 373, 374, *381*
Darnell, J. E. 571, *579*
Darnell, J. E., Philipson, L., Wall, R., Adesnik, M. 574, 575, *579*, 664, *665*
Darnell, J. E., Wall, R., Tushinski, R. 574, 575, *579*
Darnell, J. E., see Adesnik, M. 575, *579*
Darnell, J. E., see Bernhardt, D. 578, *579*
Darnell, J. E., see Jelínek, W. *669*
Darnell, J. E., see Philipson, L. *580*, 664, *667*
Darnell, J. E., see Wall, R. 574, *581*
Darnell, J. E. JR., see Levintow, L. 519, *533*
Da Rooge, M. A., see Horwitz, J. P. 273, *336*, 662, *666*
Dartnall, J. A. 707, *715*
Daržynkiewicz, E., Kuśmierek, J. T., Shugar, D. 233, *251*
Das, L., see Jaffe, N. 479, *481*, 726, 727, 730, 734, 735, *744*
Dasdia, T., see DiMarco, A. 593, 597, 605, 609, *612*
Dasdia, T., see Necco 597
Dasdia, T., see Silvestrini, R. 603, 604, 605, *613*
Datko, L. J., see Rosenthale, M. E. 408, *423*
Datta, P. R. 810, *817*
Datta, P. R., Nelson, M. J. 810, *817*
Dave, C., Caballes, L. 771, 774, 775, *784*
Dave, C., Ehrke, M. J., Mihich, E. 776, 780, 781, *784*
Dave, C., Ehrke, J., Soucek, J., Mihich, E. 771, 776, 781, *784*
Dave, C., Mihich, E. 780, 781, *784*
Dave, C., see Corti, A. 774, 775, *784*
Dave, C., see Mihich, E. 767, 780, *786*
Dave, D., see Korytnyk, W. 778, *785*
Dave, K. G., see Wenkert, E. 649, *656*
Davern, C. I. 200, *224*
Davern, C. I., see Easterbrook, K. B. 295, 302, 303, 304, 305, *332*
David, D. S., see Merkatz, I. R. 415, *422*
Davidson, E., see Ghosh, S. 493, *505*
Davidson, E. A., see Holthausen, H. S. 311, *335*
Davidson, J. D. 392, *398*
Davidson, J. D., Engle, R. R., Mancuso, R. W. *784*
Davidson, J. D., Freeman, B. B. 390, *399*
Davidson, J. D., Winter, T. S. 393, *399*, 789, *791*
Davidson, J. D., see DeVita, V. T. 69, *80*
Davidson, J. D., see Feigelson, P. 460, *465*
Davidson, J. D., see Oliverio, V. T. 770, *787*
Davidson, J. O., Oliverio, V. T., 471, 472, 473, *480*
Davidson, N., see Hyman, R. W. 583, 585, 586, *591*
Davidson, O. W., see Talwar, G. P. 113, 114, *137*
Davies, A. J. S., see Bach, J. F. 406, *419*
Davies, J., see Jiminiz, A. *569*
Davis, A. L., Skinner, C. G., Shive, W. 518, *531*
Davis, A. L., see McCord, T. J. 524, *534*
Davis, D. R., Baldwin, R. L. 293, *330*
Davis, H. L., Jr., see Ansfield, F. J. 221, *223*
Davis, J., see Thompson, R. L. 800, *807*
Davis, J. M., see Brockman, R. W. 217, *223*
Davis, J. S., Meyer, R. K., McShan, W. H. 110, *127*
Davis, J. W., see Wotiz, H. H. 106, *138*
Davis, M. E., Wiener, M., Jacobson, H. I., Jensen, E. V. 113, *127*
Davis, R. D., see Cooney, D. A. 696, 702, *715*
Davis, R. D., see Heyman, I. A. 832, *839*
Davis, R. D., see Schein, P. S. 704, 710, *720*
Davis, W., Ross, W. C. J. 42, *43*
Davis, W., see Boesen, E. 19, *30*
Davis, W. E., Schofield, R., Cole, L. J. 318, *330*
Davison, C. L., see Papirmeister, B. 13, *16*, 21, *33*, 54, *62*
Dawid, I. B., French, T. C., Buchanan, J. M. 487, 488, *504*
Dawid, I. B., see French, T. C. 487, 488, *505*
Dawson, P. J., see Reid, R. H. 417, *423*
Day, H. M., see Kenzler, C. J. 822, 824, *827*
Day, R. A., see French, T. C. 487, 488, *505*
De-Angeli, L. C., Pocchiari, F., Russi, S., Tonolo, A., Zurita, V. E., Ciaranfi, E., Perin, A. 697, *715*
De Angelo, A. B., Gorski, J. 119, 120, *127*
Dearman, H. H., see White, J. R. 634, *641*
De Asua, L. J., Rozengurt, E., Carminatti, H. 124, 125, *127*
De Barbieri, A., Astaldi, A., Jr., Micu, D., Mistretta, A. P., Astaldi, G., Burgio, G. R. 706, *715*
De Barbieri, A., Di Vittorio, P., Maugeri, M., Mistretta, P., Perrone, F., Tassi, G. C., Temelcou, O., Zapelli, P. 528, *531*
De Barros, T., Filho, M. C., Ferreira de Santana, C., Valenca, M., Pereira da Silva, M., Guedes, J., de Carvalho, A. R. L. 696, *715*
De Boer, C., see Vavra, J. J. 65, *84*
De Boer, D., Dietz, A., Lummis, N. E., Savage, G. M. 47, *60*
Debov, S. S., see Yarovaya, L. M. 489, 497, *511*
De Carli, L., see Brega, A. 566, *567*
De Carli, L., see Perani, A. 566, *569*
De Chieri, P. R., see Del Puerto, B. M. 560, *568*
De Conti, R. C., Calabresi, P. 361, *365*
De Conti, R. C., Creasey, W. A. 686, 687, *689*
De Conti, R. C., Creasey, W. A., Agrawal, K. C., Bertino, J. R., Jatlow, P. I., Mead, J. A. R., Sartorelli, A. C. 793, 800, 804, *805*

DeConti, R.C., Toftness, B. R., Agrawal, K.C., Tomchick, R., Mead, J.A.R., Bertino, J.R., Sartorelli, A.C., Creasey, W.A. 799, 800, 802, 804, *805*
DeConti, R.C., see Bertino, J.R. 477, 479, *479*
DeConti, R.C., see Capizzi, R.L. 477, *480*
DeConti, R.C., see Creasey, W.A. 233, 238, 240, 241, 242, 244, *251*
DeConti, R., see Kaplan, S. 264, *270*
DeConti, R.C., see Levitt, M. 478, *481*
DeConti, R.C., see Mitchell, M.S. 201, *228*, 237, *253*
DeConti, R.C., see Skeel, R.T. 477, *482*
DeConti, R.C., see Wagenen, G. van 357, *371*
DeCosse, J.J., see Mandel, M.A. 417, *422*
Dedella, C., see McGuire, W. L. 162, *168*
Dedrick, R.L., Forrester, D.D., Ho, D.H.W. 258, *268*
Dedrick, R.L., see Bischoff, K.B. 472, *479*
Defeo, V.J. 159, 160, *167*
Degerstedt, G., see Pontis, H. 315, 318, *342*, 352, *368*
DeGiovanni, R., see Zamenhof, S. 272, 295, 310, *347*
DeGroot, N., Lichtenstein, N. 515, *531*, 697, *715*
DeHarven, E. 674, *689*
DeHarven, E., Dustin, P., Jr. 674, *689*
DeHertogh, R., see Pearlman, W.H. 117, *134*
Deinhardt, F. 306, *330*
DeJongh, D.C., see Hanessian, S. 658, *666*
Dekker, C.A., see Roberts, W.K. 233, *254*
Dekker, C.A., see Walwick, E.R. 233, *256*
DeKloet, S.R. 207, *224*
DeKloet, S.R., Strijkert, P. J. 206, 210, 211, *224*
Delage, J.M., Simard, J., Lehner-Netsch, G., Barry, A. 735, 738, *744*
Delamore, I.W., Prusoff, W. H. 285, 301, *331*
Delamore, I.W., see Cramer, J.W. 291, *330*
DeLaTorre, C., see Gimenez-Martin, G. 662, *665*
Delhumeau-Arrecillas, G., Burris, R.H. 493, *504*
Deligianis, H., see Lynch, J.E. 564, *569*
Dellweg, H., see Wacker, A. 321, *346*
Dellweg, H., see Weygand, F. 280, 295, *346*
DeMan, J.C.H., Noorduyn, N.J.A. 583, *590*
Delmez, J.A., see Hilf, R. 124, *130*
DeLong, D.C., see Williams, R.H. 446, *457*
DelPuerto, B.M., Tato, J. C., Koltan, A., Bures, O. M., DeChieri, P.R., Garcia, A., Escary, T.I., Lorenzo, B. 560, *568*
DeMartino, L., see Boris, A. 146, *153*
Demerac, S., see Dalton, L. K. 881, *888*
Demerec, M., see Hemmerly, J. 494, *506*
Demidova, S.A., Azadova, N.B., Martynova, V.N., Galegov, G.A., Zhdanov, V.M. 354, *365*
DeMiranda, P., Chu, L.C. 412, *420*
DeMiranda, P., Beacham, L. M.III., Creagh, T., Elion, G.B. 412, *420*
Demopoulos, H.B. 524, 529, *531*
Demopoulos, H.B., see Duke, P.S. 520, *531*
Demopoulos, H.B., see Hourani, B.T. 524, *532*
DeNadai, A., see Levis, A.G. 25, *32*
Denham, C., see Adamson, R.H. 771, 772, *783*
Denham, C., see DeVita, V. T. 69, *80*
Denham, C., see Oliverio, V. T. 747, 751, 754, *764*, 770, *787*
Denham, C., see Vogel, C.L. 549, *552*, *553*
Denine, E.P., see Coffey, J.J. 523, *530*
Denman, A.M., see Denman, E.J. 416, *420*
Denman, E.J., Denman, A. M., Greenwood, B.M., Gall, D., Heath, R.B. 416, *420*
Dennis, D., see Goldin, A. 476, *481*
Dennis, E.W., see Berberian, D.A. 879, *887*
Dennis, E.W., see Hernandez, P. 880, *889*
Dennis, E.W., see Rosi, D. 879, *889*
Deodhar, S.D. 705, *715*
DePaepe, J.C. 114, *127*
DeQuattro, V., see Trams, E.G. 39, *46*
DeRatuld, Y., see Maral, R. 705, 708, *718*
Derenzo, E.C., see Ablondi, F.B. 527, *529*
DeRenzo, E.C., see Barg, W. 488, *503*
DeRepentigny, J., Sonea, S., Frappier, A. 201, *224*
Derge, J.G., see Hampar, B. 308, *334*
DeRobertis, E., Sellinger, O. Z., deL. Arnaiz, G.R., Alberici, M., Zieher, L. M., 499, *504*
DeRooij, D.G., Kramer, M. F. 37, *43*
Derr, I., see Prager, M.D. 705, 707, *720*, 733, *746*
DeRudder, J., see Boissier, J.R. 430, *432*
Desai, L., Tencer, R. 583, 584, *590*
Deshpande, N., Jensen, V., Bulbrook, R.D., Berne, T., Ellis, F. 117, *127*
Desjardins, R., Grogan, D. E., Arendell, J.P., Busch, H. 680, *689*
DeSombre, E.R., Chabaud, J.P., Puca, G.A., Jensen, E.V. 115, *127*
DeSombre, E.R., Hurst, D., Kawashima, T., Jungblut, P.W., Jensen, E.V. 115, *127*
DeSombre, E.R., Puca, G. A., Jensen, E.V. 115, 117, *127*
DeSombre, E.R., see Jensen, E.V. 85, 95, *101*, 104, 110, 114, 115, 117, 118, *131*, 164, *167*, 176, 177, 187, *190*
DeSombre, E.R., see Jungblut, P.W. 117, *131*
Dessauer, H.C., Fox, W. 120, *127*
Dessauer, H.C., Fox, W., Gilbert, N.L. 120, *128*
Dessi, P., see Cestari, A. 522, *530*
Dessi, P., see Rizzoli, C. 522, *535*
Determann, H., see Wieland, T. 517, *538*
Dethlefsen, L.A. 281, 290, 314, 315, 316, 317, *331*
Dethlefsen, L.A., Cunningham, J., Powell, E. 314, 315, *331*

Dethlefsen, L. A., Mendelsohn, M. L. 314, *331*
Dethlefsen, L. A., see Mendelsohn, M. L. 315, *340*
Dettori, R., see Calendi, E. 606, *611*
DeTorres, R. A., see Dubbs, D. R. 298, *331*
DeTorres, R. A., see Kit, S. 246, *253*, 265, *270*
Deutsch, E., Fischer, M., Frischauf, H., Honetz, N., Lechner, K., Pesendorfer, F., Stych, H., Weissmann, A. 709, *715*, 734, 735, *744*
Deutscher, M. P., see Atkinson, M. R. 660, *665*
DeVassal, F., see Mathé, G. 882, *889*
DeVassal, F., see Schwarzenberg, L. 474, *482*
DeVerdier, C. H., Potter, V. R. 291, 318, *331*
DeVita, V. T., Denham, C., Davidson, J. D., Oliverio, V. T. 69, *80*
DeVita, V. T., Hahn, M. A., Oliverio, V. T. 752, *762*
DeVita, V. T. Serpick, A. A., Carbone, P. P. 759, 760, *762*
DeVita, V. T., see Adamson, R. H. 642, *647*
DeVita, V. T., see Bray, D. A. 68, *77*, *80*
DeVita, V. T., see Chabner, B. A. 751, 752, 754, 756, *761*
DeVita, V. T., see Lowenbraun, S. 760, *763*
DeVita, V. T., see Oliverio, V. T. 747, 751, 754, *764*
DeVita, V. T., see Vogel, C. L. 478, *482*, 549, *552*, *553*
DeVita, V. T., see Young, R. C. 77, 78, *84*
DeVoe, S. E., Rigler, N. E., Shay, A. J., Martin, J. H., Boyd, T. C., Backus, E. J., Mowat, J. H., Bohonos, N. 486, 496, *504*
Devreux, S., see Chantrenne, H. 463, *465*
DeVrye, C. E., see Fahmy, O. G. 237, *251*, 297, *332*
Dewald, B., Baggiolini, M., Aebi, H. 754, *762*
Dewald, B., see Aebi, H. 751, *760*
Dewald, B., see Baggiolini, M. 751, 754, 755, *761*
DeWald, H. A., Moore, A. M. 485, *504*
Dewey, V. C., see Heinrich, M. R. 463, *465*
Dewey, V. C., see Kidder, G. W. 380, *381*, 384, *400*, 458, 459, 463, *466*
Dewey, W. C., Westra, A., Miller, H. H., Nagasawa, H. 294, *331*
Dewey, W. C., see Westra, A. 294, *346*
DeWitt, W., Helsinki, D. R. 58, *60*
DeWys, W. D., Humphreys, S. R., Goldin, A. 650, *655*
DeWys, W. D., see Mc Quitty, J. T. 844, *848*
Dexter, D. L., Heidelberger, C. 205, 222, 223, *224*
Dexter, D. L., Wolberg, W. H., Ansfield, F. J., Helson, L., Heidelberger, C. 222, 223, *224*
Dexter, D. L., see Nesnow, S. *229*
Dexter, R. N., see Temple, T. E. 811, 814, *819*
Diamond, I., Anderson, M. M., McCreadie, S. R. 38, *43*
Diamond, L. K., see Farber, S. 512, *531*
Diamond, R. D., see Farber, S. L. H. 476, *480*
Dias, C. B., see Katz, N. 879, *889*
Dibenedetto, J., see Hofer, K. G. 317, 318, *335*
Dice, J. R., see Moore, J. A. 485, *507*
Dick, D. A. T., see Bittar, E. E. 861, *871*
DiCuonzo, G., see Casazza, A. M. 597, 610, *611*
Diczfalusy, E. 107
Diczfalusy, E., see Bolte, E. 107, *126*
Diderholm, H., Fichtelius, O., Linder, O. 307, 314, *331*
Dietrich, L. S. 542, *542*
Dietrich, L. S., Friedland, I. M. 541, *542*
Dietrich, L. S., Friedland, I. M., Kaplan, L. A. 541, *542*
Dietrich, L. S., Kaplan, L. A., Friedland, I. M., Martin, D. S. 541, *542*
Dietrich, L. S., Martin, D. S. 542, *542*
Dietrich, L. S., Muniz, O., Farinas, B., Franklin, L. 541, *542*
Dietrich, L. S., see Bieber, S. 386, 393, *398*
Dietrich, L. S., see Martin, D. S. 542, *543*
Dietrich, L. S., see Shapiro, D. M. 541, *543*
Dietz, A., see Bhuyan, B. K. 557, *567*, 623, 624, 631, *631*
Dietz, A., see DeBoer, D. 47, *60*
Dietz, A., see Haňka, L. J. 351, *367*
Dietz, A., see Owen, S. P. 565, *569*
Dietz, A., see Vavra, J. J. 65, *84*
DiFronzo, G., Gambetta, R. A. 608, *612*
DiFronzo, G., Gambetta, R. A., Lenaz, L. 608, 609, *612*
DiFronzo, G., Silvestrini, R., Scarpinato, B. M. 608, *612*
DiFronzo, G., see Rusconi, A. *613*
Diggelmann, H., see Koblet, H. 758, *763*
Digiulio, W., Beierwaltes, W. H. 809, *817*
Dignam, W., see Kaufman, J. J. 415, *422*
Diluiso, G., see Verbin, R. S. 235, 236, *255*
DiMarco, A. 598, *612*
DiMarco, A., Boretti, G., Rusconi, A. 608, *612*
DiMarco, A., Gaetani, M., Orezzi, P., Scarpinato, B., Silvestrini, R., Soldati, M., Dasdia, T., Valentini, L. 593, 597, 609, *612*
DiMarco, A., Gaetani, M., Dorigotti, L., Soldati, M., Bellini, O. 593, 597, 609, *612*
DiMarco, A., Gaetani, M., Orezzi, P., Soldati, M. 593, 597, *612*
DiMarco, A., Gaetani, M., Scarpinato, B. 593, 597, 609, *612*
DiMarco, A., Lenaz, L., Casazza, A. M., Scarpinato, B. M. 597, *612*
DiMarco, A., Rusconi, A. 608, *612*
DiMarco, A., Silvestrini, R., DiMarco, S., Dasdia, T. 605, *612*
DiMarco, A., Soldati, M., Fioretti, A., Dasdia, T. 594, *612*

DiMarco, A., Terni, M., Silvestrini, R., Scarpinato, B., Biagioli, E., Antonelli, A. 607, *612*
DiMarco, A., Zunino, F., Silvestrini, R., Gambarucci, C., Gambetta, R. A. 599, 605, *612*
DiMarco, A., see Calendi, E. 598, 599, *611*
DiMarco, A., see Casazza, A. M. 597, 610, *611*
DiMarco, A., see Chandra, P. 602, 608, *611*
DiMarco, A., see Rusconi, A. 601, 603, *613*
DiMarco, A., see Sandberg, J.S. 597, *613*
DiMarco, A., see Silvestrini, R. 603, 604, 605, *613*
DiMarco, A., see Venditti, J.M. 597, *613*
DiMarco, A., see Zunino, F. 599, *614*
DiMarco, S., see DiMarco, A. 605, *612*
DiMarco, S., see Silvestrini, R. 603, *613*
Dingman, C.W., Aronow, A., Bunting, S.L., Peacock, A.C., O'Malley, B.W. 121, *128*
Dingman, C.W., Sporn, M. B. 583, 584, *590*
Dingman, E.W., see O'Malley, B.W. 121, *134*
Dinusson, W.E., Andrews, F.N., Beeson, W.M. 113, *128*
Dion, H.W., Fusari, S.A., Jakubowski, Z.L., Zora, J.G., Bartz, Q.R. 485, *504*
Dion, R.L., see Loo, T.L. 65, 69, *82*
DiPaolo, J.A. *31*, 78, *80*, 310, *331*
DiPaolo, J.A., see Givelber, H.M. 78, *80*
DiPaolo, J.A., see Pine, M. J. 776, 777, *787*
Dipple, A., Heidelberger, C. 196, *224*
Dittmer, K. 512, *531*
DiVittorio, P., see DeBarbieri, A. 528, *531*
Diwan, A., Prusoff, W.H. 282, 287, *331*
Dixon, G.J., Dulmadge, E. A., Mulligan, L.T., Mellett, L.B. 684, *689*
Dixon, G.J., see Bennett, L. L., Jr. 386, *398*
Dixon, G.J., see Miller, F.A. 428, *433*
Dixon, G.J., see Pittillo, A. F. 820, *827*
Dixon, G.J., see Sidwell, R. W. 428, *433*, 800, *807*
Dixon, G.J., see Wilkoff, L. J. 76, *84*, 235, *256*, 260, 263, *271*, 298, *347*, 494, *511*
Dixon, G.L., Sidwell, R.W., Miller, F.A., Sloan, B.J. 428, *432*
Dixon, R.L., Adamson, R. H. 235, 238, *251*, 261, *268*
Dixon, R.L., Lee, I.P. 753, *762*
Dixon, R.L., see Adamson, R.H. 682, 683, *687*
Dixon, R.L., see Loo, T.L. 65, 69, *82*
Dixon, R.L., see Woods, J. S. 708, *722*
Djaczenko, W., see Benedetto, A. 584, *589*
Djerassi, C., see McGinty, D.A. 182, *191*
Djerassi, I. 477, *480*
Djerassi, I., Rominger, C.J., Kim, J.S., Turchi, J., Suvansri, U., Hughes, D. 478, *480*
Djerassi, I., Royer, G., Treat, C., Carim, H. 478, *480*
Djerassi, I., see Jaffe, N. 479, *481*
Djordjevic, B., Kim, J.H. 59, *60*, 859, *871*
Djordjevic, B., Szybalski, W. 289, 298, 299, 301, 314, 319, *331*
Djordjevic, B., see Kim, K. H. 603, 605, *613*
Djordjevic, B., see Sutic, D. 208, *230*
Dmochowski, L.L., see Bowen, J.M. 302, 307, *328*
Dmochowski, L., see Munyon, W. 302, 304, 306, 307, *341*
DoAmaral, J.R., French, F. A., Blanz, E.J., Jr., French, D.A. 779, *784*
DoAmaral, J.R., see Blanz, E.J., Jr. 795, *805*
Dobriner, K., Liberman, S. 177, *188*
Dockerty, M.B., see Jackson, R.L. 174, *189*
Dodds, E.C., Folley, S.J., Glascock, R.F., Lawson, W. 113, *128*
Dodds, E.C., Goldberg, L., Lawson, W., Robinson, R. 105, *128*
Dodds, E.C., Lawson, W. 105, *128*
Dodds, E.C., see Cook, J.W. 105, *127*
Doering, A.M., Jansen, M., Cohen, S.S. 662, *665*
Doering, A.M., Keller, J., Cohen, S.S. 244, *251*
Doggett, R.L.S., Bagshaw, M.A., Kaplan, H.S. 324, *331*
Doggett, R.L.S., see Bagshaw, M.A. 291, 319, 324, *327*
Doggett, R.L.S., see Bagshaw, M.A. 319, 324, *327*
Dohlman, C., see Kaufman, H.E. 302, 322, *337*
Doisy, E.A., Veler, C.D., Thayer, S.A. 104, *128*, 170, *189*
Doisy, E.A., see Allen, E. 104, 108, *125*
Doisy, E.A., see MacCorquodale, D.W. 104, *133*
Doklen, A., see Feher, I. 522, *531*
Dold, U., Mielsch, M., Holzer, H. 25, *31*
Dold, U., Schmidt, C.G. 870, *871*
Dold, U., see Fussganger, R. 25, *31*
Dollinger, M.R., Burchenal, J.H., Kreis, W., Fox, J. J. 233, 239, *251*
Dollinger, M., Kreis, W., Stoll, D., Fox, J., Burchenal, J.H. 234, *251*
Dollinger, M.R., see Burchenal, J.H. 264, *268*
Dolowy, W.C., Elrod, L.M., Ammeraal, R.N., Schrek, R. 707, *715*
Dolowy, W.C., Henson, D., Cornet, J., Sellin, H. 696, *715*
Dolowy, W.C., Schrek, R., Henson, D., Cornet, J., Brown, E. 696, *715*
Dolowy, W.C., see Roberts, J. 501, *509*
Dolowy, W.C., see Schrek, R. 706, *720*, 733, *746*
Domagk, G., Behnisch, R., Mietzsch, F., Schmidt, H. 841, *848*
Dominguez, J.M., see Sterental, A. 112, *136*, 174, *191*
Dominici, C., see Lauro, V. 415, *422*

Donaldson, G.R., Atkinson, M.R., Murray, A.W. 564, *568*
Donati, L., see Bertelli, A. 705, *714*
Dondon, J., see Michelson, A.M. 272, 274, *340*
Dongorozi, C.S. 516, *531*
Donnelli, M.G., see Rosso, R. 69, *83*
Donnelly, R.B., see Stone, G.M. 113, *136*
Donnelly, T.E., Jr., see Booth, B.A. 846, 847, *848*
Donnelly, T.E., Jr., see Sartorelli, A.C. *807*
Donovan, K.L., Rowe, J.A., Moyed, H.S. 448, *453*
Donovick, R., see Hamre, D. 800, *806*
Doremus, H.M., see Jaffe, J.J. 441, *454*
Dorfman, R.I., Shipley, R.A. 139, 142, *153*
Dorfman, R.I., see Rooks, W.H. 145, *156*
Dorfman, R.I., see Savard, K. 140, *156*
Dorfman, R.I., see Shimizu, K. 139, *156*
Dorfman, R.I., see Toren, D. 139, *156*
Dorigotti, L. 594, *612*
Dorigotti, L., see DiMarco, A. 593, 597, 609, *612*
Dormont, J., see Hamburger, J. 407, 410, *421*
Dorrington, J.H., Kirkpatrick, R. 140, *153*
Dorsett, M.T., Morse, P.A., Gentry, G.A. 290, *331*
Dorsey, J.K., see Papirmeister, B. 13, *16*
Doskočil, J. *365*
Doskočil, J., Pačes, V. 351, *365*
Doskočil, J., Pačes, V., Šorm, F. 361, *365*
Doskočil, J., Šorm, F. 351, 362, *365*
Doskočil, J., see Pačes, V. 362, *368*
Dossetor, J.B., see Caplan, R.M. 415, *420*
Dost, F.N., Reed, D.J. 755, *762*
Dost, F.N., Reed, D.J., Wang, C.H. 755, *762*
Dost, F.N., see Reed, D.J. 754, *764*
Doty, P., Boedtker, H., Fresco, J.R., Haselkorn, R., Litt, M. 292, *331*
Doty, P., see Kohn, K.W. 8, *15*, 41, *44*
Dougherty, M., see Slotnick, I.J. 680, *693*
Dougherty, T.F., White, A. 86, *100*, 175, *189*
Dougherty, T.F., see Stevens, W. 87, *103*
Douglas, M., see Strong, J.A. 178, *192*
Dove, W.F., see Jones, T.C. 326, *336*
Dow, R.W., see Lindenauer, S.M. 523, *533*
Dowben, R.M., see Rabinowitz, J.C. 106, *134*
Dowling, M.D., see Clarkson, B.D. 727, 728, 730, 732, *743*
Downing, V., see Weiss, A.J. *511*
Dox, A.W. 697, *715*
Drahovsky, D., Kreis, W. 247, *251*, 265, *268*
Drahovsky, D., see Kreis, W. 247, 249, *253*
Drahovský, D., see Winkler, A. 352, *372*
Drake, E.H., see Burrows, J.H. 478, *480*
Drake, J.W. 6, *15*
Dralle, E., see Thiele, J. 766, *788*
Drane, W., see Mueller, G.A. 674, *692*
Draper, D.A., see Board, J.A. 415, *419*
Draper, R.W., see Kende, A.S. 650, *655*
Drassner, J.D., see Jondorf, W.R. 560, *569*
Draycott, C., see Stewart, S.E. 308, *345*
Drews, J. 90, *100*
Dreyer, B.B., see Cole, D.R. 642, *647*
Dreyfus, B., see Jacquillat, C. 726, 727, 728, 732, 734, 735, *744*
Driskell-Zamenhof, P.J., Adelberg, E.A. 58, *60*
Drobnik, J., Krekulova, A., Kubelkov, A. 835
Drobnik, J., see Horacek, P. 835, 837, *839*
Drobnik, J., see Rosenberg, B. 829, *840*
Drobnik, J., see Vonka, V. 838, *840*
Drobnik, J., see Zak, M. 836, *840*
Droegemueller, W., see Penn, I. 415, *423*
Drolet, B.P., see Foley, G.E. 29, *31*
Druckrey, H., Preussmann, R., Ivankovic, S. 70, *80*
Druckrey, H., Preussmann, R., Ivankovic, S., Schmähl, D., Afkham, J., Blum, G., Mennel, H.D., Müller, M., Petropoulas, P., Schneider, H. 78, *80*
Druckrey, H., Raabes, S. 180, *189*
Druckrey, H., see Preussmann, R. 70, *82*
Drummond, G.I., Powell, C.A. 438, *453*
Duane, D.D., Engel, A.G. 561, *568*
Dubbs, D.R., Kit, S. 302, 303, 316, *331*
Dubbs, D.R., Kit, S., DeTorres, R.A., Anken, M. 298, *331*
Dubbs, D.R., see Kit, S. 56, *61*, 246, *253*, 265, *270*, 298, *337*, *338*
Dubbs, D.R., see Pearson, P.M. 246, *254*
Dubois, S., see Gale, G.R. 790, *791*
Dubost, M., Ganter, P., Maral, R., Ninet, L., Pinnet, S., Preud Homme, J., Werner, G.H. 593, *612*
Duchková, H., see Rašková, H. 361, *369*
Duchková, M., see Slavík, M. *370*
Dudley, H.C. 879, *888*
Duke, P.S., Demopoulos, H.B. 520, *531*
Duke, P.S., Yuen, T.G.H., Demopoulos, H.B. 520, *531*
Dukes, B.A., see Korenman, S.G. 117, 118, *132*
Dukes, C.D., see Smith, K.O. 302, 303, 304, 305, *345*
Dukes, C.E., see Bloom, H.J.G. 175, 186, *188*
Dulaney, E.L., see Kaczka, E.A. 658, *666*
Dulbecco, R., see Smith, J.D. 302, 307, *344*
Dulin, W.E., see Wyse, B.M. 76, *84*
Dulmadge, E.A., see Bennett, L.L., Jr. 386, *398*
Dulmadge, E.A., see Dixon, G.J. 684, *689*

Dulmadge,E.A., see Wilkoff,L.J. 76, *84*, 235, *256*, 260, 263, *271*, 298, *347*, 494, *511*
Dumont,J.N., see Wallace, R.A. 120, 121, *138*
Dumont,P., see Bui,N.M. 273, *329*
Dumont,P., see Maisin,J.A. 38, *45*
Dunaway,P.B., see O'Farrel,T.P. 283, 284, 318, *341*
Duncan,G.W., Lyster,S.C., Clark,J.J., Lednicer,D. 110, *128*
Duncan,G.W., Stucki,J.C., Lyster,S.C., Lednicer, D. 110, *128*
Duncan,L.J.P., Baird,J.D. 766, *784*
Dunjic,A. 39, *43*
Dunjic,A., see Maisin,J.A. 38, *45*
Dunlap,R.B., see Huennekens,F.M. 469, *481*
Dunn,C.D.R., Elson,L.A. 38, *43*
Dunn,D.B., Smith,J.D. 272, 274, 280, 295, 303, *331*, 380, *381*
Dunn,M.S., see Levy,H.M. 521, *533*
Dunne,C.R. 23, *31*
Dunnebacke,T.H.,Reaume, M.G. 306, *331*
Dunnicliff,M.A., Eigner,E. A., Jaffe,N., Traggis,D., Rosenoer,V.M. *744*
Dunning,W.F., see Cooper, G.M. 216, *224*
Duprat,A.M., Miquel,M.T., Beetschen,J.C., Zalta, J.P. 628, *631*
Durham,J.F., Ives,D.H. 240, *251*
Durr,G.J., Hammond,S. 350, *365*
Durr,G.J., Keiser,J.F., Ierardi,P.A. 350, *365*
Durst,J., see Weitzel,G. 754, 756, *765*
Duschinsky,R., Gabriel,T., Tautz,W., Nussbaum, A., Hoffer,M., Grunberg,E., Burchenal,J. H., Fox,J.J. 197, *225*
Duschinsky,R., Pleven,E., Heidelberger,C. 195, *225*
Duschinsky,R., Walker,H., Kara,J. 273, *331*
Duschinsky,R., see Heidelberger,C. 193, 198, *226*
Duschinsky,R., see Hoffer, M. 195, *226*, 272, *335*
Duschinsky,R., see Kara,J. 273, *337*
Duschinsky,R., see Koechlin,B.A. 201, 202, *227*
Duschinsky,R., see Lozeron,H.A. 198, *228*, 321, *340*
Duschinsky,R., see Van Dyk,J.J. 197, *231*
Duschinsky,R., see Wempen,I. 196, *231*, 278, *346*
Duschinsky,R., see Kung, N.C. 196, *231*, 272, *347*
Dusonchet,L., Perbasi,F., Gebbia,N. 608, *612*
Dustin,P.,Jr. 671, 673, 674, *689*
Dustin,P.,Jr., see DeHarven,E. 674, *689*
Dustin,P.,Jr., see Eigsti, O.J. 671, 673, 675, *689*
Dutton,A.H., see Dutton, R.W. 309, *331*
Dutton,R.W., Dutton,A. H., Vaughn,J.H. 309, *331*
Dutton,R.W., Pearce,J.D. 310, *331*, 406, *420*
Dutz,W., see Heine,K.M. 416, *421*
Duval,J., Ebel,J.P. 274, *332*
Duval,J., see Yoshida,H. 273, *347*
Duvall,L.R. 485, 486,487, 500, *504*
Dvorkin,B., see Makman, M.H. 86, 87, 88, 89, 92, 93, *102*
Dvorkin,B., see Nakagawa, S. 94, *102*
Dvorkin,B., see Pena,A. 89, *102*
Dworak,J.E., see Ryan,W. L. 708, *720*
Dyck,P.J., see Gottschalk, P.G. 682, 686, *690*
Dyke,R.W., see Armstrong, J.G. 685, *688*
Dykstra,W.G., Herbst,E. J. 148, *153*
Dym,H., Becker,Y. 519, *531*
Dzelzkalns,M., see Lerner, L.J. 146, *155*

Eagle,H. 695, *715*
Eagle,H., Oyama,V.I., Levy,M., Horton,C.L., Fleischman,R. 484, *504*
Eagon,R.G., see Williams, A.K. 517, *538*
Earle,K.M., see Schochet, S.S. 677, *693*
Earnhardt,J., see Jackson, V. 825, *827*
Easterbrook,K.B., Davern, C.I. 295, 302, 303, 304, 305, *332*
Eaton,W.L. 162
Ebel,J.-P., see Beck,G. 121, *126*
Ebel,J.P., see Duval,J. 274, *332*
Ebel,J.P., see Yoshida,H. 273, *347*
Eberle,P., Hunstein,W., Perings,E. 415, *420*
Ebert,M., see Wacker,A. 26, *34*
Ebstein,B.S. 583, *590*
Eckermann,G., see Atkinson,M.R. 386, *397*
Eckhardt,S., Sellei,C., Hindy,I. 36, *43*
Eckhardt,S., see Sellei,C. 19, *33*
Eckstein,B., Villee,C.A. 123, *128*
Eddleston,A.L.W.F., see Mitchell,C.G. 413,414, *422*
Edelman,I.S., Fimognari, G. 164, *167*
Edelman,I.S., see Chu,L.L. H. *669*
Edelman,I.S., see Herman, T.S. 85, *101*, 164, *167*
Edelman,I.S., see Swaneck, G.E. 164, *168*
Edelman,J.C., Brendler, H., Zorgniotti,A.W., Edelman,P.M. 151, *153*
Edelman,P.M., see Edelman,J.C. 151, *153*
Edelman,S., see Pratt,W. B. 90, *102*
Edelson,J., Fissekis,J.D., Skinner,C.G., Shive,W. *531*
Edelson,J., Skinner,C.G., Ravel,J.M., Shive,W. 524, *531*
Edelson,J., Skinner,C.G., Shive,W. 497, *504*
Edgren,R.A., Calhoun,D. W. 110, *128*
Edlin,G., see Colby,C. 242, *250*
Edmonds,M., Vaughan,M. H., Nakazoto,N. 574, 575, *579*
Edmunds,M.E., see Hipkiss,A.R. 209, *226*

Edwards, C.L., Hayes, R.L. 879, *888*
Edwards, D.A., see Whalen, R.E. 149, *157*
Edwards, K., Craig, A.W., Jackson, H., Jones, A.R. 35, 40, *43*
Edwards, K., Jackson, H. 40, *43*
Edwards, K., Jackson, H., Jones, A.R., 40, *43*
Edwards, P.A., see Lawley, P.D. 10, *16*
Edwards, R., Brush, M.G., Taylor, R.W. 160, *167*
Egami, F., see Ikeda, K. 862, *872*
Egami, F., see Kageyama, M. 583, *591*
Egger, G., Ackman, D. 410, *420*
Eggerding, F., see Vietti, T. 199, *231*
Egami, F., see Hashimoto, J. 437, *453*
Eggler, J., see Danishefsky, S. 650, *655*
Eggler, J., see Volkmann, R. 650, *656*
Ehrenberg, L., see Ahnström, G. 314, *327*
Ehrenfeld, E.R., see Narrod, S.A. 491, *508*
Ehrhardt, J., see Fateh-Moghadam, A. 734, 735, *744*
Ehrke, M.J., see Dave, C. 771, 776, 780, 781, *784*
Ehrke, M.J., see Mihich, E. 767, 780, *786*
Ehrke, M.J., see Souček, J. 781, *787*
Ehrlich 545, 548, 606
Ehrlich, D., see Dalldorf, G. 417, *420*
Ehrlich, E.N., see Landau, R.L. 185, *190*
Ehrlich, J., see Miller, F.A. 428, *433*
Ehrlich, J., see Sloan, B.J. 428, *433*
Ehrlich, P. 18, *31*
Ehrman, L. 440, *453*
Ehrman, M., Cedar, H., Schwartz, J.H. 697, 701, *715*
Ehrman, M., see Schwartz, J.H. 515, *536*
Eickhoff, K., see Agarwal, D.P. 283, *327*
Eichelberger, L., see Huggins, C. 172, *189*
Eichhorn, J., see Halkerston, I.D.K. 139, *154*
Eidinoff, M.L., Cheong, L., Gambetta, G.E., Benua, S., Ellison, R.R. 283, 295, 314, *332*
Eidinoff, M.L., Cheong, L., Rich, M.A. 295, 314, *332*
Eidinoff, M.L., Knoll, J.E., Marano, B., Cheong, L. 490, *504*
Eidinoff, M.L., Rich, M.A. 298, *332*
Eidinoff, M.L., see Cheong, L. 272, 273, 298, *329*
Eidinoff, M.L., see Gelbard, A.-S. 354, *366*
Eidinoff, M.L., see Hampton, A. 274, 318, *335*
Eidinoff, M.L., see Hampton, E.G. 273, 282, 283, 289, 290, 291, 314, *335*
Eidinoff, M.L., see Kim, J. H. 21, *32*, 59, *61*, 233, 235, 241, 242, *253*, 261, *270*, 299, *337*
Eidinoff, M.L., see Rich, M. A. 199, *229*
Eigner, E.A., see Dunnicliff, M.A. *744*
Eigsti, O.J., Dustin, P., Jr. 671, 673, 675, *689*
Eik-Nes, K.B. 139, 140, *153*
Eik-Nes, K.B., see Connell, G.M. 140, *153*
Einarsson, M., see Kristiansen, T. *717*
Eisenberg, E., see Gordan, G.S. 91, *100*
Eisenfeld, A.J. 117, *128*
Eisenfeld, A.J., Axelrod, J. 114, 116, 117, *128*
Eisenstadt, J.M., Grossman, L., Klein, H.P. 514, *531*
Eisner, A., see Schwartz, R. S. *423*
El-Asmar, F.A., Greenberg, D.M. 485, 501, *504*
Eldareer, S.M., see Mellett, L.B. 259, *270*
Elder, C.C., see Bartz, Q.R. 485, *503*
Elford, H.L., Freese, M., Passamani, E., Morris, H.P. 793, *805*
Elger, W., see Neumann, F. 146, *155*
Eliasson, R., see Brown, N. C. 790, *791*
Eliel, L., see Condit, P.T. 477, *480*
Elion, G.B. 384, 387, 389, 392, *399*, 404, 411, 412, 413, *420*
Elion, G.B., Benezra, F.M., Carrington, L.O., Strelitz, R.A. 412, 413, *420*
Elion, G.B., Burgi, E., Hitchings, G.H. 389, *399*, 459, *465*
Elion, G.B., Callahan, S.W., Bieber, S., Hitchings, G. H., Rundles, R.W. 404, 408, 409, 410, 411, *420*
Elion, G.B., Callahan, S.W., Hitchings, G.H., Rundles, R.W., Laszlo, J. 389, *399*, 411, *420*
Elion, G.B., Callahan, S.W., Rundles, R.W., Hitchings, G.H. 384, 387, *399*, 411, *420*
Elion, G.B., Hitchings, G. H. 292, *332*, 384, 389, 392, *399*, 404, *420*, 459, *465*
Elion, G.B., Mueller, S., Hitchings, G.H. 387, *399*
Elion, G.B., see Bieber, S. 309, *328*, 386, 393, *398*
Elion, G.B., see Blancuzzi, V. 409, *419*
Elion, G.B., see Clarke, D.A. 396, *398*
Elion, G.B., see DeMiranda, P. 412, *420*
Elion, G.B., see Hitchings, G.H. 24, *32*, 384, 391, 396, *400*, 404, 407, 408, *421*
Elion, G.B., see Nathan, H. C. 407, 409, *422*
Elion, G.B., see Quinn, R. P. 410, *423*
Elion, G.B., see Thompson, R.L. 302, *346*
Elis, J., Rašková, H. 350, 360, *365*
Elis, J., Slavík, M., Rašková, H. 361, *365*
Elis, J., see Čerey, K. 350, *364*
Elis, J., see Gutová, M. 357, *366*
Elis, J., see Havelka, S. 361, *367*
Elis, J., see Jiřička, Z. 349, 358, *367*
Elis, J., see Misařová, Z. 360, *368*
Elis, J., see Myška, V. 360, *368*
Elis, J., see Rašková, H. 361, *369*
Elis, J., see Slavík, M. 361, *370*
Elis, J., see Záruba, F. 361, *372*

Elkerbout, F., Thomas, P., Zwaveling, A. 19, *31*
Elkind, M.M., Whitmore, G. F. 319, 322, *332*
Elkind, M.M., see Mohler, W.C. 298, *341*
Ellem, K.A.O., Fabrizio, A. M., Jackson, L. 709, *715*
Ellem, K.A.O., Rhode, S. L., III. 573, *579*, 628, *632*
Elliott, E.V., see Sinclair, N. R.St.C. 707, *721*
Elliot, J. 478, *480*
Elliott, A.Y., see Bowen, J.M. 302, 307, *328*
Elliott, H.W., Gale, E.F. 499, *504*
Elliott, J.A., see Ryan, W. L. 519, 529, *535*
Elliott, J.H., see Leibowitz, H.M. 410, *422*
Ellis, D.B., LePage, G.A. 387, *399*, 430, *432*, 659, *665*
Ellis, F., see Deshpande, N. 117, *127*
Ellison, R.R., Burchenal, J. H. 394, *399*
Ellison, R.R., Holland, J. F., Weil, M., Jacquillat, C., Boiron, M., Bernard, J., Sawitsky, A., Rosner, F., Gussoff, B., Silver, R.T., Karanas, A., Cuttner, J., Spurr, C.L., Hayes, D.M., Blom, J., Leone, L.A., Haurani, F., Kyle, R., Hutchison, J.L., Forcier, R.J., Moon, J.H. 260, *268*
Ellison, R.R., Karnofsky, D.A., Sternberg, S.S., Murphy, M.L., Burchenal, J.H. 500, *504*
Ellison, R.R., see Burchenal, J.H. 384, 389, *398*
Ellison, R.R., see Carey, R. W. 260, 261, *268*
Ellison, R.R., see Eidinoff, M.L. 283, 295, 314, *332*
Ellison, R.R., see Hayes, D. M. 264, *269*
Ellison, R.R., see Kreis, W. 822, 824, *827*
Ellison, R.R., see Lyman, M. 820, *827*
Ellison, R.R., see Murphy, M.L. 394, *401*
Ellison, R.R., see Pahl, H. B. 282, 283, *341*
El-Merzabani, M.M., Sakurai, Y. 36, *43*
Elmes, B.C., see Dalton, L. K. 881, *888*
El-Nakeeb, M.A., Lampen, J.O. 681, *689*
El-Nakeeb, M.A., McLellan, W.L., Jr., Lampen, J.O. 681, *689*
Elrod, L.M., see Dolowy, W. C. 707, *715*
Elslager, E.F., see Hirschberg, E. 879, *889*
Elson, L.A. 23, *31*, 37, 38, *43*
Elson, L.A., Galton, D.A. G., Till, M. 38, *43*
Elson, L.A., see Connors, T. A. 20, 28, *31*, 523, *530*
Elson, L.A., see Dunn, C.D. R. 38, *43*
Elson, L.A., see Talbot, T. R. 38, *46*
Elsworth, R., see Wade, H. E. 697, *721*
Eltringham, J.R. 408, *420*
Elves, M.W., Buttoo, A.S., Israëls, M.C.G., Wilkinson, J.F. 361, *365*
Ely, J.O., Batt, W.G. 521, *531*
Emdes, J. von der, see Goldenberg, D.M. 259 *269*
Emeliyanov, B.A., see Kaverin, N.V. 354, *367*
Emeraud, J., see Laboureur, P. 699, 700, *717*
Emmelot, P. 458, *465*
Emmens, C.W. 108, *128*
Emmens, C.W., Cox, R.I., Martin, L. 110, *128*
Emmersen, J., see Behnke, O. 676, *688*
Endo, Y., Tominaga, H., Natori, Y. 583, *590*
Eng, R., see Corbett 871
Eng, R., see Pietsch, P. 851, 853, 855, 860, 861, *874*
Engberg, J., see Frederiksen, S. *669*
Engel, A.G., see Duane, D. D. 561, *568*
Engel, L.L., see Baggett, B. 106, *125*
Engel, L.L., see Savard, K. 140, *156*
Engel, L.L., see Ryan, K.J. 107, *135*
Engel, S.L., see Lerner, L.J. 123, *132*, 147, *155*
Engle, R.R., see Davidson, J.D. *784*
English, A.R., see Lynch, J.E. 564, *569*
English, J.P., see Roblin, R.O., Jr. 458, *467*
Enimens, C.W., see Martin, L. 110, *133*
Ennis, H.L., Lubin, M. 352, *365*
Enot, K.J., see Wilson, C.B. 69, *84*
Ephrati-Elizur, E., Zamenhof, S. 308, *332*
Ephrati-Elizur, E, see Szybalski, W. 308, *345*
Erbertová, B., see Rašková, H. 361, *369*
Erdmann, V.A., Fahnestock, S., Hijo, K., Nomura, M. 566, *568*
Erdos, T. 114. 115, *128*
Erdos, T., Best-Belpomme, M., Bessada, R. 115, *128*
Erdos, T., Gospodarowicz, D., Bessada, R., Fries, J. 114, *128*
Eremenko, V.V., Evseev, L. P., Nikolaev, A.Y. 697, *715*
Erichson, S., see Velle, W. 107, *137*
Erikson, R.L., Szybalski, W. 292, 298, 319, *332*
Eriksson, G., see Bolte, E. 107, *126*
Erlanger, M., Martz, G., Ott, F., Storck, H., Rieder, J., Kessler, S. 222, *225*
Ersley, A.J., see Vivacqua, R.J. 39, *46*
Ertel, N., Omokoku, B., Wallace, S.L. 684, *689*
Ertl, H.H., Feinendegen, L. E., Heiniger, H.J. 314, *332*
Ertürk, E., see Skibba, J.L. 547, *552*
Erukhimov, L.S., Vermel, E.M. 360, *365*
Escary, T.I., see Del Puerto, B.M. 560, *568*
Escher, G.C., see Magill, G. B. 500, *507*
Essen, C.F. von, see Calabresi, P. 283, 284, 314, 319, 323, 324, *329*
Essen, C.F. von, see Cramer, J.W. 291, *330*
Estabrook, R.W., see Omura, T. 139, *155*
Estabrook, R.W., see Simpson, E.R. 140, *156*
Estborn, B., see Reichard, P. 318, *343*

Esterman, M. A., see Sweeney, M. J. 450, 451, *456*
Etcubanas, E., Tan, C., Wollner, N., Bethune, V., Krakoff, I., Burchenal, J. 793, 799, 800, *805*
Etheredge, S. J., see Danishefsky, S. 650, *655*
Etzold, G., Preussel, B., Hintsche, R., Langen, P. 289, 290, *332*
Etzold, G., Preussel, B., Langen, P. 289, 296, *332*
Etzold, G., see Langen, P. 273, 289, 290, *338*, *339*, 661, *666*
Etzold, G., see Preussel, B. 289, *342*
Evans, A., see Talwar, G. P. 113, 114, *137*
Evans, H. E., see Knight, V. *338*
Evans, H. M., see Long, J. A. 108, *132*
Evans, J. S., Bostwick, L., Mengel, G. D. *251*, 263, 264, *268*
Evans, J. S., Haňka, L. J. 362, *365*
Evans, J. S., Mengel, G. D. 235, 236, 240, *251*
Evans, J. S., Musser, E. A., Bostwick, L., Mengel, G. D. 235, 236, *251*, 259, *268*
Evans, J. S., Musser, E. A., Mengel, G. D., Forsblad, K. R., Hunter, J. H. 235, *251*
Evans, J. S., see Haňka, L. J. 351, *367*
Evans, L. H., Hähnel, R. 117, *128*
Evans, W., see Burk, D. 776, *783*
Evennett, P. J., see Nicholls, T. J. 121, *134*
Everson, R., Kessel, D., Hall, T. C. 216, *225*
Evseev, L. P., Nikolaev, A. Y. 697, *715*
Evseev, L. P., see Eremenko, V. V. 697, *715*
Ey, R. C., Hughes, W. F., Holmes, A. W. *332*
Ezell, see Moutschen, J. 40

Fabrizio, A. M., see Ellem, K. A. O. 709, *715*
Fabro, S., see Adamson, R. H. 695, 710, *713*
Fadeeva, L. L., see Leontieva, N. A. 306, *339*
Fahmy, M. J., see Fahmy, O. G. 22, 31, 41, *43*, 237, *251*, 297, *332*
Fahmy, O. G., Fahmy, M. J. 22, *31*, 41, *43*
Fahmy, O. G., Fahmy, M. J., De Vrye, C. E. 237, *251*, 297, *332*
Fahnestock, S., see Erdmann, V. A. 566, *568*
Faiferman, I., see Cornudella, L. *669*
Fairley, G. H., Malpas, J. S., Galton, D. A. G. 726, 727, 728, 730, 732, 734, *744*
Fairley, G. H., Patterson, M. J. L., Scott, R. B. 759, *762*
Fairley, G. H., see Alexander, P. 728, *742*
Fairley, G. H., see Beard, M. E. J. 726, 727, 728, 730, 734, 735, *743*
Falaschi, A., Kornberg, A. 856, 857, 860, 862, 865, *872*
Falaschi, A., see Brega, A. 566, *567*
Falco, E. A., Fox, J. J. 233, *251*
Falco, E. A., see Thompson, R. L. 302, *346*
Falco, E. A., see Wempen, I. 233, *256*
Falk, R. J., Bardin, C. W. 160, 162, *167*
Falke, D., Rada, B. 354, *365*
Falkenhaug, E. M., see Baguley, B. C. 234, 238, *249*, 262, *267*
Falkson, G. 773, *784*, 886
Falkson, G., Falkson, H. C. 525, *531*
Falkson, G., see Ohnuma, T. 726, 727, 728, 734, 735, *746*
Falkson, H. C., see Falkson, G. 525, *531*
Fallon, H. J., Frei, E. III., Block, J., Seegmiller, J. E. 352, 259, *365*
Fallon, H. J., see Handschumacher, R. E. 355, 358, 359, 360, 361, *366*
Falvey, C. F., see MacDonald, A. S. 752, *763*
Fan, H., Penman, S. 664, *665*
Fan, H., see Penman, S. 571, 575, *580*, 664, *667*
Fanelli, A., see Lauro, V. 415, *422*
Fanestil, D. 861, *872*
Fang, S., Anderson, K. M., Liao, S. 149, 150, *153*, 164, *167*
Fang, S., Liao, S. 177, *189*
Fang, S., see Liao, S. 148, *155*, 177, 187, *190*
Fanshier, L., see Levinson, W. E. 307, *339*
Fanshier, L., see McDonnell, J. P. 583, *591*, *613*
Fantes, K. H., see Sonnabend, J. A. 607, *613*
Fantini, G., see Arcamone, F. 593, *611*
Farah, A., see Hernandez, P. 880, *889*
Farber, E. 522, *531*
Farber, E., see Goldblatt, P. J. 583, *590*
Farber, E., see Magee, P. N. 71, *82*
Farber, E., see Stewart, G. A. 583, *592*
Farber, E., see Verbin, R. S. 235, 236, *255*
Farber, L. R., see Levitt, M. 478, *481*
Farber, S., Diamond, L. K., Mercer, R. D., Sylvester, R. F., Jr., Wolff, J. A. 512, *531*
Farber, S., Toch, R., Sears, E. M., Pinkel, D. 394, *399*
Farber, S., see Caspersson, T. 6, *15*, 21, *31*
Farber, S., see D'Angio, G. J. 589, *590*
Farber, S., see Jaffe, N. 479, *481*
Farber, S. L. H., Diamond, R. D., Mercer, R. F., Sylvester, J. R., Wolff, J. O. 476, *480*
Farinas, B., see Dietrich, L. S. 541, *542*
Faris, T. D., see Starzl, T. E. 410, *424*
Farkaš, J., Beránek, J., Šorm, F. 350, *366*
Farkaš, J., see Bobek, M. 349, *364*
Farmar, R. M., see Herman, E. H. 609, *612*
Farnham, G., see Cleveland, J. C. 474, 478, *480*
Farnsworth, W. E., Brown, J. R. 149, *153*
Faroog, A., see Laumas, K. R. 160, *167*
Farquhar, D. 550

Farquharson, E., see Gimlin, D. M. 308, *334*
Fastier, F. N. 767, *784*
Fateh-Moghadam, A., Lamerz, R., Schwandt, P., Hornung, B., Ehrhardt, J. 734, 735, *744*
Fauconnet, M., see Borel, Y. 407, *419*
Faulcon, F. M., see Regan, J. D. 525, *535*
Faulkner, R., see Allfrey, V. G. 824, *826*
Fecher, R., see Yung, N. C. 196, *231*, 272, *347*
Federicq, P. *60*
Feeley, E. J. 303, *332*
Feeney, R. J., see Bergmann, W. 232, *249*
Feher, I., Doklen, A., Selmeci, V. 522, *531*
Feherty, P., Robertson, D. M., Waynforth, H. B., Kellie, A. E. 116, *128*
Feherty, P., see Méšter, J. 115, *133*
Feichtmeir, T. V., see Hales, D. R. 394, *399*
Feigelson, M., Feigelson, P. 90, *100*
Feigelson, P., Davidson, J. D. 460, *465*
Feigelson, P., see Feigelson, M. 90, *100*
Feigelson, P., see Ultmann, J. E. 460, *467*
Feigin, R. D., Klainer, A. S., Beisel, W. R. 529, *531*
Feinendegen, L. E., Bond, V. P. 314, *332*
Feinendegen, L. E., Bond, V. P., Cronkite, E. P., Hughes, W. L. 314, 315, *332*
Feinendegen, L. E., Bond, V. P., Hughes, W. L. 283, 314, 315, 316, *332*
Feinendegen, L. E., see Ertl, H. H. 314, *332*
Feinendegen, L. E., see Heiniger, H. J. 314, *335*
Feinendegen, L., see Porschen, W. 315, *342*
Feingold, M. L., Koss, L. G. 39, *43*
Feit, P. W. 41, *43*
Feldman, L. A., Rapp, F. 237, *251*
Feldman, L. A., see Rapp, F. 302, 303, 304, *343*
Felicetti, L., see Colombo, B. 557, 565, *568*
Feller, W., see Stewart, S. E. 308, *345*
Fellig, J., see Barnes, J. R. 643, *647*
Felsenfeld, G., see Gellert, M. 585, 589, *590*
Ferfoglia, L., see Astaldi, G. 706, *713*, 735, *742*
Ferm, V. H. 676, *690*
Ferm, V. H., see Ruffolo, P. R. 310, *343*
Fernandes, J. F., LePage, G. A., Lindner, A. 390, *399*
Fernández-Gómez, M. E., see Giménez-Martin, G. 662, *665*, *669*
Fernández-Gómez, M. E., see González-Fernández, A. 662, *665*
Fernández-Gómez, M. E., see Stockert, J. C. 662, *667*
Fernbach, D. J., Sutow, W. W., Thurman, W. G., Vietti, T. S. 263, *268*
Fernbach, D. J., see Sullivan, M. P. 476, *482*
Ferrari, W., Gessa, G. L., Loddo, B., Schivo, M. C. 303, *332*
Ferrari, W., Loddo, B., Gessa, G. L., Spanedda, A., Brotzu, G. 769, *784*
Ferrari, W., see Loddo, B. 302, 303, *339*
Ferreira, M. T., see Katz, N. 879, *889*
Ferreira de Santana, C., see DeBarros, T. 696, *715*
Fetty, W. O., see Katchman, B. J. 25, *32*
Fetzer, V. A., see Schmid, F. A. 521, 524, *536*
Fichtelius, O., see Diderholm, H. 307, 314, *331*
Fidler, I. J. 314, 315, 317, *332*, 705, *715*
Fidler, J., see Old, L. J. 723, *746*
Field, E. O., Mauro, F., Hellmann, K. 886, *888*
Field, E. O., see Sharpe, H. B. A. 885, *889*
Field, M., Block, J. B., Oliverio, V. T., Rall, D. P. 771, 774, *784*
Field, M., see Block, J. B. 771, 774, *783*
Field, R. B., see Vogel, C. L. 549, *553*
Fielden, E. M., Lillicarp, S. C. 321, *332*
Fikus, M., Shugar, D. 321
Fikus, M., Wierzchowski, K., Shugar, D. 198, *225*, 321, *332*
Filho, M. C., see DeBarros, T. 696, *715*
Filip, J., Nejedly, Z. 273, *333*
Filiposyan, S. T., see Chorin, V. A. 617, *621*
Filler, R. S., see Jondorf, W. R. 560, *569*
Fillingame, R. H., Morris, D. R. 774, 775, *784*
Fillios, L. C., Kaplan, R., Martin, R. S., Stare, F. 109, *128*
Filogamo, G., see Barasa, A. 675, *688*
Fimognari, G. M., see Edelman, I. S. 164, *167*
Fimognari, G. M., see Herman, T. S. 85, *101*, 164, *167*
Fina, J. J., see Rosen, J. M. 86, 87, 88, 90, 91, 92, 93, *102*
Finch, S. C., see Calabresi, P. 283, 284, 314, 319, 323, 324, *329*
Findley, A., see Gillette, R. W. 527, *531*
Fine, R. N., Clarke, R. R., Shore, N. A. 687, *690*
Finean, J. B., see Gurr, M. I. 824, *827*
Finger, H., see Weitzel, G. 756, *765*
Fink, K., Cline, R. E., Henderson, R. B., Fink, R. M. 283, *333*
Fink, M., see Bertino, J. R. 473, *479*
Fink, M. E., see Creasey, W. A. 359, *365*
Fink, R. M., see Fink, K. 283, *333*
Fink, U., Begemann, H. 708, *716*, 734, 735, 738, *744*
Fink, U., see Begemann, H. 708, *713*
Finkel, S. I., see Suhadolnik, R. J. 437, 440, *456*, 659, *668*
Finkelstein, G., Gordon, A. S., Charipper, H. A. 145, *153*
Finkelstein, J. Z., Scher, J., Karon, M. 238, *251*, 258, 260, *268*
Finkelstein, J. Z., see Karon, M, 364, *367*

Finnegan, J. K., Haag, H. B., Larson, P. S. 809, *817*
Finotto, E., see Fiorentino, M. 759, *762*
Finzi, A. F., see Grignani, F. 472, *481*
Fiorentino, M., Finotto, E. 759, *762*
Fioretti, A., see DiMarco, A. 594, *612*
Fioretti, A., see Soldati, M. 566, *570*
Fioretti, A., see Verini, M. A. 608, *613*
Firket, H. 604, *612*
Firth, J. J., see Hurwitz, J. 583, *591*
Fischer, D. S., Black, F. L., Welch, A. D. 308, *333*
Fischer, D. S., Cassidy, E. P., Welch, A. D. 237, *251*, 309, 323, *333*, 356, 362, *366*
Fischer, G. A. 471
Fischer, G. A., Bertino, J. R., Welch, A. D. 471, *480*
Fischer, G. A., see Chu, M. Y. 233, 235, 240, 241, 242, 244, 245, 246, *250*, 261, 264, *268*
Fischer, G. A., see Haley, E. E. 514, *532*, 695, *716*, 723, *744*
Fischer, G. A., see Handschumacher, R. E. 515, *532*
Fischer, G. A., see Hryniuk, W. M. 469, *481*
Fischer, G. A., see Mathias, A. P. 280, 295, 298, *340*
Fischer, G. A., see Momparler, R. L. 240, 247, *253*, 265, *270*, 427, 433
Fischer, G. A., see Pasternak, C. A. 355, *368*
Fischer, G. A., see Young, R. S. K. 235, *256*
Fischer, M., see Deutsch, E. 709, *715*, 734, 735, *744*
Fischer, R., see Burchenal, J. H. 822, *826*
Fischinger, P. J., see Hirschman, S. Z. 237, *252*
Fishbein, W. N., Carbone, P. P., Owens, A. H., Jr., Kelly, M. G., Rall, D. P., Tarr, N. 521, *531*
Fisher, D. A., Panos, T. C., Melby, J. C. 811, *817*
Fisher, J. M., see Rabinovitz, M. 498, *508*, 518, *535*
Fisher, R. A., see Weston, J. K. 38, *46*
Fishman, J., see Gallagher, T. F. 178, *189*
Fishman, J., see Zumoff, B. 178, *192*
Fishman, W. H., Sie, H. 516, *531*
Fisken, R. A., see Kurtz, S. M. 428, *433*
Fissekis, J. D., see Edelson, J. *531*
Fitzgibbon, W. E., see Shealy, Y. F. 549, *552*
Fitzmaurice, M. A., see Riley, V. 704, *720*
Fiume, L., Nardi, I., Bucci, S., Mancino, G. *669*
Flaks, J. G., see Cohen, S. S. 199, 203, 204, 218, *224*, 289, *330*
Flanagan, J. F., Ginsberg, H. S. 354, *366*
Flangas, A. L., see Van Lancker, J. L. 680, *694*
Flanigan, S., see Creasey, W. A. 238, 240, 241, 242, 244, *251*
Flather, M. T., see Bratzel, R. P. 18, *30*
Fletcher, H. J., Jr., see Glaudemans, C. P. J. 427, *432*
Fleischman, R., see Eagle, H. 484, *504*
Fleischman, R. W., see Heyman, I. A. 832, *839*
Fleisher, G. A., see Kolmeier, K. H. 777, *785*
Flesher, J. W. 114, *128*
Flesher, J. W., see Jensen, E. V. 114, *131*, 176, 187, *190*
Flickinger, R. A. 236, *251*
Fliedner, T. M., see Rubini, J. R. 280, 314, *343*
Flint, S. F., see Gregory, F. J. 523, *532*
Flippin, R. S., see Mickelson, M. N. 501, *507*, 514, *534*
Floersheim, G. L. 752, *762*
Floersheim, G. L., Brune, K. 752, *762*
Floersheim, G. L., Seiler, K. 408, *420*
Floersheim, G. L., Taub, R. N., Phillips-Quagliata, J. M., Levey, R. H. 752, *762*
Florini, J. R. 434, *453*
Florini, J. R., Bird, H. H., Bell, P. H. 434, *453*
Flowers, A., see Schmidt, L. H. 18, *33*
Fluhmann, C. F., see Laqueur, G. L. 143, *154*
Flury, F., Wieland, H. 18, *31*
Folb, R. I., Trounce, J. R. 416, *420*
Folbergrova, J. 499, *504*
Folca, P. J., Glascock, R. F., Irvine, W. T. 117, *128*
Foley, G. E., Friedman, O. M., Drolet, B. P. 29, *31*
Foley, G. E., see Caspersson, T. 6, *15*, 21, *31*
Foley, H. T., Shnider, B. I., Gold, G. L., Rius, J. 500, *504*
Foley, H. T., see Vogel, C. L. 549, *553*
Folk, R. M., see St. Pierre, R. L. 706, *720*
Folkers, K., see Kaczka, E. A. 658, *666*
Folkers, K., see Kaczka, E. A. 658, *666*
Follett, B. K., Nicholls, T. J., Redshaw, M. R. 120, 121, *128*
Follett, B. K., Redshaw, M. R. 120, 121, *128*
Follett, B. K., see Nicholls, T. J. 121, *134*
Follett, B. K., see Redshaw, M. R. 120, *135*
Folley, S. J. 111
Folley, S. J., Kon, S. K. 144, *153*
Folley, S. J., see Dodds, E. C. 113, *128*
Folley, S. J., see Van Wagonen, G. 144, *157*
Folsome, C. E. 309, *333*
Folston, B., see Pilcher, K. S. 515, *535*
Fontaine, J. L., see Foucher, G. 502, *504*
Forbes, I. J., see Smith, J. L. 406, *424*
Force, E. E., Stewart, R. C. 303, 307, *333*
Forchielli, E., see Toren, D. 139, *156*
Forcier, R. J., see Ellison, R. R. 260, *268*
Ford, J. H., Klomparens, W. 561, *568*
Forer, A., see Behnke, O. 676, *688*
Forrester, D. D., see Dedrick, R. L. 258, *268*
Forsblad, K. R., see Evans, J. S. 235, *251*
Forster, W., see Zahn, R. K. 244, *256*
Foster, D. O., see Ray, P. D. 521, *535*

Foucher, G., Wuyts, J. L., Mack, G., Geisert, J., Fontaine, J. L. 502, *504*
Fournier, C., Bach, M. A., Dardenne, M., Bach, J. F. 405, *420*
Fournier, C., see Bach, J. F. 406, 414, *419*
Fouts, P. J., see Armstrong, J. G. 685, *688*
Fowden, L., Lewis, D., Tristram, H. 512, 519, 521, 529, *531*
Fowler, W. M., see Hewlett, J. S. 740
Fowst, G., see Bergamini, N. 883, *888*
Fox, B. W. 28, *31*, 35, 40, *43*
Fox, B. W., Craig, A. W., Jackson, H. 39, *43*
Fox, B. W., Fox, M. 752, *762*
Fox, B. W., Jackson, H. 35, 37, 38, *43*
Fox, B. W., Perkins, J. P., Prusoff, W. H. 289, 315, 318, *333*
Fox, B. W., Prusoff, W. H. 280, 289, 314, 315, 316 317, *333*
Fox, B. W., see Fox, M. 41, *43*
Fox, B. W., see Jackson, H. 37, *44*
Fox, B. W., see Partington, M. 37, *45*
Fox, E., Meselson, M. *333*
Fox, J. J., Miller, N., Wempen, I. 196, *225*
Fox, J. J., Watanabe, K. A., Bloch, A. 434, 435, 436, *453*, 658, *665*
Fox, J. J., Yung, N., Bendich, A. 232, *251*
Fox, J. J., see Burchenal, J. H. 198, *224*
Fox, J. J., see Cushley, R. 197, *224*
Fox, J. J., see Dollinger, M. R. 233, 234, 239, *251*
Fox, J. J., see Duschinsky, R. 197, *225*
Fox, J. J., see Falco, E. A. 233, *251*
Fox, J. J., see Hoffer, M. 195, *226*, 272, *335*
Fox, J. J., see Kim, J. H. 233, 241, *253*
Fox, J. J., see Shugar, D. 296, *344*
Fox, J. J., see Wempen, I. 195, 196, 197, 198, *231*, 233, *256*, 278, *346*
Fox, J. J., see Yung, N. C. 196, *231*, 272, *347*
Fox, K. E., Gabourel, J. D. 88, 89, *100*
Fox, K. E., see Gabourel, J. D. 89, 90, *100*
Fox, M., Fox, B. W. 41, *43*
Fox, M., Lajtha, L. 316, *333*
Fox, M., see Fox, B. W. 752, *762*
Fox, W., see Dessauer, H. C. 120, *127*, *128*
Foyt, D. C., see McCord, T. J. 524, *534*
Fradkin, R., see Schmidt, L. H. 18, *33*
Fraenkel-Conrat, H., see Singer, B. 7, 15, *17*, 71, *83*
Franceschi, F., see Arcamone, F. 593, *611*
Francis, B. F., see Allen, E. 108, *125*
Francis, D., see Kirschner, S. 836, *840*
Franco, J., see Hales, D. R. 394, *399*
Frank, B. H., Pekar, A. H., Veros, A. J., Ho, P. P. K. 699, 700, *716*
Frank, B. H., see Ho, P. P. K. 698, 699, 702, 708, 716
Frank, R. T., Klempner, E. 140, *153*
Frankel, H. H., Yamamoto, R. S., Weisburger, E. K., Weisburger, J. H. 410, 417, *421*
Frankel, S., see Roberts, E. 485, *509*
Franklin, H. A., see Moore, G. E. 90, *102*
Franklin, L., see Dietrich, L. S. 541, *542*
Franklin, R. M. 584, *590*
Franklin, R. M., see Reich, E. 53, 54, 58, *62*, 582, 583, 584, *591*
Franklin, R. M., see Shatkin, A. H. 54, *62*
Franklin, T. J., Cook, J. M. 450, 451, *453*
Franklin, T. J., see Carter, S. B. 446, 450, 451, *453*
Franzen, S., see Dahlwitz, A. 735, *743*
Franzino, A., see Colsky, J. 500, *504*
Frappier, A., see de Repentigny, J. 201, *224*
Fraser, P. E., see Meister, A. 708, *718*
Fraser, T. H., Rich, A. *669*
Fraser, T. J., see Bhuyan, B. K. 75, 76, *80*, 218, *223* 629, *631*, 802, *805*, 881, *888*
Fraser, T. J., see Li, L. H. 362, *367*, 653, *656*
Fraser, W. D., see Blondal, H. 524, *530*
Fratta, I., see Greengard, P. 542, *542*
Frauenberger, G., see Jaffe, N. 479, *481*
Frazier, J., see Howard, F. B. 293, *336*
Frazier, L. E., see Samal, B. A. 520, *535*
Frazier, L. F., see Wissler, R. W. 525, 526, *538*
Frearson, P. M., see Kit, S. 298, *338*
Frederiksen, S., see Danø, K. 573, *579*
Frederiksen, S. 658, 661, *665*
Frederiksen, S., Klenow, H. 663, *665*
Frederiksen, S., Malling, H., Klenow, H. 658, *665*
Frederiksen, S., Pedersen, I. R., Hellung-Larsen, P., Engberg, J. *669*
Frederiksen, S., Rasmussen, A. H. 660, 661. *665*
Frederiksen, S., Tønnesen, T., Hellung-Larsen, P. 663, *665*
Frederiksen, S., see Hellung-Larsen, P. 664, *666*
Frederiksen, S., see Klenow, H. 659, *666*
Frederiksen, S., see Truman, J. T. 663, *668*
Freed, J. J., Bhisey, A. N., Lebowitz, M. M. 676, *690*
Freedlander, B. L., French, F. A. 766, 767, 768, *784*
Freedlander, B. L., see French, F. A. 793, *806*, 841, 842, 844, *848*
Freele, H., see Berberian, D. A. 879, *887*
Freele, H., see Rosi, D. 879, *889*
Freeman, A., see Ohnuma, T. 514, *534*, 703, *719*, 724, 725, 733, 734, 735, *745*
Freeman, B. B., see Davidson, J. D. 390, *399*
Freeman, G., see Smith, J. D. 302, 307, *344*
Freeman, J. J., see Hilf, R. 123, *130*
Freeman, J. M., see Leonard, L. L. 354, *367*

Freeman, L., see Lubitz, J. A. 811, 814, 815, 816, *818*
Freeman, M. V. 471, *480*
Freeman, M. V., see Li, M. C. 472, *482*
Freese, E. 52, *60*, 296, *333*
Freese, E., see Benzer, S. 295, *328*
Freese, E., see Rhaese, H.-J. 8, *16*
Freese, M., see Elford, H. L. 793, *805*
Freeze, E., see Bautz, E. 11, *15*
Fregly, M. J., see Straw, J. A. 813, *819*
Frei, E, III. 266, 430
Frei, E, III, Bickers, J. N., Hewlett, J. S., Lane, M., Leary, W. V., Talley, R. W. 260, 262, *269*
Frei, E., III., Freireich, E. J. 687, *690*
Frei, E., III., Whang, J., Scoggins, R. B., Van Scott, E. J., Rall, D. P., Ben, M. 679, *690*
Frei, E., III, see Bono, V. H. 352, *364*
Frei, E., III, see Carbone, P. P. 394, *398*
Frei, E., III., see Fallon, H. J. 352, 359, *365*
Frei, E., III., see Freireich, E. J. 260, *269*, 772, *785*
Frei, E., III., see Goldin, A. 389, *399*
Frei, E., III, see Handschumacher, R. E. 355, 358, 359, 360, 361, *366*
Frei, E., III., see Hart, J. S. 265, *269*
Frei, E., III., see Ho, D. H. W. 238, *252*, 258, 259, 260, 262, 263, 266, *269*, 698, 699, 700, 702, *716*, 733, *744*
Frei, E., III., see Loo, T. L. 386, *401*, 546, *551*
Frei, E., III., see Samuels, M. L. 759, *764*
Frei, E., III., see Shirakawa, S. 77, *83*, 546, *552*
Frei, E., III., see Talley, R. W. 261, *271*
Frei, E., III., see Venditti, J. M. 393, *403*
Frei, E., III., see Lyman, M. 820, *827*
Frei, J. V. 77, *80*
Freireich, E. J., Bodey, G. P., Harris, J. E., Hart, J. S. 397, *399*
Freireich, E. J., Bodey, G. P., Hart, J. S., Rodriguez, V., Whitecar, J. P., Frei, E., III 260, *269*
Freireich, E. J., Bodey, G. P., Hart, J. S., Whitecar, J. P., Jr., McCredie, K. B. 262, 265, *269*
Freireich, E. J., Frei, E., III, Karon, M. 772, *785*
Freireich, E. J., see Bodey, G. P. 260, 261, 263, 264, *268*
Freireich, E. J., see Frei, E., III. 687, *690*
Freireich, E. J., see Gutterman, J. U. 265, *269*
Freireich, E. J., see Hersh, E. M. 264, *269*, 384, *400*, 770, *785*
Freireich, E. J., see Ho, D. H. W. *252*
Freireich, E. J., see Levin, R. H. 769, 772, *786*
Freireich, E. J., see Whitecar, J. P., Jr. 726, 727, 728, 730, 734, 735, *746*
Freireich, E. J., see Whitecar, J. P., Jr. 263, *271*
Freisheim, J. H., see Huennekens, F. M. 469, *481*
French, E. F., see Britten, R. J. 513, *530*
French, F. A., see Blanz, E. J., Jr. 795, *805*
French, F. A., see DoAmaral, J. R. 779, *784*
French, F. A., Blanz, E. J., Jr. 768, *785*, 794, 795, 797, 798, 799, *805*, *806*
French, F. A., Freedlander, B. L. 739, *806*, 841, 842, 844, *848*
French, F. A., Lewis, A. E., Sheena, A. H., Blanz, E. J., Jr. 798, *806*
French, F. A., see Blanz, E. J., Jr. 795, 799, *805*, 880, *888*
French, F. A., see DoAmaral, J. R. 779, *784*
French, F. A., see Freedlander, B. L. 766, 767, 768, *784*
French, F. A., see Podrebarac, E. G. 768, *787*
French, T. C., Dawid, I. B., Day, R. A., Buchanan, J. M. 487, 488, *505*
French, T. C., see Dawid, I. B. 487, 488, *504*
Frenkel, E. P., see Luce, J. K. 397, *401*
Frenster, J. H. 824, 825, *827*
Frenster, J. H., see Rose, H. G. 824, *828*
Fresco, J. R., see Doty, P. 292, *331*
Fretzdorff, A. M., see Weitzel, G. L. 754, 756, *765*
Freudenberg, J., see Meyer zum Büschenfelde, K. H. 407, *422*
Frey, J. R., see Brossi, A. 563, *567*
Fridhandler, L., see Palmer, W. M. 860, *874*
Friedkin, M., see Wilson, L. 678, *694*
Fridland, A., Langenbach, R. J., Heidelberger, C. 204, *225*
Fried, J., Sabo, E. F. 185, *189*
Fried, J., Thoma, R. W., Klingsberg, A. 182, *189*
Friedkin, M. 460, *465*
Friedkin, M., Roberts, D. 272, 273, 283, *333*
Friedland, I. M., see Dietrich, L. S. 541, *542*
Friedland, M., Visser, D. W. 380, *381*
Friedman, E. A., see Gelfand, M. C. 407, *421*
Friedman, H. 707, *716*
Friedman, H., see Chakrabarty, A. K. 705, *715*
Friedman, H., see Klatskin, G. 558, 561, *569*
Friedman, M., see Frohwein, Y. Z. 697, *716*
Friedman, M., see Von Furth, O. 695, 697, *721*
Friedman, O. M., Rutenburg, A. M. 520, *531*
Friedman, O. M., see Foley, G. E. 29, *31*
Friedman, P. A., see Goldberg, I. H. 582, *590*
Friedman, R. M., Cooper, H. L. 608, *612*
Friedman, R. M., see Baron, S. 607, *611*
Friedman, R. M., see Stern, R. 584, *592*
Friedman, S., see Selye, H. 143, *156*
Friedrich, G. D., see Heiniger, H. J. 314, *335*
Friedrich, U., Zeuthen, E. 415, *421*
Fries, J., see Erdos, T. *114*, *128*
Frigerio, N. A., see Coley, R. F. 836, *839*
Frisch, A. W. 526, *531*
Frisch, D. M., Visser, D. W. 272, *333*

Frischauf, H., see Deutsch, E. 709, *715*, 734, 735, *744*
Fritzson, P. 283, *333*
Froese, A., see Linford, J. H. 28, *32*
Frohardt, R. P., see Bartz, Q. R. 485, *503*
Frohardt, R. P., see Fusari, S. A. 485, *505*
Frohwein, Y. Z., Friedman, M., Reizer, J., Grossowicz, N. 697, *716*
Fromageot, P., see Darlix, J. L. 462, *465*
Fromageot, P., see Sentenac, A. 583, *592*, 629, *632*, 659, *667*
Frost, P., see Dalldorf, G. 417, *420*
Fruton, J. S., see Golumbic, C. 19, *31*
Fry, B. A. 499, *505*
Fry, D. J., see Bittar, E. E. 861, *871*
Fučík, V., Kara, J. 273, *333*
Fučík, V., Michaelis, A., Rieger, R. 362, *366*
Fučík, V., Zadražíl, S., Jurovčík, M., Šormorá, Z. *366*
Fučík, V., see Jurovčík, M. 363, *367*
Fudenberg, H., see Taylor, F. B., Jr. 527, *537*
Fugmann, R. A., see Martin, D. S. 542, *543*
Fugmann, R. A., see Shapiro, D. M. 522, *536*
Fujimoto, M., see Higuchi, M. *60*, 857, *872*
Fujimoto, N., see Nakamura, S. 870, *873*
Fujimoto, Y., see Wakaki, S. 47, *64*
Fujimura, S., see Cheng, C. J. 68, 70, *80*
Fujita, H., see Kimura, K. 870, *873*
Fujiwara, A. N., Acton, E. M., Goodman, L. 881, *888*
Fujiwara, T., see Mizuno, H. 279, *341*
Fujiwara, Y., Heidelberger, C. 205, *225*
Fujiwara, Y., Oki, T., Heidelberger, C. 205, *225*, 292, 298, *333*
Fukagawa, Y., see Sawa, T. 444, *455*
Fukagawa, Y., see Umezawa, H. 444, *456*
Fukatsu, H., Yoshida, K. 870, *872*
Fukuhara, T. K., Visser, D. W. 272, *333*, 376, *381*
Fukui, T., see Ikehara, M. 437, 443, *454*
Fukunishi, R., see Huggins, C. *131*
Fukushima, D. K., Bradlow, H. L., Hellman, L. 813, *817*
Fukuyama, T. T., Moyed, H. S. 448, *453*
Fuller, W., see Hamilton, L. 586, *590*
Fuller, W., see Ward, D. C. 441, 443, *456*, 462, 463, *467*
Fulmor, W., see Morton, G. O. 434, *455*
Fulmor, W., see Patrick, J. B. 48, *62*
Fulmor, W., see Webb, J. S. 47, *64*
Fumagalli, R., see Grafnetterová, J. 357, 358, *366*
Funk, F., see Osborn, M. 11, *16*
Funkhouser, J. T., see Yesair, D. W. 822, 823, *828*
Funkhouser, J. T., see Yesair, D. W. 823, 824, *828*
Funzle, J., see Weston, J. K. 38, *46*
Furesz, S., see Arioli, V. 883, *887*
Furlong, N. B., Gresham, C. 243, 244, *251*
Furth, J. J., Cohen, S. S. 241, 243, 244, *251*, 261, *269*, 427, *432*
Furth, R., van 384, *399*
Furusawa, E., Cutting, W., Buckley, P., Furusawa, S. 302, 307, *333*
Furusawa, S., see Furusawa, E. 302, 307, *333*
Fusari, S. A., Haskell, T. H., Frohardt, R. P., Bartz, Q. R. 485, *505*
Fusari, S. A., see Bartz, Q. R. 485, *503*
Fusari, S. A., see Dion, H. W. 485, *504*
Fusari, S. A., see Westland, R. D. 485, *511*
Fusenig, N. E., Obrecht, P., Strickstrock, K. H. 757, *762*
Fusenig, N. E., see Obrecht, P. 682, *692*, 757, *763*
Fushekawa, O., see Suzuki, M. 870, *875*
Fussel, C. P., see Smith, H. H. 380, *382*
Fussganger, R., Dold, U., Holzer, H. 25, *31*

Gabor, E. P., Scott, J. L. 410, *421*
Gabourel, J. D., Aronow, L. 86, 87, *100*
Gabourel, J. D., Comstock, J. P. 89, *100*
Gabourel, J. D., Fox, K. E. 89, 90, *100*
Gabourel, J. D., see Chung, L. 681, *688*
Gabourel, J. D., see Fox, K. E. 88, 89, *100*
Gabriel, T., see Duschinsky, R. 197, *225*
Gabriel, T., see Koechlin, B. A. 201, 202, *227*
Gabriel, T., see Lozeron, H. A. 198, *228*, 321, *340*
Gabrielder, C., see Georgatos, J. G. 280, *333*
Gabrielsen, A. E., Good, R. A. 309, *333*
Gadekar, K., see Kelly, M. G. 752, *762*, *763*
Gadjos, A., see Bariety, M. 683, *688*
Gaetani, M., see Di Marco, A. 593, 597, 609, *612*
Gaetani, M., see Silvestrini, R. *613*
Gahan, P. B., see Chayen, J. 824, *826*
Gailani, S. D., Armstrong, J. G., Carbone, P. P., Tan, C., Holland, J. F. 685, *690*
Gaines, D., see Wells, W. 352, *371*
Gaito, R. A., Prusoff, W. H. 318, *333*
Galaev, Y. V., Kharats, K. S. 698, *716*
Gale, E. F., see Elliott, H. W. 499, *504*
Gale, G. R. 74, 76, *80*
Gale, G. R., Howle, J. A., Walker, E. M., Jr. 835, *839*
Gale, G. R., Kendall, S. M., McClain, H. H., Dubois, S. 790, *791*
Gale, G. R., Morris, C. R., Atkins, L. M., Smith, A. B. 838, *839*
Gale, G. R., Ostrander, W. E., Atkins, L. M. 882, *888*
Gale, G. R., Simpson, J. G., Smith, A. B. 757, *762*

Gale, G. R., Smith, A. B. 882, *888*
Gale, G. R., see Howle, J. A. 829, 830, 831, 833, 834, 835, 838, *839*
Gale, G. R., see Thompson, H. S. 831, 835, *840*
Gale, M. M., see Daniel, P. M. 314, *330*
Galegov, G. A., Kukhar, E. E., Bikbulatova, R. M. 354, *366*
Galegov, G. A. 513, *531*
Galegov, G. A., Benyumovich, M. S. 524, *531*
Galegov, G. A., Bikbulatova, R. M., Vanag, K. A., Shen, R. M. *366*
Galegov, G. A., see Demidova, S. A. 354, *365*
Galegov, G. A., see Pravdina, N. F. 354, *368*
Galegov, G. A., see Terskikh, I. I. 354, *371*
Gall, D., see Denman, E. J. 416, *420*
Gallagher, T. F., Fishman, J., Sumoff, B., Cassouto, J., Hellman, L. 178, *189*
Gallagher, T. F., see Beer, C. T. 108, *126*
Gallagher, T. F., see Moore, C. R. 143, *155*
Gallagher, T. F., see Nelson, W. O. 144, *155*
Gallagher, T. F., see Zumoff, B. 178, *192*
Gallmeier, W., see Schmidt, C. G. 726, 727, 730, 734, 735, *746*
Gallmeier, W. M., see Stier, H. W. *746*
Gallo, R. C., Longmore, J. L., Adamson, R. H. 711, *716*
Gallo, R. C., Whang-Peng, J., Adamson, R. H. 650, 653, *655*
Gallo, R. C., see Smith, R. G. 883, *889*
Gallo, R. C., see Wu, A. M. *669*
Gallo, R. C., see Yang, S. S. 883, *890*
Galson, E. C., see Tepper, H. B. 857, *875*
Galton, D. A. G. 35, *43*
Galton, D. A. G., Till, M., Wiltshaw, E. 35, 36, 37, *43*
Galton, D. A. G., see Beard, M. E. J. 726, 727, 728, 730, 734, 735, *743*
Galton, D. A. G., see Elson, L. A. 38, *43*
Galton, D. A. G., see Fairley, G. H. 726, 727, 728, 730, 732, 734, *744*
Gambarucci, C., see Casazza, A. M. 607, 610, *611*
Gambarucci, C., see DiMarco, A. 599, 605, *612*
Gambetta, G. E., see Eidinoff, M. L. 283, 295, 314, *332*
Gambetta, R. A., see DiFronzo, G. 608, 609, *612*
Gambetta, R. A., see DiMarco, A. 599, 605, *612*
Gambetta, R. A., see Zunino, F. 599, *614*
Gang, M., see Hoffman, G. S. 263, *269*, 548, *550*
Gang, M., see Kline, I. 79, *81*, 198, *227*, 259, *270*, 545, 548, *551*, 767, *785*
Gang, M., see Tyrer, D. D. 523,, *537*, 548, *552*
Ganter, P., see Dubost, M. 593, *612*
Garapin, A. C., see McDonnell, J. P. 583, *591*, *613*
Garattini, S., see Amiel, J.-L. 752, *760*
Garattini, S., see Rosso, R. 69, *83*
Garaza, A., see Sellinger, O. Z. 499, *510*
Garcia, A., see DelPuerto, B. M. 560, *568*
Garcia, F., see Sutow, W. W. 726, 727, 732, *746*
Garcia-Ferrandiz, F., see Munoz, E. F. 554, *569*
Garcia-Giralt, E., Macieira-Coelho, A. 881, *888*
Gardner, D. G., see Wittliff, J. L. 117, *138*
Gardner, L. T., see Jacobs, N. F. 859, *873*
Gardner, R. S., see Wahba, A. J. 214, *231*
Garen, A., Siddiqi, O. 214, *225*
Garfinkel, E., see Barclay, R. K. 487, 489, *503*
Garin, A. M., see Astrakhan, V. I. 621, *621*
Garofalo, M., see Schwartz, H. S. 790, *792*
Garrett, E. R. 65, *80*
Garrett, E. R., Chermburkar, P. B., Suzuki, T. 275, 276, *333*
Garrett, E. R., Goto, S., Stubbins, J. F. 65, 66, *80*
Garrett, E. R., Suzuki, T., Weber, D. J. 275, *333*
Garrett, E. R., Yakatan, G. J. 276, 277, *333*
Garrett, H., see Pietsch, P. 859, 862, 863, 864, 865, 866, 869, *874*
Garrett, J. V., see Craig, A. W. 318, *330*
Garrison, F. E., Jr., see Rundles, R. W. 408, 412, *423*
Gaucher, G. M., see Price, C. C. 1, *5*, 19, 26, *33*
Gaulden, M. E., see Mueller, G. A. 674, *692*
Gause, G. F. 593, *612*, 616, 617, *621*
Gawadi, N. 676, *690*
Gebbia, N., see Dusonchet, L. 608, *612*
Gebhart, E. 41, *43*
Gee, M., see Bachur, N. R. 609, 610, *611*
Gee, T. S., Yu, K. P., Clarkson, B. D. *269*, 394, 397, *399*
Geeraets, W. J., Wong, G., Guerry, D. III. 298, *333*
Gehan, E. A., see Bodey, G. P. 264, *268*
Gehan, E. A., see Sutow, W. W. 726, 727, 732, *746*
Gehrke, J., see Hensen, D. 302, 304, *335*
Gehrman, G., see Putter, J. *740*
Geiduschek, P. 8, *15*
Geiger, J., see Nyman, M. A. 106, *134*
Geigy, J. R. 528, *531*
Geiling, E. M., see Kocsis, J. J. 684, *691*
Geiser, C., see Jaffe, N. 479, *481*
Geisert, J., see Foucher, G. 502, *504*
Gelbard, A. S., Kim, S. H., Eidinoff, M. L. 354, *366*
Gelbard, A. S., see Kim, J. H. 59, *61*, 299, *337*
Gelbard, A. S., see Kim, K. H. 603, 605, *613*
Gelfand, I. M., see Vasiliev, J. M. 681, *694*
Gelfand, M. C., Nowakowski, A., Friedman, E. A., Knepshield, J. H. 407, *421*
Gellert, E., Govindachari, T. R., Lakshmikantham, M. V., Ragade, I. S., Rudzuts, R., Viswanathan, N. 564, *568*

Gellert, M., Smith, C. E., Neville, D., Felsenfeld, G. 585, 589, *590*
Gellhorn, A. 459, 460, *465*
Gellhorn, A., Kream, J., Hirschberg, E. 459, 460, *465*
Gellhorn, A., Wagner, M., Richler, M., Koren, A., Benjamin, W. 822, 823, *827*
Gellhorn, A., see Booth, J. 822, 823, 824, *826*
Gellhorn, A., see Hirschberg, E. 460, *466*, 879, *889*
Gellhorn, A., see Ochoa, M., Jr. 823, 824, *827*
Gelzer, J., Loustalot, P. 747, *762*
Gelzer, J., Marxer, A., Schmid, K. 777, 780, *785*
Gelzer, J., see Marxer, A. 778, *786*
Gelzer, J., see Mihich, E. 777, *786*
Genova, R., see Astaldi, G. 526, *529*
Genova, R., see Astaldi, G. 706, *713*, 735, *742*
Gentry, G. A., see Dorsett, M. T. 290, *331*
Georgatsos, J. G., Antonoglou, O., Gabrielder, C. 280, *333*
Georgatsos, J. G., Karemfyllis, T. 681, *690*
Georgatsos, J. G., Karemfyllis, T., Symeonidis, A. 678, *690*
George, P., Journey, L. J., Goldstein, M. N. 673, *690*
George, P., see Journey, L. J. 673, 674, *691*
Georgiev, G. P. 147, *154*
Georgiev, G. P., Samarina, O. P., Lerman, M. I., Smirnov, M. N., Severtzov, A. N. 584, *590*
Geraci, G., see Scarano, E. 287, *343*
Gerber, G. B., Remy-Defraigne, J. 283, 284, *333*
Gerber, N. N. 661, *665*
Gerber, N. N., Lechevalier, H. A. 658, 660, *665*
Gerber, N. N., see Pugh, L. H. 660, *667*
Gerber, P. 308, *333*
Gerberová, J., see Šmahel, O. 361, *370*
Gerhartz, H., Begeman, H. 726, 727, 728, 734, 735, *744*
Gericke, D., see Chandra, P. 602, 608, *611*
German, J., LaRock, J. 57, *60*
Gerner, R. E., see Moore, G. E. 90, *102*
Gerone, P. J., see Knight, V. *338*
Gerroluzzi-Ames, G., see Shifrin, S. 517, 529, *536*
Gerron, G. G., see Rudman, D. 703, *720*
Gershenovich, Z. S., Krichevskaya, A. A., Koloušek, J. 499, *505*
Gershon, D., Sachs, L. 354, *366*
Gerulath, A. H., Loo, T. L. 547, *550*
Gerulath, A. H., see Loo, T. L. 547, *551*
Gerzon, K., see Sweeney, M. J. 446, 451, *456*
Gerzon, K., see Williams, R. H. 446, *457*
Gessa, G. L., see Ferrari, W. 303, *332*, 769, *784*
Gessa, G. L., see Tagliamonte, A. 519, *537*
Getz, G. S., Bartley, W. 824, *827*
Ghadially, F. N., see Wiseman, G. 517, 528, *538*
Ghione, M., see Soldati, M. 566, *570*
Ghione, M., see Verini, M. A. 608, *613*
Ghiringhelli, D., see Cardani, C. 566, *567*
Ghobar, A., see Heidelberger, C. 300, *335*
Ghosh, A. C., see Korytnyk, W. 778, *785*
Ghosh, S., Blumenthal, H. J., Davidson, E., Roseman, S. 493, *505*
Giannopoulos, G., Gorski, J. 95, *100*
Gibson, F., Pittard, J., Reich, E. 492, *505*
Gibson, H. V., see Allen, E. 108, *125*
Gichner, T., Veleminský, J. 78, *80*
Gichner, T., Veleminský, J., Křepinský, J. 78, *80*
Gichner, T., Veleminský, J., Pokorný, V. 78, *80*
Gideon, L., see Cerilli, G. J. 752, *761*
Giege, R., Weil, J. H. 210, *225*
Giese, A. C. 857, *872*
Gilbert, D. M., see Berenbaum, M. C. 706, *713*
Gilbert, N. L., see Dessauer, H. C. 120, *128*
Gilbert, P. J., see Wittliff, J. L. 117, *138*
Gilbert, W., see Gros, F. 210, *225*
Gilbert, W. R., Jr., see McCollister, R. J. 390, 395, *401*
Gilboe, D. P., see Mizuno, N. S. 636, 637, *641*
Gilead, Z., Becker, Y. 560, *568*
Giles, W. G., see Hansen, H. J. 500, 502, *505*
Gill, D. M., see Baseman, J. B. 561, *567*
Gillespie, D., see Slater, D. W. *669*
Gillespie, E., Levine, R. J., Malawista, S. E. 683, *690*
Gillett, R., see Bui, N. M. 273, *329*
Gillette, J. R., see Greene, F. E. 812, *818*
Gillette, R. W., Findley, A., Conway, H. 527, *531*
Gillibrand, P. N. 416, *421*
Gilman, A., Philips, F. S. 18, *31*
Gilot, J., see Moutschen, J. 42, *45*
Gimlin, D. M., Farquharson, E., Leach, F. R. 308, *334*
Gimlin, D. M., Hardman, S. D., Kelley, B. N., Butler, G. C., Leach, F. R. 308, *334*
Giménez-Martin, G., González-Fernández, A., De La Torre, C., Fernández-Gómez, M. E. 662, *665*
Giménez-Martin, G., de la Torre, C., Fernández-Gómez, M. E., Gonzáles-Fernández, A. *669*
Gingras, B. A., Hornal, R. W., Bayley, C. H. 841, *848*
Gingras, B. A., Somarjai, R. L., Bayley, C. H. 841, *848*
Gingras, B. A., Suprunchuk, T., Bayley, C. H. 841, *848*
Ginsberg, H. S., see Flanagan, J. F. 354, *366*
Ginsberg, T., see Heymann, H. 515, *532*

Ginsburg, H., see Berenbaum, M.C. 706, *713*
Giraldo, G., see Schulten, H.K. 705, 707, *720*, *721*
Gish, D.T., Neil, G.L., Wechter, W.J. 233, *252*
Gish, D.T., see Gray, G.D. 237, *252*, 266, *269*
Gisler, R.H., Bell, J.P. 430, *432*
Githens, J.H., Rosenkrantz, J.G., Tunnock, S.M. 415, *421*
Githens, J.H., see Rosenkrantz, J.G. 415, *423*
Gitlin, D., Commerford, S.L., Amsterdam, E., Hughes, W. 314, 318, *334*
Gitlin, D., see Commerford, S.L. 283, 318, *330*
Gitlin, D., see Hughes, W.L. 280, 281, 283, 284, 314, 315, 316, *336*
Gitlin, D., see Krueger, R.C. 283, 314, 315, *338*
Gitterman, C.O., Burg, R.W., Boxer, G.E., Meltz, D., Hitt, J. 661, *665*
Gitterman, C.O., see Kaczka, E.A. 658, *666*
Givelber, H.M., DiPaolo, J.A. 78, *80*
Giziewicz, J., Kušmierek, J.T., Shugar, D. 233, *252*
Glaeser, R.M., see Richmond, J.E. *874*
Glascock, R.F., Hoekstra, W.G. 95, *100*, 113, *129*
Glascock, R.F., see Dodds, E.C. 113, *128*
Glascock, R.F., see Folca, P.J. 117, *128*
Glasgow, L.A. 417, *421*
Glasser, S., see Balin, H. 104, *125*
Glasser, S.R. 159, 162, *167*
Glaudemans, C.P.J., Fletcher, H.J., Jr. 427, *432*
Glazko, A.J., see Ch'ien, L.T. 428, *432*
Gleichmann, E., Gleichmann, H., Schwartz, R.S. 418, *421*
Gleichmann, H., see Gleichmann, E. 418, *421*
Glickman, G., see Philipson, L. *580*, 664, *667*
Glidewell, O., see Ohnuma, T. 726, 727, 728, 734, 735, *746*
Glidewell, O.J., see Rausen, A.R. 726, 730, 732, 735, 738, *746*
Glišin, V., see Crkvenjakov, R. 363, *365*
Glock, G.E., McLean, P. 539, *542*
Gloyna, R.E., Wilson, J.D. 149, *154*
Gluckman, M.I., see Rosenthale, M.E. 523, 526, *535*
Gmelin, R., Strauss, G., Hassenmaier, G. 498, *505*
Godin, C., see Berecz, A. 521, *530*
Goedde, H.E., see Agarwal, D.P. 283, *327*
Goetsch, D.D., see Bottoms, G. 96, *100*
Götz, A., see Chandra, P. 602, 608, *611*
Goffinet, D.R., Brown, J.M., Bagshaw, M.A., Kaplan, H.S. 319, *334*
Goffinet, D.R., see Brown, J.M. 319, *329*
Gohlke 852
Golbey, R.B., see Clarkson, B.D. 727, 728, 730, 732, *743*
Golbey, R.B., see Hackethal, C.A. 638, *640*
Golbey, R.B., see Karnofsky, D.A. 500, 502, *506*
Golbey, R.B., see Oettgen, H.F. 727, 728, 730, 732, 734, 735, *745*
Gold, G.L., see Foley, H.T. 500, *504*
Gold, J. 521, *531*, *532*
Gold, M., Hurwitz, J. 583, *590*
Goldberg, B., see Goldin, A. 459, 460, *465*
Goldberg, I.H. 554, *568*, 585, *590*, 628
Goldberg, I.H., Friedman, P.A. 582, *590*
Goldberg, I.H., Mitsugi, K. 566, *568*
Goldberg, I.H., Rabinowitz, M. 352, *366*, 583, 585, *590*
Goldberg, I.H., Rabinowitz, M., Reich, E. 585, *590*
Goldberg, I.H., Stewart, M.L., Ayuso, M., Kappen, L. 557, 558, 559, 566, *568*
Goldberg, I.H., see Cerami, A. 585, *590*
Goldberg, I.H., see Reich, E. 582, 583, 585, *592*, 626, *632*
Goldberg, I.H., see Ward, D.C. 602, *614*, 625, 626, 629, *632*
Goldberg, L., see Dodds, E.C. 105, *128*
Goldberg, L.E., see Baumstein, V.E. 620, *621*
Goldberg, L.E., Kremer, V.E. 619, 620, *622*
Goldberg, N.D., Dahl, J.L., Parks, R.E., Jr. 201, *225*
Goldberg, R.C., Chaikoff, I.L. 171, *189*
Goldblatt, P.J., Sullivan, R.J., Farber, E. 583, *590*
Golde, A., see Vigier, P. 58, *63*
Golden, A., see Stewart, S.E. 308, *345*
Golden, J., see Bennett, L.L., Jr. 391, *398*
Golden, J., see Simpson, L. 392, *402*
Goldenberg, D.M. 238, *252*
Goldenberg, D.M., Schricker, K.T., von der Emdes, J., Sogtrop, H.H. 259, *269*
Goldenberg, G.J. 40, *43*
Goldenberg, G.J., Alexander, P. 40, *44*
Goldenberg, H., see Hilf, R. 119, 123, 124, *130*
Goldfinger, S.E., Howell, R.R., Seegmiller, J.E. 683, *690*
Goldie, J., Hillcoat, B.L. 469, *481*
Goldin, A., Greenspan, E.M., Goldberg, B., Schoenbach, E.B. 459, 460, *465*
Goldin, A., Humphreys, S.R., Venditti, J.M., Mantel, N. 500, *505*
Goldin, A., Sandberg, J.S., Henderson, E.S., Newman, J.W., Frei, E.III., Holland, J.F. 389, *399*
Goldin, A., Serpick, A.A., Mantel, N. 564, *568*
Goldin, A., Vendetti, J.M., Humphreys, S.R., Dennis, D., Mantel, N., Greenhouse, S.W. 476, *481*
Goldin, A., Venditti, J.M., Kline, I., Mantel, N. 301, *334*
Goldin, A., Wood, H.B., Jr. 36, *44*
Goldin, A., see DeWys, W.D. 650, *655*
Goldin, A., see Hoffman, G.S. 263, *269*, 548, *550*

Goldin, A., see Kaplan, N. O. 540, *543*
Goldin, A., see Kline, I. 198, *227*, 235, *253*, 259, 260, 262, *270*, 545, *551*, 767, *785*
Goldin, A., see Lin, Y. T. 549, 550, *551*
Goldin, A., see Narrod, S. A. 491, *508*
Goldin, A., see Pujman, V. 196, *229*
Goldin, A., see Sandberg, J. S. 36, *46*, 597, *613*
Goldin, A., see Schrecker, A. W. 234, *255*, 265, *271*
Goldin, A., see Tsukagoshi, S. 76, *84*
Goldin, A., see Tyrer, D. D. 236, *255*, *271*, 523, 537, 548, *552*
Goldin, A., see Vadlamudi, S. 362, *371*, 705, 706, *721*
Goldin, A., see Venditti, J. M. 393, 397, *403*, 597, *613*, 687, *694*, 799, *807*, 820, *828*
Goldman, L., see Weiss, A. J. *511*
Goldman, R., see Kaufman, J. J. 415, *422*
Goldner, M., see Weisenfeld, S. 814, *819*
Goldner, M. G., see Southren, A. L. 811, *819*
Goldstein, A. L., see Bach, J. F. 410, 413, 414, *419*
Goldstein, M. N., Slotnick, I. J., Journey, L. J. 583, *590*
Goldstein, M. N., see George, P. 673, *690*
Goldstein, M. N., see Journey, L. J. 583, *591*
Goldthwait, D. A. 488, *505*
Goldzieher, J. W., see Axelrod, L. R. 106, 107, *125*
Goldzieher, J. W., see Nyman, M. A. 106, *134*
Gollan, F., see Linn, B. S. 527, *533*
Goller, H., see Hartmann, G. 602, 603, *612*
Gollin, F. F., see Ansfield, F. J. 221, *223*
Gollin, F. F., see Clifton, K. H. 289, 291, *330*
Gollub, E. G., see Gots, J. S. 390, *399*, 492, 494, 495, *505*
Golomb, F. M., see Harris, M. N. 638, *640*
Golomb, F. M., see Wright, J. C. 478, *483*
Golumbic, C., Fruton, J. S., Bergmann, M. 19, *31*
Gomez, E. C., Hsia, S. L. 149, *154*
Gomori, G. 29, *32*
Gonatas, N. K., Robbins, E. 676, *690*
Gonatas, N. K., see Robbins, E. 676, *693*
Gontcharoff, M., Mazia, D. 310, *334*
Gontcharoff, M., see Mazia, D. 310, *340*
Gonzales, E. M., see Rousselot, L. M. 221, *230*
Gonzales, L., see Chun, E. H. L. 14, *15*, 28, *31*
Gonzalez, E. M., Krejczy, K., Malt, R. A. 410, *421*
Gonzalez, E. M., see Malamud, D. 410, *422*
Gonzalez, R., see Sugiura, K. 36, *46*
González-Fernández, A., Fernandez-Gomez, M. E., Stockert, J. C., Lopez-Saez, J. F. 662, *665*
González-Fernández, A., see Giménez-Martin, G. 662, *665*, *669*
Good, R. A., see Gabrielsen, A. E. 309, *333*
Good, R. A., see Lemmel, E. M. 59, *61*
Good, R. A., see Page, A. R. 384, *401*
Goodman, F. 199, *225*
Goodman, L., see Fujiwara, A. N. 881, *888*
Goodman, L., see Iwamoto, R. H. 388, *400*
Goodman, L., see Lee, W. W. 427, 429, 430, 431, *433*, 658, *666*
Goodman, L., see Marsh, J. P., Jr. 593, *613*
Goodman, L., see Reist, E. J. 426, 427, 428, 429, 430, 431, *433*
Goodman, L., see Ryan, K. J. 196, *230*
Goodman, L., see Tong, G. L. 350, *371*
Goodman, M. G., see Painter, R. B. 326, *342*
Goodridge, T. H., see Bratzel, R. P. 18, *30*
Goodwin, W. E., see Kaufman, J. J. 415, *422*
Goolsby, C. M., see Hisaw, F. L. 109, *130*
Gopalan, H. N. B. *669*
Gorbacheva, L. B., Kukushkina, G. V. 74, *80*
Gorbman, A., see Hahn, W. E. 121, *129*, 165, *167*
Gordan, G. S., Bentinck, R. C., Eisenberg, E. 91, *100*
Gordee, R. S., see Williams, R. H. 446, *457*
Gordon, A. S., see Finkelstein, G. 145, *153*
Gordon, A. S., see Steinberg, M. 109, *136*
Gordon, A. S., see Vollmer, E. P. 145, *157*
Gordon, B. M., see Schein, P. S. 704, 710, *720*
Gordon, B. S., see Rakieten, N. 860, 861, *874*
Gordon, C., see Hollander, V. P. 89, *101*
Gordon, C. N., see Shigeura, H. T. 659, 663, *667*
Gordon, C. S., see Mashburn, L. T. 709, *718*
Gordon, D. L., see Segaloff, A. 181, *191*
Gordon, G., see Southren, A. L. 811, 813, *818*
Gordon, H. C., see Thayer, P. S. 820, *828*
Gordon, J., see King, R. J. B. 113, 114, 117, *131*
Gordon, M., see Greengard, O. 120, 121, *129*
Gordon, M., see Scholler, J. 283, *344*
Gordon, M. J., see Benson, J. V., Jr. 697, *713*
Gordon, M. P., see Lozeron, H. A. 321, *340*
Gordon, M. P., see Pahl, H. B. 282, 283, *341*
Gordon, M. P., Staehelin, M. 208, *225*
Gordon, M. P., see Lozeron, H. A. 198, *228*
Gorlich, M., see Heise, E. 145, *154*
Gorman, M., see Johnson, I. S., 671, 675, 679, 682, 685, 686, 687, *691*
Gorman, M., see Williams, R. H. 446, *457*
Gorman, T. 852
Gorman, T., Pietsch, P. 867, *872*
Gorman, T., see Pietsch, P. 868, 869
Gorski, J. 119, *129*
Gorski, J., Axman, M. C. 119, *129*
Gorski, J., Morgan, M. S. 119, *129*

Gorski, J., Noteboom, W.D., Nicolette, J.A. 88, *100*, 119, *129*
Gorski, J., Notides, A.C. 115, 117, 119, *129*
Gorski, J., Shyamala, G., Toft, D.O. 115, *129*
Gorski, J., Toft, D., Shyamala, G., Smith, D., Notides, A. 115, 117, *129*
Gorski, J., see Barry, J. 119, *126*
Gorski, J., see Clark, J.H. 115, 116, *127*
Gorski, J., see DeAngelo, A.B. 119, 120, *127*
Gorski, J., see Giannopoulos, G. 95, *100*
Gorski, J., see Mueller, G.C. 119, *133*
Gorski, J., see Nicolette, J.A. 119, 124, *134*
Gorski, J., see Noteboom, W.D. 114, 119, *134*, 164, *168*
Gorski, J., see Notides, A. 120, *134*
Gorski, J., see Sarff, M. 117, *135*
Gorski, J., see Shyamala, G. 115, *136*
Gorski, J., see Smith, D.E. 93, *103*, 124, *136*
Gorski, J., see Toft, D.O. 114, 115, 117, *137*, 164, *168*
Gospodarowicz, D., see Erdos, T. 114, *128*
Goss, R.J. 527, *532*
Gosslee, D.G., see Cudkowicz, G. 314, *330*
Gostof, R., see Veselý, J. 351, 363, *371*
Gotjamanos, T. 410, *421*
Goto, K., see Higuchi, M. *60*, 857, *872*
Goto, S., see Garrett, E.R. 65, 66, *80*
Gots, J.S., Bird, T.J., Mudd, S. 494, *505*
Gots, J.S., Gollub, E.G. 390, *399*, 492, 495, *505*
Gots, J.S., see Adye, J.C. 461, *464*
Gots, J.S., see Kalle, G.P. 461, *466*
Gottesman, M.E., see Canellakis, E.S. 274, *329*
Gottlieb, D., Shaw, P.D. 554, *568*
Gottlieb, J.A. 549
Gottlieb, J.A., Guarino, A.M., Call, J.B., Oliverio, V.T., Block, J.B. 650, *655*
Gottlieb, J.A., Luce, J.K. *645*, 650, 655
Gottlieb, J.A., Serpick, A.A. 474, *481*, 545, *550*
Gotto, A.M., Belkhode, M.L., Touster, O. 216, *225*, 280, 290, 291, *334*
Gottschalk, P.G., Dyck, P.J., Kiely, J.M. 682, 686, *690*
Gottschling, H., Heidelberger, C. 199, 200, 203, 205, *225*
Gottwaldová, A., see Nouza, K. 356, *368*
Goubet, B., see Strecker, G. 448, *456*
Goudemand, M., Bauters, F. 726, 727, 728, 732, 734, 735, *744*
Gould, E.A., see Littlefield, J.W. 297, *339*
Goulian, M. 325, *334*
Goulian, M., see Rama Reddy, G.V. 242, 243, *254*
Goulian, M., see Reddy, G.V.R. 660, *667*
Gourevitch, A., see Lein, J. 57, *61*, 862, 869, *873*
Goutier, R., see Baugnet-Mahieu, L. 280, 315, *328*
Govindachari, T.R., see Gellert, E. 564, *568*
Goy, R.W., see Resko, J.A. 149, *156*
Goz, B., McCrea, J.F., Prusoff, W.H. 305, *334*
Goz, B., Prusoff, W.H. 194, 199, *225*, 305, 306, 322, 324, 325, *334*
Goz, B., see Aamodt, L. 305, *327*
Grady, H.J., Azarnoff, D.L., Creager, R., Huffman, D.H., Nichols, J. 810, *818*
Grady, H.J., see Azarnoff, D.L. 814, *817*
Grady, J.E., see Smith, C.G. 222, *230*, 683, *693*
Graf, J., see Israels, L.G. 38, *44*
Graff, G.L.A., Gueuning, C., Hildebrand, J. 682, *690*
Graffi, A., Hoffman, F., Schütt, M. 78, *80*
Graffi, A., see Wunderlich, V. 70, *84*
Grafnetter, D., Grafnetterová, J. 356, *366*
Grafnetter, D., see Grafnetterová, J. 356, 357, 358, *366*
Grafnetterová, J., Beránek, J., König, J., Šmahel, O., Šorm, F. 357, 358, 359, *366*
Grafnetterová, J., Grafnetter, D. 357, *366*
Grafnetterová, J., Grafnetter, D., Poledne, R. 356, *366*
Grafnetterová, J., Grossi, E, Fumagalli, R., Morganti, P., Grafnetter, D. 357, 358, *366*
Grafnetterová, J., Jedlička, V., Šmahel, O. 358, *366*
Grafnetterová, J., see Grafnetter, D. 356, *366*
Grafnetterová, J., see Šmahel, O. 358, *370*
Grage, T.B., Rochlin, D.B., Weiss, A.J., Wilson, W.L. 441, *453*
Grage, T., see Weiss, A.J. *511*
Graham, F.L., Whitmore, G.F. 243, 244, 245, *252*, 260, *269*
Graham, O.L., see Kit, S. 301, 302, *337*
Grahame-Smith, D.G. 519, *532*
Grahn, B., Løvtrup-Rein, H. *669*
Gralnick, H.R., Henry, P.H. 735, *741*
Gram, T.E., see Guarino, A.M. 709, *716*
Grand, L.C., see Huggins, C. 117, *131*
Grandi, M., see Bertazzoli, C. 609, 610, *611*
Grant, D.J.W., see Arden, G.M. 517, *529*
Grant, J.K., see Griffiths, K. 106, 107, *129*
Grasy, J.E., see Smith, C.G. 222, *231*
Gray, G.D., Camiener, G.W., Bhuyan, B.K. 630, 631, *632*
Gray, G.D., Nichol, R., Mickelson, M.M., Camiener, G.W., Gish, D.T., Kelly, R.C., Wechter, W.J., Moxley, T.E., Neil, G.L. 237, *252*, 266, *269*
Gray, G.D., see Smith, C.G. 437, 445, *456*
Gray, J.G., Aronow, L., Pratt, W.B. 91, *100*

Grayson, S., Berry, S. J. *669*
Green, C., see Morris, H. P. 171, *191*
Green, H., see Todaro, G. J. 302, 307, *346*
Green, H. D., see Nichols, J. 810, *818*
Green, M., Pina, M. *334*
Green, M., Pina, M., Chagoya, V. *334*
Green, R., see Whalen, R. E. 149, *157*
Green, S. 76, *80*
Greenberg, D. M., Blumenthal, G., Ramadan, M. A. 501, *505*
Greenberg, D. M., see El-Asmar, F. A. 485, 501, *504*
Greenberg, D. M., see Kasbekar, D. K. 217, *227*
Greenberg, D. M., see Rabinovitz, M. 485, 497, 499, *508*, *509*, 524, *535*
Greenberg, G., Sommerville, R. L. 277, *334*
Greenberg, J., Mandell, J. D., Woody, P. L. 494, *505*
Greenberg, J., see Curry, J. 494, *504*
Greenberg, J., see Kilgore, W. W. 79, *81*, 494, *506*
Greenberg, J., see Terawaki, A. 52, *63*, 494, *511*
Greenberg, J., see Woody, P. L. 494, *511*
Greenberg, J., see Woody-Karrer, P. 494, *511*
Greenberg, J. R., see Perry, R. P. 571, *580*
Greenberg, N. H., see Jondorf, W. R. 558, *569*
Greenberg, S. A., see Zimmerman, E. F. 463, *467*
Greenblatt, R. B., see Roy, S. 113, 114, *135*
Greene, F. E., Stripp, B., Gillette, J. R. 812, *818*
Greengard, O., Gordon, M. Smith, M. A., Acs, G. 120, 121, *129*
Greengard, O., Sentenac, A., Acs, G. 121, *129*
Greengard, P., Sigg, E. B., Fratta, I., Zak, S. B. 542, *542*
Greenhouse, S. W., see Goldin, A. 476, *481*
Greenius, H. F., McIntyre, R. W., Beer, C. T. 684, *690*
Greenlees, J., LePage, G. A. 390, 391, *399*, 487, *505*
Greenlees, J. L., see LePage, G. A. 390, *400*
Greenman, D. L., Kenney, F. T. 120, *129*
Greenman, D. L., Wicks, W. D., Kenney, F. T. 147, *154*
Greenman, D. L., see Kenney, F. T. 88, *101*
Greenman, D. L., see Wicks, W. D. 147, *157*
Greenquist, A. C., Wriston, J. C., Jr. 700, *716*
Greenspan, E. M., see Goldin, A. 459, 460, *465*
Greenspan, E. M., see Schoenbach, E. B. 766, *787*
Greenstein, J. P., Carter, C. E. 697, *716*
Greenstein, J. P., Carter, C. E., Chalkley, H. W. 238, *252*
Greenstein, J. P., Price, V. E. 698, *716*
Greenstein, J. P., see Sugimura, T. 528, *537*
Greenwood, B. M., see Denman, E. J. 416, *420*
Greenwood, F. C., see Bulbrook, R. D. 178, 179, *188*
Greer, M., Anton, A. H., Williams, C. M. 520, *532*
Greer, S. 294, 301, 319, *334*
Greer, S., Zamenhof, S. 275, 301, 319, *334*
Greer, S., see Cooper, G. M. 216, *224*, 290, *330*
Greggs, V. C., see Burchenal, J. H. 822, *826*
Gregory, F. J., Flint, S. F., Ruelius, H. W., Warren, G. H. 523, *532*
Gregušová, V., see Rada, B. 354, *369*
Gregušová, V., see Winkler, A. 352, *372*
Grein, A., see Arcamone, F. 593, *611*
Greiner, M., see Dao, T. L. 112, *127*
Gresham, C., see Furlong, N. B. 243, 244, *251*
Greslin, J. G., see Holtkamp, D. E. 105, *130*
Gribnau, A. G. M., Veldstra, H. 48, *60*
Griboff, G., see Zamenhof, S. 274, 295, *347*
Grieder, A., see Schindler, R. L. 41, *46*, 294, *344*
Griepp, R. B., see Stinson, E. B. 416, *424*
Griesbach, L., see Heidelberger, C. 193, 198, 204, 217, *226*, 300, *335*
Griesbach, W., see Purves, H. D. 171, *191*
Griffin, A. C., see Klatt, O. 29, *32*
Griffith, K. M., see Sullivan, M. P. 476, *482*
Griffith, W. R., see Knight, V. *338*
Griffiths, C. T., Tomic, M., Craig, J. M., Kistner, R. W. 175, 179, *189*
Griffiths, K., Grant, J. K., Symington, T. 106, 107, *129*
Grigg, G. W. 859, 868, 869, *872*
Grignani, F., Martinelli, M. F., Tonato, M., Finzi, A. F. 472, *481*
Grimes, P., v. Smallmann, L. 39, *44*
Grimley, E. B., see Rosenberg, B. 829, *840*
Grimley, P. M., see Kohler, P. O. 159, *167*
Grindey, G. B. 779
Grindey, G. B., Mihich, E., Nichol, C. A. 769, *785*, 799, *806*
Grindey, G. B., Nichol, C. A. 799, *806*
Grindey, G. B., Saslaw, L. D., Waravdekar, V. S. 240, *252*, 267, *269*
Grindey, G. B., see Saslaw, L. D. 267, *270*
Grinnan, E. L., see Ho, P. P. K. 698, 699, 700, 702, 708, *716*
Grisolia, S., Cardoso, S. S. 283, *334*
Grisolia, S., see Wallach, D. P. 283, *346*
Griswold, D. P., Laster, W. R., Snow, M. Y., Schabel, F. M., Jr., Skipper, H. E. 767, *785*
Griswold, D. P., Jr., Simpson-Herren, L., Schabel, F. M., Jr. 235, *252*
Griswold, D. P., Jr., see Laster, W. R., Jr. 389, *400*
Grogan, D. E., see Desjardins, R. 680, *689*
Grollman, A. P., Grollman, E. F. 559, *568*
Grollman, A. P. 558, *568*
Grollman, A. P. 558, 559, 560, 561, 562, 563, 565, *568*

Grollman, A. P., Huang, M. T. 554, 559, 565, *568*
Grollman, A. P., see Horwitz, S. B. 578, *579*, 643, 644, 646, *647*, 649, 651, 552, 653, 654, *655*, 860, *872*
Grollman, A. P., see Huang, M. T. 556, 564, *568*
Grollman, A. P., see Rao, S. S. 561, *570*
Grollman, E. F., see Grollman, A. P. 559, *568*
Gros, F., Gilbert, W., Hiatt, H. H., Attardi, G., Spahr, P. F., Watson, J. D. 210, *225*
Gros, F., Naono, S. 212, *225*
Gros, F., see Bussard, A. 212, *224*
Gros, F., see Naono, S. 211, 212, *229*
Gross, A., see Kit, S. 301, 302, *337*
Gross, C. L., see Papirmeister, B. 13, *16*
Gross, P. R. 311, *334*
Gross, R., see Coles, N. W. 56, *60*
Gross, S. R., see Hackney, J. F. 97, 99, *100*
Grossi, C. E., see Rousselot, L. M. 221, *230*
Grossi, E., see Grafnetterová, J. 357, 358, *366*
Grossman, L., see Eisenstadt, J. M. 514, *531*
Grossowicz, N., see Frohwein, Y. Z. 697, *716*
Grossowicz, N., see Halpern, Y. S. 515, *532*, 697, *716*
Grossowicz, N., see Schlesinger, M. 514, 520, *536*
Groth, D. P., D'Angelo, J. M., Vogler, W. R., Mingioli, E. S., Betz, B. 74, *81*
Grover, C. E., Chibnall, A. C. 697, *716*
Grozdanovič, J., Vích, Z., Truxová, G. 355, *366*
Grozdanovič, J., Vích, Z., Truxová, G., Kratochvíl, J. 355, *366*
Gruber, M. 120, *129*
Gruber, M., see Beuving, G. 120, *126*
Gruber, M., see Coolsma, J. W. 121, *127*
Gruber, T., see Coolsma, J. W. 121, *127*
Grünberger, D., Holy, A., Šorm, F. 464, *465*
Grünberger, D., Meissner, L., Holy, A., Šorm, F. 464, *465*
Grünberger, D., O'Neal, C., Nirenberg, M. 464, *465*
Gruenstein, M., see Hilf, R. 123, 124, *130*
Gruenstein, M., see Shay, H. 112, *136*
Gruickshank, J. G., see Barry, R. D. *328*
Grula, E. A., Smith, G. L., Grula, M. 59, *60*
Grula, M., see Grula, E. A. 59, *60*
Grunberg, E., Prince, H. N. 558, 560, *568*, 747, 748, 749, *762*
Grunberg, E., Prince, H. N., Tittsworth, E., Beskid, G., Tendler, M. D. 642, *647*
Grunberg, E., see Bollag, W. 747, 748, 749, 756, *761*
Grunberg, E., see Duschinsky, R. 197, *225*
Grunberg, E., see Heidelberger, C. 198, *226*
Grunberger, D., see Cheng, C. J. 68, 70, *80*
Grunberg-Manago, M., Michelson, A. M. 214, *225*, 325, *334*, 378, *381*
Grunberg-Manago, M., see Michelson, A. M. 272, 274, *340*
Grundmann, E., see Lauenstein, K. 705, *718*
Grunicke, H., see Puschendorf, B. 29, *33*
Grupta, G. N., see Jensen, E. V. 176, 187, *190*
Guadagni, A., see Nervi, C. 478, *482*
Gualandi, G., Bergamini, A. 521, 522, *532*
Guarino, A. J. 658, *666*
Guarino, A. J., Ibershof, M. L., Swain, R. 661, *666*
Guarino, A. J., Kredich, N. M. 661, *666*
Guarino, A. J., see Jagger, D. V. 660, *666*
Guarino, A. J., see Kredich, N. M. 658, 661, *666*
Guarino, A. J., see Rottman, F. 659, 660, 661, 663, *667*
Guarino, A. M., Schroeder, D. H., Adamson, R. H., Call, J. B., Gram, T. E. 709, *716*
Guarino, A. M., see Gottlieb, J. A. 650, *655*
Gubareff, N., see Shimkin, M. B. 36, *46*
Guedes, J., see DeBarros, T. 696, *715*
Guelstein, V. I., see Vasiliev, J. M. 681, *694*
Guerola, N., see Cerdá-Olmeda, E. 8, *15*
Guerry, D. III, see Geeraets, W. J. 298, *333*
Guess, W. L., see Watkins, W. D. 560, *570*
Guest, M. M., see Monto, R. W. 621, *622*
Gueuning, C., see Graff, G. L. A. 682, *690*
Guha, A., see Bach, J. F. 410, 413, 414, *419*
Guild, W. R., see Miller, D. S. 634, 635, 636, 637, *641*
Guin, H. W., see Shealy, Y. F. 549, *552*
Gulati, O. D., Patel, D. G. 309, *334*
Gulesich, J. J., see Ravin, L. J. 275, *343*
Gulick, Z. R., see Heymann, H. 515, *532*
Gumport, S. L., see Harris, M. N. 638, *640*
Gumport, S. L., see Wright, J. C. 478, *483*
Gundersen, L. E., see Huennekens, F. M. 469, *481*
Gunther, H., see Prusoff, W. H. 282, 283, 313, 316, *342*
Gupta, G. N., see Jensen, E. V. 114, *131*
Gupta, S., see Mukherjee, S. 109, *134*
Guroff, G. 519, *532*
Gurr, M. I., Finean, J. B., Hawthorne, J. N. 824, *827*
Gursky, G. V. 586, *590*
Guschlbauer, W., see Michelson, A. M. 293, *340*
Gussoff, B., see Ellison, R. R. 260, *268*
Gut, J., see Prystaš, M. 349, *369*
Gut, M., see Burstein, S. 139, *153*
Gut, M., see Shimizu, K. 139, *156*
Gut, M., see Wotiz, H. H. 106, *138*
Gutmann, H., see Zeller, P. 747, *765*
Gutová, M., Elis, J., Rašková, H. 357, *366*
Gutová, M., see Rašková, H. 361, *369*

Gutová, M., see Slavík, M. *370*
Gutová, M., see Welch, A. D. 357
Gutteridge, W. E., see Trigg, P. I. 660, *668*
Gutterman, J. A., Huang, A. T., Hochstein, P. 757, *762*
Gutterman, J. U., Curtis, J. E., Freireich, E. J. 265, *269*
Guttman, H. N., Tendler, M. D. 643, *647*
Guyers, R. G., see Beard, M. E. J. 726, 727, 728, 730, 734, 735, *743*
Guyonnet, J. C., see Maral, R. 705, 708, *718*

Haag, H. B., see Finnegan, J. K. 809, *817*
Haar, F., von der, see Sprinzl, M. *669*
Haar, H., see Rauen, H. M. 820, 823, *827*
Haas, R., Maass, G. 302, 306, 307, *334*
Haas, R., see Maass, G. 304, *340*
Habermann, V., Šorm, F. 352, *366*
Hacker, B. 121, *129*
Hackethal, C. A., Golbey, R. B., Tan, G. T. C., Karnofsky, D. A., Burchenal, J. H. 638, *640*
Hackett, P., Hanawalt, P. 280, *334*
Hackney, J. F., Gross, S. R., Aronow, L., Pratt, W. B. 97, 99, *100*
Hackney, J. F., Pratt, W. B. 98, *100*
Haddow, A., Timmis, G. M. 36, 37, *44*
Haddow, A., see Connors, T. A. 523, *530*
Haddow, A. L., Watkinson, J. M., Patterson, E., Koller, P. C. 183, *189*
Haddy, T. B., see Sullivan, M. P. 476, *482*
Hadfield, J. R., see Hebden, H. F. 684, *690*
Hadjiolov, A. A., see Mackedonski, V. V. 584, *591*
Hadjiolov, A. A., see Smuckler, E. A. *669*
Hadler, H. I., Claybourn, B. E., Tschang, T. P. 374, *381*
Hadler, H. I., Moreau, T. L. 374, *381*
Hähnel, R., see Evans, L. H. 117, *128*
Haerlin, R., see Lingens, F. 70, 71, *82*
Hagawara, A., see Iijima, T. 56, *60*
Hagemann, G., Pénasse, L., Teillon, J. 497, *505*
Hagemann, R. F., see Sigdestad, C. P. 642, 644, *648*
Hagen, J. J., see Ablondi, F. B. 527, *529*
Hagen, P. S., see Hewlett, J. S. 740
Hager, E. B., see Murray, J. E. 502, *508*
Hager, E. B., see Rowinski, W. A. 527, *535*
Hager, S. E., Jones, M. E. 489, 497, *505*
Haggerty, W. J., Jr., see Baiocchi, F. 768, *783*
Haggmark, A., see Bertani, L. E. 277, *328*
Haghbin, M., Tan, C., Tallal, L., Wollner, N., Rosenstock, J., Burchenal, J. H. 726, 732, *744*
Hagiwara, A., see Paul, J. 206, 211, *229*
Hahn, F. E., see O'Brien, R. L. 774, *787*
Hahn, J. D., see Neumann, F. 146, *155*
Hahn, M. A., Adamson, R. H. 877, 878, *888*
Hahn, M. A., see Adamson, R. H. 710, *713*, 878, *887*
Hahn, M. A., see DeVita, V. T. 752, *762*
Hahn, M. A., see Liegler, D. G. 473, *482*
Hahn, R. G., see Moertel, C. G. 546, *551*, 650, *656*, 793, *806*
Hahn, W. E. 120, *129*
Hahn, W. E., Church, R. B., Gorbman, A. 121, *129*
Hahn, W. E., Church, R. B., Gorbman, A., Wilmot, L. 121, *129*, 165, *167*
Hahn, W. E., Schjeide, O. A., Gorbman, A. 121, *129*
Haidaka, T., see Aizawa, S. 441, 444, *452*
Hakala, M. T. 288, 295, 297, 298, 302, *334*, 471, *481*, 680, *690*, 769, 778, 779, 780, 781, *785*
Hakala, M. T., Nichol, C. A. 391, 392, *399*
Hakala, M. T., Suolinna, E. M. R. 775, *785*
Hakala, M. T., see Mihich, E. 769, 778, 779, *786*
Hakala, M. T., see Weiss, L. 781, *788*
Halberg, F., see Haus, E. 249, *252*
Hales, D. R., Jerner, R. W., Hall, B. E., Willet, F. M., Franco, J., Feichtmeir, T. V. 394, *399*
Hales, H. B., see Hutchinson, F. 319, 321, *336*
Haley, E. E., Fischer, G. A., Welch, A. D. 514, *532*, 695, *716*, 723, *744*
Halgrimson, C. G., see Penn, I. 415, *423*
Halgrimson, C. G., see Penn, I. 417, *423*
Halkerston, I. D. K., Eichhorn, J., Hechter, O. 139, *154*
Halkerston, I. D. K.. see Hechter, O. 118, *130*
Hall, B. E., see Hales, D. R. 394, *399*
Hall, J. G. 704, *716*
Hall, J. G., Smith, M. E. 318, *334*
Hall, K., see Korenchеřsky, V. 143, *154*
Hall, P. F. 140, *154*
Hall, R. H., see Robins, M. J. 435, *455*
Hall, T. C., Kessel, D., Levine, R., Roberts, D. 265, *269*
Hall, T. C., Krant, M. J., Lloyd, J. B., Patterson, W. B., Ishibara, A., Potee, K. G., Lořina, T. O., Mullen, J. M. 459, *465*
Hall, T. C., Levine, R. 238, *252*
Hall, T. C., see Breeden, C. J. 323, *328*
Hall, T. C., see Cavins, J. A. 440, *453*
Hall, T. C., see Everson, R. 216, *225*
Hall, T. C., see Kessel, D. 216, 217, *227*, 239, 247, *253*, 265, *270*, 471, 473, *481*
Hall, T. C., see Lahiri, S. R. 220, *228*
Hall, T. C., see Reyes, P. 216, *229*
Hall, T. C., see Roberts, D. W. 242, 245, *254*, 469, *482*, 681, *693*

Hall, T. C., see Savloř, E. D. 546, *552*
Hall, T. C., see Wittliff, J. L. 117, 118, *138*
Hallahan, C., Young, D. A., Munck, A. 93, *100*
Halle, S. 363, *366*
Hallman, B. L., see Brown, J. H. U. 815, *817*
Hallum, J. V., Youngner, J. S., Arnold, N. J. 607, *612*
Halpern, Y. S., Grossowicz, N. 515, *532*, 697, *716*
Halvorson, H. 492, 495, *505*
Halvorson, H. O., Spiegelman, S. 513, *532*
Halvorson, H. O., see Spiegelman, S. 377, *382*
Hamada, M., see Umezawa, H. 444, *456*
Hamberger, L., see Ahren, D. 176, *188*
Hamburger, J., Crosnier, J., Dormont, J., Bach, J. F. 407, 410, *421*
Hamilton, A. E., see Vodopick, H. 40, *46*
Hamilton, H. E., see Hwang, Y. F. 686, *690*
Hamilton, L., Fuller, W., Reich, E. 586, *590*
Hamilton, L. D., see Philips, F. S. 389, 394, *401*
Hamilton, T. H. 118, 119, 120, *129*
Hamilton, T. H., Widnell, C. C., Tata, J. R. 119, *129*
Hamilton, T. H., Teng, C. S., Means, A. R. 119, *129*
Hamilton, T. H., see Luck, D. N. 120, *132*
Hamilton, T. H., see Means, A. R. 119, *133*
Hamilton, T. H., see Moore, R. J. 120, *133*
Hamilton, T. H., see Teng, C. S. 119, 120, *137*
Hamilton, W. C., Laplaca, S. J. 773, *785*
Hammerstein, J., Rice, B. F., Savard, K. 106, *129*
Hammond, S., see Durr, G. J. 350, *365*
Hampar, B., Derge, J. G., Martos, L. M., Walker, J. L. 308, *334*
Hamparian, V. V., Hilleman, M. R., Ketler, A. 307, *335*
Hampel, K. E., Lackner, A., Schulz, G., Busse, V. 415, *421*
Hampson, S. E., see Altmann, F. P. 824, *826*
Hampton, A. 386, 395, *399*
Hampton, A., Hampton, E. G., Eidinoff, M. L. 274, 318, *335*
Hampton, C. L., see Loveless, A. 70, 78, *82*
Hampton, E. G., Eidinoff, M. L. 273, 282, 283, 289, 290, 291, 314, *335*
Hampton, E. G., Rich, M. A., Eidinoff, M. L. *335*
Hampton, E. G., see Hampton, A. 274, 318, *335*
Hamre, D., Bernstein, J., Donovick, R. 800, *806*
Hananian, J., see Iriarte, P. V. 69, *81*
Hanafusa, H., see Kawai, S. 200, *227*
Hanawalt, P., see Hackett, P. 280, *334*
Hanawalt, P., see Kanner, L. 280, *337*
Hanawalt, P. C. 52, *60*
Hanawalt, P. C., Haynes, R. 13, *15*
Hanawalt, P. C., see Cerdá-Olmeda, E. 8, *15*
Hanawalt, P. C., see Maaløe, O. 528, *533*
Hancock, R. L., Zelis, R. F., Shaw, M., Williams-Ashman, H. G. *154*
Hancock, R. L., see Williams-Ashman, H. G. 147, *157*
Handler, A. H., see Cardinali, G. 673, *688*
Handler, P., see Klingman, J. D. 493, *507*
Handler, P., see Preiss, J. 491, *508*
Handschumacher, R. E. 349, 352, *366*, 700, *716*
Handschumacher, R. E., Bates, C. J., Chang, P. K,. Andrews, A. T., Fischer, G. A. 515, *532*
Handschumacher, R. E., Calabresi, P., Welch, A. D., Bono, V. H. Jr., Fallon, H. J., Frei, E., III 355, 358, 359, 360, 361, *366*
Handschumacher, R. E., Pasternak, C. A. 352, 355, *366*
Handschumacher, R. E., Škoda, J., Šorm, F. 349, *367*
Handschumacher, R. E., Welch, A. D. 458, *465*
Handschumacher, R. E., see, Capizzi, R. L. 705, *715*, 723, 725, 726, 733, 734, 735, *743*
Handschumacher, R. E., see Chou, T. C. 712, 713, *715*
Handschumacher, R. E., see Cooney, D. A. 501, *504*, 514, *530*, 695, 696, 701, 703, 705, 710, *715*, 725, *743*
Handschumacher, R. E., Creasey, W. A. 359, *365*
Handschumacher, R. E., see Jackson, R. C. 515, *532*, 696, 699, 701, 703, *717*
Handschumacher, R. E., see Jaffe, J. J. 355, *367*
Handschumacher, R. E., see Liu, Y. P. 700, *718*
Handschumacher, R. E., see Pasternak, C. A. 352, 355, *368*
Handschumacher, R. E., see Peterson, R. G. 705, *720*, 735, 738, *746*
Handschumacher, R. E., see Rubin, R. J. 352, *369*
Handschumacher, R. E., see Summers, W. P. 515, *537*
Handschumacher, R. E., see Wagenen, G. van 357, *371*
Hanessian, S., De Jongh, D. C., McCloskey, J. A. 658, *666*
Hanham, I. W. F., see Hellmann, K. 886, *889*
Hanisch, J., Vajda, G., Bertha, I. 568
Haňka, L. J. 448, *453*
Haňka, L. J., Evans, J. S., Mason, D. J., Dietz, A. 351, *367*
Haňka, L. J., Kuentzel, S. L., Neil, G. L. 234, *252*
Haňka, L. J., see Evans, J. S. 362, *365*
Haňka, L. J., see Vavra, J. J. 65, *84*
Hann, H. W., see Jaffe, N. 726, 727, 730, 734, 735, *744*
Hanna, C. *335*
Hanna, C., Wilkinson, K. P. 306, *335*
Hannonen, P., see Holtta, E. 775, *785*

Hano, K., Akashi, A., Suzuki, Y., Yamamoto, I., Narumi, S., Iwata, H. 547, *550*
Hano, K., Akashi, A., Yamamoto, I., Narumi, S., Horri, Z., Ninomiya, I. 545, *550*
Hansen, H. H., see Haskell, C. M. 704, *716*, 734, 735, *744*
Hansen, H. H., see Muggia, F. M. 650, *656*
Hansen, H. J., Bennett, S. J., Nadler, S. B. 386, *399*
Hansen, H. J., Nadler, S. B. 386, *399*
Hansen, H. J., Vandevoorde, J. P., Bennett, K. J., Giles, W. G. 500, 502, *505*
Hansen, H. J., see Vandevoorde, J. P. 495, *511*
Hansen, K., see Lindberg, B. 658, 659, 661, 662, *666*
Hanson, C. V. 869, *872*
Hanson, R. L., see Ray, P. D. 521, *535*
Hanušovská, T., see Rada, B. 355, *369*
Hanze, A. R. 239, *252*, 259, 266, *269*
Hanze, A. R., see Smith, C. G. 437, 445, *456*
Hara, I., see Kato, S. 870, *873*
Harada, F., see Ikehara, M. 443, 444, *454*
Harbers, E., Chaudhuri, N. K., Heidelberger, C. 202, 203, 206, 208, 211, *225*
Harbers, E., Müller, W. 583, *590*
Harbers, E., Vogt, M. 583, *590*
Harbers, E., see Bosch, L. 203, 204, 206, *223*
Harbers, E., see Heidelberger, C. *226*
Harder, H. C. 834, *839*
Harder, H. C., Rosenberg, B. 834, *839*
Hardesty, B., see McKeehan, W. 559, 561, 565, *569*
Hardesty, B., see Obrig, T. C. 561, *569*
Hardesty, C. T., Chaney, N. A., Mead, J. A. R. 881, *888*
Harding, H. R., Rosen, F., Nichol, C. A. 88, *101*
Harding, N. G. L., see Huennekens, F. M. 469, *481*
Hardisty, R. M., McElwain, T. J. 732, *744*
Hardman, S. D., see Gimlin, D. M. 308, *334*
Hargrove, W. W., see Johnson, I. S. 671, *691*
Harley, E. M., see Cohen, A. 607, *611*
Harley, J. B., see Hayes, D. M. 394, 397, *399*, 500, *505*
Harmath, A., see Cseh, G. 94, *100*
Harper, A. A., see Baseman, J. B. 561, *567*
Harper, C., see Andrews, F. N. 113, *125*
Harpootlian, H., see Smith, C. G. 437, 440, 441, 445, *456*
Harrap, K. R., see Hill, B. T. 28, *32*
Harris, A. W., see Baxter, J. D. 97, 99, *100*
Harris, C., see Shay, H. 112, *136*
Harris, C., see Svoboda, D. 589, *592*
Harris, D. N., Lerner, L. J., Hilf, R. 123, *130*
Harris, D. N., see Hilf, R. 152, *154*
Harris, D. N., see Lerner, L. J. 123, *132*, 147, 152, *155*
Harris, D. R., MacIntyre, W. M. 197, *225*
Harris, J., see Pagé, D. 416, *423*
Harris, J. E. 708, *716*
Harris, J. E., see Freireich, E. J. 397, *399*
Harris, J. E., see Ohno, R. *719*
Harris, J. E., see Whitecar, J. P., Jr. 726, 727, 728, 730, 734, 735, *746*
Harris, M. N., Medrek, T. J., Golomb, F. M., Gumport, S. L., Postel, A. H., Wright, J. C. 638, *640*
Harris, N., see Benedict, W. F. 236, *249*, 261, *267*
Harris, P. 676, *690*
Harris, P. N., see Johnson, I. S. 671, *691*
Harris, P. N., see Sweeney, M. J. 446, 451, *456*
Harrison, J. H., see Murray, J. E. 415, *422*, 502, *508*
Harrold, B. P. 39, *44*
Hart, J. S., Ho, D. H. W., Salem, P., Frei, E. III. 265, *269*
Hart, J. S., see Bodey, G. P. 263, *268*
Hart, J. S., see Freireich, E. J. 260, 262, 265, *269*, 397, *399*
Hart, J. S., see Whitecar, J. P., Jr. 263, *271*
Hart, L. G., Call. J. B., Oliverio, V. T. 650, *655*
Hart, L. G., see Adamson, R. H. 642, *647*
Hart, M. M., Adamson, R. H. 879, *888*
Hart, M. M., Reagan, R. L., Adamson, R. H. 811, *818*
Hart, M. M., Smith, C. F., Yancey, S. T., Adamson, R. H. 879, *888*
Hart, M. M., Swackhamer, E. S., Straw, J. A. 812, *818*
Hart, M. M., Straw, J. A. 810, 811, 812, *818*
Hart, M. M., see Arseneau, J. 879, *887*
Hartley, B., see Kihlman, B. A. 859, *873*
Hartley, J. W., see Lowy, D. R. 308, *340*, 355, *368*
Hartline, E. J. H., see Coleman, J. R. 311, *330*
Hartman, A. C., see Rogers, W. I. 219, *229*
Hartman, P. E., see Levin, A. P. 517, *533*
Hartman, P. E., see Simoni, R. D. 93, *103*
Hartman, S. C. 486, 488, 489, *505*
Hartman, S. C., Levenberg, B., Buchanan, J. M. 486, 487, *505*
Hartmann, D., see Wacker, A. 380, *383*
Hartmann, G., Coy, U., Kniese, G. 583, *591*
Hartmann, G., Goller, H., Koschel, K., Kersten, W., Kersten, H. 602, 603, *612*
Hartmann, G., see Behr, W. 616, 617, *621*
Hartmann, K. U., Heidelberger, C. 289, 301, *335*
Hartmann, K. U., Heidelberger, C. 203, 204, 216, *225*
Hartroft, P., see Kaminsky, N. 811, *818*
Hartwell, J. L., Abbott, B. J. 654, *655*, 881, *888*

Hartwell, J.L., see Kelly, M. G. 671, *691*
Hartwick, J., see Rosenberg, B. 829, *840*
Harvey, S.C., see Clermont, Y. 23, *31*
Harzewski, E., see Pine, M. J. 820, 823, 824, *827*
Haschenmeyer, A.E.V., Rich, A. 441, *453*
Hasegawa, K., see Suzuki, M. 870, *875*
Hasegawa, M., see Kageyama, M. 583, *591*
Hasegawa, Y., Irikura, T., Mizuno, D. 856, *872*
Haselkorn, R. 585, *591*
Haselkorn, R., see Doty, P. 292, *331*
Hassenmaier, G., see Gmelin, R. 498, *505*
Hashiguchi, T., see Nakamura, S. 870, *873*
Hashimoto, J., Uchida, T., Egami, F. 437, *453*
Hashimoto, K., see Oka, S. 870, *874*
Haskell, C.M., Canellos, G. P. 491, *505*, 514, *532*, 711, *716*, 733, *744*
Haskell, C.M., Canellos, G. P., Cooney, D.A., Hansen, H.H. 704, *716*
Haskell, C.M., Canellos, G. P., Leventhal, B.G., Carbone, P.P., Serpick, A.A., Hansen, H.H. 734, 735, *744*
Haskell, C.M., see Canellos, G.P. 709, 711, *714*, 733, 735, *743*
Haskell, C.M., see Carbone, P.P. 726, 727, 728, 730, 732, 734, 735, *743*
Haskell, J., see Sweat, M.L. 106, *136*
Haskell, T.H., see Bartz, Q. R. 485, *503*
Haskell, T.H., see Fusari, S. A. 485, *505*
Hassel, O., Romming, C. 286, 335
Hasselberger, F.X., Brown, H.D., Chattopadhyay, S.K., Mather, A.N., Stasiw, R.O., Patel, A. B., Pennington, S.N. 724, 735, *744*
Hata, T., Nomura, S., Umesawa, I. 47, *60*
Hata, T., Sano, Y., Sugawara, R., Matsuma, A., Kanamori, K., Shima, T., Hoshi, T. 47, *60*
Haurani, F., see Ellison, R. R. 260, *268*
Haurani, I., see Vivacqua, R.J. 39, *46*
Haus, E., Halberg, F., Scheving, L.E., Pauly, J. E., Cardoso, S., Kühl, J. F.W., Sothern, R.B., Shiotsuka, R.N., Hwang D.S. 249, *252*
Haut, A.B., see Bodey, G. P. 264, *268*
Haut, W.F., see Taylor, J. H. 200, *230*
Havelka, S., Pěgřimová, E. Trnavský, K., Slavík, M., Elis, J. 361, *367*
Hawk, W.A., see Roenigk, H.H. 475, *482*
Hawkins, R., Owen, L.N., Danielli, J.F. 28, *32*
Hawthorne, J.J., see Armstrong, J.G. 685, *688*
Hawthorne, J.N., see Gurr, M.I. 824, *827*
Haxhe, J.J., Alexandre, G. P.J., Kestens, P.J. 410, *421*, 502, *505*
Haxhe, J.J., see Alexandre, G.P.J. 502, *503*
Hayaishi, O., see Honjo, T. 561, *568*
Hayano, M., see Shimizu, K. 139, *156*
Hayat, M., see Mathé, G. 726, 727, 728, 732, 734, 735, *745*, 882, *889*
Hayat, M., see Schwarzenberg, L. 474, *482*
Hayes, D.M., Costa, J., Moon, J.H., Hoogstraten, B., Harley, J.B. 394, 397, *399*, 500, *505*
Hayes, D.M., Ellison, R.R. 264, *269*
Hayes, D.M., see Ellison, R. R. 260, *268*
Hayes, E.F., see Vredevoe, D.L. 417, *425*
Hayes, J., see Berman, L.D. 78, *79*
Hayes, R.L., Carlton, J.E., Byrd, B.L. 879, *888*
Hayes, R.L., Nelson, B., Swartzendruber, D.C., Carlton, J.E., Byrd, B. L. 879, *888*
Hayes, R.L., see Edwards, C.L. 879, *888*
Haynes, G.R., see Klemperer, H.G. *338*
Haynes, R., see Hanawalt, P. 13, *15*
Haynes, R.C., Jr., Sutherland, III, E.W. 87, *101*
Haynes, R.H., see Brendel, M. 41, *42*
Hayon, E., see Danziger, R. M. 319, *330*
Hayslett, J.P., see Kaplan, S.R. 502, *506*
Hayward, J.L., Bulbrook, R.D. 179, *189*
Hayward, J.L., see Bulbrook, R.D. 179, *188*
Hayward, S.K., see McElwain, T.J. 706, *718*, 735, *745*
Hazlett 583
Heald, P.J., McLachlan, P. M. 121, *130*
Heard, B.E., Cooke, R.A. 39, *44*
Heard, R.D., Bligh, E.G., Cann, M.C., Jellinck, P. H., O'Donnell, V.J., Rao, B.G., Webb, J.L. 106, *130*
Heath, R.B., see Denman, E.J. 416, *420*
Heathcote, J.G., Pace, J. 499, *505*
Hebborn, P., Danielli, J.F. 29, *32*
Hebborn, P., see Bardos, T. J. 20, 29, *30*
Hebden, H.F., Hadfield, J. R., Beer, C.T. 684, *690*
Heby, O., Russell, D.H. 774, 775, *785*
Heby, O., Sauter, S., Russell, D.H. 775, *785*
Hecht, A., see Weisenfeld, S. 814, *819*
Hecht, S.M., see Leonard, N.J. 435, *454*
Hecht, T., Summers, D.F. 855, 859, *872*
Hechter, O., Halkerston, I. D.K. 118, *130*
Hechter, O., see Halkerston, I.D.K. 139, *154*
Hedegaard, J., Maspero-Segre, S., Thoai, N.-V., Roche, J. 492, *506*
Hedegaard, J., see LeGal, M.-L. 489, *507*
Hedgcoth, C., see Kaiser, I.I. 209, 210, *227*
Heene, D.L., Löffler, H. 709, *716*, *744*
Heer, J., Billeter, J.R., Miescher, K. 106, *130*
Heftmann, E. 140, *154*
Hegedus, B., see Zeller, P. 747, *765*

Heidelberger, C. 193, 199, 207, 208, 216, 219, *225*, *226*, 289, *335*
Heidelberger, C., Anderson, S.W. 198, 219, *226*
Heidelberger, C., Ansfield, F.J. 193, 219, *226*
Heidelberger, C., Birnie, G. D., Boohar, J., Wentland, D. 203, 215, *226*
Heidelberger, C., Boohar, J., Kampschroer, B. 202, 203, 205, 219, *226*
Heidelberger, C., Chaudhuri, N.K., Danneberg, P., Mooren, D., Griesbach, L., Duschinsky, R., Schnitzer, R.J., Pleven, E., Scheiner, T. 193, 198, *226*
Heidelberger, C., Griesbach, L., Cruz, O., Schnitzer, R.J., Grunberg, E.G. 198, *226*
Heidelberger, C., Griesbach, L., Ghobar, A. 300, *335*
Heidelberger, C., Griesbach, L., Montag, B.J., Mooren, D., Cruz, O., Schnitzer, R.J., Grunberg, E. 198, *226*
Heidelberger, C., Kaldor, G., Mukherjee, K.L., Danneberg, P.B. 204, 217, *226*
Heidelberger, C., Keller, R. A. 390, *399*
Heidelberger, C., Leibman, K.C., Harbers, E., Bhargařa, P.M. *226*
Heidelberger, C., Parsons, D.G., Remy, D.C. 196, *226*
Heidelberger, C., Sunthankar, A.V., Griesbach, L., Randerson, S. 198, 204, 217, *226*
Heidelberger, C., see Birnie, G.D. 203, 215, *223*, 315, 318, *328*
Heidelberger, C., see Bosch, L. 203, 204, 206, *223*
Heidelberger, C., see Bujard, H. 208, 214, *224*
Heidelberger, C., see Chaudhuri, N.K. 202, 207, 208, 215, 219, *224*, 283, *329*
Heidelberger, C., see Clifton, K.H. 289, 291, *330*
Heidelberger, C., see Curreri, A.R. 220, *224*
Heidelberger, C., see Danneberg, P.B. 204, 205, *224*
Heidelberger, C., see Dexter, D.L. 205, 222, 223, *224*
Heidelberger, C., see Dipple, A. 196, *224*
Heidelberger, C., see Duschinsky, R. 195, *225*
Heidelberger, C., see Fridland, A. 204, *225*
Heidelberger, C., see Fujiwara, Y. 205, *225*, 292, 298, *333*
Heidelberger, C., see Gottschling, H. 199, 200, 203, 205, *225*
Heidelberger, C., see Harbers, E. 202, 203, 206, 208, 211, *225*
Heidelberger, C., see Hartmann, K.U. 203, 204, 216, *225*, 289, 301, *335*
Heidelberger, C., see Huberman, E. 200, 205, *226*
Heidelberger, C., see Kaufman, H.E. 199, *227*
Heidelberger, C., see Kent, R.J. 196, 203, 215, 216, *227*
Heidelberger, C., see Khwaja, T.A. 196, 200, 215, *227*
Heidelberger, C., see Mukherjee, K.L. 196, 202, 215, *228*
Heidelberger, C., see Nesnow, S. *229*
Heidelberger, C., see Nizhizawa, Y. 197, *229*
Heidelberger, C., see Oki, T. 205, *229*
Heidelberger, C., see Remy, D.C. 196, *229*
Heidelberger, C., see Reyes, P. 203, 204, *229*
Heidelberger, C., see Umeda, M. 199, 216, 217, *230*, *231*
Heidelberger, C., see Wagner, N.J. 206, 209, *231*
Heilman, F.R., Kendall, E. C. 175, 187, *189*
Heim, H.C., see Appelt, G. D. 560, *567*
Hein, P.E., see Clegg, R.E. 120, *127*
Heine, K.M., Stobbe, H., Klatt, R., Apostoloff, E., Dutz, W. 416, *421*
Heine, U., Langlois, A.J., Beard, J.W. 583, *591*
Heine, U.I., see Krueger, G. R.F. 417, *422*
Heinemann, B., Howard, A. J. 697, *716*, 869, *872*
Heinemann, B., see Lein, J. 57, *61*, 862, 869, *873*
Heinemann, H.O., see Muggia, F.M. 589, *591*
Heiniger, H.J., Feinendegen, L.E., Burke, K. 314, *335*
Heiniger, H.J., Friedrich, G.D., Feinendegen, L. E., Cantelmo, F. 314, *335*
Heiniger, H.J., see Ertl, H. H. 314, *332*
Heinrich, M.R., Dewey, V. C., Parks, R.E., Jr., Kidder, G.W. 463, *465*
Heinricks, W.L., see Kahwanago, I. 117, *131*
Heise, E., Gorlich, M., Bacigalupo, G. 145, *154*
Held, I., Wells, W., Koenig, H. 487, *506*
Hell, E., Cox, D.G. 679, *690*
Heller, G., see Vazquez, D. 554, 565, *570*
Heller, K.S., see Moncrief, J.W. 672, *692*
Heller, R.H., Jones, H.W. 39, *44*
Hellman, L., see Fukushima, D.K. 813, *817*
Hellman, L., see Gallagher, T.F. 178, *189*
Hellman, L., see Zumoff, B. 178, *192*
Hellman, S., Iannotti, A., Bertino, J.R. 477, *481*
Hellmann, K. 886, *889*
Hellmann, K., Burrage, K. 885, 886, *889*
Hellmann, K., Newton, K. A., Whitmore, D.N., Hanham, I.W.F., Bond, J.V. 886, *889*
Hellmann, K., see Creighton, A.M. 885, *888*
Hellmann, K., see Field, E. O. 886, *888*
Hellmann, K., see Sharpe, H.B.A. 885, *889*
Hellström, I.E., see Quadracci, L.J. 416, *423*
Hellström, K.E., see Quadracci, L.J. 416, *423*
Hellung-Larsen, P., Frederiksen, S. 664, *666*
Hellung-Larsen, P., see Danø, K. 573, *579*

Hellung-Larsen, P., see Frederiksen, S. 663, *665*, *669*
Helsinki, D. R., see De Witt, W. 58, *60*
Helson, L., Yagoda, A., McCarthy, M., Murphy, M. L., Krakoff, I. H. 219, *226*
Helson, L., see Dexter, D. L. 222, 223, *224*
Helson, L., see Tallal, L. 727, 728, 730, 732, *746*
Hemmerly, J., Demerec, M. 494, *506*
Hempel, K., Lange, H. W., Birkofer, L. 518, *532*
Hemphill, S. C., see Burchenal, J. H. 198, *224*
Hemsworth, B. N. 39, *44*
Hemsworth, B. N., Jackson, H. 38, 39, *44*
Hen, A. C., see Shiguera, H. T. 524, 528, *536*
Hendee, E. D., see Strauss, N. 561, *570*
Hendel, R. C., see Schluederberg, A. 584, *592*
Hender, S., see Baliga, B. S. 209, *223*
Henderson, E., see Levin, R. H. 769, 772, 773, *786*
Henderson, E. J., see Nagano, H. 492, *508*
Henderson, E. S. 390, *399*, 477, *481*, 884, *889*
Henderson, E. S., Adamson, R. H., Oliverio, V. T. 471, 472, 473, 474, *481*
Henderson, E. S., Burke, P. J. 261, *269*
Henderson, E. S., Samaha, R. J. 687, *690*, 799, *806*
Henderson, E. S., see Goldin, A. 389, *399*
Henderson, E. S., see Leventhal, B. G. 501, *507*, 726, 732, 734, 735 *745*
Henderson, E. S., see Liegler, D. G. 473, *482*
Henderson, E. S., see Oliverio, V. T. 770, *787*
Henderson, E. S., see Rubin, R. C. 472, *482*
Henderson, E. S., see Sandler, S. G. 686, *693*
Henderson, J. F. 389, *399*, 487, *506*
Henderson, J. F., Junga, I. G. 500, *506*
Henderson, J. F., Khoo, M. K. Y. 390, *400*, 437, 453
Henderson, J. F., Mandel, H. G. 384, *400*
Henderson, J. F., Mikoshiba, A., Chu, S. Y., Caldwell, I. C. 386, *400*
Henderson, J. F., Patterson, A. R. P., Caldwell, I. C., Hori, M. 442, 445, *453*
Henderson, J. F., see Caldwell, I. C. 386, *398*, 442, 444, *453*
Henderson, J. F., see Kandaswamy, T. S. 501, *506*
Henderson, R. B., see Fink, K. 283, *333*
Hendler, S. S., see Rama Reddy, G. V. 242, 243, *254*
Hendler, S. S., see Reddy, G. V. R. 660, *667*
Hendlin, D., see Stapley, E. W. 518, *536*
Heneen, W. K., Nichols, W. W. 236, *252*
Hengy, H., see Preussmann, R. 71, *82*, 547, *551*
Hennigar, G., see Nichols, J. 809, *818*
Henry, M. C. 429, *432*
Henry, P., see Karon, M. 241, *253*, 261, *270*, 463, *466*
Henry, P. H., see Gralnick, H. R. 735, *744*
Henry, R. A. 66, *81*
Hensen, D., Smith, R. P., Gehrke, J. 302, 304, *335*
Hensen, K., see Lindberg, B. 448, *454*
Henson, D., see Dolowy, W. C. 696, *715*
Hentzen, D., see Beck, G. 121, *126*
Hepler, P. K., see Newcomb, E. H. 676, *692*
Heppner, G. H., Calabresi, P. 237, *252*
Herbert, D., see Wade, H. E. 697, *721*
Herbst, E. J., Bachrach, V. 766, *785*
Herbst, E. J., see Dykstra, W. G. 148, *153*
Herbut, P. A., see Suld, H. M. 697, 698, 699, 702, 703, *721*
Herken, H., Senft, G., Zemisch, B. 541, *542*
Herman, E. H., Schein, P., Farmar, R. M. 609, *612*
Herman, E. H., Schein, P., Taylor, C., Waravdekar, U. S. 609, *612*
Herman, E. H., see Burka, B. 609, *611*
Herman, T. S., Fimognari, G. M., Edelman, I. S. 85, *101*, 164, *167*
Hermann, T. J., see Starzl, T. E. 410, *424*
Hernandez, K. W., see Luce, J. K. 397, *401*
Hernandez, P., Dennis, E. W., Farah, A. 880, *889*
Herr, R. R., Jahnke, H. K., Argoudelis, A. D. 65, *81*
Herranen, A. M., see Mueller, G. C. 118, *133*
Herren, T. C., see Wheeler, G. P. 69, *84*
Herrera, F. M., see Yang, S. S. 883, *890*
Herrington, K. A., see Lukens, L. N. 385, *401*
Herriot, J., see Kimball, A. P. 234, 241, *253*, 429, 430, *432*
Herrmann, E. C., Jr. 302, 322, *335*
Herrmann, E. C. 302, 307, *335*
Herrmann, E. C., see Kucera, L. S. 302, 306, *338*
Herrmann, E. C., see Person, D. A. 302, 307, *342*
Herrmann, E. C., see Rawls, W. F. 302, *343*
Herrmann, R. L., see Cooper, A. D. 309, *330*
Herrmann, W. L., see Kahwanago, I. 117, *131*
Herschberger, L. G., Shipley, E. G., Meyer, R. K. 140, *154*
Hersh, E. M. 503, *506*, 547, 707, *716*
Hersh, E. M., Bodey, G. P., Nies, B. A., Freireich, E. J. 264, *269*
Hersh, E. M., Brown, B. W. 503, *506*, 527, *532*, 707, *716*
Hersh, E. M., Carbone, P. P., Wong, V. G., Freireich, E. J. 770, *785*
Hersh, E. M., Le Page, G. A. 430, *432*
Hersh, E. M., Oppenheim, J. J. 416, *421*
Hersh, E. M., Wong, V. G., Freireich, E. J. 384, *400*

Hersh, E.M., see Ohno, R. 705, 706, 707, *719*, 735, 738, *745*
Herter, F.P., Weissman, S. G., Thompson, H.G., Jr., Hyman, G., Martin, D. S. 541, *542*
Hertig, A.T., see Wall, E. 175, *192*
Hertz, R., Larsen, C.D., Tullner, W. 121, *130*
Hertz, R., Lewis, J., Jr., Lippsett, M.B. 475, 476, *481*
Hertz, R., Lipsett, M.B., Moy, R.H. 686, *690*
Hertz, R., Ross, G.T., Lipsett, M.B. 476, *481*
Hertz, R., Sebrell, W.H. 110, *130*
Hertz, R., see Bergenstal, D. M. 811, 812, 814, *817*
Hess, A.F., Bills, C.E., Weinstock, M., Rinkin, H. 120, *130*
Hess, V.F., see Škoda, J. 349, *370*
Heuson 188
Hewett, C.L., see Cook, J. W. 105, *127*
Hewlett, J.S. 878, *889*
Hewlett, J.S., Bettle, J.D., Jr., Bishop, R.C., Fowler, W.M., Schwartz, S. O., Hagen, P.S., Louis, J. 740
Hewlett, J.S., see Bodey, G. P. 260, 261, 363, 264, *268*
Hewlett, J.S., see Frei, E.III. 260, 262, *269*
Heyman, I.A., Thompson, G.R., Schaeppi, U.H., Rosenkrantz, H., Fleischman, R.W., Ilievski, V., Cooney, D. A., Davis, R.D. 832, *839*
Heymann, H., Ginsberg, T., Gulick, Z.R., Konopka, E.A., Mayer, R.L. 515, *532*
Heyn, R.M., Brubaker, C. A., Burchenal, J.H., Cramblett, H.G., Wolff, J.A. 397, *400*, 500, *506*
Hiatt, H.H., see Gros, F. 210, *225*
Hiatt, H.H., see Revel, M. 584, *592*
Hidaka, T., see Otake, N. 441, *455*
Hidvegi, E.J., Arky, J., Antoni, F., Koteless, G.J., Ballweg, H. 518, *532*
Higashinakagawa, T., see Muramatsu, M. 564, *569*
Higgins, G.M., see Morrison, S.S. 522, *534*
Hignett, R.C. 207, 211, *226*
Higuchi, M., Goto, K., Fujimoto, M., Namiki, O., Kiguchi, G. *60*, 857, *872*
Hijmans, J.C., McCarty, K. S. 91, *101*
Hijo, K., see Erdmann, V.A. 566, *568*
Hilal, H.M., see Mizgerd, J. B. 546, *551*
Hilbert, G.E., Johnson, T. B. 272, *335*
Hildebrand, J., see Graff, G. L.A. 682, *690*
Hildebrand, J., see Kenis, Y. 759, *763*
Hilf, R. 112, 123, *130*, 144, *154*
Hilf, R., Battaglini, J.W., Delmez, J.A., Cohen, N., Rector, W.D. 124, *130*
Hilf, R., Bell, C., Michel, I. 117, 119, 123, *130*
Hilf, R., Goldenberg, H., Bell, C. 119, 123, *130*
Hilf, R., Goldenberg, H., Michel, I., Carrington, M.J., Bell, C., Gruenstein, M., Meranze, D.R., Shimkin, M.B. 123, *130*
Hilf, R., Goldenberg, H., Michel, I., Gruenstein, M., Meranze, D.R., Shimkin, M.B. 124, *130*
Hilf, R., Lerner, L.J., Harris, D.N. 152, *154*
Hilf, R., Lerner, L.J., Lang, E., Borman, A. 110, *130*
Hilf, R., McDonald, E., Sartini, J., Rector, W.D., Richards, A.H. 124, *130*
Hilf, R., Michel, I., Bell, C. 123, *130*, 144, *154*
Hilf, R., Michel, I., Bell, C., Freeman, J.J., Borman, A. 123, *130*
Hilf, R., Michel, I., Silverstein, G., Bell, C. 123, *130*
Hilf, R., Segaloff, A., Lerner, L.J. 123, *130*, 145, *154*
Hilf, R., see Harris, D.N. 123, *130*
Hilf, R., see Lerner, L.J. 122, 123, *132*, 147, 152, *155*, 182, 183, *190*
Hilf, R., see Richards, A.H. 123, 124, *135*
Hilf, R., see Wittliff, J.L. 117, 118, *138*
Hill, B.T., Jarman, M., Harrap, K.R. 28, *32*
Hill, C.S., Jr., see Whitecar, J.P., Jr. 709, *722*
Hill, D.L., Bennett, L.L., Jr. 390, 391, *400*, 437, *454*
Hill, D.L., Kirk, M.C., Struck, R.F. 29, *32*
Hill, D.L., see Brockman, R. W. 496, *503*
Hill, D.L., see Schnebli, H. P. 436, 442, *455*, 659, *667*
Hill, D.L., see Struck, R.F. 29, *33*
Hill, J.M., Loeb, E., Hill, N. O., MacLellan, A., Khan, A., Alexander, T.R., Adachi, M. 702, *716*
Hill, J.M., Loeb, E., Mac Lellan, A., Khan, A., Roberts, J., Shields, W. F., Hill, N.O. 704, *716*, 726, 728, 732, *744*
Hill, J.M., Loeb, E., Speer, R.J., MacLellan, A., Hill, N.O. 838, *839*
Hill, J.M., Roberts, J., Khan, A., Mac Lellan, A., Hill, R.W., Loeb, E. 723, 728, *744*
Hill, J.M., Roberts, J., Loeb, E., Khan, A., MacLellan, A., Hill, R.W. 696, *716*
Hill, J.M., see Khan, A. 705, 708, *717*, 735, *745*, 833, 836, 837, *839*, *840*
Hill, J.M., see Loeb, E. 726, 727, 728, 734, 735, *745*
Hill, J.M., see Tanaka, M. 689, 699, 702, *721*
Hill, J.M., see Roberts, J. 698, *720*
Hill, N.O., see Hill, J.M. 702, 704, *716*, 726, 728, 732, *744*, 838, *839*
Hill, R.H., Jr., Rowlands, D.T., Jr., Rifkind, D. 416, *421*
Hill, R.W., see Hill, J.M. 696, *716*, 723, 728, *744*
Hillcoat, B.L., see Bertino, J.R. 528, *530*, 775, *783*
Hillcoat, B.L., see Goldie, J. 469, *481*

Hillcoat, B. L., see Perkins, J.P. 469, *482*
Hilleman, M. R., see Coggin, J.H. 298, 308, *330*
Hilleman, M. R., see Hamparian, V.V. 307, *335*
Hilleman, M. R., see Nemes, M. 302, *341*
Hills, D. C., Horowitz, J. 206, 210, *226*
Hilscher, W., Reichelt, P. 753, *762*
Hilton, J., see Sartorelli, A. C. *807*
Himelstein, E. S., see Bettigole, R. E. 735, *743*
Hindy, I., see Eckhardt, S. 36, *43*
Hintsche, R., see Etzold, G. 289, 290, *332*
Hintsche, R., see Langen, P. 273, *339*, 661, *666*
Hipkiss, A. R., Arnstein, H. R. V., Edmunds, M. E. 209, *226*
Hippel, P. H. v., see Printz, M.P. 869, *874*
Hirai, T., see Tezuka, N. *456*
Hiranaka, H., see Ikekawa, T. 851, 852, 855, 869, *872*
Hirano, M., see Miura, M. 514, 515, 526, *534*, 705, 706, 707, 713, *719*, 735, 738, *745*
Hiremath, C. B., Olson, G., Rosenblum, C. 524, *532*
Hiremath, C. B., see Shiguera, H. T. 524, 528, *536*
Hirokawa, H., see Abe, M. 522, *529*
Hirokawa, I., see Ichikawa, T. 870, *872*
Hirono, I., Kachi, H., Ohashi, A. 28, *32*
Hiroyuki, A., see Hoshino, A. *613*
Hirsch, M. S., Black, P. H., Tracy, G. S., Leibowitz, S., Schwartz, R. S. 418, *421*
Hirsch, M. S., Phillips, S. M., Solnik, C., Black, P. H., Schwartz, R. S., Carpenter, C. B. 418, *421*
Hirschberg, E. 389, *400*
Hirschberg, E., Brindle, S. D., Semente, G. 880, *889*
Hirschberg, E., Gellhorn, A., Murray, M. R., Elslager, E. F. 879, *889*
Hirschberg, E., Kream, J., Gellhorn, A. 460, *466*
Hirschberg, E., Murray, M. R., Peterson, E. R., Kream, J., Schafranek, R., Pool, J. L. 460, *465*
Hirschberg, E., Weinstein, I.B. 880, *889*
Hirschberg, E., see Gellhorn, A. 459, 460, *465*
Hirschberg, E., see Ochoa, M., Jr. 6, *16*, 21, 25, 28, 29, *33*, 35, *45*
Hirschberg, E., see Weinstein, I. B. 880, *890*
Hirschhorn, K., see Weiner, M.S. 707, *722*
Hirschman, S. Z., Fischinger, P. J., O'Connor, T. E. 237, *252*
Hirschmann, W., see Weitzel, G. 754, 756, *765*
Hirschmann, W. D., see Oerkermann, H. 734, 738, *745*
Hirsh, M., Penman, S. 577, *579*
Hirt, B. 302, 308, *335*
Hirt, R., Berchtold, R. 820, *827*
Hirt, R., see Burchenal, J. H. 822, *826*
Hisaw, F. L., Velardo, J. T., Goolsby, C. M. 109, *130*
Hisaw, F. L., see Velardo, J. T. 110, *137*
Hitchcock, C. R., see Zimmerman, B. 809, *819*
Hitchings, G. H. 387, 391, *400*, 407, *421*, 469, *481*
Hitchings, G. H., Elion, G. B. 24, *32*, 384, 391, 396, *400*, 404, 407, 408, *421*
Hitchings, G. H., see Bieber, S. 309, *328*, 386, 393, *398*
Hitchings, G. H., see Burchall, J. J. 469, *480*
Hitchings, G. H., see Clarke, D.A. 396, *398*
Hitchings, G. H., see Elion, G.B. 292, *332*, 384, 387, 389, 392, *399*, 404, 408, 409, 410, 411, *420*, 459, *465*
Hitchings, G. H., see Nathan, H.C. 407, 409, *422*
Hitchings, G. H., see Scannell, J.P. 386, 390, 392, 393, *402*
Hitchings, G. H., see Sugiura, K. 459, *467*
Hitchings, G. H., see Thompson, R. L. 302, *346*, 800, *807*
Hitt, J., see Gitterman, C. O. 661, *665*
Hlad, C. L., see Starzl, T. E. 410, *424*
Ho, B. T., see Baker, B. R. 469, *479*
Ho, D. H. W. 266, *269*
Ho, D. H. W., Frei, E., III 238, *252*, 258, 259, 260, 262, 263, 266, *269*
Ho, D. H. W., Freireich, E. J. *252*
Ho, D. H. W., Whitecar, J. P., Jr., Luce, J. K., Frei, E., III. 698, 699, 700, 702, *716*, 733, *744*
Ho, D. H. W., see Dedrick, R. L. 258, *268*
Ho, D. H. W., see Hart, J. S. 265, *269*
Ho, D. H. W., see Loo, T. L. 386, *401*
Ho, H. W., see Loo, R. V. 258
Ho, M., Hohler, H. 608, *612*
Ho, P. P. K., Frank, B. H., Burck, P. J. 698, *716*
Ho, P. P. K., Milikin, E. B., Bobbitt, J. L., Grinnan, E. L., Burck, P. J., Frank, B. H., Boeck, L. D., Squires, R. W. 698, 699, 700, 702, 708, *716*
Ho, P. P. K., see Frank, B. H. 699, 700, *716*
Hoberman, H. D., see White, A. *103*
Hobik, H. P. 705, *717*
Hobik, H. P., see Lauenstein, K. 705, *718*
Hobson, J. B., see Rundles, R.W. 408, 412, *423*
Hochman, A., see Benezra, D. 706, *713*, 735, 738, *743*
Hochman, H. I., Agrawal, K. C., Sartorelli, A. C. 803, *806*
Hochstein, P., Laszlo, J., Miller, D. S. 635, *640*
Hochstein, P., see Gutterman, J. A. 757, *762*
Hochstein, P., see Miller, D. S. 634, 635, 636, 637, *641*
Hodas, S., see Young, C. W. 241, *256*, 634, *641*, 790, *792*
Hodenberg, A. v., see Preussmann, R. 70, 71, *82*, 547, *551*

Hodes, M.E., Rohn, R.J., Bond, W.H., Yardley, J. 685, *690*
Hodges, C.V., see Huggins, C. 143, *154*, 170, 172, *189*
Hoefnagel, D., see Nyhan, W.L. 414, *423*
Hoeksema, H., Slomp, G., Van Tamelen, E.E. 446, 447, *454*
Hoeksema, H., see Schroeder, W. 446, *455*
Hoekstra, W.G., see Glascock, R.F. 95, *100*, 113, *129*
Hoelscher, B., see Zimmerman, B. 809, *819*
Hoerni, B., see Amiel, J.L. 752, *760*
Hoeschele, J.D., see Cleare, M.J. 838, *839*
Hofer, K.G. 316, *335*
Hofer, K.G., Dibenedetto, J., Hughes, W.L. 317, 318, *335*
Hofer, K.G., Hofer, M. 316, *335*
Hofer, K.G., Hughes, W.L. 283, 292, 314, 315, 317, 318, *335*
Hofer, K.G., Prensky, W., Hughes, W.L. 314, 315, 316, 317, *335*
Hofer, K.G., Rosenoff, S., Prensky, W., Hughes, W.L. 315, 316, 317, *335*
Hofer, M., see Hofer, K.G. 316, *335*
Hofert, J.F., White, A. *101*
Hoffer, M., Duschinsky, R., Fox, J.J., Yung, N. 195, *226*, 272, *335*
Hoffer, M., see Duschinsky, R. 197, *225*
Hoffman, D.H., see Sweeney, M.J. 450, 451, *456*
Hoffman, F., see Graffi, A. 78, *80*
Hoffman, G.S., Kline, I., Gang, M., Tyrer, D.D., Goldin, A., Mantel, N., Venditti, J.M. 263, *269*
Hoffman, G.S., Kline, I., Gang, M., Tyrer, D.D., Venditti, J.M., Goldin, A. 548, *550*
Hoffman, H. 675, *690*
Hoffman, J., Post, J. 313, *335*
Hoffman, J., see Post, J. 313, 316, *342*
Hoffman, P.F., Ritter, H. W., Krueger, R.F. 884, *889*
Hoffmann, G.R. 298, *335*
Hofook, C., see Yesair, D.W. 822, 824, *828*
Hogeboom, G.H., Schneider, W.C. 539, *542*
Hohler, H., see Ho, M. 608, *612*
Hohorst, H.J., Ziemann, A., Brock, N. 29, *32*
Hohorst, H.J., see Brock, N. 29, *31*
Holcenberg, J.S. 697, 712, *717*
Holcenberg, J.S., Pease, J. 712, *717*
Holcenberg, J.S., see Roberts, J. 501, *509*
Holden, K., see Saunders, H. L. 146, *156*
Holland, J.F. 687, *690*, 777
Holland, J.F., Bardos, T.J., Bryant, B., Mihich, E. 769, *785*
Holland, J.F., see Costa, G. 451, *453*
Holland, J.F., see Ellison, R.R. 260, *268*
Holland, J.F., see Gailani, S.D. 685, *690*
Holland, J.F., see Goldin, A. 389, *399*
Holland, J.F., see Kung, F. 521, *533*
Holland, J.F., see Ohnuma, T. 514, 515, 529, *534*, *535*, 703, *719*, 724, 725, 726, 727, 728, 733, 734, 735, *745*, *746*
Holland, J.F., see Regelson, W. 769, 772, *787*, 843, *849*
Holland, J.F., see Senn 780
Hollander, N., Chiu, Y.W. 98, 99, *101*
Hollander, N., see Hollander, V.P. 89, *101*
Hollander, V.P., Gordon, C., Hollander, N. 89, *101*
Hollander, V.P., see Ambellan, E. 94, *100*
Hollander, V.P., see MacLeod, R.M. 94, *101*
Hollander, V.P., see Stevens, J. 90, *103*
Holler, B.W., see Zimmerman, E.F. 464, *467*
Hollingsworth, J.W., see Johns, D.G. 472, 473, *481*
Hollingsworth, J.W., see Papac, R.J. 236, 238, *254*
Hollis, C.A., see Tepper, H. B. 857, *875*
Hollunger, G. 766, *785*
Holly, F.W., see Jenkins, S. R. 661, *666*
Holly, F.W., see Walton, E. 658, 661, *668*
Holmberg, E.A.D., see Burchenal, J.H. 198, *224*
Holmes, A.W., see Ey, R.C. *332*
Holmes, R.E., see Sweeney, M.J. 446, 451, *456*
Holmes, R.E., see Williams, R.H. 446, *457*
Holmes, W.L., see Prusoff, W.H. *342*
Holmgren, A., see Dahlwitz, A. 735, *743*
Holmquist, N.D. 695, *717*
Holmstrom, E.G., see Sweat, M.L. 106, *136*
Holthaus, F.J., Jr., see Lerner, L.J. 110, *132*
Holthausen, H.S., Chacko, S., Davidson, E.A., Holtzer, H. 311, *335*
Holtkamp, D.E., Greslin, J. G., Root, C.A., Lerner, L.J. 105, *130*
Holton, C.P., see Mayer, C. M. 726, 727, 734, 735, *745*
Holton, C.P., see Pratt, C.B. 726, 727, 734, 735, *746*
Holtta, E., Hannonen, P., Pispa, J., Janne, J. 775, *785*
Holtzer, H., see Abbot, J. 311, *327*
Holtzer, H., see Anderson, H.C. 311, *327*
Holtzer, H., see Bischoff, R. 311, 312, *328*
Holtzer, H., see Chacko, S. 311, *329*
Holtzer, H., see Holthausen, H.S. 311, *335*
Holtzer, H., see Mayne, R. 311, *340*
Holtzer, H., see Okazaki, K. 311, *341*
Holtzer, H., see Sanger, J. W. 311, *343*
Holtzer, H., see Stockdale, F. 311, *345*
Holtzer, S., see Chacko, S. 311, *329*
Holtzman, E., see Penman, S. 572, *580*

Holum, L.B., see Shealy, Y.F. 544, 548, 549, *552*
Holý, A., see Grünberger, D. 464, *465*
Holý, A., see Lisý, V. 353, *368*
Holý, A., see Škoda, J. *370*
Holzer, H., see Dold, U. 25, *31*
Holzer, H., see Fussganger, R. 25, *31*
Homma, I., see Sawa, T. 444, *455*
Homma, I., see Umezawa, H. 444, *456*
Homma, M., see Ishida, N. 444, *454*
Homolka, J., see Slavík, M. 361, *370*
Honda, Y., Ohmori, K., Yoshida, K., Arai, K. 870, *872*
Honetz, N., see Deutsch, E. 709, *715*, 734, 735, *744*
Honikel, K., see Behr, W. 616, 617, *621*
Honjo, T., Nishizuka, Y., Hayaishi, O., Kato, I. 561, *568*
Hoogstraten, B., see Hayes, D.M. 394, 397, *399*, 500, *505*
Hooper, D.C., see Bieber, S. 309, *328*
Hooper, J.L., see Levintow, L. 519, *533*
Hopkins, C.E., see Marmorston, J. 178, *191*
Horacek, P., Drobnik, J. 835, 837, *839*
Horakova, K., see Tidd, D. M. 396, *403*
Hori, A., see Paterson, A.R. P. 393, *401*
Hori, M., Ito, E., Takita, T., Koyama, G., Takeuchi, T., Umezawa, H. 441, 442, *454*
Hori, M., Ito, E., Umezawa, H. 857, *872*
Hori, M., Wakashiro, T., Ito, E., Sawa, T., Takeuchi, T., Umezawa, H. 445, *454*
Hori, M., see Henderson, J. F. 442, 445, *453*
Hori, M., see Kunimoto, T. 444, *454*, 859, 860, *873*
Hori, M., see Sawa, T. 444, *455*
Hori, M., see Tsukada, I. 444, *456*
Hori, M., see Umezawa, H. 855, 870, *875*, *876*
Hori, S., see Ishizuka, M. 444, *454*
Hori, S., see Umezawa, H. *875*
Hori, S.H., Matsui, S. 124, *130*
Horiguchi, T., see Natori, S. 55, *62*
Horn, T., see Ward, D.C. 438, *456*
Horn, V., see Yanofsky, C. 9, 11, *17*
Hornal, R.W., see Gingras, B.A. 841, *848*
Horning, E.S. 175, *189*
Hornung, B., see Fateh-Moghadam, A. 734, 735, *744*
Horowitz, B., Madras, B.K., Meister, A., Old, L.J., Boyse, E.A., Stockert, E. 711, *717*
Horowitz, B., Meister, A. 712, *717*
Horowitz, B., Nelson, J.A., Meister, A. 712, *717*
Horowitz, J., Chargaff, E. 208, *226*
Horowitz, J., Kohlmeier, V. 212, *226*
Horowitz, J., Saukkonen, J. J., Chargaff, E. 206, 211, 212, *226*
Horowitz, J., see Hills, D.C. 206, 210, *226*
Horowitz, J., see Johnson, J.L. 209, 210, *227*
Horri, Z., see Hano, K. 545, *550*
Horton, C.L., see Eagle, H. 484, *504*
Horton, J., see Cavins, J.A. 440, *453*
Horton, J., see Cohen, J.L. 221, *224*
Horton, J., see Kingra, G.S. 546, *551*
Horwitt, B.N., see Segaloff, A. 181, 184, *191*
Horwitz, J.P., Chua, J., DaRooge, M.A., Noel, M., Klundt, I.L. 662, *666*
Horwitz, J.P., Chua, J., Noel, M., DaRooge, M. A. 273, *336*
Horwitz, J.P., see Nagpal, K.L. *668*
Horwitz, M.S., Brayton, C. 654, *655*
Horwitz, M.S., Horwitz, S. B. 649, 651, 652, 653, 654, *655*
Horwitz, M.S., see Horwitz, S.B. 653, *655*
Horwitz, S.B. 644, 645, 646, *647*
Horwitz, S.B., Chang, C., Grollman, A.P. 578, *579*, 644, *647*, 649, 651, 652, 653, 654, *655*
Horwitz, S.B., Chang, C., Grollman, A.P., Bořkovec, A.B. 646, *647*, 860, *872*
Horwitz, S.B., Grollman, A. P. 643, 644, 646, *647*
Horwitz, S.B., Horwitz, M. S. 653, *655*
Horwitz, S.B., see Bořkovec, A.B. 644, *647*
Horwitz, S.B., see Horwitz, M.S. 649, 651, 652, 653, 654, *655*
Hoshi, A., Kanzawa, F., Kuretani, K. 887, *889*
Hoshi, A., Kanzawa, F., Kuretani, K., Saneyoshi, M., Arai, Y. 234, *252*, 266, 267, *269*, 886, *889*
Hoshi, A., Yoshida, M., Kanzawa, F., Kuretani, K., Kanai, T., Ichino, M. 887, *889*
Hoshi, T., see Hata, T. 47, *60*
Hoshino, A., Taketoshi, K., Hiroyuki, A., Kazuo, O. *613*
Hoshino, T., Sano, K. 319, 324, *336*
Hoshino, T., see Sano, K. 291, 319, 324, *343*
Hosoi, H., see Nagao, M. 73, *82*
Hotta, Y., Stern, H. 859, *872*
Hotz, G., Reuschl, H. 319, 321, *336*
Houlabek, V. 208, *226*
Hourani, B.T., Demopoulos, H.B. 524, *532*
Housewright, R.D., see Altenbern, R.A. 697, *713*
Housholder, G.E., Loo, T.L. 546, 547, *551*
Housholder, G.E., see Loo, T.L. 546, *551*
Howard, A.J., see Heinemann, B. 697, *716*, 869, *872*
Howard, B.D., Tessman, I. 297, *336*
Howard, C.H., see Rudman, D. 703, *720*
Howard, F.B., Frazier, J., Miles, H.T. 293, *336*
Howard, F.B., see Lipkin, D. 273, 274, 277, *339*

Howard, J.G. 405, *421*
Howard, J.P., Cevik, W., Murphy, M.L. 261, *269*
Howard, J.P., see Luce, J.K. 397, *401*
Howard-Flanders, P. 11, *15*, 52, *60*
Howard-Flanders, P., see Boyce, R.P. 12, *15*, 53, 54, *60*
Howe, C.D., see Samuels, M.L. 759, *764*
Howell, D.C., see McCord, T.J. 524, *534*
Howell, D.S., see Slonim, R.R. 675, *693*
Howell, R.R., see Goldfinger, S.E. 683, *690*
Howle, J.A., Gale, G.R. 829, 830, 833, 834, 835, *839*
Howle, J.A., Gale, G.R., Smith, A.B. 838, *839*
Howle, J.A., Thompson, H.S., Stone, A.E., Gale, G.R. 833, 834, *839*
Howle, J.A., see Gale, G.R. 835, *839*
Howsden, F.L., see Sandberg, J.S. 597, *613*
Howsden, L., see Pujman, V. 196, *229*
Howse, R., see Shooter, K.V. 837, *840*
Hrada, T., see Rooks, W.H. 145, *156*
Hrodek, O., Veselý, J. 363, *367*
Hruban, Z., Wissler, R.W. 515, 519, *532*
Hruban, Z., Wissler, R.W., Slesers, A. 519, *532*
Hruban, Z., see Samal, B.A. 520, *535*
Hryniuk, W.M., Bertino, J.R. 470, 473, 475, 476, *481*
Hryniuk, W.M., Fischer, G.A., Bertino, J.R. 469, *481*
Hsia, S.L., see Gomez, E.C. 149, *154*
Hsu, D., see Krishan, A. 673, 679, *691*
Hsu, K.C., see Rosencranz, H.S. 790, *792*
Hsu, T.C., Billen, D., Levan, A. 300, *336*
Hsu, T.C., Humphrey, R.M., Somers, C.E. 200, *226*
Hsu, T.C., Somers, C.E. 300, *336*
Hsu, T.C., see Humphrey, R.M. 300, *336*
Hsu, T.C., see Kit, S. 293, 298, *338*
Hsu, T.C., see Ockey, C.H. 200, *229*
Huang, A.T., Kremer, W.B. 757, *762*
Huang, A.T., see Gutterman, J.A. 757, *762*
Huang, M.T., Grollman, A.P. 556, 564, *568*
Huang, M.T., see Grollman, A.P. 554, 559, 565, *568*
Huang, R.C., Bonner, J. 824, *827*
Huang, R.C.C., see Kleiman, L. 584, *591*
Huang, W.M., see Okamoto, K. 57, *62*
Huang, W.Y., Pearlman, W.H. 106, *130*
Huang, Y.H.J., Roy-Burman, D., Visser, D.W. 377, 378, 380, *381*
Huang, Y.H.J., see Roy-Burman, S. 375, *382*
Hubbard, S.P., see Skeel, R.T. 477, *482*
Huber, R.E., see MacLean, S.J. 521, *534*
Huberman, E., Heidelberger, C. 200, 205, *226*
Hubert-Habart, M., Cohen, S.S. 427, 429, *432*
Huebner, R.J., Lane, W.T., Welch, A.D., Calabresi, P., McCollum, R.W., Prusoff, W.H. 308, *336*
Huebner, R.J., see Klement, V. 308, *338*
Huennekens, F.M., Dunlap, R.B., Freisheim, J.H., Gundersen, L.E., Harding, N.G.L., Levison, S.A., Mell, G.P. 469, *481*
Huennekens, F.M., see Jackson, R.C. 775, *785*
Huennekens, F.M., see Mathews, C.K. 468, *482*
Huennekens, F.M., see Niethammer, D. 471, *482*
Huerga, J. de la, see Popper, H. 522, *535*
Huffman, D.H., see Grady, H.J. 810, *818*
Huggins, C., Bergenstal, D.M. 176, *189*
Huggins, C., Briziarelli, G., Sutton, H., Jr. 112, *131*, 181, *189*
Huggins, C., Clark, P.J. 170, 172, *189*
Huggins, C., Grand, L.C., Brillantes, F.P. 117, *131*
Huggins, C., Grand, L.C., Fukunishi, R. *131*
Huggins, C., Hodges, C.V. 143, *154*, 170, 172, *189*
Huggins, C., Jensen, E.V. 110, *131*
Huggins, C., Masina, M.H., Eichelberger, L., Warton, J.D. 172, *189*
Huggins, C., Scott, W.W., Hodges, C.V. 170, *189*
Huggins, C., Stevens, R.E., Jr., Hodges, C.V. 170, *189*
Huggins, C., Yang, N.P. 185, *189*
Huggins, C., see Barron, E.S.G. 151, *153*
Huggins, C., see Dao, T.L. 176, *188*
Huggins, C., see Landau, R.L. 185, *190*
Hughes, A.C., see Clegg, R.E. 120, *127*
Hughes, B., see Reynolds, R.C. 583, *592*
Hughes, D., see Djerassi, I. 478, *480*
Hughes, E.C., Rubulis, A. 122, *131*
Hughes, E.C., see Rubulis, A. 125, *135*
Hughes, J.S., see Roepke, R.R. 120, *135*
Hughes, R., see Munyon, W. 302, 304, 306, 307, *341*
Hughes, R.G., see Bowen, J.M. 302, *328*
Hughes, W.F., see Ey, R.C. *332*
Hughes, W.L., Commerford, S.L., Gitlin, D., Krueger, R.C., Schultze, B., Shah, V., Reilly, P. 280, 281, 283, 284, 314, 315, 316, *336*
Hughes, W.L., see Commerford, S.L. 283, 318, *330*
Hughes, W.L., see Cudkowicz, G. 314, *330*
Hughes, W.L., see Feinendegen, L.E. 283, 314, 315, 316, *332*
Hughes, W., see Gitlin, D. 314, 318, *334*
Hughes, W.L., see Hofer, K.G. 283, 292, 314, 315, 316, 317, 318, *335*
Hughes, W.L., see Krueger, R.C. 283, 314, 315, *338*
Hugo, R., see Vinegar, R. *424*

Huguley, C., see Vogler, W. R. 477, *482*
Hulínský, K., see Rašková, H. 361, *369*
Hull, W., White, A. 86, *101*
Hultin, T., see Magee, P.N. 72, *82*
Hume, D.M., see Board, J. A. 415, *419*
Humpherson, P.G., see Robards, A.W. 676, *693*
Humphrey, E.W., Blank, N. 638, *640*
Humphrey, E.W., see Mizuno, N.S. 74, *82*
Humphrey, R.M., Hsu, T.C. 300, *336*
Humphrey, R.M., see Barranco, S.C. 76, 77, *79*, 392, *398*
Humphrey, R.M., see Hsu, T.C. 200, *226*
Humphrey, R.R., see Callentine, M.R. 109, 110, *127*
Humphreys, J.S., see Ravel, J.M. 697, *720*
Humphreys, S.R., see Charache, S. 472, *480*
Humphreys, S.R., see DeWys, W.D. 650, *655*
Humphreys, S.R., see Goldin, A. 476, *481*, 500, *505*
Humphreys, S.R., see Kaplan, N.O. 540, *543*
Hunstein, W., Perings, E., Klose, U. 409, *421*
Hunstein, W., see Eberle, P. 415, *420*
Hunt, D.E., Pittillo, R.F. *252*
Hunt, D.E., see Pittillo, R.F. 234, *254*, 485, *508*
Hunt, T., see Kosower, N.S. 759, *763*
Hunter, J., see Burk, D. 776, *783*
Hunter, J.C. 682, *690*
Hunter, J.H. 233, *252*
Hunter, J.H., see Evans, J.S. 235, *251*
Hunter-Craig, I.D., see Alexander, P. 728, *742*
Huntress, W.T., see Bratzel, R.P. 18, *30*
Hurd, E.R. *400*
Hurlbert, R.B., Kammen, H.O. 490, *506*
Hurlbert, R.B., see Chakraborty, K.P. 490, *504*
Hurlbert, R.B., see Kammen, H.O. 490, *506*
Hurlbert, R.P. 274, *336*
Hurst, D., see DeSombre, E.R. 115, *127*
Hurst, D.J., see Jensen, E. V. 114, *131*
Hurst, J.M., see Medici, P. T. 38, *45*
Hurteau, G.D., see Morris, J.M. 357, *368*
Hurwitz, B.S., see Walker, M.D. 69, *84*
Hurwitz, J., Firth, J.J., Malamy, M., Alexander, M. 583, *591*
Hurwitz, J., see Gold, M. 583, *590*
Hurwitz, J., see Kahan, F. M. 208, *227*, 462, *466*
Hurwitz, J., see Maitra, U. 583, *591*
Husberg, B., see Aronsen, K. F. 410, *419*
Huser, H.J., Murphy, G.P. 410, *421*
Hussain, S., see Ahnström, G. 314, *327*
Hutchinson, F., Hales, H.B. 319, 321, *336*
Hutchinson, F., see Köhnlein, W. 321, *338*
Hutchinson, S.A., see Cunningham, K.G. 658, 660, *665*
Hutchison, D., see Clarkson, B. 222, *224*
Hutchison, D.J. 384, *400*, 820, *827*
Hutchison, D.J., see Brockman, R.W. 460, *465*
Hutchison, D.J., see Kreis, W. 758, *763*
Hutchison, D.J., see Salser, J.S. 392, *402*
Hutchison, D.J., see Uchida, K. 240, 247, *255*
Hutchison, J.L., see Ellison, R.R. 260, *268*
Hutter, A.M., Kayhoe, D. E. 811, 814, 816, *818*
Hwang, D.S., see Haus, E. 249, *252*
Hwang, Y.F., Hamilton, H. E., Sheets, R.F. 686, *690*
Hyánek, J., see Slavík, M. 361, *370*
Hyman, C.B., see Sullivan, M.P. 397, *403*
Hyman, G., see Herter, F.P. 541, *542*
Hyman, R.W., Davidson, N. 583, 585, 586, *591*

Iannotti, A.T., see Hellman, S. 477, *481*
Iannotti, A.T., see Johns, D.G. 196, *226*, 473, *481*
Iannotti, A.T., see Sartorelli, A.C. 771, 776, *787*
Iball, J., Morgan, C.H., Wilson, H.R. 279, *336*
Ibershof, M.L., see Guarino, A.J. 661, *666*
Ichikawa, T. 870, *872*
Ichikawa, T., Matsuda, A., Miyamoto, K., Tsubosaki, M., Kaihara, T., Sakamoto, K., Umezawa, H. 855, 870, *872*
Ichikawa, T., Nakano, I., Hirokawa, I. 870, *872*
Ichikawa, T., Umezawa, H. 855, 870, *872*
Ichino, M., see Hoshi, A. 887, *889*
Ichino, M., see Kanai, T. 233, *252*, 266, *269*
Ichino, M., see Kikugawa, K. 266, *270*
Ichinose, R.R., see Coffey, D.S. 151, *153*
Ierardi, P.A., see Durr, G.J. 350, *365*
Igarashi, N., see Aizawa, S. 441, 444, *452*
Iijima, T., Hagawara, A. 56, *60*
Iijima, T., Ikeda, Y. 862, *872*
Iijima, T., see Ikeda, Y. 862, *872*
Iizuka, N., see Kimura, K. 870, *873*
Ikeda, K., Egami, F. 862, *872*
Ikeda, T., see Kato, S. 870, *873*
Ikeda, Y., Iijima, T., Tajima, K. 862, *872*
Ikeda, Y., see Iijema, T. 862, *872*
Ikeda, Y., see Shishido, K. 326, *344*
Ikehara, M., Fukui, T. 437, 443, *454*
Ikehara, M., Murao, K., Harada, F., Nishimura, S. 443, 444, *454*
Ikehara, M., Ohtsuka, E. 438, *454*
Ikehara, M., see Mizuno, Y. 444, *455*
Ikekawa, T., Iwami, F., Hiranaka, H., Umezawa, H. 851, 852, 855, 869, *872*
Ikekawa, T., see Umezawa, H. *876*

Ilan, J., Quastel, J. H. 679, 681, *690*
Ilan, Joseph, Tokuyasu, K., Ilan, Judith 428, *432*
Ilan, Judith, see Ilan, Joseph 428, *432*
Ilievski, V., see Heyman, I.A. 832, *839*
Ilonopisov, R. L., see Alexander, P. 728, *742*
Imada, A., see Kida, M. 448, *454*
Inaba, M., Sakurai, Y. 28, *32*
Inada, Y., see Nishimura, Y. 703, *719*
Inagaki, A., Nakamura, T., Wakisaka, G. 242, 243, *252*, 261, *269*
Inagaki, A., see Kageyama, M. 583, *591*
Inagaki, J., see Kimura, K. 870, *873*
Inman, D. R., Banfield, R. E. W., King, R. J. B. 114, *131*
Inman, R. B., Baldwin, R. L. 293, 294, *336*
Inman, R. B., Schnos, M. 294, 325, *336*
Innocenti, I. R. D., see Rosso, R. 69, *83*
Inoue, H., see Čihák, A. 363, *365*
Inuyama, Y., Machukawa, J. 870, *872*
Ionesco, M., Ryter, A., Schaeffer, P. 57, *61*
Ireland, J. T., see Allan, J. D. 529, *529*
Iriarte, P. V., Hananain, J., Cortner, J. A. 69, *81*
Irikura, T., see Hasegawa, Y. 856, *872*
Irion, E., Arens, A. 702, *717*, 723, *744*
Irion, E., see Arens, A. 698, 699, 702, 703, *713*
Irion, E., see Rauenbusch, E. 699, 700, *720*
Irion, E., see Wagner, O. 698, 703, *721*, *722*
Irvin, J. L., see Wilson, J. E. 523, *538*
Irvine, E., see McCoy, T. A. 696, 711, *718*
Irvine, W. T., see Braunsberg, H. 117, *126*
Irvine, W. T., see Folca, P. J. 117, *128*
Irwin, L. E., see Bateman, J. R. 221, *223*
Isaacs, B. L., see Luce, J. K. 544, 545, 546, *551*
Isassi, A. A., see Luce, J. K. 397, *401*
Ishibara, A., see Hall, T. C. 459, *465*
Ishida, N., Homma, M., Kumagai, K., Shimizu, Y., Matsumoto, S., Izawa, A. 444, *454*
Ishida, N., Izawa, A., Homma, M., Kumagai, K., Shimizu, Y. 444, *454*
Ishihara, H., Wang, S. Y. 321, *336*
Ishii, Y., see Yüntsen, H. 446, *457*
Ishizuka, M., Sawa, T., Hori, S., Takayama, H. 444, *454*
Ishizuka, M., Sawa, T., Koyama, G., Takeuchi, T., Umezawa, H. 441, *454*
Ishizuka, M., Takayama, H., Takeuchi, T., Umezawa, H. 851, 855, 860, 861, 870, *873*
Ishizuka, M., see Umezawa, H. 444, *456*, 855, 870, *875*, *876*
Island, D. P., see Bledsoe, T. 813, *817*
Isola, J. B., see Ungar, G. 527, *537*
Isono, K., see Aizawa, S. 441, 444, *452*
Israels, L. G., Sinclair, C., Graf, J., Zipursky, A. 38, *44*
Israels, L. G., see Linford, J. H. 28, *32*
Israëls, M. C. G., see Buttoo, A.S. 352, 356, 359, *364*
Israëls, M. C. G., see Elves, M.W. 361, *365*
Iszard, D. M., see Krant, M. J. 523, *533*
Ito, E., see Hori, M. 441, 442, 445, *454*, 857, *872*
Ito, J., see Yanofsky, C. 9, 11, *17*
Ito, M., see Suzuki, M. 870, *875*
Ito, Y., see Shimazaki, J. 149, *156*
Itoga, T., see Rundles, R. W. 408, 412, *423*
Itoi, I. 200
Ivankovic, S., see Druckrey, H. 70, *80*
Ivankovic, S., see Preussmann, R. 70, *82*
Iványi, J., see Stejskalorá, V. 356, *371*
Ives, D. H., Morse, P. A., Potter, V. R. 285, *336*
Ives, D. H., see Durham, J. F. 240, *251*
Ives, D. R., see Barry, R. D. *328*
Ives, J. H., see Durham, J. F. *251*
Iwabuchi, M., Okata, E., Kono, M., Osawa, S. 210, *226*
Iwami, F., see Ikekawa, T. 851, 852, 855, 869, *872*
Iwamoto, R. H., Acton, E. M., Goodman, L. 388, *400*
Iwanaga, J., see Takeuchi, T. 444, 445, *456*
Iwanaga, J., see Umezawa, H. 855, *875*
Iwanami, Y., see Yamada, T. 28, *34*
Iwata, A., Consigli, R. H. 855, 857, 858, 862, *873*
Iwata, H., Yamamoto, I., Muraki, K. 547, *551*
Iwata, H., see Hano, K. 547, *550*
Iwata, H., see Yamamoto, I. 547, *553*
Iwatsuki, N., Okazaki, R. 285, 286, *336*
Iyer, V. N., Szybalski, W. 48, 49, 52, 54, *61*, 494, *506*, 637, *640*
Iyer, V. N., see Steinman, I. D. 494, *510*
Iyer, V. N., see Szybalski, W. 48, 49, 50, 51, 53, 58, *63*
Izawa, A., see Ishida, N. 444, *454*
Izima, H., see Suzuki, M. 870, *875*
Izutsu, K., Biesele, J. J. 300, *336*

Jacherts, D., see Wacker, A. 274, 295, *346*
Jackson, H. 23, 24, *32*, 42, *44*
Jackson, H., Craig, A. W. 38, *44*
Jackson, H., Fox, B. W., Craig, A. W. 37, *44*
Jackson, H., see Cooper, E. R. A. 37, *42*
Jackson, H., see Edwards, K. 35, 40, *43*
Jackson, H., see Fox, B. W. 35, 37, 38, 39, *43*
Jackson, H., see Hemsworth, B. N. 38, 39, *44*
Jackson, H., see Partington, M. 37, *45*
Jackson, H. L., see Vodopick, H. 40, *46*

Jackson, J., see Levinson, W.E. 307, *339*
Jackson, L., Barr, M., Weiss, A. 735, 738, *744*
Jackson, L., see Ellem, K.A. O. 709, *715*
Jackson, R.C., Handschumacher, R.E. 515, *532*, 696, 699, 701, 703, *717*
Jackson, R.C., Huennekens, F.M. 775, *785*
Jackson, R.L., Dockerty, M. B. 174, *189*
Jackson, S.M., see Craig, A. W. 318, *330*
Jackson, V., Earnhardt, J., Chalkley, R. 825, *827*
Jacob, F., see Schubert, D. 312, *344*
Jacobs, E.M., Reeves, W.J., Wood, D.A., Rugh, R., Braunwald, J., Bateman, J.R. 220, *226*
Jacobs, J., see Vogler, W.R. 477, *483*
Jacobs, N.F., Neu, R.L., Gardner, L.T. 859, *873*
Jacobs, R.D., see Rubulis, A. 125, *135*
Jacobs, S.A., see Chello, P. 469, *480*
Jacobs, S.P., Wodinsky, I., Kensler, C.J., Venditti, J. 501, *506*
Jacobs-Lorena, M., Brega, A., Baglioni, C. 567, *569*
Jacobs-Lorena, M., see Baglioni, C. 567, *567*
Jacobson, H.I., see Davis, M.E. 113, *127*
Jacobson, H.I., see Jensen, E.V. 85, 95, *101*, 113, 114, 116, 117, *131*, 149, *154*, 176, 187, *190*
Jacobson, H.I., see Lee, C. 117, *132*
Jacobson, M., see Kaiser, I. I. 209, 210, *227*
Jacquez, J.A. 495, *506*
Jacquez, J.A., Barclay, R. K., Stock, C.C. 519, *532*
Jacquez, J.A., Mottram, F. 519, *532*
Jacquez, J.A., Sherman, J. H. 500, *506*
Jacquez, J.A., Stock, C.C., Barclay, R.K. *532*
Jacquez, J.A., see Anderson, E.P. 495, *503*
Jacquez, J.A., see Krenitsky, T.A. 289, *338*
Jacquillat, C., Weil, M., Bussel, A., Loisel, J.P., Rousse, J., Larrieu, M.J., Boiron, M., Dreyfus, B., Bernard, J. 726, 727, 728, 732, 734, 735, *744*
Jacquillat, C., see Bernard, J. 260, *267*
Jacquillat, C., see Boiron, M. 773, *783*
Jacquillat, C., see Ellison, R.R. 260, *268*
Jacquillat, C., see Weil, M. 772, 773, *788*
Jae Ho Kim, Eidinoff, M.L. *32*
Jänish, W., Schreiber, D. 78, *81*
Jaffe, J. 855, *873*
Jaffe, J.J. 768, 769, 776, *785*
Jaffe, J.J., Handschumacher, R.E., Welch, A. D. 355, *367*
Jaffe, J.J., Meymarian, E., Doremus, H.M. 441, *454*
Jaffe, J.J., Prusoff, W.H. 300, 301, 313, *336*
Jaffe, J.J., see Momparler, R.L. 495, *507*
Jaffe, J.J., see Prusoff, W. H. 282, 283, 313, 316, *342*
Jaffe, J.J., see Ross, A.F. 437, 439, *455*
Jaffe, J.J., see Rubin, R.J., 352, *369*
Jaffe, N., Farber, S., Traggis, D., Geiser, C., Das, L., Kim, B.S., Frauenberger, G., Djerassi, I. 479, *481*
Jaffe, N., Traggis, D., Das, L., Moloney, W.C., Hann, H.W., Kim, B.S., Nair, R. 726, 727, 730, 734, 735, *744*
Jaffe, N., see Dunnicliff, M. A. *744*
Jagger, D.V., Kredich, N. M., Guarino, A.J. 660, *666*
Jagiello, G.M. 859, *873*
Jahnes, W.G., Li, C.P., Tauraso, N.M. *717*
Jahnke, H.K., see Herr, R. R. 65, *81*
Jahnke, H.K., see Wiley, P.F. 557, *570*
Jain, S.C., see Sobell, H.M. 573, *581*, 587, *592*
Jakubowski, Z.L., see Dion, H.W. 485, *504*
Jamara, M., see Dalldorf, G. 417, *420*
Jamazak, Z.I., see Müller, W.E.G. 243, *254*
James, D.H., Jr., see Slotnick, I.J. 680, *693*
James, R., see Montgomery, J.A. 65, 66, 67, 68, *82*
James, R.M.V. 38, *44*
James, V.H.T., see Braunsberg, H. 117, *126*
Jameson, E., Ainis, H., Ryan, R.M. 695, *717*
Jameson, E., see Kwak, K. S. 695, *717*
Janes, J.O., see Prager, M. D. 733, *746*
Janků, I., Kršiak, M., Novotný, J., Volicer, L., Čapek, R. 349, *367*
Janků, I., Kršiak, M., Volicer, L., Čapek, R., Smetana, R., Novotný, J. 359, *367*
Janků, I., see Jiřička, Z. 349, 358, *367*
Janků, I., see Plevová, J. 358, 359, *368*
Janků, I., see Šeferna, I. 359, *370*
Janne, J., see Holtta, E. 775, *785*
Janne, J., see Raina, A. 774, *787*
Jansen, C.J., Jr., see Armstrong, J.G. 685, *688*
Jansen, C.J., Jr., see Neuss, N. 671, 687, *692*
Jansen, M., see Doering, A. M. 662, *665*
Jardine, J.H., see Loo, T.L. 546, *551*
Jared, D.W., see Wallace, R.A. 120, 121, *138*
Jarman, M., see Hill, B.T. 28, *32*
Jasińska, S., Link, F., Blaškovič, D., Rada, B. 354, *367*
Jasmin, C., see Mathé, G. 882, *889*
Jasmin, C., see Schwarzenberg, L. 474, *482*
Jatlow, P.I., see De Conti, R.C. 793, 800, 804, *805*
Javid, M., see Mukhjerjee, K. L. 202, 215, 221, *228*
Jayaram, H.N., Ramakrishnan, T., Vaidyanathan, C.S. 697, 698, 699, *717*
Jayaram, H.N., see Reddy, V.V.S. 697, 698, 699, *720*

Jedeikin, L. A., Weinhouse, S. 539, *542*
Jedeikin, L. A., White, A. 91, *101*
Jedlička, V., see Grafnetterová, J. 358, *366*
Jehn, U., see Nathanson, L. 547, *551*
Jelínek, R., Rychter, Z., Klika, E. 358, *367*
Jelínek, R., Rychter, Z., Seichert, V. 358, *367*
Jelínek, R., see Rychter, Z. 358, *369*
Jelínek, U., see Buděšínsky, Z. 196, *223*
Jelinek, W., Adesnik, M., Salditt, M., Sheiness, D., Wall, R., Molloy, G., Philipson, L., Darnell, J. E. *669*
Jelliffe, A. M., Marks, J. 747, *762*
Jellinck, P. H. 108, *131*
Jellinck, P. H., see Heard, R. D. 106, *130*
Jeney, A., see Connors, T. A. 20, 28, *31*
Jenkins, S. R., Holly, F. W., Walton, E. 661, *666*
Jenkins, S. R., Walton, E. *668*
Jenkins, S. R., see Walton, E. 658, 661, *668*
Jensen, E. V. 113, 114, *131*, 164, *167*
Jensen, E. V., Block, G. E., Smith, S., Kyser, K., DeSombre, E. R. 85, 95, *101*, 117, *131*
Jensen, E. V., DeSombre, E. R., Hurst, D. J., Kawashima, T., Jungblut, P. W. 114, *131*
Jensen, E. V., DeSombre, E. R., Jungblut, P. W. 95, *101*, 114, 115, 117, 118, *131*, 176, 177, 187, *190*
Jensen, E. V., DeSombre, E. R., Jungblut, P. W., Stumpf, W. E., Roth, L. J. 164, *167*
Jensen, E. V., Jacobson, H. I. 85, 95, *101*, 113, 114, 116, 117, *131*, 149, *154*, 176, 187, *190*
Jensen, E. V., Jacobson, H. I., Flesher, J. W., Saha, N. N., Grupta, G. N., Smith, S., Colucci, V., Shiplacoff, D., Neumann, H. G., DeSombre, E. R., Jungblut, P. W. 114, *131*, 176, 187, *190*
Jensen, E. V., Numata, M., Brecher, P. I., DeSombre, E. R. 104, *131*
Jensen, E. V., Numata, M., Smith, S., Suzuki, T., Brecher, P. I., DeSombre, E. R. 110, 114, 115, *131*
Jensen, E. V., Suzuki, T., Kawashima, T., Stumpf, W. E., Jungblut, P. W., DeSombre, E. R. 114, 115, *131*, 164, *167*
Jensen, E. V., Suzuki, T., Numata, M., Smith, S., DeSombre, E. R. 114, *131*
Jensen, E. V., see Davis, M. E. 113, *127*
Jensen, E. V., see DeSombre, E. R. 115, 117, *127*
Jensen, E. V., see Huggins, C. 110, *131*
Jensen, E. V., see Jungblut, P. W. 117, *131*
Jensen, M. K. 415, *422*
Jensen, V., see Deshpande, N. 117, *127*
Jernell, K. F., see Mueller, G. C. 118, *133*
Jerner, R. W., see Hales, D. R. 394, *399*
Jetzer, T., see Shons, A. 705, *721*
Jewett, G., see Pietsch, P. 855, 871, *874*
Jimenez, L., see Bloom, B. R. 417, *419*
Jiminiz, A., Littlewood, B., Davies, J. *569*
Jirásek, J., see Vojta, M. 357, *371*
Jiřička, Z., Smetana, K., Janků, I., Elis, J., Novotný, J. 349, 358, *367*
Jobst, K. 78, *81*
Joel, W., see Condit, P. T. 473, *480*
Johannessen, D. W., see Bartz, Q. R. 485, *503*
Johansson, H., Terenius, L., Thoren, L. 117, 118, *131*
Johansson, J. G., see Skinner, W. A. 37, *46*
Johns, C. O., see Johnson, T. B. 272, *336*
Johns, D. C., see Vogel, C. L. 478, *482*
Johns, D. G., Hollingsworth, J. W., Cashmore, A. R., Plenderleith, I. H., Bertino, J. R. 472, 473, *481*
Johns, D. G., Iannotti, A. T., Sartorelli, A. C., Booth, B. A., Bertino, J. R. 473, *481*
Johns, D. G., Sartorelli, A. C., Bertino, J. R., Iannotti, A. T., Booth, B. A., Welch, A. D. 196, *226*
Johns, D. G., Spencer, R. P., Chang, P. K., Bertino, J. R. 472, *481*
Johns, D. G., Valerino, D. M. 473, *481*
Johns, D. G., see Bertino, J. R. 474, *479*, 528, *530*
Johns, D. G., see Booth, B. A. 846, 847, *848*
Johns, D. G., see Cleveland, J. C. 474, 478, *480*
Johns, D. G., see Sartorelli, A. C. 771, 776, *787*
Johns, D. G., see Sieber, S. M. 880, *889*
Johns, R. J., see Uy, Q. L. 675, 682, *694*
Johnson, A. G., see Buskirk, H. H. 24, *31*, 237, *250*, 525, *530*
Johnson, A. G., see Watson, D. W. 525, *537*
Johnson, D. E., see Bratzel, R. P. 18, *30*
Johnson, F. 561, *569*
Johnson, F., see Siegel, M. R. 562, *570*
Johnson, G., see Arseneau, J. 879, *887*
Johnson, H. G., see Renis, H. E. 237, 240, *254*
Johnson, I. S. 685, *691*
Johnson, I. S., Armstrong, J. G., Gorman, M., Burnett, J. P., Jr. 671, 675, 679, 682, 685, 686, 687, *691*
Johnson, I. S., Hargrove, W. W., Harris, P. N., Wright, H. F., Boder, G. B. 671, *691*
Johnson, I. S., Wright, H. F., Svoboda, G. H. 670, *691*
Johnson, I. S., see Neuss, N. 671, 687, *692*
Johnson, J. L., Yamamoto, K. R., Weislogel, P. O., Horowitz, J. 209, 210, *227*
Johnson, K. M., see Knight, V. *338*
Johnson, L. C., see Wall, E. 175, *192*
Johnson, R. E., see Lyons, W. R. 111, *132*

Johnson, R.K., see Jondorf, W.R. 560, *569*
Johnson, R.O., see Skibba, J.L. 71, *83*
Johnson, T.B., Johns, C.O. 272, *336*
Johnson, T.B., see Hilbert, G.E. 272, *335*
Johnson, W.J., McColl, J.D. 540, 541, *542*, 543
Johnson, W.W., see Pratt, C.B. 734, *746*
Johnston, Petering, H.G. 843
Johnston, C.G., see Allen, E. 108, *125*
Johnston, D.W., see Morris, J.M. 357, *368*
Johnston, T.P., McCaleb, G.S., Montgomery, J.A. 65, 68, *81*
Johnston, T.P., McCaleb, G.S., Opliger, P.S., Montgomery, J.A. 65, 68, *81*
Johnston, T.P., Opliger, P.S. 65, 68, *81*
Johnston, T.P., McCaleb, G.S., Opliger, P.S., Laster, W.R., Montgomery, J.A. 65, 68, *81*
Johnston, T.P., see Carter, S.K. 65, *80*
Johnston, T.P., see Montgomery, J.A. 65, 66, 67, 68, *82*
Johnston, T.P., see Schabel, F.M., Jr. 65, 68, 69, 79, *83*
Joklik, W.K. 304, *336*
Joklik, W.K., see McAuslan, B.R. *340*
Jondorf, W.R., Abbott, B.J., Greenberg, N.H., Mead, J.A.R. 558, *569*
Jondorf, W.R., Drassner, J.D., Johnson, R.K., Miller, H.H. 560, *569*
Jondorf, W.R., Filler, R.S. 560, *569*
Jondorf, W.R., Simon, D.C., Avnimelech, M. 560, *569*
Jondorf, W.R., Spector, A., Chaiken, S.J. 824, *827*
Jondorf, W.R., Szapary, D. 560, *569*
Jones, A.R., see Edwards, K. 35, 40, *43*
Jones, B.R., see Wellings, P.C. 195, 200, 219, *231*
Jones, D.F., see Carter, S.B. 446, 450, 451, *453*
Jones, D.J., see Temple, T.E. 811, 814, *819*
Jones, F.F., Mills, S.D. 446, 449, 450, *454*
Jones, H.W., see Heller, R.W. 39, *44*
Jones, I.C., see Bellamy, D. 96, *100*
Jones, J., see Chun, E.H.L. 14, *15*, 28, *31*
Jones, J.C., see Christensen, H.N. 523, *530*
Jones, K.W. 628, *632*
Jones, M., see Connors, T.A. 20, 28, *31*, 712, *715*
Jones, M., see LePage, G.A. 390, 391, 395, *400*, 487, *507*
Jones, M.E., see Hager, S.E. 489, 497, *505*
Jones, N.F., Walker, G., Ruthven, C.R.J., Sandler, M. *532*
Jones, O.W., Berg, P. 326, *336*
Jones, R., see McCullagh, E.P. 145, *155*
Jones, R.G.W., Richards, J.F., Beer, C.T. 679, *691*
Jones, R.G.W., see Richards, J.F. 679, *693*
Jones, T.C., Dove, W.F. 326, *336*
Jorda, V.V., Lenfeld, J., Rothschild, L. *569*
Jorgensen, E.C., Wiley, R.A. 520, *532*
Jost, E., Amirkhanian, J.D. 37, *44*
Journey, L.J., Burdman, J., George, P. 673, 674, *691*
Journey, L.J., Goldstein, M.N. 583, *591*
Journey, L.J., see George, P. 673, *690*
Journey, L.J., see Goldstein, M.N. 583, *590*
Joyeux, M., see Kende, A.S. 650, *655*
Juel-Jensen, B.E. 323, *336*
Juel-Jensen, B.E., see Mac Callum, F.O. 323, *340*
Julian, J.A., see McGuire, W.L. 99, *102*, 117, *133*, 177, *191*
Julou, L., see Maral, R. 705, 708, *718*
Jung, I., see Baulieu, E.E. 114, 115, *126*, 150, *153*, 164, *167*
Junga, I.G., see Henderson, J.F. 500, *506*
Junga, I.G., see LePage, G.A. 388, 395, 396, *400*, 448, *454*, 658, *666*
Jungblut, P.W., DeSombre, E.R., Jensen, E.V. 117, *131*
Jungblut, P.W., see DeSombre, E.R. 115, *127*
Jungblut, P.W., see Jensen, E.V. 95, *101*, 114, 115, 117, 118, *131*, 164, *167*, 176, 177, 187, *190*
Jurkowitz, L. 584, *591*
Jurkowitz, L., see Williams-Ashman, H.G. 147, *157*
Jurovčík, M., Raška, K., Jr., Šormová, Z., Šorm, F. 362, *367*, 574, *579*
Jurovčík, M., Zadražil, S., Fučík, V., Šormová, Z. 363, *367*
Jurovčík, M., see Fučík, V. *366*
Jurovčík, M., see Raška, K. 351, 362, *369*
Jurovčík, M., see Šorm, F. 351, *370*

Kabat, S., Visser, D.W. 380, *381*
Kaboth, W., see Begemann, H. 708, *713*
Kachi, H., see Hirono, I. 28, *32*
Kaczka, E.A., Dulaney, E.L., Gitterman, C.O., Woodruff, H.B., Folkers K. 658, *666*
Kaczka, E.A., Trenner, N.R., Arison, B., Walker, R.W., Folkers, K. 658. *666*
Kaden, P., see Bremerskov, V. 234, 241, *250*
Kadlec, O., see Šeferna, I. 359, *370*
Kääriäinen, L., see Ranki, M. *515*, *535*
Kafka, V., Musil, J., Padovec, J., Šorm, F. 360, *367*
Kagawa, T., see Tanaka, M. 698, 699, 702, *721*
Kageyama, M., Hasegawa, M., Inagaki, A., Egami, F. 583, *591*
Kahan, F.M., Hurwitz, J. 462, *466*
Kahan, F.M., see Ascoli, F. 274, *327*
Kahan, F.M., Hurwitz, J. 208, *227*

Kahwanago, I., Heinricks, W. L., Herrmann, W. L. 117, *131*
Kaihara, T., see Ichikawa, T. 855, 870, *872*
Kaiser, A., see Berneis, K. 756, *761*
Kaiser, A., see Zeller, P. 747, *765*
Kaiser, I. I. 209, 210, *227*
Kaiser, I. I., Jacobson, M., Hedgcoth, C. 209, 210, *227*
Kaiser, N., Kirkpatrick, A. F., Milholland, R. J., Rosen, F. 97, *101*
Kaiser, N., see Kirkpatrick, A. F. 98, 99, *101*, 176, 187, *190*
Kaizer, H., see Shimura, Y. 209, *230*
Kajiwara, K., Kim, U. H., Mueller, G. C. 859, *873*
Kajiwara, K., Mueller, G. C. 299, *336*
Kakimoto, Y., Akazawa, S. 518, *532*
Kakizawa, K., see Miura, M. 514, 515, 526, *534*, 705, 706, 707, 713, *719*, 735, 738, *745*
Kakudo, M., see Mizuno, H. 279, *341*
Kaldor, G., see Heidelberger, C. 204, 217, *226*
Kalle, G. P., Gots, J. S. 461, *466*
Kallman, R. F., see Brown, J. M. 319, *329*
Kamada, H., see Wakaki, S. 47, *64*
Kameda, Y., see Abe, M. 522, *529*
Kametani, T., Nemoto, H., Takeda, H., Takano, S. 650, *655*
Kaminsky, N., Luse, S., Hartroft, P. 811, *818*
Kamiya, T., Ben-Porat, T., Kaplan, A. S. 304, *336*
Kamiya, T., see Kaplan, A. S. 302, 303, 304, 305, *337*
Kammen, H. O. 290, *337*
Kammen, H. O., Hurlbert, R. B. 490, *506*
Kammen, H. O., see Canellakis, E. S. 274, *329*
Kammen, H. O., see Hurlbert, R. B. 490, *506*
Kampschroer, B., see Heidelberger, C. 202, 203, 205, 219, *226*
Kanai, T., Kojima, T., Maruyama, O., Ichino, M. 233, *252*, 266, *269*
Kanai, T., see Hoshi, A. 887, *889*
Kanamori, K., see Hata, T. 47, *60*
Kandaswamy, T. S., Henderson, J. F. 501, *506*
Kaneko, T., LePage, G. A. 431, *432*
Kang, S., see Shapiro, R. *344*
Kankel, D., see Coleman, A. W. 311, *330*
Kann, H. E., Jr., Kohn, K. W. 573, 574, 577, *580*, 644, *647*, *669*
Kann, H. E., Jr., Snyder, A. L., Kohn, K. W. 75, *81*. 574, *580*
Kann, H. E., Jr., see Kohn, K. W. 644, 645, *647*
Kann, H. E., Jr., see Snyder, A. L. 574, *581*, 881, *890*
Kanner, L., Hanawalt, P. 280, *337*
Kanno, T., Kudo, T., Nakazawa, T., Takeuchi, T., Umezawa, H. 855, 871, *873*
Kano, H., see Nakagawa, Y. 373, *382*
Kantner, V., see Rašková, H. 361, *369*
Kanzawa, F., see Hoshi, A. 234, *252*, 266, 267, *269*. 887, *889*
Kao, F.-T., Puck, T. T. 78, *81*
Kao, M. H., see Tsukagoshi, S. 76, *84*
Kaplan, A. S., Ben-Porat, T. 295, 302, 303, 304, 305, 306, *337*
Kaplan, A. S., Ben-Porat, T., Kamiya, T. 302, 303, 304, 305, *337*
Kaplan, A. S., Brown, Mck., Ben-Porat, T. 241, 242, *252*
Kaplan, A. S., see Ben-Porat T. 242, *249*
Kaplan, A. S., see Kamiya, T. 304, *336*
Kaplan, A. S., see Kasamaki, A. 300, *337*
Kaplan, H. S. 319, *337*
Kaplan, H. S., see Bagshaw, M. A. 291, 319, 324, *327*
Kaplan, H. S., see Doggett, R. L. S. 324, *331*
Kaplan, H. S., see Goffinet, D. R. 319, *334*
Kaplan, L., see Wempen, I. 196, *231*, 278, *346*
Kaplan, L. A., see Dietrich, L. S. 541, *542*
Kaplan, L. H., Reilly, H. C., Stock, C. C. 492, 494, 495, *506*
Kaplan, N. O., Goldin, A., Humphreys, S. R., Ciotti, M. R, Venditti, J. M. 540, *543*
Kaplan, N. O., see Narrod, S. A. 491, *508*
Kaplan, N. O., see Zatman, L. J. 540, *543*
Kaplan, R., see Fillios, L. C. 109, *128*
Kaplan, S. B., Wade, M., Clement, D., DeConti, R., Calabresi, P. 264, *270*
Kaplan, S. R., Hayslett, J. P., Calabresi, P. 502, *506*
Kaplan, S. R., see Creasey, W. A. 233, 238, 240, 241, 242, 244, *251*
Kappen, L., see Goldberg, I. H. 557, 558, 559, 566, *568*
Kapuler, A. M., Ward, D. C., Mendelsohn, N., Klett, H., Acs, G. 437, *454*
Kara, J. 307, *337*, 350, *367*
Kara, J., Duschinsky, R. 273, *337*
Kara, J., see Duschinsky, R. 273, *331*
Kara, J., see Fučík, V. 273, *333*
Kára, J., Šorm, F. 349, 350, *367*
Kára, J., see Sagar, P. 350, *369*
Kára, J., see Škoda, J. 350, 352, *370*
Kàra, J., see Stejskalová, V. 356, *371*
Kára, J., see Winkler, A. 352, *372*
Karam, J. D., see Speyer, J. F. 282, *345*
Karanas, A., see Ellison, R. R. 260, *268*
Karemfyllis, T., see Georgatsos, J. G. 678, 681, *690*
Kariya, T., see Blohm, T. R. 105, *126*
Karlan, D., see Abelson, H. T. 573, 574, 575, *579*
Karlan, D., see Reichman, M. 574, *580*
Karlsson, J. O., Sjöstrand, J. 675, *691*
Karnofsky, D. A. 6, *15*

Karnofsky, D.A., Basch, R. S. 310, *337*
Karnofsky, D.A., Bevelander, G. 495, *506*
Karnofsky, D.A., Clarkson, B.D. 458, *466*
Karnofsky, D.A., Clifford, G.O. 512, *532*
Karnofsky, D.A., Golbey, R.B., Li, M.C. 500, 502, *506*
Karnofsky, D.A., Lacon, C. R. 236, *252*, 261, *270*
Karnofsky, D.A., see Burchenal, J.H. 384, 389, *398*
Karnofsky, D.A., see Clarkson, B.D. 727, 728, 730, 732, *743*
Karnofsky, D.A., see Dagg, C.P. *504*, *550*
Karnofsky, D.A., see Ellison, R.R. 500, *504*
Karnofsky, D.A., see Hackethal, C.A. 638, *640*
Karnofsky, D.A., see Magill, G.B. 500, *507*
Karnofsky, D.A., see Murphy, M.L. 394, *401*, 493, *507*
Karnofsky, D.A., see Oettgen, H.F. 727, 728, 730, 732, 734, 735, *745*
Karnofsky, D.A., see Tallal, L. 727, 728, 730, 732, *746*
Karol, M.H., Simpson, M.V. 282, 295, 337, *337*
Karon, E., see Levin, R.H. 769, 772, 773, *786*
Karon, M., Benedict, W.F. 802, 803, *806*
Karon, M., Henry, P., Weissman, S., Meyer, C. 241, *253* 261, *270*
Karon, M., Shirakawa, S. 235, *253*
Karon, M., Sieger, L., Leimbrock, S., Finkelstein, J. Z., Nesbit, M.E., Swaney, J.J. 364, *367*
Karon, M., Weissman, S., Meyer, C., Henry, P. 463, *466*
Karon, M., see Benedict, W. F. 236, 237, *249*, 261, *267*
Karon, M., see Finkelstein, J.Z. 238, *251*, 258, 260, *268*
Karon, M., see Freireich, E. J. 772, *785*
Karpas, A. 302, 304, *337*
Karr, A., see Leimgruber, W. 642, *648*
Kartha, G., see Mazza, F. 197, *228*
Kasamaki, A., Ben-Porat, T., Kaplan, A.S. 300, *337*
Kasamatu, T., see Suzuki, M. 870, *875*
Kasbekar, D.K., Greenberg, D.M. 217, *227*
Kasel, J.A., see Knight, V. *338*
Kashiwada, N., see Kimura, K. 870, *873*
Kasnic, G., Jr., see Stewart, S.E. 308, *345*
Kassarich, J., see Rosenthale, M.E. 408, *423*
Katagiri, K., see Matsuura, S. 374, *382*
Katchman, B.J., Fetty, W. O., Busch, K.A. 25, *32*
Katchman, B.J., Zipf, R.E., Murphy, J.P.F. 683, *691*
Kates, J. 574, 575, *580*
Kato, E., see Wakaki, S. 47, *64*
Kato, H., see Nishimura, H. 373, 374, *382*
Kato, I., see Honjo, T. 561, *568*
Kato, J., Villee, C.A. 117, *131*
Kato, N., Okabayashi, K., Mizuno, H. 55, *61*
Kato, S., Hara, I., Abe, H., Ikeda, T., Yamagami, K., Uchiya, M., Shimomura, G. 870, *783*
Katsube, Y., see Titani, Y. 374, *382*
Katz, L., see Tomita, K.I. 197, *230*
Katz, N., Pellegrino, J., Ferreira, M.T., Oliveira, C.A., Dias, C.B. 879, *889*
Katzman, P.A., Larson, D. L., Podratz, K.C. 160, *167*
Katzman, P.A., see Podratz, K.C. 162, *168*
Kaudewitz, F., see Knolle, P. 58, *61*
Kauffman, G.B. 835, *839*
Kaufman, B.T., Pierce, J.V. 469, *481*
Kaufman, H.E. 194, 199, *227*, 302, 306, 323, *337*
Kaufman, H.E., Heidelberger, C. 199, *227*
Kaufman, H.E., Maloney, E.D. 302, *337*
Kaufman, H.E., Martola, E., Dohlman, C. 302, 322, *337*
Kaufman, H.E., Nesburn, A.B., Maloney, D.E. 302, 322, *337*
Kaufman, H.E., see Wellings, P.C. 195, 200, 219, *231*
Kaufman, J.J., Dignam, W., Goodwin, W.E., Martin, D.C., Goldman, R., Maxwell, M.H. 415, *422*
Kaufmann, W., see Arens, A. 698, 699, 702, 703, *713*
Kaufmann, W., see Rauenbusch, E. 698, 702, *720*, 723, *746*
Kaufmann, W., see Wagner, O. 698, *721*
Kaump, D.H., see Kurtz, S.M. 428, *433*
Kaump, D.H., see Sidwell, R.W. 428, *433*
Kaverin, N.V., Emeliyanov, B.A. 354, *367*
Kawai, S., Hanafusa, H. 200, *227*
Kawakami, M., see Ueda, M. 683, *694*
Kawamata, J., see Shiba, S. 53, 56, *63*
Kawashima, F., see Kida, M. 448, *454*
Kawashima, K., see Miura, M. 705, 706, *719*
Kawashima, T., see DeSombre, E.R. 115, *127*
Kawashima, T., see Jensen, E.V. 164, *167*
Kay, D., see Stickler, D.J. 57, *63*
Kay, H.E.M., see Beard, M.E.J. 726, 727, 728, 730, 734, 735, *743*
Kay, J.E., Pegg, A.E. 774, 775, *785*
Kayhoe, D.E., see Hutter, A.M. 811, 814, 816, *818*
Kazimierczuk, Z., Shugar, D. 321, *337*
Kaziwara, K., Watanabe, J., Komeda, T., Usui, T. 618, 619, 620, *622*
Kazuo, O., see Hoshino, A. *613*
Keates, R.H., see Smolin, G. 527, *536*
Keblas, S. 522, *533*
Keel, H.J., see Martz, G. 759, *763*

Keilová, H., see Šorm, F. 355, *370*
Keiser, J. F., see Durr, G. J. 350, *365*
Kekomäki, M., Rahiala, E. L., Räihä, N. C. R. 516, *532*
Keller, J., see Doering, A. 244, *251*
Keller, R. A., see Heidelberger, C. 390, *399*
Kelley, B. N., see Gimlin, D. M. 308, *334*
Kelley, D. E., see Perry, R. P. 571, *580*
Kelley, R. B., see Wiley, P. F. 557, *570*
Kelley, R. M., Baker, W. H. 186, *190*
Kelley, S. A., see Coffey, J. J. 800, 802, *805*
Kelley, W. N., Rosenbloom, F. M., Seegmiller, J. E. 414, *422*
Kellie, A. E., see Feherty, P. 116. *128*
Kellie, A. E., see Méšter, J. 115, *133*
Kellner, B., Németh, L. 36, *44*
Kellum, D. L., see Rosenkrantz, J. G. 415, *423*
Kelly, C., see Rizzo, A. J. *669*
Kelly, H. J., see Tomisek, A. J. 486, *511*
Kelly, K. H., see Bierman, H. R. 36, *42*
Kelly, M. G., Hartwell, J. L. 671, *691*
Kelly, M. G., Leiter, J., Bourke, A. R., Smith, P. K. 684, *691*
Kelly, M. G., O'Gara, R. W., Gadekar, K., Yancey, S. T., Oliverio, V. T. 752, *762*
Kelly, M. G., O'Gara, R. W., Yancey, S. T., Botkin, C. 752, *763*
Kelly, M. G., O'Gara, R. W., Yancey, S. T., Gadekar, K., Botkin, C., Oliverio, V. T. 752, *763*
Kelly, M. G., see Fishbein, W. N. 521, *531*
Kelly, M. G., see O'Gara, R. W. 752, *764*
Kelly, M. G., see Oliverio, V. T. 747, 748, 749, 751, 754, *764*
Kelly, R. B., see Bhuyan, B. K. 623, *631*
Kelly, R. B., see Wiley, P. F. 623, *632*
Kelly, R. C., see Gray, G. D. 237, *252*, 266. *269*
Kelver, O., see Van Dyk, J. J. 197, *231*
Kemp, J. D., see Rutter, W. J. 311, *343*
Kendall, E. C., see Heilman, F. R. 175, 187, *189*
Kendall, S. M., see Gale, G. R. 790, *791*
Kende, A. S., Draper, R. W., Kubo, I., Joyeux, M. 650, *655*
Kendrey, G. 36, *44*
Kenis, Y., Werli, J., Hildebrand, J., Tagnon, H. J. 759, *763*
Kennealey, G. T., Lytton, B., Ruddle, N., Mitchell, M. S. 408, *422*
Kennedy, B. J. 112, *131*, 144, *154*, 173, 181, 182, 183, *190*, 621, *622*
Kennedy, B. J., Yarbro, J. W. 793, *806*
Kennedy, B. J., Yarbro, J. W., Kickertz, V., Sandberg-Wollheim, M. *622*
Kennedy, B. J., see Brown, J. H. 621, *621*
Kennedy, B. J., see Theologides, A. 603, *613*
Kennedy, B. J., see Yarbro, J. W. 616, *622*
Kenney, F. T., Kull, F. J. 88, *101*
Kenney, F. T., Wicks, W. D., Greenman, D. L. 88, *101*
Kenney, F. T., see Greenman, D. L. 120, *129*, 147, *154*
Kenney, F. T., see Tuominen, F. W. 243, *255*
Kenney, F. T., see Wicks, W. D. 147, *157*
Kenney, F. T., see Wittliff, J. L. 120, 121, *138*
Kensler, C. J. 682, *691*, 820, 824, *827*
Kensler, C. J., Palm, P. E., Day, H. M., Battista, S. P., Rogers, W. I., Yesair, D. W., Wodinsky, I. 822, 824, *827*
Kensler, C. J., see Coffey, J. J. 523, *530*, 800, 802, *805*
Kensler, C. J., see Jacobs, S. P. 501, *506*
Kensler, C. J., see Palm, P. E. 824, *827*
Kensler, C. J., see Rogers, W. I. 219, *229*, 822, 823, *828*
Kensler, C. J., see Sivak, A. 822, 823, 824, *828*
Kensler, C. J., see Wodinsky, I. 235, *256*
Kensler, C. J., see Yesair, D. W. 682, *694*, 823, 824, 825, *828*
Kensler, C. J., see York, I. M. 822, *828*
Kent, R. J., Heidelberger, C. 196, 203, 215, 216, *227*
Kent, R. J., Khwaja, T. A., Heidelberger, C. 196, 215, *227*
Kepler, J. A., Wani, M. C., McNaull, J. N., Wall, M. E., Levine, S. G. 649, *655*
Kepler, J. A., see Wani, M. C. 649, 650, *656*
Keppie, J., see Wade, H. E. 697, *721*
Kersten, H. 54, *61*
Kersten, H., Kersten, W. 54, 55, *61*
Kersten, H., Kersten, W., Leopold, G., Schnieders, B. 54, *61*
Kersten, H., see Hartmann, G. 602, 603, *612*
Kersten, H., see Kersten, W. 599, *613*, 626, 627, *632*
Kersten, H., see Leopold, G. 54, *61*
Kersten, H., see Ogilvie, A. 56, *62*
Kersten, W., Kersten, H. 599, *613*
Kersten, W., Kersten, H., Szybalski, W. 626, 627, *632*
Kersten, W., see Hartmann, G. 602, 603, *612*
Kersten, W., see Kersten, H. 54, 55, *61*
Kersten, W., see Leopold, G. 54, *61*
Kersten, W., see Ogilvie, A. 56, *62*
Kersten, W., see Ostertag, W. 584, *591*
Kerwin, J. F., see Saunders, H. L. 146, *156*
Kessel, D. 239, 240, 246, *253*, 267, *270*, 578, *580*, 650, 653, *656*, 702, *717*
Kessel, D., Bosmann, H. B. 709, *717*
Kessel, D., Bosmann, H. B., Lohr, K. 653, *656*
Kessel, D., Botteril, V., Wodinsky, L. *613*
Kessel, D., Bruns, R., Hall, T. C. 217, *227*

Kessel, D., Hall, T.C. 216, *227*, 239, *253*
Kessel, D., Hall, T.C., Reyes, P. *227*
Kessel, D., Hall, T.C., Roberts, D. 471, *481*
Kessel, D., Hall, T.C., Roberts, D., Wodinsky, I. 471, 473, *481*
Kessel, D., Hall, T.C., Rosenthal, D. 246, 247, *253*, 265, *270*
Kessel, D., Hall, T.C., Wodinsky, I. 239, *253*, 265, *270*
Kessel, D., Shurin, S.B. 240, *253*
Kessel, D., Wodinsky, I. 216, *227*, 584, *591*
Kessel, D., see Bosmann, H. B. 701, 708, 709, *714*
Kessel, D., see Everson, R. 216, *225*
Kessel, D., see Hall, T.C. 265, *269*
Kessel, D., see Spataro, A. 653, *656*
Kessler, S., see Erlanger, M. 222, *225*
Kestens, P., see Alexandre, G.P.J. 502, *503*
Kestens, P.J., see Haxhe, J. J. 410, *421*, 502, *505*
Ketler, A., see Hamparian, V.V. 307, *335*
Key, R.L., see Bledsoe, T. 813, *817*
Keyes, P.L., see Lee, C. *132*
Khan, A., Albayrak, A., Hill, J.M. 837, *839*
Khan, A., Hill, J.M. 705, 708, *717*, 735, *745*, 833, 836, 837, *839*, *840*
Khan, A., see Hill, J.M. 696, 702, 704, *716*, 723, 726, 728, 732, *744*
Khan, A., see Loeb, E. 726, 727, 728, 734, 735, *745*
Khan, N.A., see Brendel, M. 41, *42*
Kharats, K.S., see Galaev, Y.V. 698, *716*
Khoo, M.K.Y., see Henderson, J.F. 390, *400*, 437, *453*
Khung, C.L., see Cavins, J. A. 440, *453*
Khwaja, T.A., Heidelberger, C. 196, 200, 215, *227*
Khwaja, T.A., see Kent, R. J. 196, 215, *227*
Kickertz, V., see Kennedy, B.J. *622*
Kida, M., Kawashima, F., Imada, A., Nogami, I., Suhara, I., Yoneda, M. 448, *454*
Kidd, J.G. 695, 696, *717*, 723, *745*
Kidd, J.G., see Sobin, L.H. 709, *721*
Kidder, G.W., Dewey, V.C. 380, *381*, 384, *400*, 458, 459, 460, *466*
Kidder, G.W., Dewey, V.C., Parks, R.E., Jr. 463, *466*
Kidder, G.W., Dewey, V.C., Parks, R.E., Jr., Woodside, G.L. 458, 459, 460, *466*
Kidder, G.W., see Heinrich, M.R. 463, *465*
Kidson, C. 88, 90, *101*
Kiely, J.M., see Gottschalk, P.G. 682, 686, *690*
Kies, M.W., see Vogel, C.L. 549, *553*
Kiguchi, G., see Higuchi, M. *60*
Kihlman, B.A. 6, *15*, 298, *337*
Kihlman, B.A., Nichols, W. W., Levan, A. 236, *253*, 261, *270*
Kihlman, B.A., Odmark, G. 662, *666*
Kihlman, B.A., Odmark, G., Hartley, B. 859, *873*
Kikuchi, G., see Higuchi, M. 857, *872*
Kikugawa, K., Ichino, M. 266, *270*
Kilgore, W.W., Greenberg, J. 494, *506*
Kilgore, W.W., Morris, J.E., Greenberg, J. 79, *81*
Kilgore, W.W., see Suzuki, H. 54, *63*
Killander, A., see Dahlwitz, A. 735, *743*
Killander, D., see Caspersson, T. 21, *31*
Killander, D., see Dahlwitz, A. 735, *743*
Kim, B.S., see Jaffe, N. 479, *481*, 726, 727, 730, 734, 735, *744*
Kim, B.K., see Sheen, M.R. 445, *455*
Kim, J.H., Boyse, E.A., Old, L.J., Campbell, H. A. 738, *745*
Kim, J.H., Eidinoff, M.L. 21, 235, 241, 242, *253*, 261, *270*
Kim, J.H., Eidinoff, M.L., Fox, J.J. 233, 241, *253*
Kim, J.H., Gelbard, A.S., Perez, A.G., Eidinoff, M. L. 59, *61*, 299, *337*
Kim, J.H., Stambuk, B.K. 674, *691*
Kim, J.H., see Djordjevic, B. 59, *60*, 859, *871*
Kim, J.S., see Djerassi, I. 478, *480*
Kim, J.H., see Oettgen, H. F. 696, *719*, 723, 727, 730, 733, 734, *745*
Kim, J.H., see Old, L.J. 728, 733, *746*
Kim, K.H., Gelbard, A.S., Djordjevic, B., Kim, S. H., Perez, A.G. 603, 605, *613*
Kim, S.C., see Tidd, D.M. 396, *403*
Kim, S.H., Rich, A. 197, *227*
Kim, S.H., see Gelbard, A. S. 354, *366*
Kim, S.H., see Kim, K.H. 603, 605, *613*
Kim, U.H., see Kajiwara, K. 859, *873*
Kim, U.H., see Vonderhaar, B.K. 114, *137*
Kimball, A.P., Bowman, B., Bush, P.S., Herriot, J., LePage, G.A. 234, 241, *253*, 429, *432*
Kimball, A.P., Herriot, J., Allinson, P.S. 430, *432*
Kimball, A.P., LePage, G. A., Allinson, P.S. 429, *432*
Kimball, A.P., LePage, G. A., Bowman, B. 429, *432*
Kimball, A.P., LePage, G. A., Bowman, B., Herriot, J. 430, *432*
Kimball, A.P., Wilson, M.J. 243, *253*, 261, *270*
Kimball, A.P., see Pierre, K.J. 387, 388, *402*
Kimball, A.P., see Sato, K. 430, *433*
Kimura, G., Mori, R. 304, 307, *337*
Kimura, G., Mori, R., Amaleo, K. *337*
Kimura, G., see Mori, R. 302, 307, *341*
Kimura, K., Sakai, Y., Konda, T., Kashiwada, N., Kitahara, T., Inagaki, J., Sakano, K., Fujita, H., Iizuka, N., Mikuni, M. 870, *873*
Kimura, K., see Niitani, H. 54, *62*

Kimura,K., see Sakai,Y. 887, *889*
Kimura,K., see Umezawa, H. 855, *875*
King,C.E., see MacLeod,R. M. 94, *101*
King,R.J.B., Gordon,J. 114, *131*
King,R.J.B., Gordon,J., Martin,L. 113, 114, 117, *131*
King,R.J.B., see Inman,D. R. 114, *131*
King,R.J.B., see Steggles, A.W. 115, *136*
Kingra,G.S., Comis,R., Olson,K.B., Horton,J. 546, *551*
Kinoshita,S., see Suzuki,M. 870, *875*
Kirk,J. 582, 583, *591*
Kirk,J.M. 573, *580*
Kirk,M.C., see Hill,D.L. 29, *32*
Kirk,M.C., see Struck,R.F. 29, *33*
Kirkman,H. 175, *190*
Kirkman,H., Bacon,R.L. 175, *190*
Kirkman,H., see Matthews, V.S. 175, *191*
Kirkman,H.N. 124, *132*
Kirkpatrick,A.F., Kaiser, N., Milhollan,R.J., Rosen,F. 176, 187, *190*
Kirkpatrick,A.F., Milholland,R.J., Rosen,F. 95, 97, *101*
Kirkpatrick,A.F., Kaiser, N., Milholland,R.J., Rosen,F. 98, 99, *101*
Kirkpatrick,A.F., see Kaiser,N. 97, *101*
Kirkpatrick,H.C., see Linder,R.C. 561, *569*
Kirkpatrick,J.L., see McCord,T.J. 524, *534*
Kirkpatrick,R., see Dorrington,J.H. 140, *153*
Kirschbaum,J., Wriston,J. C.,Jr., Ratych,O.T. 700, *717*
Kirschfield,S., see Wacker, A. 380, *383*
Kirschner,M.A., see Lipsett,M.B. 814, *818*
Kirschner,S., Wei,Y.-K., Francis,D., Bergman,J. G. 836, *840*
Kiryabwire,J.W.M., see Vogel,C.L. *553*
Kiseleva,O.A., see Berlin, Y.A. 615, *621*
Kishi,T., see Kusaka,T. 434, *454*
Kisken,W.A., see Blomgren,S.E. 201, *223*
Kisliuk,R.L., see Crusberg, T.C. *480*
Kisliuk,R.L., see Leary,R. 469, *481*
Kistner,R.W., see Griffiths, C.T. 175, 179, *189*
Kit,S. 292, *337*
Kit,S., Bacila,M., Barron, E.S.G. 86, *101*
Kit,S., Beck,C., Graham, O.L., Gross,A. 301, 302, *337*
Kit,S., DeTorres,R.A., Dubbs,D.R. 246, *253*, 265, *270*
Kit,S., Dubbs,D.R. *337*
Kit,S., Dubbs,D.R., Frearson,P.M. 298, *338*
Kit,S., Dubbs,D.R., Piekarski,L.J., Hsu,T.C. 298, *338*
Kit,S., Hsu,T.C. 293, *338*
Kit,S., Piekarski,L.J., Dubbs,D.R. 56, *61*
Kit,S., see Dubbs,D.R. 298, 302, 303, 316, *331*
Kit,S., see Pearson,P.M. 246, *254*
Kitahara,T., see Kimura,K. 870, *873*
Kitahara,T., see Rapp,F. 302, 303, 304, 307, *343*
Kitahara,T., see Sakai,Y. 887, *889*
Kitano,M., Mihich,E., Pressman,D. 768, *785*
Kitano,M., see Carey,T. 768, *783*
Kitano,M., see Mihich,E. 768, 778, *786*
Kitay,D., see Cohlan,S.Q. 675, 676, *689*
Kitay,J.I. 123, *132*
Kitching,D., see Melling,J. *668*
Kitto,G.B., see Allison,J. P. 697, 702, *713*
Kjaer,A., Larsen,P.O. 498, *506*
Kjellen,L. 302, 303, 307, *338*
Kjellen,L., Periera,H.G., Valentine,R.C., Armstrong,J.A. 302, 307, *338*
Kjellstrand,C.M., see Simmons,R.L. 414, *424*
Klaiber,E.L., see Burstein, S. 813, *817*
Klainer,A.S., see Feigin,R. D. 529, *531*
Klatskin,G., Friedman,H. 558, 561, *569*
Klatt,D., see Milner,A.N. 27, *33*
Klatt,O., Stehlin,J.S., McBride,C., Griffin,A. C. 29, *32*
Klatt,R., see Heine,K.M. 416, *421*
Klebe,R., see Olmsted,J.B. 678, *692*
Kleibel,F. 754, *763*
Kleibel,K., see Rašková,H. 361, *369*
Kleihues,P. 73, *81*
Kleihues,P., Patzschke,K. 69, *81*
Kleiman,L., Huang,R.C.C. 584, *591*
Klein,E., see Williams,A.C. 221, *231*
Klein,G. 417, *422*
Klein,G., see Reichard,P. 217, *229*
Klein,H.P., see Eisenstadt, J.M. 514, *531*
Kleinsmith,L.J., see Allfrey,V.G. 89, *100*
Klement,V., Nicolson,M.O., Huebner,R.J. 308, *338*
Klemperer,H.G., Haynes, G.R., Shedden,W.I.H., Watson,D.K. *338*
Klempner,E., see Frank,R. T. 140, *153*
Klenow,H. 659, 661, 662, 663, *666*
Klenow,H., Overgaard-Hansen,K. 663, *666*
Klenow,H., Frederiksen,S. 659, *666*
Klenow,H., see Frederiksen, S. 658, 663, *665*
Klenow,H., see Lindberg, B. 448, *454*, 658, 659, 661, 662, *666*
Klenow,H., see Truman, J.T. 659, 662, 663, *668*
Klett,H., see Kapuler,A.M. 437, *454*
Klieger,E., see Weygand, F. 485, *511*
Kligerman,M.M. *338*
Kligerman,M.M., see Calabresi,P. 283, 284, 314, 319, 323, 324, *329*
Klika,E., see Jelínek,R. 358, *367*
Klimas,J., see Boll,I. 405, *419*
Klimowitz,Z., see Korbecki, M. 354, *367*

Kline, I., Gang, M., Tyrer, D.D., Venditti, J.M., Artis, E.W., Goldin, A. 767, *785*
Kline, I., Tyrer, D.D., Gang, M., Venditti, J.M., Goldin, A. 259, *270*
Kline, I., Venditti, J.M., Mead, J.A.R., Tyrer, D. D., Goldin, A. 198, *227*
Kline, I., Venditti, J.M., Tyrer, D.D., Goldin, A. 235, *253*, 260, 262, *270*
Kline, I., Venditti, J.M., Tyrer, D.D., Mantel, N., Goldin, A. 260, *270*
Kline, I., Woodman, R.J., Gang, M., Venditti, J.M. 79, *81*, 548, *551*
Kline, I., Woodman, R.J., Gang, M., Waravdekar, V.S., Goldin, A., Venditti, J.M. 198, *227*, 545, *551*
Kline, I., see Goldin, A. 301, *334*
Kline, I., see Hoffman, G.S. 263, *269*, 548, *550*
Kline, I., see Saslaw, L.D. 267, *270*
Kline, I., see Sirica, A. 830, *840*
Kline, I., see Tyrer, D.D. 236, *255*, *271*, 523, *537*, 548, *552*
Klinc, I., see Venditti, J.M., 820, *828*
Klinenberg, J.R., see Levy, J. 407, *422*
Klingman, J.D., Handler, P. 493, *507*
Klingsberg, A., see Fried, J. 182, *189*
Klomparens, W., see Ford, J.H. 561, *568*
Klopotowski, T., Wiater, A. 517, *533*
Klopper, A.I., see Strong, J. A. 178, *192*
Klose, U., see Hunstein, W. 409, *421*
Klundt, I.L., see Horwitz, J.P. 662, *666*
Knapton, P.J., see Beard, M.E.J. 726, 727, 728, 730, 734, 735, *743*
Knepshield, J.H., see Gelfand, M.C. 407, *421*
Kniese, G., see Hartmann, G. 583, *591*
Knight, C.A., see McLaren, A.D. 518, *534*
Knight, P., see Murray, J.E. 502, *508*
Knight, P.R., see Chalmers, A.H. 411, 412, *420*
Knight, P.R., see Murray, J.E. 407, *422*
Knight, V., Gerone, P.J., Griffith, W.R., Caudi, R. B., Cate, T.R., Johnson, K.M., Long, D.J., Evans, H.E., Spichard, A., Kasel, J.A. *338*
Knoll, J.E., see Eidinoff, M.L. 490, *504*
Knoll, J.E., see Rich, M.A. 199, *229*
Knolle, P., Kaudewitz, F. 58, *61*
Knox, W.E., see Yip, M.C. M. 490, *511*
Koblet, H., Diggelmann, H. 758, *763*
Kobrin, S., see Ungar, G. 527, *537*
Koch, G. 40, *44*, 855, *873*
Koch, G., Verly, W.G., Bacq, Z.M. 40, *44*
Koch, G., see Moutschen, J. 40, *45*
Kochakian, C.D. 145, *154*
Kociba, R.J., Sleight, S.D. 831, *840*
Kociba, R.J., Sleight, S.D., Rosenberg, B. 830, *840*
Kocsis, J.J., Walaszek, E.J., Geiling, E.M. 694, *691*
Kodama, M. 50, *61*
Kodama, M., Kodama, T. 145, *154*
Kodama, T., see Kodama, M. 145, *154*
Koe, B.K., Weissman, A. 519, *533*
Koechlin, B.A., Rubio, F., Palmer, S., Gabriel, T., Duschinsky, R. 201, 202, *227*
Koenig, H. 219, *227*
Koenig, H., see Held, I. 487, *506*
Koenig, H., see Wells, W. 352, *371*
König, J., see Grafnetterová, J. 357, 358, 359, *366*
König, J., see Šmahel, O. 361, *370*
König, K., see Šmahel, O. 358, *370*
Kofler, M., see Berneis, K. 751, 756, *761*
Kohagura, M., see Tanaka, M. 698, 699, 702, *721*
Kohler, P.O., Grimley, P. M., O'Malley, B.W. 159, *167*
Kohler, P.O., see O'Malley, B.W. 159, 163, 165, *168*
Kohlmeier, V., see Horowitz, J. 212, *226*
Kohn, K.W., Bono, V.H., Jr., Kann, H.E., Jr. 644, 645, *647*
Kohn, K.W., Spears, C.L. 644, 645, 646, *647*
Kohn, K.W., Spears, C.L., Doty, P. 8, *15*, 41, *44*
Kohn, K.W., Steigbigel, N. H., Spears, C.L. *13*, *16*, 53, *61*
Kohn, K.W., see Kann, H. E., Jr., 75, *81*, 573, 574 577, *580*, 644, *647*, *669*
Kohn, K.W., see Snyder, A. L. 574, *581*, 881, *890*
Kohner, F.A., see Yesair, D. W. 682, *694*, 823, 824, *828*
Köhnlein, W., Hutchinson, F. 321, *338*
Kojima, T., see Kanai, T. 233, *252*, 266, *269*
Kojima, Y., Wacker, W.E. C. *717*
Kolář, V., Mechl, Z. 196, *228*
Kolc, J. 518, *533*
Koller, P.C. 21, *32*
Koller, P.C., see Haddow, A. L. 183, *189*
Kolmeier, K.H., Silverstein, M.N., Fleisher, G.A. 777, *785*
Kolosov, M.N., see Berlin, Y.A. 615, *621*
Kolosov, M.N., see Sedov, K.A. 615, 619, *622*
Koloušek, J., see Gershenovich, Z.S. 499, *505*
Koltan, A., see Del Puerto, B.M. 560, *568*
Komai, T., see Sawa, T. 444, *455*
Komai, T., see Tsukada, I. 444, *456*
Komai, T., see Umezawa, H. *875*
Komatsu, Y., Tanaka, K. 375, *381*
Komatsu, Y., see Nishimura, H. 373, 374, 375, *382*
Komeda, T., see Kaziwara, K. 618, 619, 620, *622*
Kon, S.K., see Folley, S.J. 144, *153*
Konda, C., see Sakai, Y. 887, *889*
Konda, T., see Kimura, K. 870, *873*

Kondo, A., see Mitsuya, H. 870, *873*
Kondo, H., see Okami, Y. 497, *508*
Kondo, T., Maruyama, T. 460, *466*
Koneru, P., see Price, C. C. 1, 5, *5*, 19, 26, *33*
Konikov, N., see Ward, H. N. 39, *46*
Kono, M., Osawa, S. 206, *228*
Kono, M., see Iwabuchi, M. 210, *226*
Kono, T. 93, *101*
Kono, T., Barham, F. W. 95, *101*
Konopatzky, R., see Magdon, E. 355, *368*
Konopka, E. A., see Heymann, H. 515, *532*
Koons, C. R., Sensenbrenner, L. L., Owens, A. H., Jr. 621, *622*
Kopper, L., see Szende, B. 518, *537*
Korbecki, M., Luczak, M., Klimowitz, Z. 354, *367*
Korbecki, M., Plagemann, P. G. W. 354, *367*
Korbitz, B. C., see Ansfield, F. J. 221, *223*
Korbitz, B. C., see Ansfield, F. J. 221, *223*
Koren, A., see Gellhorn, A. 822, 823, *827*
Korenchevsky, V., Hall, K. 143, *154*
Korenman, S. G. 117, *132*, *167*
Korenman, S. G., Dukes, B. A. 117, 118, *132*
Korenman, S. G., O'Malley, B. W. 159, 160, 161, *167*
Korenman, S. G., Rao, C. R. 115, *132*
Korenman, S. G., see O'Malley, B. W. 159, 163, 165, *168*
Korfsmeier, K. H. 211, *228*
Koritz, S. B. 140, *154*
Koritz, S. B., see Munck, A. 91, *102*
Korman, S., Tendler, M. D. 642, *647*
Korman, S., see Tendler, M. D. 642, *648*
Korn, D., Weissbach, A. 57, *61*
Kornberg, A., see Atkinson, M. R. 660, *665*
Kornberg, A., see Bessman, J. J. 281, *328*
Kornberg, A., see Falaschi, A. 856, 857, 860, 862, 865, *872*
Kornberg, A., see Lehman, I. R. 274, *339*
Kornberg, A., see Okazaki, T. 277, 285, 286, 320, *341*
Kornberg, A., see Trautner, T. A. 325, *346*
Korth, T., see Boch, M. 650, *655*
Korytnyk, W., Ghosh, A. C., Angelino, N., Dave, D. 778, *785*
Kosaka, H., see Maeda, K. 851, 855, *873*
Koschel, K., see Hartmann, G. 602, 603, *612*
Koshiura, R., LePage, G. A. 427, 429, 430, *433*, 658, *666*
Kosower, E. M., Kosower, N. S. 758, *763*
Kosower, E. M., see Kosower, N. S. 759, *763*
Kosower, E. M., see Tsuji, T. 751, 754, *765*
Kosower, N. S., Vanderhoff, G. A., Benerofe, B., Hunt, T., Kosower, E. M. 759, *763*
Kosower, N. S., see Kosower, E. M. 758, *763*
Koss, G. L. 21, *32*
Koss, L. G. 39, *44*
Koss, L. G., see Feingold, M. L. 39, *43*
Kostantinova, N. V., see Brachnikova, M. G. 593, *611*
Kostyanovskii, R. G., see Serebryanyi, A. M. 73, *83*
Kotani, M., see Seiki, K. 160, *168*
Koteless, G. J., see Hidvegi, E. J. 518, *532*
Kotorii, K., Mori, H., Yoshida, M. 677, *691*
Kountz, W. B., see Allen, E. 108, *125*
Kovalenko, N. A., see Mardashev, S. R. 498, *507*
Kowalczyk, R. S., see Lindenauer, S. M. 523, *533*
Kowollik, G., see Langen, P. 273, *339*, 661, *666*
Koyama, G., Nakamura, H., Muraoka, Y., Takita, T., Maeda, K., Umezawa, H. 852, *873*
Koyama, G., Umezawa, H. 441, *454*
Koyama, G., see Hori, M. 441, 442, *454*
Koyama, G., see Ishizuka, M. 414, *454*
Koyama, G., see Umezawa, H. 444, *456*
Koyama, H., Ono, T. 311, *338*
Koyama, H., see Nakagawa, Y. 373, *382*
Kozai, Y., Sugino, Y. 240, *253*
Kozaka, M., see Matsumoto, I. 54, *61*
Kozinski, A. W., Szybalski, W. 295, *338*
Kozma, C., see Moore, H. L., Jr. 415, *422*
Krakoff, I., see Burchenal, J. H. 389, *398*
Krakoff, I., see Lyman, M. 820, *827*
Krakoff, I. H. 512, *533*, 675, *691*, 793, *806*
Krakoff, I. H., Brown, N. C., Reichard, P. 790, *791*
Krakoff, I. H., Savel, H., Murphy, M. L. 789, *791*
Krakoff, I. H., see Clarkson, B. D. 727, 728, 730, 732, *743*
Krakoff, I. H., see Etcubanas, E. 793, 799, 800, *805*
Krakoff, I. H., see Helson, L. 219, *226*
Krakoff, I. H., see Miller, H. K. 703, *718*
Krakoff, I. H., see Nordenskjold, B. A. 790, *792*
Krakoff, I. H., see Oettgen, H. F. 727, 728, 730, 732, 734, 735, *745*
Krakoff, I. H., see VanDyk, J. J. 197, *231*
Kramer, G., Wittmann, H. G., Schuster, H. 200, *228*
Kramer, M., see Neumann, F. 146, *155*
Kramer, M. F., see DeRooij, D. G. 37, *43*
Kramer, W., see Bermek, E. 375, *381*
Krant, M. J., Iszard, D. M., Abadi, A., Carey, R. W. 523, *533*
Krant, M. J., see Cohen, J. L. 221, *224*
Krant, M. J., see Hall, T. C. 459, *465*
Kratochvíl, J., see Grozdanovič, J. 355, *366*

Krauth, C. A., see Shealy, Y. F. 545, 547, 548, 549, 550, *552*
Krč, J., see Astaldi, C. 526, *529*
Krč, J., see Astaldi, G. 706, *713*, 735, *742*
Krč, J., see Burgio, G. R. 706, 707, *714*, 735, *743*
Kream, J., see Gellhorn, A. 459, 460, *465*
Kream, J., see Hirschberg, E. 460, *465*, *466*
Kredich, N. M., Guarino, A. J. 658, 661, *666*
Kredich, N. M., see Guarino, A. J. 661, *666*
Kredich, N. M., see Jagger, D. V. 660, *666*
Kreis, W. 758, *763*
Kreis, W., Burchenal, J. H., Hutchison, D. J. 758, *763*
Kreis, W., Drahovsky, D., Borberg, H. 247, 249, *253*
Kreis, W., Ellison, R. R., Lyman, M. S., Burchenal, J. H., Block, R., Warkentin, D. L. 822, 824, *827*
Kreis, W., Piepho, S. B., Bernhard, H. V. 758, *763*
Kreis, W., Yen, W. 758, *763*
Kreis, W., see Burchenal, J. H. 820, *826*
Kreis, W., see Chaube, S. 237, 244, *250*, 261, *268*
Kreis, W., see Dollinger, M. R. 233, 234, 239, *251*
Kreis, W., see Drahovsky, D. 247, *251*, 265, *268*
Kreis, W., see Uchida, K. 240, 247, *255*, 265, *271*
Krejczy, K., see Gonzalez, E. M. 410, *421*
Krekulova, A., see Drobnik, J. 835
Kremer, V. E., see Goldberg, L. E. 619, 620, *622*
Kremer, W. B., Laszlo, J. 635, 639, 640, *640*
Kremer, W. B., see Huang, A. T. 757, *762*
Krenitsky, T. A. 387, *400*
Krenitsky, T. A., Barclay, M., Jacquez, J. A. 289, *338*
Krenitsky, T. A., Mellors, J. W., Barclay, R. K. 289, *338*
Křepinský, J., see Gichner, T. 78, *80*
Kretovich, W. L. 697, *717*
Kreybig, T. v. 78, *81*
Krichevskaya, A. A., see Gershenovich, Z. S. 499, *505*
Krieg, D. R. 11, *16*
Krigas, T., see Rosenberg, B. 829, 836, *840*
Krim, M., see Borenfreund, E. 790, *791*
Krisch, R. E. 314, *338*
Krishan, A. 678, *691*
Krishan, A., Hsu, D. 673, 679, *691*
Krishnan, P. S., Sitaramayya, A., Kumar, K. S. 460, *466*
Kriss, J. P., Bond, S. B. 289, *338*
Kriss, J. P., Maruyama, Y., Tung, L. A., Bond, S. B., Revesz, L. 282, *338*
Kriss, J. P., Revesz, L. 282, 283, 289, 291, *338*
Kriss, J. P., Tung, L., Bond, S. 283, 289, *338*
Kristiansen, T., Einarsson, M., Sundberg, L., Porath, J. *717*
Kroeger, H., see Birnie, G. D. 203, 215, *223*, 315, 318, *328*
Krooth, R. S., see Pinsky, L. 352, *368*
Kršiak, M., see Janků, I. 349, 359, *367*
Krüger, F. W., Ballweg, H., Maier-Borst, W. 70, *81*
Krüger, F. W., Osswald, H., Walker, G., Schelten, E. 70, 71, *81*
Krüger, F. W., Preussmann, R., Niepelt, N. 547, *551*
Krueger, G. R. F., Heine, U. I. 417, *422*
Krueger, G. R. F., Malmgren, R. A., Berard, C. W. 417, *422*
Krueger, R. C., Gitlin, D., Commerford, S. L., Stein, J., Hughes, W. L. 283, 314, 315, *338*
Krueger, R. C., see Hughes, W. L. 280, 281, 283, 284, 314, 315, 316, *336*
Krueger, R. F., see Hoffman, P. F. 884, *889*
Krueger, R. F., see Mayer, G. D. 884, *889*
Kruglyakova, K. E., see Serebryanyi, A. M. 70, 73, *83*
Krumbhaar, E. B., Krumbhaar, H. D. 18, *32*
Krumbhaar, H. D., see Krumbhaar, E. B. 18, *32*
Kruse, P. F., Jr. 516
Kruse, P. F., Jr., McCoy, T. A. 515, *533*
Kruse, P. F., Jr., Miedema, E., Carter, H. A. 525, *533*
Kruse, P. F., Jr., White, P. B., Carter, H., McCoy, T. A. 513, 515, *533*
Kruse, P. F., Jr., Whittle, W., Nash, J. 524
Kruse, P. F., Jr., see McCoy, C. T. A. 514, *534*, 695, *718*
Kruse, P. F., Jr., see Miedema, E. 516, *534*
Kruse, P. F., Jr., see Sartorelli, A. C. *509*, 516, 519, *536*
Kruse, P. F., Jr., see White, P. B. 516, 529, *538*
Krygier, V., Momparler, R. L. 427, *433*
Krzeminski, Z. 697, *717*
Krzemiński, Z., see Mikucki, J. 697, *718*
Kuang, D. T., Whittington, R. M., Spencer, H. H., Patno, M. E. 638, 639, *640*
Kubelkov, A., see Drobnik, J. 835
Kubíčková, V., see Rašková, H. 361, *369*
Kubíková, M., see Slavík, M. *370*
Kubinski, H., see Szybalski, W. 325, *345*
Kubo, I., see Kende, A. S. 650, *655*
Kucera, L. S., Herrmann, E. C. 302, 306, *338*
Kudo, S., see Wakaki, S. 47, *64*
Kudo, T., see Kanno, T. 855, 871, *873*
Kudynowski, J., see Caspersson, T. 6, *15*
Kühl, J. F. W., see Haus, E. 249, *252*
Kuentzel, S. L., see Hanka, L. J. 234, *252*
Kuenzig, W., see Bates, H. M. 644, 645, 646, *647*
Kuga, G., see Nakamura, S. 870, *873*
Kugelman, B. H., see Smith, H. H. 380, *382*, 314, *344*
Kugelman, M., see Rao, K. V. 486, 496, *509*
Kukhar, E. E., see Galegov, G. A. 354, *366*

Kukushkina, G. V., see Gorbacheva, L. B. 74, *80*
Kull, F. J., see Kenney, F. T. 88, *101*
Kumagai, K., see Ishida, N. 444, *454*
Kumaoka, S., see Sakauchi, N. 814, *818*
Kumar, A., see Wu, R. S. 574, *581*, 651, *656*
Kumar, K. S., see Krishnan, P. S. 460, *466*
Kumar, S., see Tessman, I. 11, *17*, 296, 297, *345*
Kummer, D., Ochs, H. D. 28, *32*
Kummer, D., see Weitzel, G. L., 756, *765*
Kundig, F. D., see Kundig, W. 93, *101*
Kundig, F. D., see Simoni, R. D. 93, *103*
Kundig, W., Kundig, F. D., Anderson, B., Roseman, S. 93, *101*
Kundig, W., see Simoni, R. D. 93, *103*
Kung, F., Nyhan, W. L., Rosner, F., Cortner, J. A., Cuttner, J., Moon, J. H., Holland, J. F. 521, *533*
Kunimoto, T., Hori, M., Umezawa, H. 859, 860, *873*
Kunimoto, T., Wakashiro, T., Okamura, I., Asajima, T., Hori, M. 444, *454*
Kunimoto, T., see Tsukada, I. 444, *456*
Kunrat, I. A. 620, *622*
Kuntzman, R., see Conney, A. H. 813, *817*
Kuperminc, M., see Wampler, G. L. 885, *890*
Kupfer, D., Peets, L. 813, *818*
Kupiecki, F., see Petering, H. G. 843, *849*
Kupiecki, F. P., see Smith, C. G. 222, *230*, 683, *693*
Kuramitsu, H. K., Moyed, H. S. 448, 449, *454*
Kuretani, K., see Hoshi, A. 234, *252*, 266, 267, *269*, 887, *889*
Kurihara, H., see Shimazaki, J. 149, *156*
Kurita, K., see Oka, S. 870, *874*
Kurokawa, Y., see Yamagata, S. 870, *876*
Kurrle, G. R. 35, *44*
Kurtz, H. M., see Kwak, K. S. 695, *717*
Kurtz, S. M., Fisken, R. A., Kaump, D. H., Schardein, J. L. 428, *433*
Kusaka, T., Yamamoto, H., Shibata, M., Muroi, M., Kishi, T., Mizumo, K. 434, *454*
Kusama, M., see Sakauchi, N. 814, *818*
Kušmierek, J. T., see Darżynkiewicz, E. 233, *251*
Kušmierek, J. T., see Giziewicz, J. 233, *252*
Kůta, A., see Rašková, H. 361, *369*
Kůta, A., see Záruba, F. 361, *372*
Kutinova, L., see Vonka, V. 838, *840*
Kuto, J., see Suzuki, M. 870, *875*
Kuttner, R. E., see Lorincz, A. B. 529, *533*
Kvam, D. C., Parks, R. E., Jr. 463, *466*
Kvam, D. C., see Roy, J. K. 463, *467*
Kwak, K. S., Jameson, E., Ryan, R. M., Kurtz, H. M. 695, *717*
Kwan, S. W., Webb, T. E. 463, 464, *466*
Kyalwazi, S. K., see Vogel, C. L. 478, *482*
Kyle, R., see Ellison, R. R. 260, *268*
Kyle, R. A., Schwartz, R. S., Dameshek, W. 39, *44*
Kyser, K. A. 117, *132*
Kyser, K. A., see Jensen, E. V. 85, 95, *101*, 117, *131*

Labitan, A., see Momparler, R. L. 234, 238, *253*
Laboureur, P. 695, *717*
Laboureur, P., Langlois, C., Labrousse, M., Boudon, M., Emeraud, J., Samain, J. F. 699, 700, *717*
Labow, R., Maley, G. F., Maley, F. 469, *481*
Labra, C., see Wilson, W. L. 638, *641*
Labrousse, M., see Laboureur, P. 699, 700, *717*
Lacassagne, A. 170, 173, *190*
Lackner, A., see Hampel, K. E. 415, *421*
Lacon, C., see Chaube, S. 790, *791*
Lacon, C. R., see Dagg, C. P. *550*
Lacon, C. R., see Karnofsky, D. A. 236, *252*, 261, *270*
Lacour, L. F., see Chayen, J. 824, *826*
Laetsch, W. M., see Rice, H. V. 676, *692*
La Forge, F. B., see Levene, P. A. 376, *382*
Lagerborg, D. L., see Visser, D. W. 377, 380, *382*
Lahiri, S. R., Boileau, G., Hall, T. C. 220, *228*
Laird, C. D., Bodmer, W. F. 280, *338*
Lajolo, D., Astaldi, A., Jr., Pecco, P., Bert, G., Astaldi, G. *718*
Lajtha, L., see Fox, M. 316, *333*
Lakshmikantham, M. V., see Gellert, E. 564, *568*
Laland, S. G., see Øyen, T. B. 196, *229*
Lallier, R. 515, *533*
Lamar, C., Jr. *507*
Lamar, C., Jr., Sellinger, O. Z. 499, *507*
Lambert, A., see Nagatsu, M. 859, *873*
Lamerz, R., see Fateh-Moghadam, A. 734, 735, *744*
Lampen, J. O., see El-Nakeeb, M. A. 681, *689*
Lampen, J. O., see Roblin, R. O., Jr. 458, *467*
Lampert, F., Nyhan, W. L. 521, *533*
Lampert, P. W., see Schochet, S. S. 677, *693*
Lancaster, J. E., see Morton, G. O. 434, *455*
Lancaster, J. E., see Webb, J. S. 47, *64*
Lancaster, S. P., see Burchenal, J. H. 822, *826*
Lancini, G., see Yang, S. S. 883, *890*
Landau, R. L., Ehrlich, E. N., Huggins, C. 185, *190*
Landau, R. L., Lugibihl, K. 159, *167*
Landin, L. M., see Mashburn, L. T. 699, 700, 701, 704, 710, *718*, 724, 730, *745*
Landolt, A. M. 319, *338*
Lane, D. M., see Sutow, W. W. 726, 727, 732, *746*

Lane, M., Moore, J. E., III., Levin, H., Smith, F. E. 477, *481*
Lane, M., see Frei, E., III. 260, 262, *269*
Lane, W. T., see Huebner, R. J. 308, *336*
Lang, E., see Hilf, R. 110, *130*
Lang, N., Sekeris, C. E. 88, *101*
Lang, S. 695, *718*
Langan, T. A., Jr., see Narrod, S. A. 491, *508*
Lange, H. W., see Hempel, K. 518, *532*
Langemann, A., see Berneis, K. 756, *761*
Langemann, A., see Zeller, P. 747, *765*
Langen, P., Etzold, G. 289, 290, *338*
Langen, P., Etzold, G., Barwolff, D., Preussel, B. 289, *339*
Langen, P., Etzold, G., Hintsche, R., Kowollik, G. 273, *339*, 661, *666*
Langen, P., Kowollik, G. 273, *339*
Langen, P., Kowollik, G., Schutt, M., Etzold, G. 273, *339*
Langen, P., Liss, E. 298, *339*
Langen, P., Venker, P. 290, *339*
Langen, P., see Etzold, G. 289, 290, *332*
Langen, P., see Preussel, B. 289, *342*
Langenbach, R. J., see Fridland, A. 204, *225*
Langlois, A. J., see Heine, U. 583, *591*
Langlois, A. J., see Riman, J. 440, *455*
Langlois, A. J., see Sverak, L. 574, *581*
Langlois, C., see Laboureur, P. 699, 700, *717*
Langmuir, M. E., see Danziger, R. M. 319, *330*
Langston, W. C., Robinson, B. L. 108, *132*
Lanonan, G., see Baggett, B. 106, *125*
Lanzani, P., see Mascitelli-Coriandoli, E. 683, *692*
Lapárová, V., see Trnavský, K. 359, *371*
Lapis, K. 36, *44*
Lapis, K., see Szende, B. 518, *537*
Laplaca, S. J., see Hamilton, W. C. 773, *785*
Laqueur, G. L., Fluhmann, C. F. 143, *154*
Lardy, H. A., see Ray, P. D. 521, *535*
Larionov, L. F. 19, *32*
Larionov, L. F., Spasskaya, I. G. 518, *533*
Larionov, L. F., see Spasskaya, I. G. 518, *536*
LaRock, J., see German, J. 57, *60*
Larrieu, M. J., see Jacquillat, C. 726, 727, 728, 732, 734, 735, *744*
Larsen, C. D., see Hertz, R. 121, *130*
Larsen, P. O., see Kjaer, A. 498, *506*
Larsen, S. H., see Williams, R. H. 446, *457*
Larson, D. L., see Katzman, P. A. 160, *167*
Larson, J. A. L. 175, *190*
Larson, J. E., see Wells, R. D. 585, 586, 589, *592*, 626, *632*
Larson, P. S., see Finnegan, J. K. 809, *817*
Larson, S., see Arseneau, J. 879, *887*
Larson, V. M., see Coggin, J. H. 298, 308, *330*
Larsson, A., Reichard, P. 243, *253*
La Sala, E., see Van Dyk, J. J. 197, *231*
Lasfargues, E. Y., see Lyons, M. J. 306, *340*
Lash, E., Schwartz, M. K., Tallal, L., Oettgen, H. F. 735, *745*
Lash, E. D., see Schwartz, M. K. 704, *721*, 724, 725, 735, *746*
Lasher, R., Cahn, R. D. 311, *339*
Laskowski, M. 120, *132*
Laskowski, M., see Sulkowski, E. 583, *592*
Lasnitzki, I. 176, *190*
Lasnitzki, I., Mathews, R. E. F., Smith, J. D. 463, *466*
Lasnitzki, I., see Baulieu, E. E. 161, *167*
Lasnitzki, I., see Robel, P. 160, *168*
Lassman, L. P., see Bradley, W. G. 686, *688*
Laster, W. R., Jr., Mayo, J. G., Simpson-Herren, L., Griswold, D. P., Jr., Lloyd, H. H., Schabel, F. M., Jr., Skipper, H. E. 389, *400*
Laster, W. R., Jr., see Brockman, R. W. 793, 800, *805*, 877, 878, *888*
Laster, W. R., Jr., see Griswold, D. P., Jr. 767, *785*
Laster, W. R., Jr., see Johnston, T. P. 65, 68, *81*
Laster, W. R., Jr., see Pittillo, A. F. 820, *827*
Laster, W. R., Jr., see Schabel, F. M., Jr. 65, 68, 69, 79, *83*, 391, 393, *402*, 878, *889*
Laster, W. R., Jr., see Schmidt, L. H. 264, *271*
Laster, W. R., Jr., see Shealy, Y. F. 544, 549, 550, *552*
Laszlo, J., see Elion, G. B. 389, *399*, 411, *420*
Laszlo, J., see Hochstein, P. 635, *640*
Laszlo, J., see Kremer, W. B. 635, 639, 640, *640*
Laszlo, J., see Miller, D. S. 634, 635, 636, 637, *641*
Laszlo, J., see Rundles, R. W. 408, 412, *423*
Latour, J. P. A., see Blondal, H. 524, *530*
Lauenstein, K., Grundmann, E., Hobik, H. P., Madaus, W. P. 705, *718*
Laufer, A., see Southren, A. L. 811, *819*
Laughlin, M. W., see Blohm, T. R. 105, *126*
Lauinger, C., Ressler, C. 701, *718*
Laumas, K. R., Faroog, A. 160, *167*
Laumas, K. R., see Pearlman, W. H. 117, *134*
Lauro, V., Santilli Giornelli, F. E., Dominici, C., Fanelli, A., Cucchia, G. 415, *422*
La Via, M. F., Uriu, S. A., Barber, N. D., Warren, A. E. 513, 526, *533*
Law, L. W. 387, *400*, 820, *827*
Law, L. W., see Anderson, E. P. 458, *464*
Law, L. W., see Schacter, B. 460, *467*
Lawley, P. D. 6, 7, *16*, 71, *81*

Lawley, P.D., Brookes, P. 7, 8, 13, *16*, 25, 27, *32*, 49, 50, *61*, 278, *339*
Lawley, P.D., Brookes, P., Magee, P.N., Craddock, V.M., Swann, P.F. 71, *81*
Lawley, P.D., Lethbridge, J.H., Edwards, P.A., Shooter, K.V. 10, *16*
Lawley, P.D., Orr, D.J., Shah, S.A. 7, *16*
Lawley, P.D., Thatcher, C. J. 7, *16*, 66, 70, 71, 72, *81*
Lawley, P.D., Wallick, C.A. 26, *32*
Lawley, P.D., see Brookes, P. 7, *15*, 22, 26, 27, *31*, 41, *42*
Lawson, W., see Dodds, E. C. 105, 113, *128*
Leach, F.R., see Gimlin, D. L. 308, *334*
Leach, F.R., see Gimlin, D. L. 308, *334*
Leake, E., Smith, W.G., Woodliff, H.J. 39, *44*
Leary, R., Kisliuk, R.L. 469, *481*
Leary, R., see Crusberg, T.C. *480*
Leary, W.V., see Frei, E., III. 260, 262, *269*
Leary, W.V., see Samuels, M.L. 759, *764*
LeBeau, M.C., see Baulieu, E.E. 115, *126*
Leblond, C.P., Clermont, Y. 37, *44*
Leblond, C.P., see Axelrad, A.A. 171, *188*
Lebowitz, M.M., see Freed, J.J. 676, *690*
Lechevalier, H.A., see Gerber, N.N. 658, 660, *665*
Lechevalier, H.A., see Pugh, L.H. 660, *667*
Lechner, K., see Deutsch, E. 709, *715*, 734, 735, *744*
Ledbetter, M.C., Porter, K. R. 676, *691*
Leder, P., see Nirenberg, M. 352, *368*
Ledinko, N. 302, 304, 306, *339*
Lednicer, D., see Duncan, G. W. 110, *128*
Lee, A.K.Y., Mackay, I.R., Rowley, M.J., Jap, C.Y. 416, *422*
Lee, B.K., see Wilkie, D. 561, *570*
Lee, C., Jacobson, H.I. 117, *132*
Lee, C., Keyes, P.L., Jacobson, H.I. *132*
Lee, H. 643, *647*
Lee, H.M., see Board, J.A. 415, *419*
Lee, I.P., see Dixon, R.L. 753, *762*
Lee, I.P., see Woods, J.S. 708, *722*
Lee, K.-H., Yuzuriha, Y. 495, *507*
Lee, K.L., see Wittliff, J.L. 121, *138*
Lee, K.Y., Lijinsky, W., Magee, P.N. 71, *81*
Lee, M., see Weston, J.K. 38, *46*
Lee, M.B., see Nelson, S.D. 705, 707, *719*
Lee, S., see Reel, J.R. 158, *168*
Lee, S.L., see Callentine, M. R. 110, *127*
Lee, S.Y., Mendecki, J., Brawerman, G. 574, 575, *580*
Lee, S.Y., see Mendecki, J. *580*, *669*
Lee, W.H., see Regan, J.D. 525, *535*
Lee, W.L., see Tong, G.L. 350, *371*
Lee, W.W., Benitez, A., Anderson, C.D., Goodman, L., Baker, B.R. 658, *666*
Lee, W.W., Benitez, A., Goodman, L., Baker, B. R. 427, *433*
Lee, W.W., Martinez, A.P., Blackford, R.W., Bartuska, V.J., Reist, E.J., Goodman, L. 429, 430, 431, *433*
Lee, W.W., Martinez, A.P., Tong, G.L., Goodman, L. 430, *433*
Lee, W.W., see Reist, E.J. 426, 427, *433*
Leeper, R.D., see Oettgen, H.F. 696, *719*, 723, 727, 730, 733, 734, 735, *745*
Lees, E.M., Blakeney, A.B. 697, *718*
Leese, C.L., see Connors, T. A, 20, 28, *31*
LeFèvre, R.J.W., Liddicoet, T.H. 545, *551*
Lefkowitz, E., see Bertino, J.R. 473, *479*
Lefkowitz, E.R., Creasey, W.A., Calabresi, P., Sartorelli, A.C. 389, *400*, 500, *507*
LeGal, M.-L., LeGal, Y., Roche, J., Hedegaard, J. 489, *507*
LeGal, Y., see LeGal, M.-L. 489, *507*
Leh, F., see Chan, S.C. 68, *80*
Lehman, I.R., Bessman, M. J., Simms, E.S., Kornberg, A. 274, *339*
Lehman, I.R., see Bessman, J.J. 281, *328*
Lehner-Netsch, G., see Delage, J.M. 735, 738, *744*
Leibman, K.C., see Heidelberger, C. *226*
Leibowitz, H.M., Elliott, J. H. 410, *422*
Leibowitz, S., see Hirsch, M. S. 418, *421*
Leichter, D., see Weisenfeld, S. 814, *819*
Leimgruber, W., Batcho, A. D., Czajkowski, R.C. 642, *648*
Leimgruber, W., Batcho, A. D., Schenker, F. 642, *648*
Leimgruber, W., Stefanović, V., Schenker, F., Karr, A., Berger, J. 642, *648*
Lein, J., Heinemann, B., Gourevitch, A. 57, *61*, 862, 869, *873*
Lein, J., see Price, K.E. 855, 862, *874*
Leininger, K.R., see Liao, S. 148, *155*
Leiter, J., see Kelly, M.G. 684, *691*
Leiter, J., see Schepartz, S. A. 820, *828*
Leitin, V.L., see Podobed, O.V. *669*
Lelieveld, P., see VanPutten, L.M. 21, *34*
Lemahiew, M.A., see Nicolette, J.A. 119, *134*
Lemmel, E.M., Good, R.A. 59, *61*
Lemon, H.E., Wotiz, H.H., Parsons, L., Mozden, P. 178, *190*
Lemon, H.M. 117, *132*
Lemon, H.M., see Wotiz, H. H. 106, *138*
Lenaz, L., Sternberg, S.S., Philips, F.S. 233, 241, *253*
Lenaz, L., see DiFronzo, G. 608, 609, *612*
Lenaz, L., see DiMarco, A. 597, *612*
Lenfeld, J., see Jorda, V.V. *569*

Lengyel, P., Speyer, J.F., Ochoa, S. 214, *228*
Lengyel, P., see Wahba, A. J. 214, *231*
Lenny, A.B., see Speyer, J. F. 282, *345*
Leonard, B.J., see Carter, S. B. 446, 450, 451, *453*
Leonard, L.L., ter Meulen, V., Freeman, J.M. 354, *367*
Leonard, N.J., Hecht, S.M., Skoog, F., Schmitz, R.Y. 435, *454*
Leonard, N.J., see Crist, D. R. 3, *5*
Leonard, R.A., see Bellamy, D. 96, *100*
Leonard, R.J., see Bloch, A. 436, 437, 438, 439, 444, 445, *453*
Leonard, S.L. 144, *154*
Leone, L.A., Albala, M.M., Rege, V.B. 477, *481*
Leone, L.A., see Burchenal, J.H. 384, 389, *398*
Leone, L.A., see Ellison, R. R. 260, *268*
Leontieva, N.A., Fadeeva, L.L. 306, *339*
Leopold, G., Schnieders, B., Kersten, H., Kersten, W. 54, *61*
Leopold, G., see Kersten, H. 54, *61*
LePage, G.A. 386, 388, 392, 394, 395, *400*, 427, 428, 429, 431, *433*, 435, *454*
LePage, G.A., Bell, J.P., Wilson, M.J. 429, *433*
LePage, G.A., Greenlees, J. L. 390, *400*
LePage, G.A., Jones, M. 390, 391, 395, *400*, 487, *507*
LePage, G.A., Junga, I.G. 395, 396, *400*, 448, *454*, 658, *666*
LePage, G.A., Junga, I.G., Bowman, B. 388, 396, *400*
LePage, G.A., Sato, J. 427
LePage, G.A., White, S.C. 264, *270*
LePage, G.A., Whitecar, J. P., Jr. 388, 397, *401*
LePage, G.A., see Brink, J. J. 427, 428, 429, *432*
LePage, G.A., see Ellis, D. B. 387, *399*, 430, *432*, 659, *665*
LePage, G.A., see Fernandes, J.F. 390, *399*
LePage, G.A., see Greenlees, J. 390, 391, *399*, 487, *505*
LePage, G.A., see Hersh, E. M. 430, *432*
LePage, G.A., see Kaneko, T. 431, *432*
LePage, G.A., see Kimball, A.P. 234, 241, *253*, 429, 430, *432*
LePage, G.A., see Koshiura, R. 427, 429, 430, *433*, 658, *666*
LePage, G.A., see Loo, T.L. 429, *433*
LePage, G.A., see Milton, J.D. 431
LePage, G.A., see Moore, E. C. 388, 389, 394, 395, *401*, 487, 488, *507*
LePage, G.A., see Peery, A. 388, *401*
LePage, G.A., see Pierre, K. J. 387, 388, *402*, 445, *455*
LePage, G.A., see Sartorelli, A.C. 389, 393, 394, 395, 397, *402*, 487, 500, *509*
LePage, G.A., see Sato, K. 430, *433*
LePage, G.A., see Schroeder, J.M. 394, 397, *402*, 500, *510*
LePage, G.A., see York, J. L. 427, *433*
LePera, V., see Nervi, C. 478, *482*
Lepeshkina, G.N., see Chorin, V.A. 617, *621*
Lerman, M.I. 599
Lerman, M.I., Benyumovich, M.S. 56, *61*
Lerman, M.I., see Georgiev, G.P. 584, *590*
Lerman, M.I., see Podobed, O.V. *669*
Lerner, L.J. 109, 123, *132*, 146, *154*
Lerner, L.J., Bianchi, A., Borman, A. 146, *154*, 189, *190*
Lerner, L.J., Bianchi, A., Dzelzkalns, M., Borman, A. 146, *155*
Lerner, L.J., Harris, D.N., Hilf, R., Bianchi, A., Raskin, B.K. 123, *132*
Lerner, L.J., Hilf, R. 182, 183, *190*
Lerner, L.J., Hilf, R., Harris, D.N. 147, 152, *155*
Lerner, L.J., Hilf, R., Türkheimer, A.R., Michel, I. 122, *132*
Lerner, L.J., Hilf, R., Türkheimer, A.R., Michel, I., Engel, S.L. 123, *132*, 147, *155*
Lerner, L.J., Holthaus, F. J., Jr., Thompson, C.R. 110, *132*
Lerner, L.J., Türkheimer, A.R. 110, *132*
Lerner, L.J., see Harris, D. N. 123, *130*
Lerner, L.J., see Hilf, R. 110, 123, *130*, 145, 152, *154*
Lerner, L.J., see Holtkamp, D.E. 105, *130*
Lescure, O.L., see Migeon, C.J. 107, *133*
Lesher, S., see Sigdestad, C. P. 642, 644, *648*
Lesley, J.F., see Bogart, R. 113, *126*
Lester, W. 883, *889*
Lethbridge, J.H., see Lawley, P.D. 10, *16*
Lett, J.T., Caldwell, I., Little, J.G. 319, *339*
Leung, F.C., Vas, S.I. 406, *422*
Leuthy, H., see Berneis, K. 756, *761*
Levan, A., see Hsu, T.C. 300, *336*
Levan, A., see Kihlman, B. A. 236, *253*, 261, *270*
Levenberg, B., Melnick, I., Buchanan, J.M. 486, 487, 488, 490, 496, 497, *507*
Levenberg, B., see Hartman, S.C. 486, 487, *505*
Levene, P.A., LaForge, F.B. 376, *382*
Levene, P.A., Tipson, S. 273, *339*
Levenstein, I., see Vollmer, E.P. 145, *157*
Leventhal, B.G., Henderson, E.S. 726, 732, 734, 735, *745*
Leventhal, B.G., Skeel, R. T., Yankee, R.A., Henderson, E.S. 501, *507*, 726, 732, 734, 735, *745*
Leventhal, B.G., see Carbone, P.P. 726, 727, 728, 730, 732, 734, 735, *743*
Leventhal, B.G., see Haskell, C.M. 734, 735, *744*
Levey, H.A., Szego, C.M. 151, *155*
Levey, R.H., see Floersheim, G.L. 752, *762*

Levi, I., Blondal, H., Lozinski, E. 524, *533*
Levi, I., see Blondal, H. 524, *530*
Levin, A. P., Hartman, P. E. 517, *533*
Levin, D. H. 462, 463, 464, *466*
Levin, H., see Lane, M. 477, *481*
Levin, L. 109, *132*
Levin, R. H., Brittin, G. M., Freireich, E. J. 772, *786*
Levin, R. H., Henderson, E., Karon, E., Freireich, E. J. 769, 772, 773, *786*
Levin, R. J. 528, *533*
Levin, V. A., Shapiro, W. R., Clancy, T. P., Oliverio, V. T. 69, *81*
Levin, W. C., see Monto, R. W. 621, *622*
Levine, B., see Weisberger, A. S. 522, *537*
Levine, C., Chargaff, E. 824, *827*
Levine, M. 57, *61*
Levine, M., Borthwick, M. 634, *640*
Levine, M., Tarver, H. 521, *533*
Levine, P., see Boissier, J. R. 430, *432*
Levine, P., see Smith, R. G. 883, *889*
Levine, R., see Hall, T. C. 238, *252*, 265, *269*
Levine, R. J., see Gillespie, E. 683, *690*
Levine, S. G., see Kepler, J. A. 649, *655*
Levine, S. G., see Wani, M. C. 649, 650, *656*
Levins, P., see Yesair, D. W. 822, 823, *828*
Levins, P. L., Papanastassiou, Z. B. 68, *81*
Levinson, W. E., Bishop, J. M., Quintrell, N., Jackson, J., Fanshier, L. 307, *339*
Levinson, W. E., see McDonnell, J. P. 583, *591*, *613*
Levinthal, M., see Simoni, R. D. 93, *103*
Levintow, L., Thoren, M. M., Darnell, J. E., Jr., Hooper, J. L. 519, *533*
Levintow, L. 485, *507*, 711, *718*
Levis, A. G., Danieli, G. A., Piccinni, E. 22, *32*
Levis, A. G., Spanio, L., DeNadai, A. 25, *32*
Levison, S. A., see Huennekens, F. M. 469, *481*
Levitan, I. B., Webb, T. E. 363, *367*
Levitt, M., Marsh, J. C., DeConti, R. C., Mitchell, M. S., Skeel, R. T., Farber, L. R., Bertino, J. R. 478, *481*
Levy, C. C., see Russell, D. H. 774, *787*
Levy, H. B., see Adamson, R. H. 884, *887*
Levy, H. B., see Baron, S. 607, *611*
Levy, H. M., Montanez, G., Murphey, E. A., Dunn, M. S. 521, *533*
Levy, J., Barnett, E. V., MacDonald, N. S., Klinenberg, J. R., Pearson, C. M. 407, *422*
Levy, M., see Eagle, H. 484, *504*
Levy, R. N., see Ohnuma, T. 726, 727, 728, 734, 735, *746*
Lewis, A. E., see French, F. A. 798, *806*
Lewis, C. W., see Ahearn, M. J. 236, *249*
Lewis, D., see Fowden, L. 512, 519, 521, 529, *531*
Lewis, F. S., see Chun, E. H. L. 14, *15*, 28, *31*
Lewis, J., Jr., see Hertz, R. 475, 476, *481*
Lewis, L. R., see Baiocchi, F. 768, *783*
Lewis, M. G., see Alexander, P. 728, *742*
Lewis, R. G., see Wenkert, E. 649, *656*
Ley, K. D., Tobey, R. A. 528, *533*
Ley, K. D., see Tobey, R. A. 528, *537*
Li, C. H., see Lyons, W. R. 111, *132*
Li, C. P., see Jahnes, W. G. *717*
Li, L. H., Fraser, T. J., Olin, E. J., Bhuyan, B. K. 653, *656*
Li, L. H., Olin, E. J., Buskirk, H. H., Reineke, L. M. 362, *367*
Li, L. H., Olin, E. J., Fraser, T. J., Bhuyan, B. K. 362, *367*
Li, L. H., see Bhuyan, B. K. 881, *888*
Li, M. C., Nixon, N. E., Freeman, M. V. 472, *482*
Li, M. C., see Karnofsky, D. A. 500, 502, *506*
Li, M. C., see Pearson, O. H. 183, 184, *191*
Liang, H., see Verbin, R. S. 235, 236, *255*
Liao, S. 147, 148, *155*
Liao, S., Fang, S. 148, *155*, 177, 187, *190*
Liao, S., Leininger, K. R., Sagher, D., Barton, R. W. 148, *155*
Liao, S., Williams-Ashman, H. G. 147, *155*
Liao, S., see Anderson, K. M. 149, *153*, 177, *188*
Liao, S., see Fang, S. 149, 150, *153*, 164, *167*, 177, *189*
Liao, S., see Williams-Ashman, H. G. 118, *138*, 147, *157*
Liao, T. K., Baiocchi, F., Cheng, C. C. 768, *786*
Liao, T. K., Nyberg, W. H., Cheng, C. C. 650, *656*
Liao, T. K., see Baiocchi, F. 768, *783*
Liberman, S., see Dobriner, K. 177, *188*
Libman, L., see Neal, A. L. *508*
Lichtenstein, J., see Cohen, S. S. 199, 203, 204, *224*, 289, *330*
Lichtenstein, N., see DeGroot, N. 515, *531*, 697, *715*
Lichtenstein, N., see Mor, G. 520, *534*
Lichtenstein, N., see Schlesinger, M. 514, 520, *536*
Liddicoet, T. H., see LeFèvre, R. J. W. 545, *551*
Liddle, G. W., see Bledsoe, T. 813, *817*
Liddle, G. W., see Temple, T. E. 811, 814, *819*
Liebecq, C., Peters, R. A. 193, *228*
Líeberman, I., see Adams, R. L. P. 857, *871*
Liegler, D. G., Henderson, E. S., Hahn, M. A., Oliverio, V. T. 473, *482*
Light, A. E. 39, *45*
Lijinsky, W., Loo, J., Ross, A. E. 71, *82*
Lijinsky, W., see Lee, K. Y. 71, *81*
Lilley, R. McC., see Tay, B. S. 390, 391, *403*
Lillicarp, S. C., see Fielden, E. M. 321, *332*

Lillie,M.G., Mohanty,S.B. 302, *339*
Lin,A.J., Agrawal,K.C., Sartorelli,A.C. 798, *806*
Lin,S.C., see Peters,J.H. 697, *720*
Lin,S.Y., Riggs,A.D. 326, *339*
Lin,T.M., see MacMahon, B. 178, *190*
Lin,Y.T., Loo,T.L., Vadlamudi,S., Goldin,A. 549, 550, *551*
Lindberg,B. 442, *454*, 658, 659, *666*
Lindberg,B., Klenow,H., Hansen,K. 448, *454* 658, 659, 661, 662, *666*
Lindenauer,S.M., Dow,R. W., Kowalczyk,R.S. 523, *533*
Linder,O., see Diderholm, H. 307, 314, *331*
Linder,R.C., Kirkpatrick, H.C., Weeks,T.E. 561, *569*
Lindner,A. 204, *228*
Lindner,A., see Fernandes, J.F. 390, *399*
Lindqvist,B., Sinsheimer, R.L. 58, *61*
Linevich,Yu.G., see Pravdina,N.F. 354, *368*
Lineweaver,H., Burk,D. 115, *132*
Linford,J.H. 28, *32*
Linford,J.H., Froese,A., Israels,L.G. 28, *32*
Ling,G.M., see Singhal,R. L. 123, 124, *136*, 152, *156*
Lingens,F., Haerlin,R., Süssmuth,R. 70, 71, *82*
Lingens,F., Lück,W., Müller,G. 492, 498, *507*
Lingens,F., Rau,J., Süssmuth,R. 70, *82*
Link,F., see Jasińska,S. 354, *367*
Linn,B.O., see Shen,T.Y. 302, *344*
Linn,B.S., Gollan,F. 527, *533*
Lion,M.B. 319, *339*
Lipkin,D., Howard,F.B., Nowotny,D., Sano,M. 273, 274, 277, *339*
Lipman,M.B., see McCrea, J.R. 292, 304, *340*
Lipmann,F., see Sharon,N. 521, *536*
Lipsett,M.B., Kirschner,M. A., Wilson,H., Bardin, C.W. 814, *818*
Lipsett,M.B., see Bergenstal,D.M. 811, 812, 814, *817*
Lipsett,M.B., see Hertz,R. 475, 476, *481*, 686, *690*
Lipsett,M.B., see Ross,G. T. 160, *168*
Lipsett,M.N., Weissbach, A. 49, 50, *61*
Lipsky,S.R., see Agrawal, K.C. 797, *804*
Lipton,A., see Clarkson,B. D. 727, 728, 730, 732, *743*
Liquori,A.M., see Ascoli,F. 585, *589*
Lisak,R.P., see Vogel,C.L. 549, *553*
Lisi,A.G., see Scott,D.B.M. 122, *136*
Lisiewicz,J., see Micu,D. 706, *718*
Lisio,A., see Weissbach,A. 49, *64*
Lisk,R.D., see McGuire,J. L. 115, *133*
Liss,E., Palme,G. 25, *32*
Liss,E., see Langen,P. 298, *339*
Liss,R.H., see Chadwick, M. 881, *888*
Lisý,V., Škoda,J. 349, *368*
Lisý,V., Škoda,J., Rychlík, I., Smrt,J., Holý,A., Šorm,F. 353, *368*
Lisý,V., see Škoda,J. *370*
Litman,R.M., Pardoe,A.B. 295, 296, 305, *339*
Litman,R.M., Szybalski, W. 308, *339*
Lits,F. 673, *691*
Litt,M., see Doty,P. 292, *331*
Little,J.G., see Lett,J.T. 319, *339*
Little,P.A., Oleson,J.J. 660, *666*
Littlefield,J.W. 298, *339*
Littlefield,J.W., Gould,E. A. 297, *339*
Littler,W.A., Ogilvie,C. 39, *45*
Littlewood,B., see Jiminiz, A. *569*
Littman,M.L., Taguchi,T., Shimizu,Y. 523, *533*
Liu,A., see Bachur,N.R. 608, *611*
Liu,K., see Wilson,J.E. 523, *538*
Liu,Y.P., Handschumacher,R.E. 700, *718*
Lively,D.H., see Williams, R.H. 446, *457*
Livingston,R.B., Carter,S. K. 19, *32*, 232, *253*, 261, *270*, 477, *482*, 589, *591*
Livingston,R.B., Venditti, J.M., Cooney,D.A., Carter,S.K. 485, 500, *507*
Livingston,R.B., see Carter,S.K. 261, *268*
Llacer,V., see Uyeki,E.M. 406, *424*
Llerana,L., see Pearson,O. H. 112, *134*, 174, 183, *191*
Llerana,O., see Pearson, O.H. 112, *134*
Lloyd,H.H., see Laster,W. R.,Jr. 389, *460*
Lloyd,H.H., see Skipper, H.E. 235, *255*, 798, *807*
Lloyd,H.H., see Wilkoff,L. J. 298, *347*
Lloyd,J.B., see Hall,T.C. 459, *465*
Lloyd,J.R. 558, *569*
Lockwood,D.H., see Pegg, A.E. 148, *156*
Lockwood,D.H., see Williams-Ashman,H.G. 148, *157*
Loddo,B., Schivo,M.L., Ferrari,W. 302, 303, *339*
Loddo,B., see Ferrari,W. 303, *332*, 769, *784*
Loddo,B., see Muntoni,S. 307, *341*
Loder,J.W., see Culvenor, C.C.J. 881, *888*
Loder,J.W., see Dalton,L. K. 881, *888*
Loeb,E., Hill,J.M., MacLellan,A., Khan,A., Alexander,T.R., Adachi, M. 726, 727, 728, 734, 735, *745*
Loeb,E., see Hill,J.M. 696, 702, 704, *716*, 723, 726, 728, 732, *744*, 838, *839*
Loeb,M.R., see Cohen,S.S. 199, 203, 204, 218, *224*, 289, *330*
Löffler,H., see Heene,D.L. 709, *716*, *744*
Loehr,E.V., see Roberts,D. W. 246, *254*, 469, *482*
Loewi,G., see Arinoviche, R. 408, *419*
Loftus,S., see Schein,P.S. 75, *83*
LoGerfo,P., see Wilson,D. E. 354, *371*

Loh, P.C. 354, *368*
Loh, P.C., Soergel, M. 241, *253*
Lohr, K., see Kessel, D. 653, *656*
Loisel, J.P., see Jacquillat, C. 726, 727, 728, 732, 734, 735, *744*
Long, D.J., see Knight, V. *338*
Long, J.A., Evans, H.M. 108, *132*
Longmore, J.L., see Gallo, R.C. 711, *716*
Loo, J., see Lijinsky, W. 71, *82*
Loo, R.V., Ho, H.W. 258
Loo, R.V., Brennan, M.J., Talley, R.W. 261, *270*
Loo, R.V., see Talley, R.W. 238, *255*, 258, *271*
Loo, T.L. 549
Loo, T.L., Dion, R.L., Dixon, R.L., Rall, D.P. 65, 69, *82*
Loo, T.L., Gerulath, A.H. 547, *551*
Loo, T.L., Ho, D.H.W., Blossom, D.R., Shepard, B.J., Frei, E., III. 386, *401*
Loo, T.L., Lu, K., Richards, M.B., LePage, G.A. 429, *433*
Loo, T.L., Luce, J.K., Jardine, J.H., Frei, E., III. 546, *551*
Loo, T.L., Luce, J.K., Sullivan, M.P., Frei, E., III. 386, *401*
Loo, T.L., Strasswender, E. A. *551*
Loo, T.L., Tanner, B.B., Housholder, G.E., Shepard, B.J. 546, *551*
Loo, T.L., see Gerulath, A. H. 547, *550*
Loo, T.L., see Housholder, G.E. 546, 547, *551*
Loo, T.L., see Lin, Y.T. 549, 550, *551*
Loosli, J.K., see Breuer, L. H. 711, *714*
Lopez-Saez, J.F., see González-Fernández, A. 662, *665*
Lopez-Saez, J.F., see Stockert, J.C. 662, *667*
Loppes, R., see Moutschen-Dahman, J. 42, *45*
Loraine, J.A., see Strong, J. A. 178, *192*
Lorenzo, B., see Del Puerto, B.M. 560, *568*
Lorincz, A.B., Kuttner, R. E. 529, *533*
Lorke, D., Tettenborn, D. 710, *718*
Lorkiewicz, L., see Szybalski, W. 308, *345*
Lorkiewicz, Z., Szybalski, W. 27, *32*, 289, 293, *340*
Lortholary, P., see Bernard, J. 260, *267*
Losee, K.A., see Stearns, B. 789, *792*
Loth, L., see Mihich, E. 780, *787*
Louis, J. 820, *827*
Louis, J., Taylor, H., Sutow, W., Lyman, M.S., Burchenal, J.H. 820, *827*
Louis, J., see Hewlett, J.S. 740
Loukomskaya, N., see Šeferna, I. 359, *370*
Loustalot, P., see Gelzer, J. 747, *762*
Love, R. 680, *691*
Loveless, A. 6, 10, 11. *16*, 22, 27, *32*, *33*, 41, *45*, 70, 78, *82*
Loveless, A., Hampton, C.L. 70, 78, *82*
Loveless, A., Stock, J.C. 9, *16*
Lovina, T.O., see Hall, T.C. 459, *465*
Løvtrup-Rein, H., see Grahn, B. *669*
Lowenbraun, S., De Vita, V. T., Serpick, A.A. 760, *763*
Lowenstein, L., see Vas, M. 406, *424*
Lowrie, R.J., Bergquist, P. L. 209, 210, *228*
Lowy, B., Williams, M.K. 489, *507*
Lowy, D.R., Rowe, W.P., Teich, N., Hartley, J.W. 308, *340*, 355, *368*
Lozeron, H.A., Gordon, M. P. *228*
Lozeron, H.A., Gordon, M. P., Gabriel, T., Tautz, W., Duschinsky, R. 198, *228*, 321, *340*
Lozeron, H.A., Szybalski, W. 200, 205, *228*
Lozinski, E., see Levi, I. 524, *533*
Lozzio, C.B. 218, *228*
Lu, K., see Loo, T.L. 429, *433*
Lubin, M., see Ennis, H.L. 352, *365*
Lubitz, J.A., Freeman, L., Okun, R. 811, 814, 815, 816, *818*
Luce, J.K., Frenkel, E.P., Vietti, T.J., Isassi, A.A., Hernandez, K.W., Howard, J.P. 397, *401*
Luce, J.K., Thurman, W. G., Isaacs, B.L., Talley, R.W. 544, 545, 546, *551*
Luce, J.K., see Ahearn, M. J. 236, *249*
Luce, J.K., see Gottlieb, J. A. 656, *655*
Luce, J.K., see Ho, D.H.W. 698, 699, 700, 702, *716*, 733, *744*
Luce, J.K., see Loo, T.L. 386, *401*, 546, *551*
Luck, D.N., Hamilton, T.H. 120, *132*
Luczak, M., see Korbecki, M. 354, *367*
Ludford, R.J. 675, *691*
Ludlum, D.B. 8, 15, *16*, 22, *33*
Ludlum, D.B., Wilhelm, R. C. *17*, 7, 14, 15, *16*
Ludlum, D. B. see Wilhelm, R. C. *17*
Lück, W., see Lingens, F. 492, 498, *507*
Lugibihl, K., see Landau, R. L. 159, *167*
Lukens, L.N., Herrington, K.A. 385, *401*
Lummis, N.E., see De Boer, D. 47, *60*
Lummis, W.L., see Smith, C.G. 238, *255*
Lundberg, D. 683, *691*
Lundin, P.M. *101*
Luse, S., see Kaminsky, N. 811, *818*
Lutters, B.M., see Spencer, R.P. 521, *536*
Luttge, W.G., see Whalen, R.E. 149, *157*, 160, *168*
Lutwak-Mann, C. 25, *33*
Luyckx, A., Van Lancker, J. L. 680, *691*
Lyman, M., Wollner, N., Ellison, R.R., Krakoff, I., Frei, E., III, Close, H., Burchenal, J.H. 820, *827*
Lyman, M.S., see Burchenal, J.H. 820, *826*
Lyman, M.S., see Burchenal, J.H. 820, *826*
Lyman, M.S., see Kreis, W. 822, 824, *827*
Lyman, M.S., see Louis, J. 820, *827*

Lynch, J. E., English, A. R., Bauck, H., Deligianis, H. 564, *569*
Lynch, V., Smith, M. W., Marshall, E. K. 18, *33*
Lyons, M. J., Lasfargues, E. Y., Came, P. 306, *340*
Lyons, W. R., Li, C. H., Johnson, R. E. 111, *132*
Lyons, W. R., Sako, Y. 176, *190*
Lysenko, A. M., see Pravdina, N. F. 354, *368*
Lyster, S. C., see Duncan, G. W. 110, *128*
Lytton, B., see Kennealey, G. T. 408, *422*

Maag, T. A., see Shiguera, H. T. 524, 528, *536*
Maaløe, O., Hanawalt, P. C. 528, *533*
Maass, G., Haas, R. 304, *340*
Maass, G., Müller, J., Nakanoin, K., Vogt, A., Haas, R. 302, 304, *340*
Maass, G., see Haas, R. 302, 306, 307, *334*
MacAdam, R. F., see Plowright, W. 302, *342*
MacAdam, R. F., Williamson, J. 660, *666*
MacCallum, F. O., Juel-Jensen, B. E. 323, *340*
Maccotta, V., see Barasa, A. 675, *688*
MacCorquodale, D. W., Thayer, S. A., Doisy, E. A. 104, *133*
MacDonald, A. S., Chan, C. C., Falvey, C. F. 752, *763*
MacDonald, N. S., see Levy, J. 407, *422*
Machukawa, J., see Inuyama, Y. 870, *872*
Macieira-Coelho, A., see Garcia Giralt, E. 881, *888*
MacIntyre, W. M., see Harris, D. R. 197, *225*
Mack, G., see Foucher, G. 502, *504*
Mackaness, G. B., see Tripathy, S. P. 408, *424*
MacKay, E. M., see MacKay, L. L. 145, *155*
Mackay, I. R., see Lee, A. K. Y. 416, *422*
Mackay, I. R., see Rowley, M. J. 416, *423*
MacKay, L. L., MacKay, E. M. 145, *155*
Mackedonski, V. V., Hadjiolov, A. A. 584, *591*
MacKellar, F. A., see Wiley, P. F. 623, *632*
MacKeller, F., see Wiley, P. F. 557, *570*
Mackman, S., see Ansfield, F. J., 220, *223*
MacLean, S. J., Huber, R. E. 521, *534*
MacLellan, A., see Hill, J. M. 696, 702, 704, *716*, 723, 726, 728, 732, *744*, 838, *839*
MacLellan, A., see Loeb, E. 726, 727, 728, 734, 735, *745*
MacLeod, R. M., King, C. E., Hollander, V. P. 94, *101*
MacLeod, R. M., see Wiernik, P. H. *103*, 680, *694*
MacMahon, B., Cole, P., Brown, J. B., Aoki, K., Lin, T. M., Morgan, R. W., Woo, N. C. 178, *190*
Madaus, W. P., see Lauenstein, K. 705, *718*
Madden, F. J. F., see Shaw, M. T. 709, *721*
Maddock, C. L., see D'Angio, G. J. 589, *590*
Madoc-Jones, H., Bruce, W. R. 217, 218, *228*
Madoc-Jones, H., Mauro, F. 674, *691*
Madoc-Jones, H., see Mauro, F. 629, *632*
Madras, B. K., see Horowitz, B. 711, *717*
Maeda, K., Kosaka, H., Yagishita, K., Umezawa, H. 851, 855, *873*
Maeda, K., see Koyama, G. 852, *873*
Maeda, K., see Muraoka, Y. 852, *873*
Maeda, K., see Okami, Y. 497, *508*
Maeda, K., see Takita, T. 852, *875*
Maeda, K., see Takita, T. 852, *875*
Maeda, K., see Umezawa, H. 850, 851, 852, 855, 870, *875*, *876*
Maekawa, T., see Bierman, H. R. 36, *42*
Maemgwyn-Davies, G., see Trams, E. G. 39, *46*
Mäenpää, P. H., Bernfeld, M. R. 121, *132*
Magasanik, B., see Nakada, D. 211, 212, *229*
Magdon, E., Konopatzky, R. 355, *368*
Magee, P. N. 70, *82*
Magee, P. N., Farber, E. 71, *82*
Magee, P. N., Hultin, T. 72, *82*
Magee, P. N., see Lawley, P. D. 71, *81*
Magee, P. N., see Lee, K. Y. 71, *81*
Magee, P. N., see Swann, P. F. 69, 70, 71, *84*
Magee, W. E., Miller, O. V. 54, *61*
Mahoney, A. J., see Sivak, A. 824, *828*
Mahy, B. W. J., Cox, N. J., Armstrong, S. J., Barry, R. D. *669*
Magill, G. B., Meyers, W. P. L., Reilly, H. C., Putnam, R. C., Magill, J. W., Sykes, M. P., Escher, G. C., Karnofsky, D. A., Burchenal, J. H. 500, *507*
Magill, J. W., see Magill, G. B. 500, *507*
Magnussen, B., see Oehlert, W. 313, *341*
Magnusson, P. H., see Reichard, P. 217, *229*
Magnusson, P. H., see Sköld, O. 217, *230*
Mahesh, V. B., see Roy, S. 113, 114, *135*
Mahler, I. 53, *61*
Maidhof, A., see Zahn, R. K. 244, *256*
Maier-Borst, W., see Krüger, F. W. 70, *81*
Mainwaring, W. I. P. 149, 150, *155*, 164, *167*
Maisin, J. A., Dunjic, A., Dumont, P. 38, *45*
Maitra, U., Nakata, Y., Hurwitz, J. 583, *591*
Maizel, J. V., Jr., see Summers, D. F. 558, *570*
Majumder, G. C., see Turkington, R. W. 312, *346*
Mak, S., Till, J. E. 281, 314, 317, 318, *340*
Makino, H., see Nishimura, Y. 703, *719*
Makinodan, T., Santos, G. W., Quinn, R. P. 201, *228*, 525, *534*, 752, *763*
Makman, M. H., Dvorkin, B., White, A. 86, 87, 88, 89, 92, 93, *102*
Makman, M. H., Nakagawa, S., White, A. 86, 89, 91, *102*
Makowski, E., see Penn, I. 415, *423*

Malamud, D., Gonzalez, E. M., Chiu, H., Malt, R. A. 410, *422*
Malamy, M., see Hurwitz, J. 583, *591*
Malawista, S. E. 675, 683, *691*
Malawista, S. E., Bensch, K. G. 676, *691*
Malawista, S. E., Sato, H. 677, 678, *691*
Malawista, S. E., Sato, H., Bensch, K. G. 674, *692*
Malawista, S. E., Sato, H., Creasey, W. A., Bensch, K. G. *692*
Malawista, S. E., see Bensch, K. G. 677, *688*
Malawista, S. E., see Creasey, W. A. 678, 680, 682, *689*
Malawista, S. E., see Gillespie, E. 683, *690*
Maley, F., Ochoa, S. 274, *340*
Maley, F., see Labow, R. 469, *481*
Maley, G. F., see Labow, R. 469, *481*
Malling, H., see Frederiksen, S. 658, *665*
Malmgren, R. A., see Krueger, G. R. F. 417, *422*
Maloney, D. E., see Kaufman, H. E. 302, *337*
Malpas, J. S., see Beard, M. E. J. 726, 727, 728, 730, 734, 735, *743*
Malpas, J. S., see Fairley, G. H. 726, 727, 728, 730, 732, 734, *744*
Malt, R. A., see Gonzalez, E. M. 410, *421*
Malt, R. A., see Malamud, D. 410, *422*
Malt, R. A., see Van Vroonhoven, T. J. 410, *424*
Mameroff, M., see Stockdale, F. 311, *345*
Manak, R. C., see Neil, G. L. 233, *254*, 260, 266, *270*
Mancini, V., see Da Re, P. 673, *689*
Mancino, G., see Fiume, L. *669*
Mancuso, R. W., see Davidson, J. D. *784*
Mancuso, S., see Bolte, E. 107, *126*
Mandel, Merai, Connors 26
Mandel, H. G. 28, *33*, 193, 207, *228*, 458, 463, *466*
Mandel, H. G., Alpen, E. L., Winters, W. D., Smith, P. K. 459, 460, *466*
Mandel, H. G., Altman, R. L. 463, *466*
Mandel, H. G., Markham, R. 463, *466*
Mandel, H. G., see Carlo, P. E. 459, *465*
Mandel, H. G., see Henderson, J. F. 384, *400*
Mandel, H. G., see Roodyn, D. B. 463, *467*
Mandel, M. A., DeCosse, J. J. 417, *422*
Mandell, J. D., see Greenberg, J. 494, *505*
Mandell, J. D., see Woody, P. L. 494, *511*
Mandy, W. J., see Allison, J. P. 697, 702, *713*
Mangan, F. R., Neal, G. E., Williams, D. C. 149, 150, *155*
Mangan, F. R., see Parsons, I. C. 150, *155*
Mangan, J., see Okamoto, K. 57, *62*
Mangione, G., see Bonasera, N. 491, *503*
Manly, K. F., see Verma, I. M. 660, *668*
Manson, W., see Cunningham, K. G. 658, 660, *665*
Mansour, V. H., see Rosenberg, B. 830, *840*
Mantegazza, P., see Cavallini, G. 779, *783*
Mantel, N., see Goldin, A. 301, *334*, 476, *481*, 500, *505*, 564, *568*
Mantel, N., see Hoffman, G. S. 263, *269*
Mantel, N., see Kline, I. 260, *270*
Manteuil, S., Tavitian, A., Boiron, M. 439, *454*
Mant'eva, V. L., see Podobed, O. V. *669*
Manton, I. 676, *692*
Mantsavinos, R., see Canellakis, E. S. 274, *329*
Maral, R., Guyonnet, J. C., Julou, L., De Ratuld, Y., Werner, G. H. 705, 708, *718*
Maral, R., Werner, G. H. 696, *718*
Maral, R., see Dubost, M. 593, *612*
Marano, B., see Eidinoff, M. L. 490, *504*
Marantz, R., Shelanski, M. 677, 678, *692*
Marantz, R., Ventilia, M., Shelanski, M. 678, *692*
Marantz, R., see Bensch, K. G. 678, *688*
Marbach, E. P., see Chaney, P. L. 696, *715*
Marchioro, T. L., see Quadracci, L. J. 416, *423*
Marchioro, T. L., see Rifkind, D. 416, *423*
Marchioro, T. L., see Starzl, T. E. 410, *424*
Marcker, K. A., see Monro, R. E. 565, *569*
Marcus, P. I., see Bloom, B. R. 417, *419*
Mardashev, S. R., Kovalenko, N. A. 498, *507*
Mardashev, S. R., Shao, H. W. 698, *718*
Mardashev, S. R., Sokovnina 498
Mardashev, S. R., see Yarovaya, L. M. 489, 497, *511*
Margolis, A. A., see Becker, F. F. 583, *589*
Marigo, C., see Dalldorf, G. 417, *420*
Maritz, J. C. 879. *889*
Mark, J. B. D., Calabresi, P. 313, *340*
Markey, F., see Peck, R. M. 212, *229*
Markham, R., see Mandel, H. G. 463, *466*
Markiw, M. E., see Creasey, W. A. 234, 238, 242, 244, *251*, 258, 259, *268*, 680, 682, *689*
Markulis, M. A., see Spencer, R. P. 495, *510*
Marks, J., see Jelliffe, A. M. 747, *762*
Marlborough, D. I., see Miller, D. S. 699, 700, *718*
Marmont, A. M., Damasid, E. E. 726, 727, 728, 734, 735, *745*
Marmorston, J., Crowley, L. G., Myers, S. M., Sterns, E., Hopkins, C. E. 178, *191*
Marmur, J., see Okamoto, K. 57, *62*
Marmur, J., see Seaman, E. 57, *62*
Marosvari, I., see Cseh, G. 94, *100*
Marquardt, H. *718*
Marquardt, H., Zimmermann, F. K., Schwaier, R. 78, *82*
Marquardt, R. R., see Campbell, L. D. 125, *127*
Marrian, G. F. 104, *132*

Marsh, J.C., see Capizzi, R. L. 477, *480*
Marsh, J.C., see Levitt, M. 478, *481*
Marsh, J.C., see Skeel, R.T. 477, *482*
Marsh, J.M., Savard, K. 140, *155*
Marsh, J.M., Savard, K., Baggett, B., van Wyck, J.J., Talbot, L.M. 106, 107, *132*
Marsh, J.P., Jr., Mosher, L. W., Acton, E.M., Goodman, L. 593, *613*
Marshall, E.K., see Lynch, V. 18, *33*
Marshall, G.J., see Bateman, J.R. 221, *223*
Marshall, J.A., Tompkins, L.S. 814, *818*
Marshall, J.R., see Ross, G. T. 160, *168*
Marsland, D. 674, *692*
Martel, F., Berlinguet, L. 523, *534*
Martin, D.C., see Kaufman, J.J. 415, *422*
Martin, D.S. 847, *848*
Martin, D.S., Dietrich, L.S., Fugmann, R.A. 542, *543*
Martin, D.S., see Bieber, S. 386, 393, *398*
Martin, D.S., see Dietrich, L.S. 541, 542, *542*
Martin, D.S., see Herter, F. P. 541, *542*
Martin, D.S., Jr., see Sanders, C.I. 836, *840*
Martin, E.M., see Sonnabend, J.A. 607, *613*
Martin, H.F., see Shoon, M R. 444, 445, *455*
Martin, J.H., see DeVoe, S. E. 486, 496, *504*
Martin, L. 110, 113, *132*, *133*
Martin, L., Baggett, B. 113, *133*
Martin, L., Cox, R.I., Enimens, C.W. 110, *133*
Martin, L., see Emmens, C. W. 110, *128*
Martin, L., see King, R.J.B. 113, 114, 117, *131*
Martin, L., see Stone, G.M. 113, *136*
Martin, R.S., see Fillios, L. C. 109, *128*
Martin, W.G., see Mok, C.-C. 121, *133*
Martin, W.R., see Coggin, J.H., Jr. 491, 495, *504*
Martinelli, M.F., see Grignani, F. 472, *481*
Martinez, A.P., see Lee, W. W. 429, 430, 431, *433*
Martola, E., see Kaufman, H.E. 302, 322, *337*
Martos, L.M., see Hampar, B. 308, *334*
Martynova, V.N., see Demidova, S.A. 354, *365*
Martz, F., Straw, J.A. 812, 814, *818*
Martz, G. *763*
Martz, G., D'Alessandri, A., Keel, H.J., et al. 759, *763*
Martz, G., see Erlanger, M. 222, *225*
Marumo, H., see Wakaki, S. 47, *64*
Maruo, B., see Shiio, T. 54, *63*
Maruyama, O., see Kanai, T. 233, *252*, 266, *269*
Maruyama, T., see Kondo, T. 460, *466*
Maruyama, Y. *340*
Maruyama, Y., see Kriss, J. P. 282, *338*
Marxer, A. 777, *786*
Marxer, A., Gelzer, J. 778, *786*
Marxer, A., see Gelzer, J. 777, 780, *785*
Mascitelli-Coriandoli, E., Lanzani, P. 683, *692*
Masera, G., see Morasca, L. 684, *692*
Mashburn, L.T. 501, *507*
Mashburn, L.T., Gordon, C. S. 709, *718*
Mashburn, L.T., Landin, L. M. 699, 700, 701, 704, 710, *718*, 724, 730, *745*
Mashburn, L.T., Wriston, J. C., Jr. 695, 697, 698, 710, *718*, 723, *745*
Mashburn, L.T., see Boyse, E.A. 704, *714*, 723, *743*
Mashburn, L.T., see Campbell, H.A. 698, 701, *714*, 723, *743*
Mashburn, L.T., see Stevens, J. 90, *103*
Masina, M.H., see Huggins, C. 172, *189*
Mason, D.J., see Haňka, L. J. 351, *367*
Mason, H.S. 139, *155*
Mason, J.H., see Bisel, H.F. 440, *453*
Maspero-Segre, S., see Hedegaard, J. 492, *506*
Massarani, E., see Cavallini, G. 779, *783*
Massoulie, J.A., Michelson, A.M., Pochon, F. 279, 293, *340*
Massoulie, J., see Michelson, A.M. 293, *340*
Masuda, Y., see Nakamura, S. 870, *873*
Mata, J.M., see Stapley, E. W. 518, *536*
Matagne, R. 42, *45*
Matagne, R., see Moutschen, J. 42, *45*
Matewa, V., see Russeff, C. 302, *343*
Mathé, G., Amiel, J.L., Clarysse, A., Hayat, M., Schwarzenberg, L. 726, 727, 728, 732, 734, 735, *745*
Mathé, G., Berumen, L., Schweisguth, O., Brule, G., Schneider, M., Cattan, A., Amiel, J.L., Schwarzenberg, L. 759, *763*
Mathé, G., Hayat, M., De Vassal, F., Schwarzenberg, L., Schneider, M., Schlumberger, J.R., Jasmin, C., Rosenfeld, C. 882, *889*
Mathé, G., Schneider, M., Band, P., Amiel, J.L., Schwarzenberg, L., Cattan, A., Schlumberger, J. R. 685, *692*
Mathé, G., Schneider, M., Cattan, A., Amiel, J.L., Schwarzenberg, L. 772, *786*
Mathé, G., see Amiel, J.-L. 752, *760*
Mathé, G., see Schwarzenberg, L. 474, *482*
Mathor, A. N., see Hasselberger, F.X. 724, 735, *744*
Mathews, C.K., Huennekens, F.M. 468, *482*
Mathews, R.E.F. 458, *466*
Mathews, R.E.F., see Lasnitzki, I. 463, *466*
Mathews, R.E.F., see Smith, J.D. 463, *467*
Mathias, A.P., Fischer, G.A. 298, *340*
Mathias, A.P., Fischer, G. A., Prusoff, W.H. 280, 295, 298, *340*
Matias, P.I., see Cohen, J.L. 221, *224*
Matsuda, A., see Ichikawa, T. 855, 870, *872*
Matsui, N., Plager, J.E. 91, *102*

Matsui, S., see Hori, S.H. 124, *130*
Matsuma, A., see Hata, T. 47, *60*
Matsumoto, I., Kozaka, M., Takagi, Y. 54, *61*
Matsumoto, S., see Ishida, N. 444, *454*
Matsuura, S., Shiratori, O., Katagiri, K. 374, *382*
Matthaei, H., see Bermek, E. 375, *381*
Matthews, R.E.F. 512, *534*
Matthews, T.R., see Williams, R.H. 446, *457*
Matthews, V.S., Kirkman, H., Bacon, R.L. 175, *191*
Mattingly, E. 859, *873*
Mattox, V.R., see Molnar, G.D. 811, *818*
Mauer, A., see Perrin, J. 477, *482*
Mauer, A.M., Athens, J.W., Ashenbrucker, H., Cartwright, G.E., Wintrobe, M.M. 23, *33*
Maugeri, M., see De Barbieri, A. 528, *531*
Maughan, G.B., see Caplan, R.M. 415, *420*
Murao, K., see Ikehara, M. 443, 444, *454*
Mauri, L., see Cavallini, G. 779, *783*
Mauro, F., Madoc-Jones, H. 629, *632*
Mauro, F., see Field, E.O. 886, *888*
Mauro, F., see Madoc-Jones, H. 674, *691*
Mautner, H.G., see Spencer, R.P. 523, *536*
Maw, W.A., see Vanstone, W.E. 120, *137*
Mawas, C., see Carey, T. 768, *783*
Maxwell, M., see McCoy, T. A. 514, *534*, 695, 696, 711, *718*
Maxwell, M.D., see Patterson, M.K., Jr. *535*, 709, 712, *719*
Maxwell, M.H., see Kaufman, J.J. 415, *422*
Maxwell, R.E., Nickel, V.S. 494, 495, *507*
Maxwell, R.E., see Weston, J.K. 38, *46*
Mayama, M., see Nishimura, H. 373, 374, *382*
Mayer, C.M., Holton, C.P. 726, 727, 734, 735, *745*
Mayer, D.T., see Bogart, R. 113, *126*
Mayer, G.D., Krueger, R.F. 884, *889*
Mayer, R.L., see Heymann, H. 515, *532*
Mayne, R., Sanger, J.W., Holtzer, H. 311, *340*
Mayo, J.G., see Laster, W. R., Jr. 389, *400*
Mayol, R.F., Thayer, S.A. 120, *133*
Mazia, D., Gontcharoff, M. 310, *340*
Mazia, D., see Gontcharoff, M. 310, *334*
Mazia, D., see Wilson, L. 678, *694*
Mazza, F., Sobell, H.M., Kartha, G. 197, *228*
Mazzoleni, E., see Sanfilippo, A. 593, 606, *613*
McAninch, L., see Wyatt, J. 478, *483*
McArthur, C.S., see Bergh, A.K. 825, *826*
McAuslan, B.R., Joklik, W. K. *340*
McBride, C., see Klatt, O. 29, *32*
McCaig, J.G., see O'Donnell, V.J. 106, *134*
McCaleb, G.S., see Johnston, T.P. 65, 68, *81*
McCaleb, G.S., see Montgomery, J.A. 65, 66, 67, 68, *82*
McCaleb, G.S., see Schabel, F.M., Jr. 65, 68, 69, 79, *83*
McCalla, D.R. 71, *82*
McCalla, D.R., Reuvers, A. 72, 73, *82*
McCalla, D.R., see Schulz, U. 72, *83*
McCandless, R.G., see Schjeide, O.A. 120, *135*
McCann, S.M., Ramirez, V. D. 109, *133*
McCarthy, B.J., see Church, R.H. 119, *127*
McCarthy, G.M., see Robertson, J.H. 686, *693*
McCarthy, J.R., Jr., Robins, M.J., Townsend, L.B., Robins, R.K. 662, *666*
McCarthy, J.R., Jr., Robins, R., Robins, M. 447, *454*
McCarthy, J.R., Jr., see Robins, M.J. 662, *667*
McCarthy, M., see Helson, L. 219, *226*
McCarthy, M., see Tallal, L. 727, 728, 730, 732, *746*
McCarthy, W.H., see Burke, P.J. 545, *550*
McCarty, K.S., see Hijmans, J.C. 91, *101*
McCarty, K.S., see Miller, D.S. 634, 635, 636, 637, *641*
McClain, H.H., see Gale, G. R. 790, *791*
McCloskey, J.A., see Hanessian, S. 658, *666*
McCluen, R.H., see Mersler, M.H. 825, *827*
McColl, J.D., see Johnson, W.J. 540, 541, *542*, *543*
McCollister, R.J., Gilbert, W.R., Jr., Ashton, D.M., Wyngaarden, J.B. 390, 395, *401*
McCollister, R.J., Gilbert, W.R., Jr., Wyngaarden, J.B. 390, *401*
McCollister, S.B., see Pietsch, P. 857, 858, 860, 871, *874*
McCollum, R.W., see Calabresi, P. 291, 324, *329*
McCollum, R.W., see Creasey, W.A. 238, 240, 241, 242, 244, *251*
McCollum, R.W., see Huebner, R.J. 308, *336*
McCord, T.J. 518, *534*
McCord, T.J., Booth, L.D., Davis, A.L. 524, *534*
McCord, T.J., Cook, D.E., Smith, L.G. 518, *534*
McCord, T.J., Foyt, D.C., Kirkpatrick, J.L., Davis, A.L. 524, *534*
McCord, T.J., Howell, D.C., Tharp, D.L., Davis, A.L. 524, *534*
McCord, T.J., Ravel, J.M., Skinner, C.G., Shive, W. 497, *507*, *534*
McCord, T.J., Skinner, C.G., Shive, W. 497, *507*
McCord, T.J., see Ravel, J. M. 497, *509*
McCord, T.J., see Skinner, C.G. 497, 500, *510*
McCord, T.J., see Smith, S. S. 524, *536*
McCormick, J.E., see Barry, V.C. 793, *805*, 841, *848*
McCorquodale, D.J., Mueller, G.C. 119, *133*
McCoy, R.A., see Neuman, R.A. 723, *745*
McCoy, T.A., Maxwell, M., Irvine, E., Sartorelli, A. C. 696, 711, *718*

McCoy, T.A., Maxwell, M., Kruse, P.F., Jr. 514, *534*, 695, *718*
McCoy, T.A., see Kruse, P.F., Jr. 513, 515, *533*
McCoy, T.A., see Neuman, R.E. 484, *508*, 514, *534*, 695, *719*
McCoy, T.A., see Patterson, M.K., Jr. 696, 697, *719*, *720*
McCrea, J.F., see Bakhle, Y.S. 273, 314, *327*
McCrea, J.F., see Goz, B. 305, *334*
McCrea, J.F., see Prusoff, W.H. 289, 293, 302, 303, 304, 305, *342*
McCrea, J.R., Lipman, M.B. 292, 304, *340*
McCreadie, S.R., see Diamond, I. 38, *43*
McCredie, K.B., see Bodey, G.P. 264, *268*
McCredie, K.B., see Freireich, E.J. 262, 265, *269*
McCredie, K.B., see Whitecar, J.P., Jr. 263, *271*
McCullagh, E.P., Jones, R. 145, *155*
McCulloch, E.A., see Till, J.E. 23, *33*
McCully, K.A., Common, R.H. 121, *133*
McDermott, E.E., see Pace, J. 499, *508*
McDonald, C.J., Bertino, J.R. 479, *482*
McDonald, E., see Hilf, R. 124, *130*
McDonald, M.R., Riddle, O. 120, *133*
McDonnell, J.P., Garapin, A.C., Levinson, W.E., Quintrell, N., Fanshier, L., Bishop, J.M. 583, *591*, *613*
McElhinney, R.S., see Barry, V.C. 793, *805*, 841, *848*
McElwain, T.J., Hayward, S.K. 706, *718*, 735, *745*
McElwain, T.J., see Hardisty, R.M. 732, *744*
McEwan, A., Petty, L.G. 418, *422*
McFall, E. 56, *62*
McGandy, E.L., see Abraham, D.J. 556, *567*
McGařic, J.D., see Murray, J.E. 407, *422*, 502, *508*
McGeer, E.G., see McGeer, P.L. 679, *692*
McGeer, P.L., McGeer, E.G. 679, *692*
McGinty, D.A., Djerassi, C. 182, *191*
McGrath, H., see Rabinovitz, M. 524, *535*
McGuire, J.L., Lisk, R.D. 115, *133*
McGuire, W.B., see Boyd, G.S. 109, *126*
McGuire, W.L., Dedella, C. 162, *168*
McGuire, W.L., Julian, J.A. 177, *191*
McGuire, W.L., Julian, J.A., Chamness, G.C. 99, *102*, 117, *133*
McGuire, W.L., O'Malley, B.W. 165, *168*
McGuire, W.L., see O'Malley, B.W. 159, 163, 165, *168*
McIlwain, H. 825, *827*
McIlwain, H., see Roper, J.A. 496, *509*
McIndoe, W.M. 120, *133*
McInerney, M.R., see Barry, V.C. 841, *848*
McIntyre, R.W., see Greenius, H.F. 684, *690*
McIntyre, R.W., see Noble, R.L. 672, *692*
McIver, F.A., see Curreri, A.R. 220, *224*
McKay, A.F., Wright, G.F. 66, *82*
McKay, D.G., Shapiro, S.S. 527, *534*
McKeehan, W., Hardesty, B. 559, 561 565, *569*
McKeehan, W.L., see Obrig, T.C. 561, *569*
McKenna, G.F., see Skinner, C.G. 500, *510*
McKenzie, I.F.C., see Rowley, M.J. 416, *423*
McLachlan, P.M., see Heald, P.J. 121, *130*
McLaren, A.D., Knight, C.A. 518, *534*
McLean, J.P., see Pearson, O.H. 183, 184, *191*
McLean, J.W., Jr., see Miller, F.A. 428, *433*
McLean, P., see Glock, G.E. 539, *542*
McLean, W.J., Jr., see Sloan, B.J. 428, *433*
McLellan, W.L., Jr., see El-Nakeeb, M.A. 681, *689*
McLeod, J.G., Penny, R. 686, *692*
McLeod, R.M., see Wiernik, P.H. 680, *694*
McMurray, W.J., see Agrawal, K.C. 797, *804*
McNaull, J.N., see Kepler, J.A. 649, *655*
McPhail, A.T., Sim, G.A. 649, *656*
McPhail, A.T., see Wall, M.E. 649, *656*
McPherson, J.F., see Shen, T.Y. 302, *344*
McQuitty, J.T., DeWys, W.D., Monaco, L., Strain, W.H., Rob, C.G., Apgar, J., Pories, W.J. 844, *848*
McShan, W.H., see Davis, J.S. 110, *127*
Mead, J.A.R., see Coffey, J.J. 800, 802, *805*
Mead, J.A.R., see DeConti, R.C. 793, 799, 800, 802, 804, *805*
Mead, J.A.R., see Hardesty, C.T. 881, *888*
Mead, J.A.R., see Jondorf, W.R. 558, *569*
Mead, J.A.R., see Kline, I. 198, *227*
Mead, J.A.R., see Schrecker, A.W. 265, *271*
Mead, J.A.R., see Tomchick, R. 802, 804, *807*
Meade, H., see Baglioni, C. 567, *567*
Means, A.R., Hamilton, T.H. 119, *133*
Means, A.R., see Hamilton, T.H. 119, *129*
Mechl, Z., see Kolář, V. 196, *228*
Medici, P.T., Hurst, J.M., Pillero, S.J. 38, *45*
Medina, V.J., see Russell, D.H. 774, *787*
Medrek, K.J., see Rivers, S.L. 640, *641*
Medrek, T.J., see Harris, M.N. 638, *640*
Meeker, B.E., see Bruce, W.R. 21, *31*, 218, *223*, 474, *479*, 494, *504*
Meeker, B.E., see Valeriote, F.A. 686, *694*
Meigen 643
Meisner, D.F., see Shelton, R.S. 105, *136*
Meissner, L., see Grünberger, D. 464, *465*
Meissner, W.A., Sommers, S.C., Sherman, G. 175, *191*
Meissner, W.A., see Sommers, S.C. 175, *191*
Meister, A. 484, 492, 498, *507*, 696, 698, 711, *718*

Meister, A., Sober, H. A., Tice, S. V., Fraser, P. E. 708, *718*
Meister, A., see Horowitz, B. 711, 712, *717*
Meister, A., see Ronzio, R. A. 499, *509*
Meister, A., see Rowe, W. B. 499, *509*
Meister, A., see Ubuka, T. 708, *721*
Meites, J., Cassell, E., Clark, J. 174, *191*
Meites, J., see Nicoll, C. S. 174, *191*
Melan, F., see Bonmassar, E. 528, *530*
Melby, J. C., see Fisher, D. A. 811, *817*
Melchior, E. 560, *569*
Mell, G. P., see Huennekens, F. M. 469, *481*
Mellett, L. B., Eldareer, S. M., Chen, F. P. 259, *270*
Mellett, L. B., see Dixon, G. J. 684, *689*
Mellett, L. B., see Mulligan, L. T., Jr. 238, 239, *245*, 259, 266, *270*
Mellett, L. B., see Skipper, H. E. 235, *255*, 798, *807*
Mellett, L. B., see Struck, R. F. 29, *33*
Melling, J., Belton, F. C., Kitching, D., Stones, W. R. *668*
Mellors, J. W., see Krenitsky, T. A. 289, *338*
Mellors, R. C. 417, *422*
Melnick, I., see Levenberg, B. 486, 487, 488, 490, 496, 497, *507*
Melnick, J. L., Rapp, F. 302, 307, *340*
Melnick, J. L., Stinebaugh, S. E., Rapp, F. *228*
Melnick, J. L., see Rapp, F. 302, 303, 304, 307, *343*
Melnykovych, G., Bishop, C. F. 96, *102*
Meloni, M. L., Rogers, W. I. 386, 387, 391, *401*
Meloni, M. L., see Shigeura, H. T. 659, 661, 663, *667*
Meltz, D., see Gitterman, C. O. 661, *665*
Melvin, S. L., see Oppelt, W. W. 282, *341*
Mendecki, J., Lee, S. Y., Brawerman, G. *580*, *669*
Mendecki, J., see Lee, S. Y. 574, 575, *580*
Mendelsohn, M. L., Dethlefsen, L. A. 315, *340*
Mendelsohn, M. L., see Dethlefsen, L. A. 314, *331*
Mendelsohn, N., see Kapuler, A. M. 437, *454*
Menefee, M. G., see Siminoff, P. 302, 303, 304, *344*
Mengel, G. D., see Evans, J. S. 235, 236, 240, *251*, 259, 263, 264, *268*
Mennel, H. D., see Druckrey, H. 78, *80*
Mennigmann, H., see Szybalski, W. 293, *345*
Menon, K. M. J., see Toren, D. 139, *156*
Merai, see Mandel 26
Meranze, D. R., see Hilf, R. 123, 124, *130*
Mercer, R. D., see Farber, S. 512, *531*
Mercer, R. F., see Farber, S. L. H. 476, *480*
Mercier-Bodard, C., see Baulieu, E. E. 115, *126*
Mercier-Parot, L., see Tuchmann-Duplessis, H. 415, *424*
Merckel, C. G., see Nelson, W. O. 143, *155*
Merigan, T. C., Stevens, D. A. 417, *422*
Merits, I., Cain, J. C. 284, *340*
Merkatz, I. R., Schwartz, G. H., David, D. S., Stenzel, K. H., Riggio, R. R., Whitsell, J. C. 415, *422*
Merker, P. C., Pearce, R. K., Sarino, J. S., Wooley, G. W. 633, *641*
Mermann, A. C., see Burchenal, J. H. 389, *398*
Merrifield, R. K., see Shooter, K. V. 837, *840*
Merrill, J. P. 407, 410, *422*
Merrill, J. P., see Murray, J. E. 415, *422*, 502, *508*
Merrill, J. R., see Murray, J. E. 502, *508*
Merritt, K., see Buskirk, H. H. 24, *31*, 237, *250*, *525*, *530*
Mersler, M. H., McCluen, R. H. 825, *827*
Mertes, M. P., Saheb, S. E. 196, *228*
Mery, A.-M., see Amiel, J.-L. 752, *760*
Meselson, M., Stahl, F. W., Vinograd, J. 292, *340*
Meselson, M., see Fox, E. *333*
Mess, E., see Sonnabend, J. A. 607, *613*
Messiha, F. S., see Aebi, H. 754, *760*
Messiha, F. S., see Baggiolini, M. 754, *761*
Méšter, J., Robertson, D. M., Feherty, P., Kellie, A. E. 115, *133*
Mettil, L., see Pittillo, A. F. 820, *827*
Meulen, V. ter, see Leonard, L. L. 354, *367*
Meuth, N. L., see Verma, I. M. 660, *668*
Meyer, C., see Karon, M. 241, *253*, 261, *270*, 463, *466*
Meyer, R. K., see Davis, J. S. 110, *127*
Meyer, R. K., see Herschberger, L. G. 140, *154*
Meyer, V. 18, *33*
Meyer, W. E., see Morton, G. O. 434, *455*
Meyer, W. E., see Patrick, J. B. 48, *62*
Meyer, W. E., see Webb, J. S. 47, *64*
Meyer zum Büschenfelde, K. H., Freudenberg, J. 407, *422*
Meyers, P., see Rich, M. A. 660, 663, *667*
Meyers, W. P. L., see Magill, G. B. 500, *507*
Meymarian, E., see Jaffe, J. J. 441, *454*
Mian, A. M., see Nesnow, S. *229*
Micciarelli, A., see Da Re, P. 673, *689*
Michael, R. P. 114, *133*
Michaelis, A., see Fučik, V. 362, *366*
Michaelis, A., Rieger, R. 41, *45*
Michaelis, A., see Rieger, R. 41, *45*
Michaels, R. M., Peterson, L. J., Stahl, G. L. 841, *848*
Michaud, R. L., Sartorelli, A. C. 798, *806*
Michaud, R. L., see Agrawal, K. C. 795, 798, *804*
Michaux, M., see Alexandre, G. P. J. 502, *503*
Michel, I., see Hilf, R. 117, 119, 123, 124, *130*, 144, *154*
Michel, I., see Lerner, L. J. 122, 123, *132*, 147, *155*
Michel, M. R., see Weil, R. 302, 308, *346*

Michelsen, P., see Alexandre, G.P.J. 502, *503*
Michelson, A.M. 325, *340*
Michelson, A.M., Dondon, J. Grunberg-Manago, M. 272, 274, *340*
Michelson, A.M., Massoulie, J., Guschlbauer, W. 293, *340*
Michelson, A.M., Todd, A. R. 273, *340*
Michelson, A.M., see Grunberg-Manago, M. 214, *225*, 325, *334*, 378, *381*
Michelson, A.M., see Massoulie, J.A. 279, 293, *340*
Mickelson, M.M., see Gray, G.D. 237, *252*, 266, *269*
Mickelson, M.N., Flippin, R. S. 501, *507*, 514, *534*
Micu, D., Astaldi, G., Astaldi, A., Jr., Mihailesco, E. Lisiewicz, J. 706, *718*
Micu, D., see Astaldi, G. 706, *713*
Micu, D., see Burgio, G.R. 706, 707, *714*
Micu, D., see DeBarbieri, A. 706, *715*
Miech, R.P., Parks, R.E., Jr. *466*
Miech, R.P., Parks, R.E., Jr., Anderson, J.H., Jr., Sartorelli, A.C. 388, 394, 395, *401*
Miech, R.P., York, R., Parks, R.E., Jr., 395, *401*, 461, *466*
Miedema, E., Kruse, P.F., Jr. 516, *534*
Miedema, E., see Kruse, P. F., Jr. 525, *533*
Mielsch, M., see Dold, U. 25, *31*
Miescher, K. 106, *133*
Miescher, K., see Heer, J. 106, *130*
Miescher, P.A., see Borel, Y. 407, *419*
Miescher, P.A., see Spiegelberg, H.L. 408, *424*
Mietzsch, F., see Domagk, G. 841, *848*
Migeon, C.J., Lescure, O.L., Zinkham, W.H., Sidbury, J.B. 107, *133*
Mihailesco, E., see Micu, D. 706, *718*
Mihich, E. 766, 767, 768, 769, 770, 771, 772, 773, 776, 777, 778, 779, *786*, *806*
Mihich, E., Bross, I., Mihich, R.M., Nichol, C.A. 770, *786*
Mihich, E., Dave, C., Souček, J., Mulhern, A.I., Ehrke, M.J. 767, 780, *786*
Mihich, E., Dave, C., Williams-Ashman, H.G. 775, *786*
Mihich, E., Gelzer, J. 777, *786*
Mihich, E., Hakala, M.T. 769, 778, 779, *786*
Mihich, E., Kitano, M. 768, 778, *786*
Mihich, E., Mulhern, A.I. 768, 777, 778, 779, 780, *786*, 843, *844*, *848*
Mihich, E., Mulhern, A.I., Senn, H., Dave, C., Ahrens, H. 780, *786*
Mihich, E., Nichol, C.A. 842, 843, 844, *848*
Mihich, E., Simpson, C.L. 843, *848*
Mihich, E., Simpson, C.L., Loth, L., Mulhern, A.I. 780, *787*
Mihich, E., Simpson, C.L., Mulhern, A.I. 445, *454*, 770, *787*, 843, *848*
Mihich, E., see Bloch, A. 444, 445, *453*
Mihich, E., see Carey, T. 768, *783*
Mihich, E., see Corti, A. 774, 775, *784*
Mihich, E., see Dave, C. 771, 776, 780, 781, *784*
Mihich, E., see Grindey, G. B. 769, *785*, 799, *806*
Mihich, E., see Holland, J.F. 769, *785*
Mihich, E., see Kitano, M. 768, *785*
Mihich, E., see Nichol, C.A. 445, *455*
Mihich, E., see Souček, J. 781, *787*
Mihich, R.M., see Mihich, E. 770, *786*
Mikoshiba, A., see Henderson, J.F. 386, *400*
Mikucki, J., Szarapińska-Kwaszewska, J., Krzemiński, Z. 697, *718*
Mikulecký, Z., see Rašková, H. 361, *369*
Mikuni, M., see Kimura, K. 870, *873*
Miles, C.P. 584, *591*
Miles, H.T., see Howard, F. B. 293, *336*
Milgrom, E., Atger, M., Baulieu, E.E. 162, *168*
Milgrom, E., Baulieu, E.E. 162, *168*
Milgrom, E., see Baulieu, E. E. 115, *126*
Milholland, R.J., see Kaiser, N. 97, *101*
Milholland, R.J., see Kirkpatrick, A.F. 95, 97, 98, 99, *101*, 176, 187, *190*
Milholland, R.J., see Rosen, J.M. 86, 87, 88, 90, 91, 92, 93, *102*
Milikin, E.B., see Ho, P.P. K. 698, 699, 700, 702, 708, *716*
Miller, D.S., Laszlo, J., McCarty, K.S., Guild, W.R., Hochstein, P. 634, 635, 636, 637, *641*
Miller, D.S., Marlborough, D.I., Cammack, K.A. 699, 700, *718*
Miller, D.S., see Hochstein, P. 635, *640*
Miller, E. 36, *45*, 759, *763*
Miller, F.A. 302, *340*
Miller, F.A., Dixon, G.J., Ehrlich, J., Sloan, B.J., McLean, J.W., Jr. 428, *433*
Miller, F.A., Sloan, B.J., Silverman, C.A. 428, *433*
Miller, F.A., see Dixon, G. L. 428, *432*
Miller, F.A., see Sloan, B.J. 428, *433*
Miller, H.H., see Dewey, W. C. 294, *331*
Miller, H.H., see Jondorf, W.R. 560, *569*
Miller, H.K., Balis, M.E. 493, *507*, 701, 703, 704, *718*
Miller, H.K., Krakoff, I.H., Salser, J.S., Balis, M.E. 703, *718*
Miller, H.K., Salser, J.S., Balis, M.E. 703, 704, *718*, 725, *745*
Miller, H.K., see Borek, E. 499, *503*
Miller, J.F.A.P., Basten, A., Sprent, J., Cheers, C. 405, *422*
Miller, J.F.A.P., Mitchell, G.F. 707, *718*
Miller, J.J., Cole, L.J. 408, *422*
Miller, N., see Fox, J.J. 196, *225*
Miller, N., see Wempen, I. 233, *256*

Miller, O. L., Jr., Beatty, B. R. 573, *580*
Miller, O. V., see Magee, W. E. 54, *61*
Miller, R. S., see Wahba, A. J. 214, *231*
Miller, S. P., see Carbone, P. P. 394, *398*
Miller, T. W., see Stapley, E. W. 518, *536*
Miller, Z. 91, *102*
Milligan, L. P., see Baldwin, R. L. 123, *125*
Mills, S. D., see Carter, S. B. 446, 450, 451, *453*
Mills, S. D., see Jones, F. F. 446, 449, 450, *454*
Mills, T. M., Spaziani, E. 93, *102*
Milne, M. D. 512, *534*
Milner, A. N., Klatt, D., Young, S. E., Stehun, J. S., Jr. 27, *33*
Milner, J., see Allan, J. D. 529, *529*
Milner, L., see Prusiner, S. 697, *720*
Milton 300
Milton, J. D., LePage, G. A. 431
Milton, G. W., see Burke, P. J. 545, *550*
Miner, N., Ray, W. J., Jr., Simon, E. H. 607, *613*
Minesita, T., see Ueda, M. 683, *694*
Mingioli, E. S., see Groth, D. P. 74, *81*, 264, *269*
Minton, S. A., Jr., see Thompson, R. L. 800, *807*
Miquel, M. T., see Duprat, A. M. 628, *631*
Mirsky, A. E., see Allfrey, V. G. 824, *826*
Misařová, Z., Elis, J. 360, *368*
Misoo, Y., see Suzuki, M. 870, *875*
Mistretta, A. P., see DeBarbieri, A. 528, *531*, 706, *715*
Mitchell, C. G., Eddleston, A. L. W. F., Smith, M. G. M., Williams, R. 413, 414, *422*
Mitchell, E., see Stewart, S. E. 308, *345*
Mitchell, G. F., see Miller, J. F. A. P. 707, *718*
Mitchell, J. H., see Bennett, L. L., Jr. 463, *464*
Mitchell, J. L. A., Rusch, H. P. 774, *787*
Mitchell, M. S., DeConti, R. C. 201, *228*
Mitchell, M. S., Wade, M. E., DeConti, R. C., Bertino, J. R., Calabresi, P. 237, *253*
Mitchell, M. S., see Bertino 474
Mitchell, M. S., see Kennealey, G. T. 408, *422*
Mitchell, M. S., see Levitt, M. 478, *481*
Mitchell, M. S., see Peterson, R. G. 705, *720*, 735, 738, *746*
Mitchell, M. S., see Skeel, R. T. 477, *482*
Mitchell, R. M., see Sheil, A. G. R. 502, *510*
Mitchell, S., see Pinsky, C. M. 735, 738, *746*
Mitchley, B. C. V., see Bloom, H. J. G. 175, 186, *188*
Mitrovic, M., see Barnes, J. R. 643, *647*
Mitsuhashi, S., Takahashi, H. 862, *873*
Mitsuya, H., Kondo, A., Senda, H., Yamanchi, T. 870, *873*
Mitsugi, K., see Goldberg, I. H. 566, *568*
Mittelman, A., see Chang, E. 99, *100*, 178, *188*
Mittermayer, C., see Bremerskov, V. 234, 241, *250*
Miura, M., Hirano, M., Kakizawa, K., Morita, A., Uetani, T., Yamada, K. 514, 515, 526, *534*, 707, 713, *719*, 735, 738, *745*
Miura, M., Kawashima, K., Uetani, T., Hirano, M., Kakizawa, H., Ohno, R., Morita, A., Nishiwaki, H., Yamada, K. 705, 706, *719*
Miura, Y., Wilt, F. H. 311, 312, *341*
Miyairi, N., see Tanaka, N. 449, *456*
Miyake, K., see Suzuki, Y. 855, 859, 862, 863, 869, 870, *875*
Miyamoto, K., see Ichikawa, T. 855, 870, *872*
Miyamoto, M., see Seiki, K. 160, *168*
Mizgerd, J. B., Amick, R. M., Hilal, H. M., Patno, M. E. 546, *551*
Mizumo, K., see Kusaka, T. 434, *454*
Mizuno, D., see Abe, M. 522, *529*
Mizuno, D., see Hasegawa, Y. 856, *872*
Mizuno, D., see Natori, S. 55, *62*
Mizuno, H., Nakanishi, N., Fujiwara, T., Tomita, K., Tsukihara, T., Ashida, T., Kakudo, M. 279, *341*
Mizuno, H., see Kato, N. 55, *61*
Mizuno, N. S. 634, 637, 640, *641*
Mizuno, N. S., Gilboe, D. P. 636, 637, *641*
Mizuno, N. S., Humphrey, E. W. 74, *82*
Mizuno, Y., Ikehara, M., Watanabe, K. A., Suzaki, S. 444, *455*
Mizunoya, T., see Takeno, T. 57, *63*
Mizutani, S., see Temin, H. A. 58, *63*
Mizutani, S., see Temin, H. M. 200, *230*
Mjos, K. J., see Oleson, J. J. 496, *508*, 633, *641*
Mobbs, B. G. 114, 117, *133*
Mocarelli, P., see Natale, N. 610, *613*
Mochizuki, K., see Tanaka, M. 698, 699, 702, *721*
Modest, E. J., see Caspersson, T. 6, *15*
Moen, T. H., see Uy, Q. L. 675, 682, *694*
Moertel, C. G., Reitemeier, R. J. 220, *228*
Moertel, C. G., Reitemeier, R. J., Hahn, R. G. 793, *806*
Moertel, C. G., Reitmeier, R. J., Hahn, R. G., Schutt, A. J. 546, *551*
Moertel, C. G., Schutt, A. J., Reitemeier, R. J., Hahn, R. G. 650, *656*
Moffatt, J. G., see Atkinson, M. R. 660, *665*
Moffatt, J. G., see Pfitzner, K. E. 275, *342*
Moffatt, J. G., see Russell, A. F. 662, *667*
Mohanty, S. B., see Lillie, M. G. 302, *339*
Mohler, W. C., Elkind, M. M. 298, *341*
Mok, C. C., Martin, W. G., Common, R. H. 121, *133*
Mok, C. C., see Common, R. H. 121, *127*

Molina, A., see Pearson, O. H. 112, *134*, 174, 183, *191*
Molloy, G., see Jelinek, W. *669*
Molnar, G. D., Mattox, V. R., Bahn, R. C. 811, *818*
Moloney, W. C., see Jaffe, N. 726, 727, 730, 734, 735, *744*
Momparler, R. L. 243, 245, *253*, 427, 660, *666*, *669*
Momparler, R. L., Chu, M. Y., Fischer, G. A. 247, *253*, 265, *270*
Momparler, R. L., Fischer, G. A. 240, 247, *253*, 427, *433*
Momparler, R. L., Jaffe, J. J. 495, *507*
Momparler, R. L., Labitan, A., Rossi, M. 234, 238, *253*
Momparler, R. L., see Krygier, V. 427, *433*
Monaco, L., see McQuitty, J. T. 844, *848*
Moncloa, F., see Cazorla, A. 810, 812, *817*
Moncrief, J. W., Heller, K. S. 672, *692*
Mondelli, R., see Arcamone, F. 593, *611*
Mondelli, R., see Cardani, C. 566, *567*
Monfardini, S., see Bonadonna, G. 759, *761*
Monkemeyer, H., see Bermek, E. 375, *381*
Monod, J., see Bussard, A. 212, *224*
Monro, R. E., Marcker, K. A. 565, *569*
Monro, R. E., see Vazquez, D. 554, 565, *570*
Montag, B. J., see Chaudhuri, N. K. 202, 207, 208, 219, *224*
Montag, B. J., see Danneberg, P. B. 204, 205, *224*
Montag, B. J., see Heidelberger, C. 198, *226*
Montanez, G., see Levy, H. M. 521, *533*
Montfort, M. L., see Svboda, G. H. 881, *890*
Montgillion, M. D., see Smale, B. C. 855, *874*
Montgomery, J. A. 384, 389, *401*, 458, *466*, 768, *787*
Montgomery, J. A., James, R., McCaleb, G. S., Johnston, T. P. 65, 66, 67, 68, *82*
Montgomery, J. A., Thomas, H. J. 233, 234, *254*
Montgomery, J. A., see Bennett, L. L., Jr. 386, *398*, 436, *452*
Montgomery, J. A., see Johnston, T. P. 65, 68, *81*
Montgomery, J. A., see Schabel, F. M., Jr. 65, 68, 69, 79, *83*, 322, 324, *344*, 393, *402*
Montgomery, J. A., see Schmidt, L. H. 264, *271*
Montgomery, J. A., see Shealy, Y. F. 544, 545, 548, 549, *552*
Montgomery, J. A., see Skipper, H. E. 235, *255*, 798, *807*
Montgomery, P. O., see Reynolds, R. C. 583, *592*
Monto, G., see Samal, B. A. 520, *535*
Monto, R. W., Talley, R. W., Caldwell, M. J., Levin, W. C., Guest, M. M. 621, *622*
Monto, R. W., see Bodey, G. P. 260, 261, 263, *268*
Montreuil, J., see Strecker, G. 448, *456*
Moon, J. H., see Ellison, R. R. 260, *268*
Moon, J. H., see Hayes, D. M. 394, 397, *399*, 500, *505*
Moon, J. H., see Kung, F. 521, *533*
Moon, J. H., see Ohnuma, T. 726, 727, 728, 734, 735, *746*
Mooney, P. D., Booth, B. A., Moore, E. C., Agrawal, K. C., Sartorelli, A. C. 798, *806*
Moore, A. L., see Bachur, N. R. 608, *611*
Moore, A. M., see DeWald, H. A. 485, *504*
Moore, C. R., Price, D. 143, *155*
Moore, C. R., Price, D., Gallagher, T. F. 143, *155*
Moore, E. C. 790, *791*
Moore, E. C., Booth, B. A., Sartorelli, A. C. 793, 798, 802, 803, 804, *806*
Moore, E. C., Cohen, S. S. 243, *254*
Moore, E. C., LePage, G. A. 388, 389, 394, 395, *401*, 487, 488, *507*
Moore, E. C., Zedeck, M. S., Agrawal, K. C., Sartorelli, A. C. 798, 803, 804, *806*
Moore, E. C., see Agrawal, K. C. 795, 797, 798, *804*
Moore, E. C., see Booth, B. A. 802, 804, *805*
Moore, E. C., see Mooney, P. D. 798, *806*
Moore, E. C., see Sartorelli, A. C. 389, 397, *402*, 793, 797, 802, 803, *807*
Moore, G. E. 48, *62*
Moore, G. E., Gerner, R. E., Franklin, H. A. 90, *102*
Moore, G. E., see Aoki, Y. 389, *397*
Moore, H. L., Jr., Kozma, C. 415, *422*
Moore, J. A., Dice, J. R., Nicolaides, E. D., Westland, R. D., Whittle, E. L. 485, *507*
Moore, J. E., III., see Lane, M. 477, *481*
Moore, R. H., see Bent, K. J. 671, *688*
Moore, R. J., Hamilton, T. H. 120, *133*
Moore, T. C. 527, *534*
Mooren, D., see Heidelberger, C. 193, 198, *226*
Mor, G., Lichtenstein, N. 520, *534*
Morasca, L., Rainisio, C., Masera, G. 684, *692*
Moreau, T. L., see Hadler, H. I. 374, *381*
Morelle, J., see Alexandre, G. P. J. 502, *503*
Morgan, C., see Nii, S. 790, *791*
Morgan, C., see Rosencranz, H. S. 790, *792*
Morgan, C. H., see Iball, J. 279, *336*
Morgan, J. 676, *692*
Morgan, J. F., Morton, H. J., Pasieka, A. E. 516, *534*
Morgan, J. F., see Pasieka, A. E. 485, *508*
Morgan, M. D., Wilson, J. D. 161, *168*
Morgan, M. S., see Gorski, J. 119, *129*
Morgan, R. W., see MacMahon, B. 178, *190*
Morganti, P., see Grafnetterová, J. 357, 358, *366*

Mori, H., see Kotorii, K. 677, *691*
Mori, M., see Acs, G. 436, 437, 438, 439, *452*
Mori, M., see Uretsky, S.C. 437, 438, *456*
Mori, R., Kimura, G. 302, 307, *341*
Mori, R., see Kimura, G. 304, 307, *337*
Morikawa, Y., see Nakamura, N. 701, *719*
Morita, A., see Miura, M. 514, 515, 526, *534*, 705, 706, 707, 713, *719*, 735, 738, *745*
Morita, Y., Munck, A. 86, 87, *102*
Morita, Y., see Bartlett, D. 91, *100*
Moriwaki, A., see Paterson, A.R.P. 391, *401*
Moriwaki, A., see Tidd, D.M. 396, *403*
Moriya, K., see Suzuki, M. 870, *875*
Morreal, C., see Dao, T.L. 178, 179, *188*
Morris, C.R., see Gale, G.R. 838, *839*
Morris, D.R., see Fillingame, R.H. 774, 775, *784*
Morris, H.P., Dalton, A., Green, C. 171, *191*
Morris, H.P., see Elford, H.L. 793, *805*
Morris, J.E., see Kilgore, W.W. 79, *81*
Morris, J.M., van Wagenen, G., Hurteau, G.D., Johnston, D.W., Carlsen, R.A. 357, *368*
Morris, M., see Aposhian, H.V. 523, *529*
Morris, N.R. 300
Morris, N.R., Cramer, J.W. 298, 299, *341*
Morris, N.R., see Cramer, J.W. 299, *330*
Morrison, B.H., Jr., see Ross, R.B. 523, *535*
Morrison, R.K., Brown, D.E., Oleson, J.J. 619, *622*
Morrison, S.S., Higgins, G.M. 522, *534*
Morrow, J. 712, *719*
Morse, B.S., Stohlman, F., Jr. 687, *692*
Morse, P.A., Potters, V.R. 217, *228*
Morse, P.A., see Dorsett, M.T. 290, *331*
Morse, P.A., see Ives, D.H. 285, *336*
Mortensen, E. 754, 758, *763*
Morton, G.O., Lancaster, J.E., Van Lear, G.E., Fulmor, W., Meyer, W.E. 434, *455*
Morton, H.J., see Morgan, J.F. 516, *534*
Morton, R.K. 539, *543*
Morton, R.K., see Atkinson, M.R. 392, 395, *397*
Morton, R.K., see Branster, M.V. 539, *542*
Moruzzi, G., see Caldarera, C.M. 148, *153*, 774, *783*
Moruzzi, M.S., see Calderera, C.M. 148, *153*
Moseley, R., see Murray, J.E. 407, *422*, 502, *508*
Moseley, R.V., see Sheil, A.G.R. 502, *510*
Moses, C., see Danowski, T.S. 814, *817*
Moses, R.E., see Shimura, Y. 209, 211, *231*
Mosher, L.W., see Marsh, J.P., Jr. 593, *613*
Mosher, M., see Bertino, J.R. 477, 479, *479*
Moss, A.D., see Allan, J.D. 529, *529*
Mottram, F., see Jacquez, J.A. 519, *532*
Moulton, J., Coggin, L. 302, *341*
Mountain, I.M., see Tarnowski, G.S. 501, *511*, 514, *537*
Mourad, N., Parks, R.E., Jr. 461, *467*
Moutschen, J. 41, 42, *45*
Moutschen, J. Ezell 40
Moutschen, J., Matagne, R., Gilot, J. 42, *45*
Moutschen, J., Moutschen-Dahmen, M. 41, *45*
Moutschen-Dahman, J., Moutschen-Dahmen, M., Loppes, R. 42, *45*
Moutschen, J., Moutschen-Dahmen, M., Verly, W.G., Koch, G. 40, *45*
Moutschen, J., Reekmans, M. 42, *45*
Moutschen-Dahmen, M., see Moutschen, J. 40, 41, *45*
Moutschen-Dahmen, M., see Moutschen-Dahman, J. 42, *45*
Mowat, J.H., see De Voe., S.E. 486, 496, *504*
Mowat, J.H., see Webb, J.S. 47, *64*
Moxley, T.E., see Gray, G.D. 237, *252*, 266, *269*
Moxley, T.E., see Neil, G.L. 233, *254*, 260, 266, *270*
Moy, R.H. 809, 810, 815, *818*
Moy, R.H., see Bergenstal, D.M. 811, 812, 814, *817*
Moy, R.H., see Hertz, R. 686, *690*
Moyed, H.S. 448, *455*
Moyed, H.S., see Donavon, K.L. 448, *453*
Moyed, H.S. 517, *534*
Moyed, H.S., see Fukuyama, T.T. 448, *453*
Moyed, H.S., see Kuramitsu, H.K. 448, 449, *454*
Moyed, H.S., see Udaka, S. 448, *456*
Moyed, H.S., see Zyk, N. 449, *457*
Mozden, P., see Lemon, H.E. 178, *190*
Mudd, J.A., see Okamoto, K. 57, *62*
Mudd, S., see Gots, J.S. 494, *505*
Mueller, C.D., see Clegg, R.E. 120, *127*
Mueller, G.A., Gaulden, M.E., Drane, W. 674, *692*
Mueller, G.C. 118, *133*
Mueller, G.C., Gorski, J., Aizawa, Y. 119, *133*
Mueller, G.C., Herranen, A.M., Jernell, K.F. 118, *133*
Mueller, G.C., see Aizawa, Y. 118, *125*
Mueller, G.C., see Kajiwara, K. 299, *336*, 859, *873*
Mueller, G.C., see McCorquodale, D.J. 119, *133*
Mueller, G.C., see Nicolette, J.A. 119, *134*
Mueller, G.C., see Rueckert, R.R. 21, *33*, 199, 204, *230*
Mueller, G.C., see Ui, H. 119, *137*
Mueller, G.C., see Vonderhaar, B.K. 114, *137*
Mueller, M., see Zeller, P. 747, *765*
Mueller, S., see Elion, G.B. 387, *399*
Muggia, F.M., Creaven, P.J., Hansen, H.H., Cohen, M.H., Selawry, O.S. 650, *656*

Muggia, F.M., Heinemann, H.O., Belanger, R., Weinstein, I.B. 589, *591*
Muirhead, E.C., see Smith, C.G. 437, 440, 441, 445, *456*
Mukherjee, K.L., Boohar, J., Wentland, D., Ansfield, F.J., Heidelberger, C. 221, *228*
Mukherjee, K.L., Curreri, A.R., Javid, M., Heidelberger, C. 202, 215, 221, *228*
Mukherjee, K.L., Heidelberger, C. 196, 202, 215, *228*
Mukherjee, K.L., see Chaudhuri, N.K. 202, 215, *224*, 283, *329*
Mukherjee, K.L., see Heidelberger, C. 204, 217, *226*
Mukherjee, S., Bhose, A. 109, *133*
Mukherjee, S., Gupta, S., Bhose, A. 109, *134*
Mulhern, A.I., see Mihich, E. 445, *454*, 767, 768, 770, 777, 778, 779, 780, *786*, *787*, 843, 844, *848*
Mullen, J.M., see Hall, T.C. 459, *465*
Müller, G., see Lingens, F. 492, 498, *507*
Müller, J., see Maass, G. 302, 304, *340*
Müller, M., see Druckrey, H. 78, *80*
Müller, W., Crothers, D.M. 584, 585, 586, 587, *591*
Müller, W., see Harbers, E. 583, *590*
Müller, W.E.G., Zahn, R.K., Seidel, H.J. 583, *591*
Müller, W.E.G., Jamazak, Z.I., Sögtrop, H.H., Zahn, R.K. 243, *254*
Müller, W.E.G., see Zahn, R.K. 244, *256*
Mulligan, L.T., Jr., Mellett, L.B. 238, 239, *254*, 259, 266, *270*
Mulligan, L.T., see Dixon, G.J. 684, *689*
Munavalli, S.N., see Barrett H.W. 283, *327*
Munck, A. 91, 93, 96, *102*
Munck, A., Koritz, S.B. 91, *102*
Munck, A., Wira, C. 87, 95, *102*
Munck, A., see Bartlett, D. 91, *100*
Munck, A., see Hallahan, C. 93, *100*
Munck, A., see Morita, Y. 86, 87, *102*
Munck, A., see Wira, C. 85, 96, 98, *103*, 164, *169*
Munday, K.A., Ansari, A.Q., Oldroyd, D., Akhtar, M. 121, *134*
Muniz, O., see Dietrich, L.S. 541, *542*
Munn, R., see Schjeide, O.A. 120, *135*
Munoz, E.F., Garcia-Ferrandiz, F., Vazquez, D. 554, *569*
Munro, H.N., see Baliga, B.S. 561, 564, *567*
Munson, A.E., Munson, J.A., Regelson, W., Wampler, G.L. 884, *889*
Munson, J.A., see Munson, A.E. 884, *889*
Munson, R.J., see Bridges, B.A. 41, *42*
Muntoni, S., Loddo, B. 307, *341*
Munyon, W., Hughes, R., Angermann, J., Bereczky, E., Dmochowski, L. 302, 304, 306, 307, *341*
Munyon, W., Salzman, N.P. 209, *228*
Murai, A., see Suzuki, M. 862, 863, 869, 870, *875*
Murai, J., see Suzuki, M. 870, *875*
Murakami, H. 51, *62*
Murakami, Y., see Nakamura, S. 870, *873*
Muraki, K., see Iwata, H. 547, *551*
Muramatsu, M., Shimada, N., Higashinakagawa, T. 564, *569*
Muraoka, Y., Takita, T., Maeda, K., Umezawa, H. 852, *873*
Muraoka, Y., see Koyama, G. 852, *873*
Muraoka, Y., see Takita, T. 852, *875*
Murase, M., see Takeuchi, T. 444, 445, *456*
Murase, M., see Umezawa, H. 444, *456*
Murison, P.J., see Segaloff, A. 173, 181, 183, 184, *191*
Muroi, M., see Kusaka, T. 434, *454*
Murphey, E.A., see Levy, H.M. 521, *533*
Murphy, G.P., see Huser, H.J. 410, *421*
Murphy, G.P., see Varkarakis, M.J. 837, *840*
Murphy, J.P.F., see Katchman, B.J. 683, *691*
Murphy, M.L. 310, *341*
Murphy, M.L., Chaube, S. 790, *791*
Murphy, M.L., Karnofsky, D.A. 493, *507*
Murphy, M.L., Tan, T.C., Ellison, R.R., Karnofsky, D.A., Burchenal, J.H. 394, *401*
Murphy, M.L., see Burchenal, J.H. 384, 389, *398*
Murphy, M.L., see Chaube, S. 200, *224*, 237, 244, *250*, 261, *268*, 310, *329*, 752, *761*, *762*, 790, *791*
Murphy, M.L., see Ellison, R.R. 500, *504*
Murphy, M.L., see Helson, L. 219, *226*
Murphy, M.L., see Howard, J.P. 261, *269*
Murphy, M.L., see Krakoff, I.H. 789, *791*
Murphy, M.L., see Oettgen, H.F. 727, 728, 730, 732, 734, 735, *745*
Murphy, M.L., see Sullivan, M.P. 397, *403*
Murphy, M.L., see Pearce, M.B. 560, *569*
Murphy, M.L., see Tallal, L. 727, 728, 730, 732, *746*
Murray, A.W., see Atkinson, M.R. 389, 392, 395, *397*, *398*
Murray, A.W., see Donaldson, G.R. 564, *568*
Murray, A.W., see Tay, B.S. 390, 391, *403*
Murray, J.E., Merrill, J.P., Harrison, J.H., Wilson, R.E., Dammin, G.J. 502, *508*
Murray, J.E., Reid, D.E., Harrison, J.H., Merrill, J.P. 415, *422*
Murray, J.E., Scheil, A.G.R., Moseley, R., Knight, P., McGavic, J.D., Dammin, G.J. 407, *422*, 502, *508*
Murray, J.E., Wilson, R.E., Tilney, N.L., Merrill, J.R., Cooper, W.C., Birtch, A.G., Carpenter, C.B., Hager, E.B., Dammin, G.J., Harrison, J.H. 502, *508*

Murray, J. E., see Alexandre, G. P. J. 407, 409, *419*, 502, *503*
Murray, J. E., see Calne, R. Y. 409, *420*
Murray, J. E., see Sheil, A. G. R. 502, *510*
Murray, K. 518, *534*
Murray, M. R., see Hirschberg, E. 460, *465*, 879, *889*
Murthy, Y. K. S., Thiemann, J. E., Coronelli, C., Sensi, P. 882, *889*
Musil, J., see Kafka, V. 360, *367*
Musser, E. A., see Evans, J. S. 235, 236, *251*, 259, *268*
Myers, L. S., see Zimbrick, J. D. 319, *347*
Myers, S. M., see Marmorston, J. 178, *191*
Myers, W. G., Vanderleeden, J. C. 314, *341*
Myers, W. P. L., see Burchenal, J. H. 389, *398*
Myška, V., Elis, J., Plevová, J., Rašková, H. 360, *368*

Nabors, C., see Sweat, M. L. 106, *136*
Nadkarni, M. V., see Rakieten, N. 860, 861, *874*
Nadkarni, M. V., see Ross, R. B. 523, *535*
Nadkarni, M. V., see Trams, E. G. 27, *33*
Nadkarni, M. V., Trams, E. G., Smith, P. K. 39, *45*
Nadler, S. B., see Hansen, H. J. 386, *399*
Nadler, S. B., see Vandevoorde, J. P. 495, *511*
Nadochey, G. A., see Omelchenkov, T. N. 302, 304, 307, *341*
Nagai, K. 528, *534*
Nagai, K., Yamaki, H., Suzuki, H., Tanaka, N., Umezawa, H. 862, *873*
Nagai, K., Suzuki, H., Tanaka, N., Umezawa, H. 862, 869, *873*
Nagai, K., see Suzuki, H. 862, 863, 869, 870, *874*, *875*
Nagai, M., see Sano, K. 291, 319, 324, *343*
Nagano, H., Zalkin, H., Henderson, E. J. 492, *508*
Nagao, M., Yokoshima, T., Hosoi, H., Sugimura, T. 73, *82*
Nagasawa, H., see Dewey, W. C. 294, *331*
Nagata, T., see Takeno, T. 57, *63*
Nagatsu, M., Okagaki, T., Richart, R. M., Lambert, A. 859, *873*
Nagatsu, T., see Undenfriend, S. 520, *537*
Nagel, J., see Ohnuma, T. 726, 728, 734, 735, *745*
Nagler, A. L., see Zweifach, B. W. 527, *538*
Nagpal, K. L., Horwitz, J. P. *668*
Nagpal, K. L., see Srivastava, P. C. 273, *345*
Nagy, G., Balazs, C., Petranyi, G. 36
Nahas, A., Capizzi, R. L., Bertino, J. R. 470, *482*
Nahas, A., Nixon, P. F., Bertino, J. R. 471, *482*
Nahorski, S. R. 697, *719*
Naik, S. R., see Robins, M. J. 195, *229*
Nair, R., see Jaffe, N. 726, 727, 730, 734, 735, *744*
Naito, T., see Yamamoto, N. 10, *17*
Najarian, J. S., see Shons, A. 705, *721*
Najarian, J. S., see Simmons, R. L. 414, *424*
Nakada, D., Magasanik, B. 211, 212, *229*
Nakagawa, S., Dvorkin, B., White, A. 94, *102*
Nakagawa, S., White, A. 89, *102*
Nakagawa, S., see Makman, M. H. 86, 89, 91, *102*
Nakagawa, Y., Kano, H., Tsuda, T., Koyama, H. 373, *382*
Nakahara, W., Tokuzen, R. 887, *889*
Nakai, Y., see Oka, S. 870, *874*
Nakamura, H., see Koyama, G. 852, *873*
Nakamura, N., Morikawa, Y., Tanaka, M 701, *719*
Nakamura, N., see Tanaka, M. 698, 699, 702, *721*
Nakamura, S., Murakami, Y., Hashiguchi, T., Kuga, G., Yanagi, Y., Fujimoto, N., Masuda, Y. 870, *873*
Nakamura, T., see Inagaki, A. 242, 243, *252*, 261, *269*
Nakanishi, K., see Suzuki, M. 870, *875*
Nakanishi, N., see Mizuno, H. 279, *341*
Nakano, I., see Ichikawa, T. 870, *872*
Nakanoin, K., see Maass, G. 302, 304, *340*
Nakata, K., see Nakata, Y. 54, *62*
Nakata, Y., Nakata, K., Sakamoto, Y. 54, *62*
Nakata, Y., see Maitra, U. 583, *591*
Nakazawa, T., see Kanno, T. 855, 871, *873*
Nakazoto, N., see Edmonds, M. 574, 575, *579*
Namiki, O., see Higuchi, M. *60*, 857, *872*
Nance, F. C., see Silas, D. E. 410, *424*
Nanjo, S., Suga, A. 870, *873*
Naono, S., Gros, F. 211, 212, *229*
Naono, S., see Bussard, A. 212, *224*
Naono, S., see Gros, F. 212, *225*
Napoli, P. A., see Nicolin, A. 705, *719*
Nardi, D., see Cavallini, G. 779, *783*
Nardi, I., see Fiume, L. *669*
Narkates, A. J., Pittillo, R. F. 494, *508*
Narkates, A. J., see Pittillo, R. F. 79, *82*, 494, *508*
Noroth, K., see Rauen, H. M. 820, 823, *827*
Narrod, S. A., Bonavita, V., Ehrenfeld, E. R., Kaplan, N. O. 491, *508*
Narrod, S. A., Langan, T. A., Jr., Kaplan, N. O., Goldin, A. 491, *508*
Naruke, T., see Sakauchi, N. 814, *818*
Narumi, S., see Hano, K. 545, 547, *550*
Nash, J. 516
Nash, J., see Whittle, W. 524
Nasjleti, C. E., Spencer, H. H. 634, *641*
Nasr, H., see Pearson, O. H. 174, 183, *191*
Natale, N., Mocarelli, P. 610, *613*
Natarajan, A. T., Ramanna, M. S. 41, *45*

Natarajan, A. T., see Ahnström, G. 314, *327*
Natarajan, A. T., see Ramanna, M. S. 41, *45*
Nathan, H. C., Bieber, S., Elion, G. B., Hitchings, G. H. 407, 409, *422*
Nathan, H. C., see Bieber, S. 309, *328*
Nathans, D., see Shimura, Y. 209, 211, *230*
Nathanson, J. T., Andervont, H. B. 173, *191*
Nathanson, L., Jehn, U., Schwartz, R. S. 547, *551*
Natori, S., Horiguchi, T., Mizuno, D. 55, *62*
Natori, Y., see Endo, Y. 583, *590*
Neal, A. L., Libman, L., Smulson, M. E. *508*
Neal, A. L., see Smulson, M. E. 485, 497, *510*
Neal, G. E., see Belham, J. E. 149, *153*
Neal, G. E., see Mangan, F. R. 149, 150, *155*
Neal, G. R., see Parsons, I. C. 150, *155*
Neal, R. A., see Barrett, P. A. 841, *847*
Necco, Dasdia 597
Neher, R., Wettstein, A. 140, *155*
Neil, G. L., Moxley, T. E., Manak, R. C. 260, 266, *270*
Neil, G. L., Wiley, P. F., Manak, R. C., Moxley, T. E. 233, *254*, 266, *270*
Neil, G. L., see Gish, D. T. 233, *252*
Neil, G. L., see Gray, G. D. 237, *252*, 266, *269*
Neil, G. L., see Hanka, L. J. 234, *252*
Neil, G. L., see Warner, D. T. 233, *256*
Nejedly, Z., see Filip, J. 273, *333*
Neimann, W., see Neuberg, C. 841, *848*
Nelke, J. M., see Boch, M. 650, *655*
Nelson, A. A., Woodward, G. 809, 810, *818*
Nelson, B., see Hayes, R. L. 879, *888*
Nelson, B. M., Andrews, G. A. 39, *45*
Nelson, J. A., see Horowitz, B. 712, *717*
Nelson, J. D., see Williams, R. H. 446, *457*
Nelson, M. J., see Datta, P. R. 810, *817*
Nelson, S. D., Lee, M. B., Bridges, J. M. 705, 707, *719*
Nelson, T. S., see Bagshaw, M. A. 291, 319, 324, *327*
Nelson, W. O., Gallagher, T. F. 144, *155*
Nelson, W. O., Merckel, C. G. 143, *155*
Nemes, M. 310, *341*
Nemes, M., Hilleman, M. R. 302, *341*
Németh, L., see Kellner, B. 36, *44*
Németh, L., see Sellei, C. 19, *33*
Nemoto, H., see Kametani, T. 650, *655*
Neri, M. G., see Calendi, E. 606, *611*
Nervi, C., Arcangeli, G., Casale, C., Carrese, M., Guadagni, A., Le Pera, V. 478, *482*
Nesbit, M. E., see Karon, M. 364, *367*
Nesburn, A. B., see Kaufman, H. E. 302, 322, *337*
Nesnow, S., Mian, A. M., Oki, T., Dexter, D. L., Heidelberger, C. *229*
Nesset, B. L., see Callentine, M. R. 109, *127*
Neth, R., see Vazquez, D. 554, 565, *570*
Neu, R. L., see Jacobs, N. F. 859, *873*
Neuberg, C., Neimann, W. 841, *848*
Neubert, D. 858, *873*
Neubert, D., Oberdisse, E., Bass, R. 280, *341*
Neubert, D., see Brunnemann, A. 541, *542*
Neubert, D., see Coper, H. 541, *542*
Neufahrt, A., Rolly, H., Schutz, E. 302, *341*
Neuhaus, F. C., see Reitz, R. H. 497, *509*
Neuman, R. E., McCoy, T. A. 484, *508*, 514, *534*, 695, *719*, 723, *745*
Neuman, R. E., see Tytell, A. A. 516, *537*
Neumann, F., von Berswordt-Wallrabe, R., Elger, W., Steinbeck, H., Hahn, J. D., Kramer, M. 146, *155*
Neumann, G. H., see Jensen, E. V. 176, 187, *190*
Neumann, H. G., see Jensen, E. V. 114, *131*
Neuss, N., Johnson, I. S., Armstrong, J. G., Jansen, C. J., Jr. 671, 687, *692*
Neville, D., see Gellert, M. 585, 589, *590*
Newcomb, E. H., Hepler, P. K. 676, *692*
Newell, G. W., Carman, W. W. 499, *508*
Newell, N. S., see Burchenal, J. H. 198, *224*
Newman, J. F. E., see Roberts, W. K. 578, *580*
Newman, J. W., see Goldin, A. 389, *399*
Newmark, P., Stephens, J. D., Barrett, H. W. 283, *341*
Newmark, P., see Barrett, H. W. 283, *327*
Newton, B. A. 774, 781, *787*
Newton, K. A., see Hellmann, K. 886, *889*
Newton, W., Sayers, M., Samuels, L. 478, *482*
Ng, K. K. F. 561, *569*
Ngo/Minh/Mah, see Schwarzenberg, L. 474, *482*
Nichol, C. A. *455*
Nichol, C. A., Bloch, A., Mihich, E. 445, *455*
Nichol, C. A., see Bloch, A. 436, 437, 438, 439, 444, 445, 448, 449, *453*, 660, *665*
Nichol, C. A., see Grindey, G. B, 769, *785*, 799, *806*
Nichol, C. A., see Hakala, M. T. 391, 392, *399*
Nichol, C. A., see Harding, H. R. 88, *101*
Nichol, C. A., see Mihich, E. 770, *786*, 842, 843, 844, *848*
Nichol, C. A., see Rosen, J. M. 87, 88, *103*
Nichol, R., see Gray, G. D. 237, *252* 266, *269*
Nicholis, A., see Vincent, P. C. 59, *63*
Nicholls, T. J., Follett, B. K., Evennett, P. J. 121, *134*
Nicholls, T. J., see Follett, B. K. 120, 121, *128*
Nicholls, T. J., see Redshaw, M. R. 120, *135*
Nichols, F., see Nichols, J. *818*

Nichols, J. 808, 810, 812, *818*
Nichols, J., Green, H.D. 810, *818*
Nichols, J., Hennigar, G. 809, *818*
Nichols, J., Prestley, W.F., Nichols, F. *818*
Nichols, J., see Grady, H.J. 810, *818*
Nichols, W.W., see Heneen, W.K. 236, *252*
Nichols, W.W., see Kihlman, B.A. 236, *253*, 261, *270*
Nickel, V.S., see Maxwell, R.E. 494, 495, *507*
Nicolaides, E.D., Westland, R.D., Wittle, E.L. 485, *508*
Nicolaides, E.D., see Moore, J.A. 485, *507*
Nicolette, J.A., Gorski, J. 119, 124, *134*
Nicolette, J.A., Lemahiew, M.A., Mueller, G.C. 119, *134*
Nicolette, J.A., Mueller, G.C. 119, *134*
Nicolette, J.A., see Gorski, J. 88, *100*, 119, *129*
Nicolin, A., Napoli, P.A. 705, *719*
Nicoll, C.S., Meites, J. 174, *191*
Nicolson, M.O., see Klement, V. 308, *338*
Nielson, M.N., Warren, J.C. 124, *134*
Niepelt, N., see Krüger, F.W. 547, *551*
Nies, B.A., see Hersh, E.M. 264, *269*
Niethammer, D., Huennekens, F.M. 471, *482*
Nii, S., Morgan, C., Rose, H.M., Rosencranz, H.S. 790, *791*
Niitani, H., Suzuki, A., Shimoyama, M., Kimura, K. 54, *62*
Nikolaev, A.Y., see Evseev, L.P. 697, *715*
Nikolaev, A.Y., see Eremenko, V.V. 697, *715*
Ninet, L., see Dubost, M. 593, *612*
Ninomiya, I., see Hano, K. 545, *550*
Nirenberg, M., Leder, P. 352, *368*
Nirenberg, M., see Grünberger, D. 464, *465*
Nisbet, M.A., see Bilimoria, M.H. 703, *714*
Nishimura, H., Komatsu, Y. 374, 375, *382*
Nishimura, H., Mayama, M., Komatsu, Y., Kato, H., Shimaoka, N., Tanaka, Y. 373, 374, *382*
Nishimura, S., see Ikehara, M. 443, 444, *454*
Nishimura, T., see Tanaka, N. 449, *456*
Nishimura, Y., Makino, H., Takenaka, O., Inada, Y. 703, *719*
Nishiwaki, H., see Miura, M. 705, 706, *719*
Nishizuka, Y., see Honjo, T. 561, *568*
Niskanen, E. 40, *45*
Nixon, N.E., see Li, M.C. 472, *482*
Nixon, P.F., see Nahas, A. 471, *482*
Nizhizawa, Y., Casida, J.E., Anderson, S.W., Heidelberger, C. 197, *229*
Nižňanská, J., see Rašková, H. 361, *369*
Noack, V.I., Schmidt, H. 123, *134*
Noack, V.I., see Schmidt, H. 123, *135*
Noall, M.W., Allen, W.M. 113, *134*
Noble, R.L. 143, *155*, 683, *692*
Noble, R.L., Beer, C.T., McIntyre, R.W. 672, *692*
Noel, M., see Horwitz, J.P. 273, *336*, 662, *666*
Noell, C.W., Cheng, C.C. 549, *551*
Nogami, I., see Kida, M. 448, *454*
Nolan, B., see Alexandre, G.P.J. 407, 409, *419*, 502, *503*
Noll, C.I., see Ross, R.B. 523, *535*
Nomura, H., see Suzuki, M. 870, *875*
Nomura, M., see Erdmann, V.A. 566, *568*
Nomura, S., see Hata, T. 47, *60*
Noorduyn, N.J.A., see DeMan, J.C.H. 583, *590*
Nordenskjöld, B.A., Krakoff, I.H. 790, *792*
Nordenskjöld, B.A., Skoog, L., Brown, N.C., Reichard, P. 242, *254*
Nordenskjöld, B.A., see Skoog, L. 242, *255*
Nordman, C.E., see Sobell, H.M. 587, *592*
Noriega, A., see Tamoney, H.J., Jr. 814, *819*
Norrell, H., Jr., see Wilson, C.B. 478, *483*
Norris, E.R., see Roŭsh, A. 459, 460, *467*
North, A.C.T., Wade, H.E., Cammack, K.A. 699, *719*, 724, *745*
Norton, S.J., Chen, Y.T. 515, *534*
Norton, S.J., see Ravel, J.M. 697, *720*
Notari, R.E. 237, *254*
Notari, R.E., Chin, M.L., Wittebort, R. 232, *254*
Noteboom, W.D., Gorski, J. 114, 119, *134*, 164, *168*
Noteboom, W.D., see Gorski, J. 88, *100*, 119, *129*
Notides, A.C. 115, 117, *134*
Notides, A.C., Gorski, J. 120, *134*
Notides, A.C., see Gorski, J. 115, 117, 119, *129*
Nouza, K. 356, *368*
Nouza, K., Pokorná, Z., Slavík, M., Gottwaldová, A. 356, *368*
Nouza, K., see Skopinska, E. 408, *424*
Novak, L., see Shamma, M. 650, *656*
Novikoff 663
Novikova, M.A. 518, *534*
Novotný, J., Smetana, R., Rašková, H. 349, *368*
Novotný, J., see Janků, I. 349, 359, *367*
Novotný, J., see Jiřička, Z. 349, 358, *367*
Nowakowski, A., see Gelfand, M.C. 407, *421*
Nowell, P.C. 56, *62*
Nowotny, D., see Lipkin, D. 273, 274, 277, *339*
Numata, M., see Jensen, E.V. 104, 110, 114, 115, *131*
Nunokawa, O., see Suzuki, M. 862, 863, 869, 870, *875*
Nussbaum, A., see Duschinsky, R. 197, *225*
Nutt, R.F., see Walton, E. 658, 661, *668*
Nutter, R.L., Rapp, F. 244, *254*
Nyberg, W.H., see Baiocchi, F. 768, *783*

Nyberg, W.H., see Liao, T. K. 650, *656*
Nyberg, W.H., see Podrebarac, E.G. 768, *787*
Nyden, S.I., Williams-Ashman, H.G. 151, *155*
Nygaard, O.F., see Potter, R.L. 314, 318, *342*
Nyhan, W.L., Sweetman, L., Carpenter, D.G., Carter, C.H., Hoefnagel, D. 414, *423*
Nyhan, W.L., see Kung, F. 521, *533*
Nyhan, W.L., see Lampert, F. 521, *533*
Nyman, M.A., Geiger, J., Goldzieher, J.W. 106, *134*

Oakberg, E.F. 37, *45*
Obe, G. 415, *423*
Oberdisse, E., see Neubert, D. 280, *341*
Oberfield, R.A., see Savlov, E.D. 546, *552*
Obrecht, P., Fusenig, N.E. 682, *692*
Obrecht, P., Strickstrock, K.-H., Fusenig, N. 757, *763*
Obrecht, P., Strickstrock, K. H., Weissleder, H. 759, *763*
Obrecht, P., Strickstrock, K. H., Woenckhaus, J.W. 749, *764*
Obrecht, P., see Fusenig, N. E. 757, *762*
Obrecht, P., see Schwartz, D.E. 754, *764*
O'Brien, B.R.A. 463, *467*
O'Brien, D.E., see Baiocchi, F. 768, *783*
O'Brien, O.P., see Callentine, M.R. 110, *127*
O'Brien, R.L., Olenick, J. G., Hahn, F.E. 774, *787*
O'Brien, T.F. 310, *341*
O'Brien, T.F., Coons, A.H. 310, *341*
Obrig, T.C., Culp, W.J., McKeehan, W.L., Hardesty, B. 561, *569*
O'Bryan, R.M., see Talley, R.W. 238, *255*, 258, *271*
O'Callaghan, C.N., see Barry, V.C. 793, *805*
Ochoa, M., Jr., Gellhorn, A., Benjamin, W.B. 823, 824, *827*
Ochoa, M., Jr., Hirschberg, E. 6, *16*, 21, 25, 28, 29, *33*, 35, *45*
Ochoa, S., see Lengyel, P. 214, *228*
Ochoa, S., see Maley, F. 274, *340*
Ochs, H., see Weitzel, G. 756, *765*
Ochs, H.D., see Kummer, D. 28, *32*
Ockey, C.H., Hsu, T.C., Richardson, L.C. 200, *229*
O'Connor, A., see Clarkson, B. 222, *224*
O'Connor, T.E., see Hirschman, S.Z. 237, *252*
Odaka, T., Takizawa, K., Yamaura, K., Yamamoto, T. 444, *455*
O'Dell, C.A., see Shealy, Y. F. 549, *552*
Odell, W.O., see Swerdloff, R.S. 160, *168*
Odmark, G. *669*
Odmark, G., see Kihlman, B.A. 662, *666*, 859, *873*
O'Donnell, V.J., McCaig, J. G. 106, *134*
O'Donnell, V.J., see Heard, R.D. 106, *130*
O'Dorisio, M.S., Barker, K. L. 124, *134*
Oehlert, W., Magnussen, B. 313, *341*
Oerkermann, H., Hirschmann, W.D., Cross, R. 734, 738, *745*
Oettgen, H.F., Clifford, P., Burchenal, J.H. 820, *827*
Oettgen, H.F., Old, L.J., Boyse, E.A., Campbell, H.A., Phillips, F.S., Clarkson, B.D., Tallal, L., Leeper, R.D., Schwartz, M.K., Kim, J. H. 696, *719*, 723, 727, 730, 733, 734, *745*
Oettgen, H.F., Schulten, H. K. 727, 728, 730, 733, 734, 735, *745*
Oettgen, H.F., Stephenson, P., Schwartz, M.K., Leeper, R.D., Tallal, L., Tan, C.C., Clarkson, B. D., Golbey, R.B., Krakoff, I.H., Karnofsky, D.A., Murphy, M.L., Burchenal, J.H. 727, 730, 732, 734, 735, *745*
Oettgen, H.F., Tallal, L., Tan, C.C., Murphy, M. L., Clarkson, B.D., Golbey, R.B., Krakoff, I.H., Karnofsky, D.A., Burchenal, J.H. 727, 728, 730, 732, 734, 735, *745*
Oettgen, H.F., see Bettigole, R.E. 735, *743*
Oettgen, H.F., see Burchenal, J.H. *329*
Oettgen, H.F., see Clarkson, B.D. 727, 728, 730, 732, *743*
Oettgen, H.F., see Lash, E. 735, *745*
Oettgen, H.F., see Old, L.J. 728, 733, *746*
Oettgen, H.F., see Pinsky, C.M. 735, 738, *746*
Oettgen, H.F., see Schulten, H.K. 705, 707, *721*
Oettgen, H.F., see Schwartz, M.K. 704, *721*, 724, 725, 735, *746*
Oettgen, H.F., see Tallal, L. 727, 728, 730, 732, *746*
Oettgen, H.F., see Tan, C.C. 732, *746*
O'Farrell, P.H., Daniel, J. C., Jr. 117, *134*
O'Farrel, T.P., Dunaway, P.B. 283, 284, 318, *341*
Officer, J.E., see Thompson, R.L. 800, *807*
Ofner, P. 146, 149, *155*
O'Gara, R.W., Adamson, R. H., Kelly, M.G., Dalgard, D.W. 752, *764*
O'Gara, R.W., see Kelly, M. G. 752, *762*, *763*
Ogilvie, C., see Littler, W.A. 39, *45*
Ogilvie, A., Kersten, W., Kersten, H. 56, *62*
Ohashi, A., see Hirono, I. 28, *32*
Ohkuma, K., see Yüntsen, H. 446, *457*
Ohlsson, W.G., see Sellinger, O.Z. 499, *510*
Ohmori, K., see Honda, Y. 870, *872*
Ohno, R., Harris, J.E., Hersh, E.M. *719*
Ohno, R., Hersh, E.M. 705, 706, 707, *719*, 735, 738, *745*
Ohno, R., see Miura, M. 705, 706, *719*
Ohnuma, T., Bergel, F., Bray, R.C. *534*, 697, 704, *719*

Ohnuma,T., Bosner,F., Levy,R.N., Cuttner,J., Moon,J.H., Silver,R.T., Blom,J., Falkson,G., Burningham,R., Glidewell,O., Holland,J.F. 726, 727, 728, 734, 735, *746*
Ohnuma,T., Holland,J.F., Freeman,A., Sinks,L.F. 514, *534*, 703, *719*, 724, 725, 733, 734, 735, *745*
Ohnuma,T., Holland,J.F., Nagel,J., St.Arneault, G. 726, 728, 734, 735, *745*
Oka,S., Sato,K., Nakai,Y., Kurita,K., Hashimoto, K., Oshibe,M. 870, *874*
Ohnuma,T., Waligunda,J., Holland,J.F. 515, 529, *535*
Ohtsuka,E., see Ikehara,M. 438, *454*
OJima,Y., see Anderson, L.L. 472, *479*
Oka,M., see Yamamoto,I. 547, *553*
Okabayashi,K., see Kato, N. 55, *61*
Okagaki,T., see Nagatsu,M. 859, *873*
Okami,Y., Maeda,K., Kondo,H., Tanaka,T., Umezawa,H. 497, *508*
Okami,Y., see Umezawa,H. 851, 855, *876*
Okamoto,K., Mudd,J.A., Mangan,J., Huang,W. M., Subbaiah,T.V., Marmur,J. 57, *62*
Okamoto,K., Mudd,J.A., Marmur,J. 57, *62*
Okamura,I., see Kunimoto, T. 444, *454*
Okata,E., see Iwabuchi,M. 210, *226*
Okazaki,K., Holtzer,H. 311, *341*
Okazaki,K., see Stockdale, F. 311, *345*
Okazaki,R., see Iwatsuki, N. 285, 286, *336*
Okazaki,R., Kornberg,A. 285, 286, 320, *341*
Okazaki,T., Kornberg,A. 277, *341*
Oki,T., Heidelberger,C. 205, *229*
Oki,T., see Fujiwara,Y. 205, *225*, 292, 298, *333*
Oki,T., see Nesnow,S. *229*
Okstein,C., see Rogers,W. I. 219, *229*
Okubo,S., Romig,W.R. 53, *62*
Okun,R., see Lubitz,J.A. 811, 814, 815, 816, *818*
Olansky,S., see Vogler,W. R. 361, *371*
Old,L.J., Boyse,E.A., Campbell,H.A. 696, *719*
Old,L.J., Boyse,E.A., Campbell,H.A., Brodey, R.S., Fidler,J., Teller,J. 723, *746*
Old,L.J., Boyse,E.A., Campbell,H.A., Daria, G.M. 695, 697, *719*
Old,L.J., Kim,J.H., Beth, E., Boyse,E.A., Oettgen,H.F., Campbell,H. A., Burchenal,J.H. 728, 733, *746*
Old,L.J., see Boyse,E.A. 696, 704, *714*, 723, *743*
Old,L.J., see Campbell,H. A. 698, 701, *714*, 723, *743*
Old,L.J., see Horowitz,B. 711, *717*
Old,L.J., see Kim,J.H. 738, *745*
Old,L.J., see Oettgen,H.F. 696, *719*, 723, 727, 730, 733, 734, *745*
Oldini,C., see Bonadonna, G. 759, *761*
Oldroyd,D., see Munday,K. A. 121, *134*
Olenick,J.G., see O'Brien, R.L. 774, *787*
Oleson,J.J., Calderella,L. A., Mjos,K.J., Reith,A. R., Thie,R.S., Toplin,I. 633, *641*
Oleson,J.J., Reith,A.R., Thie,R.S., Mjos,K.J., Calderella,L.A. 496, *508*
Oleson,J.J., see Little,P.A. 660, *666*
Oleson,J.J., see Morrison, R.K. 619, *622*
Olin,E.J., see Li,L.H. 362, *367*, 653, *656*
Oliver,W.F., see Vanstone, W.E. 120, *137*
Oliveira,C.A., see Katz,N. 879, *889*
Oliverio,V.T. 747, 753, *764*
Oliverio,V.T., Adamson,R. H., Henderson,E.S., Davidson,J.D. 770, *787*
Oliverio,V.T., Denham,C. 770, *787*
Oliverio,V.T., Denham,C., DeVita,V.T., Kelly,M. G. 747, 751, 754, *764*
Oliverio,V.T., Kelly,M.G. 747, 748, 749, 751, 754, *764*
Oliverio,V.T., Vietzke,W. M., Williams,M.K., Adamson,R.H. 69, 72, *82*
Oliverio,V.T., Zubrod,C.G. 28, *33*, 711, *787*
Oliverio,V.T., see Adamson,R.H. 642, *647*, 771, 772, *783*
Oliverio,V.T., see Block,J. B. 771, 774, *783*
Oliverio,V.T., see Bray,D. A. 68, 77, *80*
Oliverio,V.T., see Chabner, B.A. 751, 752, 754, 756, *761*
Oliverio,V.T., see Davidson,J.O. 471, 472, 473, *480*
Oliverio,V.T., see DeVita, V.T. 69, *80*, 752, *762*
Oliverio,V.T., see Field,M. 771, 774, *784*
Oliverio,V.T., see Gottlieb, J.A. 650, *655*
Oliverio,V.T., see Hart,L. G. 650, *655*
Oliverio,V.T., see Henderson,E.S. 471, 472, 473, 474, *481*
Oliverio,V.T., see Kelly,M. G. 752, *762*, *763*
Oliverio,V.T., see Levin,V. A. 69, *81*
Oliverio,V.T., see Liegler, D.G. 473, *482*
Oliverio,V.T., see Zaharko, D.S. 473, *483*
Olmsted,J.B., Carlson,K., Klebe,R., Ruddle,F., Rosenbaum,J. 678, *692*
Olson,G., see Hiremath,C. B. 524, *532*
Olson,K.B., Ansfield,F.J. 183, *191*
Olson,K.B., see Carbone,P. P. 394, *398*
Olson,K.B., see Cavins,J. A. 440, *453*
Olson,K.B., see Kingra, G.S. 546, *551*
Olson,K.B., see Yates,R.C. 451, *457*
Olson,M.E., see Rabinovitz,M. 485, 497, 499, *508*, *509*, 524, *535*
O'Malley,B.W. 119, 121, *134*

O'Malley, B.W., Aronow, A., Peacock, A., Dingman, E.W. 121, *134*
O'Malley, B.W., McGuire, W.L. 159, 165, *168*
O'Malley, B.W., McGuire, W.L., Kohler, P.O., Korenman, S.G. 159, 163, 165, *168*
O'Malley, B.W., Sherman, M.R., Toft, D.O. 160, 163, *168*
O'Malley, B.W., Sherman, M.R., Toft, D.O., Spelsberg, T.C., Schrader, W.T., Steggles, A.W. 160, 161, 162, 164, *168*
O'Malley, B.W., see Dingman, C.W. 121, *128*
O'Malley, B.W., see Kohler, P.O. 159, *167*
O'Malley, B.W., see Korenman, S.G. 159, 160, 161, *167*
O'Malley, B.W., see McGuire, W.L. 165, *168*
O'Malley, B.W., see Rosenfeld, M.G. 152, *156*
O'Malley, B.W., see Sherman, M.R. 85, *103*, 163, 164, *168*
O'Malley, B.W., see Spelsberg, T.C. 85, 96, 99, *103*, 165, *168*
Omelchenkov, T.N., Ciampor, F., Nadochey, G.A., Avakyan, A.A., Altshtein, A.D. 302, 304, 307, *341*
Ommaya, A.K., see Rubin, R.C. 472, *482*
Omokoku, B., see Ertel, N. 684, *689*
Omura, T., Sanders, E., Estabrook, R.W., Cooper, D.Y., Rosenthal, O. 139, *155*
O'Neal, C., see Grünberger, D. 464, *465*
Ono, T., see Koyama, H. 311 *338*
Ootake, S., see Suzuki, M. 870, *875*
Opara-Kubinska, Z., see Szybalski, W. 308, *345*
Openshaw, H.T. 558, 563, *569*
Opliger, C.E., see Shealy, Y.F. 549, *552*
Opliger, P.S., see Johnston, T.P. 65, 68, *81*
Oppelt, W.W., Clarkson, D.R., Melvin, S.L. 282, *341*
Oppelt, W.W., see Clarkson, D.R. 283, 284, *330*
Oppenheim, J.J., see Hersh, E.M. 416, *421*
Orezzi, P., see DiMarco, A. 593, 597, *612*
Orezzi, P., see Arcamone, F. 593, *611*
Orlando, R.A., see Wittliff, J.L. 117, 118, *138*
Orr, D.J., see Lawley, P.D. 7, *16*
Orr, G.R., see Patterson, M.K., Jr. 491, *508*, 514, *535*, 697, 711, 712, *719* *720*
Osawa, S., see Iwabuchi, M. 210, *226*
Osawa, S., see Kono, M. 206, *228*
Osborn, M., Person, S., Phillips, S., Funk, F. 11, *16*
Oshibe, M., see Oka, S. 870, *874*
Osoba, D. 707, *719*
Osswald, H., see Krüger, F.W. 70, 71, *81*
Osswald, H., see Schmähl, D. 199, *230*
Oštádal, B., see Rychter, Z. 358, *369*
Ostertag, W., Kersten, W. 584, *591*
Ostrander, W.E., see Gale, G.R. 882, *888*
O'Sullivan, J.F., see Barry, V.C. 793, *805*, 841, *848*
Ôtake, N., Aizawa, S., Iidaka, T., Seto, H., Yonehara, H. 441, *455*
Otake, N., see Aizawa, S. 441, 444, *452*
Otsuji, N. 57, *62*
Ott, F., see Erlanger, F. 222, *225*
Overgaard-Hansen, K. 659, 663, *667*
Overgaard-Hansen, K., see Klenow, H. 663, *666*
Owen, A.A., see Bruchovsky, N. 59, *60*, 674, *688*
Owen, L.N., see Hawkins, R. 28, *32*
Owen, S.P., Dietz, A., Camiener, G.W. 565, *569*
Owen, S.P., Smith, C.G. 439, *455*
Owens, A.H., Jr., see Carbone, P.P. 394, *398*
Owens, A.H., Jr., see Condit, P.T. 474, *480*
Owens, A.H., Jr., see Fishbein, W.N. 521, *531*
Owens, A.H., Jr., see Koons, C.R. 621, *622*
Owens, A.H., Jr., see Steuart, C.D. 247, *255*, 265, *271*
Owens, A.H., Jr., see Uy, Q.L. 675, 682, *694*
Owens, F.J., see Roenigk, H.H. 475, *482*
Oxford, A.E., Raistrick, H., Simonet, P. 670, *692*
Oyama, V.I., see Eagle, H. 484, *504*
Oyen, T.B., Laland, S.G. 196, *229*

Pace, J., McDermott, E.E. 499, *508*
Pace, J., see Heathcote, J.G. 499, *505*
Pačes, V., Doskočil, J., Šorm, F. 362, *368*
Pačes, V., see Doskočil, J. 351, 361, *365*
Packard, D.S., Jr., see Skalko, R.G. 310, *344*
Padarathsingh, M., see Vadlamudi, S. 362, *371*
Padawer, J. 675, *692*
Padovec, J., see Kafka, V. 360, *367*
Page, A.R., Condie, R.M., Good, R.A. 384, *401*
Pagé, D., Posen, G., Stewart, T., Harris, J. 416, *423*
Pahl, H.B., Gordon, M.P., Ellison, R.R. 282, 283, *341*
Paine, K.W.E. 410, *423*
Painter, R.B., Goodman, M.G., Reisner, B.L. 326, *342*
Painter, R.B., see Rasmussen, R.E. 54, *62*
Pallanza, R., see Arioli, V. 883, *887*
Pallotta, D., see Berlowitz, L. 583, 584, *589*
Palm, P.E., Rogers, W.I., Yesair, D.W., Kensler, C.J. 824, *827*
Palm, P.E., see Coffey, J.J. 523, *530*, 800, 802, *805*
Palm, P.E., see Kensler, C.J. 822, 824, *827*
Palm, P.E., see Rogers, W.I. 219, *229*
Palme, G., see Liss, E. 25, *32*
Palmer, C.G. 300, *342*
Palmer, C.G., Warren, A.K., Simpson, P.J. 673, *692*
Palmer, D.L., Rifkind, D., Brown, D.W. 416, *423*

Palmer, S., see Koechlin, B. A. 201, 202, *227*
Palmer, W. M., Fridhandler, L. 860, *874*
Palmiter, R., Christensen, A. K., Schimke, R. T. 121, *134*
Panettiere, F., Coltman, C. A. 558, *569*
Panos, T. C., see Fisher, D. A. 811, *817*
Panzica, R. P., Robins, R. K., Townsend, L. B. 233, 234, *254*, 267, *270*
Papac, R. J., Calabresi, P., Hollingsworth, J. W., Welch, A. D. 236, 238, *254*
Papac, R. J., Creasey, W. A., Calabresi, P., Welch, A. D. 236, 238, *254*
Papac, R. J., see Creasey, W. A. 234, 238, 242, 244, *251*, 258, 259, *268*
Papanastassiou, Z. B., see Levins, P. L. 68, *81*
Papanicolaou, G. N., see Shorr, E. 143, *156*
Papirmeister, B., Davison, C. L. 13, *16*, 21, *33*
Papirmeister, B., Davison, C. L. 54, *62*
Papirmeister, B., Dorsey, J. K., Davidson, C. L., Gross, C. L. 13, *16*
Pappenheimer, A. M., Vance, M. J. 18, *33*
Pappenheimer, A. M., Jr., see Baseman, J. B. 561, *567*
Pappenheimer, A. M., Jr., see Collier, R. J. 561, *568*
Paran, M., see Wu, A. M. *669*
Padarathsingh, M., see Vadlamudi, S. 705, 706, *721*
Pardee, A. B. 25, *33*
Pardee, A. B., Prestidge, L. S. 513, 521, *535*
Pardee, A. B., see Budman, D. R. 290, *329*
Pardee, A. B., see Litman, R. M. 295, 296, 305, *339*
Parham, W. E., Wilbur, J. M., Jr. 39, *45*
Parisi, B., Soller, A. 606, *613*
Parisi, B., see Perani, A. 566, *569*
Parkes, A. S. 104, *134*
Parkin, I. L., Chiga, M. 59, *62*
Parks, R. E., Jr. 458, 459, 461, *467*
Parks, R. E., Jr., see Agarwal, K. C. 461, 464, *464*
Parks, R. E., Jr., see Agarwal, R. P. *464*
Parks, R. E., Jr., see Cha, S. 461, *465*
Parks, R. E., Jr., see Cohen, L. H. 461, *465*
Parks, R. E., Jr., see Goldberg, N. D. 201, *225*
Parks, R. E., Jr., see Heinrich, M. R. 463, *465*
Parks, R. E., Jr., see Kidder, G. W. 458, 459, 460, 463, *466*
Parks, R. E., Jr., see Kvam, D. C. 463, *466*
Parks, R. E., Jr., see Miech, R. P. 388, 394, 395, *401*, 461, *466*
Parks, R. E., Jr., see Mourad, N. 461, *467*
Parks, R. E., Jr., see Ross, A. F. 460, 461, *467*
Parks, R. E., Jr., see Roy, J. K. 463, *467*
Parks, R. E., Jr., see Scholar, E. M. 391, *402*
Parks, R. E., Jr., see Sheen, M. R. 444, 445, *455*
Parks, R. E., Jr., see Way, J. L. 460, 461, *467*
Parlow, A. 109, *134*
Parmerter, S. M., see Shelton, R. S. 105, *136*
Parodi, S., see Baldini, L. 237, *249*
Parodi, S., see Brambilla, G. 527, *530*, 705, *714*
Parry, N. T., see Recher, L. 583, *591*
Parsons, D. G., see Heidelberger, C. 196, *226*
Parsons, I. C., Mangan, F. R., Neal. G. R. 150, *155*
Parsons, L., see Lemon, H. E. 178, *190*
Partington, M., Fox, B. W., Jackson, H. 37, *45*
Partridge, M. W., see Arden, G. M. 517, *529*
Partridge, M. W., see Baldwin, R. W. 517, *530*
Parulekar, M. R., see Valadares, J. R. E. 124, 125, *137*
Paschkis, K. E., see Rutman, R. J. 193, *230*, 283, *343*
Pascoe, J. M., see Roberts, J. J. 14, *16*, *17*, 70, 76, 78, *83*, 837, *840*
Pasieka, A. E., Morgan, J. F. 485, *508*
Pasieka, A. E., see Morgan, J. F. 516, *534*
Passamani, E., see Elford, H. L. 793, *805*
Pasternak, B. S., see Rousselot, L. M. 221, *230*
Pasternak, C. A., Fischer, G. A., Handschumacher, R. E. 355, *368*
Pasternak, C. A., Handschumacher, R. E. 352, *368*
Pasternak, C. A., see Handschumacher, R. E. 352, 355, *366*
Pasternak, J., Samoiloff, M. R. 855, *874*
Pasternak, L. 78, *82*
Patel, A. B., see Hasselberger, F. X. 724, 735, *744*
Patel, D. G., see Gulati, O. D. 309, *334*
Paterson, A. R. P. 386, 391, 392, 394, *401*
Paterson, A. R. P., Hori, A. 393, *401*
Paterson, A. R. P., Moriwaki, A. 391, *401*
Paterson, A. R. P., Sutherland, A. 387, 397, *401*
Paterson, A. R. P., Wang, M. C. 386, 391, *401*
Paterson, A. R. P., see Caldwell, I. C. 386, *398*, 442, 444, *453*
Paterson, A. R. P., see Henderson, J. F. 442, 445, *453*
Paterson, A. R. P., see Tidd, D. M. 396, *403*
Paterson, A. R. P., see Wang, M. C. 391, *403*
Patkowski, J. 407, *423*
Patno, M. E., see Kuang, D. T. 638, 639, *640*
Patno, M. E., see Mizgerd, J. B. 546, *551*
Patrick, J. B., Williams, R. P., Meyer, W. E., Fulmor, W., Cosulich, D. B., Broschard, R. W., Webb, J. S. 48, *62*
Patrick, J. B., see Webb, J. S. 47, *64*
Patterson, E., see Haddow, A. L. 183, *189*
Patterson, J. A., see Benson, J. V., Jr. 697, *713*
Patterson, M. J. L., see Fairley, G. H. 759, *762*
Patterson, M. K., Jr. 711, *719*

Patterson, M. K., Jr., Conway, E., Whittle, W., McCoy, T. A. 696, *719*
Patterson, M. K., Jr., Maxwell, M. D. 709, *719*
Patterson, M. K., Jr., Maxwell, M. D., Conway, E. *535*, 712, *719*
Patterson, M. K., Jr., Orr, G. 491, *508*, 697, 711, 712, *719*, *720*
Patterson, M. K., Jr., Orr, G. R., Conway, E. 514, *535*
Patterson, M. K., Jr., Orr, G. R., McCoy, T. A. 697, *720*
Patterson, W. B., see Hall, T. C. 459, *465*
Patzschke, K., see Kleihues, P. 69, *81*
Paucker, K., Cantell, K. 607, *613*
Paul, A., see Riley, M. 279, *343*
Paul, J., Hagiwara, A. 206, 211, *229*
Pauling, L. 321, *342*
Paulsen, C. A., see Rosemberg, E. 139, *156*
Pauly, J. E., see Haus, E. 249, *252*
Pavan, M., Bo, G. 566, *569*
Pavan, M., see Brega, A. 566, *567*
Peabody, A. M., see Armstrong, J. G. 685, *688*
Peacock, A. C., see Dingman, C. W. 121, *128*
Peacock, A. C., see O'Malley, B. W. 121, *134*
Pearce, G. W., see Bradley, W. G. 686, *688*
Pearce, J. D., see Dutton, R. W. 310, *331*, 406, *420*
Pearce, M. B., Bulloch, R. T., Murphy, M. L. 560, *569*
Pearce, R. K., see Merker, P. C. 633, *641*
Pearlman, M. R. J., see Pearlman, W. H. 117, *134*
Pearlman, W. H., DeHertogh, R., Laumas, K. R., Pearlman, M. R. J. 117, *134*
Pearlman, W. H., see Huang, W. Y. 106, *130*
Pearson, C. M., see Levy, J. 407, *422*
Pearson, G. D., see Zimmerman, E. F. 464, *467*
Pearson, H. A., see Sunderman, C. R. 410, *424*
Pearson, H. E., see Visser, D. W. 377, 380, *382*
Pearson, O. H. 175, *191*
Pearson, O. H., Llerana, O., Llerana, L., Molina, A., Butler, T. P. 112, *134*
Pearson, O. H., Molina, A., Butler, T. P., Llerena, L., Nasr, H. 174, 183, *191*
Pearson, O. H., West, C. D., Li, M. C., McLean, J. P., Travis, N. 183, 184, *191*
Pearson, O. H., see Butler, T. P. 112, *127*
Pearson, O. H., see Sterental, A. 112, *136*, 174, *191*
Pearson, P. M., Kit, S., Dubbs, D. R. 246, *254*
Pease, J., see Holĕnberg, J. C. S. 712, *717*
Pecco, P., see Lajolo, D. *718*
Peck, R. M., Markey, F., Yudkin, M. D. 212, *229*
Pedersen, I. R., see Frederiksen, S. *669*
Peery, A., LePage, G. A. 388, *401*
Peets, L., see Kupfer, D. 813, *818*
Pegg, A. E. 775, *787*
Pegg, A. E., Corti, A., Williams-Ashman, H. G. 775, *787*
Pegg, A. E., Lockwood, D. H., Williams-Ashman, H. G. 148, *156*
Pegg, A. E., see Kay, J. E. 774, 775, *785*
Pegg, A. E., see Williams-Ashman, H. G. 148, *157*
Pěgřimová, E., see Havelka, S. 361, *367*
Pekar, A. H., see Frank, B. H. 699, 700, *716*
Pellegrino, J., see Katz, N. 879, *889*
Pellizzari, G. 877, *889*
Pena, A., Dvorkin, B., White, A. 89, *102*
Pénasse, L., see Hagemann, G. 497, *505*
Penco, S., see Arcamone, F. 593, *611*
Peng, C. T. 39, *45*
Peng, C. T., see Vodopick, H. 40, *46*
Penman, M., see Penman, S. 571, 573, 575, *580*, 664, *667*
Penman, S., Fan, H., Perlman, S., Rosbash, M., Weinberg, R., Zylber, E. 571, 575, *580*, 664, *667*
Penman, S., Rosbash, M., Penman, M. 571, 575, *580*, 664, *667*
Penman, S., Smith, I., Holtzman, E. 572, 578, *580*
Penman, S., Vesco, C., Penman, M. 573, 578, *580*
Penman, S., Vesco, C., Weinberg, R., Zylber, E. 571, *580*
Penman, S., see Abelson, H. T. 573, 574, 575, 576, 577, 579, *579*, 651, 653, *655*, *668*
Penman, S., see Abelson, H. T. 573, 574, 575, *579*
Penman, S., see Fan, H. 664, *665*
Penman, S., see Hirsh, M. 577, *579*
Penman, S., see Perlman, S. 575, 578, *580*, 664, *667*
Penman, S., see Price, R. 576, *580*
Penman, S., see Reichman, M. 574, *580*
Penman, S., see Siev, M. *581*, 664, *667*
Penman, S., see Weinberg, R. A. 572, 578, *581*
Penman, S., see Weinberg, R. 664, *668*
Penman, S., see Zylber, E. A. 664, *668*
Penman, S., see Zylber, E. 574, 577, *581*
Penn, I., Halgrimson, C. G., Starzl, T. E. 417, *423*
Penn, I., Makowski, E., Droegemueller, W., Halgrimson, C. G., Starzl, T. E. 415, *423*
Pennington, F. C., see Beereboom, J. J. 565, *567*
Pennington, S. N., see Hasselberger, F. X. 724, 735, *744*
Penny, R., see McLeod, J. G. 686, *692*
Peraino, C., see Pitot, H. C. 213, *229*
Perani, A., Parisi, B., DeCarli, L., Ciferri, O. 566, *569*
Perbasi, F., see Dusonchet, L. 608, *612*
Pereira da Silva, M., see DeBarros, T. 696, *715*

Perez, A. G., see Kim, J. H. 59, *61*, 299, *337*
Perez, A. G., see Kim, K. H. 603, 605, *613*
Perez, J., see Colsky, J. 500, *504*
Periera, H. G., see Kjellen, L. 302, 307, *338*
Perin, A., see De-Angeli, L. C. 697, *715*
Perings, E., see Eberle, P. 415, *420*
Perings, E., see Hunstein, W. 409, *421*
Perkins, E. S., Wood, R. M., Sears, M. L., Prusoff, W. H., Welch, A. D. 302, 322, *342*
Perkins, H. R., see Rogers, H. J. 201, *229*
Perkins, J. P., Hillcoat, B. L., Bertino, J. R. 469, *482*
Perkins, J. P., see Fox, B. W. 289, 315, 318, *333*
Perlia, C. P., see Ream, N. W. 621, *622*
Perlia, C. P., see Rossof, A. H. 839, *840*
Perlík, F., see Rašková, H. *369*
Perlman, S., Abelson, H. T., Penman, S. 575, 578, *580*
Perlman, S., Penman, S. 664, *667*
Perlman, S., see Penman, S. 571, 575, *580*, 664, *667*
Perlman, S., see Zylber, E. A. 664, *668*
Perper, R. J., Alvarez, B., Colombo, C., Schroder, H. 408, *423*
Perrin, J., Mauer, A. 477, *482*
Perrone, F., see DeBarbieri, A. 528, *531*
Perry, R. P. 572, 573, *580*, 583, *591*
Perry, R. P., Greenberg, J. R., Tartof, K. D. 571, *580*
Perry, R. P., Kelley, D. E. 571, 573, *580*
Perry, R. P., see Schochetman, G. 246, *255*
Perry, S., see Breitman, T. R. 280, *328*
Person, D. A., Sheridan, P. J., Herrmann, E. C. 302, 307, *342*
Person, S., see Osborn, M. 11, *16*
Peruzzotti, G., see Rosi, D. 879, *889*
Pesendorfer, F., see Deutsch, E. 709, *715*, 734, 735, *744*
Pestka, S. 554, *569*
Petering, D. H. 841, 845, 846, *848*
Petering, D. H., see Van Giessen, G. J. 843, 844, 845, 847, *849*
Petering, H. G., Buskirk, H. H. 841, 842, *848*
Petering, H. G., Buskirk, H. H., Crim, J. A. 841, 843, 844, *848*, *849*
Petering, H. G., Buskirk, H. H., Crim, J. A., Van Giessen, G. J. 841, 843, *849*
Petering, H. G., Buskirk, H. H., Kupiecki, F. 843, *849*
Petering, H. G., Buskirk, H. H., Underwood, G. E. 841, 842, 843, *849*
Petering, H. G., Van Giessen, G. J. 844, 845, 847, *849*
Petering, H. G., Van Giessen, G. J., Crim, J. A., Buskirk, H. H. 842, *849*
Petering, H. G., see Buskirk, H. H. 24, *31*, 237, *250*, 525, *530*
Petering, H. G., see Crim, J. A. 844, *848*
Petering, H. G., see Johnston 843
Petering, H. G., see Van Giessen, G. J. 843, 844, 845, 847, *849*
Peterkofsky, B., Tomkins, G. M. 241, *254*
Peters, E. L., Tower, D. B. 499, *508*
Peters, E. L., see Tower, D. B. 698, 700, 703, *721*
Peters, J. H., Lin, S. C., Berridge, B. J., Jr., Chao, W. R., Cummings, J. G. 697, *720*
Peters, P. C., see Prager, M. D. 733, *746*
Peters, R. A., see Líebecq, C. 193, *228*
Peterson, E. R., see Hirschberg, E. 460, *465*
Peterson, L. J., see Michaels, R. M. 841, *848*
Peterson, M., see Schjeide, O. A. 120, *135*
Peterson, R., see Capizzi, R. L. 725, 726, 733, 734, *743*
Peterson, R. E., Ciegler, A. 697, 698, *720*
Peterson, R. G., Handschumacher, R. E., Mitchell, M. S. 705, *720*, 735, 738, *746*
Petranyi, G., see Nagy, G. 36
Petropoulas, P., see Druckrey, H. 78, *80*
Petty, L. G., see McEwan, A. 418, *422*
Peyk, D., see Wunderlich, F. 674, *694*
Pfau, C. J., see Buck, L. L. 354, *364*
Pfeiffer, S. E., Tolmach, L. J. 674, *692*
Pfitzner, K. E., Moffatt, J. G. 275, *342*
Philips, F. S., Sternberg, S. S., Hamilton, L. D., Clarke, D. A. 389, 394, *401*
Philips, F. S., see Clarke, D. A. 396, *398*
Philips, F. S., see Gilman, A. 18, *31*
Philips, F. S., see Lenaz, L. 233, 241, *253*
Philips, F. S., see Oettgen, H. F. 696, *719*, 723, 727, 730, 733, 734, *745*
Philips, F. S., see Schwartz, H. S. 47, 48, *62*, 790, *792*
Philips, F. S., see Sternberg, S. S. 36, 37, *46*, 609, *613*
Philipson, L., Wall, R., Glickman, G., Darnell, J. E. *580*, 664, *667*
Philipson, L., see Darnell, J. E. 574, 575, *579*, 664, *665*
Philipson, L., see Jelinek, W. *669*
Phillips, A. W., see Boyd, J. W. 697, 704, *714*
Phillips, D. M., see Phillips, S. G. 583, *591*
Phillips, J. G., see Bellamy, D. 96, *100*
Phillips, M., see Ablondi, F. B. 527, *529*
Phillips, S., see Osborn, M. 11, *16*
Phillips, S. G., Phillips, D. M. 583, *591*
Phillips, S. M., see Hirsch, M. S. 418, *421*
Phillips-Quagliata, J. M., see Floersheim, G. L. 752, *762*
Phillipps, M. A., see Barclay, R. K. 487, 489, 491, 496, *503*

Phoenix, C.H., see Resko, J. A. 149, *156*
Piccinni, E., see Levis, A.G. 22, *32*
Pickren, J.W., see Costa, G. 451, *453*
Picone, M.A., Traine, A. 608, *613*
Pidacks, C., see Webb, J.S. 47, *64*
Piekarski, L.J., see Kit, S. 56, *61*
Piekarski, L.J., see Kit, S. 298, *338*
Piepho, S.B., see Kreis, W. 758, *763*
Pierce, J.V., see Kaufman, B.T. 469, *481*
Pierce, M.I., see Sullivan, M.P. 397, *403*
Pierre, K.J., Kimball, A.P., LePage, G.A. 387, 388, *402*
Pierre, K.J., LePage, G.A. 387, *402*, 445, *455*
Piesach, Aisen, Blumberg *849*
Pietrzykowska, I., Shugar, D. 293, *342*
Pietsch, P. 851, 852, 853, 854, 855, 858, 860, 861, 862, 866, 867, 868, 869, *874*
Pietsch, P., Clapper, G. 855, 858, 863, 871, *874*
Pietsch, P., Corbett, C. 858, 863, *874*
Pietsch, P., Corbett, C., Briden, D.W., Jewett, G. 855, 871, *874*
Pietsch, P., Eng, R. 851, 853, 855, 860, 861, *874*
Pietsch, P., Garrett, H. 859, 862, 863, 864, 865, 866, 869, *874*
Pietsch, P., Gorman 868, 869
Pietsch, P., McCollister, S. B. 857, 858, 860, 871, *874*
Pietsch, P., see Corbett, C. 871
Pietsch, P., see Gorman, T. 867, *872*
Pihl, B., see Aronsen, K.F. 410, *419*
Pike, D., see Boch, M. 650, *655*
Pilcher, K.S., Soike, K.F., Smith, V.H., Trosper, F., Folston, B. 515, *535*
Pillero, S.J., see Medici, P. T. 38, *45*
Pina, M., see Green, M. *334*
Pindell, M.H., see Bradner, W.T. 855, 869, 870, *871*
Pine, E.K. 495, *508*
Pine, M.J., DiPaolo, J.A. 776, 777, *787*
Pine, M.J., Harzewski, E., Wissler, F.C. 820, 823, 824, *827*
Pinkel, D., see Farber, S. 394, *399*
Pinnet, S., see Dubost, M. 593, *612*
Pinsky, C.M., Mitchell, S., Oettgen, H.F., Schwartz, M.K. 735, 738, *746*
Pinsky, L., Krooth, R.S. 352, *368*
Pinto-Machado, J. 39, *45*
Pirofsky, B., see Reid, R.H. 417, *423*
Pískala, A., Šorm, F. 351, *368*
Pískala, A., see Šorm, F. 351, 362, *370*
Pispa, J., see Holtta, E. 775, *785*
Pister, L., see Schäfer, W. *369*
Pitaro, R., see Benezra, D. 706, *713*, 735, 738, *743*
Pitha, J., see Beránek, J. 349, *364*
Pitot, H.C., Peraino, C. 213, *229*
Pitot, H.C., see Čihák, A. 213, *224*, 363, *365*
Pitot, H.C., see Wilkinson, D.S. 206, 207, 210, 211, 213, *231*, 574, *581*
Pittard, J., see Gibson, F. 492, *505*
Pittillo, R.F., Bennett, L.L., Jr., Short, W.A., Tomisek, A.J., Dixon, G.J., Thomson, J.R., Laster, W.R., Jr., Trader, M., Mettil, L., Allan, P., Bowdon, B., Shabel, F., Jr., Skipper, H.E. 820, *827*
Pittillo, R.F. 492, *508*
Pittillo, R.F., Hunt, D.E. 234, *254*, 485, *508*
Pittillo, R.F., Narkates, A. J., Burns, J. 79, *82*, 494, *508*
Pittillo, R.F., Quinnelly, B. G. 492, *508*
Pittillo, R.F., Ray, B.J. 201, *229*
Pittillo, R.F., Schabel, F. M., Jr., Skipper, H.E. 20, *33*
Pittillo, R.F., see Brockman, R.W. 496, *503*
Pittillo, R.F., see Hunt, D. E. *252*
Pittillo, R.F., see Narkates, A.J. 494, *508*
Pitts, J., Sinsheimer, R.L. 855, 857, 860, *874*
Pizer, L.I., Cohen, S.S. 237, *254*
Pizer, L.I., see Tosa, T. 525, *537*
Plagemann, P.G. 662, 663, *667*
Plagemann, P.G.W., Renner, E.D. 91, *102*
Plagemann, P.G.W., see Korbecki, M. 354, *367*
Plager, J.E., see Matsui, N. 91, *102*
Plamer, K.H., see Wall, M. E. 649, *656*
Plant, J.E., Roberts, J.J. 77, *82*
Plant, J.E., see Roberts, J. J. 14, *16*, 70, 76, 78, *83*
Plaut, W.J., see Camargo, E.P. 583, *590*
Plattner, P.A. 747, *764*
Platz, B.B., see Chadwick, M. 881, *888*
Plenderleith, I.H., see Johns, D.G. 472, 473, *481*
Plentl, A.A., see Brown, G. B. 458, *465*
Pleven, E., see Duschinsky, R. 195, *225*
Pleven, E., see Heidelberger, C. 193, 198, *226*
Plevová, J., Janků, I., Šeda, M. 358, *368*
Plevová, J., Šeda, M., Janků, I. 359, *368*
Plevová, J., see Myška, V. 360, *368*
Pliml, J., Prystaš, M., Šorm, F. 349, *368*
Pliml, J., Šorm, F. 350, 351, *368*
Plowright, W., MacAdam, R.F., Armstrong, J.A. 302, *342*
Pocchiari, F., see De-Angeli, L.C. 697, *715*
Pochon, F., see Massoulie, J. A. 279, 293, *340*
Poddar, R.K., see Tessman, I. 11, *17*, 296, 297, *345*
Podobed, O.V., Leitin, V.L., Brykina, E.V., Mant'eva, V.L., Lerman, M.I. *669*
Podratz, K.C., Katzman, P. A. 162, *168*

Podratz, K.C., see Katzman, P.A. 160, *167*
Podrebarac, E.G., Cheng, C. C. 768, *787*
Podrebarac, E.G., Nyberg, W.H., French, F.A., Cheng, C.C. 768, *787*
Podrebarac, E.G., see Baiocchi, F. 768, *783*
Pogo, A.O., see Allfrey, V. G. 89, *100*
Pogo, A.O., see Cornudella, L. *669*
Pogo, B.G.T., see Allfrey, V. G. 89, *100*
Pokorná, Z., see Nouza, K. 356, *368*
Pokorný, V., see Gichner, T. 78, *80*
Pol, C., see Arcamone, F. 593, *611*
Polanský, F., see Rašková, H. *369*
Poledne, R., see Grafnetterová, J. 356, *366*
Pomaskova, F.A., see Brachnikova, M.G. 593, *611*
Pontis, H., Degerstedt, G., Reichard, P. 315, 318, *342*, 352, *368*
Pool, J.L., see Hirschberg, E. 460, *465*
Poore, G.A., see Svoboda, G.H. 881, *890*
Poore, G.A., see Sweeney, M.J. 446, 451, *456*
Poore, G.A., see Williams, R.H. 446, *457*
Popper, H., De la Huerga, J., Yesinick, C. 522, *535*
Porath, J., see Kristiansen, T. *717*
Pories, W.J., see McQuitty, J.T. 844, *848*
Porschen, W., Feinendegen, L. 315, *342*
Porter, D.G. 158, *168*
Porter, K.A., see Starzl, T. E. 410, *424*
Porter, K.R. 676, *692*
Porter, K.R., see Ledbetter, M.C. 676, *691*
Posen, G., see Pagé, D. 416, *423*
Post, J., Hoffman, J. 313, 316, *342*
Post, J., see Hoffman, J. 313, *335*
Postel, A.H., see Harris, M. N. 638, *640*
Potee, K.G., see Hall, T.C. 459, *465*
Potter, R.L., Nygaard, O.F. 314, 318, *342*
Potter, V.R. 280, 314, *342*, 522, *535*
Potter, V.R., see Butcher, F.R. *669*
Potter, V.R., see De Verdier, C.H. 291, 318, *331*
Potter, V.R., see Ives, D.H. 285, *336*
Potter, V.R., see Morse, P. A. 217, *228*
Potter, V.R., see Stone, J.E. 274, *345*
Powell, C.A., see Drummond, G.I. 438, *453*
Powell, D. 416, *423*
Powell, E., see Dethlefsen, L.A. 314, 315, *331*
Powell, R.G., Weisleder, D., Smith, C.R., Jr., Wolff, I.A. 556, *569*
Poynter, R.W. 28, *33*
Prager, M.D., Bachynsky, N. 711, *720*
Prager, M.D., Derr, I. 705, 707, *720*
Prager, M.D., Peters, P.C., Janes, J.O., Derr, I. 733, *746*
Prager, M.D., see Roberts, J. 698, 705, *720*
Pratt, C.B., Holton, C.P. 726, 727, 734, 735, *746*
Pratt, C.B., Johnson, W.W. 734, *746*
Pratt, C.B., see Aur, R.J.A. 726, 732, 734, 735, *742*
Pratt, D., Stent, G.S. 297, *342*
Pratt, O.E., see Daniel, P. M. 314, *330*
Pratt, W.B., Aronow, L. 87, 88, *102*
Pratt, W.B., Edelman, S., Aronow, L. 90, *102*
Pratt, W.B., see Gray, J.G. 91, *100*
Pratt, W.B., see Hackney, J.F. 97, 98, 99, *100*
Pravdina, N.F., Lysenko, A. M., Linevich, Yu.G., Galegov, G.A. 354, *368*
Preedy, J.R.K., see Brown, J.H.U. 815, *817*
Preiss, J., Handler, P. 491, *508*
Preiss, J., see Spencer, R.L. 491, *510*
Prensky, W., see Hofer, K. G. 314, 315, 316, 317, *335*
Pressman, B.C. 776, *787*
Pressman, D., see Kitano, M. 768, *785*
Prestidge, L.S., see Pardee, A.B. 513, 521, *535*
Prestley, W.F., see Nichols, J. *818*
Preud Homme, J., see Dubost, M. 593, *612*
Preussel, B., Etzold, G., Barwolf, D., Langen, P. 289, *342*
Preussel, B., see Etzold, G. 289, 290, *332*
Preussel, B., see Langen, P. 289, *339*
Preussmann, R., Druckrey, H., Ivankovic, S., Hodenberg, A.v. 70, *82*
Preussmann, R., Hodenberg, A.v. 71, *82*, 547, *551*
Preussmann, R., Hodenberg, A.v., Hengy, H. 71, *82*, 547, *551*
Preussmann, R., see Druckrey, H. 70, *80*
Přibíková, V., see Rašková, H. 361, *369*
Price, C.C. 1, 3, *5*, 19, *33*
Price, C.C., Gaucher, G.M., Koneru, P., Shibakawa, R., Sowa, J.R., Yamaguchi, M. 1, 5, *5*, 19, 26, *33*
Price, C.C., Yamaguchi, M., Sowa, J.R., Rao, K.P., Gaucher, G.M., Shibakawa, R. 1, *5*
Price, C.C., see Sowa, J.R. 2, *5*
Price, D., see Moore, C.R. 143, *155*
Price, K.E., Bradner, W.T., Buck, R.E., Lein, J. 862, *874*
Price, K.E., Buck, R.E., Lein, J. 855, *874*
Price, K.E., Buck, R.E., Schlein, A., Siminoff, P. 496, *508*
Price, R., Penman, S. 576, *580*
Price, V.E., see Greenstein, J.P. 698, *716*
Pridham, T.G., see Smale, B.C. 855, *874*
Přikryl, J., see Buděšínský, Z. 196, *223*
Prince, H.N., see Grunberg, E. 558, 560, *568*, 642, *647*, 747, 748, 749, *762*
Pringle, C.R. 363, *368*
Printz, M.P., von Hippel, P. H. 869, *874*
Privat de Garilke, M., see Boissier, J.R. 430, *432*

Pronczuk, A. W., see Baliga, B.S. 561, 564, *567*
Prough, R., Wittkop, J., Reed, D.J. 751, 754, *764*
Prough, R., see Wittkop, J.A. 754, *765*
Prusiner, S., Milner, L. 697, *720*
Prusoff, W.A., see Mathias, A.P. 280, 295, 298, *340*
Prusoff, W.H. 272, 273, 278, 280, 283, 291, 292, 295, 301, 314, 315, 321, 322, 323, 324, *342*, *369*, *806*
Prusoff, W.H., Bakhle, Y. S., McCrea, J.F. 289, 293, 302, 303, 304, 305, *342*
Prusoff, W.H., Bakhle, Y. S., Sekely, L. 292, 302, *342*
Prusoff, W.H., Chang, P.K. 282, 287, *342*
Prusoff, W.H., Holmes, W. L., Welch, A.D. *342*
Prusoff, W.H., Jaffe, J.J., Gunther, H. 282, 283, 313, 316, *342*
Prusoff, W.H., see Bakhle, Y.S. 273, 281, 285, 287, 301, 314, 315, *327*
Prusoff, W.H., see Calabresi, P. 238, *250*, 302, 323, *329*
Prusoff, W.H., see Cramer, J.W. 291, *330*
Prusoff, W.H., see Cysyk, R. 281, 320, 322, 325, *330*
Prusoff, W.H., see Delamore, I.W. 285, 301, *331*
Prusoff, W.H., see Diwan, A. 282, 287, *331*
Prusoff, W.H., see Fox, B. W. 287, 289, 314, 315, 316, 317, 318, *333*
Prusoff, W.H., see Gaito, R. A. 318, *333*
Prusoff, W.H., see Goz, B. 194, 199, *225*, 305, 306, 322, 324, 325, *334*
Prusoff, W.H., see Huebner, R.J. 308, *336*
Prusoff, W.H., see Jaffe, J. J. 300, 301, *336*
Prusoff, W.H., see Perkins, E.S. 302, 322, *342*
Prusoff, W.H., see Rupp, W. D. 319, 320, 321, *343*
Prusoff, W.H., see Sekely, L. 282, *344*
Prusoff, W.H., see Voytek, P. 281, 285, 286, 287, 302, 325, *346*
Prusoff, W.H., see Welch, A.D. 282, 283, 284, 314, 316, 319, 324, *346*
Prystaš, M., Gut, J., Šorm, F. 349, *369*
Prystaš, M., Šorm, F. 273, *342*, 349, 350, *369*
Prystaš, M., see Pliml, J. 349, *368*
Puca, G.A., Bresciani, F. 114, 117, *134*
Puca, G.A., see DeSombre, E.R. 115, 117, *127*
Puck, T.T., see Kao, F.-T. 78, *81*
Pütter, J. 704, 705, *720*
Pugh, L.H., Gerber, N.N. 660, *667*
Pugh, L.H., Lechevalier, H. A., Solotorovsky, M. 660, *667*
Pugh, R.P., see Bateman, J.R. 221, *223*
Pujman, V., Sandberg, J., Howsden, L., Goldin, A. 196, *229*
Pullman, A., see Pullman, B. 294, *342*, 541, *543*
Pullman, B., Pullman, A. 294, *342*, 541, *543*
Purple, J.R., see Burchenal, J.H. 779, *783*, 820, *826*
Purves, H.D., Griesbach, W. 171, *191*
Puschendorf, B., Wolf, H., Grunicke, H. 29, *33*
Puszkin, E., Puszkin, S., Aledort, L.M. *692*
Puszkin, S., see Puszkin, E. *692*
Putnam, R.C., see Magill, G. B. 500, *507*
Putter, J. 724, *746*
Putter, J., Gehrman, G. *746*

Quadracci, L.J., Hellström, I.E., Striker, G.E., Marchioro, T.L., Hellström, K.E. 416, *423*
Quaglino, D., see Storti, E. 408, *424*, 726, 727, 728, 730, 735, *746*
Quarck, U.C., see Barker, S. A. 493, *503*
Quastel, J.H., see Ilan, J. 679, 681, *690*
Quick, J., see Danishefsky, S. 650, *655*
Quilico, A., see Cardani, C. 566, *567*
Quinn, R.P., Elion, G.B. 410, *423*
Quinn, R.P., see Makinodan, T. 201, *228*, 525, *534*, 752, *763*
Quinnelly, B.G., see Pittillo, R.F. 492, *508*
Quintrell, N., see Levinson, W.E. 307, *339*
Quintrell, N., see McDonnell, J.P. 583, *591*, *613*

Raabes, S., see Druckrey, H. 180, *189*
Raaflaub, J., Schwartz, D. E. 754, *764*
Rabinovitz, M., Fisher, J.M. 498, *508*, 518, *535*
Rabinovitz, M., McGrath, H. 524, *535*
Rabinovitz, M., Olson, M.E., Greenberg, D.M. 485, 497, 499, *508*, *509*, 524, *535*
Rabinovitz, M., Tuve, R.K. 518, *535*
Rabinovitz, M., see Smulson, M.E. 524, *536*
Rabinowitz, J.C. 106, *134*
Rabinowitz, J.C., Dowben, R.M. 106, *134*
Rabinowitz, K.W., Shada, J.D., Wood, W.A. 440, *455*
Rabinowitz, M., see Goldberg, I.H. 352, *366*, 583, 585, *590*
Rabinowitz, M., see Reich, E. 585, *592*
Rada, B. 355, *369*
Rada, B., Altanerová, V. 355, *369*
Rada, B., Blaškovič, D. 302, 306, *342*, 354, *369*
Rada, B., Blaškovič, D., Šorm, F., Škoda, J. 354, *369*
Rada, B., Gregušová, V. 354, *369*
Rada, B., Hanušovská, T. 355, *369*
Rada, B., Shatkin, A.J. 354, *369*
Rada, B., Smidová, V., Závada, J. 354, *369*
Rada, B., Závada, J. 354, *369*
Rada, B., see Falke, D. 354, *365*
Rada, B., see Jasińska, S. 354, *367*
Radding, C.M. 634, *641*

Radunz, H., see Boch, M. 650, *655*
Radunz, H., see Winterfeldt, E. 650, *656*
Räihä, N.C.R., see Kekomäki, M. 516, *532*
Raggio, J.R., see Skalko, R. G. 310, *344*
Rahiala, E.L., see Kekomäki, M. 516, *532*
Rahman, A., Wilson, H.R. 279, *343*
Raina, A. 148, *156*
Raina, A., Janne, J., Siimes, M. 774, *787*
Raina, P.N., Rosen, F. 94, *102*
Rainisio, C., see Morasca, L. 684, *692*
Raistrick, H., see Birkinshaw, J.H. 446, *453*
Raistrick, H., see Oxford, A.E. 670, *692*
Rakieten, M.L., see Rakieten, N. 860, 861, *874*
Rakieten, N., Nadkarni, M.V., Rakieten, M.L., Gordon, B.S. 860, 861, *874*
Rakieten, N., see Schein, P. S. 704, 710, *720*
Rall, D.P., see Adamson, R. H. 682, 683, *687*
Rall, D.P., see Field, M. 771, 774, *784*
Rall, D.P., see Fishbein, W. N. 521, *531*
Rall, D.P., see Frei, E., III. 679, *690*
Rall, D.P., see Loo, T.L. 65, 69, *82*
Rall, D.P., see Rubin, R.C. 472, *482*
Rall, D.P., see Schein, P.S. 704, 710, *720*
Rall, D.P., see Shapiro, W. R. 69, *83*
Ramadan, M.A., see Greenberg, D.M. 501, *505*
Ramakrishnan, T., see Jayaram, H.N. 697, 698, 699, *717*
Ramakrishnan, T., see Reddy, V.V.S. 697, 698, 699, *720*
Ramanna, M.S., Natarajan, A.T. 41, *45*
Ramanna, M.S., see Natarajan, A.T. 41, *45*
Rama Reddy, G.V., Goulian, M., Hendler, S.S. 242, 243, *254*
Ramirez, G., see Ansfield, F. J. 219, 221, *223*
Ramirez, G., see Skibba, J. L. 545, 546, 547, *552*
Ramirez, G., see Weiss, A.J. *511*
Ramirez, V.D., see McCann, S.M. 109, *133*
Ramseier, L., see Schindler, R.L. 41, *46*
Ramseier, L., see Schindler, R. 294, *344*
Randerson, S., see Heidelberger, C. 198, 204, 217, *226*
Ranki, M., Kääriäinen, L. 515, *535*
Rao, B.G., see Heard, R.D. 106, *130*
Rao, B.R., see Wiest, W.G. 162, *169*
Rao, C.R., see Korenman, S.G. 115, *132*
Rao, K.R. 756, *764*
Rao, K.V. 439, *455*, 486, *509*
Rao, K.V., Biemann, D., Woodward, R.B. 633, *641*
Rao, K.V., Brooks, S.C., Kugelman, M., Romano, A.A. 486, 496, *509*
Rao, K.V., Cullen, W.P. 633, *641*
Rao, S.R.V., see Arora, O. P. 57, *60*
Rao, S.S., Grollman, A.P. 561, *570*
Rapp, F. 302, *343*
Rapp, F., Butel, J.S., Feldman, L.A., Kitahara, T., Melnick, J.L. 302, 303, 304, *343*
Rapp, F., Melnick, J.L., Kitahara, T. 302, 304, 307, *343*
Rapp, F., Vanderslice, D. 302, 303, 304, *343*
Rapp, F., see Feldman, L.A. 237, *251*
Rapp, F., see Melnick, J.L. *228*, 302, 307, *340*
Rapp, F., see Nutter, R.L. 244, *254*
Rapp, F., see Tevethia, F. 855, 857, 859, 865, *875*
Rappel, M., Brihaye, J. 324, *343*
Raška, K., Jurovčík, M., Šormová, Z., Šorm, F. 351, 362, *369*
Raška, K., Jr., Zedeck, M.S., Welch, A.D. 357, *369*
Raška, K., Jr., see Jurovčík, M. 362, *367*, 574, *579*
Raška, K., see Šorm, F. 351, *370*
Raška, K., Jr., see Svatá, M. 363, *371*
Raskin, B.K., see Lerner, L.J. 123, *132*
Rašková, H., Elis, J. *369*
Rašková, H., Elis, J., Gutová, M., Nižňanská, J., Mikulecký, Z., Kubíčková, V., Borč, K., Přibíková, V., Hulínský, K., Kantner, V., Belsan, I., Kůta, A., Erbertová, B., Kleibel, K., Seyček, V., Duchková, H. 361, *369*
Rašková, H., Elis, J., Perlík, F., Polanský, F., Slavík, M. *369*
Rašková, H., see Čerey, K. 350, *364*
Rašková, H., see Elis, J. 350, 360, 361, *365*
Rašková, H., see Gutová, M. 357, *366*
Rašková, H., see Myška, V. 360, *368*
Rašková, H., see Novotný, J. 349, *368*
Rašková, H., see Slavík, M. *370*
Rasmussen, A.H., see Frederiksen, S. 660, 661, *665*
Rasmussen, R.E., Painter, R.B. 54, *62*
Ratuschni, A., see Southren, A.L. 811, 813, *818*
Ratych, O.T., see Kirschbaum, J. 700, *717*
Rau, J., see Lingens, F. 70, *82*
Rauen, H.M., Haar, H., Unterberg, W. 820, 823, *827*
Rauen, H.M., Noroth, K., Unterberg, W. 820, 823, *827*
Rauenbusch, E., Bauer, K., Kaufmann, W., Wagner, O. 698, 702, *720*, 723, *746*
Rauenbusch, E., Irion, E., Arens, A. 699, 700, *720*
Rauenbusch, E., see Arens, A. 698, 699, 702, 703, *713*
Rauenbusch, E., see Wagner, O. 698, *721*
Rausen, A.R., Glidewell, O. J. 726, 730, 732, 735, 738, *746*
Rauth, A.M. 52, *62*
Ravel, J.M., McCord, T.J., Skinner, C.G., Shive, W. 497, *509*

Ravel, J.M., Norton, S.J., Humphreys, J.S., Shive, W. 697, *720*
Ravel, J.M., see Edelson, J. 524, *531*
Ravel, J.M., see McCord, T. J. 497, *507*, *534*
Ravel, J.M., see Skinner, C. G. 497, *510*
Ravin, L.S., Simpson, C.A., Zappala, A.F. 275, *343*
Ravin, L.J., Simpson, C.A., Zappala, A.F., Gulesich, J.J. 275, *343*
Rawls, W.F., Cohen, R.A., Herrmann, E.C. 302, *343*
Ray, B.J., see Pittillo, R.F. 201, *229*
Ray, P.D., Foster, D.O., Lardy, H.A. 521, *535*
Ray, P.D., Hanson, R.L. 521, *535*
Ray, W.J., Jr., see Miner, N. 607, *613*
Rayford, P.L., see Ross, G. T. 160, *168*
Raynaud, J.P., see Baulieu, E.E. 115, *126*
Raynaud-Jammet, M., Baulieu, E.E. 119, *134*
Raynaud-Jammet, M., see Baulieu, E.E. 115, *126*
Reagan, R.L., see Hart, M. M. 811, *818*
Ream, N.W., Perlia, C.P., Wolter, J., Taylor, S. G.III. 621, *622*
Reaume, M.G., see Dunnebacke, T.H. 306, *331*
Recher, L., Briggs, I.G., Parry, N.T. 583, *591*
Rector, W.D., see Hilf, R. 124, *130*
Rector, W.D., see Hilf, R. 124, *130*
Reddi, A.H., see Williams-Ashman, H.G. 115, 118, *138*, 146, 150, *157*
Reddy, G.V.R., Goulian, M., Hendler, S.S. 660, *667*
Reddy, J., see Svoboda, D. 589, *592*
Reddy, V.V.S., Jayaram, H.N., Sirsi, M., Ramakrishnan, T. 697, 698, 699, *720*
Redetzki, H.M., Alvarez-O'Bourke, F. 541, *543*
Redon, H. 870, *874*
Redshaw, M.R., Follet, B. K., Nicholls, T.J. 120, *135*
Redshaw, M.R., see Follett, B.K. 120, 121, *128*
Reed, D.J. 754, *764*
Reed, D.J., Dost, F.N. 754, *764*
Reed, D.J., see Dost, F.N. 755, *762*
Reed, D.J., see Prough, R. 751, 754, *764*
Reed, D.J., see Wittkop, J. A. 754, *765*
Reed, M.L., see Vaitkevicius, V.K. 673, *694*
Reekmans, M., see Moutschen, J. 42, *45*
Reel, J.R., Lee, S., Callantine, M.R. 158, *168*
Rees, K.R., Rowland, G.F., Varcoe, J.S. 824, *827*
Rees, K.R., see Crook, L.E. 573, *579*
Reese, W.N., see Saunders, G.F. 627, 628, *632*
Reeve, T.S., see Vincent, P. C. 59, *63*
Reeves, J.Y., see Schwartz, J.H. 697, 698, *721*
Reeves, W.J., see Jacobs, E. M. 220, *226*
Regade, I.S., see Gellert, E. 564, *568*
Regan, J.D., Vodopick, H., Takeda, S., Lee, W.H., Faulcon, F.M. 525, *535*
Rege, V.B., see Leone, L.A. 477, *481*
Regelson, W., Holland, J.F. 769, 772, *787*
Regelson, W., Holland, J.F., Talley, R.W. 843, *849*
Regelson, W., see Munson, A.E. 884, *889*
Regelson, W., see Wampler, G.L. 885, *890*
Reggiani, M., see Calendi, E. 598, 599, *611*
Reich, E. 583, *591*
Reich, E., Cerami, A., Ward, D.C. 573, *580*
Reich, E., Franklin, R.M. 53, 54, 58, *62*
Reich, E., Franklin, R.M. Shatkin, A.J., Tatum, E.L. 582, 583, 584, *591*
Reich, E., Goldberg, I.H. 582, 583, 585, *592*, 626, *632*
Reich, E., Goldberg, I.H., Rabinowitz, M. 585, *592*
Reich, E., see Acs, G. 436, 437, 438, 439, *452*
Reich, E., see Cerami, A. 585, *590*
Reich, E., see Darlix, J.L. 462, *465*
Reich, E., see Gibson, F. 492, *505*
Reich, E., see Goldberg, I. H. 585, *590*
Reich, E., see Hamilton, L. 586, *590*
Reich, E., see Shatkin, A.H. 54, *62*
Reich, E., see Uretsky, S.C. 437, 438, *456*
Reich, E., see Ward, D.C. 437, 438, 441, 442, 443, *456*, *457*, 462, 463, *467*, 602, *614*, 625, 626, 629, *632*
Reich, E., see Wiesner, R. 583, *592*
Reichard, P. 446, *455*
Reichard, P., Cannalakis, Z. N., Cannalakis, E.S. 243, *254*
Reichard, P., Estborn, B. 318, *343*
Reichard, P., Sköld, O., Klein, G., Revesz, L., Magnusson, P.H. 217, *229*
Reichard, P., see Bertani, L.E. 277, *328*
Reichard, P., see Brown, N. C. 790, *791*
Reichard, P., see Krakoff, I. H. 790, *791*
Reichard, P., see Larsson, A. 243, *253*
Reichard, P., see Nordenskjöld, B.A. 242, *254*
Reichard, P., see Pontis, H. 315, 318, *342*, 352, *368*
Reichelt, P., see Hilscher, W. 753, *762*
Reichert, M., Wollert, U. 781, *787*
Reichman, M., Karlan, D., Penman, S. 574, *580*
Reid, B.D., Walker, I.G. 14, *16*
Reid, D.E., see Murray, J.E. 415, *422*
Reid, M.R., see Tomisek, A. J. 487, 488, 496, *511*
Reid, R.H., Pirofsky, B., Dawson, P.J. 417, *423*
Reilly, H.C. 500, *509*
Reilly, H.C., see Clarke, D.A. 391, *398*, 500, 501, *504*
Reilly, H.C., see Kaplan, L. H. 492, 494, 495, *506*
Reilly, H.C., see Magill, G. B. 500, *507*
Reilly, P., see Hughes, W.L. 280, 281, 283, 284, 314, 315, 316, *336*

Reimer, Yoshida 53
Reineke, L.M., see Li, L.H. 362, *367*
Reineke, L.M., see Smith, C.G. 437, 440, 441, 445, *456*
Reiner, B., Zamenhof, S. 26, *33*
Reiner, L., see Roth, J.S. 499, *509*
Reinhard, E.H., see Ward, H.N. 39, *46*
Reis, H.E. 525, *535*
Reis, H.E., Schmidt, C.G. *746*
Reisner, B.L., see Painter, R.B. 326, *342*
Reisner, E.H., Jr. 261, *270*
Reist, E.J., Baker, B.R. 658, *667*
Reist, E.J., Bartuska, V.J., Goodman, L. 430, *433*
Reist, E.J., Benitez, A., Goodman, L., Baker, B.R., Lee, W.W. 426, 427, 429, *433*
Reist, E.J., Calkins, D.F., Goodman, L. 431, *433*
Reist, E.J., Goodman, L. 428, *433*
Reist, E.J., see Lee, W.W. 429, 430, 431, *433*
Reitemeier, R.J., see Moertel, C.G. 220, *228*, 650, *656*, 793, *806*
Reiter, H., Strauss, B. 13, *16*
Reith, A.R., see Oleson, J.J. 496, *508*, 633, *641*
Reitmeier, R.J., see Moertel, C.G. 546, *551*
Reitz, M.S., see Yang, S.S. 883, *890*
Reitz, R.H., Slade, H.D., Neuhaus, F.C. 497, *509*
Reizer, J., see Frohwein, Y.Z. 697, *716*
Rekosh, D., see Taber, R. 558, *570*
Remers, W.A., see Roth, R.H. 48, *62*
Remington, J.S., see Stinson, E.B. 416, *424*
Remy, C.N. 385, 388, *402*
Remy, D.C., Sunthankar, A.V., Heidelberger, C. 196, *229*
Remy, D.C., see Heidelberger, C. 196, *226*
Remy-Defraigne, J., see Gerber, G.B. 283, 284, *333*
Renis, H.E. 302, *343*
Renis, H.E., Johnson, H.G. 237, 240, *254*
Renner, E.D., see Plagemann, P.G.W. 91, *102*
Rennert, O.M., Anker, H.S. 524, *535*
Rennie, P.I.C., see Scott, R.S. 117, *136*
Renshaw, E., Thomson, A.J. 832, *840*
Renshaw, E., see Rosenberg, B. 829, *840*
Reppert, J.A., see Burchenal, J.H. 198, *224*, *329*
Resko, J.A., Goy, R.W., Phoenix, C.H. 149, *156*
Reslova, S. 835
Resnick, B., see Cory, J.G. 658, 664, *665*
Ress, K.E., see Cohen, A. 607, *611*
Ressler, C., see Lauinger, C. 701, *718*
Rethy, V.B., see Weinhold, P.A. 520, *537*
Reuber, M.D. 410, *423*
Reuschl, H., see Hotz, G. 319, 321, *336*
Reusser, F., Bhuyan, B.K. 628, *629*, *632*
Reusser, F., see Bhuyan, B.K. 625, 629, 631, *631*
Reuvers, A., see McCalla, D.R. 72, 73, *82*
Revel, M., Hiatt, H.H. 584, *592*
Revesz, L., see Kriss, J.P. 282, 283, 289, 291, *338*
Revesz, L., see Reichard, P. 217, *229*
Revesz, L., see Sköld, O. 217, *231*
Reyes, P. 202, 216, 217, *229*
Reyes, P., Hall, T.C. 216, *229*
Reyes, P., Heidelberger, C. 203, 204, *229*
Reyes, P., see Kessel, D. *227*
Reynolds, A.F., Jr., see Walker, M.D. 69, *84*
Reynolds, R.C., Montgomery, P.O., Hughes, B. 583, *592*
Reynolds, S.R.M. 158, *168*
Rezny, Z., see Zak, M. 836, *840*
Rhaese, H.J., Freese, H. 8, *16*
Rheins, M.S., see Barker, A.D. 884, *887*
Rhoads, C.P., see Burchenal, J.H. 384, 389, *398*
Rhode, S.L., III., see Ellem, K.A.O. 573, *579*, 628, *632*
Rhodes, J.B., Williams-Ashman, H.G. 149, *156*
Rice, B.F., see Hammerstein, J. 106, *129*
Rice, H.V., Laetsch, W.M. 676, *692*
Rice, J.M. 78, *82*
Ricevuti, G., see Bertazzoli, C. 609, 610, *611*
Rich, A., see Chandross, R. 197, *224*
Rich, A., see Fraser, T.H. *669*
Rich, A., see Haschenmeyer, A.E.V. 441, *453*
Rich, A., see Kim, S.H. 197, *227*
Rich, A., see Tomita, K.I. 197, *230*
Rich, A., see Voet, D. 197, *231*, 279, *346*
Rich, K., see Zamenhof, S. 272, 295, 310, *347*
Rich, M.A., Bolaffi, J.L., Knoll, J.E., Cheong, L., Eidinoff, M.L. 199, *229*
Rich, M.A., Meyers, P., Weinbaum, G., Cory, J.G., Suhadolnik, R.J. 660, 663, *667*
Rich, M.A., see Cheong, L. 272, 273, 298, *329*
Rich, M.A., see Cory, J.G. 658, 664, *665*
Rich, M.A., see Eidinoff, M.L. 295, 298, 314, *332*
Rich, M.A., see Hampton, E.G. *335*
Richards, A.H., Hilf, R. 123, 124, *135*
Richards, A.H., see Hilf, R. 124, *130*
Richards, J.F., Jones, R.G.W., Beer, C.T. 679, *693*
Richards, J.F., see Jones, R.G.W. 679, *691*
Richards, M., see Vincent, P.C. 59, *63*
Richards, M.B., see Loo, T.L. 429, *433*
Richardson, A.C. 593, *613*
Richardson, J.P. 583, *592*
Richardson, L.C., see Ockey, C.H. 200, *229*
Richardson, M. 832
Richart, R.M., see Nagatsu, M. 859, *873*
Richie, R., see Brossi, A. 563, *567*
Richler, M., see Gellhorn, A. 822, 823, *827*

Richmond,J.E., Glaeser,R.M., Todd,P. *874*
Richmond,M.H. 512, 519, *535*
Richter,M., see Abdou,N.I. 70, *713*
Ricke,W.O. 314, *343*
Riddle,M., see Turkington, R.W. 312, *346*
Riddle,O., see McDonald, M.R. 120, *133*
Rieder,J., see Erlanger,M. 222, *225*
Rieger,R., Michaelis,A. 41, *45*
Rieger,R., see Fučík,V. 362, *366*
Rieger,R., see Michaelis,A. 41, *45*
Riehm,H., see Biedler,J.L. 583, *590*, 606, *611*
Rifkind,D. 417, *423*
Rifkind,D., Marchioro,T.L., Waddell,W.R., Starzl,T.E. 416, *423*
Rifkind,D., see Hill,R.H., Jr. 416, *421*
Rifkind,D., see Palmer,D.L. 416, *423*
Riggio,R.R., see Merkatz, I.R. 415, *422*
Riggs,A.D., see Lin,S.Y. 326, *339*
Rigler,N.E., see DeVoe,S.E. 486, 496, *504*
Riley,M., Paul,A. 279, *343*
Riley,V. 704, *720*
Riley,V., Spackman,D.H., Fitzmaurice,M.A., *120*, 704
Riman,J., Sverak,L., Langlois,A.J., Bonar,A., Beard,J.W. 440, *455*
Ringertz,N.R., Bolund,L. 584, *592*
Rinkin,H., see Hess,A.F. 120, *130*
Rittenberg,S.C., see Slotnick,I.J. 377, *382*
Ritter,C. 151, *156*
Ritter,E.J., Scott,W.J., Wilson,J.G. 237, 241, *254*, 261, *270*
Ritter,H.W., see Hoffman, P.F. 884, *889*
Rius,J., see Foley,H.T. 500, *504*
Riva,S., Silvestri,L.G. 883, *889*
Rive,D.J., see Schoental,R. 72, *83*
Rivera,A.,Jr., see Srinivasan,P.R. 492, 496, *510*
Rivers,S.L., Whittington, R.M., Medrek,T.J. 640, *641*
Rizki,R.M., Rizki,T.M. 297, *343*
Rizki,T.M., see Rizki,R.M. 297, *343*
Rizza,C.R., see Sprunt,J.G. 39, *46*
Rizzo,A.J., Kelly,C., Webb,T.E. *669*
Rizzoli,C., Cestari,A., Dessi,P., Concilio,A. 522, *535*
Rizzoli,C., Dessi,P., Cestari,A. 522, *535*
Rizzoli,C., see Cestari,A. 522, *530*
Roane,P.R.,Jr., see Roizman,B. 302, 303, *343*
Rob,C.G., see McQuitty,J.T. 844, *848*
Robards,A.W., Humpherson,P.G. 676, *693*
Robbins,E., Gonatas,N.K. 676, *693*
Robbins,E., see Borun,T.W. 245, *250*
Robbins,E., see Gonatas,N.K. 676, *690*
Robbins,M., see Strauss,B. 13, *17*
Robel,P., Lasnitzki,I., Baulieu,E.E. 160, *168*
Robel,P., see Baulieu,E.E. 115, *126*, 161, *167*
Roberts,D., Loehr,E.V., 469, *482*
Roberts,D., see Friedkin,M. 272, 273, 283, *333*
Roberts,D., see Kessel,D. 471, 473, *481*
Roberts,D.W., Hall,T.C., Rosenthal,D. 242, 245, *254*, 469, *482*, 681, *693*
Roberts,D.W., Loehr,E.V. 246, *254*
Roberts,D.W., see Hall,T.C. 265, *269*
Roberts,E., Borges,P.R.F. 485, *509*
Roberts,E., Frankel,S. 485, *509*
Roberts,E., see Ayengar,P. 496, *503*
Roberts,J., Burson,G., Hill, J.M. 698, *720*
Roberts,J., Holcenberg,J.S., Dolowy,W.C. 501, *509*
Roberts,J., Prager,M.D., Bachynsky,N. 698, 705, *720*
Roberts,J., see Hill,J.M. 696, 704, *716*, 723, 726, 728, 732, *744*
Roberts,J.J., Brent,T.P., Crathorn,A.R. 13, *16*, 21, 25, 27, *33*
Roberts,J.J., Pascoe,J.M. 837, *840*
Roberts,J.J., Pascoe,J.M., Plant,J.E., Sturrock,J.E., Crathorn,A.R., 14, *16*, 70, 76, 78, *83*
Roberts,J.J., Pascoe,J.M., Smith,B.A., Crathorn, A.R. 14, *17*, 78, *83*
Roberts,J.J., Warwick,G.P. 39, *46*
Roberts,J.J., see Ball,C.R. 13, *15*
Roberts,J.J., see Plant,J.E. 77, *82*
Roberts,M., Visser,D.W. 376, 377, 379, 380, *382*
Roberts,R.B., see Britten, R.J. 513, *530*
Roberts,S., see Szego,C.M. 109, 110, 122, *136*, *137*
Roberts,W.K., Dekker,C.A. 233, *254*
Roberts,W.K., Newman,J.F.E. 578, *580*
Roberts,W.K., see Walwick,E.R. 233, *256*
Robertson,D.M., see Feherty,P. 116, *128*
Robertson,D.M., see Méšter,J. 115, *133*
Robertson,J.H., McCarthy, G.M. 686, *693*
Robertson,L.L., see Allen, E. 108, *125*
Robins,A.B. 837, *840*
Robins,A.B., see Shooter, K.V. 837, *840*
Robins,M., see McCarthy,J.R.,Jr. 447, *454*
Robins,M.J., Hall,R.H., Thedford,R. 435, *455*
Robins,M.J., McCarthy,J.R.,Jr., Robins,R.K. 662, *667*
Robins,M.J., Naik,S.R. 195, *229*
Robins,M.J., see McCarthy, J.R.,Jr. 662, *666*
Robins,R., see McCarthy, J.R.,Jr. 447, *454*
Robins,R.K. 548, *551*
Robins,R.K., see Darnall, K.R. 373, 374, *381*
Robins,R.K., see McCarthy,J.R.,Jr. 662, *666*

Robins, R.K., see Panzica, R.P. 233, 234, *254*, 267, *270*

Robins, R.K., see Robins, M.J. 662, *667*

Robins, R.K., see Tolman, R.L. 233, *255*

Robins, R.K., see Townsend, L.B. 441, 444, *456*

Robison, R.S., Berk, B. 698, *720*

Robinson, B.L., see Langston, W.C. 108, *132*

Robinson, R., see Dodds, E.C. 105, *128*

Roblin, R.O., Jr., Lampen, J.O., English, J.P., Cole, Q.P., Vaughan, J.R. 458, *467*

Robson, J.M. 108, 109, *135*, 143, *156*

Robson, J.M., Schonberg, A. 105, *135*

Robson, J.M., see Auerbach, C. 21, *30*

Roche, J., see Hedegaard, J. 492, *506*

Roche, J., see Le Gal, Y. 489, *507*

Rochefort, H., Baulieu, E.E. 114, *135*

Rochefort, H., see Baulieu, E.E. 115, *126*

Rochlin, D.B., see Grage, T.B. 441, *453*

Roddy, J., see Dagg, C.P. *550*

Rodenghi, F., see Verini, M.A. 608, *613*

Rodriguez, V., see Bodey, G.P. 263, *268*

Rodriguez, V., see Freireich, E.J. 260, *269*

Roe, F.J.C., see Connors, T.A. 22, *31*

Roeder, R.G., Rutter, W.J. 574, *580*

Röhrborn, G. 41, *46*

Röhrborn, G., see Vogel, F. 22, *34*

Roenigk, H.H., Bergfeld, W.F., St. Jacques, R., Owens, F.J., Hawk, W.A. 475, *482*

Roepke, R.R., Hughes, J.S. 120, *135*

Rogers, H.J., Perkins, H.R. 201, *229*

Rogers, W.I., Hartman, A.C. Palm, P.E., Okstein, C., Kensler, C.J. 219, *229*

Rogers, W.I., Sivak, A., York, I.M. 822, *828*

Rogers, W.I., Wilson, J.A. 219, *229*

Rogers, W.I., Yesair, D.W., Kensler, C.J. *828*

Rogers, W.I., York, I.M., Kensler, C.J. 822, 823, *828*

Rogers, W.I., see Kensler, C.J. 822, 824, *827*

Rogers, W.I., see Meloni, M.L. 386, 387, 391, *401*

Rogers, W.I., see Palm, P.E. 824, *827*

Rogers, W.I., see Sivak, A. 822, 823, 824, *828*

Rogers, W.I., see Yesair, D.W. 682, *694*, 823, 824, 825, *828*

Rogers, W.I., see York, I.M. 822, *828*

Rogers, W.L., see Chadwick, M. 216, *224*

Rohn, R.J., see Hodes, M.E. 685, *690*

Roizman, B., Aurelian, L., Roane, P.R., Jr. 302, 303, *343*

Roizman, B., see Wagner, E.K. 680, *694*

Roll, P.M., see Brown, G.B. 318, *328*, 458, *465*

Rollo, I.M. 559, *570*

Rollo, I.M., see Williamson, J. 660, *668*

Rolly, H., Winkelmann, E. 800, *806*

Rolly, H., see Neufahrt, A. 302, *341*

Romano, A.A., see Rao, K.V. 486, 496, *509*

Romig, W.R., see Okubo, S. 53, *62*

Rominger, C.J., see Djerassi, I. 478, *480*

Romming, C., see Hassel, O. 286, *335*

Rondestvedt, C.S., Jr., see Clarke, D.A. 544, *550*

Ronen, A. 9, *17*

Rongone, E.L., see Segaloff, A. 173, 183, *191*

Ronneberger, H., see Staerk, J. 703, *721*

Ronzio, R.A., Meister, A. 499, *509*

Ronzio, R.A., Rowe, W.B., Meister, A. 499, *509*

Ronzio, R.A., see Rowe, W.B. 499, *509*

Ronzio, R.A., see Rutter, W.J. 311, *343*

Roodyn, D.B., Mandel, H.G. 463, *467*

Rooks, W.H., Hrada, T., Abe, O., Dorfman, R.I. 145, *156*

Root, C.A., see Holtkamp, D.E. 105, *130*

Roper, J.A., McIlwain, H. 496, *509*

Rosbash, M., see Penman, S. 571, 575, *580*, 664, *667*

Rose, H.G., Frenster, J.H. 824, *828*

Rose, H.M., see Nii, S. 790, *791*

Rose, H.M., see Rosencranz, H.S. 790, *792*

Roseman, J., see Studzinski, G.P. 54, *63*

Roseman, S., see Ghosh, S. 493, *505*

Roseman, S., see Kundig, W. 93, *101*

Roseman, S., see Simoni, R.D. 93, *103*

Rosemberg, E., Paulsen, C.A. 139, *156*

Rosen, B. 214, *230*

Rosen, B., Rothman, F., Weigert, M.G. 215, *230*

Rosen, F. 86, 94, *102*

Rosen, F., see Chang, E. 99, *100*

Rosen, F., see Harding, H.R. 88, *101*

Rosen, F., see Kaiser, N. 97, *101*

Rosen, F., see Kirkpatrick, A.F. 95, 97, 98, 99, *101*, 176, 187, *190*

Rosen, F., see Raina, P.N. 94, *102*

Rosen, F., see Rosen, J.M. 86, 87, 88, 90, 91, 92, 93, *102*

Rosen, J.M., Fina, J.J., Milholland, R.J., Rosen, F. 86, 87, 88, 90, 91, 92, 93, *102*

Rosen, J.M., Milholland, R.J., Rosen, F. 87, 93, *103*

Rosen, J.M., Rosen, F., Milholland, R.J., Nichol, C.A. 87, 88, *103*

Rosenbaum, E., see Cline, M.J. 246, *250*

Rosenbaum, J.L., Carlson, K. 676, *693*

Rosenbaum, J.L., see Olmsted, J.B. 678, *692*

Rosenbaum, R.M., see Wittner, M. 880, *890*

Rosenberg, B., Renshaw, E., Van Camp, L., Hartwick, J., Drobnik, J. 829, *840*

Rosenberg, B., Van Camp, L., 830, 832, *840*
Rosenberg, B., Van Camp, L., Grimley, E.B., Thomson, A.J. 829, *840*
Rosenberg, B., Van Camp, L., Krigas, T. 829, 836, *840*
Rosenberg, B., Van Camp, L., Trosko, J.E., Mansour, V.H. 830, *840*
Rosenberg, B., see Harder, H.C. 834, *839*
Rosenberg, B., see Kociba, R.J. 830, *840*
Rosenberg, B., see Tooth-Allen, J. 832
Rosenberg, S., Calabresi, P. 502, *509*
Rosenbloom, F.M., see Kelley, W.N. 414, *422*
Rosenblum, C., see Hiremath, C.B. 524, *532*
Rosenblum, M.L., see Walker, M.D. 69, *84*
Rosencranz, H.S., Rose, H. M., Morgan, C., Hsu, K. C. 790, *792*
Rosencranz, H.S., see Nii, S. 790, *791*
Rosenfeld, C., see Mathé, G. 882, *889*
Rosenfeld, C., see Schwarzenberg, L. 474, *482*
Rosenfeld, M.G., O'Malley, B.W. 152, *156*
Rosenkrantz, H., see Heyman, I.A. 832, *839*
Rosenkrantz, J.G., Githens, J.H., Cox, S.M., Kellum, D.L. 415, *423*
Rosenkrantz, J.G., see Githens, J.H. 415, *421*
Rosenkranz, H.S., Bitoon, M., Schmidt, R.M. 73, *83*
Rosenkranz, H.S., Carr, H.S. 73, *83*
Rosenkranz, H.S., Carr, H. S., Zyroff, J. 522, *535*
Rosenoer, V.N., see Dunnicliff, M.A. *744*
Rosenoff, S., see Hofer, K.G. 315, 316, 317, *335*
Rosenstein, R.D., see Abraham, D.J. 545, *550*, 556, *567*
Rosenthal, D., see Kessel, D. 265, *270*
Rosenstock, J., see Haghbin, M. 726, 732, *744*
Rosenthal, D., see Roberts, D.W. 242, 245, *254*, 469, *482*, 681, *693*
Rosenthal, O., see Omura, T. 139, *155*
Rosenthal, P., see Kessel, D. 246, 247, *253*
Rosenthale, M.E., Datko, L. J., Kassarich, J., Schneider, F. 408, *423*
Rosenthale, M.E., Gluckman, M.I. 523, 526, *535*
Rosi, D., Peruzzotti, G., Dennis, E.W., Berberian, D.A., Freele, H., Archer, S. 879, *889*
Rosi, D., see Berberian, D. A. 879, *887*
Rosner, A., Yagil, E. 290, *343*
Rosner, F., see Ellison, R.R. 260, *268*
Rosner, F., see Kung, F. 521, *533*
Ross, A.E., see Lijinsky, W. 71, *82*
Ross, A.F., Parks, R.E., Jr. 460, 461, *467*
Ross, A.F., Jaffe, J.J. 437, 439, *455*
Ross, D.J., see Birkinshaw, J.H. 446, *453*
Ross, D.L., Skinner, C.G., Shive, W. 498, *509*
Ross, D.L., see Skinner, C. G. *510*
Ross, G.T., Cargille, C.M., Lipsett, M.B., Rayford, P.L., Marshall, J.R., Strott, C.A. 160, *168*
Ross, G.T., see Hertz, R. 476, *481*
Ross, P. 627
Ross, R., see Southren, A.L. 811, 813, *818*
Ross, R.B., Noll, C.I., Ross, W.C.J., Nadkarni, M.V., Morrison, B.H., Jr., Bond, H.W. 523, *535*
Ross, R.B., see Bratzel, R. P. 18, *30*
Ross, V.C., Solymosi, J. 56, *62*
Ross, W.C.J. 6, *17*, 19, 20, 25, 29, *33*
Ross, W.C.J., Warwick, G. P. 29, *33*
Ross, W.C.J., see Connors, T.A. 523, *530*
Ross, W.C.J., see Davis, W. 42, *43*
Ross, W.C.J., see Ross, R. B. 523, *535*
Rossi, M., see Momparler, R. L. 234, 238, *253*
Rossi, M., see Scarano, E. 287, *343*
Rosso, R., Donnelli, M.G., Innocenti, I.R.D., Garattini, S. 69, *83*
Rossof, A.H., Slayton, R. E., Perlia, C.P. 839, *840*
Rossolimo, O.K. 618, *622*
Rossolimo, O.K., see Chorin, V.A. 618, 619, 620, *621*
Rotenberg, A.D., Bruce, W. R., Baker, R.G. 289, 314, *343*
Roth, J.S., Wase, A., Reiner, L. 499, *509*
Roth, L.J., see Jensen, E.V. 164, *167*
Roth, R.H., Remers, W.A., Weiss, M.J. 48, *62*
Rothman, F., see Rosen, B. 215, *230*
Rothschild, L., see Jorda, V.V. *569*
Rothstein, H., see Stein, G. S. 59, *63*
Rott, R., Saber, S., Scholtissek, C. 58, *62*
Rottman, F., Guarino, A.J. 659, 660, 661, 663, *667*
Roush, A., Norris, E.R. 459, 460, *467*
Rousse, J., see Jacquillat, C. 726, 727, 728, 732, 734, 735, *744*
Rousselot, L.M., Cole, D.R., Grossi, C.E., Conte, A. J., Gonzales, E.M., Pasternak, B.S. 221, *230*
Rousselot, L.M., see Cole, D. R. 642, *647*
Rovera, G., Berman, S., Baserga, R. 583, *592*
Rowe, J.A., see Donovan, K.L. 448, *453*
Rowe, W.B., Ronzio, R.A., Meister, A. 499, *509*
Rowe, W.B., see Ronzio, R. A. 499, *509*
Rowe, W.P., see Lowy, D. R. 308, *340*, 355, *368*
Rowinski, W.A., Hager, E. B. 527, *535*
Rowland, G.F., see Rees, K. R. 824, *827*
Rowlands, D.T., Jr., see Hill, R.H., Jr. 416, *421*
Rowley, B., Wriston, J.C., Jr. 697, *720*
Rowley, M.J., Mackay, I. R., McKenzie, I.F.C. 416, *423*
Rowley, M.J., see Lee, A.K. Y. 416, *422*

Roy,D. 478, *482*
Roy,J.K., Kvam,D.C., Dahl,J.L., Parks,R.E., Jr. 463, *467*
Roy,S., Mahesh,V.B., Greenblatt,R.B. 113, 114, *135*
Roy,S.C., see Basu,S.K. 56, *60*
Roy-Burman,D., see Huang,Y.H.J. 377, 378, 380, *381*
Roy-Burman,P. 379, *382*, 384, *402*, 571, *580*
Roy-Burman,P., Roy-Burman,S., Visser,D.W. 373, 374, 377, 378, *382*
Roy-Burman,P., see Roy-Burman,S. 376, 377, 378, 380, *382*
Roy-Burman,P., see Smith, D.A. 380, *382*
Roy-Burman,P., see Visser, D.W. 376, *382*
Roy-Burman,S., Huang,Y. H., Visser,D.W. 375, *382*
Roy-Burman,S., Roy-Burman,P., Visser,D.W. 376, 377, 378, 380, *382*
Roy-Burman,S., see Roy-Burman,P. 373, 374, 377, 378, *382*
Roy-Burman,S., see Visser, D.W. 376, *382*, *383*
Royer,G., see Djerassi,I. 478, *480*
Rozengurt,E., see DeAsua, L.J. 124, 125, *127*
Rubbins,M., see Strauss,B. S. 54, *63*
Rubin,A.L., see Schwartz, G.H. 406, *424*, 725, 735, 738, *746*
Rubin,R.C., Ommaya,A. K., Henderson,E.S., Bering,E.A., Rall,D.P. 472, *482*
Rubin,R.J., Jaffe,J.J., Handschumacher,R.E. 352, *369*
Rubini,J.R., Cronkite,E. P., Bond,V.P., Fliedner, T.M. 280, *314*, *343*
Rubio,F., see Koechlin,B. A. 201, 202, *227*
Rubulis,A., Jacobs,R.D., Hughes,E.C. 125, *135*
Rubulis,A., see Hughes,E. C. 122, *131*
Ruby,A., see Wilson,L. 678, *694*
Rudack,D., Wallace,R.A. 121, *135*
Ruddle,F., see Olmsted,J. B. 678, *692*
Ruddle,N., see Kennealey, G.T. 408, *422*
Ruddon,R.W., see Wolpert, M.K. 28, *34*
Rudman,D., Vogler,W.R. Howard,C.H., Gerron, G.G. 703, *720*
Rudolph,G.G., Samuels,L. T. 143, 151, *156*
Rudzuts,R., see Gellert,E. 564, *568*
Rueckert,R.R., Mueller,G. C. 21, *33*, 199, 204, *230*
Ruelius,H.W., see Gregory, F.J. 523, *532*
Ruet,A., see Sentenac,A. 659, *667*
Ruffolo,P.R., Ferm,V.H. 310, *343*
Rugh,R., see Jacobs,E.M. 220, *226*
Rundles,R., see Vogler,W. R. 477, *482*
Rundles,R.W., Laszlo,J., Itoga,T., Hobson,J.B., Garrison,F.E.,Jr. 408, 412, *423*
Rundles,R.W., see Elion, G.B. 384, 387, 389, *399*, 404, 408, 409, 410, 411, *420*
Runner,M.N., Yoshida,S. *62*
Rupp,W.D., Prusoff,W.H. 319, 320, 321, *343*
Rusch,H.P., see Brewer,E. N. 774, *783*
Rusch,H.P., see Mitchell,J. L.A. 774, *787*
Ruschmann,G., see Weil,R. 302, 308, *346*
Rusconi,A., Calendi,E. 601, 602, 603, 608, *613*
Rusconi,A., DiFronzo,G., DiMarco,A. 602, *613*
Rusconi,A., DiMarco,A. 601, 602, 603, *613*
Rusconi,A., see DiMarco,A. 608, *612*
Russeff,C., Wasselewa,L., Matewa,V. 302, *343*
Russell,W.C., see Watson, D.H. 303, *346*
Russell,A.F., Moffatt,J.G. 662, *667*
Russell,A.F., see Atkinson, M.R. 660, *665*
Russell,D.H. 246, *254*
Russell,D.H., Levy,C.C. 774, *787*
Russell,D.H., Medina,V. J., Snyder,S.H. 774, *787*
Russell,D.H., see Heby,O. 774, 775, *785*
Russell,P.B., see Thompson,R.L. 302, *346*, 800, *807*
Russi,S., see De-Angeli,L. C. 697, *715*
Rutenburg,A.M., see Friedman,O.M. 520, *531*
Rutherford,J.S., see Abraham,D.J. 545, *550*
Ruthven,C.R.J., see Jones, N.F. *532*
Rutishauser,A., Bollag,W. 756, *764*
Rutman,R.J., Cantarow, A., Paschkis,K.E. 193, *230*, 283, *343*
Rutman,R.J., see Chun,E. H.L. 14, *15*, 28, *31*
Rutter,W.J., Kemp,J.D., Bradshaw,W.S., Clark, W.R., Ronzio,R.A., Sanders,T.G. 311, *343*
Rutter,W.J., see Roeder, R.G. 574, *580*
Ryan,K.J. 106, *135*
Ryan,K.J., Acton,E.M., Goodman,L. 196, *230*
Ryan,K.J., Engel,L.L. 107, *135*
Ryan,K.J., Smith,O.W. 106, 107, *135*
Ryan,R.M., see Jameson, E. 695, *717*
Ryan,R.M., see Kwak,K. S. 695, *717*
Ryan,W.L., Dworak,J.E. 708, *720*
Ryan,W.L., Elliott,J.A. 519, 529, *535*
Ryan,W.L., Sornson,H.C. 708, *720*
Rychlík,I., see Lisý,V. 353, *368*
Rychter,Z., Jelínek,R. 358, *369*
Rychter,Z., Oštádal,B., Jelínek,R. 358, *369*
Rychter,Z., see Jelínek,R. 358, *367*
Ryder,A., see Bartz,Q.R. 485, *503*
Ryter,A., see Ionesco,M. 57, *61*

Saber,S., see Rott,R. 58, *62*
Sabo,E.F., see Fried,J. 185, *189*
Sachs,F., see Waltuch,G. 323, *346*
Sachs,L., see Gershon,D. 354, *366*

Sadler, P. W., see Bauer, D. J. 800, *805*
Safferman, R. S., see Ammann, C. A. 658, 662, *664*
Sagar, P., Kára, J. 350, *369*
Sagher, D., see Liao, S. 148, *155*
Saha, N. N., see Jensen, E. V. 114, *131*, 176, 187, *190*
Saheb, S. E., see Mertes, M. P. 196, *228*
Sahiar, K., Schwartz, R. S. 407, *423*
Saiki, J. H., see Bodey, G. P. 264, *268*
Sakai, T. T., see Santi, D. V. 198, *230*
Sakai, Y., Konda, C., Shimoyama, M., Kitahara, T., Sakano, T., Kimura, K. 887, *889*
Sakai, Y., see Kimura, K. 870, *873*
Sakamoto, K., see Ichikawa, T. 855, 870, *872*
Sakamoto, M., see Yamagata, Y. 296, *347*
Sakamoto, Y., see Nakata, Y. 54, *62*
Sakano, K., see Kimura, K. 870, *873*
Sakano, T., see Sakai, Y. 887, *889*
Sakar, N. K. 583, *592*
Sakauchi, N., Kumaoka, S., Naruke, T., Abe, O., Kusama, M., Takatani, O. 814, *818*
Sako, Y., see Lyons, W. R. 176, *190*
Sakore, T. D., see Sobell, H. M. 573, *581*, 587, *592*
Sakore, T. D., see Tavale, S. S. 279, *345*
Saksena, S. K., Chaudhury, R. R. 357, *369*
Sakuchi, G., De Witt, C. W. 59, *62*
Sakurai, Y., see Inaba, M. 28, *32*
Salditt, M., see Jelinek, W. *669*
Salem, P., see Hart, J. S. 265, *269*
Salser, J. S., Balis, M. E. 392, *402*
Salser, J. S., Hutchison, D. J., Balis, M. E. 392, *402*
Salser, J. S., see Miller, H. K. 703, 704, *718*, 725, *745*
Salvador, R. A., see Trams, E. G. 39, *46*
Salzman, N. P., 199, *230*, 307, *343*
Salzman, N. P., Shatkin, A. J., Sebring, E. D. 199, *230*
Salzman, N. P., see Munyon, W. 209, *228*
Samaan, N. A., see Whitecar, J. P., Jr. 709, *722*
Samaha, R. J., see Henderson, E. S. 687, *690*, 799, *806*
Samain, J. F., see Laboureur, P. 699, 700, *717*
Samal, B. A., Frazier, L. E., Monto, G., Slesers, A., Hruban, Z., Wissler, R. W. 520, *535*
Samarina, O. P., see Georgiev, G. P. 584, *590*
Samoiloff, M. R., see Pasternak, J. 855, *874*
Sampson, S. D., see Shigeura, H. T. 448, *455*, 659, 661, 662, 663, *667*
Samuels, L., see Newton, W. 478, *482*
Samuels, L. T., see Rudolph, G. G. 143, 151, *156*
Samuels, M. L., Leary, W. V., Alexanian, R., Howe, C. D., Frei, E., III. 759, *764*
Sandberg, J., see Pujman, V. 196, *229*
Sandberg, J. S., Goldin, A. 36, *46*
Sandberg, J. S., Howsden, F. L., DiMarco, A., Goldin, A. 597, *612*
Sandberg, J. S., see Goldin, A. 389, *399*
Sandberg-Wollheim, M., see Kennedy, B. J. *622*
Sander, S. 117, *135*
Sander, S., Attramadal, A. 117, *135*
Sanders, C. I., Martin, D. S., Jr. 836, *840*
Sanders, E., see Omura, T. 139, *155*
Sanders, F. K., Burford, B. O. 78, *83*
Sanders, M. A., Wiesner, B. P., Yudkin, J. 356, *369*
Sanders, T. G., see Rutter, W. J. 311, *343*
San Diego, F. J., see Burrows, J. H. 478, *480*
Sandler, M., see Jones, N. F. *532*
Sandler, S. G., Tobin, W. E., Henderson, E. S. 686, *693*
Sandler, S. G., see Tobin, W. E. 675, 686, *693*
Saneyoshi, M., see Hoshi, A. 234, *252*, 266, 267, *269*, 886, *889*
Sanfilippo, A., Mazzoleni, E. 593, 606, *613*
Sanford, R. E., see Clegg, R. E. 120, *127*
Sanger, J. W., Holtzer, H. 311, *343*
Sanger, J. W., see Mayne, R. 311, *340*
Sankowski, A., see Skopińska, E. 408, *424*
Sano, K., Hosino, T., Nagai, M. 291, 319, 324, *343*
Sano, K., Sato, F., Hoshino, T., Nagai, M. 291, *343*
Sano, K., see Hoshino, T. 319, 324, *336*
Sano, M., see Lipkin, D. 273, 274, 277, *339*
Sano, Y., see Hata, T. 47, *60*
St. Arneault, G., see Ohnuma, T. 726, 728, 734, 735, *745*
St. Jacques, R., see Roenigk, H. H. 475, *482*
St. Pierre, R. L., Tennenbaum, J. I., Folk, R. M. 706, *720*
Santi, D. V., Sakai, T. T. 198, *230*
Santilli, Giornelli, F. E., see Lauro, V. 415, *422*
Santos, G. W., see Makinodan, T. 201, *228*, 525, *534*, 752, *763*
Sarcione, E. J., Stutzman, L. 387, *402*
Sargeant, K., see Wade, H. E. 697, *721*
Sarff, M., Gorski, J. 117, *135*
Sarino, J. S., see Merker, P. C. 633, *641*
Sartini, J., see Hilf, R. 124, *130*
Sartorelli, A. C. 397, *402*, 687, *693*, 799, 802, *806*
Sartorelli, A. C., Agrawal, K. C., Booth, B. A., Moore, E. C. 793, 802, *807*
Sartorelli, A. C., Agrawal, K. C., Moore, E. C. 797, 803, *807*
Sartorelli, A. C., Booth, B. A. 496, 500, 501, *509*
Sartorelli, A. C., Booth, B. A., Moore, E. C. 793, 802, *807*

Sartorelli, A.C., Creasey, W. A. 196, *230*, 232, 236, *254*, 671, 687, *693*, 747, *764*
Sartorelli, A.C., Hilton, J., Booth, B.A., Agrawal, K.C., Donnelly, T.E., Jr., Moore, E.C. *807*
Sartorelli A.C., Iannotti, A. T., Booth, B.A., Schneider, F.H., Bertino, J.R., Johns, D.G. 771, 776, *787*
Sartorelli, A.C., Kruse, P.F. Jr., Booth, B.A., Schoolar, E.J., Jr. 516, 519, *536*
Sartorelli, A.C., LePage, G. A. 393, 394, 395, *402*, 487, 500, *509*
Sartorelli, A.C., LePage, G. A., Moore, E.C. 389, 397, *402*
Sartorelli, A.C., Scholar, E. J., Jr., Kruse, P.F., Jr. *509*
Sartorelli, A.C., Tsunamura, S. 748, 756, 757, *764*
Sartorelli, A.C., Upchurch, H.F., Bieber, A.L., Booth, B.A. 487, 500, *509*
Sartorelli, A.C., Welch, A. D., Booth, B.A. *849*
Sartorelli, A.C., see Agrawal, K.C. 794, 795, 797, 798, 799, 801, *804*, *805*
Sartorelli, A.C., see Bertino, J.R. 468, 472, *479*
Sartorelli, A.C., see Booth, B.A. 301, *328*, 802, 804, *805*, 844, 846, 847, *848*
Sartorelli, A.C., see Cramer, G.T. 496, *504*
Sartorelli, A.C., see Cramer, J.W. 291, *330*
Sartorelli, A.C., see Creasey, W.A. 795, 799, 800, 801, 802, *805*
Sartorelli, A.C., see DeConti, R.C. 793, 799, 800, 802, 804, *805*
Sartorelli, A.C., see Hochman, H.I. 803, *806*
Sartorelli, A.C., see Johns, D.G. 196, *226*, 473, *481*
Sartorelli, A.C., see Lefkowitz, E.R. 389, *400*, 500, *507*
Sartorelli, A.C., see Lin, A. J. 798, *806*
Sartorelli, A.C., see McCoy, T.A. 696, 711, *718*
Sartorelli, A.C., see Michaud, R.L. 798, *806*
Sartorelli, A.C., see Miech, R.P. 388, 394, 395, *401*
Sartorelli, A.C., see Mooney, P.D. 798, *806*
Sartorelli, A.C., see Moore, E.C. 793, 798, 798, 802, 803, 804, *806*
Sartorelli, A.C., see Tyrsted, G. 663, *668*
Sartorelli, A.C., see Wolpert, M.K. 393, *403*
Sakurai, Y., see El-Merzabani, M.M. 36, *43*
Sarver, M.E., see Danowski, T.S. 814, *817*
Sashikata, K., see Tanaka, N. 497, *511*
Saslaw, L.D., Grindey, G. B., Kline, I., Waravdekar, V.S. 267, *270*
Saslaw, L.D., see Grindey, G.B. 240, *252*, 267, *269*
Sato, F., see Sano, K. 291, *343*
Sato, H., see Malawista, S. E. 674, 677, 678, *691*
Sato, J., see LePage, G.A. 427
Sato, K., LePage, G.A., Kimball, A.P. 430, *433*
Sato, K., see Oka, S. 870, *874*
Satoh, P.G., Constantopoulos, G., Tchen, T.T. 139, *156*
Satoh, P.S., see Constantopoulos, G. 139, *153*
Saukkonen, J.J., see Horowitz, J. 206, 211, 212, *226*
Saunders, G.F., Reese, W. N., Saunders, P.P. 627, 628, *632*
Saunders, H.L., Holden, K., Kerwin, J.F. 146, *156*
Saunders, P.P., Schultz, G. A. 547, *551*
Saunders, P.P., see Saunders, G.F. 627, 628, *632*
Sauter, S., see Heby, O. 775, *785*
Savage, G.M., see DeBoer, D. 47, *60*
Savard, K., Dorfman, R.I., Baggett, B., Engel, L.L. 140, *156*
Savard, K., see Hammerstein, J. 106, *129*
Savard, K., see Marsh, J.M. 106, 107, *132*, 140, *155*
Savel, H. 671, *693*
Savel, H., see Krakoff, I.H. 789, *791*
Savino, M., see Ascoli, F. 585, *589*
Savlov, E.D., Hall, T.C. 546, *552*
Savlov, E.D., Hall, T.C., Oberfield, R.A. 546, *552*
Savlov, E.D., see Wittliff, J.L. 117, 118, *138*
Sawa, T., Fukagawa, Y., Homma, I., Takeuchi, T., Umezawa, H. 444, *455*
Sawa, T., Fukagawa, Y., Homma, I., Wakashiro, T., Takeuchi, T., Hori, M., Komai, T. 444, *455*
Sawa, T., see Hori, M. 445, *454*
Sawa, T., see Ishizuka, M. 441, 444, *454*
Sawa, T., see Takeuchi, T. 444, 445, *456*
Sawa, T., see Umezawa, H. 444, *456*
Sawai, M., see Ueda, M. 683, *694*
Sawawa, Y., see Takeda, K. 870, *875*
Sawitsky, A., see Ellison, R. R. 260, *268*
Sawyer, B.C., see Slater, T. F. 491, *510*
Sayers, M., see Newton, W. 478, *482*
Scannell, J.P., Hitchings, G.H. 386, 390, 392, 393, *402*
Scarano, E., Geraci, G., Rossi, M. 287, *343*
Scarpinato, B., see Calendi, E. 598, 599, *611*
Scarpinato, B., see Casazza, A.M. 597, 610, *611*
Scarpinato, B.M., see DiFronzo, G. 608, *612*
Scarpinato, B.M., see DiMarco, A. 593, 597, 607, 609, *612*
Scatchard, G. 115, *135*
Schabel, F.M., Jr. 69, *83*, 236, *254*, 263, *271*, 389, *402*, 429, *433*, 545
Schabel, F.M., Jr., Johnston, T.P., McCaleb, G. S., Montgomery, J.A., Laster, W.R., Skipper, H.E. 65, 68, 69, 79, *83*
Schabel, F.M., Jr., Laster, W.R., Jr., Skipper, H.E. 391, *402*

Schabel, F. M., Jr., Laster, W. R., Jr., Trader, M. W. 878, *889*
Schabel, F. M., Jr., Montgomery, J. A., Skipper, H. E., Laster, W. R., Jr., Thomson, J. R. 393, *402*
Schabel, F. M., Jr., Skipper, H. E., Trader, M. W., Wilcox, W. S. 76, *83*, 389, *402*, 494, *509*
Schabel, F. M., Jr., Montgomery, J. A. 322, 324, *344*
Schabel, F. M., Jr., see Bennett, L. L., Jr. 386, *398*, 486, 495, *503*
Schabel, F. M., Jr., see Brockman, R. W. 793, 800, *805*, 877, 878, *888*
Schabel, F. M., Jr., see Carter, S. K. 65, *80*
Schabel, F. M., Jr., see Griswold, D. P., Jr. 235, *252*, 767, *785*
Schabel, F. M., Jr., see Laster, W. R., Jr. 389, *400*
Schabel, F. M., Jr., see Pittillo, R. F. 20, *33*
Schabel, F. M., Jr., see Schmidt, L. H. 264, *271*
Schabel, F. M., Jr., see Sidwell, R. W. 428, *433*, 800, *807*
Schabel, F. M., Jr., see Skipper, H. E. 235, 249, *255*, 260, 261, 262, *271*, 486, *510*, 798, *807*
Schabel, F. M., Jr., see Wilkoff, L. J. 76, *84*
Schacter, B., Law, L. W. 460, *467*
Schade, A. L., see Butler, W. W. S. 151, *153*
Schäfer, W., Pister, L., Schneider, R. *369*
Schaeffer, H., Thomas, H. J. 435, *455*
Schaeffer, P., see Ionesco, M. 57, *61*
Schaeppi, U. 832
Schaeppi, U. H., see Heyman, I. A. 832, *839*
Schafranek, R., see Hirschberg, E. 460, *465*
Schardein, J. L., Sidwell, R. W. 428, *433*
Schardein, J. L., see Kurtz, S. M. 428, *433*
Scharff, M. D., see Borun, T. W. 245, *250*
Schaumberg, B. P. 96, 98, *103*
Scheetz, R. W., Whelan, H. A., Wriston, J. C., Jr. 697, 699, 702, 703, 704, *720*
Scheidt, L. G., see Bhuyan, B. K. 75, 76, *80*, 218, *223*, 629, *631*, 802, *805*
Scheil, A. G. R., see Murray, J. E. 407, *422*
Schein, P., see Herman, E. H. 609, *612*
Schein, P. S. 69, 75, 76, *83*
Schein, P. S., Loftus, S. 75, *83*
Schein, P. S., Rakieten, N., Gordon, B. M., Davis, R. D., Rall, D. P. 704, 710, *720*
Scheiner, T., see Heidelberger, C. 193, 198, *226*
Scheit, K. H., see Sprinzl, M. *669*
Schelten, E., see Krüger, F. W. 70, 71, *81*
Schenker, F., see Leimgruber, W. 642, *648*
Schenone, A., see Corti, A. 774, 775, *784*
Schenone, A., see Williams-Ashman, H. G. 774, *788*
Schepartz, S. A. 767, *787*
Schepartz, S. A., Wodinsky, I., Leiter, J. 820, *828*
Scher, J., see Finkelstein, J. Z. 238, 251, 258, 260, *268*
Scheving, L. E., see Haus, E. 249, *252*
Schiek, E., see Schiek, W. 302, 303, *344*
Schiek, W., Schiek, E. 302, 303, *344*
Schimke, R. T., see Palmiter, R. 121, *134*
Schindler, R. 525, *536*
Schindler, R., Welch, A. D. 355, *370*
Schindler, R., see Burki, K. 318, *329*
Schindler, R. L., Ramseier, L., Grieder, A. 41, *46*, 294, *344*
Schinzinger, A. 111, *135*
Schivo, M. C., see Ferrari, W. 303, *332*
Schivo, M. L., see Loddo, B. 302, 303, *339*
Schjeide, O. A., Urist, M. R. 120, 121, *135*
Schjeide, O. A., Wilkens, M., McCandless, R. G., Munn, R., Peterson, M., Carlsen, E. N., 120, *135*
Schjeide, O. A., see Urist, M. R. 120, *137*
Schjeide, O. A., see Carlsen, E. N. 121, *127*
Schjeide, O. A., see Hahn, W. E. 121, *129*
Schlein, A., see Price, K. E. 496, *508*
Schlesinger, M., Grossowicz, N., Lichtenstein, N. 514, 520, *536*
Schlesinger, M. J., see Schlesinger, S. 517, *536*
Schlesinger, R. W., see Stollar, V. 354, *371*
Schlesinger, S., Schlesinger, M. J. 517, *536*
Schlosser, J. V., see Segaloff, A. 173, 181, 184, *191*
Schluederberg, A., Hendel, R. C., Chavanich, S. 584, *592*
Schlumberger, J. R., see Mathé, G. 685, *692*, 882, *889*
Schlumberger, J. R., see Schwarzenberg, L. 474, *482*
Schmähl, D., Osswald, H. 199, *230*
Schmähl, D., see Druckrey, H. 78, *80*
Schmid, F. A., Fetzer, V. A., Smol, B. A., Tarnowski, G. S. 521, 524, *536*
Schmid, F. A., Stern, B. R., Schmid, M. M., Tarnowski, G. S. 521, 524, *536*
Schmid, F. A., see Sugiura, K. 36, *46*
Schmid, K., see Gelzer, J. 777, 780, *785*
Schmid, M. M., see Schmid, F. A. 521, 524, *536*
Schmidt, C. G. 514, *536*
Schmidt, C. G., Gallmeier, W. 726, 727, 730, 734, 735, *746*
Schmidt, C. G., see Dold, U. 870, *871*
Schmidt, C. G., see Reis, H. E. *746*
Schmidt, C. G., see Stier, H. W. *746*
Schmidt, G. 238, *254*
Schmidt, H., Noack, V. I., Walther, H., Voigt, K. D. 123, *135*
Schmidt, H., Walther, H., Voigt, K. D. 123, *136*
Schmidt, H., see Domagk, G. 841, *848*

Schmidt, H., see Noack, V. I. 123, *134*
Schmidt, L. H., Fradkin, R., Sullivan, R., Flowers, A. 18, *33*
Schmidt, L. H., Montgomery, J. A., Laster, W. R., Jr., Schabel, F. M. Jr. 264, *271*
Schmidt, L. H., see Skipper, H. E. 394, *402*
Schmidt, R. M., see Rosenkranz, H. S. 73, *83*
Schmitz, R. Y., see Leonard, N. J. 435, *454*
Schnebli, H. P., Hill, D. L., Bennett, L. L., Jr. 436, 442, *455*, 659, *667*
Schnebli, H. P., see Allan, P. W. 386, *397*
Schnebli, H. P., see Bennett, L. L., Jr. 386, *398*, 436, *452*
Schneider, F., see Rosenthale, M. E. 408, *423*
Schneider, F., see Weitzel, G. L. 754, 756, *765*
Schneider, F. H., see Sartorelli, A. C. 771, 776, *787*
Schneider, H., see Druckrey, H. 78, *80*
Schneider, M., see Mathé, G. 685, *692*, 759, *763*, 772, *786*, 882, *889*
Schneider, M., see Schwarzenberg, L. 474, *482*
Schneider, R., see Schäfer, W. *369*
Schneider, W. C., see Hogeboom, G. H. 539, *542*
Schneweis, K. E. 302, 303, 304, 307, *344*
Schnieders, B., see Kersten, H. 54, *61*
Schnieders, B., see Leopold, G. 54, *61*
Schnitzer, R. J., see Heidelberger, C. 193, 198, *226*
Schnos, M., see Inman, R. B. 294, 325, *336*
Schochet, S. S., Lampert, P. W., Earle, K. M. 677, *693*
Schochetman, G., Perry, R. P. 246, *255*
Schoefl, G. I. 583, *592*
Schoenbach, E. B., Greenspan, E. M. 766, *787*
Schoenbach, E. B., see Goldin, A. 459, 460, *465*
Schoenewaldt, E. F., see Twombly, G. H. 113, *137*
Schoental, R. 71, *83*
Schoental, R., Rive, D. J. 72, *83*
Schofield, R., see Davis, W. E. 318, *330*
Scholar, E. M., Brown, P. R., Parks, R. E., Jr. 391, *402*
Scholar, E. M., see Agarwal, R. P. *464*
Scholler, J., Gordon, M., Sternberg, S. S. 283, *344*
Scholler, J., see Sternberg, S. S. 36, 37, *46*
Scholtissek, C., see Rott, R. 58, *62*
Schonberg, A., see Robson, J. M. 105, *135*
Scholar, E. J., Jr., see Sartorelli, A. C. *509*, 516, 519, *536*
Schottin, N. H., see Callentine, M. R. 110, *127*
Schrader, W. T., see O'Malley, B. W. 160, 161, 162, 164, *168*
Schrecker, A. W. 246, 247, *255*, 265, *271*
Schrecker, A. W., Goldin, A. 234, *255*, 265, *271*
Schrecker, A. W., Mead, J. A. R. 265, *271*
Schrecker, A. W., Urshel, M. J. 240, 246, *255*
Schreiber, D., see Jänish, W. 78, *81*
Schreiber, W., see Vinegar, R. *424*
Schrek, R., Dolowy, W. C. 733, *746*
Schrek, R., Dolowy, W. C., Ammeraal, R. N. 706, *720*
Schrek, R., see Dolowy, W. C. 707, *715*
Schricker, K. T., see Goldenberg, D. M. 259, *269*
Schroder, H., see Perper, R. J. 408, *423*
Schroeder, D. D., Allison, A. J., Buchanan, J. M. 496, 498, *509*
Schroeder, D. H., see Guarino, A. M. 709, *716*
Schroeder, J. M., Ansfield, F. J., Curreri, A. R., Le Page, G. A. 394, 397, *402*, 500, *510*
Schroeder, W., Hoeksema, H. 446, *455*
Schubert, D., Jacob, F. 312, *344*
Schück, O., see Šmahel, O. 358, *370*
Schütt, M., see Graffi, A. 78, *80*
Schütt, M., see Wunderlich, V. 70, *84*
Schulten, H. K. 732, *746*
Schulten, H. K., Giraldo, G. 705, *720*
Schulten, H. K., Giraldo, G., Boyse, E. A., Oettgen, H. F. 705, 707, *721*
Schulten, H. K., see Oettgen, H. F. 727, 728, 730, 733, 734, 735, *745*
Schultz, A. G., see Stork, G. 650, *656*
Schultz, G. A., see Saunders, P. P. 547, *551*
Schultze, B., see Hughes, W. L. 280, 281, 283, 284, 314, 315, 316, *336*
Schulz, G., see Hampel, K. E. 415, *421*
Schulz, U., McCalla, D. R. 72, *83*
Schuster, H., see Kramer, G. 200, *228*
Schutt, A. J., see Moertel, C. G. 546, *551*, 650, *656*
Schutt, M., see Langen, P. 273, *339*
Schutz, E., see Neufahrt, A. 302, *341*
Schwaier, R., see Marquardt H. 78, *82*
Schwandt, P., see Fateh-Moghadam, A. 734, 735, *744*
Schwartz, D. E. 756, *764*
Schwartz, D. E., Bollag, W., Obrecht, P. 754, *764*
Schwartz, D. E., Brubacher, G. B., Vecchi, M. 754, *764*
Schwartz, D. E., see Raaflaub, J. 754, *764*
Schwartz, G. H., Stenzel, K. H., Rubin, A. L. 406, *424*, 725, 735, 738, *746*
Schwartz, G. H., see Merkatz, I. R. 415, *422*
Schwartz, H. S., Garofalo, M., Sternberg, S. S., Philips, F. S. 790, *792*
Schwartz, H. S., Sodergren, J. E., Amboye, R. Y. 584, *592*
Schwartz, H. S., Sodergren, J. E., Philips, F. S. 47, 48, *62*
Schwartz, J. H., Cedar, H., Ehrman, M. 515, *536*
Schwartz, J. H., Reeves, J. Y., Broome, J. D. 697, 698, *721*

Schwartz, J. H., see Broome, J.D. 711, *714*, 733, *743*
Schwartz, J. H., see Cedar, H. 698, *715*
Schwartz, J. H., see Ehrman, M. 697, 701, *715*
Schwartz, M. K. 704, *721*, 724, *746*
Schwartz, M. K., Lash, E. D., Oettgen, H. F., Tomao, F. A. 704, *721*, 724, 725, 735, *746*
Schwartz, M. K., see Lash, E. 735, *745*
Schwartz, M. K., see Oettgen, H. F. 696, *719*, 723, 727, 730, 733, 734, 735, *745*
Schwartz, M. K., see Pinsky, C.M. 735, 738, *746*
Schwartz, R. S. 418, *423*, 502, *510*, 512, 525, *536*, 705, *721*
Schwartz, R. S., André, J. 384, *402*, 407, 410, *423*
Schwartz, R. S., Beldotti, L. 408, *423*
Schwartz, R. S., Dameshek, W. 407, *423*
Schwartz, R. S., Eisner, A., Dameshek, W. *423*
Schwartz, R. S., Stack, J., Dameshek, W. 407, *423*
Schwartz, R. S., see Borel, Y. *419*
Schwartz, R. S., see Gleichmann, E. 418, *421*
Schwartz, R. S., see Hirsch, M.S. 418, *421*
Schwartz, R. S., see Kyle, R. A. 39, *44*
Schwartz, R. S., see Nathanson, L. 547, *551*
Schwartz, R. S., see Sahiar, K. 407, *423*
Schwartz, R. S., see Swanson, M. A. 407, *416*, *424*
Schwartz, S. O., see Hewlett, J. S. 740
Schwartzbach, E., see Yesair, D. W. 608, 609, *614*
Schwarzenberg, L., see Mathé, G. 685, *692*, 726, 727, 728, 732, 734, 735, *745*, 759, *763*, 772, *786*, 882, *889*
Schwarzenberg, L., Mathé, G., Hayat, M., DeVassal, F., Amiel, J. L., Cattan, A., Schneider, M., Schlumberger, J. R., Rosenfeld, C., Jasmin, C., Ngo/Minh/Mah 474, *482*
Schweisguth, O., see Mathé, G. 759, *763*
Schweitzer, L., see Studzinski, G. P. 54, *63*
Schwendimann, R. N., see Skalko, R. G. 310, *344*
Schwenk, E., see Werthessen, N. T. 106, *138*
Schwimmer, S. 774, 776, *787*
Scoggins, R. B., see Frei, E., III. 679, *690*
Scolnick, E. M., see Aaronson, S. A. 308, *327*
Scott, D. B. M., Lisi, A. G. 122, *136*
Scott, J. L., see Gabor, E. P. 410, *421*
Scott, R. B., see Beard, M. E. J. 726, 727, 728, 730, 734, 735, *743*
Scott, R. B., see Crowther, D. 726, 732, *743*
Scott, R. B., see Fairley, G. H. 759, *762*
Scott, R. S., Rennie, P. I. C. 117, *136*
Scott, W. J., see Ritter, E. J. 237, 241, *254*, 261, *270*
Scott, W. W., Vermeulen, C. 176, *191*
Scott, W. W., see Huggins, C. 170, *189*
Seaman, E., Tarmy, E., Marmur, J. 57, *62*
Sears, E. M., see Farber, S. 394, *399*
Sears, M. L., see Perkins, E. S. 302, 322, *342*
Sebesta, K., Bauerova, J., Sormova, Z. 283, *344*
Sebesta, K., see Bauerova, J. *328*
Sebroll, W. H., see Hertz, R. 110, *130*
Sebring, E. D., see Salzman, N. P. 199, *230*
Šeda, M., see Plevová, J. 358, 359, *368*
Sedov, K. A., Sorokina, I. B., Berlin, Y. A., Kolosov, M. N. 615, 619, *622*
Seeber, S., Warnecke, P., Straub, O. C. 710, *721*
Seeber, S., Weser, U. 710, *721*
Seeber, S., see Warnecke, P. 682, *694*
Seegmiller, J. E., see Goldfinger, S. E. 683, *690*
Seegmiller, J. E., see Kelley, W. N. 414, *422*
Seegmiller, J. E., see Fallon, H. J. 352, 359, *365*
Seelye, R. N., see Cain, B. F. 783, *783*
Šeferna, I., Loukomskaya, N., Kadlec, O., Janků, I. 359, *370*
Segal, S. J., see Talwar, G. P. 113, 114, 119, *137*
Segal, S. J., see Trachewsky, D. 119, *137*
Segaloff, A. 144, *156*, 182, *191*
Segaloff, A., Bowers, C. Y., Rongone, E. L., Murison, P. J., Schlosser, J. V. 173, *191*
Segaloff, A., Carabasi, R., Horwitt, B. N., Schlosser, J. V., Murison, P. J. 184, *191*
Segaloff, A., Horwitt, B. N., Gordon, D. L., Murison, P. J., Schlosser, J. V. 181, *191*
Segaloff, A., Weeth, J. B., Rongone, E. L., Murison, P. J., Bowers, C. Y. 183, *191*
Segaloff, A., see Hilf, R. 123, *130*, 145, *154*
Seichert, V., see Jelínek, R. 358, *367*
Seidel, H. J., see Müller, W. E. G. 583, *591*
Seidenberg, J., see Zimmerman, M. 289, *347*
Seifertová, M., Čihák, A., Veselý, J. *370*
Seifertová, M., Veselý, J., Šorm, F. 358, 363, *370*
Seifertová, M., see Čihák, A. 363, *364*
Seifter, J., see Weisberger, A. S. 522, *537*
Seiki, K., Miyamoto, M., Yamashita, A., Kotani, M. 160, *168*
Seiler, K., see Floersheim, G. L. 408, *420*
Sekely, L., Prusoff, W. H. 282, *344*
Sekely, L., see Prusoff, W. H. 292, 302, *342*
Sekeris, C. E., see Beato, M. 164, *167*
Sekeris, C. E., see Lang, N. 88, *101*
Sekiguchi, M., see Amiel, J.-L. 752, *760*
Selawry, O. 476, *482*
Selawry, O. S., see Carbone, P. P. 726, 727, 728, 730, 732, 734, 735, *743*
Selawry, O. S., see Muggia, F. M. 650, *656*

Selawry, O.S., see Wang, J.J. 262, *271*
Sellei, C., Eckhardt, S., Nemeth, L. 19, *33*
Sellei, C., see Eckhardt, S. 36, *43*
Sellei, C., see Szentklaray, J. 36, *46*
Sellin, H., see Dolowy, W.C. 696, *715*
Sellinger, O.Z., Azcurra, J. M., Ohlsson, W.G. 499, *510*
Sellinger, O.Z., Garaza, A. 499, *510*
Sellinger, O.Z., Weiler, P., Jr. 499, *510*
Sellinger, O.Z., see De Robertis, E. 499, *504*
Sellinger, O.Z., see Lamar, C., Jr. 499, *507*
Sells, B.H., see Slotnick, I. J. 583, *592*
Selmeci, V., see Feher, I. 522, *531*
Selye, H. 143, *156*
Selye, H., Friedman, S. 143, *156*
Semente, G., see Hirschberg, E. 880, *889*
Senda, H., see Mitsuya, H. 870, *873*
Senft, G., see Herken, H. 541, *542*
Senn, H., Holland 780
Senn, H., see Mihich, E. 780, *786*
Sensenbrenner, L.L., see Koons, C.R. 621, *622*
Sensi, P., see Murthy, Y.K. S. 882, *889*
Sentein, P. 673, *693*
Sentenac, A., Ruet, A., Fromageot, P. 659, *667*
Sentenac, A., Simon, E.J., Fromageot, P. 583, *592*, 629, *632*
Sentenac, A., see Greengard, O. 121, *129*
Serebryanyi, A.M., Smotryaeva, M.A., Kruglyakova, K.E. 70, *83*
Serebryanyi, A.M., Smotryaeva, M.A., Kruglyakova, K.E., Kostyanovskii, R.G. 73, *83*
Serpick, A.A., see Burke, P. J. 260, 261, 262, *268*
Serpick, A.A., see DeVita, V.T. 759, 760, *762*
Serpick, A, A., see Goldin, A. 564, *568*
Serpick, A.A., see Gottlieb, J.A. 474, *481*, 545, *550*
Serpick, A.A., see Lowenbraun, S. 760, *763*
Serpick, A.A., see Slater, L. M. 683, *693*
Serpick, A.A., see Haskell, C.M. 734, 735, *744*
Serra, J.A. 712, *721*
Setlow, R.B. 52, *62*
Setlow, R.B., Carrier, W.L. 12, *17*, 52, *62*
Setlow, R.B., see Boyce, R. P. 290, *328*
Seto, H., see Otake, N. 441, *455*
Severo, N.C., see Sullivan, M.P. 397, *403*
Severtzov, A.N., see Georgiev, G.P. 584, *590*
Seyček, V., see Rašková, H. 361, *369*
Seyček, V., see Slavík, M. *370*
Seynsche, K., see Weitzel, G. 756, *765*
Shabel, F., Jr., see Pittillo, A.F. 820, *827*
Shada, J.D., see Rabinowitz, K.W. 440, *455*
Shaddix, S., see Brockman, R.W. 496, *503*, 790, *791*, 793, 800, *805*, 877, 878, *888*
Shadduck, R.K., see Cavins, J.A. 440, *453*
Shaer, J.C., see Burki, K. 318, *329*
Shaffer, J.G., see Albach, H. R. 53, 54, *60*
Shafig, A., see Wiesner, R. 583, *592*
Shah, S.A., see Lawley, P. D. 7, *16*
Shah, V., see Hughes, W.L. 280, 281, 283, 284, 314, 315, 316, *336*
Shah, V.C., see Arora, O.P. 57, *60*
Shamma, M. 649, *656*
Shamma, M., Novak, L. 650, *656*
Shani, M., Sheba, Ch. 519, *536*
Shao, H.W., see Mardashev, S.R. 698, *718*
Shapiro, D.M., Dietrich, L. S., Shils, M.E. 541, *543*
Shapiro, D.M., Fugmann, R.A. 522, *536*
Shapiro, H.A., see Zwarenstein, H. 120, *138*
Shapiro, R., Kang, S. *344*
Shapiro, S.S., see McKay, D.G. 527, *534*
Shapiro, W.R., Ausman, J. I., Rall, D.P. 69, *83*
Shapiro, W.R., see Levin, V.A. 69, *81*
Shapovalova, S.P., see Chorin, V.A. 616, *621*
Sharon, N., Lipmann, F. 521, *536*
Sharpe, H.B.A., Field, E.O., Hellmann, K. 885, *889*
Shatkin, A.H., Reich, E., Franklin, R.M., Tatum, E.L. 54, *62*
Shatkin, A.J., see Rada, B. 354, *369*
Shatkin, A.J., see Reich, E. 582, 583, 584, *591*
Shatkin, A.J., see Salzman, N.P. 199, *230*
Shaw, M., see Hancock, R. L. *154*
Shaw, M.T., Barnes, C.C., Madden, F.J.F., Bagshawe, K.D. 709, *721*
Shaw, M.W., Cohen, M.M., *62*
Shaw, M.W., see Cohen, M. M. 56, 57, *60*, *62*, 634, *640*
Shaw, P.D., see Gottlieb, D. 554, *568*
Shay, A.J., see DeVoe, S.E. 486, 496, *504*
Shay, H., Harris, C., Gruenstein, M. 112, *136*
Shealy, Y.F. 549, 550, *552*
Shealy, Y.F., Clayton, S. J. 434, *455*
Shealy, Y.F., Krauth, C.A. 545, 547, 548, 550, *552*
Shealy, Y.F., Krauth, C.A., Clayton, S.J., Shortnacy, A.T., Laster, W. R., Jr. 550, *552*
Shealy, Y.F., Krauth, C.A., Holum, L.B., Fitzgibbon, W.E. 549, *552*
Shealy, Y.F., Krauth, C.A., Montgomery, J.A. 545, 549, *552*
Shealy, Y.F., Krauth, C.A., Opliger, C.E., Guin, H. W., Laster, W.R., Jr. 549, *552*
Shealy, Y.F., Montgomery, J.A., Laster, W.R., Jr. 544, 549, *552*
Shealy, Y.F., O'Dell, C.A. 549, *552*
Shealy, Y.F., O'Dell, C.A., Clayton, S.J., Krauth, C.A. 549, *552*
Shealy, Y.F., Struck, R.F., Holum, L.B., Montgomery, J.A. 544, 548, *552*

Sheba, Ch., see Shani, M. 519, *536*
Shedden, W. I. H., see Klemperer, H. G. *338*
Sheehan, R., Shklar, G., Tennebaum, R. 417, *424*
Sheen, M. R., Kim, B. K., Parks, R. E., Jr. 445, *455*
Sheen, M. R., Martin, H. F., Parks, R. E., Jr. 444, 445, *455*
Sheena, A. H., see French, F. A. 798, *806*
Sheets, R. F., see Hwang, Y. F. 686, *690*
Sheets, R. F., see Vodopick, H. 40, *46*
Shefner, A. M., see Smith, C. G. 437, 440, 441, 445, *456*
Sheil, A. G. R., Dammin, G. J., Mitchell, R. M., Moseley, R. V., Murray, J. E. 502, *510*
Sheil, A. G. R., Moseley, R. V., Murray, J. E. 502, *510*
Sheil, A. G. R., see Murray, J. E. 502, *508*
Sheiness, D., see Jeleník, W. *669*
Sheiness, P., see Borek, E. 499, *503*
Shelanski, M. L., Taylor, E. W. 677, 678, *693*
Shelanski, M. L., Wisniewski, H. 681, *693*
Shelanski, M. L., see Adelmann, M. R. 676, *688*
Shelanski, M., see Bensch, K. G. 678, *688*
Shelanski, M., see Marantz, R. 677, 678, *692*
Sheldrick, P., see Szybalski, W. 325, *345*
Shelton, R. S., Vancampen, M. G., Jr., Meisner, D. F., Parmerter, S. M., Andrews, E. R., Allen, R. E., Wyckoff, K. K. 105, *136*
Shemyakin, M. M., see Berlin, Y. A. 615, *621*
Shen, R. M., see Galegov, G. A. *366*
Shen, T. Y., McPherson, J. F., Linn, B. O. 302, *344*
Shepard, B. J., see Loo, T. L. 386, *401*, 546, *551*
Sheridan, P. J., see Person, D. A. 302, 307, *342*
Sherman, G., see Meissner, W. A. 175, *191*
Sherman, J. H., see Jacquez, J. A. 500, *506*
Sherman, M. R., Corval, P. L. 187, *191*
Sherman, M. R., Corvol, P. L., O'Malley, B. W. 85, *103*, 163, 164, *168*
Sherman, M. R., see O'Malley, B. W. 160, 161, 162, 163, 164, *168*
Shiba, S., Terawaki, A., Taguchi, T., Kawamata, J. 53, 56, *63*
Shibakawa, R., see Price, C. C. 1, 5, *5*, 19, 26, *33*
Shibata, M., see Kusaka, T. 434, *454*
Shida, K., see Shimazaki, J. 149, *156*
Shields, W. F., see Hill, J. M. 704, *716*, 726, 728, 732, *744*
Shigeura, H. T., Boxer, G. E. 659, *667*
Shigeura, H. T., Boxer, G. E., Meloni, M. L., Sampson, S. D. 659, 661, 663, *667*
Shigeura, H. T., Gordon, C. N. 659, 663, *667*
Shigeura, H. T., Hen, A. C., Hiremath, C. B., Maag, T. A., 524, 528, *536*
Shigeura, H. T., Sampson, S. D. 448, *455*, 662, 663, *667*
Shifrin, S., Ames, B. N., Gerroluzzi-Ames, G. 517, 529, *536*
Shiio, T., Weinbaum, G., Takahashi, H., Maruo, B. 54, *63*
Shils, M. E., see Shapiro, D. M. 541, *543*
Shima, T., see Hata, T. 47, *60*
Shimada, N., see Muramatsu, M. 564, *569*
Shimaoka, N., see Nishimura, H. 373, 374, *382*
Shimazaki, J., Kurihara, H., Ito, Y., Shida, K. 149, *156*
Shimazaki, J., see Coffey, D. S. 151, *153*
Shimizu, K., Gut, M., Dorfman, R. I. 139, *156*
Shimizu, K., Hayano, M., Gut, M., Dorfman, R. I. 139, *156*
Shimizu, Y., see Ishida, N. 444, *454*
Shimizu, Y., see Littman, M. L. 523, *533*
Shimkin, M. B., Weisburger, J. H., Weisburger, E. K., Gubareff, N., Suntzeff, V. 36, *46*
Shimkin, M. B., see Hilf, R. 123, 124, *130*
Shimkin, M. B., see White, L. P. 522, *538*
Shimkin, M. B., see Yamamoto, N. 10, *17*
Shimizu, G., see Wakaki, S. 47, *64*
Shimomura, G., see Kato, S. 870, *873*
Shimoyama, M., see Niitani, H. 54, *62*
Shimoyama, M., see Sakai, Y. 887, *889*
Shimura, Y., Kaizer, H., Nathans, D. 209, *230*
Shimura, Y., Moses, R. E., Nathans, D. 209, 211, *230*
Shiotsuka, R. N., see Haus, E. 249, *252*
Shiplacoff, D., see Jensen, E. V. 114, *131*, 176, 187, *190*
Shipley, E. G., see Herschberger, L. G. 140, *154*
Shipley, R. A., see Dorfman, R. I. 139, 142, *153*
Shipley, W. U. 406, *424*
Shirakawa, S., Frei, E., III, 77, *83*, 546, *552*
Shirakawa, S., see Karon, M. 235, *253*
Shiratori, O., see Matsuura, S. 374, *382*
Shishido, K., Ikoda, Y. 326, *344*
Shive, W. 512, *536*
Shive, W., Skinner, C. G. 485, *510*, 512, 515, 516, 518, 519, 521, *536*
Shive, W., see Davis, A. L. 518, *531*
Shive, W., see Edelson, J. 497, *504*, 524, *531*
Shive, W., see McCord, T. J. 497, *507*, *534*
Shive, W., see Ravel, J. M. 497, *509*, 697, *720*
Shive, W., see Ross, D. L. 498, *509*
Shive, W., see Skinner, C. G. 497, 500, *510*
Shklar, G., see Sheehan, R. 417, *424*
Shnider, B. I., see Condit, P. T. 474, *480*
Shnider, B. I., see Cohen, J. L. 221, *224*
Shnider, B. I., see Colsky, J. 500, *504*
Shnider, B. I., see Foley, H. T. 500, *504*

Shohet, S.B., see Adamson, R.H. 682, 683, *687*
Shons, A., Jetzer, T., Najarian, J.S. 705, *721*
Shooter, E.M., see Baldwin, R.L. 294, *327*
Shooter, K.V., Howse, R., Merrifield, R.K., Robins, A.B. 837, *840*
Shooter, K.V., Merrifield, R.K. 837, *840*
Shooter, K.V., see Lawley, P.D. 10, *16*
Shore, N.A., see Fine, R.N. 687, *690*
Shorr, E., Papanicolaou, G.N., Stimmel, B.F. 143, *156*
Short, L.N., Thompson, H.W. 499, *510*
Short, R.V. 107, *136*
Short, W.A., see Pittillo, A.F. 820, *827*
Shortnacy, A.T., see Shealy, Y.F. 550, *552*
Shuck, D., see Yesair, D.W. 822, 823, *828*
Shugar, D., Fox, J.J. 296, *344*
Shugar, D., see Berens, K. 275, 296, *328*
Shugar, D., see Daržynkiewicz, E. 233, *251*
Shugar, D., see Fikus, M. 198, *225*, 321, *332*
Shugar, D., see Giziewicz, J. 233, *252*
Shugar, D., see Kazimierczuk, Z. 321, *337*
Shugar, D., see Pietrzykowska, I. 293, *342*
Shugar, D., see Szer, W. 198, *230*, 293, *345*
Shumway, N.E., see Stinson, E.B. 416, *424*
Shurin, S.B., see Kessel, D. 240, *253*
Shyamala, G., Gorski, J. 115, *136*
Shyamala, G., see Gorski, J. 115, 117, *129*
Shyamala, G., see Toft, D.O. 114, 115, *137*, 164, *168*
Sibay, T., see Berman, L.D. 78, *79*
Sibley, C.H., see Berlowitz, L. 583, 584, *589*
Sidbury, J.B., see Migeon, C.J. 107, *133*
Siddiqi, O., see Garen, A. 214, *225*
Sidgwick, N.V. 544, *552*
Sidwell, R.W., Arnett, G., Brockman, R.W. 302, *344*
Sidwell, R.W., Arnett, G., Dixon, G.J., Schabel, F.M., Jr. 800, *807*
Sidwell, R.W., Arnett, G., Schabel, F.M., Jr., 428, *433*
Sidwell, R.W., Dixon, G.J., Schabel, F.M., Jr., Kaump, D.H. 428, *433*
Sidwell, R.W., see Brockman, R.W. 793, *805*
Sidwell, R.W., see Dixon, G.L. 428, *432*
Sidwell, R.W., see Schardein, J.L. 428, *433*
Sie, H., see Fishman, W.H. 516, *531*
Sieber, S.M., Whang-Peng, J., Johns, D.G., Adamson, R.H. 880, *889*
Siegel, M.R., Sisler, H.D., Johnson, F. 562, *570*
Siegel, M.R., see Sisler, H.D. 561, *570*
Sieger, L., see Leimbrock, S. 364, *367*
Sierra, J.L., see Thomas, C. 78, *84*
Sies, H., see Bucher, T. 554, *567*
Siev, M., Weinberg, R., Penman, S. *581*, 664, *667*
Sigdestad, C.P., Hagemann, R.F., Lesher, S. 642, 644, *648*
Sigg, E.B., see Greengard, P. 542, *542*
Siimes, M., see Raina, A. 774, *787*
Silagi, S. 241, 242, 244, *255*
Silagi, S., Bruce, S.A. 311, *344*
Silas, D.E., Nance, F.C. 410, *424*
Silberberg, D.H., see Zweiman, B. 416, *425*
Silberman, H.R., Wyngaarden, J.B. 389, *402*
Silberstein, N., see Yagil, E. 211, *231*
Silver, R.T., see Ellison, R.R. 260, *268*
Silver, R.T., see Ohnuma, T. 726, 727, 728, 734, 735, *746*
Silverman, C.A., see Miller, F.A. 428, *433*
Silverman, D.A., see Williams-Ashman, H.G. 147, *157*
Silverstein, G., see Hilf, R. 123, *130*
Silverstein, J.N., see Wallace, E.Z. 811, *819*
Silverstein, M.N., see Kolmeier, K.H. 777, *785*
Silvester, D.J., White, W.D. 273, *344*
Silvestri, L.G., see Riva, S. 883, *889*
Silvestrini, R., DiMarco, A., Dasdia, T. 604, 605, *613*
Silvestrini, R., DiMarco, A., Dasdia, T., DiMarco, S. 603, *613*
Silvestrini, R., Gaetani, M. *613*
Silvestrini, R., see Casazza, A.M. 607, 610, *611*
Silvestrini, R., see DiFronzo, G. 608, *612*
Silvestrini, R., see DiMarco, A. 593, 597, 599, 605, 607, 609, *612*
Sim, G.A., see McPhail, A.T. 649, *656*
Sim, G.A., see Wall, M.E. 649, *656*
Simard, J., see Delage, J.M. 735, 738, *744*
Simard, R. 583, *592*, 604, *613*
Simard, R., Bernhard, W. 494, *510*, 628, *632*
Simberkoff, M.S., Thomas, L. 707, *721*
Simberkoff, M.S., Thorbecke, G.J., Thomas, L. 707, *721*
Siminoff, P. 302, 304, *344*
Siminoff, P., Menefee, M.G. 302, 303, 304, *344*
Siminoff, P., see Price, K.E. 496, *508*
Simmel, E., see Chaube, S. 790, *791*
Simmons, R.L., Kjellstrand, C.M., Buselmeier, T.J., Najarian, J.S. 414, *424*
Simms, E.S., see Bessman, J.J. 281, *328*
Simms, E.S., see Lehman, I.R. 274, *339*
Simon, D.C., see Jondorf, W.R. 560, *569*
Simon, E.H. 298, 299, 302, 306, *344*
Simon, E.H., see Miner, N. 607, *613*
Simon, E.H., see Toliver, A. 299, *346*
Simon, E.J., see Sentenac, A. 583, *592*, 629, *632*
Simon, M.I., Van Vunakis, H. 608, *613*

Simone, J. V., see Aur, R. J. A. 726, 732, 734, 735, *742*
Simonet, P., see Oxford, A. E. 670, *692*
Simoni, R. D., Leivnthal, M., Kundig, F. D., Kundig, W., Anderson, B., Hartman, P. E., Roseman, S. 93, *103*
Simonis, A. M., see Ariëns, E. J. 462, *464*
Simonsen, L., see Blattner, R. J. 493, *503*
Simonsson, E., see Caspersson, T. 6, *15*
Simpson, A. I., see Wang, M. C. 391, *403*
Simpson, C. A., see Ravin, L. J. 275, *343*
Simpson, C. A., see Ravin, L. S. 275, *343*
Simpson, C. L., see Mihich, E. 770, 780, *787*, 842, 843, *848*
Simpson, E. R., Cooper, D. Y., Estabrook, R. W. 140, *156*
Simpson, J. G., see Gale, G. R. 757, *762*
Simpson, L., Bennett, L. L., Jr., Golden, J. 392, *402*
Simpson, L., see Bennett, L. L., Jr. 391, *398*
Simpson, L., see Mihich, E. 445, *454*
Simpson, M. S., see Brockman, R. W. 385, *398*, 460, *465*
Simpson, M. V., see Karol, M. H. 282, 295, *337*
Simpson, P. J., see Palmer, C. G. 673, *692*
Simpson-Herren, L., Skipper, H. E., Blow, J. G. 78, *83*
Simpson-Herren, L., see Griswold, D. P., Jr. 235, *252*
Simpson-Herren, L., see Laster, W. R., Jr. 389, *400*
Sinclair, C., see Israels, L. G. 38, *44*
Sinclair, N. R. St. C., Elliott, E. V. 707, *721*
Sinclair, W. K. 59, *63*
Singer, B., Fraenkel-Conrat, H. 7, 15, *17*, 71, *83*
Singhal, R. L. 152, *156*
Singhal, R. L., Valadares, J. R. E. *136*, 152, *156*
Singhal, R. L., Valadares, J. R. E., Ling, G. M. 123, 124, *136*
Singhal, R. L., Vijayvargiya, R., Ling, G. M. 152, *156*
Singhal, R. L., see Valadares, J. R. E. 124, 125, *137*
Sinks, L. F., see Ohnuma, T. 514, *534*, 703, *719*, 724, 725, 733, 734, 735, *745*
Sinkus, A. G. 57, *63*
Sinsheimer, R. L., see Lindqvist, B. 58, *61*
Sinsheimer, R. L., see Pitts, J. 855, 857, 860, *874*
Sirica, A., Venditti, J. M., Kline, I. 830, *840*
Sirsi, M., see Reddy, V. V. S. 697, 698, 699, *720*
Sisler, H. D., Siegel, M. R. 561, *570*
Sisler, H. D., see Siegel, M. R. 562, *570*
Sitaramayya, A., see Krishnan, P. S. 460, *466*
Sivak, A., Rogers, W. I., Kensler, C. J. 823, 824, *828*
Sivak, A., Rogers, W. I., Wodinsky, I., Kensler, C. J. 822, 823, 824, *828*
Sivak, A., Mahoney, A. J., Rogers, W. I. 824, *828*
Sivak, A., see Rogers, W. I. 822, *828*
Sjoerdsma, A. J. 519, 520, *536*
Sjöstrand, J., see Karlsson, J. O. 675, *691*
Skalko, R. G., Packard, D. S., Jr., Schwendimann, R. N., Raggio, J. R. 310, *344*
Skarpa, M., Udall, V. 410, *424*
Skeel, R. T., Marsh, J. C., DeConti, R. C., Mitchell, M. S., Hubbard, S. P., Bertino, J. R. 477, *482*
Skeel, R. T., see Bertino, J. R. 473, *479*
Skeel, R. T., see Leventhal, B. G. 501, *507*, 726, 723, 734, 735, *745*
Skeel, R. T., see Levitt, M. 478, *481*
Skibba, J. L., Beal, D. D., Ramirez, G., Bryan, G. T. 546, 547, *552*
Skibba, J. L., Bryan, G. T. 546, 547, *552*
Skibba, J. L., Ertürk, E., Bryan, G. T. 547, *552*
Skibba, J. L., Johnson, R. O., Bryan, G. T. 71, *83*
Skibba, J. L., Ramirez, G., Beal, D. D., Bryan, G. T. 545, 546, *552*
Skibba, J. L., see Ansfield, F. J. 221, *223*
Skinner, C. G., McCord, T. J., Ravel, J. M., Shive, W. 497, *510*
Skinner, C. G., McKenna, G. F., McCord, T. J., Shive, W. 500, *510*
Skinner, C. G., McKenna, G. F., Ross, D. L., Shive, W. *510*
Skinner, C. G., see Davis, A. L. 518, *531*
Skinner, C. G., see Edelson, J. 479, *504*, 524, *531*
Skinner, C. G., see McCord, T. J. 497, *507*, *534*
Skinner, C. G., see Ravel, J. M. 497, *509*
Skinner, C. G., see Ross, D. L. 489, *509*
Skinner, C. G., see Shive, W. 485, *510*, 512, 515, 516, 518, 519, 521, *536*
Skinner, W. A., Johansson, J. G. 37, *46*
Skipper, H. E. 21, 23, *33*, 390, *402*, 500, *510*, 791, *792*
Skipper, H. E., Bennett, L. L., Jr. *402*, 458, *467*
Skipper, H. E., Bennett, L. L., Jr., Schabel, F. M., Jr. 486, *510*
Skipper, H. E., Schabel, F. M., Jr., Mellett, L. B., Montgomery, J. A., Wilkoff, L. J., Lloyd, H. H., Brockman, R. W. 235, *255*, 798, *807*
Skipper, H. E., Schabel, F. M., Jr., Wilcox, W. S. 235, 249, *255*, 260, 261, 262, *271*
Skipper, H. E., Schmidt, L. H. 394, *402*
Skipper, H. E., Thomson, J. R. 502, *510*, 528, *536*
Skipper, H. E., Thomson, J. R., Bell, M. 522, *536*
Skipper, H. E., see Bennett, L. L., Jr. 386, *398*, 463, *464*, 486, 495, *503*
Skipper, H. E., see Brockman, R. W. 385, *398*, 460, *465*, 793, *805*
Skipper, H. E., see Griswold, D. P., Jr. 767, *785*
Skipper, H. E., see Laster, W. R., Jr. 389, *400*
Skipper, H. E., see Pittillo, R. F. 20, *33*, 820, *827*

Skipper, H. E., see Schabel, F. M., Jr. 65, 68, 69, 76, 79, *83*, 389, 391, 393, *402*, 494, *509*
Skipper, H. E., see Simpson-Herren, L. 78, *83*
Skipper, H. E., see Tomisek, A. J. 486, 496, *511*
Škoda, J., Hess, V. F., Šorm, F. 349, *370*
Škoda, J., Kára, J., Čihák, A., Šorm, F. 350, *370*
Škoda, J., Kára, J., Šormová, Z. 352, *370*
Škoda, J., Kára, J., Šormová, Z., Šorm, F. 352, *370*
Škoda, J., Lisý, V., Smrt, J., Holý, A., Šorm, F. *370*
Škoda, J., Šorm, F. 349, 350, 352, *370*
Škoda, J., Veselý, J. 350
Škoda, J., see Čihák, A. 350, *364*
Škoda, J., see Handschumacher, R. E. 349, *367*
Škoda, J., see Lisý, V. 349, 353, *368*
Škoda, J., see Rada, B. 354, *369*
Škoda, J., see Welch, A. D. 357
Škoda, J., see Winkler, A. 352, *372*
Sköld, O. 202, 203, *230*, 352, *370*
Sköld, O., Magnusson, P. H., Revesz, L. 217, *230*
Sköld, O., see Reichard, P. 217, *229*
Skoog, F., see Leonard, N. J. 435, *454*
Skoog, L. 446, *455*
Skoog, L., Nordenskjöld, B. A., 242, *255*
Skoog, L., see Nordenskjöld, B. A. 242, *254*
Skopińska, E., Sankowski, A., Nouza, K. 408, *424*
Slade, H. D., see Reitz, R. H. 497, *509*
Slapikoff, S., Berg, P. 208, *230*
Slater, D. W., Slater, I., Gillespie, D. *669*
Slater, I., see Slater, D. W. *669*
Slater, L. M., Wainer, R. A., Serpick, A. A. 683, *693*
Slater, T. F., Sawyer, B. C. 491, *510*
Slavík, M., Elis, J., Rašková, H., Gutová, M., Duchková, M., Kubíková, M., Seyček, V. *370*
Slavík, M., Hyánek, J., Elis, J., Homolka, J. 361, *370*
Slavík, M., see Elis, J. 361, *365*
Slavík, M., see Havelka, S. 361, *367*
Slavík, M., see Nouza, K. 356, *368*
Slavík, M., see Rašková, H. *369*
Slayton, R. E., see Rossof, A. H. 839, *840*
Slechta, L. 235, 237, *255*, 448, *455*
Sleight, S. D., see Kociba, R. J. 830, 831, *840*
Slesers, A., see Hruban, Z. 519, *532*
Slesers, A., see Samal, B. A. 520, *535*
Sloan, B. J., Miller, F. A., Ehrlich, J., McLean, W. J., Jr. 428, *433*
Sloan, B. J., see Dixon, G. L. 428, *432*
Sloan, B. J., see Miller, F. A. 428, *433*
Sloan, N., see Barg, W. 488, *503*
Slomp, G., see Hoeksema, H. 446, 447, *454*
Slonim, R. R., Howell, D. S., Brown, H. E., Jr. 675, *693*
Slotnick, I. J., Dougherty, M., James, D. H., Jr. 680, *693*
Slotnick, I. J., Sells, B. H. 583, *592*
Slotnick, I. J., Visser, D. W., Rittenberg, S. C. 377, *382*
Slotnick, I. J., see Goldstein, M. N. 583, *590*
Slotwiner, P., see Anderson, P. J. 675, *688*
Šmahel, O., Černoch, A., Šorm, F., König, J., Valenta, O., Švehla, C., Švorc, J., Bláha, V., Uher, V., Gerberová, J. 361, *370*
Šmahel, O., Grafnetterová, J., König, K., Schück, O. 358, *370*
Šmahel, O., see Grafentterová, J. 357, 358, 359, *366*
Smale, B. C., Montgillion, M. D., Pridham, T. G. 855, *874*
Smallmann, L., v., see Grimes, P. 39, *44*
Šmejkal, F., Šorm, F. 354, *370*
Šmejkal, J., see Tkaczynski, T. 350, *371*
Smellie, R. M. S., see Billing, R. J. 120, *126*
Smetana, K., see Jiřička, Z. 349, 358, *367*
Smetana, R., see Janků, I. 359, *367*
Smetana, R., see Novotný, J. 349, *368*
Smidová, V., see Rada, B. 354, *369*
Smirnov, M. N., see Georgiev, G. P. 584, *590*
Smirnova, I. N. 621, *622*
Smith, A. B., see Gale, G. R. 757, *762*, 838, *839*, 882, *888*
Smith, A. B., see Howle, J. A. 838, *839*
Smith, B. A., see Roberts, J. J. 14, *17*, 78, *83*
Smith, C. E., see Gellert, M. 585, 589, *590*
Smith, C. F., see Hart, M. M. 879, *888*
Smith, C. G., Buskirk, H. H., Lummis, W. L. 238, *255*
Smith, C. G., Grady, J. E., Kupiecki, F. P. 222, *230*, 683, *693*
Smith, C. G., Gray, G. D., Carlson, R. G., Hanze, A. R. 437, 445, *456*
Smith, C. G., Reineke, L. M., Harpootlian, H., Burch, M. R., Shefner, A. M., Muirhead, E. C. 437, 440, 441, 445, *456*
Smith, C. G., see Bhuyan, B. K. 557, *567*, 573, *579*, 602, *611*, 624, 625, 629, *631*
Smith, C. G., see Camiener, G. W. 238, 239, *250*, 259, 262, 266, *268*
Smith, C. G., see Owen, S. P. 439, *455*
Smith, C. R., Jr., see Powell, R. G. 556, *569*
Smith, C. W. 516
Smith, C. W., see White, P. B. 516, 529, *538*
Smith, D. A., Visser, D. W. 377, 378, *382*
Smith, D. A., Roy-Burman, P., Visser, D. W. 380, *382*

Smith, D.B., Chu, E.H.Y. 246, 247, *255*
Smith, D.E., Gorski, J. 93, *103*, 124, *136*
Smith, D.E., see Gorski, J. 115, 117, *129*
Smith, F.E., see Lane, M. 477, *481*
Smith, G.L., see Grula, E.A. 59, *60*
Smith, G.V.S., see Wall, E. 175, *192*
Smith, H.H., Fussel, C.P., Kugelman, B.H. 380, *382*
Smith, H.H., Kugelman, B.H. *344*
Smith, H.H., Kugelman, B.H., Commerford, S.L., Szybalski, W. 314, *344*
Smith, I., see Penman, S. 572, *580*
Smith, J.D., Freeman, G., Vogt, M., Dulbecco, R. 302, 307, *344*
Smith, J.D., Mathews, R.E.F. 463, *467*
Smith, J.D., see Dunn, D.B. 272, 274, 280, 295, 303, *331*, 380, *381*
Smith, J.D., see Lasnitzki, I. 463, *466*
Smith, J.L., Forbes, I.J. 406, *424*
Smith, K.A., see Walker, M.D. 69, *84*
Smith, K.C. 319, 321, *344*
Smith, K.C., see Bagshaw, M.A. 291, 319, 324, *327*
Smith, K.O. 303, 304, 305, 306, *344*
Smith, K.O., Dukes, C.D. 302, 303, 304, 305, *345*
Smith, L.G., see McCord, T.J. 518, *534*
Smith, L.H., see Cudkowicz, G. 314, *330*
Smith, M.A., see Greengard, O. 120, 121, *129*
Smith, M.E., see Hall, J.G. 318, *334*
Smith, M.G.M., see Mitchell, C.G. 413, 414, *422*
Smith, M.S., see Bo, W. *126*
Smith, M.W., see Lynch, V. 18, *33*
Smith, O.W., see Ryan, K.J. 106, 107, *135*
Smith, P.K., see Kelly, M.G. 684, *691*
Smith, P.K., see Mandel, H.G. 459, 460, *466*
Smith, P.K., see Nadkarni, V.M. 39, *45*
Smith, R., see Barrett, P.A. 841, *847*
Smith, R.G., Whang-Peng, J., Gallo, R.C., Levine, P., Ting, R.C. 883, *889*
Smith, R.G., see Yang, S.S. 883, *890*
Smith, R.K., see Trams, E.G. 27, *33*
Smith, R.M., see Bhuyan, B.K. 623, *631*
Smith, R.P., see Hensen, D. 302, 304, *335*
Smith, S., see Burchenal, J.H. 820, *826*
Smith, S., see Jensen, E.V. 85, 95, *101*, 110, 114, 115, 117, *131*, 176, 187, *190*
Smith, S.J., Busch, H. 25, *33*
Smith, S.S., Bayliss, N.L., McCord, T.J. 524, *536*
Smith, V.H., see Pilcher, K.S. 515, *535*
Smith, W.G., see Leake, E. 39, *44*
Smith-Kielland, I. 54, *63*
Smithers, D., see Bennett, L.L. 437, *452*
Smithers, D., see Bennett, L.L., Jr. 487, *503*
Smithson, C.H., see Aposhian, H.V. 523, *529*
Smol, B.A., see Schmid, F.A. 521, 524, *536*
Smolin, G., Keates, R.H. 527, *536*
Smotryaeva, M.A., see Serebryanyi, A.M. 70, 73, *83*
Smrt, J. 233, *255*
Smrt, J., see Černěckij, V. 349, *364*
Smrt, J., see Lisý, V. 353, *368*
Smrt, J., see Škoda, J. *370*
Smrt, J., see Šorm, F. *370*
Smrt, J., see Žemlička, J. 349, *372*
Smuckler, E.A., Hadjiolov, A.A. *669*
Smulson, M.E., Neal, A.L. 485, 497, *510*
Smulson, M.E., Rabinovitz, M., Breitman, T.R. 524, *536*
Smulson, M.E., Suhadolnik, R.J. 436, *456*
Smulson, M.E., see Neal, A.L. *508*
Sneddon, J.M. *693*
Snow, M.Y., see Griswold, D.P., Jr. 767, *785*
Snyder, A.L., Kann, H.E., Jr., Kohn, K.W. 574, *581*, 881, *890*
Snyder, A.L., see Kann, H.E., Jr. 75, *81*, 574, *580*
Sobell, H.M., Jain, S.C., Sakore, T.D. 573, *581*
Snyder, S.H., see Russell, D.H. 774, *787*
Sobell, H.M. 587, 588, *592*
Sobell, H.M., Jain, S.C., Sakore, T.D., Nordman, C.E. 587, *592*
Sobell, H.M., see Mazza, F. 197, *228*
Sobell, H.M., see Tavale, S.S. 279, *345*
Sober, H.A. *874*
Sober, H.A., see Meister, A. 708, *718*
Sobin, L.H., Kidd, J.G. 709, *721*
Sodergren, J.E., see Schwartz, H.S. 47, 48, *62*, 584, *592*
Sögtrop, H.H., see Goldenberg, D.M. 259, *269*
Sögtrop, H.H., see Müller, W.E.G. 243, *254*
Soergel, M., see Loh, P.C. 241, *253*
Sogo, J.M., see Stockert, J.C. 662, *667*
Soifer, V.S., see Berlin, Y.A. 615, *621*
Soike, K.F., see Pilcher, K.S. 515, *535*
Sokolski, W.T., see Vavra, J.J. 65, *84*
Sokovnina, see Mardashev, S.R. 498
Soldati, M., Fioretti, A., Ghione, M. 566, *570*
Soldati, M., see Di Marco, A. 593, 594, 597, 609, *612*
Soller, A., see Parisi, B. 606, *613*
Solnik, C., see Hirsch, M.S. 418, *421*
Soloff, M.S., Szego, C.M. 114, *136*
Solomon, D.M., see Volkmann, R. 650, *656*
Solomons, I.A., see Beereboom, J.J. 565, *567*
Solotorovsky, M., see Pugh, L.H. 660, *667*
Solymosi, J., see Ross, V.C. 56, *62*
Somarjai, R.L., see Gingras, B.A. 841, *848*

Somers, C. E., see Hsu, T. C. 200, *226*, 300, *336*
Sommers, S. C., Meissner, W. A. 175, *191*
Sommers, S. C., see Meissner, W. A. 175, *191*
Sommerville, R. L., see Greenberg, G. 277, *334*
Sondheimer, E., see Tepper, H. B. 857, *875*
Sonea, S., see De Repentigny, J. 201, *224*
Song, S. K., see Anderson, P. J. 675, *688*
Sonnabend, J. A., Martin, E. M., Mess, E., Fantes, K. H. 607, *613*
Sopori, M. L., see Talwar, G. P. 114, *137*
Sorensen, L. B. 414, *424*
Šorm, F., Keilová, H. 355, *370*
Šorm, F., Pískala, A., Cihák, A., Veselý, J. 351, 362, *370*
Šorm, F., Smrt, J., Černěckij, V. *370*
Šorm, F., Šormová, Z., Raška, K., Jurovčík, M. 351, *370*
Šorm, F., Veselý, J. 349, 351, 355, 362, *370*
Šorm, F., see Bauerova, J. *328*
Šorm, F., see Beránek, J. 349, 350, *364*
Šorm, F., see Bobek, M. 349, *364*
Šorm, F., see Černěckij, V. 349, *364*
Šorm, F., see Čihák, A. 350, 351, 361, 362, 363, *364*, *365*
Šorm, F., see Doskočil, J. 351, 361, 362, *365*
Šorm, F., see Farkaš, J. 350, *366*
Šorm, F., see Grafnetterová, J. 357, 358, 359, *366*
Šorm, F., see Grünberger, D. 464, *465*
Šorm, F., see Habermann, V. 352, *366*
Šorm, F., see Handschumacher, R. E. 349, *367*
Šorm, F., see Jurovčík, M. 362, *367*, 574, *579*
Šorm, F., see Kafka, V. 360, *367*
Šorm, F., see Kára, J. 349, 350, *367*
Šorm, F., see Lisý, V. 353, *368*
Šorm, F., see Pačes, V. 362, *368*
Šorm, F., see Pískala, A. 351, *368*
Šorm, F., see Pliml, J. 349, 350, 351, *368*
Šorm, F., see Prystaš, M. 273, *342*, 349, 350, *369*
Šorm, F., see Rada, B. 354, *369*
Šorm, F., see Raška, K. 351, 362, *369*
Šorm, F., see Seifertová, M. 358, 363, *370*
Šorm, F., see Škoda, J. 350, 352, *370*
Šorm, F., see Šmahel, O. 361, *370*
Šorm, F., see Šmejkal, F. 354, *370*
Šorm, F., see Škoda, J. 349, *370*
Šorm, F., see Svatá, M. 363, *371*
Šorm, F., see Tkaczynski, T. 350, *371*
Šorm, F., see Veselý, J. 351, 362, 363, *371*
Šorm, F., see Wieczorkowski, J. 350, *371*
Šorm, F., see Winkler, A. 352, *372*
Šorm, F., see Žemlička, J. 349, 350, *372*
Šormova, Z., see Bauerova, J. 283, *328*
Šormová, Z., see Fučík, V. *366*
Šormová, Z., see Jurovčík, M. 362, 363, *367*, 574, *579*
Šormová, Z., see Raška, K. 351, 362, *369*
Šormová, Z., see Sebesta, K. 283, *344*
Šormová, Z., see Škoda, J. 352, *370*
Šormová, Z., see Šorm, F. 351, *370*
Sornson, H. C., see Ryan, W. L. 708, *720*
Sorokina, I. B., see Sedov, K. A. 615, 619, *622*
Sothern, R. B., see Haus, E. 249, *252*
Souček, J., Ehrke, M. J., Mihich, E. 781, *787*
Souček, J., see Dave, C. 771, 776, 781, *784*
Souček, J., see Mihich, E. 767, 780, *786*
Soules, K. H., see Wissler, R. W. 525, 526, *538*
Southren, A. L., Tochimoto, S., Strom, L., Ratuschni, A., Ross, R., Gordon, G. 811, 813, *818*
Southren, A. L., Weisenfeld, S., Laufer, A., Goldner, M. G. 811, *819*
Sowa, J. R., Price, C. C. 2, *5*
Sowa, J. R., see Price, C. C. 1, 5, *5*, 19, 26, *33*
Spackman, D. H., see Riley, V. 704, *720*
Spaet, T. H., see Biezinski, J. J. 824, *826*
Spahr, P. F., see Gros, F. 210, *225*
Spalla, C., see Arcamone, F. 593, *611*
Spanedda, A., see Ferrari, W. 769, *784*
Spanio, L., see Levis, A. G. 25, *32*
Sparks, M. C., see Brockman, R. W. 460, *465*
Spasskaya, I. G., Larionov, L. F. 518, *536*
Spasskaya, I. G., see Larionov, L. F. 518, *533*
Spataro, A., Kessel, D. 653, *656*
Spaziani, E., see Mills, T. M. 93, *102*
Spears, C. L., see Kohn, K. W. 8, 13, *15*, *16*, 41, *44*, 53, *61*, 644, 645, 646, *647*
Speck, J. F. 499, *510*
Spector, A., see Jondorf, W. R. 824, *827*
Speer, R. J., see Hill, J. M. 838, *839*
Speert, H. 176, *191*
Spelsberg, T. C., Steggles, A. W., Chytil, F., O'Malley, B. W. *168*
Spelsberg, T. C., Steggles, A. W., O'Malley, B. W. 85, 96, 99, *103*, 165, *168*
Spelsberg, T. C., see O'Malley, B. W. 160, 161, 162, 164, *168*
Spencer, H. H., see Kuang, D. T. 638, 639, *640*
Spencer, H. H., see Nasjleti, C. E. 634, *641*
Spencer, R. L., Preiss, J. 491, *510*
Spencer, R. P., Bow, T. M., Markulis, M. A. 495, *510*
Spencer, R. P., Brody, K. R., Lutters, B. M. 521, *536*
Spencer, R. P., Brody, K. R., Mautner, H. G. 523, *536*

Spencer, R. P., see Johns, D. G. 472, *481*
Speth, V., see Wunderlich, F. 676, *694*
Speyer, J. F. 282, *345*
Speyer, J. F., Karam, J. D., Lenny, A. B. 282, *345*
Speyer, J. F., see Lengyel, P. 214, *228*
Speyer, J. F., see Wahba, A. J. 214, *231*
Spichard, A., see Knight, V. *338*
Spiegelberg, H. L., Miescher, P. A. 408, *424*
Spiegelman, S., Halvorson, H. O., Ben-Ishai, R. 377, *382*
Spiegelman, S., see Halvorson, H. O. 513, *532*
Spolter, P. D., Baldridge, R. C. *536*
Spooner, B. S., Yamada, K. M., Wessells, N. K. 676, *693*
Spooner, E., see Buchenal, J. H. 822, *826*
Sporn, M. B., see Dingman, C. W. 583, 584, *590*
Sprague, P. W., see Wenkert, E. 649, *656*
Sprent, J., see Miller, J. F. A. P. 405, *422*
Spring, F. S., see Cunningham, K. G. 658, 660, *665*
Sprinzl, M., Cramer, F. *669*
Sprinzl, M., Scheit, K. H., Sternbach, H., von der Haar, F., Cramer, F. *669*
Sprunt, J. G., Rizza, C. R. 39, *46*
Spurr, C. L., see Ellison, R. R. 260, *268*
Squires, R. W., see Ho, P. P. K. 698, 699, 700, 702, 708, *716*
Srinivasan, P. R., Rivera, A., Jr. 492, 496, *510*
Srinivasan, P. R., Weiss, B. 492, *510*
Srinivasan, P. R., see Baliga, B. S. 209, *223*
Srinivasan, P. R., see Tamir, H. 492, *510*
Srivastava, P. C., Nagpal, K. L. 273, *345*
Stacey, K. A., see Atkinson, C. 235, 241, *249*
Stack, J., see Schwartz, R. S. 407, *423*
Stähelin, H. 673, 674, 681, *693*
Stähelin, H., Cerletti, A. 675, 684, *693*
Staehelin, M., see Gordon, M. P. 208, *225*
Staehelin, M., see Wehrli, W. 883, *890*
Staerk, J., Zwisler, O., Ronneberger, H. 703, *721*
Stahl, F. W., see Meselson, M. 292, *340*
Stahl, F. W., see Terzaghi, B. E. 296, *345*
Stahl, G. L., see Michaels, R. M. 841, *848*
Stambuk, B. K., see Kim, J. H. 674, *691*
Stanislavskaya, M. S., see Chorin, V. A. 617, *621*
Stapley, E. W., Miller, T. W., Mata, J. M., Hendlin, D. 518, *536*
Stare, F., see Fillios, L. C. 109, *128*
Stark, G. R. 72, *83*, *84*
Stark, W. M., see Williams, R. H. 446, *457*
Starling, K. A., see Sutow, W. W. 726, 727, 732, *746*
Starzl, T. E. 407, 410, 414, *424*
Starzl, T. E., Marchioro, T. L., Porter, K. A., Taylor, P. D., Faris, T. D., Hermann, T. J., Hlad, C. L., Waddell, W. R. 410, *424*
Starzl, T. E., see Penn, I. 415, 417, *423*
Starzl, T. E., see Rifkind, D. 416, *423*
Stasiw, R. O., see Hasselberger, F. X. 724, 735, *744*
Stearns, B., Losee, K. A., Bernstein, J. 789, *792*
Steel 314
Steensholt, G. 697, *721*
Stefanović, V. 644, 647, *648*
Stefanović, V., Ceprini, M. Q. 647, *648*
Stefanović, V., see Leimgruber, W. 642, *648*
Steffa, M., see Burchenal, J. H. 799, *805*
Steggles, A. W., King, R. J. B. 115, *136*
Steggles, A. W., see O'Malley, B. W. 160, 161, 162, 164, *168*
Steggles, A. W., see Spelsberg, T. C. 85, 96, 99, *103*, 165, *168*
Stehlin, J. S., see Klatt, O. 29, *32*
Stehun, J. S., Jr., see Milner, A. N. 27, *33*
Steigbigel, N. H., see Kohn, K. W. 13, *16*, 53, *61*
Stein, G. S., Rothstein, H. 59, *63*
Stein, J., see Krueger, R. C. 283, 314, 315, *338*
Stein, K. F., Carrier, E. 145, *156*
Steinbeck, H., see Neumann, F. 146, *155*
Steinberg, A. D. 479, *482*
Steinberg, M. 109, *136*
Steinberg, M., Tolksdorf, S., Gordon, A. S. 109, *136*
Steinman, I. D., Iyer, V. N., Szybalski, W. 494, *510*
Stejskalová, V., Iványi, J., Kára, J. 356, *371*
Stellwagen, R. H., Tomkins, G. M. 312, 325, *345*
Stempien, M. F., Jr., see Bergman, W. 435, *452*
Stenram, U. 583, *592*
Stent, G. S., see Pratt, D. 297, *342*
Stenzel, K. H., see Merkatz, I. R. 415, *422*
Stenzel, K. H., see Schwartz, G. H. 406, *424*, 725, 735, 738, *746*
Stephens, J. D., see Newmark, P. 283, *341*
Stephens, R. E. 678, *693*
Stephens, Z. H., see Wheeler, G. P. 27, *34*
Stephenson, J., see Atkinson, M. R. 386, *397*
Stephenson, P., see Oettgen, H. F. 727, 730, 732, 734, 735, *745*
Sterental, A., Dominguez, J. M., Weissman, C., Pearson, O. H. 112, *136*, 174, *101*
Stern, B. R., see Schmid, F. A. 521, 524, *536*
Stern, H., see Hotta, Y. 859, *872*
Stern, R., Friedman, R. M. 584, *592*
Stern, R., Twanmoh, A., Cooper, H. L. *669*
Sternbach, H., see Sprinzl, M. *669*
Sternberg, S. S. 610, *613*
Sternberg, S. S., Philips, F. S. 609, *613*
Sternberg, S. S., Philips, F. S., Scholler, J. 36, 37, *46*
Sternberg, S. S., see Clarke, D. A. 396, *398*
Sternberg, S. S., see Ellison, R. R. 500, *504*

Sternberg, S.S., see Lenaz, L. 233, 241, *253*
Sternberg, S.S., see Philips, F.S. 389, 394, *401*
Sternberg, S.S., see Scholler, J. 283, *344*
Sternberg, S.S., see Schwartz, H.S. 790, *792*
Sterns, E., see Marmorston, J. 178, *191*
Šterzl, J. 356, *371*
Steuart, C.D., Burke, P.J. 247, *255*, 265, *271*
Steuart, C.D., Burke, P.J., Owens, A.H., Jr. 247, *255*, 265, *271*
van Steveninck, J. 93, *103*
Stevens, D.A., see Merigan, T.C. 417, *422*
Stevens, J., Mashburn, L. T., Hollander, V.P. 90, *103*
Stevens, J.E., Willoughby, D.A. 408, *424*
Stevens, M.F.G., see Baldwin, R.W. 517, *530*
Stevens, R.E., Jr., see Huggins, C. 170, *189*
Stevens, T.M., see Stollar, V. 354, *371*
Stevens, V., see Vorys, N. 109, *137*
Stevens, W., Colessides, C., Dougherty, T.F. *103*
Stevens, W., Dougherty, T. F. 87, *103*
Stevenson, C.J., see Ashton, H. 384, *397*
Stewart, G.A., Farber, E. 583, *592*
Stewart, M.L., see Goldberg, I.H. 557, 558, 559, 566, *568*
Stewart, P.B., Bell, R. 752, *764*
Stewart, P.B., Cohen, V. 752, *764*
Stewart, R.C., see Force, E. E. 303, 307, *333*
Stewart, S.E., Kasnic, G., Jr., Draycott, C., Feller, W., Golden, A., Mitchell, E., Ben, T. 308, *345*
Stewart, S.E., Kasnic, G., Jr., Ben, T. 308, *345*
Stewart, T., see Pagé, D. 416, *423*
Stickler, D.J., Tucher, R. G., Kay, D. 57, *63*
Stier, H.W., Gallmeier, W. M., Schmidt, C.G. *746*
Stimmel, B.F., see Shorr, E. 143, *156*
Stinebaugh, S.E., see Melnick, J.L. *228*
Stinson, E.B., Bieber, C.P., Griepp, R.B., Clark, D. A., Shumway, N.E., Remington, J.S. 416, *424*
Stinson, K.K., see Creasey, W.A. 795, 799, 800, 801, 802, *805*
Stirpe, F., see Bonetti, E. 697, *714*
Stobbe, H., see Heine, K.M. 416, *421*
Stock, C.C., Sugiura, K. 380
Stock, C.C., see Burchenal, J.H. 544, 550, *550*
Stock, C.C., see Clarke, D.A. 391, 396, *398*, 500, 501, *504*, 544, *550*
Stock, C.C., see Dagg, C.P. *550*
Stock, C.C., see Jacquez, J. A. 519, *532*
Stock, C.C., see Kaplan, L. H. 492, 494, 495, *506*
Stock, C.C., see Sugiura, K. 36, *46*, 459, *467*
Stock, C.C., see Tarnowski, G.S. 391, *403*, 500, 501, *511*, 514, *537*
Stock, J.A. 384, *402*, 458, *467*, 522, *537*, 747, *764*
Stock, J.C., see Loveless, A. 9, *16*
Stockdale, F., Okazaki, K., Mameroff, M., Holtzer, H. 311, *345*
Stockert, J.C., Fernandez-Gomez, M.E., Sogo, J. M., Lopez-Saez, J.F. 662, *667*
Stockert, E., see Boyse, E. A. 696, *714*, 723, *743*
Stockert, E., see Horowitz, B. 711, *717*
Stockert, J.C., see González-Fernández, A. 662, *665*
Stoerk, H.C., see Clark, I. 86, *100*
Stohlman, F., Jr., see Morse, B.S. 687, *692*
Stoll, D., see Dollinger, M. 234, *251*
Stollar, V., Stevens, T.M., Schlesinger, R.W. 354, *371*
Stone, A.E., see Howle, J.A. 833, 834, *839*
Stone, G.M. 113, 114, *136*
Stone, G.M., Baggett, B. 113, 117, *136*
Stone, G.M., Baggett, B., Donnelly, R.B. 113, *136*
Stone, G.M., Martin, L. 113, *136*
Stone, J.E., Potter, V.R. 274, *345*
Stone, R.L., see Chan, G.Y. 405, *420*
Stone, W.E., see Tews, J.K. 499, *511*
Stoneburg, C.A. 824, *828*
Stones, W.R., see Melling, J. *668*
Storb, R., see Thomas, E.D. 479, *482*
Storck, H., see Erlanger, M. 222, *225*
Stork, G., Schultz, A.G. 650, *656*
Storti, E., Quaglino, D. 726, 727, 728, 730, 734, 735, *746*
Storti, E., Traldi, A., Quaglino, D. 408, *424*
Stothers, S.C., see Campbell, L.D. 125, *127*
Strain, W.H., see Mc Quitty, J.T. 844, *848*
Strasswender, E.A., see Loo, T.L. *551*
Straub, O.C., see Seeber, S. 710, *721*
Straub, P.W., see Burchenal, J.H. 779, *783*
Strauss, B.S. 11, *17*, 52, *63*
Strauss, B.S., Coyle, M., Robbins, M. 13, *17*
Strauss, B.S., Rubbins, M. 54, *63*
Strauss, B.S., see Reiter, H. 13, *16*
Strauss, G., see Gmelin, R. 498, *505*
Strauss, N., Hendee, E.D. 561, *570*
Strawitz, D., see Weiss, A.J. *511*
Straw, J.A., Waters, I.W., Fregly, M.J. 813, *819*
Straw, J.A., see Hart, M.M. 810, 811, 812, *818*
Straw, J.A., see Martz, F. 812, 814, *818*
Strecker, G., Goubet, B., Montreuil, J. 448, *456*
Streisinger, G., see Terzaghi, B.E. 296, *345*
Strelitz, R.A., see Elion, G. B. 412, 413, *420*

Strelzoff, E. 296, *345*
Strickstrock, K.-H., see Fusenig, N.E. 757, *762*
Strickstrock, K.-H., see Obrecht, P. 749, 757, 759, 763, *764*
Strijkert, P.J. 212, *231*
Strijkert, P.J., see DeKloet, S.R. 206, 210, 211, *224*
Striker, G.E., see Quadracci, L.J. 416, *423*
Stringer, V., see Brockman, R.W. 790, *791*
Stripp, B., see Greene, F.E. 812, *818*
Strom, L., see Southren, A. L. 811, 813, *818*
Strong, J.A., Brown, J.B., Bruce, J., Douglas, M., Klopper, A.I., Loraine, J.A. 178, *192*
Strott, C.A., see Ross, G.T. 160, *168*
Struck, R.F., Kirk, M.C., Mellet, L.B., Dareer, S., Hill, D.L. 29, *33*
Struck, R.F., see Hill, D.L. 29, *32*
Struck, R.F., see Shealy, Y. F. 544, 548, *552*
Stryer, L., see Ward, D.C. 441, 443, *457*
Stubbins, J.F., see Garrett, E.R. 65, *80*
Stucki, J.C., see Duncan, G. W. 110, *128*
Studzinski, G.P., Cohen, L. S. 54, *63*
Studzinski, G.P., Cohen, L. S., Roseman, J., Schweitzer, L. 54, *63*
Studzinski, G.P., see Cohen, L.S. 21, *31*
Stumpf, W.E. 114, *136*
Stumpf, W.E., see Jensen, E.V. 114, 115, *131*, 164, *167*
Sturgis, S.H., see Velardo, J.T. 109, *137*
Sturrock, J.E., see Roberts, J.J. 14, *16*, 70, 76, 78, *83*
Stutts, P., Brockman, R.W. 387, *403*
Stutts, P., see Brockman, R. W. 217, *223*
Stutzman, L., see Sarcione, E.J. 387, *402*
Stych, H., see Deutsch, E. 709, *715*, 734, 735, *744*
Subbaiah, T.V., see Okamoto, K. 57, *62*
Süssmuth, R., see Lingens, F. 70, 71, *82*
Suga, A., see Nanjo, S. 870, *873*
Sugár, J. 679, *693*
Sugawara, R., see Hata, T. 47, *60*
Sugawara, S., see Tanaka, N. 497, *511*
Suggs, J.E., see Wilson, J. E. 523, *538*
Sugimori, T., see Chassy, B. M. 447, *453*
Sugimura, T., Birnbaum, S. M., Winitz, M., Greenstein, J.P. 528, *537*
Sugimura, T., see Nagao, M. 73, *82*
Sugino, Y., see Kozai, Y. 240, *253*
Sugiura, K. 501, *510*
Sugiura, K., Creech, H.J. 377, *382*
Sugiura, K., Hitchings, G. H., Cavalieri, L.F., Stock, C.C. 459, *467*
Sugiura, K., Schmid, F.A., Brown, G.F., Gonzalez, R. 36, *46*
Sugiura, K., Stock, C.C. 36, *46*
Sugiura, K., see Bennett, L. L., Jr. 463, *464*
Sugiura, K., see Stock 380
Suhadolnik, R.J. 426, *433*, 435, 436, *456*, 658, *667*
Suhadolnik, R.J., Chassy, B.M., Waller, G.R. 658, 661, *667*
Suhadolnik, R.J., Finkel, S. I., Chassy, B.M. 437, 440, *456*, 659, *668*
Suhadolnik, R.J., Uematsu, T. 436, *456*
Suhadolnik, R.J., see Chassy, B.M. 440, 447, *453*, 658, 659, *665*
Suhadolnik, R.J., see Cory, J.G. 448, *453*, 658, 664, *665*
Suhadolnik, R.J., see Rich, M.A. 660, 663, *667*
Suhadolnik, R.J., see Smulson, M.E. 436, *456*
Suhadolnik, R.J., see Uematsu, T. 435, *456*
Suhara, I., see Kida, M. 448, *454*
Suhara, Y., see Umezawa, H. *876*
Suhara, Y., see Umezawa, H. 852, 855, *876*
Suhrland, L.G., see Weisberger, A.S. 522, *537*
Suit, H.D. 319, *345*
Suld, H.M., Herbut, P.A. 697, 698, 699, 702, 703, *721*
Sulimovici, S.I., Boyd, G.S. 139, *140*, *156*
Sulkowski, E., Laskowski, M. 583, *592*
Sullivan, M.P., Beatty, E. C., Jr., Hyman, C.B., Murphy, M.L., Pierce, M.I., Severo, N.C. 397, *403*
Sullivan, M.P., Vietti, T.J., Fernbach, D.J., Griffith, K.M., Haddy, T. B., Watkins, W.L. 476, *482*
Sullivan, M.P., see Loo, T.L. 386, *401*
Sullivan, R., see Schmidt, L.H. 18, *33*
Sullivan, R.D., see Anderson, L.L. 472, *479*
Sullivan, R.J., see Goldblatt, P.J. 583, *590*
Summers, D.F., Maizel, J. V., Jr. 558, *570*
Summers, D.F., see Hecht, T. 855, 859, *872*
Summers, W.P., Handschumacher, R.E. 515, *537*
Summers, W.P., see Capizzi, R.L. *480*
Sumoff, B., see Gallagher, T. F. 178, *189*
Sund, H. 540, 542, *543*
Sundaralingam, M. 197, *230*
Sundberg, L., see Kristiansen, T. *717*
Sunderland, H., see Dao, T. L. 112, *127*
Sunderman, C.R., Pearson, H.A. 410, *424*
Sunthankar, A.V., see Heidelberger, C. 198, 204, 217, *226*
Sunthankar, A.V., see Remy, D.C. 196, *229*
Suntzeff, V., see Shimkin, M. B. 36, *46*
Suolinna, E.M.R., see Hakala, M.T. 775, *785*
Suprunchuk, T., see Gingras, B.A. 841, *848*
Suter, H., see Aebi, H. 751, 754, *760*
Sutherland, A., see Paterson, A.R.P. 387, 397, *401*
Sutherland, E.W., III, see Haynes, R.C., Jr. 87, *101*
Sutic, D., Djordjevic, B. 208, *230*

Sutow, W., see Louis, J. 820, *827*
Sutow, W.W., Garcia, F., Starling, K.A., Williams, T.E., Lane, D.M., Gehan, E.A. 726, 727, 732, *746*
Sutow, W.W., see Fernbach, D.J. 263, *268*
Sutton, H., Jr., see Huggins, C. 112, *131*, 181, *189*
Suvansri, U., see Djerassi, I. 478, *480*
Suzaki, S., see Mizuno, Y. 444, *455*
Suzuki, see Arai 845
Suzuki, A., see Niitani, H. 54, *62*
Suzuki, H. *875*
Suzuki, H., Kilgore, W.W. 54, *63*
Suzuki, H., Nagai, K., Akutsu, E., Yamaki, H., Tanaka, N., Umezawa, H .862,863,869,870,*874*
Suzuki, H., Nagai, K., Yamaki, H., Tanaka, N., Umezawa, H. 862, *874*, *875*
Suzuki, H., see Nagai, K. 862, 869, *873*
Suzuki, M., Murai, A., Watanabe, A., Nunokawa, O. 862, 863, 869, 870, *875*
Suzuki, M., Nomura, H., Ito, M., Kasamatu, T., Nakanishi, K., Yamaoka, S., Misoo, Y., Takamisawa, Y., Suzuki, T., Takeda, T., Izima, H., Kuto, J., Kinoshita, S., Moriya, K., Murai, J., Hasegawa, K., Watanabe, K., Ootake, S., Fushekawa, O. 870, *875*
Suzuki, S., see Aizawa, S. 441, 444, *452*
Suzuki, T., see Garrett, E.R. 275, 276, *333*
Suzuki, T., see Jensen, E.V. 110, 114, 115, *131*, 164, *167*
Suzuki, T., see Suzuki, M. 870, *875*
Suzuki, Y., Miyake, K. 855, 859, 862, 863, 869, 870, *875*
Suzuki, Y., see Hano, K. 547, *550*
Svatá, M., Raška, K., Jr., Šorm, F. 363, *371*
Svedbergs 571
Švehla, C., see Šmahel, O. 361, *370*
Sverak, L., Bonar, R.A., Langlois, A.J., Beard, J. W. 574, *581*
Sverak, L., see Riman, J. 440, *455*
Svoboda, D., Reddy, J., Harris, C. 589, *592*
Svoboda, D.J., see Azarnoff, D.L. 814, *817*
Svoboda, G.H., Poore, G.A., Montfort, M.L. 881, *890*
Svoboda, G.H., see Johnson, I.S. 670, *691*
Švorc, J., see Šmahel, O. 361, *370*
Swackhamer, E.S., see Hart, M.M. 812, *818*
Swain, R., see Guarino, A.J. 661, *666*
Swan, J.M., see Dalton, L. K. 881, *888*
Swaneck, G.E., Chu, L.L. H., Edelman, I.S. 164, *168*
Swaney, J.J., see Karon, M. 364, *367*
Swann, P.F. 69, *84*
Swann, P.F., Magee, P.N. 70, 71, *84*
Swann, P.F., see Lawley, P. D. 71, *81*
Swanson, M.A., Schwartz, R.S. 407, 416, *424*
Swartz, M.N., see Trautner, T.A. 325, *346*
Swartzendruber, D.C., see Hayes, R.L. 879, *888*
Sweat, M.L., Berliner, D.L., Bryson, M.J., Nabors, C., Haskell, J., Holmstrom, E.G. 106, *136*
Sweeney, C.M., see Zeleznick, L.D. 629, *632*
Sweeney, M.J., Gerzon, K., Harris, P.N., Holmes, R. E., Poore, G.A., Williams, R.H. 446, 451, *456*
Sweeney, M.J., Hoffman, D. H., Esterman, M.A. 450, 451, *456*
Sweeney, M.J., see Williams, R.H. 446, *457*
Sweetman, L., see Nyhan, W.L. 414, *423*
Swerdloff, R.S., Odell, W.O. 160, *168*
Sykes, J.A., see Bowen, J. M. 302, 307, *328*
Sykes, M.P., see Burchenal, J.H. 384, 389, *398*
Sykes, M.P., see Magill, G. B. 500, *507*
Sylvester, J.R., see Farber, S.L.H. 476, *480*
Sylvester, R.F., Jr., see Farber, S. 512, *531*
Symeonidis, A., see Georgatsos, J.G. 678, *690*
Symington, T., see Griffiths, K. 106, 107, *129*
Szapary, D., see Jondorf, W. R. 560, *569*
Szarapińska-Kwaszwseka, J., see Mikucki, J. 697, *718*
Szego, C.M., Roberts, S. 109, 110, 122, *136*, *137*
Szego, C.M., see Levey, H. A. 151, *155*
Szego, C.M., see Soloff, M.S. 114, *136*
Szego, C.M., see White, A. *103*
Szende, B., Tyihak, E. 514, *537*
Szende, B., Tyihak, E., Kopper, L., Lapis, K. 518, *537*
Szentklaray, J., Sellei, C. 36, *46*
Szer, W., Shugar, D. 198, *230*, 293, *345*
Sznycer, E., see Wolpert, M. K., 393, *403*
Szybalski, W. 56, 59, *63*, 292, 293, 294, 319, *345*, 494, *510*, 634, *641*
Szybalski, W., Arneson, V. G. 48, *63*
Szybalski, W., Iyer, V.N. 48, 49, 50, 51, 53, 58, *63*
Szybalski, W., Kubinski, H., Sheldrick, P. 325, *345*
Szybalski, W., Mennigmann, H. 293, *345*
Szybalski, W., Opara-Kubinska, Z., Lorkiewicz, L., Ephrati-Elizur, E., Zamenhof, S. 308, *345*
Szybalski, W., see Clifton, K.H. 289, 291, *330*
Szybalski, W., see Djordjevic, B. 289, 298, 299, 301, 314, 319, *331*
Szybalski, W., see Erikson, R.L. 292, 298, 319, *332*
Szybalski, W., see Iyer, V.N. 48, 49, 52, 54, *61*, 494, *506*, 637, *640*
Szybalski, W., see Kersten, W. 626, 627, *632*
Szybalski, W., see Kozinski, A.W. 295, *338*
Szybalski, W., see Lorkiewicz, Z. 27, *32*, 289, 293, *340*
Szycer, E., see Wolpert, M. K. 393, *403*

Szybalski, W., see Litman, R.M. 308, *339*
Szybalski, W., see Lozeron, H.A. 200, 205, *228*
Szybalski, W., see Smith, H. H. 314, *344*
Szybalski, W., see Steinman, I.D. 494, *510*

Taber, R., Rekosh, D., Baltimore, D. 558, *570*
Tabor, C.W., see Tabor, H. 148, *156*, 774, *788*
Tabor, H., Tabor, C.W. 148, *156*, 774, *788*
Tagliamonte, A., Tagliamonte, P., Gessa, G.L., Brodie, B.B. 519, *537*
Tagliamonte, P., see Tagliamonte, A. 519, *537*
Tagnon, H.J., see Kenis, Y. 759, *763*
Taguchi, T., see Littman, M. L. 523, *533*
Taguchi, T., see Shiba, S. 53, 56, *63*
Tajima, K., see Ikeda, Y. 862, *872*
Takagi, Y. 56, *63*
Takagi, Y., see Matsunoto, I. 54, *61*
Takahashi, H., see Mitsuhashi, S. 862, *873*
Takahashi, H., see Shiio, T. 54, *63*
Takahashi, H., see Tomizawa, H. 862, *875*
Takamisawa, Y., see Suzuki, M. 870, *875*
Takano, S., see Kametani, T. 650, *655*
Takatani, O., see Sakauchi, N. 814, *818*
Takayama, H., see Ishizuka, M. 444, *454*, 851, 855, 860, 861, 870, *873*
Takeda, H., see Kametani, T. 650, *655*
Takeda, H., see Ueda, M. 683, *694*
Takeda, K., Sawawa, Y., Arakawa, T. 870, *875*
Takeda, S., see Regan, J.D. 525, *535*
Takeda, T., see Suzuki, M. 870, *875*
Takenaka, O., see Nishimura, Y. 703, *719*
Takeno, T., Nagata, T., Mizunoya, T. 57, *63*
Taketoshi, K., see Hoshino, A. *613*
Takeuchi, M., Yamamoto, T. 855, *875*
Takeuchi, T. 855, *875*
Takeuchi, T., Iwanaga, J., Aoyagi, T., Murase, M., Sawa, T., Umezawa, H. 444, 445, *456*
Takeuchi, T., Iwanaga, J., Aoyagi, T., Umezawa, H. *456*
Takeuchi, T., see Hori, M. 441, 442, 445, *454*
Takeuchi, T., see Ishizuka, M. 441, *454*, 851, 855, 860, 861, 870, *873*
Takeuchi, T., see Kanno, T. 855, 871, *873*
Takeuchi, T., see Sawa, T. 444, *455*
Takeuchi, T., see Umezawa, H. 444, *456*, 851, 855, 870, *875*, *876*
Takita, T. 851, 861, 869, *875*
Takita, T., see Hori, M. 441, 442, *454*
Takita, T., Maeda, K., Umezawa, H. 852, *875*
Takita, T., Muraoka, Y., Maeda, K., Umezawa, H. 852, *875*
Takita, T., see Koyama, G. 852, *873*
Takita, T., see Muraoka, Y. 852, *873*
Takita, T., see Umezawa, H. 852, 855, *876*
Takizawa, K., see Odaka, T. 444, *455*
Talbot, L.M., see Marsh, J. M. 106, 107, *132*
Talbot, T.R., Elson, L.A. 38, *46*
Tallal, L., Tan, C.C., Oettgen, H.F., Wollner, N., McCarthy, M., Helson, L., Burchenal, J.H., Karnofsky, D.A., Murphy, M.L. 727, 728, 730, 732, *746*
Tallal, L., see Burchenal, J. H. 799, *805*
Tallal, L., see Haghbin, M. 726, 732, *744*
Tallal, L., see Lash, E. 735, *745*
Tallal, L., see Oettgen, H.F. 696, *719*, 723, 727, 728, 730, 733, 734, 735, *745*
Talley, R.W. 830, *840*
Talley, R.W., Carlson, R.G. 451, *456*
Talley, R.W., Frei, E.III. 261, *271*
Talley, R.W., O'Bryan, R. M., Tucker, W.G., Loo, R.V. 238, *255*, 258, *271*
Talley, R.W., Vaitkevicius, V. 236, 238, *255*, 261, *271*
Talley, R.W., see Burrows, J.H. 478, *480*
Talley, R.W., see Frei, E.III., 260, 262, *269*
Talley, R.W., see Loo, R.V. 261, *270*
Talley, R.W., see Luce, J. K. 544, 545, 546, *551*
Talley, R.W., see Monto, R. W. 621, *622*
Talley, R.W., see Regelson, W. 843, *849*
Talwar, G.P., Segal, S.J. 113, 119, *137*
Talwar, G.P., Segal, S.J., Evans, A., Davidson, O. W. 113, 114, *137*
Talwar, G.P., Sopori, M.L., Biswas, D.K., Segal, S.J. 114, *137*
Tamir, H., Srinivasan, P.R. 492, *510*
Tamoney, H.J., Jr., Noriega, A. 814, *819*
Tan, C., see Burchenal, J.H. 799, *805*
Tan, C., see Etcubanas, E. 793, 799, 800, *805*
Tan, C., see Gailani, S.D. 685, *690*
Tan, C., see Haghbin, M. 726, 732, *744*
Tan, C.C., Oettgen, H.F. 732, *746*
Tan, C.C., see Oettgen, H.F. 727, 728, 730, 732, 734, 735, *745*
Tan, C.C., see Tallal, L. 727, 728, 730, 732, *746*
Tan, E., see Dao, T.L. 184, *188*
Tan, G.T.C., see Hackethal, C.A. 638, *640*
Tan, T.C., see Burchenal, J. H. 384, 389, *398*
Tan, T.C., see Murphy, M.L. 394, *401*
Tanaka, K., see Komatsu, Y. 375, *381*
Tanaka, M., Kagawa, T., Tatano, T., Mochizuki, K., Nakamura, N., Kohagura, M., Hill, J.M. 698, 699, 702, *721*
Tanaka, M., see Nakamura, N. 701, *719*
Tanaka, N. 856, 860, *875*
Tanaka, N., Miyairi, N., Umezawa, H. 449, *456*
Tanaka, N., Nishimura, T., Yamaguchi, H., Umezawa, H. 449, *456*

Tanaka, N., Sashikata, K., Wada, T., Sugawara, S., Umezawa, H. 497, *511*
Tanaka, N., Yamaguchi, H., Umezawa, H. 850, 851, 856, 857, 858, 868, 869, *875*
Tanaka, N., see Nagai, K. 862, 869, *873*
Tanaka, N., see Suzuki, H. 862, 863, 869, 870, *874*, *875*
Tanaka, N., see Umezawa, H. *876*
Tanaka, N., see Yamaki, H. 857, *876*
Tanaka, T., see Okami, Y. 497, *508*
Tanaka, Y., see Nishimura, H. 373, 374, *382*
Tannach 314
Tannenbaum, A. 528, *537*
Tanner, B.B., see Loo, T.L. 546, *551*
Tanowitz, H., see Wittner, M. 880, *890*
Tapia, R., Awapara, J. 497, *511*
Tarmy, E., see Seaman, E. 57, *62*
Tarnowski, G.S., Mountain, I.M., Stock, C.C. 501, *511*, 514, *537*
Tarnowski, G.S., Stock, C.C. 391, *403*, 500, *511*
Tarnowski, G.S., see Schmid, F.A. 521, 524, *536*
Tarnowski, G.S., see Schmid, F.A. 521, 524, *536*
Tarr, N., see Fishbein, W.N. 521, *531*
Tarr, N.A., see Burke, P.J. 260, 261, 262, *268*
Tartof, K.D., see Perry, R.P. 571, *580*
Tarver, H., see Levine, M. 521, *533*
Tassi, G.C., see DeBarbieri, A. 528, *531*
Tata, J.R., see Hamilton, T.H. 119, *129*
Tatano, T., see Tanaka, M. 698, 699, 702, *721*
Tato, J.C., see DelPuerto, B.M. 560, *568*
Tatum, E.L., see Reich, E. 582, 583, 584, *591*
Tatum, E.L., see Shatkin, A.H. 54, *62*
Taub, R.N. 318, *345*
Taub, R.N., see Floersheim, G.L. 752, *762*
Tauraso, N.M., see Jahnes, W.G. *717*
Tautz, W., see Duschinsky, R. 197, *225*
Tautz, W., see Lozeron, H.A. 198, *228*, 321, *340*
Tavale, S.S., Sakore, T.D., Sobell, H.M. 279, *345*
Tavitian, A., Uretsky, S.C., Acs, G. 439, *456*, 574, *581*
Tavitian, A., see Manteuil, S. 439, *454*
Tay, B.S., Lilley, R.McC., Murray, A.W., Atkinson, M.R. 390, 391, *403*
Taylor, A.C. *693*
Taylor, A.J., see Warner, D.T. 233, *256*
Taylor, C., see Herman, E.H. 609, *612*
Taylor, E.W. 676, 677, *693*
Taylor, E.W., see Adelmann, M.R. 676, *688*
Taylor, E.W., see Borisy, G.G. 677, *688*
Taylor, E.W., see Shelanski, M.L. 677, 678, *693*
Taylor, E.W., see Weisenberg, R.C. 677, 678, *694*
Taylor, F.B., Jr., Fudenberg, H. 527, *537*
Taylor, H., see Louis, J. 820, *827*
Taylor, J.H., Haut, W.F., Tung, J. 200, *230*
Taylor, P.D., see Starzl, T.E. 410, *424*
Taylor, R.W., see Edwards, R. 160, *167*
Taylor, S.G., III., see Ream, N.W. 621, *622*
Tchen, T.T., see Cheer, S. 56, *60*
Tchen, T.T., see Constantopoulos, G. 54, *60*, 139, *153*
Tchen, T.T., see Satoh, P.G. 139, *156*
Teich, N., see Lowy, D.R. 308, *340*, 355, *368*
Teillon, J., see Hagemann, G. 497, *505*
Teitei, T., see Dalton, L.K. 881, *888*
Telfer, M.A. *137*
Teller, J., see Old, L.J. 723, *746*
Temelcou, O., see DeBarbieri, A. 528, *531*
Temin, H.A., Mizutani, S. 58, *63*
Temin, H.M. 200, *230*, 237, *255*, 307, *345*, 607, *613*
Temin, H.M., Mizutani, S. 200, *230*
Temple, T.E., Jones, D.J., Liddle, G.W., Dexter, R.N. 811, 814, *819*
Tencer, R., see Desai, L. 583, 584, *590*
Tendler, M.D., Korman, S. 642, *648*
Tendler, M.D., see Cole, D.R. 642, *647*
Tendler, M.D., see Grunberg, E. 642, *647*
Tendler, M.D., see Guttman, H.N. 643, *647*
Tendler, M.D., see Korman, S. 642, *647*
Teng, C.S., Hamilton, T.H. 119, 120, *137*
Teng, C.S., see Hamilton, T.H. 119, *129*
Tenkoni, L.T., see Bonomi, U. 520, 529, *530*
Tennebaum, R., see Sheehan, R. 417, *424*
Tennenbaum, J.I., see St. Pierre, R.L. 706, *720*
Tepper, H.B., Hollis, C.A., Galson, E.C., Sondheimer, E. 857, *875*
Terasima, T., Umezawa, H. 855, 860, *875*
Terasima, T., see Tsuboi, A. 868, 869, *875*
Terawaki, A., Greenberg, J. 52, *63*, 494, *511*
Terawaki, A., see Shiba, S. 53, 56, *63*
Terenius, L. 113, 117, *137*, 188, *192*
Terenius, L., see Johansson, H. 117, 118, *131*
Tereshin, I.M. 52, *63*
Terni, M., see DiMarco, A. 607, *612*
Tershak, D.R. 211, *230*
Terskikh, I.I., Galegov, G.A., Chutkov, N.A., Bekleshova, A.I. 354, *371*
Terzaghi, B.E., Streisinger, G., Stahl, F.W. 296, *345*
Tessman, I., Poddar, R.K., Kumar, S. 11, *17*, 296, 297, *345*
Tessman, I., see Howard, B.D. 297, *336*
Testorelli, C., see Bonmassar, E. 527, *530*

Tettenborn, D., see Lorke, D. 710, *718*
Tevethia, F., Rapp, F. 855, 857, 859, 865, *875*
Tews, J.K., Stone, W.E. 499, *511*
Tezuka, N., Hirai, T. *456*
Tezuka, N., Tokuzo 445, *456*
Tharp, D.L., see McCord, T. J. 524, *534*
Thatcher, C.J., Walker, I.G. 76, *84*
Thatcher, C.J., see Lawley, P.D. 7, *16*, 66, 70, 71, 72, *81*
Thayer, P.S., Gordon, H.C. 820, *828*
Thayer, P.S., see Yesair, D. W. 823, 824, 825, *828*
Thayer, P.S., see Yesair, D. W. 824, 825, *828*
Thayer, S.A., see Doisy, E. A. 104, *128*, 170, *189*
Thayer, S.A., see MacCorquodale, D.W. 104, *133*
Thayer, S.A., see Mayol, R. F. 120, *133*
Thedford, R., see Robins, M. J. 435, *455*
Theil, E., Zamenhof, S. 379, 380, *382*
Theiss, E., see Bollag, W. 753, *761*
Thelander, L., see Brown, N. C. 790, *791*
Theml, H., see Begemann, H. 708, *713*
Theologides, A., Yarbro, J. M., Kennedy, B.J. 603, *613*
Theuer, R.C. 529, *537*
Thie, R.S., see Oleson, J.J. 496, *508*, 633, *641*
Thiele, J., Dralle, E. 766, *788*
Thiemann, J.E., see Murthy, Y.K.S. 882, *889*
Thiersch, J.B. 415, *424*, *482*, 493, 495, 496, *511*
Thiry, L. 381, *382*
Thoai, N.V., see Hedegaard, J. 492, *506*
Thoma, R.W., see Fried, J. 182, *189*
Thomas, C., Sierra, J.L. 78, *84*
Thomas, D.R., see Curtis, P.J. 658, *665*
Thomas, E.D., Storb, R. 479, *482*
Thomas, H. 203, 307, *345*
Thomas, H.J., see Bennett, L.L., Jr. 386, *398*
Thomas, H.J., see Schaeffer, H. 435, *455*
Thomas, H.J., see Montgomery, J.A. 233, 234, *254*
Thomas, L., see Simberkoff, M.S. 707, *721*
Thomas, P., see Elkerbout, F. 19, *31*
Thomasz, A., Borek, E. 201, *230*
Thompson, C.R., Werner, H.W. 105, *137*
Thompson, C.R., see Lerner, L.J. 110, *132*
Thompson, G.R., see Heyman, I.A. 832, *839*
Thompson, H.G., Jr., see Herter, F.P. 541, *542*
Thompson, H.S., Gale, G.R. 831, 835, *840*
Thompson, H.S., see Howle, J.A. 833, 834, *839*
Thompson, H.W., see Short, L.N. 499, *510*
Thompson, J.B., see Wani, M.C. 649, *656*
Thompson, R.L., Davis, J., Russell, P.B., Hitchings, G.H. 800, *807*
Thompson, R.L., Minton, S. A., Jr., Officer, J.E., Hitchings, G.H. 800, *807*
Thompson, R.L., Wilkin, M. L., Hitchings, G.H., Elion, G.B., Falco, E.A., Russell, P.B. 302, *346*
Thompson, U.B., see Bresnick, E. 281, 285, *328*
Thomson, A.J., see Renshaw, E. 832, *840*
Thomson, A.J., see Rosenberg, B. 829, *840*
Thomson, J.R., see Brockman, R.W. 385, *398*, 460, *465*, 793, *805*
Thomson, J.R., see Pittillo, A.F. 820, *827*
Thomson, J.R., see Schabel, F.M., Jr. 393, *402*
Thomson, J.R., see Skipper, H.E. 502, *510*, 528, *536*
Thomson, J.R., see Skipper, H.W. 522, *536*
Thorbeck, R., see Chandra, P. 602, 608, *611*
Thorbecke, G.J., see Simberkoff, M.S. 707, *721*
Thoren, L., see Johansson, H. 117, 118, *131*
Thoren, M.M., see Levintow, L. 519, *533*
Thornton, E.R. 4, *5*
Thurman, W.G., see Fernbach, D.J. 263, *268*
Thurman, W.G., see Luce, J.K. 544, 545, 546, *551*
Thurzo, V., see Winkler, A. 352, *372*
Tice, S.V., see Meister, A. 708, *718*
Tidd, D.M., Kim, S.C. 396, *403*
Tidd, D.M., Kim, S.C., Horakova, K., Moriwaki, A., Paterson, A.R.P. 396, *403*
Till, J.E., see Bruchovsky, N. 674, *688*
Till, J.E., see Mak, S. 281, 314, 317, 318, *340*
Till, J.E., McCulloch, E.A. 23, *33*
Till, J.E., see Bruchovsky, N. 59, *60*
Till, M., see Elson, L.A. 38, *43*
Till, M., see Galton, D.A.G. 35, 36, 37, *43*
Tilney, L.G. 676, *693*
Tilney, N.L., see Murray, J. E. 502, *508*
Timasheff, S., see Weisenberg, R.C. 678, *694*
Timmis, G.M., see Berenbaum, M.C. 38, *42*
Timmis, G.M., see Bierman, H.R. 36, *42*
Timmis, G.M., see Haddow, A. 36, 37, *44*
Ting, R.C., see Adamson, R. H. 884, *887*
Ting, R.C., see Smith, R.G. 883, *889*
Ting, R.C., see Wu, A.M. *669*
Ting, R.C., see Yang, S.S. 883, *890*
Tipson, S., see Levene, P.A. 273, *339*
Titani, Y., Katsube, Y. 374, *382*
Tittsworth, E., see Grunberg, E. 642, *647*
Tkaczynski, T., Šmejkal, J., Šorm, F. 350, *371*
Tobey, R.A. 235, *255*, 881, *890*
Tobey, R.A., Ley, K.D. 528, *537*
Tobey, R.A., see Ley, K.D. 528, *533*
Tobin, J.O.H., see Barton, B.W. 323, *328*
Tobin, J.O'H., see Conchie, A.F. 323, *330*
Tobin, W.E., Sandler, S.G. 675, 686, *693*

Tobin, W.E., see Sandler, S. G. 686, *693*
Toch, R., see Farber, S. 394, *399*
Tochimoto, S., see Southren, A.L. 811, 813, *818*
Todaro, G.J., Green, H. 302, 307, *346*
Todaro, G.T., see Aaronson, S.A. 308, *327*
Todd, A., Ulbricht, T.L.V. 658, *668*
Todd, A., see Brown, D.M. 886, *888*
Tood, A.R., see Brown, D. M. 273, *328*
Todd, A.R., see Michelson, A.M. 273, *340*
Todd, I.D.H. 759, *764*
Todd, P., see Richmond, J. E. *874*
Toft, D.O., Gorski, J. 114, 115, 117, *137*, 164, *168*
Toft, D.O., Shyamala, G., Gorski, J. 114, 115, *137*, 164, *168*
Toft, D.O., see Gorski, J. 115, 117, *129*
Toft, D.O., see O'Malley, B. W. 160, 161, 162, 163, 164, *168*
Toftness, B.R., see DeConti, R.C. 799, 800, 802, 804, *805*
Toji, L., Cohen, S.S. 658, 659, 661, 662, *668*
Tokuyasu, K., see Ilan, Joseph 428, *432*
Tokuzen, R., see Nakahara, W. 887, *889*
Tokuzo, see Tezuka, N. 445
Toliver, A., Simon, E.H. 299, *346*
Tolksdorf, S., see Steinberg, M. 109, *136*
Tolmach, L.J., see Pfeiffer, S.E. 674, *692*
Tolman, R.L., Robins, R.K. 233, *255*
Tomao, F.A., see Schwartz, M.K. 704, *721*, 724, 725, 735, *746*
Tomasz, M. 50, 52, *63*
Tomchick, R., Mead, J.A.R. 802, 804, *807*
Tomchick, R., see DeConti, R.C. 799, 800, 802, 804, *805*
Tomic, M., see Griffiths, C. T. 175, 179, *189*
Tominaga, H., see Endo, Y. 583, *590*
Tomioka, K., see Wakaki, S. 47, *64*
Tomisek, A.J., Kelly, H.J., Skipper, H.E. 486, *511*
Tomisek, A.J., Reid, M.R. 487, 488, *511*
Tomisek, A.J., Reid, M.R., Skipper, H.E. 496, *511*
Tomisek, A.J., see Pittillo, A.F. 820, *827*
Tomita, K., see Mizuno, H. 279, *341*
Tomita, K.I., Katz, L., Rich, A. 197, *230*
Tomizawa, H., Takahashi, H. 862, *875*
Tomizawa, J.I., see Abe, M. 300, *327*
Tomizawa, S., Aronow, L. 396, *403*
Tomkins, G.M., see Baxter, J.D. 97, 99, *100*, 164, *167*
Tomkins, G.M., see Peterkofsky, B. 241, *254*
Tomkins, G.M., see Stellwagen, R.H. 312, *345*
Tompkins, L.S., see Marshall, J.A. 814, *818*
Tonato, M., see Grignani, F. 472, *481*
Tong, G.L., Lee, W.L., Goodman, L. 350, *371*
Tong, G.L., see Lee, W.W. 430, *433*
Tønnesen, T., see Frederiksen, S. 663, *665*
Tono, H., Cohen, S.S. 237, 244, *255*
Tonolo, A., see De-Angeli, L.C. 697, *715*
Tooth-Allen, J., Rosenberg, B. 832
Toplin, I., see Oleson, J.J. 633, *641*
Topping, N.E., see Ball, C. R. 23, *30*
Toren, D., Menon, K.M.J., Forchielli, E., Dorfman, R.I. 139, *156*
Torre, C. de la, see Giménez-Martin, G. *669*
Tosa, T., Pizer, L.I. 525, *537*
Touster, O., see Gotto, A.M. 216, *225*, 280, 290, 291, *334*
Tower, D.B., Peters, E.L., Curtis, W.C. 698, 700, 703, *721*
Tower, D.B., see Peters, E. L. 499, *508*
Townsend, L.B., Robins, R. K. 441, 444, *456*
Townsend, L.B., see Darnall, K.R. 373, 374, *381*
Townsend, L.B., see McCarthy, J.R., Jr. 662, *666*
Townsend, L.B., see Panzica, R.P. 233, 234, *254*, 267, *270*
Trabucchi, E., Jr., see Bertelli, A. 705, *714*
Trachewsky, D., Segal, S.J. 119, *137*
Tracy, G.S., see Hirsch, M. S. 418, *421*
Trader, M., see Pittillo, A.F. 820, *827*
Trader, M.W., see Schabel, F.M., Jr. 76, *83*, 389, *402*, 494, *509*, 878, *889*
Traeger, L., see Wacker, A. *346*
Traggis, D., see Dunnicliff, M.A. *744*
Traggis, D., see Jaffe, N. 479, *481*, 726, 727, 730, 734, 735, *744*
Traine, A., see Picone, M.A. 608, *613*
Traldi, A., see Storti, E. 408, *424*
Trams, E.G., Nadkarni, M. V., Smith, R.K. 27, *33*
Trams, E.G., Salvador, R. A., Maemgwyn-Davies, G., De Quattro, V. 39, *46*
Trams, E.G., see Nadkarni, V.M. 39, *45*
Trautner, T.A., Swartz, M. N., Kornberg, A. 325, *346*
Travis, N., see Pearson, O. H. 183, 184, *191*
Treat, C., see Djerassi, I. 478, *480*
Trebst, A., see Wacker, A. 274, 295, *346*
Trelle, G.J., see Carlsen, E. N. 121, *127*
Trenner, N.R., see Kaczka, E.A. 658, *666*
Trezise, L.A., see Bitman, J. 125, *126*
Trigg, P.I., Gutteridge, W. E., Williamson, J. 660, *668*
Triggle, D.J. 20, *34*
Tripathy, S.P., Mackaness, G.B. 408, *424*
Tristram, H., see Fowden, L. 512, 519, 521, 529, *531*
Trmal, T., see Boris, A. 146, *153*
Trnavský, K., Lapárová, V. 359, *371*
Trnavský, K., see Havelka, S. 361, *367*

Troll,W., see Becker,F.F. 583, *589*
Troll,W., see Zweifach,B.W. 527, *538*
Trommer,P.R., see Abelson,D. 814, *817*
Trosko,J.E., see Rosenberg,B. 830, *840*
Trosper,F., see Pilcher,K.S. 515, *535*
Trotter,J., see Camerman,N. 279, 286, *329*
Trounce,J.R., see Folb,R.I. 416, *420*
Truman,J.T., Klenow,H. 659, 662, 663, *668*
Truman,J.T., Frederiksen,S. 663, *668*
Truong,H., see Baulieu,E.E. 115, *126*
Truxová,G., see Grozdanovič,J. 355, *366*
Tschang,T.P., see Hadler,H.I. 374, *381*
Tsuboi,A., Terasima,T. 868, 869, *875*
Tsubosaki,M., see Ichikawa,T. 855, 870, *872*
Tsuda,T., see Nakagawa,Y. 373, *382*
Tsuji,T., Kosower,E.M. 751, 754, *765*
Tsuji,Y. 696, *721*
Tsukada,I., Kunimoto,T., Hori,M., Komai,T. 444, *456*
Tsukagoshi,S., Kao,M.H., Goldin,A. 76, *84*
Tsukamura,M. Tsukamura,S. 56, *63*
Tsukamura,S., see Tsukamura,M. 56, *63*
Tsukihara,T., see Mizuno,H. 279, *341*
Tsunamura,S., see Sartorelli,A.C. 748, 756, 757, *764*
Tucher,R.G., see Stickler,D.J. 57, *63*
Tuchmann-Duplessis,H., Mercier-Parot,L. 415, *424*
Tucker,W.G., see Burrows,J.H. 478, *480*
Tucker,W.G., see Talley,R.W. 238, *255*, 258, *271*
Türkheimer,A.R., see Lerner,L.J. 110, 122, 123, *132*
Tullner,W., see Hertz,R. 121, *130*
Tung,J., see Taylor,J.H. 200, *230*
Tung,L., see Kriss,J.P. 283, 289, *338*
Tung,L., see Kriss,J.P. 282, *338*
Tunnock,S.M., see Githens,J.H. 415, *421*
Tuominen,F.W., Kenney,F.T. 243, *255*
Turchi,J., see Djerassi,I. 478, *480*
Türkheimer,A.R., see Lerner,L.J. 147, *155*
Turkington,R.W., Majumder,G.C., Riddle,M. 312, *346*
Turner,R.W., Calabresi,P. 361, *371*
Turner,R.W., see Calabresi,P. 361, *364*
Turner,W.B., see Carter,S.B. 446, 450, 451, *453*
Tushinski,R., see Darnell,J.E. 574, 575, *579*
Tuve,R.K., see Rabinovitz,M. 518, *535*
Tveter,K.J. 149, *157*
Tveter,K.J., Aakvaag,A. 149, *157*
Tveter,K.J., see Unhjem,O. 150, *157*
Twanmoh,A., see Stern,R. *669*
Twombly,G.H., Schoenewaldt,E.F. 113, *137*
Twomey,D., see Barry,V.C. 793, *805*
Tyihak,E., see Szende,B. 514, 518, *537*
Tyler,H.R., see Breeden,C.J. 323, *328*
Tyrer,D.D., Kline,I., Gang,M., Goldin,A., Venditti,J.M. 523, *537*, 548, *552*
Tyrer,D.D., Kline,I., Venditti,J.M., Goldin,A. 236, *255*, *271*
Tyrer,D.D., see Hoffman,G.S. 263, *269*, 548, *550*
Tyrer,D.D., see Kline,I. 198, *227*, 235, *253*, 259, 260, 262, *270*, 267, *785*
Tyrsted,G., Sartorelli,A.C. 663, *668*
Tytell,A.A., Neuman,R.E. 516, *537*

Ubuka,T., Meister,A. 708, *721*
Uchida,K., Kreis,W. 265, *271*
Uchida,K., Kreis,W., Hutchison,D.J. 240, 247, *255*
Uchida,K., see Chaube,S. 237, 244, *250*, 261, *268*
Uchida,T., see Hashimoto,J. 437, *453*
Uchiya,M., see Kato,S. 870, *873*
Udaka,S., Moyed,H.S. 448, *456*
Udall,V. 417, *424*
Udall,V., see Skarpa,M. 410, *424*
Udenfriend,S., Zaltzman-Nirenberg,P., Nagatsu,T. 520, *537*
Ueda,M., Sawai,M., Kawakami,M., Minesita,T., Takeda,H. 683, *694*
Ueda,T. 376, *382*
Uematsu,T., Suhadolnik,R.J. 435, *456*
Uematsu,T., see Suhadolnik,R.J. 436, *456*
Ueno,M. 870, *875*
Uetani,T., see Miura,M. 514, 515, 526, *534*, 705, 706, 707, 713, *719*, 735, 738, *745*
Uete,T. 89, *103*
Uher,V., see Šmahel,O. 361, *370*
Ui,H., Mueller,G.C. 119, *137*
Ui,H., see Yüntsen,H. 446, *457*
Ulbricht,T.L.V., see Todd,A. 658, *668*
Ullberg,S., Bengtsson,G. 114, *137*
Ullery,J.C., see Vorys,N. 109, *137*
Ultmann,J.E., Feigelson,P. 460, *467*
Umeda,M., Heidelberger,C. 199, 216, 217, *230*, *231*
Umesawa,I., see Hata,T. 47, *60*
Umezawa,H. 851, 852, 855, 870, *875*
Umezawa,H., Hori,M., Ishizuka,M., Takeuchi,T. 855, 870, *875*
Umezawa,H., Ishizuka,M., Hori,S., Chimura,H., Takeuchi,T., Komai,T. *875*
Umezawa,H., Ishizuka,M., Kimura,K., Iwanaga,J., Takeuchi,T. 855, *875*
Umezawa,H., Ishizuka,M., Maeda,K., Takeuchi,T. 855, 870, *875*
Umezawa,H., Maeda,K. 850, 860, 861, *876*

Umezawa, H., Maeda, K., Takeuchi, T., Okami, Y. 851, 855, *876*
Umezawa, H., Sawa, T., Fukagawa, Y., Homma, I., Ishizuka, M., Takeuchi, T. 444, *456*
Umezawa, H., Sawa, T., Fukagawa, Y., Koyama, G., Murase, M., Hamada, M., Takeuchi, T. 444, *456*
Umezawa, H., Suhara, Y., Ikekawa, T., Ishizuka, M., Hori, M., Maeda, K., Tanaka, N., Takeuchi, T. *876*
Umezawa, H., Suhara, Y., Takita, T., Maeda, K. 852, 855, *876*
Umezawa, H., see Hori, M. 441, 442, 445, *454*, 857, *872*
Umezawa, H., see Ichikawa, T. 855, 870, *872*
Umezawa, H., see Ikekawa, T. 851, 852, 855, 869, *872*
Umezawa, H., see Ishizuka, M. 441, *454*, 851, 855, 860, 861, 870, *873*
Umezawa, H., see Kanno, T. 855, 871, *873*
Umezawa H., see Koyama, G. 441, *454*, 852, *873*
Umezawa, H., see Kunimoto, T. 859, 860, *873*
Umezawa, H., see Maeda, K. 851, 855, *873*
Umezawa, H., see Muraoka, Y. 852, *873*
Umezawa, H., see Nagai, K. 862, 869, *873*
Umezawa, H., see Okami, Y. 497, *508*
Umezawa, H., see Sawa, T. 444, *455*
Umezawa, H., see Suzuki, H. 862, 863, 869, 870, *874*, *875*
Umezawa, H., see Takeuchi, T. 444, 445, *456*
Umezawa, H., see Tanaka, N. 449, *456*, 497, *511*
Umezawa, H., see Terasima, T. 855, 860, *875*
Umezawa, H., see Tanaka, N. 850, 851, 856, 857, 858, 868, 869, *875*
Umezawa, H., see Takita, T. 852, *875*
Umezawa, H., see Takita, T. 852, *875*
Umezawa, H., see Yamaki, H. 857, *876*
Underwood, G. E. 237, *255*
Underwood, G. E., see Petering, H. G. 841, 842, 843, *849*
Ungar, G., Yamura, T., Isola, J. B., Kobrin, S. 527, *537*
Unhjem, O., Tveter, K. J. 150, *157*
Unhjem, O., Tveter, K. J., Aakvaag, A. 150, *157*
Unterberg, W., see Rauen, H. M. 820, 823, *827*
Upton, A. C., see Cudkowicz, G. 314, *330*
Upchurch, H. F., see Sartorelli, A. C. 487, 500, *509*
Uretsky, S. C., Acs, G., Reich, E., Mori, M., Altwerger, L. 437, 438, *456*
Uretsky, S. C., see Tavitian, A. 439, *456*, 574, *581*
Urist, M. R., Schjeide, A. O. 120, *137*
Urist, M. R., see Schjeide, O. A. 120, 121, *135*
Uriu, S. A., see La Via, M. F. 513, 526, *533*
Urshel, M. J., see Schrecker, A. W. 240, 246, *255*
Usui, T., see Kaziwara, K. 618, 619, 620, *622*
Utz, J. P. 219, *231*
Uy, Q. L., Moen, T. H., Johns, R. J., Owens, A. H., Jr. 675, 682, *694*
Uyeki, E. M., Llacer, V. 406, *424*
Uzuka, Y., see Yamagata, S. 870, *876*

Vadlamudi, S., Padarathsingh, M., Bonmassar, E., Goldin, A. 362, *371*
Vadlamudi, S., Padarathsingh, M., Bonmassar, E., Waravdekar, V., Goldin, A. 705, *721*
Vadlamudi, S., Padarathsingh, M., Waravdekar, V. S., Goldin, A. 706, *721*
Vadlamudi, S., see Lin, Y. T. 549, 550, *551*
Vaidyanathan, C. S., see Jayaram, H. N. 697, 698, 699, *717*
Vail, M. H., see Bennett, L. L., Jr. 436, *452*
Vail, M. H., see Wheeler, G. P. 76, 77, *84*
Vaitkevicius, V. K., Reed, M. L. 673, *694*
Vaitkevicius, V. K., see Talley, R. W. 236, 238, *255*, 261, *271*
Vajda, G., see Hanisch, J. *568*
Valadares, J. R. E., Singhal, R. L., Parulekar, M. R. 124, 125, *137*
Valadares, J. R. E., see Singhal, R. L. 123, 124, *136*, 152, *156*
Valdes-Dapena, A., see Abelson, D. 814, *817*
Valenca, M., see De Barros, T. 696, *715*
Valenta, O., see Šmahel, O. 361, *370*
Valentine, R. C., see Kjellen, L. 302, 307, *338*
Valentini, L., see Calendi, E. 598, 599, *611*
Valentini, L., see Di Marco, A. 593, 597, 609, *612*
Valerino, D. M., see Johns, D. G. 473, *481*
Valeriote, F. A., Bruce, W. R., Meeker, B. E. 686, *694*
Valeriote, F. A., see Borsa, J. 234, 238, *250*
Valeriote, F. A., see Bruce, W. R. 21, *31*, 76, *80*, 218, *223*, 474, *479*, 494, *504*
Valeriote, F. A., see Vietti, T. 199, *231*
Vanag, K. A., see Galegov, G. A. *366*
Van Atta, G., see Cooney, D. A. 696, *715*
Van Camp, L., see Rosenberg, B. 829, 830, 832, 836, *840*
Vancampen, M. G., Jr., see Shelton, R. S. 105, *136*
Vance, M. J., see Pappenheimer, A. M. 18, *33*
Van den Berg, C. J., Van den Velden, J. 499, *511*
Van den Broek, A. A. 24, *34*
Van den Velden, J., see Van den Berg, C. J. 499, *511*
Vanderhoff, G. A., see Kosower, N. S. 759, *763*
Vanderleeden, J. C., see Myers, W. G. 314, *341*
Van der Meulen, P. Y. F., Bassham, J. A. 493, *511*
Vanderslice, D., see Rapp, F. 302, 303, 304, *343*
Vandevoorde, J. P., Hansen, H. J., Nadler, S. B. 495, *511*

Vandevoorde, J.P., see Hansen, H.J. 500, 502, *505*
Van Duuren, B.L. 6, *17*
Van Dyk, J.J., Clarkson, B. D., Duschinsky, R., Kelver, O., La Sala, E., Krakoff, I.H. 197, *231*
Van Giessen, G.J., Crim, J. A., Petering, D.H., Petering, H.G. 843, 844, 845, 847, *849*
Van Giessen, G.J., Petering, H.G. 845, *849*
Van Giessen, G.J., see Petering, H.G. 841, 842, 843, 844, 845, 847, *849*
Van Hoosen, B. 558, *570*
Van Lancker, J.L., Flangas, A.L., Allen, J. 680, *694*
Van Lancker, J.L., see Luyckx, A. 680, *691*
Van Lear, G.E., see Morton, G.O. 434, *455*
Van Putten, L.M., Lelieveld, P. 21, *34*
Van Rossum, J.M., see Ariëns, E.J. 462, *464*
Van Scott, E.J., see Frei, E., III. 679, *690*
Van Scott, E.S., Auerbach, R., Weinstein, G.D. 479, *482*
Van Steveninck, J., 93, *103*
Vanstone, W.E., Dale, D. G., Oliver, W.F., Common, R.H. 120, *137*
Vanstone, W.E., Maw, W. A., Common, R.H. 120, *137*
Van Tamelen, E.E., see Hoeksema, H. 446, 447, *454*
Van Vroonhoven, T.J., Malt, R.A. 410, *424*
Van Vunakis, H., see Simon, M.I. 608, *613*
Van Wagenen, G., Folley, S. J. 144, *157*
Varadarajan, S., see Brown, D.M. 273, *328*, 886, *888*
Varcoe, J.S., see Rees, K.R. 824, *827*
Varela, R., see Dao, T.L. 178, 179, *188*
Vargha, L., Balo, J. 36, *46*
Varkarakis, M.J., Murphy, G.P. 837, *840*
Vartan, C.P., see Crowther, D. 726, 732, *743*
Vas, M., Löwenstein, L. 406, *424*
Vas, S.I., see Leung, F.C. 406, *422*
Vasiliev, J.M., Gelfand, I. M., Guelstein, V.I. 681, *694*
Vasina, I.V., see Berlin, Y. A. 615, *621*
Vaughan, J.R., see Roblin, R.O., Jr. 458, *467*
Vaughan, M.H., see Edmonds, M. 574, 575, *579*
Vaughn, J.H., see Dutton, R.W. 309, *331*
Vavra, J.J., De Boer, C., Dietz, A., Hanka, L.J., Sokolski, W.T. 65, *84*
Vazquez, D., Battaner, E., Neth, R., Heller, G., Monro, R.E. 554, 565, *570*
Vazquez, D., see Carrasco, L. 567, *567*
Vazquez, D., see Munoz, E. 554, *569*
Vecchi, M., see Schwartz, D. E. 754, *764*
Vedder, E.B. 558, *570*
Velardo, J.T. 173, *192*
Velardo, J.T., Hisaw, F.L., Bever, A.F. 110, *137*
Velardo, J.T., Sturgis, S.H. 109, *137*
Velardo, J.T., see Hisaw, F. L. 109, *130*
Veldstra, H., see Gribnau, A.G.M. 48, *60*
Velemínský, J., see Gichner, T. 78, *80*
Veler, C.D., see Doisy, E.A. 104, *128*, 170, *189*
Velle, W., Erichson, S. 107, *137*
Venditti, J.M., Abbott, B.J. 650, *656*
Venditti, J.M., Abbot, J., Di Marco, A., Goldin, A. 597, *613*
Venditti, J.M., Frei, E., III., Goldin, A. 393, *403*
Venditti, J.M., Goldin, A. 397, *403*, 476, 687, *694*, 799, *807*
Venditti, J.M., Goldin, A., Kline, I. 820, *828*
Venditti, J.M., see Abraham, D. 747, *760*
Venditti, J.M., see Goldin, A. 301, *334*, *481*, 500, *505*
Venditti, J.M., see Hoffman, G.S. 263, *269*, 548, *550*
Venditti, J.M., see Jacobs, S.P. 501, *506*
Venditti, J.M., see Kaplan, N.O. 540, *543*
Venditti, J.M., see Kline, I. 79, *81*, 198, *227*, 235, *253*, 259, 260, 262, *270*, 545, 548, *551*, 767, *785*
Venditti, J.M., see Livingston, R.B. 485, 500, *507*
Venditti, J.M., see Sirica, A. 830, *840*
Venditti, J.M., see Tyrer, D.D. 236, *255*, *271*, 523, *537*, 548, *552*
Vennitt, S. 27, *34*
Venker, P., see Langen, P. 290, *339*
Ventilia, M., see Marantz, R. 678, *692*
Venuto, F. De, see Westphal, U. 96, *103*
Verbin, R.S., Diluiso, G., Liang, H., Farber, E. 235, 236, *255*
Verini, M.A., Casazza, A.M., Fioretti, A., Rodenghi, F., Ghione, M. 608, *613*
Verly, W.G., Brakier, L., *17*
Verly, W.G., see Brakier, L. 10, *15*, 41, *42*
Verly, W.G., see Koch, G. 40, *44*
Verly, W.G., see Moutschen, J. 40, *45*
Verma, I.M., Meuth, N.L., Bromfeld, E., Manly, K. F., Baltimore, D. 660, *668*
Vermel, E.M., see Erukhimov, L.S. 360, *365*
Vermeulen, C., see Scott, W. W. 176, *191*
Vermund, H., see Ansfield, F.J. 221, *223*
Vermund, H., see Clifton, K. H. 289, 291, *330*
Veros, A.J., see Frank, B.H. 699, 700, *716*
Vertogradova, T.P. 620, *622*
Vesco, C., see Penman, S. 571, 573, 578, *580*
Vesco, C., see Zylber, E. 577, *581*
Veselý, J. 349, *371*
Veselý, J., Čihák, A. *371*
Veselý, J., Čihák, A., Šorm, F. 351, 362, 363, *371*
Veselý, J., Gostof, R., Čihák, A., Šorm, F. 351, 363, *371*
Veselý, J., see Čihák, A. 362, 363, *364*, *365*
Veselý, J., see Hrodek, O. 363, *367*
Veselý, J., see Seifertová, M. 358, 363, *370*

Veselý, J., see Škoda, J. 350
Veselý, J., see Šorm, F. 349, 351, 355, 362, *370*
Vích, Z., see Grozdanovič, J. 355, *366*
Vick, J., see Burka, B. 609, *611*
Vietti, T., Eggerding, F., Valeriote, F. 199, *231*
Vietti, T.J., see Luce, J.K. 397, *401*
Vietti, T.J., see Sullivan, M. P. 476, *482*
Vietti, T.J., see Wang, J.J. 262, *271*
Vietti, T.S., see Fernbach, D.J. 263, *268*
Vietzke, W.M., see Oliverio, V.T. 69, 72, *82*
Vigier, P., Golde, A. 58, *63*
Vijayvargiya, R., see Singhal, R.L. 152, *156*
Villadolid, L.S., see Wallace, E.Z. 811, *819*
Villee, C.A., see Eckstein, B. 123, *128*
Villee, C.A., see Kato, J. 117, *131*
Vincent, P.C., Reeve, T.S., Brittle, N., Nicholis, A., Richards, M. 59, *63*
Vinegar, R. 408, 409, *424*
Vinegar, R., Schreiber, W., Hugo, R. *424*
Vinograd, J., see Meselson, M. 292, *340*
Visser, D.W. 379, 380, *382*
Visser, D.W., Lagerborg, D. L., Pearson, H.E. 377, 380, *382*
Visser, D.W., Roy-Burman, P. 376, *382*
Visser, D.W., Roy-Burman, S. 376, *383*
Visser, D.W., see Beltz, R. E. 272, *328*, 376, 379, 380, *381*
Visser, D.W., see Friedland, M. 380, *381*
Visser, D.W., see Frisch, D. M. 272, *333*
Visser, D.W., see Fukuhara, T.K. 272, *333*, 376, *381*
Visser, D.W., see Huang, Y. H.J. 377, 378, 380, *381*
Visser, D.W., see Kabat, S. 380, *381*
Visser, D.W., see Roberts, M. 376, 377, 379, 380, *382*
Visser, D.W., see Roy-Burman, P. 373, 374, 377, 378, *382*
Visser, D.W., see Roy-Burman, S. 375, 376, 377, 378, 380, *382*
Visser, D.W., see Slotnick, I.J. 377, *382*
Visser, D.W., see Smith, D. A. 377, 378, 380, *382*
Visser, D.W., see Werkheiser, W.C. 380, *383*
Viswanathan, N., see Gellert, E. 564, *568*
Vivacqua, R.J., Haurani, I., Ersley, A.J. 39, *46*
Vodopick, H., Hamilton, A. E., Jackson, H.L., Peng, C.T., Sheets, R.F. 40, *46*
Vodopick, H., see Regan, J. D. 525, *535*
Voet, D., Rich, A. 197, *231*, 279, *346*
Vogel, C.L., Adamson, R. H., DeVita, V.T., Johns, D.G., Kyalwazi, S.K. 478, *482*
Vogel, C.L., Calabresi, P. 502, *511*
Vogel, C.L., Comis, R., Ziegler, J.L., Kiryabwire, J. W.M. *553*
Vogel, C.L., Denham, C., Waalkes, T.P., DeVita, V.T. 549, *552*
Vogel, C.L., DeVita, V.T., Denham, C., Foley, H. T., Field, R.B., Carbone, P.P. 549, *553*
Vogel, C.L., DeVita, V.T., Lisak, R.P., Kies, M.W. 549, *553*
Vogel, F., Rohrborn, G. 22, *34*
Vogler, W.R. *271*
Vogler, W.R., Huguley, C., Rundles, R. 477, *482*
Vogler, W.R., Jacobs, J. 477, *483*
Vogler, W.R., Olansky, S. 361, *371*
Vogler, W.R., see Groth, D. P. 74, *81*, 264, *269*
Vogler, W.R., see Rudman, D. 703, *720*
Vogt, A., see Maass, G. 302, 304, *340*
Vogt, M., see Harbers, E. 583, *590*
Vogt, M., see Smith, J.D. 302, 307, *344*
Voigt, K.D., see Schmidt, H. 123, *135*, *136*
Vojta, M., Jirásek, J. 357, *371*
Volcani, B.E., see Ben-Ishai, R. 377, *381*
Volicer, L., see Janků, I. 349, 359, *367*
Volkmann, R., Danishefsky, S., Eggler, J., Solomon, D.M. 650, *656*
Volkmann, R., see Danishefsky, S. 650, *655*
Vollmer, E.P., Gordon, A.S., Levenstein, I., Charipper, H.A. 145, *157*
Volucci, V., see Jensen, E.V. 176, 187, *190*
Vonderhaar, B.K., Kim, U. H., Mueller, G.C. 114, *137*
VonFurth, O., Friedmann, M. 695, 697, *721*
Vonka, V., Kutinova, L., Drobnik, J., Bräuerova, J. 838, *840*
Vorherr, H., Welch, A.D. 357, *371*
Vorys, N., Ullery, J.C., Stevens, V. 109, *137*
Vos, O., see Bootsma, D. 604, *611*
Voytek, P., Chang, P., Prusoff, W.H. 281, 285, 286, 287, 320, 322, 325, *346*
Vrba, M. 354, *371*
Vredevoe, D.L., Hayes, E. F. 417, *425*
Vyska, K., see Welsh, R. 869, *876*

Waalkes, T.P., see Vogel, C. L. 549, *552*
Wacker, A. 52, *63*, 319, 321, *346*
Wacker, A., Dellweg, H., Weinblum, D. 321, *346*
Wacker, A., Ebert, M. 26, *34*
Wacker, A., Kirschfield, S., Hartmann, D., Weinblum, U.D. 380, *383*
Wacker, A., Traeger, L. *346*
Wacker, A., Trebst, A., Jacherts, D., Weygand, F. 274, 295, *346*
Wacker, A., see Cramer, J. W. 301, 302, 303, 306, *330*
Wacker, A., see Weygand, F. 274, 280, 295, *346*
Wacker, W.E.C., see Kojima, Y. *717*
Wada, T., see Tanaka, N. 497, *511*
Waddell, W.R., see Rifkind, D. 416, *423*
Waddell, W.R., see Starzl, T.E. 410, *424*

Wade, H. E., Elsworth, R., Herbert, D., Keppie, J., Sargeant, K. 697, *721*
Wade, H. E., see North, A. C. T. 699, *719*, 724, *745*
Wade, M., see Kaplan, S. R. 264, *270*
Wade, M. E., see Wagenen, G. van 357, *371*
Wade, M. E., see Mitchell, M. S. 237, *253*
Waelsch, H., see Borek, E. 499, *503*
Wagenen, G. van, DeConti, R. C., Handschumacher, R. E., Wade, M. E. 357, *371*
Wagenen, G. van, see Morris, J. M. 357, *368*
Wagh, U., see Caspersson, T. 6, *15*
Wagner, E. K., Roizman, B. 680, *694*
Wagner, M., see Gellhorn, A. 822, 823, *827*
Wagner, N. J., Heidelberger, C. 206, 209, *231*
Wagner, O., Bauer, K., Irion, E., Rauenbusch, E., Kaufmann, W., Arens, A. 698, *721*
Wagner, O., Irion, E., Bauer, K. 703, *722*
Wagner, O., see Arens, A. 698, 699, 702, 703, *713*
Wagner, O., see Rauenbusch, E. 698, 702, *720*, 723, *746*
Wahba, A. J., Gardner, R. S., Basilio, C., Miller, R. S., Speyer, J. F., Lengyel, P. 214, *231*
Wainer, R. A., see Slater, L. M. 683, *693*
Waisman, H. A., see Curreri, A. R. 220, *224*
Waithe, W. I., see Weiner, M. S. 707, *722*
Wakaki, S., Marumo, H., Tomioka, K., Shimizu, G., Kato, E., Kamada, H., Kudo, S., Fujimoto, Y. 47, *64*
Wakashiro, T., see Hori, M. 445, *454*
Wakashiro, T., see Kunimoto, T. 444, *454*
Wakashiro, T., see Sawa, T. 444, *455*
Wakisaka, G., see Inagaki, A. 242, 243, *252*, 261, *269*
Waksman, S. A. 582, 584, 589, *592*
Waksman, S. A., Woodruff, H. B. 582, *592*
Walaas, O. 122, *138*
Walaszek, E. J., see Back, A. 684, *688*
Walaszek, E. J., see Kocsis, J. J. 684, *691*
Walford, R. L. 410, 417, *425*
Waligunda, J., see Ohnuma, T. 515, 529, *535*
Walker, E. M., Jr., see Gale, G. R. 835, *839*
Walker, G., see Jones, N. F. *532*
Walker, G., see Krüger, F. W. 70, 71, *81*
Walker, H., see Duschinsky, R. 273, *331*
Walker, I. G. 14, *17*
Walker, I. G., Watson, W. J. 26, *34*
Walker, I. G., see Reid, B. D. 14, *16*
Walker, I. G., see Thatcher, C. J. 76, *84*
Walker, J. D., see Wilson, J. D. 149, *157*
Walker, J. L., see Hampar, B. 308, *334*
Walker, M. D., Hurwitz, B. S. 69, *84*
Walker, M. D., Rosenblum, M. L., Smith, K. A., Reynolds, A. F., Jr. 69, *84*
Walker, R. W., see Kaczka, E. A. 658, *666*
Wall, E., Hertig, A. T., Smith, G. V. S., Johnson, L. C. 175, *192*
Wall, M. E. 654, *656*
Wall, M. E., Wani, M. C., Cook, C. E., Plamer, K. H., McPhail, A. T., Sim, G. A. 649, *656*
Wall, M. E., see Kepler, J. A. 649, *655*
Wall, M. E., see Wani, M. C. 649, 650, *656*
Wall, R., Darnell, J. E. 574, *581*
Wall, R., see Darnell, J. E. 574, 575, *579*, 664, *665*
Wall, R., see Jelinek, W. *669*
Wall, R., see Philipson, L. *580*, 664, *667*
Wallace, E. Z., Silverstein, J. N., Villadolid, L. S., Weisenfeld, S. 811, *819*
Wallace, R. A. 121, *138*
Wallace, R. A., Dumont, J. N. 120, 121, *138*
Wallace, R. A., Jared, D. W. 120, 121, *138*
Wallace, R. A., see Rudack, D. 121, *135*
Wallace, S. L., see Ertel, N. 684, *689*
Wallach, D. P., Grisolia, S. 283, *346*
Waller, G. R., see Suhadolnik, R. J. 658, 661, *667*
Wallick, C. A., see Lawley, P. D. 26, *32*
Walther, H., see Schmidt, H. 123, *135*, *136*
Walton, E., Holly, F. W., Boxer, G. E., Nutt, R. F., Jenkins, S. R. 661, *668*
Walton, E., Nutt, R. F., Jenkins, S. R., Holly, F. W. 658, *668*
Walton, E., see Jenkins, S. R. 661, *666*
Walton, E., see Jenkins, S. R. *668*
Walton, J. N., see Bradley, W. G. 686, *688*
Waltuch, G., Sachs, F. 323, *346*
Walwick, E. R., Roberts, W. K., Dekker, C. A. 233, *256*
Wampler, G. L., Kuperminc, M., Regelson, W. 885, *890*
Wampler, G. L., see Munson, A. E. 884, *889*
Wang, C. H., see Dost, F. N. 755, *762*
Wang, J. J., Selawry, O. S., Vietti, T. J., Bodey, G. P. 262, *271*
Wang, M. C., Simpson, A. I., Paterson, A. R. P. 391, *403*
Wang, M. C., see Paterson, A. R. P. 386, 391, *401*
Wang, S. Y. 277, *346*
Wang, S. Y., see Ishihara, H. 321, *336*
Wani, M. C., Kepler, J. A., Thompson, J. B., Wall, M. E., Levine, S. G. 649, *656*
Wani, M. C., Campbell, H. F., Brine, G. A., Kepler, J. A., Wall, M. E., Levine, S. G. 650, *656*
Wani, M. C., see Kepler, J. A. 649, *655*
Wani, M. C., see Wall, M. E. 649, *656*
Wannemacher, C. F., see Wannemacher, R. W. 56, *64*
Wannemacher, R. W., Wannemacher, C. F., Yatvin, M. B. 56, *64*

Waqar, M.A., Burgoyne, L. A. 660, *668*
Waravdekar, U.S., see Herman, E.H. 609, *612*
Waravdekar, V., see Vadlamudi, S. 705, 706, *721*
Waravdekar, V.S., see Grindey, G.B. 240, *252*, 267, *269*
Waravdekar, V.S., see Kline, I. 198, *227*, 545, *551*
Waravdekar, V.S., see Saslaw, L.D. 267, *270*
Ward, D.C., Cerami, A., Reich, E. 442, 443, *456*
Ward, D.C., Fuller, W., Reich, E. 441, 443, *456*, 462, 463, *467*
Ward, D.C., Horn, T., Reich, E. 438, *456*
Ward, D.C., Reich, E. 437, 441, 443, *457*
Ward, D.C., Reich, E., Goldberg, I.H. 602, *614*, 625, 626, 629, *632*
Ward, D.C., Reich, E., Stryer, L. 441, 443, *457*
Ward, D.C., see Cerami, A. 585, *590*
Ward, D.C., see Kapuler, A. M. 437, *454*
Ward, D.C., see Reich, E. 573, *580*
Ward, H.N., Konikov, N., Reinhard, E.H. 39, *46*
Ward, J.F., see Zimbrick, J. D. 319, *347*
Waring, M.J. 587, *592*, 599, 603, *614*, 617, *622*, 627, *632*, 880, *890*
Warkentin, D.L., see Kreis, W. 822, 824, *827*
Warnecke, P., Seeber, S. 682, *694*
Warnecke, P., see Seeber, S. 710, *721*
Warneke, J., Winterfeldt, E. 650, *656*
Warner, D.T., Neil, G.L., Taylor, A.J., Wechter, W.J. 233, *256*
Warner, J.R., see Wu, R.S. 574, *581*, 651, *656*
Warner, R.G., see Breuer, L.H. 711, *714*
Warnick, C.T. 386
Warren, A.E., see La Via, M. F. 513, 526, *533*
Warren, A.K., see Palmer, C.G. 673, *692*
Warren, G.H., see Gregory, F.J. 523, *532*
Warren, J.C., see Barker, K. L. 119, 124, *126*
Warren, J.C., see Nielson, M.N. 124, *134*
Warthin, A.S., Weller, C.V. 18, *34*
Warton, J.D., see Huggins, C. 172, *189*
Warwick, G.P. 6, *17*, 19, 25, *34*
Warwick, G.P., see Roberts, J.J. 39, *46*
Warwick, G.P., see Ross, W. C.J. 29, *33*
Wase, A., see Roth, J.S. 499, *509*
Wasselewa, L., see Russeff, C. 302, *343*
Watanabe, A., see Suzuki, M. 862, 863, 869, 870, *875*
Watanabe, J., see Kaziwara, K. 618, 619, 620, *622*
Watanabe, K., see Suzuki, M. 870, *875*
Watanabe, K.A., see Fox, J.J. 434, 435, 436, *453*, 658, *665*
Watanabe, K.A., see Mizuno, Y. 444, *455*
Watanabe, M., August, J.T. 855, 859, 860, *876*
Waters, I.W., see Straw, J. A. 813, *819*
Watkins, W.D., Guess, W. L. 560, *570*
Watkins, W.L., see Sullivan, M.P. 476, *482*
Watkinson, J.M., see Haddow, A.L. 183, *189*
Watson, D.H., Wildy, P., Russel, W.C. 303, *346*
Watson, D.K., see Klemperer, H.G. *338*
Watson, D.W., Johnson, A. G. 525, *537*
Watson, J.D., see Gros, F. 210, *225*
Watson, W.B., see Bates, H. M. 644, 645, 646, *647*
Watson, W.J., see Walker, I.G. 26, *34*
Way, J.L., Dahl, J.L., Parks, R.E., Jr. 461, *467*
Way, J.L., Parks, R.E., Jr. 460, 461, *467*
Waynforth, H.B., see Feherty, P. 116, *128*
Webb, J.L., see Heard, R.D. 106, *130*
Webb, J.S., Cosulich, D.B., Mowat, J.H., Patrick, J. B., Broschard, R.W., Meyer, W.E., Williams, R.P., Wolf, C.F., Fulmor, W., Pidacks, C., Lancaster, J.E. 47, *64*
Webb, J.S., see Patrick, J. B. 48, *62*
Webb, S.J., see Bergh, A.K. 825, *826*
Webb, T.E. 463, *467*
Webb, T.E., see Kwan, S. W. 463, *466*
Webb, T.E., see Levitan, I. B. 363, *367*
Webb, T.E., see Rizzo, A.J. *669*
Weber, D.J., see Garrett, E. R. 275, *333*
Weber, G., see Williams-Ashman, H.G. 774, *788*
Weber, M.C., see Clarke, V. 879, *888*
Wechter, W.J., see Gish, D. T. 233, *252*
Wechter, W.J., see Gray, G. D. 237, *252*, 266, *269*
Wechter, W.J., see Warner, D.T. 233, *256*
Wedeking, P.W., see Babington, R.G. 408, *419*
Wedemeyer, G. 810, *819*
Weeks, T.E., see Linder, R. C. 561, *569*
Weeth, J.B., see Segaloff, A. 183, *191*
Wehrli, W., Staehelin, M. 883, *890*
Wei, Y.-K., see Kirschner, S. 836, *840*
Weigert, M.G., see Rosen, B. 215, *230*
Weil, J.H., see Giege, R. 210, *225*
Weil, M., Jacquillat, C., Boiron, M., Bernard, J. 772, 773, *788*
Weil, M., see Bernard, J. 260, *267*
Weil, M., see Boiron, M. 773, *783*
Weil, M., see Ellison, R.R. 260, *268*
Weil, M., see Jacquillat, C. 726, 727, 728, 732, 734, 735, *744*
Weil, R., Michel, M.R., Ruschmann, G. 302, 308, *346*
Weiler, P., Jr., see Sellinger, O.Z. 499, *510*

Weinbaum, G., see Rich, M. A. 660, 663, *667*
Weinbaum, G., see Shiio, T. 54, *63*
Weinberg, A., Becker, Y. 529, *537*
Weinberg, R., see Penman, S. 571, 575, *580*
Weinberg, R., see Penman, S. 664, *667*
Weinberg, R., see Siev, M. *581*, 664, *667*
Weinberg, R. A. 571, *581*
Weinberg, R. A., Penman, S. 572, 578, *581*
Weinberger, S. 695, *722*
Weinblum, D., see Wacker, A. 321, *346*, 380, *383*
Weiner, M. S., Waithe, W. I., Hirschhorn, K. 707, *722*
Weinfeld, H., see Brown, G. B. 318, *328*
Weinhold, P. A., Rethy, V. B. 520, *537*
Weinhouse, S., see Adelman, R. C. 659, *664*
Weinhouse, S., see Jedeikin, L. A. 539, *542*
Weinstein, G. D. 479, *483*
Weinstein, G. D., see Van Scott, E. S. 479, *482*
Weinstein, I. B., Hirschberg, E. 880, *890*
Weinstein, I. B., see Cheng, C. J. 68, 70, *80*
Weinstein, I. B., see Hirschberg, E. 880, *889*
Weinstein, I. B., see Muggia, F. M. 589, *591*
Weinstock, M., see Hess, A. F. 120, *130*
Weisberger, A. S., Levine, B. 522, *537*
Weisberger, A. S., Suhrland, L. G. 522, *537*
Weisberger, A. S., Suhrland, L. G., Seifter, J. 522, *537*
Weisburger, E. K., see Frankel, H. H. 410, 417, *421*
Weisburger, E. K., see Shimkin, M. B. 36, *46*
Weisburger, J. H., see Frankel, H. H. 410, 417, *421*
Weisburger, J. H., see Shimkin, M. B. 36, *46*
Weisenberg, R. C., Borisy, G. G., Taylor, E. W. 677, 678, *694*
Weisenberg, R. C., Taylor, E. W. 677, 678, *694*
Weisenberg, R. C., Timasheff, S. 678, *694*
Weisenberg, R. C., see Adelmann, M. R. 676, *688*
Weisenfeld, S., Hecht, A., Leichter, D., Goldner, M. 814, *819*
Weisenfeld, S., see Southren, A. L. 811, *819*
Weisenfeld, S., see Wallace, E. Z. 811, *819*
Weisleder, D., see Powell, R. G. 556, *569*
Weislogel, P. O., see Johnson, J. L. 209, 210, *227*
Weiss, A., see Jackson, L. 735, 738, *744*
Weiss, A. J., Ramirez, G., Grage, T., Strawitz, D., Goldman, L., Downing, V. 511
Weiss, A. J., see Grage, T. B. 441, *453*
Weiss, B., see Srinivasan, P. R. 492, *510*
Weiss, L., Hakala, M. T. 781, *788*
Weiss, M. J., see Roth, R. H. 48, *62*
Weissbach, A., Lisio, A. 49, *64*
Weissbach, A., see Korn, D. 57, *61*
Weissbach, A., see Lipsett, M. N. 49, 50, *61*
Weissleder, H., see Obrecht, P. 759, *763*
Weissmann, A., see Deutsch, E. 709, *715*, 734, 735, *744*
Weissman, A., see Koe, B. K. 519, *533*
Weissman, C., see Sterental, A. 112, *136*, 174, *191*
Weissman, S., see Karon, M. 241, *253*, 261, *270*, 463, *466*
Weissman, S. G., see Herter, F. P. 541, *542*
Weissman, S. W., see Bono, V. H. 352, *364*
Weitzel, G. L., Schneider, F., Fretzdorff, A. M. 756, *765*
Weitzel, G. L., Schneider, F., Fretzdorff, A. M., Seynsche, K., Finger, H. 756, *765*
Weitzel, G. L., Schneider, F., Fretzdorff, A., Durst, J., Hirschmann, W. 754, 756, *765*
Weitzel, G. L., Schneider, F., Kummer, D., Ochs, H. 756, *765*
Weksler, B. B., see Weksler, M. E. 707, *722*
Weksler, M. E., Weksler, B. B. 707, *722*
Welch, A. D. 291, 323, *346*
Welch, A. D., Prusoff, W. H. 282, 283, 284, 314, 316, 319, 324, *346*
Welch, A. D., Škoda, J., Gutová, M. 357
Welch, A. D., see Calabresi, P. 238, *250*, 283, 284, 291, 302, 314, 319, 323, 324, *329*
Welch, A. D., see Chang, P. K. 272, 273, 291, *329*
Welch, A. D., see Cramer, J. W. 291, 301, 302, 303, 306, *330*
Welch, A. D., see Creasey, W. A. 234, 238, 242, 244, *251*, 258, 259, *268*
Welch, A. D., see Fischer, D. S. 237, *251*, 308, 309, 323, *333*, 356, 362, *366*
Welch, A. D., see Fischer, G. A. 471, *480*
Welch, A. D., see Haley, E. E. 514, *532*, 695, *716*, 723, *744*
Welch, A. D., see Handschumacher, R. E. 355, 358, 359, 360, 361, *366*, 458, *465*
Welch, A. D., see Huebner, R. J. 308, *336*
Welch, A. D., see Jaffe, J. J. 355, *367*
Welch, A. D., see Johns, D. G. 196, *226*
Welch, A. D., see Papac, R. J. 236, 238, *254*
Welch, A. D., see Perkins, E. S. 302, 322, *342*
Welch, A. D., see Prusoff, W. H. *342*
Welch, A. D., see Raška, K., Jr. 357, *369*
Welch, A. D., see Sartorelli, A. C. *849*
Welch, A. D., see Schindler, R. 355, *370*
Welch, A. D., see Vorherr, H. 357, *371*
Welch, J. F. 561, *570*
Welch, R. W., see Conney, A. H. 813, *817*
Weller, C. V., see Warthin, A. S. 18, *34*
Wellings, P. C., Awdry, P. N., Bors, F. H., Jones, B. R., Brown, D. C., Kaufman, H. E. 195, 200, 219, *231*
Wells, R. D., Larson, J. E. 585, 586, 589, *592*, 626, *632*

Wells, W., Gaines, D., Koenig, H. 352, *371*
Wells, W., see Held, I. 487, *506*
Welsch, C.W. 830, *840*
Welsh, R., Vyska, K. 869, *876*
Wempen, I., Duschinsky, R., Kaplan, L., Fox, J.J. 196, *231*, 278, *346*
Wempen, I., Fox, J.J. 195, 197, 198, *231*
Wempen, I., Miller, N., Falco, E.A., Fox, J.J. 233, *256*
Wempen, I., see Cushley, R. 197, *224*
Wempen, I., see Fox, J.J. 196, *225*
Wenkert, E., Dave, K.G., Lewis, R.G., Sprague, P.W. 649, *656*
Wentland, D., see Heidelberger, C. 203, 215, *226*
Wentland, D., see Mukherjee, K.L. 221, *228*
Werkheiser, W.C. 468, 469, 472, *483*
Werkheiser, W.C., Winzler, R.J., Visser, D.W. 380, *383*
Werkheiser, W.C., Visser, D.W. 380, *383*
Werli, J., see Kenis, Y. 759, *763*
Werner, G.H., see Dubost, M. 593, *612*
Werner, G.H., see Maral, R. 696, 705, 708, *718*
Werner, H.W., see Thompson, C.R. 105, *137*
Werner, I., see Coleman, A.W. 311, *330*
Werner, R. 300, *346*, 868, *876*
Werthessen, N.T., Schwenk, E., Baker, C. 106, *138*
Weser, U., see Seeber, S. 710, *721*
Wessells, N.K. 311, *346*
Wessells, N.K., see Spooner, B.S. 676, *693*
West, C.D., see Pearson, O.H. 183, 184, *191*
West, R.A., see Barrett, H.W. 282, 283, *327*
Westland, R.D., Fusari, S.A., Crooks, H.M., Jr. 485, *511*
Westland, R.D., see Moore, J.A. 485, *507*
Westland, R.D., see Nicolaides, E.D. 485, *508*
Weston, J.K., Maxwell, R.E., Lee, M., Funzle, J., Fisher, R.A. 38, *46*
Westphal, U. 96, *103*
Westphal, U., De Venuto, F. 96, *103*
Westra, A., Dewey, W.C. 294, *346*
Westra, A., see Dewey, W.C. 294, *331*
Westwood, J.C.N., see Appleyard, G. 303, *327*
Wettstein, A., see Neher, R. 140, *155*
Weygand, F., Bestmann, H.J., Klieger, E. 485, *511*
Weygand, F., Wacker, A. 274, 280, 295, *346*
Weygand, F., Wacker, A., Dellweg, H. 280, 295, *346*
Weygand, F., see Wacker, A. 274, 295, *346*
Whalen, R.E., Edwards, D.A. 149, *157*
Whalen, R.E., Luttge, W.G. 160, *168*
Whalen, R.E., Luttge, W.G., Green, R. 149, *157*
Whang, J., see Block, J.B. 236, *249*, 261, *267*
Whang, J., see Frei, E., III. 679, *690*
Whang, J.J., see Bell, W.R. 236, *249*, 261, *267*
Whang-Peng, J., see Adamson, R.H. 710, *713*
Whang-Peng, J., see Gallo, R.C. 650, 653, *655*
Whang-Peng, J., see Sieber, S.M. 880, *889*
Whang-Peng, J., see Smith, R.G. 883, *889*
Wheaton, J.R., see Agrawal, K.C. 798, *804*
Wheaton, J.R., see Agrawal, K.C. 797, *804*
Wheeler et al. 310
Wheeler, G.P. 6, *17*, 21, 25, *34*, 68, *84*
Wheeler, G.P., Bowdon, B.J. 66, 68, 74, 75, *84*, 264, *271*
Wheeler, G.P., Bowdon, B.J., Adamson, D.J., Vail, M.H. 76, 77, *84*
Wheeler, G.P., Bowdon, B.J., Herren, T.C. 69, *84*
Wheeler, G.P., Chumley, S. 68, *84*
Wheeler, G.P., Stephens, Z.H. 27, *34*
Wheeler, G.P., see Bowdon, B.J. 73, *80*
Wheelock, E.F. 608, *614*
Whelan, H.A., Wriston, J.C., Jr. 698, 699, 700, 702, *722*, 723, *746*
Whelan, H.A., see Scheetz, R.W. 697, 699, 702, 703, 704, *720*
White, A. 175, *192*
White, A., Hoberman, H.D., Szego, C.M. *103*
White, A., see Bach, J.F. 410, 413, 414, *419*
White, A., see Dougherty, T.F. 86, *100*, 175, *189*
White, A., see Hofert, J.F. *101*
White, A., see Hull, W. 86, *101*
White, A., see Jedeikin, L.A. 91, *101*
White, A., see Makman, M.H. 86, 88, 89, 91, 92, 93, *102*
White, A., see Nakagawa, S. 89, 94, *102*
White, A., see Pena, A. 89, *102*
White, C.W., see Cooper, A.D. 309, *330*
White, F.R. 394, *403*, 561, *570*
White, H.L., White, J.R. 52, *64*, *641*
White, H.L., see White, J.R. 634, 636, 637, 638, *641*
White, J.G. 677, *694*
White, J.R., Dearman, H.H. 634, *641*
White, J.R., White, H.L. 634, 636, 637, 638, *641*
White, J.R., see White, H.L. 52, *64*, *641*
White, L.P., Shimkin, M.B. 522, *538*
White, P.B., Smith, C.W., Kruse, P.F., Jr. 516, 529, *538*
White, P.B., see Kruse, P.F., Jr. 513, 515, *533*
White, S.C., see Le Page, G.A. 264, *270*
White, W.D., see Silvester, D.J. 273, *344*
Whitecar, J.P., Jr., Bodey, G.P., Freireich, E.J., McCredie, K.B., Hart, J.S. 263, *271*
Whitecar, J.P., Jr., Bodey, G.P., Harris, J.E., Freireich, E.J. 723, 727, 728, 730, 734, 735, *746*
Whitecar, J.P., Jr., Bodey, G.P., Hill, C.S., Jr., Samaan, N.A. 709, *722*

Whitecar, J.P., Jr., Harris, J.E., Bodey, G.P., Freireich, E.J. 727, 734, 735, *746*
Whitecar, J.P., Jr., see Freireich, E.J. 260, 262, 265, *269*
Whitecar, J.P., Jr., see Ho, D.H.W. 698, 699, 700, 702, *716*, 733, *744*
Whitecar, J.P., Jr., see LePage, G.A. 388, 397, *401*
Whitecross, S., see Creighton, A.M. 885, *888*
Whitehouse, J.M.A., see Crowther, D. 726, 732, *743*
Whitmore, D.N., see Hellmann, K. 886, *889*
Whitmore, G.F., see Borsa, J. 234, 238, *250*, 469, 470, *479*
Whitmore, G.F., see Elkind, M.M. 319, 322, *332*
Whitmore, G.F., see Graham, F.L. 243, 244, 245, *252*, 260, *269*
Whitsell, J.C., see Merkatz, I.R. 415, *422*
Whittington, R.M., see Kuang, D.T. 638, 639, *640*
Whittington, R.M., see Rivers, S.L. 640, *641*
Whittle, E.L., see Moore, J. A. 485, *507*
Whittle, W., see Kruse, P. F., Jr. 524
Whittle, W., see Patterson, M.K., Jr. 696, 712, *719*
Wiater, A., see Klopotowski, T. 517, *533*
Wicks, W.D., Greenman, D. L., Kenney, F.T. 147, *157*
Wicks, W.D., Kenney, F.T. 147, *157*
Wicks, W.D., see Greenman, D.L. 147, *154*
Wicks, W.D., see Kenney, F.T. 88, *101*
Wide, L., see Dahlwitz, A. 735, *743*
Widnell, C.C., see Hamilton, T.H. 119, *129*
Wieczorkowski, J., Šorm, F., Beránek, J. 350, *371*
Wieland, H., see Flury, F. 18, *31*
Wieland, T., Determann, H. 517, *538*
Wiener, M., see Davis, M.E. 113, *127*
Wiernik, P.H. 94, *103*
Wiernik, P.H., MacLeod, R. M. *103*, 680, *694*
Wierzchowski, K.L., see Fikus, M. 198, *225*, 321, *332*
Wiesner, B.P., see Sanders, M.A. 356, *369*
Wiesner, R., Acs, G., Reich, E., Shafig, A. 583, *592*
Wiest, W.G. 160, 164, *169*
Wiest, W.G., Rao, B.R. 162, *169*
Wiggins, R., see Burchenal, J.H. 233, *250*
Wilbur, J.M., Jr., see Parham, W.E. 39, *45*
Wilco, L.J., see Skipper, H. E. 798, *807*
Wilcox, W.S., see Schabel, F.M., Jr. 76, *83*, 389, *402*, 494, *509*
Wilcox, W.S., see Skipper, H.E. 235, 249, *255*, 260, 261, 262, *271*
Wilcox, W.S., see Wilkoff, L.J. 235, *256*, 260, 263, *271*, 494, *511*
Wilde, C.E., Jr. 513, *538*
Wilde, J.K.H., see Barrett, P.A. 841, *847*
Wildy, P., see Watson, D.H. 303, *346*
Wiley, P.F. 623, *632*
Wiley, P.F., Caron, E.L., Jr. 623, *632*
Wiley, P.F., Jahnke, H.K., MacKeller, F., Kelley, R. B., Argoudelis, A.D. 557, *570*
Wiley, P.F., MacKellar, F. A., Caron, E.L., Kelly, R.B. 623, *632*
Wiley, P.F., see Neil, G.L. 233, *254*, 266, *270*
Wiley, R.A., see Jorgensen, E.C. 520, *532*
Wilhelm, R.C., Ludlum, D. B. 14, *17*
Wilhelm, R.C., see Ludlum, D.B. 7, 15, *16*
Wilkens, M., see Schjeide, O. A. 120, *135*
Wilkie, D., Lee, B.K. 561, *570*
Wilkin, M.L., see Thompson, R.L. 302, *346*
Wilkins, B.M. 309, *346*
Wilkinson, D.S., Čihák, A., Pitot, H.C. 206, 207, 210, 211, 213, *231*
Wilkinson, D.S., Pitot, H.C. 574, *581*
Wilkinson, D.S., see Čihák, A. 213, *224*
Wilkinson, J.F. 361, *371*
Wilkinson, J.F., see Buttoo, A.S. 352, 356, 359, *364*
Wilkinson, J.F., see Elves, M.W. 361, *365*
Wilkinson, K.P., see Hanna, C. 306, *335*
Wilkoff, L.J., Dixon, G.J., Dulmadge, E.A., Schabel, F.M., Jr. 76, *84*
Wilkoff, L.J., Lloyd, H.H., Dulmadge, E.A., Dixon, G.J. 298, *347*
Wilkoff, L.J., Wilcox, W.S., Burdeshaw, J.A., Dixon, G.J., Dulmadge, E.A. 235, *256*, 260, 263, *271*, 494, *511*
Wilkoff, L.J., see Skipper, H.E. 235, *255*
Willen, R. 206, *231*
Willet, F.M., see Hales, D. R. 394, *399*
Williams, A.C., Klein, E. 221, *231*
Williams, A.K., Cox, S.T., Eagon, R.G. 517, *538*
Williams, C.M., see Greer, M. 520, *532*
Williams, D.C., see Belham, J.E. 149, *153*
Williams, D.C., see Mangan, F.R. 149, 150, *155*
Williams, D.W. 38, *46*
Williams. M.K., see Lowy, B. 489, *507*
Williams, M.K., see Oliverio, V.T. 69, 72, *82*
Williams, R., see Mitchell, C. G. 413, 414, *422*
Williams, R.H., Boeck, L. D., Cline, J.C., DeLong, D.C., Gerzon, K., Gordee, R.S., Gorman, M., Holmes, R.E., Larsen, S. H., Lively, D.H., Matthews, T.R., Nelson, J. D., Poore, G.A., Stark, W.M., Sweeney, M.J. 446, *457*
Williams, R.H., Lively, D. H., DeLong, D.C., Cline, J.C., Sweeney, M. J., Poore, G.A., Larsen, S.H. 446, *457*
Williams, R.H., see Sweeney, M.J. 446, 451, *456*
Williams, R.P., see Patrick, J.B. 48, *62*
Williams, R.P., see Webb, J.S. 47, *64*
Williams, S.S., see Bresnick, E. 203, *223*

Williams,T.E., see Sutow, W.W. 726, 727, 732, *746*
Williams,W.L., see Zimmerman,B. 809, *819*
Williams-Ashman,H.G. 146, 150, 151, *157*
Williams-Ashman,H.G., Coppoc,G.L., Schenone, A., Weber,G. 774, *788*
Williams-Ashman,H.G., Liao,S. 118, *138*
Williams-Ashman,H.G., Liao,S., Hancock,R.L., Jurkowitz,L., Silverman,D.A. 147, *157*
Williams-Ashman,H.G., Pegg,A.E., Lockwood, D.H. 148, *157*
Williams-Ashman,H.G., Reddi,A.H. 115, 118, *138*, 146, 150, *157*
Williams-Ashman,H.G., Schenone,A. 774, *788*
Williams-Ashman,H.G., see Coffey,D.S. 151, *153*
Williams-Ashman,H.G., see Corti,A. 774, 775, *784*
Williams-Ashman,H.G., see Hancock,R.L. *154*
Williams-Ashman,H.G., see Liao,S. 147, *155*
Williams-Ashman,H.G., see Mihich,E. 775, *786*
Williams-Ashman,H.G., see Nyden,S.I. 151, *155*
Williams-Ashman,H.G., see Pegg,A.E. 148, *156*, 775, *787*
Williams-Ashman,H.G., see Rhodes,J.B. 149, *156*
Williamson,A.P., see Blattner,R.J. 493, *503*
Williamson,C.E., Witten, B. 20, *34*
Williamson,D.H. 660, *668*
Williamson,J. 660, *668*
Williamson,J., Rollo,J.M. 660, *668*
Williamson,J., see Macadam,R.F. 660, *666*
Williamson,J., see Trigg,P. I. 660, *668*
Willigerodt,B., see Boll,I. 405, *419*
Willoughby,D.A., see Stevens,J.E. 408, *424*
Wilmanns,W. *483*
Wilmot,L., see Hahn,W.E. 121, *129*, 165, *167*
Wilson,A.R., see Brockman, R.W. 385, *398*, 460, *465*
Wilson,C.B. 478, *483*
Wilson,C.B., Boldrey,E.B., Enot,K.J. 69, *84*
Wilson,C.B., Norrell,H.,Jr. 478, *483*
Wilson,D.B. 405, 406, *425*
Wilson,D.E., LoGerfo,P. 354, *371*
Wilson,E.W. 123, *138*
Wilson,H., see Lipsett,M. B. 814, *818*
Wilson,H.E., see Barker, A.D. 884, *887*
Wilson,H.E., see Bodey, G.P. 264, *268*
Wilson,H.R. 279, *347*
Wilson,H.R., see Iball,J. 279, *336*
Wilson,H.R., see Rahman, A. 279, *343*
Wilson,J.A., see Rogers,W. I. 219, *229*
Wilson,J.D., Walker,J.D. 149, *157*
Wilson,J.D., see Bruchovsky,N. 85, *100*, 149, 150, *153*, 161, *167*, 177, *188*
Wilson,J.D., see Gloyna, R.E. 149, *154*
Wilson,J.D., see Morgan, M.D. 161, *168*
Wilson,J.E., Irvin,J.L., Suggs,J.E., Liu,K. 523, *538*
Wilson,J.G., see Ritter,E. J. 237, 241, *254*, 261, *270*
Wilson,L. 678, *694*
Wilson,L., Bryan,J., Ruby, A., Mazia,D. 678, *694*
Wilson,L., Friedkin,M. 678, *694*
Wilson,M.J., see Kimball, A.P. 243, *253*, 261, *270*
Wilson,M.J., see LePage, G.A. 429, *433*
Wilson,M.L., see Beer,C.T. 684, *688*
Wilson,R.E., see Murray,J. E. 502, *508*
Wilson,W.L., Labra,C., Barrist,E. 638, *641*
Wilson,W.L., see Bisel,H. F. 440, *453*
Wilson,W.L., see Grage,T. B. 441, *453*
Wilt,F.H. 311, *347*
Wilt,F.H., see Miura,Y. 311, 312, *341*
Wiltshaw,E. 478, *483*
Wiltshaw,E., see Galton, D.A.G. 35, 36, 37, *43*
Windsor,B.L., see Callentine,M.R. 110, *127*
Winitz,M., see Sugimura,T. 528, *537*
Winkelmann,E., see Rolly, H. 800, *806*
Winkler,A., Drahovský,D., Gregušová,V., Thurzo, V., Kára,J., Škoda,J., Šorm,F. 352, *372*
Winston,L., see Clarkson, B. 222, *224*
Winter,T.S., see Davidson, J.D. 393, *399*, 789, *791*
Winterfeldt,E., Radunz,H. 650, *656*
Winterfeldt,E., see Boch, M. 650, *655*
Winterfeldt,E., see Warneke,J. 650, *656*
Winters,W.D., see Mandel, H.G. 459, 460, *466*
Wintrobe,M.M., see Mauer, A.M. 23, *33*
Wintrobe,M.N., see Clarysse,A.M. *480*
Winzler,R.J., see Werkheiser,W.C. 380, *383*
Wiqvist,N., see Bolte,E. 107, *126*
Wira,C., Munck,A. 85, 96, 98, *103*, 164, *169*
Wira,C., see Munck,A. 87, 95, *102*
Wirtanen,G.W., see Ansfield,F.J. 221, *223*
Wiseman,G., Ghadially,F. N. 517, 528, *538*
Wisniewski,H., see Bensch, K.G. 678, *688*
Wisniewski,H., see Shelanski,M.L. 681, *693*
Wissler,F.C., see Pine,M.J. 820, 823, 824, *827*
Wissler,R.W., Frazier,L. F., Soules,K.H., Barker,P., Bristow,E.C. 525, 526, *538*
Wissler,R.W., see Bristow, E.C. 519, *530*
Wissler,R.W., see Cannon, P.R. 526, *530*
Wissler,R.W., see Hruban, Z. 515, 519, *532*
Wissler,R.W., see Samal, B.A. 520, *535*
Witt,C.W.De, see Sakuchi, G. 59, *62*
Wittebort,R., see Notari,R. E. 232, *254*
Witten,B., see Williamson, C.E. 20, *34*

Wittkop, J.A., Prough, R. A., Reed, D.J. 754, *765*
Wittkop, J.A., see Prough, R. 751, 754, *764*
Wittle, E.L., see Nicolaides, E.D. 485, *508*
Wittliff, J.L., Gardner, D. G., Battema, W., Gilbert, P.J. 117, *138*
Wittliff, J.L., Hilf, R., Brooks, W.F., Jr. 117, 118, *138*
Wittliff, J.L., Hilf, R., Brooks, W.F., Jr., Savlov, E.D., Hall, T.C., Orlando, R.A. 117, 118, *138*
Wittliff, J.L., Kenney, F.T. 120, 121, *138*
Wittliff, J.L., Lee, K.L., Kenney, F.T. 121, *138*
Wittliff, J.L., see Brooks, W.F., Jr. 115, *126*
Wittliff, J.L., see Zelson, P. R. 120, 121, *138*
Wittmann, H.C., see Wittmann-Liebold, B. 200, *231*
Wittmann, H.G., see Kramer, G. 200, *228*
Wittmann-Liebold, B., Wittmann, H.C. 200, *231*
Wittner, M., Tanowitz, H., Rosenbaum, R.M. 880, *890*
Wodinsky, I. 820
Wodinsky, I., Kensler, C.J. 235, *256*
Wodinsky, I., see Jacobs, S. P. 501, *506*
Wodinsky, I., see Kensler, C.J. 822, 824, *827*
Wodinsky, I., see Kessel, D. 216, *227*, 239, *253*, 265, *270*, 471, 473, *481*, 584, *591*
Wodinsky, I., see Schepartz, S.A. 820, *828*
Wodinsky, I., see Sivak, A. 822, 823, 824, *828*
Wodinsky, I., see Yesair, D. W. 823, 824, 825, *828*
Wodinsky, L., see Kessel, D. *613*
Woenckhaus, J.W., see Obrecht, P. 749, *764*
Woese, C., see Bleyman, M. 584, *590*
Wolberg, W.H. 204, 216, 217, *231*
Wolberg, W.H., Ansfield, F. J. 217, *231*
Wolberg, W.H., see Blomgren, S.E. 201, *223*
Wolberg, W.H., see Dexter, D.L. 222, 223, *224*
Wold, F., see Brown, W.E. 73, *80*
Wolf, C.F., see Webb, J.S. 47, *64*
Wolf, H., see Puschendorf, B. 29, *33*
Wolff, I.A., see Powell, R. G. 556, *569*
Wolff, J.A., see Farber, S. 512, *531*
Wolff, J.A., see Heyn, R.M. 397, *400*, 500, *506*
Wolff, J.O., see Farber, S.L. H. 476, *480*
Wollert, U., see Reichert, M. 781, *787*
Wollert, V.U. 770, 781, *788*
Wollner, N., see Etcubanas, E. 793, 799, 800, *805*
Wollner, N., see Haghbin, M. 726, 732, *744*
Wollner, N., see Lyman, M. 820, *827*
Wollner, N., see Tallal, L. 727, 728, 730, 732, *746*
Wolpert, M.K., Damle, S.P., Brown, J.E., Sznycer, E., Agrawal, K.C., Sartorelli, A.C. 393, *403*
Wolpert, M.K., Ruddon, R. W. 28, *34*
Wolter, J., see Ream, N.W. 621, *622*
Wong, G., see Geeraets, W. J. 298, *333*
Wong, M.S.F., see Adams, J.B. 178, 179, *188*
Wong, V.G., see Hersh, E. M. 384, *400*, 770, *785*
Woo, N.C., see MacMahon, B. 178, *190*
Wood, D.A., see Jacobs, E. M. 220, *226*
Wood, H.B., Jr., see Goldin, A. 36, *44*
Wood, R.M., see Perkins, E. S. 302, 322, *342*
Wood, W.A., see Rabinowitz, K.W. 440, *455*
Woodliff, H.J., see Leake, E. 39, *44*
Woodman, R.J. 291, *347*
Woodman, R.J., see Kline, I. 79, *81*, 198, *227*, 545, 548, *551*
Woodruff, H.B., see Kaczka, E.A. 658, *666*
Woodruff, H.B., see Waksman, S.A. 582, *592*
Woods, D.D. 512, *538*
Woods, J.S., Lee, I.P., Dixon, R.L. 708, *722*
Woods, M., Burk, D. *543*
Woods, M., see Burk, D. 776, *783*
Woodside, G.L., see Kidder, G.W. 458, 459, 460, *466*
Woodward, G., see Nelson, A.A. 809, 810, *818*
Woodward, R.B., see Rao, K.V. 633, *641*
Woody, P.L., Mandell, J.D., Greenberg, J. 494, *511*
Woody, P.L., see Greenberg, J. 494, *505*
Woody-Karrer, P., Greenberg, J. 494, *511*
Woolley, D.W. 513, *538*
Wooley, G.W., see Merker, P.C. 633, *641*
Woolridge, R.L., see Cannon, P.R. 526, *530*
Worth, W.S. 410, *425*
Wotiz, H.H., Davis, J.W., Lemon, H.M. 106, *138*
Wotiz, H.H., Davis, J.W., Lemon, H.M., Gut, M. 106, *138*
Wotiz, H.H., see Lemon, H. E. 178, *190*
Wright, G.F., see McKay, A.F. 66, *82*
Wright, H.F., see Johnson, I.S. 670, 671, *691*
Wright, J.C., Gumport, S. L., Golomb, F.M. 478, *483*
Wright, J.J., see Birch, A. J. 446, *453*
Wright, J.C., see Harris, M. N. 638, *640*
Wriston, J.C., Jr. 696, 698, 699, 703, *722*
Wriston, J.C., Jr., see Greenquist, A.C. 700, *716*
Wriston, J.C., Jr., see Kirschbaum, J. 700, *717*
Wriston, J.C., Jr., see Mashburn, L.T. 695, 697, 698, 710, *718*, 723, *745*
Wriston, J.C., Jr., see Rowley, B. 697, *720*
Wriston, J.C., Jr., see Scheetz, R.W. 697, 699, 702, 703, 704, *720*
Wriston, J.C., Jr., see Whelan, H.A. 698, 699, 700, 702, *722*, 723, *746*
Wriston, J.C., Jr., see Yellin, T.O. 699, 702, *722*

Wrona, M., Czochralska, B. 321, *347*
Wu, A. M., Ting, R. C., Paran, M., Gallo, R. C. *669*
Wu, C., Yuan, L. H. 493, *511*
Wu, R. S., Kumar, A., Warner, J. R. 574, *581*, 651, *656*
Wunderlich, F., Peyk, D. 674, *694*
Wunderlich, F., Speth, V. 676, *694*
Wunderlich, V., Schütt, M., Böttger, M., Graffi, A. 70, *84*
Wuyts, J. L., see Foucher, G. 502, *504*
Wyatt, J., Mc Aninch, L. 478, *483*
Wyck, J. J. van, see Marsh, J. M. 106, 107, *132*
Wyckoff, K. K., see Shelton, R. S. 105, *136*
Wyngaarden, J. B., see Caskey, C. T. 390, *398*
Wyngaarden, J. B., see McCollister, R. J. 390, 395, *401*
Wyngaarden, J. B., see Silberman, H. R. 389, *402*
Wyse, B. M., Dulin, W. E. 76, *84*

Xeros, N. 604, *614*

Yagil, E., Silberstein, N. 211, *231*
Yagil, E., see Rosner, A. 290, *343*
Yagishita, K., see Maeda, K. 851, 855, *873*
Yagoda, A., see Helson, L. 219, *226*
Yakatan, G. J., see Garrett, E. R. 276, 277, *333*
Yamada, K., see Miura, M. 514, 515, 526, *534*, 705, 706, 707, 713, *719*, 735, 738, *745*,
Yamada, K. M., see Spooner, B. S. 676, *693*
Yamada, T., Iwanami, Y., Baba, T. 28, *34*
Yamada, T. A. 584, *592*
Yamagami, K., see Kato, S. 870, *873*
Yamagata, S., Uzuka, Y., Kurokawa, Y., Yonahara, M. 870, *876*
Yamagata, Y., Sakamoto, M. 296, *347*
Yamaguchi, H., see Tanaka, N. 449, *456*, 850, 851, 856, 857, 858, 868, 869, *875*
Yamaguchi, M., see Price, C. C. 1, 5, *5*, 19, 26, *33*
Yamaki, H., Tanaka, N., Umezawa, H. 857, *876*
Yamaki, H., see Nagai, K. 862, *873*
Yamaki, H., see Suzuki, H. 862, 863, 869, 870, *874*, *875*
Yamamoto, H., see Kusaka, T. 434, *454*
Yamamoto, I. 547, *553*
Yamamoto, I., Iwata, H. 547, *553*
Yamamoto, I., Oka, M., Iwata, H. 547, *553*
Yamamoto, I., see Hano, K. 545, 547, *550*
Yamamoto, I., see Iwata, H. 547, *551*
Yamamoto, K. R., see Johnson, J. L. 209, 210, *227*
Yamamoto, N., Naito, T., Shimkin, M. B. 10, 17
Yamamoto, R. S., see Frankel, H. H. 410, 417, *421*
Yamamoto, T., see Odaka, T. 444, *455*
Yamamoto, T., see Takeuchi, M. 855, *875*
Yamanchi, T., see Mitsuya, H. 870, *873*
Yamaoka, S., see Suzuki, M. 870, *875*
Yamashita, A., see Seiki, K. 160, *168*
Yamaura, K., see Odaka, T. 444, *455*
Yamura, T., see Ungar, G. 527, *537*
Yanagi, Y., see Nakamura, S. 870, *873*
Yancey, S. T., see Hart, M. M. 879, *888*
Yancey, S. T., see Kelly, M. G. 752, *762*, *763*
Yang, N. P., see Huggins, C. 185, *189*
Yang, S. S., Herrera, F. M., Smith, R. G., Reitz, M. S., Lancini, G., Ting, R. C., Gallo, R. C. 883, *890*
Yankee, R. A., see Leventhal, B. G. 501, *507*, 726, 732, 734, 735, *745*
Yanofsky, C., Ito, J., Horn, V. 9, 11, *17*
Yap, C. Y., see Lee, A. K. Y. 416, *422*
Yarbro, J. M., see Theologides, A. 603, *613*
Yarbro, J. W. 789, 790, *792*
Yarbro, J. W., Kennedy, B. J., Barnum, C. P. 616, *622*
Yarbro, J. W., see Kennedy, B. J. *622*, 793, *806*
Yardley, J., see Hodes, M. E. 685, *690*
Yarovaya, L. M., Mardashev, S. R., Debov, S. S. 489, 497, *511*
Yartseva, I. V., see Berlin, Y. A. 615, *621*
Yates, R. C., Olson, K. B. 451, *457*
Yatvin, M. B., see Clifton, K. H. 314, 316, 318, *330*
Yatvin, M. B., see Wannemacher, R. W. 56, *64*
Yellin, T. O., Wriston, J. C., Jr. 699, 702, *722*
Yen, W., see Kreis, W. 758, *763*
Yesair, D. W., Asbell, M. A., Bruni, R., Bullock, F. J., Schwartzbach, E. 608, 609, *614*
Yesair, D. W., Callahan 825
Yesair, D. W., Hofook, C. 822, 824, *828*
Yesair, D. W., Kohner, F. A., Rogers, W. I., Baronowsky, P. E., Kensler, C. J. 682, *694*, 823, 824, *828*
Yesair, D. W., Levins, P., Caragay, A., Shuck, D., Funkhouser, J. T. 822, 823, *828*
Yesair, D. W., Rogers, W. I., Baronowsky, P. E., Wodinsky, I., Thayer, P. S., Kensler, C. J. 823, 824, 825, *828*
Yesair, D. W., Rogers, W. I., Funkhouser, J. T., Kensler, C. J. 823, 824, *828*
Yesair, D. W., Thayer, P. S., Kensler, C. J. 824, 825, *828*
Yesair, D. W., Wodinsky, I., Rogers, W. I., Kensler, C. J. 823, 824, *828*
Yesair, D. W., see Kensler, C. J. 822, 824, *827*
Yesair, D. W., see Palm, P. E. 824, *827*
Yesair, D. W., see Rogers, W. I. *828*
Yesinick, C., see Popper, H. 522, *535*
Yip, M. C. M., Knox, W. E. 490, *511*

Yokoshima, T., see Nagao, M. 73, *82*
Yokoyama, I. *169*
Yonahara, M., see Yamagata, S. 870, *876*
Yoneda, M., see Kida, M. 448, *454*
Yonehara, H., see Aizawa, S. 441, 444, *452*
Yonehara, H., see Otake, N. 441, *455*
Yonehara, H., see Yüntsen, H. 446, *457*
York, I. M., Rogers, W. I., Kensler, C. J. 822, *828*
York, I. M., see Rogers, W. I. 822, 823, *828*
York, I. M., see Rogers, W. I. 822, 823, *828*
York, J. L., LePage, G. A. 427, *433*
York, R., see Miech, R. P. 395, *401*, 461, *466*
Yoshida, see Reimer 53
Yoshida, H., Duval, J., Ebel, J. P. 273, *347*
Yoshida, K., see Fukatsu, H. 870, *872*
Yoshida, K., see Honda, Y. 870, *872*
Yoshida, M., see Hoshi, A. 887, *889*
Yoshida, M., see Kotorii, K. 677, *691*
Yoshida, S., see Runner, M. N. *62*
Young, C. W., Hodas, S. 241, *256*, 634, *641*, *722*, 790
Young, C. W., see Brunner, K. W. 759, *761*
Young, D. A. 86, 91, 93, *103*
Young, D. A., see Hallahan, C. 93, *100*
Young, R. C., DeVita, V. T. 77, 78, *84*
Young, R. S. K., Fischer, G. A. 235, *256*
Young, S. E., see Milner, A. N. 27, *33*
Young, W. C. 104, *138*, 139, 146, *157*
Youngner, J. S., see Hallum, J. V. 607, *612*
Ypersele, C. v., see Alexandre, G. P. J. 502, *503*
Yu, K. P., see Gee, T. S. *269*, 394, 397, *399*
Yu, J. Y.-L., see Campbell, L. D. 125, *127*
Yuan, L. H., see Wu, C. 493, *511*
Yuceoglu, M., see Burchenal, J. H. 389, *398*
Yudkin, J., see Sanders, M. A. 356, *369*
Yudkin, M. D., see Peck, R. M. 212, *229*
Yuen, T. G. H., see Duke, P. S. 520, *531*
Yüntsen, H., Ohkuma, K., Ishii, Y., Yonehara, H. 446, *457*
Yüntsen, H., Yonehara, H., Ui, H. 446, *457*
Yung, N., see Fox, J. J. 232, *251*
Yung, N., see Hoffer, M. 195, *226*, 272, *335*
Yung, N. C., Burchenal, J. H., Fecher, R., Duschinsky, R., Fox, J. J. 196, *231*, 272, *347*
Yuzuriha, Y., see Lee, K.-H. 495, *507*

Zaccara, A., see Zunino, F. 599, *614*
Zacharov, B. M., see Brachnikova, M. G. 593, *611*
Zadražil, S., see Fučík, V. *366*
Zadražil, S., see Jurovčík, M. 363, *367*
Zaharko, D. S., Bruckner, H., Oliverio, V. T. 473, *483*
Zaharko, D. S., Oliverio, V. T. 473, *483*
Zaharko, D. S., see Bischoff, K. B. 472, *479*
Zahn, R. K., Müller, W. E. G., Forster, W., Maidhof, A., Beyer, R. 244, *256*
Zahn, R. K., see Müller, W. E. G. 243, *254*, 583, *591*
Zak, M., Drobnik, J., Rezny, Z. 836, *840*
Zak, S. B., see Greengard, P. 542, *542*
Zakrzewski 771
Zalkin, H., see Nagano, H. 492, *508*
Zalta, J. P., see Duprat, A. M. 628, *631*
Zaltzman-Nirenberg, P., see Udenfriend, S. 520, *537*
Zamenhof, S., DeGiovanni, R., Rich, K. 272, 295, 310, *347*
Zamenhof, S., Griboff, G. 274, 295, *347*
Zamenhof, S., see Ephrati-Elizur, E. 308, *332*
Zamenhof, S., see Greer, S. 275, 301, 319, *334*
Zamenhof, S., see Reiner, B. 26, *33*
Zamenhof, S., see Szybalski, W. 308, *345*
Zamenhof, S., see Theil, E. 379, 380, *382*
Zapelli, P., see DeBarbieri, A. 528, *531*
Zappala, A. F., see Ravin, L. S. 275, *343*
Zappala, A. F., see Ravin, L. J. 275, *343*
Záruba, F., Kůta, A., Elis, J. 361, *372*
Zatman, L. J., Kaplan, N. O., Colowick, S. P. 540, *543*
Zatman, L. J., Kaplan, N. O., Colowick, S. P., Ciotti, M. M. 540, *543*
Závada, J., see Rada, B. 354, *369*
Závada, J., see Rada, B. 354, *369*
Zbinden, G. 642, *648*
Zech, L., see Caspersson, T. 6, *15*
Zedeck, M. S., see Moore, E. C. 798, 803, 804, *806*
Zedeck, M. S., see Raška, K., Jr. 357, *369*
Zee-Cheng, K. Y., Cheng, C. C. 523, *538*
Zeleznick, L. D., Sweeney, C. M. 629, *632*
Zelis, R. F., see Hancock, R. L. *154*
Zeller, P., Gutmann, H., Hegedus, B., Kaiser, A., Langemann, A., Mueller, M. 747, *765*
Zeller, P., see Berneis, K. 756, *761*
Zelson, P. R., Wittliff, J. L. 120, 121, *138*
Zemisch, B., see Herken, H. 541, *542*
Žemlička, J., Smrt, J., Šorm, F. 349, *372*
Žemlička, J. Šorm, F. 349, 350, *372*
Zettner, A., see Booth, B. A. 846, 847, *848*
Zeuthen, E., see Friedrich, U. 415, *421*
Zhdanov, V. M., see Demidova, S. A. 354, *365*
Ziegler, J. L., see Vogel, C. L. *553*
Zieher, L. M., see DeRobertis, E. 499, *504*
Ziemann, A., see Hohorst, H. J. 29, *32*

Zimbrick, J. D., Ward, J. F., Myers, L. S. 319, *347*
Zimmer, D. E. 855, *876*
Zimmerman, B., Bloch, H. L., Williams, W. L., Hitchcock, C. R., Hoelscher, B. 809, *819*
Zimmerman, E. F. 463, *467*
Zimmerman, E. F., Greenberg, S. A. 463, *467*
Zimmerman, E. F., Holler, B. W., Pearson, G. D. 464, *467*
Zimmerman, M. 284, 318, *347*
Zimmerman, M., Seidenberg, J. 289, *347*
Zimmermann, F. K., see Marquardt, H. 78, *82*
Zinder, N. D., see Cooper, S. 58, *60*
Zinkham, W. H., see Migeon, C. J. 107, *133*
Zipf, R. E., see Katchman, B. J. 683, *691*
Zipursky, A., see Israels, L. G. 38, *44*
Zora, J. G., see Dion, H. W. 485, *504*
Zorgniotti, A. W., see Edelman, J. C. 151, *153*
Zubrod, C. G., see Oliverio, V. T. 28, *33*, 771, *787*
Zuckerman, S. 104, *138*
Zumoff, B., Fishman, J., Cassouto, J., Hellman, L., Gallagher, T. F. 178, *192*
Zunino, F., Gambetta, R. A., Zaccara, A., DiMarco, A. 599, *614*
Zunino, F., see DiMarco, A. 599, 605, *612*
Zunio, F., see Chandra, P. 602, 608, *611*
Zurita, V. E., see De-Angeli, L. C. 697, *715*
Zwarenstein, H., Shapiro, H. A. 120, *138*
Zwaveling, A., see Elkerbout, F. 19, *31*
Zweifach, B. W., Nagler, A. L., Troll, W. 527, *538*
Zweiman, B., Silberberg, D. H. 416, *425*
Zwisler, O., see Staerk, J. 703, *721*
Zyk, N., Citri, N. 449, *457*
Zyk, N., Citri, N., Moyed, H. S. 449, *457*
Zylber, E. A., Penman, S. 574, *581*
Zylber, E. A., Perlman, S., Penman, S. 664, *668*
Zylber, E. A., Vesco, C., Penman, S. 577, *581*
Zylber, E. A., see Penman, S. 571, 575, *580*, 664, *667*
Zyroff, J., see Rosenkranz, H. S. 522, *535*

Subject Index

Abortifacient effect of 6-azauridine 356—358
3-Acetylpyridine adenine dinucleotide 540
Aconitase, androgens and 151
Actinomycin D 582—592
  antagonism of androgen-induced enzyme changes 152
  assembly of actinomycin-DNA stereochemical model 588
  binding by DNA 582, 584—589
    models of binding site 586—589
    structural specificity for 585, 586
  blockade of deciduoma reaction to progesterone 159
  carcinogenicity 589
  cell-cycle specificity 59
  chemical structure and source 582
  clinical uses 589
  complex formation with DNA 627
  cross-resistance to daunoribicin 606
  differential inhibition of precursor ribosomal RNA synthesis 573, 577, 584
  effect on DNA polymerase 602
  incorporation of 5-fluorouracil into messenger RNA inhibited by 211
  inhibition of DNA-dependent RNA synthesis 583
  inhibition of progesterone-induced avidin synthesis 165
  nuclear and nucleolar changes induced by 583, 584
  site of action in mammalian cells 583, 584
  structural features required for biological activity 583—586
  synergism with ionizing radiation 589
Acute leukemia, see also acute lymphoblastic and acute myelocytic leukemia
  cortisone for 187
  guanazole for 878
  6-mercaptopurine for 389
  methotrexate for 476, 477
Acute lymphoblastic leukemia, L-asparaginase for 726, 728—731
Acute myelocytic leukemia, L-asparaginase for 726, 728, 729
  COAP regimen for 263, 264
  methylglyoxal-*bis* (guanylhydrazone) for 772, 773
  optimal schedule for arabinosylcytosine 263
Adenine, alkylation of by nitrosoureas 71
Adenosine, antibiotics resembling 434—457
  regulation of xanthosine 5′-phosphate aminase 448
Adenosine deaminase, inhibition by 8-azaguanine 460
Adenosine deaminase, substrate specificity of intestinal mucosa enzyme 658
Adenosine kinase, action on tubercidin 436
  phosphorylation of potential polynucleotide chain terminators 658, 659
S-Adenosyl-L-methionine decarboxylase, methylglyoxal-*bis*(guanylhydrazone) and 775
  stimulation of prostatic enzyme by androgen 148
Adenylosuccinate synthetase, 8-azaguanosine triphosphate as cofactor in 461, 462
  inhibition by 6-thioinosinate 392
Adrenal cortex, changes produced by o,p′-DDD 810—813
Adrenal cortical deficiency, busulfan and 39
Adrenalectomy, effect on glucocorticoid binding 97, 98
Adrenocortical carcinoma, o,p′-DDD for 814—816
Adriamycin 593—614
  antitumor activity 597
  chemistry 593, 594
  complex with DNA 599
  cross-resistance to daunorubicin 606
  effect on thymidine incorporation 605
  excretion 608, 609
  inhibition of RNA dependent DNA polymerase 608
  mitotic effects 597
  neoplasms induced by 610
  pharmacological disposition of 608, 609
  toxicity 609, 610
Alanine transaminase, cortisol effect on 94
Alanosine; L(—) 2-amino-3-nitrosohydroxyl aminopropionic acid 882
Alazopeptin, DON analog 496
  chemical structure 486
Albizziin; β-ureido-L-alanine, chemical structure 485
  isolation, synthesis and activity 498
Aldehyde oxidase, action on azathioprine 412
  action on methotrexate 473
Aldosterone, depressed secretion during o,p′-DDD treatment 811, 812
Alkaline phosphatase, enhanced activity in resistance to 6-mercaptopurine 393
  increased rate of synthesis of in *E. coli* amber mutants exposed to 5-fluorouracil 214, 215
  properties of enzyme induced in presence of 5-fluorouracil 212
  selective inhibition by L-homoarginine 516
Alkyl diazohydroxides, intermediates in nitrosourea alkylations 66, 67

Alkylating agents, action on bacteriophage 9—11
action on DNA 25—27, 29, 30
activation of 29
amino acid derivatives 516—518, 522, 524
antineoplastic effects 22, 23
2-chloroethylamine derivatives, mechanism of action 18—34
cytological damage produced by 21
cytotoxicity and the cell cycle 20—22
distribution and metabolism 28, 29
GC to AT transitions caused by 11
hematopoietic effects 23
historical aspects of 18, 19
immune response and 24
isophosphamide 886
long-term effects of 22
methanesulfonates 35—46
mitomycins 47—64
nicotinamide adenine dinucleotide and 25
nitrogen mustards 2
nitrosoureas 65—84
1-phenyl-3,3-dialkyltriazenes 71
showdomycin 373—376
sulfur mustards 2, 5
transport of and resistance to 28
Alkylation, carbenium ions in 1—3
chemistry of 1—5
DNA bases and 7, 8, 25—27, 29, 30
esterification of phosphate groups in DNA 8
interstrand crosslinks in DNA 8
leaving-group constants, relation to pK_a 4
mechanisms of 19, 20
molecular biology of 6—17
nucleophilic constants 4
repair of damage produced in DNA by 13, 14
Allopurinol, inhibition of xanthine oxidase by 387
Amethopterin, see methotrexate
Amino acid analogs, see cytotoxic amino acid analogs, glutamine antagonists
Amino acids, alkylation by nitrosoureas 72
changes in levels during L-asparaginase treatment 725
effect of L-asparagine on serum levels of 703
possible dependence of tumors on, therapeutic implications 528, 529
ε-Aminocaproic acid, in suppression of homograft rejection 527
L-2-Amino-2-carboxyethane sulfonamide 515
Aminochlorambucil, hematopoietic effects 23
1-Aminocyclopentanecarboxylic acid, immunosuppression by 526
synthesis, activity and clinical trial 523
3′-Amino-3′-deoxyadenosine, antimitotic effect 662
chemical structure 657
inhibition of cell growth 660
synthesis and isolation 658
uptake and metabolism 662, 663
5-Aminodeoxyuridine, synthesis and activity 379, 380
5-Aminoimidazole-4-carboxamide, formation from DIC 545—547
1-Amino-3-methylcyclopentanecarboxylic acid 523
2-Amino-6-methylthiopurine, catabolite of 6-thioguanine 389
6-Aminonicotinamide, biological activity and conversion to NAD analogs 540—542
Aminopterin 468
4-Aminopyrrolo[2,3-d]pyrimidine, aglycone of tubercidin 436
5-Aminouridine, action on pyrimidine and phospholipid synthesis 380
biological activity of aminouridine and derivatives 379, 380
efficiency of triphosphate as substrate for RNA polymerase 380
inhibition of orotidylate decarboxylase by 380
sensitization of viruses to nitrous acid by 380, 381
synthesis 379
5-Aminouridine diphosphate glucose 380
Androgen receptor proteins 149—151, 177
properties 150
Androgens, see also androstenedione, testosterone
action on ovaries and female accessory sex organs 143
action on testis and male accessory sex organs 142, 143
anabolic (myotrophic) agents 142
anabolic effects 145
antagonists 145, 146
antiestrogenic effects 173, 174
assays for 142, 146
biosynthesis 139—142
cyclic-3′,5′-AMP stimulation of 140
breast cancer and 144, 145
breast development and 144
direct effect on prostatic epithelium and mammary gland tissue 176
effects on cofactor nucleotides 151
effects on enzymes in mammary tumors 144, 145
effects on glycine incorporation into mammary tumors 145
effects on pituitary 143, 144
effects on prostatic enzyme activities 148, 149
effects on respiration 151
hematopoietic effects 145
increased RNA induced by 147, 148
mechanism of action 139—157
metabolism of in patients with breast cancer 179
progesterone-like effects 143
properties of receptor proteins for 150
prostatic acid phosphatase and 143
relationship with polyamines 148, 149
relative potency of 142
specific uptake of and antagonism by antiandrogens 149
stimulation of heterogeneous RNA formation by 147

Androgens, structure-activity relationships 142
Androstanolone, see 5α-dihydrotestosterone
Androstenediol, chemical structure 141
Androstenedione, chemical structure 141
conversion to estrogens 106, 107
selective uptake by prostate and seminal vesicles 149
Angustmycin A, see decoyinine
Angustmycin C, see psicofuranine
Anhydroanthramycin 642, 643
Anisomycin, chemical structure and biological activity 564, 565
inhibition of peptide bond formation 559
mechanism of action and structure-activity relationships 565
Anthramycin 642—648
antibacterial activity 642, 643
antitumor properties 642
chemical structure 643
chemosterilant properties 643, 644
complex formation with DNA 644—646
determination of 647
inhibition of DNA polymerase 643
inhibition of nucleic acid synthesis 644
inhibition of RNA polymerase 643, 645, 646
inhibition of RNA synthesis 573, 577
structure-activity relationship 646, 647
Antiandrogens 145, 146
Antibiotics resembling adenosine 434—457
Antibodies, effect of 6-mercaptopurine and azathioprine on formation 407
inhibition of production by halogenated deoxyribonucleosides 309, 310
inhibition of production by mitomycins 59
sequence of formation 407
Antiestrogens 109—111
1-β-D-Arabinofuranosylcytosine, see arabinosylcytosine
9-β-D-Arabinofuranosylguanine 428, 429
9-β-D-Arabinofuranosylhypoxanthine 429
9-β-D-Arabinofuranosyl-6-thioguanine, synthesis and activity 430
Arabinosides, diphosphates, synthesis of 233
monophosphates, synthesis of 233
purine 426—433
structure-activity relationships 233, 234
substrates and inhibitors of pyrimidine nucleoside deaminase 238, 239
synthesis 232, 233
Arabinosyladenine; adenine arabinoside; 9-β-D-arabinofuranosyladenine; ara-A
antibacterial and antitumor activity 234, 427
antiviral activity 428
chemical structure 426
conversion to nucleotides 427
deaminase: kinase ratio as determinant of sensitivity to 427, 428
inhibition of DNA biosynthesis 241
inhibition of ribonucleoside diphosphate reductase by triphosphate of 243
isolation and synthesis 427
pharmacokinetics in man 428
Arabinosyladenine, radioactivity from in RNA 427
toxicity 428
5′-triphosphate as inhibitor of DNA polymerase 427
Arabinosylcytosine; 1-β-D-arabinofuranosylcytosine; cytosine arabinoside; ara-C 232—256
activity against experimental tumors 235
antagonism by 2′-deoxycytidine 235
synergism with other agents 236
acyl-0-esters, activity and synthesis 233
5′-adamantoate, activity in L 1210 266
antitumor activity 233
administration into the lateral ventricles 238
antagonism by 2′-deoxycytidine 235—237
antiviral effects 237
assay methods for 234, 235
cell cycle phase specificity 235, 236, 249
chromosome aberrations and teratogenesis induced by 261
chromosome damage induced by 236, 237
clinical pharmacology 238, 257—271
effects of dose and schedule on 262, 263
effects on histone synthesis 245, 246
in COAP regimen 263, 264
combination therapy involving 263, 264
combined with BCNU 264
combined with cyclophosphamide 263
combined with 6-mercaptopurine or 6-thioguanine 264
combined with porfiromycin (methylmitomycin C) 264
combined with 6-thioguanine for acute myelogenous leukemia 397
deamination 237—239
inhibitors of 239
deoxycytidine kinase and 240
deoxyribonucleotide pools and 242
effects of dose and schedule on clinical toxicity 261, 262
effects of dose and schedule on pharmacologic findings 262—263
effects on histone synthesis 245, 246
effects of nucleotides on ribonucleoside diphosphate reductase 242, 243
L-enantiomer, synthesis and activity 233
gastrointestinal toxicity 261
genetic and developmental abnormalities induced by 236, 237
half-life of 258
immunosuppressive effects 237
incorporation into nucleic acids 244, 245
incorporation into RNA correlated with acute cell death 245
inhibition of DNA polymerase by triphosphate 243, 244
inhibition of RNA dependent DNA polymerase by triphosphate 243
intramuscular and subcutaneous administration 260
intrathecal administration in man, pharmacokinetics of 260
intravenous administration 257—259

Arabinosylcytosine, intraventricular administration 238
location of incorporated analog in DNA 244, 245
megaloblastosis produced by 236
metabolism 237—239
metabolism and excretion in man 259
5′-monophosphate, activity against L 1210 234
myelosuppression by 260, 261
optimal schedule for acute myeloblastic leukemia 263
oral administration in man 259
3-N-oxide, activity of 234, 267
synthesis 233
5′-palmitate, clinical pharmacology 266
plasma half-life 238
polyamines and 246
pyrimidine nucleoside deaminase and 238, 239
resemblance of cytotoxicity to thymineless death 235
resistance to 246—249
related to intracellular ribonucleotide concentrations 246, 264, 265
relation to kinase : deaminase ratios 247, 265
S-phase dependence of 249
stability during storage 232
stimulation of phosphorylation by uridine 240, 241
5-substituted derivatives, synthesis of 233
synthesis 233
unbalanced growth induced by 261
uptake and phosphorylation 239—241
volume of distribution 257
Arabinosyl-5-fluorocytosine, see also 5-fluorocytosine arabinoside
antitumor activity 198
cytotoxic activity 233
DNA synthesis inhibited by 233, 241
Arabinosyl-5-fluorouracil, activity of 234
Arabinosylguanine 428, 429
activity 234
Arabinosylhypoxanthine 234
Arabinosyl-6-mercaptopurine; 9-β-D-arabinofuranosyl-6-mercaptopurine 429, 430
antitumor activity 234
chemical structure 426
immunosuppressive effects 430
inhibition of DNA biosynthesis 241
inhibition of ribonucleoside diphosphate reductase 429
metabolism and distribution 429
synthesis 429
teratogenic effects 429
Arabinosyl-6-thioguanine 426
Arabinosylthymine, occurrence and synthesis 232
Arabinosyluracil, derivation by metabolism of arabinosylcytosine 237, 238
induction of megaloblastic marrow by 133
occurrence 232
synthesis 233
Aristeromycin 434
L-Asparaginase, L-asparagine amidohydrolase 695—746
amino acid composition 702, 703
amino acid levels in plasma after treatment with 725
amino acid sequence studies 703
anaphylactic reaction to 739
antibody formation and 705—707
antitumor activity 696—698
antiviral activity 696
asparagine synthetase related to resistance to 711
assay of 696, 697
basic aspects 695—722
blood levels 724, 725
central nervous system leukemia and 732
clinical evaluation 723—746
clinical pharmacokinetics 724, 725
clinical toxicity 734—739
combination therapy with 732, 733
combined with glutamine antagonists 501, 514
delayed increase in RNA polymerase of regenerating liver 710
distribution 697
dose and route of administration 725
effects on electrophoretic mobility of lymphocytes 708
effects on lymphocyte blastogenesis 706, 707
effects on serum lipids 737
effects on serum proteins 736, 737
embryotoxicity 710
hematologic changes 737
immunogenicity 705
immunological mechanism for plasma clearance 704, 705
immunosuppression by 526, 705—708, 738
increased RNase levels after treatment 710
increased toxicity of other agents during treatment with 739
inhibition of glycoprotein synthesis 709
inhibition of nucleic acid synthesis 709, 710
inhibition of protein synthesis 709
isolation and purification 698, 699
pharmacological effects 703—705
plasma half-life 704, 705
properties and structure 699, 700, 723, 724
relation of remission to dose and schedule 730—732
resistance 733, 734
serum amino acids during treatment 703
skin grafts and 705, 706
spectrum of tumor response 725—730
stabilization by glycine and polyethylene glycol 702
substrates for 700—702
thymus-derived lymphocytes and 707, 708
toxicity 710

D-Asparagine, as substrate for L-asparaginase 700
L-Asparagine, metabolic fate 708
tumors requiring 695, 723
Asparagine synthetase 711—713
L-asparagine-tRNA as corepressor for 711, 712, 734
derepression of enzyme synthesis 711, 712
increase during development of resistance to L-asparaginase 733, 734
inhibition by glutamine antagonists 491
kinetic properties 712
relation to L-asparaginase sensitivity 711
Aspartate transcarbamylase, androgens and 145
increase levels in cells exposed to 6-azauridine 352
Aspartic acid, antitumor activity 513, 514
Aspartic acid-β-hydrazide, antitumor activity 514, 515
β-Aspartylhydroxamic acid, antitumor activity 514, 515
substrate for L-asparaginase 701
ATP, androgen effects on levels of 151
glucocorticoids and intracellular levels of 93
reduction of mitotic arrest by 674
Avidin, biochemical marker for progesterone activity in the chicken 159
effect of inhibitors on progesterone-induced synthesis of 165
induction of synthesis by 5 α-pregnane-3,20-dione 161
5-Azacytidine 361—364
accumulation of orotidine and orotic acid during treatment with 362
biochemical changes accompanying resistance 363
bone marrow depression by 362
chromosome damage due to 362, 363
clinical use 363, 364
destruction of liver polyribosomes by 363
disturbed formation of bacterial ribosomes 362
effects on RNA synthesis 361, 362
embryotoxic effects 363
incomplete cross-resistance to 5-aza-2′-deoxycytidine 351, 363
incorporation into nucleic acids 362
induction of mouse leukemia by 363
inhibition of β-galactosidase by 361, 362
inhibition of hormonal induction of tryptophan pyrrolase 363
inhibition of processing of 45S to ribosomal RNA 574, 577
mechanism of action 361, 362
synthesis 351
6-Azacytidine 349, 350
6-Azacytosine arabinoside 350
5-Aza-2′-deoxycytidine 351
6-Aza-2′-deoxycytidine 349, 350
8-Azaguanine 384, 458—467
antitumor activity 459
chemical structure 458
coding efficiency of 464
8-Azaguanine
conversion to nucleotides 460, 461
degradation 459, 460
early investigations 458, 459
effects on protein synthesis 463
effects on ribosomes 463, 464
incorporation into nucleic acids 463, 464
intervention in enzyme systems 459—463
nucleic acid metabolism and 462, 463
nucleoside monophosphate as substrate for guanylate kinase 461
nucleoside triphosphate as substrate for important enzyme systems 461, 462
resistance 460, 461
toxicity 459
6-Azapseudouridine 349
Azapyrimidine nucleosides 348—372
with anomalous sugar moieties 350
Azaserine; O-diazoacetyl-L-serine, antagonism by aromatic amino acids 495, 496
chemical structure 485
effects on carbamylphosphate synthetase 489, 490
effects on purine biosynthesis 486, 487
effects on transamination 493
inhibition of amidination of α-N-formylglycinamide ribonucleotide 390, 486—488
inhibition of PRPP amidotransferase 488, 489
inhibitor of xanthosine 5′-phosphate aminase 489
isolation and biological activity 485, 486
mutagenicity of 494
possible inhibition of histidine synthesis 492
synergistic cytotoxic effect with 6-mercaptopurine 391, 397
Azathioprine; 6-[(1-methyl-4-nitro-5-imidazolyl)thio]purine; imuran 404—425
activation of viral infections by 417
aldehyde oxidase action on 412
anti-inflammatory effects 408
antitumor effects in man and mouse 408, 409
biochemical effects due to 6-mercaptopurine released by 404
biochemical effects due to methylnitroimidazole moiety 405
blood levels 413
measurement of rosette inhibitory activity for determining 413, 414
carcinogenesis associated with 417, 418
cell mediated immune reactions suppressed by 407, 408
chemical structure 404
chromosome damage produced by 415
cytotoxicity *in vitro* 405, 406
immunosuppressive effects compared with 6-mercaptopurine 409
infections in patients receiving 416, 417
inhibition of dimethylbenzanthracene-induced tumors 417
inhibition of DNA synthesis in lymphocytes 406

Azathioprine, inhibition of DNA synthesis in regenerating liver 410
inhibition of the mixed lymphocyte reaction 406
inhibition of protein synthesis 405, 406
inhibition of rosette formation 406
metabolism 411—415
effect of gout on 414
effect of renal insufficiency on 414
Lesch-Nyhan syndrome and 414
liver disease and 414
nucleophilic attack on the 5-position of nitroimidazole 411
reaction with sulfhydryl ion 404
selective effect on T-cells 405
suppression of antibody formation by 407
teratogenesis 415, 416
tests for immunological reactivity in patients receiving 416
tissue distribution 411
toxicity in various species 409, 410
urinary metabolites of 411, 412
virally-induced leukemia in mice and 417
6-Azathymidine, biosynthesis of 348, 349
5-Azauridine, decomposition to ribosyl-1-formylbiuret and ribosylbiuret 350
synthesis and activity 351
6-Azauridine 351—361
accumulation of orotidine and orotic acid due to action of 352, 359
antineoplastic effects 355
augmented enzyme levels in cells exposed to 352
biosynthesis 349
clinical use in neoplastic and hyperplastic conditions 360, 361
clinical use in psoriasis 361
clinical use in viral infections 360
combined with uracil mustard 355
distribution 358—360
effects on the central nervous system 358, 359
embryotoxicity 356—358
immunosuppressive effects 356
incorporation into RNA but lack of coding activity 352, 353
increased biosynthesis of UMP in cells exposed to 352
3- and 5-methyl derivatives 349
5′-phosphate esters, biochemical effects of 352
phosphorylation 351, 352
reduction in plasma lipids produced by 356
sequence-dependent interaction with ionizing radiation 355
toxicity 358, 359
virostatic effects 354, 355
6-Azauridine-2′,3′,5′-triacetate, clinical uses 361
distribution and metabolism 358—360
embryotoxicity 357
hyperaminoaciduria during treatment with 361
immunosuppressive effects 356
Aziridine derivatives, mechanism of alkylation by 19
5-Aziridino-2,4-dinitrobenzamide, see CB 1954
Azoprocarbazine 750, 753, 754
Azotomycin; duazomycin B, chemical structure 486
conversion to DON by pronase action 496
immunosuppression by 502, 503

Bacterial cell walls, effects of 5-fluorouracil on 201
Bacteriophage, alkylating agent action on 9—11
5-iodo-2′-deoxyuridine and 305, 306
B-cells 405
BCNU; 1,3-*bis*(2-chloroethyl)-1-nitrosourea
antitumor activity synergistic with arabinosylcytosine 236, 264
carbamoylation of proteins by 73
cell cycle phase specificity 76, 77
chemistry 66—68
combined with arabinosylcytosine 264
DNA nucleotidyltransferase and 74, 75
effects on nicotinamide adenine dinucleotide metabolism 76
effects on nucleic acid and protein synthesis 74
effects on processing of HnRNA 575
interference with processing of 45S to ribosomal RNA 574, 577
metabolism 69
p-Benzoquinone-*bis*(guanylhydrazone) 778, 779
N-Benzylglutamine 497
BFNU; 1,3-*bis*(2-fluoroethyl)-1-nitrosourea 67, 68
BIC; 5-[3,3-*bis*(2-chloroethyl)-1-triazeno] imidazole-4-carboxamide
antitumor activity 548, 549
chemical structure 545
pharmacokinetics 549
5-*Bis*(2-chloroethyl)aminomethyluracil, see uracil mustard
p-[*Bis*(2-chloroethyl)amino]phenylacetylhistidine methyl ester hydrochloride 517
N^2-*Bis*(2-chloroethyl)carbamoyl-L-arginine 516
1,3-*Bis*(2-chloroethyl)-1-nitrosourea 66—68, see also BCNU
5-[3,3-*Bis*(2-chloroethyl)-1-triazeno]imidazole-4-carboxamide, see BIC
Bis-dehydrodoisynolic acid 105
1,2-*Bis*(3,5-dioxopiperazin-1-yl)propane, see ICRF 159
1,3-*Bis*(2-fluoroethyl)-1-nitrosourea; BFNU, chemistry 67, 68
Bis-guanylhydrazones 766—788, see also methylglyoxal-*bis*(guanylhydrazone) and 4,4′-diacetyldiphenylurea-*bis*(guanylhydrazone)
aliphatic derivatives 766—777
structure-activity relationships 768

Bis-guanylhydrazones
aromatic derivatives 777—782
structure-activity relationships 778, 779
comparison between 782
specificity of uptake process 771
N,N-*Bis*(methanesulfonyloxyacetal)-1,10-diaminodecane, spermatogenesis and 37
Bis-thiosemicarbazones, antitumor activity 841—845
metal chelating properties 841, 842
Bladder cancer, methotrexate for 478
Bleomycin 850—876, see also phleomycin
arrest of mitosis without effects on DNA synthesis 859
biological activity 855, 856
cancer chemotherapy with 869—871
composition 851, 852
distribution and excretion 855
inhibition of DNA synthesis 856
physical and spectral properties 852—855
pulmonary fibrosis from 870
reactions with DNA 862—869
cleavage of DNA 868, 869
toxicity 860, 861, 870
transcription and 860
variations in receptivity of target sites 858, 859
Brain tumors, methotrexate for 478
Breast, hormonal control of growth 111
Breast cancer, adrenalectomy for 111, 112
compared with cortisone 184
androgens for 144, 145, 181—183
4-androstene-3β, 17α-diol diacetate for 183
combined 5-fluorouracil, vincristine, methotrexate, cyclophosphamide and prednisone for 221
diethylstilbestrol for 184
dihydrotestosterone for 181
estradiol for 184
estrogens for 183, 184
in postmenopausal women 112
estrogen receptor proteins and 117, 118
9α-fluoro-glucocorticoids for 185
9α-fluoro-11-keto-17α-methyltestosterone for 183
5-fluorouracil for 220
glucocorticoids for 176
glucose-6-phosphate dehydrogenase to α-glycerophosphate dehydrogenase ratios and hormone dependence 112
hormonal dependence of induction by carcinogens 112
metabolism of estrogens in patients with 177—179
methotrexate for 477
17α-methyltestosterone for 182
19-nor-testosterone derivatives for 182
progestational steroids for 185, 186
role of estrogens in 111, 112
synthesis of steroid hormones by 178, 179
Δ^1-testololactone for 183
testosterone for 181
urinary estriol in relation to 178
Breast cancer, urinary etiocholanolone and testosterone metabolites in responsive patients 179
5-Bromo-2′-deoxycytidine 5′-triphosphate, allosteric activation and inhibition of thymidine kinase 286, 287
5-Bromo-2′-deoxyuridine, see also halogenated pyrimidine deoxyribonucleosides
abnormal viral particles formed in presence of 304
adenine-bromouracil rich regions of DNA and activity of RNA polymerase 325, 326
biochemical effects 301, 302
cells tolerant to in culture 299
chromosome abnormalities produced by 300
hydrolytic degradation 275, 276
immunosuppression by 309, 310
inhibition of vital replication 302—307
interaction with oncogenic viruses 307, 308
pK_a of 278
preferential induction of thymine to cytosine and adenine to guanine transitions 297
radiosensitization by 319
selective inhibition of some embryonic processes, theories of 312, 313
sensitivity of cloning during the course of the S-phase 299
sensitization of P815Y to dimethylbusulfan 41
synthesis 272, 273
toxicity in embryonic development at the histological and biochemical levels 310—312
6α-Bromo-17β-hydroxy-17α-methyl-4-oxa-5α-androstan-3-one, antiandrogenic and antipituitary gonadotrophin activity 146
Bromoketoprogesterone, breast cancer and 185
5-Bromouracil, mispairing of in DNA 296, 297
mutagenic effects on bacteriophage 295—297
photochemistry of 321, 322
Busulfan; myleran, antitumor effects 35
chemical structure 36
effects on bacteriophage 10, 11
hemopoietic effects 37, 38
immunosuppression by 38
metabolism and distribution 39, 40
miscellaneous toxic effects 39
mutagenic effects 41
reaction with DNA 41
spermatogenesis and 37
teratogenic effects 38, 39
tritiated, synthesis of 40

Calcium metabolism, estrogens and 113
Camptothecin 649—656
antitumor activity 650, 651
antiviral activity 654

Camptothecin
chemical structure 649
induction of single-strand breaks in DNA 653
inhibition of nucleic acid synthesis 651 to 654
lactol 649, 654
mechanism of action 654
methyl amide 649, 654
pharmacokinetics 650
preferential inhibition of precursor ribosomal RNA synthesis 573, 574, 577
premature termination of HnRNA transcription 574—576
specificity for ribosomal RNA synthesis 651—653
structure-activity relationships 654
synthesis 649, 650
toxicity 650, 651
L-Canaline 516
L-Canavanine; 2-amino-4-guanidinoxybutyric acid, antitumor activity 515, 516
conversion to toxic L-canaline 516
Carbamoylation 72, 73
S-Carbamyl-L-cysteine, activity of 497, 498
chemical structure 485
Carbamylphosphate synthetase, inhibition by glutamine antagonists 489, 490
O-Carbamyl-L-serine, chemical structure 485
effect on carbamylphosphate synthetase 489, 490
synthesis and activity of 497
O-Carbazyl-L-serine 497
chemical structure 485
Carbenium ions, see carbonium ions
Carbobenzoxy-L-aspartate, antitumor activity 514
Carbobenzoxy-L-phenylalanine, antitumor activity 520
Carbohydrate metabolism, abnormalities associated with fertility problems or abortion 122
estrogens and 122—125
Carbonium ions 1—3
production from nitrosoureas 67, 68
5-Carboxyuracil, derivation from trifluorothymine 198, 202
Carcinogenesis, actinomycin D and 589
after azathioprine therapy 417, 418
procarbazine and 752
Carcinoid syndrome 519
Castration, biological changes induced by 143—145
elevated urinary 17-ketosteroids after 176
enzyme changes induced by 148, 151, 152
inhibition of mammary tumor growth mediated by reduced prolactin 174
Catharanthine 671, 672
CB 1954; 5-aziridino-2,4-dinitrobenzamide, action on protein and nucleic acid synthesis 26
CCNU; 1-(2-chloroethyl)-3-cyclohexyl-1-nitrosourea
alkylation of nucleic acids and proteins by 70
CCNU
carbamoylation of proteins by 72, 73
cell cycle phase specificity 76, 77
chemistry 67, 68
DNA nucleotidyltransferase and 74, 75
interference with processing of 45S to ribosomal RNA 574
metabolism 69
selective inhibition of precursor ribosomal RNA synthesis 573, 577
Cell cycle kinetics, alkylating agents and 20—22
problems in reutilization of labeled markers 314—316
thymidine and 5-iodo-2′-deoxyuridine as markers, advantages and disadvantages 314—318
Cellular immunity, L-asparaginase and 705, 706
suppression by azathioprine and 6-mercaptopurine 407, 408
Cephalotaxine 556, 557
Charge transfer bonds, and activation of thymidine kinase by 5-iodo-2′-deoxyuridine triphosphate 286
Chinese hamster cells, repair of damaged DNA in 14
sensitivity to alkylating agents compared to HeLa cells 77, 78
Chlorambucil, action at cell surface 28
Chlormadinone acetate; 6-chloro-1,4,6-pregnatrien-17α-ol-3,20-dione acetate, antiandrogenic activity 146
2-Chloro-4′4″-*bis*(2-imidazolin-2-yl)terephthalanilide, chemical structure 778, 821
effects of combinations with halogenated nucleosides on mouse tumors 300
inhibition of *bis*(guanylhydrazone) uptake 781
toxicity 820, 822
5-Chloro-2′-deoxyuridine, pK_a of 278
synthesis 272
teratogenic effects 310
2-Chloroethylamine derivatives, antineoplastic effects 22, 23
effects on hematopoietic tissue 23
effects on immune response 24
effects on spermatogenesis 23, 24
long-term effects 22
mechanism of action at a cellular level 20—24
mechanism of action at the macromolecular level 24—29
enzymes and coenzymes 25
nucleic acids 25—29
mechanism of alkylation by 19, 20
1-(2-Chloroethyl)-3-cyclohexyl-1-nitrosourea 67, 68, see also CCNU
β-Chloroethyl diethylamine 2
p-Chlorophenylalanine, inhibition of tryptophan hydroxylase and use in the carcinoid syndrome 519
1-(o-Chlorophenyl)-1-(p-chlorophenyl)-2,2-dichloroethane, see o,p′-DDD

Chlorotrianisene; TACE, chemical structure 105
prostatic cancer and 180
Chlorouracil, photochemistry 321
Cholesterol, estrogen effects on blood levels 109
Choriocarcinoma, actinomycin D for 589
methotrexate for 476
Chromomycin A_3 615—622
antitumor activity 618, 619
blood levels 620
chemical structure 615
cross-resistance to olivomycin and mithramycin 616
inhibition of RNA polymerase 626
mode of complex formation with DNA 617
toxicity 619, 620
Chromomycinone, aglycone of chromomycin A and mithramycin 616
Chromosome damage, arabinosylcytosine and 236, 237, 261
5-azacytidine and 362, 363
azathioprine and 415
5-bromo-2′-deoxyuridine and 300
daunorubicin and 594—597
fluorinated pyrimidines and 200
phleomycin and 863—866
Chronic lymphocytic leukemia, L-asparaginase for 727, 729
streptonigrin for 639
Chronic myelocytic leukemia, L-asparaginase for 726, 727, 729
busulfan for 35
dimethylbusulfan for 36
hydroxyurea for 789
streptonigrin for 639
Cinerubin, effects on DNA polymerase 602, 603
Cis-dichlorodiammineplatinum (II); *cis*-Pt 830—839
chemical structure 830
clinical trials 838, 839
comparison with *cis*-dichloro(dipyridine)-platinum (II) 835
distribution in mice 832
effects on bone marrow 836
effects on properties and conformation of DNA and reaction with bases 837, 838
immunosuppressive effects 832, 833, 836, 837
inhibition of biosynthesis of macromolecules 833, 834
toxicity 831, 832, 838
tumor-inhibitory activity 830, 831
Cis-dichloro(dipyridine)platinum (II), comparison with *cis*-Pt 835
complex formation with biomolecules 835
distribution and excretion 835, 836
transport and binding by cells 838
Citrovorum factor; N^5-formyltetrahydrofolic acid; leukovorin
methotrexate transport and 471, 472
Clinical evaluation, criteria for rating response 740—742
Clomiphene 105
blockade of estrogen binding by 114
CN-55945-27, antiestrogenic action and chemical structure 110, 111
COAP regimen 263, 264
Coding and translational errors due to 5-fluorouracil 213—215
Coformycin, inhibitor of adenosine deaminase 444
Colcemid; deacetyl-N-methylcolchicine; demecolcine
chemical structure 672
effects on DNA synthesis 679
reversible dissolution of meiotic spindle 674
Colchicinamide derivatives 672, 673
Colchicine 670—694, see also colcemid
anti-inflammatory action 675
antitumor effects 675
binding to DNA 681
binding by microtubule protein 677—679
chemical structure 672
deacetylamino derivative, structure 672
disappearance of microtubules from cells exposed to 676
effects on respiration and phagocytosis in leukocytes 682, 683
effects on RNA synthesis 680
effects on sympathetic nerves 683
inhibition of DNA synthesis 679, 680
interference with motility, chemotaxis and phagocytosis 675
metabolism and distribution 684
mitotic arrest by 673, 674
neurological toxicity 675
source and history 670
structure-activity relationships 672, 673
Colchicine binding protein, see microtubule system
Colchicum 670
Colicinogenic factors 58
Combination therapy, see under individual drugs
Cordycepin; 3′-deoxyadenosine 435, 657—669
3′-acetamido derivative 661
antitrypanosomal effects 660
chemical structure 657
deamination and phosphorylation 658, 659
differential inhibition of synthesis of RNA fractions 663, 664
effects of phosphorylated derivatives on enzymes 659, 660
incorporation into nucleic acids 664
inhibition of cell growth 660
inhibition of formation of poly(A) termination of HnRNA 575
inhibition of mitochondrial transcription by 577
mitotic and chromosomal effects 662
N_1-oxide, inhibitory effects 661
selective inhibition of precursor ribosomal RNA synthesis 573, 574
synthesis and isolation 658

Cordycepin
  uptake and metabolism 662, 663
Cortical stromal hyperplasia, association with endometrial cancer 174, 175
Corticosterone, distribution of 96
Cortisol, changes in nucleic acid precursor pools induced by 87, 90
  depressed secretion during o,p'-DDD treatment 811, 812
  distribution of 96
  DNA synthesis and 87, 88
  effects on macromolecular synthesis in thymocytes 175, 176
  hexose transport and 93
  thymidine transport and 87
Cortisone, antagonism of colchicine action 674
  breast cancer and 184
  prostatic cancer and 180
  toxicity 185
Cross-resistance of methanesulfonates and radiation 41
Cushing's disease, o,p'-DDD for 814
L-β-Cyanoalanine, substrate and inhibitor of L-asparaginase 701
5-Cyanouracil, inhibitor of dihydrouracil dehydrogenase 290
Cyclic-3',5'-AMP, mediation of gonadotropin effects by 140
  production of testosterone-like enzyme increases 152
2,2'-O-Cyclocytidine, activity of 234, 266, 267
  antitumor activity, chemistry and clinical trial 887
  synthesis 233, 886
Cycloheximide, acetoxy derivative 561, 563
  antagonism of androgen-induced enzyme changes 152
  biological activity and toxicity 561
  changes accompanying resistance to 561
  chemical structure 558
  effects on RNA synthesis 563, 564
  inhibition of estrogen-induced changes in glucose-6-phosphate dehydrogenase 124
  inhibition of progesterone-induced avidin synthesis 165
  mechanism of action 561
  structure-activity relationships of derivatives 562
  topological similarities to emetine and the ipecac alkaloids 562, 563
Cyclophosphamide; cytoxan; endoxan, see also alkylating agents
  activation 29
  combined with arabinosylcytosine 263
  combined with vincristine, 5-fluorouracil, methotrexate and prednisone for breast cancer 221
  immunosuppression by 24
  metabolism 29
Cyproterone acetate; 6-chloro-1α,2α-methylene-4,6-pregnadien-17α-ol-3,20-dione acetate, antiandrogenic activity 146
Cyproterone acetate; competition for androgen binding sites 149, 150
Cysteine, potentiation of immunosuppression by busulfan 38
Cytarabine, see arabinosylcytosine
Cytidine deaminase, see pyrimidine nucleoside deaminase
Cytosar, see arabinosylcytosine
Cytosine, alkylation of by nitrosoureas 71
  selective alkylation by mitomycins 49—51
Cytotoxic amino acid analogs 512—538
  aromatic amino acid derivatives 519—521
  aspartic acid and asparagine analogs 513—515
  basic amino acids 515—518
  immunosuppression by 525—528
  sulfur-containing amino acids 521—523
Cytotoxic inhibitors of protein synthesis 554—570
  classification 554—556
Cytotoxic pyridine nucleotide analogs 539—543
Cytoxan, see cyclophosphamide

Daunorubicin; daunomycin; rubidomycin 593—614
  N-acetyl derivative, activity of 605
  actions during cell cycle 604, 605
  aglycone 593, 610
  antitumor activity 597
  antiviral activity 606—608
  carcinomas induced by 610
  chemistry 593, 594
  complex with DNA 598—602
  cross-resistance to other agents 606
  13-dehydro derivative 593
  effects on nucleic acid synthesis 601—605
  excretion 608, 609
  increased thymidine kinase and dCMP deaminase after treatment with 603
  inhibition of DNA polymerase 602, 603
  inhibition of RNA dependent DNA polymerase 608
  inhibition of RNA polymerase 602, 626
  interaction with A-T base pairs 602
  mechanism of action and biochemical effects 597—605
  metabolism 608—610
  mitotic and nuclear effects of 594—597
  pharmacological disposition 608, 609
  photodynamic inactivation of viruses 608
  selective inhibition of precursor ribosomal RNA synthesis 573, 577
  toxicity 609, 610
  uptake 599—601, 605
Daunorubicinol; 13-dihydrodaunorubicin
  aglycone 610
  chemical structure 610
  cytotoxic activity 609
  metabolite of daunorubicin 609, 610
Daunosaminyl-daunomycin 593
o,p'-DDD; 1-(o-chlorophenyl)-1-(p-chlorophenyl)-2,2-dichloroethane 808—819
  absorption 809
  chemical structure of analogs 808, 809

o,p'-DDD; clinical studies with 814—817
distribution 809
effects on drug metabolism 813, 814
effects on steroid metabolism 813
effects on steroid production 811, 812
effects on thyroxine binding globulin 814
enzyme induction by 813, 814
histologic and ultrastructural changes induced in adrenocortical tissue 810, 811
mechanism of adrenocorticolytic action 812, 813
metabolism and excretion 810
mitochondrial effects 812
reduced barbiturate metabolism during treatment with 814
toxicity 817
DDT; 1,1-*bis*(p-chlorophenyl)-2,2,2-trichloroethane 808
DDUG, see 4,4'-diacetyldiphenylurea-*bis*-(guanylhydrazone)
Deacetyl-N-methylcolchicine, see colcemid
7-Deazaadenosine, see tubercidin
7-Deazainosine; 4-hydroxy-7-(β-D-ribofuranosyl)-7H-pyrrolo[2,3-d]pyrimidine
chemical structure 442
formation of monophosphate by deamination of tubercidin 5'-phosphate 444
need for activation by phosphorylation and amination 445
primary distribution in plasma 445
Decoyinine; 6-amino-9-(β-D-5,6-psicofuranoseenyl)purine; angustmycin A
biological and biochemical effects 449
chemical structure 447
isolation 446, 447
Dehydroepiandrosterone, chemical structure 141
conversion to estrogens 106, 107
2',3'-Dehydro-5-fluoro-2'-deoxyuridine 196
Delalutin, see 17 α-hydroxyprogesterone caproate
Demecolcine, see colcemid
4'-Demethylepipodophyllotoxin thenylidene glucoside, see VM-26
3'-Deoxyadenosine 657—659, see also cordycepin
5'-Deoxyarabinosylcytosine, synthesis 233
3'-Deoxy-3'-chlorothymidine 661
Deoxycorticosterone, glucose oxidation and 91
2'-Deoxycytidine, antagonist of uptake and phosphorylation of arabinosylcytosine 235—237, 240
3'-Deoxycytidine, selective inhibition of precursor ribosomal RNA synthesis 573, 574, 577
Deoxycytidine kinase, decreased levels in resistance to 5-azacytidine 363
properties of and action on arabinosylcytosine 240, 241
reduced levels in 5-aza-2'-deoxycytidine resistant cells 351
reduced levels in cells resistant to arabinosylcytosine 246, 247
Deoxycytidine kinase, UTP as phosphate donor for arabinosylcytosine 240, 241, 267
Deoxycytidylate deaminase, activation by 6-aza-2'-deoxycytidine 350
dCTP interactions with 287
inhibition by 5-iodo-2'-deoxyuridine 5'-triphosphate 287, 288
3'-Deoxy-3'-fluorothymidine 661, 662
3'-Deoxyinosine, inhibitory effects of 661
7-Deoxynogalarol, DNA binding specificity 630
inhibition of growth and macromolecular synthesis 625
structure 624
4-Deoxypyridoxine, antitumor activity 515, 519
Deoxyribonuclease; DNase, cortisol-induced increase in 94
inhibition by nogalomycin 629
Deoxyribonucleotide pools 242
$\alpha(\beta)$-2'-Deoxythioguanosine, antitumor activity 396
delayed cytotoxicity 396
isolation from DNA of 6-mercaptopurine-treated cells 390, 392
phosphorylation and incorporation into DNA 388
2'-Deoxyuridine, pK_a of 278
α-Desoxycamptothecin 649, 654
Desoxycorticosterone acetate, DNA metabolism and 88
4,4'-Diacetyldiphenylurea-*bis*(guanylhydrazone); DDUG 777—782
antitumor activity 777, 778
combined with other agents 779, 780
comparison with methyl-GAG 782
disposition and cellular uptake 780, 781
effects of terephthalanilides on 781
mechanism of action 781, 782
toxicity 780
1,4-Dialdehydobenzene-*bis*(guanylhydrazone) 778, 779
2,6-Diaminopurine 384
N-Diazoacetylglycine, antitumor and immunosuppressive action 527
O-Diazoacetyl-L-serine, see azaserine
5-Diazoimidazole-4-carboxamide; DZC, activity and photochemical formation from DIC 544, 545
reactivity of 547, 548
Diazomethane, selectivity for DNA bases 5
6-Diazo-5-oxo-L-norleucine, see DON
5-Diazo-4-oxo-L-norvaline; DONV, antitumor activity 514, 515
binding to asparaginase 699
reaction with L-asparaginase 701
5-Diazouracil, inhibitor of pyrimidine dehalogenation 290
DIC; 5-(3,3-dimethyl-1-triazeno)imidazole-4-carboxamide
absorption, distribution and excretion 546
antitumor activity, clinical and preclinical 545, 546

DIC; chemistry 544, 545
cross-resistance to alkylating agents 79
effects on xanthine oxidase 547
formation of methyl carbonium ion from 547
metabolism and decomposition 547, 548
photochemical decomposition to DZC 545
prolongation of G_2 period by 546
toxicity 546
N-Dichloroacetyl-DL-serine, antitumor activity 524, 525
Di-(2-chloroethyl)sulfide, see sulfur mustard
Dichloromethotrexate, chemical structure 468
excretion 473
for head and neck cancer and hepatomas 478
2',3'-Dideoxyribonucleosides 662
Diepoxybutane, derivation from L-threitol-1,4-dimethane sulfonate 42
Diethylstilbestrol, breast cancer and 184
chemical structure 105
glycogen synthetase and 125
influence of cycloheximide 125
in prostatic cancer 179, 180
reduction of vinblastine toxicity by 674
serine-specific transfer RNA and 121
Dihydrofolate reductase, arabinosylcytosine and 246
interaction with folate antagonists 468, 469
two forms in mammalian tissues 469
5α-Dihydrotestosterone, breast cancer and 181
effects on urinary steroids and gonadotrophin 181
formation from testoterone 149
specific binding in prostate tissue 177
Dihydrouracil dehydrogenase, 5-cyanouracil as inhibitor of 290
Dimethyl busulfan 36
activity in cell culture systems 40, 41
hematopoietic effects 38
7,12-Dimethylbenzanthracene, hormone dependence of carcinogenesis induced by 112
Dimethylethylallenoic acid 105
Dimethylnitrosamine, alkylation of amino acids and protein by 72
alkylation of nucleic acids by *in vitro* 71
3,4-Dimethylpyrazolo(3,2-c)-*as*-triazine, histidine antagonist with antitumor activity 517
Dimethylstilbestrol, antiestrogenic effects 110
5-(3,3-Dimethyl-1-triazeno)imidazole-4-carboxamide, see DIC
4,4'-Diphenyl-*bis*(guanylhydrazone) 778, 779
Diphtheria toxin, cardiotoxicity and inhibition of protein synthesis 561
Divinyl sulfone, alkylating action 5
DNA, alkylation 6—9, 26, 27, 29, 30
alkylation by nitrosoureas 70, 71
binding of actinomycin D 528, 584—589
DNA, binding of adriamycin 599
binding of anthramycin 644—646
binding of *bis*(guanylhydrazones) 776, 781, 782
binding of daunorubicin 598—602
binding of streptonigrin 636, 637
bridges formed across diester bonds by bleomycin and phleomycin 869
5-bromouracil substituted, radiation-induced loss of bromine 319, 320
retention of transforming activity 308, 309
complex formation with olivomycin, mithramycin and chromomycin 616, 617
degradation produced by streptonigrin 634
denaturation of, effect of incorporated halogenated pyrimidines on heat sensitivity 294
reduction in needed pH with halogen substitution 294
increased density of material containing halogenated bases 292
induction of single-strand breaks by camptothecin 653
interaction with *cis*-dichlorodiammineplatinum(II) 837
intercalation by hycanthone 880
interstrand crosslinks in 8, 41
mitomycins and 48—50
lability of material with halogenated bases 292
melting temperature (T_m), effect of halogenated bases on 292—294
mitochondrial, alkylation by nitrosoureas 70
photochemistry of halogenated pyrimidine containing 319—322
reactions of bleomycin and phleomycin with 862—869
repair of mitomycin-induced damage 52, 53
template capacity after alkylation 14, 15
template capacity after androgen treatment 148
DNA polymerase; DNA nucleotidyltransferase
altered properties in cells resistant to arabinosylcytosine 247
arabinosylcytosine and 243, 244
arabinosylcytosine triphosphate as substrate for 244, 245
cinerubin and 602, 603
4,4'-diacetyldiphenylurea-*bis*(guanylhydrazone) and 781
equivalent utilization of triphosphates of thymidine and 5-iodo-2'-deoxyuridine 281, 282
5-fluoro-2'-deoxyuridine triphosphate as substrate for 277
increased levels in resistance to 5-azacytidine 363
inhibition by anthramycin 643

DNA polymerase; inhibition by arabinosyladenine triphosphate 427
inhibition by daunorubicin 602, 603
inhibition by 2′,3′-dideoxyadenosine triphosphate 659, 660
inhibition by 5-iodo-2′-deoxyuridine 301
inhibition by nogalamycin 628, 629
inhibition by phleomycin 856, 857
inhibition by rifamycin SV and derivatives 883
methylglyoxal-*bis*(guanylhydrazone) and 776
nitrosoureas and 74, 75
RNA dependent, inhibition by adriamycin and daunorubicin 608
inhibition by arabinosylcytosine triphosphate 243
inhibition by 2′,3′-dideoxythymidine triphosphate 660
utilization of 5-iodo-2′-deoxyuridine triphosphate 285

DNA repair 11—14
insensitivity of repair enzyme polymerase I to arabinosylcytosine 243
mitomycin-induced damage and 52, 53
steps involved in 12

DNA synthesis, activation by 6-aza-2′-deoxycytidine 350
alkylating agents and 25, 26
effects of camptothecin 651, 653
effects of colchicine and the vinca alkaloids 679—681
effects of glucocorticoids 86—88
effects of nitrosoureas 73—75
effects of VM-26 681
estrogens and 118
in murine tumors treated with arabinosyladenine 428
inhibition by anisomycin 565
inhibition by arabinosylcytosine 241, 242
inhibition by 5-aza-2′deoxycytidine 351
inhibition by azathioprine 410
inhibition by fluorinated pyrimidines 230, 204
inhibition by heterocyclic carboxaldehyde thiosemicarbazones 802
inhibition by hycanthone 880
inhibition by hydroxyurea 790, 791
inhibition by ICRF 159 885
inhibition by mycophenolic acid 450
inhibition by nogalamycin and derivatives 624, 625
inhibition by phleomycin and bleomycin 856—858
mitomycin and 53
procarbazine and 756, 757
relative sensitivity of different species to arabinosylcytosine 241, 242
selective sensitivity to platinum compounds 833—835

DNA viruses, fluorinated pyrimidines and 199, 200

DON; 6-diazo-5-oxo-L-norleucine, chemical structure 485

DON; effect on carbamylphosphate synthetase 489, 490
inhibition of amidination of formylglycinamide ribonucleotide 486—488
inhibition of conversion of uridine to cytidine nucleotides 490
inhibition of glucosamine synthesis 491
inhibition of PRPP amidotransferase 488, 489
inhibition of xanthosine 5′-phosphate aminase 489
isolation and biological activity 485, 486
synergistic cytotoxic effect with 6-mercaptopurine 391

Dromostanolone, see 2α-methyldihydrotestosterone

Drosophila, mutagenesis by halogenated analogs 297

Duazomycin A; N-acetyl-DON, chemical structure 486
conversion to DON by acylase action 496

Durabolin; 4-estren-17β-ol-3-one phenylpropionate, anabolic androgen 142

Echinomycin, inhibition of RNA polymerase 626

Ehrlich ascites carcinoma, incorporation of 5-fluorouracil into RNA of 207, 208
inhibition by arabinosyl-6-mercaptopurine 234
repair of damaged DNA in 14

Efudex, topical 5-fluorouracil 221

Ellipticine, active and inactive analogs 881
chemical structure, activity and source 881
distribution and excretion 881, 882
effect on nucleic acid synthesis 881
preferential inhibition of percursor ribosomal RNA synthesis 573, 577

Embryo toxicity, 5-azacytidine 363
6-azauridine 356—358

Emetine, basis of toxicity 560, 561
chemical structure and biological activity 558, 559
effect on RNA synthesis 560
mechanism of action 559, 560
structure-activity relationship of derivatives 560

Endoxan, see cyclophosphamide

Enzyme induction, blockade by 5-bromo-2′-deoxyuridine 312

Enzyme synthesis, inhibition by mitomycins 56

Epianthramycin 642, 642

Epidermoid cancers, bleomycin for 870

Epoxides, mechanism of alkylation by 19

Esophageal cancer, methylglyoxal-*bis*(guanylhydrazone) for 773

Estradiol, binding of 113—117, see also estrogens
biosynthesis 106—108
breast cancer and 184
chemical structure 104, 105
effects on glucose transport 93

Estradiol, effects on macromolecular synthesis 118—120
  glucose-6-phosphate dehydrogenase levels and 122, 123
  glucose phosphate isomerase levels and 123
  increased glucose metabolism induced by 124
  increased hexokinase and phosphofructokinase induced by 124
  increased pyruvate kinase induced by 124, 125
  metabolism of in men and women with breast cancer 178
Estriol, chemical structure 105
  urinary levels in relation to breast cancer 178
Estrogen, see also diethylstilbestrol, estradiol, estriol and estrone
  actions on accessory sex organs 108
  antagonists 109—111
  antiandrogenic effect 172, 173
  bioassay 108
  biochemical basis of action 113—125
  biosynthesis 106—108
  biphasic effects on breast cancer 174, 183
  body growth and 113
  calcium metabolism and 113
  carbohydrate metabolism and 122—125
  chemical structures 104—106
  cholesterol biosynthesis and 109
  dependence on folate for full effects 110
  direct effects on mammary gland epithelium 176
  effects on breast cancer in postmenopausal women 112
  effects on chicken oviduct 121
  effects on macromolecular synthesis 118—121
  effects on prolactin levels 174
  effects on uterine chromatin template capacity 119, 120
  follicle-stimulating hormone levels and 109
  formation from androgens 106, 107
  glucose phosphate isomerase levels and 123
  glycogen synthetase and 125
  hexokinase and phosphofructokinase levels and 124
  induction of renal cell cancer by 175
  induction of serum vitellogenic changes by 120, 121
  induction of specific acidic proteins by 120
  inhibition of hypothalamic prolactin inhibitory factor by 174
  interaction with target cells 115, 116
  interconversions of 107, 108
  levels of glucose-6-phosphate dehydrogenase and 122—124
    isozyme responses in mammary tumors 124
    regulatory role of NADP 124
    related to response of mammary tumors 123
  levels of NADP-malate and isocitrate dehydrogenases 122, 123
  luteinizing hormone levels and 108, 109
  mechanism of action 104—138
  metabolism of in women with breast cancer 177—179
  prostatic acid phosphatase and 172
  prostatic cancer and 113
  pyruvate kinase and 124, 125
  resistance to and steroid receptors 99
  role in breast cancer 111, 112
  role in breast development 111
  serine specific transfer RNA and 121
  specific binding proteins 113—118
  stimulation of chick oviduct growth 159
  stimulation of processing of precursor RNA 120
  synthesis 105, 106
  theca interna cells as source 106, 107
Estrogen receptor proteins 95, 96, 113—118, 176, 177
  blockade of estrogen binding sites by antiestrogens 114
  nucleo-cytoplasmic transfers 115, 116
  relation to breast cancer 117, 118
  relationship to therapeutic response in breast cancer 117, 118
  sedimentation characteristics 114, 115
  stimulation of RNA synthesis by steroid-protein complex 96
  tissue concentrations 115—117
  transfer of complex to nucleus 95
Estrone, biosynthesis 106
  chemical structure 105
  isolation of and induction of mammary cancer by 170
Ethamoxytriphetol; MER-25, antagonism of estrogen binding by 95, 114
  antiestrogenic effects 110
  chemical structure 111
  prevention of estrogen-induced enzyme elevations 123
Ethidium bromide, inhibition of mitochondrial RNA synthesis 577
  inhibition of RNA polymerase 626
Ethionine, biological activity 521, 522
3-Ethoxy-2-oxobutyraldehyde-*bis*(thiosemicarbazone) metal chelates; KTS chelates 841—849
  antineoplastic activity 842, 843
    relation to metal chelation 843—845
  effects of copper chelate on energy transport systems 847
  inhibition of biosynthetic pathways 846, 847
  kinetics of chelation 845
  mechanism of action 845—847
  reaction of copper chelates 846
  role as delivery system for metal ions 847
Ethyl α-acetamido-α-cyano-β-(3,5-dimethyl-4-methoxyphenyl) propionate
  antitumor activity 520
Ethyl methanesulfonate, effects on bacteriophage 9—11
3-Ethylcytosine, base-pairing properties 15

Ethylene dibromide, metabolism 40
Ethylene dimethanesulfonate, antitumor effects 35
chemical structure 36
hemopoietic effects 38
metabolism 40
spermatogenesis and 37
Ethyleneimine derivatives, mechanism of alkylation by 19
1-Ethyl-1-nitrosourea; ENU, alkylation of nucleic acids by 70
teratogenic effects 78
O-Ethyl-L-threonine, effects on MAREK'S disease 524
Experimental allergic encephalomyelitis, azathioprine and 408

Feminizing ovarian neoplasms, association with endometrial cancer 175
Fetuin, glycoprotein substrate for L-asparaginase 701
Fish scale homografts, assay system for immunosuppressive action of amino acid analogs 527
Fluorinated pyrimidines and their nucleosides 193—231, see also individual agents
antifungal activity 201
antiviral activity 199, 200
base-pairing of 197
cleavage of the nucleosides 203
clinical pharmacology 221—223
clinical use 219—221
effects on enzyme induction 212, 213
effects on protein synthesis 211
genetic, mutagenic and teratogenic activities 200
inhibition of cells in culture 199
inhibition of DNA synthesis 203, 204
inhibition of experimental tumors 188, 199
inhibition of RNA synthesis 205, 206
physical, chemical and conformational properties 197, 198
rationale 193—195
synthesis 195—197
5-Fluorocytosine, chemical structure and synthesis 195
arabinoside, see also arabinosyl-5-fluorocytosine
chemical structure 195
synthesis 196
clinical use 219
deamination as necessary step for inhibition of yeast growth 210
fungal infections and 194, 201
5-Fluoro-2′-deoxycytidine, chemical structure and synthesis 195, 196
5-Fluoro-2′-deoxyuridine; FUdR
antiviral activity 199
chemical structure and synthesis 195, 196
chromosome breaks induced by 200
clinical pharmacology 221, 222
clinical use 219—221
conformation 197
5-Fluoro-2′-deoxyuridine;
deletion of thymidine kinase in cells resistant to 217
DNA synthesis inhibited by 203, 204
immunosuppression by 201
inhibition of transplantable tumors by 198
photoreactivity of 321
pK_a of 278
5′-triphosphate, inhibitor of thymidine kinase 286
substrate for DNA polymerase 277
5-Fluoroorotic acid, chemical structure and synthesis 195, 196
DNA synthesis inhibited by 203, 204
increased activity of cortisol-induced tyrosine aminotransferase 213
inhibition of induction of rat liver threonine dehydratase, histidase, and tryptophan oxidase 213
inhibition of ribosomal maturation 213
selective incorporation into ribosomal RNA 210
4-Fluorophenylalanine, activity of 519
9 α-Fluoroprednisolone, RNA synthesis and 90
5-Fluoropyrimidine-2-one-2′-deoxyribonucleoside 196
5-Fluoro-4-pyrimidinol 196
5-Fluorouracil; 5-FU, action on bacterial cell wall 201
breast cancer and 220
chemical structure, pKa and ultraviolet absorbance 194, 195
clinical pharmacology 221, 222
clinical use 219—221
coding properties 213, 214
combined with DIC 198
combined with methotrexate 198
combined with vincristine, methotrexate, cyclophosphamide and prednisone for breast cancer 221
conversion to deoxyribonucleotides 203
conversion to 5-fluoro-5-hydroxy-5,6-dihydrouracil by ultraviolet light 198
conversion to ribonucleotides and incorporation into RNA 202
cycle specificity 217, 218
distribution and metabolism in man 221, 222
distribution and metabolism in mice 219
DNA synthesis inhibited by 203, 204
effects on properties of induced alkaline phosphatase 212
enzymes involved in activation 216, 217
errors of base-pairing in RNA 208
immunosuppression by 201
incorporation into messenger RNA 210, 211
incorporation into nucleic acid as index of sensitivity 217
incorporation into phage DNA 204, 205
incorporation into ribosomal RNA 210
incorporation into RNA 207—211
incorporation into transfer RNA 209, 210

5-Fluorouracil;
incorporation into viral RNA 208, 209
induction of β-galactosidase inhibited by 212
inhibition of serine dehydratase induction 212
inhibition of transplantable tumors 198, 199
mechanism of resistance 217
metabolic degradation 202
mutagenic activity in RNA viruses 200
oral administration for hepatic metastases 220, 221
photochemistry 321
physical properties 197
plasma half-time 222
preclinical pharmacology 219
properties of phage RNA containing 209
resistance related to lack of inhibition of thymidylate synthetase 204
reversal of inhibition of DNA synthesis in the presence of BUdR 298
ribosomes synthesized after treatment with 206, 207
RNA synthesis inhibited by 205, 206
role of catabolism in chemotherapeutic activity 215, 216
stimulation of constitutive enzyme synthesis in *E. coli* 212
synergism with x-ray in inhibition of mouse lymphoma 198, 199
synthesis 195, 196
topical administration for keratoses and superficial skin cancers 221
toxicity 219, 220
translational errors produced by 214, 215
6-Fluorouracil 195
5-Fluorouridine, chemical structure and synthesis 195
correlation of uridine phosphorylase with cytotoxicity 217
DNA synthesis inhibited by 203, 204
inhibition of processing of 45S to ribosomal RNA 574, 577
5-Fluorouridylate, inhibition of thymidylate synthetase 204
Fluoxidine 196
Fluoxymesterone 142
remissions in breast cancer induced by 173
remissions in hypophysectomized cancer patients 144
therapeutic efficacy and toxicity 182
Folate antagonists 468—483, see also methotrexate, dichloromethotrexate
absorption and transport 471
clinical uses 475—479
distribution 472
excretion 473
mechanism of cell death 469—471
metabolism 472, 473
resistance mechanisms 473
structure and mechanism of action 468, 469
toxicity 474, 475
transport 471
Follicle stimulating hormone, androgens and 143
estrogen effects on 109
Formycin; 7-amino-3-(β-D-ribofuranosyl)-pyrazolo[4,3-d] pyrimidine
anticancer, antiviral and immunosuppressive effects 444
chemical structure 442
conformational transitions in polymers containing 441
conversion to nucleotides 442
deamination to formycin B 444
inhibition of nucleotide and nucleic acid biosynthesis 442
inhibition of processing of 45S to ribosomal RNA 574, 577
isolation 441
NAD analogs derived from 438
properties of biopolymers containing 443, 444
replacement of adenosine nucleotides in enzymatic reactions 442, 443
selective inhibition of the synthesis of 4S and 5S RNA 576
Formycin B; 7-hydroxy-3-(β-D-ribofuranosyl)pyrazolo[4,3-d]pyrimidine
amination to formycin 444
conversion to oxoformycin B by aldehyde oxidase 444
formation by deamination of formycin 444
nucleoside uptake and metabolism in relation to 445
Formylglycinamide ribonucleotide amidination, inhibition by azaserine and DON 486—488
1-Formylisoquinoline thiosemicarbazone; IQ-1, see also heterocyclic carboxaldehyde thiosemicarbazones
antitumor activity of derivatives 794, 796, 797
chemical structure 794
in combination chemotherapy 799
effects on ribonucleoside diphosphate reductase 803
metabolism and excretion 800—802
2-Formylpyridine thiosemicarbazone, antitumor activity 793
antitumor activity of derivatives 795
chemical structure 794
inhibition of ribonucleoside diphosphate reductase 803
Fructose-1,6-diphosphatase, estrogens and 125
Fumarase, androgens and 151
Fungal infections, 5-fluorocytosine for 201

β-Galactosidase, effects of mitomycin on synthesis of 56
inhibition of induction by 5-fluorouracil 212
inhibition of induction in *E. coli* by 5-hydroxyuridine 377
Gallium, tissue distribution and possible therapeutic use 879
Giant cells, formation by alkylation 21

Glucocorticoids, acute changes induced in lymphoid tissues by 175, see also steroids
antianabolic effects 86
ATP levels and 93
biochemical actions on lymphoid tissues 86—94
breast cancer and 176
carbohydrate metabolism and 91—94
chromatin template and 87, 89
comparative effects on liver and lymphoid tissues 88
distribution 96
DNA metabolism and 86—88
effects on glucose uptake and metabolism 91, 92
enzyme changes induced by 94
for lymphomas and leukemias 187
mechanism of action 85—103
microsomal protein synthesis and 89, 90
modulation of effects on macromolecular biosynthesis by glucose 92, 93
nuclear metabolism and 89
protein metabolism and 88—91
receptors for 94—98
partially purified component 98
properties of 96—98
sedimentation characteristics 97
studies in animals 96
studies in broken cell systems 98
studies in whole cells *in vitro* 96—98
resistance mechanisms 99
resistance related to effects on RNA and protein synthesis 90
RNA metabolism and 88—91
RNA polymerase and 88, 89
serum binding globulin (transcortin) 96
temperature-dependence of intracellular binding and distribution 96—98
Glucosamine, effects of DON on synthesis of 491
Glucose, active transport system for 93
glucocorticoid effects on uptake and metabolism of 91, 92
increased metabolism induced by estradiol 124
modulation of glucocorticoid effects on macromolecular biosynthesis 92, 93
Glucose-6-phosphate dehydrogenase, androgens and 144, 145, 151, 152
estrogen effects on levels of 122—124
regulatory role of NADP 124
isozymes in mammary tumors 124
Glucose phosphate isomerase, estrogen effects on levels of 123
β-Glucuronidase, cortisol-induced increase in 94
Glutamic acid, antagonism of biological actions of the vinca alkaloids 674, 675
antagonism of vinca alkaloid inhibition of RNA synthesis 680
protection against cytotoxic effects of vinca alkaloids 679
Glutaminase, antitumor activity 501, 502
inhibition by azaserine and DON 493
Glutaminase, inhibition by S-carbamyl-L-cysteine 497, 498
Glutamine, metabolic role of 484, 485
role in histidine biosynthesis 493
substrate for L-asparaginase 701
Glutamine antagonists 484—511, see also azaserine, DON, duazomycin
antitumor action 499—502
chemical structures 485
combined with other agents 500, 501
combined with 6-thiopurines 397
cross-resistance with alkylating agents and radiation 79
different actions of azaserine and DON 494, 495
effects on asparagine synthesis 491
effects on glutaminase and glutamine synthetase 492, 493
effects on synthesis of anthranilic and p-aminobenzoic acids 492
immunosuppression by 502, 503
inhibition of NAD biosynthesis 491
inhibition of purine biosynthesis 486—489
inhibition of pyrimidine biosynthesis 489, 490
mechanism of growth inhibition by azaserine and DON 494—496
teratogenic effects 493
Glutamine-5-phosphoribosylpyrophosphate amidotransferase, inhibition by 6-thiopurine 5′-monophosphates 390, 391, 395
Glutamine synthetase 484, 485
inhibitors 498, 499
γ-Glutamylhydrazide, chemical structure 485
synthesis and biological activity 496, 497
Glutarimide antibiotics 561—564
topological similarity to ipecac alkaloids 562, 563
α-Glycerol phosphate dehydrogenase, androgens and 152
Glycogen levels in human endometrium during the menstrual cycle 125
Glycogen synthetase, estrogens and 125
Gouty arthritis, colchicine, vinblastine and griseofulvin for 675
Graft-versus-host reaction, inhibition by mitomycin C 59
Griseofulvin, anti-inflammatory action 675
binding by microtubule protein 678
binding by RNA of sensitive fungi 681
chemical structure 672
inhibition of nucleic acid synthesis 681
reversible dissolution of the meiotic spindle 674
Guanase, action on 8-azaguanine and guanine 459, 460
action on 6-thioguanine 389
Guanazole; 3,5-diamino-1,2,4-triazole, activity in acute leukemia 878
chemical structure and antitumor activity 877
distribution and excretion 878
selective action on DNA synthesis 878

Guanine, alkylation by nitrosoureas 70, 71
role in binding of actinomycin D by DNA 585, 586
selective alkylation by mitomycins 49—51
Guanosine 5'-diphosphate kinase, inhibition by mycophenolic acid 450
Guanosine 5'-phosphate kinase, inhibition by 6-thioguanylate 395
Guanosine 5'-phosphate synthetase, inhibition by S-carbamylcysteine and S-methylcarbamylcysteine 497
Guanosine 5'-triphosphate, binding by microtubule protein 678
Guinea pig serum, antitumor effect of 695

Halogenated nucleic acid, synthesis 274, 275
Halogenated polyuridylic acid, failure of halogen to alter attack by degradative enzymes 274, 275
Halogenated pyrimidine deoxyribonucleosides 272—347, see also individual agents
anabolism 279—282
augmentation of utilization 288—292
by modified means of administration 291, 292
by use of a deoxyribose-1'-phosphate donor 290
inhibition of nucleoside phosphorylase and 289, 290
inhibition of thymidylate synthetase and 288, 289
polycation complexes in 291
with 5-cyanouracil and 5-diazouracil to inhibit degradation 290, 291
base pairing errors and miscoding due to 325
biological effects of incorporation into DNA 295—314
catabolism 282—284
clinical use 322—325
effects on bacterial conjugation and recombination 309
effects on embryonic development and differentiation 310—313
enzymes inhibited by 285—288
greater lability than ribonucleosides 275
halogen electronegativity and hydrogen bonding in DNA 279
incorporation into DNA 295
increased sensitivity to pH and heat denaturation of DNA containing 294
inhibition and activation of thymidine kinase by triphosphates of 285—287
inhibition of cell division in culture 297—300
inhibition of viral replication 302—307
mediated by effects on assembly of particles 303, 304
interactions with oncogenic viruses 307, 308
ionization of 277, 278
mode of inhibition 325, 326
molecular configuration and crystal structure 278, 279
Halogenated pyrimidine deoxyribonucleosides; mutagenic effects 295—297
photochemistry 320—322
physical effects on DNA of incorporation into 292—294
radiosensitization by 318—322
resistance associated with deleted thymidine kinase 298
specificity of antiviral action 306, 307
stability 275—277
steric effects of halogens 277
synthesis 272—275
with halogenated sugar moieties 273
with radioactive label 273
Halogens, stabilizing effects in synthetic polynucleotides 293
Halotestin, see fluoxymesterone
Harringtonine and isomers, structure and mechanism of action 556, 557
Head and neck cancer, methotrexate for 477
HeLa cells, alkylating agent action and the cell cycle in 21, 22
G_1 phase sensitivity to mitomycin 59
repair of damaged DNA in 13, 14
sensitivity to alkylating agents compared with Chinese hamster cells 77, 78
S phase sensitivity to actinomycin D in 59
Hematopoiesis, androgens and 145
effects of alkylating agents on 23
methanesulfonates and 37, 38
Herpes infections, halogenated pyrimidine nucleosides for 322—324
inhibition by xylofuranosyladenine 430
α-(N)-Heterocyclic carboxaldehyde thiosemicarbazones 793—807, see also 1-formylisoquinoline thiosemicarbazone; 5-hydroxy-2-formylpyridine thiosemicarbazone
alkylation of ribonucleoside diphosphate reductase by 797
antineoplastic activity 793—800
antiviral activity 800
chemical structures 794—796
combination therapy involving 799
correlation of chelating potential with antitumor activity 798, 799
distribution and metabolism 800—802
inhibition of ribonucleoside diphosphate reductase 802, 803
inhibition of RNA biosynthetic pathways in bacteria 803, 804
mechanism of action 802—804
Hexestrol 105
Hexokinase, estrogen effects on levels of 124
Histidine, role of glutamine in biosynthesis of 493
Histidine analogs 517
Histone acetylation, cortisol and 89
Histones, effects of arabinosylcytosine on synthesis of 245, 246
HN2, see nitrogen mustard
HODGKIN's disease, L-asparaginase for 727—729
procarbazine for 759, 760
streptonigrin for 638, 639
vinca alkaloids for 685, 687

L-Homoarginine, selective action on phosphatases 516
Homocitrullylaminoadenosine 661
Honvan, see diethylstilbestrol
Hormone binding proteins 85
Hormones, disturbed feedback control of and neoplastic transformation 171
 early demonstration of tumors influenced by 170
 pharmacology and clinical utility 170 to 192
Hycanthone; hydroxymethyllucanthone, active metabolite of lucanthone 879, 880
 antischistosomal action 879
 antitumor action 880
 mechanism of action, distribution and excretion 880
2-Hydrazino-3-(4-imidazoyl) propionic acid, biological activity 517
Hydrocortisone, breast cancer and 184
 effects on glucose oxidation 91
 protein synthesis and 89
8-Hydroxyazathioprine, metabolite of azathioprine 412
6-β-Hydroxycortisol, increased excretion during treatment with o,p′-DDD 813
5-Hydroxycytidine 376
14-Hydroxydaunomycin, see adriamycin
5-Hydroxy-2′-deoxyuridine 376
S-(2-Hydroxyethyl)cysteine-N-acetate 40
 S-oxide 40
5-Hydroxy-2-formylpyridine thiosemicarbazone; 5-HP, see also heterocyclic carboxaldehyde thiosemicarbazones
 antitumor activity 795, 798, 799
 chemical structure 795
 clinical studies with 799, 800
 factors reducing clinical potency 804
 iron excretion increased by 799
 metabolism and excretion 802
1-Hydroxylaminocyclopentane carboxylic acid, antitumor activity 523
δ-Hydroxylysine 498, 499
7-Hydroxyporfiromycin 47
3α-Hydroxy-5α-pregnan-20-one, metabolite of progesterone 162
3α-Hydroxy-5β-pregnan-20-one, metabolite of progesterone 161
3β-Hydroxy-5α-pregnan-20-one, metabolite of progesterone 161
3β-Hydroxy-5β-pregnan-20-one, metabolite of progesterone 161
20β-Hydroxy-5α-pregnan-3-one, metabolite of progesterone 161
20β-Hydroxy-4-pregnen-3-one, metabolite of progesterone 161
17α-Hydroxypregnenolone, chemical structure 141
17α-Hydroxyprogesterone caproate, breast cancer and 185
 chemical structure 141
 uterine cancer and 186
4-Hydroxypyrazolo[3,4-d]pyrimidine, see allopurinol
Hydroxystilbamidine, chemical structure 778
 synergistic antitumor effects with *bis*-(guanylhydrazones) 779, 780
3-Hydroxy-tetrahydrothiophene-1,1-dioxide, urinary metabolite of busulfan 39
Hydroxyurea 789—792
 absorption and distribution 789
 cell cycle specificity 791
 clinical use 789
 effects on ribonucleoside diphosphate reductase 790
 first-order rate equation for cell kill in L1210 by 298
 mechanism of action 790, 791
 teratogenic effects 790
 viral replication and 790, 791
5-Hydroxyuridine, chemistry 376, 377
 deoxyribose triphosphate and DNA polymerase 378
 diphosphate glucose, preparation and enzymatic interactions of 377, 378
 growth inhibition by 377
 inefficient coding for phenylalanine 378
 inhibition of orotidylate decarboxylase by 5′-phosphate 378
 inhibition of RNA and protein synthesis by 377
 synthesis of nucleotides and their glucose and glucuronate conjugates 376, 377
 triphosphate as substrate for RNA polymerase 377, 378
Hypoxanthine-guanine phosphoribosyltransferase, action on 8-azaguanine and other guanine analogs 460, 461
 anabolism of 6-mercaptopurine 385
 anabolism of 6-thioguanine 387
 deficiency in Lesch-Nyhan syndrome 414
 inhibition by 6-mercaptopurine 389
 reduction or deletion in resistance to 6-mercaptopurine 393

Ibenzmethyzin, see procarbazine
ICRF 159; 1,2-*bis*(3,5-dioxopiperazin-1-yl)-propane
 biological activity and structure 885
 clearance from blood 885, 886
 clinical trial 886
Ifosfamide 886
Immunosuppressive agents, arabinosides 237
 L-asparaginase 526, 705—708
 azathioprine 404—425
 azathioprine combined with azaserine 502
 6-azauridine and its triacetate 356
 cis-dichlorodiammineplatinum (II) 832, 833
 cytotoxic amino acid analogs 525—528
 DIC and BIC 547, 549
 fluorinated pyrimidines 201
 formycin 444
 glutamine antagonists 502, 503
 halogenated pyrimidine deoxyribonucleosides 309, 310

Immunosuppressine agents;
6-mercaptopurine combined with duazomycin 502
methotrexate 479
procarbazine 752
6-thiopurines 384
Imuran, see azathioprine
Inosinate dehydrogenase, action on 6-thioinosinate 386
inhibition by mycophenolic acid 450
inhibition by 6-thioinosinate 392
inhibition by 6-thioinosinate and 6-thioguanylate through disulfide bond formation 395
Inosine kinase, action on 6-thioinosine 387
Interferon, induction by tilorone hydrochloride 884
mechanism of action 884
Interstitial cell stimulating hormone, interrelationship with testosterone 173
Iodoaminopterin-^{131}I 472
5-Iodo-2′-deoxycytidine, biological activity and deamination of 324
deamination 238
rationale for and metabolic fate of 291
5-Iodo-2′-deoxyuridine, see also halogenated pyrimidine deoxyribonucleosides
abnormal viral particles formed in presence of 304
catabolism 282—284
clinical pharmacokinetics 284
clinical use in neoplastic disease 324, 325
clinical use in viral infections 322—324
compared with thymidine as precursor for DNA synthesis 280, 281
crystal and molecular structure 279
effects on T_4-directed synthesis of proteins 305, 306
effects on thymidylate kinase 285
effects on utilization of precursors for DNA synthesis 301
enzyme kinetic factors compared with those for thymidine 281
formation of deoxyuridine free radical after ultraviolet irradiation 320
Gompertzian kinetics of inhibition of L 1210 by 298
hydrolytic degradation 275—277
incorporation into embryonic DNA 310, 311
increased fragility of viral DNA containing 292
induction of mouse leukemia by 363
inhibition of DNA viral replication 194, 199
inhibition of experimental mouse neoplasms alone or with other agents 300, 301
inhibition of thymidylate synthetase in L 5178 Y cells 285
inhibition of viral replication 302—307
interaction with oncogenic viruses 307, 308
ionic and molecular species and the pK_a of 278
5-Iodo-2′-deoxyuridine; pharmacokinetics after intracisternal administration 284
potentiation of antitumor effects by uracil mustard 301
radiobiological damage produced by radiolabeled analog in DNA 314, 315, 317
sensitization of thymidine kinase to ultraviolet light by 320, 322
synthesis 272, 273
thymidine used to modulate toxicity of 313, 314
tissue characteristics in inhibition of DNA polymerase and thymidine kinase 301
5′-triphosphate, activator or inhibitor of thymidine kinase 286—288
compared with dTTP as allosteric or feedback inhibitor 282
inhibition of deoxycytidylate deaminase 287, 288
substrate for DNA polymerase 282, 285
use of radio-labeled drug as marker for cell kinetics 314—318
factors involved in preferential use 318
5-Iodo-2′-deoxyuridine 5′-phosphate esters, synthesis 274
5-Iodouracil, lack of correlation of mutagenesis and lethality due to 326
mispairing in DNA 296
photochemistry of 320, 321
5-Iodouracil-2′-deoxyribonucleoside, see 5-iodo-2′-deoxyuridine
5-Iodouracil ribonucleoside; 5-iodouridine
crystal and molecular structure 279
hydrolytic degradation 277
synthesis 272
5-Iodouridine 5′-phosphate esters, synthesis 274
Isocitrate dehydrogenase, androgens and 144, 145, 151
Isocyanates, formation from nitrosoureas during alkylation 66—68
possible role in biological action of nitrosoureas 68
Isopentenyladenosine 435
Isophosphamide; 3-(2-chloroethyl)-2-(2-chloroethylamine)tetrahydro-2H-1,3,2,-oxaphosphorine-2-oxide 886
Isopropylidine azastreptonigrin, chemical structure 633
comparison with streptonigrin 640
N-Isopropyl-α-(2-methylhydrazino)-p-toluamide monohydrochloride, see procarbazine
N-Isopropylterephthalamic acid, major urinary metabolite of procarbazine 753,754

Kidney, androgen effects on 145
effects of phleomycin on 851, 861
toxic effects of pyrrolopyrimidine nucleosides 440
Kidney transplant patients, increased incidence of lymphoma in 417
KTS 841—849, see also 3-ethoxy-2-oxobutyraldehyde-*bis*(thiosemicarbazone)

L cells, repair of damaged DNA in 14
Lactation, inhibition by androgens 144
Leaving-group constants 4
Lesch-Nyhan syndrome, lack of hypoxanthine-guanine phosphoribosyltransferase 414
Leukemia, see also acute and chronic leukemia
activation by graft-versus-host disease 418
effects of 5-azacytidine alone or combined with prednisone 363, 364
L 1210, growth inhibition by arabinosides 233—236
6-mercaptopurine for 384
6-thioguanine for 394
Leukosarcoma, L-asparaginase for 727, 729
Leukovorin, see citrovorum factor
Lipids, complexes with phthalanilides 823—825
effects of colchicine and vinca alkaloids 682
Liver, degradation of halogenated pyrimidine analogs by 284
toxic effects of L-asparaginase 735, 736
Liver regeneration, effects of mitomycin 59
Liver tumors, methotrexate for 478
Lucanthone; miracil D, hycanthone as active metabolite 879, 880
Lung cancer, methotrexate for 477, 478
Luteinizing hormone, estrogen effects on 109
progesterone in control of 160
Lymphocytes, classification and interactions of 405
effects of L-asparaginase on blastogenesis 706, 707
Lymphoid tissues, effects of glucocorticoids 86—94
Lymphoma, comparison of 5-fluorouracil sensitivity to normal mouse hematopoietic cells 218
glucocorticoids for 187
increased incidence in kidney transplant patients 417
methotrexate for 478
procarbazine for 759
streptonigrin for 639
Lymphoma L5178Y, effects of arabinosylcytosine on 235
Lymphosarcoma, regressions in mice induced by adrenal corticosteroids 175
Lymphosarcoma P1798, biochemical action of glucocorticoids on 86—94
Lysepsin, nitrogen mustard derivative of lysine 518
Lysine, selective carbamoylation of in proteins by nitrosoureas 72, 73
Lysine analogs 518
Lysodren, see o,p′-DDD
9-β-D-Lyxofuranosyladenine, chemical structure 426
synthesis, activity and metabolism 431
9-β-D-Lyxofuranosyl-6-mercaptopurine 431

Malic dehydrogenase, androgens and 151, 152
Malignant melanoma, L-asparaginase for 727, 729
Mannitol myleran; D-mannitol-1,6-dimethanesulfonate; mannogranol
antitumor effects 36
excretion 28
Marek's disease, O-ethyl-L-threonine and 524
Matulane, see procarbazine
Mechlorethamine, see nitrogen mustard
Megaloblastic marrow, arabinosylcytosine and 236, 261
MER-25, see ethamoxytrophetol
5-Mercapto-1-methyl-4-nitroimidazole, formation from azathioprine 404
6-Mercaptopurine, action on protein and nucleic acid synthesis 26
anabolism 385—387
anti-inflammatory effects 408
antineoplastic activity and toxicity 389
antitumor activity synergistic with arabinosylcytosine 236
arabinoside 426, 429, 430
catabolism 385, 387
cell mediated immune reactions suppressed by 407, 408
delayed cytotoxicity 396
direct dethiolation to hypoxanthine 387
enzyme inhibition by free base 389
immunosuppressive effects compared with azathioprine 409
in DNA as deoxythioguanosine 386
incorporation into DNA 392, 393
inhibition of glutamine-PRPP amidotransferase by 5′-monophosphate 390, 391
inhibition of purine ribonucleotide interconversions 392
inhibition of purine ribonucleotide synthesis *de novo* 390, 391
leukemia treated with 384
mechanisms of resistance 393
metal mercaptide formation with RNA 386
self-enhancement effect of related to 6-thioinosinate 391
suppression of antibody formation by 407
synergistic cytotoxic effect with glutamine analogs 391
6-Mercaptopurine riboside, see 6-thioinosine
Merophan, hematopoietic effects 23
Methanesulfonates, cross resistance to radiation 41
immunosuppression by 38
mechanism of action 35—46
metabolism and distribution 39, 40
nitrogen mustard derivatives 36
Methicillin, mechanism of resistance 449
L-Methionine sulfoxide 499
L-Methionine sulfoximine, antitumor activity in combination therapy 501
chemical structure, convulsant activity and inhibition of glutamine synthetase 498, 499
Methotrexate; amethopterin, see also folate antagonists

Methotrexate; absorption and transport 471
affinity for dihydrofolate reductase 468, 469
for autoimmune diseases 479
for breast cancer 221
cell cycle phase specificity 469, 470
chemical structure 468
clinical uses 475—479
combinations for acute myelocytic leukemia 477
combined with L-asparaginase 470, 471
combined with vincristine, 5-fluorouracil, cyclophosphamide, and prednisone
distribution 472
effect on thymidylate synthetase 469
increased thymidylate synthetase after 246
intrathecal use 472, 476
metabolism and excretion 472, 473
renal toxicity 473
resistance through impaired transport 471, 473
retention of 472
site of action 470
thymineless and purineless death 470
toxicity 474, 475
10-Methoxycamptothecin 649, 654
9-Methoxyellipticine, chemical structure and source 881
clinical use 882
N-Methyl mitomycin A 47
reaction with DNA 49
β-Methyl-L-aspartate, substrate for L-asparaginase 701
3-Methylcytosine, base-pairing properties 15
Methyldiazine, formation from procarbazine 753, 755
2α-Methyldihydrotestosterone, antitumor action and androgenic effects 181
propionate for breast cancer 144
remissions in breast cancer induced by 173
Methylene dimethanesulfonate, antitumor effects 35
chemical structure 36
hemopoietic effects 38
metabolism 40
spermatogenesis and 37
3′-O-Methyl-5-fluoro-2′-deoxyuridine, cytotoxic activity 215
synthesis and activity 196
Methylglyoxal-*bis*(guanylhydrazone); 1,1′-[(methylethanediylidene)-dinitrilo] diguanidine; methyl-GAG 766—777
antitumor activity 767, 768
antiviral activity 769
chemical structure 767
combined with other agents 768, 769
comparison with DDUG 782
disposition and cellular uptake 770—772
effects on microorganisms 769
effects on mitochondrial functions 776, 777
mechanism of action 773—777
nucleic acids and 776
Methylglyoxal-*bis*(guanylhydrazone);
polyamine metabolism and 774—776
putrescine stimulated S-adenosylmethionine decarboxylase and 775
spermidine antagonism of uptake 771, 773
structure-activity relationships 768
therapeutic effects in man 772, 773
toxicity 769, 770
7-Methylguanine, base-pairing properties 14, 15
Methylhydrazine derivatives 747—749, see also procarbazine
metabolism 755
6α-Methyl-17α-hydroxyprogesterone acetate; medroxyprogesterone, see Provera
6-C-Methyllysine 518
6-Methylmercaptopurine ribonucleoside, see 6-methylthioinosine
O-Methylnogalarol, antitumor activity 631
DNA binding specificity 630
inhibition of growth and macromolecular synthesis 625
structure 624
1-Methyl-4-nitro-5-N-acetyl-2-cysteinyl-imidazole, metabolite of azathioprine 412
1-Methyl-4-nitro-5-carboxymethylamino-imidazole, metabolite of azathioprine 412
1-Methyl-3-nitro-nitrosoguanidine; MNNG, alkylation of amino acids and proteins 72
alkylation of nucleic acid derivatives 70, 71
chemistry 66
1-Methyl-4-nitro-5-thioimidazole, urinary excretion during azathioprine therapy 412
1-Methyl-1-nitrosourea; MNU, alkylation of nucleic acids 70
carcinogenic effects 78
cell cycle phase specificity 77, 78
chemistry 66—68
effects on nicotinamide adenine dinucleotide metabolism 75
inhibition of macromolecular biosynthesis 73, 74
metabolism 69
17α-Methyl-β-nortestosterone, antiandrogenic activity 146
Methyl streptonigrin 633
activity and toxicity compared with streptonigrin 639, 640
6-Methylsulfinyl-8-hydroxypurine, urinary metabolite of 6-thiopurines 387
17α-Methyltestosterone, breast cancer and 182
renotropic activity 145
6-Methylthioguanylate, anabolite of 6-thioguanine 388
6-Methylthioinosinate, derived from 6-mercaptopurine and 6-methylthioinosine 385, 386
persistence in cells 386
6-Methylthioinosine; 6-methylmercaptopurine ribonucleoside; MMPR, anabolism 385—387
catabolism 385, 387

6-Methylthioinosine;
inhibition of glutamine-PRPP amidotransferase by 5'-monophosphate 390, 391
synergistic cytotoxic effects with 6-mercaptopurine 391
6-Methylthiopurine in rat urine after 6-mercaptopurine administration 387
Methyltransferase, in methylation of 6-thiopurine derivatives 385, 386, 388
Microtubule system 676, 677
binding of antimitotic agents by tubulin 677—679
binding of guanosine 5'-triphosphate by tubulin 678
crystals 676, 677
subunit protein; tubulin 677—679
isolation 678
Miracil D; lucanthone 879
Mithramycin 615—622
antitumor activity 619
chemical structure 615
cross-resistance to chromomycin and olivomycin 616
mode of interaction with DNA 617
selective inhibition of precursor ribosomal RNA synthesis 573, 577
toxicity 619—621
Mitochondria, inhibition of RNA synthesis in by ethidium bromide 577
Mitomycins, activation of 50, 51
antitumor activity synergistic with arabinosylcytosine 236
biological effects 48
cell cycle specificity 59
chemical structure 47
chromosome breakage by 56, 57
degradation of ribosomes induced by 54, 55
depolymerization of DNA and 53, 54
relation to phage-like particle formation 58
relation to repair 54
immunosuppression by 59
induction of phage-like particles in bacteria by 57
inhibition by chloramphenicol 58
relation to colicinogenic factors 58
inhibition of DNA synthesis 53
relation to phage-like particle formation 58
inhibition of induced enzyme synthesis 56
inhibition of RNA viruses 58
interaction with DNA in intact cells 52, 53
interaction with DNA *in vitro* 48—52
comparison with nitrogen mustard and triethylenemelamine 50
mechanism of action 47—64
mechanism of activation 50—52
mutagenicity 56
reaction with guanine-cytosine base pairs 50, 51
repair of DNA damaged by 52, 53
RNA metabolism and 54—56
sources 47
Mitosis, inhibition by colchicine and the vinca alkaloids 673—675
inhibition by mitomycins 59
Mitotane, see o,p'-DDD
Mitotic arrest 673—675
MMPR, see 6-methylthioinosine
MNNG, see 1-methyl-3-nitro-1-nitrosoguanidine
MNU, see 1-methyl-1-nitrosourea
Moloney sarcoma virus, daunorubicin and 607
Monomethylhydrazine, formation from procarbazine 751
Mutagenesis, induced by halogenated analogs in *Drosophila* 297
methanesulfonates and 41, 42
mitomycins and 56
D-Mycarose 616
Mycophenolic acid; 6-(4-hydroxy-6-methoxy-7-methyl-3-oxo-5-phthalanyl)-4-hexenoic acid
biochemical effects 450
biochemistry of resistance to 451
chemical structure 447
glucuronide formation 451
isolation and anticancer activity 446
structural specificity of 449, 450
Mycosis fungoides, 6-azauridine for 361
methotrexate for 478

NAD; nicotinamide adenine dinucleotide, alkylating agents and 25
analogs of 540—542
androgen effects on levels of 151
catalytic oxidation of reduced form by streptonigrin 635
effects of nitrosoureas 75, 76
glycohydrolase 540
inhibition of biosynthesis by azaserine and DON 491
NADP; nicotinamide adenine dinucleotide phosphate, androgen effects on levels of 151
reduced form as cofactor in converting cholesterol to pregnenolone 139, 140
regulatory role in estrogen-induced changes in glucose-6-phosphate dehydrogenase 124
NADP-isocitrate dehydrogenase, estrogen effects on levels of 122, 123
NADP-malate dehydrogenase, estrogen effects on levels of 122, 123
Nafoxidine; U11100A, antagonism of estradiol binding 95
antiestrogenic action and chemical structure 110, 111
blockade of estrogen binding by 114, 187
breast cancer and 187, 188
Natulan, see procarbazine
Nebularine; 9-β-D-ribofuranosylpurine 434
Neoplasia, role of hormonal feedback regulation in induction of 171
Nicotinamide mononucleotide adenyltransferase, action of testosterone in 151

Nilevar; 17α-ethyl-4-estren-17β-ol-3-one, anabolic androgen 142
Nitrilase activity of L-asparaginase 701, 702
Nitriles as toxic agents in phleomycin preparations 860
Nitrogen metabolism, androgen effects on 145
Nitrogen mustard; HN2, alkylation reactions 2
cell cycle and sensitivity to 21, 22
immunosuppression by 24
mechanism of alkylation by 19, 20
preferential inhibition of precursor ribosomal RNA synthesis 573, 574, 577
premature termination of HnRNA transcription 574, 575
Nitrosoureas, see also individual agents BCNU, CCNU
alkyl diazohydroxides as intermediates in alkylation by 66, 67
blood-brain barrier and 69
carbamoylation of proteins by 72, 73
carbonium ions derived from 67, 68
cell cycle phase specificity 76—78
chemistry 65—68
comparative alkylating ability 68
cross-resistance with other agents 79
deactivation of DNA nucleotidyltransferase by 74, 75
effects on nucleic acid synthesis 73—75
genetic effects 78, 79
isocyanates derived from 66—68
mechanism of action 65—84
metabolism and distribution 69
stability in aqueous solution 65, 66
L-3-Nitrotyrosine, antitumor activity 521
Nogalamycin 623—632
antibacterial activity 623, 624
antitumor activity 631
cell cycle phase specificity 629
chemistry 623
comparative biological activity of derivatives 629, 630
cytotoxicity to mammalian cells 624
effects on nucleic acid synthesis 624, 625
inhibition of DNA polymerase 628, 629
inhibition of DNase 629
inhibition of enzyme synthesis in regenerating liver 630, 631
inhibition of RNA polymerase 626, 628, 630
interaction with DNA 624—628
intercalation 627
preference for native state, base composition and sequence 625, 626, 628
N-oxide 624
inhibition of growth and macromolecular synthesis 625
selective inhibition of precursor ribosomal RNA synthesis 573, 577
specificity for inhibition of nucleic acid synthesis 628
structure 624
whole animal toxicity 631
Nogalarene, DNA binding specificity 630
inhibition of growth and macromolecular synthesis 625
structure 624
Nogalarol, antitumor activity 631
DNA binding specificity 630
inhibition of growth and macromolecular synthesis 625
structure 624
C-Nor-D-homo-17α-epitestosterone acetate, antiandrogenic activity 146
Norlutin 182
A-Norprogesterone, antagonism of androgen-induced enzyme changes 152
antiandrogenic activity 146
19-Nortestosterone derivatives, breast cancer and 182
Nuclear heterogeneous RNA; HnRNA 574—576
steps in synthesis and processing of 576
Nucleic acids, methylation by procarbazine 758, see also DNA, RNA
Nucleocidin; 9-(4′-fluoro-5′-O-sulfamoyl-pentofuranosyl)adenosine 434
Nucleolus as site of precursor ribosomal RNA synthesis 572
Nucleophilic constants 4
Nucleoside phosphorylase, action on psicofuranine 448
deoxyglucosylthymine as inhibitor 289
reduction in effectiveness of fluorinated pyrimidine nucleosides by 215
thymine ribonucleoside as inhibitor 289
Nucleosides, halogenated in sugar moiety, synthesis of 273
non-specificity of antagonism of showdomycin effects 375
Nucleus, lipids of 824, 825

Ocular toxicity, busulfan and 39
Oliose 616
Olivomose 616
Olivomycin 615—622
antitumor activity 617—619
blood levels and excretion 620
chemical structure 615
clinical use 621
cross-resistance to chromomycin and mithramycin 616
toxicity 619—621
Olivomycose 616
Olivose 616
Ommaya reservoir 238
Oncovin, see vincristine
L-Ornithine, effects of L-canaline on metabolism 516
L-Ornithine decarboxylase, stimulation of prostatic enzyme by testosterone 148
Orotidylate decarboxylase, augmented levels in cells exposed to 6-azauridine 352
inhibition by 5-aminouridylate 380
inhibition by 5-azacytidine 5′-phosphate 362
inhibition by 6-azacytidine 5′-phosphate 349

Orotidylate decarboxylase, inhibition by 6-azauridine 5′phosphate 352, 353
inhibition by 5-hydroxyuridine 5′-monophosphate 378
Orotidylate pyrophosphorylase, augmented levels in cells exposed to 6-azauridine 352
showdomycin inhibition of 374
Osteogenic sarcoma, methotrexate for 479
Ovalbumin, estrogen-induced synthesis 121
Ovarian dysgenesis, busulfan and 39
Ovarian tumors, depressed gonadal function as a factor in induction of 171
Oxylone acetate; fluorometholone, for breast cancer 185, 186

Pactamycin, chemical structure 557
mechanism of action 557, 558
use in determining gene order 558
Paederin, biological activity and mechanism of action 566
chemical structure 567
L-Penicillamine, antibacterial and antitumor activity 523, 524
Pentanedial-*bis*(guanylhydrazone) 767
Peptidyl transferase, sparsomycin and 566
Phage-like particles, induction by mitomycins 57, 58
relation to colicinogenic factors 58
Phenoty picreversion in presence of 5-fluorouracil 214, 215
Phenylalanine analogs 519, 520
1-Phenyl-3,3-dimethyltriazene, alkylation of nucleic acids by 71
Phenylselenocysteine 522
Pheochromocytoma 520
Phleomycin 850—876, see also bleomycin
arrest of mitosis in absence of effects on DNA synthesis 859
biological activity 855, 856
cholinergic effects 861
composition 851, 852
distribution and excretion 855
effects on chromosomes 863—866
genetic effects 862
inhibition of DNA synthesis 856—858
relationship with A-T content 857
inhibition of replication of RNA viruses 859
possible relation to nitriles in drug preparations 860
kidney toxicity 851, 861
nitriles related to toxicity 860
physical and spectral properties 852—855
reactions with DNA 862—869
cleavage of DNA 868, 869
formation of nodules on chromosomes 863—866
polyphleomycin model 866—868
relationship of A-T content to sensitivity 856, 857, 865, 866
toxicity 860, 861
transcription and 860
variations in receptivity of target sites 858, 859
Phosphatase, corticosteroid-induced changes in 94
Phosphofructokinase, estrogen effects on levels of 124, 125
Phosphoglucomutase, androgens and 144, 145
Phosphoribosylpyrophosphate amidotransferase, inhibition by glutamine antagonists 488, 489
inhibition by phosphate esters of 3′-deoxyadenosine 659, 663
Phosvitin, relation to serum phosphoproteins 121
Photochemistry of halogenated pyrimidine derivatives 319—322
Phthalanilides 820—828
anionic metabolites 823
binding to cell components 823, 824
chemical structures 821
effects on biosynthetic pathways 824
effects of suramin on kidney and liver drug concentrations 822
intracellular distribution 824, 825
mechanism of action 823—825
metabolism 822—823
tumor-inhibitory activity 820
Pituitary, androgens and 143, 144
busulfan and insufficiency of 39
role in breast growth 111
Platinum compounds 829—840, see also *cis*-dichlorodiammine platinum (II); *cis*-dichloro(dipyridine)platinum (II)
chemical structures 830
distribution 832
filamentous growth of *Escherichia coli* exposed to 829
mechanism of action 833—836
reactions in aqueous solution 836
toxicity 831, 832, 838
tumor-inhibitory activity 830, 831, 838
Podophyllic acid ethyl hydrazide, binding by nucleic acids 681
binding by soluble protein 678
chemical structure 672
distribution 684
inhibition of nucleic acid synthesis 681
Podophyllotoxin, antitumor effects of derivatives 675
chemical structure 672
incomplete recovery of spindle after exposure to 674
metabolism and distribution 684
Podophyllum resin 670
Poly(A) termination of nuclear heterogeneous and messenger RNA 575
Polyamines, effects of arabinosylcytosine on 246
methylglyoxal-*bis*(guanylhydrazone) and 773—776
relationship with androgens 148, 149
Polycythemia vera, 6-azauridine for 361
Polyfluorouridylic acid, conformation of 198
Polynucleotide chain terminators 657—669
Polynucleotide phosphorylase, action on tubercidin diphosphate 437

Polynucleotide phosphorylase, altered properties in cells resistant to showdomycin 376
inhibition by arabinosylcytosine diphosphate 243
inhibition by 6-azauridine 5'-diphosphate 352
Porfiromycin, chemical structure 47
combined with arabinosylcytosine 264
Prednisolone, glucose uptake and 91
Prednisone, breast cancer and 185
combined with vincristine, 5-fluorouracil, methotrexate and cyclophosphamide for breast cancer 221
in COAP regimen 263, 264
for prostatic cancer 180
toxicity 185
5 α-Pregnane-3,20-dione, binding to progesterone receptor protein 163
biological activity 161
metabolite of progesterone 161, 162
5 β-Pregnane-3,20-dione, metabolite of progesterone 161
Pregnenolone, chemical structure 141
conversion to estrogens 106
NADPH as cofactor in synthesis from cholesterol 139, 140
synthesis as rate-limiting step in steroid formation 140
Procarbazine; N-isopropyl-α-[2-methylhydrazino]-p-toluamide monohydrochloride 747—765
chemistry 747, 749—751
clinical aspects 759, 760
combination therapy with 760
degradation 750
effects on cellular nucleic acid and protein synthesis 756—758
HODGKIN's disease and 759, 760
immunosuppression by 752
mechanism of action 756—759
metabolism 753—756
microsomal enzymes and 754, 755
methylation of nucleic acids 758
methyldiazine as possible active intermediate 755, 756
pharmacology 751—753
structural formula 750
teratogenesis 752, 753
toxicity 751—753
tumor inhibition by 747, 748, 749
Progesterone, binding of 162—164
biological responses to 158, 159
breast cancer and 185
chemical structure 141
conversion to estrogens 106, 107
deciduoma reaction 159
distribution 159, 160
effects on renal cell cancer induction by estrogen 175
effects on RNA polymerase 165
increased conversion of amino acids to urea induced by 159
induction of avidin synthesis in estrogen-stimulated chick oviduct 159, 165
Progesterone, inhibition of gonadotrophin secretion 160
luteinized granulosa cells as source of 107
mechanism of action 158—169
metabolism 160—162
myometrial blocking action 158
natriuresis induced by 159
sequence of events in action of 163—167
stimulation of uptake by estrogen 160
toxicity 186
uptake by brain regions and pituitary 160
uterine cancer and 186
Progesterone receptor protein 160, 162, 163
differentiation from transcortin 162—164
increased concentration of by prior estrogen treatment 162
nuclear chromatin binding sites for hormone-receptor complex 164, 165
properties 163, 164
transfer to nucleus 164
Prolactin, dependence of breast cancer growth on 112
estrogen and progesterone effects on levels of 174
1-Propyl-1-nitrosourea, effects on nucleic acid synthesis 74
Prostate, androgens and 143
Prostate cancer, chlorotrianisene for 180
diethylstilbestrol for 179, 180
estrogens for 113
glucocorticoids for 176, 180
hormonal steroids for 179, 180
Protamine, complex formation with halogenated nucleosides producing greater uptake into DNA 291
Protein synthesis, cytotoxic inhibitors of 554—570
classification 554—556
effects of 5-fluorouracil and its deoxyribonucleoside 211
effects of mitomycin 55, 56
effects of paederin 567
effects of tylocerebrine 564
effects of vinca alkaloids 681, 682
glucocorticoids and 88—91
inhibition by anisomycin 565
inhibition by azathioprine 405, 406
inhibition by diphtheria toxin 561
inhibition by emetine 561
inhibition by nogalomycin and derivatives 625
procarbazine and 757
reactions involved in 554, 555
sites of action of sparsomycin 566
Provera with cortisone for hamster renal cell tumors 186
Psicofuranine; 6-amino-9-(β-D-psicofuranosyl)purine; angustmycin C
chemical structure 447
chemotherapy with 451
conversion to decoyinine 447
enzymes acting on 448
inhibition of xanthosine 5'-phosphate aminase 448, 449
isolation 446, 447

Psicofuranine; resistance to 449
Psoriasis, 6-azauridine for 361
hydroxyurea for 789
methotrexate for 472, 479
Pulmonary fibrosis, busulfan and 39
Purine arabinosides 426—433
Purine 3′-deoxyribonucleosides 657—669
Purine lyxosides 426—433
Purine nucleoside phosphorylase, action on 8-azaguanine 460
action on 6-thioinosine (MPR) 387
inhibition by formycin B 445
Purine ribonucleotides, biosynthesis 487
feedback regulation 390, 391
inhibition by glutamine antagonists 486—489
inhibition by 6-thiopurines 390, 391, 394, 395
Purine xylosides 426—433
Puromycin, reaction with peptidyl-tRNA to cause termination 559
Putrescine, increased prostatic levels induced by testosterone 148
Pyridine nucleotide coenzymes, see also NAD, NADP
6-aminonicotinamide analogs 540—542
cytotoxic analogs 539—543
metabolism and concentration in neoplastic tissue 539, 540
Pyrimidine nucleoside deaminase; cytidine deaminase, properties 238, 239
role in resistance to arabinosylcytosine 247, 248
Pyrimidine ribonucleotides, biosynthesis 490
inhibition by glutamine antagonists 489, 490
Pyrophosphate and the configuration of xanthosine 5′-phosphate aminase 449
Pyrophosphokinase, effects of decoyinine on 449
Pyrrolopyrimidine nucleosides 435—441
clinical chemotherapy and toxicity 440, 441
comparative cytotoxicity and biochemistry 439, 440
Pyruvate kinase, estradiol and 124, 125

Quinones, inhibition of RNA synthesis 55
reversal by amino acids 56

Radiation, see also ultraviolet light, x-radiation
sensitization by halogenated pyrimidine deoxyribonucleosides 318—322
sequence-dependence in interaction with 6-azauridine for tumor inhibition 355
synergism with actinomycin D 589
Renal cell tumors, Provera and cortisone for 186
Reverse transcriptase, see DNA polymerase, RNA dependent
Ribonuclease; RNase, action on poly-8-azaguanylate 462, 463
Ribonuclease; 9 α-fluoroprednisolone-induced increase 94
5-fluorouracil-induced increase 94
increase after treatment with L-asparaginase 710
methotrexate-induced increase 94
vinblastine-induced increase 94
Ribonucleoside diphosphate reductase, action on tubercidin nucleotide 437
arabinosylcytosine and 242, 243
hydrophobic region 797, 798, 803
hydroxyurea and 790
inhibition by arabinosyladenine nucleotides 427
inhibition by arabinosyl-6-mercaptopurine 429
inhibition by guanazole 878
inhibition by heterocyclic carboxaldehyde thiosemicarbazones 802, 803
interaction of heterocyclic carboxaldehyde thiosemicarbazones with 797, 798
pyrrolopyrimidine nucleotides in study of regulatory site 440
role in resistance to arabinosylcytosine 247
Ribosomes, degradation induced by mitomycin 54, 55
effects of 5-azacytidine 362, 363
effects of emetine 559
effects of 5-fluorouracil on synthesis of 206, 207
interaction with cycloheximide 561
interaction with pactamycin 557, 558
interaction with paederin 567
interaction with sparsomycin 566
loss following castration 148
synthesis and processing of RNA of 572
agents interfering with 573, 574
Rifamycin SV derivatives, chemical structure 883
clinical trial 883, 884
effects on DNA polymerase 883
source and biological activity 882, 883
RNA, alkylation by nitrosoureas 70, 71
altered base composition produced by showdomycin 375, 376
complex with daunorubicin compared to DNA complex 608
derivation of ribosomal species 147
estrogens and 120, 121
heterogeneous form induced by androgens 147
incorporated arabinosylcytosine and acute cell death 245
incorporation of 6-azauridine after intracerebral injection in the cat 352
incorporation of 5-fluorouracil into 202
messenger fraction, incorporation of 5-fluorouracil and 5-fluoroorotic acid 210, 211
nuclear heterogeneous form 574—576
ribosomal fraction, agents interfering with synthesis of 573, 574
estrogen and 120

RNA, ribosomal fraction, incorporation of 5-fluorouracil into 210
inhibition of maturation by ellipticine 881
synthesis and processing of 572
transfer fraction, effects of fluorinated pyrimidines on 206
effects of 5-fluorouracil on base composition and properties 209. 210
estrogen and 121
incorporation of 5-fluorouracil into 209, 210
RNA polymerase; RNA nucleotidyl transferase
altered enzyme induced by 5-fluorouracil-containing poliovirus 211
androgens and 148
8-azaguanosine triphosphate as substrate for 462
estrogens and 119
formycin triphosphate as substrate for 443
glucocorticoids and 88, 89
increased levels induced by progesterone 165
increased levels in resistance to 5-azacytidine 363
inhibition by actinomycin D 573, 583
inhibition by anthramycin 643, 645, 646
inhibition by 6-azauridine 5′-triphosphate 352
inhibition by bleomycin and phleomycin 860
inhibition by daunorubicin 602
inhibition by nogalamycin 626, 628, 630
inhibition by triphosphates of cordycepin and 3′-amino-3′-deoxyadenosine 659
inhibition by vincristine 681
inhibition related to binding of actinomycin and nogalamycin to polydeoxynucleotides 625
reduced specific activity of in *E. coli* mutants resistant to showdomycin 376
separate enzyme for transcription of 4S and 5S RNA 576
tubercidin triphosphate as substrate for 437, 438
two forms in uterine nuclei 119
types of 574
RNA synthesis, agents causing selective inhibition 571—581
examples of the use of 578, 579
table of 577
effects of alanosine 882
effects of camptothecin 651—653
effects of colchicine and the vinca alkaloids 681, 690
effects of cycloheximide 563, 564
effects of 3′-deoxyadenosine 663, 664
effects of emetine 560
effects of nitrosoureas 73—75
estrogens and 118—121
glucocorticoids and 88—91
inhibition by actinomycin D 582—584
RNA synthesis, inhibition in bacteria by heterocyclic carboxaldehyde thiosemicarbazones 803, 804
inhibition by daunorubicin 601, 602, 604, 605
inhibition by fluorinated pyrimidines 205, 206
inhibition by hycanthone 880
inhibition by 5-hydroxyuridine 377
inhibition by nogalamycin and derivatives 624—626, 628, 630
inhibition by olivomycin, chromomycin and mithramycin 616, 617
inhibition of viral RNA synthesis by 6-azauridine 354
mitochondrial, inhibited by ethidium bromide 577
mitomycin effects on 54—56
structural requirements for 55
procarbazine and 756—758
RNA directed form not inhibited by nogalamycin 629
steps involved in for ribosomal RNA 572
agents interfering with 572—574
RNA viruses, fluorinated pyrimidines and 200
inhibition by mitomycin 58
Rosette formation, inhibition by azathioprine 406
inhibition of as assay of azathioprine levels 413, 414
Rous sarcoma virus, daunorubicin and 607
Rubidomycin, see daunorubicin

Sangivamycin; 4-amino-5-carboxamide-7-(D-ribofuranosyl)-7H-pyrrolo[2,3-d] pyrimidine
biosynthesis 435, 436
chemical structure 436
chemotherapy with 440
cytotoxic activity compared with tubercidin and toyocamycin 439
inhibition of processing of 45S to ribosomal RNA 574, 577
toxicity 440
Selective interruption of RNA metabolism by drugs 571—581
L-Selenocysteine 522
Seminal vesicles, testosterone and 143
L-Serine dehydratase, inhibition of induction of by 5-fluorouracil 212
L-Serine hydroxamate, antibacterial action and inhibition of seryl-tRNA synthetase 525
Serotonin, metabolism in carcinoid syndrome 519
Showdomycin, alkylating action of maleimide moiety 373, 374
altered base composition of RNA in cells resistant to 375, 376
altered polynucleotide phosphorylase in cells resistant to 376
antibacterial and cellular inhibitory action 374
changes in *E. coli* resistant to 375, 376

Showdomycin, chemistry 373
effects on transport of sugars and amino acids 375
enzymes inhibited by 374, 375
metabolism 373, 374
non-specific protection of *E. coli* by nucleosides 375
Skin graft survival, azathioprine 407, 408
S_N1 and S_N2 reactions 1—5
Sparsomycin, biological and biochemical activity 565, 566
chemical structure 566
inhibition of peptide bond formation 559
Spermatogenesis, effects of alkylating agents 23, 24
methanesulfonates and 37
Spermidine, antagonism of methylglyoxal-*bis*(guanylhydrazone) 769, 771, 773—776
chemical structure 767
increased prostatic levels induced by testosterone 148
Spermine, stimulation of prostatic RNA polymerase 148, 149
Spongosine; 9-β-D-ribofuranosyl-2-methoxyadenine 435
Stanolone, see 5α-dihydrotestosterone
Stein-Leventhal syndrome, association with endometrial cancer 174
Steroid 11β- and side chain hydroxylations 139, 140
Steroid 17α-dehydrogenase 141
Steroid 17β-dehydrogenase 107
Steroid 17α-hydroxylase, action on pregnenolone 140
Steroid 3β-ol dehydrogenase complex 140, 141
Steroid 5α-reductase, action on testosterone 149, 150
Steroids, see also androgens, cortisol, cortisone, estradiol, estrogens, glucocorticoids and testosterone
abnormal metabolism of in patients with cancer 177—179
effects of o,p'-DDD on production of 811, 812
non-specific binding 96
specific binding proteins 94—98
Streptonigrin 633—641
biological properties 634
catalytic oxidation of NADH and NADPH 635
chemical structure 53, 633
clinical uses 638, 639
degradation of DNA induced by 634
effects on nucleic acid synthesis 634
effects on oxygen consumption and ATP content 636
interaction with DNA 636, 637
isopropylidene aza-derivative 633
methyl derivative 633
Streptovitacin A 561, 563
Streptozotocin, chemical structure 65
effects on enzymes and cofactors 75
mutagenic effects 78
Streptozotocin, specific inhibition of DNA synthesis 73, 74
Succinate: cytochrome c dehydrogenase, decrease induced by castration 151
Sulfate, metabolite of azathioprine 412
release during catabolism of 6-thiopurines 387, 389
Sulfur mustards, effects on HeLa cells 13
effects on T_7 phage 10
Suramin, effects on retention of phthalanilides 822
Synchronization of cells, colchicine and vinblastine for 674
5-fluoro-2'-deoxyuridine and thymidine for 199
Synthalin; decamethylene-*bis*(guanidine), chemical structure 767
effects on mitochondrial functions 776
Synthetic halogenated polynucleotides, stabilizing effect of halogens seen by T_m values 293

TACE, see chlorotrianisene
T-cells 405
L-asparaginase and 707, 708
TEM; triethylenemelamine, effects on spermatogenesis 24
immunosuppression by 24
Teratogenesis, 6-aminonicotinamide and 542
azaserine and DON as agents inducing 493
azathioprine and 415, 416
busulfan and 38, 39
colchicine and vinca alkaloids 675, 676
halogenated pyrimidine deoxyribonucleosides and 310
hydroxyurea and 790
methylenemethanesulfonate and 39
procarbazine and 752
Teslac, see Δ'-testololactone
Testicular tumors, actinomycin D for 589
effects of olivomycin and mithramycin 621
methotrexate for 478
Δ'-Testololactone, antitumor activity 183
breast cancer and 144
lack of hormonal activity 182
Testosterone, see also androgens
17α-alkyl derivatives with oral activity 142
biosynthesis 139—142
breast cancer and 181
chemical structure 141
conversion to 5α-dihydrotestosterone (17β-hydroxy-5α-androstane-3-one) 149
conversion to estrogens 106, 107
in breast cancer patients 179
effects on glucose and amino acid transport 93
effects on tolerance to vinblastine 685
independent functions for metabolites 160
inhibition of gonadotrophin production 173

Testosterone, renotropic activity 145
selective uptake by the hypothalamus and pituitary 149
selective uptake by prostate and seminal vesicles 149
Tetrahydrouridine, enhancement of efficacy of oral arabinosylcytosine 259, 260, 266
inhibitor of deamination of arabinosylcytosine 234, 239, 259, 266
1,2,5,6-Tetramethanesulfonyl-D-mannitol 36
Thalicarpine, inhibition of RNA synthesis 573
Thecomas, association with endometrial cancer 175
Thioarabinosylcytosine, activity of 234
inhibition of DNA biosynthesis 241
6-Thioguanine, anabolism 387, 388
anticancer activity 393, 394
catabolism 389
effect of disease on 389
combined with arabinosylcytosine 264
competition with guanine for hypoxanthine-guanine phosphoribosyltransferase 394
conversion to 6-thioguanylate 394
delayed cytotoxicity of 396
direct dethiolation to guanine 389
incorporation into DNA 388, 395, 396
inhibition of purine ribonucleotide interconversions 395
inhibition of purine ribonucleotide synthesis *de novo* 394, 395
toxicity 394
6-Thioguanosine and di- and triphosphate esters 388
6-Thioguanylate, derived from 6-thioguanine 387
formation from 6-thioguanine and slow turnover 394
intracellular levels of and inhibition of amidotransferase 395
6-Thioinosinate, derived from 6-mercaptopurine 385
inhibition of glutamine-PRPP amidotransferase by 390, 391
intracellular pools of 392
6-Thioinosine, action of inosine kinase on 387
substrate for purine nucleoside phosphorylase 387
Thiophenealanine, suppression of antibody formation by 525, 526
6-Thiopurines 384—403 see also individual agents
combination chemotherapy with 397
combined with glutamine antagonists 500, 501
comparison of inhibitory effects of nucleotides on glutamine-PRPP amidotransferase 395
delayed cytotoxicity of 396
immunosuppressive and anti-inflammatory effects 384
6-Thiopurines, metabolism 384—389
ThioTEPA; N,N′,N″-triethylene thiophosphoramide, immunosuppression by 24
6-Thiouric acid, action of uricase on 387
catabolite of 6-mercaptopurine 387
catabolite of 6-thioguanine 389
metabolite of azathioprine 411
6-Thioxanthine, derived from 6-thioguanine by guanase activity 389
6-Thioxanthylate 386
L-Threitol-1,4-dimethane sulfonate, mutagenic effects of 41, 42
Threonine dehydrase, allosteric activity of pyrrolopyrimidine nucleotides 440
Thymidine, as marker for cell kinetics 314
cortisol effect on transport 87, 88
modulation of toxicity of 5-iodo-2′-deoxyuridine 313, 314
pK_a of 278
Thymidine kinase, activated synthesis of by mitomycin 56
activation and inhibition by halogenated nucleoside triphosphates 285—288
comparison of K_m for thymidine and 5-iodo-2′-deoxyuridine 281
effects of arabinosylcytosine therapy on 246
effects of ultraviolet light on activity in the presence of thymidine or 5-iodo-2′-deoxyuridine 320
interactions of dCTP and dTTP with 285—287
loss of in cells resistant to 5-fluorodeoxyuridine and trifluorothymidine 217
resistance to 5-bromo- and 5-iodo-2′-deoxyuridine of cells lacking 298
Thymidine phosphorylase, see also nucleoside phosphorylases
resistance to deoxyglucosylthymine 289
synthesis of 5-iodo-2′-deoxyuridine by 272
Thymidylate kinase, 5-iodo-2′-deoxyuridine and 285
Thymidylate synthetase, competitive inhibition by 5-fluorouridylate 204
effects of arabinosylcytosine therapy 245, 246
effects of methotrexate 469
increased utilization of 5-bromo(iodo)-2′-deoxyuridine after inhibition of 288, 289
inhibition by 5-amino-deoxyuridine 380
inhibition by 5-fluoro-2′-deoxyuridylate 203
inhibition by trifluorothymidylate 204
inhibition in L5178Y by 5-iodo-2′-deoxyuridine 285
methotrexate effect on 246
Thymine, chemical structure, pK_a and uv absorbance 194, 195
Thymineless death, compared with arabinosylcytosine lethality 235
Thyroid tumors, hypothyroidism as initial step in induction of 171
Tilorone hydrochloride, biological activity and chemistry 884
clinical trial 884, 885
interferon induction by 884

T_m of DNA, effect of halogenated bases on 292—294
Tobacco mosaic virus, incorporation of 5-fluorouracil into RNA of 208
  iodination of RNA in 274
Tonsillar tumors, olivomycin and mithramycin for 621
Toyocamycin; 4-amino-5-cyano-7-(D-ribofuranosyl)-7 H-pyrrolo[2,3-d]pyrimidine
  biosynthesis of 435, 436
  chemical structure 436
  cytotoxic activity compared with tubercidin and sangivamycin 439
  inhibition of maturation of nucleolar into cytoplasmic ribosomal RNA 439
  inhibition of processing of 45S to ribosomal RNA 574, 577
Toyomycin, effect on DNA polymerase 603
Transcortin 96
Triamcinolone acetonide, reduced binding of by resistant rat lymphosarcoma 176
  specific binding of 97, 98
Triazenoimidazole derivatives 544—553, see also DIC, BIC
  chemistry 544, 545
  structure-activity relationships 549, 550
2,3,6-Trideoxy-3-amino-L-lyxohexose; daunosamine, component of daunorubicin 593
DL-5,5,5-Trifluoroleucine, antitumor activity 524
5-Trifluoromethyl-6-aza-2′-deoxyuridine 196
5-Trifluoromethyluracil, see trifluorothymidine
Trifluorothymidine, activity against transplantable tumors 198
  antiviral activity 199, 200
  chemical structure, pK_a and uv absorbance 194, 195
  clinical pharmacology 223
  clinical use 219
  distribution and metabolism in mice 219
  herpes infection of the eye and 195
  incorporation into DNA 205
  inhibition of thymidylate synthetase by 203
  metabolites 222, 223
  method for analysis 219
  preclinical pharmacology 219
  reduced size of substituted DNA polymer 292
  serum levels and half-times, including metabolites 222
  specificity of incorporation into viral DNA 205
  synthesis 196
Trifluorothymine, conversion to 5-carboxyuracil 202
  hydrolysis of 198
Trimethylene dimethanesulfonate, spermatogenesis and 37
Triparinol 105
Triphenylethylene 105
Triphosphatase, increased levels in resistance to 5-azacytidine 363
L-Tryptophan, antitumor activity 521
Tryptophan analogs 521
Tubercidin; 4-amino-7-(D-ribofuranosyl)-7H-pyrrolo[2,3-d]pyrimidine; 7-deazaadenosine
  action on schistosomes 441
  aglycone 436
  biosynthesis 435, 436
  chemical structure 436
  chemotherapy with 440, 441
  conversion to 7-deazaadenosine deoxynucleotide 437
  conversion to nucleotides 436, 437
  3′,5′-cyclic phosphate 438
  cytotoxic activity compared with toyocamycin and sangivamycin 439
  formation of a diphosphopyridine nucleotide from 437, 438
  glucose utilization and 437, 439
  incorporation into nucleic acids 436—438
  inhibition of macromolecular synthesis 438
  inhibition of phosphoribosylpyrophosphate amidotransferase 437
  nucleotides as active forms of 7-deazainosine 445
  resistance to adenosine deaminase and phosphorylase 436
  toxicity 440
  triphosphate as substrate for tRNA pyrophosphorylase 437, 438
Tubulin, see microtubule system
Tubulosine, chemical structure and biological activity 563
Tumors, therapeutic implications of amino acid dependence 528, 529, see also individual tumor types
Tylocerebrine, chemical structure, activity and mechanism of action 564
Tyrosinase, inhibitors of 520
Tyrosine analogs 520, 521
Tyrosine hydroxylase, inhibitors of 520

U11100A, antiestrogenic action and chemical structure 110, 111, see also Nafoxidine
U11555A, antiestrogenic action and chemical structure 110, 111
Ultraviolet light, effects on fluorinated pyrimidines 198
  effects on 5-iodouracil 320
  liberation of deoxyuridine radical from 5-iodo-2′-deoxyuridine 320
  sensitivity of *Escherichia coli* mutants to 11, 12
Uracil, chemical structure, pK_a and uv absorbance 194, 195
  preferential utilization by tumors 193
Uracil mustard, combined with 6-azacytidine 349
  combined with 6-azauridine in EHRLICH ascites tumor 355
  potentiation of antitumor effect by 5-iodo-2′-deoxyuridine 301

Uracil phosphoribosyltransferase, correlation between levels and antitumor effects of 5-fluorouracil 216
deletion accompanying resistance to 5-fluorouracil 217
Uricase, action on 6-thiouric acid 387
Uridine, potentiating effects on phosphorylation of arabinosylcytosine 240, 241, 267
Uridine-deoxyuridine phosphorylase, deoxyglucosylthymine as inhibitor 289, 290
Uridine 5'-diphosphate-α-D-glucose dehydrogenase, inhibition by showdomycin 374
Uridine kinase, decreased activity accompanying resistance to 5-fluorouracil 217
decreased levels accompanying resistance to 5-azacytidine 363
effects of arabinosylcytosine therapy on 245, 246
increased levels in infected cells as a factor in antiviral action of 6-azauridine 354, 355
phosphorylation of 6-azauridine by 352
Uridine 5'-monophosphokinase, showdomycin as inhibitor of 374
Uridine phosphorylase, role in activation of 5-fluorouracil 216, 217
showdomycin as inhibitor 374
Uterine cancer, estrogen-dependent induction by 3-methylcholanthrene 175
17α-hydroxyprogesterone caproate for 186
progesterone for 175
role of failure of ovulation in endometrial malignancy 174, 175
Uterine cervix cancer, methotrexate for 478
Uterus, androgen effects on 143
estrogen receptor proteins in 113, 115, 116, 117
transformation of endometrial cell by progesterone 158, 159

Vagina, estrogen receptor proteins in 113
Velban, see vinblastine
Vinblastine; velban, see also vinca alkaloids
aggregation of ribosomes and erythrocyte membranes 678
anti-inflammatory action 675
binding by microtubule protein 678
cell cycle phase specificity 674
chemical structure 672
competition with glutamate for transport 682
dosage and administration 685, 686
effects on amino acid transport 682
effects on neurons 675
effects on RNA synthesis 680
effects on serum copper and iron 683
effects of testosterone on tolerance to 685
inhibition of DNA synthesis 679, 680
metabolism and distribution 683, 684
mitotic arrest 673, 674
antagonism by glutamic acid and tryptophan 674, 675
reduction in 4-amino-5-imidazolecarboxamide excretion produced by 679
Vinblastine, reversible dissolution of meiotic spindle 674
toxicity 686, 687
Vinca alkaloids 670—694, see also vinblastine, vincristine, vinleurosine and vinrosidine
acylating activity 672
clinical considerations 684—687
cross-resistance to daunorubicin 606
diseases treated with 687
effects on coenzyme A metabolism 683
effects on experimental tumors 675
effects on respiration 682, 683
immunosuppression by 676
interrelation with the histaminic and adrenergic systems 683
lack of correlation between mitotic and cytotoxic effects 679
nucleoside transport and 681
place in cancer chemotherapy 687
protection against mitotic and cytotoxic effects by glutamic acid 679
source and history 670
structure-activity relationships 671, 672
structures 672
teratogenesis and 676
toxicity 686, 687
Vincristine; oncovin, see also vinca alkaloids
chemical structure 672
combined with 5-fluorouracil, methotrexate, cyclophosphamide and prednisone
cross-resistance with terephthalanilides 682
different spectrum of activity from vinblastine 687
dosage and administration 685, 686
effects on DNA synthesis 680, 681
effects on enzyme parameters during treatment 681
effects on lipids and lipid synthesis 682
effects on RNA synthesis 680, 681
for breast cancer 221
hyponatremia from 683, 687
in COAP regimen 263, 264
incomplete reversibility of mitotic effects 673, 674
inhibition of brain RNA synthesis 681
inhibition of RNA polymerase 681
metabolism and distribution 683, 684
mitotic arrest 673, 674
neurotoxicity 675, 686
photochemical inactivation 680
toxicity 686, 687
Vindolin 671, 672
Vinglycinate, chemical structure 672
clinical use 685
Vinleurosine, chemical structure 672
clinical use 685
inhibition of phospholipid synthesis 682
Vinrosidine, chemical structure 672
clinical trial 685
Viruses, see also DNA and RNA viruses
activation of viral infections in transplant patients receiving azathioprine 417

Viruses, effects of camptothecin 654
effects of daunorubicin 607, 608
effects of emetine on viral RNA synthesis 560
growth inhibition by daunorubicin 606—608
inhibition by arabinosyladenine 428
inhibition by formycin 444
inhibition of growth by heterocyclic thiosemicarbazones 800
inhibition of herpes by xylofuranosyladenine 430
inhibition of replication by 5-bromo- and 5-iodo-2′-deoxyuridine 302—307
oncogenic, effects of halogenated pyrimidine deoxyribonucleosides 307, 308
properties of particles synthesized in presence of halogenated nucleoside analogs 303—305
pseudorabies, non-infectious particles synthesized in presence of 5-bromo-2′-deoxyuridine 304, 305
sensitivity of different varieties to halogenated deoxyribonucleosides 302, 303, 306, 307
Vitellogenesis, estrogens and 120, 121
VM-26; 4′-demethyl-epipodophyllotoxin thenylidene glucoside
chemical structure 672
inhibition of DNA synthesis in P-815 cells 681
preprophase effect 673

Walker 256 tumor, effects of arabinosylcytosine 235

Wilm's tumor, actinomycin D for 589

Xanthine oxidase, action on 6-mercaptopurine 387
action on 6-thioxanthine 389
inhibition by 8-azaguanine 460
inhibition by 6-mercaptopurine free base 389
inhibition by triazeneimidazole derivatives 547
Xanthosine 5′-phosphate aminase, adenine glycoside binding site 448
inhibition by decoyinine 449
inhibition by glutamine antagonists 489
inhibition by mycophenolic acid 450
inhibition by psicofuranine 448, 449
regulation by adenosine 448
X-radiation, potentiation of effects by 5-iodo-2′-deoxyuridine 301, see also radiation
9β-D-Xylofuranosyladenine, chemical structure 426
inhibition of 5-phosphoribosyl-1-pyrophosphate formation 430
inhibition of RNA and DNA synthesis 430
synthesis 430
9β-D-Xylofuranosyl-6-mercaptopurine, synthesis, activity and metabolism 430, 431
9β-D-Xylofuranosyl-6-thioguanine 431

Yolk protein formation, estrogens and 120, 121
Yoshida cells, repair of damaged DNA in 13, 14

Zitostop, R52; 1,2,5,6-tetramethanesulfonyl-D-mannitol 36

Recent Results in Cancer Research

Sponsored by the Swiss League against Cancer
Editor-in-chief: P. Rentchnick

Vol. 1 R. Schindler
Die tierische Zelle in Zellkultur

Vol. 2 Neuroblastomas – Biochemical Studies
Edited by C. Bohuon

Vol. 3 W. C. Hueper
Occupational and Environmental Cancers of the Respiratory System

Vol. 4 L. Goldman
Laser Cancer Research

Vol. 5 D. Metcalf
The Thymus

Vol. 6 Malignant Transformation by Viruses
Edited by W. H. Kirsten

Vol. 7 Ch. G. Moertel
Multiple Primary Malignant Neoplasms

Vol. 8 New Trends in the Treatment of Cancer
Edited by L. Manuila, S. Moles, and P. Rentchnick

Vol. 9 J. Lindenmann and P. A. Klein
Immunological Aspects of Viral Oncolysis

Vol. 10 R. S. Nelson
Radioactive Phosphorus in the Diagnosis of Gastrointestinal Cancer

Vol. 11 R. G. Freeman and J. M. Knox
Treatment of Skin Cancer

Vol. 12 H. T. Lynch
Hereditary Factors in Carcinoma

Vol. 13 Tumours in Children
Edited by H. B. Marsden and J. K. Steward

Vol. 14 N. Odartchenko
Production Cellulaire Erythropoiétique

Vol. 15 B. Sokoloff
Carcinoid and Serotonin

Vol. 16 M. L. Jacobs
Malignant Lymphomas and their Management

Vol. 17 Normal and Malignant Cell Growth
Edited by R. J. Fry, M. L. Griem, and W. H. Kirsten

Vol. 18 E. Anglesio
The Treatment of Hodgkin's Disease

Vol. 19 P. Bannasch
The Cytoplasm of Hepatocytes during Carcinogenesis

Vol. 20 Rubidomycin
Edited by J. Bernard, R. Paul, M. Boiron, C. Jacquillat, and R. Maral

Vol. 21 Scientific Basis of Cancer Chemotherapy
Edited by G. Mathé

Vol. 22 P. Koldovsky
Tumor Specific Transplantation Antigen

Vol. 23 W. A. Fuchs, J. W. Davidson, and H. W. Fischer
Lymphography in Cancer

Vol. 24 J. Hayward
Hormones and Human Breast Cancer

Vol. 25 P. Roy-Burman
Analogues of Nucleic Acid Components

Vol. 26 Tumors of the Liver
Edited by G. T. Pack and A. H. Islami

Vol. 27 J. Szymendera
Bone Mineral Metabolism in Cancer

Vol. 28 E. S. Meek
Antitumour and Antiviral Substances of Natural Origin

Vol. 29 Aseptic Environments and Cancer Treatment
Edited by G. Mathé

Vol. 30 Advances in the Treatment of Acute (Blastic) Leukemias
Edited by G. Mathé

Vol. 31 P. Denoix
Treatment of Malignant Breast Tumors

Vol. 32 R. S. Nelson
Endoscopy in Gastric Cancer

Vol. 33 Experimental and Clinical Effects of L-Asparaginase
Edited by E. Grundmann and H. F. Oettgen

Vol. 34 Chemistry and Biological Actions of 4-Nitroquinoline 1-Oxide
Edited by H. Endo, T. Ono, and T. Sugimura

Vol. 35 I. Penn
Malignant Tumors in Organ Transplant Recipients

Vol. 36 Current Concepts in the Management of Leukemia and Lymphoma
Edited by J. E. Ultmann, M. L. Griem, W. H. Kirsten, and R. W. Wissler

Vol. 37 S. Chiappa, R. Musumeci, and C. Uslenghi
Endolymphatic Radiotherapy in Malignant Lymphomas

Vol. 38 P. C. Koller
The Role of Chromosomes in Cancer Biology

Vol. 39 Current Problems in the Epidemiology of Cancer and Lymphomas
Edited by E. Grundmann and H. Tulinius

Vol. 40 F. A. Langley and A. C. Crompton
Epithelial Abnormalities of the Cervix Uteri

Vol. 41 Tumours in a Tropical Country
Edited by A. C. Templeton

Vol. 42 Breast Cancer: A Challenging Problem
Edited by M. L. Griem, E. V. Jensen, J. E. Ultmann, and R. W. Wissler

Vol. 43 Nomenclature, Methodology and Results of Clinical Trials in Acute Leukemias
Edited by G. Mathé, P. Pouillart, and L. Schwarzenberg

Vol. 44 Special Topics in Carcinogenesis
Edited by E. Grundmann

Vol. 45 P. Koldovsky
Carcinoembryonic Antigens

Vol. 46 Diagnosis and Therapy of Malignant Lymphoma
Edited by K. Musshoff

Special Supplement
Biology of Amphibian Tumors
Edited by M. Mizell

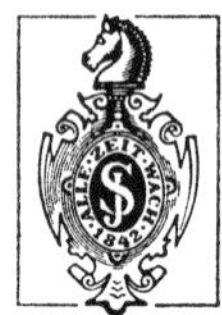

**Springer-Verlag
Berlin
Heidelberg
New York**

München Johannesburg London Madrid New Delhi Paris Rio de Janeiro Sydney Tokyo Utrecht Wien